Roberts and Hedges'
Clinical Procedures
in Emergency Medicine

Roberts and Hedges'
Clinical Procedures
in Emergency Medicine

SIXTH EDITION

EDITOR-IN-CHIEF

James R. Roberts, MD, FACEP, FAAEM, FACMT

Professor of Emergency Medicine
Vice Chair, Department of Emergency Medicine
Senior Consultant, Division of Toxicology
The Drexel University College of Medicine
Chairman, Department of Emergency Medicine
Director, Division of Medical Toxicology
Mercy Catholic Medical Center
Philadelphia, Pennsylvania

SENIOR EDITOR

Catherine B. Custalow, MD, PhD

Associate Professor, Retired
Department of Emergency Medicine
University of Virginia School of Medicine
Charlottesville, Virginia

ILLUSTRATION EDITOR

Todd W. Thomsen, MD

Department of Emergency Medicine
Mount Auburn Hospital
Cambridge, Massachusetts
Instructor in Medicine
Harvard Medical School
Boston, Massachusetts

EDITOR EMERITUS

Jerris R. Hedges, MD, MS, MMM

Professor and Dean
John A. Burns School of Medicine
University of Hawaii—Manoa
Honolulu, Hawaii
Professor and Vice-Dean, Emeritus
Department of Emergency Medicine
Oregon Health & Science University School of Medicine
Portland, Oregon

ELSEVIER
SAUNDERS

1600 John F. Kennedy Blvd.
Ste 1800
Philadelphia, PA 19103-2899

ROBERTS AND HEDGES' CLINICAL PROCEDURES
IN EMERGENCY MEDICINE

ISBN: 978-1-4557-0606-8

Notices

Knowledge and best practice in this field are constantly changing. As new research and experience broaden our understanding, changes in research methods, professional practices, or medical treatment may become necessary.

Practitioners and researchers must always rely on their own experience and knowledge in evaluating and using any information, methods, compounds, or experiments described herein. In using such information or methods, they should be mindful of their own safety and the safety of others, including parties for whom they have a professional responsibility.

With respect to any drug or pharmaceutical products identified, readers are advised to check the most current information provided (i) on procedures featured or (ii) by the manufacturer of each product to be administered to verify the recommended dose or formula, the method and duration of administration, and contraindications. It is the responsibility of practitioners, relying on their own experience and knowledge of their patients, to make diagnoses, to determine dosages and the best treatment for each individual patient, and to take all appropriate safety precautions.

To the fullest extent of the law, neither the Publisher nor the authors, contributors, or editors assume any liability for any injury and/or damage to persons or property as a matter of products liability, negligence, or otherwise or from any use or operation of any methods, products, instructions, or ideas contained in the material herein.

Library of Congress Cataloging-in-Publication Data
Clinical procedures in emergency medicine.
  Roberts and Hedges' clinical procedures in emergency medicine / editor-in-chief, James R. Roberts ; senior editor, Catherine B. Custalow ; illustration editor, Todd W. Thomsen ; editor emeritus, Jerris R. Hedges.—Sixth edition.
    p. ; cm.
  Clinical procedures in emergency medicine
  Preceded by Clinical procedures in emergency medicine / editors, James R. Roberts, Jerris R. Hedges ; associate editors, Catherine B. Custalow ... [et al.]. 5th ed. c2010.
  Includes bibliographical references and index.
  ISBN 978-1-4557-0606-8 (hardcover : alk. paper)
  I. Roberts, James R., 1946- editor of compilation. II. Custalow, Catherine B. editor of compilation. III. Thomsen, Todd W. editor. IV. Hedges, Jerris R. editor. V. Title. VI. Title: Clinical procedures in emergency medicine.
  [DNLM: 1. Emergencies. 2. Emergency Medicine—methods. 3. Emergency Treatment—methods. WB 105]
  RC86.7
  616.02'5—dc23
                                                           2013017645

Senior Content Strategist: Stefanie Jewell-Thomas
Senior Content Specialist: Dee Simpson
Publishing Services Manager: Anne Altepeter
Senior Project Manager: Doug Turner
Designer: Lou Forgione

Printed in the People's Republic of China

Last digit is the print number: 9 8 7 6 5 4 3 2 1

To Lydia, Matthew, Martha, and, of course, Jeanne.

J.R.R.

To my son, Nicholas, and to the memory of my daughter, Lauren.

C.B.C.

To my wonderful wife, Karen—thank you for your inspiration, support, and remarkable partnership; to Sydney, William, and Nathan, who will always be reminders of what is truly important; to my parents, who helped to foster the passion of medical education as a public service. To Cathy Custalow, MD, for her many, many hours and dedication to this book. And finally to those who practice and teach emergency medicine—may this book serve you well.

A.S.C.

To Marcy … my wife, my best friend, and my soul mate.

C.R.C.

To my wife, Karen, and my sons, Joshua and Zachary—thank you for your unlimited patience and encouragement while I pursued this educational passion. None of this could happen without your love. To our residents, peer faculty, nurses, and patients at LSU and Charity Hospital— your example and inspiration for patient care keep me focused on the mission of "care for all."

P.M.C.D.

To my wife, Sejal, and my three children, Nikhil, Eleena, and Kamran, for giving me purpose and inspiration. To my colleagues and my mentors for all that they have taught me through the years. To Jim Roberts, for continuing to be a driving force behind this text. And to emergency physicians around the world, who continually care and advocate for their patients despite the toughest of times and circumstances.

A.M.

To my amazing wife, Joyce; my supportive parents; the students and residents of the Keck School of Medicine; and the gracious patients of Los Angeles County–USC Medical Center.

S.P.S.

To Jim Roberts and Cathy Custalow, for the opportunity to collaborate on this project. To Gary Setnik, for your mentorship throughout the years. To my parents, Alfred and Beverly Thomsen, for everything. And most importantly, to my beautiful wife, Cristine, and wonderful sons, Henry and Cole, for your love and patience during the many months that this book took me away from you.

T.W.T.

HOW THIS MEDICAL TEXTBOOK SHOULD BE VIEWED BY THE PRACTICING CLINICIAN AND THE JUDICIAL SYSTEM

The editors and authors of this textbook strongly believe that the complex practice of medicine, the vagaries of human diseases, the unpredictability of pathologic conditions, and the functions, dysfunctions, and responses of the human body cannot be defined, explained, or rigidly categorized by any written document. *Therefore it is neither the purpose nor the intent of our textbook to serve as an authoritative source on any medical condition, treatment plan, or clinical intervention; nor should our textbook be used to rigorously define a standard of care that should be practiced by all clinicians.*

Our written word provides the physician with a literature-referenced database and a reasonable clinical guide that is combined with practical suggestions from individual experienced practitioners. We offer a general reference source and clinical roadmap on a variety of conditions and procedures that may confront clinicians who are experienced in emergency medicine practice. This text cannot replace physician judgment; cannot describe every possible aberration, nuance, clinical scenario, or presentation; and cannot define rigid standards for clinical actions or procedures. *Every medical encounter must be individualized, and every patient must be approached on a case-by-case basis.* No complex medical interaction can possibly be reduced to the written word. The treatments, procedures, and medical conditions described in this textbook do not constitute the total expertise or knowledge base expected to be possessed by all clinicians. Finally, many of the described complications and adverse outcomes associated with implementing or withholding complex medical and surgical interventions may occur, even when every aspect of the intervention has been performed correctly and as per any textbook or currently accepted standards.

The editors and authors of *Roberts and Hedges' Clinical Procedures in Emergency Medicine*, Sixth Edition

Contributors

Benjamin S. Abella, MD, MPhil
Clinical Research Director
Department of Emergency Medicine
Center for Resuscitation Science
University of Pennsylvania
Artificial Perfusion during Cardiac Arrest

Bruce D. Adams, MD
Professor
Chief of Emergency Medicine
Center for Emergency Medicine
University of Texas School of Medicine
San Antonio, Texas
*Central Venous Catheterization and
Central Venous Pressure Monitoring*

Erik H. Adler, MD
Senior Resident
Department of Emergency Medicine
Denver Health
Denver, Colorado
Thoracentesis

Pablo F. Aguilera, MD
Instructor of Emergency Medicine
Department of Internal Medicine
Emergency Medicine Program
Pontificia Universidad Católica de
  Chile
Santiago, Chile
Emergency Medicine Program
  Coordinator
Hospital Dr. Sótero del Río
Puente Alto, Región Metropolitana
Puente Alto, Chile
Venous Cutdown

**James T. Amsterdam, DMD,
MD, MMM, FACEP, FACPE**
Chair/Service Line Director
Department of Emergency Medicine
York Hospital
York, Pennsylvania
Professor of Clinical Emergency
  Medicine
Department of Emergency Medicine
Penn State University College of
  Medicine
Hershey, Pennsylvania
Adjunct Professor of Emergency
  Medicine
Department of Emergency Medicine
Drexel University College of Medicine
Philadelphia, Pennsylvania
Regional Anesthesia of the Head and Neck

Jennifer Avegno, MD
Clinical Assistant Professor
Department of Medicine
Section of Emergency Medicine
Louisiana State University Health
  Sciences Center
New Orleans, Louisiana
*Educational Aspects of Emergency
  Department Procedures*

David K. Barnes, MD, FACEP
Assistant Professor
Residency Program Director
Department of Emergency Medicine
University of California Davis Health
  System
Sacramento, California
*Extensor and Flexor Tendon Injuries in the
  Hand, Wrist, and Foot*

Steven J. Bauer, MD, MS
Staff Physician
Department of Emergency Medicine
Meritus Medical Center
Hagerstown, Maryland
*Alternative Methods of Drug
  Administration*

Jason P. Becker, MD
Undergraduate Medical Education
  Director
Emergency Medicine Residency
  Program
Albert Einstein Medical Center
Philadelphia, Pennsylvania
*Treatment of Bursitis, Tendinitis, and
  Trigger Points*

Lance B. Becker, MD, FAHA
Director
Center for Resuscitation Science
Professor
Department of Emergency Medicine
Perelman School of Medicine
University of Pennsylvania Health
  System
Philadelphia, Pennsylvania
Artificial Perfusion during Cardiac Arrest

Kip R. Benko, MD, FACEP
Clinical Assistant Professor of
  Emergency Medicine
University of Pittsburgh School of
  Medicine
Faculty, Presbyterian University
  Hospital
University of Pittsburgh Medical
  Center
Pittsburgh, Pennsylvania
Emergency Dental Procedures

Edward S. Bessman, MD, MBA
Chairman and Clinical Director
Department of Emergency Medicine
Johns Hopkins Bayview Medical
  Center
Assistant Professor
Department of Emergency Medicine
The Johns Hopkins School of
  Medicine
Baltimore, Maryland
Emergency Cardiac Pacing

Barbara K. Blok, MD
Associate Professor
Department of Emergency Medicine
University of Colorado School of
    Medicine
Aurora, Colorado
Associate Program Director
Denver Health Residency in
    Emergency Medicine
Denver, Colorado
Thoracentesis

Heather A. Borek, MD
Attending Physician
Department of Emergency Medicine
Division of Medical Toxicology
Albert Einstein Healthcare Network
Philadelphia, Pennsylvania
Decontamination of the Poisoned Patient

Eduardo Borquez, MD
Staff Physician
Department of Emergency Medicine
Kaiser Permanente San Diego Medical
    Center
San Diego, California
Noncardiac Implantable Devices

Sudip Bose, MD, FACEP, FAAEM
Associate Clinical Professor
Department of Emergency Medicine
University of Illinois
Chicago, Illinois
Attending Emergency Medicine
    Physician
Partner, Basin Emergency Physicians,
    LLC
Department of Emergency Medicine
Medical Center Hospital
Odessa, Texas
*Cricothyrotomy and Percutaneous
    Translaryngeal Ventilation*

William J. Brady, MD
Professor of Emergency Medicine and
    Medicine
Chair, Medical Emergency Response
    (Formerly Resuscitation) Committee
Medical Director, Emergency
    Management
University of Virginia Medical Center
Charlottesville, Virginia
Medical Director
Allianz Global Assistance
United States and Canada
Basic Electrocardiographic Techniques

G. Richard Braen, MD, FACEP
Professor and Chairman
Department of Emergency Medicine
Assistant Dean of Graduate Medical
    Education
School of Medicine and Biomedical
    Sciences
University at Buffalo
Buffalo, New York
Culdocentesis

Christine Butts, MD
Clinical Assistant Professor of
    Emergency Medicine
Director of Division of Emergency
    Ultrasound
Louisiana State University Health
    Sciences Center
New Orleans, Louisiana
Ultrasound

Sharon K. Carney, MD
Clinical Assistant Professor of
    Emergency Medicine
Drexel University College of Medicine
Chief Medical Officer
Mercy Catholic Medical Center
Philadelphia, Pennsylvania
Intravenous Regional Anesthesia

Merle A. Carter, MD
Residency Director
Department of Emergency Medicine
Albert Einstein Medical Center
Philadelphia, Pennsylvania
Compartment Syndrome Evaluation

Theodore C. Chan, MD
Professor
Department of Emergency Medicine
University of California, San Diego
    Health Sciences
San Diego, California
Basic Electrocardiographic Techniques

Carl R. Chudnofsky, MD
Professor
Department of Emergency Medicine
Jefferson Medical College
Chair, Department of Emergency
    Medicine
Albert Einstein Healthcare Network
Philadelphia, Pennsylvania
*Alternative Methods of Drug
    Administration*
Splinting Techniques

Ilene Claudius, MD
Assistant Professor
Department of Emergency Medicine
Los Angeles County and University of
    Southern California
Los Angeles, California
*Pediatric Vascular Access and Blood
    Sampling Techniques*

Joseph E. Clinton, MD
Professor and Head
Department of Emergency Medicine
University of Minnesota Medical
    School
Chief of Service
Department of Emergency Medicine
Hennepin County Medical Center
Minneapolis, Minnesota
*Basic Airway Management and Decision
    Making*
Tracheal Intubation

Wendy C. Coates, MD
Professor of Clinical Medicine
David Geffen School of Medicine at
    University of California, Los Angeles
Los Angeles, California
Director, Medical Education
Director, Fellowship in Medical
    Education
Department of Emergency Medicine
Harbor-UCLA Medical Center
Torrance, California
Anorectal Procedures

Jonathan E. Davis, MD
Associate Professor
Department of Emergency Medicine
Georgetown University School of
    Medicine Program Director
Emergency Medicine Residency
    Program
Georgetown University Hospital/
    Washington Hospital Center
Washington, District of Columbia
Urologic Procedures

Anthony J. Dean, MD
Associate Professor of Emergency
    Medicine
Associate Professor of Emergency
    Medicine in Radiology
Director, Division of Emergency
    Ultrasonography
Department of Emergency Medicine
University of Pennsylvania Medical
    Center
Philadelphia, Pennsylvania
*Bedside Laboratory and Microbiologic
    Procedures*

Kenneth Deitch, DO
Research Director
Department of Emergency Medicine
Albert Einstein Medical Center
Philadelphia, Pennsylvania
Intraosseous Infusion

William R. Dennis, MD, MPH
Chair of EMS
Assistant Professor of Emergency
  Medicine
University of Missouri
Columbia, Missouri
Ophthalmologic Procedures

Denis J. Dollard, MD
Clinical Assistant Professor
Department of Emergency Medicine
Drexel University College of Medicine
Director, Department of Emergency
  Medicine
Mercy Hospital of Philadelphia
Philadelphia, Pennsylvania
*Radiation in Pregnancy and Clinical Issues
  of Radiocontrast Agents*

**Timothy B. Erickson, MD,
FACEP, FACMT, FAACT**
Professor
Department of Emergency Medicine
Division of Medical Toxicology
University of Illinois
Chicago, Illinois
*Procedures Pertaining to Hypothermia and
  Hyperthermia*

Brian D. Euerle, MD
Associate Professor
Department of Emergency Medicine
University of Maryland School of
  Medicine
Baltimore, Maryland
*Spinal Puncture and Cerebrospinal Fluid
  Examination*

Michael T. Fitch, MD, PhD
Associate Professor
Department of Emergency Medicine
Wake Forest University School of
  Medicine
Winston-Salem, North Carolina
Abdominal Hernia Reduction

Molly Furin, MD, MS
Attending Physician
Associate Fellowship Director Division
  of EMS/Disaster Medicine
Department of Emergency Medicine
Albert Einstein Medical Center
Philadelphia, Pennsylvania
Prehospital Immobilization

Robert T. Gerhardt, MD, MPH
Chief Medical Officer, Tactical Combat
  Casualty Care Research Program
U.S. Army Institute of Surgical
  Research
Associate Professor
Department of Military and Emergency
  Medicine
Uniformed Services University of the
  Health Sciences
Bethesda, Maryland
Adjunct Faculty
San Antonio Uniformed Services
  Health Education Consortium
Emergency Medicine Residency
  Program and EMS/Disaster
  Fellowship
San Antonio Military Medical Center
Joint Base San Antonio–Fort Sam
  Houston
Houston, Texas
Assessment of Implantable Devices

Kevin B. Gerold, DO, JD
Assistant Professor
Departments of Anesthesiology and
  Critical Care Medicine and
  Emergency Medicine
The Johns Hopkins School of
  Medicine
Director, Critical Care Medicine
Department of Anesthesiology
Johns Hopkins Bayview Medical
  Center
Baltimore, Maryland
Burn Care Procedures

Mariana R. Gonzalez, BA
Department of Emergency Medicine
Hospital of the University of
  Pennsylvania
Philadelphia, Pennsylvania
Artificial Perfusion during Cardiac Arrest

Diane L. Gorgas, MD
Associate Professor and Residency
  Director
Department of Emergency Medicine
The Ohio State University
Columbus, Ohio
Vital Sign Measurement
*Transfusion Therapy: Blood and Blood
  Products*

Steven M. Green, MD
Professor of Emergency Medicine and
  Pediatrics
Department of Emergency Medicine
Loma Linda University Medical Center
  and Children's Hospital
Loma Linda, California
*Systemic Analgesia and Sedation for
  Procedures*

John C. Greenwood, MD
Chief Resident
Clinical Instructor Department of
  Emergency Medicine
University of Maryland School of
  Medicine
Baltimore, Maryland
Tracheostomy Care

Richard A. Harrigan, MD
Professor
Department of Emergency Medicine
Temple University School of Medicine
Philadelphia, Pennsylvania
Basic Electrocardiographic Techniques

Jeffrey Harrow, MD
Emergency Medicine Physician
Department of Emergency Medicine
The Johns Hopkins School of
  Medicine
Baltimore, Maryland
Incision and Drainage

Micelle Haydel, MD
Associate Clinical Professor
Program Director
Section of Emergency Medicine
Louisiana State University Health
  Sciences Center
New Orleans, Louisiana
*Medications and Equipment for
  Resuscitation*

Randy B. Hebert, MD
Clinical Assistant Professor
Department of Emergency Medicine
Advocate Illinois Masonic Medical
  Center
Chicago, Illinois
*Cricothyrotomy and Percutaneous
  Translaryngeal Ventilation*

Eveline Hitti, MD, MBA
Assistant Professor in Clinical
  Emergency Medicine
Interim Chair
Department of Emergency Medicine
American University of Beirut Medical
  Center
Beirut, Lebanon
Incision and Drainage

Christopher P. Holstege, MD
Associate Professor
Department of Emergency Medicine
  and Pediatrics
Chief, Division of Medical Toxicology
University of Virginia School of
  Medicine
Medical Director
Blue Ridge Poison Center
University of Virginia Health System
Charlottesville, Virginia
Decontamination of the Poisoned Patient

Liam C. Holtzman, DO, FACEP
Assistant Professor
Department of Emergency Medicine
The Johns Hopkins University School
  of Medicine
Senior Medical Officer
Center for Law Enforcement Medicine
The Johns Hopkins Medical
  Institutions
Baltimore, Maryland
Incision and Drainage

Amanda E. Horn, MD
Assistant Professor
Assistant Residency Director
Department of Emergency Medicine
Temple University Hospital
Philadelphia, Pennsylvania
Management of Common Dislocations

J. Stephen Huff, MD
Professor of Emergency Medicine and
  Neurology
Department of Emergency Medicine
University of Virginia
Charlottesville, Virginia
Special Neurologic Tests and Procedures

Charlene Irvin Babcock, MD
Department of Emergency Medicine
University of Michigan Hospital
Ann Arbor, Michigan
Autotransfusion

Paul Jhun, MD
Assistant Professor of Clinical
  Emergency Medicine
Assistant Residency Director
Department of Emergency Medicine
University of Southern California
Los Angeles, California
Noncardiac Implantable Devices

Russell F. Jones, MD
Assistant Professor
Department of Emergency Medicine
University of California Davis Health
  System
Sacramento, California
Resuscitative Thoracotomy

Colin G. Kaide, MD
Associate Professor
Department of Emergency Medicine
The Ohio State University
Columbus, Ohio
*Transfusion Therapy: Blood and Blood
  Products*

Eric D. Katz, MD
Associate Professor
Department of Emergency Medicine
University of Arizona College of
  Medicine—Phoenix Campus
Program Director and Vice-Chair for
  Education
Department of Emergency Medicine
Maricopa Integrated Health Center
Phoenix, Arizona
*Commonly Used Formulas and
  Calculations*

John J. Kelly, DO
Associate Chair
Department of Emergency Medicine
Albert Einstein Medical Center
Professor of Emergency Medicine
Jefferson Medical College
Philadelphia, Pennsylvania
*Nerve Blocks of the Thorax and
  Extremities*

Kevin P. Kilgore, MD
Assistant Professor
Department of Emergency Medicine
University of Minnesota School of
  Medicine
Minneapolis, Minnesota
Senior Staff Physician
Department of Emergency Medicine
Regions Hospital
St. Paul, Minnesota
Regional Anesthesia of the Head and Neck

Hyung T. Kim, MD
Assistant Professor of Clinical
  Emergency Medicine
Department of Emergency Medicine
University of Southern California
Los Angeles, California
Arterial Puncture and Cannulation

Thomas D. Kirsch, MD, MPH
Associate Professor
Department of Emergency Medicine
The Johns Hopkins School of
  Medicine
Department of International Health
The Johns Hopkins Bloomberg School
  of Public Health
Baltimore, Maryland
Tube Thoracostomy

Brian C. Kitamura, BS, MD
Resident Physician
Department of Emergency Medicine
Maricopa Integrated Health Center
Phoenix, Arizona
*Commonly Used Formulas and
  Calculations*

Anne Klimke, MD, MS
EMS Faculty
Assistant Director of EMS Fellowship
Department of Emergency Medicine
Albert Einstein Medical Center
Philadelphia, Pennsylvania
Prehospital Immobilization

Kevin J. Knoop, MD, MS
Commanding Officer
Medical Treatment Facility
USNS Comfort
Norfolk, Virginia
Ophthalmologic Procedures

J. Michael Kowalski, DO
Medical Director, Observation Unit
Attending Physician
Division of Medical Toxicology
Department of Emergency Medicine
Einstein Medical Center
Consulting Toxicologist
Poison Control Center at Children's
  Hospital of Philadelphia
Philadelphia, Pennsylvania
Physical and Chemical Restraint

Baruch Krauss, MD, EdM
Senior Associate Physician in Medicine
Division of Emergency Medicine
Children's Hospital Boston
Associate Professor of Pediatrics
Department of Pediatrics
Harvard Medical School
Boston, Massachusetts
*Devices for Assessing Oxygenation and
  Ventilation*
*Systemic Analgesia and Sedation for
  Procedures*

Diann M. Krywko, MD
Associate Professor
Division Director of Faculty
  Development and Mentoring
Division of Emergency Medicine
Department of Medicine
Medical University of South Carolina
Charleston, South Carolina
*Indwelling Vascular Devices: Emergency
  Access and Management*

Richard L. Lammers, MD
Assistant Dean for Simulation
Professor of Emergency Medicine
Research Director
Department of Emergency Medicine
Western Michigan University School of
    Medicine
Kalamazoo, Michigan
Principles of Wound Management
Methods of Wound Closure

David C. Lee, MD
Department of Emergency Medicine
North Shore University Hospital
Manhasset, New York
Bedside Laboratory and Microbiologic
    Procedures

George H. Lew, MD, PhD
Associate Professor
Department of Emergency Medicine
Loyola University Medical Center
Maywood, Illinois
Emergency Childbirth

Shan W. Liu, MD, SD
Instructor
Department of Surgery
Harvard Medical School
Attending Physician
Department of Emergency Medicine
Massachusetts General Hospital
Boston, Massachusetts
Peripheral Intravenous Access

**Sharon E. Mace, MD, FACEP,
FAAP**
Professor of Medicine
Department of Emergency Medicine
Cleveland Clinic
Director of Research
Director of Observation Unit
Director of Pediatric Education/
    Quality Improvement
Emergency Services Institute
Cleveland Clinic
Faculty, Emergency Medicine
    Residency
MetroHealth Medical Center/
    Cleveland Clinic
Cleveland, Ohio
Cricothyrotomy and Percutaneous
    Translaryngeal Ventilation

Haney A. Mallemat, MD
Assistant Professor
Department of Emergency Medicine
    and Critical Care
University of Maryland School of
    Medicine
Baltimore, Maryland
Pericardiocentesis

David E. Manthey, MD
Professor
Vice Chair of Education
Department of Emergency Medicine
Wake Forest University School of
    Medicine
Winston-Salem, North Carolina
Abdominal Hernia Reduction

**Joshua E. Markowitz, MD,
RDMS, FACEP**
Assistant Professor
Department of Emergency Medicine
Thomas Jefferson Medical School
Director of Emergency Ultrasound
Albert Einstein Healthcare Network
Philadelphia, Pennsylvania
Treatment of Bursitis, Tendinitis, and
    Trigger Points

†John A. Marx, MD
Chair Emeritus
Department of Emergency Medicine
Carolinas Medical Center
Adjunct Professor
Department of Emergency Medicine
University of North Carolina-Charlotte
    Campus
Charlotte, North Carolina
Peritoneal Procedures

Phillip E. Mason, MD
Emergency Medicine Physician
San Antonio Military Medical Center
San Antonio, Texas
Basic Airway Management and Decision
    Making

**Anthony S. Mazzeo, MD, FACEP,
FAAEM**
Clinical Assistant Professor
Department of Emergency Medicine
Drexel University College of Medicine
Philadelphia, Pennsylvania
Attending Physician
Medical Director
Department of Emergency Medicine
Mercy Fitzgerald Hospital
Darby, Pennsylvania
Burn Care Procedures

Douglas L. McGee, DO, FACEP
Associate Professor
Chief Academic Officer
Albert Einstein Healthcare Network
Department of Emergency Medicine
Albert Einstein Medical Center
Philadelphia, Pennsylvania
Local and Topical Anesthesia
Podiatric Procedures

John W. McGill, MD
Associate Professor
Department of Emergency Medicine
University of Minnesota School of
    Medicine
Senior Associate Faculty
Department of Emergency Medicine
Hennepin County Medical Center
Minneapolis, Minnesota
Tracheal Intubation

Jillian L. McGrath, MD
Assistant Professor
Department of Emergency Medicine
Associate Residency Program Director
The Ohio State University Wexner
    Medical Center
Columbus, Ohio
Vital Sign Measurement

Christopher R. McNeil, MD
Assistant Professor
Residency Program Director
Center for Emergency Medicine
University of Texas School of Medicine
San Antonio, Texas
Central Venous Catheterization and
    Central Venous Pressure Monitoring

Bohdan M. Minczak, MD, PhD
EMS Division Head
EMS Fellowship Director
Department of Emergency Medicine
Drexel University College of Medicine
Philadelphia, Pennsylvania
Medical Director
MidAtlantic MedEvac
Hahnemann University
Pottstown, Pennsylvania
Techniques for Supraventricular
    Tachycardias
Defibrillation and Cardioversion

Dean Moore II, MD
Attending Physician
Emergency Department
Albert Einstein Medical Center
Philadelphia, Pennsylvania
Management of Amputations

Aimee Moulin, MD, FACEP
Assistant Professor
Department of Emergency Medicine
University of California Davis Medical
    Center
Sacramento, California
Standard Precautions and Infectious
    Exposure Management

---

†Deceased.

David W. Munter, MD, MBA
Associate Clinical Professor
Department of Emergency Medicine
Eastern Virginia Medical School
Norfolk, Virginia
Associate Clinical Professor
Department of Emergency Medicine
Edward Via College of Osteopathic
  Medicine
Blacksburg, Virginia
Esophageal Foreign Bodies

Joshua Nagler, MD
Assistant Professor
Department of Pediatrics
Harvard Medical School
Fellowship Director
Division of Emergency Medicine
Children's Hospital Boston
Boston, Massachusetts
*Devices for Assessing Oxygenation and
  Ventilation*

Mark J. Neavyn, MD
Clinical Faculty
Department of Emergency Medicine
St. John Hospital and Medical Center
Wayne State University School of
  Medicine
Detroit, Michigan
Autotransfusion

**Jessica L. Osterman, BS, MS,
MD**
Assistant Residency Director
Assistant Professor of Clinical
  Emergency Medicine
Emergency Department
University of Southern California
  Medical Center
Los Angeles, California
*Management of Increased Intracranial
  Pressure and Intracranial Shunts*

Edward A. Panacek, MD, MPH
Professor
Department of Emergency Medicine
University of California Davis Medical
  Center
Sacramento, California
*Balloon Tamponade of Gastroesophageal
  Varices*

Margarita E. Pena, MD, FACEP
Associate Professor of Emergency
  Medicine
Wayne State University School of
  Medicine
Assistant Residency Director and
  Medical Director, Clinical Decision
  Unit
Department of Emergency Medicine
St. John Hospital and Medical Center
Detroit, Michigan
Autotransfusion

James A. Pfaff, MD
Staff Emergency Physician
San Antonio Uniformed Services
  Health Education Consortium
Emergency Medicine Residency
San Antonio Military Medical Center
Joint Base San Antonio–Fort Sam
  Houston
Houston, Texas
Assessment of Implantable Devices

**Heather M. Prendergast, MD,
MPH**
Associate Professor
Vice Chair Academic Affairs
Department of Emergency Medicine
University of Illinois
Chicago, Illinois
*Procedures Pertaining to Hypothermia and
  Hyperthermia*

Leigh Ann Price, MD
Assistant Professor
Department of Plastic and
  Reconstructive Surgery
The Johns Hopkins University School
  of Medicine
Director, Burn Fellowship Program
Director, Burn Residency Training
The Johns Hopkins Burn Center
Baltimore, Maryland
Burn Care Procedures

**Michael S. Pulia, MD, FAAEM,
FACEP**
Assistant Professor
Division of Emergency Medicine
University of Wisconsin School of
  Medicine and
  Public Health
Madison, Wisconsin
Emergency Childbirth

Robert F. Reardon, MD
Associate Professor
Department of Emergency Medicine
University of Minnesota
Faculty Physician
Department of Emergency Medicine
Hennepin County Medical Center
Minneapolis, Minnesota
*Basic Airway Management and Decision
  Making*
Tracheal Intubation

Salim R. Rezaie, MD
Assistant Program Director of
  Emergency Medicine
Assistant Clinical Professor of
  Emergency Medicine
Assistant Clinical Professor of Internal
  Medicine
Center for Emergency Medicine
University of Texas School of Medicine
San Antonio, Texas
*Central Venous Catheterization and
  Central Venous Pressure Monitoring*

Megan L. Rischall, MD
Resident
Department of Emergency Medicine
Hennepin County Medical Center
Minneapolis, Minnesota
*Management of Increased Intracranial
  Pressure and Intracranial Shunts*

Emanuel P. Rivers, MD, MPH
Clinical Professor
Department of Emergency Medicine
  and Surgery
Wayne State University
Vice Chairman and Research Director
Senior Staff Attending
Department of Emergency Medicine
  and Surgical Critical Care
Henry Ford Hospital
Detroit, Michigan
Resuscitative Thoracotomy

**Ralph J. Riviello, MD, MS,
FACEP, FAAEM**
Associate Professor
Department of Emergency Medicine
Drexel University College of Medicine
Attending Physician
Hahnemann University Hospital
Philadelphia, Pennsylvania
Otolaryngologic Procedures

James R. Roberts, MD, FACEP, FAAEM, FACMT
Professor of Emergency Medicine
Vice Chair, Department of Emergency Medicine
Senior Consultant, Division of Toxicology
The Drexel University College of Medicine
Chairman, Department of Emergency Medicine
Director, Division of Toxicology
Mercy Catholic Medical Center
Philadelphia, Pennsylvania
Intravenous Regional Anesthesia

Adam K. Rowden, DO
Assistant Professor of Emergency Medicine
Jefferson Medical College
Director of Operations
Department of Emergency Medicine
Associate Director, Fellowship in Medical Toxicology
Einstein Medical Center
Consulting Toxicologist
Children's Hospital of Philadelphia
Philadelphia, Pennsylvania
Physical and Chemical Restraint

Michael S. Runyon, MD
Associate Professor and Research Director
Department of Emergency Medicine
Carolinas Medical Center
University of North Carolina—Charlotte Campus
Charlotte, North Carolina
Peritoneal Procedures

Brent E. Ruoff, MD
Chief
Division of Emergency Medicine
Washington University School of Medicine
St. Louis, Missouri
Commonly Used Formulas and Calculations

Carolyn Joy Sachs, MD, MPH
Professor of Clinical Medicine
Department of Emergency Medicine
University of California, Los Angeles
Los Angeles, California
Medical Advisor
Forensic Nurse Specialists, Inc.
Long Beach, California
Examination of the Sexual Assault Victim

Leonard E. Samuels, MD
Assistant Professor
Department of Emergency Medicine
Drexel University College of Medicine
Philadelphia, Pennsylvania
Nasogastric and Feeding Tube Placement

Stewart O. Sanford, MD
Attending Physician
Department of Emergency Medicine
Albert Einstein Medical Center
Philadelphia, Pennsylvania
Arthrocentesis

Jairo I. Santanilla, MD
Clinical Assistant Professor of Medicine
Department of Medicine
Sections of Emergency Medicine and Pulmonary/Critical Care Medicine
Louisiana State University Health Sciences Center
Department of Pulmonary/Critical Care Medicine
Ochsner Medical Center
New Orleans, Louisiana
Mechanical Ventilation

Genevieve Santillanes, MD
Assistant Professor
Department of Emergency Medicine
Keck School of Medicine of USC
University of Southern California
Los Angeles, California
Pediatric Vascular Access and Blood Sampling Techniques

Jordan Sax, MD
Resident
Department of Emergency Medicine
The Johns Hopkins University
Baltimore, Maryland
Tube Thoracostomy

Richard B. Schwartz, MD
Professor and Chairman
Department of Emergency Medicine
Georgia Regents University
Augusta, Georgia
Pharmacologic Adjuncts to Intubation

David J. Scordino, MD
Resident
Department of Emergency Medicine
The Johns Hopkins University
Baltimore, Maryland
Foreign Body Removal

Greene Shepherd, PharmD
Clinical Professor
Eshelman School of Pharmacy
University of North Carolina
Asheville, North Carolina
Pharmacologic Adjuncts to Intubation

Michael A. Silverman, MD
Chairman
Department of Emergency Medicine
The Virginia Hospital Center
Arlington, Virginia
Instructor
Department of Emergency Medicine
The Johns Hopkins University School of Medicine
Baltimore, Maryland
Urologic Procedures

Zachary E. Smith, MMS, PA-C
Senior Physician Assistant
Departments of Anesthesiology/Critical Care and Emergency Medicine
The Johns Hopkins School of Medicine
Baltimore, Maryland
Principles of Wound Management
Methods of Wound Closure

Peter E. Sokolove, MD, FACEP
Professor
Vice Chair for Academic Affairs
Department of Emergency Medicine
University of California Davis Health System
Sacramento, California
Extensor and Flexor Tendon Injuries in the Hand, Wrist, and Foot
Standard Precautions and Infectious Exposure Management

Mark Spektor, DO, MBA, FACEP
President and CEO
Bayonne Medical Center
Bayonne, New Jersey
Nerve Blocks of the Thorax and Extremities

Daniel B. Stone, MD, MBA
Clinical Assistant Professor
Department of Medicine
Florida International University
Herbert Wertheim College of Medicine
Miami, Florida
Regional Medical Director
TeamHealth SouthEast
Fort Lauderdale, Florida
Foreign Body Removal

Amita Sudhir, MD
Assistant Professor
Department of Emergency Medicine
University of Virginia
Charlottesville, Virginia
Educational Aspects of Emergency Department Procedures

Semhar Z. Tewelde, MD
Clinical Instructor/Emergency
    Cardiovascular Fellow
Department of Emergency Medicine
University of Maryland Medical Center
Baltimore, Maryland
Pericardiocentesis

Jacob W. Ufberg, MD
Professor
Department of Emergency Medicine
Temple University School of Medicine
Residency Director
Department of Emergency Medicine
Temple University Hospital
Philadelphia, Pennsylvania
Management of Common Dislocations

Veronica Vasquez, MD
Assistant Professor
Director of Quality Improvement
Department of Emergency Medicine
Keck School of Medicine of USC
University of Southern California
Los Angeles, California
Venous Cutdown

**Malinda Wheeler, RN, MN, FNP,
SANE**
Director
Forensic Nurse Specialists, Inc.
Long Beach, California
Examination of the Sexual Assault Victim

**Michael E. Winters, MD, FACEP,
FAAEM**
Associate Professor of Emergency
    Medicine and Medicine
Co-Director, Combined Emergency
    Medicine/Internal Medicine/Critical
    Care Program
Director, Combined Emergency
    Medicine/Internal Medicine Program
University of Maryland School of
    Medicine
Medical Director, Adult Emergency
    Department
Department of Emergency Medicine
University of Maryland Medical Center
Baltimore, Maryland
Tracheostomy Care
*Balloon Tamponade of Gastroesophageal
    Varices*

Scott H. Witt, MD
Resident Physician
Department of Medicine
Division of Emergency Medicine
Medical University of South Carolina
*Indwelling Vascular Devices: Emergency
    Access and Management*

Richard D. Zane, MD
Professor and Chair
Department of Emergency Medicine
University of Colorado School of
    Medicine
Aurora, Colorado
Peripheral Intravenous Access

Video Contributors

Carlo Astini, MD, FRCS
Chief Consultant Surgeon
General Surgery
Hopital Italien de Balbala
Balbala, Djibouti

Anna Bargren, MD
Emergency Medicine
University of Chicago
Chicago, Illinois

Joe Bellezo, MD
Emergency Medicine
Sharp Memorial Hospital
San Diego, California

Darren Braude, MD
Department of Emergency Medicine
University of New Mexico
Albuquerque, New Mexico

James Bryant, RN, VA-BC
Clinical Coordinator
Vascular Access Department
Chesapeake Regional Medical Center
Chesapeake, Virginia

Adam Bystrzycki, MBBS, FACEM
Senior Lecturer
Department of Medicine
Monash University
Melbourne, Victoria, Australia

Lance Carter, BS, MSA, AA-C
UMKC MSA Assistant Program
  Director, Allied Health
UMKC School of Medicine
Kansas City, Missouri

Kevin Chason, DO
Department of Emergency Medicine
Mount Sinai School of Medicine
New York, New York

Panna Codner, MD
Division of Trauma and Critical Care
Department of Surgery
Medical College of Wisconsin
Milwaukee, Wisconsin

Daniel Cook, MD
President, Cookgas LLC
St. Louis, Missouri

Neil Cunningham, MBBS, FACEM
Honorary Senior Fellow
Faculty of Medicine, Dentistry and
  Health Sciences
University of Melbourne
Melbourne, Victoria, Australia

Matt Dawson, MD, RDMS, RDCS
Assistant Professor
Director of Emergency Ultrasound
Emergency Medicine
University of Kentucky
Lexington, Kentucky

George Douros, BMBS, AFCEM
Emergency Department
Austin Health
Melbourne, Australia

James DuCanto, MD
Clinical Assistant Professor
Department of Anesthesiology
Medical College of Wisconsin
Milwaukee, Wisconsin

David K. Duong, MD MS
Assistant Professor
Emergency Medicine
University of California, San Francisco
San Francisco, California

Anton J. Fakhouri, MD, FACS, FICS
Assistant Clinical Professor
Department of Orthopaedic Surgery
University of Illinois College of
  Medicine
Chicago, Illinois

Gerard Fennessy, MD
Honorary Senior Fellow
Faculty of Medicine, Dentistry and
  Health Sciences
University of Melbourne
Melbourne, Victoria, Australia

Whit Fisher, MD
Department of Emergency Medicine
The Westerly Hospital
Westerly, Rhode Island

William Fleischman, MD
Department of Emergency Medicine
Mount Sinai School of Medicine
New York, New York

Daniel Gromis, MD, RDMS
Emergency Medicine Physician
Advocate Christ Medical Center
Oak Lawn, Illinois
St Joseph's Hospital
Orange, California
Long Beach Memorial Medical Center
Long Beach, California

Fayaz Gulamani, RRT
BOMImed
Bensenville, Illinois

Mel Herbert, MD
Professor of Emergency Medicine
Keck School of Medicine of the
  University of Southern California
Los Angeles County–USC Medical
  Center
Los Angeles, California

Scott A. Joing, MD
Emergency Department
Hennepin County Medical Center
Minneapolis, Minnesota

Randy Kardon, MD, PhD
Director of Neuro-Ophtalmology
University of Iowa
Iowa City, Iowa

Raashee Kedia, MD
Department of Emergency Medicine
Mount Sinai School of Medicine
New York, New York

Heidi Harbison Kimberly, MD
Instructor
Harvard Medical School
Emergency Department
Brigham and Women's Hospital
Boston, Massachusetts

Najeeb Layyous, FRCOG
Consultant
Obstetrics and Gynecology
IVF Department
Amman, Jordan

Tim Leeuwenburg, MD
Adjunct Senior Lecturer
School of Rural Medicine
Flinders University
Adelaide, South Australia, Australia

Dan Lemkin, MD
University of Maryland School of
Medicine
Baltimore, Maryland

Michelle Lin, MD
Associate Professor of Clinical
Emergency Medicine
Academy Endowed Chair for
Emergency Medicine Education
University of California, San Francisco
San Francisco, California

Joseph Maddry, MD
Rocky Mountain Poison Center
Denver, Colorado

Michael Mallin, MD
Assistant Professor
Department of Surgery
University of Utah
Salt Lake City, Utah

Gary Marks, DO
Chief Resident
Department of Emergency Medicine
Los Angeles County–USC Medical
Center
Los Angeles, California

Joe Mayerle, MD
Emergency Medicine
St. Francis Regional Medical Center
Shakopee, Minnesota

**Larry B. Mellick, MS, MD, FAAP,
FACEP**
Vice Chairperson of Emergency
Medicine
Professor of Emergency Medicine
Georgia Regents Health Center
Augusta, Georgia

Siamak Moayedi, MD
Assistant Professor
Emergency Medicine
University of Maryland School of
Medicine
Baltimore, Maryland

Bret Nelson, MD, RDMS
Associate Professor
Director of Emergency Ultrasound
Icahn School of Medicine at Mount
Sinai
New York, New York

Jared Novack, MD
Northshore University Health System
Evanston, Illinois

Thomas A. Oetting, MD
University of Iowa Health Care
Iowa City, Iowa

Robert Orman, MD
Department of Emergency Medicine
Valley View Hospital
Glenwood Springs, Colorado

Andrew Pendley, MD
Department of Emergency Medicine
Emory University School of Medicine
Atlanta, Georgia

**Phillips Perera, MD, RDMS,
FACEP**
Clinical Associate Professor
Emergency Medicine
Division of Emergency Medicine
Department of Surgery
Stanford University School of
Medicine
Stanford, California

Adam Petersen, MSA, AA-C
Ozark Anesthesia Associates
Cox Health System
Springfield, Missouri

Ronald Pirrallo, MD
Section of Out-of-Hospital & Disaster
Medicine
Department of Emergency Medicine
Medical College of Wisconsin
Milwaukee, Wisconsin

Avital Porat, MD
Department of Emergency Medicine
Mount Sinai School of Medicine
New York, New York

Melanie M. Randall, MD
Pediatric Emergency Medicine Fellow
Department of Emergency Medicine
Loma Linda University Medical Center
Loma Linda, California

Cliff Reid, BM, FACEM
Senior Staff Specialist in Prehospital &
Retrieval Medicine
Greater Sydney Area Helicopter
Emergency Medical Service
Sydney, New South Wales, Australia

Joshua Rempell, MD
Instructor
Emergency Medicine
Brigham and Women's Hospital
Harvard Medical School
Boston, Massachusetts

William H. Rosenblatt, MD
Professor, Anesthesiology
Yale University School of Medicine
New Haven, Connecticut

Alfred Sacchetti, MD, FACEP
Chief of Emergency Medicine
Our Lady of Lourdes Medical Center
Camden, New Jersey

Zachary Shinar, MD
Emergency Medicine
Sharp Memorial Hospital
San Diego, California

Neil Singh, MD
Department of Emergency Medicine
Mount Sinai School of Medicine
New York, New York

Benjamin H. Slovis, MD
Department of Emergency Medicine
Mount Sinai School of Medicine
New York, New York

Mike Stone, MD, FACEP
Division Chief, Emergency Ultrasound
Fellowship Director, Emergency
Medicine
Brigham and Women's Hospital
Boston, Massachusetts

Chrissa Strumpe, RN
Northshore University Health System
Evanston, Illinois

Tammar Taddei, MD
Assistant Professor of Medicine
Yale University School of Medicine
New Haven, Connecticut

Felipe Teran, MD
Department of Emergency Medicine
Mount Sinai School of Medicine
New York, New York

Jack Vander Beek, RN
Neuraxiom, LLC
Olympia, Washington

Ernest Wang, MD
Northshore University Health System
Evanston, Illinois

Scott D. Weingart, MD, FCCM
Associate Clinical Professor
Division of ED Critical Care
Mount Sinai School of Medicine
New York, New York

Tim Young, MD
Assistant Professor of Emergency
    Medicine and Pediatrics
Department of Emergency Medicine
Loma Linda University Medical Center
Loma Linda, California

John Zangmeister, MD
Family Medicine Physician
Department of Family Medicine
Cleveland Clinic
Cleveland, Ohio
Vice Chairman, Family Medicine
Fairview Hospital
Cleveland, Ohio

Steven Zils, MD, FACEP
Section of Out-of-Hospital & Disaster
    Medicine
Department of Emergency Medicine
Medical College of Wisconsin
Milwaukee, Wisconsin

The sixth edition of *Roberts and Hedges' Clinical Procedures in Emergency Medicine* continues the book's original concept of providing complete, detailed, and up-to-date descriptions of many common, and some uncommon, procedures encountered during emergency medical practice. The novice may find the discussions and figures devoted to the many procedures somewhat daunting or overwhelming at first; but it is hoped that most will eventually appreciate the simple discussion and complex verbiage contained in the text. The goal is to describe clinical procedures—from simple Steri-Strip application, to loop drainage of an abscess, to skull trephination—as though each were the nascent clinician's first exposure to the concept, but with a depth and attention to detail that the seasoned operator would also deem helpful.

In previous editions it was difficult to find figures or photographs that conveyed the details or elucidated the vagaries to the extent one might want. The newly added color photographs, mostly digital quality, and a cornucopia of additional figures were a much needed update and morphed this edition into an obvious improvement over previous iterations. To make the text more user friendly, procedure boxes have been created, comprising a mini-atlas that allows the clinician to see the entire procedure at a glance. One can even bring the text to the bedside, viewing a single page of sequential images, the quintessential teaching tool for house staff and students. Many of the photographs were taken by me over 42 years of emergency department shifts or created or supplied by Todd W. Thomsen, MD. Some illustrations were borrowed from other sources, such as the wonderful text by Catherine B. Custalow, MD, PhD. This edition has more than 3500 images, half of which are new. More than 70 percent of the new images are the result of the artistic genius of graphics editor Dr. Thomsen. Frank Netter, watch out for Dr. Thomsen; he is rapidly attaining your status and may have already surpassed it in emergency medicine parlance. No doubt Dr. Thomsen has found his calling, blending amazing original art and electronic and digital prowess with equally impressive clinical medicine expertise.

The addition of the ultrasound-guided sections, presented in easily found and readily deciphered boxes, is the result of a gargantuan effort from our new ultrasound editor, Catherine Butts, MD, an ultrasonographer extraordinaire. One of the greatest achievement of this edition is the addition of a video procedures library, expertly crafted by Rob Orman, MD, and Scott Weingart, MD. Only wished for in past editions, many sections now reference online content that allows the reader to view videos of the procedures actually being performed. "See one, do one, teach one" has taken on new meaning with this text. This edition is now available electronically on such devices as the Kindle and iPad and is still fully searchable online at expertconsult.com.

There are, of course, many ways to approach any patient or any procedure, so this text is not a dictum. This book does not attempt to define standard of care. It is a compendium of self-proclaimed techniques—some tried and some true, but occasionally prospectively tested—practical hints, and successful tactics gleaned from the literature and by years of practice, adeptly described by skilled clinicians. As with prior editions, this version also significantly incorporates the personal opinions of the authors and editors. This book is intended to help the clinician and the patients who rely upon them. But it is simply a clinical guide, not a legal document. Do not reference this book if you testify in court, for either the defense or the plaintiff. Today's dogma too often becomes tomorrow's heresy, and physician hubris is worse than incompetence. Simply stated, emergency medicine and the human body too often defy the written word, personal opinion, or local custom and humble even the venerable and the universally praised gray-haired professor.

Many new authors have been added, as well as a number of new concepts and approaches. All procedures have been tweaked. Trigger point injection has been resurrected, as well as skull trephination; both were mistakenly removed from the previous edition. You will not find the novel loop abscess drainage technique so nicely described elsewhere.

My personal thanks are hereby conveyed to those who contributed to previous editions. The updated chapters often merely refine or further manipulate the scholarly work of others who originally assisted us. The current contributors include an enviable blend of friends and colleagues, former students of mine, up-and-coming rising stars in their own right, and my prior mentors and role models—all are accomplished physicians and leaders in their own milieu. We have added three new associate editors, names well known to anyone who reads the literature or attends a continuing medical education activity. All the associate editors portray and embody the pinnacle of emergency medicine excellence. Most of the contributors, and all the associate editors, probably know more than I know, and most are likely infinitely more capable and facile with procedures. All are capable of writing a text themselves, and some have already done so; however, some are now enlightened and eschew that primal urge since they now know how difficult it is to write even a single chapter. My able and erudite associate editors, all from prestigious academic teaching programs in emergency medicine, are Arjun S. Chanmugam, MD, MBA; Carl R. Chudnofsky, MD; Peter M.C. DeBlieux, MD; Amal Mattu, MD; Stuart P. Swadron, MD, FRCPC; and Dr. Thomsen. They provided the bulk of the original editing, but senior editor, Dr. Custalow, read every single word and reviewed every table and chart. Dr. Custalow is a more tenacious editor than the proverbial honey badger in regard to dealing with details, grammar, organization, and style. In the end, my personal bias may be evident, but Dr. Custalow was the fire and fuel for the book's framework. As already stated, Dr. Thomsen made the text come to life with images.

If any of our editing changed, altered, or misinterpreted the original thoughts of the contributors (and I know in some instances it must have), we apologize; but hard decisions had to be made, and waffling was rarely an option. Our book simply tells you what to do and how and when to do it, but no book can always fit every individual situation. We attempted to squarely address such omnipresent vague topics as prophylactic antibiotics, local customs, and variations in style, and accepted the fact that not all foreign bodies or tendon lacerations will be identified in the heat of the moment by even the most skilled. The prescient and sagacious clinician knows that the ability to practice medicine from a book is limited, and one learns best from past experiences; and, for certain, the most instructive past experience is one that was not always textbook perfect.

James R. Roberts, MD, FACEP, FAAEM, FACMT

Foreword

Fear! There, I said it. Procedures scare me. Not all of them, but many of them. Never in the practice of a health care professional have we had more opportunity to do direct, obvious, "no hiding from it" damage to a patient. It is even possible to kill a patient with the various blades and objects we use to treat them. If that does not strike fear into your heart, then you have a problem.

Three basic attributes are required of a successful emergency medicine practitioner:

1. Knowledge: knowing a little about a LOT of things
2. Professionalism: learning how to interact with patients, families, hospital staff, and the world around you
3. Procedural skills: knowing how and when to perform a procedure

Mastering procedural skills is what this book is all about. Learning the motor skills necessary to actually perform the procedures late at night under very stressful conditions is what formal training is for. I cannot emphasize enough how being good at the entire range of procedures affects the poise, confidence, and job satisfaction of the emergency medicine professional. It is a cornerstone of the life of an emergency practitioner. Fear of doing procedures can destroy an otherwise great doctor. Knowing the myriad causes of bradycardia will not help you when you need to drop an IV pacemaker in a dying patient at 3 AM. You need to know how to do it, immediately, without hesitation. Emergency medicine is a procedural specialty; accept it and get damn good at performing these procedures. It is our responsibility to our patients and to ourselves.

I was first introduced to the now legendary *Roberts and Hedges' Clinical Procedures in Emergency Medicine* as an intern in Australia. The fear of doing harm was more acute during that year than any other. A sage and wise senior resident saw that look of panic in my eye and directed me to The Book. "Read it, learn it, be one with it; it is the best, most practical textbook in emergency medicine," he told me. He was right then, and five editions later, *Roberts and Hedges' Clinical Procedures in Emergency Medicine* is still the best book in emergency medicine. It is a remarkable piece of practical wisdom wrapped in an academic blanket. Standard procedure texts give you the usual list of indications and contraindications, a written description of how to perform the procedure and a few pictures. The Roberts and Hedges book goes far beyond this with clear, in-depth literature reviews, finely crafted illustrations, and images that are packaged in a seamless flow. The chapters include approaches to the various procedures, including the pharmacology of sedation and analgesia, historical perspectives, and the philosophical underpinning of what, when, and how to act in the chaos of the emergency department. A perfect example of the practical wisdom of this treasured textbook comes in the section on foreign body removal. The authors encourage the practitioner to set a time limit by setting a stopwatch. Only practicing clinicians understand the profound nature of this advice. Only those who actually work on the front line and in the chaos of emergency departments realize that the "I've *almost* got it" phenomenon can result in literally hours stuck at one patient's bedside, as well as lots of pain, blood, and tissue damage that can be avoided by giving yourself a time limit and then going to Plan B.

Emergency medicine is a remarkable specialty. Comprising literally 24/7 nonstop action, anything can come in the door and you have to know how to deal with it—from the newborn who needs an umbilical line, to the 90-year-old who needs a suprapubic catheter, to the 8-year-old who needs jet ventilation or her parents will never see that perfect smile again. This is your job. Do it well. This book will help you to be confident and competent in one of the three fundamental aspects of your work. "Read it, learn it, be one with it; it is the best, most practical book in emergency medicine!"

Mel Herbert, MD, MBBS, BMedSci, FACEP, FAAEM
Professor of Emergency Medicine
Keck School of Medicine of USC
University of Southern California
Los Angeles County–USC Medical Center
Los Angeles, California

Acknowledgments

Gargantuan efforts, clairvoyant and perceptive suggestions, and decidedly prescient contributions of many individuals have brought this work to fruition. Not the least of whom were the individual authors who toiled over tedious manuscripts and answered countless queries about the vagaries and vicissitudes of seemingly straightforward clinical procedures.

All of the initially submitted work was culled, corrected, and collated by Dee Simpson; the overall concepts and layouts were tweaked and strategized by Stefanie Jewell-Thomas; and every comma and period was laboriously scrutinized by Doug Turner. My gratitude to them is warmly extended with this acknowledgment. If any reader is contemplating developing their own textbook, snag this team of publishing aficionados if you can.

Of course, the entire work was infused with vim and vigor from Catherine B. Custalow, MD, PhD, and every image was created, beautified, or otherwise superbly orchestrated by Todd W. Thomsen, MD. The final editing of Arjun S. Chanmugam, MD, MBA; Carl R. Chudnofsky, MD; Peter M.C. DeBlieux, MD; Amal Mattu, MD; and Stuart P. Swadron, MD, FRCPC, completed the task. Apparently these guys have a lot of free time on their hands or, more likely, they burned gallons of midnight oil for the project. Scott D. Weingart, MD; Robert Orman, MD; Christine Butts, MD; and Mel Herbert, MD, MBBS, BMedSci, FACEP, FAAEM, completed the lineup of stellar contributors. One could not wish for, or even fantasize about, a cadre of more gifted clinicians and eloquent editors.

Thank you all for accomplishing a goal that was once thought, even by me, to be nothing more than a seemingly good idea, but a task too difficult to even contemplate, let alone wantonly attempt.

James R. Roberts, **MD, FACEP, FAAEM, FACMT**

Contents

†Deceased.

Video Contents

VIDEO EDITORS

Robert Orman, MD
Department of Emergency Medicine
Valley View Hospital
Glenwood Springs, Colorado

Scott D. Weingart, MD, FCCM
Associate Clinical Professor
Division of ED Critical Care
Mount Sinai School of Medicine
New York, New York

Vital Signs and Patient Monitoring Techniques

CHAPTER 1

Vital Signs Measurement

Diane L. Gorgas and Jillian L. McGrath

Measuring the temperature, pulse, respiratory rate (RR), blood pressure, and pulse oximetry is generally recommended for all emergency department (ED) patients, in addition to assessment of pain in the appropriate patient population. For very minor problems or for some fast-track patients (e.g., suture removal), a full set of vital signs may not be required, but this is best decided on a case-by-case basis rather than by strict protocol. Vital signs may not only indicate the severity of illness but also dictate the urgency of intervention. Although a single set of abnormal values suggests pathology, findings on triage or the initial vital signs may be spurious and simply be related to stress, anxiety, pain, or fear. *It would be incorrect and not standard of care to attribute initial triage blood pressure, RR, or pulse rate to specific pathology or to retrospectively assume that diagnostic or treatment interventions should have been initiated based solely on these readings. The greatest utility of vital signs, therefore, is their observation and trends over time.* Deteriorating vital signs are an important indicator of a compromised physiologic condition, and improving values provide reassurance that the patient is responding to therapy. When a patient undergoes treatment over an extended period, it is essential that the vital signs be repeated as appropriate to the clinical scenario, particularly those that were previously abnormal. In some clinical circumstances it is advisable to monitor the vital signs continuously.[1]

Vital signs should be measured and recorded at intervals as *dictated by clinical judgment or the patient's clinical state or after any significant change in these parameters.* Adhering to protocols or disease categories may not be useful or productive. An abnormal vital sign may constitute the patient's entire complaint, as in a febrile infant, or it may be the only indication of the potential for serious illness, as in a patient with resting tachycardia.[2]

Emergency medical service (EMS) personnel begin assessment of the patient's status and vital signs in the prehospital setting. Surges of epinephrine and norepinephrine commonly occur during transport by the EMS, and these hormones are known to alter vital signs and lead to increases in the heart rate of greater than 10%.[3] Vagal influences may also influence EMS-derived vital signs. *Prehospital vital signs should always be interpreted with the entire clinical scenario in perspective.*

Blood pressure and pulse are frequently evaluated together as a measure of blood volume. Capillary refill is discussed as an assessment of overall perfusion, circulatory volume, and blood pressure. Although body temperature is usually the last vital sign measured during resuscitation, it has special importance for patients suffering from thermal regulatory failure. With these considerations in mind, the current chapter is organized according to the priorities of patient resuscitation and evaluation. Assessment of pain as a vital sign is gaining acceptance and is discussed briefly at the end of this chapter.

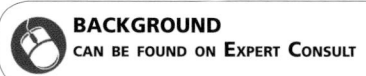

BACKGROUND
CAN BE FOUND ON EXPERT CONSULT

NORMAL VALUES

The range of normal resting vital signs for specific age groups must be recognized by the clinician to enable identification of abnormal values and their clinical significance. The normal ranges for vital signs are also influenced by gender, race, pregnancy, and residence in an industrialized nation. These ranges have not been validated in ED patients, who have many reasons for abnormalities in vital sign, including anxiety, pain, and altered physiology from their disease states. *Ranges of normal vital signs,* commonly quoted as normal or abnormal in other settings, serve only as a guide and not an absolute criterion for diagnosis, treatment, further observation, or intervention in the ED.

Published vital sign norms for children are not as well accepted as those for adult patients. Table 1-1 and Table 1-2 report normal vital signs for children by age group as means and standard deviations. In Table 1-1, the values for pulse and blood pressure for 0- to 2-month-olds are adapted from studies of newborn populations (i.e., <7 days).[8-10] During the newborn period, normal arterial blood pressure rises rapidly. Values for pulse and respiration in children older than 3 years reflect an average of male and female values for 0- to 1-, 3-, 9-, and 16-year-old populations. The values for blood pressure reflect an average of male and female values for the 1- to 6-month-old and the 3-, 9-, and 16-year-old populations.[11] Newer studies have reassessed the reference values for RR in children.[12-14] Table 1-2 reflects age-related changes and the effect of the state of wakefulness on RR in children up to 3 years of age.[14] A study evaluating resting RRs in pediatric ED

TABLE 1-1 Normal Values for Vital Signs in Infants and Children (Means ± SD)

	AGE				
PARAMETER	0-2 mo	3-12 mo	1-6 yr	7-12 yr	13-18 yr
Breaths/min	—*	—*	24 ± 3	19 ± 2	17 ± 3
Pulse/min	126 ± 20	131 ± 20	88 ± 9	70 ± 8	64 ± 7
Systolic BP†	72 ± 10	95 ± 15	93 ± 13	100 ± 10	112 ± 12
Diastolic BP	51 ± 9	53 ± 10	55 ± 10	63 ± 10	67 ± 10

BP, blood pressure; *SD*, standard deviation.
*For data on children 0 to 36 moths, see Table 1-2.
†As an estimate, for children 1 to 10 years of age, (2 × age [yr]) + 90 mm Hg = 50th percentile for systolic BP.

TABLE 1-2 Normal Respiratory Rates (Breaths/min) in Children Up to 3 Years of Age (Means ± SD)

AGE (mo)	AWAKE	ASLEEP
0-<2	48.0 ± 9.1	39.8 ± 8.7
2-<6	44.1 ± 9.9	33.4 ± 7.0
6-<12	39.1 ± 8.5	29.6 ± 7.0
12-<18	34.5 ± 5.8	27.2 ± 5.6
18-<24	32.0 ± 4.8	25.3 ± 4.6
24-<30	30.0 ± 6.2	23.1 ± 4.6
30-36	27.0 ± 4.1	21.5 ± 3.7

Adapted from Rusconi F, Castagneto M, Gagliardi L, et al. Reference values for respiratory rate in the first 3 years of life. *Pediatrics*. 1994;94:351.
SD, standard deviation.

TABLE 1-3 Vital Signs during Pregnancy in the Lateral Decubitus Position (Means ± SD)

	TRIMESTER		
PARAMETER	1st	2nd	3rd
Pulse rate (beats/min)	77 ± 2	85 ± 2	88 ± 2
Systolic BP (mm Hg)	98 ± 2	91 ± 2	95 ± 2
Diastolic BP (mm Hg)	53 ± 2	49 ± 2	50 ± 2

Adapted from Katz R, Karliner JS, Resnik R. Effects of a natural volume overload state (pregnancy) on left ventricular performance in normal human subjects. *Circulation*. 1978;58:434. By permission of the American Heart Association.
BP, blood pressure; SD, standard deviation.

patients up to the age of 18, however, indicated considerable patient variability and somewhat higher RRs than those shown in Table 1-2.[12]

For the adult population, normal blood pressure values have been established. Although systolic blood pressure increases with age, *normotensive or normal systolic blood pressure* is defined as 90 to 140 mm Hg, and *normotensive or normal diastolic blood pressure* is defined as 60 to 90 mm Hg. The recent literature suggests defining an "optimal" blood pressure as 115/75 because values at or below this level have been associated with minimal vascular mortality.[15] It has been suggested that the definition of hypertension be further expanded to integrate a global cardiovascular risk assessment.[16,17] Although most patients have similar blood pressure in both arms, Pesola and coworkers found that 18% of their hypertensive population[18] and 15% of their normotensive population *had a difference of greater than 10 mm Hg in systolic blood pressure between arms.*[19]

Within the adult population, optimal definitions for normal systolic blood pressure probably vary by age, and particular differentiation should be made in regard to geriatric patients in the emergency setting. The recent literature suggests redefining values representative of hypotension in the elderly, especially in the setting of trauma. Systolic blood pressure readings ranging from approximately 90 to 120 mm Hg have been associated with occult hypoperfusion and increased mortality in geriatric trauma patients.[20-22]

In 1928 the New York Heart Association, by consensus, established the normal limits for the resting heart rate as 60 beats/min and 100 beats/min. More recent data indicate that 45 beats/min and 95 beats/min may better define the heart rate limits of normal sinus rhythm in adults of all ages. Spodick recommended that the operational definition for the limits of the resting heart rate in adults be 50 beats/min and 90 beats/min.[23,24] This view is widely supported among cardiologists,[25,26] but these ranges have not been validated in the ED setting. *There is currently no consensus on what constitutes a normal adult RR; however, an RR range of 12 to 24 breaths/min is generally accepted in the existing literature as the norm for adults.*[27,28]

Pregnancy results in alterations in the normal adult values for pulse and blood pressure. The RR is unchanged, although the physiologic hyperventilation of pregnancy is well recognized and results from increased tidal volume and decreased residual and expiratory reserve volume.[29] The resting pulse rate increases throughout pregnancy to 10% to 15% over baseline values. The norms for systolic and diastolic blood pressure are dependent on patient positioning. When a pregnant patient is sitting or standing, systolic pressure is essentially unchanged. Diastolic pressure declines until approximately 28 weeks' gestation, at which time it begins to rise to nonpregnant levels. When a pregnant patient is in the lateral decubitus position, both systolic and diastolic pressure declines until the 28th week and then begins to rise to nonpregnant levels (Table 1-3).[30]

RESPIRATION

Breathing is initiated and primarily controlled in the medullary respiratory center of the brainstem. The respiratory center is modulated by the pneumotaxic center, which limits the length of the inspiratory signal and greatly influences the RR and apneustic center in the pons.[31] Respiratory frequency reveals only a glimpse of the entire clinical picture. The pattern, effort, and volume of respiration may be more indicative of altered respiratory physiology. An abnormality in respiration may be a primary complaint or a manifestation of other systemic diseases. Increased RRs may be seen in patients with a variety of pulmonary or cardiac diseases, but acidosis, anemia, temperature, stress, and drugs (such as stimulants and salicylates) can significantly alter the RR in the absence of cardiopulmonary dysfunction.

Indications and Contraindications

The only contraindications to careful measurement of RR are the scenarios of respiratory distress, apnea, and upper airway obstruction, which require immediate therapeutic intervention. RR and respiratory effort should be measured as soon as patient care demands allow.

The respiratory status of both adults and children plays a crucial role in determining the overall assessment of illness. Although it is a sensitive yet nonspecific indicator of respiratory dysfunction, the RR can also predict nonpulmonary morbidity. Several prehospital and hospital-based illness or injury severity scores feature the RR as a cardinal value. A prehospital RR of less than 10 or greater than 29 breaths/min is associated with major injury in 73% of children.[32] Using tachypnea alone as a predictor of pulmonary pathology, infants with an RR higher than 60 are found to be hypoxic 80% of the time.[33] Pediatric studies have linked abnormal RRs to in-hospital mortality and the level of care required in the ED.[34,35] In a retrospective study exploring predictors of critical care admission for adult ED patients who were initially triaged as having low to moderate acuity, an abnormal RR at the first nursing assessment increased the odds of critical care admission by a factor of 1.66.[36] An RR higher than 25 breaths/min in prehospital trauma patients was associated with increased mortality.[37] Pre-arrest respiratory insufficiency (RR >36 breaths/min or pulse oximetry <90%) was an independent predictor of mortality (odds ratio [OR], 4.2) in patients with EMS-witnessed cardiac arrest.[38] Although some studies have associated abnormal RRs in adult ED patients with increased mortality,[39,40] a recent large prospective cohort study of adult patients found that an initial abnormal RR on triage in the ED was not an independent predictor of hospital mortality.[41]

Procedure

To measure RR (inspirations per minute), count the respirations when the patient is unaware that his or her breathing is being observed. Count for a full minute to most accurately determine the RR. The frequency of breathing is less regular than the pulse, and inaccurate measurement is more likely to occur if the count is taken for a shorter interval. An infant's RR can easily be determined by observing or palpating the excursion of the chest or the abdominal wall.[42] Infants should be observed for grunting respirations, which are produced by expiration against a partly closed glottis (an attempt to maintain positive airway pressure).

Interpretation

Respiratory Rate

The reproducibility of RR measurements may be limited by significant interobserver variability.[43,44] Clinicians should recognize this inherent variability and interpret the RR with caution. Rates obtained by nurses versus medical students varied significantly, as did those obtained by medical students versus residents and attending clinicians.[45] Interobserver variability may account for a difference of up to 6 breaths/min, and variability in the same observer may account for up to 5 breaths/min.[45] A study comparing RRs obtained by triage nurses with an electronic monitor found that neither provided an accurate measurement of the RR in the ED, thus suggesting that new clinical strategies for obtaining this vital sign may be necessary.[46]

Current texts vary considerably in their definition of a normal RR and cite published values that range from 8 to 24 breaths/min. In a study that specifically investigated normal RRs in an ED (afebrile ambulatory patients without respiratory complaints), females had a mean RR of 20.9 breaths/min and males had a mean RR of 19.4 breaths/min. *The researchers concluded that a normal RR in the adult patient population was 16 to 24 breaths/min.*[45] Other studies have provided additional information on normal resting and sleep-state RRs in children younger than 7 years.[9-14] RRs obtained with a stethoscope were higher than those obtained by observation (mean difference, 2.6 breaths/min in awake and 1.8 breaths/min in asleep children). Smoothed percentile curves demonstrated a larger dispersion at birth (5th percentile, 34 breaths/min; 95th percentile, 68 breaths/min), whereas dispersion was less at 36 months of age (5th percentile, 18 breaths/min; 95th percentile, 30 breaths/min).

The RR will generally increase in the presence of fever. It is often difficult to determine whether tachypnea is a primary finding or is simply associated with hyperpyrexia. A study of children younger than 2 years in whom pneumonia was subsequently diagnosed found that age-appropriate limits for resting tachypnea in the presence of fever could be defined. A sensitivity of 74% and specificity of 77% for pneumonia were found when children 6 months of age had an RR higher than 59 breaths/min, when those aged 6 to 11 months had an RR higher than 52 breaths/min, and when those 1 to 2 years old had an RR higher than 42 breaths/min.[47] Even in the face of physiologic compensation for fever, interpretation of the RR alone can help predict the presence of pulmonary disease.

Respiratory Pattern and Amplitude

Hyperventilation and hypoventilation can result from an extensive variety of disorders and may be related to pulmonary or extrapulmonary pathology. Abnormal respiratory patterns can be characteristic of metabolic or central nervous system pathologic conditions (Fig. 1-1) and may aid in the differential diagnosis. Kussmaul respirations describe the hyperventilation pattern seen in diabetics with ketoacidosis. Hyperpnea, or a normal RR but clinically significant hyperventilation secondary to increased tidal volume, may be seen with salicylate poisoning.[48]

Recognition of subtle tachypnea can be difficult in the emergency setting, although it can be the solitary indicator of disease. Another instance of pathology that can confuse routine measurement of the RR is diaphragmatic breathing or retractions. The variability in counting respiratory effort

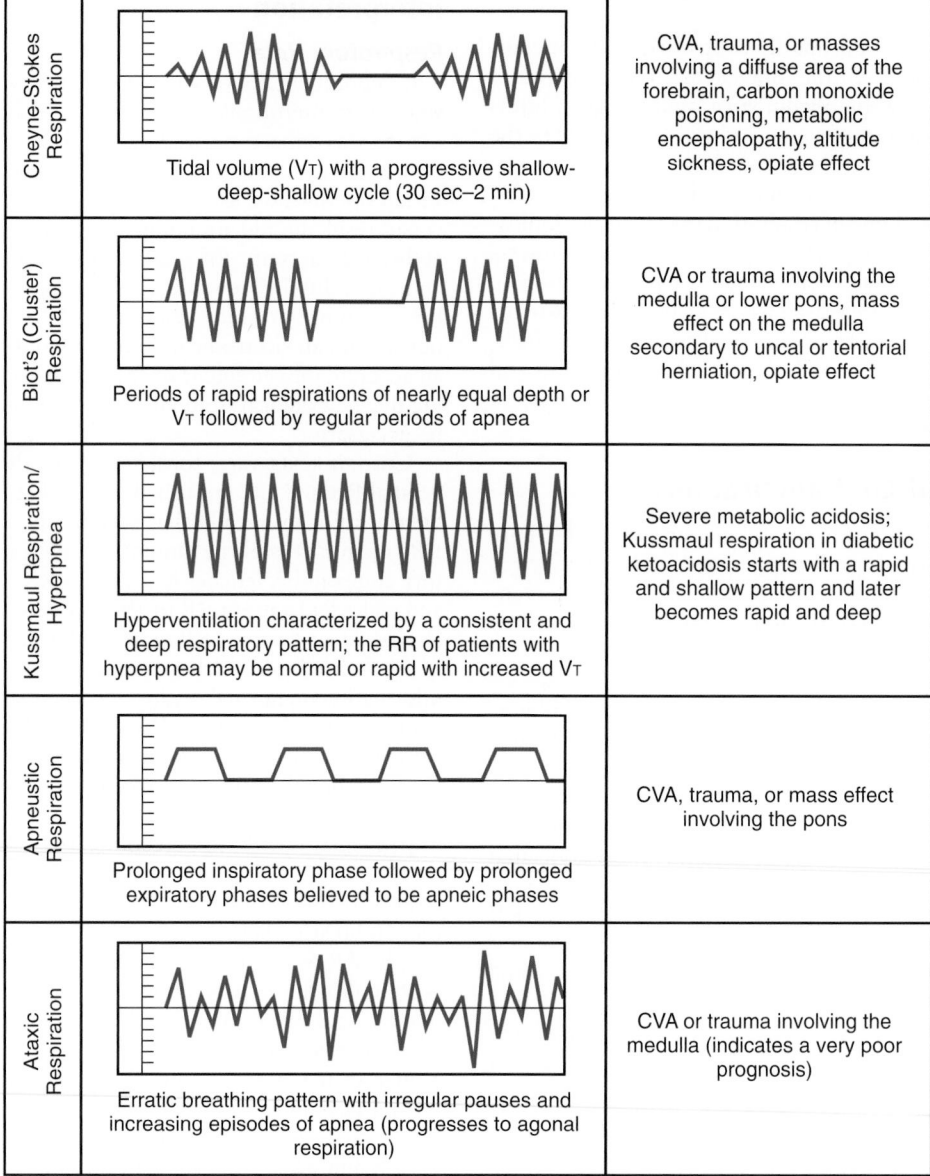

Figure 1-1 Abnormal respiratory patterns. *CVA,* cerebrovascular accident; *RR,* respiratory rate. (*Adapted from Breathing Patterns. © 2011—D'Urbano J—Breath Sounds. Available at http://www.BreathSounds.org.*)

versus effective respirations is not generally appreciated in a single recorded value.

Observe the respiratory patterns carefully in children. In infants it is essential to distinguish normal periodic breathing from apnea. By definition, *periodic breathing* consists of three or more respiratory pauses longer than 3 seconds in duration with less than 20 seconds between pauses. There is no associated bradycardia or cyanosis. This contrasts with apnea, which is a particular problem in preterm infants. *Apnea* is defined as a respiratory pause longer than 20 seconds. It may be associated with bradycardia and hypoxia.[42] Periodic breathing and apnea are believed to be disorders on a continuum, both stemming from abnormal physiologic control of respiration. Periodic breathing is considered a benign disorder, but infants with symptomatic apneic episodes that result in apparent life-threatening events are thought to be at increased risk for sudden infant death syndrome.[49]

PULSE

Examine the pulse to establish the cardiac rate and regularity of rhythm. Though rarely diagnostic, peripheral pulses may yield clues about cardiac disease, such as aortic insufficiency, and information about the integrity of the peripheral vascular supply. Doppler ultrasound has utility in locating a pulse, assessing fetal heart tones beyond the first trimester of pregnancy, evaluating peripheral lower extremity vascular insufficiency, and assessing blood pressure in infants or in patients with low-flow states.

Physiology

Blood flowing into the aorta with each cardiac cycle initiates a pressure wave. Blood flows through the vasculature at approximately 0.5 m/sec, but pressure waves in the aorta move at 3 to 5 m/sec. Therefore, palpated peripheral pulses represent pressure waves, not blood flow.

Indications and Contraindications

Assessment of blood flow by palpation of the pulse can be used to gauge the presence of cardiac contractility and not just the electrical rhythm. Caution should be taken to not over-generalize the presence or strength of a pulse in predicting blood pressure. The necessity for repeated pulse evaluations is dictated by the clinical complaint and the status of the patient. Continuous monitoring is not routine but may be helpful when the clinical situation may predict significant variability in heart rate, as in the setting of sepsis.[50] An association between absence of a radial pulse or absence of both radial and femoral pulses and hypotension has been demonstrated in hypovolemic trauma patients. The variability in individual response prohibits the use of this parameter as an absolute gauge of blood pressure.[51]

No contraindications exist to assessment of the pulse rate, but keep in mind a few cautionary notes about examination of the carotid pulse. Avoid concurrent bilateral carotid artery palpation because this maneuver could endanger cerebral blood flow. Massage of the carotid sinus, found at the bifurcation of the external and internal carotid arteries at the level of the mandibular angle, may result in reflex slowing of the heart rate. To avoid inadvertent carotid sinus massage, palpate the carotid pulse at or below the level of the thyroid cartilage. In adults with atherosclerotic disease, there is a rare risk of precipitating a cerebrovascular event by vigorous palpation of the carotid artery. Minimize this risk by prior auscultation of the carotid artery. If a bruit is present, gently palpate the carotid pulse while avoiding vigorous palpation.

Procedure

Depending on the clinical scenario, pulses are palpable at numerous sites, although for convenience the radial pulse at the wrist is routinely used. Use the tips of the first and second fingers to palpate the pulse. The two advantages of this technique are that (1) the fingertips are quite sensitive, thereby enabling the pulse to be located easily and counted, and (2) the examiner's own pulse may be erroneously counted if the thumb is used instead of the first and second fingers. Pulses are also easily palpated at the carotid, brachial, femoral, posterior tibial, and dorsalis pedis arteries. Palpate the pulse at the brachial artery to appreciate its contour and amplitude. Locate the pulse at the medial aspect of the elbow and note that it is more easily palpated when the elbow is held slightly flexed.[52] Determine the pulse rate by counting for 1 minute, particularly if any abnormality is present. Common convention in the acute care setting is to count a regular pulse for 15 seconds and multiply the resulting number by 4 to determine the beats per minute.

In newborns, use direct heart auscultation and umbilical palpation as the methods of choice to determine the heart rate. Instantaneous changes in newborn heart rates are best indicated to the resuscitation team by the clinician tapping out each heartbeat.[53] In unstable children, palpate the central arteries, particularly the femoral and brachial pulses, instead of the more peripheral arteries. In a comparison of four methods of determining the heart rate in infants, listening at the apex of the heart was found to be more accurate than palpation of the brachial, carotid, or femoral pulses.[54] Of the sites for palpation of the heart rate, the femoral artery has proved most valuable, especially in hypotensive infants.[55]

Interpretation

Pulse Rate

Consider the individual's physiology when interpreting the pulse. In infants and children, interpret the pulse rate with reference to age (See Table 1-1). Pulse varies with respiration: it increases with inspiration and slows with expiration. This is known as sinus dysrhythmia and is physiologic.

Although *bradycardia* is defined as a heart rate lower than 60 beats/min in adults, a well-conditioned athlete may have a normal resting heart rate of 30 to 40 beats/min.[56,57] As discussed earlier, a redefinition of bradycardia to less than 45 beats/min and tachycardia to greater than 95 beats/min has been proposed based on a normal healthy population.[24,58] Such definitions include 95% of the population and do not address any given individual's normal baseline rate.

Consider whether a patient's abnormal pulse rate is a primary or secondary condition. Examine the entire set of vital signs when attempting to discern the cause of the abnormal rate. For example, hyperthermia causes sinus tachycardia. Drug fever, typhoid fever, and central neurogenic fever are suggested when no corresponding tachycardia is found in a patient with elevated body temperature. This condition is called temperature-pulse disassociation. Hypothermia, with its reduced metabolic demands, may be associated with bradycardia.

Consider the medications that the patient may be taking or the presence of a mechanical pacemaker. Digitalis compounds, β-blockers, and antidysrhythmics may alter the normal heart rate and the ability of this vital sign to respond to a new physiologic stress. These cardioactive medications may be causing the abnormality in the patient's heart rate.

Heart Rhythm

In addition to determining the pulse rate, obtain information about the regularity of the pulse by palpation. An irregular pulse suggests atrial fibrillation or flutter with variable block, and accurate assessment of the pulse should be done by auscultation of the apical cardiac sounds. The apical pulse is frequently greater than the peripheral pulse because of inadequate filling time and stroke volume, with resultant nontransmitted beats. A greater pulse deficit generally reflects more severe disease.[59]

Pulse Amplitude and Contour

Accurate examination and description of pulse amplitude and contour can provide additional clinical information and aid in decision making. Superimposition of one pathophysiologic state on another may modify the pulse. For example, sepsis may result in variable pulse amplitudes, depending on the stage in the development of the disease at initial evaluation of the patient. Early in sepsis, cardiac output increases and vascular resistance decreases, which causes bounding pulses. In advanced sepsis or septic shock, falling cardiac output and increased vascular resistance are seen, and pulses are diminished.[60] Definable age-related changes in pulse amplitude and contour can be identified. Such changes are due to an increase in arterial stiffness, which results in increased pulse wave velocity and progressively earlier wave reflection. This leads to increased pulse amplitude in the elderly at all commonly measured sites (carotid, femoral, and radial).[60] In addition to these age-related changes, pulse wave analysis may be useful in determining arterial stiffness and the likelihood of atherosclerotic disease in a vascular laboratory setting.[61] Weak pulses can be a significant finding in patients with hypotension if present globally or an indication of limb ischemia if isolated to one extremity. Bounding pulses can be seen with a widened pulse pressure, which is discussed later in the section on blood pressure. Routine measurement of pulse amplitude is not reproducible by simple palpation and requires instrumentation not available in EDs.

Pulses during Cardiopulmonary Resuscitation

Palpated "femoral pulses" during chest compression may represent either forward arterial blood flow or "to-and-fro" movement of blood from the right side of the heart to the venous system. A carotid pulse is preferred when assessing the adequacy of chest compressions during cardiopulmonary resuscitation (see Chapter 17).

ARTERIAL BLOOD PRESSURE

Changes in arterial blood pressure over time may indicate success of treatment or worsening of the patient's overall condition. An abrupt reduction in a patient's arterial blood pressure usually indicates the need for immediate intervention or reconsideration of therapy. The current section discusses indirect blood pressure monitoring, and intraarterial techniques are considered elsewhere. Discussion of the specific use of the Doppler device for measurement of pulse and blood pressure and for measurement of orthostatic blood pressure and changes in pulse follow this section. Despite an association between the absence of hypotension and a radial pulse or between hypotension and the absence of both radial and femoral pulses, in the setting of trauma, the variability in individual response prohibits the use of this parameter as an absolute gauge of blood pressure.[52]

Physiology

Arterial blood pressure indicates the overall state of hemodynamic interaction between cardiac output and peripheral vascular resistance. Arterial blood pressure is the lateral pressure or force exerted by blood on the vessel wall. It indirectly measures perfusion, and blood flow equals the change in pressure divided by resistance. Because peripheral vascular resistance varies, a normal blood pressure does not confirm adequate perfusion.[62] Mean arterial blood pressure (MAP) can be estimated by adding one third of the pulse pressure (i.e., the difference between systolic and diastolic blood pressure) to diastolic pressure or by using the following measure.[63]

$$MAP = \frac{Diastolic\ pressure \times 2 + Systolic\ pressure}{3}$$

Indications and Contraindications

Patients with minor ambulatory complaints unrelated to the cardiovascular system may not necessarily need their blood pressure measured in the ED, but those with hemodynamic instability need frequent monitoring of blood pressure. In children there is a significant amount of variability regarding standard situations that require measurement of blood pressure. In general, the younger the patient, the less likely blood pressure will be measured.[64,65] In newborns, infants, and even toddlers, capillary refill is sometimes substituted for standard blood pressure measurement, although viewing these tests as equivalent can lead to significant errors.

In low-flow states, Doppler measurement of blood pressure may be obtained rapidly. Repeated measurements will provide an evaluation of the adequacy of resuscitation in patients whose blood pressure cannot be auscultated by standard techniques and in those in whom intraarterial blood pressure measurements are either contraindicated or technically unobtainable.[66,67] Placing a catheter for direct intraarterial measurement of blood pressure has a higher risk for complications, but it may be performed safely in the ED. In particular, direct measurement of arterial pressure during pulseless electrical rhythms may help discriminate between severe shock and otherwise nonresuscitatable status.[68] Alternative noninvasive devices for continuous blood pressure measurement (CBPM) have been introduced clinically, with varying success. One common method of CBPM uses finger cuffs equipped with infrared (IR) photoplethysmography and sophisticated technology for quantification of finger blood pressure levels. Finapres (Ohmeda, Madison, WI) was the first commercial product using this technique, and several newer products are on the market today. A number of commercial systems use an alternative method of arterial applanation tonometry to measure CBPM. Further study is needed for solid validation of devices using these techniques.[69,70]

Relative contraindications to specific extremity blood pressure measurement include an arteriovenous fistula, ipsilateral mastectomy, axillary lymphadenopathy, lymphedema, and circumferential burns over the intended site of cuff application.

Equipment

Two types of blood pressure monitoring equipment are currently available and used in EDs: cuff-type and noninvasive waveform analysis.

Cuff Type

The equipment required for indirect blood pressure measurement includes a sphygmomanometer (cuff with an inflatable bladder, inflating bulb, controlled exhaust for deflation, and manometer) and a stethoscope, Doppler device (for auscultation), or oscillometric device.[71-74] A common practice in the prehospital and interhospital transport setting is to forego auscultatory blood pressure measurements with a stethoscope and instead obtain systolic values only by palpation of the first Korotkoff sound. This practice, though sometimes the only feasible method of obtaining any value in a noisy environment, poses a significant potential for error. In a study of critically ill patients transferred between hospitals, palpated systolic blood pressure values underestimated manometric values by nearly 30%.

According to the American Heart Association guidelines, the sphygmomanometer cuff should be an appropriate size for the patient to ensure an accurate reading. The width of the bladder should be at least 40% of the distance of the limb's midpoint (i.e., from the acromion process to the lateral epicondyle). This published figure of the ideal width, when studied in a validation review, may be higher, up to approximately 50%.[75] The length of the bladder should be 80% of the midarm circumference or twice the recommended width.[66] Discrepancies in matching upper arm size with cuff size have been demonstrated to produce significant errors in critically ill populations when compared with invasive intraarterial blood pressure measurements.[76] The availability of appropriately sized cuffs appears to be a pervasive problem, especially since about 80% of patients do not fit the standard 12-cm large cuffs.[77] In one study, 90% of aneroid devices had only one size of cuff available.[78] A second study phase from this group showed no marked improvement in agreement of oscillatory and invasive measurements despite correct cuff size.[79]

The manometers in common use are either aneroid, digital, or mercury gravity column. All three types of manometers are convenient for bedside use, although the mercury gravity column must be placed vertically to ensure accurate measurements. An aneroid manometer uses a metal bellows that elongates with the application of pressure. This elongation is mechanically amplified and transmits the motion to the indicator needle.

Manometers require annual servicing. Mercury columns may require the addition of mercury to bring the edge of the meniscus to the zero mark. The air vent or filter at the top of the mercury column should also be checked for clogging. An aneroid manometer should be calibrated against a mercury column at least yearly. If the aneroid indicator is not at zero at rest, the device should not be used.[80] Digital manometers may not be validated for all patient groups and could give inaccurate readings.

Automatic sphygmomanometers may improve physiologic monitoring with their alarm and self-cycling capabilities. They offer indirect arterial blood pressure measurement with little pain and without the risks associated with invasive arterial lines.[81] Accuracy of measurements does not suffer during rapid cycling, but the potential for vascular injury from nearly continuous arterial compression dictates that most automated blood pressure units will revert back to less frequent (i.e., every 15 to 20 minute) cycling as a safety precaution. Oscillometric blood pressure monitors detect motion of the blood pressure cuff transmitted from the underlying artery. A sudden increase in the amplitude of arterial oscillations occurs with systolic pressure and MAP, and an abrupt decrease occurs with diastolic pressure.[82]

There appears to be less variability with the oscillometric blood pressure method than with the auscultatory method in children. These results are not generalizable to the neonatal population, and errors are commonly encountered even when exhaustive measures are taken to control the environment.

In adult patients, numerous studies have focused on the reliability of auscultatory versus automated blood pressure measurements. Mercury column versus Dinamap readings showed increased disparity with systolic blood pressure greater than 140 mm Hg, the range at which accuracy should be most rigorously sought to correctly identify hypertension. In general, automated blood pressure devices yield higher systolic and lower diastolic blood pressure.[83] The range of error in automated devices was, on average, 4.0 to 8.6 mm Hg.[84,85] Unfortunately, these studies represent populations without critical illness and do not reflect the accuracy of readings at the extremes of hypertension and hypotension, thus making generalization to an ED population difficult.[85,86]

Procedure

Obtain indirect blood pressure measurements at the patient's bedside by palpation, auscultation, Doppler, or oscillometric methods. The technique is straightforward and accurate when the equipment is well maintained, calibrated, and used by clinicians who follow accepted standards. The patient may be lying or sitting, as long as the site of measurement is at the level of the right atrium and the arm is supported.[66,74] Unless the arm is kept perpendicular to the body with the elbow resting on a desk, measurements will be 9 to 14 mm Hg higher, regardless of body position.[75,87] Allowing the arm to be parallel to the body when supine but supporting the arm perpendicular to the body when measuring blood pressure may create a pseudo-drop in blood pressure. These changes are thought to be dependent on the mechanical properties of the arteries themselves and not associated with hydrostatic pressure alone.[88]

To palpate arterial blood pressure, inflate the cuff to 30 mm Hg above the level at which the palpable pulse disappears. Once properly inflated, palpate directly over the artery and deflate the cuff at a rate of 2 to 3 mm Hg/sec. Report the initial appearance of arterial pulsations as the palpable blood pressure. This practice, known as the Riva-Rocci palpatory technique, has shown mixed results in yielding accurate estimations of blood pressure. One study determined that the average underestimation of systolic blood pressure was 6 mm Hg.[89] Another operative study looking at the combination of palpated systolic blood pressure and observed visual return of continuous pulse oximetry reported an underestimation of 10 to 20 mm Hg.[85] The same technique is used with the Doppler device, but the palpated pulse is replaced with the Doppler auditory signal. Measurement of arterial pressure by palpation and Doppler yields only estimates of systolic blood pressure. The Doppler method is preferred when determining blood pressure in infants.[86]

When auscultating blood pressure at the brachial artery, apply the blood pressure cuff about 2.5 cm above the antecubital fossa with the center of the bladder over the artery.[74] Apply the bell of the stethoscope directly over the brachial artery with as little pressure as possible.[90] *Systolic arterial blood pressure* is defined as the first appearance of faint, clear, tapping sounds that gradually increase in intensity (Korotkoff phase I). *Diastolic blood pressure* is defined as the point at which the sounds disappear (Korotkoff phase V).[74-91] In children, phase IV defines diastolic blood pressure (Fig. 1-2).[7] Phase IV is marked by a distinct, abrupt muffling of sound when a soft, blowing quality is heard.

It is best to measure by auscultation over the brachial artery because of accepted standardization of the measured values. Alternative sites include the radial, popliteal, posterior tibial, or dorsalis pedis arteries, although any fully compressible extremity artery may be used. Studies evaluating direct and indirect blood pressure measurements have demonstrated good correlation between these methods.[92,93]

It may not be feasible to obtain upper extremity blood pressure measurements because of patient access issues, particularly those encountered in the prehospital setting. Forearm measurements may be obtained more easily and show fair correlation to standard upper extremity values (within 20 mm Hg in 86% of systolic measurements and 94% of diastolic measurements).[94] Alternatively, noninvasive finger blood pressure measurements have shown promise when

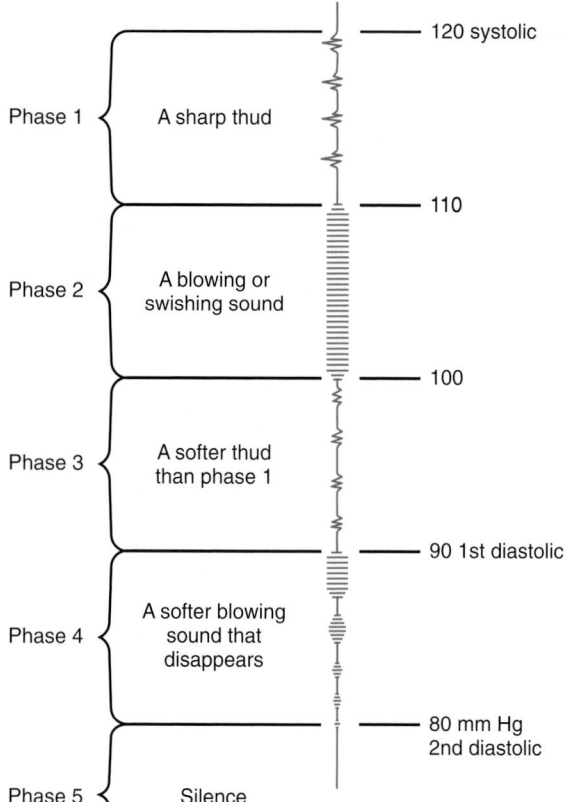

Phase 1 — A sharp thud
Phase 2 — A blowing or swishing sound
Phase 3 — A softer thud than phase 1
Phase 4 — A softer blowing sound that disappears
Phase 5 — Silence

120 systolic
110
100
90 1st diastolic
80 mm Hg 2nd diastolic

Figure 1-2 Korotkoff sounds. The first audible sound occurs in systole, and the sound disappears in diastole. *(From Burnside JW, McGlynn TJ. Physical Diagnosis. 17th ed. Baltimore: Williams & Wilkins; 1986.)*

compared with standard upper extremity readings. The overall discrepancy in an ED study was 0.1 mm Hg with a standard deviation of ±5.02 mm Hg when comparing finger blood pressure and invasive MAP via radial artery cannulation.[95]

Novel noninvasive continuous finger cuff technology offers the benefit of uninterrupted monitoring and has the advantage over invasive techniques of being safer and immediately available. Noninvasive finger cuff measurements have shown reasonable correlation, even in critically ill populations in the ED.[70] Wrist blood pressure has shown to have good average accuracy in the surgical environment when compared with oscillometric devices. Patient comfort is reported to be greater with these devices. The typically stated contraindications to the acquisition of upper arm blood pressure (limitation after mastectomy, etc.) may not apply.[96]

The accuracy of the palpatory, Doppler, and oscillometric methods has also been investigated.[97-99] When phase I and V Korotkoff sounds are used, indirect methods typically underestimate systolic and diastolic pressure by several millimeters of mercury.[97-100] During shock, the palpatory and auscultatory methods underestimate simultaneous direct arterial pressure measurements.[101] The flush method, in which return of color after deflation of the cuff is used to estimate blood pressure in infants, may underestimate systolic blood pressure by up to 40 mm Hg.[102] This method is unreliable and not recommended.

Complications

Complications of indirect blood pressure measurements are minimal when the proper procedure is followed. Inadvertent prolonged application of an inflated blood pressure cuff may result in falsely elevated diastolic pressure and ischemia distal to the site of application.[76] Invasive blood pressure monitoring is associated with a number of potential problems (see Chapter 20).

Interpretation

Normal blood pressure increases with decreasing distance from the heart and aorta. Blood pressure tends to increase with age and is generally higher in males. Individual factors that influence blood pressure include body posture, emotional or painful stimuli, environmental influences, vasoactive foods or medications, and the state of muscular and cerebral activity. Exercise and sustained isometric muscular contraction increase blood pressure in proportion to the strength of the contraction. A normal diurnal pattern of blood pressure consists of an increase throughout the day with a significant, rapid decline during early, deep sleep.[103]

Normal lower limits of systolic blood pressure in infants and children can be estimated by adding 2 times the age (in years) to 70 mm Hg. The 50th percentile for a child's systolic arterial blood pressure from 1 to 10 years of age can be estimated by adding 2 times the age (in years) to 90 mm Hg. Children older than 2 years are considered hypotensive when systolic blood pressure is less than 80 mm Hg.[104] Children are able to maintain MAP until very late during shock.[105] The finding of a normal blood pressure in a child with signs of poor perfusion should not dissuade the clinician from appropriate treatment. Most adults are considered hypotensive if systolic blood pressure is lower than 90 mm Hg, but some individuals normally exhibit a systolic pressure in that range. In the elderly, the presence of normotension within defined or published limits may not be reassuring. When considering systolic blood pressure cutoffs for trauma patients, 85 mm Hg for patients aged 18 to 35, 96 mm Hg for patients aged 36 to 64, and 117 mm Hg for those older than 65 have been proposed as new standards for hypotension.[20] When accompanied by signs of shock, immediate treatment is indicated. In patients with shock, blood flow cannot be reliably inferred from heart rate and blood pressure values.[106,107]

Hypertension

Adults are hypertensive if either systolic or diastolic pressure consistently exceeds 140 or 90 mm Hg, respectively.[108,109] A meta-analysis showed strong correlation of blood pressure to vascular and overall mortality down to at least 115/75.[110] Some authors have suggested altering the blood pressure definitions to include an "optimal" blood pressure of 115/75.[15] Other authors have suggested incorporating blood pressure into a global cardiovascular risk assessment that includes other associated risk factors.[16,17] The applicability of population norms for hypertension in a stressful emergency situation is controversial. *One should not make diagnostic or therapeutic decisions based solely on an abnormal initial measurement.* Patients with hypertension require repeated measurements to assess whether therapy is required in the ED. Because sustained hypertension may be seen in more than a third of initially hypertensive ED patients, careful evaluation and follow-up are required.[111] The phenomenon of *white coat hypertension* (WCH) is defined as a persistent elevation in blood pressure in the clinical setting only. The prevalence of WCH is between 20% and 94%, depending on the frequency of reassessment of the clinical setting.[112] It is unclear whether patients who have isolated hypertension in the clinical setting (WCH) are at increased risk for the development of hypertension and subsequent end-organ damage.[113]

Measurement Errors

Erroneous blood pressure measurements may result from several factors.[114] Falsely low blood pressure may be caused by using an overly wide cuff, by placing excessive pressure on the head of the stethoscope, or by rapid cuff deflation.[115,116] Falsely high blood pressure may be caused by the use of an overly narrow cuff, anxiety, pain, tobacco use, exertion, an unsupported arm, or slow inflation of the cuff.[117] There appears to be a statistically significant difference in the error rate associated with patients weighing more than 95 kg, whether from obesity or as a result of muscular upper arms from body building.[118,119]

Of note, 41% of adults observed at the University of Pittsburgh required non–standard-sized cuffs, and the use of small cuffs was associated with a mean error of 8.5 and 4.6 mm Hg in systolic and diastolic pressure, respectively.[116] Other studies have confirmed relatively high rates of inappropriately diagnosed hypertension in obese patients based on erroneous cuff size.[118] Other specific study populations in this area have been critically ill patients, in whom disparate cuff size can lead to significant inaccuracies based on arm circumference.[82]

Hypotensive patients have unreliable Korotkoff sounds, but Doppler measurements are well correlated with direct arterial systolic pressure measurements in hypotensive patients.[120] An auscultatory gap can be appreciated in hypertensive patients and may mislead the clinician. It is heard during the latter part of phase I and should not be confused with diastolic readings. Auscultation until the manometer reading approaches zero should prevent misinterpretation. In patients with aortic insufficiency or hyperthyroidism, in those who have just finished exercising, and in children younger than 5 years, measurement of diastolic blood pressure should occur at Korotkoff phase IV. Extremes of blood pressure, both hypotension and hypertension, have been found to be factors contributing to measurement errors in critically ill pediatric patients. Predictably falsely high readings for noninvasive versus invasive measurements have been obtained in hypotensive patients and falsely low values in hypertensive states.[121]

Irregular heart rates may also interfere with accurate determination of blood pressure. Take a second or third reading, with 2 minutes of deflation between recordings, and obtain an average when premature contractions or atrial fibrillation is present.

Hemiplegic patients may exhibit different blood pressure in the affected and unaffected arms.[122] A flaccid extremity tends to yield lower systolic and diastolic pressure, whereas a spastic extremity tends to yield higher values than the extremity with normal motor tone. Although these differences are generally small, it is preferable to monitor blood pressure in the unaffected limb.

Numerous errors may occur in the accurate measurement of blood pressure. The only way to combat them is to first be cognizant of practices contributing to them. Unfortunately,

few nurses can identify causes of potentially erroneous readings. In a study examining nurses' ability to obtain accurate readings, proper technique in determining systolic blood pressure could be identified 61% of the time; diastolic blood pressure, 71% of the time; and an auscultatory gap, 54% of the time. Nurses were able to correctly identify faulty equipment 58% of the time, assess cuff size 57% of the time, determine appropriate inflation pressure 29% of the time, note the appropriate deflation rate 62% of the time, and determine correct arm positioning 14% of the time.[123]

With the increasing number of patients with heart failure, those receiving bridging measures to transplantation, or those treated with long-term circulatory augmentation devices in the form of left ventricular assist devices (LVADs), it useful to understand the difficulty in interpreting blood pressure measurements in these patients. All types of VADs fit into two categories: (1) pulsatile and (2) nonpulsatile. Pulse and blood pressure readings in patients with pulsatile VADs (Thoratec, HeartMate IP and VE, Novacor) are comparable to values in the general non-VAD population. Nonpulsatile VADs (Levitronix Centri Mag, Tandem Heart, Impella, DeBakey LVAD, HeartMateII) function by either centrifugal or axial blood flow, and this has a significant impact on the ability to detect pulses.[124] Typically, these patients appear to be perfusing well with adequate skin warmth and capillary refill even though pulses may be absent. Blood pressure readings can be obtained with these nonpulsatile flow devices, but diastolic blood pressure, pulse pressure values, and MAP vary significantly depending on the speed of the pump.[125]

Pulse Pressure

The difference between systolic and diastolic pressure is termed pulse pressure. Increased pulse pressure (i.e., ≥60 mm Hg) is commonly observed with anemia, exercise, hyperthyroidism, arteriovenous fistula, aortic regurgitation, increased intracranial pressure, and patent ductus arteriosus. A narrowed pulse pressure (≤20 mm Hg) may be a manifestation of hypovolemia, increased peripheral vascular resistance as seen in early septic shock, or decreased stroke volume.

Differential Brachial Artery Pressure

The presence of a systolic blood pressure differences of 10 to 20 mm Hg between the arms suggests a normal condition. If greater, it may indicate advanced focal atherosclerosis, coarctation of the aorta proximal to the left subclavian artery, type A aortic dissection, aortic arch syndromes, or other vascular processes preferentially affecting one extremity. The utility of upper extremity bilateral blood pressure measurements has recently come into question. One study found a 10-mm Hg systolic or diastolic difference in 53% of patients in the emergency setting and a 20-mm Hg or higher difference in 19% of patients.[126] Although these numbers have not generally been found to be of this magnitude in metaanalysis,[127] the unique setting of the study in the ED makes correlation particularly salient for the emergency physician. The reliability of peripheral pulse deficits in diagnosing or excluding type A aortic dissection is a frequently cited reason for evaluating blood pressure in both arms. In a metaanalysis, Teece and Hogg noted that the absence of a clinical pulse deficit to exclude thoracic dissection in patients with chest pain was just 31%, and the authors concluded that peripheral pulse deficits are far too insensitive to warrant their use as a means of excluding thoracic aortic dissection in patients with chest pain.[128] Given that many in the general population have significant differences in blood pressure in each arm, the diagnostic value of this frequently cited indication for obtaining bilateral brachial blood pressure is unproven. Essentially, most patients with a type A aortic dissection will not have a measurable blood pressure discrepancy between the arms, and most of those who do have such a finding will not have dissection.

Brachial pressure differences did not appear to be linked to age, gender, race, MAP, cardiovascular risk, or final discharge diagnosis. Smaller interarm differences have been reported in the ED setting (18% in hypertensive patients and 15% in normotensive patients when a cutoff greater than 10 mm Hg was used).[18,19] Though not tested, a method proposed to minimize these differences in the ED is to take simultaneous blood pressure readings from both the left and right extremities with two calibrated automated blood pressure units.[129]

Pulsus Paradoxus

Normal respiration briefly decreases systolic blood pressure by approximately 10 mm Hg during inspiration. Pulsus paradoxus occurs when there is greater a than 12–mm Hg decrease in systolic blood pressure during inspiration. Pulsus paradoxus may occur in patients with chronic obstructive pulmonary disease, pneumothorax, severe asthma, or pericardial tamponade.[101]

To measure a paradoxical pulse, have the patient lie comfortably in the supine position at a 30- to 45-degree angle and breathing normally in an unlabored fashion (which are unusual conditions in a patient suspected of having cardiac tamponade, severe asthma, chronic obstructive pulmonary disease, or pneumothorax).[130] Inflate the blood pressure cuff well above systolic pressure and slowly deflate it until the systolic sounds that are synchronous with expiration are first heard (Fig. 1-3). Initially, the arterial pulse will be heard only during expiration and will disappear during inspiration. Deflate the cuff further until arterial sounds are heard throughout the respiratory cycle. Palpation at the radial or femoral arteries may yield complete disappearance during inspiration. When present, this technique is a quick bedside confirmation of the possibility of severe tamponade.

An alternative method for determination of pulsus paradoxus is by visually observing loss of the pulse oximetry waveform and then its reappearance.[131] The plethysmographic method has been validated in intensive care unit settings.

If the difference between inspiratory and expiratory pressure is greater than 12 mm Hg, the paradoxical pulse is abnormally wide.[130,131] Most patients with proven tamponade have a difference of 20 to 30 mm Hg or greater during the respiratory cycle.[130-132] This may not be true of patients with very narrow pulse pressures (typical of advanced tamponade), who have a "deceptively small" paradoxical pulse of 5 to 15 mm Hg.[132-134]

Pulsus paradoxus has been correlated with the amount of impairment of cardiac output by tamponade. In an uninjured patient with pericardial effusion, a pulsus paradoxus greater than 25 mm Hg (in the absence of relative hypotension) is both sensitive and specific for moderate or severe versus mild tamponade.[130,135] An echocardiographic study found that an abnormal pulsus paradoxus had a sensitivity of 79%, a specificity of 40%, a positive predictive value of 81%, and a negative predictive value of 40% for right ventricular diastolic

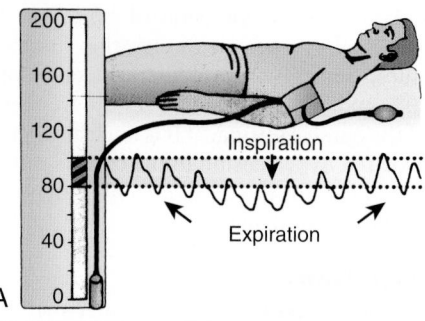

PROCEDURE FOR THE MEASUREMENT OF PULSUS PARADOXUS

The patient should be reclining at a 30° to 45° angle and instructed to breathe normally.

1. Inflate a standard blood pressure cuff until Korotkoff sounds over the brachial artery disappear.
2. Lower pressure in the cuff a few millimeters of mercury per second until the first Korotkoff sounds appear during expiration.
3. Maintain pressure at this level and observe the disappearance of sounds during inspiration. Record this cuff pressure.
4. Very slowly lower cuff pressure until Korotkoff sounds are heard throughout the respiratory cycle. Record this cuff pressure.
5. The difference between pressures recorded in the two previous steps is then recorded as the measurement (in millimeters of mercury [mm Hg]) of pulsus paradoxus. A pulsus paradoxus >12 mm Hg is abnormal but nonspecific (see text).

Figure 1-3 A, Measurement of pulsus paradoxus. Note that systolic pressure varies during the respiratory cycle. **B,** Technique for measurement of pulsus paradoxus. (*A, From Stein L, Shubin H, Weil M. Recognition and management of pericardial tamponade. JAMA. 1973;225:504. Copyright 1973, American Medical Association. Reproduced by permission.*)

collapse.[135-137] The absence of a paradoxical pulse does not rule out tamponade.

In the pediatric population, pulsus paradoxus has been studied to determine the severity of obstructive and restrictive pulmonary disease,[136] most commonly asthma. A value of 15 mm Hg or greater correlates well with the clinical score, peak expiratory value, flow rate, oxygen saturation, and subsequent need for admission.[137]

Despite the disease entities that a widened pulsus paradoxus may suggest, it is a difficult test to perform adequately with only a sphygmomanometer. Because it is a useful clinical tool, new aids should be developed and used to reliably predict this important vital sign.[138]

Shock Index

The ratio of pulse rate to systolic blood pressure has been suggested as a measure of clinical shock. The shock index (SI) has a normal range of 0.5 to 0.7. Although calculating the SI is not standard of care in the ED, a number of clinical scenarios have been studied in which the SI can be used as a predictor of severe illness or injury. An SI above 0.85 to 0.90 suggests acute illness in medical patients and a marked increase in the potential for gross hemodynamic instability in trauma patients.[139-142] The SI has been studied for use in a variety of clinical scenarios from severe pneumonia to first-trimester risk for ectopic pregnancy to sepsis. It has been found to be a valid gauge of the severity of illness.[143-145] Some studies, however, have found that the initial pulse rate alone had nearly the same predictive power as the SI for the severity of illness. Although the SI appears to correlate with the left ventricular stroke work index, it has little correlation with systemic oxygen transport in patients with hemorrhagic and septic shock.[146]

DOPPLER ULTRASOUND FOR EVALUATION OF PULSE AND BLOOD PRESSURE

Principles of Doppler Ultrasound

Doppler ultrasound is based on the Doppler phenomenon. The frequency of sound waves varies depending on the speed of the sound transmitter in relation to the sound receiver. Doppler devices transmit a sound wave that is reflected by flowing erythrocytes, and the shift in frequency is detected. Frequency shift can be detected only for blood flow greater than 6 cm/sec.

Indications and Contraindications

Doppler ultrasound is commonly used in the ED for the measurement of blood pressure in low-flow states, evaluation of lower extremity peripheral perfusion, and assessment of fetal heart sounds after the first trimester of pregnancy. Doppler's sensitivity allows detection of systolic blood pressure down to 30 mm Hg in the evaluation of a patient in shock. In a patient with peripheral vascular disease in whom there is concern about the adequacy of peripheral perfusion, the ankle-brachial index provides a rapid, reproducible, and standardized assessment.[145] Fetal heart sounds provide a baseline assessment of any pregnant patient with 12 weeks' gestation or longer in the setting of abdominal trauma or fetal distress as a result of a complication of pregnancy. The use of Doppler ultrasound for the evaluation of deep venous thrombosis is a valuable tool, but specific training and experience are required to attain proficiency. Discussion of this topic is beyond the scope of this chapter.

Equipment

A nondirectional Doppler device has a probe that houses two piezoelectric crystals. One crystal transmits the signal and the other receives it. Reflected signals are converted to an electrical signal and fed to an output that transforms them to an audible sound.

Probes with a frequency of 2 to 5 MHz are best for detecting fetal heart sounds. Frequencies of 5 to 10 MHz are appropriate for limb arteries and veins. The probes should be monitored periodically for electrical damage and integrity of the crystals. The sphygmomanometers used in conjunction with the Doppler device should be calibrated periodically, as described in the section on evaluation of blood pressure.

Procedure

Place the Doppler probe against the skin with an acoustic gel used as an interface. The gel ensures optimal transmission and reception of the ultrasound signal and protects the crystals. In an emergency, water-soluble lubricant (e.g., Surgilube or K-Y jelly) may be substituted for commercial acoustic gel.

Figure 1-4 A, Handheld Doppler device with a speaker. Devices with an attached stethoscope are also used. **B,** Peripheral vascular testing is performed in a vascular laboratory, but an approximation of the integrity of the peripheral arterial circulation can be gleaned in the emergency department by using Doppler to determine systolic blood pressure in the foot and arm and calculate the ankle-brachial index.

Angle the probe at 45 degrees along the length of the vessel to optimize frequency shifts and signal amplitude.

To evaluate peripheral perfusion, place a sphygmomanometer cuff proximal to the arterial pulse and inflate it. Place the probe over the arterial pulse and slowly deflate the cuff. The pressure at which flow is first heard is the systolic pressure *under the cuff.*

In the evaluation of peripheral vascular disease, one may determine the ankle-brachial index. It is standard for this procedure to be performed in a formal vascular laboratory. However, an approximation of pressures can be determined in the ED (Fig. 1-4). Usually, only the ankle-brachial index is considered for ED purposes. Examine both brachial arteries at the medial aspect of the antecubital fossa. Angle the probe until the most satisfactory signal is obtained. Inflate the cuff and slowly deflate it until the systolic pulse is heard. Repeat the procedure for the posterior tibial and dorsalis pedis arteries of both lower extremities. This procedure may be done with oscillometric devices but lacks sensitivity in identifying disease.[146]

In evaluating fetal heart tones, because of variable positioning of the fetus, an examination of several locations and angles over the uterus must be performed in search for the optimal signal. It is best to begin in the mid-suprapubic area and then explore the uterus via angulation of the probe. Once tones are located, move the probe along the abdomen to reach a position closer to the origin of the sound. Distinguish fetal heart tones from placental flow by differentiating the quality of the fetal heart tones, which will not match the maternal pulse. The placental flow and maternal pulse should be identical.

Interpretation

As noted earlier, in low-flow states, Doppler ultrasound can detect blood pressure as low as 30 mm Hg. Calculate the ankle-brachial index of each limb by dividing the higher systolic pressure of the posterior tibial or the dorsalis pedis artery of the limb by the higher of the systolic pressures in the brachial arteries. In normal individuals the index should be greater than 1.0 (Fig. 1-5). Patients with claudication have values between 0.6 and 0.8. Values lower than 0.5 indicate severe impairment and are consistent with rest pain or gangrene.[147] When the lower extremity has been amputated or injured, brachial-brachial indices can be used (i.e., comparison of systolic blood pressure in the injured or diseased upper extremity with the other extremity). Patients with ankle-brachial index values of 0.9 or lower have increased cardiovascular morbidity and mortality.[148] One study of 323

penetrating extremity wounds found that an ankle-brachial index (or brachial-brachial index) lower than 0.9 was 72.5% sensitive and 100% specific for vascular injuries.[149] Segmental lower extremity pressure measurements may help identify the level of the obstruction (Table 1-4).[150] Obese patients, diabetic patients, or those with calcified vessels that are not compressible may have abnormally high systolic pressure (e.g., 250 to 300 mm Hg) and indices that do not accurately reflect flow. Normal fetal heart tones should be between 120 and 140 beats/min. Fetal heart tones may be heard as early as the 12th week of gestation.

VITAL SIGN DETERMINATION OF VOLUME STATUS

Many techniques have been advocated to assess volume status. Unfortunately, *most procedures lack a database against which to judge their reliability.* Recommended methods include evaluation of skin color; skin turgor; skin temperature; supine, serial, and orthostatic vital signs; neck vein status; transcutaneous oximetry; and hemodynamic monitoring (e.g., monitoring of central venous pressure). Serial vital sign measurements have been used for assessing blood loss, but they do not reliably detect small degrees of blood loss.[147,151,152] Up to 15% of the total blood volume can be lost with minimal hemodynamic changes or any alteration in supine vital signs.[153] A decrease in pulse pressure occurs with acute blood loss,[154] but the patient's baseline blood pressure values are often unknown. Clinical examination of neck veins adds useful information but is less precise than measurement of central venous pressure. Most clinicians use skin color, temperature, and

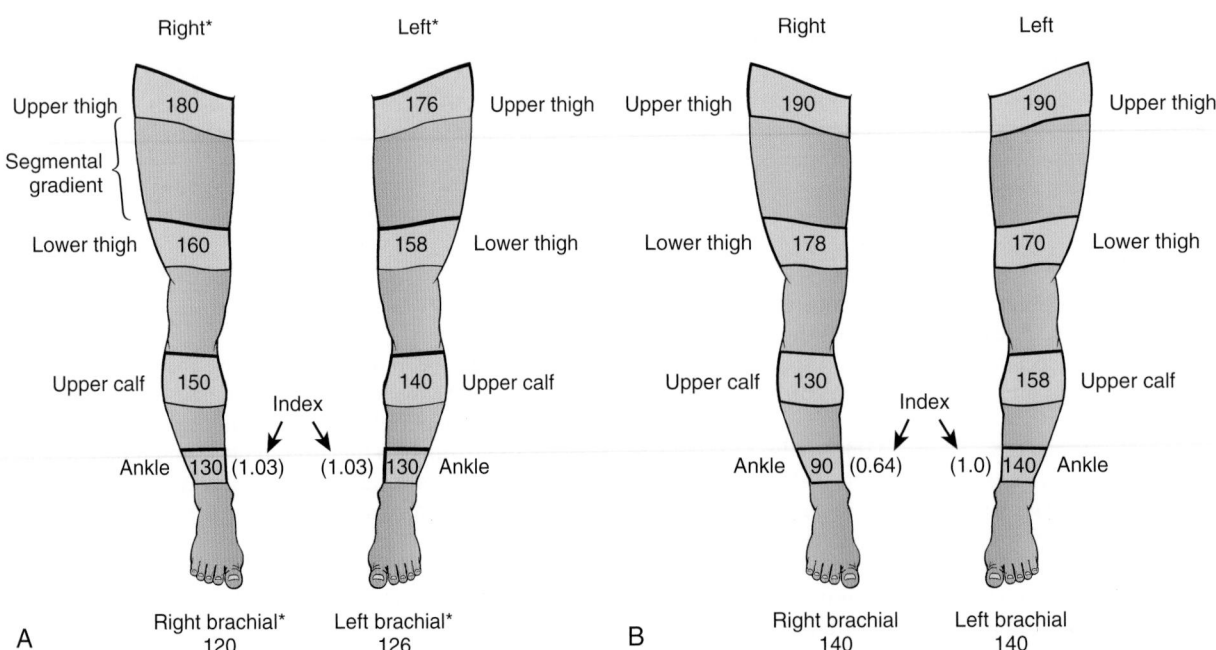

Figure 1-5 A, Typical pressures in a normal subject. Findings, based on resting pressure, show no evidence of occlusive disease of the large or medium-sized arteries. Normal findings are as follows: (1) ankle-to-brachial pressure index of 1.0 or higher, (2) all segmental pressure gradients lower than 30 mm Hg, and (3) upper thigh pressure at least 40 mm Hg above brachial pressure. *Systolic pressure in mm Hg.
B, Typical pressures in a patient with obstruction of the right popliteal or tibial arteries. Significant findings are as follows: (1) ankle-to-brachial pressure index less than 0.9 in the right leg, (2) abnormally high gradient from the ankle to below the knee and again from below to above the knee in the right leg, and (3) upper thigh pressure 50 mm Hg higher than brachial pressure, consistent with normal flow at the aorta-iliac level. Findings are suggestive of right popliteal occlusion or right anterior and posterior tibial occlusion, or both. (*From* Doppler Evaluation of Peripheral Arterial Disease: A Clinical Handbook, 5th ed. *Fredericksburg, VA: Sonicaid, Inc. Reproduced by permission.*

moisture as a reflection of skin perfusion and sympathetic tone. This is not an accurate guide to circulatory volume because the vasomotor tone of the skin is affected by numerous diseases, as well as by emotional and environmental factors. Capillary refill has been advocated as a noninvasive test for hypovolemia, but it has been found to be inaccurate in adults (see the following discussion regarding its use in children).[155] The ideal test for determining volume status would rapidly and accurately detect 5% or greater depletion of volume with a noninvasive technique. At present, no such test exists.

ORTHOSTATIC VITAL SIGNS MEASUREMENT

Orthostatic vital signs have historically been used to evaluate patients with fluid loss, hemorrhage, syncope, or autonomic dysfunction. They are also used to assess the patient's response to therapy. The clinician is often concerned with accurate

TABLE 1-4 Use of Segmental Lower Extremity Pressure to Identify the Level of Obstruction

	UPPER THIGH	LOWER-THIGH	UPPER CALF	ANKLE
Normal*				
Right	180	160	150	130
Left	176	158	140	130
Arm	124	124	124	124
ABI	1.45	1.29	1.21	1.05
Obstruction at the Right Popliteal Artery†				
Right	190	178	130	90
Left	190	176	158	140
Arm	140	140	140	140
ABI	1.36	1.27	R 0.92 L 1.12	R 0.64 L 1.0
Obstruction at the Abdominal Aorta or Bilateral Iliac Obstruction‡				
Right	140	126	112	94
Left	130	120	110	100
Arm	135	135	135	135
ABI	1.03	0.91	0.82	0.71

ABI, ankle-brachial index.
*Typical pressures in a normal subject. The findings, based on resting pressures, show no evidence of occlusive disease of the large or medium-sized arteries. Normal findings are as follows: (1) ABI of 1.0 or higher, (2) all segmental pressure gradients lower than 30 mm Hg, and (3) upper thigh pressure at least 40 mm Hg above brachial pressure.
†Typical pressures in a patient with obstruction of the right popliteal or tibial arteries. Significant findings are as follows: (1) ABI less than 0.9 in the right leg, (2) abnormally high gradient from the ankle to below the knee and again from below to above the knee in the right leg, and (3) upper thigh pressure 50 mm Hg higher than brachial pressure, consistent with normal flow at the aorta-iliac level. The findings are suggestive of right popliteal occlusion or right anterior and posterior tibial occlusion, or both.
‡Typical pressures in a patient with obstruction of the abdominal aorta or bilateral iliac obstruction. Significant findings are as follows: (1) ABI of less than 0.9 in both legs, (2) all segmental gradients lower than 30 mm Hg, and (3) both upper thigh pressures relatively low with respect to brachial pressure. The findings are suggestive of severe aortoiliac occlusive disease.

detection of acute blood loss or volume depletion. When the clinical syndrome of shock exists, assessment of a deficit in blood volume poses little difficulty. It is preferable that loss of volume be detected before loss of physiologic compensation and clinical shock occur.

Although orthostatic testing is commonly cited as a method to detect hypovolemia, *it is frequently misleading and has less clinical value than often touted.* The medical literature is inconsistent regarding values representative of a positive or negative orthostatic test, and its value for estimating volume status is probably overstated. In patients with an acute loss of less than 20% of total blood volume, orthostatic vital signs have been shown to lack both sensitivity and specificity.[156]

Physiologic Response to Hypovolemia

Acute blood loss or severe hypovolemia related to dehydration decreases venous return.[157] This can be seen with acute blood loss (usually greater than 20% of blood volume), severe burns, or prolonged vomiting or diarrhea that depletes body fluids. As a result, cardiac output falls and clinical manifestations of shock ensue. Several compensatory mechanisms are initiated by acute hypovolemia (Box 1-1). The dominant compensatory mechanism in shock is a reduction in carotid sinus baroreceptor inhibition of sympathetic outflow to the cardiovascular system. This increased sympathetic outflow results in several effects: (1) arteriolar vasoconstriction, which greatly increases peripheral vascular resistance; (2) constriction of venous capacitance vessels, which increases venous return to the heart; and (3) an increase in the heart rate and force of contraction, which helps maintain cardiac output despite significant loss of volume.[153]

The value of sympathetic reflex compensation is illustrated by the fact that 30% to 40% of blood volume can be lost before death occurs. When sympathetic reflexes are absent, loss of only 15% to 20% of blood volume may cause death.[158] Increased sympathetic nerve activity results in the commonly recognized physical signs of shock, including pallor, cool clammy skin, rapid heart rate, muscle weakness, and venous constriction. An inadequate immediate compensatory response will result in dizziness, altered mental status, or loss of consciousness.[159] The central nervous system response to ischemia further stimulates the sympathetic nervous system

BOX 1-1 Homeostatic Mechanisms in Hemorrhagic Shock

Sympathetic reflex compensation
  Arteriolar vasoconstriction
  Venous capacitance vasoconstriction
  Increased inotropic and chronotropic cardiac activity
  Central nervous system ischemic response
Selective increase in cerebral and coronary perfusion by means of
  local autoregulation
Increased oxygen unloading in tissues
Restoration of blood volume
  Renin-angiotensin-aldosterone axis activation
  Antidiuretic hormone secretion
  Transcapillary refill
  Increased thirst resulting in increased fluid intake
  Increased erythropoiesis

after arterial pressure falls below 50 mm Hg.[128] Subsequent compensatory mechanisms that work to restore blood volume to a normal level include the release of angiotensin and antidiuretic hormone (vasopressin). This causes arteriolar vasoconstriction, conservation of salt and water by the kidneys, and a shift in fluid from the interstitium to the intravascular space.[159]

Several investigators have examined the changes in blood pressure and pulse that occur in supine patients with blood loss.[153,154,160] Collectively, these studies have shown variable individual hemodynamic responses to acute blood loss of up to 1 L. The frequent inability to detect significant loss of volume with supine vital signs and the observation that syncope frequently develops in patients with acute volume loss on rising led to investigation of the use of orthostatic vital signs to detect occult hypovolemia.

Physiologic Response to Changes in Posture

When an individual assumes the upright posture, complex homeostatic mechanisms compensate for the effects of gravity on the circulation to maintain cerebral perfusion with minimal change in vital signs. These responses include (1) baroreceptor-mediated arteriolar vasoconstriction, (2) venous constriction and increased muscle tone in the legs and the abdomen to augment venous return, (3) sympathetic-mediated inotropic and chronotropic effects on the heart, and (4) activation of the renin-angiotensin-aldosterone system.[159] These compensatory mechanisms preserve cerebral perfusion in the upright position with minimal changes in vital signs. When a normal subject stands, the pulse increases by an average of 13 beats/min, systolic blood pressure falls slightly or does not change, and diastolic pressure rises slightly or does not change.[160] In patients with vasodepressor syncope, the normal compensatory reflexes that preserve cerebral perfusion with changes in posture are altered. The normally increased sympathetic tone on standing is paradoxically inhibited, and an exaggerated enhancement of parasympathetic activity (bradycardia) occurs and can lead to syncope.[154]

Few data exist regarding the true effect of acute blood loss on postural vital signs, and this parameter varies greatly among individuals experiencing hypovolemia. One study of 23 young adult volunteers from whom 500 to 1200 mL of blood was withdrawn found no reliable change in postural blood pressure, but a consistent postural increase in pulse of 35% to 40% was noted after 500-mL blood loss.[161] Of the six subjects from whom approximately 1000 mL of blood was withdrawn, only two were able to tolerate standing, and each had a postural increase in pulse of greater than 30 beats/min. The other four subjects experienced severe symptoms on standing, followed by marked bradycardia and syncope if they were not allowed to lie down.

Following phlebotomy of 450 to 1000 mL of blood from healthy volunteers, the criterion of an increase in pulse of 30 beats/min or the presence of severe symptoms (syncope or near-syncope) during a supine-to-standing test accurately distinguished between 1000-mL blood loss and no blood loss. The sensitivity and specificity of using the aforementioned criteria for detecting 1000-mL blood loss (Box 1-2) were both 98%, for an accuracy of 96% (2% false-negative results and 2% false-positive results). The investigators were unable to consistently detect blood loss of 500 mL with these criteria, though.[162] In a similar study, the change in heart rate with postural changes after 500-mL phlebotomy was more

discriminatory for blood loss than were changes in blood pressure or a change in the bioimpedance-based stroke index. Of note, these authors found that a change in heart rate of 30 beats/min or greater was 13.2% sensitive and 99.5% specific for 500-mL blood loss and that a change in heart rate of 20 beats/min or greater was 44.7% sensitive and 95.4% specific. The finding of a significant rise in pulse, though insensitive for 500-mL blood loss, was relatively specific in these healthy adult blood donors.[161] In the most recent meta-analysis of orthostatic vital signs, the authors concluded that a large postural pulse change (>30 beats/min) or severe postural dizziness precluding the completion of vital sign measurements is required to clinically diagnose hypovolemia secondary to acute blood loss. The analysis demonstrated that orthostatic vital signs are often absent after moderate amounts of blood loss, thus significantly limiting the test's sensitivity (22%) in this scenario.[162] A consensus statement defined orthostatic hypotension as a reduction in systolic blood pressure of at least 20 mm Hg or a reduction in diastolic blood pressure of at least 10 mm Hg within 3 minutes of standing but appropriately reinforces that this is a physical finding rather than a disease process.[159]

Variables Affecting Orthostatic Vital Signs

Many conditions affect the compensatory mechanisms that allow patients to assume the upright posture (Box 1-3).[158] Most of the conditions that affect postural blood pressure regulation involve a pathologic condition that affects the sympathetic nervous system. Orthostatic hypotension caused by autonomic insufficiency is not usually accompanied by tachycardia, but the orthostatic hypotension produced by acute volume depletion is commonly accompanied by a pronounced reflex tachycardia. Even in normal subjects, passive tilting generates a high incidence of orthostatic syncope.[163]

Because of decreased vasomotor tone, limited chronotropic response, and other factors, the elderly have a higher incidence of orthostatic hypotension leading to syncope and fall-related injuries.[164] Carotid sinus hypersensitivity may play

---

BOX 1-2   Summary of Orthostatic Tilt Testing*

TEST PROCEDURE

1. Blood pressure and pulse are recorded after the patient has been supine for 2 to 3 minutes.
2. Blood pressure, pulse, and symptoms are recorded after the patient has been standing for 1 minute; the patient should be permitted to resume a supine position immediately if syncope or near-syncope develop.

POSITIVE TEST

1. Increase in pulse of 30 beats/min or more in adults *or*
2. Presence of symptoms of cerebral hypoperfusion (e.g., dizziness, syncope)

*The predictive ability of orthostatic vital signs to assess volume status is often overestimated in clinical practice. This suggested guide is based on the ability of the change in pulse and patient symptoms to distinguish between no acute blood loss and 1000-mL acute blood loss in healthy, previously normovolemic volunteers (sensitivity of 98% for detecting 1000-mL acute blood loss).[162] This guide may not be applicable to elderly patients, sick children, medicated patients, and those with autonomic dysfunction.

BOX 1-3	Classification of Disorders of Postural Blood Pressure Regulation

I. Poor postural adjustment
   A. Tall, asthenic habitus
   B. Advanced age
   C. Physical exhaustion
   D. Prolonged recumbency
   E. Prolonged weightlessness
   F. Pregnancy
   G. Gastrectomy
II. Orthostatic hypotension
   A. Secondary orthostatic hypotension
      1. Endocrinologic-metabolic disorders
         a. Diabetes mellitus
         b. Dopamine α-hydroxylase deficiency
         c. Primary amyloidosis
         d. Primary and secondary adrenal insufficiency
         e. Pheochromocytoma
         f. Primary aldosteronism with marked hypokalemia
         g. Porphyria
      2. Central and peripheral nervous system disorders
         a. Intracranial tumors (parasellar and posterior fossa)
         b. Idiopathic paralysis agitans
         c. Wernicke's encephalopathy
         d. Multiple cerebral infarctions

   e. Brainstem lesions
   f. Tabes dorsalis
   g. Syringomyelia
   h. Traumatic and inflammatory myelopathies
   i. Guillain-Barré syndrome
   j. Chronic inflammatory polyradiculoneuropathy
   k. Peripheral neuropathies
   l. Familial dysautonomia (Riley-Day syndrome)
      3. Miscellaneous disorders
         a. Ciguatera fish poisoning
         b. Electrolyte disturbance
         c. Hypochromic anemia
         d. Hypovolemia
         e. Medications
            i. Alcohol
            ii. Antihypertensives with central effects (methyldopa, clonidine)
            iii. Antihypertensives with peripheral effects (prazosin, hydralazine, guanethidine)
            iv. Calcium channel blockers
            v. Diuretics
            vi. Insulin

            vii. Levodopa
            viii. Marijuana
            ix. Narcotic agents
            x. Nitrates
            xi. Psychotropic agents (tricyclic antidepressants, phenothiazines, monoamine oxidase inhibitors, minor tranquilizers)
            xii. Sympatholytics
            xiii. Sympathomimetic agents (prolonged use)
            xiv. Vasodilators
            xv. Vincristine sulfate
         f. Extensive surgical sympathectomy
         g. Chronic hemodialysis
         h. Anorexia nervosa
         i. Hyperbradykininism
   B. Primary or idiopathic orthostatic hypotension
      1. Idiopathic orthostatic hypotension (Bradbury-Eggleston syndrome)
      2. Idiopathic orthostatic hypotension with somatic neurologic deficit (Shy-Drager syndrome)

Adapted from Thomas JE, Schirger A, Fealey RD, et al. Orthostatic hypotension. Mayo Clin Proc. 1981;56:117. Reproduced by permission.

a greater role than orthostasis in geriatric syncope.[165] Note that drugs that antagonize the normal autonomic compensatory mechanisms can also produce orthostatic changes. These changes can be severe enough to produce frank syncope, especially in the elderly. A study of patients with syncope seen in an ED found that orthostatic hypotension was considered to be the cause of the syncope in 24% and that the largest proportion of these cases were drug related. Patients with orthostatic hypotension as the cause of syncope were older, had more comorbid conditions, and were found to be more frequently taking antihypertensive medications.[166] Advanced patient age is an independent risk factor for orthostatic blood pressure changes but does not appear to have a direct correlation to the presence of chronic cardiovascular disease, disability, or body mass index.[167]

Patients with hypertension may also have abnormal vasomotor responses to tilt testing and demonstrate more instability.[168] Chronic anemia patients, who exhibit compensated blood volume, seem to have the same postural response as normal subjects do.[169] Ethanol ingestion exaggerates postural pulse changes and mimics the hemodynamic changes seen with acute blood loss.[170]

The utility of orthostatic vital signs in children has been questioned. Healthy adolescents had changes in heart rate of 21.5 ± 21.2 beats/min and variable changes in systolic blood pressure (+19 to −17 mm Hg) after 2 minutes of standing.[171]

A study comparing mildly dehydrated children with normal children found a significant difference in the orthostatic rise in pulse, but no difference in orthostatic blood pressure. The investigators concluded that an orthostatic increase in pulse of greater than 25 beats/min constitutes a positive tilt test and less than 20 beats/min constitutes a negative test (sensitivity of 75%, specificity of 95%, and predictive value of 92% when using near-syncope or an increase in heart rate greater than 25 beats/min).[172]

Another complicating factor in interpreting orthostatic vital signs is the development of paradoxical bradycardia in the presence of blood loss. Bradycardia in the face of hemorrhage has generally been considered a preterminal finding of irreversible shock, but bradycardia has been documented in hypovolemic, yet conscious trauma patients as well. It has been reported that when orthostatic syncope occurs, it is accompanied by hypotension and often bradycardia.[149,151] Many central nervous system factors can contribute to vagally mediated syncope in ED patients with acute traumatic blood loss, including pain, the sight of blood, anxiety, and nausea. This paradoxical bradycardia may be more frequently associated with rapid and massive bleeding. Patients with more gradual blood loss tend to have a more typical tachycardic response. When the patient's clinical findings are consistent with loss of volume or shock, the clinician should not allow the absence of tachycardia to change the assessment.

Indications and Contraindications

When the volume status of a patient is assessed with use of orthostatic vital signs, several points should be remembered. Many factors influence orthostatic blood pressure, including age, preexisting medical conditions, medications, and autonomic dysfunction (see Box 1-3). Data relating the effect of blood loss to orthostatic vital signs are limited to phlebotomized healthy volunteers. Great care must be used when extrapolating these data to patients with anemia, dehydration, or painful trauma. The clinician must consider the patient's clinical condition coupled with the orthostatic vital signs when evaluating a patient for volume depletion.

Orthostatic vital signs can be considered an adjunct for the evaluation of any patient with known or suspected loss of blood volume or a history of syncope. Contraindications to orthostatic measures include supine hypotension, the clinical syndrome of shock, severely altered mental status, the setting of possible spinal injuries, and lower extremity or pelvic fractures.

The use of medications that block the normal vasomotor and chronotropic response to orthostatic tests is also a contraindication to using this test for the assessment of volume status. However, when the patient's volume status is believed to be adequate and the clinician seeks to determine whether specific medications may have affected the patient's ability to respond to postural changes, the test may be useful. In these situations the primary finding may be the feeling of near-syncope with little or no change in vital signs.

Orthostatic vital signs are often used to assess a patient's response to therapy. In patients receiving intravenous rehydration therapy, serial orthostatic vital signs are widely used to judge the end point of therapy before release. In one study, individual orthostatic vital sign response to saline infusion in women with hyperemesis gravidarum was associated with other measures of rehydration, including weight gain and decreased urine specific gravity.[173] Although the individual improvement in orthostatic vital signs in response to rehydration was of clinical value, the initial orthostatic vital signs were considered insufficient as the sole indicator of clinical dehydration in this population.

Technique

To obtain orthostatic vital signs, record the blood pressure and pulse after the patient has been in the supine position for 2 to 3 minutes (see Box 1-2). Allow the patient to rest quietly and do not perform any painful or invasive procedures during the test.

Next, ask the patient to stand and be prepared to assist if severe symptoms or syncope develop. A supine-to-standing test is more accurate than a supine-to-sitting one. If severe symptoms develop on standing, defined as syncope or extreme dizziness requiring the patient to lie down, the test is considered positive and should be terminated. If not symptomatic, allow the patient to stand for 1 minute and then record the blood pressure and pulse. A 1-minute interval resulted in the greatest difference between control and 1000-mL phlebotomy groups in one study.[162]

A number of studies have been conducted on normotensive, normovolemic patients to assess end points for orthostatic vital sign parameters. Such studies have included sitting-to-standing methods and varying rates of postural changes,[174] including lying times of 5 to 10 minutes and standing times of 0 to 2 minutes.[175] Arm position may affect postural changes in blood pressure and should be held constant to accurately assess orthostatic change.[176] Complications include syncope with resulting falls and injuries.

Interpretation

The most sensitive criteria for orthostasis is tachycardia or symptoms of cerebral hypoperfusion (e.g., near-syncope). Although changes in blood pressure may be seen, they are too variable to be an indicator of loss of blood volume. Specific population-based thresholds for changes in pulse rate and blood pressure have some value in identifying patients at high risk for significant loss of blood volume, but great individual variability limits the use of this technique as a screening test. That is, a loss of 500 mL, and occasionally more, may be associated with a negative orthostatic vital sign assessment.[165,177] The use of serial measurements to ascertain the response to therapy of patients considered to be at risk for loss of volume appears to have clinical utility.[178]

In the setting of suspected blood loss, if the patient has a rise in pulse of 30 beats/min or manifests severe symptoms and other complicating factors have been excluded, blood loss is highly likely (2% false-positive rate). The presence of a negative test indicates only that acute blood loss of 1000 mL is unlikely (2% false-negative rate) and that blood loss of 500 mL cannot be excluded (43% to 87% false-negative rate).[162,165-177,179] Orthostatic changes in the shock index were no more sensitive than established tilt test criteria in discriminating normal individuals from those with moderate acute blood loss (450 mL).[178]

Criteria for significant orthostatic changes in blood pressure cannot be definitively set for the following reasons: (1) large variability in postural blood pressure has been found in the adult ED population[180-185]; (2) the results of studies using passive tilt tables cannot be extrapolated to the bedside use of orthostatic vital signs; (3) studies using healthy patients with acute blood loss may not reflect the orthostatic changes seen in the elderly or those with chronic bleeding, dehydration, and other medical problems; and (4) many studies of orthostatic changes never used a criterion standard in their determinations.

In summary, orthostatic vital sign testing in common in the ED, but in reality, this procedure has limited proven value, and clinical interpretation of orthostatic changes in blood pressure and pulse varies widely. Although this intervention may occasionally yield information not obtained through other means, the authors do not consider orthostatic blood pressure testing a standard of care in the evaluation of ED patients.

CAPILLARY REFILL

The capillary refill test is a measurement of the interval of time from the release of nail bed or soft tissue pressure sufficient to blanch the nail bed or superficial soft tissue until the return to normal coloration. Delayed capillary refill is an indication of reduced skin turgor, often as a result of volume depletion or limited perfusion. Measurement of capillary refill time (CRT) appears to be *somewhat accurate* in children, *but its accuracy in assessing dehydration and reduced perfusion in adults is highly suspect.*[158,159,161-181] Skin elasticity is the characteristic that allows skin to spring back to its original shape after it has been deformed, and the speed of refilling the capillary bed after compression is responsible for the return of color to the skin.

Indications and Contraindications

CRT should not be determined from a dependent extremity, from a recently burned or injured extremity, or at the site of an infection or acute injury. Because CRT can be used without additional equipment and takes only a few seconds to perform, it can be a useful bedside assessment of perfusion and dehydration when used in conjunction with other objective signs of the adequacy of perfusion. It should not be considered accurate as a stand-alone tool. *Capillary refill is not an appropriate alternative to measuring blood pressure in pediatric patients.*

Procedure

The preferred sites for determining CRT are the nail bed, the thenar surface of the palm, and the heel. Alternative sites may have different CRTs, and the current standards are best developed for capillary refill determined at the nail bed.[186] Regardless of the site chosen, position the extremity at about the level of the right atrium. The minimum pressure necessary to produce blanching yields the most reproducible values. Release the nail bed and begin timing with a stopwatch or simply by counting out "one-thousand-one, one-thousand-two" for an approximation of the interval. Stop the clock when the nail bed becomes pink again. Interobserver reliability has been shown to be moderate, with kappa values less of than 0.5 in the evaluation of both adults and children.[182,183]

Interpretation

The normal CRT increases with age and is slightly longer in female patients. It is further increased by degrees of dehydration or hypoperfusion. Hypothermia, hyponatremia, congestive heart failure, malnutrition, and edema all increase CRT. Environmental conditions such as ambient air temperature can falsely alter capillary refill.[182] Fever alone did not appear to prolong or shorten CRT in children,[183] but a study of healthy adults found a 5% decrease in CRT for each degree Celsius rise in patient temperature.[187,188]

The main difficulty in interpreting CRT is that normal values in healthy patients fall into a wide range. In 30 normal infants 2 to 24 months of age, mean CRT was 0.8 ± 0.3 second. Measurements obtained from the nail bed were more reproducible than those from the heel. Combined results from four studies evaluating capillary refill revealed a pooled sensitivity of 0.60 (95% confidence interval [CI], 0.29 to 0.91) and a specificity of 0.85 (95% CI, 0.72 to 0.98) for detecting 5% dehydration in children.[189] The presence of a 2-second or longer delay in CRT when combined with any two or more of the findings of absent tears, dry mucous membranes, or ill general appearance predicted clinical dehydration (>5% deficit in body weight) in children (1 month to 5 years of age) with 87% sensitivity and 82% specificity.[190-192]

Frequent monitoring of capillary refill may be useful in assessing responses to rapid fluid resuscitation in children. A normal CRT of 2 seconds or less has recently been shown to correlate with superior vena cava oxygen saturation ($Svco_2$) of 70% or higher in critically ill children.[186,192] The role of serial CRT measurements for assessing the response to rehydration in adults is unknown, but it does not appear to be useful for assessing acute loss of blood volume. Lima and colleagues[193] studied the prognostic value of the subjective assessment of peripheral perfusion in critically ill patients following initial resuscitation. When an abnormal CRT was defined as greater than 4.5 seconds, coupled with extremity coolness, these parameters identified patients who had been hemodynamically stabilized but continued to have more severe organ dysfunction and higher lactate levels. In adults, CRT was found to be less sensitive and less specific than orthostatic vital signs in detecting 450-mL blood loss during blood donation.[161]

In summary, assessment of CRT is a common technique used in the ED, but in reality this procedure has limited proven value, clinical interpretation is very subjective, and use varies widely. Although this intervention may occasionally yield information not obtained through other means, predominantly in children, the authors do not consider such testing an absolute standard of care in the evaluation of ED patients.

TEMPERATURE

Detection of abnormal body temperature may facilitate proper diagnosis and evaluation of complaints of patients in the ED. An inability to maintain normal body temperature is indicative of a vast number of potentially serious disorders, including infections, neoplasms, shock, toxic reactions, and environmental exposures.[192,194-197] Fever in neutropenic, immunocompromised, or intravenous drug–abusing patients may be more reliable than laboratory tests or clinician assessment in diagnosing serious illness.[187,194] Infants are particularly sensitive to thermal stress and may demonstrate lower body temperatures during critical illness.[188,195] In one study, although higher rates of serious bacterial infection were found in neonates who had documented fever (OR, 3.23) on admission, in only 8.4% of neonates with historical fever was serious bacterial infection later diagnosed.[196] Pre-triage or home assessment of body temperature is fraught with difficulty and unreliability. *Whether taken by the oral, rectal, or tympanic routes, reports of fever at home are very difficult to interpret in the clinical setting.*[194,197] Some studies report rates as low as 13% in frequency when measuring temperature in the critically ill or injured.[198]

Physiology

Under normal conditions, the temperature of deep central body tissues (i.e., core temperature) remains at $37°C \pm 0.6°C$ ($98.6°F \pm 1.08°F$).[199] Core body temperature can be maintained within a narrow range while environmental temperature varies from as much as 13°C to 60°C (55°F to 140°F),[199] but surface temperature rises and falls with the environmental and other influences. Mean oral temperature is $36.8°C \pm 0.4°C$ ($98.2°F \pm 0.7°F$).[200] Maintenance of normal body temperature requires a balance of heat production and heat loss. Heat loss occurs by radiation, conduction, and evaporation. Approximately 60%, 18%, and 22% of heat loss, respectively, occurs by these methods. Heat loss is increased by wind, water, and lack of insulation (e.g., clothing). Sweating, vasodilation, and decreased heat production serve to decrease temperature. Piloerection, vasoconstriction, and increased heat production serve to increase body temperature. Heat production is increased by shivering, fat catabolism, and increased thyroid hormone production.

Temperature is controlled by feedback mechanisms operating through the preoptic area of the hypothalamus. Heat-sensitive neurons in this area increase their rate of firing during experimental heating. Receptors in the skin, spinal cord, abdominal viscera, and central veins primarily detect cold and provide feedback to the hypothalamus that signals an increase in heat production. Stimuli that change core body temperature result in reflex changes in mechanisms that increase either heat loss or heat production.[197-206]

Indications and Contraindications

Clinicians generally measure body temperature to determine whether it is outside the normal range and as an indication of pathologic conditions that can affect core body temperature. Measurement of actual core body temperature requires the placement of invasive monitors, such as an esophageal or pulmonary artery probe. Clinicians commonly use estimates of core body temperatures to conveniently and safely assess abnormalities in core temperature. All noncore body sites and methods have inherent limitations in accuracy, and clinicians have come to accept these shortcomings in assessing most patients.

Measurement of oral temperature requires a cooperative adult or child. Patients who are uncooperative, hemodynamically unstable, septic, or in respiratory distress (with an RR >20 beats/min) require a method of measuring temperature other than the traditional oral route.[201] This group includes children younger than 5 years and patients who are intubated. Recent ingestion of hot or cold beverages can alter oral temperature readings for 5 to 30 minutes and can falsely elevate a normal temperature or mask a fever.[202]

Special techniques of measuring core body temperature may be indicated in certain patients (e.g., those with profound hypothermia, frostbite, or hyperthermia). Measurement of core body temperature is indicated in these individuals because it accurately measures the effects of treatment. This is the group of patients who will benefit the most from continuous temperature measurements.[203]

Measurement Sites

Core Body Temperature

The following sites accurately reflect core body temperature and changes in it: the distal third of the esophagus, the tympanic membrane (TM) (with a direct thermistor in contact with the anterior inferior quadrant of the TM),[204,205] and the pulmonary artery.[206,207] Other sites may represent core body temperature under certain conditions, for example, (1) the rectum when the temperature is obtained at least 8 cm from the anus with an indwelling thermistor and the body temperature is relatively constant and (2) the bladder when measured with an indwelling thermistor.[208]

Rectal temperature is often considered the criterion standard for body temperature in ambulatory patients and it is often used routinely in children younger than 3 years.[209] Its

advantages include accuracy, sensitivity, and availability. One intensive care unit study found that rectal probe temperatures demonstrated limited variability or bias when compared with pulmonary artery temperatures.[210] Disadvantages include longer intervals for measurement, safety concerns, and inconvenience. Neutropenia and recent rectal surgery represent relative contraindications to measurement of rectal temperature. Thermistor probes (i.e., small thermocouples with instantaneous readouts) for esophageal and vascular temperature measurement provide continuous temperature readouts when attached to a potentiometer. Thermistor probes are available for measurement of esophageal, bladder, and rectal temperature with appropriate monitors.

Peripheral Body Sites Approximating Core Temperature

A body temperature measurement by IR radiation can be detected from the ear, including the auditory canal and TM, and is easy to use, hygienic, convenient, and quick. It can be used as a general screening technique, particularly in cases in which temperature is not of great importance, such as in minor trauma. Though clearly superior to axillary temperature readings,[211] controversy remains regarding the sensitivity and specificity of IR TM readings in the ED. More work is being done in the pediatric population, with an overall sensitivity of between 50% and 80% and a specificity of 85%. The lower sensitivities are found in newborns and infants younger than 3 years.[212-214] Systematic reviews of pediatric studies have pooled data suggesting 65% sensitivity, but this is likely to be unacceptable in the clinical setting.[215] A recent study found that neither TM nor skin thermometers could reliably predict rectal temperature, and it concurred that these methods could not replace rectal temperature measurement as the "gold standard" for detecting fever in the pediatric population.[216] Adult studies, though generally more favorable in recommending TM temperatures, have shown gaps in reliability as well.[217] However, a recent systematic review suggested that TM and oral thermometry provides an accurate measure of core temperature in critically ill adults with fever.[218] Temporal artery scanning to detect fever is increasingly being examined. In general, these devices show better sensitivity in detecting fever in infants than TM thermistors do (66% versus 49% sensitivity) and may be useful in excluding fever,[219] defined as a rectal temperature higher than 38.3°C if the temporal artery readings are lower than 37.7°C.[220] The point can be argued that a sensitivity of 60% in any population lacks the required sensitivity to be useful clinically. A theoretical disadvantage of TM temperatures might be a falsely elevated estimate of the core temperature in the presence of otitis media. In one study, TM thermometers accurately reflected oral temperatures in children with otitis media.[221]

Although probably not a concern in the ED, prehospital providers who might wish to measure IR TM temperature at low ambient temperatures should be aware that below 24.6°C, the TM readings will greatly underestimate core temperatures.[222] EMS personnel should also be aware that in a cohort of exhausted marathon runners, rectal and IR TM temperatures have only moderate correlation.[223] When hyperthermia or hypothermia is clinically suspected and the IR TM temperature does not confirm an abnormal temperature, a rectal temperature should be obtained.

Axillary and tactile temperature assessments have been demonstrated to be unreliable and insensitive. They should not be used as screening methods for core temperature abnormalities in the ED.[224-226] Single-use Tempa-DOT thermometers show progressive temperature dot darkening with increasing temperature, and these thermometers have been adopted by many EDs. These temperature devices have been shown to have 100% sensitivity and approximately 80% specificity for identification of fever when temperature was obtained orally in both adults and children.[227] The most rudimentary method for temperature measurement, parental assessment by tactile touch, is associated with a measured fever approximately 75% of the time.[228] Clinician estimation of fever is almost identical (70%).[229]

Procedure

Begin the temperature measurement by selecting the body site. Consider the accuracy of using a certain site to reflect core temperature, the sensitivity of the site to changes in temperature, the convenience, the time required, the safety, and the availability of the site.[230] Insert the temperature probe and allow the probe to equilibrate with the temperature of the local body tissues.

Proper placement of the temperature probes significantly influences the results of oral, rectal, esophageal, and vascular temperature.[231-233] Obtain sublingual oral temperatures in either the right or the left posterior sublingual pocket with the mouth closed.[234] Though anxiety-producing for parents, biting and breaking a mercury thermometer is generally inconsequential with regard to ingestion of either glass or mercury. Obtain a rectal temperature with the patient in the left or right lateral decubitus position and advance the probe gently to a depth of 3 to 5 cm to ensure accurate, atraumatic results.[235] Complications associated with rectal temperature measurements are extremely rare but include rectal perforation, pneumoperitoneum, bacteremia, dysrhythmias, and syncope.[236] Falsely low but supranormal rectal temperature measurements may be seen during shock.[237] Rectal temperature may also lag behind changes in core temperature.

An esophageal catheter or pulmonary artery probe can be placed for measurement of core body temperature, but these techniques are not used in the ED.

Though not commonly used, measurement of the temperature of a freshly voided urine specimen can validate measurement of temperature at other body sites.[238] Urinary bladder temperature measurement has been demonstrated to be similar to pulmonary artery catheter temperature.[239]

Digital electronic probes are commonly used for the measurement of oral temperature in ambulatory patients.[236] Electronic methods of temperature measurement are based on the thermocouple principle. Modern electronic thermometers signal once extrapolation of the temperature-time curve occurs. Current in vitro standards call for an accuracy of ±0.1°C (±0.18°F) over the range of 37°C to 39°C (98.6°F to 102.2°F). Disadvantages include factors that affect clinical accuracy and sensitivity. Disposable single-use oral thermometers are now available and are as reliable as mercury or TM thermometers.[234] In the pediatric population, pacifier thermometers record supralingual readings in infants. The average time needed to record a reading with a pacifier thermometer is 3 minutes and 23 seconds, thus making its application in emergency medicine limited, although its sensitivity (72%) and specificity (98%) rival that of alternative methods.[240] Various IR ear thermometers are available

commercially with varying operating temperature ranges, features, and reported accuracy.[241] Complications associated with axillary, oral, ear IR, and liquid crystal thermometers are rare or unreported. TM perforation and pain have been reported as complications of placement of the thermistor probe in the auditory canal.

Interpretation

Normal values for body temperature are affected by the following variables: (1) site and methods used for measurement, (2) perfusion, (3) environmental exposure, (4) pregnancy, (5) activity level, and (6) time of day. Clinicians must interpret body temperature with knowledge of the range of normal values at the intended site of measurement. Although core body temperature remains nearly constant (37.0°C ± 0.6°C or 98.6°F ± 0.18°F), surface temperature rises and falls with changes in ambient temperature, exercise, and time of day. The definition of *fever* varies by the site of measurement and is defined by a temperature greater than 2 standard deviations above the mean. *Fever has been defined as an oral temperature of 37.8°C or higher (100.0°F),*[235] *a rectal temperature of 38.0°C or higher (100.4°F),*[242] *or an IR ear temperature of 37.6°C or higher (99.6°F).*[235] Based on measurement of temperatures in normal, healthy infants, it is recommended that fever be defined as a rectal temperature of 38°C or higher in infants younger than 30 days, 38.1°C or higher in infants 30 to 60 days (1 to 2 months), and 38.2°C or higher in infants 60 to 90 days old (2 to 3 months).[243] *Hypothermia* has been defined as a core body temperature lower than 35°C (<95°F), and *hyperthermia* has been defined as a core body temperature higher than 41°C (>105.8°F) with accompanying symptoms and signs.[207,244] A useful nomogram and formulas for conversion of centigrade to Fahrenheit are provided in Figure 1-6.

Figure 1-6 Temperature conversion scale. To change Celsius (centigrade) to Fahrenheit, multiply the Celsius temperature by 9/5 and add 32. To change Fahrenheit to Celsius, subtract 32 from the Fahrenheit number and multiply by 5/9. *100.4°F.

TABLE 1-5 Normal Ranges and Suggested Febrile Thresholds for Human Body Temperature (in Healthy Resting Patients)

BODY SITE	TYPE OF THERMOMETER	NORMAL RANGE (°C)	FEVER (°C)
Core*	Electronic	36.4-37.9	38.0
Oral	Mercury in glass, electronic	35.5-37.7	37.8
Rectal	Mercury in glass, electronic	36.6-37.9	38.0
Ear	Infrared emission	35.7-37.5	37.6†

*Temperature obtained with a properly positioned pulmonary artery, esophageal, or tympanic membrane thermistor.
†For unadjusted ear temperature using the Thermoscan Pro-1 (Thermoscan, Inc., San Diego, CA).

Temperature probes that depend on transfer of heat energy from local tissues to the probe require a period of equilibration and reliable tissue contact at the intended body site. Acceptable equilibration times for mercury-in-glass thermometers in oral, rectal, and axillary sites are 7, 3, and 10 minutes, respectively. Used in a predictive mode, electronic digital thermometers generally require 30 seconds for oral or rectal temperature equilibration. The predictive mode uses temperature changes versus time to predict an equilibration temperature.

Normal ranges and suggested febrile thresholds for common body sites and methods should be considered in the interpretation of temperature values (Table 1-5). Interpretation of temperature measurements during clinical assessment must consider the use of antipyretics, level of activity, pregnancy, environmental exposure, and patient age. Body temperature is increased during sustained exercise, pregnancy, and the luteal phase of the menstrual cycle. Temperature also increases in the late afternoon because of diurnal variation. Body temperature is generally reduced with advanced age, and age may have an impact on the magnitude of fever. Axillary temperatures have low sensitivity but a high specificity for fever. Axillary temperatures should not be used to screen for fever.

Oral temperature measurements are affected by the ingestion of hot or cold liquids,[218] tachypnea,[245] and cold ambient air.[246] Before taking an oral temperature, the examiner should inquire about these features and possibly delay taking the temperature. A 2.7°C (4.9°F) reduction in oral temperature measurement was found when the probe was placed under the tip of the tongue instead of under the posterior sublingual pocket.[234] Given the extrapolation that occurs with rapidly reading thermocouple devices and IR detectors, it is not surprising that the sensitivity of these devices for detection of fever is only 86% to 88%.[247] Many clinicians have adopted the adage that when an elevated temperature is suspected or crucial in decision making but not evident with an oral thermocouple probe or IR TM thermometer, measurement with a mercury-in-glass thermometer is indicated.

When rapid changes in body temperature occur, oral and TM temperature measurements appear to be more reliable than rectal temperature. In 20 adults examined during open heart surgery, oral temperatures showed a better correlation with blood temperature during rapid cooling and rewarming.[240]

Infrequently, ED patients require constant monitoring of temperature (e.g., in cases of profound hypothermia or hyperthermia). This can usually be performed by using a bladder or esophageal probe attached to a potentiometer. Patients with indwelling central venous or pulmonary arterial catheters may have electronic thermistors inserted into the central circulation to measure core body temperature. As noted earlier, rectal temperature measurements are less desirable for monitoring patients undergoing rapid changes in core temperature. Periodic IR TM temperature monitoring may represent one useful option in a hypothermic patient.[248]

Interpretation of ear IR temperatures requires knowledge of the mode of thermometer operation and ambient temperature. Occlusion of the ear canal by cerumen may produce a falsely low reading.[249] Most IR ear thermometers have different modes that allow users to predict the equivalent temperature at other body sites. IR ear thermometers appear to be moderately sensitive for fever.[250] If these devices are used, the clinician must be aware of the potential for a falsely low temperature. When in doubt, the measurement should be repeated with a more standard method.

Patients, parents, and caregivers often misinterpret the significance of a fever, and the term "fever phobia" has been coined to describe the ubiquitous and unsubstantiated fear that fever, by itself, is harmful or has diagnostic or prognostic significance.[197] Some of the highest fevers are the result of benign viral infections. Fever has been demonstrated to increase the body's immune response, thus making aggressive fever reduction counterproductive. Most individuals, especially children, feel better when a high fever is lowered. However, uninitiated medical personnel may contribute to the incidence of fever phobia. Routine administration of antipyretics in the ED for any fever, regardless of the degree of discomfort, has fueled unwarranted concern and may result in potentially harmful interventions, unnecessary testing and treatments, avoidable side effects of medications, and additional patient anxiety. Mandatory medical evaluation for any fever, the use of alcohol sponge baths, waking a sleeping child to administer antipyretics, alternating ibuprofen with acetaminophen, around-the-clock use of antipyretics, and misconceptions about fever causing brain damage are some of the myths that are still extant in some EDs and throughout the general population. An ED protocol stating that any child be afebrile or demonstrate a significant decrease in hyperpyrexia or even have a temperature reading repeated before discharge has no scientific validity.

PAIN AS A VITAL SIGN

Background

For centuries, the goal of physicians has been alleviation of pain. Albert Schweitzer called pain "the most terrible of all the lords of mankind," and appropriately, one of the goals of modern medicine has been to understand and accurately assess pain in the hope of designing better methods to treat it. A paradigm shift has occurred in which pain is viewed as a mechanism to provide a mechanical warning of actual or potential damage to cells and tissues in a specific area.

There is no question that at least temporary pain relief is one intervention that any clinician can usually accomplish with relative ease, but the concept of using pain as "the fifth vital sign" has not met with universal agreement.[251] *Literal interpretation of this concept can be fraught with problems, and because of the subjective nature of pain, measurement and interpretation are, by nature, imprecise.* Initiatives mandating documentation of pain as the fifth vital sign have not been associated with improvement in pain management.[252] A prospective, multi-center study evaluating the current state of ED pain management practices concluded that there is high pain intensity as demonstrated by intense pain on arrival (median rating, 8 of 10) and suboptimal pain management practices, with assessment of pain occurring in 83%, 40% receiving no analgesics, lengthy delays in analgesic administration, and a large proportion of patients reporting moderate to severe pain at discharge (74%).[253] Assuming weight-based dosing for acute pain management, analgesic regimens did not conform to the recommended regimens in a study of ED patients.[254] Simply mandating the recording of a triage pain score has been shown to improve time to initial analgesic treatment.[255]

Pain can cause sympathetically mediated changes in vital signs. With regard to the quantitative effect of pain, it is well established that standard vital signs (pulse, respiration, blood pressure) do not meaningfully correlate with the level of perceived pain, even in patients with substantial pain, regardless of age, gender, or diagnosis.[256] A recent retrospective study of patients with confirmed painful diagnoses showed no clinically significant associations between self-reported triage pain scores and heart rate, blood pressure, or RR.[257] Contentions that the judicious use of analgesics will obscure a clinical condition or otherwise adversely affect clinical care are antiquated, unscientific, and inhumane. In short, pain control facilitates the overall ED encounter for both the patient and clinician.

Two types of pain are of concern to ED clinicians. *Acute pain* is defined as the normal predicted physiologic response to a noxious chemical or thermal stimulus. It is generally time limited. *Chronic pain* is defined as persistent or episodic pain of a duration or intensity that adversely affects the function or well-being of the patient. Pain of either variety is the most common chief complaint of more than 50% of ED patients, with the figure approaching 75% in some studies.[258] Special focus should be placed on pain based on goals of the Joint Commission on Accreditation of Healthcare Organizations (JCAHO), which mandates that all hospitals develop comprehensive programs for the measurement, treatment, and documentation of pain.[259]

Reliably quantifying pain should be the goal of ED clinicians and is an appropriate step in the triage process. The discrete cognitive process that signals the sensation of pain is inherently influenced by culture, personality, experiences, and the patient's underlying emotional state. The ideal pain measurement continues to depend on methods that can use or control for subjective experience.

Procedure/Interpretation

Although JCAHO has required organizations to assess the nature and intensity of pain in all patients, there is no perfect measurement tool suitable for the wide variety of patients and clinical settings experienced in EDs. Pain is a complex, subjective, multifaceted, personal experience that is difficult to easily quantify in all individuals. The perfect pain assessment tool for the ED setting would be simple and rapid to administer while providing a precise, reliable, and valid measure of pain regardless of a patient's age, cultural background, and cognitive or physical impairments. Although numerous instruments to measure acute pain have been proposed, none meets all the criteria necessary to satisfy this definition. Regardless of the instrument chosen to measure pain, the primary focus should be to allow patients to personally report their pain and to rate it from a personal viewpoint. It is widely accepted that health professionals cannot rate pain intensity as accurately as patients themselves.[260,261] Even though a patient's reporting of pain intensity can be frustrating to the clinician, a patient's self-report of the pain is considered the gold standard for the initial assessment of pain and tracking of a response to interventions. Such patient reporting is not necessarily a gold standard to mandate specific interventions.[262]

Multiple unidimensional acute pain measurement instruments have been published, and many have been independently validated. These tools are limited to quantifying pain severity only and may overlook the other multidimensional aspects of an individual's pain experience. Common unidimensional pain instruments include the verbal rating scale (VRS), numerical rating scale (NRS), visual analog scale (VAS), and graphic rating scales (Fig. 1-7). A systematic review recently evaluated a variety of graphic scales in pediatric patients and supported use of the Faces Pain Scale (FPS), the Faces Pain Scale-Revised (FPS-R), the Oucher Pain Scale, and the Wong-Baker Faces Pain Rating Scale (WBFPRS).[263] Clinicians need to be aware of the possibility of misinterpreted application of self-reported pain intensity measurement tools that use facial expression.[264] The VRS is administered by asking the patient to rate the severity of the pain by using a set of descriptors such as "none," "mild," "moderate," or "severe." These tests are rapid and easy to use but may be less responsive to changes in severity of pain because of the small number of categories.[265] Language and cultural barriers can also limit effectiveness. In the prehospital setting, the verbal NRS appears to be the most appropriate pain measure to administer to adult patients. It is practical and valid. The Oucher scale or the FPS is suitable to assess pain in children.[266]

The NRS consists of numbers on a line, and patients are asked to score their pain after explanation of the scale.[267] For example, 1 means no pain and 10 means the worst pain ever experienced. The NRS has been validated for verbal administration but may be difficult to use in cognitively impaired patients, who may have difficulty translating pain into numbers.[262]

Probably the most used pain scale in the ED is the 1 to 10 VAS. The VAS uses a 10-cm line bounded on each end by perpendicular stops and descriptors. Zero equates to no pain, and 10 equates to the worst pain ever experienced. The initial score is not as important as change during treatment. Generally, a change in VAS scores has been shown to be valid and reliable if self-completion is appropriate.[268] *There is wide variability in this technique, and at least a 13- to 30-mm (1.3- to 3-cm) change on the scale is required to validate clinically relevant worsening or relief.*[262] Low completion rates may be seen in patients with visual or cognitive impairment. In one ED study, failure rates with the VAS were 15% versus 0% with the NRS.[269] Graphic rating scales are useful for patients with limited cognitive and expressive ability, especially children. They may also be helpful to overcome language or cultural differences.

Figure 1-7 Pain rating scales. *(Modified from Turk DC, Burwinkle TM. Assessment of chronic pain in rehabilitation: outcomes measures in clinical trials and clinical practice. Rehabil Psychol. 2005;50:56-64.)*

In an ED survey, the WBFPRS was the most common (81.7% of responding facilities) pain measurement tool used for pediatric pain assessment.[267] The FPS-R was developed to overcome potential cultural differences in how patients perceive tears or the act of smiling.

Multidimensional pain measurement tools attempt to provide more insight by incorporating affective, sensory, and cognitive aspects of the pain experience into the measurement process. Multidimensional measurement tools require more time to administer and are mostly impractical for routine use in the ED. One exception may be the short-form McGill Pain Questionnaire (SF-MPQ), which is reported to take only 2 to 5 minutes to complete.[270] The SF-MPQ has been shown to be reliable and valid,[267] but little study has been performed in the ED setting. These tools may be difficult to administer in patients with hearing or visual difficulty and in those with limited cognitive ability, such as children or the elderly.

Overview of Visual Analog Pain Scales

The patient's use of the commonly applied 1 to 10 VAS, though perhaps helpful to monitor progress of pain control or lack thereof, often overestimates the level of pain from the clinician's standpoint. Conversely, it may underestimate the pain in certain stoic individuals or certain cultural groups. A rating of 10 was designed to indicate the "worst pain ever experienced," but this level is commonly chosen by patients with problems clearly of a minor nature. A rating of 10 may be patients' understanding of their level of pain and be used to describe the worst pain that *they have personally experienced.* This rating does not mandate a specific pain reduction approach and is better driven by clinician evaluation and consideration of the entire scenario. It is not uncommon for patients to rate their pain a 12 on a scale of 1 to 10 in an attempt to emphasize their personal experience, anxiety, or fear of receiving inadequate analgesia. It may be a patient's perception that a higher rating will expedite treatment, prompt higher doses of narcotics, or otherwise engender more compassionate care. *A common erroneous tactic or subterfuge of litigation proceedings is to incriminate a clinician's diagnosis, treatment, or disposition based on the patient's rendition of the pain scale.* Many benign kidney stones rightly garner a pain rating of 10, but some aortic dissections are totally painless, hardly rendering any pain report equal to the seriousness of the medical condition.

Overall Goal of Pain Relief

The goal of EP pain management is to adequately relieve or control pain without compromising diagnosis, treatment plans, or the safety of the patient and population. The ideal objective is to totally relieve pain (0 on the pain scale). This goal is difficult to consistently achieve in the complex ED milieu. It is best accomplished by combining clinician experience, real-time clinical judgment, repeated evaluation, and discussion with the patient and family. Concerns about the abuse potential of addictive pharmaceuticals often weigh into the decision-making process for emergency physicians, and universal prescriptive reporting services can be used to assist in patient care and safe prescribing practices.[270,271] Strict adherence to protocols, patient self-reporting on any pain scale, or reliance on a dogmatic approach to relief of a patient's pain can be fraught with peril. It is best to treat the patient, not the pain scale.

In summary, although the routine use of patient-reported pain scales may facilitate the administration of analgesics and be somewhat useful in trending response to analgesia, experienced clinicians and the authors view such pain scales with skepticism. With certainly, the vagaries and vicissitudes of pain in the ED do not allow one to scientifically conclude that any specific pain scale has any diagnostic or prognostic value. Pain scales are best used to raise awareness that pain—and prudent efforts to relieve it—should be aggressively addressed in the ED.

References are available at www.expertconsult.com

CHAPTER 2

Devices for Assessing Oxygenation and Ventilation

Joshua Nagler and Baruch Krauss

SPIROMETRY

For patients with acute exacerbations of asthma and chronic obstructive pulmonary disease (COPD), accurately estimating the severity of airflow obstruction is a critical component of their care. A focused history plus physical examination is the cornerstone of this assessment in the practice of emergency medicine. The history and physical examination alone, however, cannot reliably quantify airflow obstruction during acute attacks.[1-5] In patients with COPD, wide variation exists in the ability to accurately diagnose airway obstruction, and up to 15% of patients with marked airflow obstruction will not be dyspneic.[6-9] This blunted perception of disease severity may be a contributor to fatal and near-fatal asthma attacks.[10] After therapy for acute exacerbations of asthma, patients may experience subjective resolution of their symptoms even while severe airflow obstruction is still present.[11] Given these difficulties in recognizing airflow obstruction, objective measurement provides valuable information.

Spirometry is measurement of the volume of air exhaled during forced expiration.[12] It can be interpreted as a function of time to determine the flow rate. Spirometry gives the most complete picture of lung mechanics and is the centerpiece of pulmonary function testing. Many parameters can be derived from a spirogram, the most useful of which are forced vital capacity (FVC), which is the total volume exhaled during a forced expiratory maneuver, and forced expiratory volume in 1 second (FEV_1), which is the average flow rate during the first second of the forced expiratory maneuver (Fig. 2-1).

The advent of small handheld devices allows convenient spirometric evaluation in the emergency department (ED). The most common objective measurement of respiratory mechanics used in the ED is peak expiratory flow rate (PEFR). PEFR is the maximum flow of gas achieved during a forced expiratory maneuver. It correlates well with standard spirometry and has been studied extensively in the ED setting.[13-15]

Indications

Evaluation of Acute Asthma Attacks

Currently, no standards exist for the measurement of pulmonary function parameters in ED patients, and practices vary widely. Most patients with asthma exacerbations can be evaluated, treated, and given a disposition with no further pulmonary function testing other than PEFR if quantitative assessment is deemed prudent. Several consensus guidelines recommend obtaining an objective measure of airflow obstruction in all patients seen in the ED with an acute exacerbation of asthma.[16-18] Others have proposed that the decision to measure PEFR in patients with acute asthma should be individualized.[19] It is reasonable that mild and easily reversible disease be evaluated and treated according to clinical judgment, but if any pulmonary function parameters are to be used, their use is optimized if measured at arrival, after initial treatment, and periodically thereafter.[16-18]

Evaluation of Exacerbations of COPD

PEFR and spirometry testing can yield objective data on airflow obstruction during the ED evaluation of COPD exacerbations. Though used by some ED practitioners, consensus guidelines do not recommend routine use of these tests in the acute setting.[20-22]

Differentiating Causes of Dyspnea

PEFR has been studied for its ability to differentiate between COPD and congestive heart failure (CHF).[23] Insufficient data exist to recommend its routine use for this purpose in the ED.

Evaluation of Neuromuscular and Chest Wall Disease

Diseases of the chest wall and neuromuscular system can cause respiratory compromise. Though not commonly done in the ED, pulmonary function testing and assessment of negative inspiratory force can quantify the degree of impairment and help determine the level of admission needed.

Contraindications

Need for Immediate Intervention

Patients with severe respiratory compromise should receive aggressive therapy without delaying care for pulmonary function testing. Formal pulmonary function testing has limited value for acute exacerbations, and such assessments are most predictive when patients are at their baseline functional status.

Conditions That May Be Worsened by Increased Intrathoracic Pressure

Significant elevations in intrathoracic pressure will develop in patients performing a forced expiratory maneuver. Pneumothorax, pneumomediastinum, aneurysms of the aorta, or aneurysms of the cerebral vasculature may be exacerbated by the forced expiratory maneuver. The presence of these conditions should be considered a relative contraindication to pulmonary function testing.

Equipment

Spirometers can be divided into two categories. Volume spirometers measure the amount of gas exhaled as a function of time. These devices, however, tend to be cumbersome and are not ideally suited to the ED. Flow spirometers measure the flow of gas past a certain point and use that information to extrapolate volume and time data. These machines are smaller, simpler to use, and more portable. Flow spirometers determine gas flow by measuring the difference in pressure between two points in a tube (pneumotachograph), cooling of a heated wire (hot wire anemometer), or revolutions of a rotating vane. Most handheld spirometers also measure PEFR.

The most commonly used device to measure PEFR is the "mini-Wright" peak-flow flowmeter (Fig. 2-2). These meters provide accurate and reproducible measurements of PEFR.[24] The mini-Wright peak-flow flowmeter retains its accuracy for at least 5 years.[25] There is significant variation between types and brands of peak-flow flowmeters, so measurements recorded with the same brand of peak-flow flowmeter are most useful when comparing a patient's baseline PEFR.[11,26,27]

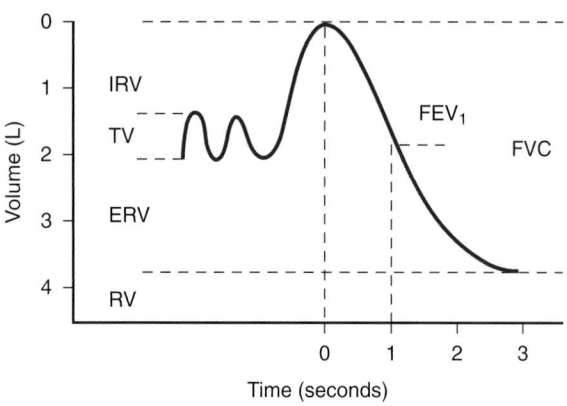

Figure 2-1 Diagrammatic representation of spirometry values. *ERV,* expiratory reserve volume; *FEV₁,* forced expiratory volume in 1 second; *FVC,* forced vital capacity; *IRV,* inspiratory reserve volume; *RV,* residual volume; *TV,* tidal volume.

Figure 2-2 The "mini-Wright" peak flow meter.

Procedure

Calibrate the spirometer in accordance with the manufacturer's directions and examine the peak-flow flowmeter to ensure that the measurement bar is resting at the zero line before beginning the procedure. For multipatient devices, attach a disposable mouthpiece to the input orifice.

Before starting the test, explain the procedure and allow unfamiliar patients to practice a few times. Ideally, the patient should be in the standing position or, if not feasible, be seated upright in bed. Ask the patient to elevate the chin and hold the neck in a slightly extended position. A nose clip is not required for PEFR measurements but may be useful when performing formal spirometry testing.

After a period of normal breathing, ask the patient to take a maximal inspiration with the lips sealed around the mouthpiece while taking care to keep the tongue from partially obstructing the mouthpiece. Request the patient to initiate a rapid, forceful expiration as soon as possible after reaching maximal inspiration (Fig. 2-3). Coach the patient throughout the procedure and remind the patient to continue to make a forceful and complete exhalation. The PEFR usually occurs during the first 100 msec of expiration. In contrast, when performing spirometry, it is essential that the patient exhale fully. With both tests it is important to have a rapid, forceful exhalation rather than a slow, sustained one. Obtain three separate measurements for both spirometry and PEFR.[28,29]

PEFR measurements are very sensitive to technique and patient effort. Even a small decrease in effort can lead to considerable degradation of results.[11,30] Because airflow is greatest when the lung volumes are highest and the airways are larger, the test is accurate only if performed after a maximal inspiration.

Interpretation

Obstructive diseases are characterized by a disproportionate decrease in airflow (FEV₁) in relation to the volume of gas

Figure 2-3 Measurement of the peak expiratory flow rate (PEFR) with a portable disposable peak flow meter. Ask the patient to take a maximal inspiration with the lips sealed around the mouthpiece and then initiate a rapid, forceful expiration immediately afterward. Three separate measurements should be obtained. Be sure to zero the device before each test. PEFR is the easiest and most common pulmonary function test used to evaluate asthma in the emergency department. Trends are more important than actual values because individual baselines vary widely. PEFR alone cannot be used to make accurate clinical decisions on admission or discharge.

TABLE 2-1 Approximate Values			
	FEV₁ (L)	**FVC (L)**	**FEV₁/FVC Ratio (%)**
Male	3.0-5.0	3.5-6.0	75-85
Female	2-3.5	2.5-4.0	75-85

Based on Hankinson JL, Odencrantz JR, Fedan KB. Spirometric reference values from a sample of the general U.S. population. *Am J Respir Crit Care Med.* 1999;159:179.
FEV₁, forced expiratory volume in 1 second; *FVC,* forced vital capacity.

exhaled (FVC).[31] A decreased FEV₁/FVC ratio with preservation of FVC indicates the presence of airflow obstruction. Restrictive diseases decrease total lung capacity and therefore decrease FVC to a greater degree than FEV₁. Decreased FVC with a normal or increased FEV₁/FVC ratio is indicative of restriction. It is useful to consider the FEV₁/FVC ratio when attempting to determine whether a patient has airflow obstruction. In patients with an established diagnosis of obstructive disease, FEV₁ is the test that best reflects changes in lung function. Typical values are shown in Table 2-1. These values are dependent on age, gender, ethnicity, and height and can be predicted from mathematical equations.[32]

Isolated measurements of PEFR are not reliable in making the diagnosis of asthma because of significant variation between individuals. However, it is appropriate to use PEFR to monitor the degree of airflow obstruction in known asthmatics.

Although measures of airflow obstruction are not standalone tests, when considered along with other clinical factors, they can guide decisions regarding the disposition of patients with acute asthma exacerbations. The highest of three PEFR or FEV₁ measurements should be used and, whenever possible, compared with the patient's personal best.[16-18] In one study of inner-city patients, only 29% knew their personal best PEFR, and even when known, this number may be unreliable.[33] In circumstances in which previous best values are unknown or thought to be inaccurate, comparison with predicted values is appropriate. Normal PEFR values for adults are shown in Figure 2-4. Values for children are presented in Tables 2-2 and 2-3. The National Asthma Education and

PREDICTED PEFR
CAUCASIAN PATIENTS

PREDICTED PEFR
AFRICAN AMERICAN PATIENTS

PREDICTED PEFR
MEXICAN AMERICAN PATIENTS

Figure 2-4 Predicted peak expiratory flow rate (PEFR) for adults. **A,** Caucasian patients. **B,** African American patients. *C,* Mexican American patients. *(Based on equations from Hankinson JL, Odencrantz JR, Fedan KB. Spirometric reference values from a sample of the general U.S. population.* Am J Respir Crit Care Med. *1999;159:179.)*

Figure 2-5 Pulse oximeter sensors. **A,** Reusable adult sensor attached to a finger. **B,** Single-use adult sensor attached to a finger. **C,** Single-use pediatric sensor attached to a toe. Note that the light source is centered over the nail, not the fat pad. See text for various parameters that affect pulse oximetry readings.

TABLE 2-4 Severity of Asthma Exacerbations according to Objective Measures of Airflow Obstruction

% OF PERSONAL BEST OR PREDICTED (FEV₁ OR PEFR)	SEVERITY OF EXACERBATION
≤30	Life-threatening
31-50	Severe
51-80	Moderate
>80	Mild

FEV₁, forced expiratory volume in 1 second; *PEFR*, peak expiratory flow rate.

Figure 2-6 Factors influencing light absorption through a pulsatile vascular bed. *(From McGough EK, Boysen PG. Benefits and limitations of pulse oximetry in the ICU. J Crit Illness. 1989;4:23.)*

Prevention Program has used the results of FEV_1 and PEFR testing to classify the severity of asthma exacerbations (Table 2-4).[16]

Table 2-2 Predicted Peak Expiratory Flow Rate in Males 8-20 Years of Age CAN BE FOUND ON EXPERT CONSULT

Table 2-3 Predicted Peak Expiratory Flow Rate in Females 8-18 Years of Age CAN BE FOUND ON EXPERT CONSULT

Multiple guidelines and articles have advocated specific cutoff values for PEFR and FEV_1 to guide decisions on disposition.[16-18] There is variation across these guidelines and no consensus that absolute cutoffs should exist.[16] When these values are obtained, they should be viewed as additional data points to be considered, along with other clinical variables, in determining the disposition of asthmatics seen in the ED. At the extremes, data may be useful. For example, asthmatic patients with an initial PEFR greater than 70% of personal best or the predicted value will probably be discharged and those below 35% will probably need admission. Beyond the degree of initial airflow obstruction, the response to inhaled bronchodilators is a useful gauge of suitability for outpatient asthma management. A poor response argues in favor of admission, whereas recovery of PEFR or FEV_1 to greater than 70% of personal best is a favorable sign.

NONINVASIVE OXYGENATION MONITORING: PULSE OXIMETRY

Pulse oximetry, or noninvasive measurement of the percentage of hemoglobin bound to oxygen, provides real-time estimates of arterial saturation in the range of 80% to 100% and gives early warning of diminished capillary perfusion while avoiding the discomfort and risks associated with arterial puncture. As a result, it has become the standard of care in a wide variety of clinical settings.

Technology

Oximetry is based on the Beer-Lambert law, which states that the concentration of an unknown solute dissolved in a solvent can be determined by light absorption. Pulse oximetry combines the principles of optical plethysmography and spectrophotometry. The probe, set into a reusable clip or a disposable patch, is made up of two photodiodes, which produce red light at 660 nm and infrared light at 900 to 940 nm, and a photodetector, which is placed across a pulsatile vascular bed such as the finger or ear (Fig. 2-5). These particular wavelengths are used because the absorption characteristics of oxyhemoglobin and reduced hemoglobin are quite different at the two wavelengths. The majority of the light is absorbed by connective tissue, skin, bones, and venous blood. The amount of light absorbed by these substances is constant with time and does not vary during the cardiac cycle. A small increase in arterial blood occurs with each heartbeat, thereby resulting in an increase in light absorption (Fig. 2-6). By comparing the ratio of pulsatile and baseline absorption at these two wavelengths, the ratio of oxyhemoglobin to reduced hemoglobin is calculated.

Because the pulse oximeter uses only two wavelengths of light, it can distinguish only two substances. As a result, pulse oximeters measure "functional saturation," which is the concentration of oxyhemoglobin divided by the concentrations of

Figure 2-7 Oxyhemoglobin dissociation curve. Measurements of Sao_2 are relatively insensitive in detecting significant changes in Pao_2 at high levels of oxygenation because these Sao_2 values fall on the plateau portion of the curve (labeled). Hence, oxygen saturation is an insensitive way of detecting early compensation in patients with asthma.

oxyhemoglobin plus reduced hemoglobin. The disadvantage of functional saturation is that the denominator *does not include other hemoglobin species that may be present, such as carboxyhemoglobin and methemoglobin.* The advantage of using only two wavelengths in the oximeter is that the cost, size, and weight of the device are reduced. The CO-oximeter, one example of a commercially available in vitro oximeter and the standard by which pulse oximetry is calibrated, uses four or more wavelengths, measures "fractional saturation," and is able to quantify additional hemoglobin species.

Physiology

Arterial O_2 saturation (Sao_2) measures the large reservoir of O_2 carried by hemoglobin, 20 mL of O_2/100 mL of blood, whereas arterial O_2 partial pressure (Pao_2) measures only the relatively small amount of O_2 dissolved in plasma, approximately 0.3 mL of O_2/100 mL of blood. Sao_2 correlates well with Pao_2, but the relationship is nonlinear and is described by the oxyhemoglobin dissociation curve (Fig. 2-7). In hypoxemic patients, small changes in Sao_2 represent large changes in Pao_2 because these Sao_2 values fall on the steep portion of the curve. Conversely, measurements of Sao_2 are relatively insensitive in detecting significant changes in Pao_2 at high levels of oxygenation because these Sao_2 values fall on the plateau portion of the curve.

Currently available pulse oximeters are accurate and precise when saturation ranges from 70% to 100%. This range is satisfactory because for most patients an O_2 saturation of 80% is as much an urgent warning as is one lower than 70%. Testing of pulse oximeters has shown that at 75% saturation, bias is scattered uniformly, with 7% underestimation and 7% overestimation.

Clinical Utility

Pulse oximetry offers an advantage in assessing the adequacy of oxygenation over arterial blood gas analysis by providing continuous estimated Sao_2 measurements. Direct

measurement of Sao_2 is determined from blood gas values coupled with knowledge of the actual hemoglobin levels in a patient's blood. Sao_2 measurement is estimated with pulse oximetry (Spo_2). In this chapter we equate Sao_2 and Spo_2.

Data on the clinical efficacy of routine pulse oximetry monitoring in the ED are limited, so clinical value has been extrapolated from anesthesia studies.[34-36] These studies have demonstrated that continuous monitoring of saturation decreases the incidence and duration of desaturation episodes, thereby resulting in fewer adverse events during recovery and shortening the time to discovery of hypoxia. It follows logically that use in critically ill patients should result in similar benefits, including more rapid recognition of adverse physiologic events and fewer episodes of severe arterial desaturation. Patient outcomes should be improved by initiation of therapeutic interventions following immediate notification of an unfavorable Sao_2.[37]

Indications

Recommended uses for pulse oximetry fall into two broad categories: (1) as a real-time indicator of hypoxemia, continuous oximetry monitoring can be used as a warning system because many adverse patient events are associated with arterial desaturation,[38] and (2) as an end point for titration of therapeutic interventions to avoid hypoxia (Box 2-1).

Pulse oximetry can also be used to assess peripheral perfusion and evaluate for possible ischemia in the extremities. Such use is not standardized, and although clinical experience validates its use, minimal data are available for such utilization in the ED. Vascular surgeons will use a pulse oximetry probe on a finger or toe to assess the results of vascular surgery on the arm or leg. Peripheral artery occlusion from peripheral artery disease may be suggested by comparison of pulse oximetry readings in the extremities. Decreased peripheral oxygenation may be detected in patients with compartment syndrome, traumatic arterial injury, and external compression of the proximal circulation (Fig. 2-8).[39,40]

Procedure

The location for the probe is determined by the clinical situation and the probes available. A reusable clip-on probe works well on digits that are easily accessible. Other sites include the earlobe, the nasal bridge, the septum, the temporal artery, and the foot or palm of an infant. A newer probe developed for use on the forehead may provide better readings in cold

Figure 2-8 Pulse oximetry can be used to assess the distal circulation after vascular surgery for trauma and to initially evaluate other causes of decreased peripheral perfusion. **A,** This patient had a markedly swollen and ischemic finger from a tight ring. **B,** Although the need for immediate removal of the ring is clinically obvious, a pulse oximetry probe confirmed ischemia with an oxygen saturation of 61%. The uninvolved fingers registered 99%. Following ring removal the saturation returned to normal, thus suggesting that fasciotomy need not be performed. **C,** When a discharged EpiPen caused a pale finger, injection of phentolamine was considered. **D,** When pulse oximetry demonstrated a saturation of 96% (97% to 98% in the other fingers), injection was not performed and the circulation spontaneously normalized over a period of 30 minutes.

ambient temperature or during movement.[41] Tape and splints can also be used to secure oximetry probes and minimize motion.

The computer analyzes the incoming data to identify the arteriolar pulsation and displays this parameter as beats per minute. Newer devices also display a pulse plethysmograph (Fig. 2-9). Simultaneously, O_2 saturation is displayed on a beat-to-beat basis. Some machines have hard-copy capability and can provide paper documentation of the patient's status. Machines differ in their display when a pulsatile flow is not detected. Either the reading will not display at all, or the Sao_2 value will be given along with a poor-signal quality warning. It is important to evaluate serial measurements and to verify that the measurements correlate with other clinical markers.

Interpretation

Patients with normal physiologic gas exchange have an O_2 saturation between 97% and 100%. When Sao_2 falls below 95%, hypoxemia may be present, although this may be base-line for some patients with cardiac or lung disease. Oxygen saturation below 90% represents significant hypoxemia. As with spirometry, an isolated, low early measurement of Sao_2 does not mandate admission because of the potential for rapid response to therapy. Low Sao_2 readings should be heeded as

Figure 2-9 Patient monitor displaying a pulse plethysmograph (*arrow*). The patient's heart rate (84) and oxygen saturation (95) are also displayed (blue numbers).

important clinical warning signs. Pulse oximetry may be affected by numerous extrinsic factors, but a decline in oxygen saturation with serial measurements should always prompt an evaluation of respiratory status and adequacy of circulation.

Although pulse oximetry represents a significant advance in noninvasive monitoring of oxygenation, clinicians must recognize and understand its limitations.[42] Pulse oximetry measures only O_2 saturation. In contrast to arterial blood gas determination or capnography, pulse oximetry provides no direct information on pH or the arterial partial pressure of CO_2 ($Paco_2$). Witting and Lueck[43] empirically demonstrated that a room-air Sao_2 value of 97% or higher strongly rules against hypoxemia and moderate to severe hypercapnia. Their validated study of patients with respiratory complaints undergoing arterial blood gas analysis found good discrimination with a room-air Sao_2 value of 96% or less. For hypoxemia (Pao_2 <70 mm Hg), this value was 100% sensitive and 54% specific. For hypercapnia ($Paco_2$ >50 mm Hg), this value was 100% sensitive and 31% specific. Kelly and colleagues[44] found a cutoff value of 92% or less for room-air Sao_2 to be more accurate in identifying hypoxemia in patients with COPD.

Pulse oximetry is not a substitute for monitoring ventilation because of the variable lag time between the onset of hypoventilation or apnea and a change in oxygen saturation.[45] Therefore, during procedural sedation, monitoring of ventilation is a more desirable goal for prevention of hypoxemia and hypercapnia than simple pulse oximetry is (see "Procedural Sedation and Analgesia" under "Carbon Dioxide Monitoring" later in this chapter). Hypoventilation and the resultant hypercapnia may precede a decrease in hemoglobin O_2 saturation by many minutes. Furthermore, supplemental O_2 may mask hypoventilation by delaying the eventual O_2 desaturation that pulse oximetry is designed to monitor and recognize. In preoxygenated animals, airway obstruction was detected within 10 seconds with capnography, but Sao_2 values did not change during the 180-second study periods.[45] Other limitations of pulse oximetry are summarized in Box 2-2.

BOX 2-2 Factors Affecting Pulse Oximetry Readings

Severe anemia: Satisfactory readings obtained down to a hemoglobin level of 5 mg/dL

Motion artifact: See text regarding probe sites

Dyes: Transient effect unless resulting in methemoglobinemia

Light artifact: Minimize by covering the probe with opaque material

Hypoperfusion: An inadequate pulse signal will be displayed

Electrocautery: Minimize by increasing the distance of the sensor from the surgical site

Deep pigmentation: Use the fifth finger, earlobe, or other area with lighter pigmentation

Dark nail polish: Remove with acetone or place a sensor sideways on the digit

Dyshemoglobinemias (e.g., carboxyhemoglobin and methemoglobin): Falsely elevate true oxygen saturation readings

Elevated bilirubin: Accurate up to a bilirubin level of 20 mg/dL in adults; no problem reported in jaundiced children

High saturation: Pulse oximetry not useful for monitoring hyperoxemia in neonates

Fetal hemoglobin: No effect on pulse oximetry; falsely reduced co-oximetry readings

Venous pulsations: Artificially lower O_2 saturation; choose a probe site above the heart

Dialysis graft (arteriovenous fistula): No difference from the contralateral extremity unless the fistula is producing distal ischemia

---

Sources of Interference

Effects of Dyshemoglobinemias

In patients with methemoglobinemia or elevated carboxyhemoglobin levels, pulse oximetry does not accurately depict quantitative changes in hemoglobin O_2 saturation.[46,47]

Carboxyhemoglobin results in falsely elevated Sao_2 estimates of hemoglobin O_2 saturation. Low quantities of methemoglobin will reduce pulse oximetry readings by about half the actual methemoglobin percentage. Large quantities of methemoglobin (>10%) can result in a stable pulse oximetry reading of 85% regardless of the actual Sao_2. Because pulse oximetry will variably underestimate the percentage of abnormal hemoglobin, a CO-oximeter or blood gas sample is required for confirmation of these conditions and quantitative analysis.

Fetal Hemoglobin

Full-term newborns can have up to 75% of total hemoglobin in the form of fetal hemoglobin and up to 5% in the form of carboxyhemoglobin. Although fetal hemoglobin interferes with the spectrophotometric method, pulse oximetry will remain accurate. However, a CO-oximeter may erroneously interpret the carboxyhemoglobin level as elevated and the oxyhemoglobin level as artificially reduced. Therefore, when fetal hemoglobin levels are high, CO-oximetry readings should not be used to confirm pulse oximetry readings.

Low Perfusion

To function properly, pulse oximeters require a pulsating vascular bed. Vasoconstriction related to hypotension, hypothermia, or the administration of vasoconstricting drugs may reduce the pulsatile component to less than 0.2% of the total signal. At this level the true signal cannot be distinguished from background noise. Under these conditions, pulse oximeters may display a message indicating an inadequate pulse signal. Changing the location of the sensor to an area with higher perfusion, such as an earlobe or the forehead, may improve the pulse signal.

Intravenous Dyes

A number of dyes and pigments interfere with the accuracy of pulse oximetry.[48] Methylene blue, the treatment of methemoglobinemia, absorbs light at 660 nm, which is similar to the absorption of reduced hemoglobin, and can significantly decrease pulse oximeter saturation readings to as low as 1%. Low readings can also be seen with other intravenous dyes such as indigo carmine, indocyanine green, and fluorescein, although the rapid clearance of these agents minimizes this phenomenon.

Bilirubin

Hyperbilirubinemia does not affect the accuracy of pulse oximetry, but it may have an effect on absorption at the lower wavelengths used by CO-oximeters and result in a discrepancy between pulse oximeter and CO-oximeter readings.

Skin Pigmentation

The accuracy of pulse oximeters is somewhat reduced by darkly pigmented skin. This effect is probably due to a shift in the light-emitting diode's output spectrum as the light output is increased. This effect is small and results in only a slight decrease in accuracy. Placing the probe on an area of lighter pigmentation, such as the fifth finger or an earlobe, is suggested to minimize this effect.

Nail Polish

Conflicting data exist about the effect of nail polish on the accuracy of pulse oximetry.[49,50] Mounting the probe side to side on the finger was found to correspond to readings on uncovered nails.[51] This technique also circumvents the problem of only partial placement of the probe because of very long fingernails, which may cause a low O_2 saturation reading. An alternative solution to the problem of nail polish is to remove it with acetone. The accuracy of Sao_2 readings in the setting of synthetic nails is unknown. If a poor signal is obtained through a synthetic nail, either the nail should be removed or an alternative site should be used for placement.

High Saturation

Because the O_2 dissociation curve plateaus at saturation levels greater than 90%, a large increase in Pao_2 results in only a small increase in saturation. Therefore, an error of a few percentage points could represent a large error in Pao_2. This is inconsequential for most adult patients but is of extreme importance for neonates, who are at risk for retinopathy caused by hyperoxemia.

Venous Pulsations

The increased venous pulsations resulting from right heart failure and tricuspid regurgitation can interfere with accurate readings and lead to artificially lower O_2 saturation because the pulse oximeter interprets any pulsatile measurement as arterial. Placing the probe on a site above the heart may improve accuracy. Some pulse oximeters have the capability of synchronizing pulsations at the probe site to electrocardiographic (ECG) signals, thus enhancing the signal-to-noise ratio.

Anemia

Because pulse oximetry depends on light absorption by hemoglobin, it becomes less accurate and less reliable in conditions of severe anemia. Studies suggest that a hemoglobin content below 5 mg/dL is likely to affect oximetry readings.[52,53]

Ambient Light

Because the pulse oximeter's photodetector is nonspecific, high-intensity ambient light can produce interference. Surgical, fluorescent, and heating lamps are common sources of light interference. This problem can be corrected by wrapping the probe with a light barrier, such as a dark cloth or other opaque material.

Motion

Motion of the probe can produce considerable artifact and inaccurate readings. Correlating a pulse oximetry signal with an ECG waveform or using alternative probe sites, such as the ear or toe, may reduce motion artifact. Newer-generation pulse oximetry signal–processing technology has greatly reduced the effect of motion artifact.

Probe Site

The finger is the most common probe site used for adult pulse oximetry. If the finger is inaccessible or unsuitable, other probe sites, such as the earlobe, nose, and forehead (using reflectance instead of transmittance), may be used. It should be noted, though, that forehead and nasal bridge probes may be less accurate than finger and ear probes. In infants and small children, an adhesive sensor unit is preferred and frequently placed on the fingers and toes. Probes can also be secured in place over the palm, heel, or lateral aspect of the foot with a gauze or Coban wrap.

Electrocautery

Electrical interference from devices such as electrocautery can also impair the accuracy of pulse oximetry. Such interference can be reduced by increasing the distance between the surgical site and the probe.

Conclusions

Pulse oximetry is a widely available technology that provides an easy, noninvasive, and generally reliable method of monitoring oxygenation. Because measurements are continuous, pulse oximetry allows earlier detection of hypoxic episodes than intermittent arterial blood gas analysis does. Frequent measurements can lead to earlier corrective measures and prevention of adverse consequences.

CO_2 MONITORING

Capnography is a noninvasive measurement of the partial pressure of CO_2 in an exhaled breath. Measurement of CO_2 at the airway can be displayed as a function of time (CO_2 concentration over time) or as an exhaled tidal volume (CO_2 concentration over volume). This chapter discusses the use of time-based capnography because this is the only form of CO_2 monitoring used by the emergency medical service (EMS) and the predominant form used in the ED. In addition, volume-based capnography is not easily adaptable to nonintubated subjects and therefore not applicable in the majority of patients.

The relationship of CO_2 concentration to time is graphically represented by the CO_2 waveform or capnogram (Fig. 2-10). The maximum CO_2 concentration at the end of each tidal breath is the end-tidal CO_2 pressure ($Petco_2$). Changes in the shape of the capnogram are diagnostic of disease conditions, whereas changes in $Petco_2$ can be used to assess disease severity and response to treatment.

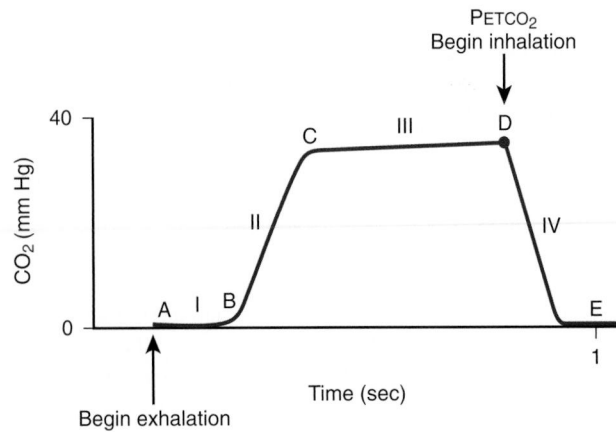

Figure 2-10 Normal capnogram. The maximum CO_2 concentration at the end of exhalation of each tidal breath and at the beginning of inhalation is the *end-tidal CO_2 pressure* ($Petco_2$), depicted by *D* on this graph. CO_2 pressure at *D* will be displayed numerically on the screen. See text for further explanation of the physiology of this graph. (*From Krauss B, Hess DR. Capnography for procedural sedation and analgesia in the emergency department. Ann Emerg Med. 2007; 50:172.*)

Oxygenation and ventilation are distinct physiologic functions that are assessed in both intubated and spontaneously breathing patients. Pulse oximetry provides real-time feedback about oxygenation, whereas capnography provides breath-to-breath information about all of the following: ventilation (how effectively CO_2 is being eliminated by the pulmonary system), perfusion (how effectively CO_2 is being transported through the vascular system), and metabolism (how effectively CO_2 is being produced by cellular metabolism).

Terminology

The ancient Greeks believed there was a combustion engine inside the body that gave off smoke (*capnos* in Greek) in the form of a breath. A capnometer is a CO_2 monitor that displays a number (i.e., P_{ETCO_2}). A capnograph is a CO_2 monitor that displays a number and a waveform (i.e., the capnogram).

Technology

Capnography became a routine part of anesthesia practice in Europe in the 1970s and in the United States in the 1980s.[54] Capnography was incorporated into the American Heart Association (AHA) guidelines in 2000 and the American College of Emergency Physicians (ACEP) guidelines in 2001 and has become the standard of care for verification of endotracheal (ET) tube placement in the operating room, the ED, and the prehospital setting.

Most capnography technology is built on infrared (IR) radiation techniques. These techniques are based on the fact that CO_2 molecules absorb IR radiation at a very specific wavelength (4.26 μm), with the amount of radiation absorbed having a close to exponential relationship to the CO_2 concentration present in the breath sample. Detecting these changes in IR radiation levels by using appropriate photodetectors sensitive in this spectral region allows the CO_2 concentration in the gas sample to be calculated.

CO_2 monitors measure gas concentration or partial pressure by using one of two configurations, depending on the location of the sensor: mainstream or sidestream (Fig. 2-11). Mainstream devices measure CO_2 directly from the airway, with the sensor located at the proximal end of the ET tube. Sidestream devices measure CO_2 by aspirating a small sample from the exhaled breath through tubing and a sensor located inside the monitor. Mainstream systems are configured only for intubated patients because the sensor is located on the ET tube. Sidestream systems do not require an ET tube because the sensor is located inside the monitor and may therefore be used in either intubated or nonintubated patients. The airway interface for intubated patients is an airway adapter placed on the hub of the ET tube. For spontaneously breathing patients, a nasal-oral cannula is used. This allows concomitant CO_2 sampling and delivery of low-flow oxygen to the patient.

Sidestream systems can be high flow (requiring 150 mL/min of CO_2 in the breath sample to obtain an accurate reading) or low flow (requiring 50 mL/min of CO_2). Low-flow sidestream systems have a lower occlusion rate (from moisture or patient secretions) and are more accurate in patients with low tidal volumes (neonates, infants, and patients with hypoventilation and low–tidal volume breathing).[55]

CO_2 monitors can be either quantitative or qualitative (Fig. 2-12). Quantitative devices measure the precise P_{ETCO_2} as either a number (capnometry) or a number and a waveform

Figure 2-11 End-tidal CO_2 sensors. **A,** Mainstream sensor. This device measures CO_2 directly from the proximal end of an endotracheal tube. **B,** Sidestream sensor. This cannula-type device allows concomitant CO_2 sampling and low-flow oxygen delivery to the patient.

Figure 2-12 CO_2 monitors. **A,** Quantitative monitor. A capnography waveform (*arrow*) is displayed, as is a capnometry numerical reading (37). **B,** Qualitative device. This simple colorimetric detector is used to verify endotracheal tube position and changes color when exposed to CO_2.

(capnography). Qualitative devices measure the range in which P_{ETCO_2} falls (e.g., 0 to 10 mm Hg, >35 mm Hg) as opposed to a precise value (e.g., 38 mm Hg). The most commonly used qualitative device is the colorimetric P_{ETCO_2} detector, which consists of a piece of specially treated litmus paper that turns color when exposed to CO_2. Its primary use is for verification of ET tube position. If the tube is in the trachea, the resultant exhalation of CO_2 will change the color of the litmus paper; if the tube is in the esophagus with no CO_2 in the breath, no change in color will take place.

Physiology

The capnogram, which corresponds to a single tidal breath, consists of four phases (ascending phase, alveolar plateau, inspiratory limb, dead space ventilation) (see Fig. 2-10). Each phase has conventionally been approximated as a straight line.[54-56] Phase I (dead space ventilation, A to B) represents the beginning of exhalation in which dead space is cleared from the upper airway. Phase II (ascending phase, B to C) represents the rapid rise in CO_2 concentration in the breath stream as CO_2 from the alveoli reaches the upper airway. Phase III (alveolar plateau, C to D) represents the CO_2 concentration reaching a uniform level in the entire breath stream (from alveolus to nose) and concludes with a point of maximum CO_2 pressure (P_{ETCO_2}). *This is the number that appears on the monitor display.* Phase IV (D to E) represents the inspiratory cycle in which the CO_2 concentration drops to zero as atmospheric air enters the airway.

A normal capnogram, for patients of all ages, is characterized by a specific set of elements: it includes the four distinct phases just described, the CO_2 concentration starts at zero and returns to zero (i.e., there is no rebreathing of CO_2), a maximum CO_2 concentration is reached with each breath (i.e., P_{ETCO_2}), the amplitude is dependent on P_{ETCO_2}, the width is dependent on the expiratory time, and there is a characteristic shape for all subjects with normal lung function.

Patients with normal lung function, irrespective of age, will have a characteristic rectangular- or trapezoidal-shaped capnogram and a narrow P_{ETCO_2}-P_{CO_2} gradient (0 to 5 mm Hg), with P_{ETCO_2} accurately reflecting P_{aCO_2}.[57] Patients with obstructive lung disease will have a more rounded ascending phase and an upward slope in the alveolar plateau (Fig. 2-13).[58] In patients with abnormal lung function from $\dot{V}/\dot{Q}$ mismatch, the gradient will widen, depending on the severity of

A Normal patient: Trapezoidal capnogram

B COPD patient: Rounded capnogram, upward sloping alveolar plateau (arrow)

Figure 2-13 Capnogram shape in normal subjects and patients with chronic obstructive pulmonary disease (COPD). *(From Krauss B, Deykin A, Lam A, et al. Capnogram shape in obstructive lung disease. Anesth Analg. 2005;100:884.)*

the lung disease, and P_{ETCO_2} will be useful only for trending ventilatory status over time and not as a spot check because it may not correlate with P_{aCO_2}.[59,60]

Indications for Intubated Patients

- Verification of ET tube placement
- Continuous monitoring of tube location during transport
- Gauging the effectiveness of resuscitation and prognosis during cardiac arrest
- Titrating P_{ETCO_2} levels in patients with suspected increases in intracranial pressure
- Determining prognosis in patients after trauma
- Determining the adequacy of ventilation

Verification of ET Tube Placement

Unrecognized misplaced intubation (UMI) is placement of an ET tube in a location other than the trachea that is not recognized by the clinician. This life-threatening condition has been extensively documented in the EMS literature, with early studies reporting a 0.4% to 8% UMI rate. Katz and Falk[61] in 2001 were the first to perform a study with the primary outcome of identifying the rate of UMI and noted an alarming rate of 25%. More recent EMS studies have reported UMI rates of 7% to 10%.[62,63]

After intubation, the presence of a waveform with all four phases indicates that the ET tube is through the vocal cords. A flatline waveform following intubation indicates esophageal placement except in selected conditions, including obstruction of the ET tube, complete airway obstruction distal to the tube, tracheal placement with inadequate pulmonary blood flow as a result of poor chest compressions, or prolonged cardiac arrest with no circulating CO_2 because of cessation of cellular metabolism.

The accuracy of P_{ETCO_2} in confirming the tracheal location of an ET tube varies according to the type of CO_2 technology used. In patients who are not in cardiac arrest, qualitative colorimetric P_{ETCO_2} and quantitative capnography studies have demonstrated 100% sensitivity and specificity for tracheal placement.[64] In marked contrast, the use of clinical signs for verification has been shown to be unreliable. Fogging or condensation of the tube occurs in 80% of esophageal tubes,[65] chest wall movement can be produced by tracheal or esophageal tubes,[66] and anesthesiologists under ideal operating room conditions, using breath sounds as the sole means of verification, incorrectly identified tube location in 16% of cases.[67]

Although the accuracy of P_{ETCO_2} in verifying ET tube placement is 100% in patients with spontaneous circulation or low-perfusion states, sensitivity for tracheal placement in cardiac arrest patients ranges from 62% to 100%, depending on the type of CO_2 monitoring used and the duration of the arrest.[64,68] The specificity of capnography for esophageal intubation in patients in cardiac arrest is uncertain because of the small number of esophageal intubations in cardiac arrest studies. When a waveform is present in an intubated patient in cardiac arrest, the ET tube can be assumed to be in the trachea. However, absence of a waveform may result from esophageal intubation or a correctly placed ET tube in a patient with insufficient pulmonary blood flow.

Colorimetric studies have shown variable sensitivity because the exhaled CO_2 concentration can fall below the detection threshold. Therefore, it is particularly important when

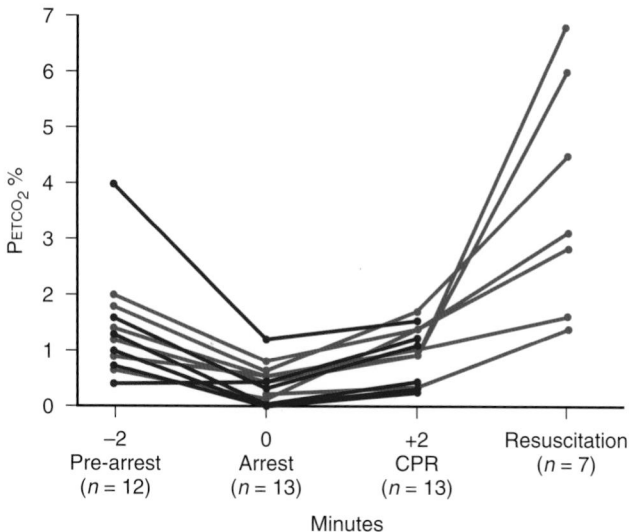

Figure 2-14 End-tidal carbon dioxide concentration (P_{ETCO_2}) pattern during cardiac arrest. *CPR*, cardiopulmonary resuscitation. (*Adapted from Falk JL, Rackow ED, Weil MH. End-tidal carbon dioxide concentration during cardiopulmonary resuscitation.* N Engl J Med. *1988; 318:607.*)

evaluating P_{ETCO_2} studies to distinguish those involving qualitative colorimetric detection from those using capnography.

Monitoring Tube Position during Transport

UMI (as a result of either initial misplacement of the ET tube or subsequent dislodgment during transport) can have catastrophic consequences. However, UMI is largely preventable. Continuous monitoring of tube position during transport (prehospital to hospital, interhospital, or intrahospital) is essential for patient safety. P_{ETCO_2} confirmation of initial ET tube placement with continuous monitoring of tube position is an accepted standard of care by the American Society of Anesthesiologists and is recommended by other national organizations as well.[69] In 2005, Silvestri and coworkers[70] studied the impact of continuous P_{ETCO_2} monitoring on the UMI rate and found a 23% UMI rate in the group that did not use continuous P_{ETCO_2} monitoring and a 0% UMI rate in the group that did.

Gauging the Effectiveness of Cardiopulmonary Resuscitation

In the 1980s, studies in animal models demonstrated that P_{ETCO_2} levels reflect cardiac output during cardiopulmonary resuscitation (CPR) and can be used as a noninvasive measure of cardiac output. A landmark study in 1988 demonstrated this principle in humans (Fig. 2-14).[71] During cardiac arrest, when alveolar ventilation and metabolism are essentially constant, P_{ETCO_2} reflects the degree of pulmonary blood flow. Therefore, P_{ETCO_2} can be used as a gauge of the effectiveness of cardiac compressions. Effective cardiac compression leads to higher cardiac output, and the resultant increase in perfusion corresponds to a rise in P_{ETCO_2} from baseline. Additional prehospital- and intensive care-based studies found P_{ETCO_2} levels lower than 3 mm Hg at the onset of cardiac arrest, with higher levels being generated during cardiac compressions and a mean peak greater than 7.5 mm Hg occurring ust before return of spontaneous circulation (ROSC).[71,72]

Indicator of ROSC

A peak in P_{ETCO_2} is the earliest sign of ROSC and may occur before palpable or measurable hemodynamic signs (pulse or blood pressure).[71] When the heart is restarted, the dramatic increase in cardiac output and the resulting increase in perfusion lead to a rapid increase in P_{ETCO_2} from baseline as the CO_2 that has built up in the blood during cardiac arrest is effectively transported to the lungs and exhaled.

The AHA guidelines emphasize the importance of continuing chest compressions without interruption until a perfusing rhythm is reestablished. Experimental evidence indicates that interruptions in chest compressions are followed by sustained periods during which flow gradually returns to pre-interruption levels. Capnographic monitoring virtually eliminates the need to "stop pumping" for the purpose of checking for pulses. Reestablishment of a perfusing rhythm will be immediately accompanied by a dramatic increase in P_{ETCO_2}, at which point chest compressions can safely be stopped while ECG rhythm and blood pressure are reassessed.[64]

The 2010 AHA guidelines further emphasize the importance of capnography for both verification of ET tube placement (class I) and management of cardiac arrest (monitoring CPR quality class IIb, indicating ROSC class IIa).[73]

Assessing Prognosis after Initiation of Cardiac Arrest Resuscitation

P_{ETCO_2} can be used as a prognostic indicator of survival in adult cardiac arrest patients. In multiple studies, P_{ETCO_2} levels of 10 mm Hg or lower measured 20 minutes after the initiation of advanced cardiac life support accurately predicted death in patients with cardiac arrest. This prognostic value of measuring P_{ETCO_2} has been demonstrated in both animal and human studies.

Identifying the Cause of Cardiac Arrest

Though not generally used clinically, P_{ETCO_2} may be useful in determining the cause of the cardiac arrest. Animal studies reported higher P_{ETCO_2} values at the onset of cardiac arrest caused by primary asphyxia than after arrest caused by ventricular fibrillation. A prehospital cardiac arrest study found similar results: higher P_{ETCO_2} was reported for the asphyxia group (initial rhythm of asystole or pulseless electrical activity secondary to conditions such as a foreign body in the airway, aspiration, asthma, or drowning) than for the ventricular tachycardia/fibrillation group (initial rhythm of ventricular tachycardia/fibrillation associated with acute myocardial infarction).

Titrating E_TCO_2 in Patients with Suspected Increased Intracranial Pressure

P_{ETCO_2} monitoring has been shown to play a role in controlled ventilation in patients with head injury and suspected increased intracranial pressure. CO_2 levels affect blood flow to the brain, with high CO_2 levels resulting in cerebral vasodilation and low CO_2 levels resulting in cerebral vasoconstriction. Sustained hypoventilation (P_{ETCO_2} ≥ 50 mm Hg) is detrimental to patients with increased intracranial pressure because it results in increased cerebral blood flow and potential worsening of intracranial pressure.

Sustained hyperventilation is also detrimental and associated with worse neurologic outcome in severely brain-injured patients. Consequently, unless a patient is actively herniating, ventilation with CO_2 monitoring to achieve normocapnia is recommended.[74,75] The benefit of $P_{ET}CO_2$ monitoring for this indication has been demonstrated in two prehospital-based studies. Severely head-injury patients monitored with continuous $P_{ET}CO_2$ had a lower incidence of inadvertent hyperventilation than did those without $P_{ET}CO_2$ monitoring and were more likely to arrive at the ED appropriately ventilated.[76,77]

$P_{ET}CO_2$ monitoring has also demonstrated prognostic value in determining outcome in trauma victims. In a study of blunt trauma patients requiring prehospital intubation, $P_{ET}CO_2$ levels were able to distinguish survival from nonsurvival groups.[78]

Indications for Capnography in Spontaneously Breathing Patients

In spontaneously breathing, nonintubated patients, capnography can be used for

- Rapid assessment of critically ill, injured, or seizing patients through assessment of the airway, breathing, and circulation (ABCs)
- Assessment and triage of victims of chemical terrorism and mass casualty
- Gauging the severity and response to treatment in patients with acute respiratory distress
- Determining the adequacy of ventilation in patients with altered mental status
- Detecting metabolic acidosis in diabetic patients and children with gastroenteritis

Assessment of Critically Ill, Injured, or Seizing Patients

The ABCs of critically ill or injured patients can be assessed rapidly by using the capnogram and $P_{ET}CO_2$. The presence of a normal waveform denotes a patent airway and spontaneous breathing.[79] Normal $P_{ET}CO_2$ (35 to 45 mm Hg) signifies adequate perfusion.[71,80]

Capnography can be used to assess and triage critically ill or injured patients and actively seizing patients.[81] Unlike pulse oximetry, capnography is not affected by motion artifact and provides reliable readings in low-perfusion states.

Capnography is a reliable, accurate monitoring modality for actively seizing patients. Capnographic data (respiratory rate [RR], $P_{ET}CO_2$, and capnogram) can be used to distinguish among

- Seizing patients with apnea (flatline waveform, no $P_{ET}CO_2$ readings, and no chest wall movement)
- Seizing patients with ineffective ventilation (small waveforms, low $P_{ET}CO_2$)
- Seizing patients with effective ventilation (normal waveform, normal $P_{ET}CO_2$)

Assessment and Triage of Victims of Chemical Terrorism and Mass Casualty

EDs and EMS systems have focused on training to identify and effectively manage mass casualty and chemical terrorism events. Capnography can serve as a noninvasive assessment tool to quickly identify the common life-threatening complications of chemical terrorism.[82] It can rapidly detect the common airway, respiratory, and central nervous system adverse events associated with nerve agents, including apnea, upper airway obstruction, laryngospasm, bronchospasm, respiratory failure, seizures, and coma (Table 2-5).

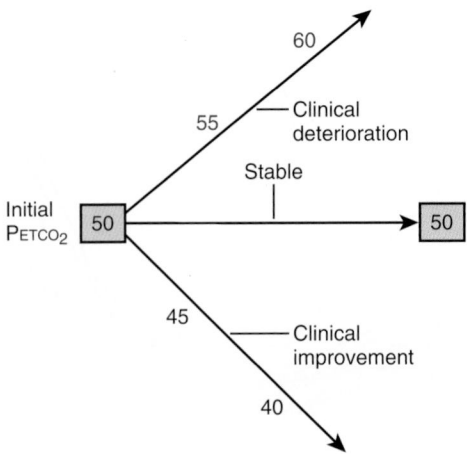

Figure 2-15 $P_{ET}CO_2$ trending in patients with acute respiratory distress. The dynamic ventilatory information provided by $P_{ET}CO_2$ trends can be used to gauge response to treatment in patients with acute respiratory distress. Trends show worsening despite treatment (increasing $P_{ET}CO_2$), stabilized (stable $P_{ET}CO_2$) ventilatory status, or improving (decreasing $P_{ET}CO_2$) ventilatory status.

 Table 2-5 Capnographic Identification of Life-Threatening Complications of Nerve Agents
CAN BE FOUND ON EXPERT CONSULT

Gauging Severity and Response to Treatment of Patients in Acute Respiratory Distress

Capnography provides dynamic monitoring of ventilatory status in patients with acute respiratory distress from any cause, including asthma, bronchiolitis, COPD, CHF, croup, and cystic fibrosis. By measuring $P_{ET}CO_2$ and RR with each breath, capnography provides immediate information on the clinical status of the patient. RR is measured directly from the airway (nose and mouth) with an oral-nasal cannula and provides a more reliable reading than does impedance respiratory monitoring. In upper airway obstruction and laryngospasm, impedance monitoring detects chest wall movement, interprets this as valid breathing, and displays an RR even though the patient is not ventilating. In contrast, capnography will detect absence of air movement and therefore shows a flatline waveform.

$P_{ET}CO_2$ trends can be assessed rapidly, especially in tachypneic patients. For example, a patient with an RR of 30 breaths/min will generate 150 $P_{ET}CO_2$ readings in 5 minutes. This provides sufficient information to determine whether the patient's ventilation is worsening despite treatment (increasing $P_{ET}CO_2$), stabilizing (stable $P_{ET}CO_2$), or improving (decreasing $P_{ET}CO_2$) (Fig. 2-15).

Procedural Sedation and Analgesia

Pulse oximetry is the standard technique for monitoring procedural sedation in the ED, but capnography can also detect the common adverse airway and respiratory events associated with procedural sedation and analgesia.[83] Capnography is the earliest indicator of airway or respiratory compromise and will show an abnormally high or low $P_{ET}CO_2$ well before pulse oximetry detects a falling oxyhemoglobin saturation, especially in patients receiving supplemental oxygen (Fig. 2-16). In addition, as discussed earlier, capnography provides a non–impedance-based RR directly from the airway, which is more accurate than impedance-based respiratory monitoring, especially in patients with obstructive apnea or laryngospasm.

Figure 2-16 Capnographic detection of apnea.

Figure 2-17 P_{ETCO_2}-HCO_3 correlation in patients with diabetes. *(From Fearon DM, Steele DW. End-tidal carbon dioxide predicts the presence and severity of acidosis in children with diabetes.* Acad Emerg Med. *2002;9:1373.)*

Both central and obstructive apnea can be detected almost instantaneously by capnography (Table 2-6). Loss of the capnogram, in conjunction with no chest wall movement and no breath sounds on auscultation, confirms the diagnosis of central apnea. Obstructive apnea is characterized by loss of the capnogram with continued chest wall movement but absent breath sounds. Response to airway alignment maneuvers can further distinguish upper airway obstruction from laryngospasm.

Capnography may be more sensitive than clinical assessment of ventilation in detecting apnea. In one study, 10 of 39 patients (26%) experienced 20-second periods of apnea during procedural sedation and analgesia. All 10 episodes of apnea were detected by capnography but not by the anesthesia providers.[84]

Because the amplitude of the capnogram is determined by P_{ETCO_2} and the width is determined by the expiratory time, changes in either of these parameters affect the shape of the capnogram. Hyperventilation (increased RR, decreased P_{ETCO_2}) results in a low-amplitude and narrow capnogram, whereas classic hypoventilation (decreased RR, increased P_{ETCO_2}) results in a high-amplitude and wide capnogram (see Table 2-6). Acute bronchospasm results in a capnogram with a curved ascending phase and an up-sloping alveolar plateau (see Fig. 2-13). A P_{ETCO_2} reading higher than 70 mm Hg in patients without chronic ventilation problems indicates respiratory failure.

Two types of drug-induced hypoventilation occur during procedural sedation and analgesia (see Table 2-6).[83] Bradypneic hypoventilation (type 1), commonly seen with opioids, is characterized by increased P_{ETCO_2} and increased $Paco_2$. RR is depressed proportionally greater than tidal volume, which results in bradypnea, an increase in expiratory time, and a rise in P_{ETCO_2}, graphically represented by a high-amplitude, wide capnogram (see Table 2-6).

Bradypneic hypoventilation follows a predictable course, with P_{ETCO_2} increasing progressively until respiratory failure and apnea occur. Although there is no absolute threshold at which apnea occurs, patients with acute increases in P_{ETCO_2} to above 80 mm Hg are at significant risk.

Hypopneic hypoventilation (type 2), commonly seen with sedative-hypnotic drugs, is characterized by normal or decreased P_{ETCO_2} but increased $Paco_2$ because airway dead space remains constant (e.g., 150 mL in the normal adult lung) and tidal volume decreases. Tidal volume is depressed proportionally greater than RR, thereby resulting in low-tidal volume breathing and leading to an increase in the fraction of airway dead space (dead space volume/tidal volume). As tidal volume decreases, the airway dead space fraction increases, which in turn results in an increase in the $Paco_2$-P_{ETCO_2} gradient. Even though $Paco_2$ is increasing, P_{ETCO_2}

may remain normal or be decreasing, graphically represented by a low-amplitude capnogram.

Hypopneic hypoventilation follows a variable course. Three possibilities exist: (1) ventilation may remain stable with the low–tidal volume breathing resolving over time as drug levels in the central nervous system decrease following redistribution, (2) hypoventilation may progress to periodic breathing with intermittent apneic pauses (which may resolve spontaneously or progress to central apnea), or (3) hypoventilation may progress directly to central apnea.

The low–tidal volume breathing that characterizes hypopneic hypoventilation increases dead space ventilation as a result of inhibition of the normal compensatory mechanisms by drug effects. Minute ventilation, which normally increases to compensate for an increase in dead space, does not change or may decrease. As minute ventilation decreases, arterial oxygenation decreases. However, P_{ETCO_2} may initially be high (bradypneic hypoventilation) or low (hypopneic hypoventilation) without significant changes in oxygenation, particularly if supplemental oxygen is given. Therefore, a drug-induced increase or decrease in P_{ETCO_2} does not necessarily lead to oxygen desaturation and may not require intervention.

Determining the Adequacy of Ventilation in Patients with Altered Mental Status

Patients with altered mental status, including those with alcohol intoxication or intentional or unintentional drug overdose and postictal patients (especially those treated with benzodiazepines), may have impaired ventilatory function. Capnography can differentiate between patients with effective ventilation and those with ineffective ventilation, as well as provide continuous monitoring of ventilatory trends over time to identify patients at risk for worsening respiratory depression.

Detection of Metabolic Acidosis

In addition to its established uses for assessment of ventilation and perfusion, capnography is a valuable tool for assessing metabolic status by providing information on how effectively CO_2 is being produced by cellular metabolism.

Recent studies have shown that P_{ETCO_2} and serum bicarbonate (HCO_3) are well correlated in patients with diabetes and gastroenteritis. P_{ETCO_2} can be used as an indicator of metabolic acidosis in these patients (Fig. 2-17).[85-87] As the

TABLE 2-6 Capnographic Airway Assessment for Procedural Sedation and Analgesia

DIAGNOSIS	WAVEFORM	FEATURES		INTERVENTION
Normal	[CO2] 40 / 0 — Time	SpO2 PETCO2 Waveform RR	Normal Normal Normal Normal	No intervention required Continue sedation
Hyperventilation	[CO2] 40 / 0 — Time	SpO2 PETCO2 Waveform RR	Normal → Decreased amplitude and width ↑	Reassess patient Continue sedation
Bradypneic hypoventilation (type 1)	[CO2] 40 / 0 — Time	SpO2 PETCO2 Waveform RR	Normal ↑ Increased amplitude and width ↓↓	Reassess patient Continue sedation
		SpO2 PETCO2 Waveform RR	→ ↓ ↑ Increased amplitude and width ↓↓↓	Reassess patient Assess for airway obstruction Supplemental oxygen Cease drug administration or reduce dosing
Hypopneic hypoventilation (type 2)	[CO2] 40 / 0 — Time	SpO2 PETCO2 Waveform RR	Normal ↓ Decreased amplitude →	Reassess patient Continue sedation
		SpO2 PETCO2 Waveform RR	→ ↓ ↓ Decreased amplitude →	Reassess patient Assess for airway obstruction
Hypopneic hypoventilation with periodic breathing	[CO2] 40 / 0 — Time	SpO2 PETCO2 Waveform RR Other	Normal or ↓ ↓ Decreased amplitude → Apneic pauses	Reassess patient Assess for airway obstruction Supplemental oxygen Cease drug administration or reduce dosing
Physiologic variability	(waveform)	SpO2 PETCO2 Waveform RR	Normal Normal Varying* Normal	No intervention required Continue sedation

Condition	Waveform	Parameter	Finding	Response
Bronchospasm		Spo₂: Normal or ↓ Petco₂: Normal, ↑, or ↓† Waveform: Curved RR: Normal, ↑, or ↓† Other: Wheezing		Reassess patient Bronchodilator therapy Cease drug administration
Partial airway obstruction		Spo₂: Normal or ↓ Petco₂: Normal Waveform: Normal RR: Variable Other: Noisy breathing and/or inspiratory stridor	Full airway patency restored with airway alignment / Noisy breathing and stridor resolve	Reassess patient Establish IV access Supplemental O₂ (as needed) Cease drug administration
Partial laryngospasm			Airway not fully patent with airway alignment / Noisy breathing and stridor persist	
Apnea		Spo₂: Normal or ↓‡ Petco₂: Zero Waveform: Absent RR: Zero Other: No chest wall movement or breath sounds		Reassess patient Stimulation Bag-mask ventilation Reversal agents (as appropriate) Cease drug administration
Complete airway obstruction		Spo₂: Normal or ↓‡ Petco₂: Zero Waveform: Absent RR: Zero Other: Chest wall movement and breath sounds present	Airway patency restored with airway alignment Waveform present	
Complete laryngospasm			Airway not patent with airway alignment / No waveform	Positive pressure ventilation

Petco₂, end-tidal carbon dioxide pressure; RR, respiratory rate; Spo₂, oxygen saturation as measured by pulse oximetry.
*Varying waveform amplitude and width.
†Depending on the duration and severity of bronchospasm.
‡Depending on the duration of the episode.

patient becomes acidotic (i.e., HCO_3 decreases), a compensatory respiratory alkalosis develops with an increase in minute ventilation and a resultant decrease in $PETCO_2$. By increasing minute ventilation, these patients are able to lower arterial CO_2 tension to help correct the underlying acidemia. The more acidotic, the lower the HCO_3, the higher the RR, and the lower the $PETCO_2$.

$PETCO_2$ can be used to distinguish diabetics in ketoacidosis (metabolic acidosis, compensatory tachypnea, low $PETCO_2$) from those who are not (nonacidotic, normal RR, normal $PETCO_2$). In a study of diabetic children encountered in the ED, a $PETCO_2$ reading of less than 29 mm Hg identified 95% of the patients with ketoacidosis with 83% sensitivity and 100% specificity. Conversely, no ketoacidosis was detected in patients with $PETCO_2$ greater than 36 mm Hg.[85]

A similar association between $PETCO_2$ and HCO_3 was demonstrated in children with gastroenteritis, with maximal sensitivity occurring at a $PETCO_2$ of 34 mm Hg or lower (sensitivity of 100%, specificity of 60%) and optimal specificity without compromise of sensitivity occurring at a $PETCO_2$ of 31 mm Hg or lower (sensitivity of 76%, specificity of 96%).[87]

As a potential triage tool to determine the need for oral versus intravenous rehydration, a $PETCO_2$ reading of 31 mm Hg or lower can identify patients with clinically significant acidosis, with a positive likelihood ratio (LR) of 20.4 for detecting an HCO_3 level of 15 mmol/L or less and an LR of 14.1 for detecting an HCO_3 level of 13 mmol/L or less.

Limitations

Significant technical problems have historically restricted the effective clinical use of capnography. Such problems include interference with the sensor by condensed water and patient secretions in both mainstream and high-flow sidestream devices, cross-sensitivity with anesthetic gases in conventional CO_2 sensors, lack of ruggedness for intrahospital and interhospital transport, and power consumption issues related to portable battery operation time. These issues have largely been resolved in the newer-generation capnography monitors.

Problems with accuracy continue to affect high-flow sidestream systems. When the tidal volume of the patient drops below the flow rate of the system (e.g., neonates, infants, hypoventilating patients with low–tidal volume breathing), the monitor will entrain room air, thereby falsely diluting $PETCO_2$ and slurring the ascending phase of the waveform.[88-90]

Early capnography airway interfaces (i.e., nasal cannula) had difficulty providing consistent measurements in mouth-breathing patients and those who alternated between mouth and nose breathing. The newer oral-nasal interface has addressed these problems.

Capnography is most effective when assessing a pure ventilation, perfusion, or metabolism problem. Capnographic findings in patients with mixed ventilation, perfusion, or metabolism problems are difficult to interpret. For example, in patients with complex pathophysiology, a ventilation problem may elevate $PETCO_2$, whereas a perfusion problem may simultaneously lower $PETCO_2$. Absolute values and even trends over time may be difficult to interpret in these situations.

Although capnography in patients in cardiac arrest is 100% specific for tracheal placement of the ET tube, its sensitivity for esophageal placement is uncertain.

CONCLUSION

Capnography is a versatile noninvasive diagnostic modality for monitoring ventilation, perfusion, and metabolic status in both intubated and nonintubated patients. Clinical applications include verification and continuous monitoring of ET tube placement; determination of the efficacy of CPR in cardiac arrest; ventilatory monitoring of head-injured patients; assessment of vital signs in patients who are critically ill, injured, or seizing or have altered mental status; evaluation of patients in acute respiratory distress; and detection of metabolic acidosis.

Suggested Readings

Pulse Oximetry

McMorrow RC, Mythen MG. Pulse oximetry. *Curr Opin Crit Care.* 2006;12:269.

New W. Pulse oximetry. *J Clin Monit.* 1985;1:126.

Sinex JE. Pulse oximetry: principles and limitations. *Am J Emerg Med.* 1999;17:59.

The Technology Assessment Task Force of the Society of Critical Care Medicine. A model for technology assessment applied to pulse oximetry. *Crit Care Med.* 1993;21:615.

Witting MD, Lueck CH. The ability of pulse oximetry to screen for hypoxemia and hypercapnia in patients breathing room air. *J Emerg Med.* 2001;20:341.

CO_2 Monitoring

Falk JL, Rackow EC, Weil MH. End-tidal carbon dioxide concentration during cardiopulmonary resuscitation. *N Engl J Med.* 1988;318:607.

Krauss B. Capnography as a rapid assessment and triage tool for chemical terrorism. *Pediatr Emerg Med.* 2005;21:493.

Krauss B, Deykin A, Lam A, et al. Capnogram shape in obstructive lung disease. *Anesth Analg.* 2005;100:884.

Krauss B, Hess DR. Capnography for procedural sedation and analgesia in the emergency department. *Ann Emerg Med.* 2007;50:172.

Silvestri S, Ralls GA, Krauss B, et al. The effectiveness of out-of-hospital use of continuous end-tidal carbon dioxide monitoring on the rate of unrecognized misplaced intubation within a regional emergency medical services system. *Ann Emerg Med.* 2005;45:497.

(**References are available at www.expertconsult.com**)

Respiratory Procedures

CHAPTER 3

Basic Airway Management and Decision Making

Robert F. Reardon, Phillip E. Mason, and Joseph E. Clinton

Basic airway procedures are often overlooked in favor of more exciting intubation devices and techniques, but basic procedures are critically important and often lifesaving. Establishment of a patent airway, oxygenation, and bag-mask ventilation (BMV) remain the cornerstones of good emergency airway management.[1,2] These techniques can be used quickly and in any setting. They allow practitioners to *keep apneic patients alive until a definitive airway can be established*.[3]

Extraglottic devices, such as laryngeal mask airways (LMAs) and the King Laryngeal Tube (LT), have also become important for the initial resuscitation of apneic patients and for rescue ventilation when intubation fails.[4-6] Another commonly used device is the esophageal-tracheal Combitube, which will be discussed and compared with the King LT. Noninvasive positive pressure ventilation (NPPV) is widely available in both prehospital and emergency department (ED) settings and can be used to optimize oxygenation before intubation or to avoid intubation in carefully selected patients.[7,8]

This chapter describes basic airway skills, including opening the airway, O_2 therapy, BMV, and extraglottic airway (EGA) devices. These are the skills that providers can rely on when other airway techniques are difficult or impossible. Mastery of these skills and use of an airway algorithm help providers manage difficult, anxiety-provoking emergency airways.

Pulse oximetry (SpO_2) has greatly improved our ability to monitor the oxygenation of patients at risk for airway or ventilatory compromise.[9] These monitors are accurate under most conditions[10] and allow clinically subtle deterioration to be recognized quickly (see Chapter 2). SpO_2 monitors are standard equipment in all emergency airway settings. The use of waveform capnography in the emergency setting is rapidly increasing but is not yet universally available or applied. This trend should be encouraged because capnography can improve patient safety by rapidly detecting hypoventilation, impending airway obstruction, and risk for apnea before these conditions occur.[11]

THE CHALLENGE OF EMERGENCY AIRWAY MANAGEMENT

Although other specialists are sometimes available, most emergency airways are managed by emergency medicine providers.[12] Airway management in the ED is quite unique and much different from airway management in the controlled setting of an operating room. Likewise, conventional airway management tools may be ineffective in the uncontrolled emergency environment. Major challenges include an incomplete historical database, hypoxia, shock, full stomach, and the presence of vomit, blood, or excessive secretions in the airway. Many patients are uncooperative and combative, thus making it impossible to properly examine their airway before choosing an intubation technique. Medical history, allergies, and even the current diagnosis are often unknown before emergency airway management begins. Time constraints, lack of patient cooperation, and risk for vomiting limit the use of some techniques, such as awake intubation. In trauma patients, the risk for cervical spine injury limits optimal head and neck positioning for BMV and laryngoscopy. All these factors increase the risk for complications from emergency airway management,[12,13] and about 1% of all emergency airways require a surgical approach.[14] The popularity of video laryngoscopy and other video airway devices may further reduce the incidence of emergency surgical airways.

BASIC AIRWAY MANAGEMENT TECHNIQUES
Opening the Airway

The first concern in the management of a critically ill patient is *patency of the airway*. Upper airway obstruction most commonly occurs when patients are unconscious or sedated. It can also be due to injury to the mandible or muscles that support the hypopharynx. In these situations, the tongue moves posteriorly into the upper airway when the patient is in a supine position (Fig. 3-1*A*). Upper airway obstruction caused by the tongue can be relieved by positioning maneuvers of the head, neck, and jaw; the use of nasopharyngeal or oropharyngeal airways; or the application of continuous positive airway pressure (CPAP).

Manual Airway Maneuvers

Airway obstruction in unconscious patients may be due to posterior displacement of the tongue, but research in patients with obstructive sleep apnea using CPAP supports the concept that the airway collapses like a flexible tube.[3,15] Upper airway

MANUAL AIRWAY MANEUVERS

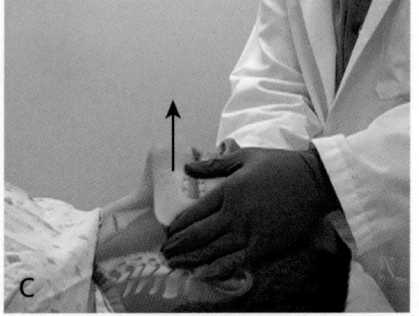

Figure 3-1 Manual airway maneuvers. **A,** The most common cause of airway obstruction in an unconscious patient is the tongue. Initial maneuvers for opening the airway include head tilt/chin lift (**B**) and jaw thrust (**C**).

obstruction may cause obvious snoring or stridor, but it may be difficult to appreciate in some patients. All unconscious patients are at high risk for upper airway obstruction.

More than 35 years ago, Guildner[16] compared different techniques for opening obstructed upper airways and found that the head-tilt/chin-lift and jaw-thrust techniques were both effective (Fig. 3-1B and C). Modern airway textbooks still describe the head-tilt/chin-lift and jaw-thrust maneuvers but also use the term "triple airway maneuver," which is a combination of head tilt, jaw thrust, and mouth opening.[3,17] Many airway experts believe that the jaw-thrust maneuver (anterior mandibular translation to bring the lower incisors anterior to the upper incisors) is the most important technique for opening the upper airway (Fig. 3-1C).[3,18,19]

It is widely accepted that the jaw-thrust-only (without head tilt) maneuver should be performed in patients with suspected cervical spine injury,[17] but there is no evidence that it is safer than the head-tilt/chin-lift maneuver.[20] In 2005, the American Heart Association (AHA)[21] concluded that airway maneuvers are safe during manual in-line stabilization of the cervical spine but highlighted evidence that all airway maneuvers cause some spinal movement. Both the chin-lift and the jaw-thrust maneuvers have been shown to cause similar substantial movement of the cervical vertebrae.[22-26] The AHA recommended that "in a victim with a suspected spinal injury and an obstructed airway, the head-tilt/chin-lift or jaw-thrust (with head-tilt) techniques are feasible and may be effective for clearing the airway" and emphasized that "maintaining an airway and adequate ventilation is the over-riding priority in managing a patient with a suspected spinal injury."[21]

Importantly, the addition of CPAP may relieve airway obstruction when simple manual positioning maneuvers fail. Meier and colleagues[15] showed that adding CPAP to the chin-lift and jaw-thrust maneuvers decreased stridor and improved the nasal fiberoptic view of the glottic opening in anesthetized children.

The Head-Tilt/Chin-Lift Maneuver

To perform the head-tilt/chin-lift maneuver, place the tips of the index and middle fingers beneath the patient's chin (Fig. 3-1B). Lift the chin cephalad and toward the ceiling. The upper part of the neck will naturally extend when the head tilts backward during this maneuver. Apply digital pressure on only the bony prominence of the chin and not on the soft

tissues of the submandibular region. The final step in this maneuver is to use the thumb to open the patient's mouth while the head is tilted and the neck is extended.

The Jaw-Thrust Maneuver

To perform the jaw-thrust maneuver, place the tips of the middle or index fingers behind the angle of the mandible (Fig. 3-1C). Lift the mandible toward the ceiling until the lower incisors are anterior to the upper incisors. This maneuver can be performed in combination with the head-tilt/chin-lift maneuver or with the neck in the neutral position during in-line stabilization.

The Triple Airway Maneuver

The "triple airway maneuver" is described by many authors as the best manual method for maintaining a patent upper airway.[3,17] The most common description of this maneuver is head tilt, jaw thrust, and mouth opening.[3,17] Other authors describe the triple maneuver differently—as a combination of upper cervical extension (head tilt), lower cervical flexion, and jaw protrusion (jaw lift).[19] The triple airway maneuver has been described as a technique for providers with advanced airway skills.[17] No studies exist to support the assertion that this technique is more effective than the head-tilt/chin-lift or jaw-thrust maneuvers, but the triple maneuver is commonly mentioned in the anesthesia literature as a valuable technique.

Patient Positioning

The best way to position a patient's head and neck for opening the upper airway is to mimic how patients position themselves when they are short of breath, with the neck flexed relative to the torso and with atlanto-occipital extension.[2] This is known as the "sniffing position" and was described by Magill almost 100 years ago.[27] In normal-sized supine adults, this is accomplished by elevating the head about 10 cm while tilting the head back so that the plane of the patient's face tilts slightly toward the provider at the head of the bed (see Chapter 4, Fig. 4-8).[2,3,28-30] Morbidly obese patients require much more head elevation to achieve the proper sniffing position. This can be accomplished by building a ramp of towels and pillows under the upper torso, head, and neck or by using a Troop Elevation Pillow (Mercury Medical, Clearwater, FL)

Figure 3-2 The best position for opening the upper airway in morbidly obese patients is elevation of the head, neck, and shoulders so that the external auditory meatus is aligned with the sternum. The Troop Elevation Pillow (Mercury Medical, Clearwater, FL) is shown here; however, similar results may be achieved with other devices or a ramp of towels and pillows. *Note:* The device is demonstrated here on a nonobese patient.

or similar device (Fig. 3-2).[31-34] Horizontal alignment of the external auditory meatus with the sternum is the best position for opening the upper airway in morbidly obese patients.[33-36]

The sniffing position is contraindicated in patients with cervical spine injuries. The best technique for opening the airway in this situation is a simple jaw-thrust maneuver with anterior mandibular translation to bring the lower incisors anterior to the upper incisors (Fig. 3-1*C*).[3,18,19]

In young children, this position is often achieved without lifting the head because the occiput of a child is relatively large, so the lower cervical spine is normally flexed when the child is lying supine on a flat surface.

Airway management is usually easiest when patients are in the supine position, but the lateral position may be best for patients who are actively vomiting and those with excessive upper airway bleeding or secretions. Some evidence suggests that rotating patients to the lateral position may not prevent aspiration.[37] Patients with suspected cervical spine injury should have their head immobilized with in-line stabilization if they need to be rolled to the lateral position. Airway management maneuvers may be limited or difficult when patients are in the lateral position.

Foreign Body Airway Obstruction

Awake patients with partial airway obstruction can usually clear a foreign body on their own. Intervention is required when the patient is not moving air or has altered mental status. Some patients with upper airway obstruction can be ventilated and oxygenated with aggressive high-pressure BMV, so always try this if standard BMV fails. Massive aspiration of vomitus, however, is often a fatal event because of inability of the patient and clinician to adequately clear the airway.

Abdominal Thrusts (Heimlich Maneuver), Chest Thrusts, and Back Blows (Slaps)

The 2010 International Consensus Conference on Cardiopulmonary Resuscitation and Emergency Cardiopulmonary

Care[4] evaluated the evidence for different techniques to clear foreign body airway obstruction. They found good evidence for the use of chest thrusts, abdominal thrusts, and back blows or slaps. Insufficient evidence exists to determine which technique is the best and which should be used first. Some evidence indicates that chest thrusts may generate higher peak airway pressure than the Heimlich maneuver does.

The technique of subdiaphragmatic abdominal thrusts to relieve a completely obstructed airway was popularized by Dr. Henry Heimlich and is commonly referred to as the "Heimlich maneuver."[38] The technique is most effective when a solid food bolus is obstructing the larynx. In a conscious patient, stand behind the upright patient. Circle the arms around the patient's midsection with the radial side of a clenched fist placed on the abdomen, midway between the umbilicus and xiphoid. Then grasp the fist with the opposite hand and deliver an inward and upward thrust to the abdomen (Fig. 3-3*A*). A successful maneuver will cause the obstructing agent to be expelled from the patient's airway by the force of air exiting the lungs. Abdominal thrusts are relatively contraindicated in pregnant patients and those with protuberant abdomens. Potential risks associated with abdominal thrusts include stomach rupture, esophageal perforation, and mesenteric laceration, thus compelling the rescuer to weigh the risks and benefits of this maneuver.[39-44] Use a chest position for pregnant patients (Fig. 3-3*B*).

If a choking patient loses consciousness, use chest compressions in an attempt to expel the obstructing agent (Fig. 3-3*C*).[4] The theory is the same as the Heimlich maneuver, with high intrathoracic pressure created to push the obstruction out of the airway. Some data suggest that chest compressions may generate higher peak airway pressure than the Heimlich maneuver.[45] After 30 seconds of chest compressions, remove the obstructing object if you see it, attempt 2 breaths, and then continue cardiopulmonary resuscitation (CPR; 30 compressions to 2 breaths). Every time you open the airway to give breaths, look for the object and remove it if possible, and then continue CPR if necessary.

Back blows are recommended for infants and small children with a foreign body obstructing the airway. Some authors have argued that back blows may be dangerous and may drive foreign bodies deeper into the airway, but there is no convincing evidence of this phenomenon.[46,47] As with the other techniques, anecdotal evidence suggests that back blows are effective.[48-50] No convincing data, however, indicate that back blows are more or less effective than abdominal or chest thrusts. Back blows may produce a more pronounced increase in airway pressure, but over a shorter period than with the other techniques. The AHA guidelines suggest back blows in the head-down position (Fig. 3-3*D*) and head-down chest thrusts in infants and small children with foreign body airway obstruction (Fig. 3-3*E*).[4] The AHA does not recommend abdominal thrusts in infants because they may be at higher risk for iatrogenic injury. From a practical standpoint, back blows should be delivered with the patient in a head-down position, which is more easily accomplished in infants than in larger children.

Any patient with a complete airway obstruction may benefit from chest compressions, abdominal thrusts, or back blows. It is important to realize that more than one technique is often required to clear obstruction of the airway by a foreign body, so multiple techniques should be applied in a rapid sequence until the obstruction is relieved.[21] Perform a finger sweep of the patient's mouth only if a solid object is seen in the airway. It is recommended that suction be performed on newborns rather than giving them back blows or abdominal thrusts.[51]

Perform CPR on all unconscious patients with airway obstruction. Try aggressive high-pressure BMV in this setting. In cases in which obstructive foreign bodies cannot be removed under direct visualization and aggressive positive pressure ventilation has failed, practitioners with advanced airway skills and proper equipment can try to push a subglottic foreign body beyond the carina.

Suctioning

Patient positioning and airway-opening maneuvers are often inadequate to achieve complete airway patency. Ongoing hemorrhage, vomitus, and particulate debris frequently require suctioning. Several types of suctioning tips are available. A large-bore dental-type suction tip is the most effective in clearing vomitus from the upper airway because it is less likely to become obstructed by particulate matter. The tonsil tip (Yankauer) suction device can be used to clear hemorrhage and secretions. Its rounded tip is less traumatic to soft tissues,

but the tonsil tip device is not large enough to effectively suction vomitus.

A large-bore dental-type tip device, such as the HI-D Big Stick suction tip, should be readily available at the bedside during all emergency airway management (Fig. 3-4). The large-bore tip allows rapid clearing of vomitus, blood, and secretions.

A limiting feature of many suction catheters is the diameter of the tubing. Vomitus may obstruct the standard $\frac{1}{4}$-inch-diameter catheter.[52] A $\frac{5}{8}$- or $\frac{3}{4}$-inch-diameter suction tube (Kuriyama Tubing, $\frac{5}{16}$-inch inner diameter, 0.44-inch outer diameter, clear; www.grainger.com) has been shown to significantly decrease suction time for viscous and particulate material (see Fig. 3-4).[53]

Keep suctioning equipment connected and ready to operate. Everyone participating in emergency airway management should know how to use it. Interposition of a suction trap close to the suction device prevents clogging of the tubing with particulate debris. A trap that fits directly onto a tracheal tube has been described, and use of this device allows effective suctioning during intubation.[54]

No specific contraindications to airway suctioning exist. Complications of suctioning may be avoided by anticipating

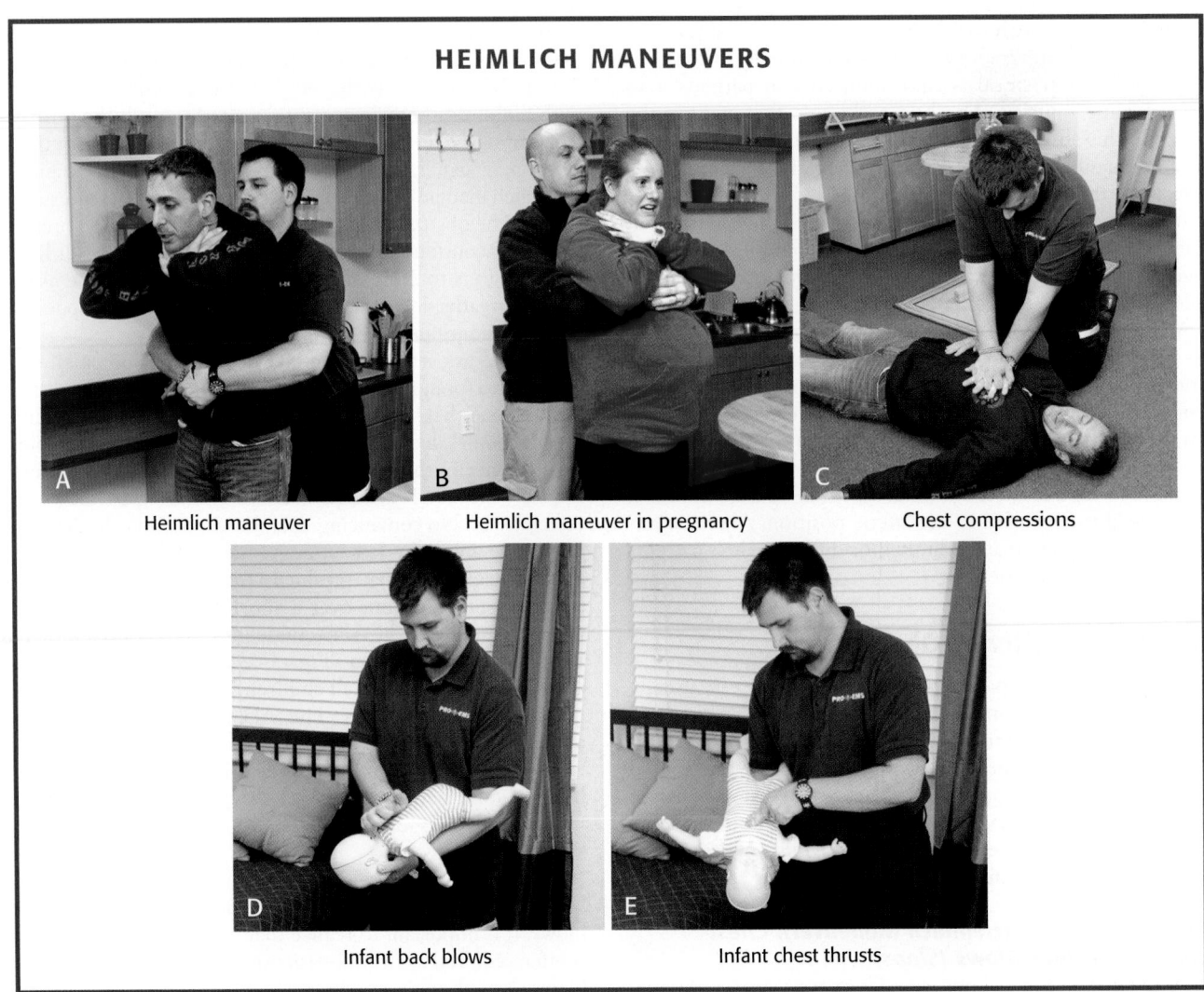

HEIMLICH MANEUVERS

A — Heimlich maneuver

B — Heimlich maneuver in pregnancy

C — Chest compressions

D — Infant back blows

E — Infant chest thrusts

Figure 3-3 A-E, Heimlich maneuvers (see text).

problems and providing appropriate care before and during suctioning maneuvers. Nasal suction is seldom required, except in infants, because most adult airway obstruction occurs in the mouth and oropharynx.

Avoid prolonged suctioning because it may lead to significant hypoxia, especially in children. Do not exceed 15 seconds for suctioning intervals and administer supplemental O_2 before and after suctioning. Naigow and Powasner[55] found that suctioning consistently induced hypoxia in dogs and that it was best avoided by hyperventilation with high-concentration O_2 before and after suctioning.

When feasible, perform suctioning under direct vision or with the aid of the laryngoscope. Forcing a suction tip blindly into the posterior pharynx can injure tissue or convert a partial obstruction to a complete obstruction.

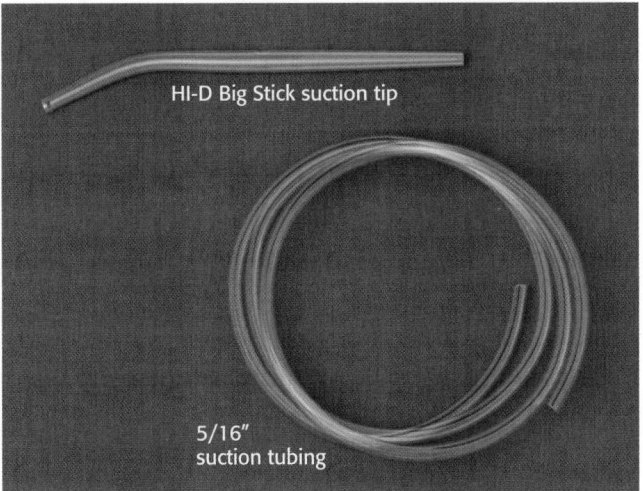

Figure 3-4 HI-D Big Stick suction tip (SSCOR, Inc., Sun Valley, CA) and ⁵⁄₁₆-inch tubing.

Oropharyngeal and Nasopharyngeal Artificial Airways

Indications and Contraindications

Once the airway has been opened with manual maneuvers and suctioning, artificial airways, such as nasopharyngeal and oropharyngeal airways, can facilitate both spontaneous breathing and BMV. In semiconscious patients who require a head-tilt/chin-lift or jaw-thrust maneuver to open their airways, hypoxia may develop because of recurrent obstruction if these maneuvers are discontinued. Oxygen supplementation and a nasopharyngeal airway may be all the support that is necessary to maintain a functional airway.

Patients who are unresponsive or apneic are usually easier to ventilate with a bag-mask device when an oropharyngeal airway is in place. In the ED, patients who tolerate an oropharyngeal airway should probably be intubated.

Artificial Airway Placement

The simplest and most widely available artificial airways are the oropharyngeal and nasopharyngeal airways (Fig. 3-5). Both are intended to prevent the tongue from obstructing the airway by falling back against the posterior pharyngeal wall. The oral airway may also prevent teeth clenching. In cases of severe upper airway edema, such as angioedema caused by an angiotensin-converting enzyme inhibitor, these devices may not function properly or be able to adequately bypass the obstruction. The oropharyngeal airway may be inserted by either of two procedures. One approach is to insert the airway in an inverted position along the patient's hard palate (Fig. 3-5, *step 2*). When it is well into the patient's mouth, rotate the airway 180 degrees and advance it to its final position along the patient's tongue, with the distal end of the artificial airway lying in the hypopharynx (Fig. 3-5, *step 3*). A second approach is to open the mouth widely, use a tongue blade to displace the tongue, and then simply advance the artificial

Oropharyngeal and Nasopharyngeal Airways

Indications
Facilitation of spontaneous breathing and bag-valve-mask ventilation in patients requiring head-tilt/chin-lift or jaw-thrust maneuvers

Contraindications
Nasopharyngeal
Significant facial and basilar skull fractures

Complications
Oropharyngeal
Vomiting (in patients with an intact gag reflex)
Airway obstruction (if the tongue is pushed against the posterior pharyngeal wall during insertion)
Nasopharyngeal
Epistaxis
Deterioration requiring intubation (semiconscious patient)

Equipment

Review Box 3-1 Oropharyngeal and nasopharyngeal airways: indications, contraindications, complications, and equipment.

OROPHARYNGEAL AIRWAY INSERTION

For oropharyngeal airway insertion, first measure. An airway of correct size will extend from the corner of the mouth to the earlobe or the angle of the mandible.

Open the patient's mouth with your thumb and index finger, then insert the airway in an inverted position along the patient's hard palate.

When the airway is well into the mouth, rotate it 180°, with the distal end of the airway lying in the hypopharynx. It may help to pull the jaw forward during passage.

Alternatively, open the mouth widely and use a tongue blade to displace the tongue inferiorly, and advance the airway into the oropharynx. No rotation is required with this method.

NASOPHARYNGEAL AIRWAY INSERTION

For nasopharyngeal airways, a device of correct size will extend from the tip of the nose to the earlobe.

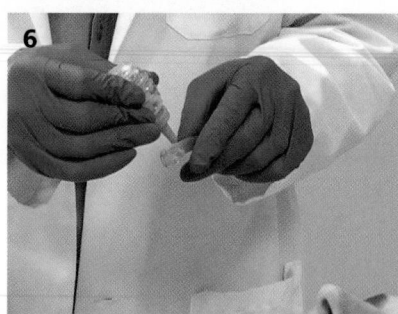

Generously lubricate the airway prior to insertion.

Advance the airway into the nostril and direct it along the floor of the nasal passage in the direction of the occiput. Do *not* advance in a cephalad direction!

Advance the airway fully until the flared external tip of the device is at the nasal orifice.

Figure 3-5 Oropharyngeal and nasopharyngeal airway insertion.

airway into the oropharynx (Fig. 3-5, *step 4*). No rotation is necessary when the airway is placed in this manner. This technique may be less traumatic, but it takes longer.

The nasopharyngeal airway is very easy to place. It may be easiest to place it on the patient's right so that the bevel is facing the septum on insertion. Be sure to lubricate the device before insertion (Fig. 3-5, *step 6*). Some clinicians use a nasopharyngeal airway to dilate the nasal passages for 20 to 30 minutes before nasotracheal intubation. Simply advance it

into the nostril and direct it along the floor of the nasal passage in the direction of the occiput, not cephalad (Fig. 3-5, *step 7*). *Advance it fully until the flared external tip of the airway is located at the nasal orifice* (Fig 3-5, *step 8*).

Both oropharyngeal and nasopharyngeal airways are available in multiple sizes. To find the correct size of either device, estimate its size by measuring along the side of the patient's face before insertion. An oropharyngeal airway of the correct size will extend from the corner of the mouth to the tip of the earlobe (Fig. 3-5, *step 1*); a nasopharyngeal airway of the correct size will extend from the tip of the nose to the tip of the earlobe (Fig. 3-5, *step 5*).

Both oropharyngeal and nasopharyngeal airways provide airway patency similar to that achieved with the head-tilt/chin-lift maneuver. The nasal airway is better tolerated by semiconscious patients and is less likely to induce vomiting in those with an intact gag reflex.

Complications

The nasopharyngeal airway may cause epistaxis and may be dangerous in patients with significant facial and basilar skull fractures. Semiconscious patients with nasopharyngeal airways may deteriorate and require intubation, so they should be monitored closely.

The oropharyngeal airway may induce vomiting when placed in patients with an intact gag reflex. It may also cause airway obstruction if the tongue is pushed against the posterior pharyngeal wall during insertion. The oropharyngeal airway should not be used as a definitive airway.

OXYGEN THERAPY

Adequate O_2 delivery depends on the inspired partial pressure of O_2, alveolar ventilation, pulmonary gas exchange, oxygen-carrying capacity of blood, and cardiac output. The easiest factor to manipulate is the partial pressure of inspired O_2, which is accomplished by increasing the fraction of inspired oxygen (FIO_2) with supplemental O_2.

Indications and Contraindications

Resuscitate all patients in cardiac or respiratory arrest with 100% O_2. The most certain indication for supplemental O_2 is the presence of arterial hypoxemia, defined as a PaO_2 lower than 60 mm Hg or arterial oxygen saturation (SaO_2) less than 90%.[56] Normal subjects will begin to experience memory loss at an arterial oxygen partial pressure (PaO_2) of 45 mm Hg, and loss of consciousness occurs at a PaO_2 of 30 mm Hg.[57-59] Chronically hypoxemic patients can adapt and function with a PaO_2 of 50 mm Hg or lower.[60]

When tissue hypoxia is present or suspected, give O_2 therapy.[56,61] Shock states resulting from hemorrhage, vasodilatory states, low cardiac output, and obstructive lesions can all lead to tissue hypoxia and benefit from supplemental O_2. Whatever the cause of the shock state, administration of O_2 is indicated until the situation can be thoroughly evaluated and cause-specific therapy instituted.

Respiratory distress without documented arterial hypoxemia is a common indication for O_2 administration, although no evidence exists to support this practice.[62] Oxygen therapy is often recommended for acute myocardial infarction, but there is *no difference in outcomes between patients receiving O_2 and those receiving room air after myocardial infarction*. The AHA has given a class I recommendation for O_2 only in patients with hypoxemia, cyanosis, or respiratory distress.[56,61,63-65]

Although O_2 is routinely administered to acute stroke patients, *there is no convincing evidence that this practice is beneficial without documented hypoxia*, and it is not recommended by current guidelines.[66-68] It is reasonable to administer O_2 to hypotensive patients and those with severe trauma until tissue hypoxia can definitively be excluded.[62]

Administer 100% O_2 to patients with carbon monoxide poisoning. The half-life of carboxyhemoglobin is 4 to 5 hours in a subject breathing room air but can be decreased to approximately 1 hour by the administration of 100% O_2 by non-rebreather face mask at atmospheric pressure.[69]

There are no contraindications to O_2 therapy when a definite indication exists. The risks associated with hypoxemia are grave and undeniable. Never withhold oxygen therapy from a hypoxemic patient for fear of complications or clinical deterioration. Carbon dioxide retention is not a contraindication to O_2 therapy. Rather, it demands that the clinician administer O_2 carefully and recognize the potential for respiratory acidosis and clinical deterioration. Although the mechanism for the development of respiratory acidosis in patients with chronic obstructive pulmonary disease (COPD) who are administered O_2 is debated, its occurrence is not.[70,71] Use caution when administering supplemental O_2 to hypoxic patients with arterial carbon dioxide pressure ($PaCO_2$) higher than 40 mm Hg, but do not withhold it.

Oxygen Administration during Cardiac Arrest and Neonatal Resuscitation

The 2010 American Heart Association Guidelines for Cardiopulmonary Resuscitation and Emergency Cardiovascular Care[4] address the potential harm of oxygen therapy and hyperoxemia following cardiac arrest and during neonatal resuscitation. Excerpts from this document are shown in Box 3-1. Although it is still prudent to administer oxygen in the prehospital and ED setting as discussed earlier, additional research may alter current recommendations. See also "Complications of Oxygen Therapy" in this chapter. As a general guideline, fear of oxygen toxicity should not prevent the use of O_2 when there is an indication but should encourage the clinician to use the minimum concentration of O_2 necessary to achieve the therapeutic goals.

Oxygen Delivery Devices

High-flow delivery systems provide an FIO_2 that is relatively constant despite changes in the patient's respiratory pattern. The Venturi mask is the high-flow delivery device that is most widely available (Fig. 3-6). Room air is entrained into the system through entrainment ports and mixes with the O_2 provided from the O_2 source. The proportion of entrained air—and therefore FIO_2—is constant and determined by the velocity of the O_2 jet and the size of the entrainment ports. Because the total gas flow (O_2 plus air through the entrainment ports) meets or exceeds the patient's inspiratory flow rate, no additional entrainment of air occurs around the mask, thereby minimizing changes in FIO_2 as the patient's respiratory pattern changes.[72,73] The mask is continuously flushed by the high flow of gas, which prevents the accumulation of exhaled gas in the mask. Venturi masks are packaged with multiple inserts, each with a different size orifice for O_2 inflow. FIO_2 is determined by selecting the appropriate colored insert and O_2 flow rate according to the manufacturer's instructions. The inspiratory flow rate for a resting adult is about 30 L/min, a rate matched by the total gas flow provided by the Venturi mask at all settings. A patient in respiratory distress may have an inspiratory flow rate of 50 to 100 L/min.[73] If the inspiratory flow rate exceeds the total gas flow delivered by the mask, additional air will be entrained around

BOX 3-1 | **Potential Adverse Effects of Oxygen Administration during Adult and Neonate Resuscitation: Excerpts from the 2010 Guidelines of the American Heart Association**

OVERVIEW OF POST-CARDIAC ARREST CARE AND THE USE OF SUPPLEMENTAL OXYGEN

Although 100% oxygen may have been used during initial resuscitation, providers should titrate inspired oxygen to the lowest level required to achieve an arterial oxygen saturation of ≥94%, so as to avoid potential oxygen toxicity. It is recognized that titration of inspired oxygen may not be possible immediately after out-of-hospital cardiac arrest until the patient is transported to the emergency department or, in the case of in-hospital arrest, the intensive care unit (ICU). The optimal FIO_2 during the immediate period after cardiac arrest is still debated. The beneficial effect of high FIO_2 on systemic oxygen delivery should be balanced with the deleterious effect of generating oxygen-derived free radicals during the reperfusion phase. Animal data suggests that ventilations with 100% oxygen (generating $PaO_2 > 350$ mm Hg at 15 to 60 minutes after ROSC) increase brain lipid peroxidation, increase metabolic dysfunctions, increase neurological degeneration, and worsen short-term functional outcome when compared with ventilation with room air or an inspired oxygen fraction titrated to a pulse oximeter reading between 94% and 96%.[82-87]* One randomized prospective clinical trial compared ventilation for the first 60 minutes after ROSC with 30% oxygen (resulting in $PaO_2 = 110 \pm 25$ mm Hg at 60 minutes) or 100% oxygen (resulting in $PaO_2 = 345 \pm 174$ mm Hg at 60 minutes).[88]* This small trial detected no difference in serial markers of acute brain injury, survival to hospital discharge, or percentage of patients with good neurological outcome at hospital discharge but was inadequately powered to detect important differences in survival or neurological outcome.

Once the circulation is restored, monitor systemic arterial oxyhemoglobin saturation. It may be reasonable, when the appropriate equipment is available, to titrate oxygen administration to maintain the arterial oxyhemoglobin saturation ≥94%. Provided appropriate equipment is available, once ROSC is achieved, adjust the FIO_2 to the minimum concentration needed to achieve arterial oxyhemoglobin saturation ≥94%, with the goal of avoiding hyperoxia while ensuring adequate oxygen delivery. Since an arterial oxyhemoglobin saturation of 100% may correspond to a PaO_2 anywhere between ~80 and 500 mm Hg, in general it is appropriate to wean FIO_2 when saturation is 100%, provided the oxyhemoglobin saturation can be maintained ≥94% (Class I, LOE C).

ASSESSMENT OF OXYGEN NEED AND ADMINISTRATION OF OXYGEN IN THE NEONATE

There is a large body of evidence that blood oxygen levels in uncompromised babies generally do not reach extrauterine values until approximately 10 minutes following birth. Oxyhemoglobin saturation may normally remain in the 70% to 80% range for several minutes following birth, thus resulting in the appearance of cyanosis during that time. Other studies have shown that clinical assessment of skin color is a very poor indicator of oxyhemoglobin saturation during the immediate neonatal period and that lack of cyanosis appears to be a very poor indicator of the state of oxygenation of an uncompromised baby following birth.

Optimal management of oxygen during neonatal resuscitation becomes particularly important because of the evidence that either insufficient or excessive oxygenation can be harmful to the newborn infant. Hypoxia and ischemia are known to result in injury to multiple organs. Conversely there is growing experimental evidence, as well as evidence from studies of babies receiving resuscitation, that adverse outcomes may result from even brief exposure to excessive oxygen during and following resuscitation.

ADMINISTRATION OF SUPPLEMENTARY OXYGEN IN NEONATAL RESUSCITATION

Two meta-analyses of several randomized controlled trials comparing neonatal resuscitation initiated with room air versus 100% oxygen showed increased survival when resuscitation was initiated with air.[44,45]† There are no studies in term infants comparing outcomes when resuscitations are initiated with different concentrations of oxygen other than 100% or room air. One study in preterm infants showed that initiation of resuscitation with a blend of oxygen and air resulted in less hypoxemia or hyperoxemia, as defined by the investigators, than when resuscitation was initiated with either air or 100% oxygen followed by titration with an adjustable blend of air and oxygen.[46]†

In the absence of studies comparing outcomes of neonatal resuscitation initiated with other oxygen concentrations or targeted at various oxyhemoglobin saturations, it is recommended that the goal in babies being resuscitated at birth, whether born at term or preterm, should be an oxygen saturation value in the interquartile range of preductal saturations measured in healthy term babies following vaginal birth at sea level (Class IIb, LOE B). These targets may be achieved by initiating resuscitation with air or a blended oxygen and titrating the oxygen concentration to achieve an SpO_2 in the target range as described above using pulse oximetry (Class IIb, LOE C). If blended oxygen is not available, resuscitation should be initiated with air (Class IIb, LOE B). If the baby is bradycardic (HR <60 per minute) after 90 seconds of resuscitation with a lower concentration of oxygen, oxygen concentration should be increased to 100% until recovery of a normal heart rate (Class IIb, LOE B).

*Citations 82-88 are from Peberdy MA, Callaway CW, Neumar RW, et al. Part 9: post-cardiac arrest care: 2010 American Heart Association Guidelines for Cardiopulmonary Resuscitation and Emergency Cardiovascular Care. *Circulation.* 2010;122(18 suppl):S768. Available at http://circ.ahajournals.org/content/122/18_suppl_3.toc. Accessed November 3, 2012.
†Citations 44-46 are from Kattwinkel, J, Perlman JM, Aziz, K, et al. Part 15: neonatal resuscitation: 2010 American Heart Association Guidelines for Cardiopulmonary Resuscitation and Emergency Cardiovascular Care. *Circulation.* 2010;122(18 suppl):S909. Available at http://circ.ahajournals.org/content/122/18_suppl_3.toc. Accessed November 3, 2012.

the mask, and FIO_2 will decrease. Masks with higher FIO_2 ratings entrain less outside air and therefore provide less total flow. Caution should be used with masks rated above 35% in patients with respiratory distress because FIO_2 may be significantly reduced with high inspiratory flow rates.

Low-flow delivery devices provide gas flow that is less than the patient's inspiratory flow rate. The difference between the patient's inspiratory flow and the flow delivered by the device is met by a variable amount of room air being drawn into the system. Patients with normal respiratory rates and tidal

Figure 3-6 The Venturi mask, also known as an air entrainment mask, delivers a known oxygen concentration to patients requiring controlled oxygen therapy. Venturi mask kits include multiple color-coded interchangeable oxygen dilution jets that are selected and placed in the base of the mask tubing to provide a specific FIO_2. Marked on each jet is the flow rate of wall oxygen required to deliver the specific FIO_2 associated with that diluter. For example, a blue jet provides 24% FIO_2 when 2 L/min is delivered from the wall oxygen source. There are stepwise increments, from the white jet providing 28% FIO_2 at 4 L/min, up to the green jet providing 60% FIO_2 at 15 L/min. *(Photo courtesy of Dr. Ronan O'Driscoll.)*

Figure 3-7 This patient suffered serious facial burns when she smoked a cigarette while oxygen was being delivered through a nasal cannula.

volumes will require less outside air than those in respiratory distress, who typically receive a higher FIO_2. As a patient's inspiratory flow changes, so will the FIO_2 that they receive from a low-flow device.[72,73]

The prongs of a nasal cannula deliver a constant flow of O_2 that accumulates in the nasopharynx and provides a reservoir of oxygen-enriched air for inspiration. The FIO_2 delivered by nasal cannulas is determined by many factors, including the respiratory rate, tidal volume, pharyngeal geometry, and O_2 flow. Most importantly, at a constant O_2 flow rate, FIO_2 varies inversely with the respiratory rate. Despite this limitation, nasal cannulas are very comfortable for patients and are the most common low-flow O_2 delivery device. Although it may seem intuitive, patients using a nasal cannula should be reminded that they should not smoke while oxygen is being delivered (Fig. 3-7).

Simple masks receive a constant flow of O_2 from the O_2 source and have multiple vent holes. During inspiration, the oxygen-enriched air that has accumulated in the mask, along with room air entrained through the vent holes, is inhaled. During expiration, 200 mL (the approximate volume of the mask) of exhaled gas is deposited in the mask with the rest exiting through the vent holes. The continuous flow of O_2 then partially washes out the mask before the next inspiration. The mask itself provides the reservoir of oxygen-rich gas for inhalation. A complex interplay between mask volume, tidal volume, respiratory rate, and O_2 flow determines the FIO_2 delivered to the patient.

A partial rebreathing mask incorporates a bag-type reservoir to increase the amount of O_2 available during inspiration, thereby requiring less outside air to be entrained. Non-rebreathing masks are similar to partial rebreathing masks but have a series of one-way valves. One valve lies between the mask and the reservoir and prevents exhaled gas from entering the reservoir. Two valves in the side of the mask permit exhalation while preventing the entry of outside air. In practice, one of these valves is often removed to permit inhalation in the event of interruption of flow of O_2 to the mask. A variable amount of air can still leak around the mask. This outside air and the exhaled gas remaining in the mask dilute the O_2 from the reservoir and prevent the mask from providing 100% O_2. Oxygen flow to the mask should be sufficient to prevent collapse of the bag during inspiration. As with all low-flow devices, the FIO_2 delivered varies with the patient's respiratory pattern. Many clinicians have the misconception that a non-rebreathing mask can provide an FIO_2 near 100%. In practice, a non-rebreathing mask usually delivers an FIO_2 of about 70%.

Procedure

In selecting the proper delivery device, consider the clinical condition of the patient and the amount of O_2 needed. High-flow systems should generally be used for patients who need precise control of FIO_2, such as COPD patients with chronic respiratory acidosis. Low-flow masks are appropriate for patients who need supplemental O_2 but do not require precise control of FIO_2. Nasal cannulas are traditionally used in patients who do not require a high FIO_2 and will not be harmed by the lack of precise control. An oxygen flow rate of 1 to 3 L/min by nasal cannula will result in an FIO_2 of 23% to 35%. Patients with significant hypoxemia, end-organ dysfunction, or respiratory distress require a higher FIO_2 delivery system.

An initial FIO_2 of 24% to 28% delivered by Venturi mask is indicated for patients with hypoxemia and chronic respiratory acidosis.[62,70]

Frequent clinical assessment and SpO_2 monitoring are needed in all patients receiving O_2 therapy. Periodic blood gas analysis or capnography is imperative for those at risk for respiratory acidosis.[74-76] Equilibration of SaO_2 after changes in supplemental O_2 occurs within 5 minutes.[77]

FIO_2 should be titrated to achieve therapeutic goals while minimizing the risk for complications. An SaO_2 of 90% to 95% ($PaO_2 \approx 60$ to 80 mm Hg) is an appropriate target for most patients receiving supplemental O_2.[62] Increases above these levels do not add appreciably to the O_2 content of blood and are unlikely to confer an additional benefit. One may exceed these parameters in patients with shock and end-organ dysfunction, but the added risk and small potential benefit should be considered on an individual basis. In patients with COPD-associated hypercapnia, an SaO_2 of 90% ($PaO_2 \approx$ 60 mm Hg) should be the goal of O_2 therapy.[74-76] Mechanical ventilation should be considered when oxygenation goals cannot be achieved without progressive respiratory acidosis.

Preoxygenation for Rapid-Sequence Intubation

Preoxygenation is one of the most important aspects of emergency airway management. Preoxygenation before rapid-sequence intubation (RSI) provides much more time for intubation before desaturation occurs and thus significantly increases the chance of successful intubation on the first attempt. Failure to preoxygenate before RSI is often a critical factor when a straightforward emergency airway becomes an airway disaster. Preoxygenation is usually accomplished by providing the maximal FIO_2 with a non-rebreather mask for 3 to 5 minutes before intubation. Alternatively, eight vital capacity breaths from a maximal FIO_2 system, such as a non-rebreather mask or a bag-valve-mask device, is acceptable when there is no time for standard preoxygenation.[78] When using a bag-valve-mask device for preoxygenation, it is important that the exhalation port have a one-way valve so that room air is not drawn into the mask when the patient inhales.

The purpose of preoxygenation is not just to maximize oxygen saturation but to wash out nitrogen from the patient's lungs and replace it with oxygen. This provides the maximum safe apneic time during RSI. Those at greatest risk for rapid desaturation include obese, pregnant, critically ill, and pediatric patients, and they will benefit the most from good preoxygenation. Most studies addressing preoxygenation have been conducted under ideal conditions in relatively healthy individuals. It is far more challenging to effectively preoxygenate critically ill patients.[79]

Morbidly obese patients are best preoxygenated in a 25-degree head-up position because significantly higher oxygen tension can be achieved in this position.[80] Patients who are hypoxic despite maximal oxygen delivery have been shown to benefit from 3 minutes of NPPV (with 100% O_2) just before intubation.[81,82]

Sometimes patients who need preoxygenation the most are uncooperative with a face mask because of delirium from hypoxia, hypercapnia, or other factors. These patients may benefit from delayed-sequence intubation—careful sedation without blunting of respirations to allow oxygenation with a face mask or NPPV for 2 to 3 minutes before administering a paralytic agent.[82] Ketamine (1 to 1.5 mg/kg by slow intravenous push) has been suggested for this technique. Delayed-sequence intubation is a practical way to deal with a difficult problem, but it has not been well studied, and providers using this method should be prepared for clinical deterioration, hypoventilation, or apnea.

Oxygen Therapy during Apnea

Another method to delay desaturation during RSI is nasopharyngeal oxygen insufflation during apnea. Many studies have shown that providing oxygen therapy during apnea is much more beneficial than one might imagine.[83-86] During apnea, oxygen continues to be absorbed through the alveoli, and air with a low oxygen concentration is left in the lower airways.

Supplying oxygen to the nasopharynx during apnea allows air with a higher oxygen concentration to passively replenish oxygen in the alveoli. Multiple studies, in normal and morbidly obese patients, have shown that nasopharyngeal oxygen insufflation results in a significant delay in desaturation after the onset of apnea.[83,86,87] In these studies, nasopharyngeal oxygen insufflation was accomplished by inserting a 10-Fr catheter into the nasopharynx to a distance equal to the distance from the mouth to the tragus of the ear and delivering oxygen at a flow rate of 5 L/min when apnea occurred.[83] Using a standard nasal cannula with a nasopharyngeal airway is simpler and would probably provide the same benefit. Also, it is important to keep the upper airway open by using a jaw thrust or artificial airway for this technique to be most beneficial.

Nasal High-Flow Oxygen

High-flow nasal oxygen is a relatively new concept that may have some utility for optimizing oxygenation in critically ill children and adults.[88] At lower flow rates, FIO_2 is somewhat dependent on the patient's respiratory rate, but at very high flow rates, FIO_2 is consistently very high. In one study, the FIO_2 delivered by nasal cannula ranged from about 25% at 1 L/min to 70% to 80% at 15 L/min.[89] Commercially available humidified high-flow nasal cannula (HHFNC) systems use flow rates of 5 to 40 L/min and deliver an FIO_2 of close to 100%. High-flow oxygen by nasal cannula is not well tolerated unless it is humidified, so commercially available systems (Vapotherm 2000i, Fisher and Paykel Nasal High Flow, AquinOx) deliver oxygen with nearly 100% humidity. HHFNC devices are popular in neonatal and pediatric intensive care units and are commonly used for respiratory support after extubation and for management of respiratory disease.[90,91] Some evidence suggests that high-flow nasal oxygen may provide low-grade CPAP.[92,93] Several adult studies have shown that high-flow nasal oxygen systems are well tolerated and deliver a higher FIO_2 than a high-flow mask in patients with respiratory failure or simulated respiratory failure.[94-96]

Complications of Oxygen Therapy

Worsening of CO_2 retention leading to progressive respiratory acidosis and obtundation in patients with COPD is the complication most likely to be seen in the ED. This phenomenon is well documented and was first described by Barach in 1937.[97] It has been attributed to several mechanisms, including loss of hypoxic respiratory drive, ventilation-perfusion ($\dot{V}/\dot{Q}$) mismatch, and decreased hemoglobin affinity for CO_2 (Haldane effect). This avoidable complication is best prevented by administering O_2 to chronic CO_2 retainers only when there is an indication, administering it at the smallest effective dose, and carefully monitoring clinical, capnographic, and arterial blood gas parameters.

Exposing the brain and lung to excessive concentrations of O_2 can lead to toxicity and, in severe cases, can cause acute respiratory distress syndrome. Injury to the pulmonary parenchyma occurs as a result of the formation of reactive oxygen species. Oxygen toxicity is of special concern in premature neonates, in whom prolonged hyperoxemia can lead to retinopathy. No data describe what concentration or duration of exposure to O_2 leads to toxicity, but presumably both these factors and individual patient characteristics determine the likelihood of toxicity. The benefits of O_2 therapy in the ED usually outweigh the risk for O_2 toxicity. Fear of toxicity should not prevent the use of O_2 when there is an indication but should encourage the clinician to use the minimum concentration of O_2 necessary to achieve therapeutic goals. High concentrations of O_2 are well tolerated over short periods and may be lifesaving.

In patients receiving high concentrations of supplemental O_2, nitrogen in the alveoli is largely replaced by O_2. If this O_2 is then absorbed into the blood faster than it can be replaced, the volume of the alveoli will decrease and absorptive atelectasis can occur. Airway obstruction potentiates this problem by preventing the rapid replacement of absorbed gas.

BAG-MASK VENTILATION

BMV is the single most important technique for emergency airway management.[1,19,98] Bag-mask devices are widely available and are standard equipment in all patient care settings. Although the bag-mask method of ventilation appears to be simple, it can be difficult to perform correctly. Having good BMV skills is a prerequisite to more advanced methods of emergency airway management.[1] Manually opening the airway, properly positioning the head and neck, placing an oropharyngeal airway device, and achieving a tight face mask seal are the keys to good BMV.

Indications and Contraindications

BMV is the most common initial technique for ventilation of apneic patients and for rescue ventilation after failed intubation.[1,2] Many authors note that BMV is relatively contraindicated in patients with a full stomach, those in cardiac arrest, and those undergoing RSI.[2,3] These patients have a high risk for stomach inflation and subsequent aspiration. Unfortunately, these are the patients for whom ED providers most commonly use BMV. In ED situations, the need for ventilation and oxygenation always takes priority over potential aspiration.[2]

The only contraindication to attempting BMV is when application of a face mask is impossible. It is often impossible to achieve an effective face mask seal on patients with significant deforming facial trauma and those with thick beards. An intermediate ventilation device, such as an LMA, is a better choice for initial ventilation in such patients.

Bag-Mask Ventilation Technique

Achieving adequate ventilation with a bag-mask device requires an open upper airway and a good mask seal. Overly aggressive BMV causes stomach inflation and increases the risk for aspiration. The goal is to achieve adequate gas exchange while keeping peak airway pressure low. Squeezing the bag forcefully creates high peak airway pressure and is more likely to inflate the stomach. Several studies have shown that increased tidal volume is associated with higher peak airway pressure and increased gastric inflation.[66,98-101] Data also show that decreased inspiratory time increases peak airway pressure and gastric inflation.[102,103] Therefore, the best method of BMV is to provide a tidal volume of about 500 mL delivered over a period of 1 to 1.5 seconds.[103] Using a ventilator (instead of a resuscitation bag) to provide the proper tidal volume and inspiratory time is a novel alternative to using a bag-valve device.[82] Effective ventilation and oxygenation should be judged by chest rise, breath sounds, SpO_2, and capnography.

A variety of mask configurations are available to facilitate a tight seal. The most common mask used in ED situations is a transparent disposable plastic mask with a high-volume, low-pressure cuff. This type of mask eliminates the need for an anatomically formed mask and can be used for a wide variety of patients with different facial features. Various mask sizes are available.

Bag-Mask Ventilation

Indications
Initial ventilation technique in apneic patients
Rescue ventilation after failed intubation

Contraindications
Situations when application of a face mask is impossible
  (e.g., deforming facial trauma, thick beards)

Complications
Inability to ventilate
Gastric inflation

Equipment

Bag ventilator with reservoir attached to supplemental O_2

Oropharyngeal airway

Nasopharyngeal airway

Mask

Review Box 3-2 Bag-mask ventilation: indications, contraindications, complications, and equipment.

For a single rescuer, only one hand can be used to achieve the seal because the other must squeeze the bag. The rescuer must apply pressure anteriorly while simultaneously lifting the jaw forward. The thumb and index finger provide anterior pressure while the fifth and fourth fingers lift the jaw. The C-E clamp technique is often the most effective: the thumb and index finger form a "C" to provide anterior pressure over the mask, whereas the third, fourth, and fifth fingers form an "E" to lift the jaw (Fig. 3-8, steps 1 and 2). Generally, well-fitting intact dentures should be left in place to help ensure a better seal with the mask.

In the ED setting it is best to hold the face mask with two hands and have an assistant squeeze the bag. If face mask ventilation is difficult, the most experienced provider should hold the face mask while the less experienced provider squeezes the bag.

There are two different methods for two-handed face mask control. The traditional technique is the double C-E method, where the thumb and index finger of both hands encircle the top of the mask (Fig. 3-8, step 3) and the third, fourth, and fifth fingers of both hands form an "E" to lift both sides of the mandible to meet the mask (Fig. 3-8, step 4). The problem with the double C-E technique is that it is difficult to perform a good jaw lift with the hands in this position. Having an assistant lend a third or fourth hand to help lift the jaw is an option, but this can be awkward unless the assistant is a very experienced provider. A better two-handed method is to hold the mask in place with the thenar eminence of both hands (Fig. 3-8, step 5) and use the long fingers under the angle of the mandible to perform a jaw lift while also pressing the mask firmly against the face (Fig. 3-8, step 6). This technique allows the operator to perform a good jaw lift (create mandibular protrusion or an "underbite") and create a good mask seal with the strongest muscles of the hands.[104,105] This method is best for patients with difficult mask ventilation, and it also allows inexperienced providers and those with small hands to do a better job with face mask ventilation.[105] In addition, it is important to remember to use oropharyngeal or

BAG-MASK VENTILATION

ONE-HANDED TECHNIQUE

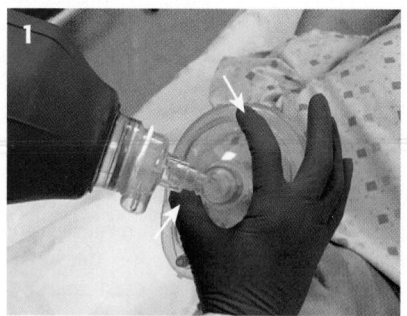

The "C-E" clamp technique provides the most effective seal.

Use your thumb and index finger to form a letter "C" and provide anterior pressure on the mask.

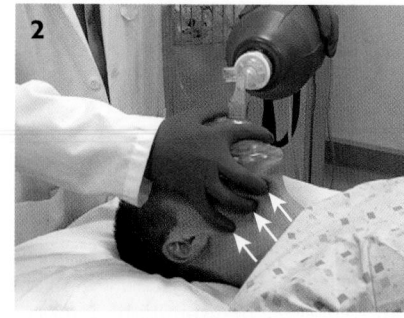

Use your third, fourth, and fifth fingers to lift the mandible up into the mask. It may be possible to place the fifth finger behind the mandible and perform a jaw thrust.

TWO-HANDED TECHNIQUE

The traditional technique is the "double C-E" method.

Use the thumb and index fingers of both hands to encircle the top of the mask.

Use the third, fourth, and fifth fingers of each hand to lift both sides of the mandible to meet the mask. It is difficult to do a good jaw lift with this method.

A better two-handed method is to hold the mask in place with the thenar eminences of both hands.

Use the long fingers under the mandible to do a jaw lift while also pressing the mask firmly against the face. This allows the operator to do a good jaw lift and create a good seal with the strongest muscles of the hands.

Figure 3-8 Bag-mask ventilation. It is best to hold the face mask with two hands and have an assistant squeeze the bag. If face mask ventilation is difficult, the most experienced provider should hold the mask while the less experienced provider squeezes the bag.

nasopharyngeal airways (or both) whenever face mask ventilation is difficult.

All bag-mask devices should be attached to a supplemental O_2 source (with a flow rate of 15 L/min) to avoid hypoxia. A significant problem with the bag-mask method is the low percentage of O_2 achieved with some reservoirs. The amount of O_2 delivered is dependent on the ventilatory rate, the volumes delivered during each breath, the O_2 flow rate into the ventilating bag, the filling time for reservoir bags, and the type of reservoir used. A 2500-mL bag reservoir and a demand valve are preferred for O_2 supplementation during BMV.[106]

Pediatric bag-mask devices should have a minimum volume of 450 mL. Pediatric and larger bags may be used to ventilate infants with the proper mask size, but care must be maintained to administer only the volume necessary to effectively ventilate the infant. Avoid pop-off valves because airway pressure under emergency conditions may often exceed the pressure of the valve.[107]

BMV may be the best method of prehospital airway support in trauma patients and children. Murray and coworkers[108] performed a large retrospective study suggesting that patients with severe head injury had a higher risk for mortality if they were intubated in the prehospital setting. In the same year, Gausche and associates[109] reported that neurologic outcomes and ultimate survival rates after prehospital pediatric resuscitation with BMV by emergency medical service (EMS) providers were as good as those with tracheal intubation.

Complications

The main complications of the bag-mask technique are an inability to ventilate and gastric inflation. Langeron and colleagues[110] performed a large prospective study of adults undergoing general anesthesia and reported a 5% incidence of difficult mask ventilation. The incidence is obviously much higher in the emergency setting. Risk factors for difficult BMV include presence of a beard, obesity, lack of teeth, age older than 55 years, history of snoring, short thyromental distance, and limited mandibular protrusion (Box 3-2).[110-113] Patients who are not spontaneously breathing but awake enough to interfere with the procedure can also be difficult to bag-mask ventilate. A recent study showed that most patients with difficult BMV became easier to ventilate after paralytic agents were administered and none were more difficult to ventilate after paralytics.[114]

When mask ventilation is technically difficult, higher peak airway pressure is often required to provide adequate tidal volume. In these situations, gastric inflation is more likely and aspiration may occur. Be vigilant to recognize complications early and take corrective action. Even when BMV is easy and good technique is used, some gastric dilation will generally occur. Minor gastric distention should not be considered substandard in the setting of prolonged BMV.

Cricoid Pressure: Sellick's Maneuver

In 1961, B.A. Sellick described the use of cricoid pressure to prevent regurgitation during anesthesia, and this technique has since become known as Sellick's maneuver.[115] The purpose of this technique is to apply external force to the anterior cricoid ring to push the trachea posteriorly and compress the esophagus against the cervical vertebrae. In theory, cricoid pressure compresses the distensible upper esophagus but not the airway because the cricoid ring is fairly rigid.

There are no good data that Sellick's maneuver prevents regurgitation,[116,117] but there are data that cricoid pressure prevents gastric inflation during BMV,[115,116,118-121] thereby reducing the risk for subsequent regurgitation and vomiting. Several studies have confirmed that Sellick's maneuver reduces tidal volumes, increases peak inspiratory pressure, and prevents good air exchange when applied during BMV.[118,120-129] Sellick's maneuver also decreases successful insertion of and intubation through LMAs.[130-137]

BMV can produce gastric inflation, especially if high volume and high pressure are used. To avoid gastric inflation it is best to ventilate with a small volume (500 mL or 6 to 8 mL/kg) and avoid high peak pressure by using a long inspiratory time (1 second). Applying Sellick's maneuver during BMV may further decrease the risk for gastric inflation and is still recommended by most airway experts.[138,139] It should be noted that *the routine use of cricoid pressure during BMV of patients in cardiac arrest is not recommended in the 2010 American Heart Association Guidelines for Cardiopulmonary Resuscitation and Emergency Cardiovascular Care.*[6] It is recommended that cricoid pressure be released immediately if there is any difficulty ventilating with a face mask in an emergency setting.[117] In addition, it is reasonable to release or relax cricoid pressure during insertion of an LMA and if ventilation with the LMA is difficult.[116,117,136] It may be reasonable to release cricoid pressure during laryngoscopy and tracheal intubation, and this is discussed in Chapter 4.

Some authors believe that improper technique is to blame for the many reported failures of Sellick's maneuver.[116] The proper technique for applying Sellick's maneuver is to place the thumb and middle finger on either side of the cricoid cartilage with the index finger in the center anteriorly.[115] Apply 30 N (6.7 lb) of force to the cricoid cartilage in the posterior direction.[116,139] As a reference, about 40 N of digital force on the bridge of the nose will usually cause pain.[116]

EXTRAGLOTTIC AIRWAY DEVICES

EGAs are devices that are blindly placed above or posterior to the larynx to allow rapid ventilation and oxygenation. These are good rescue devices for patients who are difficult or impossible to ventilate and oxygenate with a face mask, especially morbidly obese patients and those with large beards or significant facial trauma. In the emergency setting, EGAs can provide temporary rescue ventilation until tracheal intubation or a surgical airway can be performed. It is important to have at least one of these devices immediately available when managing emergency airways. EGAs can be divided into two groups, LMAs and retroglottic devices.

BOX 3-2	Risk Factors for Difficult Mask Ventilation
Presence of a beard	History of snoring
Obesity	Short thyromental distance
Lack of teeth	Limited mandibular protrusion
Age older than 55 years	

LMAs

The first LMA, the LMA Classic (Laryngeal Mask Company, Singapore; www.lmaco.com) became available in 1988. Since then it has been used more than 200 million times and has been described in more than 2500 academic papers.[136,140] LMAs are widely considered to be essential adjuncts for rescue ventilation and difficult intubation.[141,142] LMAs are primary rescue adjuncts in the difficult airway guidelines put forth by the American Society of Anesthesiologists[141] and the Difficult Airway Society in Europe.[142] Advanced Cardiac Life Support guidelines suggest that the LMA provides a more secure and reliable means of ventilation than a face mask does.[4,6] Pediatric Advanced Life Support guidelines acknowledge the LMA as a potential backup device for difficult pediatric airways.[143,144] Several manufacturers now make LMAs since the patent on the LMA Classic expired in 2003. It is important to recognize that all LMAs are not the same and that some of the newer devices have not been well studied.

Either an intubating LMA (ILMA) or a nonintubating LMA can be used in the "cannot-intubate/cannot-ventilate" scenario when face mask ventilation is difficult because of a beard, massive facial trauma, or obesity. Both devices can be inserted in less than 30 seconds and provide effective ventilation in more than 98% of patients.[136] In the emergency setting, where obtaining a definitive airway (i.e., tracheal intubation) is the eventual goal, it is more practical to use an ILMA. In addition, the LMA Fastrach (Laryngeal Mask Company, Singapore; www.lmaco.com), the most widely used and well-studied ILMA, is easier to insert than the LMA Classic.[145-149] Finally, when the head is in the neutral position, the LMA Fastrach is more likely to allow successful ventilation than the LMA Classic during in-line stabilization of the cervical spine.[150-152]

The LMA Supreme (Laryngeal Mask Company, Singapore; www.lmaco.com) is the latest offering from the Laryngeal Mask Company; it has a new mask shape that may allow a better mask seal and a gastric evacuation tube. It features a firm curved shape and a bite block handle, so ease of insertion may be similar to that of the Fastrach, and it is available in all sizes from neonate to large adult.[153-162] Drawbacks are that it has not been extensively studied and does not facilitate tracheal intubation.

The Cookgas air-Q (Mercury Medical, Clearwater, FL), i-gel (Intersurgical, Berkshire, UK), and Ambu Aura-I (Ambu, Glen Burnie, MD) are promising new LMAs that can facilitate tracheal intubation and are available in pediatric sizes. The air-Q features a large-bore flexible airway tube and an inflatable mask that is stiffer than other LMAs. A few studies in adults and children show that it provides adequate ventilation in nearly all patients, but it has not been extensively tested.[163-170] i-gel features a thermoplastic elastomer cuff that does not need inflation, so it may be easier to insert than other LMAs, but it has not been extensively tested.[160,171-177] The Ambu Aura-I has some attractive features, but it is very new and almost completely untested.

This chapter describes how to insert the LMA Fastrach and use it for rescue ventilation. Details about intubation with the Fastrach are described in Chapter 4. Use of the LMA Unique (the disposable version of the LMA Classic) and LMA Supreme will also be described because they are cheap, disposable, well tested, and widely available.

Background

The LMA Classic has been available since 1988 and has changed the practice of anesthesia in the last 20 years. In anesthesia practice LMAs are now used for a large percentage of cases in which an endotracheal (ET) tube may have been used in the past. The LMA Classic has been used more than 200 million times worldwide and has been tested more than any other airway device in history.

Anatomy and Physiology

All the LMA devices consist of an airway tube attached to an oval mask, rimmed by an inflatable cuff. The cuffed mask is

---

Laryngeal Mask Airway Insertion

Indications
Failed rapid-sequence intubation
Difficult bag-mask ventilation
Difficult intubation
Facial trauma
Obesity
Primary airway in cardiac arrest or use by emergency medical services

Contraindications
Limited mouth opening (<2 cm)
High airway pressure
Inadequate paralysis or sedation

Complications
Inability to ventilate (rare)
Inability to intubate
Aspiration (rare)

Equipment

Intubating LMA (ILMA/"Fastrach")

LMA unique

60-mL syringe

Review Box 3-3 Laryngeal mask airways: indications, contraindications, complications, and equipment.

designed to form a seal around the glottis when the device is placed properly. The ILMA has a handle that allows the operator to increase seal pressure by lifting the entire device toward the ceiling, like lifting a frying pan (see Review Box 3-3). This is called "Chandy's" maneuver (see Fig. 3-9, *steps 7 and 8*). The tip of the LMA sits in the proximal esophagus when it is placed properly. It is common for the epiglottis to become down-folded by the tip of the LMA device on insertion. When using the LMA Fastrach, epiglottic down-folding can be corrected with the "up-down maneuver" (see Fig. 3-9, *steps 9 and 10*).

Pathophysiology

The cannot-intubate/cannot-ventilate scenario is one reason for using an LMA in the ED. In this situation, failure to adequately ventilate and oxygenate with the LMA occurs in about 6% of cases. Another 6% of patients with difficult airways suffer episodes of hypoxia during attempts to intubate through the LMA.[136] There is evidence that the ILMA performs better in the cannot-intubate/cannot-ventilate situation.[136] Failure to ventilate with the ILMA occurs in only about 2% of cases, and hypoxia after ILMA placement is very rare. In addition, for difficult airway management, there are more technical difficulties with the LMA than with the ILMA. This is probably due to the fact that the LMA requires more skill for proper insertion and was not specifically designed to facilitate tracheal intubation.

Indications

The LMA Fastrach is indicated as an alternative to BMV or as a conduit for intubation of difficult airways.[178] In the cannot-intubate/cannot-ventilate scenario it is a reliable rescue device. In this situation, adequate ventilation with the ILMA is possible in nearly all cases.[5,114,136] Ventilation with the ILMA is probably superior to face mask ventilation with inexperienced providers.[179] The ILMA can also be used as a primary ventilation and intubation device for patients with difficult airways.[178] Tracheal intubation through the ILMA can be accomplished by using a blind technique, with a light-wand, or under fiberoptic guidance (see Chapter 4 for tracheal intubation through the ILMA). Studies of difficult airway management with the ILMA show that almost all patients can be adequately ventilated with the ILMA and 94% to 99% can be intubated through the device.[5,136,178,180-187]

The LMA Fastrach is especially useful in patients with difficult face mask ventilation caused by a beard, severe facial trauma, or obesity because none of these factors inhibit ILMA placement. When brisk bleeding above the glottis makes ventilation and intubation difficult, the ILMA can prevent aspiration of blood and facilitate blind or fiberoptic intubation. In patients requiring urgent cricothyrotomy or percutaneous needle insertion into the trachea, the ILMA can be used to counteract anterior neck pressure. In this capacity, the ILMA provides temporary ventilation and stabilizes the cervical spine during the surgical airway procedure.

The LMA Classic (or single-use LMA Unique) is the most extensively tested LMA for children. It may provide a more secure and reliable means of ventilation than a face mask.[4] The LMA allows adequate ventilation in 98% of adults with known difficult airways and in 90% to 95% of those with unexpectedly difficult airways.[136,188-191] It is also useful as a rescue device in difficult pediatric airways.[136] Two descriptive studies and 86 case reports describe use of the LMA for difficult pediatric airways.[136,192-198] In these reports, ventilation

was adequate with the LMA in nearly all pediatric patients.[136,196,198,199] Intubation of pediatric patients through the LMA is usually possible with a small fiberoptic scope.[196,198] Case series and case reports also suggest that the LMA can provide an effective rescue airway during neonatal resuscitation if BMV and ET intubation fail.[200]

Contraindications

The ILMA is contraindicated in patients with less than 2 cm of mouth opening because it requires 2 cm of space between the upper and the lower incisors to be inserted. The ILMA is relatively contraindicated in awake patients, especially those with a full stomach. Insertion of the ILMA in an awake patient will cause coughing, gagging, or vomiting. If the ILMA is inserted when the patient is awake and the stomach is full, there is a high likelihood of emesis and aspiration. In the ED, the ILMA should be used only if the patient is unconscious or after a paralytic agent has been given. Once the ILMA is inserted and ventilation is established, the patient should not be allowed to wake up or gag. Consider giving a long-acting paralytic agent or multiple doses of succinylcholine after the ILMA is placed and ventilation is adequate.

Although several studies have shown that the ILMA is safe and effective for ventilation and intubation during in-line cervical spine stabilization, some evidence shows that the ILMA causes posterior pressure on the midportion of the cervical spine.[183,201-204] The clinical importance of cervical spine pressure caused by the ILMA is unknown, and the device is generally considered safe in patients with an unstable cervical spine injury. Nevertheless, providers should be aware of this concern and make every effort to stabilize the ILMA in these situations.

Procedure
LMA Fastrach

The first step is to select the appropriate size of ILMA. The ILMA is available in three sizes: size 3 for children weighing 30 to 50 kg, size 4 for small adults weighing 50 to 70 kg, and size 5 for adults weighing 70 to 100 kg (Table 3-1). When there is doubt about which size is appropriate, it is probably better to use the larger size.

After choosing the correct ILMA, completely deflate the cuff while pushing it posteriorly so that it assumes a smooth wedge shape without any wrinkles (Fig. 3-9, *step 1*). Place a small amount of water-based lubricant onto the posterior surface of the ILMA just before insertion (Fig 3-9, *step 2*). Open the patient's mouth and position the posterior mask tip so that it is flat against the hard palate, immediately posterior to the upper incisors (Fig. 3-9, *step 3*). Advance the airway straight into the mouth along the hard palate without rotation until the curved part of the airway tube is in contact with the patient's chin. Then rotate the ILMA completely into the hypopharynx by advancing it along its curved axis. Keep the posterior of the mask firmly applied to the soft palate and posterior pharynx until firm resistance is felt (Fig. 3-9, *step 4*). Cricoid pressure impedes proper placement of the ILMA, so consider briefly releasing cricoid pressure while the device is rotated into its final position, wedged into the proximal esophagus.[133,134,205] After insertion, the airway tube should emerge from the mouth directed somewhat caudally. Without holding the tube or handle, inflate the mask cuff (Fig. 3-9, *step 5*). The entire device will normally slide backward a bit when the cuff is inflated. Frequently, only half the maximum

INTUBATING LARYNGEAL MASK AIRWAY INSERTION

1
Completely deflate the cuff while pushing it posteriorly, so that it assumes a smooth wedge shape without any wrinkles.

2
Place a small amount of water-based lubricant onto the posterior surface of the ILMA just before insertion.

3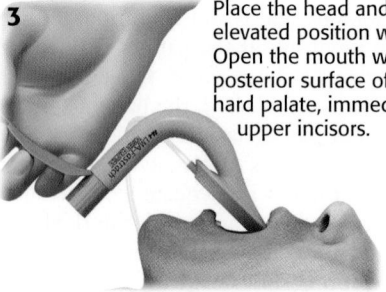
Place the head and neck in a slightly elevated position with minimal extension. Open the mouth widely and place the posterior surface of the device against the hard palate, immediately posterior to the upper incisors.

4
Advance the ILMA straight into mouth until the curved part of the airway tube contacts the chin. Then, rotate the ILMA into the hypopharynx until firm resistance is felt. Release cricoid pressure during this step.

5
Let go of the handle and inflate the cuff. Initially inflate the cuff with only half of the maximum volume, and increase inflation as needed. Do not overinflate the cuff. (See product manual for maximum volumes.)

6
Attach a bag and ventilate the patient. Use chest rise, breath sounds, and capnography to confirm adequate gas exchange. If bagging is easy and ventilation is good, the LMA is probably correctly aligned over the glottis.

7
CHANDY MANEUVER
Step 1
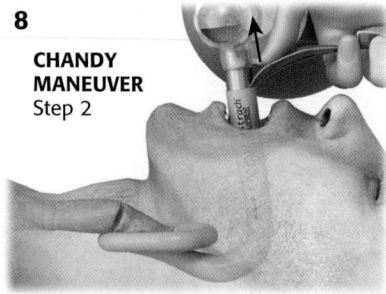
If adjustment is needed, try the Chandy maneuver. First, gently rotate the ILMA farther into the hypopharynx.

8
CHANDY MANEUVER
Step 2

Next, lift the handle upwards, toward the ceiling above the patient's feet.

This manuever aligns the mask with the glottis and may provide for better ventilation.

9
If these manuevers fail, the epiglottis may be folded down over the glottis (*asterisk*).

Perform the "up-down" manuever, by first rotating the ILMA out of the hypopharynx along its curvature about 5–6 cm.

10
Next, slide the ILMA back into position while pressing it against the posterior pharynx.

(Note, the cuff should remain inflated during this maneuver.)

Figure 3-9 Intubating laryngeal mask airway (ILMA or "Fastrach") insertion.

TABLE 3-1 Laryngeal Mask Airway, Disposable Laryngeal Mask Airway, and Intubating Laryngeal Mask Airway Size Recommendations Based on Weight*

WEIGHT (kg)	LMA	DISPOSABLE LMA	ILMA
<5	1	—	—
5-10	1.5	—	—
10-20	2	—	—
20-30	2.5	—	—
30-50	3	3	3
50-70	4	4	4
70-100	5	5	5
>100	6	—	—

ILMA, intubating laryngeal mask airway; *LMA*, laryngeal mask airway.
*Note that only a standard LMA is available for patients less than 30 kg.

cuff volume is sufficient to obtain a good mask seal. Do not overinflate the cuff because this may make the seal worse. See the instruction manual for maximum cuff volumes. Attach a bag and ventilate the patient while using chest rise, breath sounds, and capnography to confirm adequate gas exchange. If bagging is easy and ventilation is good, the aperture of the ILMA is probably aligned correctly over the vocal cords.

If optimal ILMA placement is not accomplished initially, adjusting maneuvers can be attempted. The purpose of adjusting maneuvers is to align the aperture of the ILMA with the glottic opening. Proper positioning of the ILMA aperture with the glottic opening allows optimal ventilation and facilitates tracheal intubation. Before adjusting the ILMA, consider the patient's position and degree of relaxation because both may affect ILMA function. The ILMA works best in the neutral or sniffing position; cervical extension may interfere with proper placement. The patient should not react to ILMA placement with coughing or gagging because this may interfere with proper placement. Have a single operator perform the adjustment maneuvers by gripping the ILMA handle with one hand, in a "frying pan" grip, and providing bag ventilation with the other hand. After each adjustment maneuver, assess the quality of bag ventilation and mask seal. Easy bag ventilation, good chest rise, and absence of an audible mask leak are indications of good ILMA alignment with the glottis (Fig. 3-9, step 6).

To adjust the position of the ILMA, first gently pull the handle toward you without rotation along the ILMA's curvature. Next, gently push the handle toward the patient's feet without rotating it. Finally, try the "Chandy maneuver," which consists of gently rotating the ILMA farther into the hypopharynx and then lifting the handle toward the ceiling above the patient's feet (Fig. 3-9, steps 7 and 8). If these simple maneuvers do not result in adequate ventilation, consider the "up-down maneuver" (Fig. 3-9, steps 9 and 10). This technique is used to correct down-folding of the epiglottis, which is common with insertion of the ILMA and may interfere with ventilation or intubation. The up-down maneuver is accomplished by rotating the ILMA out of the hypopharynx along its curvature about 5 to 6 cm while the cuff remains inflated and then sliding it back into position while pressing it against the posterior of the pharynx. Do not use excessive force when placing or adjusting the ILMA.

If adjusting maneuvers do not result in adequate ventilation, it is likely that the wrong size ILMA has been used. Incorrect ILMA size is more likely to be a problem if the device is too small; attempting insertion of a larger ILMA is a reasonable first approach. If another ILMA size is not available, external anterior neck manipulation or downward pressure may bring the glottis and ILMA cuff into proper alignment. If the size of the ILMA is not in question, consider completely removing and carefully reinserting the device (see Chapter 4 for intubation through the ILMA and ILMA removal).

LMA Classic (or Single-Use LMA Unique)

The first step is to select the appropriate size LMA. The LMA is available in a wide range of sizes, from size 1 for neonates weighing less than 5 kg to size 6 for adults weighing more than 100 kg. The disposable version is available in sizes 1 through 5, but not size 6. After selecting the proper size, completely deflate the LMA cuff while pushing it posteriorly so that it forms a smooth wedge shape without any wrinkles (Fig. 3-10, step 1). Place a small amount of water-based lubricant onto the posterior surface of the LMA just before insertion (Fig 3-10, step 2). The best patient position for insertion of the LMA is the sniffing position, with the neck flexed and the head extended. The LMA may be inserted via two different techniques, depending on access to the patient. The most common method is the index finger insertion technique. This is accomplished by holding the LMA like a pen, with the index finger at the junction of the airway tube and the cuff (Fig. 3-10, step 3). Have an assistant open the patient's mouth and insert the LMA with the posterior tip pressed against the hard palate just behind the upper incisors (Fig. 3-10, step 4). Under direct vision, use the index finger to slide the LMA along the hard palate and into the oropharynx (Fig. 3-10, step 5). As the LMA is inserted farther, extend the index finger and push the posterior cuff along the soft palate and posterior pharynx. Exert counterpressure on the back of the patient's head during insertion. Continue to push the LMA into the hypopharynx until resistance is felt. Use the other hand to hold the proximal end of the LMA tube while removing your index finger from the patient's mouth (Fig. 3-10, step 6).

An alternative method is the thumb insertion technique. Use this technique when you have limited access to the patient from behind (see www.lmana.com for details). Hold the LMA with your thumb at the junction of the cuff and the airway tube. Place the mask against the hard palate under direct vision as with the index finger technique. Use the thumb to push the LMA into the mouth along the palate and posterior pharynx. Hold the end of the airway tube with the other hand while removing your thumb from the patient's mouth.

After the LMA is fully inserted, let go of the proximal end of the airway tube and inflate the cuff enough to achieve a good seal over the glottis (Fig. 3-10, step 7). This may require only half the maximum cuff volume. Be careful to not overinflate the LMA cuff (see the product packaging for maximal cuff volumes). Attach a bag and ventilate the patient, with chest rise, breath sounds, and capnography used to confirm adequate gas exchange (Fig. 3-10, step 8). If bagging is easy and ventilation is good, the aperture of the LMA is probably aligned correctly over the glottic opening. Proper positioning of the LMA aperture with the glottic opening allows optimal ventilation.

Several tips or techniques should be considered if LMA ventilation is inadequate. The best way to ensure proper ventilation is to optimize the insertion technique by carefully following the aforementioned directions. Position the patient's head and neck properly and ensure that the patient is deeply anesthetized or paralyzed. Listen for an audible cuff leak to make sure that a good mask seal has been achieved. Adjust the cuff volume if necessary to improve the mask seal and ensure optimal ventilation. Simply adding more air to the cuff will not necessarily improve the seal of the mask with the glottis. Cuff overinflation may cause a leak, but deflation and repositioning may improve the seal.

Sometimes adjusting the patient's head and neck position is easier than trying to change the position of the LMA. Move the patient into a better sniffing position or into the chin-to-chest position to see whether this improves the LMA cuff seal. If these positions do not help or are not possible, try a jaw-thrust or a chin-lift maneuver. Also, apply anterior neck pressure to help manipulate the glottis into improved contact with the LMA mask. This technique can be used in combination with any of the maneuvers just discussed.

If mask seal and ventilation are still not optimal after simple repositioning maneuvers, withdraw, advance, or rotate the LMA cuff. Another alternative is to completely remove

LARYNGEAL MASK AIRWAY INSERTION

1 After selecting the appropriate size LMA, completely deflate the cuff while pushing it posteriorly so that it forms a smooth wedge shape without any wrinkles.

2 Place a small amount of water-soluble lubricant onto the posterior surface of the LMA just before insertion.

3 Hold the LMA like a pen, with the index finger at the junction of the airway tube and the cuff.

4 Insert the LMA with the posterior tip pressed against the hard palate and into the oropharynx.

5 Advance the LMA further by extending the index finger and pushing the posterior cuff along the soft palate and posterior pharynx. Exert counterpressure on the occiput during insertion.

6 When resistance is felt, carefully remove the index finger while holding the proximal end of the tube with the other hand.

7 Let go of the airway tube and inflate the cuff with enough air to achieve a good seal. This may require only half of the maximum cuff volume. *Do not overinflate the cuff!*

8 Attach a bag and ventilate while using chest rise, breath sounds, and capnography to confirm adequate gas exchange.

Figure 3-10 Laryngeal mask airway insertion. The LMA Unique is shown in this sequence.

and reinsert the LMA while paying careful attention to the details just described. If unsuccessful, change the size of the LMA. A larger LMA will usually improve ventilation even if it is more difficult to insert. It is much more common to need to increase the LMA size than to decrease it. Finally, consider using the ILMA, placing a King LT, or performing a surgical airway when ventilation with the LMA is not adequate.

Aftercare

If the LMA or ILMA will remain in place without tracheal intubation, it can be secured like an ET tube. Removal of the ILMA after tracheal intubation is easy, but more difficult than insertion of the device (see Chapter 4).

Complications

The most important complications associated with using the LMA are aspiration of gastric contents and hypoxia. The LMA does not protect against aspiration and may actually cause vomiting if the patient gags during placement of the device. In fasted anesthetized patients, the incidence of aspiration is very low, about 2 per 10,000 cases.[136] There are many descriptive studies and case reports of the use of an LMA for difficult airways with no mention of significant aspiration.[136] Although the risk for aspiration is surely higher than 2 per 10,000 when using the LMA in the ED, there is evidence that it provides some protection from passive regurgitation and produces less gastric inflation than BMV does.[206]

Retroglottic Airway Devices

King LT

The King LT (King Airway-LTS-D EMS, King Systems, Noblesville, IN; www.kingsystems.com) is a retroglottic device that functions similar to the esophageal-tracheal Combitube (see later). Like the Combitube, the LT is designed to isolate the glottic opening between an oropharyngeal cuff and an esophageal cuff (see Review Box 3-4). Unlike the Combitube,

the King LT has only one airway lumen and a simplified cuff system, so both cuffs can be inflated from a single port. The literature regarding the King LT is a bit confusing in that many versions of the device have been clinically tested during the last decade. The latest disposable versions are the LT-D and the LTS-D. The LTS-D has an 18-Fr gastric suction port at the tip. The modern LTS-D has been available since 2004 and is also called the LTS II in some literature.[207,208]

Like the Combitube, the King LT is designed for blind placement and has a large proximal cuff and small distal cuff. Unlike the Combitube, the tip of the King LT is designed to be placed in the esophagus only. The shape of the King LT and the size of the tip in previous versions made it unlikely to be placed into the trachea.[209] However, the latest design of the LTS-D has a narrower tip and in one study had a 10% incidence of tracheal placement.[210] Interestingly, most patients with tracheal placement of the LTS-D were still able to be adequately ventilated.[210]

Popularity of the LTS-D has grown rapidly in EMS systems, and it is now widely used by EMS agencies in the United States. Several studies have shown that the LTS-D has a high rate of successful ventilation in the operating room setting.[211-213] In addition, there are several case reports of the LT being used as a rescue device for the cannot-intubate/cannot-ventilate scenario and when placement of an LMA failed.[214,215] Some data suggest that the LTS-D may be useful in neonates and small infants when direct laryngoscopy fails.[216] In the EMS setting, the LT-D has a high success rate (95%) when used for ventilation of out-of-hospital cardiac arrest.[217] Finally, an out-of-hospital study by Frascone and colleagues showed that the rate of successful insertion and ventilation with the LTS-D is essentially equivalent to that of standard ET intubation in the hands of paramedics.[218]

Intubation through the King LT devices is possible with fiberoptics or a bougie, but many who have tried this maneuver in clinical practice have been disappointed. The reason is that the aperture does not necessarily directly align with the

Retroglottic Airway Devices

Indications
Primary airway in the emergency medical services setting
Primary airway in cardiac arrest
Failed rapid-sequence intubation
Difficult bag-mask ventilation
Difficult intubation
Facial trauma
Obesity

Contraindications
Limited mouth opening
High airway pressure
Inadequate paralysis or sedation

Complications
Inability to ventilate
Aspiration (rare)
Specifically for the King LT device:
  Tracheal placement
  Tongue edema

Equipment

The King LTS-D (left) and the Combitube (right).

Review Box 3-4 Retroglottic airway devices: indications, contraindications, complications, and equipment.

glottis, even when the device is ventilating properly.[210] In one study the glottis was visualized in only 51% of patients when a fiberscope was passed through the King LT.[212]

Many EMS agencies that have used the King LT extensively have noticed cases of tongue edema, especially with prolonged use of the device. One case of massive tongue swelling has been reported in the literature.[219] Moreover, there is some concern that the large oropharyngeal balloon of the King LT might compress the carotid arteries and be detrimental in patients undergoing CPR, but there is currently no evidence to support this concern.

Indications and Contraindications

In the ED, indications for using the King LT are the same as those for the Combitube. It appears to be a good rescue ventilation device for failed BMV or failed intubation.[209,220,221] Because the King LT is a supraglottic airway and is designed to be placed blindly, it is relatively contraindicated in patients with obstruction of the upper airway by a foreign body.

Placement of the King LT

The first step is to choose the proper size King LT. It is available only in adolescent and adult sizes in the United States. Size 3 is yellow and designed for patients 4 to 5 feet in height, size 4 is red and designed for patients 5 to 6 feet in height, and size 5 is purple and designed for patients taller than 6 feet. Several pediatric sizes are available in Europe, but not in the United States.

After determining the appropriate size King LT, check the cuffs and then completely deflate them before placement. Lubricate the device with a water-based lubricant. The best patient position for insertion of the King LT is the sniffing position, but it can be placed with the head in the neutral position if necessary. Hold the LT at the connector with the dominant hand, and hold the mouth open by grasping the chin with the nondominant hand. Introduce the tip of the device into the corner of the mouth while rotating the tube 45 to 90 degrees so that the blue orientation line on the tube is touching the corner of the mouth. Pass the tip of the device into the mouth and under the tongue. As the tip passes under the base of the tongue, rotate the tube back to the midline so that the blue orientation line faces the ceiling. Without exerting force, advance the King LT until the connector is aligned with the teeth. Inflate the cuffs with the minimum volume necessary to create a good seal (see the product brochure for maximum cuff volumes). Ventilate with a bag-valve system and confirm placement with chest rise, breath sounds, and capnography (Fig. 3-11).

Complications

It is hard to assess the complication rate of the King LT because the device has been modified several times in the last decade and there is no organized surveillance of out-of-hospital airway devices.[222] The current LT-D and LTS-D devices have been available since 2004. The LTS-D is referred to as the LTS II in some studies. The most serious complication is tracheal placement, which occurred in 10% of cases in one study and is probably significantly underappreciated and underreported.[210] Another complication that is not uncommon and certainly underreported is tongue edema. There is one case report of massive tongue edema occurring 3 hours after placement of the King LT,[219] and mild tongue edema is relatively common and not reported in the literature. Finally,

Figure 3-11 King LTS-D. The device is properly placed posterior to the larynx, with the distal end in the proximal esophagus. The distal cuff is inflated in the proximal esophagus and the larger proximal cuff is inflated at the base of the tongue. The proximal portion of the tube is at the lip line and the distal aperture (between the cuffs) is aligned with the glottic opening; oxygen flow from the device to the glottis is depicted by the *white arrows.*

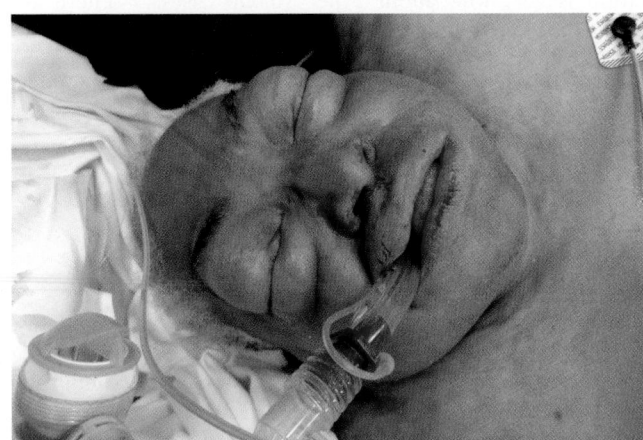

Figure 3-12 Massive neck and facial edema following cardiopulmonary resuscitation with a King LT airway in place. The exact pathology was not determined but was thought to be a pharyngeal or esophageal perforation.

there is some concern that the large oropharyngeal balloon of the King LT might compress the carotid arteries and be detrimental in patients undergoing CPR, but no evidence currently supports this concern. Figure 3-12 depicts probable pharyngeal or esophageal perforation, with massive subcutaneous neck and face emphysema following prehospital placement of a King LT. Because an autopsy was denied, the exact injury was never confirmed and may have been related to other interventions during resuscitation.

Combitube and EasyTube

The esophageal-tracheal Combitube (Nellcor, Pleasanton, CA; www.nellcor.com) and the EasyTube (Teleflex Medical–Rusch, Durham, NC) are retroglottic airway devices designed as rescue devices for difficult and emergency airways and can be placed blindly and rapidly.[223,224] The EasyTube is very similar to the Combitube and may have some minor advantages,[224] but it has not been as well studied. The discussion here will concentrate on the Combitube.

The Combitube has two parallel lumens, a small distal cuff, and a large proximal cuff. When it is placed blindly, the tip will

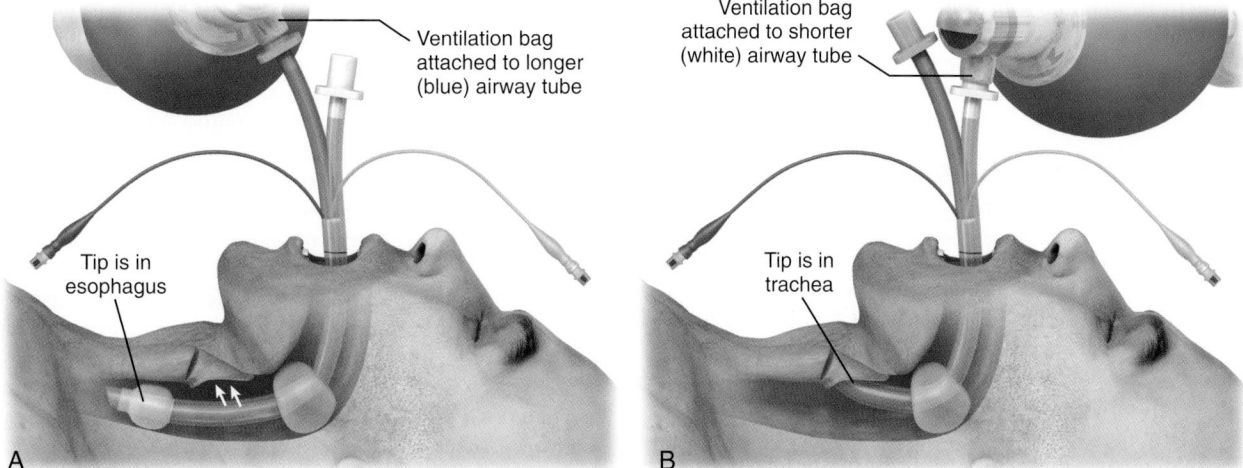

Figure 3-13 Combitube. **A,** About 95% of placements are esophageal, so begin ventilation through the longer (*blue*) airway tube. Use chest rise, breath sounds, and capnography to assess for proper placement. When the distal tip is in the esophagus, ventilation occurs through the vent holes between the distal and proximal cuffs (*white arrows*). **B,** If the tip of the Combitube is in the trachea, ventilation cannot be accomplished via the long (*blue*) airway tube. It is essential to recognize this quickly and use the short (*white*) tube for ventilation.

end up in the esophagus in about 95% of cases and in the trachea in about 5% (Fig. 3-13). The longer lumen or tube is used for ventilation when the tip is in the esophagus. It is perforated at the level of the pharynx and occluded at the distal end. The shorter lumen or tube is used for ventilation when the tip is in the trachea. It is open at the distal end, like a standard ET tube. The large proximal cuff or balloon is designed to occlude the pharynx by filling the space between the base of the tongue and the soft palate. The small distal cuff serves as a seal in either the esophagus or the trachea.[225-230]

The Combitube provides adequate ventilation in about 95% of patients when placed by prehospital providers.[225,229,230] When the Combitube is placed by physicians, the success rate approaches 100%.[231] It compares favorably with the ET tube with respect to ventilation and oxygenation in cardiac arrest situations.[223,228] In unconscious patients, the Combitube may provide protection from aspiration.[232]

Indications and Contraindications

The Combitube is a good choice as a primary airway in patients who are unresponsive or in cardiac arrest, especially in the uncontrolled prehospital environment. The Combitube can also be used in any emergency airway setting for rescue ventilation after failed BMV or failed intubation. In cases of failed intubation with an unexpectedly difficult airway, the Combitube may be used to provide adequate ventilation and allow time for other methods of intubation or a controlled surgical airway.[233,234] The Combitube should not be used in patients with an intact gag reflex and is not recommended in patients shorter than 4 feet. It is contraindicated in patients with suspected caustic poisoning or proximal esophageal disorders.

Placement of the Combitube

The Combitube is available in two sizes. The manufacturer recommends the smaller 37-Fr device for patients 4 feet to 5 feet 6 inches tall and the larger 41-Fr device for patient taller than 5 feet 6 inches. Studies suggest that the smaller 37-Fr Combitube can be used safely in patients up to about 6 feet tall.[235,236] The larger 41-Fr device is appropriate for patients taller than 6 feet.

To insert the Combitube, hold the device in the dominant hand and gently advance it caudally into the pharynx while grasping the tongue and jaw between the thumb and index finger of the nondominant hand. Pass the tube blindly along the tongue to a depth that places the printed rings on the proximal end of the tube between the patient's teeth and the alveolar ridge.[237] If resistance is met in the hypopharynx, remove the tube and bend it between the balloons for several seconds to facilitate insertion.[237] After insertion, fill the pharyngeal balloon with 100 mL of air and the distal cuff with 10 to 15 mL of air. The large pharyngeal balloon serves to securely seat the Combitube in the oropharynx and create a closed system in the case of esophageal placement. Because about 95% of placements are esophageal, begin ventilation through the longer (blue) airway tube.[230]

Use chest rise, good breath sounds, and capnography, without gastric inflation, to confirm proper ventilation. Alternatively, use a Wee-type aspirator device on the shorter (clear) lumen to confirm that the tip is in the esophagus before ventilation through the longer (blue) lumen.[238] An inability to easily aspirate air confirms esophageal placement. Easy aspiration with the Wee-type device indicates tracheal positioning of the tube and requires changing the ventilation to the shorter (clear) tracheal lumen.

If there is confusion about the location of the Combitube tip, use capnography to ensure that the correct airway tube is being ventilated. Capnography may be confusing in cases of cardiac arrest.

If the Combitube is in the esophageal position, suction the stomach by passing a catheter through the shorter (clear) lumen into the stomach while the patient is being ventilated via the longer (blue) lumen.[230]

Complications

Inappropriate balloon inflation and incorrect Combitube placement can lead to air leaks during ventilation. The most common placement error is an improper insertion angle. Use a more caudal, longitudinal direction of insertion as opposed to an anteroposterior direction of insertion. The Combitube must also be maintained in the true midline position during insertion to avoid blind pockets in the supraglottic area, which can prevent passage of the tube.[230] Attention to aligning the ring markings on the tube at the level of the incisors ensures proper positioning of the tube.

DECISION MAKING IN EMERGENCY AIRWAY MANAGEMENT

The airway provider must have many tools readily available to deal with an acutely compromised airway. It is important to be proficient in a number of different techniques and to tailor their use to the needs of the individual patient. Rescuers should practice potential scenarios before facing patients with a compromised airway. Failure to do so may lead to unnecessarily aggressive management in some situations or to irreversible hypoxic injury as a result of hesitation in others. Deciding who requires a definitive airway and who needs only supportive measures is a formidable task for even the most skilled clinician.

The following parameters should be assessed before the decision is made to establish a definitive airway:

- Adequacy of current ventilation
- Potential for hypoxia
- Airway patency
- Need for neuromuscular blockade (uncooperative, full stomach, teeth clenching)
- Cervical spine stability
- Safety of the technique and skill of the operator

Consideration of these factors should guide the clinician in selecting the optimal technique. Choosing the initial approach is often straightforward. Difficulty arises precipitously when the initial approach fails. Time becomes critical as the risk for irreversible hypoxic injury and cardiac arrest rises. Anxiety then increases and the potential for error increases. Forethought and practice are invaluable when managing these situations.

Rapid-Sequence Intubation

RSI in anesthesia has evolved since the introduction of succinylcholine in 1951. RSI was initially used as an abbreviation for rapid-sequence induction but is now synonymous with rapid-sequence intubation. Initially, the main purpose of RSI was to decrease the risk for aspiration in patients with full stomachs who needed emergency intubation. RSI has now become the most common method of emergency airway management because it provides optimal conditions for direct laryngoscopy.[14,239-243] Providers using RSI must appreciate the importance of basic skills such as preoxygenation, patient positioning, and BMV.

Emergency providers should be very careful to not use RSI in a cavalier manner. When giving a paralytic agent, the provider takes complete responsibility for airway maintenance, ventilation, and oxygenation of the patient. Consider awake intubation in patients with known difficult airways. RSI is contraindicated in patients who cannot be orally intubated. It should be avoided in patients with laryngotracheal abnormalities caused by tumors, infection, edema, or a history of cervical radiation therapy.

One of the most important concepts to appreciate when using RSI is that of optimal laryngoscopy to maximize first-pass success.[244-246] Preparation, preoxygenation, proper patient positioning, anterior neck maneuvers, and good laryngoscopy skills are all important components of optimal laryngoscopy (see Chapter 4). Just as important as optimal laryngoscopy is the ability to recognize when laryngoscopy (or any technique) has failed and it is time to move to a different approach. It is easier to take a different approach when you follow a simple preconceived algorithm. Patient safety during RSI depends on the provider's ability to maintain ventilation and oxygenation if the first attempt at intubation fails.[246] In this situation, BMV restores oxygenation and keeps the patient stable enough for further intubation attempts. Therefore, the importance of BMV skills cannot be overstated, and mastery of this skill alleviates much of the anxiety associated with difficult emergency airways and improves the chance for successful RSI.[3] Also, it is critical to have an EGA device immediately available during every RSI in the event that BMV is difficult or impossible. Finally, all providers who perform RSI should be prepared to perform a surgical airway when all other procedures and devices fail.

Difficult Airways, Failed Intubation, and When to Avoid Rapid-Sequence Intubation

The term *difficult airway* is popular, but there is no standard definition of this term. It is most commonly used to describe patients who are difficult to intubate with direct laryngoscopy. Subsequently, there has been a significant amount of literature dedicated to predicting difficult direct laryngoscopy. However, even in the best circumstances only about half the instances of difficult laryngoscopy can be predicted.[247] Many factors such as Mallampati scoring and measurement of thyromental distance have not been found to accurately predict difficult laryngoscopy, especially in the emergency setting.[247-250] Only obvious anatomic and pathologic abnormalities and a history of difficult intubation are accurate predictors of difficult laryngoscopy (see Chapter 4).[248]

In the emergency setting it is more useful to think of difficult airways as situations in which our usual methods of ventilation and intubation fail. Our goal should be to avoid RSI in patients who cannot be ventilated with a bag-mask device and cannot be intubated by direct or video laryngoscopy. Risk factors for difficult or impossible BMV have been well studied and include the presence of a beard, obesity, lack of teeth, age older than 55 years, a history of snoring, short thyromental distance, and limited mandibular protrusion (see Box 3-2).[110-113] Interestingly, one recent study showed that patients who were difficult to ventilate with a face mask usually became easier to ventilate when paralytic agents were administered and that none had worsened ventilation quality when paralyzed.[114] Regardless, the realization that we cannot predict all cases of failed BMV and failed laryngoscopy mandates the need for a simple preconceived algorithm that uses proven rescue techniques that are applicable to a broad range of clinical scenarios, such as the bougie and the LMA Fastrach. The value of the bougie is indisputable, and it is clear that use of the LMA Fastrach after failed RSI has decreased the frequency of failed airways and the need for surgical airways (Fig. 3-14).* Finally, if RSI is our usual method of intubation, we must be prepared to perform a surgical airway when laryngoscopy, BMV, and backup devices fail.[2,5]

---

*References 5, 114, 180, 182, 186, 251-254.

Figure 3-14 A, This morbidly obese patient was found asystolic by the emergency medical service. She could not be intubated in the field with multiple attempts and did not survive bag-mask resuscitation. This patient is a candidate for a laryngeal mask airway (LMA). **B-D,** The LMA is inserted by depressing the jaw, introduced, advanced, inflated, and attached to an Ambu bag. Postmortem ventilation with the LMA was very easy. In retrospect, the LMA device *should have been the first airway adjunct chosen* by EMS (and in the ED), totally bypassing attempts with other methods likely to fail.

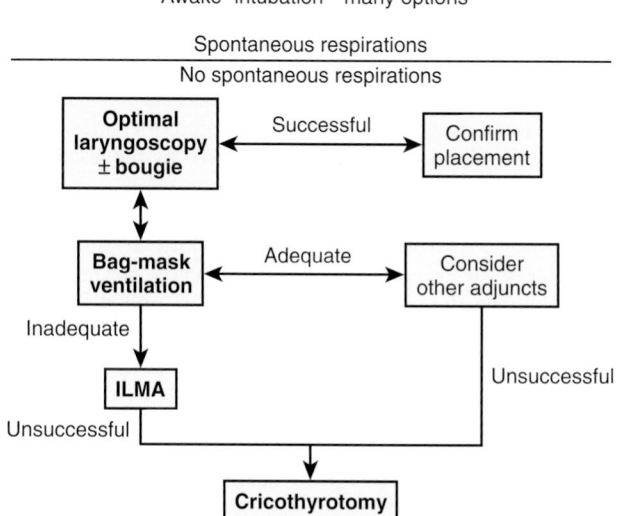

Figure 3-15 Emergency airway management algorithm used at Hennepin County Medical Center. The end point of the algorithm is successful tracheal intubation. This algorithm is presented as an example. Individuals and institutions should formulate their own algorithms based on technical skills and the availability of resources.

Emergency Airway Management Algorithm

The algorithm presented here summarizes the general approach used in the Department of Emergency Medicine at Hennepin County Medical Center (Fig. 3-15, Box 3-3). This algorithm is presented as an example. Individual providers and institutions should determine their own algorithms based on the availability of skills and resources. There are many similarities between this algorithm and those put forth by the American Society of Anesthesiologists and the Difficult Airway Society.[141,142] However, this algorithm is simpler and more applicable to emergency airway management. Most published airway algorithms are not ideal for emergency airway management because they do not account for the

BOX 3-3	Intubation Methods for Emergency Airway Management
Flexible fiberoptics (bronchoscope)	Intubating laryngeal mask airway
Video laryngoscope	Optical stylet
Video/optical laryngoscope with a tube channel	Blind nasal
	Retrograde

conditions that are commonly encountered: patients with full stomachs who are critically ill and often uncooperative, and intubations that cannot be canceled if the airway is too difficult. Also, many algorithms resemble wish lists of equipment and skills that are simply not available to many emergency airway providers. Our algorithm is based on the concept that oxygenation, not intubation, is the key.[255] It stresses well-proven concepts, procedures, and devices, and it is modeled after a simple algorithm developed by Combes and colleagues that was validated in a large prospective study.[5,180,254]

CONCLUSION

Good basic airway skills, a clear preconceived plan, and availability of proven rescue devices are the keys to emergency airway management. There are many techniques and devices that can be used to manage emergency airways. In difficult situations, providers will probably have the best success with procedures and devices with which they have familiarity and comfort.

Acknowledgment

The authors would like to thank Robb Poutre for his assistance with this chapter.

References are available at www.expertconsult.com

CHAPTER 4

Tracheal Intubation

Robert F. Reardon, John W. McGill, and Joseph E. Clinton

Intubation is often the pivotal procedure in the emergency management of critically ill patients. There are several new devices that can improve the likelihood of successful intubation, but it is important to understand that intubation is just one aspect of airway management. The primary objective of airway management is to maintain adequate oxygenation. Intubation allows oxygenation once it is completed, but not during the procedure.[1] A comprehensive approach, such as the algorithm described in Chapter 3, is crucial (see Fig. 3-15).[2] In the emergency setting it is important to use intubation techniques that have a high likelihood of success, critically recognizing when a given approach has failed and quickly moving to a different technique.

This chapter describes nearly every possible means of tracheal intubation, with emphasis on widely used techniques. The most common means of intubation in the emergency setting is rapid-sequence intubation (RSI), but this approach must be considered very carefully.[3] If a difficult intubation is anticipated, awake intubation may be preferred. With good topical anesthesia, nearly any intubating technique can be used for awake intubation, although flexible fiberoptic devices are commonly used. Because many difficult airways cannot be predicted, it is essential to have a well-defined backup plan and appropriate resources. The intubating laryngeal mask airway (LMA Fastrach) is an ideal backup device for failed RSI because it provides ventilation and oxygenation and facilitates tracheal intubation in a high percentage of patients with failed RSI.[2]

GENERAL APPROACH TO EMERGENCY INTUBATION

Preplanning is the key to successful emergency airway management. Providers should follow a clear, preconceived, practiced airway algorithm that uses readily available and familiar equipment and techniques. When encountering a difficult airway, it is more important to be comfortable with a few well-proven devices and techniques than to try new or unfamiliar devices.[2,4] It is important to know when to abandon one approach and move on to the next. *No single approach is mandated. The best technique is the one chosen by the clinician at the bedside based on one's individual experience and expertise and the specific clinical scenario.*

A critical aspect of preparation is making sure that all essential equipment required to perform the airway maneuvers is immediately available and within easy access. This may be accomplished by wall-mounting essential equipment in the emergency department (ED) resuscitation room.[5] Alternatively, equipment can be placed in dedicated adult and pediatric airway carts or tackle boxes in an open, organized, and labeled manner, and the carts and boxes checked regularly and stocked (Fig. 4-1).[6] Essential equipment that is seldom used

but is potentially lifesaving should be clearly identified and placed in an easily accessible location such as a dedicated difficult airway cart. The importance of this concept cannot be overstated. Technical expertise cannot substitute for the lack of essential equipment. In airway management, failure has ominous consequences. Mental, physical, and equipment preparation maximizes the chance of success.

AIRWAY ANATOMY

An understanding of airway anatomy and its terminology is requisite for any discussion of airway management procedures (Fig. 4-2). The following terms are used frequently in this chapter:

Pharynx: the upper part of the throat posterior to the nasal cavity, mouth, and larynx
1. *Nasopharynx*: base of the skull to the soft palate
2. *Oropharynx*: soft palate to the epiglottis
3. *Hypopharynx*: epiglottis to the cricoid ring (posteriorly), including the piriform sinus/recess/fossa

Piriform sinus/recess/fossa: the pockets on both sides of the laryngeal inlet separated from the larynx by the aryepiglottic folds

Larynx: the anterior structures of the throat (commonly called the voice box) from the tip of the epiglottis to the inferior border of the cricoid cartilage, including the laryngeal inlet

Laryngeal inlet: the opening to the larynx bounded anterosuperiorly by the epiglottis, laterally by the aryepiglottic folds, and posteriorly by the arytenoid cartilage

Arytenoid/posterior cartilage: the posterior aspect of the laryngeal inlet separating the glottis (anterior) from the esophagus (posterior)
1. *Corniculate cartilage*: the medial portion of the arytenoid/posterior cartilage
2. *Cuneiform cartilage*: the lateral prominence of the arytenoid/posterior cartilage
3. *Interarytenoid notch*: the notch between the posterior cartilage

Glottis: the vocal apparatus, including the true and false cords and the glottic opening

Vallecula: the space between the base of the tongue and the epiglottis

Hyoepiglottic ligament: anterior midline ligament connecting the epiglottis to the hyoid bone

PREPARATION

Intubation is best accomplished with two operators, one to perform the intubation and the other to handle equipment, help with positioning, observe the monitor, and keep track of time. *Unfortunately, the ideal scenario and adequate time for preparation are not always available to the clinician, who has to make calculated adjustments based on the situation at hand.* Before intubating, it is preferable to take the following steps in chronologic order: (1) attach the necessary monitoring devices and administer oxygen, (2) establish intravenous access, (3) draw up essential medications and label them if time permits, (4) confirm that the intubation equipment is available and functioning, (5) reassess oxygenation and maximize preoxygenation, (6) position the patient correctly, and (7) make sure that all team members are aware of the primary

Figure 4-1 A, Adult airway cart. Equipment and materials are visible, labeled, and accessible. **B,** Labeling is especially important because it lets you know what is missing. *(Concept of Dr. Ernest Ruiz, Department of Emergency Medicine, Hennepin County Medical Center, Minneapolis.)*

Nasal septum
Nasopharynx
Soft palate

Hard palate
Oral cavity

Palatine tonsil
Body of tongue
Oropharynx
Lingual tonsil

Epiglottis
Mandible

Hyoid bone

Thyrohyoid membrane
Laryngeal inlet (aditus)
Thyroid cartilage
Vocal fold
Cricoid cartilage
Trachea
Esophagus
Thyroid gland

Manubrium of sternum

Base of tongue
Vallecula
Epiglottis
Vocal cord
Aryepiglottic fold
Piriform fossa
Cuniform cartilage
Corniculate cartilage
Arytenoid cartilage
Posterior

Figure 4-2 A, Anatomy of the upper airway. **B,** View of the larynx, epiglottis, and vocal cords seen with a laryngoscope. *(A, Netter illustration used with permission of Elsevier, Inc. All rights reserved.)*

BOX 4-1 **Suggested Preintubation Checklist**

1. Ask an assistant to monitor O_2 saturation and vital signs and to remind the intubator how much time has elapsed without ventilation.
2. Be sure that an intravenous infusion is running properly. Administer oxygen to the patient.
3. Draw up the necessary drugs (e.g., lidocaine, paralyzing agent, induction agent).
4. Attach the bag-valve-mask device to an oxygen source (rate of 15 L/min).
5. Insert a stylet into the tracheal tube and have a "straight to cuff" shape with a 35-degree distal bend.
6. Check the integrity of the balloon and cuff on the tracheal tube.
7. Have tape, twill tape, or a commercial tube stabilizer available.
8. Check the laryngoscope light source. Have a second light source, a selection of blades, and additional endotracheal (ET) tubes available.
9. Turn on the oral suction device and place it so that it is immediately available near the clinician's right hand. Prepare the catheter suction for postintubation use.
10. Place a syringe, to inflate the ET tube balloon, on the bed to the right of the patient's head.
11. If the patient is not pharmacologically paralyzed, restrain the hands.
12. Remove the patient's dentures (delay this action until immediately before intubation if the patient is undergoing bag-mask ventilation).
13. Position the patient in the sniffing position (conditions permitting). Facilitate this by placing a towel under the patient's occiput to raise it 10 cm. Obese patients usually require significantly more elevation of the occiput.
14. Have waveform capnography on and ready to connect immediately after intubation or an aspiration device for detection of the esophagus if capnography is not available.

---

procedural approach and the most likely backup plan. In the haste of the moment, it is a common error to forget to preoxygenate or to position the patient optimally. Simple omissions, such as failing to restrain the patient's hands or remove the patient's dentures or misplacing the suction tip, can seriously hamper the success of the procedure. One suggested preintubation checklist is presented in Box 4-1. In addition, be sure to use universal precautions by wearing gloves, a gown, and eye and mouth protection.

PREOXYGENATION

Preoxygenation is one the most important aspects of emergency airway management. Preoxygenation before RSI provides much more time for intubation before desaturation occurs and thus significantly increases the chance for successful intubation on the first attempt. Failure to preoxygenate before RSI is often a critical factor when a straightforward emergency airway becomes an unexpected airway problem. Preoxygenate by providing the maximal fraction of inspired oxygen (FIO_2) with a non-rebreather mask for 3 to 5 minutes before intubation. Alternatively, give eight vital capacity breaths from a maximal FIO_2 system, such as a non-rebreather mask or a bag-valve-mask device, if there is not enough time for standard preoxygenation.[7] When using a bag-valve-mask device for preoxygenation it is important for the exhalation port to have a one-way valve so that room air is not drawn into the mask when the patient inhales.

The purpose of preoxygenation is not solely to maximize oxygen saturation, but also to wash out nitrogen from the patient's lungs and replace it with oxygen. This provides the maximum safe apneic time during RSI. Those at greatest risk for rapid desaturation include obese, pregnant, critically ill, and pediatric patients, and they will benefit the most from appropriate preoxygenation. Most studies addressing preoxygenation have been conducted under ideal conditions on relatively healthy individuals. It is far more challenging to effectively preoxygenate critically ill patients.[8]

Morbidly obese patients are best preoxygenated in a 25-degree head-up position because significantly higher oxygen tension can be achieved with this position.[9] Patients who are hypoxic despite maximal oxygen delivery have been shown to benefit from 3 minutes of noninvasive positive pressure ventilation (NPPV) with 100% O_2 just before intubation.[10,11]

Sometimes patients who will benefit the most from preoxygenation are uncooperative with a face mask because of delirium from hypoxia, hypercapnia, or other factors. These patients may benefit from delayed-sequence intubation: careful sedation without suppression of respirations, and oxygenation with a face mask or NPPV for 2 to 3 minutes before administration of a paralytic agent.[11] Ketamine (1 to 1.5 mg/kg by slow intravenous push) has been suggested for this technique. Delayed-sequence intubation is a commonsense way to deal with a difficult problem, but it has not been well studied and providers using this method should be ready for hypoventilation or apnea.

Another method to delay desaturation during RSI is nasopharyngeal oxygen insufflation during apnea. Many studies have shown that providing oxygen therapy during apnea is much more beneficial than previously considered.[12-15] During apnea, oxygen continues to be absorbed through the alveoli, and thus air with a low oxygen concentration remains in the lower airways. Supplying oxygen to the nasopharynx during apnea allows air with a higher oxygen concentration to passively replenish oxygen in the alveoli. In two studies of patients undergoing RSI, nasopharyngeal oxygen insufflation significantly delayed desaturation after the onset of apnea in both normal and morbidly obese patients.[12,15] In these studies, nasopharyngeal oxygen insufflation was accomplished by inserting a 10-Fr catheter into the nasopharynx to a distance equal to that from the mouth to the tragus of the ear and delivering oxygen at a flow rate of 5 L/min when apnea occurred.[12] Using a standard nasal cannula with a nasopharyngeal airway is simpler and would probably provide the same benefit. It is important to keep the upper airway open with a jaw thrust or artificial airway for this technique to be most beneficial.

ASSESSING FOR A DIFFICULT AIRWAY

When trying to predict whether there will be difficulty during emergency intubation, it is important to understand that most of the literature on prediction of difficult laryngoscopy does not apply very well in the emergency setting. A study by Levitan and colleagues in 2004 showed that two thirds of patients who were intubated in their ED via RSI could not be assessed with the most common difficult airway prediction tests (Mallampati scoring, measurement of thyromental distance, and neck mobility testing) because of altered mental status or cervical spine immobilization.[16] Even in the best circumstances, only about half of cases of difficult laryngoscopy can be predicted.[17] Many factors such as Mallampati scoring and measurement of thyromental distance have not been found to accurately predict difficult laryngoscopy, especially in the emergency setting.[16-19] Only obvious anatomic and pathologic abnormalities and a history of difficult intubation are accurate predictors of difficult laryngoscopy.[16] The American Society of Anesthesiology Difficult Airway Guidelines state that "in patients with no gross upper airway pathology or anatomic anomaly, there is insufficient published evidence to evaluate the effect of a physical examination on predicting the presence of a difficult airway."[20] This does not mean that emergency providers should ignore factors that are known to be associated with difficult laryngoscopy, but these must be placed in perspective.

No examination finding alone can predict difficult laryngoscopy, but a combination of multiple factors makes difficulty more likely. The classic predictors of difficult intubation include a history of previous difficult intubation, prominent upper incisors, limited ability to extend at the atlanto-occipital joint,[21] poor visibility of pharyngeal structures when the patient extends the tongue (Mallampati classification or the tongue-pharyngeal ratio) (Fig. 4-3A),[22] limited ability to open the mouth (suggested by a space less than three fingerbreadths between the upper and lower incisors),[23] short thyromental distance (<6 cm from the thyroid notch to the chin with the neck in extension) (Fig. 4-3B),[24] and a limited direct laryngoscopic view of the laryngeal inlet (Fig. 4-4).[23] A relatively new test is the upper lip bite test, which has been shown in some studies to be more accurate and specific than older tests.[25-27] It is essentially a test of anterior mandibular mobility, and the less mobility, the more difficult it is to intubate the patient. Upper lip bite criteria are as follows: class I, the lower incisors can bite the upper lip above the vermillion line; class II, the lower incisors can bite the upper lip below the vermillion line; and class III, the lower incisors cannot bite the upper lip.[25] Interestingly, a 2008 study by Tremblay and associates identified factors predictive of difficult GlideScope intubation, which included a high Cormack-Lehane grade during direct laryngoscopy, short thyromental distance, and high upper lip bite test score.[28]

As noted earlier, many of these predictors cannot be assessed in the emergency setting.[16] Fortunately, some of the key predictors are apparent simply by observing the external appearance of the patient's head and neck. Patients with neck tumors, thermal or chemical burns, traumatic injuries involving the face and anterior aspect of the neck, angioedema, infection of pharyngeal and laryngeal soft tissues, or previous operations in or around the airway suggest a difficult intubation because distorted anatomy or secretions may compromise visualization of the vocal cords. Facial or skull fractures may further limit airway options by precluding nasotracheal

Figure 4-3 A, The Mallampati classification predicts intubation difficulty based on the visibility of intraoral structures. Classes III and IV predict difficult intubation. **B,** A short thyromental distance (less than 6 cm or 3 fingerbreadths) *when the head is extended* predicts difficult intubation. *(A, From Kryger MH. Sleep breathing disorders: examination of the patient with suspected sleep apnea. In: Kryger MH, ed: Kryger Atlas of Clinical Sleep Medicine. Philadelphia: Elsevier; 2010.)*

(NT) intubation. Patients with ankylosing arthritis or developmental abnormalities such as a hypoplastic mandible or the large tongue of Down's syndrome are difficult to intubate because neck rigidity and problems of tongue displacement can obscure visualization of the glottis.

Besides these obvious congenital and pathologic conditions, the presence of a short, thick neck is one of the more

Figure 4-4 Cormack and Lehane grading of laryngeal views during laryngoscopy. **A**, Grade I. Most of the glottis is visible. **B**, Grade II. The posterior aspect of the glottis is visible. **C**, Grade 3. Only the epiglottis is seen; no part of the laryngeal inlet is visible. **D**, Grade IV. The epiglottis is not visible. Patients with grades I and II are usually easy to intubate with direct laryngoscopy, whereas those with grades III and IV are often difficult; the ability to see the arytenoid cartilage is the important difference.

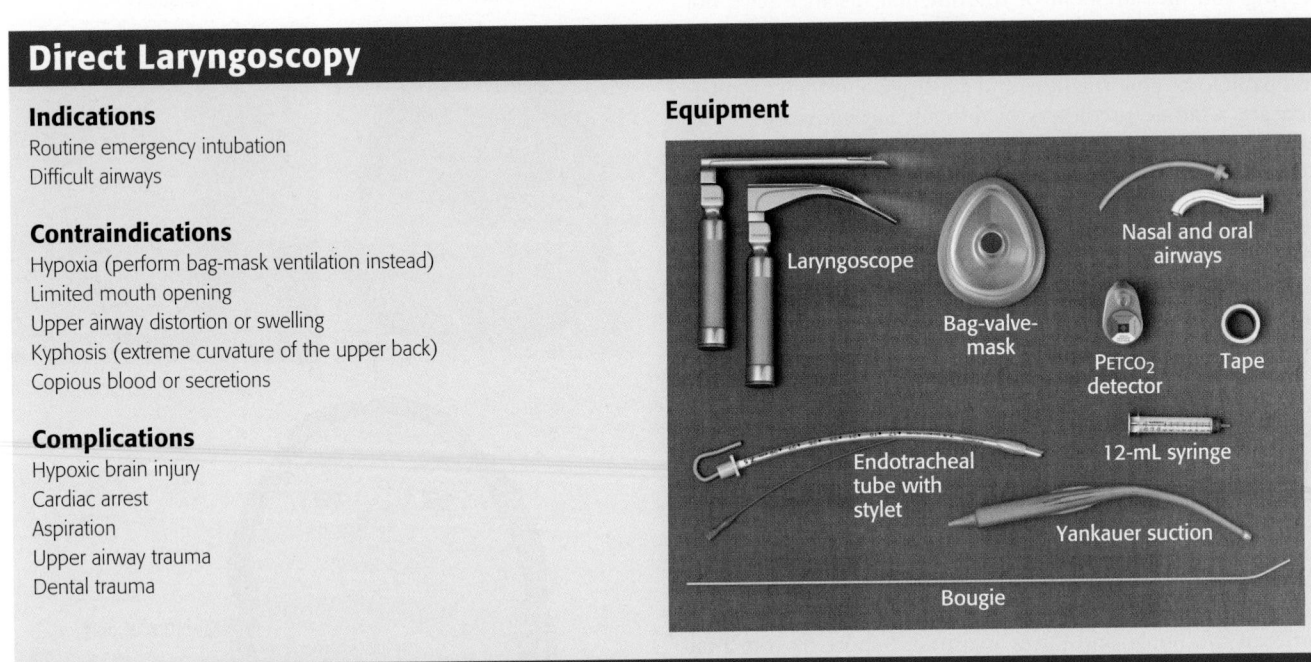

Direct Laryngoscopy

Indications
Routine emergency intubation
Difficult airways

Contraindications
Hypoxia (perform bag-mask ventilation instead)
Limited mouth opening
Upper airway distortion or swelling
Kyphosis (extreme curvature of the upper back)
Copious blood or secretions

Complications
Hypoxic brain injury
Cardiac arrest
Aspiration
Upper airway trauma
Dental trauma

Equipment
Laryngoscope
Bag-valve-mask
Nasal and oral airways
PETCO$_2$ detector
Tape
Endotracheal tube with stylet
12-mL syringe
Yankauer suction
Bougie

Review Box 4-1 Direct laryngoscopy: indications, contraindications, complications, and equipment.

common predictors of a difficult airway. Such individuals are easily identifiable by observing the head and neck in profile. Obesity alone may not be an independent predictor of difficult intubation, but obese patients with large-circumference necks are likely to be difficult to intubate.[29] Facial hair can complicate a difficult airway by rendering bag-mask ventilation ineffective because of the lack of a good mask seal. One patient type that does not immediately stand out as a difficult intubation—but can be surprisingly so—is a patient with an unusually long mandibulohyoid distance (the thyroid prominence appearing low in the neck) and a short mandibular ramus.[30] Visualization of the larynx is difficult because of the distance to the larynx and the relative hypopharyngeal location of the tongue.

Knowledge of the poor performance of difficult airway predictors should not make emergency providers more cavalier about using RSI; it should create more concern. The solution is not to avoid RSI, because lack of paralysis makes every intubation more difficult. Instead, it is essential to appreciate the critical importance of having a clear backup plan when intubation with RSI fails.[16,31] This situation mandates the need for a preconceived algorithm that uses proven rescue techniques applicable to a broad range of clinical scenarios, such as the bougie (flexible intubating stylet) and the LMA Fastrach.[2] The value of the bougie is indisputable, and it is clear that using the LMA Fastrach after failed RSI has decreased the frequency of failed airways and the need for surgical intervention.[2,4,32-38] Finally, if RSI is the "go to" method for emergency intubation, providers must be prepared to perform a surgical airway when laryngoscopy, bag-mask ventilation, and backup devices fail.[2,39]

DIRECT LARYNGOSCOPY

Despite the proliferation of approaches and devices designed to secure a definitive airway, direct laryngoscopy remains the mainstay of tracheal intubation. The equipment is simple and the approach direct. Visual confirmation of the tube going through the vocal cords is usually possible.

Indications and Contraindications

Direct laryngoscopy is indicated in any clinical situation in which a definitive emergency airway is necessary, including

Figure 4-5 Macintosh (**A**) and Miller (**B**) laryngoscope blades.

TABLE 4-1 Tracheal Tube Sizes for Average Patients*

AGE	INTERNAL DIAMETER (mm)	EQUIVALENT TRACHEOTOMY TUBE SIZE
Children		
Newborn	2.5	00
6 mo	3.5	00-0
1 yr	4.5	0-1
2 yr	5.0	1-2
4 yr	5.5	2
6 yr	6.0	3
8 yr	6.5	4
10 yr	7.0	4
12 yr	7.5	4
14 yr	8.0	5
Adults		
Female	7.0-8.0	5
Male	7.5-9.0	6
Special cases		8-10

Modified from Applebaum EL, Bruce DL, eds. *Tracheal Intubation*. Philadelphia: Saunders; 1976.
*A slightly smaller size may be required for nasotracheal intubation.

routine and difficult airways. Relative contraindications to direct laryngoscopy include limited mouth opening, upper airway distortion or swelling, severe kyphosis, or copious blood or secretions.

Equipment

Laryngoscope

There are two basic blade designs for direct laryngoscopy, curved (Macintosh) and straight (Miller) (Fig. 4-5). Each comes in various adult and pediatric blade sizes. Slight variations in laryngoscopic technique follow from the choice of blade design, and it is often a matter of personal preference. The tip of the straight blade goes under the epiglottis and lifts it directly, whereas the curved blade fits into the vallecula and indirectly lifts the epiglottis via engagement of the hyoepiglottic ligament to expose the larynx.

Each blade type has advantages and disadvantages. The straight blade is often a better choice in pediatric patients, in patients with an anterior larynx or a long floppy epiglottis, and in individuals whose larynx is fixed by scar tissue. It is less effective, however, in patients with prominent upper teeth, and it is more likely to damage dentition. Use of the straight blade is also more often associated with laryngospasm because it stimulates the superior laryngeal nerve, which innervates the undersurface of the epiglottis. A straight blade may inadvertently be advanced into the esophagus and initially reveal unfamiliar anatomy until it is withdrawn. The blade has a lightbulb at the tip, which may slightly hamper vision. The wider, curved blades are helpful in keeping the tongue retracted from the field of vision and allowing more room for passing the tube through the oropharynx, and they are generally preferred for uncomplicated adult intubations. Aside from patient considerations, some clinicians prefer the curved blade because they find that it requires less forearm strength than the straight blade does.

The illumination provided by the laryngoscope can make a big difference in the ability to visualize the laryngeal inlet. The importance of these factors is underappreciated, as demonstrated by Levitan[40] in a survey of the Macintosh blades used in 17 Philadelphia EDs. It was found that only 24% of all blades provided the brightness necessary for fine inspection. This finding was largely explained by the fact that the majority of EDs used the A-Mac (American) as opposed to the clearly superior brightness design of the G-Mac (German) or the intermediate brightness of the E-Mac (English).

Tracheal Tubes

The standard adult endotracheal (ET) tube measures approximately 30 cm in length. Tube size is typically printed prominently on the tube and is based on the internal diameter (ID) and measured in millimeters. The range is 2.0 to 10.0 mm in increments of 0.5 mm. The outer tube diameter is 2 to 4 mm larger than the internal diameter.[41] Tubes are also imprinted with a scale in centimeters that indicates the distance from a tube's distal tip.

Adult men can generally accept a 7.5- to 9.0-mm orotracheal tube, whereas women can usually be intubated with a 7.0- to 8.0-mm tube. Larger tubes are theoretically desirable because airway resistance increases as tube size decreases, but in practice, a 7.5-mm tube is adequate for almost all patients. In emergency intubations, particularly if a difficult intubation is anticipated, many clinicians choose a smaller tube and change to a larger tube later if necessary. Though generally an acceptable practice, this should be avoided in burn patients because swelling may prohibit subsequent tube placement. For nasal intubation, a slightly smaller (by 0.5 to 1.0 mm) tube may be easier to advance through the nasal passages.

Correct tube size is important in the pediatric population. It is especially important when using an uncuffed tube because a good seal is needed between the ET tube and the upper part of the trachea (Table 4-1). Since tube size is based on the ID, a cuffed tube should generally be a half size (0.5 mm) smaller than an uncuffed tube. The smaller ID of an appropriately sized, small cuffed tube could theoretically make it more prone to plugging from secretions. Cuffed tubes are available down as small as 3-mm ID, although indications for these tubes in neonates and infants are rare. A cuffed tube is used in children with decreased lung compliance who may require

Figure 4-6 Pediatric endotracheal (ET) tube size estimation using the fingernail width of the little finger. In children, a cuffed or uncuffed ET tube may be used. If an uncuffed ET tube is used for emergency intubation, it is reasonable to select a tube 3.5 mm in internal diameter (ID) for infants up to 1 year of age and a 4.0-mm-ID tube for patients between 1 and 2 years of age. If a cuffed tube is used for emergency intubation of an infant younger than 1 year, it is reasonable to select a 3.0-mm-ID tube. For children between 1 and 2 years of age, it is reasonable to use a cuffed ET tube with an ID of 3.5 mm After age 2, ET tube size can be estimated by the following formulas: estimated size of an *uncuffed* ET tube in millimeters = [4 + age]/4 and estimated size of a *cuffed* tube in millimeters = [3 + age]/4.

Figure 4-7 Comparison of the standard tracheal tube tip with the Parker Flex-Tip Tracheal Tube. *Note:* When a standard tube is inserted in the normal fashion, the bevel is oriented vertically and toward the patient's left. The Parker tube tip bevel faces posteriorly and may avoid getting caught on laryngeal structures. The flexible tip of the Parker tube also provides a closer fit on an introducer.

prolonged mechanical ventilation. In a child, the smallest airway diameter is at the cricoid ring rather than at the vocal cords, as in adults. Hence, a tube may pass the cords but go no farther. If this should occur, the next smaller size tube should be passed.

In children 2 years or older, the following formula is a highly accurate method for determining correct uncuffed and cuffed ET tube size:

$$\text{Uncuffed tube size (mm)} = [4 + \text{Age (yr)}]/4$$

$$\text{Cuffed tube size (mm)} = [3 + \text{Age (yr)}]/4$$

For most clinical situations, using the width of the nail of the little (fifth) finger as a guide is sufficiently accurate and has been shown to be more precise than finger diameter (Fig. 4-6).[42] A standard tracheal tube uses a high-volume, low-pressure cuff to avoid pressure necrosis the tracheal lining. A clinical test for determining correct cuff inflation is to slowly inject air until no air leak is audible while the patient is receiving bag-tube ventilation. This usually occurs with 5 to 8 mL of air if the proper size tracheal tube has been selected. Many clinicians use the tension of the pilot balloon as a guide to cuff inflation. Slight compressibility with gentle external pressure indicates adequate inflation for most clinical situations. For long-term use, cuff pressure should be measured and maintained at 20 to 25 mm Hg. Capillary blood flow is compromised in the tracheal mucosa when cuff pressure exceeds 30 mm Hg. In emergency situations, the balloon may simply be inflated with 10 mL of air and adjusted when the patient's condition has stabilized.

Interest in design of the tip of the tracheal tube has grown as the Seldinger technique is increasingly being applied to intubation. When a tracheal tube is passed over a smaller-caliber introducer (Seldinger technique), regardless of whether it is a tracheal tube introducer or a fiberoptic scope, there is a reasonable chance that the tube will get hung up on the laryngeal soft tissue.[43] A tracheal tube that has been designed to overcome this problem has a bevel oriented posteriorly and

a flexible tip that decreases the distance between the tube and whatever it is being passed over (Fig. 4-7).

Check the ET tube cuff for leaks by inflating the pilot balloon before attempting intubation. Prepare the tube for placement by passing a malleable stylet down the tube to increase its stiffness and enhance control of the tip of the tube. Do not extend the stylet beyond the eyelet of the tube. Bend the tube and stylet to create a "straight-to-cuff" shape with a 35-degree distal bend. Lubricate the tip and cuff of the tube with viscous lidocaine or a water-soluble gel.

Optimal Patient Positioning for Direct Laryngoscopy

The sniffing position, with the head extended on the neck and the neck flexed relative to the torso, has traditionally been considered the best head position for direct laryngoscopy.[44,45] This position aligns the oral, pharyngeal, and laryngeal axes (Fig. 4-8*A-C*). Horton and colleagues described the ideal sniffing position for normal patients as neck flexion of 35 degrees and atlanto-occipital extension such that the plane of the face is −15 degrees to the horizontal position (Fig. 4-8*C*).[46] In supine patients, neck flexion is achieved by head elevation. Depending on the size and shape of the patient, the amount of head elevation may differ significantly, and the end point should be horizontal alignment of the external auditory meatus with the sternum.[44,47-49] In normal-size adults it is usually possible to achieve the sniffing position with 7 to 10 cm of head elevation.[50,51] Morbidly obese patients require much more head elevation to achieve the proper sniffing position. In these patients, aligning the external auditory meatus with the sternum requires elevation of the head and neck, as well as the upper part of the back (Fig. 4-8*D*).[3,48,49,52] This can be accomplished by building a ramp of towels and pillows under the upper torso, head, and neck or by using a Troop Elevation Pillow (Mercury Medical, Clearwater, FL) or similar device (see Fig. 3-2).[3,48,49,52] Alternatively, elevating the head to a 25-degree backup position may achieve the same purpose.[53]

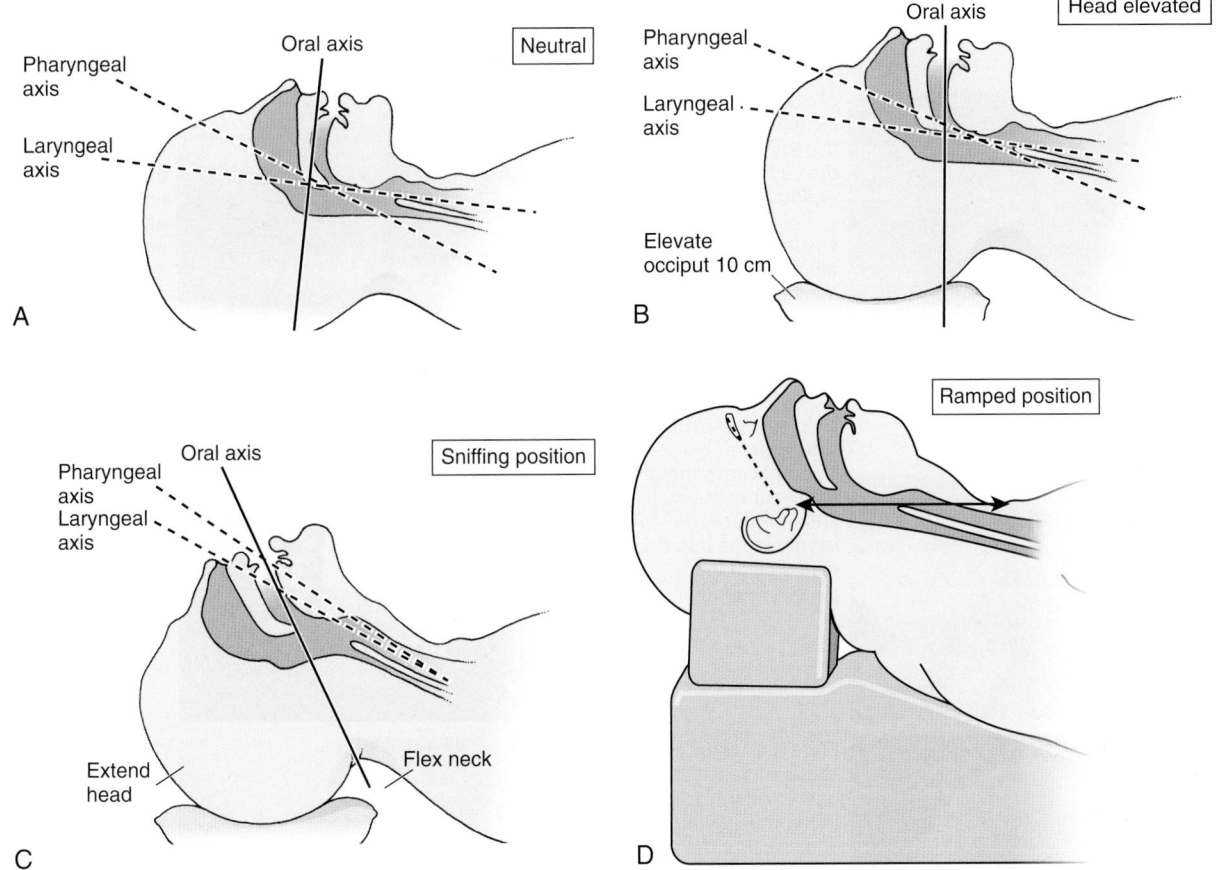

Figure 4-8 Head positioning for tracheal intubation. **A,** Neutral position. **B,** Head elevated. **C,** "Sniffing" position with a flexed neck and extended head. Note that flexing the neck while extending the head lines up the various axes and allows direct laryngoscopy. **D,** Morbidly obese patients are best intubated in a ramped position with elevation of the upper part of the back, neck, and head; the ideal position aligns the external auditory canal and the sternum.

Two studies have shown that elevating the head (flexing the neck) beyond the sniffing position often improves visualization of the glottis.[48,54] Because the amount of head elevation needed for optimal laryngoscopy varies depending on individual patient anatomy, it is important to make laryngoscopy a dynamic procedure. This is best accomplished by putting your right hand behind the patient's head to lift, flex, and extend the head as needed to bring the glottis into view.[55] Optimal positioning of the head and neck is not possible in trauma patients who require in-line stabilization of the cervical spine. This is one of the aspects that makes trauma airways so challenging and makes other maneuvers, such as external laryngeal manipulation, even more important in these patients.[55]

Procedure and Technique of Direct Laryngoscopy

Adults
Place the patient in the supine position with the head at the level of the lower part of the intubator's sternum (Fig. 4-9, *step 2*). To maintain the best mechanical advantage, keep your back straight and do not hunch over the patient; bend only at the knees (Fig. 4-10). Keep the left elbow relatively close to the body and flex it slightly to provide better support. In a severely dyspneic patient who cannot tolerate lying down, perform direct laryngoscopy with the patient seated semierect and the clinician on a step stool behind the patient.[56]

Grasp the laryngoscope in the left hand with the back end of the blade pressed into the hypothenar aspect of your hand. Draw the patient's lower lip down with your right thumb, and introduce the tip of the laryngoscope into the right side of the patient's mouth (Fig 4-9, *step 3*). Slide the blade along the right side of the tongue while gradually displacing the tongue toward the left as you move the blade to the center of the mouth (Fig. 4-9, *step 4*). If you initially place the blade in the middle of the tongue, it will fold over the lateral edge of the blade and obscure visualization of the airway. Placing the blade in the middle of the tongue and failing to move the tongue to the left are two common errors that prevent visualization of the vocal cords (Fig. 4-11).

As you move the tip of the blade toward the base of the tongue, exert force along the axis of the laryngoscope handle by lifting upward and forward at a 45-degree angle (Fig. 4-9, *step 6*). The direction of this force is critical because if the force is too horizontal or too vertical, poor visualization will result. The epiglottis should come into view with this maneuver. It may help to have an assistant retract the cheek laterally to further expose the laryngeal structures. Avoid bending the wrist because it can result in dental injury if the teeth are used as a fulcrum for the blade.

The step after visualization of the epiglottis depends on which laryngoscope blade is being used. With the curved blade, place the tip into the vallecula, the space between the base of the tongue and the epiglottis (Fig. 4-11*D*). Continued

DIRECT LARYNGOSCOPY

Check all equipment, including the light on the laryngoscope and the cuff on the endotracheal tube.

Ensure that suction and difficult airway devices are within reach.

Place patient in the sniffing position, elevate the bed so that the patient's head is at the level of the lower part of your sternum, and preoxygenate.

Hold laryngoscope with your left hand. Open patient's mouth with your right hand and introduce the laryngoscope into the right side of the patient's mouth.

Push the tongue to the left side of the mouth, slowly advance the blade, and progressively identify the base of the tongue, the epiglottis, and the posterior cartilages.

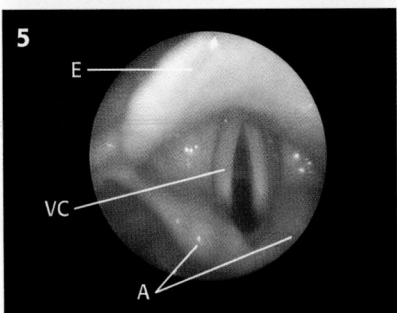

Place the Macintosh blade in the vallecula, or the Miller blade under the epiglottis (E), and visualize the vocal cords (VC) and arytenoid cartilages (A).

Do not take your eyes off of the cords once they are identified!

Lift in the direction of the laryngoscope handle.

Manipulate the thyroid cartilage to achieve optimal laryngeal exposure. Have an assistant maintain that position during intubation.

Instruct an assistant to retract the right cheek for better visualization. Pass the tube on the right side of the patient's mouth. *Do not allow the tube to obstruct your view of the vocal cords during advancement!*

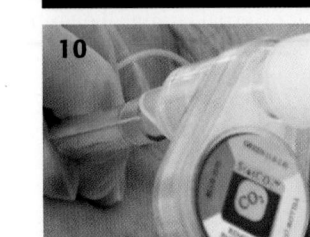

Under direct visualization, pass the tube 3–4 cm beyond the vocal cords.

Remove the stylet and inflate the pilot balloon.

Confirm proper placement with end-tidal CO_2 detection, ausculation, and a chest radiograph.

Figure 4-9 Direct laryngoscopy.

Assistant to watch the monitor, keep track of time, and monitor the patient's vital signs

Head far enough away to have binocular vision

Lift this way— aim to the junction of the ceiling and the far wall

Back straight

Left arm straight, not bent

Leads to the cardiac monitor

Essential drugs drawn and ready for use (syringes/medications)

Head elevated to 10 cm to flex neck

Patient's hands restrained

Connect to pulse oximetry

Bag-valve-mask device attached to oxygen—15 L/min

Suction tip under the mattress to the left side of the patient's head

Patient's head elevated to the level of the lower part of the intubator's sternum

Syringe for the tube cuff on the bed to the right of the patient's head

Figure 4-10 Proper positioning of the clinician, patient, and assistant for tracheal intubation. The following points are demonstrated: the difficult airway cart is adjacent to the patient, the suction device is at the head of the bed, the patient is in the "sniffing position" with the occiput elevated and the clinician's right hand ready for additional adjustment if necessary, the bed is elevated and the clinician is at the appropriate distance from the patient, and the laryngoscope handle is angled at 45 degrees.

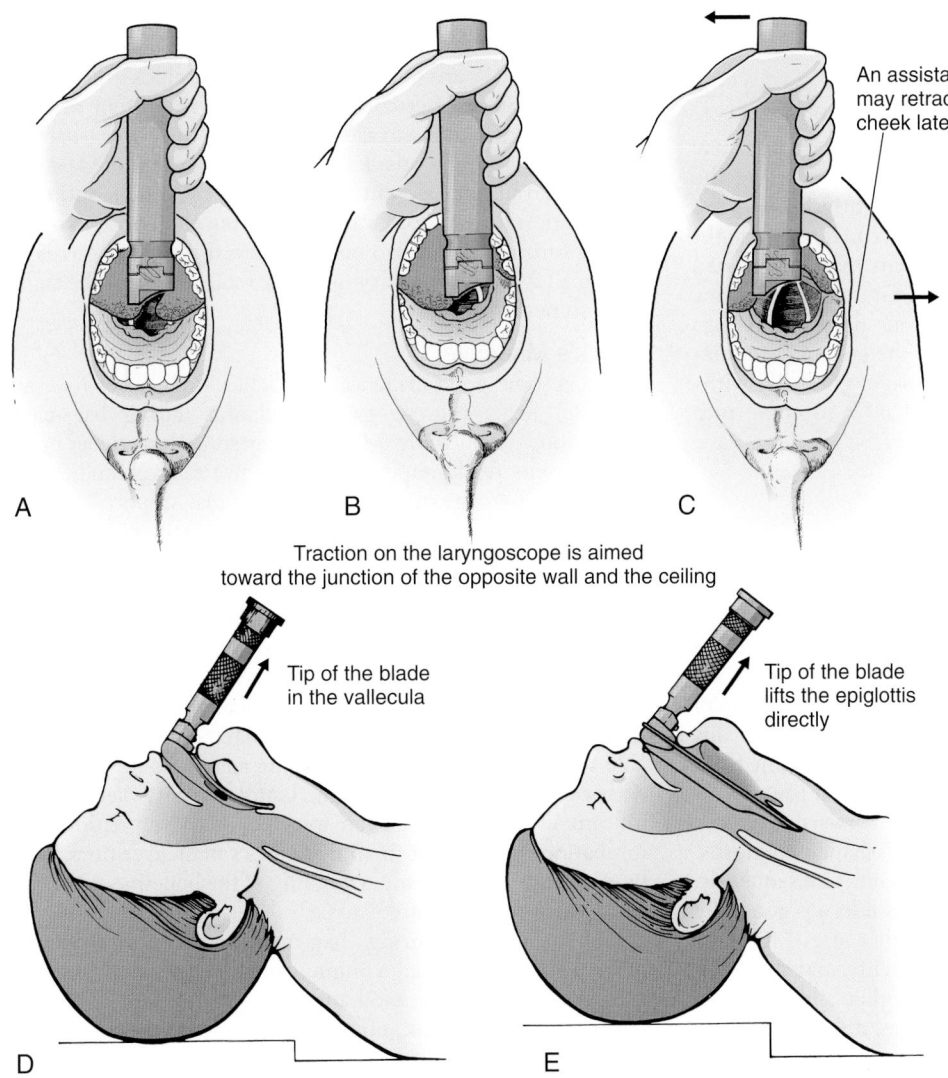

An assistant may retract the cheek laterally

A   B   C

Traction on the laryngoscope is aimed toward the junction of the opposite wall and the ceiling

Tip of the blade in the vallecula

Tip of the blade lifts the epiglottis directly

D   E

Anatomy

Figure 4-11 Common problems encountered when using a laryngoscope. **A,** The laryngoscope blade is under the middle of the tongue, with the sides of the tongue hanging down and obscuring the glottis. **B,** The tongue is not pushed far enough to the left and is obscuring the glottis. **C,** Correct blade position with the tongue elevated and to the left. **D,** Use of the curved (Macintosh) laryngoscope blade. **E,** Use of the straight (Miller) blade.

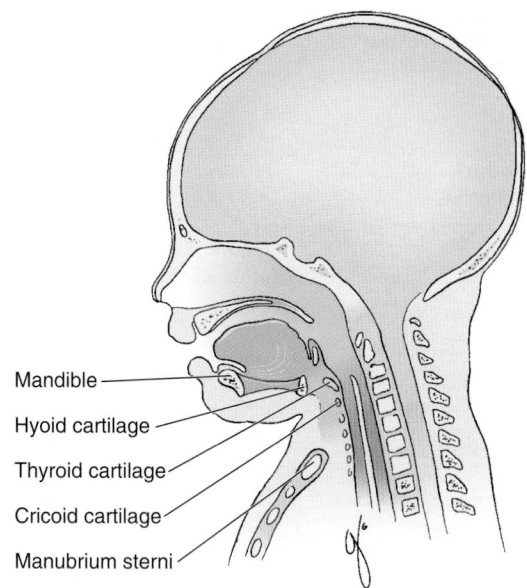

Figure 4-12 Sagittal section of the neck of an infant. Note that in small children, the neck is shorter and the larynx is located more cephalad. *(From Snell RS, Smith MS, eds.* Clinical Anatomy for Emergency Medicine. *St Louis: Mosby–Year Book; 1993:16.)*

anterior elevation of the base of the tongue and the epiglottis will expose the vocal cords. If the tip of the blade is inserted too deeply into the vallecula, the epiglottis may be pushed down and obscure the glottis.[22] When using the straight blade, insert the tip under and slightly beyond the epiglottis and directly lift it up (Fig. 4-11*E*). If the straight blade is placed too deeply, the entire larynx may be elevated anteriorly and out of the field of vision. Gradually withdraw the blade to allow the laryngeal inlet to drop down into view. If the blade is deep and posterior, the lack of recognizable structures indicates esophageal passage; gradually withdraw the blade to permit the laryngeal inlet to come into view.

Infants and Children
It is helpful to appreciate the anatomic differences between children and adults when intubating pediatric patients (Fig. 4-12 and Table 4-2). Children's proportionately larger heads naturally place them in the sniffing position, so a towel under the occiput is rarely necessary (Fig. 4-13). The large head of newborns can result in a posterior positioning of the larynx that prevents visualization of the vocal cords. A small towel under the infant's shoulders should correct this problem. The head may also be floppy and may benefit from stabilization by an assistant. The child's increased tongue-to-oropharynx ratio and shorter neck hinder forward displacement of the tongue and, coupled with a U-shaped epiglottis, can make visualization of the glottis difficult. Consequently, direct laryngoscopy in infants and young children is generally best performed with a straight blade: Miller size 0 for premature infants, size 1 for normal-sized infants, and size 2 for older children. The infant's larynx lies higher and relatively more anterior. If no laryngeal structures are visible after laryngeal pressure, gradually withdraw the blade. Inadvertent advancement of the blade into the esophagus is a common error.

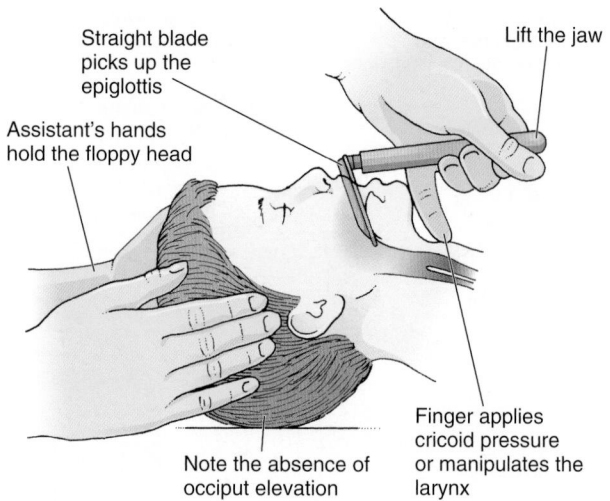

Figure 4-13 Oral intubation in a child with a straight blade. The proportionately large floppy head of a child may present some difficulty, and an assistant may be required to hold the child's head straight.

Sellick's Maneuver, External Laryngeal Manipulation, Bimanual Laryngoscopy, and BURP
The differences between Sellick's maneuver, external laryngeal manipulation (ELM), and backward, upward, rightward pressure (BURP) are often misunderstood. Sellick's maneuver is the application of cricoid pressure with the intent of preventing regurgitation and aspiration, not to improve visualization during laryngoscopy. ELM is the application of pressure on the thyroid cartilage during laryngoscopy to help optimize visualization of the glottis. BURP is often the best combination of forces that need to be applied to the thyroid cartilage during ELM. Bimanual laryngoscopy refers to use of the right hand to perform ELM.

Sellick's Maneuver
There is some good evidence that Sellick's maneuver (cricoid pressure) helps prevent gastric inflation during bag-mask ventilation.[57-62] The only evidence suggesting that cricoid pressure prevents regurgitation consists of five cadaver studies,[62-66] one small human study,[67] and some case reports[68]—poor evidence by today's standards of evidence-based medical practice.[57,69] Furthermore, there are many reports of significant regurgitation and aspiration regardless of the application of Sellick's maneuver.[70-73] Despite the lack of evidence, many experts believe that Sellick's maneuver is critical during RSI.[74-77]

Because aspiration has dire consequences and Sellick's maneuver has traditionally been considered integral to patient safety during emergency airway management,[69] it is reasonable to apply cricoid pressure as long as it does not interfere with ventilation and intubation. Unfortunately, there is significant evidence that it can interfere with ventilation and intubation, so it is best to apply Sellick's maneuver on a case-by-case basis with full understanding of the benefits and drawbacks of cricoid pressure.[69]

When applied during bag-mask ventilation, Sellick's maneuver reduces tidal volume, increases peak inspiratory pressure, and prevents good air exchange.[58,60,61,78-85] There are mixed data about the effects of cricoid pressure during laryoscopy,[86] but several studies have shown that it worsens visualization of the larynx.[87-89] Cricoid pressure also decreases successful insertion of and intubation through LMAs.[90-97]

TABLE 4-2   Comparison of the Airway in Adults and Children

COMPARISON	CHILD	ADULT	CLINICAL CONSEQUENCES OR ADJUSTMENTS FOR CHILDREN
Head	Proportionately larger (up to about age 10 yr)	Proportionately smaller	A child is naturally in the sniffing position when supine. Do not place a towel under the occiput; a child may benefit from elevation of the shoulders. The large head may be "floppy" and require the assistant to hold the head still during intubation.
Teeth	Easily knocked out	Stable unless decay or trauma is a factor	Teeth may be knocked out and aspirated or forced into trachea.
Tonsils or adenoids	Large and friable	Generally not a problem	Nasotracheal intubation in a child may cause excessive bleeding and is not recommended. Adenoid or tonsil tissue may plug the endotracheal tube or cause airway obstruction from aspiration.
Tongue	Relatively larger	Relatively smaller	The tongue is difficult to displace anteriorly in a child. Consider using a straight blade.
Larynx	Opposite C2-3	Opposite C4-6	A more superiorly located larynx or an "anterior" larynx is more difficult to visualize. Consider using a straight blade.
Epiglottis	U shaped, shorter, stiffer	Flatter, more flexible	The epiglottis is more difficult to manipulate in a child; it may fold down and obstruct the view with use of a curved blade. Consider using a straight blade.
Vocal cords	Concave upward; anterior attachment of the cords lower than posterior, thereby creating a slant	Horizontal	A concave shape does not affect intubation, but it may affect ventilation. For partial airway obstruction or to break laryngospasm, consider positive pressure ventilation with a jaw-lift maneuver to open the arytenoids. The anterior superior slant of the vocal cords may cause the endotracheal tube to hang up on the anterior commissure as it passes into larynx. Rotate the tube 90° counterclockwise. Overextension of neck may cause partial airway obstruction as a result of airway collapse.
Length of the trachea	Relatively shorter	Relatively longer	A short trachea increases the likelihood of main stem bronchus intubation. Follow the formula for correct depth of placement (cm depth = 0.5 age [yr] + 12) measured from the corner of the mouth. The double black line on the endotracheal tube should pass just beyond the cords.
Airway diameter	Relatively smaller; smallest diameter at the cricoid ring	Relatively larger; smallest diameter between the vocal cords	Laryngoscope-induced trauma, edema, and foreign material will significantly alter the diameter of the airway. Be gentle. Extremes of flexion or extension may kink the airway. If trouble with bag-valve-mask ventilation occurs, reassess the degree of head flexion or extension. Cricoid pressure may cause complete airway obstruction. The endotracheal tube may pass through the cords but be too large to pass through the cricoid ring. If unable to pass into the trachea, use the next smaller tube.
Residual lung capacity	Relatively smaller	Relatively larger	A child becomes hypoxic more quickly than an adult does. Closely monitor O_2 saturation and avoid prolonged periods without ventilation.

Figure 4-14 External laryngeal manipulation (ELM) (or bimanual laryngoscopy). **A,** ELM step 1. The laryngoscopist optimizes view of the larynx by reaching around to the patient's neck with the right hand and manipulating the thyroid cartilage while performing laryngoscopy. **B,** ELM step 2. The assistant's hand replaces the laryngoscopist's hand on the anterior aspect of the neck and maintains the position of the larynx while the laryngoscopist places the tracheal tube.

Because of lack of evidence of the utility of Sellick's maneuver and evidence of adverse effects, routine use of cricoid pressure during bag-mask ventilation of patients in cardiac arrest is not recommended in the 2010 American Heart Association Guidelines for Cardiopulmonary Resuscitation and Emergency Cardiovascular Care.[98] Also, it is recommended that cricoid pressure be released immediately if there is any difficulty either intubating or ventilating a patient in an emergency setting.[69,73,81,99,100] In addition, it is reasonable to release or relax cricoid pressure during insertion of an LMA, during intubation with an intubating LMA (ILMA), or if ventilation with the LMA is difficult.[57,69,96]

Some authors believe that improper technique is to blame for the many reported failures of Sellick's maneuver.[57] The proper technique for applying Sellick's maneuver is to place the thumb and middle finger on either side of the cricoid cartilage and the index finger in the center anteriorly.[62] Apply 30 N (6.7 lb) of force to the cricoid cartilage in the posterior direction.[57,77] As a reference, about 40 N of digital force on the bridge of the nose will usually cause pain.[57]

External Laryngeal Manipulation, Bimanual Laryngoscopy, and BURP

ELM is the application of pressure on the thyroid cartilage in an attempt to improve the view of the larynx during laryngoscopy. Multiple studies have shown that ELM performed by the laryngoscopist (bimanual laryngoscopy) is superior to having an assistant apply anterior neck pressure.[88,101] Bimanual laryngoscopy is best because the direction and amount of force that will optimize laryngeal exposure is variable. BURP is sometimes optimal, but it often worsens the laryngoscopic view,[88] so it is best to move the larynx in a variety of directions to determine the optimal ELM. The best way to quickly apply a variety of different forces to the larynx to determine the optimal ELM is by manipulation of the larynx with the laryngoscopist's right hand (Fig. 4-14).[101]

Operator-directed posterior displacement of the larynx during laryngoscopy was described by Brunnings in 1912.[102] After Sellick described the use of cricoid pressure to avoid regurgitation in 1961, it became common to have an assistant apply anterior neck pressure during laryngoscopy.[62] In 1993 Knill reported that having an assistant apply BURP to the cricoid or thyroid cartilage improved visualization of the

Figure 4-15 The epiglottis is elevated and visualization of the vocal cords is improved by applying pressure on the hypoepiglottic ligament and external laryngeal manipulation. (*Courtesy of Richard M. Levitan, MD, Airway Cam Technologies, Inc., Wayne, PA. Used with permission.*)

glottis during two cases of difficult laryngoscopy.[103] In 1993 Takahata and coworkers performed a prospective study of 630 intubations and found that BURP produced better laryngeal exposure than just backward pressure did in patients with difficult laryngoscopy.[104] However, a 2005 prospective crossover trial by Snider and colleagues found no benefit with routine application of the BURP maneuver.[105]

Studies by Benumof, Levitan, and colleagues have demonstrated that it is best to apply pressure on the thyroid cartilage (not the cricoid cartilage) and suggested that ELM should be applied by the laryngoscopist's right hand, not by an assistant.[88,101,106] They also found that the direction of force required for optimal ELM was not always upward and rightward and that the amount of backward pressure was variable.[88] In a 1996 study of 181 patients, Benumof and Cooper found that external manipulation was optimal when applied to the thyroid cartilage in 88% of patients and to the cricoid cartilage in only 11% of patients.[101] In a 2006 cadaveric study of 1530 laryngoscopies by 104 laryngoscopists, Levitan and associates found that bimanual laryngoscopy was more effective than both BURP and cricoid pressure for optimizing laryngeal exposure (Figs. 4-15 and 4-16; see also Fig. 4-14).[88] In addition, they found that cricoid pressure worsened the view

Figure 4-16 Note the assistant manipulating the anterior part of the neck and retracting the cheek for better visualization.

Figure 4-17 Several types of tracheal tube introducers. The classic introducer, the gum elastic bougie (**A**), is reusable and comes in curved- and straight-tipped adult forms and a straight pediatric form. The straight bougies (**B**) are 70 cm long and the curved-tipped bougies are 60 cm long. The blue introducer (**C**, Flextrach ET Tube Guide) is polyethylene and designed for single use and comes only in a curved-tipped adult form (60 cm). **D**, Create a 60-degree bend in the distal portion of the introducer if the laryngeal inlet cannot be seen on laryngoscopy.

of the larynx in 29% of cases and BURP worsened it in 35%.[88] Finally, in a 2002 study of eight first-year emergency medicine residents performing 271 intubations in an operating room setting, Levitan and colleagues found that bimanual laryngoscopy (ELM performed by the laryngoscopist) consistently improved laryngeal exposure by novice intubators (see Fig. 4-12).[106]

Passing the Tube

Once the vocal cords have been visualized, the final step is to pass the tube under direct vision through the vocal cords and into the trachea. It is best to use a malleable stylet for all emergency intubations. The best stylet shape is straight with a 35-degree hockey-stick bend at the proximal cuff ("straight-to-cuff"). In a 2006 study, Levitan and colleagues showed that stylet bend angles greater than 35 degrees made ET tube passage more difficult.[107]

Hold the tube in your right hand and introduce it from the right side of the patient's mouth. *Distraction of the cheek may greatly aid overall visualization.* Advance the tube toward the patient's larynx below the line of sight with the bend facing upward. When advanced in this manner the tube does not obstruct the view of the larynx until the last possible moment before the tube enters the larynx. If the patient is not chemically paralyzed, pass the tube during inspiration, when the vocal cords are maximally open. It enters the trachea when the cuff disappears through the vocal cords. Advance the tube 3 to 4 cm beyond this point. It is not enough to see the tube and the cords; watch the tube pass through the vocal cords to ensure tracheal placement. *Directly observing the tube pass through the cords is the best way to immediately confirm correct placement.* If part of the glottis is visualized but it is difficult to pass the tube, consider using a bougie (tracheal tube introducer).

Tracheal Tube Introducer (Bougie)

If direct laryngoscopy does not bring the vocal cords fully into view, a tracheal tube introducer may be used to facilitate intubation. This adjunct is a long, thin, semirigid introducer that, with the aid of a laryngoscope, is passed through the laryngeal inlet and over which an ET tube is advanced through the cords and into the trachea. The technique, originally described more than 60 years ago by Macintosh,[108] was recommended for patients in whom visualizing the vocal cords

was difficult. It has also been shown to be effective when the laryngeal inlet cannot be visualized at all.[109] It is the most common airway adjunct used in British EDs for complicated intubations.[110] Its efficacy has been demonstrated prospectively during difficult intubations in the operating room, as a pivotal component of a difficult airway algorithm in the operating room, and when compared with conventional laryngoscopy in the ED.[33,111,112]

A variety of tracheal tube introducers are available today (Fig. 4-17). The original adjunct was called the gum elastic bougie, or simply "the bougie," and is currently available in a reusable form for both adult and pediatric patients (Eschmann Tracheal Tube Introducer, Portex Sims, Kent, UK). The adult size comes in two forms, a 60-cm (15-Fr) version with a short, 40-degree hockey-stick curve at the end and a straight one that is 70 cm. The adult version can accommodate a 5.5-mm ET tube. The pediatric version is 70 cm (10 Fr) and straight and can accommodate a 4.0-mm tube. A polyethylene introducer designed for single use is also available and comes only in the 60-cm version (Flextrach ET Tube Guide, Greenfield Medical Sourcing, Austin, TX). A variation of this concept is the FROVA Introducer (Cook Critical Care, Bloomington, IN), a plastic introducer with a similar profile to the others except that it has a hollow lumen through which the patient can be ventilated when an accompanying adapter is attached.

Consider using a tracheal tube introducer when a difficult airway is anticipated; it can also be helpful in all intubations when visualization of the laryngeal inlet is limited. A trauma patient with cervical spine precautions is a typical example. The presence of blood and vomitus is rarely a significant complicating factor. Its safety record is impressive despite decades of use, and only two complications have been reported, perforation of the pharyngeal wall after recent head and neck surgery[113] and atelectasis from blood clots after mild bronchial trauma.[114]

Shaping the introducer may not be necessary in many cases, but with difficult laryngeal views, create a 60-degree bend in the distal introducer (see Fig. 4-17*D*).[115] Ideally, tracheal tube introducer-assisted intubation is a two-person procedure (Fig. 4-18). Use the laryngoscope in the normal fashion to obtain the best possible view of the larynx. If the cords are in full view, proceed with intubation with a styletted ET tube. If the view is suboptimal, an assistant can pass the tracheal tube introducer to the operator for placement anterior to the arytenoids and into the larynx. If only the epiglottis is visible, place the introducer, with a 60-degree distal bend, just under the epiglottis and direct it anteriorly. With the laryngoscope still in place and the introducer stabilized by the operator, the assistant slides the ET tube over the introducer. Pass the tube through the larynx. Just before entering the larynx, rotate the tube 90 degrees counterclockwise to avoid having the tip of the ET tube get caught on the laryngeal structures (Fig. 4-19).[43] Withdraw the laryngoscope and confirm proper tube placement. While securing the ET tube, ask the assistant to remove the introducer.

There are a number of confirmatory findings after successful introducer placement. If any portion of the arytenoids is visible and the introducer was seen to pass anterior to them without resistance, the introducer is in the airway. Unlike seeing an ET tube "go through the cords" when in fact the laryngeal inlet may have been momentarily obscured by the tube or balloon, the smaller-caliber introducer does not obscure the view of the glottis and thus avoids this potential pitfall. In addition to better visual confirmation, successful passage is indicated, up to 90% of the time, by feeling clicks produced by the angled tip of the introducer as it strikes against the tracheal rings.[116] An assistant will also usually feel confirmatory movement in the airway if the anterior aspect of the neck is palpated. If there is still any question whether the introducer is in the airway, advance it at least 40 cm, at which point resistance should be felt as the introducer passes the carina and into a main bronchus. If this is not felt, the introducer is most likely in the esophagus. Withdraw it and reattempt placement.

Several technical points should be emphasized. The first is that it is important to create a curve in the distal portion of the introducer when the laryngeal inlet is not visible. This is not uniformly appreciated, even in England where the bougie is used commonly.[111] It is a mistake to think that the

Figure 4-18 Two-person tracheal tube introducer technique. The introducer is handed to the clinician after the best glottic view has been obtained. **A,** The clinician places the introducer (the black line positioned at the teeth indicates the proper introducer depth to ensure stable positioning within the trachea while providing enough length to grasp the end of the introducer before passing the tube). **B,** An assistant passes the tracheal tube over the introducer as the clinician holds the introducer steady. **C,** The clinician passes the tracheal tube with a 90-degree counterclockwise rotation as the tube approaches the glottis, and the assistant withdraws the introducer.

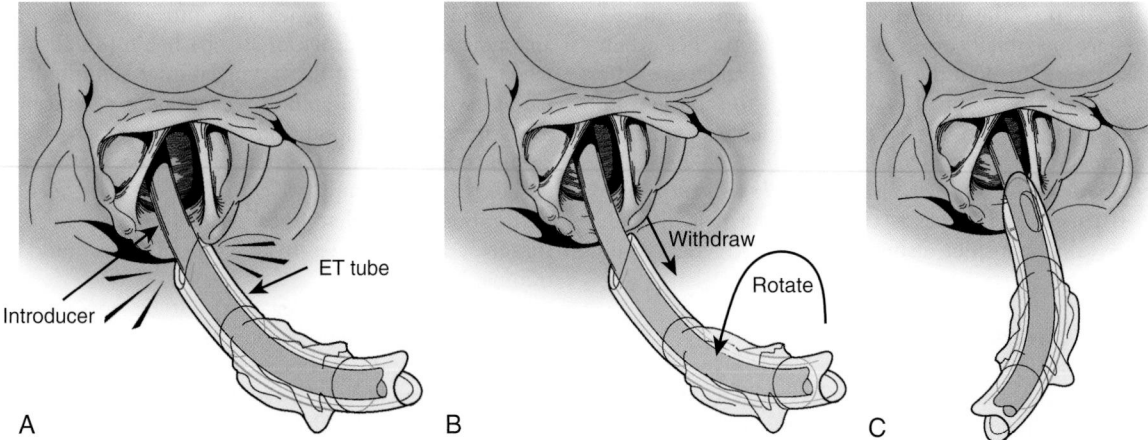

Figure 4-19 A common cause of difficulty when railroading an endotracheal (ET) tube over a tracheal tube introducer. **A,** The tip of the ET tube is caught on the right arytenoid as it is being railroaded over the introducer. **B,** Corrective maneuvers: (1) withdrawal of the ET tube 2 cm to disengage the arytenoids and (2) counterclockwise 90-degree rotation of the ET tube to orient the bevel posteriorly. **C,** The bevel of the ET tube is facing posteriorly and allows smooth passage through the glottis. (*A-C, Courtesy of Department of Emergency Medicine, Hennepin County Medical Center, Minneapolis.*)

factory-formed curve at the tip will be sufficient to access the glottis in these situations. Although there may be some benefit to lubricating the distal end of the introducer, in emergency intubations, lubricating the full length of the introducer makes it slippery and hard to handle without conferring any obvious advantage. Lubricating the ET tube, conversely, remains critical for smooth passage through the vocal cords. A common error when first using the tracheal tube introducer is to remove the laryngoscope before passing the ET tube over the introducer. This often results in difficulty placing the tube because it is displaced posteriorly by the weight of the pharyngeal soft tissues and gets hung up on the laryngeal structures. Reinsert the laryngoscope. Pull the tube back 2 cm to disengage the soft tissue. Rotate the tube 90 degrees counterclockwise and then readvance it. In instances in which it is difficult to get the introducer sufficiently anterior to access the laryngeal inlet, make sure that the introducer lines up with the operator's line of vision. If the introducer enters the mouth at a significant angle above this line, most often when the clinician is too close to the patient, it may be deflected posteriorly by the lip or intraoral structures and escape the attention of the operator. This creates the impression that the introducer is "too floppy."

In the prehospital setting, where assistance might not be available, the laryngoscope should be removed to mount the ET tube onto the introducer. Once the tube is on the introducer, reinsert the laryngoscope and advance the introducer through the glottic opening. Advance the ET tube while rotating it 90 degrees counterclockwise to ensure successful passage into the trachea. Mounting the tube onto the introducer to insert them as a unit is not advised because it is often difficult to direct the introducer into the laryngeal inlet as it moves within the ET tube.

Laryngospasm

If the patient is not paralyzed, laryngospasm, or persistent contraction of the adductor muscles of the vocal cords, may prevent passage of the tube. Inadequate anesthesia is often the cause. Pretreat with topical lidocaine to decrease the likelihood of laryngospasm occurring. Lidocaine, 2% or 4%, can be sprayed directly onto the vocal cords. An infrequent but effective means of achieving tracheal anesthesia is transtracheal puncture and injection of a bolus of 3 to 4 mL of lidocaine through the cricothyroid membrane. Laryngospasm is usually brief and often followed by a gasp. Be ready to pass the tube at this moment. Occasionally, the spasm is prolonged and needs to be disrupted with sustained anterior traction applied at the angles of the mandible, the jaw-lift maneuver. Do not force the tube at any time because it could cause permanent damage to the vocal cords. Consider using a smaller tube. Prolonged, intense spasm may ultimately require muscle relaxation with a paralyzing drug (see Chapter 5). Pediatric patients are far more prone to laryngospasm than adults are.[117] In a child, if vocal cord spasm prevents passage of the tube, a chest-thrust maneuver may momentarily open the passage and permit intubation.[118]

Positioning and Securing the Tube

Secure the ET tube in a position that minimizes both the chance of inadvertent, main stem endobronchial intubation and the risk for extubation. The tip should lie in the midtrachea with room to accommodate neck movement. Because tube movement with both neck flexion and extension averages 2 cm, the desired range of tip location is between 3 and 7 cm above the carina.[119]

The average tracheal length is between 10 and 13 cm. On a radiograph, the tip of the tube should ideally be 5 ± 2 cm above the carina when the head and neck are in a neutral position. On a portable radiograph, the adult carina overlies the fifth, sixth, or seventh thoracic vertebral body. If the carina is not visible, it can be assumed that the tip of the tube is properly positioned if it is aligned with the third or fourth thoracic vertebra. In children, the carina is more cephalad than in adults, but it is consistently situated between T3 and T5. In children, T1 is the reference point for the tip of the ET tube.[120]

Estimate the proper depth of tube placement before radiographic confirmation by using the following formulas, in which length represents the distance from the tip of the tube to the upper incisors in children[121,122] and from the upper incisors[123] or the corner of the mouth[124] in adults:

Children:	Tracheal tube depth (cm) = [age (yr)/2] + 12
Adults:	Tracheal tube depth (cm) = 21 cm (women)
	Tracheal tube depth (cm) = 23 cm (men)

In adults, this method has been shown to be more reliable than auscultation in determining the correct depth of placement.[123] One can anticipate that tall male patients will often require deeper placement, to 24 or 25 cm, and that short women will often require a shallower placement of 19 or 20 cm.

Inflate the cuff to the point of minimal air leak with positive pressure ventilation. In an emergency intubation, inflate with 10 mL of air and adjust the inflation volume after the patient is stabilized.

After placement of the tracheal tube, auscultate both lungs under positive pressure ventilation. Take care to auscultate posterolaterally because auscultation anteriorly can reveal sounds that mimic breath sounds but arise from the stomach. With the tube in position and the cuff inflated, secure the tube in place. Attach commercial ET tube holders, adhesive tape, or umbilical (nonadhesive cloth) tape securely to the tube and around the patient's head (Figs. 4-20 and 4-21). Position the tube at the corner of the mouth, where the tongue is less likely to expel it. This position is also more comfortable for the patient and allows suctioning. A bite block or oral airway to prevent crimping of the ET tube or damage from biting is commonly incorporated into the system used to secure the tube.

Unintentional extubation can have disastrous consequences, particularly if the patient was difficult to intubate initially. Secure the ET tube immediately after correct placement has been confirmed. Orotracheal intubation is associated with a higher rate of unplanned extubation than NT intubation is.[125] During transport, moving the intubated patient, or taking radiographs, *designate one person to tend to the ET tube to avoid unplanned extubation.* Inadequate sedation is another risk factor for unplanned extubation.[125] If long-acting paralytics have not been administered, consider sedation or physical restraints to prevent self-extubation by an agitated or confused patient.

Confirmation of Tracheal Tube Placement
Clinical Assessment

Confirm tracheal placement clinically *by seeing the tube pass through the vocal cords* (Table 4-3). If any question remains,

TAPING AN ENDOTRACHEAL TUBE

1 Prepare a piece of 1-inch tape to wrap around the patient's neck.

Split each side of the tape for 6 to 8 inches.

Apply a second piece of tape (sticky side down) to the center of the long piece of tape. This prevents the tape from sticking to hair.

2 Place the center of the tape behind the neck.

Bring one side of the tape forward.

Place one split end across the top of the mouth while avoiding the lips.

3 Wrap the other split end around the endotracheal tube.

4 Bring the other end of the tape forward.

Secure one split end across the top of the mouth, again avoiding the lips.

5 Wrap the remaining split end around the tube.

A companion oral airway/bite block (not shown) may be used.

Note that the tape completely encircles the head for maximum security.

Figure 4-20 Technique for taping an endotracheal tube. The method illustrated can be replaced by using a commercial holder or tracheostomy cloth tie. Avoid taping the lips.

Figure 4-21 A, A commercial disposable tube holder is ideal and preferred to secure an endotracheal (ET) tube without the use of messy tape. **B,** A plastic disposable ET holder firmly secures the ET tube with a small clamp. **C,** When positioning a patient for transfer to another bed or for a chest radiograph, ensure the integrity of the ET tube by placing the right hand firmly against the right side of the face while holding the tube securely with the same hand. The other hand immobilizes the neck. (**B,** *Courtesy of Laerdal Medical, Wappingers Falls, NY.*)

TABLE 4-3   Assessing Proper Tube Placement

TEST	INTERPRETATION
Observe the tube pass through the vocal cords	Accurate way to ensure placement; if in doubt, look again after intubation
Auscultation of breath sounds over the chest	May be misleading, especially if only the midline is examined; listen in both axillae
Auscultation over the stomach	Gurgling indicates esophageal placement
Condensation (fog) forms inside the tube with each breath	Quite reliable
Observe the chest rise with positive pressure and fall with release	Generally reliable if good chest rise is present; may be absent in patients with a small tidal volume or severe bronchospasm
Feel air exiting from the end of the tube after inflation	Reliable
Air remains in the lung after the end of the tube is occluded and exits when the occlusion is removed	Reliable, but one may "ventilate" a closed area of the esophagus
Ask the patient to speak; listen for moaning or other sounds	If the tube is in proper place, no sound is possible
Chest radiograph	Generally reliable but can be misleading
End-tidal CO_2 measurements	Reliable if a good persistent waveform is present; can be misleading with nasotracheal intubation if the tip is curled supraglottically: it will give a positive CO_2 reading
Aspiration technique	Tracheal location with a patent tube if 30-40 mL of air is aspirated without resistance; probable esophageal location if unable to aspirate the syringe easily or delayed bulb refill occurs; can be misleading with nasotracheal intubation if the tube has curled supraglottically
Fiberoptic bronchoscope	Reliable if tracheal rings are seen down the endotracheal tube
Lighted stylet down the endotracheal tube	Reliable if transillumination seen in the low midline portion of the neck
Ultrasound detection of tracheal tube location	Appears to be reliable but not well studied

apply posterior pressure on the ET tube while the laryngoscope is still in place and expose the tube by altering the angle as it passes between the cords.[126] Absent or diminished breath sounds, any sound or vocalization, increased abdominal size, and gurgling sounds during ventilation are clinical signs of esophageal placement. *If the patient can moan or groan, the tube is not in the trachea!* Critically, esophageal placement is not always obvious. One may hear "normal" breath sounds if only the midline of the thorax is auscultated. The presence of condensation of the ET tube as a means of confirming tracheal placement may also be misleading. Blinded observers noted condensation of the ET tube during ventilation in 23 of 27 esophageal intubations in an animal model.[127] One way to clinically assess tracheal placement after several ventilations or during spontaneous respiration is to note whether air is felt or heard to exit through the tube after cuff inflation. If tidal volume is adequate, the exit of air should be obvious. It is important to note that when an appropriately sized tube is placed in the trachea, the patient cannot groan, moan, or speak. Vocalization strongly suggests esophageal placement.

Asymmetric breath sounds indicate probable main stem bronchus intubation. Because of the angles of takeoff of the main bronchi and the fact that the carina lies to the left of midline in adults, right main stem intubation is most common and is indicated by decreased breath sounds on the left side. When asymmetric sounds are heard, deflate the cuff and withdraw the tube until equal breath sounds are present. Bloch and coworkers[128] reported accurate pediatric tracheal positioning if after noting asymmetric breath sounds the tube is withdrawn a defined distance beyond the point at which equal breath sounds are first heard: 2 cm in children younger than 5 years and 3 cm in older children.

Esophageal Detector Device

An aspiration technique used to determine ET tube location was first described by Wee in 1988.[129] The technique takes advantage of the difference in tracheal and esophageal resistance to collapse during aspiration to locate the tip of the tracheal tube. After intubation, attach a large syringe to the end of the ET tube and withdraw the plunger of the syringe. If the tube is placed in the trachea correctly, the plunger will pull back without resistance as air is aspirated from the lungs. If the tracheal tube is in the esophagus, resistance is felt when the plunger is withdrawn because the pliable walls of the esophagus collapse under the negative pressure and occlude the end of the tube. Another device that uses the same principle as syringe aspiration is the self-inflating bulb (e.g., Ellick device).

In the initial study conducted in an operating room, tube placement was identified correctly in 99 of 100 cases (51 esophageal, 48 tracheal).[129] The result was considered equivocal in the remaining case. That tube was removed and found to be nearly totally occluded with purulent secretions. Slight resistance was noted in one patient with right main stem intubation; the resistance decreased when the tube was pulled back. Before use, always check the esophageal detector device for air leaks. If any connections are loose, the leak may allow the syringe to easily be withdrawn, thereby mimicking tracheal location of the tube.

When using the aspiration technique, apply constant, slow aspiration to avoid occlusion of the tube from tracheal mucosa drawn up under the high negative pressure. If the tracheal tube is placed correctly, 30 to 40 mL of air can be aspirated without resistance. If air was initially aspirated and some resistance is then encountered, the tracheal tube should be pulled back between 0.5 and 1.0 cm and rotated 45 degrees. This takes the tube out of the bronchus if it has been placed too deeply and changes the orientation of the bevel if the tube has been temporarily occluded with tracheal mucosa. Air is easily aspirated if the tube was in the trachea, but repositioning it will make no difference if the tube was in the esophagus. The syringe aspiration technique can be used before or after ventilation of the patient. Apply continuous cricoid pressure pending confirmation of proper tube placement. Inflation of the tube cuff has no effect on the reliability of the test.[130] This device is reliable, rapid, inexpensive, and easy to use.[130]

A squeeze-bulb aspirator is an alternative to the syringe technique. Attach the bulb to the ET tube and squeeze; if the tube is in the esophagus, it is accompanied by a flatus-like sound followed by absent or markedly delayed refilling. Insufflation of a tube in the trachea is silent with instantaneous refill. An early study with the Ellick evacuator bulb device reported that 82% of esophageal intubations were identified.[131] A later study using a slightly different bulb device (Respironics, Murrysville, PA) found that all 45 esophageal intubations were detected.[132] The device is cheap, easy to use, and operated single-handedly in less than 5 seconds.[131] The bulb should not be used in freezing temperatures because of loss of elasticity. Confusion may occur if the esophageal tube is tested more than once because subsequent inflations may be silent. With repeated assessments, false-positive refilling of the bulb may occur as a result of instillation of air during the first attempt. This observation has led to a recommendation that the bulb be compressed before it is attached to the ET tube. Delayed, though complete refilling of the bulb may occur with bronchial tube placement or placement in the more pliable pediatric airway. The bulb suction modification of the aspiration technique has not been studied as thoroughly as the syringe technique.

A significant number of false positives occur with esophageal detection devices (the tube is correctly placed in the trachea, but the device suggests that it is in the esophagus). These patients are almost uniformly obese. Fiberoptic evaluation found that the tracheal wall was invaginated into the ET tube because of the negative pressure.[133] In such circumstances, if the intubation was felt to be successful, visually confirm that the ET tube went through the cords. Alternatively, if the patient has a perfusing rhythm and an expired CO_2 device is available, it should be used. To date, there has been one reported case of unrecognized esophageal intubation undetected by the syringe aspiration technique.[134] In this case there was marked gastric distention from forceful bag-mask ventilation. The esophageal detection device is not reliable in confirming tracheal tube depth and position after intubation because easy aspiration of air will occur if the tip of the tube is located supraglottically (expired CO_2 will also be misleading).

End-Tidal CO_2 Detector Devices

A high level of CO_2 in exhaled air is the physiologic basis for capnography and the principle on which end-tidal CO_2 pressure (P_{ETCO_2}) detectors were developed (see Chapter 2). Continuous waveform capnography is recommended by the American Heart Association guidelines as the most reliable method of confirming and monitoring correct placement of an ET tube (class I, level of evidence [LOE]). This recommendation is based on multiple studies showing 100% accuracy of waveform capnography for detecting correct ET tube placement.[98] Continuous waveform capnography is accurate even in cardiac arrest. Patients with prolonged cardiac arrest will still have a typical square waveform but a low P_{ETCO_2} value.

When waveform capnography is not available, emergency providers may have to rely on colorimetric CO_2 indicators, which correspond to CO_2 levels flowing through the device when placed on the tracheal tube adapter (Fig. 4-9, *step 10*). The typical device displays opposite colors (e.g., yellow and purple) to indicate low levels of CO_2 in esophageal gas versus the high levels of CO_2 exhaled from the respiratory tree. Handheld quantitative or semiquantitative electronic CO_2 monitors are also available. Eventually, all prehospital defibrillators will have advanced monitoring capability that includes capnography.

A multicenter study of a colorimetric device demonstrated an overall sensitivity of 80% and a specificity of 96%.[135] In patients with spontaneous circulation and an inflated tracheal tube cuff, the sensitivity and specificity were 100%. The poor sensitivity (69%) noted in patients in cardiac arrest was due to the fact that low exhaled CO_2 levels were seen with both very-low-flow states and esophageal intubation. The device must be used with caution in cardiac arrest victims. CO_2 levels return to normal after return of spontaneous circulation. Furthermore, colorimetric changes may be difficult to discern in situations with reduced lighting, and secretions can interfere with the change in color. Regardless of the monitoring device, patients should be ventilated for a minimum of six breaths before taking a reading. Otherwise, recent ingestion of carbonated beverages can result in spuriously high CO_2 levels with esophageal intubation.[136] Colorimetric changes do not rule out glottic positioning of the tip of the ET tube. Adequate ventilation and oxygenation may be achieved in the glottic position, but there is still a risk for aspiration in the absence of a protected airway and the potential for further tube dislodgment. Glottic positioning may be difficult to detect clinically. The only signs may be persistent cuff leak or diminished chest rise with ventilation. Radiographic evidence or direct visualization confirms the diagnosis.[137]

Ultrasound Detection of Tracheal Tube Location
Some early data suggested that ultrasound may play a future role in identifying tube location after intubation. There are two reports and both are small. The first study, performed with cadavers, had a sensitivity of 100% and a specificity of 97%.[138] The second study, which was conducted in the operating room, had both a sensitivity and specificity of 100%.[139]

Comparison of Detector Devices
In the setting of spontaneous circulation, both syringe aspiration and P_{ETCO_2} detection are highly reliable means of excluding esophageal intubation. An animal study comparing these techniques with clinical assessment and measuring the speed and accuracy of determining tube placement demonstrated that both the syringe esophageal detector device and P_{ETCO_2} detection were highly accurate, approaching 100%.[140] The esophageal detector device was more rapid, with determination in 13.8 seconds versus 31.5 seconds for P_{ETCO_2} detection. The detector device remained accurate when air was insufflated into the esophagus for 1 minute, thus simulating unrecognized esophageal placement. Clinical assessment alone yielded an alarming 30% rate of failure to identify esophageal

intubation. In the setting of cardiac arrest, the aspiration method is more reliable than CO_2 detection because its accuracy is not dependent on the presence of blood flow.

An unequivocal method for determining tracheal tube location uses the fiberoptic scope. Passage of the scope through the tube with visualization of the tracheal rings confirms ET placement and position within the trachea. Placement of a lighted stylet down the tracheal tube and successful transtracheal illumination can also be used to determine correct ET placement.[141]

At present, there is no perfect device for confirmation of ET tube placement in all situations. Be aware of the limitations of each device and ideally rely on input from multiple means of confirmation to ensure tracheal placement of the ET tube.

Complications of Intubation
Failure to achieve adequate ventilation and oxygenation is the most serious complication of tracheal intubation. The potential for hypoxia exists just before intubation as more conservative oxygenation methods are attempted and then fail, during difficult intubation when ventilation is halted for an attempt at intubation, and after intubation when esophageal intubation goes undetected. Because irreversible cerebral anoxia occurs within minutes, conservative airway management maneuvers should be limited to 2 to 3 minutes; failure to achieve adequate oxygenation should lead to a quick decision to intubate.

As a guide, limit intubation attempts to the amount of time that a single deep breath can be held. This is especially important in a child because the functional residual capacity of a child's lungs is less than that of an adult. Historically, the maximum recommended duration of an intubation attempt in an apneic patient has been 30 seconds, followed by a period of bag-mask ventilation before intubation is attempted again. However, longer attempts at intubation are permissible when guided by accurate data from an oxygen saturation monitor because oxygen saturation may remain in the normal range for much longer in patients who have been preoxygenated. As a general rule, intubation attempts may continue if oxygen saturation is above 90% and should be interrupted for bag-mask ventilation when oxygen saturation drops below 90%.

Assessment of tube location is the top priority immediately after placement. The best assurance of tracheal placement is to see the tube pass through the vocal cords. Techniques to assess tube placement were discussed earlier. If esophageal intubation is discovered, *removal of the tube may be followed by emesis.* Apply cricoid pressure during tube removal and maintain it until the intubation is successful. Keep a large-bore suction tip readily available should vomiting occur. Alternatively, leave the first tube in the esophagus to serve as a temporary gastric-venting device and as a guide to intubation until tracheal intubation is achieved.

Though seldom associated with serious complications, unrecognized placement of the tip of the ET tube in the right main stem bronchus may cause hypoxia, atelectasis, pneumothorax, and unilateral pulmonary edema.[142] Obtain a chest radiograph soon after intubation to confirm tube positioning. Endobronchial intubation was clinically unrecognized without a chest film in 7% of prehospital intubations in one study.[143] Persistent asymmetric breath sounds after correct tube positioning suggests unilateral pulmonary pathology (e.g., main stem bronchus obstruction, pneumothorax, hemothorax).

Prolonged efforts to intubate can also cause cardiac decompensation. Pharyngeal stimulation can produce profound bradycardia or asystole, thereby confirming the need for *an assistant to monitor cardiac rhythm throughout the intubation.* Keep atropine available to reverse the vagal-induced bradycardia that may occur secondary to suctioning or laryngoscopy. Prolonged pharyngeal stimulation may also result in laryngospasm, bronchospasm, and apnea.

Generally, dentures are removed for intubation but kept in place for bag-mask ventilation. Check for loose or missing teeth before and after orotracheal intubation. Look for any avulsed teeth not found in the oral cavity on the postintubation chest film. Broken teeth are the most common complication of laryngoscopy.[144] Laceration of the mucosa of the lips, especially the lower lip, may occur. Tracheal or bronchial injuries are rare but serious and usually occur in infants and the elderly as a result of their decreased tissue elasticity.[145]

Vomiting with aspiration of gastric contents is another serious complication that can occur during intubation. Case reports of both adult respiratory distress syndrome and chronic lung disease are thought to be due to aspiration of activated charcoal.[145,146] In patients who are obtunded or who are at high risk for seizures or vomiting, consider tracheal intubation before the administration of activated charcoal.

There are ongoing concerns that direct laryngoscopy may cause or worsen spinal cord injury in a patient with an unstable cervical spine injury. *These concerns are essentially theoretical, with no credible data to prove or disprove a true effect.* Many anesthesiologists prefer awake fiberoptic intubation in this setting, but no data support one approach over another. A cadaveric study of intubation during fluoroscopy showed that direct laryngoscopy with in-line immobilization in the setting of complete C4-5 ligamentous instability did not result in clinically significant movement.[147] The greatest degree of motion occurs at the atlanto-occipital junction and decreases with each sequential interspace, and studies of cervical spine instability at these higher levels have not been performed.[148] It can also be argued that cadaveric studies do not accurately depict the trauma setting, and yet this model is probably going to remain the best one available. Unless new information emerges regarding the risks of orotracheal intubation with direct laryngoscopy, *it appears to be a safe approach when performed in conjunction with in-line immobilization.*

Intubation can be complicated by a persistent air leak. This is generally caused by failure of either the cuff or the pilot balloon or by positioning the cuff balloon between the vocal cords. If the cuff balloon is leaking, replace the tracheal tube (see "Changing Tracheal Tubes" later in this chapter). If the pilot balloon is determined to be leaking, this can usually be remedied without changing the tube.[149] An incompetent one-way balloon valve can be fixed by placing a stopcock in the inflating valve. Reinflate the cuff and shut off the stopcock to solve the problem. If the leak involves the pilot balloon or if the distal inflation tube has been inadvertently severed, cut off the defective part and slide a 20-gauge catheter into the inflation tube. Then connect the stopcock to the catheter, inflate the cuff, and close the stopcock.

Tracheal stricture used to be a significant late complication of long-term intubation with low-volume, high-pressure cuffs. The use of high-volume, low-pressure cuffs has markedly decreased the incidence of this complication.[150] Tubes with high-pressure cuffs are obsolete and should be avoided.

Conclusion

Direct laryngoscopy is the most common means of securing a definitive airway. With adequate preparation and emphasis on preoxygenation and positioning, it is usually successful. RSI has rendered patients much more amenable to direct laryngoscopy for emergency airway management (see Chapter 5). Once the patient is paralyzed, it becomes the clinician's supreme responsibility to ventilate, oxygenate, and protect the patient's airway. Mastery of direct laryngoscopy fulfills part of this obligation. Being prepared for failure and having a successful backup plan fulfills this responsibility. The remainder of this chapter is devoted to adjuncts and alternatives to direct laryngoscopy.

VIDEO AND OPTICAL LARYNGOSCOPES

Several video and optical laryngoscopes are transforming airway management. These devices are all somewhat similar in that they use video, fiberoptics, or mirrors to visualize the larynx. They provide a better view of the glottis with less effort and have a shorter learning curve than direct laryngoscopy does. Only the Macintosh shaped video laryngoscopes are designed to sweep the tongue aside and allow either a direct or video view of the larynx. The other devices are made to look around the curve of the tongue rather than lifting it or pushing it aside, so they are more angulated. The drawback of more angulated devices is that getting an excellent view of the vocal cords does not always correlate with easy intubation[151,152] because it can be difficult to manipulate the ET tube around the sharp curve of the blade. Adding a tube channel to the blade obviates the need to manipulate the ET tube around the sharp curve but may add other complexities.[151] Because expense is a major impediment to the widespread use of video laryngoscopy, the relatively inexpensive Airtraq device (see category 3 below) may be a good choice in settings in which difficult intubation is rare and funding is limited.[4]

Video and optical laryngoscopes can be divided into three broad categories[152]:

1. Video laryngoscopes with standard Macintosh blades (Storz C-MAC, GlideScope Direct Intubation Trainer, McGrath MAC, Venner A.P. Advance Mac Blade)
2. Video laryngoscopes with angulated blades (GlideScope, McGrath Series 5, Storz D-Blade)
3. Video or optical laryngoscopes with a tube channel (Airtraq, Pentax AWS, KingVISION)

See the following sections for pictures and manufacturers of each device.

Video Laryngoscopes with Standard Macintosh Blades

These devices have blades that are exactly the same or very similar to a standard English or German Macintosh direct laryngoscope. They all have a digital camera adjacent to the light source a few centimeters proximal to the tip. Each of these devices can be used for either conventional direct laryngoscopy or video laryngoscopy. The Storz C-MAC is the only device in this group that has been sufficiently tested (Fig. 4-22).[153-161] The laryngeal view obtained on the video monitor is better than the direct view in most patients.[154,156] The

Video and Optical Laryngoscopy

Indications
Routine emergency intubation
Teaching of direct laryngoscopy skills to novices
Difficult airways
Failed direct laryngoscopy
Morbid obesity
Trauma patients with cervical spine immobilization

Contraindications
Limited mouth opening
Severe kyphosis
Copious blood or secretions

Complications
Dental trauma
Oropharyngeal trauma

Equipment

Ancillary equipment (endotracheal tubes, etc) not depicted

Review Box 4-2 Video laryngoscopy: indications, contraindications, complications, and equipment.

Figure 4-22 The Storz C-MAC video laryngoscope.

improved laryngeal view provided by the camera is especially helpful in morbidly obese patients and in trauma patients who require cervical spine immobilization.[153,160]

Background
The Storz Video Macintosh Laryngoscope was introduced into clinical practice by Kaplan, Berci, and colleagues in 2002.[159] The latest version of this device, the Storz C-MAC, is smaller, more portable, and cheaper.[152] It also has a wider field of view because the camera is on the blade instead of in the handle.[162] The C-MAC consists of a one-piece blade, a cable, and a monitor. It can record digital video or still images onto a Secure Digital memory card. Older versions of this device were referred to as the Storz Video Macintosh Laryngoscope, Storz BERCI DCI Video Laryngoscope, Storz V-MAC BERCI DCI, and Storz Berci-Kaplan Videolaryngoscope.[154,156,161,163] The GlideScope Direct Intubation Trainer,

McGrath MAC, and Venner A.P. Advance Mac Blade appear similar in design, but they are all very new and untested.

Anatomy and Physiology
When the tip of the Storz C-MAC is advanced into the vallecula, it gives an 80-degree-wide field of view and offers a panoramic view of the glottis. Moving slowly and using a progressive visualization technique to find the tongue, epiglottis, posterior cartilages, and vocal cords (as with direct laryngoscopy) is the best approach to performing laryngoscopy with the C-MAC.

Pathophysiology
There is limited research but some data that the Storz C-MAC provides better glottic visualization and decreases the number of intubation attempts in patients with cervical spine immobility and morbid obesity.[153,160]

Indications
The Storz C-MAC may be a good option for routine intubations at academic institutions that are teaching novice intubators. In 2008, Howard-Quijano and coauthors published a prospective, randomized, crossover study of 37 novice intubators (medical students and residents) who performed 222 intubations with the Storz Video Macintosh system.[155] The novice intubators performed only direct laryngoscopy and were not allowed to see the video monitor in any case. Intubations were randomized so that either the instructors could see the video monitor or it was covered by a drape. Novice intubators were given 2 minutes to intubate before the instructor took over. When instructors were allowed to see the video monitor, the novice intubators had a 69% success rate and a 3% rate of esophageal intubation. When instructors were blinded to the video monitor, the novice intubators had a 55% success rate and a 17% rate of esophageal intubation. Also, a 2008 manikin study by Low and associates showed that novices who learned

direct laryngoscopy skills via the Storz Video Macintosh system found it easier to intubate, had more confidence, and exhibited improved knowledge of airway anatomy.[163]

Use of the C-MAC may also be indicated when direct laryngoscopy is difficult. In 2006, Kaplan and coauthors published a prospective multicenter trial in which the direct laryngoscopy view was compared with the video view during 865 intubations with the Storz Video Macintosh system.[157] They reported 7 cases in which the direct view of the larynx was easy and the video view was difficult and 100 cases in which the direct view was difficult and the video view was easy. In 2009, Jungbauer and colleagues studied 200 patients with Mallampati class III or IV anatomy.[156] They randomized patients to intubation with direct laryngoscopy or with the Storz Video Macintosh system. The success rate with direct laryngoscopy was 92% and the success rate with the Storz Video Macintosh system was 99%. Finally, in 2010 Cavus and coworkers published a report of three patients in whom there was unexpected difficulty with direct laryngoscopy but good glottic visualization and successful intubation on the first attempt with the Storz C-MAC.[162]

Two studies compared the Storz C-MAC with the Glide-Scope and McGrath systems. A 2009 study of 450 patients with normal airways by van Zundert and colleagues showed that those intubated with the Storz C-MAC were intubated more quickly and had a higher first-pass success rate than did those intubated with the GlideScope or McGrath MAC.[161] Another study compared the C-MAC with the GlideScope and McGrath in 150 morbidly obese patients and found that those intubated with the C-MAC had significantly fewer intubation attempts and a shorter intubation time.[160]

In addition, the C-MAC may be useful in trauma patients with cervical spine immobilization. Two studies suggest that the C-MAC provides better visualization of the glottis and decreases the number of intubation attempts in manikins with a stiff cervical spine.[163]

Contraindications

Contraindications to use of the C-MAC are rare. Like other video laryngoscopes, the lens on the video camera is susceptible to obscuration by secretions or blood. Unlike other video devices, the C-MAC facilitates direct visualization of anatomic structures, so this is much less of a concern.

Procedure

Much of the procedure for laryngoscopy with the C-MAC is similar to that for direct laryngoscopy. Keep in mind that the tip of the C-MAC is usually placed in the vallecula, but when laryngoscopy is difficult, it may help to directly lift the epiglottis with the tip of the blade; this is known as the "straight-blade technique."[162]

Complications

A complication that may be encountered is blind passage of the ET tube into the mouth while fixating on the video monitor. This can result in damage to oral and pharyngeal structures. It is less common with the C-MAC than with the GlideScope and McGrath.

Video Laryngoscopes with Angulated Blades

The GlideScope (Verathon, Bothell, WA), McGrath Series 5 (Aircraft Medical Ltd., Edinburgh, United Kingdom), and

Storz D-Blade (Karl Storz, Tuttlingen, Germany) video laryngoscopes are similarly shaped devices that have sharply angulated, nonchanneled, and narrow-flanged blades.[151,152,164,165] All of these devices have a distal angulation of about 60 degrees and a digital camera a few centimeters proximal to the tip. These blades do not allow laryngoscopy by direct visualization. They are designed to follow the natural curvature of the upper airway and look around the tongue rather than displace it. Excellent visualization of the glottis is nearly always achieved when the distal tip of the blade is in or near the vallecula. Because the point of reference is from the location of the camera near the distal tip of these devices, they reliably provide a panoramic view of the larynx that cannot be achieved with direct laryngoscopy. Both the Glide-Scope and the McGrath allow easy visualization of the larynx, even with inexperienced providers or difficult airway anatomy.[160,161,164,166-171] However, maneuvering the ET tube around the severe angle of the blade and into the trachea is more difficult, and this is where problems can occur.[151] In one large trial involving inexperienced GlideScope operators, the device was abandoned in 3.7% of intubations despite the fact that an excellent view of the glottis was achieved in most of these cases.[164]

Background

In 2001 the original GlideScope video laryngoscope became the first commercially available video laryngoscope. The first report of its use was a case report of management of a difficult airway.[172] Three GlideScope models are now available: the GVL, which has a reusable plastic handle and a mountable monitor; the Cobalt AVL, which uses disposable plastic blades to cover a reusable video baton with a mountable monitor; and the Ranger, which has a small portable monitor and the choice of a reusable blade or a video baton with disposable blades (Ranger Single Use). All GlideScope models have a lens antifog mechanism and digital recording capability.

The McGrath portable video laryngoscope is another device with similar characteristics but is more compact. It became available in 2005, and the current model is called the McGrath Series 5 (Fig. 4-23). The shape of the blade is very similar to that of the GlideScope, but it has a small video

Video monitor

Disposable plastic blade

Adjustable-length, detachable, angulated blade

Figure 4-23 The McGrath Series 5 video laryngoscope.

monitor (1.7 inches diagonally) on the end of the handle. It also has an adjustable-length, detachable metal blade (camera stick) that is covered by a disposable plastic blade during use, so no part of the handle or metal blade makes contact with the patient. It has no recording capability.

The Storz D-Blade became available in 2010 and also has a blade shape similar to that of the GlideScope. It is an optional blade for use with the Storz C-MAC system and has the same functionality as the other C-MAC blades but does not allow the option of direct visualization of the larynx. It was designed specifically for difficult intubations.

The GlideScope and its use are discussed as representative of this class of indirect video-assisted laryngoscopes with thin, sharply angulated and unchanneled blades.

Indications

The GlideScope, McGrath Series 5, and Storz D-Blade may be especially useful when direct laryngoscopy is difficult or fails. In 2010, Noppens and coauthors reported a series of 61 patients with failed direct laryngoscopy, all with Cormack-Lehane grade III and IV views, who subsequently had good laryngoscopic views and 95% were successfully intubated with a McGrath video laryngoscope.[173] In 2011, Cavus and colleagues published a very similar series of 20 patients with grade III and IV views who had failed direct laryngoscopy but subsequently had good laryngoscopic views and were all successfully intubated with the Storz D-Blade.[174] There are many case reports of easy intubations with the GlideScope and McGrath video laryngoscopes after failed direct laryngoscopy.[172,175] In addition, several case reports show that the GlideScope and McGrath can facilitate successful awake intubation in patients with known or suspected difficult airways.[176-178]

A significant advantage of the more angulated video laryngoscopes is that they can provide a good view of the larynx when the neck is in the neutral position. Not surprisingly, there are several small studies and case reports demonstrating that the GlideScope and McGrath provide good laryngoscopic views and a high rate of successful intubation in patients with cervical spine immobilization.[179-181] In 2006, Lai and associates published a series of 12 patients with ankylosing spondylitis and difficult direct laryngoscopy. Eight of these patients were able to be *intubated nasotracheally* with the GlideScope.[182] There is also a case report of a patient with severe ankylosing spondylitis who was easily intubated on the first attempt with the McGrath.[183]

Finally, the GlideScope is useful for routine intubations by inexperienced or novice intubators. In a 2009 study by Nouruzi-Sedeh and coworkers, 20 novices each intubated five patients with direct laryngoscopy and five patients with the GlideScope. They had a 51% success rate with direct laryngoscopy and a 93% success rate with the GlideScope.[169]

Contraindications

Contraindications to using angulated video laryngoscopes are not well described in the literature. As with any video or optical device, blood or secretions on the lens may decrease visualization of the larynx. Fogging was a problem with older fiberoptic devices, but this problem is rare with the newer video devices. Limited mouth opening (<2 cm) can make insertion of these devices more challenging. The biggest contraindication is probably lack of experience or absence of a rigid stylet to allow the operator to maneuver the ET tube around the sharp angle of the blade.[151]

Procedure and Technique

Grasp the video laryngoscope in the left hand and place it in the patient's mouth with the scissor technique. *Under direct vision*, advance it through the oropharynx along the midline of the tongue (Fig. 4-24, *step 4*). Then look up at the monitor while continuing to advance the blade down the midline of the tongue, progressively identifying the base of the tongue and the epiglottis. With a gentle lifting motion, place the tip of the blade in the vallecula. Elevate the epiglottis and expose the laryngeal inlet (Fig. 4-24, *step 5*). If the glottis is not well visualized, tilt the handle back slightly to enhance exposure. Manipulate the neck externally to enhance visualization. If more exposure is required, place the tip of the blade under the epiglottis and gently lift and tilt back. While attempting to optimize the laryngeal view, be careful to not place the blade too close to the laryngeal inlet because it may tip the larynx anteriorly and inferiorly and thus make it more difficult to access the laryngeal inlet and pass the tube through it.

Use a rigid steel GlideRite stylet, which has the same 60-degree curve as the blade of the GlideScope, McGrath, and D-Blade. Alternatively, a malleable stylet with a 60-degree distal bend or a bougie may be acceptable, but these devices may fail if tube passage is challenging. Pass the ET tube through the oropharynx under direct vision until it passes under the curve of the blade, and then look for it on the monitor (Fig. 4-24, *step 6*). Decrease the chance of soft tissue injury by carefully passing the ET tube along the side of the GlideScope.[184] When the tip of the ET tube comes into view, direct it into the glottis and advance it to the appropriate depth (Fig. 4-24, *step 8*). If a malleable stylet or bougie is used, it may be difficult to get the tube to go anterior enough. If a malleable stylet must be used, try introducing the tube from the right side of the patient and rotating it 90 degrees and vertically into a midline position behind the tongue. This will help the tip of the stylet maintain its shape as it passes through the oropharynx. Another option is to use a Parker Flex-It intubation stylet to direct the tip of the ET tube anteriorly.[164] It is important to realize that the fixed steel (GlideRite) stylet needs to be withdrawn as the ET tube is passed through the vocal cords because the tip of the stylet will be essentially pointing toward the ceiling as it approaches the laryngeal inlet (Fig. 4-24, *step 9*). The large knob on the proximal end of the GlideRite stylet is designed to be pushed up by the tip of the intubator's thumb, thus making ET tube advancement and stylet withdrawal a one-handed procedure.

Complications

Several relatively minor complications have been reported with use of the GlideScope. There are case reports of injury to the soft palate and tonsillar pillars, as well as two cases of puncture of the right palatopharyngeal arch, one requiring surgical repair.[184-186]

Summary

Video-assisted laryngoscopy is a major advancement in visualization of the laryngeal inlet. These devices are very promising because they provide an improved laryngeal view and have a shorter learning curve than direct laryngoscopy does. The majority of intubation failures are due to an inability to pass the tube through the larynx despite excellent glottic views.[164] Using a fixed steel stylet (GlideRite stylet) helps, but does not eliminate this problem.[151] Advancements need to be made in achieving tracheal intubation once the glottis is seen. The

VIDEO LARYNGOSCOPY (GLIDESCOPE)

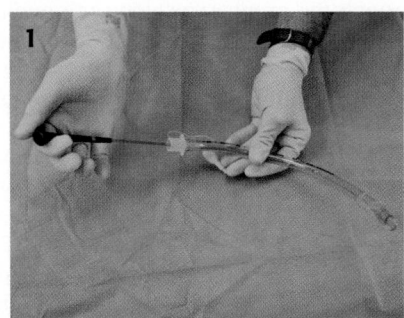

Prepare the endotracheal tube.

Depending on the system that you are using, insert a rigid stylet or preload the tube onto the device.

Check the rest of your equipment, including the light source and video monitor.

Preoxygenate and premedicate the patient as clinically indicated.

Place the blade into the mouth under direct visualization (don't look at the video monitor yet).

Keep the blade in the midline of the tongue throughout the procedure.

Slowly advance the blade while watching the video monitor. Progressively identify the tongue and epiglottis.

Place the blade in the vallecula or under the epiglottis, gently lift, and identify the vocal cords.

Under direct visualization (don't look at the monitor), pass the styleted tube through the mouth and into the posterior pharynx.

Look up at the video monitor and watch for the tip of the tube to appear.

Direct the tube through the vocal cords under direct visualization on the video monitor.

While the operator firmly secures the endotracheal tube, an assistant removes the stylet as the tube is passed through the vocal cords.

NOTE: This image sequence depicts video laryngoscopy using the Glidescope. The procedure sequence may vary with the use of other devices. Refer to text for additional information.

Be familiar with the equipment used at your institution prior to use.

Figure 4-24 Video laryngoscopy (GlideScope). Note that there are times when the operator *does not look at the screen* but rather uses direct vision (*steps 4* and *6*).

addition of a tube channel obviates the need to maneuver the ET tube around the sharp angle of the blade, and channeled devices are described in the next section.

Video and Optical Laryngoscopes with a Tube Channel

Four devices allow indirect video or optical visualization of the larynx and also provide a channeled blade to guide the ET tube through the vocal cords. The Airtraq (Prodol Meditec S.A., Vizcaya, Spain) and Pentax AirWay Scope (AWS) (Pentax, Tokyo) are the only devices in this group that have been sufficiently tested (Figs. 4-25 and 4-26). The KingVISION (King Systems, Noblesville, IN) and Venner A.P. Advance Difficult Airway Blade (DAB) (Venner Medical, Singapore) are very new and essentially untested. The ET tube is inserted into the channel before the device is placed

Figure 4-25 The Airtraq intubation device. The device pictured uses prisms and mirrors so that the larynx can be visualized via the eyepiece. There is also an optional video system available (not pictured) that can project the image to a wireless display recorder.

Figure 4-26 The Pentax AWS (Air Way Scope).

in the airway, and the channel guides the ET tube into the trachea once the glottis is visualized. This design helps alleviate the most common problem associated with video and optical laryngoscopy, difficulty placing the ET tube despite an excellent view of the glottis. Several small studies have demonstrated the utility of the Airtraq and Pentax AWS, but the KingVISION is very new and untested.

Background
The concept of a laryngoscope shaped like the natural curvature of the upper airway and containing a channel to guide the ET tube is not new, but the addition of optics and video just recently made this concept a reality.[187-190] The advantage of these devices is that they provide an excellent view of the glottis with little need for maneuvering and they eliminate the requirement for the hand-eye coordination needed to pass the ET tube around an acute curve.[191-193]

Anatomy and Physiology
All three of the channel-guided devices have the same curvature as the normal upper airway. They allow visualization of the glottis by looking around the tongue instead of trying to straighten the airway and push the tongue out of the way. They consistently provide a better view of the glottis and may lead to less airway trauma and hemodynamic stimulation than occurs with direct laryngoscopy.[188,194,195]

Indications
Difficult intubation with direct laryngoscopy is an indication for using a channel-guided optical or video device. The Airtraq and Pentax AWS have a high rate of success in patients with known or predicted difficult airways.[168, 188,194] In 2009, a study by Asai and colleagues reported 270 patients with difficult airways by direct laryngoscopy (grade III and IV views) and found that 268 of these patients (99.3%) had good glottic visualization and were easily intubated with the Pentax AWS.[194] In a 2009 trial of patients with expected difficult airways, Malik and coworkers randomized 75 patients to direct laryngoscopy, the Pentax AWS, or the GlideScope.[168] The rate of successful intubation was 84% with direct laryngoscopy, 96% with the GlideScope, and 100% with the Pentax AWS.

The Airtraq and Pentax AWS are particularly useful for difficult airways because of cervical spine immobilization and morbid obesity.[196-199] In 2007, Ndolo and coauthors published a study of 106 morbidly obese patients who were randomized to intubation with direct laryngoscopy or the Airtraq.[200] All patients randomized to the Airtraq were successfully intubated, but six patients in the direct laryngoscopy group required rescue intubation with the Airtraq. In 2007, Maharaj published a study of 40 patients with cervical spine immobilization who were randomized to direct laryngoscopy or the Airtraq.[198] All patients randomized to the Airtraq group were intubated on the first attempt and were intubated faster and with less difficulty than the direct laryngoscopy group. Dhonneur, Ndoko, and their colleagues described alternative techniques for insertion of the Airtraq into the mouths of morbidly obese patients.[199,200] They rotated the device 90 to 180 degrees for initial insertion of the distal tip into the patient's mouth and then rotated it into the normal orientation before advancing it into the hypopharynx.

In 2008, Enomoto and associates studied 203 patients with manual in-line neck stabilization who required intubation.[197]

They randomized these patients to intubation with direct laryngoscopy or the Pentax AWS. The intubation success rate with direct laryngoscopy was 89% versus 100% with the Pentax AWS. A similar study by Liu and coworkers in 2009 included 70 patients with manual in-line stabilization of the cervical spine and randomized them to intubation with the Pentax AWS or the GlideScope.[166] They reported a 100% rate of successful intubation with the Pentax AWS and 89% with the GlideScope. In addition, two studies used fluoroscopy to compare cervical spine motion during intubation with direct laryngoscopy versus intubation with the Pentax AWS.[201,202] Both studies found that intubation with the Pentax AWS caused less movement of the upper cervical spine than direct laryngoscopy did.

The Airtraq is generally used during RSI but may also be used for awake intubation of patients with difficult airways.[203,204] When compared with direct laryngoscopy, both the Airtrach and Pentax AWS consistently provide better visualization of the glottis and have a higher rate of successful intubation.[168,188,189,194,197] Most impressively, two small studies and one large trial have shown that the Airtraq has a very high rate of success after failed direct laryngoscopy.[4,188,189] In 2011, Amathieu and coauthors reported the results of a large prospective trial in which they used an algorithm that specified use of the Airtraq as a backup for all cases of failed RSI with direct laryngoscopy.[4] They had 28 patients who could not be intubated with direct laryngoscopy after multiple attempts, including the use of a bougie. Intubation with the Airtrach was successful in 27 of 28 of these patients (97%), and the other patient was intubated with an ILMA.[4]

Contraindications

The greatest drawback of channeled video and optical devices is that copious amounts of blood or secretions can obscure the view. Because they do not allow a direct line of sight to the larynx, visualization and intubation are dependent on the video or optical image. If blood or fluid covers the tip of the lens, the image is obscured. This problem can be minimized by aggressively suctioning the hypopharynx before placing the device in the mouth.

Inability to open the mouth or severely limited mouth opening is a contraindication to using the channel-guided devices just described. However, if the patient's mouth opening is more than about 2 cm, these devices can succeed in cases in which direct laryngoscopy would be impossible. The normal adult-size Airtraq requires 18 mm of mouth opening, and the pediatric and infant sizes require 12.5 mm. The Pentax AWS requires about 20 mm of mouth opening.

Procedure

Before beginning the procedure check that you are using the correct size device, make sure that it is functioning properly, and choose the correct size ET tube for the device and the patient. Insert the ET tube into the channel of the device and position it in the channel so that it is not covering the video or optical lens. Insert the tip of the blade into the mouth vertically so that the handle of the device is pointed toward the patient's feet. Rotate it into the pharynx and hypopharynx along the midline of the tongue until the tip is in the vallecula. If the glottis is not visualized immediately, try backing the blade out 1 to 2 cm and lift the device gently in the direction of the handle (toward the ceiling). A common mistake is to insert the blade too deep initially, which offers a narrower

view of the glottis and may make intubation difficult. When the vocal cords are well visualized in the center of the video or optical image, advance the ET tube through the cords by sliding it forward within the channel. If the ET tube does not go through the cords, pull it back and realize that you need to adjust the position of the entire device to change the trajectory of the tube. If the tube tends to go posterior to the vocal cords, lift the device toward the ceiling and tip the handle back slightly (while avoiding contact with the upper teeth), and then advance the tube again. Alternatively, pass a bougie through the ET tube and direct the curved tip up and through the vocal cords.

When using the Pentax AWS, it is important to know that the ET tube leaves the channel in line with the tip of the blade (more anterior than the Airtraq). Therefore, when the tip of the AWS blade is in the vallecula, the tube often strikes the epiglottis when it is advanced. To avoid this problem, advance the tip of the AWS blade posterior to the epiglottis (as with straight-blade laryngoscopy), and lift the epiglottis out of the way before advancing the ET tube.

Dhonneur, Ndoko, and colleagues described alternative techniques for insertion of the Airtraq in morbidly obese patients.[199,200] They rotate the device 90 to 180 degrees for initial insertion of the distal tip into the patient's mouth and then rotate it into the normal orientation (handle toward the patient's feet) before advancing it into the hypopharynx. This helps alleviate problems with the handle of the device striking the patient's chest during insertion.

Aftercare

A common mistake when using laryngoscopes with a tube channel is to quickly remove the laryngoscope after the ET tube is advanced into the trachea. Because the ET tube is already inside the trachea, it is best to attach a resuscitation bag and start ventilating the patient. After giving several breaths, stabilizing oxygenation, and confirming tracheal placement with capnography, slowly and carefully remove the device while providing ongoing ventilation. It is appropriate to leave the laryngoscope in place for a few minutes after intubation to allow visual reconfirmation of proper tracheal placement, particularly if there is a problem with ventilation or oxygenation immediately following intubation. When removing the tube from the channel of these devices, hold the end of the ET tube firmly in the right hand and carefully wiggle the laryngoscope to the left. When the tube slides out of the channel, slowly rotate the laryngoscope out of the patient's mouth. Reconfirm tracheal placement with capnography and adjust the depth of the ET tube as needed.

Complications

No significant complications have been reported with the tube channel video and optical devices. Because the blades of these devices are rigid and cannot be directly visualized after entering the mouth, they have potential for soft tissue damage. Complications of other video laryngoscopes are primarily a result of blind ET tube placement through the mouth and pharynx, and the tube channel devices eliminate this problem.

INTUBATING LARYNGEAL MASK AIRWAYS

ILMAs are unique devices because they are easy to insert, provide excellent ventilation and oxygenation (better than

Intubating Laryngeal Mask Airway

Indications
Failed rapid-sequence intubation
Cannot-intubate cannot-ventilate scenario
Difficult mask ventilation
Expected difficult intubation

Contraindications
Unable to open mouth
Awake patient

Complications
Laryngeal or esophageal injury from blind intubation
Aspiration (rare)

Equipment

Intubating LMA (ILMA) Fastrach

Large-volume syringe

ILMA endotracheal tube

ILMA stabilizer rod

10-mL syringe

Standard endotracheal tube (optional)

Review Box 4-3 Intubating laryngeal mask airway: indications, contraindications, complications, and equipment.

bag-mask ventilation), and also provide a reliable means of tracheal intubation.[35,205-208] Many clinicians who have used the Fastrach ILMA in an emergency setting insist on having this device in their difficult airway tool kit.* It is impossible to overstate the value of this device for failed emergency RSI, and unlike other rescue devices, a large volume of data support its use in general and in the setting of failed RSI.† Subsequently, it has become the primary rescue device for failed RSI in many emergency departments.

There are many different LMAs and other extraglottic devices on the market, and this can cause confusion. Although several extraglottic devices (see Chapter 3) can be used for rescue ventilation or oxygenation, only the devices discussed here can also provide a reliable means of tracheal intubation. The Fastrach is the only device in this group that has been extensively tested and the only ILMA that can reliably facilitate blind intubation (without fiberoptic guidance).‡

Indications

The LMA Fastrach is indicated as an alternative to bag-mask ventilation or as a conduit for intubation of difficult airways.[212] In the cannot-intubate/cannot-ventilate scenario it is a reliable rescue device. In this situation, adequate ventilation with the ILMA is possible in nearly all cases.[2,4,96] The ILMA is more successful for ventilation and intubation of difficult airways than the LMA Classic.[96] For inexperienced providers, ventilation with the ILMA is usually superior to face mask ventilation.[219]

The ILMA can also be used as a primary ventilation and intubation device in patients with difficult airways.[212] Studies of difficult airway management with the ILMA show that almost all patients can be adequately ventilated with the

ILMA and 94% to 99% can be intubated through the device.§ Patients who are difficult to intubate by direct laryngoscopy are often easy to intubate with the ILMA because many anatomic factors that cause difficult direct laryngoscopy do not affect placement or function of the LMA Fastrach.[35,36]

The LMA Fastrach is especially useful in patients with difficult face mask ventilation because of a beard, severe facial trauma or obesity, since none of these factors inhibit Fastrach placement. When brisk bleeding above the glottis makes ventilation and intubation difficult, the Fastrach can prevent aspiration of blood and facilitate blind or fiberoptic intubation. In patients requiring urgent cricothyrotomy or percutaneous needle insertion into the trachea, the ILMA can be used to counteract anterior neck pressure. In this capacity, the Fastrach provides temporary ventilation and aids in stabilization of the cervical spine during the surgical airway procedure.

Contraindications

One limitation of the ILMA is that it cannot be used in infants and small children because the smallest size, a No. 3, is not suitable for patients smaller than 30 kg. The LMA is the preferred rescue device for these patients.

LMAs are contraindicated in patients with less than 2 cm of mouth opening. They are unlikely to be successful in patients with grossly distorted supraglottic anatomy from disease processes or postradiation scarring. They are also relatively contraindicated in awake patients because of the high risk for emesis when the gag and airway reflexes are intact.

Intubation through the LMA Fastrach

The majority of intubations through the ILMA are performed blindly by using either the designated LMA ET tube or a

*References 2, 33, 37, 207, 209, 210.
†References 2, 33, 36-38, 210-214.
‡References 2, 33, 35, 206-208, 215-218.

§References 2, 33, 35, 37, 96, 206-208, 212, 220, 221.

standard ET tube. Regardless of the tube used, it is critical that the ILMA be optimally adjusted before attempting blind intubation through the device.

The LMA ET tube, also known as the LMA Fastrach, *is designed specifically for the ILMA.* There are two versions of the LMA ET tube: a reusable and a single-use disposable. The reusable version is made of silicone and the single-use version is made of polyvinyl chloride (PVC). The specialized LMA ET tubes are soft and straight and have a midline-beveled tip. These features are designed to allow the LMA ET tubes to emerge from the ILMA mask at an acute angle and to minimize potential injury to the vocal cords and esophagus. The drawback of the specialized Fastrach ET tubes is that they have low-volume high-pressure cuffs, which could potentially cause ischemic damage to the trachea, and there are no clinical data on how long these tubes can remain in place.[222] Use of a standard ET tube for intubation through the LMA Fastrach has been well studied and is the current practice in many EDs.[223-225] Another option is to use a Parker Flex-Tip ET tube (see Fig. 4-7).[226]

Procedure and Technique

Before intubation through the ILMA, make sure that the patient is ventilating optimally through the device. Determine this by manually ventilating the patient while holding the ILMA handle with a "frying-pan" grip. If any resistance is felt, adjust the handle by slight rotation in the sagittal plane and then lift the entire device toward the ceiling (see the "Chandy maneuver," Fig. 4-27, *step 3*).

Before inserting the ET tube, lubricate it generously. Advance the ET tube with the curve opposite that of the LMA Fastrach curve (Fig. 4-27, *step 5*). When the tube has advanced to 15 cm, the tip will start to emerge from the LMA Fastrach mask. Just before advancing the tube, use the frying-pan grip and apply a slight anterior lift (not a tilt) to further align the aperture of the ILMA with the glottis (second part of the "Chandy maneuver," Fig. 4-27, *step 6*). Do not use a levering action. While holding the handle in this position, gently pass the tracheal tube to about 16.5 cm. In this position the ET tube will push the epiglottic elevating bar up and may now come in contact with the larynx or esophagus. If cricoid pressure is being applied, decrease it because it may interfere with passage of the ET tube through the glottis. If no resistance is encountered, advance the tube into the trachea until the tracheal tube adapter comes in contact with the proximal end of the ILMA tube (Fig. 4-27, *step 7*). Do not use force when advancing the tube.

If the ET tube does not pass into the trachea easily, withdraw the ET tube to the 15-cm mark and readjust the position of the LMA Fastrach. If the tube meets resistance at about 17 cm, this may indicate a fully down-folded epiglottis or impaction of the tip of the tube against the anterior laryngeal wall. Rotating the tube may overcome impaction of the tip. To correct a down-folded epiglottis, remove the ET tube and perform the "up-down maneuver" by rotating the ILMA outward 5 to 6 cm without deflating the mask and then sliding it back into the hypopharynx (see Chapter 3, Fig. 3-9, *steps 9 and 10*). If these maneuvers are unsuccessful, it is likely that the wrong size LMA Fastrach is being used. Consider using a fiberoptic scope to guide intubation (also see the "Insertion Technique and Maneuvers Guide," on the company website: www.lmana.com).

Once the LMA ET tube has passed into the trachea, inflate the tube cuff and attempt to ventilate the patient. Check for proper tube placement with a PETCO$_2$ detector. If the tube is in the trachea, deflate the cuff of the ILMA. There is no rush to remove the ILMA; it can remain in place for an hour or longer if more pressing patient care issues need to be addressed first.

Using a Standard ET Tube

Use of a standard ET tube is not recommended by the manufacturer, but it is a well-studied and common practice.[224,227-229] The manufacturer warns that using a standard ET tube may be associated with a greater likelihood of laryngeal trauma, but there are no reports of such trauma in the literature. The only report of significant trauma with blind intubation through the LMA Fastrach is a case report of esophageal perforation and subsequent death caused by use of the specialized LMA ET tube.[230] A laboratory study showed that a standard PVC ET tube exerts 7 to 10 times more pressure on distal structures than the silicone LMA ET tube does, but the clinical relevance of this finding is unknown.[223,231] Some experts suggest warming the tip of a standard PVC ET tube (to soften it) before insertion through the LMA Fastrach.[224,227,229]

Because of the potential for injury with blind intubation through the ILMA, use fiberoptic guidance if there is any difficulty. If using a standard ET tube, insert the ET tube with its curvature opposite the curvature of the LMA Fastrach tube (Fig. 4-27, *step 5*). This allows the ET tube to exit the Fastrach at a less acute angle and then to advance into the trachea more easily.[213,229]

If intubation through the LMA Fastrach fails, the device can still be used to provide ventilation and oxygenation during more invasive airway procedures, such as retrograde intubation or cricothryotomy.[232]

Fiberoptic Intubation through the LMA Fastrach

A fiberoptic bronchoscope (FOB) can be used to verify the position of the larynx either before or during intubation. When intubating through the ILMA over an FOB, a standard ET tube is sufficient and there is no reason to use the specialized LMA ET tube. Before passing the FOB through the ILMA, advance the ET tube through the ILMA to 15 cm. At a 15-cm depth the view through the FOB should show the glottis beyond the epiglottic elevating bar. Advance the ET tube 1.5 cm before advancing the FOB. This protects the fiberoptic elements from being damaged by the epiglottic elevating bar. The view at 16.5 cm should show the vocal cords and trachea. Advance the FOB into the trachea and then pass the ET tube over the FOB. If the vocal cords are not visualized immediately, see the LMA Fastrach "Insertion Technique and Maneuvers Guide," described previously.

LMA Fastrach Removal

To remove the ILMA, deflate the cuff (Fig. 4-27, *step 8*), but be careful to not deflate the ET tube cuff. Start by removing the ET tube adapter. Then hold the proximal end of the ET tube in place while rotating the ILMA out of the hypopharynx. As the ILMA passes over the ET tube and out of the mouth, hold the ET tube in place with the stabilizer rod provided with the ILMA (see Fig. 4-27, *step 9*). When the ET tube pilot balloon comes in contact with the stabilizer rod, remove the stabilizer rod to allow the pilot balloon to travel

ENDOTRACHEAL INTUBATION WITH THE ILMA (FASTRACH)

1

Insert the ILMA by sliding the posterior surface of the mask along the palate and posterior pharynx until firm resistance is felt (see Chapter 3).

2

Inflate the ILMA cuff and begin ventilations through the device as you prepare for intubation.

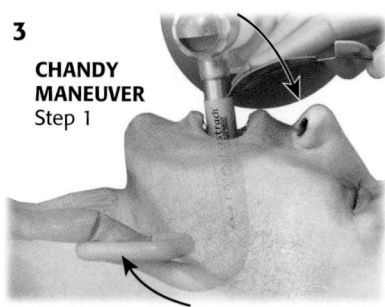

3

CHANDY MANEUVER
Step 1

Rotate handle in the sagittal plane to move the cuff forward against the larynx.

This maneuver provides a good seal and optimal ventilations.

4

Insert the LMA Fastrach ET tube to the 15-cm mark.

At this point, the tip of the tube will begin to emerge from the LMA.

5
Correct

Incorrect

If using a standard ET tube, align the curve so that it is opposite of the LMA curve.

This allows the tube to exit the mask at an angle more conducive to tracheal entry.

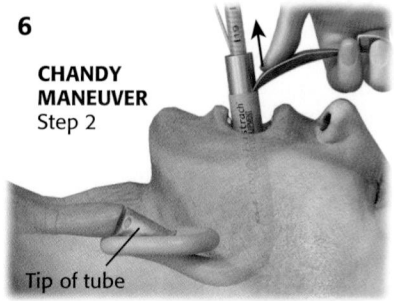

6

CHANDY MANEUVER
Step 2

Tip of tube

Prior to passing the tracheal tube, lift the handle anteriorly (not tilted) to better align the cuff and larynx for smooth ET tube passage.

7

Adapter

If no resistance is felt, advance the tube into the trachea until the adapter comes into contact with the ILMA airway tube.

Do not use force!

8

Inflate the ET tube cuff, ventilate, and check tube position with PETCO$_2$.

If the tube is properly positioned, deflate the LMA cuff.

9

Adapter

Stabilizer rod

To remove the LMA, deflate the LMA cuff and removes the adapter from the tube.

Rotate the LMA out of the mouth while using the stabilizer rod to keep the tube in place.

10

Remove the stabilizing rod when the mask is clear of the mouth, and complete removal of the LMA.

Reattach the adapter and resume ventilation.

Figure 4-27 Endotracheal (ET) intubation with the intubating laryngeal mask airway (ILMA) (Fastrach).

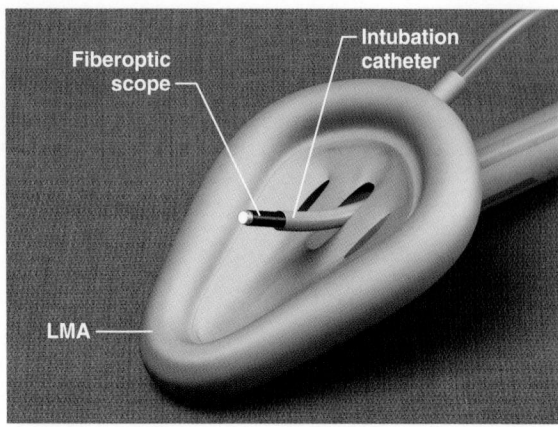

Figure 4-28 Laryngeal mask airway (LMA) as a conduit for intubation. A hollow introducer (Aintree Intubation Catheter, 60 cm) is placed though an LMA and into the trachea with the help of a fiberoptic scope. The LMA is then withdrawn while leaving the introducer in place. The tracheal tube is then railroaded over the introducer into the trachea.[233,234]

through the ILMA tube. Then reattach the ET adapter and resume ventilation. Adjust the depth of the ET tube as needed.

Intubation through the LMA Classic

The recommended technique for tracheal intubation through the LMA Classic uses an FOB and has a high success rate but requires a smaller ET tube and some adjustment maneuvers.[233,234] Blind intubation through a nonintubating LMA (LMA Classic or LMA Unique) has a poor success rate and is not recommended.[235-237] Using a tracheal tube introducer as a guide through the LMA is also unlikely to be successful and is not recommended.[238,239]

Fiberoptic Intubation through the LMA Classic

After ensuring that the LMA is ventilating properly, place a well-lubricated ET tube into the LMA tube and advance it to a depth of 24 cm (No. 5 LMA), so that the tip of the ET tube has just passed the fenestrations. Pass a lubricated FOB through the ET tube and advance it through the vocal cords. If the epiglottis is deflected downward, manipulate the tip of the FOB under the epiglottis until the vocal cords come into view. Pass the ET tube over the FOB and into the trachea, and then inflate the ET tube cuff and ventilate the patient. Check for correct ET tube placement with a PETCO$_2$ detector.

Alternatively, place a hollow introducer, such as an Aintree Intubation Catheter (Cook Critical Care, Bloomington, IN; www.cookmedical.com), in conjunction with an FOB, through the LMA and into the trachea (Fig. 4-28). Remove the LMA while leaving the exchange catheter as an introducer for the ET tube, much like a conventional tracheal tube introducer.

Cricoid pressure may impede placement and intubation through the LMA.[93,94] Release cricoid pressure, if necessary, to accomplish these procedures.

Complications When Intubating through LMAs

Although most patients can be safely intubated blindly through the ILMA, there is a small chance of injury to the larynx or esophagus, especially with multiple blind attempts. There is one case report of a death caused by esophageal perforation during blind intubation through the ILMA. Consider using fiberoptic guidance if blind intubation is difficult or if the clinician is inexperienced. Intubation through a nonintubating LMA is not recommended unless facilitated by an FOB.

Summary

LMAs provide an excellent means of oxygenation and ventilation when face mask ventilation is difficult or impossible. In addition, the LMA Fastrach is particularly useful when managing patients who are difficult to intubate with direct laryngoscopy. By facilitating the management of difficult or failed ventilation and difficult or failed intubation, the LMA Fastrach is an indispensable component of the difficult airway algorithm.

FLEXIBLE FIBEROPTIC INTUBATION

Flexible fiberoptic intubation with an FOB is the most common technique used by anesthesiologists for known difficult airways. Physicians who perform fiberoptic intubations daily have a success rate of nearly 100% when using this technique for difficult intubations.[240] In the ED, with more difficult intubating conditions and less experienced fiberoscopists, the success rate is 50% to 90%.[241-244] The most common reason cited for failure of flexible fiberoptic intubation in the operating room is clinician inexperience.[245] In the ED, failure is most often attributed to poor visibility from blood, vomitus, and other secretions.[241-243] Mlinik and colleagues[243] found that successful ED fiberoptic intubations averaged 2 minutes whereas failures averaged 8 minutes. They recommended consideration of alternative approaches if intubation attempts take more than 3 minutes. ED clinicians have the opportunity to develop fiberoptic laryngoscopy skills when performing diagnostic nasopharyngoscopy on ambulatory patients.

Flexible fiberoptic intubation is often the best method for intubating awake patients with a known difficult airway. It can be accomplished via the nasal or oral route and is better tolerated than direct laryngoscopy. It usually provides excellent visualization of the airway and permits evaluation of the airway before placement of the tube. The expense of the equipment, its fragility, and the length of time required to both achieve and maintain technical proficiency are drawbacks.

FOBs are graded according to their external diameter (in millimeters). FOBs specifically designed for ET intubations are available from several companies (Pentax, Olympus, Machida, Storz, and Fujinon). A practical size for an intubating scope is about 4 mm. Although it is physically possible to pass a 4.5-mm (0.5 mm larger) tracheal tube over the scope, the fit is tight. As a rule, the tracheal tube should be about 1 mm larger than the intubating scope. The size of the working channel, the port that allows suction, administration of oxygen, and passage of fluid or catheters, is another important dimension when evaluating FOBs. A working channel of about 2 mm is desirable to allow adequate suction of secretions. Very thin nasopharyngoscopes, with diameters of 3.0 to 3.5 mm, have no working channel but can be used for pediatric tracheal intubation.

Indications and Contraindications

Patients with known or suspected difficult airways are good candidates for awake or semi-awake fiberoptic intubation.

Flexible Fiberoptic Intubation

Indications

Known or suspected difficult airway
Distorted airway anatomy
  Swelling
  Abscess/infection
  Morbid obesity
  Trauma
  Tumors/previous radiation therapy

Contraindications

Nasal approach
  Severe midface trauma
  Coagulopathy
Relative
  Active airway bleeding
  Vomiting

Complications

Hypoxia from prolonged intubation attempts
Vomiting
Laryngospasm
Soft tissue trauma

Equipment

Flexible fiberoptic bronchoscope (FOB)

Endotracheal tube

Review Box 4-4 Flexible fiberoptic intubation: indications, contraindications, complications, and equipment.

Patients with distorted airway anatomy, including swelling of the mouth or tongue, upper airway abscess or infection, morbid obesity, cervical spine injury, trismus, and penetrating and blunt neck trauma, are all good candidates for awake fiberoptic intubation. Patients with laryngeal tumors, especially those with a history of radiation therapy encompassing the cervical region, may be impossible to intubate by any other nonsurgical method. An FOB can also be helpful when assessing and intubating patients with airway obstruction from presumed foreign body aspiration. Flexible fiberoptic intubation is best used as the initial approach to tracheal intubation, but it may be used as a rescue device when other methods fail.[246] Flexible fiberoptic intubation can also be performed through an ILMA or LMA after difficult ventilation or failed intubation.

Contraindications to the nasal approach are severe midface trauma and coagulopathy. Patients who are likely to receive thrombolytics should also be excluded. Although there are no clear contraindications to fiberoptic orotracheal intubation, active airway bleeding and vomiting are relative contraindications because successful fiberoptic intubation is rarely achieved in these settings. If the clinician is inexperienced in fiberoptic intubation, significant hypoxia is another relative contraindication.

Procedure and Technique

Preparation of the upper airway is important for successful awake or semi-awake fiberoptic intubation. Deliver local anesthetic to the upper airway by one of several methods. Nebulized lidocaine (4 to 6 mL of a 4% solution) can be used to anesthetize the entire upper airway if time permits. Lidocaine (3 mL of a 4% solution) can also be injected percutaneously through the cricothyroid membrane via a 20-gauge needle, thereby providing anesthesia to the larynx and trachea. Some laryngeal and tracheal anesthesia can also be achieved by transoral spray with a laryngeal tracheal anesthetic set. Finally, lidocaine (4%) can be sprayed through the working channel of the fiberoptic scope during the procedure via the "spray as you go" technique. The maximum dose of lidocaine for airway anesthesia is 3 to 4 mg/kg (about 200 mg in an adult). Sedation for fiberoptic intubation can be accomplished with ketamine, etomidate, propofol, fentanyl, alfentanil, or midazolam (see Chapter 5). The goal of sedation is to preserve spontaneous respiration but limit patient movement and reaction to the procedure. A combination of good topical anesthesia and mild sedation allows the best chance for successful intubation.

The optimal position of the neck is extension, as opposed to the slight cervical flexion desired when using direct laryngoscopy. Extension allows better visualization of the glottis by elevating the epiglottis off the posterior pharyngeal wall. This is especially pertinent in a comatose patient who lacks the muscle tone necessary to maintain an open airway. If problems arise with the tongue and soft tissues falling back and obscuring the view of the FOB, apply a jaw-lift maneuver or grasp the tongue and pull it forward and away from the soft palate and posterior pharyngeal wall. This also moves the epiglottis away from the posterior pharyngeal wall and facilitates exposure of the cords. Extend the head to accomplish the same objective.

Fiberoptic intubation may be performed with the patient in the upright, semi-upright, or supine position. Stand facing the patient or at the patient's head, depending on personal preference. The upright and semi-upright positions help keep pharyngeal soft tissue from obstructing the airway. The upright position may be more familiar to emergency clinicians who are skilled at diagnostic nasopharyngoscopy.

The greatest impediment to successful fiberoptic intubation is an inability to visualize the larynx because blood or secretions have covered the optical element and cannot be removed. Suction actively just before introduction of the FOB. Once the scope is in place, suction minor secretions through the fiberoptic suction port. Significant blood and secretions are best removed by high-flow oxygen through the suction port, which serves simultaneously to remove blood and secretions, defog the tip, and increase the inspired O_2 content. The setup required for oxygen insufflation should be available immediately, if not already attached to the suction port before the scope is inserted. Once the scope has entered the trachea, difficulty advancing the ET tube may be encountered. The tip of the tube most commonly catches on the right arytenoid cartilage or vocal cord. To fix this, withdraw the tube 2 cm, rotate it counterclockwise 90 degrees, and readvance the tube to remedy the problem (see Fig. 4-19).

Nasal Approach

The nasal approach is technically easier than the oral approach because the angle of insertion allows better visualization of the larynx with minimal manipulation of the FOB. Patient cooperation is also less critical with this approach. In an unconscious patient, the tip of the scope is also less likely to impinge on the base of the tongue with a nasal approach.

If conditions permit, choose the most patent nostril. In a cooperative patient, determine this by simply occluding each nostril and asking the patient to identify the nostril that is easiest to breathe through. Identify the most patent nostril by direct vision or by gently inserting a gloved finger that is lubricated with viscous lidocaine into the nostrils. If time is not an issue, an effective method to dilate the nasal cavity and administer an anesthetic is to pass a lidocaine gel–lubricated nasopharyngeal airway (nasal trumpet) into the selected nostril. Leave this airway in place for several minutes, and introduce progressively larger trumpets.

To prepare the nose and upper airway, administer vasoconstrictors, topical anesthetics, and lubricants. Vasoconstrictors such as 0.25% or 1.0% phenylephrine drops, oxymetazoline (Afrin) spray, or 4% cocaine spray can limit epistaxis. Ample 2% lidocaine gel in the nasal cavity helps the tube negotiate the nasopharynx without complication. Hypopharyngeal anesthesia, as described previously, minimizes gagging and laryngospasm. Place the well-lubricated ET tube in the nostril first to a depth of about 10 cm and then pass the scope through it. Alternatively, mount the ET tube over the scope and first pass the scope through the nostril (Fig. 4-29). Either sequence is acceptable. The advantage of first passing the tracheal tube through the nose is that it avoids the possibility of secretions covering the scope and positions the scope just above the laryngeal inlet. Its disadvantages are that NT placement may cause bleeding and, in some patients, the tube may not pass easily into the nasopharynx. In some patients the mouth is not accessible at all because of trismus, swelling, or trauma (e.g., angioedema caused by an angiotensin-converting enzyme [ACE] inhibitor), so the nasal route is the only option for fiberoptic intubation (Fig. 4-30).

Prepare the most patent nostril and advance the ET tube until it makes the bend into the nasopharynx. If negotiating this bend is difficult, place a well-lubricated FOB through the tube and into the oropharynx to serve as a guide for the ET tube. Once the tracheal tube is in the oropharynx, perform thorough oropharyngeal suctioning before introducing the scope into the ET tube. Advance the FOB toward the larynx.

Figure 4-29 Fiberoptic intubation. Note that the tracheal tube is first premounted on the scope. The fiberoptic scope enters the trachea and then serves as a guide over which the tracheal tube is passed. *Larger image*, The nasal approach. *Inset*, Use of an oral intubating airway via the oral approach. (*Courtesy of Department of Emergency Medicine, Hennepin County Medical Center, Minneapolis.*)

The epiglottis and vocal cords are seen with little or no manipulation of the tip of the FOB in 90% of patients.[236] Advance the scope and keep the cords in view by making frequent minor adjustments of the tip of the scope.

In a comatose or obtunded patient, the tongue and other soft tissues may obscure the view of the larynx. This can be alleviated by asking an assistant to pull the tongue forward or apply a chin- or jaw-lift maneuver. Advance the scope through the larynx to the carina and pass the ET tube over the firmly held FOB into the trachea. Remember that in adults, the average distance from the naris to the epiglottis is 16 to 17 cm. If the scope has been advanced much beyond this distance and the glottis is still not seen, the scope is probably in the esophagus.[247] If the scope meets resistance at about this same level and only a pink blur is visible, the tip of the scope is probably in a piriform sinus. Transillumination of the soft tissues may confirm this and indicate the necessary corrective maneuvers.

Oral Approach

Oral fiberoptic intubation is indicated when nasal intubation is contraindicated, most commonly because of severe midface trauma or clinician inexperience. Skilled fiberoscopists often find the oral approach just as easy as the nasal approach. For the less experienced, though, the oral approach may be more difficult because the path of the scope is less defined by the surrounding soft tissue and the tip of the scope is more likely to impinge on the base of the tongue or vallecula. Keeping the scope in the midline and elevating the soft tissue by pulling the tongue forward or applying the jaw-lift maneuver will minimize this difficulty. Because the oropharyngeal axis is not as well aligned with the larynx as the nasopharyngeal

Figure 4-30 A, This patient with life-threatening angiotensin-converting enzyme inhibitor-induced angioedema is in severe distress, and oral intubation is impossible. **B,** Fiberoptic nasotracheal intubation is a good choice, but it is very difficult, if not impossible, in a struggling patient. Ketamine anesthesia allowed patient cooperation and administration of supplemental oxygen. A less ideal option is blind nasotracheal intubation. Tracheostomy may be required. *Note:* In this case the tracheal tube was premounted on the scope before the scope was passed into the patient's nose. Alternatively, the tube may be first passed about 10 cm through the nose, and then the scope passed through the tube and into the trachea.

Figure 4-31 Examples of oral intubating airways. The Williams Airway Intubator (*left*) cradles the endotracheal (ET) tube in an open, curved guide, whereas the Ovassapian Fiberoptic Intubating Airway (*right*) positions the ET tube on the posterior surface of the intubation airway.

axis is, more scope manipulation is required when using the oral approach.

Difficulty with the oral approach can be minimized by using an oral intubating airway (Fig. 4-31). This adjunct resembles an oropharyngeal airway but is longer and has a cylindrical passage through which the FOB and tracheal tube are passed. The tip of this airway lies just cephalad to the epiglottis and ensures midline positioning. Make sure that the patient is either adequately anesthetized or obtunded before the oral airway is placed to minimize gagging or vomiting. Place a well-lubricated FOB, premounted with an ET tube, through the oral intubating airway and fiberoptically intubate the trachea (Fig. 4-29, *upper right inset*). Advance the ET tube over the scope and into the trachea. This may require the same counterclockwise maneuver as described with the nasal approach. After successful intubation, the oral airway can be

Figure 4-32 Two-person fiberoptic intubation for difficult intubation. The laryngoscopist obtains the best hypopharyngeal exposure and directs the fiberoptic tip in the direction of the glottis. The second clinician, who manipulates the tip of the fiberoptic scope, directs the laryngoscopist to slowly advance the tip until it has successfully passed through the cords.

left in place as a bite block or may be removed over the ET tube after removal of the tube adapter. Some oral intubating airways can be removed from the mouth without disconnecting the ET tube adapter.

An alternative approach to the traditional oral fiberoptic intubation for an anticipated difficult airway requires two clinicians. One performs direct laryngoscopy, places the tip of the fiberoptic scope under the epiglottis, and blindly advances it while the second clinician, holding the body of the scope, directs the tip fiberoptically through the cords (Fig. 4-32).

Complications

Complications of fiberoptic orotracheal intubation include hypoxia from prolonged intubation attempts, emesis, and laryngospasm. Oxygen saturation monitoring should alert the clinician to hypoxia. Most complications seen with fiberoptically guided NT intubation are associated with passing the ET tube through the nasopharynx. Epistaxis is the most common, followed by other nasopharyngeal injuries. A rare but potentially significant complication may result if on blind advancement of the fiberoptic scope through the ET tube the tip of the scope exits through Murphy's eye (distal side port of the ET tube).[248] Attempts at passing the ET tube through the larynx will fail because the tip of the tube, now extending off the midline, will catch on the laryngeal structures. To avoid this complication, introduce the scope before placing the ET tube.

Summary

The primary advantages of fiberoptic intubation are the ability to visualize upper airway abnormalities, to negotiate difficult airway anatomy, and to carefully perform tracheal intubation under visual guidance. Fiberoptic intubation is noninvasive and well tolerated. Its major limitation as an emergency airway is poor visibility because of blood and secretions; in this setting it is best to avoid the FOB. Procedural time can be another limitation. Fiberoptic intubation requires more practice than many other methods of airway management, and considerable experience should be obtained before using the FOB in an airway emergency. Fiberoptic intubation is more likely to be successful if used early in the management of a difficult airway rather than as a last resort after repeated failure with direct laryngoscopy.

OPTICAL STYLETS

A class of devices that incorporates fiberoptics into a semirigid metal or metal-reinforced stylet was introduced in the late 1990s. These devices can be used in conjunction with direct laryngoscopy or as stand-alone intubating devices. They have been shown to require direct laryngoscopic assistance in 8% to 20% of cases and in general are more successful when used in this way.[249,250] Pass the tip of the fiberoptic stylet, with its overlying ET tube, under the epiglottis and direct it through the glottis and into the trachea. Visibility can be hampered by blood and secretions, but less so than with flexible fiberoscopy.[251] These devices are far more intuitive and require less practice than an FOB does. The Shikani Optical Stylet and Levitan FPS Scope (Clarus Medical, Minneapolis) are examples of these malleable optical stylets (Fig. 4-33). The Shikani Optical Stylet is most often used similarly to the Trachlight, with the added feature of fiberoptic visualization of anatomic structures lying just beyond the tip of the tube. The Levitan FPS Scope is designed to be used with a laryngoscope and serves as a stylet for the tracheal tube while providing fiberoptic visualization if required. The Bonfils Retromolar Intubation Fiberscope (Storz Endoscopy, Culver City, CA) is rigid but otherwise structurally and functionally similar to the Shikani. The distal end of the Bonfils has a fixed curve of 40 degrees, whereas the other scopes are malleable up to 120 degrees. Power for the Shikani and Bonfils stylets may be supplied by either an external source or batteries. Video

Figure 4-33 Examples of semirigid fiberoptic stylets: the Levitan (*top*) and Shikani (*bottom*). The recommended bends when used with a direct laryngoscope (*top*) and when used alone (*bottom*) are demonstrated. The sliding adapter on the Shikani allows various lengths of tracheal tubes.

cameras can be attached to the eyepiece of all of these devices but have the drawback of making them less maneuverable. The Bonfils is available with an integrated video module. The Levitan stylet is shorter than the other devices, and although it conforms more to the normal length of a stylet, it currently requires that the tube be cut at 27.5 to 28 cm before mounting it on the stylet. It can accommodate down to a 5.5-mm-ID tube. The Shikani stylet comes in two sizes, the adult, which accommodates a 5.5-mm-ID tube, and a pediatric version, which goes down to a 3.5-mm-ID tube. An adjustable plastic ET tube stop is located proximally on the stylet, secures the tube at the desired length, and provides a means for oxygen supplementation during the procedure.

The Video-Optical Intubation Stylet (VOIS; Acutonic Medical Systems AG, Baar, Switzerland) is a semirigid fiberoptic scope that is used like a malleable stylet and attaches to the ET tube via a sliding adapter located on the more distal aspect of a 2-m length of fiberoptic cable. An external light source is required. The image is transmitted to a monitor but can also be viewed through an eyepiece. Direct laryngoscopy is used routinely with the VOIS. Mannequin studies of the VOIS versus the Bullard scope and the Shikani scope versus the gum elastic boogie demonstrated greater success with Cormack-Lehane grade III views (Fig. 4-4C) with the semirigid fiberoptic stylets.[252,253]

Indications and Contraindications

Semirigid fiberoptic stylets are useful when the glottis cannot be seen readily. Blood and secretions may complicate their use, but less so than with flexible fiberoscopy. The Bonfils stylet, with its fixed 45-degree curve, is not recommended for patients with severely limited neck extension or limited mouth opening.[254]

Procedure and Technique

The semirigid fiberoptic stylet can be used with or without direct laryngoscopy. In either case, place the patient in the sniffing position. Load an ET tube onto a lightly lubricated stylet so that the ET tube extends 1 to 2 cm beyond the end of the stylet.

If the device is used alone, create an accentuated curve of between 70 and 80 degrees at the proximal aspect of the cuff of the tube so that it can negotiate the oropharynx. Deliver high-flow oxygen down the ET tube to decrease the chance of getting blood and secretions on the optical element. Suction the oropharynx well before attempting intubation. Grasp the mandible with the left hand. Next, raise the jaw to lift the tongue and epiglottis off the posterior hypopharyngeal wall. Ask an assistant to apply a jaw-thrust maneuver or grasp the tongue with gauze and retract it anteriorly. Place the device into the mouth, and while following the curve of the tongue, bring it up under the epiglottis with fiberoptic guidance. To identify landmarks, you may need to use a rocking action, similar to that used with the lighted stylet. On seeing the laryngeal inlet, direct the tip into the larynx. Advance the ET tube as you withdraw the stylet. If resistance is met while advancing the tube, the tip may be catching on the anterior larynx or trachea. Rotate the tube clockwise 120 degrees at the proximal end, which will result in 90-degree rotation at the tip. With the bevel now anterior, allow the tube to advance without catching. It is important to remember that the direction of rotation of the ET tube is *clockwise* if resistance is encountered *after* going through the cords. For resistance encountered *before* the cords, such as occurs with tracheal tube introducers, fiberoptic scopes, and NT intubation, rotate the tube *counterclockwise*.

Semirigid optical stylets can be used with direct laryngoscopy, either primarily or after encountering difficulty while using the device alone. With this approach, make the angle of the distal stylet less acute, at about 35 degrees, and introduce the device only after obtaining maximal visualization with the laryngoscope. If the epiglottis can be seen, advance the tip of the stylet just underneath it via direct vision. Be careful to not embed the tip of the ET tube in the supraglottic soft tissue because it will obscure visibility. At this point, fiberoptically guide the stylet–ET tube unit into the glottis and advance the tube off the stylet.

There have been no reported complications with semirigid fiberoptic stylets other than the failures or prolonged attempts usually related to poor visibility from blood and secretions.[249]

Summary

Semirigid fiberoptic stylets combine the features of direct and indirect laryngoscopy and provide a valuable tool when approaching a difficult airway. They can be used alone or in conjunction with a laryngoscope. They are considerably less expensive than rigid fiberoptic devices and are easier to use than flexible scopes. The supporting literature exists as case reports and relatively small series. There are no head-to-head clinical trials with other devices, but experience suggests that semirigid fiberoptic stylets may play an increasing role in managing difficult intubations.

LIGHTED STYLET INTUBATION

This technique uses a battery-operated lighted stylet that is placed in an ET tube and used to guide the tube into the trachea by transilluminating the soft tissues of the neck. First described in 1957 by Macintosh and Richards,[255] it was designed for the difficult airway. It can also be useful in determining the position of the tracheal tube.[141] Early models suffered from insufficient illumination to function well in

Figure 4-34 Trachlight and related stylets. The malleable stylet is bent at a 90-degree angle, 6.5 to 8.5 cm from the tip (marked on stylet). The smallest stylet accommodates a 2.5-mm–internal diameter tube.

ambient light and had equipment failures that rendered them commercial failures. The Trachlight (Laerdal Medical Corp., Wappengers Falls, NY), introduced in 1995, had a brighter light source, enclosed bulb, and adjustable length, which successfully addressed these problems (Fig. 4-34). It is the only lighted stylet, among several available, that has a proven track record. The Trachlight compared favorably with direct laryngoscopy in a randomized study of 950 surgical patients, with a 99% overall success rate and 92% on the first attempt, and reduced lighting was necessary 21% of the time.[256] In another large series the device was 99% successful in intubating patients with difficult airways.[257] The Trachlight has a handle and a malleable optical stylet that is composed of an inner stiff wire stylet and an outer flexible optical element. The stylets come in adult, pediatric, and infant sizes and can accommodate down to a 2.5-mm-ID tube.

Indications and Contraindications

An excellent candidate for light-guided tracheal intubation is a patient with a difficult airway and failed intubation with direct laryngoscopy as a result of excessive blood and secretions. A multiple-trauma patient with airway bleeding is a good example. A patient who has been pharmacologically paralyzed and cannot be intubated with direct laryngoscopy is another example. It can also be used for routine intubations, depending on the experience and skill set of the clinician. The lighted stylet may be helpful in successfully completing a difficult NT intubation. One advantage of this technique over blind NT intubation is that it can be used in an apneic patient.

Because lighted stylet intubation is a semiblind approach, avoid using it in patients with expanding neck masses, oropharyngeal trauma, and or airway compromise presumably caused by a foreign body. Massive obesity is the most common cause of failure of this device because of difficulty transilluminating the anterior portion of the neck.

Procedure and Technique

Place the patient's head and neck in the neutral or slightly extended position. If the patient is awake, spray the oropharynx and hypopharynx with lidocaine and administer sedation as indicated. Check the function of the bulb on the lighted stylet before use. Ideally, lubricate the inner wire stylet, optical stylet, and ET tube with a water-soluble agent to prepare the device for use. If the device is used primarily for rescue, it will be preassembled and only the ET tube will be lubricated. Check to make sure that the wire insert is snapped into the adjustable guide rail connector on the handle; otherwise, the wire will turn freely from side to side, and the tip of the tube will not be controllable as it is maneuvered within the hypopharynx.

With the Trachlight unit assembled, bend the distal tip into the shape of a hockey stick with a 90-degree curve beginning just proximal to the tube cuff. Obese patients with a short thyromental distance may require a bend of up to 110 degrees. Mark the bend distance on the stylet as a 2-cm line, corresponding to 6.5 to 8.5 cm from the end of the ET tube. Use a shorter bend point in patients with short thyromental distances.[258] Stand at the patient's head. If this is not possible, approach the patient from either side. Grasp the patient's jaw near the corner of the mouth, between the thumb, index, and middle finger. Lift to elevate the tongue and epiglottis (Fig. 4-35). Turn the light on and insert the unit into the mouth in the midline by following the curve of the tongue into the oropharynx. With a rocking motion, gently advance the tip. A transilluminating glow indicates the location of the tip of the tube. Applying cricoid pressure may enhance the transillumination.[141] Dim the overhead lights to see the glow better in an obese patient. Positioning is optimal when a lightbulb-like glow emanates from the midline just below the level of the thyroid prominence. If a more diffuse glow is seen just above this prominence, the tip may be in the vallecula. A more lateral position suggests placement in the piriform fossae. In this case, withdraw the unit 2 cm or cock it back and reposition it as indicated by the light. If you do not see a light, the tube is in the esophagus and should be pulled back. Apply external laryngeal pressure, and if necessary, extend the head

slightly. In a very thin patient it is possible to observe transillumination and still be in the esophagus. The clue is that the glow will be diffuse if the tip is in the esophagus, as opposed to the well-circumscribed glow of intralaryngeal placement. Once the tube is in the larynx, withdraw the stiff wire stylet 10 cm and advance the tube to the level of the sternal notch. Release the tube from the Trachlight, withdraw the lighted stylet, and confirm the tube's position.

Complications

Earlier reports noted complications with lighted stylets that resulted from equipment failure and lost bulbs. These technical problems have ceased since the advent of the Trachlight. No other complications attributable to the Trachlight have been reported. The clear instructions to avoid using the device in patients with upper airway distortion from tumor, infection, and hematoma may be responsible for this clean record. A study of pathologic specimens showed no evidence of burn injury in the tracheal mucosa in cats intubated with the Trachlight.[259]

Summary

Lighted stylet intubation is a safe, rapid, and highly successful method that has a definite place in the management of difficult airways. Because it is placed with the patient in a neutral position and blood and secretions are not an impediment to success, it is especially amenable to the trauma setting. A patient who is most likely to fail lighted stylet intubation is one who is morbidly obese with a short thyromental distance. Though not overly challenging technically, practice under controlled intubating conditions is advised. Improvements in the device have made its use more practical in emergency airway management settings.

BLIND NASOTRACHEAL INTUBATION

Blind NT intubation can be one of the more technically demanding airway approaches, with the outcome being heavily dependent on the skill and experience of the clinician and a certain amount of luck. The primary advantage of the blind technique is that it minimizes neck movement and does not require mouth opening. In extenuating circumstances, it can be accomplished without an intravenous line.

General Indications and Contraindications

NT intubation is technically more difficult than oral intubation, but it has definite advantages. Blind NT intubation is possible with the patient in the sitting position, a distinct advantage when intubating a patient with congestive heart failure who cannot tolerate lying flat. In fact, patients in respiratory distress are the easiest to intubate blindly because their air hunger results in increased abduction of the vocal cords, which facilitates entry of the tube into the trachea.

An NT tube has advantages that extend beyond the immediate difficulties of airway control. The patient cannot bite the tube or manipulate it with the tongue. Oral injuries may be cared for without interference from the tube. An NT tube is more easily stabilized and generally easier to care for than an orotracheal tube. It is better tolerated by the patient,

Figure 4-35 Lighted stylet intubation. The Trachlight is used for endotracheal intubation with transillumination of the soft tissues as a guide to placement. *(Courtesy of Department of Emergency Medicine, Hennepin County Medical Center, Minneapolis.)*

permits easier movement in bed, and produces less reflex salivation than an orotracheal tube.

Blind Placement

Blind NT intubation is the most common form of NT intubation in the emergency setting. Danzl and Thomas[260] reported a success rate of 92% in a large series of ED patients, but success rates are highly dependent on clinician skill.

Indications and Contraindications

Patients requiring airway control who have spontaneous respirations can be considered for blind NT intubation. The typical patient is one with an anticipated difficult airway and persistently low oxygen saturation despite preoxygenation. Patients with severe chronic obstructive pulmonary disease (COPD) or asthma who have high airway pressures and may be difficult to ventilate with a face mask are another group to consider for NT intubation. Some other common examples of a difficult airway to consider for NT intubation are patients with short thick necks, trismus, neck immobility, and oral injuries. Other conditions that preclude successful orotracheal intubation include severe arthritis, fixed deformities of the cervical spine, or ACE inhibitor-induced angioedema.

Avoid nasal intubation in patients with severe nasal or midface trauma. In the presence of a basilar skull fracture, an NT tube may inadvertently enter the cranial cavity.[261,262] Avoid this technique in patients in whom thrombolytic therapy is being considered. Nasal intubation is also relatively contraindicated if the patient is taking anticoagulants, has a known coagulopathy, or has recently been administered thrombolytics. Apnea is the major contraindication to blind NT intubation because attempts to place the tube without respirations as a guide are futile. Blind NT intubation should be avoided in patients with expanding neck hematomas and oropharyngeal trauma. Patient combativeness, if not controlled with sedation, is another relative contraindication. Inability to open the mouth (such as a wired jaw) is a relative contraindication because emesis may be induced and it may be impossible to clear the vomitus. Exercise judgment in each individual case and be prepared to use neuromuscular blocking agents or to bypass the upper airway with a surgical technique if such a complication develops.

Procedure and Technique

Place the patient in the sniffing position with the proximal part of the neck slightly flexed and the head extended on the neck. In preparation for intubation, constrict the nasal mucosa of both nares with 0.25% to 1.0% phenylephrine drops, oxymetazoline (Afrin) spray, or 4% cocaine spray. Topical anesthesia of the nares, oropharynx, and hypopharynx with lidocaine spray (4%) is also indicated if time permits. If available, cocaine is ideal because it is both a vasoconstrictor and an anesthetic, but caution is necessary in hypertensive patients. Choose the most patent nostril. In a cooperative patient, simply occlude each nostril and ask the patient which one is easier to breathe through. The most patent nostril can also be identified by direct vision or by gently inserting a gloved finger lubricated with viscous lidocaine into the nostrils. If time permits, pass a nasal airway first and allow it to remain in place to physically dilate the passage. Some

clinicians preemptively place nasal airways in patients for prognostication of subsequent intubation if other interventions fail (such as in exacerbations of COPD).

After preparation of the nostril, insert a well-lubricated 7.0- or 7.5-mm ET tube along the floor of the nasal cavity. Do not direct the tube cephalad, as one might expect from the external nasal anatomy, but rather direct it straight backward toward the occiput and along the nasal floor. Twist the tube gently to bypass any soft tissue obstruction in the nasal cavity. It is sometimes recommended that the tube's bevel be oriented toward the septum to avoid injury to the inferior turbinate. At 6 to 7 cm, one usually feels a "give" as the tube passes the nasal choana and negotiates the abrupt 90-degree curve required to enter the nasopharynx. This is the most painful and traumatic part of the procedure and must be done gently. If resistance persists despite continued gentle pressure and twisting of the tube, pass a suction catheter down the tube and into the oropharynx to allow successful passage of the tube over the catheter.[263] If this attempt fails, try the other nostril. To avoid this difficulty from the outset, use a controllable-tip tracheal tube (Endotrol, Mallinckrodt Medical, Inc., St. Louis). The tube allows you to increase the flexion of the tube, thereby facilitating passage past this tight curve. One study found that the Endotrol tube enhanced first-attempt success with blind NT intubation.[264] A study of paramedic-performed blind NT intubation reported success rates of 58% with standard ET tubes versus 72% with ET tubes with a directional controllable tip.[265]

As the tube advances through the oropharynx and hypopharynx, it approaches the vocal cords, and breath sounds from the tube typically become louder. Fogging of the tube may also occur. At the point of maximal breath sounds, the tube is lying immediately in front of the laryngeal inlet. The tube is most easily advanced into the trachea during inspiration, when the vocal cords are maximally open. As the patient begins to breathe in, advance the tube in one smooth motion. If a cough reflex is present, the patient usually coughs and becomes stridulous during this maneuver, which suggests successful tracheal intubation. The absence of such a response should alert the clinician to probable esophageal passage. If there is a delay in advancing the tube, add oxygen to the end of the tube to increase the inspired oxygen concentration. Once the tube is in the trachea, vocalization should cease. Persistent vocalizations suggest esophageal intubation. Breath sounds coming from the tube and tube fogging are other signs of correct ET tube placement. Reflex swallowing during blind NT intubation may direct the tube posteriorly toward the esophagus. If this occurs, direct conscious patients to stick out their tongue to inhibit swallowing and prevent consequent movement of the larynx. Application of laryngeal pressure may also help avoid esophageal passage.

After intubation, auscultate over both lungs while applying positive pressure ventilation. If only one lung is being ventilated, withdraw the tube until breath sounds are heard bilaterally. The optimum distance from the external nares to the tip of the tube is about 28 cm in males and 26 cm in females.[266] After verification of tracheal placement, inflate the cuff and secure the tube.

Technical Difficulties

The NT tube may slide smoothly through the hypopharynx and into the trachea on the first pass. Unfortunately, such is not always the case; in an operating room series, the first attempt was successful in less than 50% of instances.[267] When the initial pass is unsuccessful, there are four potential locations of the tip of the tube: anterior to the epiglottis in the vallecula, on the arytenoids or vocal cords, in a piriform sinus, or in the esophagus.

Observation and palpation of the soft tissues of the neck during attempted passage of the NT tube are helpful in finding the misplaced tube. Before reattempting placement, withdraw the tube slightly. Do not remove it from the nose because this will create additional trauma to the nasal soft tissues. Contemplate the possibility of spinal injury when considering corrective maneuvers. Any cervical maneuver that moves the neck significantly should not be used if alternatives are available. Methods to achieve success when difficulties with tube placement are encountered include the following.

Anterior to the Epiglottis
Difficulty advancing the tube beyond 15 cm or palpation of the tip of the tube anteriorly at the level of the hyoid bone suggests an impasse anterior to the epiglottis in the vallecula. Withdraw the tube 2 cm, decrease the degree of neck extension, and readvance the tube.

Arytenoid Cartilage and Vocal Cord
Contrary to the classic teaching,[268] studies have demonstrated a propensity for an NT tube, when placed through the right nares, to lie posteriorly and to the right as it approaches the larynx.[269,270] It is not surprising that the most common obstacles to advancement of the NT tube are the right arytenoid and the vocal cords. No data are available on common obstacles encountered if the tube is placed in the left nares. If the tube appears to be hanging up on firm, cartilaginous tissue, withdraw the tube 2 cm, rotate it 90 degrees counterclockwise, and readvance it. This maneuver orients the bevel of the tube posteriorly and frequently results in successful passage (Fig. 4-36). When evaluated in the ED, this maneuver was successful 73% of the time.[271] Another technique is to pass a suction catheter down the tube. It will often pass through the larynx without difficulty, and the tube can then be advanced over the catheter (Fig. 4-37).[272,273]

Piriform Sinus
Bulging of the neck lateral and superior to the larynx indicates tube location in a piriform sinus. Withdraw the tube 2 cm, rotate it slightly away from the bulge, and then readvance it. An alternative method is to tilt the patient's head toward the side of the misplacement and then reattempt placement.[274]

Esophageal Placement
Esophageal placement is indicated by a smooth passage of the tube and the loss of breath sounds. The larynx may be seen or felt to elevate as the tube passes under it. Assisted ventilation will usually produce gurgling sounds when the epigastrium is auscultated. Withdraw the tube until breath sounds are clearly heard, and reattempt passage while applying pressure to the cricoid. Increase extension of the head on the neck during placement. If attempts continue to result in esophageal misplacement, the following maneuver may result in successful tracheal intubation. From the precise point at which breath sounds are lost, withdraw the ET tube 1 cm and inflate the cuff with 15 mm of air, which results in elevation of the tube off the posterior pharyngeal wall. Angle it toward the larynx.

Figure 4-36 Common problem with blind tracheal tube passage through the larynx. **A,** The tip of the tube is caught on the arytenoid cartilage. **B,** Rotation of tube 90 degrees counterclockwise orients the bevel of the tip posteriorly and allows passage into the larynx. *(Courtesy of Department of Emergency Medicine, Hennepin County Medical Center, Minneapolis.)*

Figure 4-37 Use of suction catheter to aid in passage of a nasotracheal tube caught at laryngeal inlet. The suction catheter is passed down the tracheal tube and into the trachea. The tracheal tube is then passed over the suction catheter, and the catheter is removed. *(Courtesy of Department of Emergency Medicine, Hennepin County Medical Center, Minneapolis.)*

Advance the tube 2 cm. Continued breath sounds indicate a probable intralaryngeal location. At this point, deflate the cuff and advance the ET tube into the trachea (Fig. 4-38). This technique may be particularly useful in patients with cervical spine injury because it requires no manipulation of the head or neck.[275] This maneuver, when used on the first pass in 20 patients in the operating room, was successful in 75% of cases.[267] One should bear in mind that these patients were paralyzed and did not experience the laryngospasm that may be encountered in a breathing patient. The use of topical anesthesia is recommended. Alternatively, if a controllable-tip ET tube (Endotrol) is used, flex the tip anteriorly to help avoid esophageal placement.[264] Remember that the tip is very responsive to pulling on the ring. A common mistake is exerting too much force on the ring, which can result in the tube

Figure 4-38 Much skill and a lot of luck are involved in successful blind nasotracheal intubation. Use of tracheal tube cuff inflation may aid in nasotracheal intubation. **A,** The tracheal tube is pulled back after passage through the esophagus. **B,** Once breath sounds are heard, the cuff is inflated with 15 mL of air and readvanced into the laryngeal inlet. Once seated in the inlet, the cuff is deflated and the tube advanced into the trachea. *(Courtesy of Department of Emergency Medicine, Hennepin County Medical Center, Minneapolis.).*

curling up before the larynx and prevent advancement. There has been a case report of an Endotrol tube "kinking" at the point of sharpest curvature and causing difficulty with suctioning but no problems with ventilation.[276] Another device that allows flexion of the distal ET tube is the Parker Flex-Tip stylet (Parker Medical, Engelwood, CO).

Laryngospasm

Laryngospasm is a common problem that arises when NT intubation is attempted. It is usually transient. Withdraw the tube slightly and wait for the patient's first gasp to advance the tube. This is frequently successful because the vocal cords are widely abducted during inhalation. Assess laryngeal anesthesia, and if topical and nebulized lidocaine has already been administered without success, consider transcricothyroid anesthesia (e.g., 2 mL of 4% lidocaine).[277] Occasionally, a jaw lift is necessary to break prolonged spasm. Another option is to use a smaller tube.

Complications

Epistaxis is the most common complication of blind NT intubation. Severe epistaxis was encountered in only 5 of 300 cases reported by Danzl and Thomas.[260] Tintinalli and Claffey[278] reported severe bleeding in 1 of 71 patients and less serious bleeding in 12 others. Bleeding is not usually a problem unless it provokes vomiting or aspiration, which is a serious potential problem in obtunded patients with trismus or a decreased gag reflex. Other immediate complications include turbinate fracture, intracranial placement through a basilar skull fracture, retropharyngeal laceration or dissection, and delayed or unsuccessful placement.[261,279,280] Complications may be minimized by selecting a smaller tube and using a gentle technique.

Sinusitis in patients with an NT tube is common and can be an unrecognized cause of sepsis.[281] Rare but potentially fatal delayed complications include mediastinitis after retropharyngeal abscess[282] and massive pneumocephalus.[283]

Because most complications occur during tube advancement through the nasal passage and proximal nasopharynx, the complications of blind NT intubation and placement

under direct vision are largely the same. Retropharyngeal laceration and esophageal intubation are more of a threat with blind placement techniques because they are more likely to go unrecognized.[278]

Summary

Blind NT intubation is being used less frequently than in the past because clinicians are increasingly becoming comfortable performing oral intubation in patients with potential cervical spine injuries. In addition, emergency physicians frequently use paralytics to facilitate orotracheal intubation. Nevertheless, blind NT intubation remains an effective and potentially lifesaving approach to a difficult airway.

DIGITAL INTUBATION

Digital intubation uses the index and middle fingers to blindly direct the ET tube into the larynx. It is particularly well suited to the prehospital situation, such as when a trapped victim cannot be positioned for intubation. A prehospital series of 66 digitally intubated patients demonstrated an 89% success rate.[284]

Indications and Contraindications

Digital intubation is indicated in a deeply comatose patient whose larynx cannot be visualized and who has a contraindication to NT intubation. Advantages include speed and ease of placement, immunity to constraints visualizing the larynx, and little neck movement. Contraindications are primarily precautions to protect the clinician. Digital intubation should not be attempted in any patient with a significant risk of biting. This includes calm, awake patients and agitated patients.

Procedure and Technique

Place the patient's head and neck in the neutral position. Stand at the patient's right side, facing the patient. Introduce your left index and middle fingers into the right angle of the patient's

Figure 4-39 Digital intubation. The tracheal tube is cradled between the index and middle fingers and guided into the glottic opening. *(Courtesy of Department of Emergency Medicine, Hennepin County Medical Center, Minneapolis.)*

Figure 4-40 Digital intubation in a neonate. The tube is guided by using only the index finger to palpate the epiglottis and laryngeal inlet. A stylet is optional. *(Courtesy of Department of Emergency Medicine, Hennepin County Medical Center, Minneapolis.)*

mouth and slide them along the surface of the tongue until the epiglottis is felt. The tip of the epiglottis should be palpated 8 to 10 cm from the corner of the mouth in average adults. Use of a stylet in the tube is optional, but the largest reported series had good success without a stylet.[284] For a clinician with short fingers or a patient with an anterior larynx, a stylet is advantageous. If a stylet is used, place it in the tube and bend it into the form of an open J with the distal end terminating in a gentle hook. Introduce a lubricated tube from the patient's left side between the tongue and the rescuer's two fingers (Fig. 4-39). Cradle the tube between two fingers and guide the tip beneath the epiglottis. Apply gentle anterior pressure to direct the tube into the larynx. If the clinician has sufficiently long fingers, place them posterior to the arytenoids to act as a "backstop" for the tube, to both avoid esophageal passage and assist in laryngeal placement.[285] If a stylet has been used, withdraw it at this time while simultaneously advancing the tube. An alternative to using a stylet for directing the tube anteriorly is to select an ET tube with a controllable tip (Endotrol, Mallinckrodt Medical, Inc., St. Louis).

A variation of the technique of digital intubation has been described for intubating a newborn.[286] In this technique, only the index finger is used to guide the tube into the larynx. Bend the end of the tube and moisten both the tube and the finger with sterile water. Use the index finger of the nondominant hand to follow the tongue posteriorly and palpate the epiglottis and paired arytenoids. Use the thumb of the same hand to apply cricoid pressure and steady the larynx. Hold the ET tube in the dominant hand and advance it with the nondominant index finger used as a guide (Fig. 4-40). The tube will encounter subtle resistance as it enters the trachea, and palpation of the tube through the trachea provides further confirmation of correct placement. A styletted tube, shaped in the form of a J, is usually desired until familiarity with the procedure is achieved.

Complications

The risk associated with esophageal intubation is always present, and the potential for esophageal misplacement is increased in comatose or cardiac-arrested patients. If used in patients with a gag reflex, induction of emesis with aspiration is a risk. A high incidence of left main stem intubation was noted in a cadaveric study,[287] but clinical confirmation is lacking. The greatest risk seems to be to the clinician, whose fingers may be bitten.

Summary

Although the most recent experience with digital intubation in adults has been prehospital use, there is no reason why it should be confined to this setting. The majority of moribund ED patients who defy orotracheal intubation are never given a trial of digital intubation. This omission undoubtedly deprives some patients of expeditious airway management.

RETROGRADE INTUBATION

Retrograde orotracheal intubation is a technique of guided ET intubation that involves the use of a wire or catheter placed percutaneously through the cricothyroid membrane or high trachea and exiting through the mouth or nose. An ET tube is then passed over this guide and advanced through the vocal cords into the trachea. Introduced by Butler and Cirillo in 1960,[288] the technique has undergone several recent modifications that have enhanced its value as a means of establishing a definitive airway when more conventional techniques have failed.

Indications and Contraindications

Retrograde intubation is indicated when definitive airway control is required and less invasive methods have failed. Indications include trismus, ankylosis of the jaw or cervical spine, upper airway masses, unstable cervical spine injuries, and maxillofacial trauma. It can be used to convert transtracheal needle ventilation (see Chapter 6) into a definitive airway. It was used successfully in a 1-month-old with developmental abnormalities.[289] It can be particularly helpful in trauma patients with airway bleeding that prevents visualization of the glottis.[290]

Contraindications to retrograde intubation include the availability of a less invasive means of airway control and inability to open the mouth. A relative contraindication is an apneic patient who cannot be effectively ventilated with a

Retrograde Intubation

Indications
Need for a definitive airway when other methods have failed
Trismus
Ankylosis of the jaw or cervical spine
Upper airway masses
Unstable cervical spine fractures
Maxillofacial trauma

Contraindications
Availability of less invasive means of airway control
Inability to open the mouth

Complications
Hemorrhage
Subcutaneous emphysema
Soft tissue infection
Failure to achieve intubation

Equipment

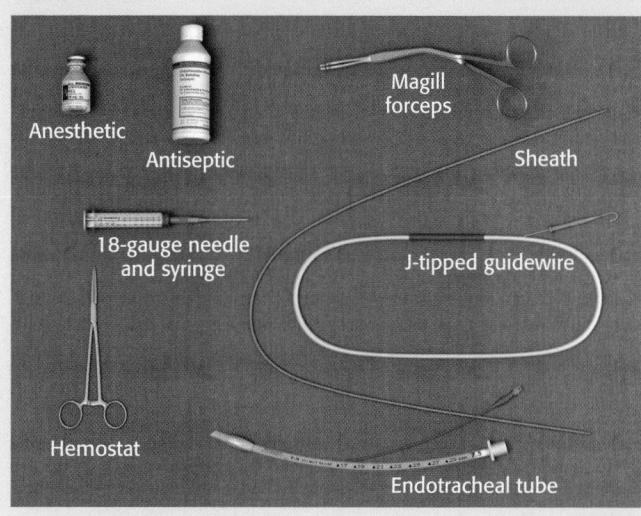

Review Box 4-5 Retrograde intubation: indications, contraindications, complications, and equipment.

bag-valve-mask device. In this setting, it is advisable to first establish transtracheal needle ventilation (see Chapter 6) before attempting retrograde intubation or to proceed directly to cricothyrotomy.

Equipment

Materials include (1) local anesthetic and skin preparation material, (2) an 18-gauge needle, (3) a 60-cm epidural catheter-needle combination or an 80-cm (0.88-mm-diameter) spring guidewire (J tip preferred), (4) a hemostat, (5) long forceps (e.g., Magill) for grasping the wire in the pharynx, (6) an ET tube of appropriate size, (7) a syringe for the tube cuff, and (8) material for securing the tube. A prepackaged alternative is the Cook Retrograde Intubation Set (Cook Critical Care, Bloomington, IN), which also contains a sheath.

Procedure and Technique

Locate the three important anatomic landmarks by palpation: hyoid bone, thyroid cartilage, and cricoid cartilage. Prepare the skin overlying the cricothyroid membrane and anesthetize it. Maintain a cephalad orientation of the needle bevel, and puncture the lower half of the cricothyroid membrane. Direct the needle slightly cephalad. Aspirate air to confirm position of the tip of the needle within the lumen of the larynx. An alternative entry point is the high trachea, usually through the subcricoid space, with the same steps being used as described for the cricothyroid membrane.

Remove the syringe and pass the wire through the needle. Advance it until it is seen in the patient's mouth or until it exits the nose. A laryngoscope may facilitate this process. If the wire is found in the hypopharynx, grasp it with the Magill forceps and draw it out through the mouth. Remove the needle from the neck and secure the end of the wire at the puncture site with a hemostat. Thread the oral end of the wire in through the ET tube side port (not the end of the tube), and advance it up the tube until it can be grasped with

a second hemostat. Threading the wire through the side port allows the tip of the tube to protrude 1 cm beyond the point at which the wire enters the larynx. Pull the wire taut and move it back and forth to ensure that no slack remains.

Advance the ET tube over the wire until resistance is met. This is the most critical point in the procedure. Because retrograde intubation is a blind technique, it may be difficult to determine whether the tube has entered the trachea or is impeded by more proximal structures. If the ET tube has successfully passed through the vocal cords and it is being restricted by the guidewire as it traverses the anterior laryngeal wall, the clinician should feel some caudally directed tension on the wire at its laryngeal insertion point. If this does not occur, the tip of the ET tube may be proximal to the vocal cords, in the vallecula, in a piriform sinus, or abutting the narrow anterior aspect of the vocal cords. If in doubt, pull the tube back 2 cm, rotate it 90 degrees counterclockwise, and then readvance the tube. This will usually result in successful passage through the larynx.[247] When satisfied that the tube has entered the trachea, stabilize the tube and pull the guidewire out through the mouth. Then advance the tube farther into the trachea.

The classic method of retrograde intubation, as described earlier, has undergone modifications that facilitate passage of the ET tube through the glottis. A significant advance has been the addition of a plastic sheath that is passed antegradely over the wire until it meets resistance where the wire penetrates the laryngeal mucosa (Fig. 4-41).[291] This sheath needs to be stiff enough to effectively guide an ET tube, yet small enough to easily pass through the vocal cords without impinging on any supraglottic or glottic structures. When the sheath comes to rest against the anterior laryngeal wall, withdraw the wire from the mouth and advance the sheath. Once the sheath is well within the trachea, pass the ET tube over the sheath. If you encounter any resistance at the arytenoids or vocal cords, pull the tube back 1 to 2 cm and rotate it 90 degrees counterclockwise. One advantage of the antegrade sheath is that it lies freely in the larynx, which allows more posterior passage through the widest distance between the cords. In

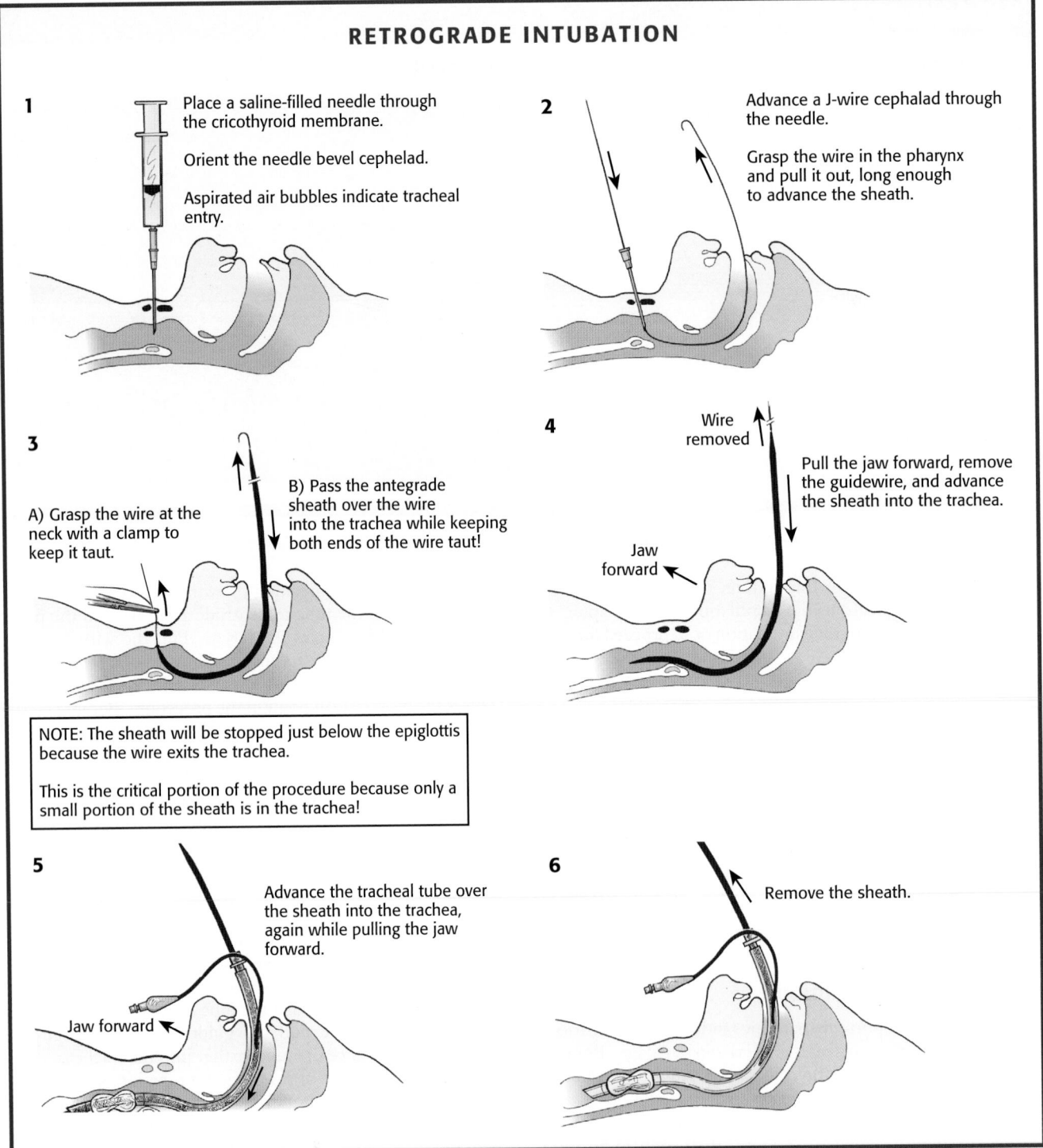

RETROGRADE INTUBATION

1 Place a saline-filled needle through the cricothyroid membrane.

Orient the needle bevel cephelad.

Aspirated air bubbles indicate tracheal entry.

2 Advance a J-wire cephalad through the needle.

Grasp the wire in the pharynx and pull it out, long enough to advance the sheath.

3 A) Grasp the wire at the neck with a clamp to keep it taut.

B) Pass the antegrade sheath over the wire into the trachea while keeping both ends of the wire taut!

4 Wire removed

Pull the jaw forward, remove the guidewire, and advance the sheath into the trachea.

Jaw forward

NOTE: The sheath will be stopped just below the epiglottis because the wire exits the trachea.

This is the critical portion of the procedure because only a small portion of the sheath is in the trachea!

5 Advance the tracheal tube over the sheath into the trachea, again while pulling the jaw forward.

Jaw forward

6 Remove the sheath.

Figure 4-41 Retrograde intubation using a guidewire and antegrade sheath. *(Courtesy of Department of Emergency Medicine, Hennepin County Medical Center, Minneapolis).)*

contrast, the wire pulls the ET tube anteriorly toward the narrow commissure of the vocal cords and is more likely to result in impingement of the tube on the cords. Also, use of the sheath permits unrestricted advancement of the ET tube, but a wire entering the larynx 1.0 to 1.5 cm below the vocal cords prevents the tube from advancing more than this distance before removal of the wire.

If no sheath is available, consider placing the needle inferiorly in the trachea, thereby increasing the distance that the

ET tube can be advanced before being stopped by the wire.[292] This will decrease the likelihood of dislodging the tip of the ET tube when the guidewire is withdrawn.

Complications

The complications of retrograde intubation are largely related to puncture of the cricothyroid membrane (see Chapter 6). The potential for hemorrhage is minimized by taking care to puncture the cricothyroid membrane in its lower half to avoid the cricothyroid artery. Subcutaneous emphysema may occur, but it is of no clinical significance because no air is insufflated during this technique. A small incidence of soft tissue infection is reported with translaryngeal needle procedures, but ensuring that the wire is withdrawn from the mouth rather than the neck can minimize this problem. The final complication, failure to achieve intubation, has been mitigated by addition of the antegrade sheath over the wire.

Summary

Retrograde intubation is an underused technique for achieving tracheal intubation in a patient who cannot be intubated by less aggressive means. It is more invasive than fiberoptic intubation but requires less skill. Retrograde intubation usually takes several minutes to complete,[285] and the patient can undergo bag-mask ventilation throughout much of the procedure. Recent modifications in the technique guarantee this method a prominent place in the management of difficult airways, particularly when active bleeding compromises the airway.

TRACHEAL INTUBATION WITH A LARYNGEAL TUBE OR COMBITUBE IN PLACE

Patients presenting to the ED with a King LT (or Combitube) in place need to have it replaced with an ET tube at some point. Placement of a bougie through the King LT is not usually successful. Direct laryngoscopy with the King LT in place is difficult. In contrast, video laryngoscopy usually allows excellent visualization of the glottis and placement of an ET tube while the King LT remains in place (with the balloons deflated). This approach allows providers to avoid the risk of removing a functional airway in a patient who may be difficult to intubate.

CHANGING TRACHEAL TUBES

A tracheal tube with a leaking cuff is a vexing problem, especially if the original intubation was difficult. A method of replacing the tube without losing control of the tracheal lumen is preferred. This can be achieved by passing a guide down the defective tube, withdrawing the tube while leaving the guide in place, and introducing a new tube over the guide and into the trachea.

A number of different guides have been described (e.g., simple nasogastric tubes, 18-Fr Salem sump tubes, feeding tubes), but they are poor substitutes for a designated tube exchanger such as the Tracheal Tube Exchanger (Hudson Respiratory Care, Inc., Temecula, CA) or a similar commercially available device. Advantages of the designated tube exchanger include the following: it is long enough to allow deep placement within the airway while allowing easy exchange of the ET tubes, it is stiff enough to prevent dislodgment when the ET tube is introduced, it is ready to use without modification, it has a printed scale to aid in determining the depth of placement, and if replacement is prolonged, the patient may be oxygenated through the exchanger with wall oxygen.

Procedure and Technique

Before the procedure, sedate and restrain the patient properly. Hyperventilate the patient before placing the guide through the existing tube. Lubricate the guide and advance it into the defective tube so that it is well within the tracheal lumen (adults, 30 cm). While applying cricoid pressure (Sellick's maneuver), withdraw the defective tube over the guide, and take care to not dislodge the guide when removing the tube. Slide the replacement tube over the guide and gently advance it into the trachea (Fig. 4-42). At this juncture it may be helpful to perform a jaw-thrust or chin-lift maneuver to facilitate passage through the pharynx. Resistance may be encountered at the laryngeal inlet or vocal cords. If this occurs, withdraw the tube 1 to 2 cm, rotate it 90 degrees counterclockwise, and then readvance it. With the tube clearly in the trachea, remove the guide, inflate the cuff, and ventilate the patient. After correct placement has been verified, secure the new tube.

Benumof[293] described a technique in which a bronchoscope with an ET tube jacketed over the proximal end is first passed into the trachea with the defective ET tube still in place. A tube exchanger capable of jet ventilation is then passed through the defective tube. The defective tube can then be withdrawn and the new ET tube passed over the bronchoscope and adjacent to the exchange catheter. The tube exchanger can be withdrawn once placement of the new tube is confirmed. This technique permits direct visualization of placement of a new tube and a failsafe means of ventilating the patient should difficulties arise.

Complications are related to the time required to change the tube. A successfully performed procedure can be accomplished within 30 seconds. Laryngeal injury from forcing the exchange guide or the new ET tube is a possibility to consider when replacing a tube.

PREVENTING UNPLANNED EXTUBATION

Unplanned extubation is undesirable and can be medically disastrous if unrecognized or if the medical condition requires immediate reintubation. Not all extubations can be prevented. They most often occur when patients suddenly pull out their own tube or during transport. It is not uncommon for a deceased patient to arrive at the medical examiner with a tube in an incorrect position that was dislodged during transit. Unplanned extubation is best prevented with the use of physical and chemical restraints, aggressive sedation of intubated patients, and careful attention to the integrity of the ET tube during procedures, such as positioning for postresuscitation chest radiographs or transfer to another bed (Fig. 4-21C.).

CONCLUSION

Emergency airway management in critically ill or injured patients with acute airway compromise is one of the greatest challenges for clinicians. Although the definition of a difficult airway will change as our ability to visualize the laryngeal inlet continues to improve, the challenge of emergency airways will persist. Mastery of the basics of airway management and direct laryngoscopy, competency in a number of guided or indirect intubation techniques, and the ability to perform a surgical airway are all necessary skills for emergency airway

REPLACING A MALFUNCTIONING ENDOTRACHEAL TUBE

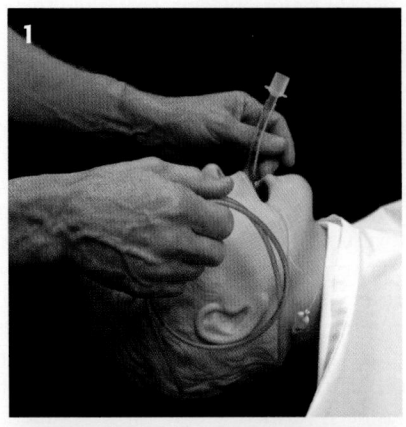

Pre-oxygenate and sedate the patient as clinically indicated.

The procedure here is demonstrated with an 80-mm TTX tube exchanger (Hudson Respiratory Care).

Pass the tube exchanger through the defective ET tube deep into the airway.

Remove the defective tube and leave the tube exchanger in place as a guiding stylet.

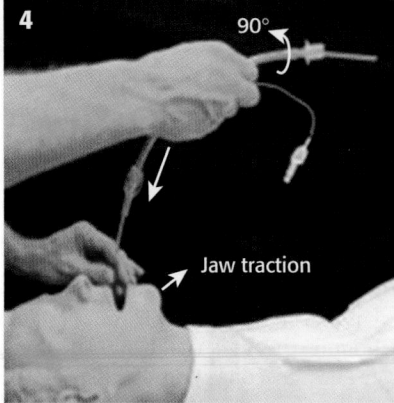

Pass a new ET tube over the tube exchanger and into the airway.

A 90° counterclockwise tube rotation and jaw traction will help the tube pass into the laryngeal inlet.

Use a laryngoscope to elevate soft tissues if necessary.

Place the ET tube into the trachea to the desired depth.

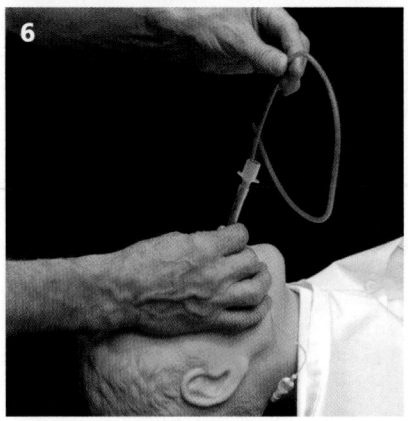

Remove the tube exchanger.

Confirm ET tube position.

Figure 4-42 Replacing a malfunctioning endotracheal (ET) tube. **1,** Commercial tube exchangers are preferred, although other devices are possible (see text). Shown here is an 80-cm TTX (Tracheal Tube Exchanger; Hudson Respiratory Care). Before tube exchange, the patient should be hyperoxygenated and sedated if necessary. **2,** The tube exchanger is passed through the defective ET tube and placed deep in the airway. **3,** The defective tube is removed and the tube exchanger is left in place as a guiding stylet. **4,** The new ET tube is placed over the tube exchanger and passed into the airway. A 90-degree counterclockwise rotation of the tube and traction on the jaw will help the tube pass into the laryngeal inlet; insertion of the laryngoscope may be necessary to elevate the hypopharyngeal soft tissues and facilitate passage of the tube. **5,** The ET tube is placed to the desired depth. **6,** The tube exchanger is removed. ET tube position is then confirmed.

management. Mastery of technique, advance preparation of equipment, and experience in clinical decision making are essential. Scenario visualization and advanced simulation models can provide an excellent means of practicing the difficult decision making and technical maneuvers necessary for effective emergency airway management.

Acknowledgment

The authors would like to thank Robb Poutre and Ben Dolan for their assistance with this chapter.

References are available at www.expertconsult.com

CHAPTER 5

Pharmacologic Adjuncts to Intubation

Richard B. Schwartz and Greene Shepherd

Endotracheal (ET) intubation in the emergency setting presents a challenge distinct from that associated with intubation of fasted, premedicated patients in the operating room (OR). Patients in the emergency department (ED) are frequently uncooperative and unstable and may have medical problems that are completely unknown to the treating clinician. It is challenging that within a matter of minutes and with scant data the clinician must assess and control the airway while diagnosing and managing the patient's other life-threatening problems.

In 1979, Taryle and coworkers[1] reported that complications occurred in more than half the patients intubated in a university hospital ED. They called for improved house officer training in ET intubation, including "more liberal use of the procedures and agents used in the operating room (OR), including sedatives and muscle relaxers."[1] Since this report, the use of neuromuscular blockade and rapid-sequence intubation (RSI) has become the standard for emergency medicine practice.[2,3] In addition to RSI, emergency physicians now use airway devices such as videoscopes and flexible fiberoptic bronchoscopes to manage difficult and complex airways.

Clinicians must concentrate not only on the manual skills of airway management but also on selection of the appropriate drugs to achieve specific objectives. These objectives include (1) immediate airway control, including induction of unconsciousness and muscle paralysis; (2) analgesia and sedation in awake patients; and (3) minimization of the adverse physiologic effects of intubation, including systemic and intracranial hypertension.

This chapter reviews the mechanisms and strategic use of the drugs that are currently available to facilitate intubation in the ED.

OVERVIEW OF RAPID-SEQUENCE INTUBATION

The sequential process for quickly intubating a patient in an emergency situation is referred to as *rapid-sequence intubation*. The steps in performing RSI are often described by the six "P's": preparation, preoxygenation, pretreatment and induction, paralysis, placement of the tube, and postintubation management (Fig. 5-1). This sequential technique of rapidly inducing unconsciousness (induction) combined with muscular paralysis and optimal conditions for intubation has gained broad acceptance among ED clinicians. Obviously, many patients do not afford the clinician the time or opportunity to comply with the ideal scenario of tracheal intubation described in this chapter. RSI, as described in this chapter, is the ideal method of emergency airway management for intubations *not anticipated to be difficult.*

Preparation occurs before and during preoxygenation. Assess the airway to determine the likelihood of a difficult intubation. Simultaneously, establish an intravenous (IV) line and connect the patient to cardiac, pulse oximetry, and end-tidal CO_2 monitors when available. Assemble all necessary drugs and equipment for oral intubation and the desired backup equipment for airway control, such as cricothyrotomy.

Begin RSI preoxygenation as soon as possible by administering 100% oxygen. The intent is to displace nitrogen from the lungs and replace it with an oxygen reserve that will last several minutes. Under optimal conditions, breathing 100% oxygen for 3 minutes has been demonstrated to *maintain acceptable oxygen saturation for up to 8 minutes in previously healthy apneic individuals.*[4] Another method is to give four maximal breaths of 100% oxygen from a face mask, which can also maintain *acceptable saturation for 6 minutes.*[4] Comparable results may not be expected in the ED setting, though, because of differences in the underlying health and cooperation of the patient population.

Pretreatment consists of the administration of medications to mitigate the potential untoward responses to intubation. Pretreatment during RSI usually occurs 2 to 3 minutes before induction of unconsciousness or muscular paralysis. Although preoxygenation should be maintained for as long as practical before beginning intubation, the ideal situation and circumstances are not always present, and clinical judgment is the deciding factor for this portion of RSI.

Paralysis and induction involve the induction of a state of unconsciousness with a sedative agent, followed immediately by muscle paralysis. A protocol for ED-based RSI is summarized in Box 5-1. ET intubation and RSI have also expanded beyond the ED into the prehospital setting. Prehospital RSI protocols use a sedative plus a paralytic for patients not in cardiac arrest, with success rates as high as 92% to 98% being demonstrated.[5-9] As in the ED setting, without a full complement of medications, prehospital intubation becomes significantly more difficult, and success rates drop to approximately 60%.[10] Rates of misplaced ET tubes and complications by paramedics may be much higher than previously reported.[11,12] Recent studies indicate that outcomes may be worse for patients with traumatic brain injury intubated in the prehospital setting than in the ED.[13] For these reasons many prehospital systems have moved away from the use of RSI.

The technique for proper ET tube placement is discussed in Chapter 2.[1-3] Postintubation monitoring should assess for proper tube placement, adequate tissue oxygenation, and response to previously administered drugs. After laryngoscopy, the clinician should ensure ongoing analgesic and anxiolytic therapy.

PRETREATMENT: PREVENTING THE COMPLICATIONS OF INTUBATION

Numerous reports have highlighted the physiologic responses to tracheal intubation and attempted to define their immediate or long-term adverse effects and to offer interventions to ameliorate potential organ injury. It is certain that intubation and adjunctive medications have the potential to alter reflexes, intracranial pressure (ICP), blood pressure, and the pulse rate and may induce disturbances in cardiac rhythms, but the *actual clinical consequences of these commonly observed changes are largely unknown.* Clinical experience suggests that

RAPID-SEQUENCE INTUBATION: the 6 "P's"

1   Preparation

Preparation occurs prior to and during oxygenation. Assess the airway for difficulty. Establish an IV line, place the patient on the monitors, and assemble all required medications and equipment.

2   Preoxygenation

Begin RSI preoxygenation as soon as possible by placing the patient on 100% oxygen. Oxygen will displace nitrogen from the lungs and provide an oxygen reserve that will last several minutes.

3   Pretreatment

Consider pretreating with medications such as lidocaine, atropine, and/or fentanyl (depending on the clinical scenario) 2 to 3 minutes prior to induction and paralysis.

4   Paralysis and Induction

Administer a sedative agent to induce loss of consciousness (induction). After induction, administer a paralytic agent to achieve muscle relaxation, which greatly facilitates intubation.

5   Placement of the Tube

Once the patient is sedated and paralyzed, place the endotracheal tube. Intubation techniques are reviewed in Chapter 4.

6   Post-Intubation Management

Confirm proper tube position with a Petco$_2$ detector, auscultation, and chest radiograph. Assess for adequate tissue oxygenation and response to previously administered drugs.

Figure 5-1 The 6 "P's" of rapid sequence intubation. *IV,* intravenous; *RSI,* rapid-sequence intubation.

| **BOX 5-1** | **Rapid-Sequence Intubation Protocol** |

1. Preoxygenate (denitrogenate) the lungs by providing 100% oxygen by mask.
2. Assemble the equipment required:
   - Bag-valve-mask device connected to an oxygen delivery system
   - Suction with a Yankauer tip
   - ET tube with an intact cuff, stylet, syringe, and tape
   - Laryngoscope and blades, in working order
   - Back up airway equipment
3. Check to be sure that a functioning, secure intravenous line is in place.
4. Continuously monitor cardiac rhythm and oxygen saturation.
5. Premedicate as appropriate:
   - Fentanyl: 2 to 3 μg/kg given at a rate of 1 to 2 μg/kg/min intravenously for analgesia in awake patients
   - Atropine: 0.01 mg/kg by intravenous push for children or adolescents (minimum dose of 0.1 mg recommended)
   - Lidocaine: 1.5 to 2 mg/kg intravenously over a period of 30 to 60 seconds
6. Induce anesthesia with one of the following agents administered intravenously: thiopental, methohexital, fentanyl, ketamine, etomidate, or propofol. Apply cricoid pressure.
7. Give succinylcholine, 1.5 mg/kg by intravenous push (use 2 mg/kg for infants and small children).
8. Apnea, jaw relaxation, and/or decreased resistance to bag-mask ventilation (use only when oxygenation before rapid-sequence intubation cannot be optimized by spontaneous ventilation) indicates that the patient is sufficiently relaxed to proceed with intubation.
9. Perform ET intubation. If unable to intubate during the first 20-second attempt, stop and ventilate the patient with the bag-mask device for 30 to 60 seconds. Monitor pulse oximetry readings as a guide.
10. Treat bradycardia occurring during intubation with atropine, 0.5 mg by intravenous push (smaller dose for children; see item 5).
11. Once intubation is completed, inflate the cuff and confirm ET tube placement by auscultating for bilateral breath sounds and checking the pulse oximetry and capnography readings.
12. Release cricoid pressure and secure the ET tube.

ET, endotracheal.

most transient alterations in physiology occurring with ED intubation produce *no specific or readily documented long-term sequelae* or are often consequences that cannot easily be monitored or prevented. Prudent clinicians are aware of the potential adverse effects of intubation and are cognizant of potential methods to minimize them. Careful monitoring of the postintubation condition will guide specific interventions. Overzealous attempts to suppress the physiologic responses that normally accompany airway manipulation may be counterproductive. It would be desirable to provide airway control under the best of circumstances and with the least amount of injury to the patient, but the ideal approach to the physiologic responses to intubation is simply unknown. Most information has been extrapolated from experimental animal models or from the anesthesia experience, and similar issues may not apply to the milieu of the ED experience. The following discussion serves as a general clinical guide to alterations in the physiologic response to intubation.

The Pressor Response

In addition to the ubiquitous sinus tachycardia, a number of dysrhythmias have been reported after intubation. They are primarily ventricular in origin and include ectopic beats, bigeminy, and short runs of ventricular tachycardia. Bradyarrhythmias have been reported uncommonly. Electrocardiographic changes suggestive of ischemia have been documented, particularly in patients with dramatic increases in blood pressure.[14,15] In 1977, Fox and colleagues[16] reported two patients, both of whom deteriorated after induction of anesthesia and orotracheal intubation. This report has been widely quoted as evidence that the pressor response should be prevented. No studies have reported comparative data, and none have established a direct relationship between the response and subsequent clinical deterioration in a large patient population. It is also unclear whether attenuation of the pressor response will prevent dysrhythmias or electrocardiographic evidence of ischemia, although it is prudent to avoid sudden increases in blood pressure in unstable patients with acute cardiac or vascular disease.

Multiple studies have evaluated procedures to pharmacologically block the pressor response. Lidocaine has been the most extensively evaluated, but the results of these studies are inconclusive.[17-23] No standards are universally accepted. Although it appears that administration of lidocaine, 1.5 to 2 mg/kg intravenously before intubation, may blunt the response, it is not clear that the reductions reported (10 to 15 mm Hg and 20 beats/min) are of any clinical significance. Other drugs, including thiopental, sodium nitroprusside, labetalol, nitroglycerin, verapamil, nifedipine, clonidine, fentanyl, sufentanil, etomidate, and magnesium, have shown variable responses.[24-33]

Of these drugs, fentanyl may be the most effective. It completely suppresses the pressor response at large anesthetic doses of 50 μg/kg,[34-36] but considerably smaller doses may be effective. Two studies have shown marked suppression of the pressor response at doses of 5 to 6 μg/kg, although in both studies patients also received 5 mg/kg of thiopental.[18,37] Fentanyl has blunted the pressor response when administered in conjunction with etomidate.[32] The 1998 SHRED (Sedatives and Hemodynamics during Rapid-Sequence Intubation in the Emergency Department) study evaluated the pressor response to RSI and compared thiopental, fentanyl, and midazolam as induction agents.[38]

Midazolam, which is associated with the poorest intubating conditions and the most attempts required for intubation, showed a mean increase in heart rate of 17 beats/min. Thiopental, probably because of its direct myocardial depressant and venodilatory effects, decreased mean arterial pressure by about 40 mm Hg. Fentanyl recipients maintained a relatively neutral hemodynamic profile during intubation. Use of paralytics during intubation did not appear to alter the hemodynamic response associated with each sedative agent. One study isolated the effect of laryngoscopy from the effect of tube passage into the trachea. Adachi and colleagues[39] found that pretreatment with 2 μg/kg of fentanyl could blunt the hemodynamic effects of tracheal tube passage, but not the hemodynamic effects of laryngoscopy.

It is important to note that even studies demonstrating blunting of the pressor response failed to show that this provided any real benefit to patients. It is likely that the pressor response is innocuous in the vast majority of patients, but it may be exaggerated and potentially harmful in those with preexisting hypertension, cardiovascular disease,[40] or other vascular comorbid conditions, in whom sudden changes in hemodynamics may be detrimental.[41] The pressor response may contribute to the rise in ICP that follows laryngoscopy, and it is potentially harmful in patients with intracranial pathology. Administration of lidocaine or fentanyl to blunt the pressor response may be appropriate in these subsets of patients, but no universal standards exist.

Intracranial Hypertension

Physical stimulation of the respiratory tract by maneuvers such as laryngoscopy, tracheal intubation, and ET suctioning is commonly associated with a brief rise in ICP. The exact mechanism responsible for this rise is unknown. One potential mechanism is the coughing and gagging that frequently follow manipulation of the upper airway and subsequent transmission of intrathoracic pressure to the cerebral circulation. An alternative explanation is the release of catecholamine that accompanies laryngoscopy, which causes a rise in mean arterial pressure and cerebral perfusion pressure. A small rise in ICP has been reported after the administration of succinylcholine. The value of pretreatment with defasciculating doses of neuromuscular blockers (NMBs) to prevent rises in ICP is unknown.[42]

Although the exact significance of a transient rise in ICP is not known, it is logical to assume that it may be detrimental in patients with head trauma or intracranial hypertension. A number of drugs, including lidocaine, succinylcholine, and the majority of the anesthesia induction agents, have been studied to determine whether their use prevents this response. Many of the existing clinical data are not particularly relevant to the ED setting because they are derived from patients in various stages of general anesthesia, which often incorporates a wide variety of drug combinations and doses.

Good evidence suggests that deep general anesthesia prevents the rise in ICP associated with intubation. Depending on the drug used, anesthesia may compromise cardiovascular performance and critically reduce cerebral blood flow.[43-45] Consequently, the ideal anesthetic agents to facilitate intubation of patients with acute intracranial pathology may be those that have minimal effects on cardiovascular performance, such as etomidate or fentanyl. Etomidate has been demonstrated to prevent changes in both cerebral perfusion pressure and ICP after tracheal intubation of patients with space-occupying intracranial lesions.[46]

At the present time the clinical consequences of intubation-induced physiologic changes are not thoroughly understood. The role of drugs in preventing these changes is equally unclear. Despite this lack of data, it may be intuitively reasonable to attempt to protect patients at theoretical risk. The approach outlined in Box 5-2 is recommended.

INDUCTION AGENTS

After premedication, a sedative agent is used to induce loss of consciousness. A number of diverse drugs are available in the ED to induce unconsciousness before intubation, including

---

BOX 5-2 **Sample Protocol for Intubation of a Head-Injured Adult Patient***

1. Preoxygenate with 100% O_2 for 2 to 3 minutes.
2. Administer lidocaine, 1.5 to 2 mg/kg intravenously.
3. Administer 0.01 mg/kg (up to 1 mg max) of vecuronium or pancuronium (1 mg) (optional).
4. Sedate with fentanyl, 3 to 5 μg/kg.
5. Induce anesthesia with etomidate, 0.3 mg/kg.
6. Paralyze with succinylcholine, 1.5 mg/kg.
7. Apply cricoid pressure and perform intubation.
8. Maintain postintubation analgesia and sedation.
9. Maintain paralysis if indicated (vecuronium, 0.1 mg/kg).

The benefit of this traditional protocol is unproved but can be supported if contraindications do not exist.

---

barbiturates, benzodiazepines, etomidate, ketamine, opiates, and propofol. The choice of a particular induction agent depends on the experience and training of the clinician, the patient's clinical status, drug characteristics, and institutional protocols (Box 5-3).

Considerable evidence indicates that the sedative agent selected influences the quality of intubation conditions and the rapidity of their attainment. These effects persist even when paralytic agents are used. Commonly used drugs and their doses are summarized in Table 5-1.

Barbiturates: Thiopental and Methohexital

The barbiturates, particularly thiopental, have been the traditional agents used for induction in the OR setting, but their use in the ED is minimal. The ultrashort-acting barbiturates thiopental and methohexital are the most suited for ED RSI, but, their potential hemodynamic effects require cautious use in the ED setting. Barbiturates are central nervous system (CNS) depressants capable of producing effects ranging from mild sedation to deep coma. They do not block afferent sensory input to a significant extent and should be used in conjunction with an analgesic agent such as fentanyl if a painful procedure is to be performed. It is common practice to intubate patients who have received only barbiturates as the induction agent without an analgesic.

The barbiturates rapidly cross the blood-brain barrier and induce unconsciousness in less than a minute. They are rapidly redistributed and then ultimately degraded in the liver. After a single IV dose of thiopental, anesthesia lasts 5 to 10 minutes, as compared with 4 to 6 minutes for methohexital.[47,48] The recommended dose of thiopental is 3 to 5 mg/kg intravenously administered over a 60-second period. Methohexital is dosed at 1 to 1.5 mg/kg intravenously over a 30- to 60-second period.

Advantages of barbiturates as induction agents include their high potency, rapid onset, and short duration of action. They reduce cerebral metabolism, oxygen consumption, cerebral blood flow, and ICP.[49,50] For this reason, thiopental is considered the agent of choice for induction of anesthesia and maintenance of long-term anesthesia in patients with elevated ICP. Short-term use of barbiturates during RSI has not been shown to have a protective effect on the CNS. Barbiturate use in hypovolemic patients may lead to systemic

BOX 5-3 **Recommendations for Sedation of Patients Undergoing Rapid-Sequence Intubation in Specific Circumstances**

The most appropriate medications for sedation before rapid-sequence intubation are based on evaluation of the clinical scenario, and no specific recommendations are appropriate for all circumstances. Different situations, too complex to list here, lend themselves to the use of certain agents (see text). There are no specific standards that must be followed, and the medical literature can be confusing, contradictory, or inadequate. The following conditions and sedation agent recommendations may guide the clinician. *Note that appropriate paralytic drugs should also be used.*

HEAD INJURY OR POTENTIALLY ELEVATED INTRACRANIAL PRESSURE

Pretreatment with the various medications described in text are appropriate but of unproven value. Adequate cerebral perfusion pressure should be maintained to prevent secondary brain injury. Etomidate is suggested for induction of these patients. For hypotensive patients, etomidate or ketamine may be used. Ketamine should probably be avoided in patients with severe hypertension or if elevated intracranial pressure is caused by spontaneous cerebral hemorrhage.

STATUS EPILEPTICUS

Midazolam or thiopental may be used for induction. Reduced doses should be used in the unusual circumstance of seizure with hypotension. Etomidate may be used when the patient is hemodynamically compromised. Propofol is acceptable. Ketamine has been reported for the treatment of status epilepticus.

HEMODYNAMICALLY STABLE PATIENT WITH SEVERE BRONCHOSPASM

Induction with ketamine or propofol is suggested. Etomidate and midazolam are acceptable alternatives. In hemodynamically unstable patients with severe bronchospasm, ketamine or etomidate is suggested. Thiopental should *not* be used in these patients because it provokes release of histamine and can induce or exacerbate bronchospasm.

PATIENTS WITH CARDIOVASCULAR COMPROMISE

Etomidate is suggested because of the hemodynamic stability that it provides. If the patient is in shock or severely hypotensive, ketamine and/or etomidate is suggested. If etomidate is used in a patient with sepsis who has associated hypotension refractory to treatment with fluid resuscitation and a vasopressor, a single dose of hydrocortisone (100 mg intravenously) may be given (value unproven).

FOR AN "AWAKE LOOK" BEFORE INTUBATION

Ketamine is suggested, but it may not be appropriate when these patients have cardiovascular disease or hypertension.

Adapted from Caro D, Walls RM, Grayzel J. Sedation or induction agents for rapid sequence intubation in adults. Up To Date. Based on Literature through February 2012. Queried 4/12/12.

hypotension and impaired cerebral perfusion pressure, which may offset any cerebral-protective characteristics.[38] Some evidence indicates that for ED RSI, thiopental may produce the best intubating conditions when used in conjunction with succinylcholine.[51]

The most significant complication of barbiturate therapy is depression of the vasomotor center and myocardial contractility, which can lead to significant hypotension. One study showed the average decrease in mean arterial pressure during RSI with thiopental to be 40 mm Hg.[38] This is particularly pronounced in the presence of hypovolemia or cardiovascular disease.

Barbiturates also depress the brainstem respiratory centers when given rapidly or in large doses. This effect may be accelerated by simultaneous treatment with opioids. Patients with asthma or chronic bronchitis may experience bronchospasm. Laryngospasm may occur in patients who were anesthetized lightly with barbiturates during manipulation of the upper airway. This complication usually responds to positive pressure ventilation or neuromuscular blockade. The high pH of the barbiturate solution can cause tissue necrosis after extravascular administration and severe pain, vessel spasm, and thrombosis after intraarterial infusion.

Etomidate

Etomidate is an ultrashort-acting nonbarbiturate hypnotic agent that has been used successfully as an anesthesia induction agent in Europe since the mid-1970s and in the United

TABLE 5-1 Recommended Anesthetic Dosing for Rapid-Sequence Intubation and Clinical Considerations

DRUG*	DOSE	PREFERRED IN	AVOID IN
Thiopental	3-5 mg/kg IV	↑ ICP, SE	Hypotension, RAD
Methohexital	1-1.5 mg/kg IV	↑ ICP, SE	Hypotension, RAD
Fentanyl	5-15 µg/kg IV		
Midazolam	0.1-0.3 mg/kg IV		Hypotension
Ketamine	1-2 mg/kg IV	RAD	
Etomidate	0.3 mg/kg IV	Hypotension	
Propofol	2 mg/kg IV	↑ ICP, SE	Hypotension

ICP, intracranial pressure; *IV,* intravenously; *RAD,* reactive airway disease; *SE,* status epilepticus.
*Any of these can drugs be used before the administration of a neuromuscular blocking agent to induce anesthesia (see text).

States since 1983. A significant benefit of etomidate in the emergency setting is its lack of cardiodepressant effects.[52,53] Several case series have now demonstrated its safety and effective use in ED RSI.[54-58] Extensive experience with this agent now exists in both pediatric[59] and adult patients, and it is an agent of choice for most ED intubations.

Etomidate is a carboxylated imidazole that is both water and lipid soluble. The drug reaches peak brain concentrations within 1 minute of IV infusion[60] and induces unconsciousness within 30 seconds of administration. Its effects last less than 10 minutes after a single bolus dose.[10] Redistribution of the drug is quite rapid, which accounts for its short duration of action. Etomidate is rapidly hydrolyzed in the liver and plasma and forms an inactive metabolite excreted primarily in urine.[60] The recommended dose is 0.3 mg/kg via rapid IV bolus. There is virtually no accumulation of the drug, and anesthesia may be maintained through repeated doses; however, etomidate should not be used as an infusion or in repeated bolus doses for maintenance of sedation after intubation in the ED.[61]

Etomidate acts on the CNS by stimulating γ-aminobutyric acid (GABA) receptors and depressing the reticular activating system. It produces electroencephalographic changes similar to those produced by barbiturates as patients pass rapidly through light to deep levels of surgical anesthesia. Because etomidate has no analgesic activity,[60] it should be used in conjunction with a parenteral analgesic when painful conditions are being treated, although it is most commonly used as a sole induction agent for intubation. Etomidate decreases cerebral oxygen consumption, cerebral blood flow, and ICP but appears to have minimal effects on cerebral perfusion pressure.[46] Most importantly in the ED setting, etomidate is characterized by hemodynamic stability without significant changes in mean arterial pressure,[53,54,57] although a slightly increased heart rate may be observed.[61] Etomidate is suggested for induction of patients with significant cardiovascular disease requiring RSI. The hemodynamic stability that it provides and the absence of induced hypertension make it preferable to other sedatives. This hemodynamic stability persists even in patients with preexisting hypotension.[62] The most common immediate side effects of etomidate are pain on injection, nausea, vomiting, and myoclonic jerks.[63] Pain on injection is reported in up to two thirds of patients. Use of a large vein, simultaneous saline infusion, and opioid premedication can reduce the discomfort in appropriate situations.[64] Myoclonic activity has been reported in about one third of cases and is believed to be caused by disinhibition of subcortical activity rather than CNS stimulation and *does not represent seizure activity*.[60] This sometimes dramatic effect can be avoided through the use of NMBs and is rarely seen in the ED, where paralytic agents are regularly used with RSI. No treatment of myoclonus is usually necessary, and it is generally of no clinical significance. If persistent, an intravenous benzodiazepine may be administered. Etomidate need not be avoided in patients with seizure disorders, status epilepticus, head injury, or stroke.

Some degree of altered adrenal function has been demonstrated even after a single dose of etomidate.[65,66] The true clinical effect is unknown, but because the alteration in adrenal function appears to persist for 12 to 24 hours, there is theoretical concern about potential clinical consequences.[10,67,68] Etomidate is a reversible inhibitor of 11β-hydroxylase, the enzyme that converts 11-deoxycortisol to cortisol. Although cortisol levels do not fall below the normal physiologic range, even a single induction dose of etomidate causes a measurable decrease in the level of circulating cortisol that occurs in response to the administration of exogenous adrenocorticotropic hormone (ACTH). Despite concerns regarding the safety of etomidate in the specific setting of adrenal insufficiency related to sepsis, no well-designed, prospective trial has shown adverse effects from a single dose of etomidate used for intubation in patients with sepsis or septic shock. Overall, however, the literature on this subject provides conflicting results.[69-86]

When comparing etomidate with ketamine, a multicenter randomized trial of critically ill patients requiring emergency intubation found no significant difference in organ failure score, 28-day mortality, or intubating conditions between patients given etomidate for induction and those given ketamine.[83] No serious, drug-related adverse events were reported with either medication. Even though adrenal insufficiency occurred at a higher rate in the etomidate group (86%), it also developed in approximately 48% of patients receiving ketamine.

Although historically no individual study is sufficiently powered to detect differences in mortality from the adrenal effects of etomidate, a systematic review of 20 studies in which etomidate was given in a bolus dose as part of induction for tracheal intubation found that etomidate does not have a significant proven effect on mortality.[84] Declines in serum cortisol concentration were more prevalent in etomidate recipients than in those who did not receive etomidate in the large majority of studies, but the effect did not persist beyond 5 hours. When intubating a critically ill patient with possible adrenal insufficiency, the clinician must weigh the theoretical risk of cortisol suppression against the hemodynamic instability that may be caused by alternative induction agents. Overall, the mixed results in the current literature do not justify recommendations to avoid using etomidate for induction in patients with sepsis. Pending more definitive studies and subject to change as additional evidence is forthcoming, etomidate is an acceptable induction agent for patients with severe sepsis.[87]

Clinicians performing ACTH stimulation testing should be aware that the results may be affected by prior administration of etomidate. The empirical administration of glucocorticoids for the first 24 hours after a dose of etomidate has been given to patients with sepsis is not supported by outcome studies. However, some clinicians treating patients with sepsis who have received etomidate for RSI will administer a single dose of glucocorticoid (e.g., hydrocortisone, 100 mg intravenously) if the hypotension is refractory to treatment with aggressive fluid resuscitation and vasopressors. Though yet unproven and seemingly an ever-changing recommendation, this approach is consistent with that used for septic patients who have not received etomidate.

Ketamine

Unique among anesthetic agents and probably underused in the ED, ketamine produces a dissociative anesthesia characterized by excellent analgesia and amnesia despite the appearance of wakefulness. As a drug that is potent and relatively safe with a rapid onset and brief duration of action, ketamine fits the profile of an agent that could be used effectively to facilitate intubation. Ketamine has also been advocated for pharmacologic control of undifferentiated agitated and violent patients with excited delirium. It does possess some pharmacologic properties that theoretically limit its use in selected circumstances.

Ketamine is a water- and lipid-soluble drug that rapidly penetrates into the CNS. Like the barbiturates, ketamine accumulates rapidly and then undergoes redistribution with subsequent degradation in the liver.[88] The recommended dose of ketamine before intubation is 1 to 2 mg/kg administered intravenously over a 1-minute period. Anesthesia occurs within 1 minute of completing the infusion and lasts 5 to 10 minutes. A smaller additional dose (0.5 to 1 mg/kg) may be given 5 minutes after the initial dose if needed to maintain anesthesia. Simultaneous administration of succinylcholine and midazolam is recommended to provide adequate muscle relaxation and to decrease the incidence of postanesthesia emergence reactions, respectively. The intramuscular dose for intubation has not been well studied, but a suggested dose is 4 to 5 mg/kg. Onset of action occurs within 2 to 3 minutes. Because of its good vascularity, the anterior thigh muscle is theoretically the preferred site for administration.

Unlike other anesthetic agents that depress the reticular activating system, ketamine acts by interrupting association pathways between the thalamocortical and limbic systems. Characteristically, the eyes remain open, and patients exhibit spontaneous, though not purposeful movements. Increases in blood pressure, heart rate, cardiac output, and myocardial oxygen consumption are seen, most likely mediated through the CNS. In vitro studies indicate that ketamine is a myocardial depressant, but the CNS-mediated pressor effects generally mask the direct cardiac effects,[89,90] thus making it potentially useful in patients with hemorrhagic shock or hypotension. Respirations are initially rapid and shallow after ketamine administration, but they soon return to normal.

Other features of ketamine anesthesia include increased skeletal muscle tone, preservation of the laryngeal and pharyngeal reflexes, hypersalivation, and relaxation of bronchial smooth muscle. Discussions exist regarding the use of ketamine in patients with head injury or potentially elevated ICP. Ketamine can cause a rise in ICP through sympathetic stimulation, thereby potentially exacerbating the condition of such patients with elevated ICP. When ketamine is used with a GABA agonist, however, this rise in ICP may not occur. Ketamine may benefit patients with a neurologic injury by increasing cerebral perfusion.

In one study, eight patients with traumatic brain injury and elevated ICP who were sedated with propofol were given different doses of ketamine (1.5, 3, or 5 mg/kg).[91] Ketamine did not alter cerebral hemodynamics at any time. In another study, researchers randomly assigned 25 patients with traumatic brain injury to sedation with either ketamine and midazolam or sufentanil and midazolam.[85]

Other studies suggest that ketamine does not interfere with cerebral metabolism or increase cerebral oxygen consumption and does not reduce regional glucose metabolism.[86] Ketamine can also offset any decrease in mean arterial pressure caused by fentanyl, a drug commonly used as part of RSI in patients with a head injury.[92]

Overall, evidence suggesting that ketamine elevates ICP to any significant clinical extent is weak, and evidence that harm might ensue is weaker. Based on current evidence it is reasonable to conclude that ketamine is an appropriate induction agent for RSI in patients with suspected elevated ICP and normal blood pressure or hypotension. In patients with hypertension and suspected ICP elevation, ketamine should be avoided because of its tendency to further increase blood pressure.

The most promising use of ketamine as an intubation adjunct has been in the setting of acute bronchospastic disease. Ketamine relaxes bronchial smooth muscle either directly through enhancement of sympathomimetic effects or indirectly through inhibition of vagal effects. Ketamine also increases bronchial secretions and may decrease the incidence of mucous plugging, which is commonly seen in decompensating asthmatic patients.[93] Clinical reports have demonstrated a reduction in airway resistance and an increase in pulmonary compliance within minutes of ketamine administration.[88,94] *Bronchospastic patients struggling to breathe and unable to tolerate oxygen masks or bronchodilators because of hypoxic encephalopathy will continue to breath deeply and rapidly with ketamine anesthesia, thereby allowing the maximum delivery of oxygen before a more elective intubation* (Fig. 5-2).

A potential side effect that has raised some concern about the use of ketamine for RSI is its tendency to produce postanesthesia emergence reactions, a characteristic that it shares with the structurally similar drug phencyclidine. The reemergence phenomenon, such as disturbing dreams as patients emerge from ketamine-induced anesthesia, is much less of a concern when the drug is used for RSI. In fact, there are no convincing data indicating that when used for RSI, ketamine produces unpleasant reemergence reactions that are significant or common enough to limit its use for this purpose. One study found that although dreams occurred frequently following sedative doses of ketamine, they were generally pleasant and the frequency of reemergence phenomena and delirium was markedly reduced by the concomitant use of a benzodiazepine.[95] Rarely, reactions may be marked and distressing, with symptoms including floating sensations, dizziness, blurred vision, out-of-body experiences, and vivid dreams or nightmares. The true incidence of emergence reactions following RSI is unknown, and clinical experience suggests that it is not an issue for RSI in the ED. Such reactions are less common in children than in adults and may be suppressed

Figure 5-2 This asthmatic is diaphoretic, confused, and agitated and cannot tolerate inhaled bronchodilators. He is about to suffer respiratory arrest and cannot be preoxygenated before intubation. Pulse oximetry shows an oxygen saturation of 82% to 84%. Within 60 seconds following intravenous administration of ketamine (100 mg), he stopped fighting but kept breathing rapidly. A non-rebreathing oxygen mask was tolerated and oxygen saturation rose to 98%, after which he was electively intubated under controlled preoxygenated conditions. A ketamine infusion (1 mg/kg/hr) was maintained for a few hours.

with benzodiazepines. Both diazepam and lorazepam appear to be useful in adults, but the latter is more effective, most likely because of its enhanced amnestic effect. Midazolam is effective in adult patients at doses of 0.07 mg/kg[96] and may be the preferred agent because it has potent amnestic effects and a short duration of action. Studies in children have failed to show a reduction in the rate of emergence reactions in those treated with both ketamine and midazolam.[97,98]

Despite preservation of pharyngeal and laryngeal reflexes in patients sedated with ketamine, aspiration can still occur.[99,100] Ketamine does not relax skeletal muscles, and production of the desired intubating conditions requires the simultaneous administration of a paralytic agent, thereby removing all upper airway reflexes.

Propofol

Propofol is a popular drug among anesthesiologists for OR-based induction and is ideal for ED use. Multiple reports have demonstrated the safety and efficacy of propofol for ED procedural sedation.[101,102] Although some ED clinicians now intubate only with propofol, eschewing longer-acting agents and paralysis, its role as an adjunct to intubation in the ED is undergoing evolution.

Propofol is an alkylphenol sedative-hypnotic used for induction and maintenance of general anesthesia. The drug has no analgesic activity, but it does exert a powerful amnestic effect. Propofol also tends to decrease vomiting through an unknown antiemetic effect. It produces dose-dependent depression of consciousness ranging from light sedation to coma. Propofol is a highly lipophilic, water-insoluble compound that undergoes rapid uptake by vascular tissues, including the brain, followed soon afterward by redistribution to muscle and fat. The drug is metabolized by the liver and excreted in urine.[103,104] After an induction dose of 2 mg/kg intravenously, unconsciousness occurs within 1 minute and lasts for 5 to 10 minutes. A smaller dose (1 to 1.5 mg/kg) is recommended in the elderly and when simultaneously administering other CNS depressants. Because propofol has a short duration of action and patients rapidly regain consciousness, repeat boluses are not a practical way to maintain a desired level of sedation.[103,104] Therefore, a slow drip infusion of 3 to 5 mg/kg/hr titrated to effect is preferred.

Propofol reduces airway resistance, which renders it a useful induction agent for patients with bronchospasm. Its neuroinhibitory effects make propofol a good induction agent for patients with intracranial pathology, provided that they are hemodynamically stable. The propofol-induced decrease in mean arterial pressure, generally about 10 mm Hg, can reduce cerebral perfusion pressure, thereby theoretically exacerbating CNS injury.

Propofol does not prolong the QT interval. Although the manufacturer lists egg or soybean allergy as a contraindication to the use of propofol, significant allergic reactions to the newer preparation of the drug are extremely rare.

Propofol suppresses sympathetic activity, thereby causing myocardial depression and peripheral vasodilation, particularly in the elderly or hypovolemic patients and when administered simultaneously with opioids. Hypotension can be minimized with fluid loading or reversal with 5 to 10 mg of IV ephedrine. Propofol reduces cerebral blood flow and may cause mild CNS excitatory activity (e.g., myoclonus, tremors, hiccups) during induction. Pain on injection occurs commonly, even when the drug is infused slowly.[103,104] Pretreating the infusing vein with 3 mL of 1% lidocaine (30 mg) injected over a 30-second period or choosing a large antecubital vein will ameliorate this pain.

Benzodiazepines (Midazolam)

The benzodiazepines are a widely used class of drugs characterized by anxiolytic, hypnotic, sedative, anticonvulsant, muscle relaxant, and amnestic effects. Several of these properties make the benzodiazepines appealing adjuvant agents for intubation, particularly when used in combination with opioids. It is important to remember that benzodiazepines do not have analgesic effects. Although they may produce excellent sedation and impair the patient's memory of an unpleasant experience, they will not prevent the pain associated with intubation.

Midazolam has replaced diazepam as a preoperative sedative agent, even in elderly patients.[105-109] When compared with diazepam, the primary advantages of midazolam include a twofold increase in potency, shorter half-life, and decreased potential for cardiorespiratory depression. Midazolam is water soluble in an acid medium and does not require suspension in propylene glycol like other benzodiazepines. It is rarely associated with phlebitis and can be given intramuscularly when a very rapid onset of action is not required. At physiologic pH, midazolam is lipophilic and rapidly accumulates in the CNS, with onset of sedation occurring in as little as 1 to 2 minutes. Outside the CNS it accumulates in fatty tissue and extensively binds to plasma, which accounts for the paucity of non-CNS side effects. Its half-life of elimination is 1 to 4 hours and is dependent on release of the drug from adipose tissue and protein-binding sites. The period of sedation after a single IV dose is considerably shorter. Emergence from a 0.15-mg/kg dose occurs in 15 to 20 minutes.[110]

Clinical experience using midazolam with or without fentanyl for procedural sedation is considerable, and it is considered both safe and effective in the ED setting. The recommended dose for moderate sedation with midazolam is 0.05 to 0.1 mg/kg given in 1-mg boluses and not exceeding 2.5 mg over a period of 2 minutes. Doses upward of 0.1 mg/kg are often needed to produce good conditions for intubation.[38,06]

The potential for adverse effects with midazolam is similar to that with other benzodiazepines. A small increase in heart rate is seen frequently, as is a small decrease in systolic blood pressure.[111] Changes in blood pressure may be exaggerated in the presence of hypovolemia.[112] An ED-based study reported a mean 10% decrease in systolic blood pressure, with 19% of intubated patients having systolic blood pressure lower than 90 mm Hg.[111] The cardiac index and coronary artery blood flow are not generally affected. In the prehospital setting, hypotension with midazolam was found to be dose related,[113] and it should be used cautiously in patients with hypovolemia or traumatic brain injury. Respiratory depression may occur even at standard doses, but it most often follows rapid administration of an excessive dose. Respiratory depression is also more likely to occur in debilitated or elderly patients and in those simultaneously receiving opioids. The effects of midazolam are rapidly reversed by administration of the benzodiazepine antagonist flumazenil. A study of various induction agents for ET intubation suggested that the use of midazolam alone for RSI may be associated with suboptimal intubating conditions and increased difficulty.[51] Other induction agents may be preferred over midazolam alone during RSI.

Opioids (Fentanyl)

Although any of several opioids administered intravenously could be used to induce unconsciousness, fentanyl has significant advantages over other opioid agents. A synthetic opioid, it has been widely used since its introduction in 1968. Its favorable pharmacologic properties include rapid serum clearance, high potency, and minimal release of histamine.[114-117] Fentanyl quickly crosses the blood-brain barrier and produces analgesia in as little as 1 to 2 minutes. Serum levels decline rapidly from peak concentrations because of extensive tissue uptake.[118,119] Unlike morphine, the brain concentration of fentanyl falls in conjunction with the serum level. The duration of analgesic action is 30 to 40 minutes, although at high doses a second peak of activity may be seen several hours later because of release of the bound drug from tissue stores. Fentanyl is about 50 to 100 times as potent as morphine.[120] This unique combination of potency and short half-life permits the administration of numerous small doses that can be titrated to the desired clinical effect. Similar to other opioids, fentanyl is competitively reversed with naloxone.

The relative safety of fentanyl permits considerable latitude in dosing. When used as a primary anesthetic agent for major surgical procedures, doses ranging from 50 to 100 μg/kg produce minimal side effects.[121] Comparatively tiny doses produce sedation, and 3 to 5 μg/kg, given at a rate of 1 to 2 μg/kg/min, is generally an effective analgesic dose. More rapid administration will cause greater depression of the level of consciousness. Mostert and coworkers[114] reported successful awake intubation in 99 of 103 patients who were administered an average cumulative dose of 3.7 μg/kg. Most of these patients were able to follow commands, and many recalled events surrounding the intubation. A small percentage could not be intubated even after receiving 500 μg of fentanyl.

Larger doses, perhaps up to 25 μg/kg, may be needed to produce ideal intubating conditions, although if given rapidly, 10 μg/kg is usually adequate. Even this lower dose is more likely to produce unconsciousness than a lesser depth of sedation, and it may cause a longer period of unresponsiveness than is desirable. It is preferable to use a low dose of fentanyl (2 to 3 μg/kg) for analgesia combined with a paralytic agent (e.g., succinylcholine) to produce adequate muscle relaxation and a sedative (e.g., midazolam) to reduce anxiety and produce amnesia for the event.

Unlike other opioids, fentanyl causes little or no release of histamine, and its use is seldom associated with emesis or hypotension. It is probably the safest opioid to use in hypovolemic patients. Fentanyl also has significantly fewer emetic effects than other opioids do. Adverse effects that have been reported with fentanyl are few and primarily follow the rapid IV infusion of very large doses. Like other opioids, fentanyl may cause rigidity of the skeletal musculature, including the chest wall and diaphragm. Rigidity occurs with doses in excess of 15 μg/kg, but it has also been reported with doses as low as 10 μg/kg and may also be related to rapid administration.[114,122] The muscular rigidity may be prevented or treated with standard doses of succinylcholine or naloxone.[123] The most common significant complication with fentanyl is respiratory depression, and it generally occurs when fentanyl is given in combination with other CNS depressants or in excessive amounts.[124]

NEUROMUSCULAR BLOCKING AGENTS

NMBs are used to achieve muscle relaxation for intubation. They permit complete airway control and greatly simplify visualization of the vocal cords. This is particularly important when intubation must be performed quickly under less than ideal circumstances. Sedatives may provide some muscle relaxation, but this requires rapid administration of large doses, which poses a risk for depression of the cardiovascular system. The combination of a paralytic agent and a sedative or analgesic agent is generally superior to the use of either agent alone. A 1999 report showed an 18% failure-to-intubate rate with a sedative alone versus a 0% failure rate for sedatives plus paralytics.[125] Procedural complication rates such as significant airway trauma and aspiration were also markedly higher in the group receiving sedation only.

The only absolute contraindication to the use of NMBs is the inability to manage the airway once the patient becomes apneic. Though not absolutely contraindicated, it is considered inhumane to paralyze and intubate an alert patient. A sedative or an analgesic agent should always be administered simultaneously if the patient is able to perceive pain.

NMBs are classified as either depolarizing or nondepolarizing. Depolarizing agents mimic the action of acetylcholine (ACh) and produce sustained depolarization of the neuromuscular junction, during which time muscle contractions cannot occur. Nondepolarizing agents competitively block the action of ACh at the neuromuscular junction and prevent depolarization and therefore muscle contractions. Commonly used NMBs and their dosages and characteristics are listed in Table 5-2.

Succinylcholine

The standard depolarizing agent currently in use is succinylcholine.[126] It has a chemical structure similar to that of ACh and depolarizes the postjunctional neuromuscular membrane. Administration is followed by a brief period of muscle fasciculations that correspond to the initial membrane depolarization and muscle fiber activation. Unlike ACh, which is released in minute amounts and hydrolyzed in milliseconds,

TABLE 5-2 Commonly Used Neuromuscular Blocking Agents

AGENT	DOSE (mg/kg)	ONSET (min)	DURATION (min)
Succinylcholine	1.5	1	3-5
Pancuronium	0.1	2-5	40-60
Vecuronium	0.1	3	30-35
	0.25	1	60-120
Atracurium	0.5	3	25-35
Mivacurium	0.15	2-3	15-20
Rocuronium	1.0	1-1.5	30-110

succinylcholine requires several minutes for breakdown to occur. During this time the neuromuscular junction remains depolarized, but the muscles relax and will not contract again until the neuromuscular end plate and adjacent sarcoplasmic reticulum return to the resting state and are again depolarized. Relaxation proceeds from the small, distal, rapidly moving muscles to the proximal, slowly moving muscles. The diaphragm is one of the last muscles to relax.[127]

Succinylcholine is rapidly degraded in serum by the enzyme pseudocholinesterase, and the duration of action of a single dose is 3 to 5 minutes. Relaxation may be maintained by repeated IV injections. Prolonged or repeated use of the drug enhances its vagal stimulatory effects, thereby resulting in bradycardia, hypotension, and other muscarinic effects. These effects may be seen even at normal doses, particularly in children.[128] For this reason, atropine pretreatment at a dose of 0.02 mg/kg has been recommended in all small children and for adults receiving multiple doses, although the need and optimal dose are still in question.[128] Repeated dosing of succinylcholine may produce a desensitization blockade and create a scenario in which the neuromuscular membrane returns to the resting state and becomes resistant to further depolarization by succinylcholine.[129,130] In general, there is little need for repeated doses of succinylcholine if appropriately dosed the first time. If paralysis in excess of 3 to 5 minutes is desired, longer-acting, nondepolarizing agents such as vecuronium or pancuronium should be used.

The recommended dose of succinylcholine is 1 to 1.5 mg/kg given intravenously. Dosages at the upper end of this range are suggested to guarantee complete relaxation and avoid the need for repeated dosing. Dosage calculations should also be based on actual, not lean body mass because of alterations in both volume of distribution and pseudocholinesterase activity.[131] Neonates and infants require a slightly higher dose of succinylcholine (2 mg/kg intravenously) as a result of their higher volume of distribution.[61,132] It is crucial that succinylcholine be administered as a rapid bolus because slow administration may lead to incomplete relaxation. Use of a rapid 20- to 30-mL saline flush after IV administration may enhance its desired effect.

There are a number of potential adverse effects of the use of succinylcholine ranging from minor to life-threatening. Muscle fasciculations accompany the initial depolarization of the neuromuscular membrane. Fasciculations are most prominent in muscular patients and create deep, aching muscle pain that may last for days.[133] It is unclear whether any regimen will totally prevent the succinylcholine-induced fasciculations (seen in 73% to 100% of patients) and myalgias (seen in 10% to 83% of patients), with varying effects reported after numerous interventions.[134] Interestingly, higher doses of succinylcholine may be associated with less myalgia. Traditionally, fasciculations have been prevented by the preadministration of a defasciculating dose (0.01 mg/kg) of pancuronium or vecuronium. The evidence available does not suggest that succinylcholine worsens outcomes in at-risk patients, nor does any evidence suggest that defasciculation improves outcomes in at-risk patients.[135]

A major consideration in the use of succinylcholine is its propensity to cause hyperkalemia. This electrolyte disturbance is believed to occur secondary to asynchronous depolarization of muscle cells and resulting cellular injury. Elevation in serum potassium occurs in normal patients after standard doses but is typically clinically inconsequential, with increases of less than 0.5 mmol/L (mEq/L).[136] Increases in potassium are not prevented with defasciculating doses of nondepolarizing agents. Marked hyperkalemia is associated with increased extrajunctional muscle ACh receptors, which develop in patients with prolonged diseases of the neuromuscular system. Susceptibility may occur within as little as 5 to 7 days and persist indefinitely. In these cases the hyperkalemic response may be as much as 5 mmol/L (mEq/L). Such conditions include late severe burns,[137] major muscle trauma,[138] spinal cord injury, muscular dystrophy, multiple sclerosis, and other upper motor neuron diseases[139,140] such as amyotrophic lateral sclerosis. These large elevations occur only in patients who have had significant tissue injury or muscle denervation for several days or weeks before the use of succinylcholine. Importantly, succinylcholine is not contraindicated in the initial management of patients with *acute injuries*, including burns, major crush injuries, and spinal cord injuries. Succinylcholine is also not contraindicated in normokalemic patients with renal failure because the magnitude of the rise in serum potassium is the same as in patients with normally functioning kidneys.[141] A retrospective review of the use of succinylcholine in 38 operative cases with moderate pre-RSI hyperkalemia (5.6 to 7.6 mmol/L) suggested that the risk for hyperkalemia-related complications may be lower than feared.[142] In a review of more than 41,000 intubations (38 patients had hyperkalemia with a mean serum potassium level of 5.9 mmol/L), Schow and colleagues[142] concluded that it is safe to administer succinylcholine to patients with a potassium level of 5.5 to 6.0 mEq/L. Regardless, succinylcholine is best avoided (if other equally effective pharmacologic options such as rocuronium exist) in the setting of known or suspected preexisting hyperkalemia (e.g., renal failure patients not receiving regular dialysis or demonstrating a wide QRS complex). Concern has also been raised over the use of succinylcholine in the pediatric population because of rare case reports of hyperkalemic cardiac arrest after administration to children with undiagnosed myopathies. Succinylcholine is currently recommended for use in pediatric patients only under emergency circumstances when the airway must be secured rapidly.[132]

Malignant hyperthermia is a rare complication with an autosomal dominant inheritance pattern that is triggered by multiple anesthetic agents, including succinylcholine. Most provocative agents, such as halothane, are not used in the ED setting, and it is extremely rare for the ED physician to encounter this complication. It occurs in approximately 1 in 15,000 children and 1 in 50,000 adults.[143] The clinical syndrome consists of high fever, tachypnea, tachycardia, cardiac arrhythmias, hypoxia, acidosis, myoglobinuria, and impaired coagulation. Unabated muscle contractions mediated by abnormal calcium channels are the physiologic basis for this condition.[144] Treatment includes aggressive cooling measures, volume replacement, and correction of hypoxia and acid-base and electrolyte abnormalities. Dantrolene sodium, a direct-acting skeletal muscle relaxant, is thought to be effective in reducing the muscle hypermetabolism that causes the dramatic hyperpyrexia.[145] An associated abnormal response to succinylcholine is isolated masseter spasm,[146] but it can occur in isolation or portend the subsequent development of malignant hyperthermia. Though rare, it has been reported in the emergency medicine literature.[147] In this condition, forcible sustained contraction of the masseter muscles occurs and prevents mouth opening and oral intubation. Management is controversial, with recommendations ranging from use of a bag valve mask, securing a surgical airway until the contraction abates, to attempting to suppress the contractions through administration of a nondepolarizing NMB.

Prolonged paralysis after the administration of succinylcholine may occur in clinical conditions that result in decreased pseudocholinesterase levels and subsequent decreased metabolism of succinylcholine. Physiologic states associated with this condition include hepatic disease, anemia, renal failure, organophosphate poisoning, pregnancy, chronic cocaine use, advanced age, bronchogenic carcinoma, and connective tissue disorders. Patients with these conditions experience a twofold to threefold increase in the duration of apnea.[148] Patients with cocaine intoxication may also experience prolonged muscle relaxation because cocaine is competitively metabolized by the cholinesterases. An inherited deficiency of pseudocholinesterase is also present in about 0.03% of the population and can lead to prolonged paralysis from the administration of succinylcholine.[145]

Succinylcholine can also result in an increase in ICP, but the magnitude and significance of the increase in ICP remains controversial.[149-153] Increases in the range of 5 to 10 mm Hg have been reported by several investigators, but other researchers have shown no increase. There is no evidence of neurologic deterioration associated with these transient elevations in ICP. Mechanisms that have been proposed to explain the elevated ICP include (1) a direct effect of fasciculations, (2) an increase in cortical electrical activity with a resultant increase in cerebral blood flow and blood volume, and (3) sympathetic postganglionic stimulation. Limited studies have been performed to evaluate the significance of this rise in ICP in a brain-injured human patient population. These studies have shown no significant change in electroencephalographic activity or ICP with succinylcholine, but the small size of the studies limits the ability to draw conclusions about clinical outcomes.[132,154,155]

Questions concerning the safety of succinylcholine in the setting of acute intracranial pathology do not have clear answers. The drug has been used widely and successfully in this setting, and its continued use is supported by this experience. The very real risk for airway compromise and secondary cerebral insult because of hypoxia from delayed or failed intubation must always be weighed against the theoretical harmful effects. Succinylcholine, despite its many potential side effects, is currently the most frequently used agent for neuromuscular blockade with RSI because of its rapid onset and offset and reliable muscle relaxation characteristics.

Nondepolarizing Agents

Nondepolarizing agents act in a competitive manner to block the effects of ACh at the neuromuscular junction. Drugs in this class include pancuronium, atracurium, vecuronium, mivacurium, and rocuronium. These drugs, particularly the intermediate-acting agents, have fewer side effects than succinylcholine does and the potential for reversal. They generally have a longer onset and duration of action than succinylcholine does, thus making them less attractive choices for RSI because of the delay in muscle relaxation. In most instances, succinylcholine remains the agent of choice to facilitate emergency intubation, and nondepolarizing agents are indicated to maintain paralysis after intubation. Knowledge of appropriate nondepolarizing NMBs is important for situations when succinylcholine may be contraindicated.

Because nondepolarizing agents act competitively at neuromuscular junction receptors, increasing the concentration of ACh may reverse their effects. Cholinesterase inhibitors such as neostigmine or edrophonium may be used but will not be effective until some spontaneous signs of reversal are seen. The concept of reversal is of limited clinical importance in the ED with rare exceptions, such as performance of a neurologic examination on a previously paralyzed patient. When reversal is required, neostigmine, 0.02 to 0.04 mg/kg, is given by slow IV push. An additional dose of 0.01 to 0.02 mg/kg may be given in 5 minutes if reversal is incomplete, but the total dose should not exceed 5 mg in adults. Atropine, 0.01 mg/kg (with a minimum dose of 0.1 mg in children and a maximum dose of 1 mg in adults), should be given concurrently with neostigmine to block its systemic cholinergic effects.[156-158] Another potential reversing agent, sugammadex, binds directly to the aminosteroid NMB rather than to cholinesterases.[159] For reversal of shallow or profound neuromuscular blockade, 2 or 4 mg/kg intravenously, respectively, is recommended. Unfortunately, no studies currently address its use in emergency situations. It is approved for use in Europe but not the United States.

Long-Acting Agents: Pancuronium

Pancuronium is an aminosteroid that is primarily excreted in urine within 1 hour of IV administration.[159] Classified as a long-acting agent, its onset and duration of action are dose related. After a typical IV dose of 0.1 mg/kg, paralysis occurs within 2 to 5 minutes and lasts approximately 60 minutes. Paralysis may be maintained safely by repeated bolus or drip infusion. Because the effects of the drug are cumulative, repeating the original dose significantly lengthens the duration of paralysis.

Relatively few adverse effects are associated with the use of pancuronium. Many patients experience an increase in heart rate, blood pressure, and cardiac output because of the vagolytic effect of the drug. Ventricular tachycardia and severe hypertension have been reported but are quite rare.[160,161] Pancuronium may cause release of histamine resulting in bronchospasm or anaphylactic reactions.[162] Prolonged paralysis may occur, primarily in patients with myasthenia gravis or with significant impairment in renal function. One consensus panel recommended pancuronium for maintaining paralysis, except in patients with cardiac disease or hemodynamic instability, for whom they recommended vecuronium.[163]

Intermediate-Acting Agents: Vecuronium, Atracurium, Mivacurium, and Rocuronium

Vecuronium and atracurium are intermediate-acting agents with an onset of action of approximately 3 minutes and a duration of action of 30 minutes. Mivacurium has an onset of action of 2 to 3 minutes and a duration of action of 15 to 20 minutes. Rocuronium has an onset of action within 1 to 1.5 minutes and a duration of action of 20 to 75 minutes (longer in geriatric patients). These drugs have minimal cardiovascular effects, cause little release of histamine (with the exception of mivacurium),[132] and lack cumulative effects.[164]

The recommended doses of vecuronium, atracurium, mivacurium, and rocuronium are listed in Table 5-2. Use of larger doses hastens the onset of action but greatly prolongs the period of paralysis. For example, vecuronium at a dose of

0.25 mg/kg intravenously will cause paralysis in as little as 1 minute, but the period of paralysis will last 1 to 3 hours.[165,166] Because a rapid onset of action comparable to that of succinylcholine is achieved at high doses of intermediate-acting agents, they may be used as the sole agents to facilitate intubation, particularly if a long period of paralysis is desired after intubation. The use of succinylcholine before intubation and an intermediate-acting agent at a normal dose after intubation provides rapid intubating conditions and better control over the duration of paralysis. The paralysis induced by vecuronium or atracurium may be maintained by repeated boluses or drip infusion. Unlike both pancuronium and succinylcholine, these agents have no side effects specifically related to repeated dosing in the ED. A repeated dose of 0.01 to 0.02 mg/kg of vecuronium will extend the period of paralysis 12 to 15 minutes.

Rocuronium, a structural analogue of vecuronium, is emerging as a desirable alternative agent for RSI when succinylcholine is contraindicated. At doses of 0.6 to 1.2 mg/kg, rocuronium consistently provides good to excellent intubating conditions within 1 minute of administration. Its duration of action is dose dependent and ranges from 20 to 75 minutes.[167,168] Smaller anesthesia and ED-based studies have demonstrated its clinical utility and safety in RSI protocols.[55,167-173] However, a 2003 Cochrane review[174] found that except when used in conjunction with propofol, the intubation conditions produced by rocuronium tend to be inferior to those produced by succinylcholine for RSI.

THE "SEDATED LOOK" EVALUATION OF THE AIRWAY BEFORE RAPID-SEQUENCE INTUBATION

In selected stable patients, conditions may exist that preclude the immediate use of RSI, and the more prudent approach would be to assess the airway and intubation needs or potential complications before using paralytics. Examples are patients with angiotensin-converting enzyme inhibitor–induced angioedema or smoke inhalation, where clinical issues of RSI and intubation can be assessed by directly visualizing the larynx. This approach, referred to as a "sedated look" or "awake look," is used when the clinician suspects a difficult intubation. This approach allows the clinician to verify that the laryngeal structures are indeed visible and accessible before committing to paralysis. This technique allows the patient to maintain respiratory drive during analysis of the airway. This approach is distinct from the practice of intubation with sedation alone or non-paralytic RSI, in which the patient receives a full induction dose of a sedative agent but no neuromuscular blocking agent. This older practice may create a vulnerable and compromised patient in whom intubating conditions are then problematic.

Traditionally in the OR, topical anesthesia (e.g., nebulized 4% lidocaine) along with moderate sedation has been used to allow a view into the airway while enabling the patient to maintain respiratory drive and protective airway reflexes. Although more research is needed to determine which medications are best for sedated looks in the ED, ketamine may be ideal in this circumstance by allowing the patient to maintain respiratory drive while providing analgesia, amnesia, and sedation. Ketamine's analgesic properties allow it to be used as the sole agent in patients with a bloody traumatized airway,

for which topical anesthesia is unlikely to work effectively. Other options are discussed in the following section.

AWAKE INTUBATION

An alternative to induction of unconsciousness in patients requiring intubation is the use of local anesthetic and sedative agents in conscious patients. The availability of relatively effective and safe induction agents makes this a less attractive alternative than in the past, but these techniques may be desirable in specific patients, such as for fiberoptic intubation of a predicted difficult airway. Awake intubation offers a number of potential advantages over RSI. The natural airway is maintained along with spontaneous respiration and a degree of protection from aspiration. The use of sedative agents to produce a state of mild or moderate sedation and adequate topical anesthesia are the principal components needed for awake intubation.

Thomas[175] likened standard laryngoscopy in an awake patient to the "mouth being held open with a wrench." Awake nasotracheal intubation and fiberoptic intubation can also be an extremely unpleasant experience. The upper airway is richly innervated by sensory branches of the 5th, 7th, 9th, and 10th cranial nerves. In addition to pain fibers, there are stretch receptors that stimulate the coughing and gagging reflexes with even minor airway manipulation. It is essential that adequate analgesia be provided before intubation in all but the most extreme circumstances. Treatment options include topical application of anesthetic agents to the pharyngeal and tracheal mucosa and IV infusion of analgesic or sedative agents.

Local or topical anesthesia techniques may be used in patients who are awake, either in place of or as a supplement to IV analgesia or sedation. They are particularly useful as adjuncts to nasotracheal and fiberoptic intubation but do not generally provide the degree of analgesia or relaxation desirable for traditional laryngoscopy. In addition, the time required to achieve good topical anesthesia may limit the usefulness of these techniques in emergency situations. Topical anesthesia may be achieved by direct application, by cricothyroid membrane puncture, or by inhalation of a nebulized anesthetic.

Direct Application

Achieving anesthesia of the oral and pharyngeal mucosa is a relatively simple procedure that involves the use of commonly available agents such as 4% lidocaine or a combination such as 14% benzocaine, 2% butamben, and 2% tetracaine (Cetacaine). Achieving anesthesia of the hypopharynx is more difficult because optimal results require application of the anesthetic to the epiglottis and vocal cords.

This procedure begins with spraying the tongue and pharynx with a topical agent. Use of atomization devices that attach to standard syringes (e.g., Mucosal Atomization Device [MAD], Wolfe Tory Medical, Inc., Salt Lake City) can provide effective drug dispersal without a forceful spray (Fig. 5-3). The more forceful pressurized canister sprays commonly provoke a cough reflex. After allowing at least 2 to 3 minutes to achieve numbing of the tongue and pharynx, the epiglottis and vocal cords can be sprayed with the MAD device. A malleable extension tube allows the tip of the MAD to pass around the base of the tongue, thereby permitting direct

Figure 5-3 The Mucosal Atomization Device. *(Courtesy of Wolfe Tory Medical, Inc., Salt Lake City.)*

Lidocaine 4%
(2 mL)

Cricothyroid
membrane

Figure 5-4 Cricothyroid membrane puncture. Prepare the skin with an antiseptic and then puncture the cricothyroid membrane in the midline. Advance the needle until air can be aspirated and then rapidly inject 2 mL of 4% lidocaine. Alternatively, 3 to 4 mL of 2% lidocaine can be used.

spraying of the epiglottis and vocal cords. This is generally well tolerated. An alternative method is to visualize the epiglottis and vocal cords with a laryngoscope and directly spray with the anesthetic agent. The use of a laryngoscope to visualize the vocal cords is much more stimulating to the patient and often not well tolerated. Another alternative is percutaneous injection of an anesthetic agent into the trachea at the level of the cricothyroid membrane.[176,177]

Cricothyroid Membrane Puncture

Direct application of topical anesthetics to the subglottic region can also be achieved through cricothyroid membrane puncture (Fig. 5-4). In this procedure, identify the cricothyroid membrane immediately below the thyroid cartilage. After antiseptic skin preparation, puncture the overlying

tissue and membrane with a 22-gauge needle in the midline and just above the superior border of the cricoid cartilage. Take care to maintain the needle in the midline at all times to avoid injury to the recurrent laryngeal nerves. Advance the needle until air can be aspirated, which indicates placement of the tip in the trachea. Inject a 2-mL volume of 4% lidocaine rapidly. If the 4% concentration is not available, use 3 to 4 mL of 1% to 2% lidocaine. Typically, this will precipitate a cough and distribute the anesthetic over the upper part of the trachea, vocal cords, and epiglottis.

Nebulized Anesthesia

Nebulized anesthesia is a simple and painless technique that can be used to facilitate awake intubation when the patient's condition is stable enough to permit a several-minute delay. Deliver the anesthetic via a standard nebulizer and face mask connected to an oxygen source that delivers 4 to 8 L/min. Nebulize a 4-mL volume of a 4% lidocaine solution over a period of about 5 minutes. Bourke and associates[178] reported achieving consistently good topical anesthesia with this technique, although their patients were often premedicated with combinations of opioids and sedatives.

Sedation for Awake Intubation

Many patients can be intubated while awake with adequate topical anesthesia, but anxiolysis and mild to moderate sedation may be helpful for selected patients. The use of propofol in low doses (0.2 to 0.3 mg/kg) may be helpful. If time allows, anticholinergic agents such as glycopyrrolate may be helpful to reduce airway secretions. A new sedative agent, dexmedetomidine (an α_2-adrenoreceptor agonist), has been described for use in awake intubation. Dexmedetomidine produces sedation and anxiolysis with minimal respiratory depression. Patients become sleepy but, if stimulated, can easily be aroused and are generally cooperative. These properties make it seem like an ideal agent for awake intubation, but its use is limited in emergencies by a requisite 10-minute loading dose followed by a maintenance infusion. Propofol may also cause hypertension with high doses because of direct stimulation of α_2 receptors on the vasculature and can cause hypotension when given as a low-dose infusion[179,180] because of inhibition of release of norepinephrine from sympathetic terminals. Future studies will be needed before this medication can be recommended for use in the ED.

Acknowledgment

The editors and authors wish to acknowledge the contribution of Laura R. Hopson to this chapter in previous editions.

References are available at www.expertconsult.com

CHAPTER 6

Cricothyrotomy and Percutaneous Translaryngeal Ventilation

Randy B. Hebert, Sudip Bose, and Sharon E. Mace

Few clinical scenarios are as critical as when a patient's airway cannot be controlled with traditional endotracheal (ET) intubation. Although cricothyroidotomy is rarely required,[1-4] the incidence of surgical airways has decreased even further since the advent of adjunctive intubation techniques.[5,6] The conditions accompanying an airway emergency are often stressful and chaotic and require the emergency department (ED) physician to be intimately familiar with this procedure.

When ET intubation has failed or is contraindicated, cricothyrotomy is often the procedure of last resort. Both surgical cricothyrotomy and needle cricothyrotomy entail puncture of the cricothyroid membrane through the overlying skin to gain access to the airway.

Surgical cricothyrotomy is a procedure in which an incision is made in the cricothyroid membrane and a tracheostomy tube or modified ET tube is placed into the airway to ventilate the patient. *Tracheostomy* differs from cricothyrotomy in that the incision is made between two of the tracheal rings. *Needle cricothyrotomy* refers to insertion of a catheter via percutaneous needle puncture of the cricothyroid membrane to allow *percutaneous translaryngeal ventilation* (PTLV). The term *transtracheal jet ventilation* is often used interchangeably with PTLV in conjunction with needle cricothyrotomy, but PTLV is more accurate because the cricothyroid membrane is part of the larynx and not the trachea. PTLV is sometimes provided by bag insufflation instead of jet ventilation. The term *jet ventilation* usually refers to low-frequency jet ventilation with oxygen from a wall source as opposed to high-frequency jet ventilation from a dedicated jet ventilator.

ANATOMY

The central structure of importance is the cricothyroid membrane, an elastic membrane located anteriorly and midline in the neck. The membrane is bordered superiorly by the thyroid cartilage and inferiorly by the cricoid cartilage. The lateral aspects of the cricothyroid membrane are partially covered by the cricothyroid muscles, but the central triangular portion is subcutaneous, which makes it an ideal location to access the airway.

Identify the cricothyroid membrane by locating the prominent thyroid cartilage superior to it. The thyroid cartilage consists of two lateral laminae that join at an acute angle in the midline to form the laryngeal prominence and is more pronounced in males. It is commonly known as the "Adam's apple." The internal aspect of the anterior body of the thyroid cartilage provides the attachment for the vocal ligaments.

Superior to the thyroid cartilage and connecting it to the hyoid bone is the thyroid membrane, which allows passage of the superior laryngeal vessels and the internal branch of the superior laryngeal nerve through its laterally located foramina.

The cricoid cartilage forms the inferior border of the cricothyroid membrane and is the only completely circumferential cartilaginous structure of the larynx. It is composed of a broad posterior segment that tapers laterally to form a narrow anterior arch. The tracheal rings descend inferiorly to the cricoid cartilage.

Identify the cricothyroid membrane between the previously mentioned structures as a shallow depression measuring about 9 mm longitudinally and 30 mm transversely. If the depression is obscured by soft tissue swelling, estimate the location of the cricothyroid membrane at about 2 to 3 cm inferior to the laryngeal prominence or four fingerbreadths above the sternal notch.[7-9]

The area overlying and immediately adjacent to the cricothyroid membrane is relatively avascular and free of other significant anatomic structures. The cricothyroid arteries branch from the superior thyroid arteries and may form a small anastomotic arch traversing the superior aspect of the cricothyroid membrane. The external branch of the superior laryngeal nerve runs along the lateral aspect of the larynx and innervates the cricothyroid muscles inferior to the membrane. The isthmus of the thyroid gland most often overlies the second and third tracheal rings, although an aberrant pyramidal lobe of the gland may extend just superior to the cricothyroid membrane. The anterior attachments of the vocal cord structures are protected by the thyroid cartilage[10,11] (Fig. 6-1).

In children, the larynx is positioned more superiorly than in adults.[12] There is also more overlap between the thyroid cartilage and the cricoid cartilage, thus making the cricoid membrane proportionally smaller[13] (Fig. 6-2).

SURGICAL CRICOTHYROTOMY

Indications and Contraindications

The chief indication for surgical cricothyrotomy is an inability to secure the airway with less invasive techniques in a patient with impending or ongoing hypoxia.[14]

Surgical cricothyrotomy, like any invasive procedure, is associated with significant complications and should not be attempted until less invasive measures have failed. No simple algorithm fits all cases. When time and the clinical situation allow, it may be appropriate to attempt to intubate multiple times with traditional laryngoscopy or to try alternative intubation techniques. Emergency decisions are subject to controversy and differ on a case-by-case analysis, but alternatives to cricothyrotomy include bag-valve-mask ventilation, the gum elastic bougie, and laryngeal mask airways. At some point, further attempts at intubation become futile and the benefits of a surgical airway outweigh the risks associated with ongoing hypoxia.[15]

When approaching a patient with a compromised airway, the clinician must have a clear potential algorithm in mind with a well-defined plan that shifts the airway approach from laryngoscopy to alternative techniques to cricothyrotomy.[16] The first step in deciding whether cricothyrotomy is indicated is anticipating a possible difficult intubation.[17]

Cricothyrotomy

Indications
Inability to maintain >90% saturation between intubation
  attempts or after three attempts
Inability to bag-mask-valve ventilate the patient between
  intubation attempts or after three attempts
Multiple attempts at endotracheal intubation fail to secure the airway
After failed rescue maneuvers (e.g., gum elastic bougie
  intubation, intubating laryngeal mask airway)

Contraindications
Age younger than 5–12 years (depending on the source)
Tracheal transection, fracture, or obstruction below the
  cricothyroid membrane

Complications
Acute
  Bleeding
  Tube malposition
  Bronchial intubation
  Laryngotracheal injury
  Tension pneumothorax
  Tube obstruction
Late
  Subjective voice changes
  Difficulty swallowing
  Infections
  Persistent shortness of breath
  Persistent stoma
  Subglottic or glottic stenosis

Equipment
Traditional surgical cricothyrotomy

Melker technique

Review Box 6-1 Cricothyrotomy: indications, contraindications, complications, and equipment.

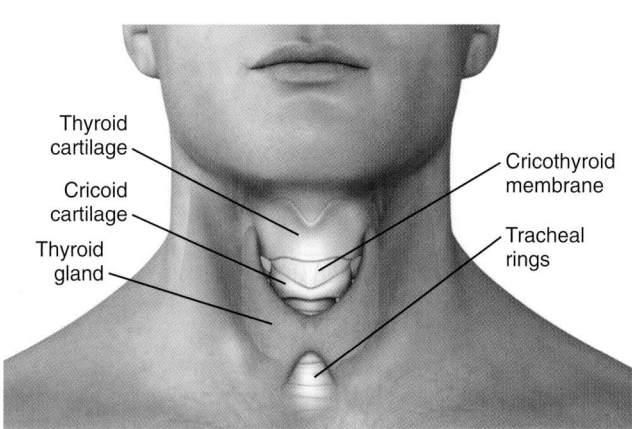

Figure 6-1 Normal adult larynx.

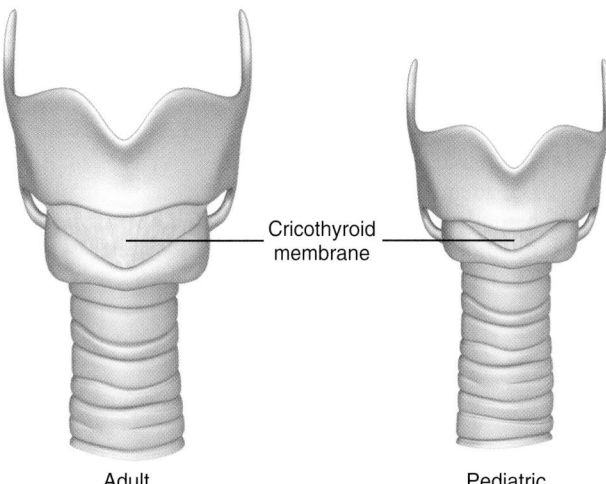

Figure 6-2 Adult larynx compared with a pediatric larynx.

| Class I | Class II |
| Class III | Class IV |

Figure 6-3 Modified Mallampati classes. *(From Kryger MH. Sleep breathing bisorders: examination of the patient with suspected sleep apnea. In: Kryger MH, ed: Kryger Atlas of Sleep Medicine. Philadelphia: Elsevier; 2010.)*

THE LEMON LAW

EVALUATION CRITERIA	POINTS
L = Look externally	
Facial trauma	1
Large incisors	1
Beard or mustache	1
Large tongue	1
E = Evaluate the 3-3-2 rule	
Incisor distance—3 fingerbreadths	1
Hyoid-mental distance—3 fingerbreadths	1
Thyroid-to-mouth distance—2 fingerbreadths	1
M = Mallampati (Mallampati score >3)	1
O = Obstruction (presence of any condition such as epiglottitis, peritonsillar abscess, trauma)	1
N = Neck mobility (limited neck mobility)	1
Total	10

Figure 6-4 The LEMON law can be used to quickly assess for potentially difficult airways. Higher scores are associated with poor glottic visualization and difficult intubation. *(Modified from Soyuncu S. Determination of difficult intubation in the ED. Ann J Emerg Med. 2009;8:905.)*

BOX 6-1   Clinical Indicators of a Difficult Airway

High Mallampati score
Thyroid-to-hyoid distance <2 fingerbreadths
Obesity
Large incisors
Limited neck mobility
Airway obstruction (partial or complete)
    Nontraumatic
        Oropharyngeal edema
        Laryngospasm
        Mass effect (cancer, tumor, polyp, web, or other mass)
    Traumatic
        Oropharyngeal edema
        Foreign body obstruction
        Laryngospasm
        Obstruction secondary to a mass effect or displacement
        Stenosis
Traumatic injuries making oral or nasal endotracheal intubation difficult or potentially hazardous (relative)
    Maxillofacial injuries
    Cervical spine instability

Several studies in the anesthesia and emergency medicine literature have attempted to identify predictors of a difficult airway. A Mallampati score can be determined in cooperative patients who are able to sit upright. It classifies the degree that the faucial pillars, soft palate, and uvula can be visualized (Fig. 6-3). A higher score predicts a more difficult ET intubation.[18] A Mallampati score can be obtained only in a limited number of ED patients requiring intubation.[19] A modified LEMON score, when excluding the Mallampati score, is more easily applied to ED patients for prediction of more difficult ET intubation[20] (Fig. 6-4). Additional indicators of a difficult airway include obesity, oropharyngeal edema, hemorrhage, and laryngospasm[21-24] (Box 6-1).

Cricothyrotomy is indicated when a difficult airway becomes a "failed airway," and this is somewhat difficult to define in emergency medicine. The American Society of Anesthesiologists suggests defining a failed airway as an inability to maintain oxygen saturation greater than 90%, signs of inadequate ventilation (cyanosis, absent breath sounds, hemodynamic instability) with positive pressure bag-mask ventilation, or more than three failed attempts at ET intubation or failure to intubate after 10 minutes by an experienced operator.[25] As more rescue airway adjunctive devices such as the laryngeal mask airway, gum elastic bougie, or lighted stylet become available, it is reasonable to continue beyond three attempts at ET intubation if adequate ventilation and oxygen saturation greater than 90% can be maintained.[26,27]

Because of the anatomic differences between children and adults, including a smaller cricothyroid membrane and a rostral, funnel-shaped, and more compliant pediatric larynx, surgical cricothyrotomy has been contraindicated in infants and young children. The exact age at which surgical cricothyrotomy can be done is controversial and not well defined. Various textbooks list the lower age limit from 5 years[28] to 10 years[29] or 12 years.[30] The advanced cardiac life support (ACLS) and pediatric advanced life support (PALS) define an infant airway as age up to 1 year and a child airway as age 1 to 8 years.

Some authors also identify tracheal transection or low tracheal obstruction (below the cricoid) as absolute contraindications to cricothyrotomy because of the need to secure the airway below the injury[31] (Box 6-2).

Indications for and Contraindications to Surgical Cricothyrotomy

INDICATIONS

Inability to maintain >90% oxygen saturation between intubation attempts or after three attempts

Inability to ventilate the patient with a bag-valve-mask device between intubation attempts or after three attempts

Multiple attempts at endotracheal intubation fail to secure the airway

CONTRAINDICATIONS

Age younger than 5-12 years (depending on the source)

Tracheal transection, fracture, or obstruction below the cricothyroid membrane

Figure 6-5 Standard Shiley tracheostomy tube with removable trocar and inner cannula.

Equipment

The equipment necessary to perform a traditional surgical cricothyrotomy includes a scalpel with a No. 11 blade, a Trousseau dilator, a tracheal hook, and a tracheostomy tube or modified ET tube (see Review Box 6-1). Bent 18-gauge needles may substitute for tracheal hooks. In addition, the sterile tray may include a syringe and lidocaine with epinephrine for local anesthesia, sterile drapes or towels, antiseptic preparation solution, 4 × 4-cm sterile gauze, scissors, hemostats, and suture material. The average adult's cricothyroid membrane is about 9 mm longitudinally and 30 mm horizontally. Familiarity with the dimensions of several standard tracheostomy and ET tubes is essential when selecting the appropriate size for surgical airways. Cuffed tracheostomy tubes are recommended, and they come in various sizes. Shiley tracheostomy tubes are commonly available in most EDs. The No. 4 tube has an inner diameter (ID) of 5.0 mm and an outer diameter (OD) of 9.4 mm, and the No. 6 tube has an ID of 6.4 mm and an OD of 10.8 mm. Shiley tracheostomy tubes come with three parts: a cuffed outer cannula, a removable inner cannula, and a removable obturator that is solid and removed after insertion (Fig. 6-5). ET tubes are often used temporarily in place of a tracheostomy tube. With respect to ID, ET tube OD can vary with the manufacturer.

As an example, the Mallinckrodt TaperGuard Evac Endotracheal Tube with IDs of 6.0 and 8.0 mm have ODs of 9.0 and 11.8 mm, respectively.[32] Although a No. 11 scalpel blade is most commonly used, a No. 20 blade is recommended in some variations of the technique. Commercially available kits include the Melker Cricothyrotomy Kit (Cook Critical Care, Bloomington, IN) for percutaneous cricothyrotomy, which uses the Seldinger technique to insert a cuffed or uncuffed airway catheter.

Procedure

Positioning plays a critical role in success, but the ideal patient position may be impossible because of clinical parameters. For example, hypoxic patients often cannot recline. Ketamine anesthesia does not suppress the respiratory drive and may aid in patient cooperation and positioning. When feasible, use the supine position with the neck exposed. Unless the patient has a known or suspected cervical spine injury, it is important to *hyperextend the neck to more readily identify the landmarks*. Surgical cricothyrotomy can safely and successfully be performed with minimal cervical spine movement.[33] Preoxygenate the patient by bag-mask ventilation. Prepare the skin of the anterior aspect of the neck with antiseptic solution and create a sterile field with the use of drapes or towels. If the patient is awake or responding to pain, give a subcutaneous and translaryngeal injection of lidocaine with epinephrine as a local anesthetic. Test the integrity of the balloon on the tracheostomy or ET tube by injecting it with 10 mL of air. Wear sterile gloves and take standard precautions by wearing a mask, goggles, and gown. All preparatory steps are optional and depend on the urgency of the procedure.

Traditional Technique

The "traditional" (open) cricothyrotomy technique (Fig. 6-6) has changed little since the original description of elective cricothyroidotomy by Brantigan and Grow in 1976.[34] McGill and colleagues[35] described the addition of a tracheal hook for emergency cricothyrotomy in 1982. In a follow-up report in 1989, Erlandson and colleagues[36] emphasized the importance of making an initial *vertical skin incision and using a relatively small (No. 4 Shiley) tracheal tube*. These modifications have generally been accepted and are commonly described as part of the traditional technique.[37]

If you are right hand dominant, stand on the patient's right side. Stabilize the larynx with the nondominant hand by grasping both sides of the lateral thyroid cartilage with the thumb and middle finger. Palpate the depression over the cricothyroid membrane with the index finger. Control the larynx throughout the procedure by stabilizing it in this manner (Fig. 6-6, *step 1*). If the laryngeal landmarks are not easily identifiable because of obesity or swelling, bedside ultrasonography may assist in identifying the cricothyroid membrane[38,39] (Fig. 6-7).

While holding the scalpel with a No. 11 blade in the dominant hand, make an approximately 2- to 3-cm *vertical incision* through the skin and subcutaneous tissue (Fig. 6-6, *step 2*). With the index finger of the nondominant hand, palpate the cricothyroid membrane through the incision. It is important to understand that the remainder of the procedure should be performed by palpation of the anatomy, not visualization, because bleeding may obscure the field and there is no time to delay while trying to achieve hemostasis. If the

SURGICAL CRICOTHYROTOMY: TRADITIONAL TECHNIQUE

1 Extend the neck whenever possible for better access to the trachea. Immobilize the larynx with your nondominant hand and palpate the cricothyroid membrane with your index finger.

2 Make a 3- to 5-cm *vertical* midline incision through the skin and subcutaneous tissues.

Palpate the membrane through the skin to confirm the anatomy.

3 Make a <1-cm *horizontal* incision through the cricothyroid membrane. *Note that the skin incision is vertical, but the membrane incision is horizontal.*

4 Insert the tracheal hook in the opening of the membrane, and rotate it cephalad, while grasping the inferior border of the thyroid cartilage. Ask an assistant to provide upward traction on the hook.

5 Place the tips of the Trousseau dilator into the opening in the membrane and spread in the longitudinal (vertical) plane.

6 Rotate the handle 90° until the handle is vertical or parallel to the neck

7 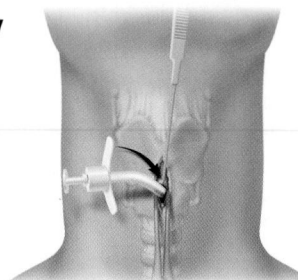 Insert the tube between the blades of the dilator until the flanges rest against the skin of the neck.

Keep your thumb on the obturator during tube insertion.

8 Carefully remove the Trousseau dilator and the obturator.

9 Replace the inner cannula of the tracheostomy tube and inflate the balloon.

10 Ventilate and confirm tube position by auscultation and end-tidal CO_2.

Secure the tube in place.

Figure 6-6 Surgical cricothyrotomy: traditional technique. (*Adapted from Custalow CB. Color Atlas of Emergency Department Procedures. Philadelphia: Saunders; 2005.*)

Figure 6-7 As an option, use the linear ultrasound probe to locate the cricothyroid membrane.

Cut proximal to the inflation device

Figure 6-8 A, Modify the standard endotracheal (ET) tube for use in surgical cricothyrotomy as a temporary alternative to a tracheostomy tube. Cut the proximal end of the ET tube but be careful to not cut the balloon inflation apparatus. **B,** Replace the adapter on the cut end of the tube.

cricothyroid membrane cannot be palpated, extend the initial incision superiorly and inferiorly and try to palpate again. Using the stabilizing index finger as a guide, make a *horizontal* incision of less than 1.0 cm in length through the cricothyroid membrane (Fig. 6-6, *step 3*). *Note that the skin incision is vertical but the membrane incision is horizontal.* Place the index finger into the stoma momentarily to exchange the scalpel for the tracheal hook.[40]

Using the dominant hand, place the tracheal hook into the opening in the cricothyroid membrane. Rotate the handle cephalad while grasping the inferior border of the thyroid cartilage with it. Ask an assistant to provide upward traction or provide traction yourself by passing the handle of the hook to the nondominant hand (Fig. 6-6, *step 4*). Use the tracheal hook to stabilize the larynx and keep it in place throughout the remainder of the procedure.

With the dominant hand, place the tips of the Trousseau dilator into the opening in the membrane with the *spreading action oriented initially in the longitudinal or vertical plane* so that the handle is facing horizontal or perpendicular to the direction of the neck (Fig. 6-6, *step 5*). This instrument works opposite that of most ordinary instruments, such as hemostats. Squeezing the handles opens rather than closes the blades. This can be confusing the first time you use this instrument, and it is worth practicing before you need it in an emergency. If this instrument is not available in an emergency, Mayo scissors, a hemostat, or even the blunt end of a scalpel handle can be used to dilate the incision in the cricothyroid membrane.[41]

Dilate the incision vertically with the Trousseau dilator. Hold the handles of the Trousseau dilator with the nondominant hand and *rotate the handle 90 degrees until the handle is vertical or parallel to the neck* (Fig. 6-6, *step 6*). Perform this rotation because if the dilator is still horizontal, the blades of the dilator prevent passage of the tracheostomy tube into the trachea. Prepare the tracheostomy tube by testing the balloon, removing the inner cannula, and inserting the solid white obturator. While holding the dilator with the nondominant hand, take the tube in the dominant hand and *insert it between the blades of the dilator* until the flanges rest against the skin of the neck (Fig. 6-6, *step 7*). Keep the thumb on the obturator throughout the procedure. Carefully remove the Trousseau

dilator (Fig. 6-6, *step 8*). Remove the obturator and insert the inner cannula. Inflate the balloon (Fig. 6-6, *step 9*). Remove the tracheal hook while being especially careful to not puncture the cuff.[42,43]

If a tracheostomy tube is not available or if there is difficulty placing the tracheostomy tube into the opening in the cricothyroid membrane, try using a 6-0 cuffed ET tube cut to a shorter length. The ID/OD ratios of tracheostomy tubes are comparable to those of ET tubes. Use of a gum elastic bougie may facilitate and even hasten placement of an ET tube through the cricothyroid membrane into the trachea.[44] The advantage of using the bougie is that you can get immediate confirmation that the device is inside the trachea because of the "washboard" vibration that the curved tip makes as it contacts the tracheal rings.[45] Modify the ET tube by cutting the distal end and replacing the adapter to the cut end (Fig. 6-8). Be careful to not cut the pilot balloon or inflation port. If the ET tube is shortened, it is less likely to kink once it is attached to a ventilator. Advance the ET tube only about 5 cm from the tip to avoid main stem intubation. Keep in mind that standard ET tubes do not have centimeter markings at the distal end. Inserting the ET tube so that the distal cuff is about 2 cm beyond the cricothyroid membrane usually ensures proper placement.

Confirm proper placement in the same manner as with ET tube placement: end-tidal CO_2, bilateral chest movement, and breath sounds. Secure the tracheostomy tube with a circumferential tie around the neck or with sutures (Fig. 6-6, *step 10*). Order a postprocedure portable chest radiograph.

Rapid Four-Step Technique (Brofeldt)

Brofeldt and colleagues[46] developed a rapid four-step technique (RFST) to decrease the amount of time required to establish an airway and reduce complications of hypoxia. It combines aspects of traditional cricothyroidotomy and ET intubation. For right hand–dominant operators, stand at the bedside to the patient's left. Palpate the depression over the cricothyroid membrane with the nondominant hand (Fig. 6-9, *step 1*). With the dominant hand, make a single horizontal stab incision with a No. 20 scalpel blade approximately 1.5 cm in length through the skin, subcutaneous tissue, and

SURGICAL CRICOTHYROTOMY: RAPID FOUR-STEP TECHNIQUE

1

If possible, extend the neck to better expose the trachea. Palpate the depression over the cricothyroid membrane with your nondominant hand.

2

Make a 1.5-cm single horizontal stab incision through the skin, subcutaneous tissue, and cricothyroid membrane.

3

Using the scalpel blade as a guide, pick up the cricoid cartilage with the tracheal hook and provide traction in the caudal direction to stabilize the trachea.

4

Place a No. 4 cuffed tracheostomy tube or a 6.0 cuffed endotracheal tube through the opening.

Figure 6-9 Surgical cricothyrotomy: rapid four-step technique. Extension of the neck (if clinically feasible) facilitates the procedure. (*Redrawn from Brofeldt BT, Panacek EA, Richards JR. An easy cricothyrotomy approach: the Rapid Four Step Technique.* Acad Emerg Med. *1996;3:1060.*)

cricothyroid membrane (Fig. 6-9, *step 2*). With the scalpel blade as a guide, pick up the cricoid cartilage with the tracheal hook and provide traction in the caudal direction to stabilize the trachea (Fig. 6-9, *step 3*). Place a No. 4 cuffed tracheostomy tube or a 6-0 cuffed ET tube through the opening (Fig. 6-9, *step 4*).

Because this technique omits dilating the stoma with the Trousseau dilator, it may be more difficult to pass a tracheostomy tube. A gum elastic bougie, using the Seldinger technique, may assist in this step.[46]

Bair and colleagues[47] modified this technique further by introducing a new device called a "Bair Claw" to replace the tracheal hook. The technique is similar to the four-step method except for positioning the operator at the head of the bed instead of the patient's side and the use of a double-hook device rather than a single hook. By replacing the single hook with the double hook, they found a decrease in the incidence of cricoid ring fractures in cadavers (Fig. 6-10).

Melker Percutaneous Cricothyrotomy Technique

The Melker Cricothyrotomy Kit (Cook Critical Care, Bloomington, IN) is a prepackaged commercial kit that uses the Seldinger technique to place a tracheostomy tube over a

Figure 6-10 Bair Claw.

guidewire. The kit comes supplied with a 6-mL syringe, an 18-gauge needle with an overlying tetrafluoroethylene (TFE) catheter (the TFE catheter is not included in some kits), a guidewire, a tapered dilator, and a Melker airway catheter in lieu of a tracheostomy tube. Similar to retrograde intubation or needle cricothyrotomy with PTLV, the cricothyroid membrane must be easy to identify because no initial skin incision will be made. Anatomic distortion will make locating the cricothyroid membrane with a needle more difficult.

Preparation for this technique is similar to that for the other techniques. Palpate the cricothyroid membrane with

MELKER PERCUTANEOUS CRICOTHYROTOMY

1

Palpate the cricothyroid membrane and advance the needle at a 45° angle in a caudal direction. Aspirate on the saline-filled syringe as you advance; air bubbles will enter the syringe when the trachea is entered.

2

Advance the catheter over the needle and then remove the needle. Thread the guidewire through the catheter into the trachea. Once the guidewire is in place, remove the catheter.

3

Make a small incision at the point of guidewire entry to facilitate passage of the dilator and airway catheter.

4

Place the dilator into the airway catheter and thread them over the wire as a unit until it is flush with the skin. Remove the guidewire and dilator, confirm placement, and secure.

Figure 6-11 Melker percutaneous cricothyrotomy. As with other cricothyrotomy techniques, extension of the neck (if clinically feasible) exposes the trachea and facilitates the procedure.

the nondominant hand. With the dominant hand, attach the needle to the syringe and insert it through the cricothyroid membrane pointing caudally at a 45-degree angle relative to the skin surface (Fig. 6-11, *step 1*). Be careful to not advance the needle too far because this may result in perforation of the posterior aspect of the trachea. To help recognize when the trachea has been entered, place a small amount of saline in the syringe before the procedure. Apply gentle negative pressure while advancing the syringe. When the membrane is pierced and the trachea is entered, air will be aspirated into the syringe and air bubbles will appear in the saline.

When the needle is in the trachea, pull the syringe and needle back and advance the flexible TFE catheter through the distal end of the trachea to its hub. If the needle does not have an overlying catheter, leave the needle in place and remove the syringe. Thread the guidewire through the needle or the catheter (Fig 6-11, *step 2*). Once the guidewire is placed securely in the trachea, remove the needle or catheter. With a disposable No. 15 scalpel, make a small incision in the skin at the point of guidewire entry to facilitate passage of the dilator and airway catheter (Fig. 6-11, *step 3*).

Place the gray-tipped dilator into the airway catheter and thread it over the wire as one unit (Fig. 6-11, *step 4*). Once it is through the skin and into the trachea, advance the airway catheter to its hub until it is flush against the neck. Remove the guidewire and dilator. Confirm placement in the trachea by standard methods. Secure the kit in place with "trach tape."

Melker kits on the market differ with respect to airway catheter ID and whether the airway catheter is cuffed. Some kits do not contain a needle with an overlying catheter.[48]

Complications

Surgical cricothyrotomy is performed infrequently and usually under circumstances that are inherently chaotic. These patients often have confounding medical issues, as well as high morbidity and mortality rates. Evaluation of short- and long-term complications in this population is also difficult.[49]

Regardless of which technique is used, surgical cricothyrotomy has been studied to assess the periprocedure and short-term complications that occur with significant frequency. Acute complication rates have been reported to be between 8.7%[50] and 40%.[36] The most frequent complications are uncontrollable bleeding and misplacement of the tube.[35,51] Most bleeding is from small superficial vessels that can be controlled, but significant bleeding can also occur as a result of the procedure. The cricoid arteries branch from the superior thyroid arteries and anastomose at the anterior superior aspect of the cricothyroid membrane. The laterally running superior thyroid arteries are more often damaged when the initial incision is broad and horizontal. To prevent hemorrhage from these vessels, make the initial skin incision longitudinally as in the traditional technique and maintain careful awareness of the landmarks.[52] When making the horizontal incision in the cricothyroid membrane, avoid the cricoid artery by incising the membrane at its inferior aspect. Misplacement of the tracheostomy or ET tube during cricothyrotomy is a concern, just as esophageal intubation is a concern with ET intubation. If the opening in the cricothyroid membrane is not carefully stabilized during the procedure, the tube may inadvertently be inserted into subcutaneous tissue. This complication can be recognized by the presence of subcutaneous emphysema when attempting to ventilate the patient. It is essential to recognize this immediately to prevent the development of hypoxia and obliteration of anatomic landmarks. In addition, failure to detect end-tidal CO_2 and absence of breath sounds by auscultation should alert the physician to a misplaced tube. If suspected, remove the tube and reassess the airway. A misplaced tube can pass into any location other than through the cricothyroid membrane, but the most crucial locations are those that do not enter the airway because this will lead to hypoxia and death if not recognized.

Many other occult complications have been reported less frequently or have been described in case reports, such as main stem bronchial intubation,[53] laryngotracheal injury,[54] tension pneumothorax,[55] and obstruction of the tracheostomy tube with blood or secretions.[56] Slobodkin and colleagues[57] reported one case of retrograde pharyngeal intubation (Box 6-3).

BOX 6-3 | **Complications of Surgical Cricothyrotomy**

ACUTE COMPLICATIONS

More common
  Bleeding
  Malposition of the tube
Less common

  Bronchial intubation
  Laryngotracheal injury
  Tension pneumothorax
  Obstruction of the tube

LATE COMPLICATIONS

More common
  Subjective voice changes
  Difficulty swallowing
  Infections
  Persistent shortness of breath
  Persistent stoma
Infrequent
  Subglottic or glottic stenosis

Chevalier Jackson's 1921 report[58] highlighted the concern that subglottic stenosis was a major and frequent complication of cricothyrotomy. It was later refuted by Brantigan and Grow's 1976 study,[34] which reported not only an overall complication rate of just 6.1% but also no occurrence of chronic subglottic stenosis as a long-term complication. Since the publication of this latter report, numerous other studies have corroborated their findings that chronic subglottic stenosis is an infrequent long-term complication of surgical cricothyrotomy.[59-63] Factors that increase the likelihood of development of subglottic stenosis include concurrent laryngotracheal pathology, prolonged time until decannulation, old age, and diabetes.[64,65]

Long-term complications resulting in "minor airway problems" have been reported more frequently than subglottic stenosis.[66] Of these complications, subjective voice change is the most frequently reported.[67] Other reported complications include difficulty swallowing, subjective shortness of breath, wound infections, and "noisy breathing."[68]

To decrease the morbidity and mortality associated with prolonged hypoxia and other factors inherent in an airway emergency, researchers have attempted to determine whether any of the techniques is superior with regard to complication rate and time needed to secure the airway. When comparing Brofeldt and colleagues' RFST with the traditional five-step technique, Davis and colleagues[54] found an increased incidence of cricoid ring fracture when the single hook was used for caudal traction on the cricoid cartilage and concluded that the traditional technique produced a lower complication rate. A study by Holmes and coworkers[40] in which the same two techniques were performed by inexperienced medical students and residents on human cadavers concluded that the single-hook RFST was executed significantly faster than the traditional technique. They noted that there were more complications with the RFST but that the difference in complication rates failed to reach statistical significance. Davis and colleagues[69] revisited this comparison in a later study and replaced the single hook in the RFST with the double-hooked Bair Claw. The revised study showed that the airway could be secured faster with the RFST and that the complication rate was comparable; they also observed that the Bair Claw did not cause any fractures of the cricoid cartilage. Bair and colleagues' retrospective report[70] of ED cricothyrotomy showed a lower complication rate with the RFST than with the traditional technique.

Consensus cannot be drawn from the literature comparing the traditional method with the percutaneous Seldinger (Melker kit) method. Some studies show no difference in time to ventilation or complication rate when the traditional technique is compared with the Seldinger technique.[71] Some studies report that the surgical method is faster than the Seldinger method,[72-76] whereas others conclude the opposite.[77,78]

Many complications of cricothyrotomy are relatively minor in comparison to those caused by prolonged hypoxia. Be aware of these potential complications and prepare for them, but do not delay performing the procedure out of fear of them. Reduce complication rates by maintaining a sterile field and being familiar with the techniques and anatomy.

When deciding which surgical cricothyrotomy technique to use, consider the advantages and disadvantages of each technique, the clinical scenario, availability of equipment, and comfort and familiarity with each individual technique.

Success Rates

Success rates for first-attempt ET intubation in the ED are quite high (90% success for all ED intubators, including residents; 98% success rate if an attending), with the "rescue" cricothyrotomy rate reported to be just 0.7% according to the National Emergency Airway Registry.[3] A study including more than 6000 trauma patients reported a 0.3% cricothyrotomy rate in those requiring airway management within the first hour after arrival.[79] In pediatric patients, the success rate with the first attempt for all ED intubators is slightly less at 85%, with rescue cricothyrotomy performed less than 1% of the time (1 of 156 patients).[80] As an overview, few emergency physicians have the opportunity to gain extensive experience with surgical airways, and no standards of care have been developed that define the exact role of cricothyrotomy in clinical practice. In reality, it is difficult to successfully perform an emergency surgical airway, and even with proper training and standard experience, not all attempts with this technically difficult procedure will be successful. Although the reported success rate for cricothyrotomy has been quite high (89% to 100%) in most studies,* one study found only a 62.5% success rate.[82] In a community hospital setting, the rather optimistic success rate reported from trauma centers probably cannot be duplicated. In one ED study, the incidence of failed cricothyrotomy (e.g., tube misplacement into the pretracheal space or failed attempts) was 3.6%,[70] with earlier ED studies being in the 7.9% to 10% range.[35,36] In the prehospital setting, the reported failure rates are 6% to 12% for paramedics,[24,49,81] 0% for physicians,[60] and 0% to 38% for air transport medics.[82,83] In a cadaver model, the first-time performance of cricothyrotomy by intensive care unit clinicians, versus standard surgical cricothyrotomy with the Seldinger technique, resulted in successful tracheal placement in only 70% with the standard technique and 60% with the Seldinger technique.[71] In an animal model, paramedics had a 90.9% success rate with a percutaneous technique and a 100% success rate with the open surgical technique.[73]

*References 24, 35, 36, 49, 56, 60, 70, 81.

Percutaneous Translaryngeal Ventilation

Indications

Similar to surgical cricothyrotomy

Failed attempts at endotracheal intubation with an inability to bag-mask ventilate to an oxygen saturation >90%

Airway obstruction above the level of the cricothyroid membrane

Preferred method of securing a crash airway in infants and children

Contraindications

Ability to secure the airway through less invasive means

Laryngeal transection or fracture

Complications

Associated with needle placement

Subcutaneous emphysema

Kinking of the catheter

Bleeding

Malposition of the catheter

Posterior tracheal wall perforation

Pneumothorax

Associated with ventilation

Barotrauma, pneumothorax, pneumomediastinum

Hypercapnia, respiratory acidosis

Equipment

For cricothyroid membrane puncture:

For attachment to bag-valve device:

- or -

3-mL syringe and 7.0 ETT adapter

Cut IV tubing and 2.5 ETT adapter

14-gauge angiocatheter

Saline-filled 5-mL syringe

For attachment to wall oxygen source:

Transtracheal jet ventilation kit

Review Box 6-2 Percutaneous translaryngeal ventilation: indications, contraindications, complications, and equipment.

PERCUTANEOUS TRANSLARYNGEAL VENTILATION

PTLV is a procedure in which oxygen is delivered through a 12- to 14-gauge catheter inserted through the cricothyroid membrane via needle cricothyrotomy. Needle cricothyrotomy does not differ greatly from the Seldinger technique variation of surgical cricothyrotomy. Administer oxygen by bag insufflation for pediatric patients younger than 5 years, but use jet ventilation in older children and adults. For jet ventilation, supply the oxygen from a high-flow source and deliver it to the percutaneous translaryngeal catheter through a relatively small-caliber tube. The method for controlling jet ventilation has evolved over recent years. The initial use of continuous oxygen flow provided adequate oxygenation but not ventilation,[84] so the technique has advanced to giving shorter bursts of oxygen followed by a longer passive exhalation to resemble a more physiologic respiratory state.

Indications and Contraindication

The indications for and contraindications to needle cricothyrotomy with PTLV are similar to those for surgical cricothyrotomy. Indications include failed attempts at ET intubation, inability to bag-mask ventilate to an oxygen saturation greater than 90%, or airway obstruction above the level of the cricothyroid membrane. Based on the operator's experience, needle cricothyrotomy may be relatively indicated over surgical cricothyrotomy in adult patients. Much of the otolaryngology literature supports the use of PTLV as a means of nonemergency ventilation during head and neck surgery because the smaller ventilation catheter provides a relatively unobstructed field in which to work.[85-87] In an emergency airway situation, needle cricothyrotomy is a successful bridge to establishing an airway via the ET route.[88] Case reports describe PTLV to be relatively indicated over the more invasive surgical cricothyrotomy when ET intubation has failed as a result of copious oropharyngeal secretions. Providing temporary ventilation through the needle catheter may allow sufficient time to clear the upper airway of secretions or obstructions and give the operator more time to establish ET intubation.[89,90]

Surgical cricothyrotomy is contraindicated in infants and young children. The contraindication arises from the fact that the cricothyroid membrane is too small to insert a tracheostomy tube and there is a significant risk for injury to surrounding structures. Therefore, needle cricothyrotomy is the preferred method of securing the airway in crash airway situations in infants and young children.[91]

An absolute contraindication to needle cricothyrotomy is the ability to secure the airway without difficulty through less invasive means.[92] Similar to surgical cricothyrotomy, needle cricothyrotomy is contraindicated in cases of laryngotracheal transection or fracture because the airway needs to be established below this level.[31] It has been suggested that in cases of complete upper airway obstruction, needle cricothyrotomy is relatively contraindicated in comparison to surgical cricothyrotomy. This concern, which is debatable, is due to the fact that the PTLV catheter theoretically does not permit adequate expiration volumes and results in hypercapnia and barotrauma.[93]

Equipment

The essential material needed for PTLV includes a needle with an overlying catheter, oxygen tubing, an oxygen source

Figure 6-12 ENK oxygen flow modulator set available as separate kit. *(Courtesy of Cook Critical Care, Bloomington, IN.)*

with a means of regulating the pressure, and a means to connect them together.

Commercial kits are available, but a standard 12- or 14-gauge Angiocath attached to a 3- or 5-mL syringe can be used to make the puncture through the cricothyroid membrane. The catheter can be left in place to serve as the conduit for oxygen delivery. The larger the diameter of the catheter, the greater the oxygen flow, depending on the method of oxygen delivery.[94] Commercial catheters such as wire-coiled nonkinking catheters and fenestrated catheters are available as part of prearranged kits (Fig. 6-12). Larger-caliber, 3.0- to 4.0-mm-ID percutaneous tracheal catheter devices are also available.

There are two different basic means and therefore armories of equipment to choose from to deliver oxygen through the transtracheal catheter. One method uses a standard ventilation bag to supply oxygen through the needle. This requires the constant effort of manual bag insufflation as long as the patient is being oxygenated and ventilated. Attach the bag to the adapter of a 7.0-mm ET tube and insert it into the back of a plungerless 3-mL syringe connected to the translaryngeal catheter (Fig. 6-13). Alternatively, attach the bag directly to the catheter with the adapter of a 3.5-mm pediatric ET tube.[95] An inherent problem with this setup is the rigidity of the system. Although the translaryngeal catheter itself is flexible, there is no flexibility from the hub of the catheter to the bag. Thus, slight movements of the bag relative to the patient may cause dislodgment of the catheter. To ameliorate this obstacle, connect standard intravenous infusion tubing directly to the translaryngeal catheter and attach the distal cut end of a 2.5-mm ET tube to the bag.

In an alternative method, supply oxygen from a standard 50-psi wall source. Connect the high-pressure oxygen tubing to the wall source. Then connect the oxygen tubing to a manual on/off valve that is connected to the hub of the catheter. The on/off valve controls the inspiratory-to-expiratory ratio. This valve can be a separate component that is pushed down and released, the third arm of a three-way stopcock open to the atmosphere (Fig. 6-14), or holes placed at the end of the oxygen tubing. A pressure gauge connected to a hand-triggered jet injector may also be used to control the amount of air pressure reaching the catheter[96] (Fig. 6-15). Commercial kits are available that contain prepackaged systems already assembled. Otherwise, assemble the apparatus in the ED. In

Figure 6-13 Homemade ventilation setup for transtracheal catheter ventilation using a ventilation bag, a standard endotracheal tube adapter, a 3-mL syringe, and a 14-gauge angiocatheter. *ETT,* endotracheal tube; *IV,* intravenous.

Figure 6-14 Three-way stopcock connecting the oxygen tubing to the hub of the catheter with the third arm open to the atmosphere.

an emergency situation, it is unlikely that one would be able to assemble an apparatus for PTLV from individual components in a timely manner. If a prepackaged PTLV kit is not available, prepare the appropriate components from the ED ahead of time and place them with other airway supplies for easy access.

Assemble additional material such as antiseptic preparation solution, sterile drapes, sterile gauze, and suture material or trach tape in the kit.

Procedure

As with the surgical cricothyrotomy technique, place the patient in the supine position with the neck exposed. Prepare the skin of the anterior aspect of the neck. Wear appropriate protective equipment, including sterile gloves, gown, protective eyewear, and a face shield. Hyperextend the patient's neck unless a suspected cervical spine injury prohibits it. Infiltrate the skin with local anesthetic.

Similar to the needle insertion technique used for guidewire-assisted surgical cricothyrotomy, locate the cricothyroid membrane with the nondominant hand. Locate the thyroid cartilage and cricoid cartilage and palpate the cricothyroid membrane in the depression between the two while keeping in mind that this depression will be proportionately smaller in children (Fig. 6-16, *step 1*).

Attach a 12- to 14-gauge Angiocath to a 3- or 5-mL syringe filled with 1 to 2 mL of saline or lidocaine. Once the cricothyroid membrane has been located, insert the catheter through the overlying skin, subcutaneous tissue, and membrane directed at a 30- to 45-degree angle caudally (Fig. 6-16,

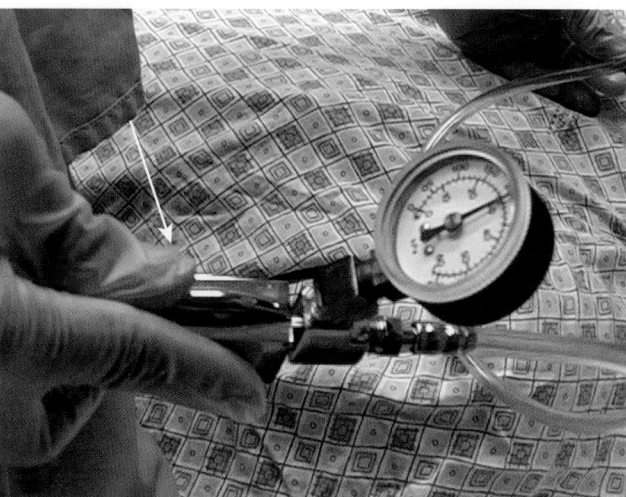

Figure 6-15 Hand-triggered jet injector. Depressing the lever with the thumb (*arrow*) delivers oxygen to the patient.

step 2). While doing so, aspirate gently with the syringe. The cricothyroid membrane has been pierced and the airway entered when air bubbles are seen in the fluid or there is an increase in the ease of air aspiration (Fig. 6-16, *step 3*). Once through the membrane, hold the needle in place, advance the catheter to the hub, and then remove the needle (Fig 6-16, *steps 4 and 5*). Hold the catheter by hand until the oxygen supply is connected and appropriate placement is confirmed (Fig. 6-16, *step 6*). Make sure that the hub of the catheter is flush against the skin to avoid an air leak and then secure it with a circumferential tie around the neck. To prevent the

PERCUTANEOUS TRANSLARYNGEAL VENTILATION

1

Hyperextend the patient's neck if possible. Locate the cricothyroid membrane with your nondominant hand.

2

Attach a 14-gauge angiocatheter to a saline-filled syringe. Insert the needle through the skin, subcutaneous tissue, and membrane directed at a 30° to 45° angle caudally.

3

Air bubbles

Aspirate the syringe as you advance the needle; air bubbles will be seen in the syringe when the trachea is entered.

4

Once the trachea is entered, advance the catheter over the needle until the hub is flush with the skin.

5

Remove the needle.

6

Attach the oxygen supply and begin to ventilate the patient.

Figure 6-16 Percutaneous translaryngeal ventilation.

tube from being dislodged, keep one hand on the hub of the catheter until the entire procedure is completed and the airway is secured.

Oxygen can be supplied to the catheter through several different conduits. With the resuscitation bag setup, manually ventilate the lungs through the catheter by squeezing and releasing the bag. When coupled with a 14-gauge Angiocath, ventilation with a resuscitation bag produces low maximal tidal volumes, approximately 100 mL per 1 second of inspiratory time in one study.[97] Children, especially those younger

than 5 years, have small total lung capacities and need smaller tidal volumes. In these cases, use the bag instead of the jet ventilator. To use this setup, control the volume of air inspired and adjust it breath by breath based on chest wall motion and pulse oximetry. This method is not appropriate for adults because the operator cannot provide adequate tidal volumes and allow enough time for exhalation.[98,99]

If using high-flow oxygen supplied from a wall source, attach the oxygen tubing to the wall source and secure the distal end of the tubing apparatus to the hub of the translaryngeal catheter. The flow rate recommended for children is 1 L/min per year of age, with titration upward in increments of 1 L/min based on chest wall movement.[100] Most wall-mounted oxygen flowmeters have a maximum flow rate marked at 15 L/min. Pressures generated at this flow rate have been shown to be inadequate to sustain ventilation in adults.[101,102] To provide the additional pressure necessary to ventilate an adult, *open the oxygen flowmeter to full output.*[103] Ventilate the patient by alternating between allowing and inhibiting airflow through the catheter. This is done by occluding and then releasing the hole or holes if using a stopcock or the ENK oxygen flow modulator or by pushing and releasing a trigger if using this type of modulator. Watch for chest wall rise and fall, and make sure to allow enough time for exhalation before the next cycle. A pressure gauge, if attached, can help guide inspiration time.

Complications

Complications reported with needle cricothyrotomy are similar to those associated with surgical cricothyrotomy: bleeding, misplacement of the catheter, subcutaneous emphysema, and pneumothorax.[104,105] Complications more specific to needle cricothyrotomy include catheter kinking[106] and perforation of the posterior aspect of the trachea.[107]

One would assume that a translaryngeally placed catheter would not afford any airway protection against aspiration because the diameter of the catheter is not nearly large enough to occlude the lumen of the trachea. A few studies, though, have shown a decreased rate of aspiration in dogs that were ventilated with PTLV versus control animals who were not ventilated, thus suggesting some airway protection with this mode of ventilation.[108,109]

The potential complications more specific to PTLV than to ventilation through a tracheostomy tube stem from the idea that especially in cases of complete upper airway obstruction, egress of inspired gas is limited through the relatively small translaryngeal catheter. It has been reported that PTLV inevitably causes retention of CO_2 in adults. This leads to poor ventilation despite adequate oxygenation. This assumption may be a remnant of earlier oxygenation techniques in which continuous low-flow "apneic oxygenation" was used without ventilation.[110] Many animal studies have shown that adequate ventilation, normal blood pH, and normal arterial CO_2 partial pressure can be maintained with PTLV for 30 or even 60 minutes.[111-116] Factors that seem to improve ventilation are increased expiratory time[117] and a high-flow oxygen source.[118] Even with partial or nearly complete oropharyngeal obstruction, adequate ventilation has been achieved.[119,120] Unfortunately, none of these studies looked at ventilation for extended periods. Barotrauma is a significant risk associated with PTLV and occurs when upper airway obstruction is preventing air from being exhaled. This causes an increase in lung volume and pressure and leads to lung injury.[122,123] Lenfant and colleagues[124] found that use of a lower respiratory rate and the ENK oxygen flow modulator versus the Manujet

---

BOX 6-4   Complications of Percutaneous Translaryngeal Jet Ventilation

COMPLICATIONS ASSOCIATED WITH NEEDLE PLACEMENT

Subcutaneous emphysema
Kinking of the catheter
Bleeding
Malposition of the catheter
Posterior tracheal wall perforation
Pneumothorax

COMPLICATIONS ASSOCIATED WITH VENTILATION

Barotrauma (more common with complete upper airway obstruction)
Pneumothorax
Pneumomediastinum
Hypercapnia, respiratory acidosis

---

decreases pulmonary pressure, which theoretically reduces the likelihood of barotrauma. The ENK oxygen flow modulator may also be superior to a three-way stopcock for similar reasons.[125] Use of a bidirectional valve or an expiratory ventilation assistance ejector device has been shown to improve ventilation dynamics and decrease the complications associated with PTLV in patients with complete upper airway obstruction[126,127] (Box 6-4).

CONCLUSION

The majority of crash airway scenarios are controlled successfully with ET intubation. The development of airway aids such as the gum elastic bougie, laryngeal mask airway, and fiberscopic laryngoscope has obviated the need to convert efforts to an invasive surgical technique. Situations arise when an airway cannot be secured with one of these aids or the patient cannot be ventilated via bag-mask-valve ventilation, and then a surgical approach is indicated.

Researchers have attempted to delineate which method of gaining emergency airway access is superior by comparing all techniques across the spectrum from traditional surgical cricothyrotomy to needle cricothyrotomy to commercially available kits such as the QuickTrack. Given the variety of equipment and techniques to choose from and the advantages and disadvantages reported about each throughout the literature, it would be difficult for an inexperienced physician to know which to choose in a critical situation. Aside from being familiar with the equipment available in the ED, research shows that overall success rates increase if physicians are trained in simulated situations before an actual airway emergency.[126,127]

References are available at www.expertconsult.com

CHAPTER 7

Tracheostomy Care

John C. Greenwood and Michael E. Winters

INTRODUCTION

Placement of a tracheostomy tube is a common procedure in critically ill patients. Common indications for this procedure include upper airway obstruction, head or neck trauma, and prolonged respiratory failure.[1,2] Approximately one fourth of patients in the intensive care unit (ICU) will require a tracheostomy tube for prolonged respiratory support or weaning from mechanical ventilation.[3] Advances in health care allow many patients with tracheostomies to live at home or in other relatively low-technology environments such as rehabilitation facilities and nursing homes. As a result, tracheostomy care is often provided by a variety of caregivers, including family members, home health care nurses, and patient care technicians.[4,5]

Patients with tracheostomies are seen in emergency departments (EDs) for a variety of problems related to the tracheostomy.[6] Common complaints include difficulty breathing as a result of tube obstruction, tube displacement, or equipment failure; poor oxygenation from infection or altered patient anatomy; and bleeding. In some cases, complications can be life-threatening. Emergency physicians must be knowledgeable regarding the evaluation and management of patients with tracheostomies. This chapter reviews the relevant tracheal anatomy and essential tracheostomy equipment, discusses pertinent tracheostomy care, provides a systematic approach to the evaluation and management of selected complications, and identifies high-risk patient populations.

BACKGROUND

Most tracheostomies are performed electively. For elective tracheostomies, the surgical site is between the first and second or the second and third tracheal rings. With an open, or surgical, tracheostomy, the anterior aspect of the trachea is generally left sutured to the skin until the tract matures, approximately 4 to 5 days after the procedure. In recent years, percutaneous dilational tracheostomy has become the preferred technique for many ICU patients. It can be performed at the bedside and eliminates the risks associated with transporting critically ill patients to an operating room. Postoperative complications vary and depend on the timing and insertion technique (Box 7-1). Early postoperative complications tend to arise in days to weeks. Sixteen percent to 20% of patients experience early complications, and 6% to 8% experience late complications.[7] Although elective and emergency tracheostomies are generally performed with the same technique, the complication rate associated with emergency procedures may be higher than the rate for elective tracheostomies.[8-10]

TRACHEAL ANATOMY AND PHYSIOLOGY

The lower respiratory tract begins at the vocal cords. Inferior to the vocal cords lies the cricoid cartilage, which encases the 1.5- to 2-cm subglottic space. Inferior to the cricoid cartilage is the trachea (Fig. 7-1). The typical adult trachea is 10 to 12 cm in length. The anterior and lateral walls of the trachea are supported by 18 to 22 incomplete cartilaginous rings. A fibromuscular sheet lying anterior to the esophagus completes the posterior wall. The interior diameter of the adult trachea is 12 to 25 mm, and it is lined with mucosa covered by respiratory epithelium.[8] Blood is supplied to the trachea by branches of the inferior thyroid, innominate (brachiocephalic), bronchial, and subclavian arteries. Critically, the innominate artery (IA) lies in close proximity to the tracheostomy stoma. From its origin at the aortic arch, the IA courses between the sternum and the anterior aspect of the trachea and veers right at the sternomanubrial joint. The location of the IA is important because erosion of the anterior tracheal wall can lead to life-threatening bleeding. The recurrent laryngeal nerve innervates the intrinsic laryngeal muscles and mucosa below the vocal cords. Efferent vagal fibers stimulate bronchoconstriction, mucosal secretions, and vasodilation. Efferent sympathetic fibers of the pulmonary plexus stimulate tracheal bronchodilation and vasoconstriction.

The upper airway, including the oropharynx and nasal passages, filters particulate matter, humidifies inspired air, and aids in the expectoration of secretions. These functions are reduced in patients with a tracheostomy.[8] Placement of a tracheostomy bypasses humidification and results in the formation of thick, dry secretions.[11] In the absence of humidification, squamous metaplasia and chronic inflammatory changes develop in the trachea.[12] Bronchoconstriction resulting in reduced airflow can occur if the inspired air temperature is below room temperature. Normal mucociliary clearance is also impaired because of the increased viscosity of respiratory secretions, which underlies chronic illness and respiratory infections, particularly with *Mycoplasma* or viral pathogens.[13]

The tracheostomy procedure weakens the anterior tracheal wall and blunts the normal cough mechanism, an important component for clearance of secretions by the trachea.[13] Normally, the epiglottis and vocal cords close to trap air in the lungs and raise intrathoracic pressure before a cough. Patients with a tracheostomy tube are generally unable to generate sufficient pressure to initiate a strong cough and facilitate airway clearance.[14] In addition to an impaired cough mechanism, immune responses are often blunted in patients with tracheostomies as the result of underlying illnesses, chronic lung disease, chemotherapy, or acquired immunosuppression.

EVALUATION OF TRACHEOSTOMY PATIENTS

Every ED patient with a tracheostomy who has a respiratory complaint or a complaint related to the tracheostomy should be seen and evaluated promptly. Begin the primary assessment with a review of the patient's vital signs and evaluation of the airway. Examine the tracheostomy and consider dislodgement, obstruction, and fracture of the tube. Next assess the patient's respiratory status. If the patient is receiving mechanical ventilation on arrival and is in acute distress, remove the patient from the ventilator and replace it with manual

EARLY COMPLICATIONS (DAYS TO WEEKS)

Hemorrhage—postoperative
Tube dislodgment or obstruction
Subcutaneous emphysema
Soft tissue infection
Pneumothorax, pneumomediastinum

LATE COMPLICATIONS (>3 WEEKS)

Tracheal stenosis or malacia (granulation tissue)
Tube dislodgment or obstruction
Equipment failure
Tracheoinnominate artery fistula
Tracheoesophageal fistula
Infection—pneumonia, aspiration

Figure 7-2 Suggested equipment for tracheostomy care.

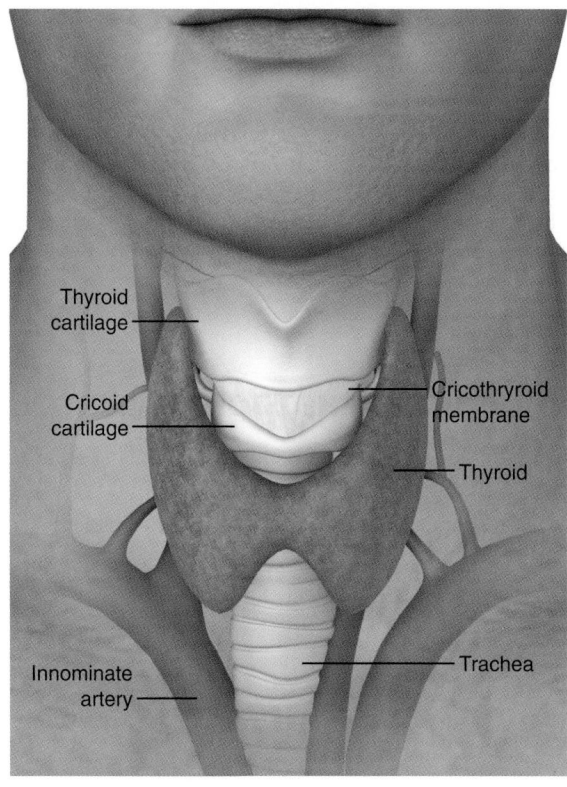

Figure 7-1 Tracheal anatomy.

ventilation with a bag-valve-mask device. Initiate continuous cardiac monitoring, pulse oximetry, and capnography, if available, in all tracheostomy patients in respiratory distress.

In the history of the present illness, include the indications for placement of a tracheostomy, the length of time from placement to arrival at the ED, and any previous complications. Discuss any planned or existing voice prosthesis, previous bleeding complications or strictures, and whether a permanent tracheostomy or decannulation of the tracheostomy is anticipated. Ask whether there have been any recent changes in ventilator settings or tracheostomy care, including increased oxygen use, increased suctioning, equipment failure, or changes in equipment.

After the primary assessment and focused history, perform a thorough physical examination to differentiate between

tracheostomy complications and other causes of the patient's respiratory complaint. The differential diagnosis may include pneumonia, exacerbation of chronic obstructive pulmonary disease, congestive heart failure, pulmonary embolism, pneumothorax, and acute coronary syndrome. During the secondary evaluation, evaluate the patient's stoma for signs of bleeding, infection, or skin breakdown. Make a note of the specific type and model of equipment used in the event that a replacement tube is needed.

GENERAL EQUIPMENT FOR TRACHEOSTOMY PATIENTS

Before performing any procedure on the tracheostomy tube, it is important that the emergency physician ensure that essential equipment is readily available at the patient's bedside. These items are shown in Figure 7-2. Adequate preparation is crucial in preventing a poor outcome should complications arise. Most of this equipment can be placed in a designated airway box that can easily be accessed within the room or ED.

ROUTINE TRACHEOSTOMY MAINTENANCE

Routine tracheostomy maintenance involves (1) regular cleaning of the tube, (2) frequent stomal care, and (3) periodic monitoring of cuff pressure. There are many different types of tracheostomy tubes, but the focus of this section is on the most common types of tracheostomy tubes, those with a removable inner cannula (Fig. 7-3*A*). Regular cleaning of the tracheostomy tube and inner cannula can prevent the accumulation of dried secretions. *Lack of cleaning and maintenance of the inner cannula is the primary cause of tube obstruction* (Fig. 7-3*B*). Under normal circumstances the inner cannula should be in place. It sits snugly within the tracheostomy tube and can easily be removed without disturbing the tube itself. *The inner cannula should be cleaned daily.* Soak it in a half-strength hydrogen peroxide solution for 10 to 15 minutes and remove encrustations with a soft-bristle tracheostomy brush.[15] Clean dried debris and blood from the tracheostomy tube flanges as well. To prevent damage to the tracheal mucosa, rinse all

Figure 7-3 Shiley tracheostomy tube. **A,** The obturator is placed inside the tube (while the inner cannula is removed) to facilitate insertion through the stoma. The inner cannula must be inserted into the tube to ventilate the patient. **B,** The inner cannula should always be in place and removed only for daily cleaning. An inner cannula clogged with mucus and debris is the most common cause of respiratory distress in patients in the emergency department.

airway equipment with sterile saline before reinsertion.[16] Important stomal wound care includes changing contaminated tube ties, cleaning the tube flanges regularly, and using pre-cut tracheostomy gauze. Loose fibers from hand-cut gauze may induce inflammatory changes at the stomal site.[14]

The tracheostomy cuff provides a tight seal to allow positive pressure ventilation and prevent aspiration. Cuff pressure should ideally be maintained below 25 mm Hg.[16] Overinflation is common and can cause disastrous injury to the tracheal wall and mucosa and lead to tracheomalacia, tracheal stenosis, or the development of a fistula between surrounding anatomic structures.[17] It is a good practice to regularly check and document cuff pressure with a handheld pressure manometer to document inflation volumes. If an air leak occurs at the maximum recommended cuff pressure, the tube may have become dislodged, which requires further evaluation.

It is essential that adequate air humidification be provided to patients with a tracheostomy. Inadequate humidification can result in obstruction of the tube from thick secretions, sputum retention, keratinization or ulceration of the tra-

Figure 7-4 Close-up of a Shiley tracheostomy tube. Note that only the *inner* cannula has a 15-mm adapter that will accept an Ambu bag or a ventilator; the *outer* cannula will not. *The inner cannula MUST be in place to ventilate the patient.*

cheal mucosa, and impaired gas exchange as a result of lung atelectasis. Ambulatory patients and those who require low-flow oxygen can be fitted with a heat-moisture exchanger that attaches to the external opening of the tracheostomy tube. Patients receiving long-term ventilation or high-flow oxygen require regular saline nebulizer treatments delivered by an in-line humidification system.

VENTILATING TRACHEOSTOMY PATIENTS

To properly ventilate ED patients with a tracheostomy, it is important to determine the make, model, and type of tube (Fig. 7-4). For proper ventilation, a 15-mm adapter must be present, either on the tube itself or on the end of an inner cannula that has an inflatable cuff. The inner cannula adapter will accept an Ambu bag or ventilator tubing, and the cuff will allow positive pressure ventilation. If the patient requires manual or mechanical ventilation and the tracheostomy tube is not suitable for ventilatory support, immediately replace it with a 6-0 cuffed endotracheal (ET) tube for ventilation.

TRACHEAL SUCTIONING

Tracheal suctioning is required to remove secretions or aspirated material from the upper airway in patients whose cough is impaired or in whom an artificial airway is in place. Tracheal suctioning can be performed through an ET tube, a tracheostomy tube, a minitracheostomy placed in the cricothyroid membrane, or the nasopharynx. The indications, equipment, procedure, and complications are similar for each technique.

Indications

The primary indications for tracheal suctioning are to remove secretions, enhance oxygenation, or obtain samples of lower respiratory tract secretions for diagnostic tests. In the ED, tracheal suctioning should be performed to enhance oxygenation in any tracheostomy patient in respiratory distress. In

Tracheostomy Suctioning

Indications

Removal of excess secretions
Worsening dyspnea
Decreased oxygenation in the presence of
  rales, rhonchi, or tubular breath sounds
Arterial oxygen desaturation
Respiratory distress

Contraindications

Absolute
  None
Relative
  Severe bronchospasm
  Persistently elevated intracranial pressure

Complications

Hypoxemia   Atelectasis
Increased intracranial pressure   Mucosal injury
Dysrhythmias   Bleeding
Patient agitation   Infection/tracheitis

Equipment

Review Box 7-1 Tracheal suctioning: indications, contraindications, complications, and equipment.

addition, tracheal suctioning should be performed when the patient has coarse rales, rhonchi, or tubular breath sounds; acute or worsening dyspnea; or arterial oxygen desaturation. It is important to emphasize that tracheal suctioning should be performed only when it is clinically indicated; frequent, routine suctioning is not recommended.[18,19]

There are no absolute contraindications to tracheal suctioning. Relative contraindications include severe bronchospasm, which may worsen with suctioning, and persistently elevated intracranial pressure (ICP), which is exacerbated by suctioning.[20] Bronchodilators, sedatives, and paralytics may alleviate these symptoms. Tracheal suctioning should be undertaken with caution in patients with cardiovascular instability because of an increased risk for associated dysrhythmias.[21]

Equipment

A suction catheter and vacuum system, open or closed, is required to perform tracheal suctioning (Fig. 7-5). It is recommended that the diameter of the suction catheter be no larger than half the inner diameter of the tracheostomy tube.[22,23] The size of the suction catheter in French gauge (Fg) can be calculated as follows:

$$\text{Size (Fr)} = 2 \times (\text{Size of the tracheostomy tube} - 2)$$

For example, a 7-0 tracheostomy tube will require a 10-Fg suction catheter because $2 \times (7 - 2) = 10$ Fg. If the catheter is too small, it will not remove excess secretions adequately. If the catheter is too large, it can obstruct airflow during insertion and cause alveolar collapse with resultant hypoxemia.

In adults, the suction catheter should be inserted only 10 to 15 cm, depending on the length of the tracheostomy tube.

Figure 7-5 Closed-system suction catheter.

The goal of suctioning is to remove secretions only from the proximal airways. *Shallow suctioning* occurs when the catheter is placed just beyond the hub of the tracheostomy tube to remove proximal secretions. *Premeasured suctioning* occurs when a catheter is inserted such that the distal side ports are beyond the caudal end of the tracheostomy tube. *Deep suctioning* occurs when the suction catheter is advanced until resistance is met. It is used for clearing excess secretions in the lower airways.[19] Deep suctioning has not been shown to be more beneficial than shallow suctioning and should not be performed routinely because it might damage the mucosal epithelium and lead to an increase in granulation tissue.[24,25]

A number of suction catheter tips have been designed to maximize removal of secretions without causing mucosal

TRACHEAL SUCTIONING

Place the patient on a pulse oximeter, cardiac monitor, and continuous capnography (if available). Preoxygenate with 100% O_2.

Insert the suction catheter through the inner cannula in situ.

Closed-system suction catheter

Tracheostomy tube

Advance the catheter to the desired depth.

Apply suction while slowly removing the catheter; gently rotate the catheter to facilitate removal of the secretions.

Figure 7-6 Tracheal suctioning.

injury. Tips may have a single or multiple side ports proximal to the distal tip. Directional or Coude tip catheters are available for selective suctioning of the main stem bronchi.

A closed-system airway encases a suction catheter in a sterile sheath attached to ventilator tubing. This prevents the suction catheter from being contaminated by contact with the outside environment and allows tracheal suctioning to be performed without interrupting ventilatory support. The vacuum should be set to the lowest possible pressure to reduce atelectasis. Vacuum pressure should not exceed 80 mm Hg in infants or 150 mm Hg in adults.[22]

Procedure and Technique

Before tracheal suctioning, continuous pulse oximetry, cardiac monitoring, and continuous capnography, if available, should be initiated (Fig. 7-6, *step 1*). Awake and alert patients should be sitting upright with their head in a neutral position. For mechanically ventilated patients, the head of the bed should be elevated to 30 degrees to improve respiratory mechanics. Aseptic technique should be used throughout all suctioning procedures to prevent the introduction of bacteria. Backup airway equipment should be readily available (see Fig. 7-2). Preoxygenate the patient for at least 30 to 60 seconds. For

mechanically ventilated patients, increase the fraction of inspired oxygen (FIO_2) to 100%. For nonventilated patients, provide 10 to 15 L of high-flow oxygen. Humidify the air before suctioning to reduce the viscosity of respiratory secretions. Routine instillation of normal saline has not been shown to provide regular clinical benefit and is no longer recommended.[22,26]

Once the patient has been adequately preoxygenated, insert the suction catheter through the inner cannula in situ (Fig. 7-6, *step 2*). If the carina is irritated during deep suctioning, a vigorous cough reflex will be activated. After reaching the desired depth, withdraw the suction catheter 1 to 2 cm and then apply suction while slowly removing the catheter (Fig. 7-6, *steps 3 and 4*). Gently rotate the catheter as it is withdrawn to facilitate removal of secretions. The duration of suctioning should not exceed 10 to 15 seconds.[27]

Monitor the patient throughout the procedure for signs of cardiac dysrhythmia, hypoxia, or a rise in end-tidal CO_2. Immediately stop suctioning if any of these signs develop (see "Complications of Suctioning"). If marked respiratory distress is presumed to be secondary to significant tracheal obstruction, continue with expeditious suctioning to remove the obstruction (see "Obstruction and Complications from Tube Changes").

Complications of Suctioning

Complications that occur during or after suctioning are relatively common and can result in significant morbidity. Fortunately, most complications can be anticipated and simple maneuvers can reduce their incidence and severity.

Hypoxemia from suctioning may cause increased ICP, dysrhythmias, or even death. In neonates, hypoxia during suctioning may contribute to spontaneous intracerebral hemorrhage.[28] A number of factors contribute to suctioning-related hypoxia, including interruption of mechanical ventilation, aspiration of air from the respiratory tract, and suctioning-related atelectasis.[29] Use in-line suction catheters for ventilator-dependent patients to allow continuous oxygen delivery and positive pressure ventilation. Select the catheter size carefully to reduce the evacuation of airway gases during suctioning and help prevent atelectasis. Limit the duration of suctioning to 10 to 15 seconds and perform no more than three passes in succession. Measurement of arterial oxygen saturation may not be sufficient to assess hypoxia after suctioning. Oxygen consumption increases during suctioning despite insignificant changes in oxygen saturation. This increase in oxygen consumption is more prevalent in patients who possess a vigorous cough, are agitated, or resist suctioning.[30]

Dysrhythmias associated with suctioning may be caused by hypoxia, increased myocardial oxygen consumption, vagal stimulation, hypoventilation, or catecholamine release. Vagal stimulation caused by suctioning can cause bradycardia and hypotension.[31] Bradycardia in the setting of hypoxia potentiates ventricular dysrhythmias, including ventricular fibrillation. Nebulized or intravenous atropine is recommended for bradycardia and can be used as pretreatment in patients at risk for bradycardia, particularly infants. Digoxin enhances vagal activity and may potentiate the vagal stimulation of ET suctioning.[32] Sympathetic stimulation may occur as a result of hypoxia, pain, or stress of the procedure. Pain medications, anxiolytics, and preparation of the patient for the procedure may blunt the sympathetic response. Suctioning should be stopped immediately if a dysrhythmia develops.

Increases in ICP during suctioning are well documented.[33-35] ET suctioning can induce a strong cough reflex, which is thought to contribute to the increased ICP by raising intrathoracic pressure, reducing cerebral perfusion pressure, and increasing systemic blood pressure. In susceptible patients, increases in ICP can lead to devastating outcomes.[28,34,36] If there is concern that increases in ICP could harm the patient, several preventive steps should be taken before initiating ET suctioning. The most important interventions are providing adequate sedation and maximizing oxygenation.[20] Hyperventilation before and between passes of the suction catheter can transiently lower ICP by reducing systemic CO_2.[34] One minute before suctioning, hyperventilate the patient by increasing the respiratory rate to approximately 30 breaths/min. If not heavily sedated, most patients will cough vigorously when suctioned. Lidocaine can be instilled into the trachea to blunt the cough reflex, thereby preventing an increase in ICP. To anesthetize the trachea locally, instill 1.5 to 2.0 mg/kg of 2% lidocaine into the tracheal tube. After administering the medication, prepare the patient for suctioning by ensuring that sedation and oxygenation are adequate. After 10 minutes to allow the lidocaine to produce its local effect, begin tracheal suctioning. This method has been shown to prevent increases in ICP and changes in cerebral hemodynamics.[37]

Atelectasis can occur when airway gases are suctioned too rapidly. To reduce this complication, choose a suction catheter that is less than half the inner diameter of the tracheostomy tube and minimize the duration and suction pressure. Atelectasis can be minimized by using a closed suction system and providing positive end-expiratory pressure after suctioning.[38] Hyperventilation should not be performed routinely to resolve suction-related atelectasis.[29]

Mucosal injury is a common complication of tracheal suctioning. Invagination of the mucosa into the side ports of the catheter occurs during suctioning and causes the tracheal mucosa to become denuded, edematous, and predisposed to bleeding. Mucosal damage also interferes with mucociliary transport. Tracheitis can occur as a result of frequent or improperly performed suctioning.

Minitracheostomy Suctioning Procedure

The minitracheostomy ("minitrach") was designed to improve tracheal hygiene in patients with intact cough reflexes, normal ventilatory function, and vocalization. The minitrach serves as a small port solely for suctioning secretions. Commonly, a 4-mm indwelling cuffless cannula is inserted through the cricothyroid membrane into the trachea. Patients who are suctioned through a minitrach are at lower risk for gagging and aspiration because they are able to maintain laryngeal and glottic function.[39] The minitrach device is seldom used in children because they have smaller airway diameters.

The technique used to suction through a minitrach is the same as that for tracheal suctioning. The smaller port size may require that smaller catheters be used. Most patients with minitrachs are decannulated before discharge from the ICU and are rarely seen in EDs.

CHANGING A TRACHEOSTOMY TUBE

Indications

Maturation of the tracheostomy tract is generally completed by postoperative day 7.[40] Most ED patients with a tracheostomy are seen after the stomal tract has matured, so routine changes of the tracheostomy tube can be done safely in the ED.[41] Indications for exchange of the tracheostomy tube include cuff rupture or leak, leakage around the tube caused by tracheomalacia, other changes in tracheal anatomy, complete or partial tube occlusion, and conversion to an alternative tube style.[42] There are no absolute contraindications to exchanging a tracheostomy tube in the ED as long as the stomal tract has matured. Before undertaking the exchange, consider whether further tissue trauma or hemorrhage might occur as a result of it[42] or whether anatomic abnormalities could make the exchange difficult.

There is conflicting evidence on how frequently tracheostomy tubes should be changed.[43] Do not perform tube changes on a predetermined schedule, but rather as the patient's clinical condition dictates. There is some evidence that tubes left in place longer than 3 months are at higher risk for infection.[44] Most manufacturers recommend that tracheostomy tubes be changed about 30 days after placement.

Changing a Tracheostomy Tube

Indications
Complete or partial tube obstruction
Mechanical failure
    Peritubal leak
    Cuff rupture
Conversion to an alternative tube style (only with a mature
    stomal tract)

Contraindications
Absolute: None
Relative: Tracheostomy placement <7 days earlier

Complications
Hemorrhage
False passage
Obstruction
Prolonged procedure time
Tract closure
Hypoxia
Subcutaneous emphysema
Aspiration

Equipment

Red rubber catheter (optional)

Tracheostomy tube:
    Outer cannula   Obturator   Inner cannula

Lubricating jelly

10-mL syringe

Review Box 7-2 Changing a tracheostomy tube: indications, contraindications, complications, and equipment.

Table 7-1   Common Tracheostomy Tube Sizes with Dimensions

Portex Cuffed D.I.C. Tracheostomy Tubes				Shiley Tracheostomy Tubes*			
TUBE SIZE (mm) AND COLOR CODE	INTERNAL DIAMETER (mm)	OUTER DIAMETER (mm)	LENGTH (mm)	TUBE SIZE (JACKSON)	INTERNAL DIAMETER (mm)	OUTER DIAMETER (mm)	LENGTH (mm)
6.0 (orange)	6.0	8.5	64.0	4	5.0	9.4	62
7.0 (green)	7.0	9.9	70.0	6	6.4	10.8	74
8.0 (white)	8.0	11.3	73.0	8	7.6	12.2	79
9.0 (blue)	9.0	12.6	79.0	10	8.9	13.8	79
10.0 (yellow)	10.0	14.0	79.0				

Adapted from *Standards for the Care of Adult Patients with a Temporary Tracheostomy*. London: The Intensive Care Society; 2008:53.
*Shiley also offers tracheostomy tubes with both distal and proximal (relative to the cuff) extended lengths for patients with large necks or other abnormal anatomy.

Equipment

When changing a tracheostomy tube, familiarize yourself with the resources and equipment available in the ED. Keep the equipment readily available, if not at the patient's bedside. The necessary equipment is depicted in Figure 7-2.

Tracheostomy tubes may be made from metal or other synthetic material such as plastic. Plastic tubes are either polyvinyl chloride, which softens at body temperature, or silicon, which is naturally soft and unaffected by temperature. Metal tubes are constructed of silver or stainless steel and lack both a cuff and a 15-mm connector for attachment to a ventilator or Ambu bag.

Sizing

To determine the appropriate size of tube, consider the internal diameter (ID), outside diameter (OD), length, and curvature of the tube. The Chevalier Jackson sizing system indicates the length and tapering of the OD. This sizing method applies to metal tubes and most Shiley dual-cannula tracheostomy tubes. Table 7-1 lists common tracheostomy tubes and their dimensions. For dual-cannula tracheostomy tubes, the inner cannula has a 15-mm connection for a ventilator. Note that tracheostomy tubes with the same ID can have very different ODs and lengths. Consider the pretracheal distance before selecting a replacement tube of the appropriate size for obese patients (see "Special Populations").

Single-cannula tracheostomy tubes are sized by the ID of the tube at its smallest dimension. The size of the tube is usually stamped on the flange. Before changing a tube, have the appropriate size of tube at the bedside along with tubes that are one or two sizes smaller. As a rule of thumb, most women can accommodate a tube with an OD of 10 mm, and most men can accommodate a tube with an OD of 11 mm.[45] Table 7-1 lists the recommended sizes of tracheostomy tubes.

Components

Most tracheostomy tubes have three standard components: an outer cannula, an obturator, and an inner cannula (Fig. 7-3A). The outer cannula is the permanent portion of the tracheostomy tube and should not be removed unless complications arise or a tube change is needed. Attached to the outer cannula is a flange on either side with eyelets used to tether the tube to the patient's neck. The obturator is a white rounded or cone-shaped object that is used to facilitate insertion of the tube. When inserted into the outer cannula, it extends several millimeters beyond the distal end of the tube.

Tracheostomy tubes can be cuffed or uncuffed. Cuffed tracheostomy tubes are used for patients on long-term mechanical ventilation and those at risk for aspiration. Cuffed tubes also prevent loss of volume during positive pressure ventilation while preventing air leaks across the vocal cords. As a result, speech is not possible for patients with a cuffed tube. Most tubes have a high-volume, low-pressure cuff that reduces mucosal injury and the risk for tracheal erosion or stenosis.[46] Low-volume, low-pressure cuffs may be more effective in preventing aspiration.[47,48] Inflate the tracheostomy cuff and deflate it by attaching a syringe to the Luer-Lok port at the proximal end of the pilot balloon and either injecting or removing approximately 10 mL of air. Determine cuff pressure by connecting the Luer-Lok port to a handheld manometer.

Uncuffed and metal tubes are used in patients with adequate ventilatory effort who are alert and at low risk for aspiration. Depending on the size of the tracheostomy tube and how much of the tracheal diameter is filled by the tube itself, the patient may be able to speak. Air must be able to bypass the tube and be transmitted across the vocal cords. Digital occlusion of the tracheostomy tube or the use of specialized speaking valves can occlude expired air from the tracheostomy and facilitate voice production. Fenestrated tubes also allow air to be transmitted across the vocal cords. The fenestrations are generally located at the superior, posterior arch of the tube but can also be found on the inner cannula in some models.

During weaning from tracheostomy, tracheal buttons can be used to maintain patency of the stoma in patients who do not require mechanical ventilation. They can be retained permanently if decannulation is not possible. Tracheal buttons have a hollow outer cannula and a solid inner cannula and extend from the outer skin into the tracheal lumen. Tracheal buttons can become displaced into the tracheal lumen if it is not tethered correctly and may become clogged with secretions.[49] They may also have a speaking valve, such as the Passy-Muir (Passy-Muir, Inc., Irvine, CA) or the Shiley Phonate (Mallinckrodt Medical, St. Louis). These devices generally clip or twist onto the 15-mm coupling of the tracheostomy tube or inner cannula. Remove the speaking valve before changing the tracheostomy tube.

Procedure

As discussed previously, it is essential to ensure that all airway equipment is at the patient's bedside before performing the tube exchange. In addition to having airway equipment ready, place the patient on continuous pulse oximetry, cardiac monitoring, and capnography, if available, to confirm tube placement. Identify the tracheostomy tube model and determine its size. Have this size and two other tubes that are one or two sizes smaller in the event that tube replacement is difficult. Inspect all equipment for proper function, including the replacement tube cuff for leaks and the obturator for ease of insertion and removal (Fig. 7-7, *step 1*). Coat the replacement tracheostomy tube with a water-based lubricant (Fig. 7-7, *step 2*).

Place the patient in a semirecumbent position with the neck slightly extended to ensure proper alignment of the external stoma and the tracheostomy tract. Do not flex the neck because this may misalign the tissues and make tube replacement more difficult. Remove the old tracheostomy dressing and clean the stomal site. If awake, preoxygenate the patient by placing a non-rebreather oxygen mask over the tracheostomy site for 3 minutes and then suction the oropharynx. If the patient is ventilator dependent, increase the F_{IO_2} to 100% for at least 1 minute before beginning the tube exchange to ensure adequate oxygenation. If needed, provide the patient with soft restraints or anxiolytic medication to improve compliance.

The tracheostomy tube can be changed by either of two methods. If the tracheostomy tract is well matured, the tube can be exchanged with an obturator. To remove the old tracheostomy tube, first deflate the cuff completely (if present) (Fig. 7-7, *step 3*). Remove the existing tube with an "out-then-down" movement while the patient exhales (Fig. 7-7, *step 4*). Next, with the obturator in place, insert the new tube into the stoma at a 90-degree angle to the cervical axis (Fig. 7-7, *step 5*). If two experienced providers are available, one can be responsible for deflating the cuff and removing the old tube while the other inserts the new device.[50] Next, gently push the tube downward in a fluid, sweeping motion so the external flange is flush against the neck. If necessary, use a tracheal hook to hold the stoma open. Remove the solid obturator immediately, insert the hollow internal cannula, inflate the cuff, return the patient's head to the neutral position, and secure the external flange (Fig. 7-7, *steps 6 to 8*).

The second technique involves exchanging the tube with a modified Seldinger technique using a red rubber catheter, nasogastric tube, or a gum elastic bougie (Fig. 7-8).[45,51] This technique is preferable if the tracheostomy tract is not well defined or if there is concern that tube exchange could be difficult. To exchange tubes with this method, first premeasure the distance needed to extend the guidewire device beyond the distal tip of the old tracheostomy tube. Advance the guide to the premeasured distance, deflate the cuff, and remove the tube as described previously. Next, without the obturator in place, advance the new device over the guide until it is seated securely in the trachea. Remove the guide and secure the new tube. Weinmann and Bander developed a modified Seldinger technique involving the use of an airway exchange catheter to allow jet or bag ventilation into the trachea during tube exchange. This adjunct delivers intratracheal oxygen and is helpful if hypoxemia is likely to occur.[42]

Confirm proper placement of the tube within the trachea with one of several possible techniques. Traditionally, the patient is ventilated and correct tube placement confirmed by observation of equal chest rise and auscultation of bilateral breath sounds. Although both signs are important to confirm correct placement, quantitative waveform capnography is now a class I American Heart Association recommendation for confirmation of ET intubation.[52] It should be used for tracheostomy tube placement, if available. Multiple studies have shown quantitative capnography to be a highly sensitive tool for confirming correct placement of airway devices.[53,54]

CHANGING A TRACHEOSTOMY TUBE

Inspect the tube for proper function; check for a cuff leak.

Apply a water-based lubricant to the tube.

Deflate the cuff on the old tube completely.

Remove the old tube during exhalation.

Insert the new tube (with the obturator in place) into the stoma at a 90-degree angle; push the tube downward in a fluid, sweeping motion.

Remove the obturator, and insert the inner cannula.

Attach the ventilator to the tracheostomy tube.

Inflate the cuff.

Figure 7-7 Changing a tracheostomy tube. Maintain the neck in the same position (slightly extended) for removal and insertion so that the tract is not lost. If the tube is already out, and the specifics of the tract are unknown, *extending the neck to align the stoma with the tissue tract is the first best position for tube replacement.*

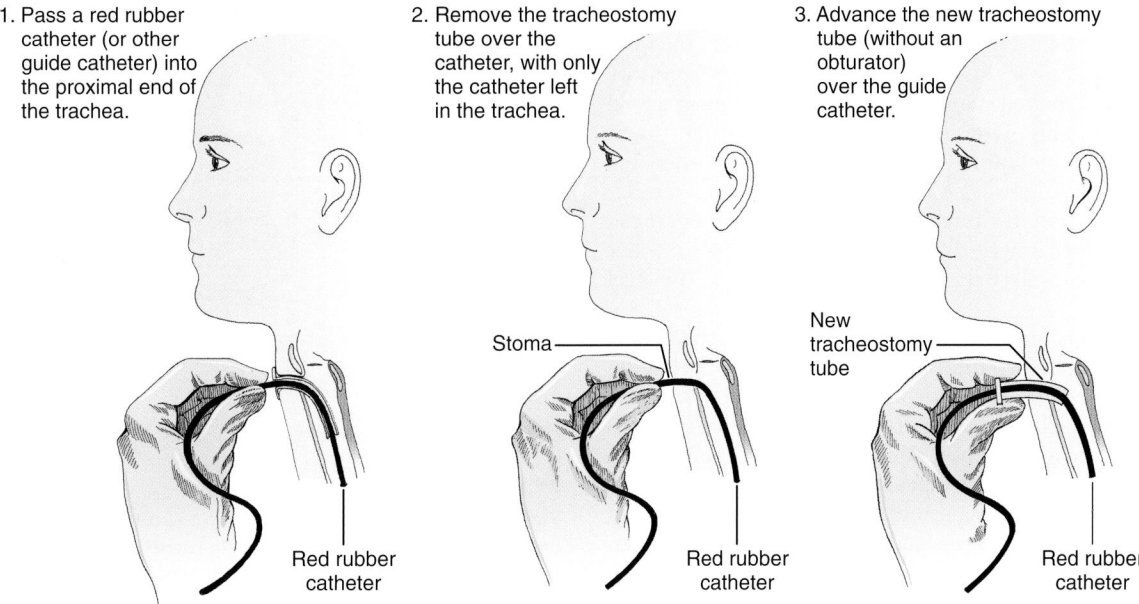

1. Pass a red rubber catheter (or other guide catheter) into the proximal end of the trachea.

2. Remove the tracheostomy tube over the catheter, with only the catheter left in the trachea.

3. Advance the new tracheostomy tube (without an obturator) over the guide catheter.

Stoma

New tracheostomy tube

Red rubber catheter

Red rubber catheter

Red rubber catheter

Figure 7-8 Changing a tracheostomy tube over a guide catheter.

Correct tube placement can also be confirmed by direct visualization of the tracheal rings with a fiberoptic scope.

COMPLICATIONS OF TRACHEOSTOMY

Complications related to tracheostomy placement are common and sometimes life-threatening. This section addresses the emergency development of late postoperative complications (occurring more than 3 weeks after the operation). Patients with immediate and early postoperative complications are usually still hospitalized and are less likely to be seen in the ED.[55] Late postoperative tracheostomy complications encountered in ED patients include obstruction, dislodgement, equipment failure, infection, anatomic disruption, and hemorrhage. Management of the patient varies depending on the type of complication that the patient is experiencing. Rapid recognition of the problem is paramount and can drastically affect the outcome.

Obstruction and Complications from Tube Changes

Obstruction of the tracheostomy tube is a common complication and can occur at the external opening of the tube, within the inner cannula, or at the distal end of the outer cannula. In one review, 30% of ED visits for respiratory distress were due to an obstructed tube.[41] Obstruction is caused most commonly by dried respiratory secretions and, less often, by blood, aspirated material, or granulation tissue. The obstructing object may act as a ball valve and allow air to enter but restricts expiration.[8] Such obstruction is easily remedied in the ED by removing the inner cannula and then cleaning and replacing it.

Preparation

First, assess the patient's airway for patency and respiratory status. Place the patient on a cardiorespiratory monitor, a pulse oximeter, and continuous capnography. Gather appropriate airway equipment at the bedside. Be sure to have a large-bore suction catheter available in case the appropriate size of catheter is inadequate. Examine the tracheostomy tube to see whether the inner cannula is obstructed or any obvious external obstruction is present.

Interventions

Administer high-flow oxygen and encourage patients who can breathe spontaneously to cough. Manually remove any obstruction seen at the external tracheal tube opening. If there is no obvious external obstruction, remove the inner cannula and suction the secretions. Inspect the inner cannula and remove any obstructing objects. If the patient's tracheostomy does not have an inner cannula, suction the tracheostomy tube to remove obstructing plugs. Thick secretions can be loosened in a *critically ill* patient by instilling normal saline into the tracheostomy tube, but this is no longer recommended for routine suctioning.[26]

If the obstruction persists, evaluate the distal tip of the tracheostomy tube. First, deflate the tracheostomy cuff and supply high-flow oxygen via face mask if the patient is breathing spontaneously or via a bag-valve-mask device if the patient is unable to breathe without assistance. If the tracheostomy cuff is inflated, you will *not* be able to provide oxygen or ventilatory support from above the tracheostomy tube. If the patient is still in respiratory distress despite these interventions, remove the outer tube and replace it. If these maneuvers are ineffective, consider more distal causes of airway obstruction, such as granulation tissue, a mass, or a clot. Be sure to have a surgical airway kit available at the patient's bedside.

Dislodgment

Displacement of the tracheal tube is a serious complication that can have a disastrous outcome if not recognized and corrected quickly. Patients at highest risk for poor outcomes from a dislodged tube are those who are obese, who have a recently inserted or changed tube, who have anatomic anomalies, and who are difficult to ventilate or were difficult to intubate in the past.[56-58] Evidence of tube dislodgment is usually obvious. Signs and symptoms include hypoxemia, agitation, respiratory distress, altered mental status, subcutaneous emphysema, and high airway pressure. Dislodgement can occur during patient transfers, when traction is placed on the tube, or when the tube is manipulated for bag-valve-mask ventilation or ventilator tube connection. If a tracheostomy tube is too long, it can become dislodged inferiorly, which causes the tip to either abut the mucosal wall of the trachea or obstruct it at the level of the carina.

It is important to know when and why the tracheostomy was placed because such information will influence evaluation and management of the patient.[59] If a tracheostomy tube becomes dislodged within the first 7 days after initial placement, the stoma can close rapidly and make reinsertion difficult. Blind, forceful attempts at reinsertion of the tracheostomy tube in the early postoperative period can result in the creation of a false passage and possible respiratory arrest. If accidental decannulation occurs before the tract has time to form, orotracheal intubation is the safest approach in the ED. Reinsertion of the tracheostomy tube is possible, but the patient will most likely require ET intubation to secure the airway.[59] Patients with abnormal neck anatomy or other causes of a "difficult airway" may not benefit from reinsertion in the ED. In these cases, the procedure may need to be performed in the operating room. Seek emergency surgical consultation for complicated cases.

Preparation

As for all patients with tracheostomy complications, begin with a quick primary assessment and place the patient on appropriate monitoring devices. Continuous waveform capnography can be invaluable in determining whether the tracheostomy tube is placed properly. Absence of a waveform or end-tidal CO_2 partial pressure less than 10 mm Hg is an indication that the airway device has become dislodged or was placed inappropriately.[60] It is essential to have advanced airway equipment at the bedside, including two replacement tracheostomy tubes (each with an inner cannula). A fiberoptic bronchoscope, if available, can be helpful. Position the patient with the neck in extension to maximize alignment of the stoma and trachea. Neck flexion can cause downward displacement of the tube by as much as 3 to 4 cm.[16]

Interventions

First, determine that the tube flanges rest snugly at the skin. Lateral neck x-ray films may reveal that the opening of the tracheostomy tube is abutting the anterior tracheal wall or obstructing the tracheal lumen. If the tracheostomy tube appears to be minimally displaced, attempt to reposition the tube by gentle manipulation. If the tracheostomy tube is completely dislodged or no waveform is present on capnography, tube replacement should be attempted.

If the tracheostomy stoma was created less than 7 days earlier, be prepared to orally intubate the patient. First, cut any flange sutures and remove the tracheostomy tube (Fig. 7-9). Stay sutures may be placed to hold the stoma open and better visualize the tracheal opening. If the patient is stable, attempt to reinsert the tracheostomy tube with the assistance of a gum elastic bougie or fiberoptic bronchoscope.[45] If the patient is unstable with an obstructed tracheostomy tube, cut the flange sutures, remove the tube, and orally intubate the patient.

Figure 7-9 Newly inserted tracheostomy tube. Replacement under emergency conditions can be difficult, particularly if the event occurs soon after the tube is initially placed and before a tract has formed (usually about 5 days after the procedure). Blind forceful attempts at reinsertion in this circumstance can be associated with the creation of a false passage and respiratory arrest. Orotracheal intubation is another option for accidental decannulation occurring before tract formation. In patients with surgical tracheostomies, traction on stay sutures placed circumferentially around the tracheal rings (which are generally cut long and often taped to the anterior chest wall—not shown here) will facilitate reintubation.

If the tracheostomy stoma was created 7 to 30 days earlier, remove the tube and any other cause of obstruction from the stoma. If the patient can ventilate independently, allow the patient to oxygenate and then reinsert the tube when ready. If the patient is unstable, occlude the stoma with moist gauze or other occlusive device and provide bag-valve-mask ventilation for oxygenation. Once the patient is stabilized, replace the tracheostomy tube. If a replacement tube is not available, a cuffed ET tube of equal size (or at minimum, 6-0) may be used as a substitute.

If the tracheostomy is more than 30 days old, the tube may not need to be replaced. If the patient is unstable, prepare as described for reinsertion or ET intubation. However, if the patient is stable and ventilating spontaneously without any signs of distress, contact the appropriate specialty care physician to discuss the need for emergency reinsertion.

Once the tube is reinserted, confirm correct placement with auscultation and waveform capnography. Tube position can also be confirmed by direct visualization with a fiberoptic bronchoscope.

False Passage

A false lumen can be created during replacement of a tracheal tube or during repositioning of a dislodged tube. Obese patients are at high risk for false passage because of their redundant neck tissue (see "Special Populations"). Subcutaneous air, crepitus, or distortion of anterior neck landmarks may indicate placement of the tracheostomy tube into a false passage. Absence of a waveform on capnography confirms misplacement of the tracheostomy tube. Abdominal distention after bag-valve-mask ventilation may indicate placement of the tracheal tube through a tracheoesophageal fistula

(TEF). If a false passage is suspected, remove and replace the tracheostomy tube expeditiously.

Equipment Failure

Fracture

Tracheostomy tubes do not fracture frequently. When fractures do occur, they are most often located at the juncture of the flange and the tube connection.[61,62] A fractured tube fragment may migrate inferiorly and obstruct the tracheal lumen. Patients may have acute respiratory complaints such as cough, dyspnea, choking, or wheezing. Prolonged retention of a foreign body can result in chronic respiratory symptoms such as wheezing, coughing, or recurrent bouts of pneumonia or bronchiectasis. To manage this problem, replace the tube if possible and consider bronchoscopy for retrieval of the tube fragment.[63]

Tracheal Cuff Complications

Complications related to the tracheal tube cuff include perforation, which results in a poor seal and increased risk for aspiration; overinflation, which causes pressure on or impingement of the esophageal lumen; and distention of the cuff distal to the tracheal tube, which results in obstruction of the tracheal tube opening. Mucosal injury is less common since the use of low-pressure cuffs has become standard practice. Pain with ventilation or swallowing, inadequate oxygenation, or the presence of gastric secretions in the tracheostomy tube may indicate cuff problems. Verify inflation pressure with a manometer (target range, 18 to 25 mm Hg) and appropriate cuff position. Replacement of the tube is indicated if the symptoms persist.

Infection

Patients who require long-term tracheostomy and mechanical ventilation are at high risk for nosocomial pneumonia, ventilator-associated pneumonia (VAP), and tracheobronchitis. In general, the frequency of infection increases with the duration of mechanical ventilation, but the risk for infection is highest in the first week following intubation. Nonventilated tracheostomy patients are also at increased risk for pneumonia, tracheobronchitis, stomal infections, and other soft tissue infections.

Risk factors for systemic infection include impairment of host defenses and exposure to large numbers of bacteria that bypass the upper airway defense systems. In healthy patients, the upper respiratory tract is colonized by normal oropharyngeal flora. In tracheostomy patients, the normal flora can be replaced by virulent pathogens such as enteric gram-negative bacteria.[64] The organisms most commonly cultured from tracheostomy stomas and tubes are *Pseudomonas aeruginosa*, *Acinetobacter*, and *Staphylococcus aureus*.[65] Colonization rates are high in these patients, even in the absence of systemic infection. The tracheostomy tube bypasses the natural protective barriers of the upper airway. Suctioning a colonized tracheostomy tube can introduce bacteria into the lower respiratory tract. Underlying medical conditions, prolonged hospitalization, impaired host defense mechanisms, and poor nutrition all increase susceptibility to infection.

Ventilator-associated tracheobronchitis (VAT) is the result of colonization of the upper airway and can eventually progress to VAP.[66] Patients with VAT have fever, production of purulent sputum, and positive respiratory cultures but no evidence of a new infiltrate on chest radiography.[66] VAT is frequently caused by multidrug-resistant organisms. Therefore, when choosing antimicrobial therapy, consider recent hospitalizations, previous infections, recent antibiotic use, and the hospital's antibiogram.

Tracheostomy patients on long-term ventilation are also at risk for VAP. These patients are similar to those with VAT, except that they have an infiltrate on chest radiography. A common cause of VAP is aspiration. Patients become predisposed to aspiration if they have altered neurologic function, have an abnormal swallowing mechanism, or are mechanically ventilated and kept in the supine position for a prolonged time. Some degree of aspiration occurs in 33% to 61% of all patients with tracheostomies.[67,68] To reduce the risk for aspiration, keep patients requiring mechanical ventilation in a semi-recumbent position. It is generally recommended that 30 to 45 degrees is adequate to reduce the risk for VAP.[69-71]

Stomal infections and cellulitis are also common.[41] The bacteria cultured most frequently from patients with tracheostomy-related cellulitis are *S. aureus*, *Pseudomonas* species, and *Monilia*. Consider *Candida albicans* infection in patients previously treated with antibiotics and those who have an underlying immunocompromised state. Peristomal cellulitis can usually be treated with good wound care and oral antibiotics. The most dangerous complications from cellulitis are mediastinitis, mediastinal abscess, necrotizing fasciitis, and paratracheal abscess. Consider these complications in patients who have pain with breathing, pain with swallowing, or signs of systemic infection. Strongly consider a deep neck infection in diabetic patients.[72] β-Hemolytic streptococci or coagulase-positive staphylococci are the cause in 90% of patients with craniocervical necrotizing fasciitis.[73] Sputum samples, obtained via tracheal suctioning, should be analyzed when infectious complications are suspected. Radiologic studies, namely, a chest radiograph, cervical computed tomography (CT), and chest CT, should be ordered as indicated.

Antimicrobial treatment in the ED should cover the most common organisms for the suspected site of tracheostomy-related infection. Broad-spectrum systemic antimicrobials, along with adjuvant aerosol therapy, should be given urgently to high-risk patients.[74] Depending on the patient's condition, surgical evaluation may be needed.[41]

Tracheal Stenosis and Tracheomalacia

Tracheal stenosis and tracheomalacia are late complications of a tracheostomy, often occurring weeks to months after decannulation. Its overall incidence is unknown, but clinically significant stenosis has been estimated to develop in 10% of all tracheostomy patients.[75] Tracheal stenosis occurs most often at the level of the stoma but can develop proximal (suprastomal) or distal to the stoma as a result of a poorly fitting tube or cuff. Pressure on the tracheal lumen from the tube or cuff can cause epithelial destruction, tracheitis, ulceration, persistent inflammation, and subsequent stenosis. Stenosis at the stoma can occur from rigid tube systems with excessive motion and pressure points.[16] Symptoms become evident when the tracheal diameter is narrowed by 50% to 60%.[76] Stridor typically occurs when the tracheal lumen is narrower than 5 mm.[16] Respiratory symptoms such as cough, retained secretions, and progressive dyspnea with exertion are indications of clinically significant stenosis.

Figure 7-10 **A** and **B,** Tracheomalacia. (*From Patterson AG, Cooper JD, eds. Pearson's Thoracic and Esophageal Surgery. Philadelphia: Elsevier, 2008.*)

Tracheomalacia is weakening of the tracheal cartilage from pressure necrosis and results in luminal widening. A loose tracheostomy tube with excessive mobility can cause air leaks or tracheal collapse (Fig. 7-10). Patients with significant tracheomalacia experience tracheal collapse on expiration. This can result in air trapping and retained respiratory secretions. Pediatric patients are less able to tolerate cartilaginous weakening and tracheomalacia.

Interventions

Relief of respiratory compromise is problematic because a high-grade stenosis may make ET intubation difficult or impossible. To treat a patient with respiratory distress secondary to tracheal stenosis, first attempt to improve ventilation by elevating the head of the bed and placing the patient on high-flow humidified oxygen. Nebulized bronchodilators or racemic epinephrine may also be helpful. Keep a cricothyrotomy kit readily available in the event that ET intubation is impossible. Tracheal stenosis can be diagnosed definitively by laryngoscopy and flexible fiberoscopy.[41] Other imaging modalities, such as CT, are not sensitive enough to detect stenosis. Treatment of tracheal stenosis involves operative dilation or resection of granulomatous tissue in the operating room.

Tracheoesophageal Fistula

TEF is an uncommon, late complication of tracheostomy. It occurs in 1% of tracheostomy patients as a result of injury to the posterior tracheal wall.[77] Early TEF can occur if a puncture wound or small laceration is made in the anterior esophageal wall during placement of the tracheostomy. The most common cause of a TEF is a poorly fitted tracheostomy tube or an overinflated cuff.[77] Injury to the esophageal mucosa from a nasogastric or orogastric tube can also cause a TEF.

Most patients with a TEF have increased secretions, recurrent pneumonia, or aspiration of gastric contents while receiving mechanical ventilation. The most frequent sign of a TEF is cough after swallowing. A persistent cuff leak or abdominal distention may also indicate a TEF. The clinician may be able to auscultate breath sounds over the lung fields and the epigastrium simultaneously, but this finding is unreliable. Bronchoscopy, barium esophagography, or mediastinal CT can aid in making the diagnosis.

Interventions

Once a TEF is diagnosed, the immediate goal should be to reduce the amount of tracheal and pulmonary soilage by inflating a cuff below the level of the fistula. If the current tracheostomy tube is not long enough to allow placement of a cuff distal to the TEF, exchange it with a longer tracheostomy tube or an ET tube. An orogastric or nasogastric tube can also be inserted to prevent gastric contents from further contaminating the respiratory tract. Early consultation with an otolaryngologist or thoracic surgeon is appropriate because the definitive treatment is surgical.[77] TEF is not usually an immediately life-threatening complication, and tube exchange can be performed in conjunction with the surgical team.

Bleeding

Major Bleeding

Major bleeding is one of the most feared complications of tracheostomy. A history of bleeding or minor bleeding that has stopped spontaneously cannot automatically be attributed to minor irritation or skin erosion. It may not be possible to fully evaluate bleeding from a tracheostomy site in the ED without consultation or specialized equipment such as a fiberoptic endoscope. Sources of bleeding include the thyroid vessels, anterior jugular veins, brachiocephalic (innominate) artery, carotid artery, and aortic arch.[78,79] Bleeding from esophageal or gastric sources may occur if a TEF is present or if the patient has aspirated blood. Erosion of a major vessel from the cuff or tip of the tube is responsible for 10% of all tracheostomy hemorrhages and is a devastating complication. The IA is the vessel most commonly involved.[80]

A tracheoinnominate artery fistula (TIF) is a late complication of tracheostomy that usually occurs within the first 4 weeks after insertion, but it can happen at any time.[12,81] The mortality rate associated with a TIF approaches 100%.[82] The anatomic proximity of the IA to the trachea places it at higher risk for fistulization if the tracheal wall is injured. The vessel crosses from left to right as it moves superiorly and lies immediately anterior to the trachea at the level of the superior thoracic inlet. Risk factors for TIF include placement of the stoma below the third tracheal ring, caudal migration of the tracheal tube, and the presence of a cephalad-coursing IA.

A single episode of hemoptysis or tracheal bleeding may be the only warning sign of a TIF. Any amount of bleeding or hemoptysis exceeding 10 mL within 48 hours after placement of the tube should be considered a "sentinel bleed" and an indication that a fatal hemorrhage may be imminent. Some patients report only a new cough or retrosternal pain.[83] Presume that a history or evidence of 10 mL or more of blood is from an arterial source.

Preparation
When evaluating a patient with a suspected TIF, place advanced airway equipment at the bedside. Emergency surgical consultation is mandatory. Position the patient with the head of the bed elevated and the neck in slight extension. Secure adequate intravenous access, and prepare the patient to go to the operating room. In addition to the equipment noted in Figure 7-2, have a scalpel with a No. 10 or 11 blade and a 50-mL syringe at the bedside.

Interventions
If the patient is stable, attempt to visualize the bleeding site. Look for the IA in the anterior tracheal wall at or below the sternal notch. If significant tracheal bleeding is present, hyperinflate the tracheostomy tube cuff with the 50-mL syringe to compress the artery against the posterior sternal wall. Inflate the balloon slowly to prevent rupture of the cuff. Depending on the make and model of the tube, inflating the cuff with the entire 50 mL may not be possible. If a TIF has been caused by cuff erosion, this procedure should tamponade the bleeding. If the patient's tracheostomy tube does not have a cuff, replace it with a cuffed ET or tracheostomy tube.

If cuff hyperinflation is unsuccessful, the TIF may be located at or beyond the distal tip of the tracheostomy tube. In this circumstance, the current tracheostomy tube must be removed and replaced with either an oral ET tube or an ET tube inserted through the stoma. If ET intubation is not possible, advance the ET tube through the tracheostomy site.

Position the cuff of the ET tube below the stoma at the level of the upper part of the sternum and hyperinflate it. If the patient continues to bleed despite this maneuver, apply digital pressure through the tracheal stoma to compress the anterior tracheal wall against the sternum. Digital pressure is considered the most reliable technique to stop hemorrhage and can provide control of bleeding during transport to the operating room (Fig. 7-11).[41] Extension of the stoma with a vertical incision to the jugular notch may be necessary if the provider cannot reach the TIF through the original stoma.

Minor Bleeding
All bleeding from a tracheostomy site must be evaluated for a potentially life-threatening event. Seemingly minor or self-limited bleeding may be a harbinger of subsequent severe hemorrhage. Sentinel hemorrhages frequently precede massive bleeding. Consider endoscopic examination for complete evaluation unless a superficial bleeding site is confirmed.

Minor bleeding is most likely the result of irritated granulation tissue and is usually confined to the skin surrounding the stoma. Bloody secretions from the tracheostomy tube may represent tracheitis, bleeding running down from the skin or thyroid, or superficial tracheal ulceration from tracheal suctioning or tracheal tube pressure.

Examine the stoma site and tube first in an attempt to locate the source and quantify the volume of blood loss. If the source of bleeding is within the stoma or from within the trachea, remove the tracheostomy tube if it was placed more

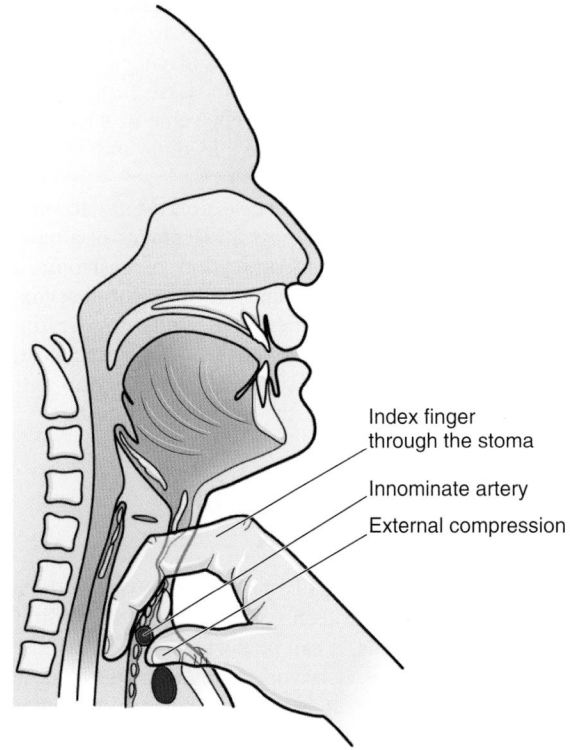

Figure 7-11 Control of innominate artery bleeding by digital compression.

than 7 days before the current event. Visualize the tracheal lumen, proximal end of the trachea, and inner stoma with a nasopharyngoscope or a small pediatric laryngoscope. It is important to differentiate superficial erosions from active bleeding. Do not attempt to remove clots in the trachea because this may increase the rate of hemorrhage. Consider obtaining a basic metabolic panel, complete blood count, and coagulation studies to evaluate for other factors complicating bleeding such as uremia, thrombocytopenia, or coagulopathy.

Preparation
Prepare patients with minor tracheostomy bleeding in the same way that you would those with major bleeding. Gather the appropriate airway equipment at the bedside. In addition to the standard equipment shown in Figure 7-2, obtain the following:
- Sterile gauze
- Sterile saline for irrigation
- 22-gauge needle with syringe
- 1% lidocaine with 1:100,000 epinephrine
- Absorbable hemostat (e.g., Surgicel)
- Suture kit with suturing material
- Electrocauterization or chemical cauterization supplies, if available

Interventions
For external or stomal bleeding, begin with local irrigation to find the source of the bleeding. Most incisional or stomal bleeding can be stopped by applying direct pressure for 3 to 5 minutes. Application of absorbable hemostatic material may improve the outcome of direct pressure application. If an

external bleeding site continues to ooze, consider adjunctive treatment. Options include injecting 0.5 to 1.0 mL of lidocaine with epinephrine near the source, placing a single suture for hemostasis, or using cauterization. Last, replace the tracheostomy tube. Following tube replacement, suction carefully to confirm resolution of the bleeding and to identify secondary sources of bleeding.

If stomal bleeding or intratracheal sites do not account for the bleeding, consider other causes. Placement of a nasogastric tube will help in the identification of gastrointestinal bleeding. Examine the nasopharynx and oropharynx for bleeding sources. If the patient has undergone radiation therapy, examine the area above the level of the tracheostomy stoma, where mucosal injury secondary to radiation damage may be the cause of blood in the tracheal secretions.

TRANSESOPHAGEAL PUNCTURE FOR VOICE RESTORATION

Transesophageal puncture (TEP) has become one of the most widely used and accepted techniques for voice rehabilitation. Developed in the 1980s, it can be performed as a primary or secondary procedure after laryngectomy or other pharyngeal surgeries. A puncture site is created through the anterior esophagus and posterior tracheal wall, where the TEP prosthesis is later inserted. The mucosa in segments of the pharyngeal esophagus vibrates in response to airflow, thereby creating speech.

Complications

Operative and immediate postoperative complications of TEP are infrequent.[84] Long-term complications include stomal stenosis, aspiration of the prosthesis, fistula leakage, TEP necrosis, and swallowing impairment. Reported infectious complications associated with TEP include deep neck abscess, aspiration pneumonia, and cervical cellulitis.[85]

The emergency care provider should be aware of the most common complications, few of which are life-threatening. Accumulation of thick or inspissated secretions or food above the TEP can cause upper airway obstruction. Prosthesis dislodgment, occlusion, or erosion secondary to infection should be considered in all patients with acute changes in voice production or decreased ability to speak.[86] Esophageal edema causing dysphagia and loss of TEP speech has been reported and should be differentiated from other causes of esophageal obstruction.[86]

When evaluating patients with a TEP, review the medical records, assess airway and esophageal patency, and determine whether the patient has experienced changes or difficulty in voice production. In stable patients, management of prosthesis complications should be referred to a specialist, most commonly an otolaryngologist.

TRANSTRACHEAL OXYGEN DELIVERY SYSTEMS

Low-flow oxygen is prescribed for patients who have adequate ventilatory function but chronic hypoxia. Many patients with chronic obstructive pulmonary disease, pulmonary fibrosis, sleep apnea, lung cancer, and α_1-antitrypsin deficiency are candidates for outpatient use of supplemental oxygen.[87-89] Traditionally, supplemental oxygen has been delivered by nasal cannula. Although nasal cannula oxygenation is easy to administer, it has several side effects, including drying of the nasal mucosa, epistaxis, ear discomfort, contact dermatitis from the oxygen tubing, and dry throat.[87,89] Use of a nasal cannula is inefficient because it delivers oxygen only during inspiration and the oxygen must traverse the anatomic dead space of the nares and hypopharynx.

Transtracheal oxygen (TTO) delivery systems enhance the efficiency of oxygenation by administering oxygen directly to the lower respiratory tract. These systems reduce complications, improve patient comfort, and increase compliance.[90] Oxygen is delivered through all phases of the respiratory cycle and directly into the trachea, thereby bypassing dead spaces in the upper airway.[88] As a result, the required oxygen flow rate is commonly reduced by at least 50%.[90] Gas mixture in the distal end of the trachea is more effective in eliminating CO_2. Clinically, TTO systems usually reduce the patient's work of breathing and exertional dyspnea.[89] Physiologic benefits include reduced erythrocytosis, decreased pulmonary vascular resistance, improved cor pulmonale, improved arterial oxygen tension, and increased exercise capacity.[91]

TTO catheters are small tubes that deliver oxygen directly to the lumen of the trachea. The catheter is held in place by a subcutaneous tract, and the catheter is inserted into the lower part of the trachea. Low-flow oxygen (2 to 10 L/min) is supplied directly to the trachea by a narrow (7- to 11-Fr) catheter. Typically, an 11-cm catheter sits in the trachea with its tip 1 to 2 cm above the carina.[89] It can have a single or multiple distal ports for oxygen flow. The catheter is held in place by a thin band or necklace through two openings in the flange.

The surgical procedure is often done in an outpatient setting with the patient under local anesthesia. Initially, a small stent is placed percutaneously into the anterior aspect of the neck; it is then replaced with a TTO catheter in 1 to 2 weeks after the tract matures.[89] Dislodgment of the catheter during this time can result in closure of the tract within a matter of minutes. Once the tracheocutaneous fistula has epithelialized, the catheter may be inserted. Early catheter changes should be done in the clinician's office via a modified Seldinger technique if the integrity of the stoma is questionable. After the tract has fully matured, most patients can change their catheter at home.

Regular maintenance includes cleaning and changing the TTO catheter. One milliliter of sterile saline is instilled into the catheter, and a cleaning rod is inserted as far as possible. The cleaning rod is inserted and extracted three times to remove secretions and encrustations from the lumen of the catheter. Catheters are usually changed according to the manufacturer's recommendations, from twice daily to once every 2 weeks. The stoma should be cleaned twice each day and inspected thoroughly for signs of infection. All patients should be given supplemental oxygen by nasal cannula during catheter maintenance procedures. Adequate humidification, cleaning, and systemic hydration will help reduce the incidence of mucus blockage.

Early complications (developing within 3 weeks after the procedure) occur in approximately 30% of patients and include bleeding, infection, pneumothorax, costochondritis, and dislodgement (which can be caused by coughing).[87,92] Pneumomediastinum and sudden death have been reported as possible, yet rare complications.[93] Late complications occur in about 40% of patients and include mucus plugging, bleeding, infection, and hemoptysis.[91] A mucus ball is an accumulation of inspissated mucus that adheres to the outer surface of the TTO catheter tip. It can cause coughing, wheezing, and dyspnea. Life-threatening airway obstruction resulting from the formation of a large mucus ball has been reported.[94]

Dyspnea or increased coughing may indicate that the TTO catheter is obstructed by a mucus ball, that the tube is kinked, or that the tip of the catheter is positioned cephalad to the stoma. Obstruction within the catheter tubing may cause a whistling sound from the oxygen tank humidifier. Always examine the patient for signs of subcutaneous air and catheter dislodgement.

If routine broad-spectrum antibiotics are used by the patient, *Candida* infections can develop at the stoma. Such infections are more common in patients receiving systemic antibiotics or long-term corticosteroids or those with diabetes. Tracheal chondritis may result from bacterial infection of the cartilage. Many patients with chondritis have a deep, indurated, nonfluctuant lump around the tract that may be tender to palpation. A 3-week course of an oral antibiotic that specifically covers *S. aureus* should be prescribed as treatment.

Interventions

If obstruction is suspected while the patient is in the ED, clean and replace the catheter. If the stoma tract has not healed or appears to be infected, change the catheter via a modified Seldinger technique. Use a water-soluble lubricant for the catheter change. If changing the catheter does not relieve the obstruction and the patient's airway is intact, encourage the patient to perform maneuvers that raise intrathoracic pressure to increase the force of the cough. Ask the patient to sit upright, hold a pillow to the abdomen, and cough forcefully after three deep inspirations. This maneuver may help mobilize secretions or small mucus plugs in the airway. Dyspnea and coughing should lessen with effective removal of the obstruction.

Manage minor bleeding at the catheter site with gauze packing or cauterization. If significant bleeding is identified or suspected, consult a specialist on an emergency basis and manage the airway definitively as clinically indicated (see the section "Major Bleeding"). Manage skin and pulmonary infections with the techniques discussed for tracheostomy care.

Stents

Tracheal stenosis and tracheomalacia are known complications of artificial airways. Management options include surgery and placement of silicone stents in the trachea. Patients who have had their tracheostomy tubes successfully decannulated may need stents if symptomatic stenosis or tracheomalacia occurs. Indications for and complications of tracheal stents are beyond the scope of this chapter, but the clinician should be aware of the possibility that these indwelling devices may be present in patients who have undergone head and neck surgery or previous tracheostomies.[57,95]

TRANSTRACHEAL NEEDLE ASPIRATION

Transtracheal needle aspiration was first described in the late 1950s as a means of obtaining sterile sputum for culture from patients with recurrent pneumonia or lower respiratory tract infections. In theory, the risk of sample contamination is reduced by introducing a collection device beyond the oropharynx. This procedure has largely fallen out of favor with many clinicians because of patient noncompliance, the risk for complications, and the belief that the procedure is unnecessary.[96] Alternative sampling methods such as bronchoalveolar lavage have become more widely accepted and used. At present, transtracheal needle aspiration is no longer recommended[97] and should not be performed in the ED.

SPECIAL POPULATIONS

Obese Patients

The prevalence of obesity (body mass index [BMI] ≥30) and morbid obesity (BMI ≥40) has increased dramatically over the past few decades.[98,99] Obesity increases the patient's risk for cardiovascular and metabolic comorbidity, and obese patients have a higher risk for ventilatory dysfunction secondary to altered respiratory mechanics.[100] Lung compliance, functional residual capacity, and expiratory reserve volume in an obese patient are reduced exponentially in relation to BMI.[101,102] As weight increases, vital capacity and total lung capacity decrease.[101] Ultimately, obese patients have decreased pulmonary reserve, which can cause a rapid onset of hypoxia if they become critically ill.

Morbidly obese patients are particularly at risk for life-threatening complications related to tracheostomy.[103] Tube obstruction and accidental dislodgement appear to be more common in obese patients. Dislodgement is specifically associated with increased rates of morbidity and mortality.[58] Delayed recognition of tube dislodgment because of abnormal neck anatomy accounts for nearly 30% of tracheostomy-related deaths in the obese population.[58,103]

Preparation

For the management of an obese patient with a tracheostomy-related complaint, it is important to have all advanced airway equipment at the bedside (Fig. 7-2). In addition to standard equipment, attempt to obtain an extra long or adjustable-flange tracheostomy tube to span the elongated pretracheal distance that is common in morbidly obese patients.[104] In obese patients, standard tracheostomy tubes may be too short proximal to the cuff and have a higher risk for malposition.

In addition to standard monitoring, use continuous capnography, if available, to prevent delay in the recognition of tube dislodgement.[58] Physical signs, such as reduced breath sounds and subcutaneous air, may be more difficult to recognize in obese patients. Fiberoptic bronchoscopy may be needed to confirm correct tube placement. The patient should be positioned with the neck in slight extension, and the head of the bed should be elevated to approximately 30 degrees.

Interventions

Approach an obese patient with the same protocols outlined previously in this chapter for the applicable complication. If the tube is obstructed, deflation of the tracheostomy cuff may not be sufficient to allow adequate ventilation because external compression caused by abnormal neck anatomy may occur. If tube dislodgement is suspected, ET intubation may be preferred over blind reinsertion because of the increased risk for false passage.[103] Tube placement can be confirmed with direct visualization via fiberoptic bronchoscopy.

Pediatrics

Most considerations for pediatric patients follow adult guidelines and are discussed in the appropriate sections of this chapter, but some specific considerations should be mentioned. The tracheostomy-related mortality rate in pediatric patients ranges from 0.5% to 6%.[105] The main causes of death are accidental dislodgement and obstruction of the tracheostomy tube.[106] Complication rates are highest in patients requiring tracheostomy for airway obstruction. In comparison, patients with central nervous system disorders, respiratory distress syndrome, and congenital heart disorders are less likely to experience complications.[24]

Equipment

When replacing a tracheostomy tube in a child, always have at least two tracheostomy tubes available: the current size and a size smaller. Pediatric tubes generally have a much smaller diameter than adult tracheostomy tubes, and many of them do not have an inner cannula. Pediatric tracheostomy tubes rarely have inflatable cuffs, except for those used for certain special indications.[107] Suction catheters, a bag-valve-mask device, ET tubes, resuscitation medication, and equipment appropriate for the pediatric population should be available when treating pediatric tracheostomy patients. Continuous capnography may detect certain tracheostomy complications and is recommended.[108]

Sizing

Pediatric tracheostomy tubes share most of the same components of the tubes used in adults. The ID of the tube is stamped on the outer cannula flange, and that information should guide the clinician's choice of replacement tubes. Recommended tube sizes according to age are listed in Table 7-2. Age guidelines can be helpful, but they may not be reliable in pediatric patients because of complex medical problems.

Table 7-2 Tracheostomy Tube Sizes Based on Patient Age

AGE	SIZE	INNER DIAMETER (mm)	OUTER DIAMETER (mm)
Premature	00	3.1	4.5
Newborn-3 mo	0	3.4	5.0
3-10 mo	1	3.7	5.5
10-12 mo	2	4.1	6.0
13-24 mo	3	4.8	7.0
2-9 yr	4	5.0	8.5
10-11 yr	6	7.0	10
≥12 yr	8	8.5	12.0
	10	9.0	13.0

Adapted from Mullins JB, Templer JW, Kong J, et al: Airway resistance and work of breathing in tracheostomy tubes. *Laryngoscope.* 1993;103:1367.

Premature infants may be small for their age and weight, thus making estimation of tube size even more difficult.

Like ET tubes, tracheostomy tubes are sized by the tube's ID. When the tracheostomy tube is seated correctly in a pediatric patient, it should extend at least 2 cm beyond the stoma and no closer than 1 to 2 cm above the carina. Its curvature should be such that when the tube is placed appropriately, the distal portion of the tube is concentric and collinear with the trachea. After replacing a tracheostomy tube, confirm its position by auscultating breath sounds, using capnography, and confirming the location of the distal tip with a chest radiograph.

Cuff

The general rule that cuffed ET tubes should not be used in patients younger than 6 years is under a great deal of debate and does not universally apply to tracheostomy patients. If a patient requires high-pressure ventilation or only nocturnal ventilation or is at risk for aspiration, a cuffed tube may be appropriate. Cuffed tubes are also used in patients with a tracheal anomaly. Replacement of these tubes should ensure that the individual's anatomic and physiologic needs are met.

Cuff pressure recommendations for pediatric patients are less than 20 cm H_2O.[109] With few exceptions, low-pressure, high-volume cuffs should be used.[24]

Humidifiers

Humidifiers for pediatric tracheostomy tubes attach to the external port. Some humidifiers have lithium-coated moisture exchangers. Systemic absorption of lithium is unlikely to cause clinical symptoms in adults but may be a consideration in children. Use humidifiers regularly to keep secretions loose and help prevent obstruction of the tube.

Suctioning

Suctioning recommendations in pediatric patients clearly support the use of a premeasured suction catheter to reduce the rate of mucosal irritation and to limit the development of granulation tissue. The premeasured technique uses an exact depth of insertion, which reduces epithelial damage if the catheter is inserted too deeply and inadequate suctioning if the catheter is not inserted deeply enough. Depth of insertion can be estimated by measuring a similar tube before inserting the suction catheter. In children with fenestrated tracheostomy tubes, suction catheters may accidentally go through the fenestrations and cause mucosal irritation. If this happens repeatedly, granulation tissue may develop at the site.[24]

Complications

Pediatric tracheostomy complications are similar to those in the adult population. Their incidence is estimated to be between 5% and 49%.[105] Late complications most likely to be seen in the ED include obstruction, dislodgement, bleeding, pneumothorax, infection, pneumomediastinum, TEF, and TIF. Chronic respiratory complications include tracheomalacia, tracheal stenosis, vocal cord paralysis, and vocal cord fusion.

Granuloma formation is common in pediatric patients. It often occurs in the tracheal lumen either at the superior margin of the tracheostomy or at the level of the tip of the tube. The development of granulation tissue is the result of persistent mucosal irritation and inflammation. Any patient with a clinically significant granuloma should be evaluated by a pediatric specialist for definitive care.

Pneumomediastinum and pneumothorax are generally thought to be early complications of tracheostomy, but they should always be considered in a pediatric tracheostomy patient. In children, the pleural apices rise higher than in adults and can even extend into the lower part of the neck. These complications can be caused by a dislodged tube positioned in a false passage or a malpositioned tube that causes an increase in intrathoracic pressure.[106]

The most common bacterial species that colonize pediatric tracheostomies are *P. aeruginosa* and *S. aureus*. As in adults, colonization does not require treatment unless signs of acute infection are present.[106] Suprastomal collapse of the anterior tracheal wall is very common in pediatric patients and can cause air trapping. A tracheostomy tube that places excessive pressure on the tracheal rings will cause inflammation, chondritis, and weakening of the cartilaginous rings. Significant collapse can hamper subsequent decannulation success.

Management of major bleeding in pediatric patients follows the same recommendations given for adults. However, the smaller stoma size may prevent the application of digital pressure to the site of hemorrhage. If the clinician is unable to reach the source of the bleeding, expeditious ET intubation followed by cuff overinflation may temporize the bleeding until the patient can be taken to the operating room.

SUMMARY

A tracheostomy emergency can be one of the most high-risk scenarios in the ED. The emergency physician must be well prepared for a variety of tracheostomy complications and should approach the patient in an organized, stepwise fashion so that interventions can be initiated in timely fashion. Tube dislodgement and obstruction are common and associated with an extremely high mortality rate, especially in obese patients. Always ensure correct tube position, have backup airway equipment readily available, and obtain surgical support early if the patient needs to go to the operating room.

References are available at www.expertconsult.com

CHAPTER 8

Mechanical Ventilation

Jairo I. Santanilla

INTRODUCTION

Mechanical ventilation (MV) is an important tool for resuscitation of critically ill patients in the emergency department (ED). It is vital that ED practitioners have a thorough understanding of the basics of MV and to know when to apply these principles and how to support patients in respiratory or cardiac failure. Hospital overcrowding has led to a delay in transfer of mechanically ventilated patients out of the ED, and ventilator management often falls on the emergency medicine physician. Also, during nights and weekends in some facilities, the ED physician may be called on to troubleshoot or stabilize mechanically ventilated patients in the intensive care unit (ICU). The traditional view of MV as a prescription that fits virtually all patients equally should be discarded as a gross misunderstanding of pulmonary pathophysiology. Increasing evidence has shown that the mechanism of lung ventilation by MV may be as deleterious as it is helpful.[1] *Because patients remain in the ED while mechanically ventilated, ED clinicians should embrace the established paradigm of pulmonary-protective MV strategies as a cornerstone of care.*

BASIC PHYSIOLOGY

Understanding basic pulmonary physiology is essential to understanding how to initiate MV. This ensures that the method of gas delivery meshes with the patient's underlying physiology to avoid ventilator-induced lung injury.

Minute Volume and Alveolar Ventilation

The volume of air that moves in and out of a patient's lungs per minute is termed *minute volume* ($\dot{V}E$). $\dot{V}E$ is the product of tidal volume (VT) and respiratory frequency or rate (f):

$$\dot{V}E = VT \times f$$

Normal $\dot{V}E$ is 7 to 10 L/min. VT can be further broken down into alveolar volume (VA) and dead space volume (VDS):

$$VT = VA + VDS$$

In healthy young persons, the anatomic dead space is accounted for by the trachea and the larger airways and is approximately 2.2 mL/kg lean body weight. In disease states, in addition to the anatomic dead space, there is a variable amount of "pathologic" dead space, which corresponds to ventilated alveoli and respiratory bronchioles that are not adequately perfused. The sum of anatomic and pathologic dead space is often referred to as *physiologic dead space*.

Alveolar minute ventilation ($\dot{V}A$) is the product of rate times VT minus dead space:

$$\dot{V}A = (VT - VDS) \times f$$

$\dot{V}A$ and the rate of CO_2 production by the body determine the partial pressure of CO_2 in the alveoli ($PACO_2$), which is approximately equal to systemic arterial CO_2 tension.

Volume-Pressure Relationship

Volume and pressure are related for a given respiratory system. A given volume (V) will create a certain pressure (P) relative to the compliance (C) of the respiratory system. The respiratory system consists of the ventilator tubing, endotracheal (ET) tube, trachea, airways, lung parenchyma, chest wall, and diaphragm tension. For example, a 500-mL volume will create a certain pressure based on the compliance of the respiratory system. Increasing the volume will increase the pressure in the system. Decreasing the volume will result in lower pressure. Decreasing the compliance (i.e., making the system "stiffer") will increase the pressure in the system. Increasing the compliance will decrease the pressure in the system.

$$P = V/C$$

Conversely, this relationship also holds for volume. For example, a pressure of 20 cm H_2O will create a certain volume based on the compliance of the system. Increasing pressure will result in higher volume. Decreasing pressure will result in lower volume. Decreasing compliance will result in lower volume. Increasing compliance will result in higher volume.

$$V = P \times C$$

Airway Pressures

Plateau Pressure

Plateau pressure is measured at the end of inspiration with a short breath-hold (Fig. 8-1). At this point no airflow should be occurring. This is considered a static pressure. By understanding the aforementioned volume-pressure relationship, one can easily deduce how plateau pressure is inversely related to respiratory system compliance and directly related to volume. Anything that decreases compliance will increase plateau pressure. Increasing compliance will decrease plateau pressure. Decreasing volume will decrease plateau pressure (a major tenet in lung-protective ventilation).

Peak Airway Pressure

Peak airway pressure is derived during inspiration and thus incorporates airflow. Because there is air movement during this measurement, it is considered a dynamic pressure. It reflects the dynamic compliance of the entire respiratory system and incorporates static compliance and airflow. Peak airway pressure can never be lower than plateau pressure. In addition, because its main distinction is that it incorporates airflow, it is reflective of resistance to airflow. Anything that decreases compliance or increases resistance to airflow will increase peak airway pressure. Increasing compliance or decreasing resistance to airflow will decrease peak airway pressure.

A physiologically appropriate means of detecting and monitoring bronchospasm is the peak-plateau gradient. A normal gradient is less than 4 cm H_2O pressure, and elevated values indicate increased airway resistance. The efficacy of treatment with β_2-agonists, steroids, intravenous magnesium, or diuresis

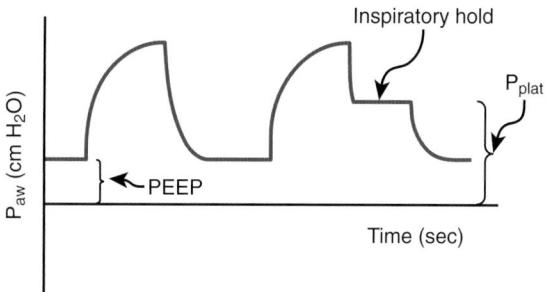

Figure 8-1 Schematic of a pressure-time curve showing an inspiratory breath-hold and subsequent plateau pressure (P$_{plat}$) measurement. *P$_{aw}$*, airway pressure; *PEEP*, positive end-expiratory pressure.

Figure 8-2 Schematic of two superimposed pressure-time curves showing an isolated decrease in peak inspiratory pressure (P$_{peak}$) with no change in plateau pressure (P$_{plat}$) as airflow resistance improves. *P$_{aw}$*, airway pressure.

Figure 8-3 Alveolar interdependence. Note that alveoli are not round in shape; instead, they are polygons. Polygons have corners and may have two opposing surfaces that may adhere to one another via surface tension. Surfactant works to reduce this surface tension and allow alveoli to open with reduced shear stress at the junction of closed and open alveoli. Alveoli are connected via the pores of Kohn. These pores allow opening alveoli to pull a relatively closed alveolus open while equalizing pressure between adjacent alveoli. The central alveolus on the right is fairly closed in the upper part of the diagram, but it is pulled open by its neighbors as they expand and accept gas.

may be assessed by monitoring the changes in this gradient (Fig. 8-2).

Positive End-Expiratory Pressure

Positive end-expiratory pressure (PEEP) is the pressure in the airway at the end of exhalation. PEEP helps keep the large noncartilaginously supported airways and the smaller alveoli open to prevent collapse, atelectasis, and ensuing hypoxia. The ventilation required to compensate for this triad commonly worsens lung compliance and is associated with ventilator-induced lung injury. Progressive increases in PEEP result in elevations in both total lung pressure and total lung volume. For example, serial elevations in PEEP often result in increased plateau pressure and elevated functional residual capacity (FRC; i.e., lung volume).

Extrinsic PEEP

When discussing MV and PEEP, most often authors are referring to extrinsic PEEP (PEEP$_e$). This is also referred to as applied PEEP. It is the PEEP that is extrinsically applied by the ventilator. When PEEP is used without a subscript in this chapter, it refers to PEEP$_e$. The useful PEEP range is from 3 to 20 cm H$_2$O.[2] PEEP is used to increase FRC and move the zero pressure point of each alveolar unit more proximally in the airway and thereby prevent early alveolar collapse.[3] By so doing, PEEP increases the available number of alveolar units that can participate in gas exchange. The primary effect of PEEP on gas exchange is improvement in oxygenation, not removal of CO$_2$. CO$_2$ clearance is rather efficient and will be well preserved, even in hypoxic situations. By opening one alveolar unit, the tendency of adjacent units is to open as well (i.e., alveolar codependency) (Fig. 8-3).[4]

Excessive PEEP will compromise hemodynamics. There are two primary questions to ask when using PEEP to augment oxygenation: (1) What is the "optimal PEEP" and (2) Is the current amount of PEEP compromising the patient's hemodynamics?

PEEP is not without untoward side effects, and increased levels of PEEP can lead to lung injury and hemodynamic compromise.[5] Increased intrathoracic pressure can result in cardiac compression and collapse, principally of the right atrium. It is imperative that the patient be adequately volume-resuscitated because preload depletion compounds this problem. Desired levels of PEEP simply may not be possible because of deleterious effects on cardiac output.

Optimal PEEP can be determined in several ways. One is to increase PEEP until there are no longer increases in Po$_2$. However, this method may result in several untoward events. First, oxygen tension may increase steadily, but carbon dioxide pressure (Pco$_2$) may increase as a result of alveolar overdistention. With overdistention, alveolar pressure may exceed pulmonary arteriolar pressure and actually decrease pulmonary blood flow and clearance of CO$_2$. Second, alveolar overdistention may increase total intrathoracic pressure and result in diminished venous return and cardiac output. Third, decreased venous return may cause cerebral venous hypertension. The optimal PEEP for one organ system may be deleterious for another. For example, the optimal PEEP for ideal oxygenation may be the worst PEEP for cerebral venous drainage.

An alternative is to increase PEEP until a complication of PEEP occurs (e.g., elevation in Pco$_2$, hypotension) and then reduce PEEP if needed (inability to tolerate hypercapnia) or expand the patient's intravascular volume to combat the decreased venous return.

Another excellent method of determining the optimal PEEP is guided by assessing changes in plateau pressure with changes in PEEP. As PEEP is increased from a minimal level, the patient's peak airway pressure and plateau pressure will increase by the amount of $PEEP_e$. When the optimal PEEP for the lung units is achieved, plateau pressure will no longer increase. As the lung is optimally recruited, peak and plateau pressure may decrease because more volume of lung is available to receive a set V_T. Once this level is exceeded, there will be further increases in plateau pressure beyond the incremental increase in PEEP as the units overdistend. Therefore, the clinician must readily identify the plateau in this plateau pressure trend. The same relationship may be displayed graphically in the dynamic pressure-volume loop (Fig. 8-4). The lower limb of the loop represents the pressure required to open the alveolar units.[6,7] In the absence of PEEP (or inadequate PEEP), this limb is prolonged and flattened and has an inflection point far to the right of the origin of the loop (Fig. 8-5). As PEEP is progressively increased, the inflection point travels to the left. When the optimal PEEP is achieved, there will be a rapid upstroke of the loop because the vast majority of the functional lung units are already open and ready to be ventilated (see Fig. 8-4). This strategy is known as the *open lung model* of MV.[6]

Irrespective of what technique is used, it is currently widely agreed that plateau pressure should not exceed 30 cm H_2O. If respiratory system compliance is so low that plateau pressure exceeds 30 cm H_2O, either PEEP or V_T has to be decreased. If this is not possible because of either recalcitrant hypoxia or acidosis, rescue therapies may need to be used (see the section "Acute Lung Injury and Acute Respiratory Distress Syndrome").

Intrinsic PEEP

Intrinsic PEEP ($PEEP_i$) is additional pressure that is generated within the airways from trapped gas that should have been exhaled but for various reasons (commonly obstruction to exhalation such as in chronic obstructive pulmonary disease [COPD]) was not. $PEEP_i$ is also referred to as auto-PEEP, dynamic hyperinflation, and breath stacking. For the remainder of this chapter it will be referred to as $PEEP_i$.

$PEEP_i$ can cause hemodynamic instability secondary to decreased venous return, just like high levels of PEEP.[7] $PEEP_i$ may be detected in two ways: (1) evaluation of the flow-time trace or (2) disconnection of the patient from the ventilator and listening for additional exhaled gas after an exhalation should have occurred.[6] The flow-time trace will demonstrate that the exhalation is not yet completed before the next breath has been initiated (Fig. 8-6).[8]

INDICATIONS FOR MECHANICAL VENTILATION

There are wide-ranging reasons for patients to require MV in the ED, and there are no absolute contraindications. Many time-honored indications for invasive ventilation are now identified as appropriate indications for noninvasive ventilation and are addressed later. Indications for MV range from loss of airway anatomy (edema, direct or indirect trauma, burns, infection), loss of protective airway mechanisms (intoxicants, brain injury, stroke), inability to ventilate, inability to oxygenate, or the expected clinical course. Indications for ET intubation may be separated into several

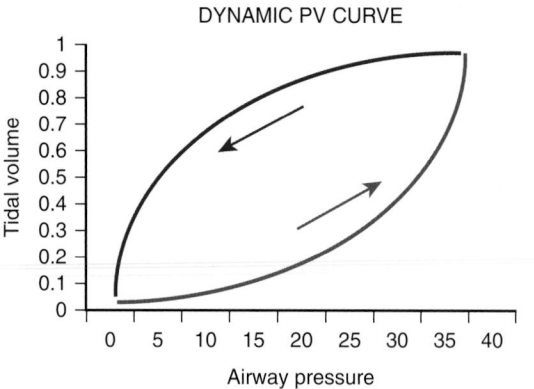

Figure 8-4 Dynamic pressure-volume (PV) loop. Note that as soon as pressure is delivered to the airway, there is an increase in measured tidal volume. The *lower arrow* denotes inspiration and the upper arrow indicates exhalation. This indicates that the airways are open and do not need to be forced open by increasing the pressure in the airway. If this latter case were true, the PV loop would initially be flat along the x-axis.

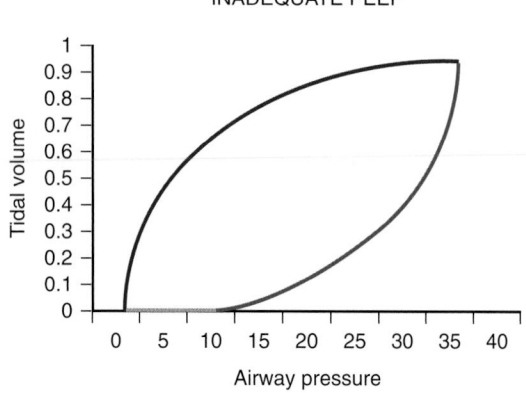

Figure 8-5 Inadequate positive end-expiratory pressure (PEEP) and the pressure-volume loop. Compare this curve with that in Figure 8-4. Note that the loop is initially flat (*lower segment*) along the x-axis. Once airway pressure is high enough to open the alveolar units, each increase in airway pressure is matched by a corresponding increase in tidal volume.

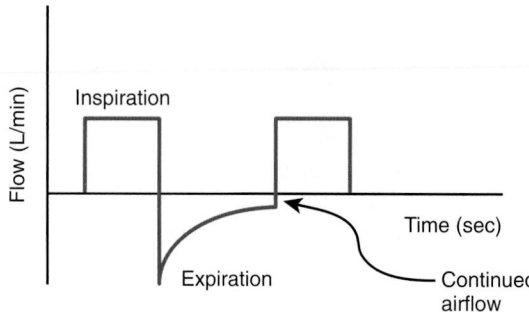

Figure 8-6 Schematic of a flow-time curve showing potential air trapping. Note that full exhalation has not occurred before initiation of the next breath. This is seen by the fact that flow has not reached zero when the next breath is given. A square waveform is being used in this example. Continuation of this state can lead to intrinsic positive end-expiratory pressure.

categories—emergency, urgent, delayed, and elective—based on the urgency of establishing a definitive airway.

EQUIPMENT—STANDARD OPTIONS

Perhaps one of the most confusing aspects of MV is the plethora of terms and acronyms that are used. Understanding the basic terminology helps clarify this subject. The following discussion explores machine features and settings. Regardless of which ventilator is used, a limited number of standard features are common to each (Fig. 8-7).

Set Respiratory Rate

Most ventilators allow the clinician to set a respiratory rate. The respiratory rate and actual V_T determine a patient's minute ventilation. Patients intubated for airway protection because of trauma or toxicosis often do well with a normal minute ventilation. Initially setting the respiratory rate at 10 to 14 breaths/min and V_T at 7 to 8 mL/kg ideal body weight (IBW) is usually sufficient. Adjustments can be made based on arterial blood gas (ABG) analysis, end-tidal CO_2, or venous blood gas and pulse oximetry. Patients who are septic or have severe acidosis often require higher minute ventilation. Respiratory rates can be increased, as can V_T, but volumes higher than 10 mL/kg IBW should not be used because of the risk of inducing ventilator-associated lung injury. In special scenarios such as acute lung injury (ALI) and acute respiratory distress syndrome (ARDS), initial V_T values should be lowered

to 6 mL/kg IBW within 2 hours of intubation. Some of these specific scenarios are discussed later.

Fraction of Inspired Oxygen

All ventilators can deliver an adjustable fraction of inspired oxygen (F_{IO_2}). Recommendations are to set it initially at 1.0 because the act of transitioning from negative pressure ventilation (normal physiologic breathing) to positive pressure ventilation (PPV) may unpredictably alter ventilation-perfusion ($\dot{V}/\dot{Q}$) matching. Although initially an F_{IO_2} of 100% is optimal, it is beneficial to quickly titrate F_{IO_2} down because of the theoretical risk for oxygen toxicity. Make adjustments based on ABG analysis or pulse oximetry, with a goal of keeping arterial P_{O_2} higher than 60 mm Hg or arterial oxygen saturation at 88% to 92% to avoid potential oxygen toxicity (see Table 3-3 in Chapter 3). Such adjustments may best be accomplished in the ICU rather than the ED, after the entire clinical scenario can be analyzed and all interventions are appropriately adjusted.

Positive End-Expiratory Pressure

$PEEP_e$ is typically set at 5 to 8 cm H_2O. Most patients should be started at a PEEP of 5 cm H_2O, which is considered a physiologic level. It is used to offset the gradual loss of functional residual volume (FRC) in supine, mechanically ventilated patients. PEEP can be increased by 2 cm H_2O every 10 to 15 minutes as needed or tolerated by patients who remain hypoxic. The initial goal is to reduce F_{IO_2} to nontoxic levels. This goal is coming under increasing scrutiny as new information challenges the time frame and concept of O_2-induced lung injury at F_{IO_2} levels greater than 0.6.[9] Exercise care when using PEEP levels higher than 8 cm H_2O in the setting of elevated intracranial pressure (ICP),[10] unilateral lung processes, hypotension, hypovolemia, or pulmonary embolism. High PEEP can potentially lead to hypotension as it increases intrathoracic pressure and decreases venous return and subsequently cardiac output.

Flow Rate

The flow rate is the speed, in liters per minute, that the ventilator is delivering gas. It is found in volume-targeted modes, but not pressure-targeted modes. The flow rate is typically set at 60 L/min, which means that a set V_T will be delivered at that speed. Patients wanting higher flow rates will not receive them and may display air hunger. Increase flow rates to deliver the set volume faster and shorten the inspiratory time (thereby increasing the inspiratory-to-expiratory [I/E] time ratio).

Waveform

The waveform determines how the ventilator delivers the flow of gas. It is traditionally set to a "decelerating waveform" in an effort to optimize recruitment because of different time constants in the lung.

Decelerating (Ramp)

Once the maximal inspiratory flow is reached, the rate of gas delivery immediately begins to slow in a preprogrammed fashion. When compared with the square waveform, longer time is spent in inhalation to deliver the set V_T or achieve the

Figure 8-7 The Nellcor Puritan Bennett 840 Ventilator system (Mansfield, MA). Selected features common to all ventilators include the respiratory rate (*A*), F_{IO_2} (*B*), positive end-expiratory pressure (PEEP) (*C*), waveform (*D*), inspiratory-to-expiratory ratio (I/E) (*E*), and trigger (*F*).

target pressure and allow improved oxygenation. This waveform also achieves lower peak airway pressure and higher mean airway pressure.

Square

Once the maximal inspiratory flow rate is achieved, gas flow is constant until the set volume is delivered. When that point is reached, gas flow is terminated. This waveform is best for patients with asthma, COPD, and head injury because gas delivered with this waveform allows a longer expiratory time (T_e, thereby increasing the I/E time ratio) and lower mean airway pressure. The longer T_e is beneficial for patients with restrictive airway disease such as asthma or COPD. Spending a longer time in exhalation allows improved venous drainage from the brain and greater loss of trapped V_T. The drawback with this waveform is increased peak airway pressure, which often requires lower V_T. This can lead to inadequate alveolar recruitment in patients with ALI.

I/E Time Ratio

The ratio of inspiratory time (the time that it takes to take a breath) to expiratory time (the time that it takes to exhale a breath) is automatically reported in some modes, whereas in others it is dialed in.

The normal I/E ratio in a spontaneously breathing, nonintubated patient is 1:4.[11] Intubated patients commonly achieve I/E ratios of 1:2. Shorter ratios may lead to decreased exhalation by compromising T_e. In its extreme form, inverse ratio ventilation (IRV), the normal pattern of breathing is reversed. A longer time is spent in inhalation to allow more time for oxygenation and recruitment. The decrease in T_e can lead to air trapping, elevated mean airway pressure, and rising P_{CO_2}. These problems lead to hypercapnia, respiratory acidosis, and $PEEP_i$[12] (Fig. 8-8).

Trigger

The trigger is the aspect that initiates a machine-generated breath. The trigger can be set to detect either a pressure or a flow gradient. It should be set so that the patient can trigger the ventilator without great effort.

Sensitivity

This refers to the sensitivity of the trigger. If the trigger is set too high (not sensitive enough), the work of breathing incurred by the patient can be substantial. Some providers have been known to set the sensitivity at a high level if the patient is markedly overbreathing the set rate. This is not recommended because it causes an undue increase in the work of breathing. Many ventilators are set to a pressure trigger with a sensitivity of 1 to 3 cm H_2O.[13] If the sensitivity is set too low (too sensitive), the ventilator can "auto-trigger" (inappropriate initiation of machine-generated breaths) because of oscillating water in the ventilator tubing, hyperdynamic heartbeats, or patient movement.

MODES OF VENTILATION

Once some of the standard features are understood, the next step is determining the ventilator's target. Most ventilators can be set to achieve spontaneous breathing, volume-targeted ventilation, pressure-targeted ventilation, or some combination. In volume-targeted ventilation, the ventilator is set to reach a determined volume regardless of the pressure required to do so. Pressure-targeted modes are set to reach a determined pressure regardless of the volume generated. Dual modes combine the benefits of both strategies (Fig. 8-9).

Spontaneous Breathing

Spontaneously breathing patients can be supported on the ventilator by pressure support ventilation (PSV). In this mode the ventilator provides a supplemental inspiratory pressure to each of the patient-generated breaths. The clinician sets F_{IO_2} and PEEP. The patient dictates the respiratory rate and generates the desired flow rate. The applied pressure is turned off once the flow decreases to a predetermined percentage. V_T is dictated by the pressure support given, patient effort, and compliance of the respiratory system. There is no set respiratory rate, although most modern ventilators have a backup apnea rate.

FLOW RATE: IMPACT ON T_i AND T_e

Equal V_T but different T_i and T_e

Figure 8-8 Effect of flow rate on inspiratory (T_i) and expiratory (T_e) time. Note that as the flow rate changes, there are corresponding alterations in the effective times for inspiration and exhalation. Deflections above the x-axis (time) indicate inspiration, and those below indicate exhalation. The tidal volume (V_T) delivered for each cycle is the same, but T_i and T_e are different.

Initial Ventilator Settings for Standard Patient
VCV: AC, RR 10–14, V_T 7–8 mL/kg IBW, PEEP 5, F_{IO_2} 100% Flow rate 60 L/min, Decelerating waveform
PCV: AC, RR 12–16, pressure high 20, PEEP 5, F_{IO_2} 100% • Monitor size of V_T obtained with this pressure, adjust pressure to obtain a V_T around 7–8 mL/kg IBW
• SIMV can be picked for either VCV or PCV. If SIMV is picked, add PSV at a sufficient level to obtain an adequate V_T
• Adjust F_{IO_2} based on PO_x or PaO_2 • Adjust PEEP based on hypoxia • Adjust minute ventilation based on blood pH (remember that on AC, decreasing the RR does not change minute ventilation in a patient breathing over the set rate)

Figure 8-9 Initial ventilator settings for standard patients. *AC,* assist/control mode; *F_{IO_2},* fraction of inspired oxygen; *IBW,* ideal body weight; *PEEP,* positive end-expiratory pressure; *PCV,* pressure-cycled ventilation; *PSV,* pressure support ventilation; *RR,* respiratory rate; *SIMV,* synchronized intermittent mandatory ventilation; *VCV,* volume-cycled ventilation; *V_T,* tidal volume.

Volume-Cycled Ventilation

Volume-cycled ventilation (VCV) may also be termed volume-limited, volume-control, volume-assist, or volume-targeted ventilation. Volume-targeted modes are the most commonly used and the most familiar mode of MV in adults. As its name implies, "volume"—in this case V_T—is the ventilator's targeted parameter. With this target, the ventilator seeks to deliver a preset amount of gas. The ventilator will generate the necessary driving pressure to reach this "target." In addition to V_T, the clinician sets the desired respiratory rate, F_{IO_2}, and PEEP. It should be noted that other important aspects of the mechanical ventilator can be controlled in this setting, such as waveform (decelerating or square), I:E ratio, flow rate, trigger, and sensitivity.

The time of gas flow is determined by the set volume, flow rate, and waveform of gas delivery. When the set volume is reached, gas flow is terminated and expiration passively begins. An advantage is that VCV delivers a reliable volume, but it does not take into account dynamic changes in lung compliance, which may alter the ability of the lung to accept delivered gas in gas-exchanging alveoli.

Pressure-Cycled Ventilation

Pressure-cycled ventilation (PCV) may also be termed pressure-limited, pressure-control, pressure-assist, or pressure-targeted ventilation. As its name implies, "pressure" is the ventilator's targeted parameter. The ventilator will generate an inspiratory pressure that has been set by the clinician. With this target, the ventilator alters gas flow to achieve and maintain a preset airway pressure for the duration of a preset inspiratory time (T_i). Gas flow is terminated when the preset pressure is achieved. The volume delivered is determined by the compliance of the patient's respiratory system, airway resistance, T_i, and the pressure target. In addition, the clinician sets the desired PEEP, respiratory rate, F_{IO_2}, T_i, I:E ratio, and trigger mode. Pressure is maintained with a variable or intermittent flow rate for the set T_i. In the setting of hypoxemia, T_i may be increased quite precisely to increase mean airway pressure and oxygenation. This strategy is much more difficult, if not impossible, to manipulate with VCV.

An advantage of PCV is that airway pressure is tightly managed to limit or eliminate alveolar overdistention and to reduce ventilator-induced lung injury.[14] It should be noted that the clinician does not control waveform or peak inspiratory flow. Patients can generate their desired flow rate and thus reduce air hunger. Pressure-targeted modes, which are growing in popularity, might have better pressure distribution, improved dissemination of airway pressure, and greater distribution of ventilation.[14]

One problem with PCV is that the volume received by the patient is potentially variable. Any change in system compliance or resistance (or both) will affect the V_T generated. For example, if the patient bites on the ET tube or a mucus plug develops, the set pressure that was generating an adequate volume will no longer do so. In contrast, a sudden increase in system compliance might result in the generation of V_T that may be considerably larger than desired. Instead of the traditional pressure alarm limits, one must adjust and be cognizant of V_T and minute ventilation alarm settings. Uncertainties such as these have led many clinicians to favor volume-targeted strategies or dual controlled strategies in the acute care setting.

Modes of Ventilation Commonly Used in the ED

Assist/control (AC) and synchronized intermittent mandatory ventilation (SIMV) are the ventilation modes most commonly used in the ED. Both are acceptable, and no data have demonstrated a better outcome with either mode. Other modes are also acceptable based on clinician preference.

Assist/Control Ventilation

Here, ventilator-initiated breaths, known as *machine breaths* (i.e., control breaths), are provided at a preset rate. Every breath is fully supported by the ventilator, regardless of whether the breath is initiated by the patient or the ventilator. The clinician sets the base ventilation rate, but if the patient tries to breathe faster than the set rate, additional breaths can be initiated by the patient, known as *spontaneous breaths* (i.e., assist breaths). A potential downside is inappropriate hyperventilation.

AC modes may be either volume or pressure cycled. Both assist breaths and control breaths will reach the set target, be it a set volume (in a volume-targeted mode) or a set pressure (in a pressure-targeted mode). In VCV, the spontaneous breath receives the same V_T that is set for the machine breath. In PCV, the spontaneous breath receives the same *pressure* that is set for the machine breath. To be more specific, in the *volume-targeted mode*, the clinician sets V_T, as well as the inspiratory flow rate, flow waveform, sensitivity to the patient's respiratory effort (i.e., trigger), and the basal ventilatory rate. In the *pressure-targeted mode*, the clinician determines the basal ventilatory rate and how sensitive the ventilator will be to the patient's respiratory effort and also selects pressure levels and T_i. Hence in this mode V_T is not set by the ventilator but is dependent on the compliance of the lung and chest wall and airway pressure. This helps avoid pressure-induced lung injury, but a specific V_T is not guaranteed.

For the patient to trigger the ventilator and initiate flow for a spontaneous breath, mean airway pressure must decrease by a preset amount below PEEP if set on a pressure trigger or flow to be generated if set on a flow trigger. The amount necessary to open the inflow valve is the sensitivity setting.

Caution should be exercised *to avoid auto-PEEP* (also known as breath stacking) when using volume-targeted AC modes. Because each mechanically delivered breath is given at full V_T, patients with a high actual respiratory rate on AC may not have sufficient time to completely exhale between breaths. This results in progressive air trapping, which leads to an increase in auto-PEEP ($PEEP_i$) (see Fig. 8-6). This is of clinical concern in patients with asthma, in whom auto-PEEP can significantly reduce cardiac output and even promote cardiovascular collapse.

Synchronized Intermittent Mechanical Ventilation

SIMV provides breaths at a preset rate (machine breath), similar to the AC mode. The patient can *initiate an additional spontaneous breath* between the mandated or preset number of ventilator-supported breaths. Such spontaneous breaths above the preset ventilatory rate *are not supported by the ventilator*, and the patient receives only a spontaneous V_T that reflects the depth and time spent in the patient-controlled inspiration. For each of these nonmandatory (i.e., spontaneous) breaths, the patient has a high work of breathing. SIMV is typically partnered with PSV to aid in spontaneous breathing support and to overcome the intrinsic resistance associated with MV. This mode was initially recommended by those who thought that as a patient's need for mechanical ventilatory support decreased, the set respiratory rate could be decreased and the patient "weaned" to PSV alone and ensuing extubation. Subsequent data have shown that this method of liberation actually increases the number of ventilator days.[15] The synchronized version of intermittent MV allows the ventilator to attempt to coordinate spontaneous and machine breaths to prevent it from delivering a scheduled breath on top of a spontaneous breath or during exhalation after a spontaneous breath. This could lead to elevated mean airway pressure, alveolar overdistention, and biotrauma.[16]

Both volume-targeted ventilation and pressure-targeted ventilation modes can be set to either an AC or SIMV mode to achieve the desired minute ventilation. In a chemically paralyzed patient with no intrinsic respiratory drive, AC and SIMV look virtually identical. Both will reach their target (volume or pressure) at the set rate. If a patient triggers the ventilator at a rate greater than the set rate, these two strategies diverge. In AC, each breath above the set respiratory rate will result in a full mechanically supported breath to reach either the set volume or pressure target. In SIMV, the ventilator will give only the set number of breaths that the clinician has selected. Each additional breath will require the patient to generate a spontaneous V_T without mechanical assistance. This patient-generated breath must overcome any resistance caused by the artificial airway and ventilator circuitry. Pressure support should be added to SIMV for patient-generated breaths to reduce any increase in the work of breathing related to the resistance imposed by the ventilator circuit and ET tube.

Advanced Modes of Mechanical Ventilation

Dual Control Modes

Advanced modes of mechanical ventilation use a closed-loop ventilator logic that combines the features of volume- and pressure-targeted ventilation (Box 8-1). These modes automatically alter control variables, either breath to breath or within a breath, to ensure a minimum V_T or minute ventilation.[17] Detailed explanation of these modes is beyond the scope of this chapter. If these modes are encountered, one should discuss options with a respiratory therapist and critical care medicine specialist.

Other Modes

High-Frequency Ventilation

High-frequency ventilation (HFV) attempts to achieve adequate gas exchange by using asymmetric velocity profiles when combining very high respiratory rates with V_T levels that are smaller than the volume of anatomic dead space. It is used more commonly in neonates and infants with neonatal respiratory failure. There has been renewed interest in using HFV in adult patients with ALI or ARDS under the rationale that the small V_T may cause less ventilator-associated lung injury. More trials are necessary to determine whether HFV can improve mortality outcomes in these patients.[18]

BOX 8-1	Advanced Modes of Mechanical Ventilation

BREATH TO BREATH

Pressure-regulated volume control (PRVC)
Auto flow
Volume control plus (VC+)
Adaptive pressure ventilation (APV)
Variable-pressure control (VPC)

WITHIN A BREATH

Volume-assured pressure support ventilation (VAPSV)
Pressure augmentation

OTHER

High-frequency ventilation (HFV)
Airway pressure release ventilation (APRV)
Bilevel
Proportional assist ventilation

Airway Pressure Release Ventilation and Bi-Level Ventilation

Both these modes are proprietary names yet function in essentially the same manner. The clinician sets a pressure high, a pressure low, and a time at each level (time high and time low). Although at first glance this appears to be similar to PCV, it differs markedly in that the majority of time is spent at pressure high with brief periods at pressure low. The patient typically spends 4 to 6 seconds in time high. Pressure high may be as high as 40 cm H_2O or greater. Ventilation occurs during the release from pressure high to pressure low. Time low is typically 0.2 to 0.8 second in restrictive lung disease and 0.8 to 1.5 seconds in obstructive lung disease. It is probably prudent to start at 0.8 and titrate to meet individual patient requirements. Time low is also referred to as the release phase.[19] The long time that high-level pressure is maintained achieves oxygenation, and the short release period achieves clearance of CO_2 (Fig. 8-10). The long time at high-level pressure results in substantial recruitment of alveoli from markedly different regional time constants at rather low gas flow rates. The establishment of $PEEP_i$ by the short release time enhances oxygenation. CO_2 clearance is aided by recruitment of the patient's lung at close to total lung capacity. Elastic recoil creates large-volume gas flow during the release period.

In a paralyzed patient, airway pressure release ventilation and bilevel ventilation (APRV/Bi-Level) are identical to pressure-targeted IRV. For these reasons, some have described this mode as *inverse ratio ventilation*. A major difference between APRV/Bi-Level and IRV is that IRV typically requires chemical paralysis or heavy sedation. APRV/Bi-Level is a fundamentally different mode from cyclic ventilation. This mode allows the patient to spontaneously breathe during all phases of the cycle, thus making it relatively more comfortable and reducing the level of sedation or paralysis needed. This mode is enabled to succeed by having a floating valve that is responsive to the patient's needs, regardless of the location within the respiratory cycle. The patient is allowed to breathe in or out during the pressure high phase and during the release phase. Accordingly, the sequence is called a *phase*

Figure 8-10 Airway pressure release ventilation (APRV)—airway pressure-time and flow-time traces. Note that peak airway pressure (P$_{aw}$ high) is maintained for a long period. This phase establishes oxygenation (T$_{high}$). There is a short period of release when most CO$_2$ is cleared (T$_{low}$). The bottom trace indicates flow over time. The combined time for T$_{high}$ and T$_{low}$ is known as a *phase cycle*. Note that the number of phase cycles is not the respiratory rate because patients breathe within the entirety of T$_{high}$. As the release phase is initiated, the flow rate is identified as negative and is of a high rate (here, ≈7.5 L/min), consistent with significant alveolar recruitment. During the high continuous positive airway pressure (CPAP) phase, the patient is allowed to exhale (negative deflections on the flow-time trace). Thus, APRV is quite dissimilar from traditional cyclic ventilation. This unique mode is made possible by a floating valve system.

Figure 8-11 Continuous positive airway pressure (CPAP) mask (Vital Signs, Inc., Totowa, NJ). The device shown provides continuous positive airway pressure and is run simply by attaching the mask tubing to a wall oxygen source. The amount of CPAP delivered can be adjusted by changing the threshold resistor valve (*arrow*).

cycle. There is no T$_i$ or T$_e$ and no readily identifiable respiratory rate in the traditional sense. During the pressure high phase, patients may exhale 50 to 200 mL or more of gas as the lung volume becomes full of gas. This is not a full exhalation, and the release of excess gas should not be counted as a breath. APRV has been used successfully for neonatal, pediatric, and adult forms of respiratory failure. It is considered an alternative open–lung model approach to MV.[19]

Given the spontaneous nature of the mode, there should be virtually no need for continuous infusion of neuromuscular blocking drugs in patients placed on this mode of ventilation. This may result in a shorter length of ICU stay and a reduced incidence of prolonged neuromuscular blockade syndrome. The need for sedatives is reduced because patients are more comfortable on this spontaneous mode than on cyclic ventilation.[20] APRV/Bi-Level has gained popularity in patients with hypoxemic respiratory failure because it improves oxygenation by optimizing alveolar recruitment and $\dot{V}/\dot{Q}$ matching.[21]

A common mistake with this mode is setting time low too long. This essentially mimics a pressure-targeted SIMV strategy. Transport of patients on APRV with pressure high greater than 20 cm H$_2$O should occur with the patient attached to the ventilator instead of being hand-ventilated.[22] Hand ventilation is unable to match the manner of gas delivery and pressure dynamics that the patient requires. Attempts at hand ventilation, even with an appropriately set PEEP valve, are frequently complicated by unexpected hypoxemia and hemodynamic instability.

Noninvasive Positive Pressure Ventilation

Noninvasive ventilation is defined as the provision of ventilatory assistance without an invasive artificial airway. Noninvasive ventilators consist of both negative and positive pressure ventilators. Because negative pressure ventilation is so rarely used today, our discussion is limited to PPV.

Before the 1960s, the use of negative pressure ventilation in the form of a tank ventilator (the "iron lung") was the most common form of MV outside the anesthesia suite. It was not until the 1952 polio epidemic in Copenhagen that anesthesiologist Bjorn Ibsen showed that he could improve the survival of patients with respiratory paralysis by using invasive PPV.

Nonetheless, negative pressure or "iron lungs" were the mainstay of ventilatory support for patients with chronic respiratory failure until as late as the mid-1980s. In the early 1980s, nasal continuous positive airway pressure (CPAP) was introduced to treat obstructive sleep apnea. These tightly fitting masks proved to be an effective means of assisting ventilation, and noninvasive positive pressure ventilation (NPPV) quickly displaced traditional negative pressure ventilation as the treatment of choice for chronic respiratory failure in patients with neuromuscular and chest wall deformities. Current NPPV devices are able to provide a set respiratory rate, set V$_T$, and set F$_{IO_2}$. The use of NPPV has also been integrated into the acute inpatient setting, where it is now used to treat acute respiratory failure.[23]

Definitions

The current literature uses different definitions for NPPV. Although some authors use NPPV as an umbrella term that includes CPAP and bilevel positive airway pressure, more recently, authors have used the term NPPV as synonymous with bilevel and consider CPAP a separate entity. The terms NPPV and noninvasive intermittent positive pressure ventilation (NIPPV) are often used interchangeably with bilevel.

As its name suggests, CPAP supplies continuous positive pressure via a tightly fitting face mask (Fig. 8-11). NPPV or bilevel provides an inspiratory positive airway pressure (IPAP)

Figure 8-12 Bilevel positive airway pressure (BiPAP) S/T noninvasive ventilation system (Philips Respironics, Inc, Andover, MA). Adjustable parameters include inspiratory positive airway pressure, expiratory positive airway pressure, and breaths per minute. Both BiPAP and continuous positive airway pressure are used to support ventilation in patients with decompensated congestive heart failure, chronic obstructive pulmonary disease, pneumonia, and asthma, but neither mode has a clear benefit over the other.

in addition to end-expiratory positive airway pressure (EPAP), and breaths are usually triggered by the patient (Fig. 8-12). On many such devices, backup rates may be set that deliver bilevel pressure, even if patients fail to initiate a breath.

Rationale for Using NPPV

The most important advantage of NPPV is avoiding the complications associated with invasive MV. It has been well documented that invasive MV increases the incidence of airway and lung injury and augments the risk for nosocomial pneumonia. NPPV avoids these complications by keeping the upper airway defense mechanisms intact and allows the patient to retain the ability to eat, clear secretions, and communicate normally when NPPV is used intermittently (NIPPV).[23] NPPV has the potential to reduce the mortality of a selected group of patients with acute respiratory failure and may shorten hospital stays, thereby reducing cost. Specific to the ED, appropriate initiation of NPPV may avoid unnecessary intubation of certain patients, hence avoiding ICU admission, reducing cost, decreasing complications, and improving mortality.

Pathophysiologic Effects of NPPV

CPAP increases alveolar recruitment and size, thereby enhancing the area available for gas exchange, and improves the $\dot{V}/\dot{Q}$ relationship. The term CPAP is synonymous with $PEEP_e$ and bilevel EPAP. It can also negate the effects of $PEEP_i$. In patients with dynamic hyperinflation (such as asthma or COPD), an escalating $PEEP_i$ increases the magnitude of the drop in airway pressure that the patient must generate to trigger a breath. This causes increased work of breathing for the patient. Careful application of $PEEP_e$ can reduce this gradient and decrease the patient's work of breathing. PPV also creates an increase in intrathoracic pressure. This causes preload to decrease as a result of diminished venous return and also decreases transmural pressure, which reduces afterload.[24]

In NPPV, IPAP is similar to pressure support and, when combined with EPAP, further augments alveolar ventilation,

thereby allowing some rest of the respiratory muscles during the inspiratory phase (Box 8-2).

Acute Exacerbation of Chronic Obstructive Pulmonary Disease

Numerous studies have shown that NPPV can reduce the need for intubation, length of hospital stay, and in-hospital mortality in patients with acute exacerbations of COPD.[25,26] NPPV should be initiated early and along with standard medical therapy. If it is started late, after the failure of medical treatment, the benefits conferred by NPPV (hospital mortality, length of ICU stay, number of days on the ventilator, overall complications) are eliminated.[27] Early implementation of NPPV in patients seen in the ED with an acute exacerbation of COPD and without contraindications should be considered the standard of care.

Acute Cardiogenic Pulmonary Edema

CPAP has been shown to produce a reduction in the rate of intubation and a trend toward decreasing mortality.[28] CPAP and NPPV both reduce the risk of intubation in the ED.[29] An early article described an increased rate of acute myocardial infarction in patients with acute cardiogenic pulmonary edema treated with NPPV,[30] but several subsequent trials have refuted this increased risk for myocardial infarction.

Hypoxemic Respiratory Failure

Although some of the literature suggests that NPPV may be beneficial in the setting of acute hypoxemic respiratory failure, doubt still exists. A large multicenter trial of NPPV in patients with acute hypoxemic respiratory failure that excludes patients with cardiogenic pulmonary edema and COPD may help clarify the use of NPPV in this setting.

NPPV has been used increasingly in the ICU for hypoxemic respiratory failure. It can be considered for patients who are hemodynamically stable with single-organ (i.e., pulmonary) failure, but extremely close monitoring is required.

Immunosuppressed Patients

When faced with a severely immunosuppressed patient with acute hypoxemic respiratory failure in the ED, early initiation of NPPV may be beneficial in avoiding the serious complications of ET intubation. NPPV can keep upper airway defenses intact and minimize the risk for ventilator-associated pneumonia, which is universally fatal in these patients.[31] NPPV has been shown to be associated with a lower rate of ET intubation, shorter ICU stay, and lower ICU mortality. In-house mortality did not differ significantly.[32]

"Do-Not-Intubate/Do-Not-Resuscitate" Patients

In do-not-intubate/do-not-resuscitate (DNR/DNI) patients willing to undergo NPPV, success would be measured by

Properly fit face mask
Explain the procedure to the patient
Encourage the patient

Initial NPPV Settings

Low-High Approach:
 IPAP 10, EPAP 5, F_{IO_2} 100%

High-Low Approach:
 IPAP 20–25, EPAP 5, F_{IO_2} 100%

Start with an EPAP of 8 if morbid obesity or intrisic PEEP

- Titrate IPAP up (low-high) or down (high-low) based on dyspnea, decreased respiratory rate, increased tidal volume, and patient-ventilator synchrony
- Increase PSV (IPAP-EPAP) if hypercapnic
- Titrate F_{IO_2} to keep PO_x at 86–92%
- Increase EPAP if hypoxic

Figure 8-13 Initiation of noninvasive positive pressure ventilation (NPPV). *EPAP,* end-expiratory positive airway pressure; *IPAP,* inspiratory positive airway pressure; *PEEP,* positive end-expiratory pressure; *PSV,* pressure support ventilation.

improved ventilation, oxygenation, and comfort. NPPV can provide support for the patient while the underlying cause of the respiratory failure is being treated. NPPV should be discontinued if it is not producing the desired response or if the patient is unable to tolerate this therapy. In these circumstances it should be a joint decision between the health care team, the patient, and the family to limit NPPV and transition toward comfort measures.

In patients who have chosen to forego any life-sustaining therapy and are receiving comfort care measures, NPPV might be used as a form of palliative care in an attempt to reduce the associated dyspnea. In this circumstance, the use of NPPV is considered successful if it alleviates the patient's symptoms. If it causes any discomfort to the patient, it should be discontinued. This use of NPPV is controversial, and no studies have assessed the benefits of NPPV in these patients.[33] Another use of NPPV in patients who have chosen comfort care measures is a time-limited trial to achieve the goal of survival until the arrival of family and friends. In this situation, NPPV would be used to provide life support until friends and family can achieve closure.

Even if a patient with a known do-not-intubate advance directive arrives at the ED with acute respiratory failure of reversible etiology, it can be beneficial discussing the use of NPPV with the patient and family. In this situation, communication about the expectations and goals of care is of utmost importance.

Initiation of NPPV

There is no standard approach to the initiation of NPPV. Different methods have been used in clinical trials, yet these methods have never been compared. There are two main strategies: a high-low approach and a low-high approach (Fig. 8-13).

Emphasis should be placed on the importance of close follow-up of patients in whom NPPV is started in the ED. It is important to serially assess patient response as soon as 30 minutes after the initiation of NPPV. Those who are persistently tachypneic and acidemic should be considered for intubation sooner rather than later. It is imperative to

BOX 8-3 Contraindications to Noninvasive Positive Pressure Ventilation

Impending cardiovascular collapse or respiratory arrest
Severe upper gastrointestinal bleeding
Facial surgery, trauma, or deformity limiting placement of the mask
Upper airway obstruction
Inability to cooperate or protect the airway, altered mental status
Inability to clear respiratory secretions
High risk for aspiration

closely observe patients for deterioration. ABGs should be checked within 1 to 2 hours after initiation of NPPV to assess treatment success or failure. Patients who do not improve clinically should be considered for intubation.

Cautions with the Use of NPPV

Most studies involving NPPV have excluded patients who were hemodynamically unstable, had an altered level of consciousness, or were unable to protect their airway. This was based on the concern that a depressed sensorium would predispose the patient to aspiration. The International Consensus Conference in Intensive Care Medicine on Noninvasive Positive Pressure Ventilation in Acute Respiratory Failure held in April 2000 considered the presence of severe encephalopathy, as manifested by a Glasgow Coma Scale score lower than 10, to be a contraindication to NPPV.[34]

Other accepted contraindications to NPPV are listed in Box 8-3.

Recently, studies have looked specifically at the use of NPPV in patients with hypercapnic coma secondary to acute respiratory failure. This was based on the observation that some do-not-intubate patients who declined intubation had successful outcomes with NPPV therapy despite their initial comatose state. Diaz and colleagues conducted an observational study and found that success rates were comparable between the comatose and noncomatose group.[35] Scala and coworkers performed two studies, both showing that NPPV could be used successfully in treating patients with exacerbations of COPD and hypercapnic encephalopathy. Their 2007 study showed that performance of NPPV by an experienced team led to similar short- and long-term survival, fewer nosocomial infections, and shorter durations of hospitalization than in patients who underwent MV.[36,37] Of note, these studies were conducted in the ICU[35] or specialized respiratory care units[37] with a nursing ratio of at least 1:3. The patients were very closely monitored by staff while they received NPPV. This high nursing-to-patient ratio may not be feasible in a busy ED, however.

The other key point in these studies was the rapid improvement in neurologic status that occurred 1 to 2 hours after the initiation of NPPV. The importance of close monitoring of patients in whom NPPV is started is crucial in identifying those who will fail this therapy.

High-Flow Nasal Cannula

The high-flow nasal cannula (HFNC) is a relatively new oxygen delivery system. A conventional nasal cannula uses a low-flow system and at higher flow (>6 L/min) can cause nasal dryness, epistaxis, and patient discomfort. The HFNC system (Fig. 8-14) is a novel device that combines oxygen, pressurized

Figure 8-14 High-flow nasal cannula system. *A,* High-flow flowmeter; *B,* oxygen blender; *C,* low-flow flowmeter; *D,* nasal cannula; *E,* low compliance, heated-wire circuit; *F,* high-flow humidifier; *G,* water reservoir; *H,* air/O_2 supply. *(From Yeow ME, Santanilla JI. Noninvasive positive pressure ventilation in the emergency department. Emerg Med Clin North Am. 2008;26:835-847).*

air, and warm humidification to deliver tolerable flow of up to 40 L/min through a nasal cannula. FIO_2 and flow rates can be adjusted. With higher flow, less room-air entrainment occurs, and the higher flow rates match the dyspneic patient's increased minute ventilation.

Its use has been studied more extensively for neonatal respiratory care, where ongoing studies suggest that HFNC may be as effective as nasal CPAP in preterm neonates.[38] One study looked at the effect of HFNC on exercise performance in adults with COPD.[39] Currently, there are no published studies that have investigated the use of HFNC in patients with acute respiratory failure. Anecdotally, this system has been used with some success in adults in the ICU, with immunosuppressed patients being targeted in the hope of avoiding intubation. It seems to be better tolerated than NPPV, and at higher flow it is believed to provide a certain amount of continuous positive pressure. More studies will have to be performed before this technology becomes a mainstay of treatment in patients with acute respiratory failure.

Conclusions
NPPV has been shown to work well in patients with reversible conditions and acts as a bridge while allowing medical therapy (e.g., bronchodilators, steroids, diuretics) to take effect, thereby potentially avoiding the need for ET intubation.

Those with less reversible causes of their acute respiratory failure (ARDS, pneumonia) may be less likely to respond. With careful patient selection, NPPV can be safely initiated in the ED, give time for medical treatment to work, and potentially avoid ICU admission. Patients being considered for intubation should be evaluated for the potential use of NPPV.

Close monitoring and follow-up of patients placed on NPPV is crucial in determining whether the therapy has been successful or whether further intervention is needed. In EDs in which the staff has been adequately trained, selected patients, even those in a hypercapnic coma, can be considered for a short trial of NPPV. Extreme diligence in monitoring these patients must be used, and if improvement is not seen in 1 to 2 hours, intubation should not be delayed.

NEUROMUSCULAR BLOCKADE/PARALYZING AGENT FOR MECHANICALLY VENTILATED PATIENTS

The short-term administration of paralyzing agents, in addition to sedation and analgesia, for mechanically ventilated patients in the ED is appropriate to improve patient-ventilator synchrony, enhance gas exchange, diminish the risk for barotrauma, decrease muscle oxygen consumption, facilitate short procedures, and prevent movement in patients with elevated ICP. Importantly, *neuromuscular blocking agents (NMBAs) have no sedative, amnestic, or analgesic properties, and all patients administered such an agent must receive concomitant sedation and analgesia.* After proper sedation and analgesia, short-term administration of paralyzing agents may be considered to improve patient-ventilator synchrony, enhance gas exchange, diminish the risk for barotrauma, decrease muscle oxygen consumption, facilitate short procedures, and prevent movement in patients with elevated ICP.

The long-term use of chemical paralysis in the ICU has greatly diminished because of prolonged recovery secondary to drug and metabolite accumulation. Cases of prolonged paralysis, also known as critical illness myopathy, postparalysis syndrome, polyneuropathy of critical illness, and acute quadriplegic myopathy syndrome, lead to protracted ICU stays.[40] In the ICU, daily discontinuation of NMBAs for a few hours or avoiding their use entirely has been recommended to potentially decrease the incidence of these conditions. When clinically feasible, it is advisable to stop administration of the NMBA in the ED and reassess the need for continued paralysis.

A number of drugs are available, but the nondepolarizing agents vecuronium and pancuronium are the most commonly prescribed agents for short-term paralysis in the ED.[41] Both are given by intermittent bolus administration as needed. Continuous infusion, though potentially useful, is rarely used or indicated in the ED. Nondepolarizing NMBAs can be reversed by neostigmine at a dose of 0.035 to 0.07 mg/kg.

Vecuronium has an intermediate duration of action with a half-life of 80 to 90 minutes, slightly longer in the elderly but not affected by renal or hepatic failure. Minimal adverse cardiovascular side effects have been reported, and there is minimal risk for hypotension. Vecuronium has minimal adverse cardiovascular effects and is the drug of choice for patients with cardiovascular disease or hemodynamic instability. The dose for intermittent bolus administration is 0.1 mg/kg.

SEDATIVES

Propofol, 5-80 μg/kg/min

Dexmedetomidine, 0.2-1.5 μg/kg/hr

Lorazepam, 1-5 mg IV prn; infusion at 0.5-7 mg/hr if multiple doses required

Midazolam, 1-6 mg IV prn

Haloperidol, 2-10 mg IV every 20-30 minutes until stable, then 25% of the loading dose q6h prn

Remifentanil infusion: 0.025-0.2 μg/kg/hr (no bolus used, provides both sedation and analgesia)

ANALGESICS

Fentanyl, 25-100 μg IV q15-30min prn

Hydromorphone, 0.2-1 mg IV prn

Morphine, 2-5 mg IV prn

Fentanyl infusion: 50-200 μg/hr if more than 2-3 boluses per hour of above agents are needed

prn, *as needed.*

Pancuronium is long acting with a half-life of 100 to 130 minutes. Its duration of action is prolonged in patients with renal or hepatic failure. There is a moderate risk for adverse cardiovascular effects associated with pancuronium, such as tachycardia, hypertension, and increased cardiac output secondary to vagal blockade. The dose for intermittent bolus administration is 0.05 to 0.1 mg/kg.

SEDATION

See Box 8-4 for common sedatives and analgesics. It is recommended that only the minimal amount needed to achieve comfort be used. Sedation should be targeted to a specific sedation scale (such as the Richmond Agitation Sedation Scale). Agents with a quick offset are preferable to improve spontaneous awakening and for breathing trials once the patient is a candidate for extubation. Benzodiazepines should be avoided if possible. If paralyzing drugs are used for neuromuscular blockade, it is imperative to provide aggressive sedation because pain and anxiety in paralyzed patients cannot be evaluated. *It is prudent to conclude that a paralyzed ventilated patient is awake and can hear and feel unless sedated.*

SPECIFIC DISEASE PROCESSES

Asthma and COPD (Fig. 8-15)

As asthma and COPD treatment (β-agonists, steroids) takes effect, peak pressure will begin to lower, the peak expiratory flow rate should increase, and the expiration flow time should shorten (Fig. 8-16). It is necessary to adequately sedate these patients because their hypercapnic state is a powerful stimulus to breath rapidly. Opiates such as fentanyl and sedatives such as propofol and ketamine have gained increased roles in these patients. Occasionally, one will be required to chemically weaken these patients with the use of paralytics to keep their respiratory rate and expiratory time controlled. This should

---

Peri-intubation

Monitor the rate of BVM ventilation
Provide an IVF bolus
Consider Ketamine as an induction agent if available
$NaHCO_3$ bolus if known to have a pH <7 before RSI

Initial Ventilator Settings

Volume targeted (VCV), AC, RR 8–10, VT 6 mL/kg IBW, PEEP 5, FIO_2 100%
Flow rate 80 L/min, square waveform
• These strategies may worsen hypercapnia (termed permissive hypercapnia) because of a decrease in minute ventilation and is tolerated if pH >7.15
• $NaHCO_3$ infusion or the administration of THAM (tris[hydroxymethyl] aminomethane) may be required to keep arterial pH above 7.15 to 7.20

After Intubation

Adequate sedation and analgesia. Consider the use of Propofol, Ketamine, or opiates
Monitor flow-time curves and pressure-time curves
Follow peak pressure and plateau pressure
Consider chemical weakening as a last resort (goal TOF 2–4)
Consider heliox if available

Figure 8-15 Initial ventilator settings for exacerbation of asthma. *AC,* assist/control mode; *BVM,* bag-valve-mask ventilation; *FIO_2,* fraction of inspired oxygen; *IBW,* ideal body weight; *IVF,* intravenous fluid; *PEEP,* positive end-expiratory pressure; *RR,* respiratory rate; *RSI,* rapid sequence induction; *TOF,* train of four; *VCV,* volume-cycled ventilation; *VT,* tidal volume.

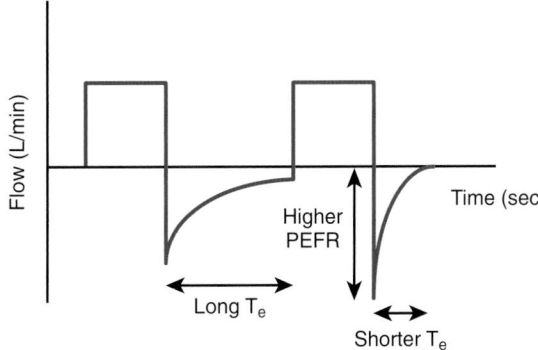

Figure 8-16 Schematic of a flow-time curve showing improvement in an obstructive process. Note that the peak expiratory flow rate (PEFR) increases and the expiratory time (T_e) decreases with improvement and flow reaches zero before the next breath is given.

be a final option and be done with the understanding that the side effects of steroids and paralytics can be quite devastating,[42,43] but paralysis cannot be avoided in certain cases. In the ICU, paralysis is commonly titrated to an effect monitored by a peripheral nerve monitor applied over the ulnar or other peripheral nerve distribution.[44] No blockade results in four twitches of the adductor pollicis muscle causing four supramaximal triggering stimuli; complete blockade yields no response. A common goal of blockade is to use enough of the agent to result in two twitches out of a "train of four." A peripheral nerve monitor is not commonly used in the ED and is not a standard intervention during resuscitation and interim ED care.

Valuable information can be gained from flow-time curves and pressure-time curves. Improvement (Fig. 8-16) or worsening of airway obstruction and air trapping (see Fig. 8-6) can often be evident in these curves before becoming clinically apparent. In ideal situations, $PEEP_i$ can be measured with an end-expiratory hold. This measurement is often inconsistent and difficult to obtain. Some authors have recommended that $PEEP_e$ be applied at 80% of the measured $PEEP_i$.[45] Because of the difficulty in accurately measuring $PEEP_i$ and the potential hazard of adding too much $PEEP_e$,[46] others have suggested that it should be set at 50% of the measured $PEEP_i$. If $PEEP_i$ becomes severe enough, it will begin to affect plateau pressure. Current recommendations for obstructive airway disease are to keep plateau pressure below 35 cm H_2O,[47,48] but many clinicians follow the ALI/ARDS recommendations and maintain plateau pressure at less than 30 cm H_2O.

$PEEP_e$ can be used to decrease some of the negative pressure that the patient has to generate to initiate a breath. For example, a patient with a $PEEP_i$ of 10 cm H_2O and a set pressure trigger of –2 cm H_2O (and no applied PEEP) has to generate an alveolar pressure of 12 cm H_2O to produce a breath. Adding a $PEEP_e$ of 5 cm H_2O means that the ventilator will trigger a breath when alveolar pressure is 3 cm H_2O. The patient has to generate a decrease of only 7 cm H_2O (instead of 12 cm H_2O), thereby reducing the inspiratory effort required.

Though seemingly counterintuitive, decreasing the respiratory rate and V_T in a critically ill asthmatic may be beneficial and result in an acceptable elevation in Pco_2, termed permissive hypercapnia.[49] Hence, it may not be advisable to meet arbitrary Pco_2 levels in a ventilated asthmatic but rather concentrate on maintaining acceptable oxygenation (Po_2 >60 mm Hg, oxygen saturation of 88% to 92%) while minimizing $PEEP_i$ and optimizing plateau pressure.

If cardiovascular collapse occurs in a ventilated asthmatic with either pulseless electrical activity or sudden hypotension, a first step in troubleshooting is to remove the patient from the ventilator. This is both a diagnostic and a therapeutic maneuver for air trapping. Some clinicians also advocate fluid loading and rapid and deep chest compressions while the patient is disconnected from the ventilator to expel the excess volumes of air trapped by prior aggressive ventilation (Fig. 8-17).[50] Tension pneumothorax must also be considered (see below).

ALI and ARDS

Initial ventilator settings for patients with ALI and ARDS can be found in Figure 8-18.

A common finding in lung-protective ventilation is the occurrence of patient-ventilator dyssynchrony. This is thought to be due to the patient wanting a higher flow rate than the ventilator is providing while on a volume-targeted strategy. This occasionally leads to double or triple cycling of the ventilator. It should be noted that in this situation the patient is actually receiving a higher V_T and not benefiting from lung-protective ventilation. Sedation needs to be optimized, and at times different modes, such as pressure-targeted modes, may be attempted. Temporarily weakening the patient with paralytics may be considered.

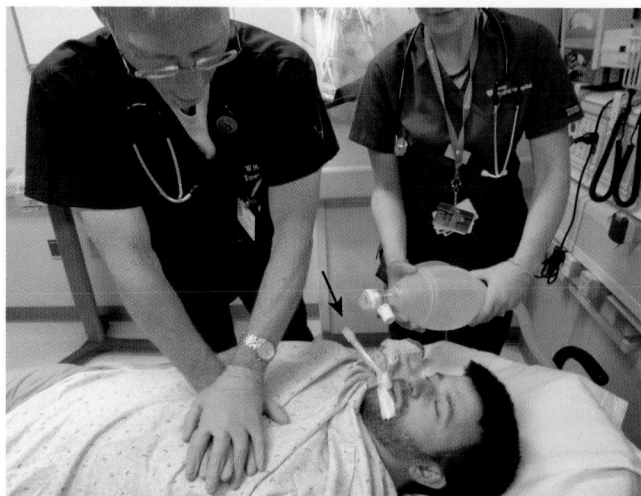

Figure 8-17 The crashing asthmatic. Once a struggling asthmatic is intubated, the temptation is to rapidly hyperventilate with deep breaths, but this may cause cardiovascular collapse because of exacerbating previous auto–positive end-expiratory pressure (PEEP)/breath stacking. A hyperinflated asthmatic lung severely diminishes venous return, which leads to a marked decrease in cardiac output, even pulseless electrical activity. If a recently intubated asthmatic suffers these consequences, stop ventilating the patient entirely (*arrow*), compress the chest until no more air is exhaled, and then continue ventilating as per discussion in text. Acceptable permissive hypercapnia may ensue.

ALI/ARDS/Diffuse Lung Injury Initial Ventilator Settings
VCV, AC, RR 20, VT 8 mL/kg IBW, PEEP 8, FIO2 100%
Titrate FIO2 and PEEP based on oxygenation (goal PaO2 ≥≈60, POX 88–92%). An ARDSNet PEEP table is helpful
Titrate VT down to 6 mL/kg IBW over the first 2 hours (may need to increase RR if minute ventilation is not adequate to keep pH >7.2)

Monitor plateau pressures (keep below 30)
• If >30, incrementally lower VT to 4 mL/kg IBW

Monitor blood pH
• Permissive hypercapnia expected and tolerated at pH >7.2
• NaCO3 infusion or administration of THAM may be required to keep pH above 7.15 to 7.20.

Insert a central venous catheter:
  If not in shock, follow a fluid conservation strategy

Figure 8-18 Initial ventilator settings for acute lung injury (ALI), acute respiratory distress syndrome (ARDS), and diffuse lung injury. *AC,* assist/control mode; *FIO2,* fraction of inspired oxygen; *IBW,* ideal body weight; *PEEP,* positive end-expiratory pressure; *THAM,* tris(hydroxymethyl)aminomethane; *RR,* respiratory rate; *VCV,* volume-cycled ventilation; *VT,* tidal volume.

There are several areas of uncertainty with MV in patients with ALI or ARDS. Patients with traumatic brain injury, intracranial hemorrhage, fulminant hepatic failure, and elevated ICP in whom ARDS develops must be managed carefully because lung-protective ventilation may induce hypercapnia. Acutely, this may lead to cerebral vasodilation and an increase in ICP. There is little evidence to support the recommendation for any particular rescue therapy in patients with severe refractory hypoxia, such as recruitment maneuvers, high-dose albuterol, IRV, HFV, prone ventilation, and extracorporeal membrane oxygenation. In dire circumstances, these modalities may be used on the basis of clinician preference and expertise and consultation with a critical care specialist.

COMPLICATIONS OF MV

Though necessary to sustain life, MV is associated with a number of pathophysiologic derangements that can lead to morbidity and mortality, including pulmonary barotrauma, ventilator-associated lung injury, hemodynamic compromise, PEEP$_i$, and elevated ICP.

Pneumothorax

Pneumothorax that is not associated with trauma in a mechanically ventilated patient typically stems from alveolar overdistention (continuous or episodic) and leads to alveolar rupture and escape of gas into the pleural space.[51] In patients receiving PPV, it is wise to drain the pleural space to prevent a simple pneumothorax from progressing to tension pneumothorax with hemodynamic compromise. Loculated pneumothoraces may be successfully drained percutaneously under ultrasound or computed tomography (CT) guidance. Successful drainage of air space disease leads to enhanced liberation from MV.[52] Pneumothorax or tension pneumothorax may also result from aggressive bag-valve-mask ventilation. Patients with intrinsic lung disease such as COPD or asthma are more prone to the development of pneumothorax than the average patient is.[53]

A simple pneumothorax can be drained by surgical tube thoracostomy with a small-bore tube (24 Fr), a commercially available pneumothorax kit (Arrow), or a pigtail catheter placed into the pleural space via the Seldinger technique (see Chapter 9). Each of these catheters should be placed into a chest drainage collection unit that incorporates a water seal chamber and variable suction control. Treat persistent air leaks initially with continuous suction (usually suction at 20 cm H$_2$O) to evacuate the pleural space and promote coaptation of the visceral and parietal pleurae. Reduce suction and place the chest tube on water seal only after resolution of any air leak. Remove the chest tube directly from the water seal if no pneumothorax is apparent on a chest film or after a test period of tube clamping and subsequent radiographic evaluation. The author favors a 4-hour period of clamping because recurrent pneumothorax is easier to treat by unclamping a tube than by placing a new one. Not all patients with a pneumothorax require invasive techniques to evacuate air from the pleural space. It is important to recognize that small pneumothoraces occurring in *spontaneously breathing patients* (i.e., negative pressure ventilation) may be reevaluated in 4 to 6 hours with a repeated chest radiograph and drained only if they are expanding. This option is *not* advised for patients who are on any form of PPV because a simple pneumothorax can rapidly become a tension pneumothorax with subsequent hypotension and death. Tension pneumothoraces may be recognized by tachycardia, hypotension, elevated peak airway pressure (if mechanically ventilated, tachypnea if not), jugular venous distention, thoracic resonance by percussion *on* the affected side, diminished or absent breath sounds *on* the affected side, and tracheal deviation *away from* the affected side. Because not all signs or symptoms are present in all patients, treatment should be dictated by the patient's clinical condition.

Loculated pneumothoraces or fluid collections develop in certain patients. If the collections are either single or immediately adjacent to one another and readily identified, they may be drained under ultrasound guidance at the bedside.[54] Loculations are frequently in inaccessible areas or are difficult to image with ultrasound. CT scanning of the thorax can provide precise anatomic definition of the presence and number of loculated collections and be used as a guide for the interventional radiologist. Successful treatment involving CT-guided drainage of loculated pleural collections (air and fluid) to assist in weaning of patients from mechanical ventilator support has been reported.[52]

Ventilator-Induced Lung Injury

There are several causes of ventilator-induced lung injury, including biotrauma, volutrauma, barotrauma, and atelectasis-related trauma. *Biotrauma* refers to the self-sustaining process of lung injury from MV that follows alveolar overdistention or rupture, alveolar hypoperfusion, and repetitive shear stress across alveolar walls. Originally, this problem was thought to be caused by too much pressure (barotrauma).[55] Current principles hold that elevated airway pressure is a straightforward reflection of excess volume delivered to a lung that cannot accept excess gas (i.e., in volutrauma, excess volume is delivered).[56] Lung injury is an inhomogeneous process with areas of normal lung immediately adjacent to diseased and injured segments.[57] The healthy and compliant segments with shorter regional time constants will readily accept gas, but their neighbors with reduced compliance and longer regional time constants will not. The end result is overdistention of the compliant segments, alveolar injury, liberation of inflammatory cytokines and chemokines, activation of endothelin and arachidonic acid pathways, and the expression of adhesion molecules along the vascular endothelium.[58] This leads to infiltration of inflammatory cells, release of destructive lysosomal enzymes, and induction of toxic oxygen metabolites. Avoiding this inflammatory cascade is an intelligent means of protecting a patient's lungs from volume-induced lung injury. Such a notion has given rise to lung-protective ventilator strategies based on low-V$_T$ ventilation (6 mL/kg IBW) and low plateau pressure (<30 cm H$_2$O).[59] Several studies have reported the development within hours of ventilator-induced lung injury in patients with normal lungs that were ventilated with larger V$_T$ (12 mL/kg).[60-64] Current recommendations are for all MV to be conducted with lower V$_T$ than the once-standard 12 to 15 mL/kg. Patients with abnormal lungs (interstitial lung disease, lung resection, severe pneumonia, edema) or the presence of an ALI risk factor (sepsis, aspiration, transfusion) should be ventilated at a V$_T$ of 6 mL/kg IBW. These patients may initially be markedly acidotic and may require starting V$_T$ at 8 mL/kg IBW and titrating down to 6 mL/kg IBW within 2 hours. Those with normal lungs and no ALI risk factors should be started at a V$_T$ of less than 10 mL/kg IBW.[64]

Hemodynamic Compromise

In all circumstances, the volume of venous return exactly matches the volume of cardiac output. Any process that impedes venous return will decrease the available volume that establishes cardiac output. For patients receiving PPV, each gas delivery increases intrathoracic pressure, and exhalation decreases that pressure. Venous return principally occurs during exhalation. If the ventilator settings lead to increased intrathoracic pressure during exhalation, venous return will be reduced. Variables that can lead to this circumstance are increased PEEP, auto-PEEP, and IRV. Venous return not only depends on a relatively negative pressure within the thoracic cavity but also relies on a sufficient amount of time for flow into the thoracic vasculature and right side of the heart. Significantly high respiratory rates may compromise venous return. An additional untoward side effect of impaired venous return is cerebral venous hypertension from impeded venous drainage. Because of the absence of valves between the cerebral parenchyma and the right atrium, increased pressure on the right atrium reduces cerebral venous flow and may contribute to cerebral ischemia in patients with traumatic brain injury or stroke, especially in those with compromised systemic hemodynamics. These patients are prone to watershed infarction, and cerebral venous hypertension may increase this risk.

Intrinsic PEEP

Maneuvers directed at elimination of $PEEP_i$ result in a decrease in inspiratory time and an increase in expiratory time. Decreasing the respiratory rate and V_T and increasing the inspiratory flow rate (IFR) effectively accomplish this goal. Frequently, this cannot be achieved without sedation and possibly requires the addition of pharmacologic paralysis.

Difficulty Triggering the Ventilator

To trigger a ventilator, a patient must cause either a drop in pressure or an increase in airflow at the proximal airway, depending on the type of settings used. The magnitude of change required to trigger the ventilator is adjusted by setting the sensitivity, usually in the range of -1 to -2 cm H_2O below the level of $PEEP_e$. Difficulty triggering the ventilator is often hard to detect. When it becomes obvious by physical examination that the patient is using the accessory muscles of respiration to trigger the ventilator, the problem may be severe. The condition can be detected earlier by inspecting the pressure-volume time curve on the ventilator display, if available. A large negative deflection at the beginning of inhalation suggests that ventilator sensitivity needs to be increased.

More commonly, high $PEEP_i$ is the cause. The patient must first lower intrathoracic pressure enough to overcome $PEEP_i$ before airway pressure can drop to the threshold sensitivity. The solution to this problem is to raise $PEEP_e$ to a level $\frac{1}{2}$ to $\frac{3}{4}$ of $PEEP_i$, which allows the patient to perform less work to trigger each inhalation. This process mandates frequent reassessment of $PEEP_i$ and manipulation of the ventilator during this dynamic period.

Auto-Cycling

Auto-cycling refers to a phenomenon when the ventilator set in AC mode begins to rapidly trigger without the patient initiating respiration. The cause is usually vacillations in airway pressure that the ventilator "interprets" as patient effort. Tremors, shivering, voluntary motion, convulsions, and oscillating water in the ventilator circuit are all potential causes. Auto-cycling should prompt immediate disconnection from the ventilator circuit and ventilation with a bag-valve device until the problem is resolved.

Rapid Breathing

When attempting to ventilate a patient with an obstructive process, the goal is to eliminate $PEEP_i$. Permissive hypercapnia is best achieved at low respiratory rates, but at the same time hypercapnia is a powerful stimulus to breathe. This can typically be quelled with a combination of sedation with high-dose opiates, ketamine, or propofol. Neuromuscular blockade should be considered a last resort undertaken only after careful consideration of the risk of prolonged paralysis and potential development of neuropathy in critical illness. If undertaken, the goal should be to weaken the patient sufficiently to inhibit dyssynchrony with the ventilator. Other common causes of rapid breathing include sepsis, pulmonary embolism, pregnancy, hepatic encephalopathy, intracranial hypertension, stroke or hemorrhage, and hypercapnia.

Outstripping the Ventilator and Double Cycling

Hypercapnia will develop in patients receiving low-V_T ventilation for ARDS or for an obstructive process and generate an increased respiratory drive. Outstripping the ventilator refers to the patient's effort to draw a higher V_T than set while in a volume-targeted mode. This can be detected by observing the exhaled V_T or by finding a negative deflection at the end of inhalation on the pressure-volume time plot. Double cycling occurs when the patient desires a larger V_T than is set and continues to inspire despite the delivery of a breath. The ventilator will then provide a second breath almost immediately after the first. This is especially problematic because the actual V_T delivered is twice the set volume. As with controlling rapid breathing, the solution is sedation and analgesia, particularly with opiates. Switching to a pressure-targeted mode or increasing the set V_T may alleviate this issue.

Straining over the Ventilator

Straining over the ventilator indicates that the patient on a volume-targeted mode is attempting to inhale at a flow rate in excess of the set IFR. On the pressure-volume time plot, the rise in pressure during inhalation will be concave rather that convex. Potential solutions are to raise the IFR, switch to a pressure-targeted mode or PSV, or use sedation and analgesia.

Coughing

Coughing is a common problem that arises from increased secretions, airway foreign body (ET tube), or an underlying pulmonary disease process. Coughing can lead to auto-cycling, poor patient comfort, dislodgment of the ET tube, and rarely airway injury. Accurate placement of the ET tube above the carina should be confirmed. Suctioning and provision of warmed, humidified air are often helpful. If these simple measures fail to provide relief, aerosolized lidocaine or suppression with opiates may increase patient comfort.

Equipment Failure

Whenever a patient decompensates while undergoing MV, consideration should be given to equipment failure as the cause. Interruption of the oxygen supply, erroneous settings, disconnected ventilator circuitry, and obstructed tubes are all potential culprits. Immediate action should include disconnection from the ventilator and bag ventilation with 100% O_2. The mnemonic made popular by the American Heart Association Pediatric Advanced Life Support Course is useful for recalling the causes of unexpected decompensation: DOPE (*D*islodgment of the ET tube, *O*bstruction of the tube, *P*neumothorax, and *E*quipment failure). Confirmation of ET tube placement, suctioning via the ET catheter, auscultation, chest radiography, and equipment troubleshooting are necessary actions.

TROUBLESHOOTING

Critically ill patients are encountered in the ED every day. Some of them required intubation in the prehospital setting, whereas others are intubated on arrival or during ED evaluation. After their airway has been secured and their condition stabilized, patients may remain in the ED because of a lack of critical care beds. In some hospitals, a dedicated intensivist will take charge of these patients, but in others, this type of coverage may not be available. Acute complications or deterioration must be handled by the emergency physician.

This section provides a framework for managing crashing, mechanically ventilated patients. The information provided

will assist the practitioner in determining whether the patient's condition is related to the underlying pathology that necessitated MV or whether it is being caused by MV itself.

Determine Hemodynamic Stability

The initial step in managing a crashing ventilated patient is to determine the patient's hemodynamic stability. A ventilated patient is, by definition, critically ill. The patient can fall anywhere on the spectrum from being ventilated for airway protection, with normal vital signs, blood pressure, and oxygen saturation, to being ventilated and in cardiac arrest. Determining where the patient is on this spectrum, including assessment for hypotension and hypoxia, will dictate how much time that the practitioner has to implement rescue strategies. In addition, it is important to anticipate the patient's clinical course. The approach to a patient who is intubated for hypoxia stemming from pneumonia and whose blood pressure and oxygenation gradually trend down over a period of hours or days is different from the approach to a patient who is declining over a span of minutes (Fig. 8-19).

As a general rule, the following evaluation should be performed on patients with new unexplained hypotension (systolic blood pressure [SBP] <90 mm Hg), new unexplained hypoxia (Sao_2 <90%), or a new marked change in vital signs (a drop in SBP by more than 20 mm Hg or a drop in Sao_2 by

Figure 8-19 Troubleshooting algorithm for respiratory distress and hemodynamic instability in critically ill ventilated patients. *CXR*, chest x-ray; *ET*, endotracheal; *PEEP*, positive end-expiratory pressure; *US*, ultrasound.

more than 10%) within an hour. Patients with *stable* SBP between 80 and 90 mm Hg and Sao$_2$ between 80% and 90% should be evaluated expeditiously in the hope of halting the decline. Those with SBP lower than 80 mm Hg or Sao$_2$ less than 80% and those who continue to decline rapidly should be evaluated quickly, with consideration given to entering the cardiac arrest/near arrest algorithm. These values are arbitrary demarcation points and do not take precedent over bedside clinical judgment.

Cardiac Arrest and Near Arrest Patients

Time is of the essence in a patient with cardiac arrest or near arrest. Advanced cardiac life support should be implemented quickly, and there are some key points to remember in a ventilated patient in cardiac arrest or one who becomes acutely hemodynamically unstable. The ED practitioner should develop a stepwise approach in this situation. During each step, the practitioner should "look, listen, and feel" to run through the differential diagnosis.

During stabilization of these patients it is important to keep in mind the original pathology that necessitated intubation. Sudden decompensation in an asthmatic is a common example of physician intervention worsening the scenario unless the pathophysiology of the arrest is appreciated (see Fig. 8-17). A crashing ventilated patient may simply be worsening from the primary pathology. A multitrauma patient may have an intrathoracic or intraabdominal catastrophe, and a septic patient may be deteriorating clinically from lack of source control.

It is also important to determine and address special circumstances that the ventilator can precipitate, the most significant of which are tension pneumothorax and severe auto-PEEP. Tension pneumothorax can lead to marked hypotension as a result of decreased cardiac output and marked hypoxia from $\dot{V}/\dot{Q}$ mismatch.[63] Auto-PEEP (also referred to as PEEP$_i$, breath stacking, or dynamic hyperinflation) is caused by trapped volume in the pulmonary system. If severe enough, it will eventually lead to increased intrathoracic pressure. This can cause hypotension and decreased cardiac output from decreased venous return and marked hypoxia from $\dot{V}/\dot{Q}$ mismatch.[64]

In critically ill ventilated patients with respiratory distress who are hemodynamically unstable, the following steps will assist the ED physician in determining the cause of the decompensation.

Step 1: Disconnect the Patient from the Ventilator

This is perhaps the easiest step to perform. It can be both diagnostic and therapeutic in a crashing ventilated patient. A quick rush of air or prolonged expiration of trapped air from the ET tube can be diagnostic of ventilator-induced auto-PEEP. A few seconds of observation can determine whether this entity is present. Return of hemodynamic stability implies that the maneuver was successful.

Patients undergoing cardiopulmonary resuscitation (CPR) should not be connected to a ventilator. The variations in intrathoracic pressure caused by CPR will trigger ventilator breaths at high rates if set on AC mode. Patients treated with inhaled nitric oxide (iNO) should not be removed from iNO abruptly, and effort should be made to quickly establish this supply through the bag-valve system. In addition, care should be taken when disconnecting patients who are on high

PEEP, such as those with ARDS. While disconnecting the ventilator it is important to address auto-PEEP because derecruitment can occur and hypoxia may be worsened. Once auto-PEEP has been ruled out, PEEP valves may be used to maintain PEEP levels and thus avoid derecruitment. PEEP valves may be problematic in a markedly hypotensive patient. They may increase intrathoracic pressure and decrease venous return.

Step 2: Breathing—Hand-Ventilate with 100% Oxygen

Ensure that 100% oxygen is being delivered and limit the respiratory rate to 8 to 10 breaths/min. Particular attention should be paid to the delivery of hand ventilation. Inadvertent rates as high as 40 breaths/min are often used in codes.[65,66] Excessive rates will increase intrathoracic pressure and lead to a decrease in venous return and cardiac output.[67] Look at both sides of the chest to determine whether there is equal chest rise. Unequal chest rise can signify main stem intubation, pneumothorax, or a mucus plug. Listen for air escaping from the mouth or nose (a sign of an air leak). Listen over the epigastric area and in both axillae. Decreased breath sounds may provide clues regarding main stem intubation, pneumothorax, or an atelectatic lung. Feel for subcutaneous crepitus (a sign of pneumothorax) and assess for difficulty in hand ventilating (a sign of low dynamic or static respiratory system compliance).

Step 3: Airway—Determine That the ET Tube Is Functioning and in the Proper Position

The ET tube functions by providing a conduit to the lower part of the trachea. Its cuff attempts to create a seal between it and the inner wall of the trachea. To determine whether the ET tube is functioning properly, pass the suction catheter and listen for an air leak (Fig. 8-20). Easy passage of the suction catheter does not guarantee that the ET tube is in the trachea because the catheter may be passing down the esophagus. If it is difficult or not possible to pass the suction catheter, the ET tube is either dislodged or obstructed. Attempt to correct this by repositioning the head in the case of a twisted or bent ET tube or inserting a bite block if the patient is biting on the tube. Dislodged or obstructed ET tubes require reintubation. Patients with dislodged ET tubes should be treated as difficult intubations because unplanned extubations are notorious for causing trauma to the glottis and for leading to vocal cord edema.[68]

In a cardiac arrest or near-arrest patient, the best choice for determining that the ET tube is in the proper position is direct visualization of the ET tube passing through the cords. This step is often omitted in a crashing ventilated patient because of the belief that the ET tube has not migrated. Unfortunately, unrecognized ET tube migration can occur during routine care of a critically ill patient. Patients are frequently moved in and out of emergency medical service vehicles, transferred to and from stretchers for imaging studies, and turned for procedures or bathing, all of which are capable of dislodging the tube. This visualization step can be performed while providing hand ventilation.

Other simple techniques may be used to confirm that the ET tube is in the trachea. Direct visualization of the carina with a fiberoptic scope is an option, but this device is not typically readily available to the ED practitioner. Another quick and readily available technique is to pass an intubating stylet (gum elastic bougie or Eschmann introducer).[69] The

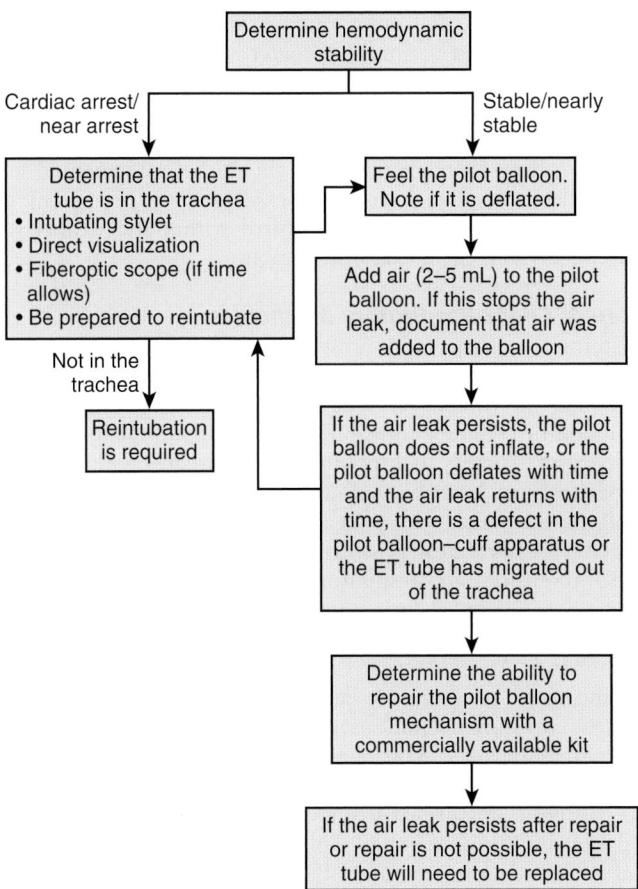

Figure 8-20 Troubleshooting an air leak. *ET,* Endotracheal.

Figure 8-21 Ultrasound image of a lung slide ("seashore sign") in M-mode. This patient does not have a pneumothorax.

Figure 8-22 Ultrasound image of the "bar code" sign in M-mode, indicative of pneumothorax. See the Ultrasound Box in Chapter 10 for additional details.

stylet is passed gently through the ET tube. If resistance is met at 30 cm, the ET tube is in the trachea. If the stylet passes beyond 35 cm without resistance, the ET tube is probably in the esophagus. If resistance is met too soon, the intubating stylet may be catching on the ET tube.

At least one of these techniques to determine proper positioning should be used early enough in the resuscitation to correct any airway issues. In addition, proper positioning should be confirmed before simply removing the ET tube and reintubation, particularly if the patient is deemed to have a difficult airway (unless it is glaringly evident that the patient is extubated).

Step 4: Special Procedures

If the patient is still in cardiac arrest or near arrest after being disconnected from the ventilator, ensuring proper placement of the ET tube, and hand-ventilating with 100% oxygen, a clinical decision will be required regarding needle decompression of the chest. If time permits, a focused history from the bedside nurse, respiratory therapist, or paramedic and a focused physical examination will indicate which side of the chest to decompress. In addition, depending on the urgency of the situation, bedside ultrasound and chest radiography may be used. Bedside ultrasound has been shown to exclude pneumothorax in the presence of "lung slide." This is depicted in M-mode as the "seashore sign" (Fig. 8-21) and, in its absence, as the "stratosphere sign/bar code sign" (Fig. 8-22).[70-72]

At times, the clinical situation does not allow imaging studies, and the focused history and physical examination may

not be helpful. In these cases, needle decompression of both sides of the chest should be considered if other more likely causes of acute decompensation are not found. It is important to remember that chest tube placement is required in patients after needle decompression.[73-75]

Stable and Nearly Stable Patients

If the patient is deemed stable or near stable or quickly regains stability after disconnection from the ventilator and hand ventilation, the event should be approached in a systematic manner. The patient should be placed on 100% oxygen during this evaluation.

Step 1: Obtain a Focused History

A focused history should be obtained from the practitioners most involved in the patient's care (bedside nurse, respiratory therapist, resident, paramedic). Valuable information includes the indication for intubation, difficulty of the intubation, depth of the ET tube, ventilator settings, and recent procedures or moves (central line insertion; chest tube placement; removal or transition to a water seal; thoracentesis; ET tube manipulation; transport off the stretcher; rotation for cleaning, a procedure, or chest radiography).

Step 2: Perform a Focused Physical Examination

Take a general survey of the patient. Observe for agitation, attempts to pull at the ET tube and lines, gasping for breath (the patient will have the mouth open and appear dyspneic), and tearing of the eyes.

Airway

Look at the ET tube and determine whether it has migrated from its previous position. It is possible that the ET tube has migrated out of the trachea or into a main bronchus. Adjust if necessary. Listen for escaping air (an air leak) from the mouth or nose (see Fig. 8-20). This typically signifies that the tube has lost its seal with the trachea and occurs with extubation or cuff failure. Feel the pilot balloon. If it is deflated, the cuff is deflated. Add air to the pilot balloon. If this stops the air leak, make a note that air was added to the balloon. If the pilot balloon does not inflate or deflates with time, there is a defect in the pilot balloon-cuff apparatus, and the ET tube will probably need to be exchanged. Occasionally, it may be possible to repair the pilot balloon mechanism with commercially available kits. This is a good option in patients who are difficult to intubate.

Determine that the ET tube is functioning properly by passing the suction catheter. If it is difficult or not possible to pass the suction catheter, the ET tube is either dislodged or obstructed. Attempt to correct by repositioning the head in the case of a twisted or bent ET tube or inserting a bite block if the patient is biting on the tube. Dislodged or obstructed ET tubes require reintubation.

Determine that the ET tube is in proper position if at any point in the evaluation it is suspected that extubation has occurred. Any of the techniques discussed in the previous section may be used.

Breathing

Look at both sides of the chest to determine whether there is equal chest rise. Unequal chest rise can signify main stem intubation, pneumothorax, or a mucus plug. Look at the ventilator tubing and determine whether there is an oscillating water collection. Listen for air escaping from the mouth or nose (a sign of an air leak). Listen over the epigastric area and in both axillae. Decreased breath sounds may provide clues regarding main stem intubation, pneumothorax, or an atelectatic lung. Feel for subcutaneous crepitus (a sign of pneumothorax).

Circulation

Check for pulses and cycle the blood pressure cuff frequently. If the patient has an arterial line, make sure that the transducer is level. Determine the need for fluid bolus or vasopressors.

Step 3: Assess Gas Exchange

Hypoxia can be diagnosed with pulse oximetry if the waveform is reliable. The waveform should not be highly variable and the frequency of the waveform should match the heart rate on the cardiac monitor. In a few instances, such as carbon monoxide poisoning, pulse oximetry is not reliable.[76] In these cases or if the pulse oximeter is not picking it up, an ABG sample should be obtained. Patients with a Pao_2/Fio_2 ratio of less than 200 should be evaluated for ARDS. Those with a ratio between 200 and 300 should be evaluated for ALI.[77] A lung-protective strategy should be implemented in those determined to have ALI or ARDS (see Fig. 8-18).[78] Hypoventilation cannot be identified with pulse oximetry. ABG analysis is beneficial in this event.

Step 4: Check Respiratory Mechanics

Determine whether peak pressure and plateau pressure have changed from their previous values. These values should be obtained on volume-targeted modes. Airway pressure is a function of volume and respiratory system compliance. The respiratory system incorporates the ventilator circuit, ET tube, trachea, bronchi, pulmonary parenchyma, and chest wall. A set volume with a set system compliance results in a specific pressure. Peak pressure is a function of volume, resistance to airflow, and respiratory system compliance. Plateau pressure is obtained during an inspiratory pause, thus eliminating airflow, and therefore reflects only respiratory system compliance. An isolated increase in peak pressure is indicative of increased resistance to airflow. An isolated increase in plateau pressure is indicative of a decrease in respiratory system compliance. Note that plateau pressure can never be higher than peak pressure and that if plateau pressure rises, so will peak pressure. It is important to keep in mind the Δ relationship (peak pressure − plateau pressure). These measurements assume a comfortable patient, and peak pressure and plateau pressure values are not reliable in a "bucking" patient.[79,80]

Step 5: Observe Ventilator Waveforms

The two most helpful ventilator waveforms are the flow-time curve and the pressure-time curve. The flow-time curve can be used to detect air trapping. The pressure-time curve can be used to determine plateau pressure with an inspiratory hold (see Fig. 8-1).

A notching in the pressure-time curve during inspiration can signify air hunger. In this situation the patient desires a higher flow rate than the ventilator is delivering. It is commonly seen in volume-targeted modes. Increasing the flow rate will often alleviate this phenomenon. Another solution is to change to a pressure-targeted mode.

Double cycling can also be seen on ventilator waveforms. This occurs when the patient desires a higher V_T than the ventilator is set to deliver. The patient is still inspiring when the first breath has finished cycling and the ventilator immediately gives a second mechanical breath. This is frequently seen with low-V_T ventilation, which is used in patients with ARDS and status asthmaticus. It is important to recognize because the actual V_T being provided is essentially twice the set V_T. This has important ramifications for patients with ARDS and obstructive processes such as asthma and COPD, for whom the goal is lower V_T. Typically, improved sedation with emphasis on blunting the respiratory drive with opiates alleviates double cycling. Other adjustments that may prove helpful are increasing the flow rate, increasing V_T by 1 mL/kg of predicted body weight up to 8 mL/kg, or changing from a volume-targeted mode to a pressure-targeted mode.

Step 6: Imaging Studies—Chest Radiograph and Bedside Ultrasound

Evaluate the chest radiograph for ET tube position, main stem intubation, lung atelectasis, pneumothorax, and a worsening parenchymal process. Bedside ultrasound, if available, is typically quicker in evaluating for pneumothorax, but it will not provide information on the location of the ET tube, lung atelectasis, or parenchymal processes (see Figs. 8-21 and 8-22).

Step 7: Evaluate Sedation

Patients requiring MV often need sedation and analgesia to make the ET tube and ventilation tolerable. Some patients, such as those with drug overdoses or traumatic head injuries, may not require any sedation. Others may tolerate intubation quite well while almost fully awake. The majority of patients require some form of sedation or analgesia. *Note that a plethora of non–MV-associated conditions, such as unrecognized bladder obstruction, alcohol or drug withdrawal, occult fractures or compartment syndrome, or bowel ischemia, can cause significant agitation that can mistakenly be attributed to the stress of intubation and ventilation.*

Selection of agents should be based on the desired effect. If a patient appears agitated, sedative-hypnotics should be used. Such drugs include benzodiazepines, propofol, dexmedetomidine, and haloperidol. It is important to note that these agents do not provide an analgesic component. If a patient is being given adequate sedative doses and still appears agitated, consider pain as a cause. Typical opiates that can be used are fentanyl, hydromorphone, and morphine. A remifentanil infusion is ultrashort acting and can provide both sedation and analgesia. Remifentanil does not accumulate in patients with renal or hepatic insufficiency. Prompt reversal of analgesia and sedation are seen on discontinuation. Remifentanil is an alternative to fentanyl for patients requiring frequent neurologic assessment or those with multiorgan failure.

The goal of sedation and anesthesia in ventilated patients who are not being evaluated for extubation is one in which the patient will arouse with gentle stimulation but will return to a sedated state when left alone. Patients who are being sedated and require deep stimulation to get a response are oversedated.

Patients who display air hunger and have a high respiratory rate can be given a trial of opiates to relieve their symptoms. Proper sedation and analgesia are paramount in patients being treated with a strategy that allows or permits hypercapnia, such those with as status asthmaticus, and in patients being treated with lung-protective strategies, such as those with ARDS. Hypercapnia is a powerful stimulus to the respiratory drive, and opiates are often required to control respiratory rates. Patients who tend to be difficult to control (besides those with status asthmaticus and ARDS) include patients with hepatic encephalopathy or intracranial processes such as a mass effect and hemorrhage. Chemical weakening with intermittently dosed paralytics may be required if patients have undergone a good trial of sedation, analgesia, and ventilator changes and are still markedly tachypneic. Careful consideration should be given before this step because prolonged paralysis has been implicated in critical illness polyneuropathy.[81,82] In addition, expert consultation should be obtained before prolonged paralysis of a neurosurgical patient. The goal in chemical paralysis in these patients is to weaken them enough to control their interaction with the ventilator. Usually, this does not require a full dose of the paralytic.

Hemodynamic instability in mechanically ventilated and sedated patients may be a result of medications because sedatives and analgesics can precipitate or worsen hypotension. As a general rule, continuous infusions should be withheld in these cases. Patients who are hypoxic and agitated but not hypotensive may benefit from improved sedation. It is possible that their pulmonary status is so tenuous that they are agitated from the hypoxia and their condition is worsened by the oxygen consumption caused by their agitation. Patients who are agitated and hypotensive may respond well to a low-dose benzodiazepine and opiate if the agitation is a precipitant of hypotension. In all these cases, it is imperative to determine whether sedation is a factor in the decompensation. Chemical paralysis should be reserved as a final option. It is important to remember that without continuous electroencephalographic recordings, seizure activity cannot be monitored if the patient is paralyzed.

SPECIAL SCENARIOS

Two special scenarios should be mentioned. One is a crashing intubated pediatric patient and the second is a patient with a tracheostomy. The approach described earlier can be used in pediatric patients, but there are a few caveats that may improve the approach. The first is to recognize that migration of the ET tube is common with small movements of the head and neck. A simple solution is to use a cervical collar for immobilization. Second, small ET tubes are often uncuffed and do not have a pilot balloon. Air leaks in this scenario should prompt the clinician to consider that the ET tube is either dislodged or too small. Finally, specialized equipment such as intubating stylets and fiberoptic scopes are typically not available in pediatric sizes.

Important questions that have ramifications in the care of a crashing ventilated patient with a tracheostomy are the following: (1) Does the patient have a laryngectomy? (2) Why does the patient have a tracheostomy? and (3) How old is the tracheostomy? These are important questions because patients with a laryngectomy cannot be intubated orally, patients with a tracheostomy secondary to anatomic considerations or difficult or failed airways may be difficult to intubate orally, and the tract in a patient with a recent tracheostomy (less than a week old) may not have matured enough to safely reintroduce a tracheostomy tube.

LIBERATION FROM THE VENTILATOR

Occasionally, patients can be considered for extubation while still in the ED. Before extubating a patient, several questions should be answered in the affirmative (Fig. 8-23). Common scenarios include resolution of exacerbations of COPD or asthma, exacerbation of congestive heart failure, and metabolism of intoxicants. Patients who were difficult intubations or required multiple attempts should have a planned extubation. It may be prudent to allow the edema from a traumatic intubation to subside.

Once these screening questions have been answered in the affirmative, one should perform an awakening trial followed

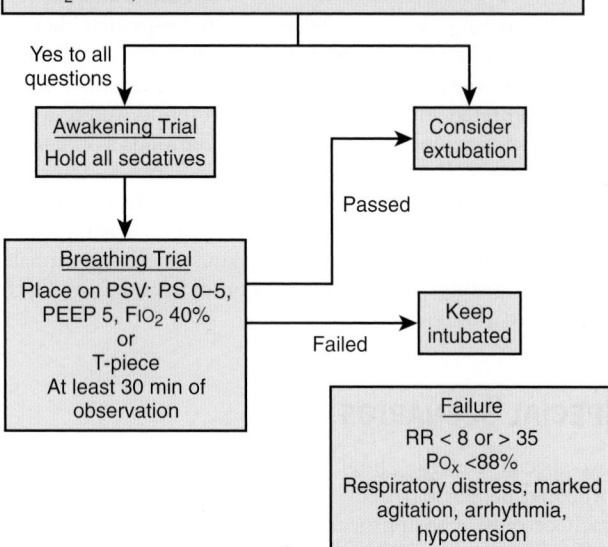

1. Resolution of the reason for intubation?
2. Presence of adequate mental status to protect the airway?
3. "Easy" intubation; will I be able to reintubate the patient if needed?
4. Are there sufficient resources to manage an extubation in the ED?
5. Hemodynamically stable, oxygenating, ventilating properly?
6. Is the patient on minimal settings? No vasopressors, FIO₂ ≤40%, PEEP≤8

Yes to all questions

Awakening Trial
Hold all sedatives

Consider extubation

Passed

Breathing Trial
Place on PSV: PS 0–5,
PEEP 5, FIO₂ 40%
or
T-piece
At least 30 min of observation

Failed

Keep intubated

Failure
RR < 8 or > 35
PO$_x$ <88%
Respiratory distress, marked agitation, arrhythmia, hypotension

Figure 8-23 Liberation from ventilator. *ED*, emergency department; *FIO₂*, fraction of inspired oxygen; *PEEP*, positive end-expiratory pressure; *PSV*, pressure support ventilation; *RR*, respiratory rate.

by a spontaneous breathing trial. Extubation should be considered if the patient does not fail the breathing trial.

For patients intubated for exacerbation of COPD, NPPV should be considered. For patients with COPD who failed a spontaneous breathing trial, extubating to NPPV decreases mortality, hospital length of stay, the incidence of ventilator-associated pneumonia, and the total duration of mechanical ventilation.[83]

CONCLUSION

Mechanically ventilated patients are typically the most critically ill patients that the ED practitioner will manage. The underlying disease process that required intubation is typically life-threatening. When patients become unstable, the physician should take a stepwise approach toward determining whether the patient is deteriorating because of the underlying disease process or because of interaction with the ventilator. It is hoped that the approach presented here will assist practitioners with a framework to evaluate and stabilize crashing ventilated patients. For further information, Wood and Winters present an up-to-date review of the care of ventilated patients in the ED and evaluation of potential problems.[84]

References are available at www.expertconsult.com

CHAPTER 9

Thoracentesis

Erik H. Adler and Barbara K. Blok

Thoracentesis is a word derived from the Greek *thorakos* (chest) and *kentesis* (to pierce). Classically, this refers to any maneuver whereby a sharp object is inserted into the chest to make a conduit between the intrathoracic cavity and the atmosphere that allows air or fluid to exit. Clinically, *thoracentesis* refers to the removal of fluid from the pleural space for diagnostic or therapeutic purposes. This chapter concentrates on the identification and management of fluid accumulations in the chest of patients seen in the emergency department (ED).

ANATOMY AND PHYSIOLOGY OF THE PLEURAL SPACE

During embryologic development, the lung buds grow out of a median mass of mesenchymal tissue into the future thoracic cavities. This process results in the development of two linings: the visceral pleura, which wraps around the lungs, and the parietal pleura, which lines the inner surface of the thoracic cavities and meets the visceral pleura at the root of the lungs in the mediastinum. The space between the two linings is called the *pleural space*.

Understanding this basic anatomy is important because it underlines the similarities and differences between the two linings, which in turn determines the physiology and pathophysiology of the pleural space. Both the visceral and parietal pleurae are thin layers of connective tissue through which both fluid and protein can leak. Embedded in each membrane are capillary beds that generate both hydrostatic and oncotic pressure. The visceral pleura is supplied by the bronchial arteries and empties into the pulmonary veins, whereas the parietal pleura is supplied by the intercostal arteries and empties into the intercostal veins. In the healthy state there is a small net movement of fluid across the pleural and parietal capillary beds into the low-pressure pleural space. Over the course of a day, the lymphatic system maintains a minimum pleural space outflow of 0.01 mL/kg/hr, with a 30-fold capacity of 3 mL/kg/hr.[1,2] Overall, in a healthy state a small amount of fluid, estimated at 0.26 mL/kg of body mass, is present in the pleural space at any given time.[3]

It is believed that in most instances, the development of a pleural effusion requires both an increase in fluid entry into the pleural space and a decrease in its removal.[4]

ETIOLOGY OF PLEURAL EFFUSIONS

The most common causes of pleural effusion in adults are congestive heart failure (CHF), pneumonia, malignancy, pulmonary embolism (PE), and viral disease.[4,5] The most common cause of pleural effusions in children is pneumonia, followed by congenital heart disease, malignancy, renal disease and trauma.[6] Pleural effusions can be classified as either transudates or exudates. Distinguishing between transudates and exudates narrows the differential diagnosis and directs management and therapy. A comprehensive list of causes can be found in Box 9-1. The most common are discussed in the following sections.

Transudates: Overwhelming the System

Transudates are caused by either an increase in intravascular hydrostatic pressure or a decrease in intravascular oncotic pressure, which generates a net flow of fluid into the pleural space. These effusions are typically straw colored and serous with very low cellular and protein content.

The most common cause of a transudate is CHF. The increased hydrostatic pressure in patients with CHF results in a net flow of fluid into the pulmonary interstitium. This fluid readily moves across the leaky visceral pleura into the pleural space,[7] and when the volume of fluid exceeds the capacity of the lymphatics for drainage, a pleural effusion develops. In addition, the elevated systemic hypertension associated with CHF also increases fluid flow across the parietal pleura and decreases lymphatic flow out of the thorax. Any process that results in compromised left ventricular outflow can result in a pleural effusion, including myocardial infarction, cardiomyopathy, and valvular disease.

Patients with cirrhosis are frequently hypoalbuminemic, which leads to a chronic state of decreased plasma oncotic pressure. The imbalance between the hydrostatic and oncotic forces across the pleural membrane results in an effusion.[8] In addition, experiments have shown that high volumes of ascites can stretch the diaphragm enough to allow fluid to pass through preexisting microdefects.

Similarly, renal diseases such as the hypoalbuminemic state of patients with nephrotic syndrome or the intraabdominal fluid associated with peritoneal dialysis or obstructive uropathy can cause transudative pleural effusions.

Exudates: Pathology of Tissues, Destroying the System

Exudates are caused by pleural inflammation, increased pleural membrane permeability, or lymphatic obstruction. More than 90% of exudative effusions are due to malignancy, pneumonia, PE, and gastrointestinal diseases (e.g., pancreatitis, esophageal perforation).

The main mechanism of cancer-related pleural effusion is obstruction. Neoplasms can either damage functional lymphatic stomata in the parietal pleura or prevent outflow more distally via involvement of the mediastinal lymph nodes. Other mechanisms involving neoplasm include metastasis to the visceral pleura, increasing capillary permeability, and obstruction of the thoracic duct with consequent chylothorax.[9]

A pleural effusion associated with pneumonia (bacterial or viral) or a lung abscess is termed a *parapneumonic effusion*. In the first stage of a parapneumonic effusion, called the *exudative stage*, sterile fluid flows across the visceral pleura secondary to increased pulmonary interstitial fluid. When the infection and resultant inflammation continue unchecked, a simple uncomplicated parapneumonic effusion becomes *complicated*. This occurs initially by deposition of fibrin on the visceral and parietal pleurae, which results in loculations (the

BOX 9-1 **Causes of Pleural Effusion**

TRANSUDATES
Most Common
- Congestive heart failure

Less Common
- Cirrhosis
- Nephrotic syndrome
- Peritoneal dialysis
- Pericardial disease
- Central venous obstruction
- Myxedema
- Acute atelectasis
- Bone marrow transplantation
- Urinothorax

EXUDATES
Most Common
- Malignancy
- Pneumonia

Less Common
- Pulmonary embolism
- Trauma
- Esophageal perforation
- Pancreatitis
- Intraabdominal abscess
- Abdominal surgery
- Collagen vascular disease
- Drug induced
- Chylothorax
- Asbestosis
- Coronary artery bypass surgery
- Sarcoidosis
- Uremia
- Meigs' syndrome
- Ovarian hyperstimulation syndrome
- Radiation therapy

fibrinopurulent stage), and finally, by growth of fibroblasts along the pleural surfaces, which results in a tough peel that encases the lung (the organizational stage).

A pleural effusion develops in at least 30% of those with PE.[10] Therefore, when the cause of the effusion is unclear, PE should be strongly considered. The effusions associated with PE are often too small to require thoracentesis, but recent studies have shown them to be uniformly exudative, probably resulting from ischemia- and infarction-induced increases in pulmonary capillary permeability.[11]

Traumatic Effusions: Acute and Catastrophic Destruction of the System

Esophageal rupture can result from forceful vomiting, as in the case of Boerhaave's syndrome, or from instrumentation, as in the case of endoscopy, Blakemore-Sengstaken tube placement, or rigid nasogastric tube placement. Hemothorax can result from sharp traumatic injuries, cannulation of

the subclavian vein or artery, PE, aortic aneurysm, and supratherapeutic levels of anticoagulant. Chylothorax develops from acute disruption of the thoracic duct, usually in the setting of trauma or malignancy. These effusions are usually large-volume collections that accumulate over an extremely short period and rapidly compromise both oxygenation and the circulation.

DIAGNOSIS OF PLEURAL EFFUSION

Clinical Diagnosis

The three most common symptoms related to pleural effusions are chest pain, cough, and dyspnea. The chest pain may be of several types, depending on the underlying pathology. Chest pain solely from the fluid collection is often described as a "dull ache." Pleuritic chest pain is more indicative of localized irritation of the parietal pleura, which has abundant nerve fibers. Because of innervation by the phrenic nerve, involvement of the mediastinal pleura results in chest pain with ipsilateral shoulder pain. Pain can often be referred to the abdomen also via innervation of the intercostals. Cough may be due to bronchial irritation from compression of the lung parenchyma.

Because pleural effusions result from a large list of disease processes, be sure to cover all systems in the history and physical examination of the patient while searching for clues to the underlying etiology. Perform the lung examination both as an evaluation of lung pathology and to determine the extent of the effusion. Large effusions can result in an increase in the size of the hemithorax, as well as bulging intercostal spaces on the side of the effusion. On palpation, tactile fremitus is either reduced or completely absent over the effusion because the fluid separates the lung from the thoracic wall and absorbs the vibrations from the lung. Percussion over the effusion produces a characteristic dullness, which shifts when the patient changes position if the fluid is free flowing. In general, auscultation reveals decreased to absent breath sounds, depending on the size of the effusion. Egophany can occasionally be appreciated at the superior border of the effusion as a result of underlying atelectatic lung tissue. Pleural rubs may be appreciated if pleural irritation is present, but they are often difficult to auscultate until after evacuation of fluid. Palpation, percussion, auscultation, and bedside ultrasound (US) are all useful in determining the upper extent of the effusion.

Radiologic Diagnosis

Chest Radiograph

Because pleural fluid is denser than air-filled lung, a free-flowing effusion will first accumulate in the most dependent parts of the thoracic cavity, the subpulmonic space and the lateral costophrenic sulcus. Pleural effusions are usually visible on an upright posteroanterior chest radiograph if 200 to 250 mL of fluid is present. A lateral radiograph may reveal an effusion of 50 to 75 mL.

The earliest recognized sign of a pleural effusion on an upright chest radiograph is *blunting of the lateral costophrenic angle*, which may be seen on either the frontal or the lateral view (Fig. 9-1). With larger free-flowing effusions, the pleural fluid appears as a *meniscus* that curves downward toward the mediastinum in the frontal view and appears "lowest" midway

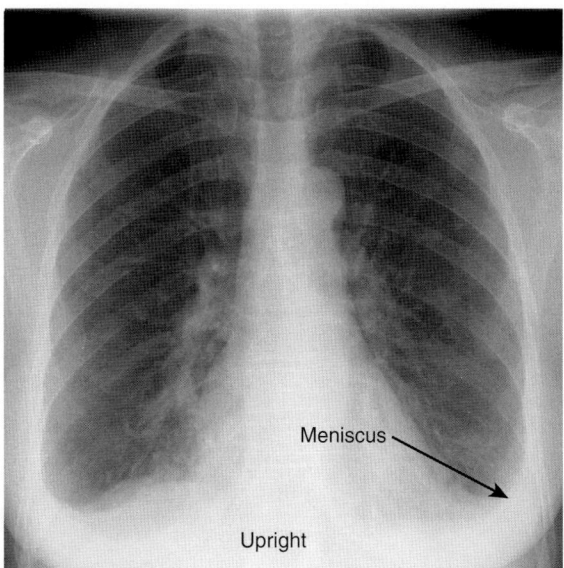

Figure 9-1 Posteroanterior upright chest radiograph indicating a moderate pleural effusion with a bilateral meniscus at the costophrenic angles. The pleural effusion has a curvilinear upper margin concave to the lung and is higher laterally than medially.

Figure 9-2 Left-sided pleural effusion seen on posteroanterior (**A**) and lateral (**B**) radiographs. The meniscus can be visualized on both views (*arrows*). The meniscus is the highest point of the effusion for thoracentesis purposes.

through the thoracic cavity on the lateral view (Fig. 9-2). The true height of an effusion corresponds to the highest portion of the meniscus. The presence of a pneumothorax or abscess may alter the appearance of the meniscus to more of a straight line (air-fluid level).

Occasionally, up to 1000 mL of fluid can collect in the subpulmonic space and cause neither blunting of the costophrenic angles nor a meniscus appearance on the upright radiograph. This is called a *subpulmonic effusion* (Fig. 9-3) and should be suspected if the hemidiaphragm is elevated and the dome peaks more laterally than expected on the anteroposterior radiograph.

Pleural effusions are more challenging to identify on a chest radiograph in a supine patient. If the effusion is large enough, a diffuse haziness may be appreciated (Fig. 9-4). Other findings include apical capping, obliteration of the hemidiaphragm, partial opacification of a hemithorax, and a widened minor fissure.

Obtain bilateral decubitus radiographs when a pleural effusion is seen or suspected. With the side of the effusion down, a simple pleural effusion will follow gravity and layer between the floating lung and the chest wall (Fig. 9-5). Unusual shapes reflect the presence of loculations, contained abscesses, or masses. A lateral decubitus view on the opposite side draws the fluid toward the mediastinum and allows visualization of the lung parenchyma to determine whether infiltrates or masses are present.

With diseased or scarred lung, tissue adhesions can trap pleural fluid within the parietal, visceral, or interlobar surfaces. Because these adhesions anchor the fluid collection, *loculated effusions* are often described as "D-shaped" (Fig. 9-6). Fluid loculated in the fissures assumes a lenticular shape.

In the case of a massive pleural effusion, the entire hemithorax is opacified (Fig. 9-7). On such films, identification of mediastinal shift is a key to identifying the underlying process. In the absence of a diseased lung or mediastinum, large fluid accumulations push the mediastinum contralaterally. When the mediastinum is shifted toward the effusion, the lungs and

main stem bronchi are diseased or obstructed (or both). When the mediastinum is fixed midline, it is likely that it is invaded by a tumor.[12,13] As discussed later, differentiation of these disease processes is best done with computed tomography (CT). CHF often produces bilateral pleural effusions, which is generally first evident on the right side (Fig. 9-8).

CT

Although thoracentesis is usually performed on the basis of findings on plain radiography, CT is more sensitive than plain films in detecting very small effusions and can readily assess the extent, number, and location of loculated pleural effusions. Loculated lesions can appear vague on plain films. In the distinct anatomic relationships shown on cross-sectional CT views, free-flowing pleural fluid will form a sickle shape in the most dependent regions (see Fig. 9-4), whereas loculated fluid collections will remain lenticular and relatively fixed in space. In addition, CT can be used to assess pleural thickening, irregularities, and masses that are suggestive of malignancy and other diseases that result in exudative effusions. With intravenous contrast dye, CT differentiates lung parenchymal disease, such as a lung abscess. Pulmonary emboli can also be detected with the use of intravenous contrast enhancement. CT is also useful in identifying

Figure 9-3 Right-sided subpulmonary pleural effusion. On erect posteroanterior (**A**) and lateral (**B**) radiographs, the effusion simulates a high hemidiaphragm. It is also seen with ultrasound (**C**) and computed tomography (**D**).

Figure 9-4 A, Supine radiograph of a patient with a large pleural effusion. Note the generalized homogeneous ("ground glass") increase in radiopacity of the right side of this patient because of posterior layering of a pleural effusion. Also note the difference in the appearance of the pleural effusion when the patient is supine. As opposed to the upright radiograph (see Fig. 9-2), there is minimal blunting of the costophrenic angles and the vascular opacities are preserved in the overlying lung. **B,** A chest computed tomography (CT) scan of the same patient confirms the presence of a right-sided pleural effusion. Note the typical sickle-shaped appearance of the effusion on CT.

Figure 9-5 Left lateral decubitus chest radiograph demonstrating the presence of free pleural fluid. The amount of pleural fluid can be semiquantified by measuring the distance between the *two arrows*. Thoracentesis may be difficult to perform if the fluid distance is less than 1 cm on the lateral decubitus radiograph. This view may also differentiate simple effusions from loculated effusions.

mediastinal pathology and in differentiating ascites from loculated subpulmonic pleural fluid.

Ultrasound

There are definite advantages to using US for assessment of pleural effusions as well. In particular, it is easy and noninvasive and can be performed at the bedside. US is superior to chest radiographs in diagnosing effusions[14-16] and can detect effusions as small as 5 mL.[17] Although some details can be seen only with CT, US can identify fluid loculations, separate fluid from pleural thickening, and distinguish solid from fluid pleural lesions. US can also be used to identify both pulmonic and abdominal causes of the pleural effusion (Fig. 9-9). Furthermore, US is a useful bedside tool when performing thoracentesis because it allows rapid identification of both the diaphragmatic location and the intercostal level that correlates with the superior margin of the effusion.

INDICATIONS

Diagnostic Thoracentesis

During diagnostic thoracentesis, a sample of pleural fluid is obtained to evaluate the cause of a pleural effusion. It requires the removal of 50 to 100 mL of pleural fluid for laboratory studies. Most new effusions that measure greater than 10 mm on a decubitus radiograph, CT, or US require diagnostic

Figure 9-6 Loculated pleural effusion. **A,** A posteroanterior radiograph demonstrates the D-shaped appearance of a right-sided loculated pleural effusion (*arrows*) in the midchest region. **B,** Occasionally, pleural effusions (*arrows*) may become loculated in the fissures.

Figure 9-7 Massive pleural effusion before (**A**) and after (**B**) thoracentesis. Notice the underlying mass that is seen following thoracentesis. A computed tomography scan would have prospectively confirmed this radiograph.

Figure 9-8 Effusion from congestive heart failure. **A,** A frontal chest radiograph in a patient with pulmonary edema shows cardiomegaly, bilateral pleural effusions (*arrows*), and central interstitial thickening, including Kerley's A lines. Note that the right effusion is slightly larger than the left effusion. **B,** High-resolution computed tomography scan in a patient with pulmonary edema shows interstitial edema with bilateral, basilar, centrilobular ground-glass opacity nodules (*arrowheads*) and smooth interlobular septal thickening (*arrow*). Bilateral pleural effusions are also present. *(Courtesy of Michael B. Gotway, MD, Department of Radiology, University of California, San Francisco.)*

Figure 9-9 Ultrasound image of a patient with a large right-sided pleural effusion. Note the dark appearance of the pleural effusion with a free-floating lung. Ultrasound is also useful for identifying the diaphragm (*right of the screen*) and the top of the effusion (*left of the screen*). Ultrasound can be used during the procedure itself if a sterile probe cover is used, which enables the operator to view the tip of the needle entering the effusion and to avoid vital structures, such as the lung or diaphragm. *(From Thomsen T, Setnik G, eds.* Procedures Consult—Emergency Medicine Module. *Copyright 2008 Elsevier Inc. All rights reserved.)*

thoracentesis. An exception would be a new pleural effusion with a clear clinical diagnosis (e.g., CHF) and no evidence of a superimposed pleural space infection.

Therapeutic Thoracentesis

The usual goal of therapeutic thoracentesis is to help relieve the dyspnea associated with a large pleural effusion and typically requires removing a much larger volume of pleural fluid.

CONTRAINDICATIONS

There are no absolute contraindications to thoracentesis. Recent studies indicate that if performed under real-time US guidance, thoracentesis is safe despite abnormal coagulation parameters.[18] Closely watch all patients with coagulation abnormalities, including those with renal failure, for signs of bleeding after the procedure. Avoid skin puncture through a site of cellulitis or herpes zoster by choosing an alternative insertion site or patient position. Use real-time US guidance when performing thoracentesis on patients who are undergoing mechanical or manual ventilation because the positive pressure associated with mechanical ventilation may place the patient at increased risk for the development of a pneumothorax.

PROCEDURE

Thoracentesis is generally an elective procedure. Obtain and document informed consent, according to hospital policy, before initiation of the procedure. Follow sterile technique throughout the entire procedure to avoid the introduction of infection.

Choosing a Technique

The specific technique and equipment for thoracentesis are a matter of personal choice and experience, and no specific device has been proved to be superior. Use of a simple 21-gauge needle for thoracentesis has mostly been supplanted by various catheters and kits. The catheter technique uses a catheter that is inserted over a needle and subsequently left in the pleural space during removal of fluid. A standard 16- to 18-gauge intravenous catheter, three-way stopcock, and syringe are still frequently used. There are many advantages of commercial thoracentesis catheters (Fig. 9-10). A one-way valve prevents entry of air into the catheter during removal of the needle. A blunt spring-loaded safety cannula extends beyond the sharp needle tip once the pleural space is entered to protect the lung from puncture or laceration. There is a built-in side port for drainage of fluid, which obviates the need for a three-way stopcock. Numerous kits are marketed for both thoracentesis and paracentesis and can be used for either of these procedures.

Studies have attempted to determine the relative safety of the needle and catheter techniques, with varied results.[19] It is generally recommended that clinicians use the smallest possible needle. For diagnostic procedures, in which only

small volumes of fluid are being withdrawn, the needle technique is recommended. For therapeutic maneuvers, either technique is generally believed to be safe; however, the catheter technique avoids prolonged insertion of a needle in the pleural space when large volumes of fluid are being removed.

Real-time US guidance is recommended for small or loculated effusions, especially when adhesions are suspected. It is also recommended in patients with relative contraindications or in whom iatrogenic pneumothorax may cause significant respiratory compromise, such as those with severe underlying lung disease or mechanical ventilation. US-guided thoracentesis is associated with a significantly lower rate of complications.[20]

Equipment and Patient Preparation

Gather and organize all necessary equipment before the procedure (see Review Box 9-1 for a list of recommended equipment). Confirm the patient's identification and verify the correct side of the pleural effusion by physical examination and chest radiography. If the procedure is diagnostic, use a red-topped tube for serum protein and lactate dehydrogenase (LDH) to send to the laboratory. Keep atropine available at the bedside in case the patient has a vasovagal reaction during the procedure. Monitor oxygen saturation by pulse oximetry and administer supplemental oxygen as needed. Take time immediately before the procedure to verify the correct patient, procedure, side, and site.

Termination of the Procedure

Understand the end points of a procedure before its initiation. The most common indication for termination of thoracentesis is removal of the desired volume of fluid. For diagnostic thoracentesis, terminate the procedure after removal of 50 to 100 mL of fluid. For therapeutic thoracentesis, terminate the

Figure 9-10 The Safe-T-Centesis needle, which is available in a prepackaged kit. Safety features of this device include a blunt-tipped obturator needle, a color-changing indicator, a pigtail catheter, and an attached three-way valve. The blunt-tipped obturator retracts with pressure to expose the sharp needle tip. This causes the color in the device to change from white to red. Once the pleural space is entered and there is no longer pressure on the tip, the spring-loaded obturator covers the sharp needle tip to prevent damage to the lung. This will cause its color to revert back to white.

Thoracentesis

Indications
Suspected pleural space infection
New effusion without a clear clinical diagnosis
Relief of dyspnea associated with a large effusion

Contraindications
Absolute
 None
Relative
 Severe clotting abnormality

Complications
Pneumothorax	Reexpansion pulmonary edema
Cough	Air embolism
Infection	Catheter fragment in the pleural space
Hemothorax	Intraabdominal hemorrhage

Equipment

Review Box 9-1 Thoracentesis: indications, contraindications, complications, and equipment.

procedure on relief of dyspnea or when up to 1500 mL of fluid has been withdrawn. The recommended maximum of 1500 mL is suggested to help avoid significantly negative pleural pressure, which has been associated with both symptomatic hypovolemia and the potentially fatal complication of reexpansion pulmonary edema. Larger volumes may be removed if pleural pressure is monitored, but this is not typically done in the ED setting. Terminate the procedure if aspiration of air occurs, which indicates lung puncture or laceration. Finally, a change in patient symptoms, including abdominal pain and worsening shortness of breath, should raise suspicion for a complication and the procedure should be terminated.

Insertion Site and Patient Position

Figure 9-11 illustrates various patient positions for thoracentesis. Upright positioning is the desired technique for draining most pleural effusions. With this technique, have the patient sit erect on the edge of the bed with the arms extended on a bedside table or Mayo stand (Fig. 9-12). If the effusion is sufficiently large, allow the patient to lean forward slightly while supported by the bedside table. Locate the height of the effusion clinically by dullness to percussion and a decrease in tactile fremitus. US can be a valuable tool in identifying the height of the effusion and location of the diaphragm (Fig. 9-13 and see Ultrasound Box). Use a sterile US probe during real-time US guidance and ask an assistant to hold it if possible. Position the patient and then identify

A

B

C

Figure 9-11 A-C, Various patient positions for thoracentesis. Note the midscapular line when the patient is sitting upright. This anatomic line is important in that thoracentesis should not be performed medial to this marker because of the increased incidence of trauma to the neurovascular bundle.

Figure 9-12 Preferred positioning for thoracentesis by the posterior approach is with the patient sitting upright and leaning over an adjacent Mayo stand.

Figure 9-13 Ultrasound image of a right-sided pleural effusion. Ultrasound can be used during the procedure itself if a sterile probe cover is used. This enables the operator to view the tip of the needle entering the effusion and to thus avoid vital structures such as the lung or diaphragm. Note the superior, inferior, and medial landmarks that are used during the procedure itself.

ULTRASOUND: Thoracentesis

by Christine Butts, MD

Ultrasound is an excellent tool for both identifying and directing the aspiration of pleural effusions. It can be used to both "mark the spot" for thoracentesis and directly guide the procedure.

Equipment

A 3.5- to 5-mHz transducer will reliably identify most pleural effusions. A higher-frequency transducer should be used when direct visualization of the procedure is desired.

Interpretation of Images

A normal lung is filled with air and will typically appear as a hazy gray area when viewed by ultrasound (Fig. 9-US1). Reverberation or comet tail artifacts may also be seen (Fig. 9-US2). When pleural fluid is present, it will typically be seen in the most dependent area of the thorax, typically in the recesses above the diaphragm. Pleural fluid will appear as anechoic (black) collections of varying size (Fig. 9-US3). Depending on the consistency of the fluid, it may appear heterogeneous, with areas of lighter gray representing more solid components (such as clotted blood).

Procedure and Technique

Once a pleural effusion is known or suspected to be present, scan the area over the posterior aspect of the thorax with a low-frequency transducer (Fig. 9-US4). Identifying the abdominal organs (such as the kidney, liver, and spleen) and diaphragm first will often help orient the sonographer (Fig. 9-US5). Assess the recess superior to the diaphragm for the presence and size of the effusion. If the procedure is to be performed blindly (such as with a very large effusion), mark a location several rib spaces above the diaphragm to avoid any possible intraabdominal injury. The procedure can then proceed in the usual fashion. If the procedure is to be performed under direct ultrasound guidance (such as with smaller effusions), cover the high-frequency transducer with a sterile sheath. Once the field has been prepared, use the sterile transducer again to locate the fluid pocket. At this time, introduce the needle alongside the transducer (see the basic ultrasound chapter for more on direct needle guidance).

Figure 9-US2 This image demonstrates two key artifacts seen in a normal lung. As with the previous image, the pleura is recognized as a hyperechoic horizontal line deep to the ribs (at the *far right and left* of the image). A comet tail, or a small vertical line, can be seen extending deep to the pleura (*arrow*). This is a normal artifact created by the pleura. A-lines, or a series of horizontal lines extending deep to the pleura, can also be seen (*arrowhead*). These artifacts are created by reverberation and may be seen in a normal aerated lung.

Figure 9-US1 Ultrasound images of a normal lung. **A,** High-frequency image. In this view the pleura can be seen as a brightly echogenic (*white*) horizontal line deep to the ribs and corresponding rib shadows (*arrow*). **B,** Low frequency. In this image, less of the pleura is visible. However, abnormalities such as effusions may be recognized more easily.

Figure 9-US3 Large pleural effusion seen on ultrasound with a low-frequency transducer. In this longitudinal image the thorax is seen on the left side of the image, and a large anechoic (*black*) fluid collection can also be seen (*arrow*). Within the thorax the lung can be seen as the hypoechoic (*dark gray*) mass on the left of the image.

Continued

ULTRASOUND: Thoracentesis, cont'd

Figure 9-US4 Placement of the ultrasound transducer over the posterior of the thorax to identify a pleural effusion.

Figure 9-US5 Longitudinal image of the lower part of the thorax and upper part of the abdomen demonstrating a large pleural effusion. The *bright white* (hyperechoic) *line* arcing over the kidney (*arrow*) is the diaphragm, which is an important landmark in planning the location of aspiration.

Complications

Most complications occur when the sonographer incorrectly interprets the image or the anatomy. Special care should be taken during the initial evaluation to identify the diaphragm and to direct any attempts at aspiration superior to this point to avoid injury to the abdominal cavity. Effusions that are loculated may not be gravity dependent and may be found in varying areas of the thorax.

the location of the diaphragm and the superior aspect of the effusion with US. Avoid relying solely on the chest radiograph to determine the level of effusion because the radiographic level changes with patient positioning and respiration. Insert the thoracentesis catheter one to two intercostal spaces below the highest level of effusion in the midscapular or posterior axillary line (Fig. 9-14). *In all cases, the lowest level recommended is the space between the eighth and the ninth ribs, which is at the eighth intercostal space.* Below the eighth intercostal space, the risk for diaphragmatic or hepatic/splenic injury increases. Medial to the midscapular line the neurovascular bundle is located more centrally in the intercostal space, and the risk for neurovascular injury increases. Mark the designated site. If the patient is too ill to sit upright, perform the procedure with the patient in the lateral decubitus position, the side of the effusion down, and the back at the edge of the bed. Insert the needle at the posterior axillary line in this position. Alternatively, position the patient supine with the head elevated as much as possible. Use the midaxillary line as the point of needle insertion for this position. For both these alternative positions, determine the fluid level clinically by physical examination or bedside US and make sure that the selected site is not lower than the eighth intercostal space. Once the insertion site is identified, prepare the skin with antiseptic in a wide area around the thoracentesis site via sterile technique. Place sterile towels or a sterile drape around the site.

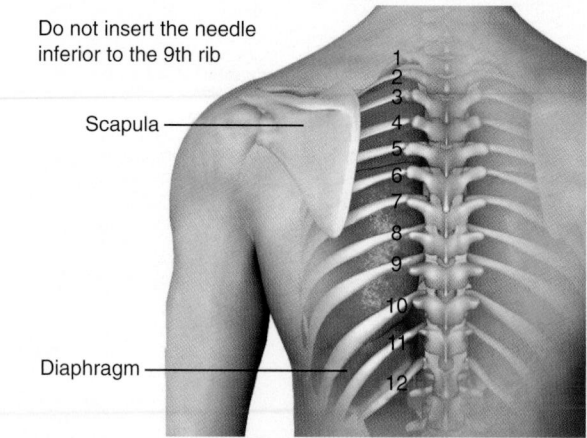

Figure 9-14 The inferior tip of the scapula is at the seventh rib. Do not insert the thoracentesis needle below the ninth rib. *(From Thomsen T, Setnik G, eds.* Procedures Consult—Emergency Medicine Module. *Copyright 2008 Elsevier Inc. All rights reserved.)*

Anesthesia and Pleural Fluid Localization

Use a 25-guage needle attached to a syringe containing 5 to 10 mL of 1% lidocaine or an equivalent anesthetic. Raise a skin wheal at the upper edge of the rib just below the marked intercostal space. Use the upper edge of the rib to avoid accidental trauma to the neurovascular bundle, which runs

Figure 9-15 A, Anatomy of the neurovascular bundle. The intercostal nerve, artery, and vein typically run inferior to the rib. **B,** The proper approach mandates walking the needle up and over the rib to avoid these vital structures. *(From Thomsen T, Setnik G, eds.* Procedures Consult— Emergency Medicine Module. *Copyright 2008 Elsevier Inc. All rights reserved.)*

along the inferior margin of each rib. With each 1 to 2 mm of needle advancement, aspirate and then infiltrate the subcutaneous tissue and muscle with 1 to 2 mL of anesthetic. While the aspiration-infiltration process is continued, "walk" the needle above the superior edge of the rib and advance it through the intercostal space until the pleural space is entered (Fig. 9-15). Hold the needle perpendicular to the chest wall to avoid inadvertent trauma to the neurovascular bundle of the adjacent rib. On entering the pleural space, a pop may sometimes be felt. Aspirate fluid to ensure that the pleural space has been reached. It is important to properly anesthetize the parietal pleura because it contains abundant sensory nerve fibers. Once fluid is aspirated, *grasp the needle at the skin with the thumb and index finger and withdraw it. This allows measurement of the proper depth of penetration needed during subsequent needle insertion.* If no fluid is encountered, this is consistent with a dry tap. A *dry tap* in the setting of a free-flowing pleural effusion indicates that either the needle is too short or the site chosen is too high or too low. If air bubbles are encountered, the lung parenchyma may have been entered and the chosen site is probably too high. If no fluid or air is encountered, the chosen site is probably too low. If a dry tap occurs during fluid localization and the patient has no new symptoms, reevaluate the patient's position and fluid level, administer local anesthetic as needed, and reattempt to aspirate fluid with the needle. If the repeated attempt is unsuccessful, obtain fluid under direct visualization with sterile US guidance.

Over-the-Needle-Catheter Insertion Technique

This technique is preferred and uses an 8-Fr catheter mounted on an 18-gauge introducer needle. Attach the needle-catheter unit to a 10-mL syringe (Fig. 9-16). Pierce the skin with a scalpel at the selected insertion site to ease entry of the catheter through the skin. Mark the depth of the pleural space that was determined from the anesthetic needle by gently grasping the shaft of the needle-catheter unit with the index finger and thumb of the nondominant hand. *This stabilizes the*

device and controls the advance. "Walk" the needle-catheter unit over the rib through the anesthetized area and into the pleural space while applying constant, gentle negative pressure with the syringe. As fluid is encountered, angle the needle-catheter unit slightly caudally. Advance the catheter off the needle into the pleural space while holding the needle steady. Withdraw the needle and cover the exposed lumen of the catheter hub with a finger to prevent entry of air. Attach a three-way stopcock with a 60-mL syringe and drainage tubing to the catheter hub. Aspirate fluid with the syringe. Turn the stopcock lever to prevent passage of fluid into the catheter (off to the catheter/patient), and expel the fluid through the drainage tube into a sterile container or sterile vacuum bottle, where it can subsequently be transferred into appropriate specimen tubes. Repeat this process of aspirating and expelling fluid until an adequate amount of fluid is obtained. Alternatively, allow the fluid to drain directly from the needle and three-way stopcock through high-pressure tubing into a vacuum bottle. Turn the stopcock lever to prevent entry of air or fluid back into the catheter when changing bottles. If the catheter tip has multiple side ports for the entry of fluid, be careful to avoid withdrawing the catheter from the chest during the removal of fluid, which might expose a side port and allow air to enter the pleural space. Once an indication for discontinuing the procedure has been met, remove the catheter and cover the entry site with a sterile bandage.

The procedure is simplified by using a commercial needle-catheter kit. Some kits, such as the Safe-T-Centesis Kit, have a spring-loaded blunt obturator that extends over the needle tip. This obturator retracts when pressure is applied to it, thereby exposing the needle tip and causing a color indicator in the hub to appear red. Once the pleural space is reached, the obturator extends back over the tip and the indicator returns to white. In addition, a self-sealing valve automatically prevents air from entering the catheter hub as the needle is removed. Many of these commercial products have a built-in stopcock that is located either on the base of the catheter or at the end of a built-in drainage tube (see Fig. 9-10), thus obviating the need for the three-way stopcock described earlier.

THORACENTESIS

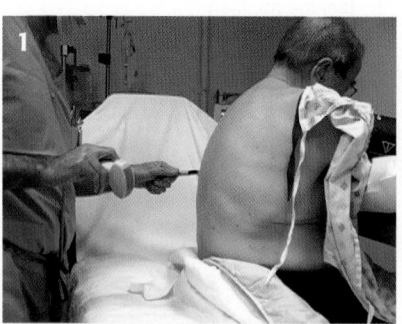

Position the patient, and then identify and mark the insertion site. The insertion site is best chosen after ultrasound evaluation.

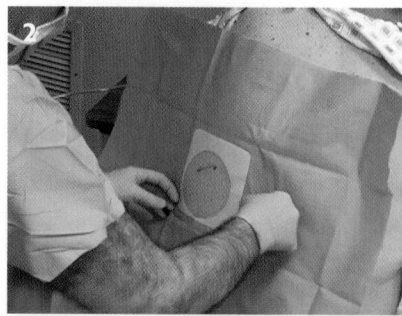

Prepare the area with antiseptic and apply a sterile drape.

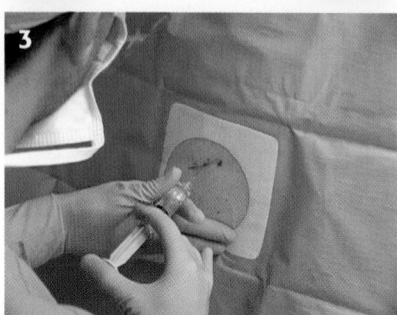

Anesthetize the skin and underlying tissues; "walk" the needle above the superior rib surface.

Pierce the skin with a scalpel or large-gauge needle.

Advance the catheter over the rib into the pleural space. Stabilize and control the shaft with the left hand during advancement.

Aspirate and stop advancing once pleural fluid is obtained.

Slide the catheter over the needle into the pleural space.

Collect diagnostic specimen with a 60-mL syringe.

Remove the pleural fluid with an evacuated container or a syringe and stopcock assembly.

Remove the catheter and apply an occlusive dressing.

Figure 9-16 Steps in the thoracentesis procedure. (*From Thomsen T, Setnik G, eds.* Procedures Consult—Emergency Medicine Module. *Copyright 2008 Elsevier Inc. All rights reserved.*)

Preprocedure

Postprocedure

Figure 9-17 Chest radiographs before and after thoracentesis. Postprocedure films are not always routine but should be performed if air was aspirated, the patient has postprocedure chest pain or dyspnea, multiple attempts were made, or the patient is on a ventilator. *(From Thomsen T, Setnik G, eds. Procedures Consult—Emergency Medicine Module. Copyright 2008 Elsevier Inc. All rights reserved.)*

PEDIATRIC PATIENTS

The indications for and contraindications to performing thoracentesis are much the same in children as in adults. Positioning is also similar but will probably require an assistant to help hold the patient and prevent movement. Sedation may be helpful when respiratory distress is minimal. Determine the effusion level clinically by dullness to percussion, a decrease in tactile fremitus, and bedside US. Make sure that the needle insertion site is not lower than the eighth intercostal space in the posterior axillary line. Any technique described for an adult patient may be used, and the smallest possible needle or needle-catheter unit is recommended.

Postprocedure Radiograph

In many centers, chest radiographs are routinely obtained after thoracentesis to evaluate for procedure-related pneumothorax (Fig. 9-17). This has been shown to be unnecessary in patients who require a single needle pass, have no risk for adhesions, and experience no new symptoms during or after thoracentesis.[21,22] Obtain a chest radiograph in patients who require multiple needle passes, if air is aspirated, in those at risk for adhesions, or in those in whom any new symptoms (chest pain, dyspnea) develop during or after thoracentesis. In addition, it is reasonable to obtain a postprocedure radiograph in patients at risk for future decompensation from expansion of a small asymptomatic pneumothorax, including those with severe underlying lung disease and patients receiving *mechanical ventilation*. Notably, the postprocedure radiograph rarely shows new findings that aid in identifying the cause of the effusion, such as an underlying mass or infiltrate.[23]

PLEURAL FLUID ANALYSIS

Pleural fluid should be analyzed in an organized and thoughtful manner based on clinical suspicion for a disease process. The most cost-effective approach is to perform an initial evaluation to determine whether the fluid is transudative or exudative and obtain other tests only if the fluid is an exudate. Many laboratories are comfortable performing all required tests from the initial 60-mL syringe, so dividing the specimens into individual tubes at the bedside is often unnecessary. An

exception is that pleural fluid sent for cell count with differential should be transferred to an anticoagulant-containing tube (e.g., lavender top) to prevent clumping of cells because this has been shown to significantly affect the results.[24] Analyze the fluid within 4 hours when possible, but results remain accurate for much longer if the samples are collected and refrigerated at 4°C.[24,25] One exception is pleural fluid pH, where delays in analysis result in clinically significant increases in pH measurements.[26] Transfer samples for pleural fluid pH immediately to a blood gas syringe, place it on ice, and analyze it within 1 hour. Because of differences in laboratory preference, consult your individual laboratory for its policies on specimen collection and delivery.

Visual Inspection

Identifying a cause based on pleural fluid appearance alone is inaccurate, but certain findings are suggestive. The presence of blood suggests trauma, malignancy, pulmonary infarction, or pneumonia.[27] White or milky fluid suggests the presence of lipids, whereas purulent, malodorous fluid indicates empyema. Pleural effusion containing food particles is highly suggestive of esophageal rupture.

Distinguishing Transudate from Exudate: Light's Criteria

The next step in evaluation of pleural fluid is categorization of the fluid as exudative or transudative. As discussed earlier, exudates are caused by pleural inflammation, increased pleural membrane permeability, or lymphatic obstruction and therefore contain high levels of either LDH or protein. Light and coworkers[28] published criteria for distinguishing transudates from exudates in 1972 based on measurements of serum and pleural fluid protein and LDH. The value for LDH was subsequently changed to accommodate variations in assay conditions.[29] These criteria have since become known as *Light's criteria* (Box 9-2). An exception to using Light's criteria for differentiating transudates from exudates is in the setting of CHF treated with diuretics. Effusions in patients with CHF are due to increased capillary hydrostatic pressure and are therefore transudates. However, it has been shown that use of diuretics increases pleural fluid protein and LDH concentrations, thus making the fluid appear exudative by Light's criteria.[30-32] This is hypothesized to be due to diuretic-induced shifting of fluid out of the pleural space. In the diuretic-treated CHF population with an exudate by Light's criteria, measuring the level of N-terminal pro–brain natriuretic peptide (NT-proBNP) is recommended.[33] A pleural fluid or serum NT-proBNP level of 1500 pg/mL or higher indicates a diagnosis of CHF.

BOX 9-2   **Transudate versus Exudate: Light's Criteria**

If at least one of the following three criteria is present, the fluid is virtually always an exudate; if none is present, the fluid is virtually always a transudate:

- Pleural fluid-serum protein ratio >0.5
- Pleural fluid lactate dehydrogenase (LDH) level greater than two thirds the upper limit of the serum reference range
- Pleural fluid-serum LDH ratio >0.6

Once a fluid is classified as transudative, it typically requires no further fluid analysis, and therapy is directed at the underlying cause of the effusion (e.g., CHF, cirrhosis, nephrotic syndrome).

In the presence of an undiagnosed exudative effusion, however, more extensive fluid evaluation is required.

Evaluation of Exudates

For all undiagnosed exudates, at a minimum pleural fluid should be sent for cell count with differential, glucose, adenosine deaminase (ADA), and cytologic evaluation (Table 9-1).[34-39] Clinical suspicion of an underlying disease process should guide additional fluid assessment.

Cell Count with Differential

In general, the presence or absence of red blood cells (RBCs) is not useful in determining the cause of the effusion because it takes only a small amount of blood to impart a blood-tinged appearance. A grossly bloody pleural effusion or RBC count greater than 100,000 cells/mm³ is suggestive of trauma, malignancy, pneumonia, or pulmonary infarction,[27,40] but a lack of

---

TABLE 9-1   Exudates: Evaluation of an Undiagnosed Exudative Effusion

PLEURAL FLUID ASSAY	RESULT	PROBABLE DIAGNOSIS (DIFFERENTIAL DIAGNOSIS)
Standard Testing: Perform on All Exudative Effusions		
CBC with differential		
RBC count	Grossly bloody or >100,000 cells/mm³	Trauma, malignancy, PE, pneumonia
WBC count	>10,000 cells/mm³	Parapneumonic effusion
Neutrophils	>50%	Acute pleural process: infection, pulmonary infarct
Lymphocytes	>50%	Chronic pleural process: malignancy, TB
Eosinophils	>10%	Air or blood in the pleural space
Glucose	<60 mg/dL	Parapneumonic infection, malignancy, TB, rheumatoid arthritis
Cytology	Abnormal cells	Malignancy
Adenosine deaminase	>40 IU/L	TB (lymphoma, empyema)
Selective Testing: Order If High Clinical Suspicion for Diagnosis		
Gram stain and culture	Presence of organism	Pleural space infection
Amylase[34,35]	>100 U/L	Pancreatitis, esophageal rupture (malignancy, TB, cirrhosis)
Triglycerides[36]	>110 mg/dL (>50 if fasting or malnourished)	Chylothorax (intrathoracic TPN infusion)
Creatinine (with serum measurement)	Pleural fluid-serum creatinine ratio >1	Urinothorax with elevated LDH[37]
N-terminal pro-brain natriuretic peptide	≥1500 pg/mL	Congestive heart failure after diuretics
pH	<7.2	Complicated parapneumonic effusion (malignancy, TB, esophageal rupture, collagen vascular disease)
Rheumatoid factor[4]	≥1:320	Rheumatoid pleuritis
ANA[38,39]	≥1:160	SLE (malignancy, parapneumonic effusion)

ANA, antinuclear antibody; *CBC*, complete blood count; *LDH*, lactate dehydrogenase; *PE*, pulmonary embolism; *RBC*, red blood cell; *SLE*, systemic lupus erythematosus; *TB*, tuberculosis; *TPN*, total parenteral nutrition; *WBC*, white blood cell.

RBCs does not exclude these diagnoses. Grossly bloody pleural fluid with a hematocrit greater than 50% of the peripheral hematocrit often requires tube thoracostomy.

Exudates typically have a pleural fluid white blood cell count greater than 1000 cells/mm^3, and counts may reach levels higher than 10,000 cells/mm^3, most commonly with parapneumonic effusions.[40] The differential cell count can be useful in identifying the cause of an exudative pleural effusion. A predominance of neutrophils indicates an acute process affecting the pleural surface, such as acute infection or pulmonary infarction. A predominance of lymphocytes is consistent with a more chronic pleural process, including malignancy, tuberculosis (TB), CHF, and effusion after coronary artery bypass graft surgery.[40] Eosinophil counts greater than 10% often have no clear etiology but have traditionally been associated with blood or air in the pleural space.

Culture

If bacterial infection is a concern, culture the pleural fluid by both bedside inoculation of blood culture bottles and standard laboratory culture. The addition of blood culture bottles increases the overall yield of identifiable pathogens in parapneumonic effusions by 20%, from a baseline of a 40% yield with standard laboratory culture alone.[41] As little as 2 mL of fluid can be used in each bottle without affecting the results.

Glucose

The concentration of glucose in exudates is extremely variable and, in general, does not correlate with any specific disease process. Routine measurement of pleural fluid glucose for exudative effusion is recommended because a low glucose concentration (<60 mg/dL) narrows the differential diagnosis to parapneumonic effusion, malignancy, TB, rheumatoid effusion, and the uncommonly seen paragonimiasis or Churg-Strauss syndrome.[4] Keep in mind, however, that these diagnoses are not *excluded* by a high or normal pleural fluid glucose level. Of note, patients with active rheumatoid arthritis and rheumatoid pleural effusion will commonly have an extremely low pleural fluid glucose concentration (<20 to 30 mg/dL).[42] Comparatively, with systemic lupus erythematosus, pleural fluid glucose levels are usually normal.[43]

Adenosine Deaminase

Pleural fluid ADA is an important screening tool for TB. In populations with a high prevalence, a pleural fluid ADA concentration above 40 U/L is highly suggestive of the diagnosis,[44,45] and further testing to demonstrate the organism in sputum, pleural fluid, or pleural biopsy specimens is warranted. In populations with a low prevalence, the positive predictive value of ADA is also low, but it maintains a high negative predictive value. A normal level in this setting is useful in excluding the diagnosis. Of note, extremely high ADA levels (>250 U/L) are more likely to be due to lymphoma or empyema than to TB.

Cytology

Perform cytologic analysis on all undiagnosed effusions or when malignancy is suspected. The sensitivity for diagnosing pleural malignancy hovers around 55%, regardless of whether small or large (>50 mL) volumes are analyzed.[46] Obtaining repeated pleural samples increases the yield of malignant cells.[47]

BOX 9-3 | **Indications for Surgical Management of Parapneumonic Effusions**

Effusion >50% of the hemithorax
Loculated effusion
Pleural thickening seen on a computed tomography scan
Aspiration of frank pus
Pleural fluid pH <7.2
Pleural fluid glucose <60 mg/dL
Positive Gram stain or culture of pleural fluid

Parapneumonic Effusions

Patients with suspected parapneumonic effusions warrant rapid evaluation and outcomes risk assessment based on pleural anatomy, pleural fluid bacteriology, and pleural fluid chemistry.[48] All parapneumonic effusions require at least diagnostic thoracentesis with the goal of identifying patients with complicated parapneumonic effusions. Indications for tube thoracostomy or other surgical procedures include large or loculated effusions, pleural thickening on CT (the pleural peel), aspiration of frank pus (indicating empyema), pleural fluid pH lower than 7.20, pleural fluid glucose concentration lower than 60 mg/dL, and positive Gram stain or culture (Box 9-3).

Pleural pH measurement gives useful information regarding pleural inflammation. Normal pleural fluid pH is approximately 7.64, and a pH lower than 7.20 indicates a significant inflammatory process. The differential diagnosis of pleural fluid acidosis includes not only complicated parapneumonic effusion but also malignancy, TB, esophageal rupture, and collagen vascular disease.[49] Measurement of pleural pH is important in the evaluation of patients with suspected parapneumonic effusions because pH has the highest diagnostic accuracy of pleural fluid tests in identifying effusions that require surgical drainage.[50,51] The fluid may be transferred from the initial 60-mL syringe into a heparinized blood gas syringe[52] and then left at room temperature for up to 1 hour before laboratory analysis[53] without affecting the accuracy of the results. Avoid introduction of air or lidocaine into the sample because it may significantly alter the results.[26] Because of these specifics regarding the collection and evaluation of pleural fluid pH, transfer the pleural fluid to a heparinized blood gas syringe and place it on ice while awaiting the decision for pH testing. When pH testing is not possible, a reasonable alternative is to use pleural fluid glucose levels. Though slightly less accurate than pH in identifying complicated parapneumonic effusions, measurement of pleural fluid glucose does not have the collection challenges of pleural fluid pH, and levels lower than 60 mg/dL indicate a need for surgical drainage.

COMPLICATIONS

Pneumothorax

The most frequently reported complication of thoracentesis is pneumothorax, with an overall rate of 6% in a recent meta-analysis.[20] Pneumothorax can develop in some patients with even the most pristine and seemingly uncomplicated procedure. It is a known complication and does not necessarily denote poor technique. Thoracostomy tubes are required in less than 50% of post-thoracentesis pneumothoraces.[19,23,54] The mechanism for this complication is puncture of the lung or inadvertent entry of air through the needle or catheter during the procedure. Suspect pneumothorax if air is aspirated during removal of fluid or if new symptoms develop during or after the procedure.[20] Procedure-related factors that appear to contribute to pneumothorax include an inexperienced operator, multiple needle insertion attempts, therapeutic taps, and the use of needles larger than 20 gauge. Risk for pneumothorax is increased in patients with mechanical ventilation[20] and underlying chronic obstructive pulmonary disease.[55] Conversely, risk for pneumothorax is significantly lower when performed under US guidance.[20]

Cough

Cough is another complication that is frequently encountered. Although it is typically considered a minor complication that results only in patient discomfort, it may be associated with the creation of an iatrogenic pneumothorax.[20] Terminate the procedure if persistent coughing occurs.

Infection

As with all procedures, there is a potential risk for infection, which is estimated at 2%. Keep the risk low with careful patient preparation and sterile technique.

Uncommon Serious Complications

Other serious complications have been reported but occur in less than 1% of procedures. Such complications include hemothorax, splenic rupture, abdominal hemorrhage, unilateral pulmonary edema, air embolism, and catheter fragments left in the pleural space.

Hemothorax may be suspected by rapid accumulation or reaccumulation of pleural fluid or by a change in the patient's vital signs after the procedure. Hemothorax may be due to laceration of the lung or the diaphragmatic, intercostal, or internal mammary vessels. Pay careful attention to technique, such as *avoiding the superior portion* of the intercostal space, never puncturing medial to the midscapular line, and not penetrating too deeply into the thorax during needle insertion. Hemothorax requires appropriate surgical consultation and drainage via a thoracostomy tube.

Puncture of the spleen or liver through the diaphragm may result in localized organ hematoma or hemoperitoneum. Clinically, this is suspected when the needle pass does not yield pleural fluid (dry tap) and is followed by a patient's complaint of abdominal pain. If this diagnosis is suspected, appropriate resuscitation is the initial treatment, followed by a diagnostic imaging study, preferably a CT scan. If the patient is hemodynamically unstable, obtain bedside US and immediately consult a surgeon.

Reexpansion pulmonary edema is a complication associated with rapid reexpansion of the lung. Symptoms include dyspnea, tachypnea, tachycardia, cough, and frothy sputum.[56] It is believed that this problem can be avoided by discontinuing the procedure when pleural pressure is greater than −20 mm Hg, which is suspected to occur after 1500 mL of fluid has been acutely removed.[57] Because pleural pressure is rarely measured in the ED, 1500 mL of fluid is typically viewed to be the maximum amount that can be safely withdrawn at one time. There is no proven way to be sure that reexpansion pulmonary edema will not occur, however.

References are available at www.expertconsult.com

CHAPTER 10

Tube Thoracostomy

Thomas D. Kirsch and Jordan Sax

Tube thoracostomy is a procedure used to evacuate an abnormal accumulation of fluid or air from the pleural space and can be performed on an elective, urgent, or emergency basis. Air or fluid can accumulate in the pleural space as a result of spontaneous or traumatic pneumothorax, pleural fluid accumulation of blood, malignancy, infection (empyema), or lymph (chylothorax). The first modern methods to evacuate the contents of the pleural space were developed in the 19th century, but these techniques did not become widespread until 1918, when they were used to treat postinfluenza empyema. Military experience demonstrated that thoracic drainage combined with antiseptics and antibiotics reduced mortality related to thoracic trauma from 62.5% during the Civil War, to 24.6% in World War I, and to 12% in World War II.[1]

PATHOPHYSIOLOGY

The lung is surrounded by two layers, the parietal pleura, which lines the interior of the chest wall, and the visceral pleura, which covers the lungs. They are separated by a thin layer of lubricating fluid within the "pleural space." A small negative pressure within the pleural space helps keep the lung inflated and the two layers closely apposed. With inspiration, the negative intrathoracic pressure increases and leads to expansion of the lung from an influx of air. If the pleural space is disrupted, air, blood, or other fluid can accumulate in between the two layers of the pleura and the normal pressure gradient is compromised. This interferes with normal inspiratory-induced inflation and leads to "collapse" of the lung. As the amount of fluid or air increases, respiratory function worsens and symptoms of dyspnea are produced, often with pleuritic chest pain and anxiety. The degree of respiratory compromise depends on the volume of fluid or air in the pleural space, the patient's age, baseline pulmonary status, and the integrity of the chest wall. The positive pressure accumulation of air associated with tension pneumothorax leads to severe respiratory dysfunction and cardiovascular compromise.

Pneumothorax

A pneumothorax is caused by the presence of air in the pleural space and the loss of negative pressure (Fig. 10-1). Air can enter the pleural space from the outside as a result of a penetrating injury or internally from a ruptured lung bleb or damaged trachea. Iatrogenic causes from needle procedures such as subclavian venous cannulation, transthoracic biopsy, thoracentesis, positive pressure ventilation (PPV), or cardiopulmonary resuscitation (CPR) are also common (Fig. 10-2). Pneumothoraces are commonly divided into "open" and "closed." An open pneumothorax indicates that the skin and underlying soft tissue sustained an injury that penetrated into at least the pleural space.

Spontaneous (Closed) Pneumothorax

Spontaneous pneumothorax is caused by rupture of a subpleural lung bleb with little or no trauma and can be categorized as either primary or secondary based on the presence of underlying lung disease. *Primary spontaneous pneumothorax* occurs in a patient *without* overt lung disease. The typical patient with

Tube Thoracostomy

Indications
Spontaneous and traumatic pneumothorax
Hemothorax
Empyema
Patients with penetrating chest trauma undergoing positive
  pressure ventilation or long-distance transport

Contraindications
Absolute
  None
Relative
  Presence of multiple pleural adhesions
  Presence of emphysematous blebs
  Coagulopathy

Complications
Infection
Laceration of an intercostal vessel
Pulmonary injury
Intraabdominal or solid organ tube placement
Failure of reexpansion of pneumothorax
Reexpansion pulmonary edema

Equipment

Review Box 10-1 Tube thoracostomy: indications, contraindications, complications, and equipment.

Figure 10-1 Pneumothorax. **A,** Anteroposterior chest radiograph of a right-sided, seemingly small, simple pneumothorax (PTX). Note the absence of peripheral lung markings on the right side and the distinct line indicating the edge of the collapsed lung (*arrow*). Although this appears to be a small PTX, it produced significant dyspnea in this patient with chronic obstructive pulmonary disease and therefore required a chest tube. **B,** Computed tomography scan showing the extent of the collapse. Adhesions kept part of the lung expanded.

Figure 10-2 A, After successful cardiopulmonary resuscitation and intubation, this patient began to deteriorate, with a precipitous drop in blood pressure and decreasing oxygen saturation. *It was believed that the cause of the initial cardiac arrest was returning.* Marked subcutaneous air was noted in the scrotum and abdominal wall, but little air was noted in the chest wall tissue. The subcutaneous air had curiously tracked via tissue planes, a distinctly unusual place for air to accumulate. **B,** A chest tube (*arrow*) quickly reversed the decompensation. **C,** This patient suffered respiratory arrest from heroin injected into a neck vein (note the extensive scar). After bag-mask resuscitation the respiratory depression returned, he was unresponsive to naloxone, and he was very difficult to ventilate. He had a small pneumothorax (PTX) from a nick in the lung from the neck injection.

spontaneous pneumothorax is a tall, thin, 20- to 40-year-old male smoker (Fig. 10-3). *Secondary spontaneous pneumothoraces* occur in patients with underlying lung or pleural disease, including emphysema, chronic bronchitis, asthma, Marfan's syndrome, infection, and neoplasm. The morbidity, mortality, and long-term complications associated with pneumothorax increase in patients with underlying lung disease. Whereas a primary pneumothorax may be selectively observed or simply

aspirated, a secondary pneumothorax often requires a more aggressive approach to management.

The sudden onset of pleuritic chest pain and dyspnea with exertion or at rest is the most common finding. More subtle manifestations occur with little or no pain and only mild dyspnea on excursion that the patient may ignore for days. A person with a small spontaneous pneumothorax may never seek medical attention, and the process will resolve without

Figure 10-3 Spontaneous pneumothorax. **A,** Spontaneous pneumothorax in a young male patient. There is nearly total collapse of the right lung, and lung markings are absent lateral to the visible pleural reflection (*arrow*). Note also the slight deviation of the mediastinum to the contralateral side. **B,** The patient was treated with a pigtail catheter inserted in the second intercostal space in the midclavicular line (*arrow*). Note that the lung has totally reexpanded and the mediastinum has shifted back to the midline.

treatment. The signs and symptoms do not always correlate well with the size or cause of the collapsed lung. Tube thoracostomy is the most common treatment, but new trials suggest that conservative management or aspiration of first-time primary pneumothoraces results in similar outcomes as traditional tube thoracostomy, though with fewer complications, shorter hospital stay, and lower cost. Conservative management and aspiration are both reasonable initial interventions in clinically stable patients. However, to date no high-quality clinical trials have definitely demonstrated that aspiration is a superior treatment methodology.[2-4] Rarely, a spontaneous pneumothorax may be bilateral or progress to tension pneumothorax, a potentially life-threatening condition that is described in more detail later in this chapter.

Traumatic Closed Pneumothorax

A closed pneumothorax may also result from an injury without penetration of the chest wall, usually from a rib fracture that penetrates the lung, but also when an alveolus or bleb ruptures after blunt trauma. The air leak from a closed pneumothorax is generally self-limited but can rarely progress to a tension pneumothorax.

Traumatic Open Pneumothorax

An open pneumothorax occurs when the chest wall is penetrated and the negative intrapleural pressure is lost. Each breath can increase intrapleural pressure. If the diameter of the chest wound is greater than the diameter of the trachea, with each respiratory attempt, air moves preferentially through the chest wall opening rather than down the trachea and thus prevents meaningful ventilation of the involved lung.

Tension Pneumothorax

An open pneumothorax can occasionally be manifested as a tension pneumothorax, which is a life-threatening condition that requires immediate intervention. A tension pneumothorax occurs when an injury creates a one-way "flap valve" mechanism that allows air into the pleural space with inspiration but then closes with expiration and traps the air (Fig. 10-4). The progressive accumulation of air in the pleural space leads to ipsilateral complete lung collapse and then impingement on the mediastinum with a shift of the heart toward the uninvolved side, which restricts ventricular filling and subsequently decreases cardiac function. This severe disruption in both respiratory and cardiac function can lead to hypotension and reduced ventilation (both hypoxia and CO_2 retention) and eventually to cardiopulmonary collapse.

A tension pneumothorax is usually caused by penetrating chest injuries but can result from fracture of the trachea or bronchi, a ruptured esophagus, the presence of an occlusive dressing over an open pneumothorax, and PPV. *Patients with chest or lung injuries who are treated with PPV are at much greater risk for the development of a tension pneumothorax.* Consequently, any patient with a penetrating thoracic injury (even without immediate evidence of a hemothorax or pneumothorax) may be a candidate for a "prophylactic" chest tube before mechanical ventilation. A pneumothorax may also develop in patients with asthma or emphysema from the high pressure required for ventilation, followed by a tension pneumothorax.

Hemothorax

Hemothorax is an accumulation of blood in the pleural space as a result of injury to the heart, great vessels, or vessels of the lungs, mediastinum, or chest wall. Bleeding from the lung parenchyma is low pressure and usually self-limited or ceases when a chest tube is inserted. On the other hand, bleeding from an intercostal artery, a pulmonary artery, or the internal mammary artery can be profuse and often requires surgical intervention.

Empyema and Effusions

An empyema is an accumulation of pus in the pleural space, usually from a parapneumonic infectious effusion (Fig. 10-5). An empyema can also be caused by violation of the thoracic space by surgical procedures (e.g., tube thoracostomy), trauma, and esophageal perforation. Pleural infection rates have increased 3% per year in the United States in the last 2 decades. The bacteriology of pleural infections appears to track closely with classification of pneumonia as community or hospital acquired. Nearly 60% of cases of community-acquired pneumonia are caused by *Streptococcus*

Figure 10-4 Traumatic tension pneumothorax. **A** and **B**, Pathophysiology of a tension pneumothorax. During inspiration, air enters the pleural space through a one-way valve either from the outside or from the lung itself. On expiration, the injury/valve closes and traps increasing amounts of air in the pleural space. Eventually, the mediastinum shifts and cardiac filling and ultimately cardiac output are compromised. **C,** This elderly patient sustained a tension hemopneumothorax after slipping and falling on ice. The left hemithorax is very dark (radiolucent) because of total collapse of the left lung (*large white arrow*). Note the dramatic shift of the mediastinum to the right, indicative of tension. Multiple posterior rib fractures are present but are difficult to appreciate on this film (*small white arrows*). The air-fluid level (*black arrow*) indicates the presence of fluid in the pleural cavity in addition to air. **D,** A computed tomography scan of the same patient redemonstrates the findings seen on the conventional radiograph.

Figure 10-5 Empyema. This 34-year old patient with a history of alcoholism had fever, cough, pleuritic chest pain, and hypoxia. **A,** Posteroanterior chest radiograph demonstrating nearly total opacification of the right hemithorax. The presence of a meniscus (*large arrow*) suggests a pleural effusion. However, small lucent areas (*small arrows*) can be seen throughout the opacity, which may represent air bronchograms in consolidated lung parenchyma. Thus, a computed tomography (CT) scan was performed. **B,** CT revealed nearly total collapse of the right lung with only a small portion of the apex remaining inflated (*white arrow*). A massive pleural collection was found with gas bubbles throughout (*black arrows*), suggestive of pyogenic empyema. Tube thoracostomy was performed and more than 1700 mL of purulent fluid was drained. Fluid cultures grew *Streptococcus anginosus*.

pneumoniae species, whereas *Staphylococcus* species account for nearly 45% of hospital-acquired infections.[5]

Chylothorax

Chylothorax results from injury to the thoracic duct during placement of a central line, operative injury, or chest trauma. Primary thoracic duct injury is usually asymptomatic because the chyle initially collects extrapleurally and may not begin to fill the pleural cavity for 2 to 10 days. As the fluid accumulates, respiratory symptoms slowly develop. The chest radiograph demonstrates a pleural effusion, and the diagnosis is made when thoracentesis reveals a milky fluid with a high fat and lymphocyte content and 4 to 5 g/dL of protein. Definitive treatment is either repeated thoracentesis or tube thoracostomy combined with parenteral alimentation until the volume of chyle decreases.

DIAGNOSIS

Symptoms

The symptoms of patients with abnormal collections in the pleural space range widely depending on the size of the pneumothorax, the rapidity of accumulation, the age of the patient, and the presence of an underlying lung disease. Specific symptoms range from mild dyspnea with exercise and pleuritic chest pain with small disruptions to hypotension or severe dyspnea in those with tension pneumothorax. With a spontaneous pneumothorax, 95% of patients complain of the sudden onset of sharp, pleuritic chest pain, shoulder pain, or both. Sixty percent of patients experience dyspnea, and 12% have a mild cough. Dyspnea and anxiety are more common in older patients.

Tension pneumothorax must be considered in any patient with sudden respiratory or cardiac deterioration and in intubated patients who become difficult to ventilate because of increased airway pressure, hypotension, or elevated central venous and pulmonary artery pressure. Severe dyspnea, restlessness, agitation, and a feeling of impending doom will develop rapidly in conscious patients with tension pneumothorax. They are usually tachycardic and tachypneic and can quickly become hypotensive.

The symptoms of hemothorax can be similar to those of pneumothorax but may be accompanied by hypotension as blood accumulates in the pleural space. The onset of symptoms with effusions is usually much more gradual, with increasing shortness of breath and dyspnea on exertion occurring over a period of days to weeks.

Physical Examination

Unstable Patients

During the initial phase of resuscitation (airway, breathing, circulation, disability), consider the diagnosis of pneumothorax in patients who are tachycardic, hypotensive, and dyspneic. Similar symptoms occur with pulmonary embolism, pericardial tamponade, and severe pneumonia. Conduct multiple examinations because the diagnosis of tension pneumothorax by physical examination can be very subtle. Use the phrase "look, listen, and feel" as your guideline. Observe the chest wall, which may reveal asymmetric chest expansion, and the neck and forehead veins, which may be distended, even if the patient is hypotensive. The trachea may be deviated away from the side of the pneumothorax. When percussing the chest wall, hyperresonance on the affected side and subcutaneous emphysema may be present. Auscultation may demonstrate diminished breath sounds on the injured side. In one prospective study, the sensitivity, specificity, and diagnostic accuracy of auscultation for hemothorax and pneumothorax were 84%, 97%, and 89%, respectively.[6] A false-negative auscultation is more likely than a false-positive one.[6] *Pulsus paradoxus* may be evident. For intubated patients, an early sign of tension pneumothorax is difficulty ventilating because of increased airway pressure.

In injured patients with apnea, hypotension, or cardiopulmonary arrest, diagnose and treat a tension pneumothorax by immediate needle or catheter decompression thoracentesis; do not take the time taken to obtain and review a radiograph because delay can lead to increased morbidity and mortality in patients with this emergency condition. Confirm the diagnosis of tension pneumothorax by observing rapid improvement in vital signs and a rush of air through the needle.

Stable Patients

In more stable patients (and those with smaller accumulations) the findings on physical examination are less sensitive, and a chest radiograph or even a computed tomography (CT) scan is usually necessary to make a definitive diagnosis. Physical findings may include unilaterally decreased breath sounds, tachypnea, tachycardia, decreased tactile fremitus, increased resonance with percussion, or subcutaneous emphysema, but the examination may reveal little to no abnormalities with a small pneumothorax. Patients with a pneumothorax involving less than 20% of the hemithorax will often have completely normal findings on chest examination, including equal breath sounds (Fig. 10-6). Pleural fluid collections are difficult to detect by physical examination, particularly with less than 500 mL of fluid in the pleural space. Breath sounds may be decreased and percussion of the bases may be dull.

Figure 10-6 Smaller pneumothoraces such as this (note the faintly visible pleural reflection [*arrow*], absence of lung markings at the left apex, and relative crowding of vessels at the left hilum) can be difficult to see on radiographs and even harder—if not impossible—to appreciate on physical examination. Patients with a pneumothorax of less than 20% will often have completely normal findings on chest examination, including equal breath sounds.

Parapneumonic empyemas are often accompanied by fever, cough, chest pain, dyspnea, and purulent sputum (see Fig. 10-5). Physical examination may reveal diminished breath sounds, dullness on percussion, egophony, and diminished tactile fremitus on the involved side. Fever will often develop in patients with an indwelling chest tube and empyema. The pleural fluid drainage may be copious and purulent, and respiratory symptoms may worsen.

Radiography

Plain Radiographs

A chest radiograph is an essential tool for diagnosing a pneumothorax in stable patients. In unstable patients with a potential tension pneumothorax the diagnosis should be made clinically, but in rare cases a portable radiograph may be obtained in the resuscitation room if carefully monitored by a clinician. The best plain radiographs for hemothorax or pneumothorax are traditional *upright inspiratory* posteroanterior and lateral chest radiographs. Diagnostic sensitivity is not increased with an *expiratory* upright chest radiograph. Upright is preferable to a supine chest radiograph, particularly for a hemothorax, because even with large amounts of blood there may only be slight *differences in the density of the lung fields* since the blood may layer out evenly. With an upright chest radiograph, 300 to 500 mL of fluid is needed to cause blunting of the costophrenic angle (Fig. 10-7).[7] When CT is not available, other useful views include a bilateral decubitus chest radiograph, with the pneumothorax expected to be seen on the side away from the table as gravity pulls the affected lung down.

On a chest radiograph the partially collapsed lung of a pneumothorax appears as a visceral pleural line with no pulmonary markings beyond it (see Figs. 10-1, 10-3, 10-6, and 10-7). *It is easy to initially mistake large blebs for a pneumothorax or to identify the scapular border, skin folds, or indwelling lines as a pneumothorax,* but a CT scan quickly resolves the issue (Fig. 10-8). Other radiographic findings include hyperlucency of the affected hemithorax, a double diaphragm contour,

increased visibility of the inferior cardiac border, better visualization of pericardial fat at the cardiac apex, and possibly a depressed diaphragm. *If subcutaneous air is noted on the chest radiograph of a patient with blunt chest trauma, it can be assumed that the air came from an injured lung and that a pneumothorax exists.*

It is difficult to accurately predict the size of a pneumothorax on plain radiographs. Greater accuracy in predicting size can be accomplished with a CT scan. With a tension pneumothorax, the chest radiograph reveals lung collapse, a depressed hemidiaphragm on the affected side, and a shift of the mediastinum and trachea to the opposite side (see Fig. 10-4). With a bilateral pneumothorax, no mediastinal shift may be seen.

Figure 10-7 Hydropneumothorax. This radiograph is an excellent example of a hydropneumothorax. When accumulated fluid in the chest cavity is seen as a *straight line on a radiograph* (an air-fluid level [*black arrow*]) with no meniscus up the side, air must be present in the pleural space. In this patient the pneumothorax is readily visualized, with no lung markings seen lateral or superior to the pleural reflection (*white arrows*).

Figure 10-8 Pneumothorax and bullous emphysema. This patient had a history of severe chronic obstructive pulmonary disease and arrived at the emergency department in respiratory distress. **A,** On the chest radiograph, both apices are relatively radiolucent, and faint lines can be seen coursing through that are not clearly blebs or pleural reflections (*arrows*). **B,** A computed tomography scan was obtained and defined the pathology in detail. In the right apex there is no pneumothorax, but rather large blebs are present (*small white arrows*). On the left a pleural reflection is clearly visible (*large white arrow*), indicative of pneumothorax. Subcutaneous air is also noted in the thoracic soft tissues (*black arrows*), thus further supporting the diagnosis of pneumothorax. (This finding is also evident on the chest radiography but was overlooked on the initial interpretation.)

Thoracic CT

The gold standard for diagnosis is a thoracic CT scan, which can detect a pneumothorax not easily visible on a plain radiograph. CT scans of the chest are much more sensitive than plain radiographs in detecting hemothorax and pneumothorax. They are also more accurate for estimating the size and other characteristics of a pneumothorax (see Figs. 10-1, 10-4, and 10-8). CT scans are not routine for diagnosis of a pneumothorax but are more useful for hemothoraces and other fluid collections. They also offer invaluable information on the cause of such abnormalities. A CT scan may be useful when the diagnosis is unclear or when looking for small amounts of pleural fluid. CT scans are particularly helpful in determining whether an empyema is loculated or draining successfully. About 10% of trauma patients with normal findings on a chest radiograph will demonstrate a small hemothorax or pneumothorax.[7-9] The clinical significance of a small, previously undetected occult injury is probably not great, and it has been suggested that a small pneumothorax seen only on CT may be left untreated and simply observed in otherwise stable patients. Some patients with a pneumothorax seen only on CT may also safely undergo PPV without placement of a chest tube.[9]

Ultrasound

Ultrasound is useful in diagnosing both hemothoraces and pneumothoraces, and its use is reviewed in the Ultrasound Box.[10,11]

INDICATIONS FOR TUBE THORACOSTOMY

Pneumothorax

Tube thoracostomy is by far the most common treatment of all types of pneumothoraces, but controversy exists over the treatment of small traumatic and spontaneous primary pneumothoraces. However, the American College of Chest Physicians has developed useful guidelines for the management of primary and secondary spontaneous pneumothoraces (Box 10-1).[12]

Chest tube placement is probably not necessary in healthy patients with small primary spontaneous or isolated small traumatic pneumothoraces in the absence of respiratory compromise or concomitant injuries or when PPV will not be required. With no intervention, a small pneumothorax will resolve over a period of days to weeks. Supplemental oxygen will speed the process of lung reexpansion by increasing the rate of pleural air absorption. No controlled studies have been conducted to compare the various interventions for primary spontaneous pneumothorax, and there is wide variation in treatment approaches. In particular, no significant difference has been found between simple aspiration and tube drainage with regard to the immediate success rate, early failure rate, duration of hospitalization, and 1-year success and pleurodesis.[13] Needle aspiration is associated with reduced analgesia requirements, lower pain scores, and a lower percentage of patients being hospitalized. Recent studies have shown excellent short- and long-term outcomes after video-assisted

ULTRASOUND: Recognizing Pneumothorax
by Christine Butts, MD

To evaluate for pneumothorax, a high-frequency transducer should be used to ensure a high degree of resolution. In a supine patient the transducer should be placed on the anterior chest wall in the midclavicular line at approximately the second to third intercostal space (Fig. 10-US1). The depth of the image should be adjusted until the ribs are seen as brightly echogenic (white) arcs with acoustic shadows behind them. The pleural line can be found just deep to the ribs and is

represented as a horizontal, echogenic line (Fig. 10-US2). In a normal lung the visceral and parietal pleural layers are directly opposed to one another (save for a thin layer of pleural fluid). When the patient breathes in and out, the layers "slide" past each other to allow the lungs to expand. When this is viewed with ultrasound, the pleural line can be seen to slide back and forth with patient respiration. This is referred to as the "slide sign." In cases in which this interface is disrupted (such as by a

Figure 10-US1 Proper positioning of the probe for evaluation of pneumothorax.

Figure 10-US2 Ultrasound image of the pleura as seen with a high-frequency transducer. The pleura can be recognized as a hyperechoic (*white*) line (*arrow*) that normally moves back and forth with respiration. Identifying the rib, along with its accompanying shadow (*arrowhead*), often aids in identifying the pleura because it will lie immediately deep to the rib.

Continued

ULTRASOUND: Recognizing Pneumothorax, cont'd

Figure 10-US3 This image demonstrates two key artifacts seen in a normal lung. As with the previous image, the pleura is recognized as a hyperechoic horizontal line deep to the ribs (at the *far right and left* of the image). A comet tail, a small vertical line, can be seen extending deep to the pleura (*arrow*). This is a normal artifact created by the pleura, and its presence aids in ruling out a pneumothorax. A-lines, or a series of horizontal lines extending deep to the pleura, can also be seen (*arrowhead*). These artifacts may be seen both in normal lung and in the presence of pneumothorax.

Figure 10-US4 Seashore sign seen in a normal lung. This M-mode image shows movement of the pleura. The solid lines at the top of the image represent the immobile skin, soft tissue, and muscle. The hazy lines at the bottom of the image represent the back-and-forth movement of the normal pleura.

pneumothorax), the sliding is lost. When these patients are evaluated with ultrasound, the pleural line will be seen as a static echogenic line that does not change with respiration.

Although the slide sign carries significant sensitivity for ruling out a pneumothorax, other secondary confirmatory findings should be sought as well.[1]

Comet tail artifacts may be seen in a normal lung. These are hyperechoic vertical lines that extend deep to the pleural interface

Figure 10-US5 Bar code sign consistent with a pneumothorax. This M-mode image shows lack of movement of the pleura. Unlike the previous image, the solid lines can be seen to continue past the point of the pleural line. Because the presence of the pneumothorax causes the pleura to appear stationary, no movement is seen in this image.

(Fig. 10-US3). Typically, they will be seen in small numbers in a normal lung. Patients in whom a pneumothorax is present are noted to lack comet tails because this artifact arises from the normal pleural interface, which is disrupted. The presence of comet tails may be used by the sonographer to further rule out a pneumothorax.[2,3]

M-mode may also be used to further evaluate for the presence of a pneumothorax. M-mode is used to evaluate objects in motion and plots a linear representation of motion on screen. Objects that move toward the surface (or toward the transducer) are represented by an upward deflection. Objects that move away from the transducer are represented by a downward deflection. Objects that are not in motion are represented by a solid line.

In a normal patient, the pleura will slide back and forth as the patient breathes. Because this motion is neither toward nor away from the transducer but instead is parallel, the motion will be seen as a series of hazy lines deep to the pleura. The overlying soft tissue is not in motion and will be seen as a series of clear, flat lines. This typical appearance is described as the "seashore" sign (Fig. 10-US4).

In patients in whom a pneumothorax is present, no motion is detected by ultrasound. Therefore, the M-mode tracing will show clear, flat lines throughout the frame. This is referred to as the "stratosphere" or "bar code" sign (Fig. 10-US5).

REFERENCES:

1. Blaivas M, Lyon M, Duggal S. A prospective comparison of supine chest radiography and bedside ultrasound for the diagnosis of traumatic pneumothorax. *Acad Emerg Med*. 2005;12:844-849.
2. Lichtenstein D, Meziere G, Biderman P, et al. The comet-tail artifact: an ultrasound sign ruling out pneumothorax. *Intensive Care Med*. 1999; 25:383-388.
3. Chan SS. Emergency bedside ultrasound to detect pneumothorax. *Acad Emerg Med*. 2003;10:91-94.

BOX 10-1 **Guidelines of the American College of Chest Physicians for the Management of Primary and Secondary Spontaneous Pneumothoraces**

PRIMARY SPONTANEOUS PNEUMOTHORAX (NO UNDERLYING LUNG DISEASE)

A clinically stable patient must have all of the following present: respiratory rate lower than 24 breaths/min, heart rate higher than 60 beats/min or less than 120 beats/min, normal blood pressure, room-air O_2 saturation higher than 90%, and the ability to speak in whole sentences between breaths.

CLINICALLY STABLE PATIENTS WITH SMALL PNEUMOTHORACES (<3-CM APEX-TO-CUPOLA DISTANCE)

Clinically stable patients with small pneumothoraces (PTXs) should be observed in the emergency department (ED) for 3 to 6 hours and be discharged home if a repeated chest radiograph excludes progression of the PTX (good consensus). Patients should be provided with careful instructions for follow-up within 12 hours to 2 days, depending on the circumstances. A chest radiograph should be obtained at the follow-up appointment to document resolution of the PTX. Patients may be admitted for observation if they live distant from emergency services or follow-up care is considered unreliable (good consensus). Simple aspiration of the PTX or insertion of a chest tube is not appropriate for most patients (good consensus) unless the PTX enlarges. The presence of symptoms for longer than 24 hours does not alter the treatment recommendations.

CLINICALLY STABLE PATIENTS WITH LARGE PNEUMOTHORACES (≥3-CM APEX-TO-CUPOLA DISTANCE)

Clinically stable patients with large PTXs should undergo a procedure to reexpand the lung and should be hospitalized in most instances (very good consensus). The lung should be reexpanded by using a small-bore catheter (≤14 Fr) or placement of a 16- to 22-Fr chest tube (good consensus). Catheters or tubes may be attached either to a Heimlich valve (good consensus) or to a water seal device (good consensus) and may be left in place until the lung expands against the chest wall and the air leaks have resolved. If the lung fails to reexpand quickly, suction should be applied to a water seal device. Alternatively, suction may be applied immediately after placement of a chest tube in all patients managed with a water seal system (some consensus).

Reliable patients who are unwilling to undergo hospitalization may be discharged home from the ED with a small-bore catheter attached to a Heimlich valve if the lung reexpanded after the removal of pleural air (good consensus). Follow-up should be arranged within 2 days. The presence of symptoms for longer than 24 hours does not alter management recommendations.

SECONDARY SPONTANEOUS PNEUMOTHORAX
Clinically Stable Patients with Small Pneumothoraces

Clinically stable patients with small PTXs should be hospitalized (good consensus). Patients should not be managed in the ED with observation or simple aspiration without hospitalization (very good consensus). Hospitalized patients may be observed (good consensus) or treated with a chest tube (some consensus), depending on the extent of their symptoms and the course of their PTX. Some of the panel members argued against observation alone because of a report of deaths with this approach. Patients should not be referred for thoracoscopy without prior stabilization (very good consensus). The presence of symptoms for longer than 24 hours did not alter the panel members' recommendations.

Clinically Stable Patients with Large Pneumothoraces

Clinically stable patients with large PTXs should undergo placement of a chest tube to reexpand the lung and should be hospitalized (very good consensus). Patients should not be referred for thoracoscopy without prior stabilization with a chest tube (very good consensus). The presence of symptoms for longer than 24 hours did not alter the panel members' recommendations.
This is meant to be a guide, and clinical judgment should always be used.

From Baumann MH, Strange C, Heffner JE, et al, for the AACP Pneumothorax Consensus Group. Management of spontaneous pneumothorax: an American College of Chest Physicians Delphi consensus statement. Chest. *2001;119:590.*

thoracoscopic treatment (VATS) of primary and secondary spontaneous pneumothorax, and rates of recurrence are lower than after other treatment modalities. However, VATS continues to have a higher complication rate than simple tube thoracostomy does, with 4.6% of patients with spontaneous pneumothorax experiencing serious side effects as a result of the procedure.[14,15]

In patients with a simple pneumothorax, prolonged suction is rarely required, and the tube can simply be attached to a Heimlich valve or underwater seal.[16-18]

Treatment is different for patients with a secondary spontaneous pneumothorax because the presence of underlying disease leads to more serious compromise and more frequent complications. In patients with chronic obstructive pulmonary disease, malignancy, cystic fibrosis, pneumonia, and tuberculosis, a chest tube cannot usually be avoided.

The underlying lung pathology of a patient with a spontaneous pneumothorax is best initially evaluated with CT.

Frequently, this is followed by diagnostic or therapeutic visual inspection of the lung and pleural space by fiberoptic thoracoscopy. Extensive evaluation is not, however, usually recommended for the first episode of a small primary pneumothorax. When patients have recurrent spontaneous pneumothoraces, further evaluation (CT, thoracoscopy) and evaluation for surgical treatment are indicated. Patients who have had one spontaneous pneumothorax have a 30% to 50% chance of recurrence within 2 years, and after the second pneumothorax there is a 50% to 80% chance of a third developing. Surgery may be recommended for a first pneumothorax in the following situations: life-threatening tension pneumothorax, massive air leaks with incomplete reexpansion, an air leak persisting 4 days after a second tube has been placed, associated hemothorax with complications, identifiable bullous disease, or failure of easy reexpansion in patients with cystic fibrosis.

In patients with *traumatic causes*, the urgency and type of treatment depend primarily on the stability of the patient; a hypotensive patient with a tension pneumothorax requires immediate decompression with a chest tube or needle thoracostomy, whereas a patient with normal vital signs and a small pneumothorax may be observed initially. Emergency needle thoracostomy is only a temporary solution for a compromised patient with a pneumothorax. Once done, needle thoracostomy necessitates an ipsilateral tube thoracostomy. Other factors that modify treatment include the patient's age, the size of the pneumothorax, whether bilateral pneumothoraces are present, and whether the current episode represents a recurrence. A chest tube is usually indicated for a pneumothorax.

Because of the risk for tension pneumothorax, a chest tube should be considered in all patients with a penetrating chest injury if PPV will be used or if they will be transported a long distance for definitive care. However, CT scans of trauma victims have demonstrated that many patients with small pneumothoraces that would have escaped detection with standard radiographs have safely undergone PPV without clinically evident pneumothorax developing. Close observation for signs of tension pneumothorax is necessary for patients in whom a chest tube is not placed *and* PPV is used.

Hemothorax

Tube thoracostomy is the treatment of hemothorax, but it is also used to monitor the amount and rapidity of blood output, which determines the need for additional interventions, including video-assisted thoracoscopy or open thoracotomy. About three fourths of patients with a traumatic hemothorax can be managed by tube thoracostomy and volume replacement alone. The remaining patients will require immediate or delayed elective thoracotomy. The indications for surgery after an acute hemothorax vary somewhat between authors but are summarized in Box 10-2. Early institution of blood replacement is recommended for patients with massive hemothoraces (>2000 mL) because they are often associated with continuing hemorrhage. Autotransfusion of the shed blood is desirable whenever possible. For patients with active blood loss but stable hemodynamics, VATS can be used to locate and stop the bleeding, evacuate blood clots, and break down adhesions.

BOX 10-2 **Indications for Surgery after Tube Thoracostomy Based on Results of Thoracostomy**

Massive hemothorax, >1000- to 1500-mL initial drainage
Continued bleeding
>300 to 500 mL in the first hour
>200 mL/hr for the first 3 or more hours
Increasing size of the hemothorax on a chest film
Persistent hemothorax after two functioning tubes are placed
Clotted hemothorax
Large air leak preventing effective ventilation
Persistent air leak after placement of a second tube or inability to fully expand the lung

This is meant to be a guide, and clinical judgment should always be used.

Empyema

Treatment of empyema depends on the severity of the infection and the patient's underlying condition. Some patients with empyema can be treated with serial thoracentesis, but most will require continuous drainage with a chest tube (see Fig. 10-5). Thoracoscopic decortication represents definitive therapy for severe cases. Usually, diagnostic thoracentesis is performed first to assess the fluid for signs of infection. Thick pus on thoracentesis, positive Gram stain, fluid glucose level lower than 60 mg/dL, pH less than 7.20, or elevated lactate dehydrogenase is associated with infection and an effusion that requires chest tube drainage. Once an empyema is detected, therapy should not be delayed because the fluid can quickly become loculated. Generally, the tube is left in place until the pleural drainage fluid becomes clear yellow and accumulates less than 150 mL in 24 hours. An empyema that fails to resolve on chest radiography within 48 hours requires chest CT and a careful review of antibiotic choice. Multiloculated effusions are best managed by thoracoscopic decortication.

CONTRAINDICATIONS

For unstable trauma patients with a pneumothorax or hemothorax, there are no absolute contraindications to tube thoracostomy. In critical patients, placement of a chest tube is often performed empirically. In stable patients, relative contraindications include anatomic problems such as the presence of multiple pleural adhesions, emphysematous blebs, or scarring. Coagulopathic patients should be evaluated for replacement of clotting factors before any invasive procedure.

TREATMENT

Treatment of a Possible Tension Pneumothorax in an Unstable Patient

Immediate decompression of the chest must be considered in all injured patients with unexplained hypotension or tachypnea, particularly those with penetrating chest injuries. The goal is to open the pleural space quickly to allow any accumulated air to escape and decompress the chest cavity. This can be accomplished with a scalpel and forceps, as is done at the beginning stages of a thoracostomy (Fig. 10-9), or more commonly, decompression can be achieved with a large-bore needle/angiocatheter combination (minimum of 16 gauge) (Fig. 10-10). Place the catheter in the second intercostal space at the midclavicular line on the side with diminished breath sounds or on both sides if the diagnosis is unclear. Remove the needle, but leave the angiocatheter in place to create a simple pneumothorax. Regardless of whether this is successful in improving the patient's vital signs, perform a standard tube thoracostomy immediately following the decompression. If the needle decompression is not effective, an open thoracostomy can be started, even without the immediate availability of a chest tube, to help create an exit for the air so that the patient's respiratory and cardiovascular function can normalize.

Prehospital Treatment

Emergency needle decompression thoracostomy may be used in the prehospital setting or when a patient suspected of

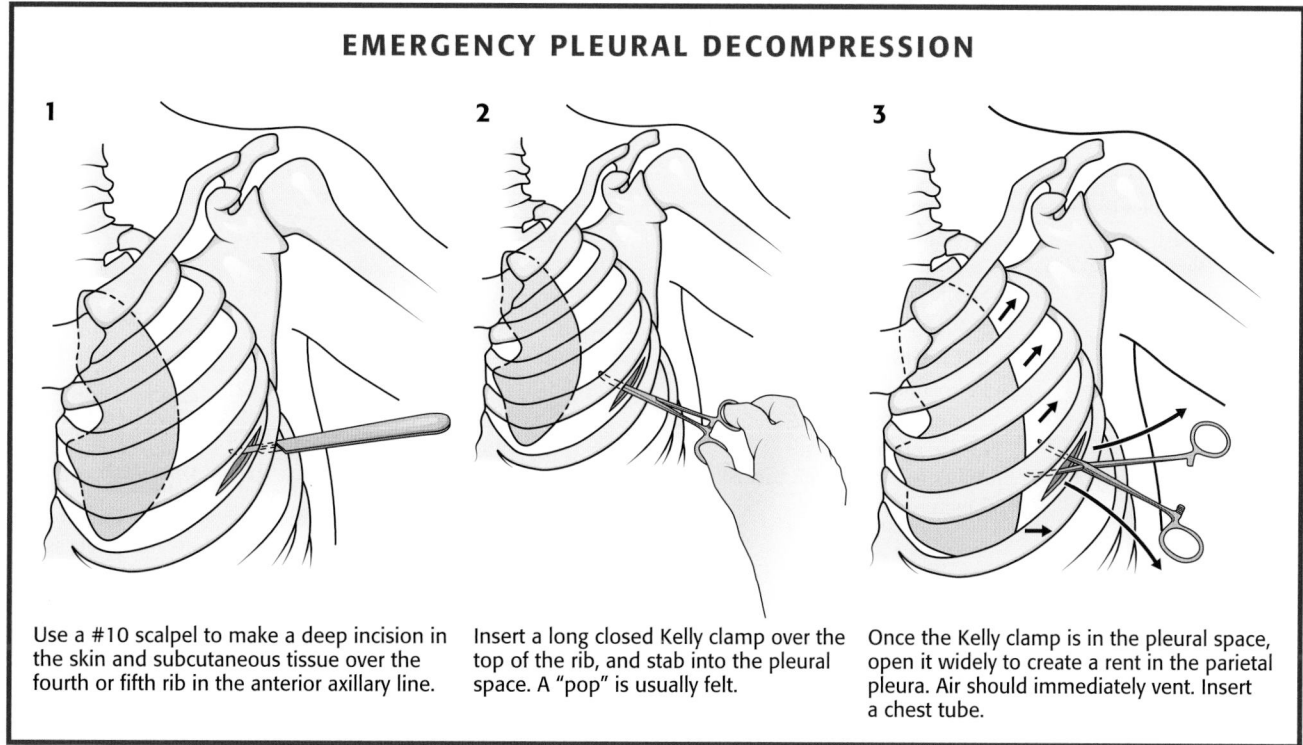

EMERGENCY PLEURAL DECOMPRESSION

1

Use a #10 scalpel to make a deep incision in the skin and subcutaneous tissue over the fourth or fifth rib in the anterior axillary line.

2

Insert a long closed Kelly clamp over the top of the rib, and stab into the pleural space. A "pop" is usually felt.

3

Once the Kelly clamp is in the pleural space, open it widely to create a rent in the parietal pleura. Air should immediately vent. Insert a chest tube.

Figure 10-9 Emergency pleural decompression. During resuscitation of a patient with a tension pneumothorax, there may be no time for a chest tube, and needle decompression may not be effective rapidly enough. Under these circumstances, the pleural cavity can be vented in seconds. This assumes that the patient is intubated.

having a pneumothorax rapidly deteriorates or is initially seen in extremis. In such cases, attach the needle (or catheter) to a one-way (Heimlich) valve, underwater seal, or even a flutter valve (fashioned from the fingers of a surgical glove) so that the air can continue to escape during expiration but cannot enter during inspiration.

When a patient has an open chest wound in the prehospital setting, use a three-sided occlusive dressing to cover the wound. Similar to the one-way valve mechanisms, this dressing also acts as a one-way valve to allow air to escape but prevents air from entering the chest cavity. Use a sterile dressing, such as petrolatum-impregnated gauze, that extends 6 to 8 cm beyond the wound in all directions. Tape down only three sides of the dressing. Instruct the patient to deeply inhale, perform a Valsalva maneuver, or cough while you place the dressing.

Emergency Department Treatment

Equipment

The standard instruments for a tube thoracostomy tray are listed in Box 10-3 and depicted in Review Box 10-1. The most basic needs are a scalpel, a large (Kelly) clamp, and the thoracostomy (chest) tube.

Thoracostomy tubes are clear plastic tubes of various diameter that are open at both ends (Fig. 10-11). There is a radiopaque strip along the length of the tube that is interrupted by a series of holes along the distal length of the tube. The strip allows visualization of the tube's location on the postprocedure radiograph and ensures that the side ports are within the pleural cavity. Tube sizes vary from 12 to 42 Fr, with smaller tubes being used for smaller pneumothoraces and larger (a minimum of 36 Fr) tubes for hemothorax and

Second intercostal space, midclavicular line

14-gauge angiocatheter attached to a syringe

Figure 10-10 Needle decompression. A large-bore needle/catheter combination is used to puncture the parietal pleura and establish the presence of blood or air in the pleural space. The needle can be placed anywhere in the pleural space, but traditionally at the same sites used for tube thoracostomy: the anterior second intercostal space in the midclavicular line or the anterior axillary line in the fourth or fifth interspace. The needle is placed so that it enters over the rib to avoid neurovascular injury. The needle is then withdrawn while leaving the catheter behind to create a simple open pneumothorax. The procedure can be done either with or without the syringe attached to the catheter. This is only a temporary therapeutic maneuver for a tension pneumothorax, and a chest tube must also be inserted.

| BOX 10-3 | Recommended Equipment for Tube Thoracostomy |

PROCEDURE

Sterile drapes

10- to 20-mL syringe and assorted needles (for local anesthesia)

Local anesthetic (1% to 2% lidocaine)

Antiseptic solution

Scalpel with a No. 10 blade

Large clamps (Kelly)

Needle holder

Chest tubes (size appropriate)

No. 0 or 1-0 silk or similar suture

Forceps

Straight (suture) scissors

Large, curved (Mayo) scissors

Soft arm restraints

DRAINAGE SYSTEM AND TUBING

Drainage apparatus with sterile water for the water seal

Hard plastic serrated connectors

Sterile tubing

DRESSING

Petrolatum gauze or similar occlusive dressing

Gauze or similar pads

Adhesive tape—cloth backed

Tincture of benzoin

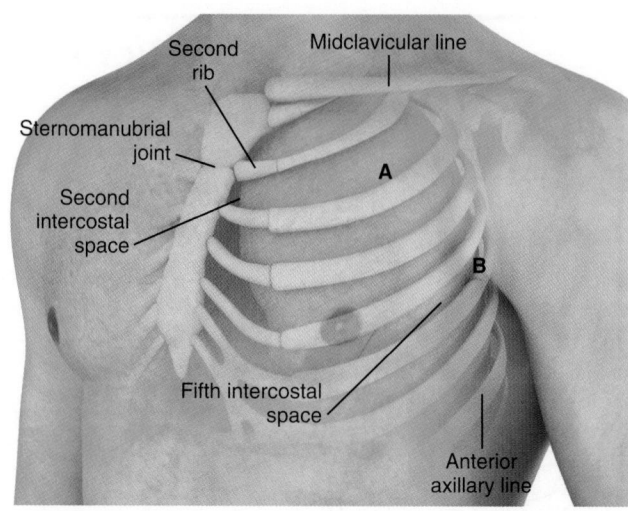

Figure 10-12 Entry sites for tube thoracostomy. The second intercostal space, midclavicular line, is the preferred site for needle aspiration or catheter insertion (*A*). To find the second intercostal space, first palpate the sternomanubrial joint. The second rib articulates with this structure. The second intercostal space is found *below* the second rib. The fourth or fifth intercostal space, midaxillary to anterior axillary line (lateral to the pectoralis muscle and breast tissue), is preferred for a chest tube (*B*). The fifth intercostal space is usually at the level of the nipple. In an obese woman an assistant has to retract the breast upward to identify landmarks and avoid low placement.

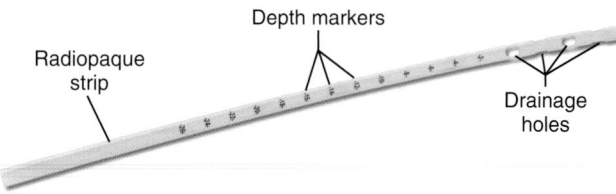

Figure 10-11 Thoracostomy tube.

empyema. For pediatric patients, 14-, 16-, 20-, and 24-Fr tubes are adequate.

PROCEDURE

Conduct the procedure as sterilely as possible and wear a gown, glove, mask, and goggles. When possible, obtain consent.

Tube Insertion Site

Insert the tube over the top of the rib rather than near the bottom to avoid the neurovascular structures located on the inferior aspect of the ribs. The most common location for a chest tube is the midaxillary to anterior axillary line, usually in the fourth or fifth intercostal space (Fig. 10-12). This approach is cosmetically preferable and better tolerated than the anterior chest wall approach in the second intercostal space of the midclavicular line. The fifth intercostal space is approximately at the level of the nipple or the inferior scapular border in most patients, although the position of the female breast mass leads to variance. To avoid penetrating the abdominal cavity, choose a more superior insertion site because the external landmarks can be misleading. The diaphragm of a supine patient who is not taking a deep breath is much higher than expected.

Hold the tube next to the chest wall with the tip of the tube at the level of the clavicle to estimate the distance that the tube needs to be advanced from the incision site to the apex of the lung. Place a clamp on the tube to mark the maximum length that the tube should be inserted to prevent the tube from advancing too far. Confirm that the last drainage hole is within the pleural space at the level of the insertion site to ensure that the tube has been advanced sufficiently far. In markedly obese patients, it is common to fail to advance the tube far enough, with the last hole being left in fatty tissue rather than in the pleural space.

Patient Preparation

If indicated clinically, start oxygenating and monitoring the patient continuously with cardiac and pulse oximetry. When possible, elevate the head of the bed 30 to 60 degrees (Fig. 10-13) to lower the diaphragm and decrease the risk for injury to the diaphragm, spleen, and liver. Abduct the arm on the affected side, place it over the patient's head, and restrain it in that position. Clean the skin with a standard surgical scrub and drape the field with sterile towels.

Anesthesia

Tube thoracostomy can be extremely painful, so give parenteral analgesics or procedural sedation to stable patients before the procedure. A common problem is inadequate systemic analgesia and local anesthesia. Use generous local anesthesia, such as up to 5 mg/kg of locally injected 1% lidocaine with or without epinephrine. Slowly inject local anesthetic over the superior aspect of the rib; through the muscle, periosteum, and parietal pleura; and along the *entire anticipated tract of passage of the tube* (Fig. 10-14). Intermittently aspirate for air or fluid with the needle to find the pleural cavity. If air or fluid is not found, change the insertion site.

Figure 10-13 To insert a chest tube, position the patient semi-erect with the ipsilateral arm abducted as far as possible and preferably restrained. Supplemental oxygen and monitoring are recommended.

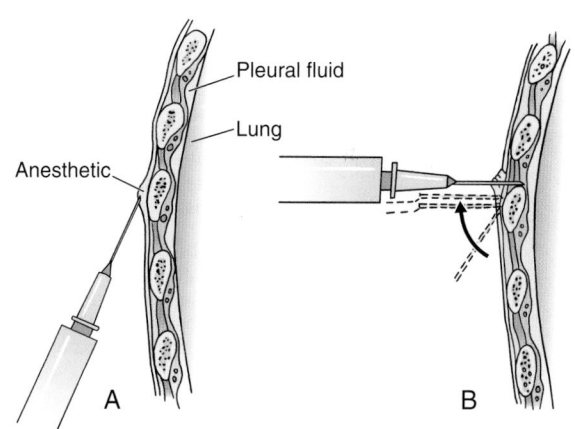

Figure 10-14 Local anesthesia is essential to reduce the pain from insertion of a chest tube. Both the skin and pleura should be infiltrated with a generous amount of local anesthetic. **A,** The anesthetic is first infiltrated over the rib at the site of the incision. **B,** The needle is then advanced slowly over the top of the rib while intermittently infiltrating and aspirating until the pleura is breeched and air is withdrawn. Anesthetic is then injected liberally (maximum of 5 mg/kg of lidocaine) to cover the pleural lining. (*A and B, Redrawn from Hughes WT, Buescher ES.* Pediatric Procedures. *2nd ed. Philadelphia: Saunders; 1980:234.*)

Once the tube is in place, administer local anesthetic through the chest tube into the pleural space to reduce pain caused by the tube rubbing against the pleura. In a stable patient, add 10 mL of 0.5% bupivacaine through the chest tube while the patient is lying on the contralateral side.[19] After 5 minutes without drainage of the thorax, reinitiate standard gravity or vacuum drainage. Use parenteral analgesic agents as needed to control pain.

Insertion

The incision site should be lateral to the edge of the pectoralis major and breast tissue and not through these structures. A common problem is that the skin incision is too short to create and maintain an adequate tract to insert the thoracostomy tube. Make sure that the incision is no less than 3 to 5 cm long (Fig. 10-15, *step 1*). Make a transverse incision through the skin and subcutaneous tissue with a No. 10 blade over the rib. Some authors advocate making the initial skin incision over a rib lower than the intended intercostal space through which the tube will enter and then "tunneling" the tube under the skin and up over the next rib. This is theoretically done to prevent air leaks, but there is no good evidence to support this practice. It is more common to simply make the incision so that there is a straight path to the pleural cavity, but over the appropriate rib. This avoids the problem of losing the entrance point or increasing damage to soft tissue, both issues in obese patients. After the incision is made, insert a large Kelly clamp to push and spread the deeper tissues. Bluntly dissect a tract over the rib while avoiding the intercostal vessels and nerve on the inferior margin of each rib (Fig. 10-16; also see Fig. 10-15, *step 2*). Firm resistance will usually be felt when the tough parietal pleura is met. Close the clamp and push it forward with firm pressure to penetrate the pleura and enter the cavity. Considerable force may be needed. To prevent the clamp from penetrating too deeply, hold it at the midshaft a few centimeters distal to the incision and rest the tip against the pleura before pushing through (Fig. 10-17). *Penetrating the pleura is usually the most painful portion of the procedure,* so consider injecting extra anesthetic or analgesic at this point. On entering the pleural cavity, a palpable pop may be felt and a rush of air or fluid may occur. With only the tips of the clamp in the pleural cavity, spread the clamp to make an adequate hole in the pleura and then withdraw it (see Fig. 10-15, *step 3*). *Make the opening in the parietal pleura wide enough to comfortably insert both a finger and the tube, but avoid a larger pleural opening to reduce the risk for an air leak* (Fig. 10-18).

Another common problem occurs at this point, particularly in obese patients: *the dissected tract and pleural opening can be lost when the clamp is withdrawn.* To prevent this problem, slide a sterile gloved finger over the clamp and into the pleura before withdrawing the clamp (Fig. 10-19). *This is done to further define the tract and to verify that the pleura has been entered and that no solid organs have been penetrated.* Whenever possible, *leave the finger in the pleural space* so that the hole is not lost (see Fig. 10-15, *step 4*) and then pass the tube over, under, or beside the finger into the pleural space, with the fingertip being used to guide the course of the tube (Fig. 10-20). This step allows the clinician to feel the tube passing into the pleural cavity, avoids subcutaneous dissection by the tube, and enhances proper direction of the tube. Pass the tube alone or hold onto a large curved clamp with the tip of the tube protruding beyond the tip of the clamp (Fig. 10-21; also see Fig. 10-15, *step 5*). Normally, the tube should pass with little resistance. If resistance is met, the tube may not be in the pleural cavity and instead is passing subcutaneously, is in a fissure, or is abutting against the mediastinum (Fig. 10-22). Still using the finger that remains in the pleural space, direct the tube posteriorly, medially, and superiorly until the last hole of the tube is clearly in the thorax, the marker clamp that was previously attached touches the chest wall, or resistance

TUBE THORACOSTOMY

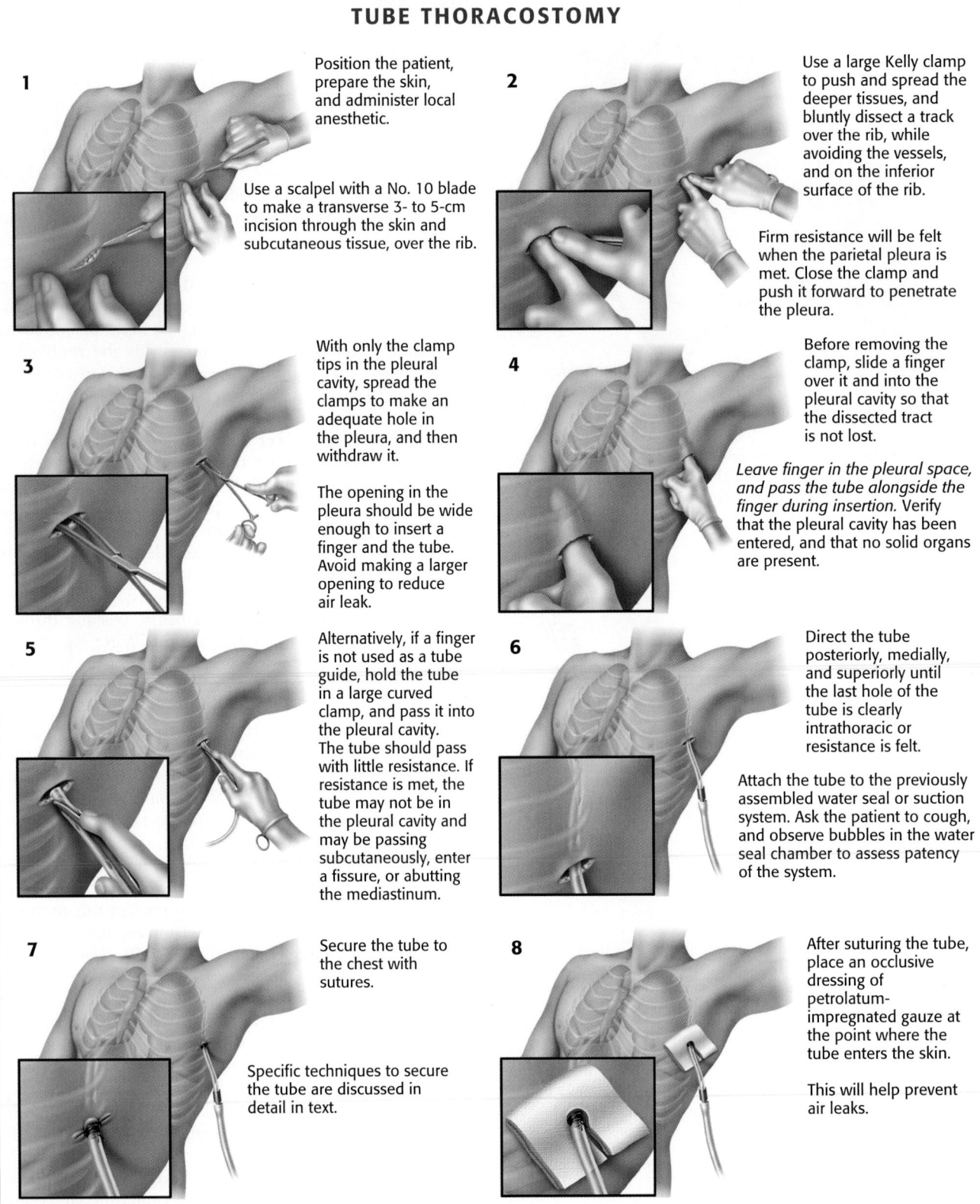

1 Position the patient, prepare the skin, and administer local anesthetic.

Use a scalpel with a No. 10 blade to make a transverse 3- to 5-cm incision through the skin and subcutaneous tissue, over the rib.

2 Use a large Kelly clamp to push and spread the deeper tissues, and bluntly dissect a track over the rib, while avoiding the vessels, and on the inferior surface of the rib.

Firm resistance will be felt when the parietal pleura is met. Close the clamp and push it forward to penetrate the pleura.

3 With only the clamp tips in the pleural cavity, spread the clamps to make an adequate hole in the pleura, and then withdraw it.

The opening in the pleura should be wide enough to insert a finger and the tube. Avoid making a larger opening to reduce air leak.

4 Before removing the clamp, slide a finger over it and into the pleural cavity so that the dissected tract is not lost.

Leave finger in the pleural space, and pass the tube alongside the finger during insertion. Verify that the pleural cavity has been entered, and that no solid organs are present.

5 Alternatively, if a finger is not used as a tube guide, hold the tube in a large curved clamp, and pass it into the pleural cavity. The tube should pass with little resistance. If resistance is met, the tube may not be in the pleural cavity and may be passing subcutaneously, enter a fissure, or abutting the mediastinum.

6 Direct the tube posteriorly, medially, and superiorly until the last hole of the tube is clearly intrathoracic or resistance is felt.

Attach the tube to the previously assembled water seal or suction system. Ask the patient to cough, and observe bubbles in the water seal chamber to assess patency of the system.

7 Secure the tube to the chest with sutures.

Specific techniques to secure the tube are discussed in detail in text.

8 After suturing the tube, place an occlusive dressing of petrolatum-impregnated gauze at the point where the tube enters the skin.

This will help prevent air leaks.

Figure 10-15 Tube thoracostomy. *(From Custalow CB. Color Atlas of Emergency Department Procedures. Philadelphia: Saunders; 2005.)*

is felt (see Fig. 10-14, *step 6*). *Ensure that all the holes in the tube are within the pleural space.* Rotate the tube 360 degrees to reduce the likelihood of kinking.

Attach the tube to the previously assembled water seal or suction before releasing the clamp. Ask the patient to cough and look for bubbles in the water seal chamber to check for patency of the system.

Confirmation of Tube Placement

There are many ways to confirm the location of the tube. Slide a finger along the tube to verify that it has entered the pleural cavity. Look for condensation on the inside of the tube and listen for air movement, which is audible during respirations. Observe free flow of blood or fluid. Check to be sure that the tube rotates freely after insertion. A chest radiograph is used for definitive assessment of tube placement (Fig. 10-23). If the tube and most proximal hole are not completely

within the pleural space and *if the field has remained sterile,* advance the tube. If the tube is kinked or dysfunctional or the sterile field has been lost and advancement is required, place a new tube in sterile fashion through the same tract. If the tube has been advanced too far, simply withdraw it to the correct depth.

Securing the Tube

Once the position of the tube has been verified with a radiograph, secure it. There are numerous methods to secure a tube. The usual one is to sew the tube to the skin with large 0 or 1-0 silk or nylon sutures. Nylon sutures are acceptable but must be tied tightly or they will slip on the surface of the tube. One common method is to use a "stay" suture in which the same suture that closes the skin incision is used to hold the tube (Fig. 10-24, *plate 1*). After this suture is used to close the skin incision at the site of insertion of the tube, wrap

Figure 10-16 Direct the Kelly clamp *over the top of the rib* to avoid the intercostal neurovascular bundle that courses along the inferior portion of the rib. Do not use excessive tunneling. (*From Millikan JS, Moore EE, Steiner E. Complications of tube thoracostomy for acute trauma. Am J Surg. 1980;140:739.*)

Figure 10-18 Right-sided subcutaneous emphysema after chest tube placement *secondary to making too large a hole in the pleura with a subsequent air leak (arrows)*. It is usually benign and self-limited, but with positive pressure ventilation, it can be problematic. Because there is no way to close the pleura, making just the right-sized hole is the key to success.

Figure 10-17 A and **B,** Use the right hand to push the clamp through the pleura (*white arrows*). Firmly encircle the midportion of the clamp with the fingers of the left hand to serve as a safety stop measure to avoid penetrating too deeply.

Figure 10-19 After puncturing the pleural lining and spreading with the clamp, slide a gloved finger over the clamp to ensure that the pleural space has been reached and that no solid masses are present. Then withdraw the clamp and use the finger as a guide for the chest tube to ensure entry into the pleural cavity.

Figure 10-20 Leave your finger in the pleural space and use it to guide the course of the tube.

Tube tip protruding beyond the clamp

Chest tube

Kelly clamp

Figure 10-21 Hold the tube with the tip of the tube protruding beyond the tip of the clamp to reduce the risk for pulmonary injury.

Figure 10-22 Subcutaneous placement of a chest tube (*arrows*) can occur because the tube can dissect through tissue planes with relative ease. If this tube had been directed posteriorly, the radiograph would erroneously "confirm" intrapleural placement despite the tube being subcutaneous throughout its entire course. A computed tomography scan would settle the issue of a misplaced tube.

Figure 10-23 Definitive assessment of chest tube placement is with a chest radiograph. This patient has two chest tubes in place, and the radiopaque marking lines on the tubes (*large arrows*) are readily visible. Chest tubes are manufactured so that these radiopaque lines are interrupted at the level of the last drainage hole (*small arrows*). *The gap in the line must be within the pleural cavity on the radiograph* to ensure that the tube has been placed deep enough.

the ends tightly and repeatedly around the chest tube and tie it securely. *Tie the sutures tightly enough to indent the chest tube slightly and avoid slippage.* If the skin incision is especially long, use additional simple sutures to close it completely.

Another optional suture technique can both help close the skin around the tube and completely close the incision once the chest tube is removed. To do this, place a *horizontal mattress suture* approximately 1 cm across the incision on either side of the tube, essentially encircling it (Fig. 10-24, *plate 2*). Secure it with a simple knot that can easily be untied so that it can be opened and retied to close the incision after the tube has been removed.

SECURING A THORACOSTOMY TUBE

1

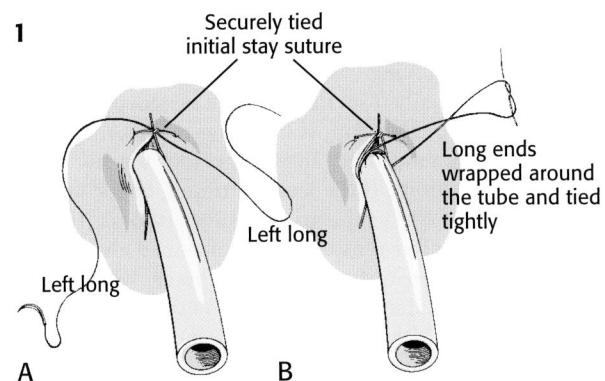

Securely tied
initial stay suture

Long ends
wrapped around
the tube and tied
tightly

Left long

Left long

A   B

A, To secure the tube, first close the skin incision with a "stay" suture near the tube. **B**, Tie the knot securely and leave the suture ends long for wrapping around and tying the tube. Wrap the suture tightly at least twice around the tube, enough to indent the tube slightly, and tie securely.

2

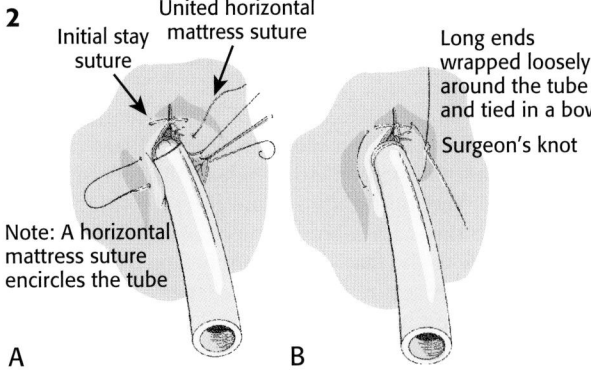

United horizontal
mattress suture

Initial stay
suture

Long ends
wrapped loosely
around the tube
and tied in a bow

Surgeon's knot

Note: A horizontal
mattress suture
encircles the tube

A   B

Another method to close the wound and secure the tube is with a horizontal mattress suture combined with a stay suture. **A**, A horizontal mattress suture is placed on either side (above and below) of the tube and held only with a surgeon's knot. **B**, The loose ends are also wrapped around the tube and tied loosely in a bow to identify the suture. This suture will be untied and used to close the skin incision after removal of the tube.

3

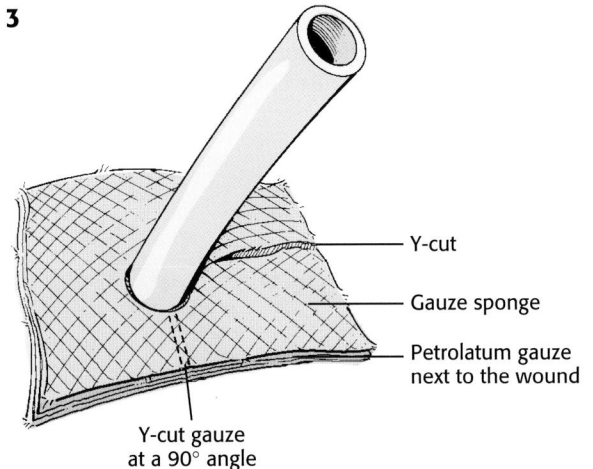

Y-cut

Gauze sponge

Petrolatum gauze
next to the wound

Y-cut gauze
at a 90° angle

To dress the wound and reduce the risk for air leaks, an occlusive dressing should be applied. First wrap the base of the tube at the skin incision with a petroleum-impregnated dressing. A two-layer dressing of gauze sponges with a Y-shaped cut centered at the tube is shown. Place the second layer at a 90° angle to the first.

4

Wide tape

To skin on one side of the tube

To wrap around the chest tube

To skin on the other side of the tube

Half length of tape torn
into 3 pieces

A

Middle strip of
the torn tape

Torn tape

Tape secures
the anchoring
tape

B

One method to further secure the tube is to use wide, split cloth tape. **A**, The distal half of a 15- to 20-cm-long, wide piece of tape is longitudinally split into three pieces. The two outside pieces are placed on the skin on either side of the tube, and the center strip is wrapped around the chest tube itself. **B**, This process may be repeated with a similar piece of tape placed at a 90° angle. The tape is securely anchored to the skin (benzoin is optional, but the skin must be clean and dry), and the torn tape is wrapped around the tube. Each anchoring piece is covered by another piece of tape.

5

The tube can be further secured with an additional anchor system further down on the tube. Wrap a 20- to 25-cm piece of tape or elastic, adhesive dressing around the tube and seal at least 3 cm of the tape together on the side of the tube nearest the chest wall. Spread the remaining tape against the dry skin of the chest wall and secure with additional tape.

Figure 10-24 Methods of securing a thoracostomy tube.

After suturing the tube in place, apply an occlusive dressing of petrolatum-impregnated gauze at the point where the tube enters the skin to help reduce air leaks. Cover the skin with two or more gauze pads with a Y-shaped cut from the middle of one side to the center (Fig. 10-24, *plate 3*). Secure this dressing with wide (8- to 9-cm) cloth or elastic adhesive tape with or without benzoin.

Use approximately 10 to 12 cm of tape split into three pieces and extending halfway along its length. Place the two outside pieces on the skin on either side of the tube site, and wrap the center section tightly around the tube (Fig. 10-24, *plate 4*). Repeat this with a second piece of tape placed at a 180-degree angle to the first. Also securely tape the tube connections. To further secure the tube, use tape to create a loop or stalk by wrapping it around the tube. Then press the tape together for 1 to 2 cm before applying the tape to the chest wall (Fig. 10-24, *plate 5*).

Drainage and Suction Systems

A basic understanding of chest tube drainage systems is necessary to prevent life-threatening complications associated with their use. All drainage systems have two essential components: a one-way valve to allow air or fluid to drain out of the pleural space without allowing air back into the pleural space and a suction mechanism to increase the rate of drainage. The simplest drainage device is just a one-way valve without suction. This can be accomplished with either an underwater seal or a flutter (Heimlich) valve attached to the end of the chest tube (Fig. 10-25). Normal respiration and coughing are often sufficient to create the pressure necessary to remove excess air from the pleural space and allow the lung to expand. The Heimlich valve does not require suction and can be used for outpatient therapy.

With a one-bottle underwater seal system, the intrapleural fluid or air exits under a small amount of water. It collects in the single reservoir and mixes with the water (Fig. 10-26*A*). The water above the tube *acts as a seal* because it is too heavy to be drawn back into the chest. For drainage to occur, intrathoracic pressure must be greater than the water pressure at the distal end of the immersed tube. This pressure is determined by the height of the water above the exit port of the tubing. When the height is too great (the tube is too deep in the water), even coughing may not raise intrapleural pressure sufficiently to drain the chest. Place the collecting bottle below the patient, usually on the floor, to prevent inspiration from generating enough negative pressure to pull the contents of the collection bottle into the chest cavity.

Use suction initially to treat patients with pneumothorax or hemothorax, but replace it with a water seal once drainage and expansion are satisfactory and no persistent air leaks are present. The suction device should have high suction flow (≤20 L/min) and be able to keep the suction constant. Wall suction of 10 to 20 cm H_2O is normally used, but *the amount of suction in the chest tube depends on the depth of water in the water seal reservoir, not on the suction from the wall valve.* When negative pressure from the suction source exceeds the depth of the water in the chamber, air enters from the top of the third tube and causes continuous bubbling (see Fig. 10-26*B*). This prevents a further increase in pressure in the chest tube. The wall suction dial can be turned down until only occasional bubbling can be detected. Vigorous bubbling does not equate with more suction.

The bottle combinations example is provided to illustrate the principles but is rarely used now. Many types of commercial, enclosed systems are available that essentially combine a two-bottle method that can be connected to suction, but with the addition of an "air leak chamber" (see Fig. 10-26*C*). Bubbling in this chamber indicates the presence of an air leak, usually from the drainage system itself as a result of a loose tube connection. If bubbling is present, first check the drainage system, tube, and connectors for any problems or loose connections. If the leak continues, check whether all the holes of the chest tube are within the thorax. If the bubbling continues after these steps, a continued air leak may be due to a large hole in the lung parenchyma, which is usually seen only with expiration or with coughing. A continuous air leak or a leak during inspiration indicates a larger and possibly more significant lung injury.[20] Surgical intervention is indicated if an air leak persists for longer than 72 hours or if the lung is not completely reexpanded.

The drainage reservoir must remain below the level of the chest to prevent the fluid in the collection system from reentering the chest. Place the reservoir on the floor or hang it from the edge of the bed. Simple respirations do not generate enough negative intrathoracic pressure to pull the water in the reservoir up to the height of the chest if the reservoir is kept on the floor and the patient is either sitting or lying at standard chair or bed height. The length of the tubing should

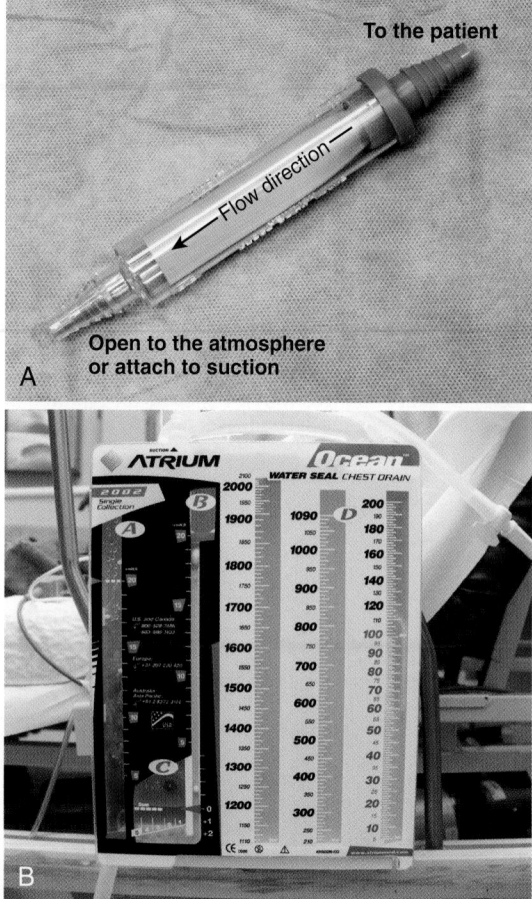

Figure 10-25 Pleural drainage devices. **A,** A one-way Heimlich valve alone is often sufficient to treat a pneumothorax, but it cannot be used to treat a hemothorax. **B,** Disposable water seal chest drain set.

be long enough so that the reservoir can be kept below the level of the patient, but not long enough to cause it to form dependent loops of fluid or kinks. Dependent loops collect fluid and create an additional water seal that if large enough, can require greater intrapleural pressure to drain. If these pressures become high enough (15 to 25 cm H_2O), a tension pneumothorax may result.

When the drainage system is functioning properly, the height of the fluid level in the drainage tube fluctuates with inspiration and expiration. Absence of respiratory fluctuation or a decrease in drainage may indicate that the system is blocked or that the lung is fully expanded. If the tube is blocked, the chest tube or collecting tubing, or both, can be

Figure 10-26 A, A single-bottle (water seal) collection device. **B,** A two-bottle system. The trap reservoir proximal to the water seal keeps the accumulating drainage from affecting the water seal pressure. **C,** This has now been replaced by a disposable system that mimics the two-bottle system. *(Courtesy of Thora Klex System, Davol, Inc., Warwick, Rhode Island)*

changed or "stripped" to dislodge clots. Replacing the tube is a complicated process associated with risks, but the stripping procedure is controversial because of concern that the potentially high negative pressure from the procedure could damage lung tissue.[21] For *stripping*, clamp the tube proximally and progressively compress it distally and then release it to allow the tube to spring open. The sudden increase in negative pressure may extract clots and fluid from a more proximal location. If the blockage is within the thorax, the tube can be cleared by forcing air or fluid back into the chest. The tube must be clamped distally and then compressed and stripped to force the contents proximally.

Perform occlusive clamping of a chest tube only with close monitoring because a tension pneumothorax can result in rare cases. Patients with chest tubes in place are best transported with a Heimlich valve or water seal only, not with the tube clamped. Avoid clamping the chest tube as a trial maneuver before removing it.

Prophylactic Antibiotics

The use of prophylactic antibiotics after placement of a chest tube in the emergency department (ED) is common, but no specific standards exist. It appears reasonable to provide short-term antibiotic prophylaxis since analyses of many studies have shown that antibiotics reduce the incidence of chest tube-associated empyema or pneumonia.[22] Guidelines from the Eastern Association of Surgeons of Trauma recommend the use of first-generation cephalosporins during the first 24 hours for patients undergoing chest tube drainage for hemothorax.[23]

Tube Removal

Chest tubes are rarely removed by emergency clinicians. The usual indication for removal of a chest tube is after a chest radiograph demonstrates complete resolution of the pneumothorax and there is no evidence of an ongoing air leak. Before removal, discontinue suction and establish a water seal. The literature is not clear about the use of a chest radiograph after suction is discontinued and after pulling the tube. Textbooks continue to recommend such practice, but studies have show that it is not necessary for postoperative patients.[24,25]

To remove the chest tube, ask the patient to sit upright at about a 45-degree angle. Use sterile technique, clean the skin, and drape the insertion site. Suturing equipment is needed to close the wound after the tube is removed except when a pursestring suture was placed at the time of insertion, in which case only sterile scissors are needed to cut the suture. Keep additional equipment available to reinsert a chest tube if the lung collapses. Prepare a petrolatum- or antibiotic-impregnated gauze dressing to cover the wound.

If a purse-string suture was placed previously, loosen it and prepare it for closing the wound. Cut the skin loop of the suture holding the tube to the skin and remove it from the skin. With the tube clamped, it has traditionally been advised to ask the patient to inhale fully and perform a mild Valsalva maneuver. Although this is theoretically beneficial in minimizing residual air following tube removal, it is of no proven value and many clinician use no special protocols for removal of the tube. Pull the tube out in one swift motion. Quickly tie the purse-string suture or suture the wound closed, and then cover it with an occlusive dressing. If no purse-string suture is present, once the tube is removed, suture the skin as quickly as is prudent for the physician. Observe the patient for 2 to 6 hours and obtain a chest radiograph before discharge. Any increase in symptoms requires prompt reevaluation. After 48 hours the patient may remove the dressing. Remove the sutures in 7 to 10 days.

OTHER TECHNIQUES

Small-Bore Tube Thoracostomy

Since the advent of common pleural drainage techniques in the early 20th century, physicians have preferred large-bore pleural drainage catheters (PDCs) inserted via blunt dissection for thoracic drainage and decompression. This preference for tubes greater than 16 Fr in diameter was born largely of concern for fibrin blockage, inadequate drainage capability, and the perception of frequent dislodgement of small-bore PDCs. To date, no quality randomized clinical trials have compare the use of large- versus small-bore PDCs, mainly because of the difficulty of conducting comparative studies in critically ill patients.

Despite these impediments, recent studies have hinted at the adequacy of small-bore PDCs for the treatment of many conditions. Review of the data available suggests that the rate of blockage and dislodgement is similar with large- and small-bore PDCs and that drainage capability is comparable in all but the most extreme circumstances.[26-29] Another study has shown that large-bore PDC placement is associated with significantly more pain and slightly increased rates of empyema.[30]

Review of the current pulmonology and critical care literature reveals no consensus on the appropriate use of small-bore PDCs; however, recent review articles have attempted to establish rough guidelines for their use. The current literature suggests that patients with malignant effusion, simple pneumothorax without penetrating injury, or a suspected air leak, as well as those with simple or complex parapneumonic effusions, are good candidates for small-bore PDCs. Patients with empyema, penetrating injury, traumatic hemothorax, or complex pneumothorax and those on mechanical ventilation require large-bore PDCs because of the potential for large-volume air leaks in such patients and the need for rapid evacuation of the pleural space.[31,32]

Many protocols are available for use of catheter aspiration as the first step in treating simple pneumothoraces. In general, patients with successful aspiration are observed in the ED for 4 to 6 hours after catheter insertion, and if a repeated radiograph shows no reaccumulation of air, the catheter is removed. After 2 more hours, another chest radiograph is obtained, and the patient is released if there is no recurrent pneumothorax. Patients with continued residual pneumothorax often receive a conventional chest tube.

Guidewire Technique for Catheter Aspiration

Catheters designed specifically for aspirating a pneumothorax are made of flexible, thrombosis-resistant radiopaque material with multiple distal side ports to reduce the risk for occlusion. Commercially available small-bore catheter systems are ideal for this procedure.

The catheters are placed via a standard "over-the-wire" (Seldinger) technique. The most common insertion site is the second intercostal space in the midclavicular line, but either of the standard locations (the midaxillary to anterior axillary line, usually in the fourth or fifth intercostal space, or the midclavicular line, second intercostal space) can be used. Place the patient in a semi-upright position. Clean the skin with an antiseptic solution and drape the area. Infiltrate locally with lidocaine for anesthesia. Advance the guide needle *in a straight line* at a 60 degrees angle cephalad over the top of the rib (Figs. 10-27 and 10-28). Unless a straight tract is created, it will be difficult to advance the floppy catheter, so a tunneling approach cannot be used. When the pleural space is identified by intermittent aspiration, halt advancement of the needle. Feed a guidewire through the needle and into the pleural space. Remove the needle while stabilizing the guidewire to keep it in the pleural space. Make a small incision in the skin with a No. 11 blade at the base of the wire to allow passage of the catheter through the skin. Some systems use a dilator over the wire to open the path through the soft tissue. Then thread the minicatheter over the guidewire and into the pleural space. Remove the wire and dilator while leaving the catheter in the pleural space. Advance the catheter through the subcutaneous tissue with a twisting motion. Secure the catheter to the skin with a suture and dress the incision site. The catheter may be removed after a period of observation, or suction may be maintained for a few days. If the catheter becomes clogged with mucus or blood, inject sterile saline through the device to clear it.

To aspirate the pneumothorax, attach a three-way stopcock to the catheter and slowly aspirate air with a 60-mL syringe until resistance is felt. Gentle wall suction can also be used because a number of aspirations may be required until all the air exits. Take a chest radiograph to determine whether the lung is fully expanded. If residual pneumothorax is present, attempt further aspirations. If the residual pneumothorax persists and air cannot be aspirated, the catheter may be kinked or blocked with soft tissue. To relieve the blockage, place the patient in the full upright position and have the patient cough or take a deep breath. Alternatively, the catheter can be twisted or rotated gently.

TUBE THORACOSTOMY IN PEDIATRIC PATIENTS

Pneumothoraces can occur in the neonatal population. They are often associated with resuscitative measures (such as mechanical ventilation) for meconium aspiration or prematurity. For the rest of the pediatric population, trauma is the most common cause. A pneumothorax will develop in approximately one third of children with thoracic trauma. As in adults, physical examination of newborns and infants with pneumothorax can be highly variable, thus necessitating the use of a chest radiograph for diagnosis. Ideally, both anteroposterior and cross-table lateral projections are used because small pneumothoraces may be seen only on the lateral view. A chest CT is more sensitive and specific.

In general, tube thoracostomy is the treatment of choice once a symptomatic pneumothorax is detected in infants. When signs of tension pneumothorax are present, immediately aspirate with a plastic catheter-over-the-needle device. Small pneumothoraces (<20% of the hemithorax) in relatively asymptomatic infants (e.g., those without other problems who do not require positive airway pressure) can be observed.

CATHETER ASPIRATION OF PNEUMOTHORAX: SELDINGER TECHNIQUE

The Seldinger-type catheter kit contains a pigtail catheter and all necessary equipment, including local anesthesia, introducing needle and syringe, scalpel, guidewire, and dilator.

After generous local anesthesia, advance the introducing syringe in a straight line over the top of the fifth rib until air is aspirated. Unless a straight tract is created, it will be difficult to advance the floppy catheter, and a tunneling approach cannot be used.

Advance the guidewire through the introducing needle into the pleural space, and then remove the needle. The procedural steps are analogous to initiating a central venous catheter via the Seldinger technique.

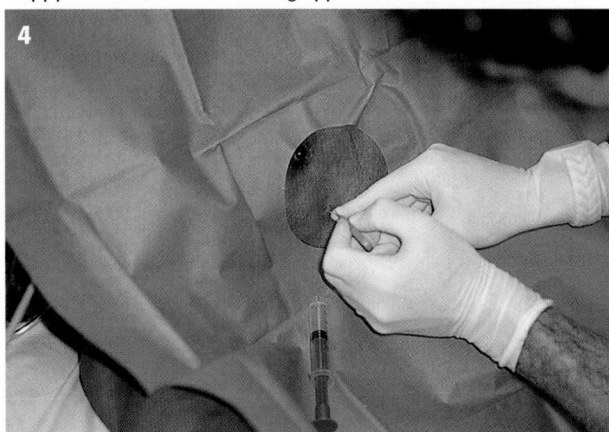

Puncture the skin at the site of wire insertion with a scalpel. Make the incision large enough to accept the dilator and pigtail catheter.

Advance the dilator over the wire to create a tract for the catheter. Remove the dilator while leaving the wire in place. Again, this is analogous to establishing a central venous line.

Advance the pigtail catheter over the wire through the dilated tract. It will assume its pigtail configuration when it is in the pleural space. A twisting motion may be needed to advance the catheter through subcutaneous tissue. Advance the catheter to the hilt and secure to suction. This catheter may be removed after a period of observation, or the suction may be maintained for a few days.

Figure 10-27 Aspiration of a pneumothorax with an Arrow 14-French Percutaneous Cavity Drainage Catheterization Kit. This 23-cm pigtail multihole catheter is ideal for such purposes. Air can be aspirated from the catheter with a syringe, or the catheter can be attached to suction or a Heimlich valve. This catheter is not used for patients on a ventilator, those with continuing air leaks, or those with a hemothorax. It is ideal for stable patients who have a primary pneumothorax or a collapse that can be expected to be stable if the lung is reexpanded (such as induced by intravenous drug use, minor blunt trauma, or insertion of a central venous catheter). If used for a few days, the catheter will become clogged with mucus or blood, which may be cleared by injecting sterile saline through the device.

ASPIRATION OF PNEUMOTHORAX: CATHETER-OVER-THE-NEEDLE TECHNIQUE

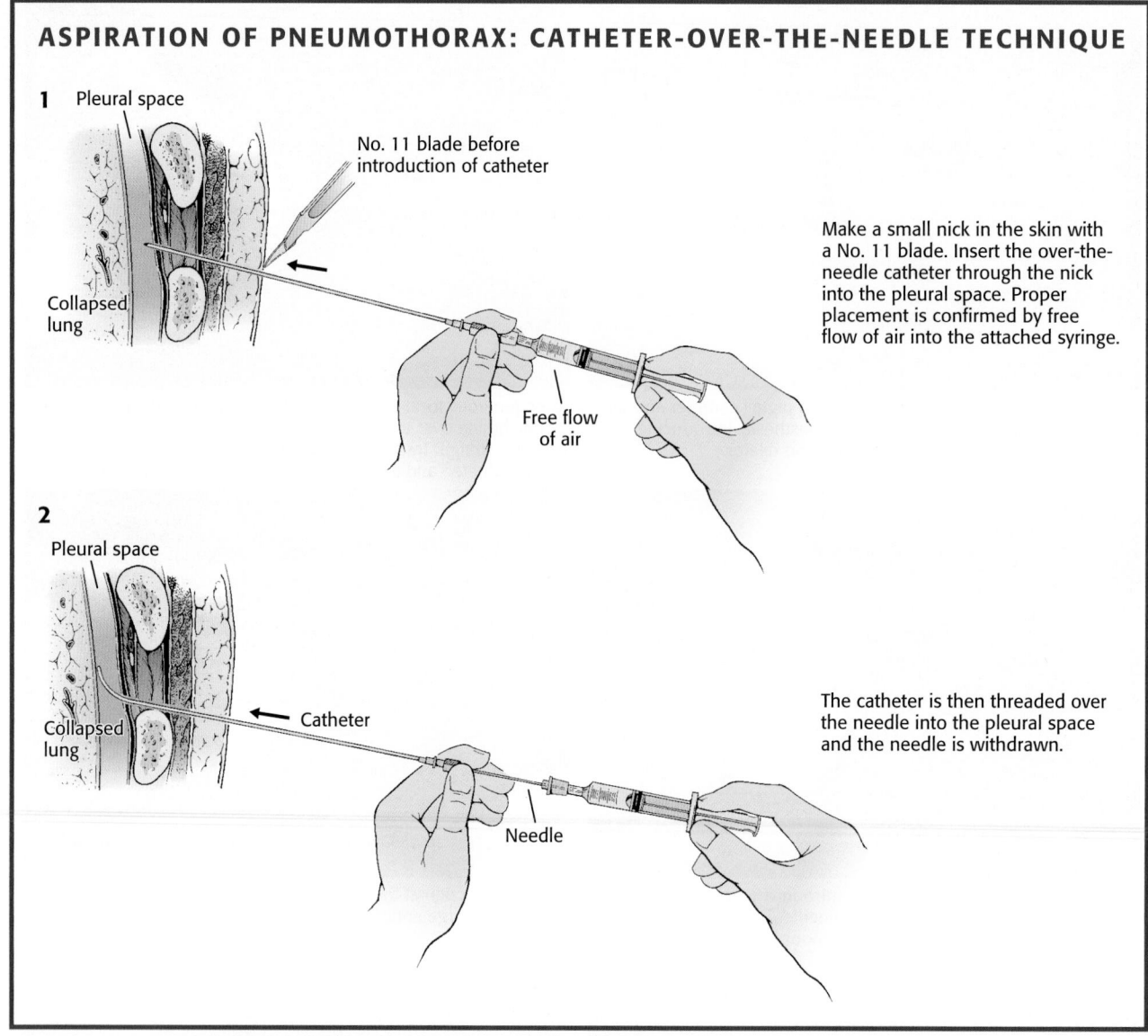

1 Pleural space

No. 11 blade before introduction of catheter

Collapsed lung

Free flow of air

Make a small nick in the skin with a No. 11 blade. Insert the over-the-needle catheter through the nick into the pleural space. Proper placement is confirmed by free flow of air into the attached syringe.

2 Pleural space

Collapsed lung

Catheter

Needle

The catheter is then threaded over the needle into the pleural space and the needle is withdrawn.

Figure 10-28 Catheter-over-the-needle technique for aspiration of a pneumothorax.

TABLE 10-1   Approximate Pediatric Chest Tube Size by Weight

WEIGHT (kg)	CHEST TUBE (Fr)
<3	8-10
3-5	10-12
6-10	12-16
11-15	17-22
16-20	22-26
21-30	26-32
>30	32-40

The technique of tube thoracostomy in pediatric patients is essentially the same as that in adults, but the body size and small spaces between the ribs make the procedure more difficult. The size of the tube increases with the patient's weight, starting with 8- to 10-Fr catheters for premature infants (Table 10-1). *Because of the risk for future breast deformities, avoid the midclavicular approach.* Instead, use the anterior axillary line through the fifth intercostal space for newborns and infants.[33]

COMPLICATIONS

The most common complications include infection, laceration of an intercostal vessel, laceration of the lung, and intraabdominal or solid organ placement of the chest tube (Boxes 10-4 and 10-5). Local infection at the insertion site is

BOX 10-4	Physical Complications of Tube Thoracostomy

INFECTION
Pneumonia
Empyema
Local infection of the incision
Osteomyelitis
Necrotizing fasciitis

PHYSIOLOGIC
Allergic reactions to the surgical preparation or anesthesia
Pulmonary atelectasis
Reexpansion pulmonary edema
Reexpansion hypotension

INJURIES—BLEEDING
Local incision hematoma
Intercostal artery or vein laceration
Internal mammary artery laceration (with midclavicular line placement)
Pulmonary vein or artery injury
Great-vessel injury

INJURIES TO SOLID ORGANS OR NERVES
Lung, liver, spleen, diaphragm, stomach, colon; long thoracic nerve, intercostal nerve

MISCELLANEOUS
Subcutaneous or mediastinal emphysema
Persistent pneumothorax
Retained hemothorax
Recurrence of pneumothorax after removal of the chest tube

BOX 10-5	Mechanical Complications of Tube Thoracostomy

MECHANICAL PROBLEMS
Dislodgment of the chest tube from the chest wall
Incorrect tube position
Subcutaneous placement
Intraabdominal placement

AIR LEAKS
Leaks within the drainage system (tubing or drainage device)
Last tube port not within the pleural space
Leaks from a skin site

BLOCKED DRAINAGE
Flow of drainage contents into the chest from elevation of the drainage bottles
Kinked chest tube or drainage tubes
Occlusion of the tube by clots

common and often related to the emergency nature of the procedure. Subcutaneous emphysema is a frequent, usually benign complication that is self-limited and generally caused by an excessively large opening in the pleura. Subcutaneous air may be a result of the incident that caused the pneumothorax in the first place. The development of palpable subcutaneous air is another complication of chest tube placement. It is usually limited to the insertion site but can become massive with PPV in a patient with continued air leak or an occluded tube.

Intercostal arteries or veins may be lacerated, but this can be minimized by using blunt dissection and carefully directing the tube just above the rib. The tube may adequately tamponade such bleeding. If the bleeding persists, extend the incision to ligate the bleeding vessel. If the bleeding continues, consult a thoracic surgeon.

Failure of a pneumothorax to reexpand may be due to a mechanical air leak, but it may also indicate a bronchopleural fistula, a continued parenchymal lung leak, or a bronchial injury. Tension pneumothorax can occur if a blockage in the drainage system at any point is associated with a continued air leak from the lung. Reinsertion or placement of a second tube may be indicated if the first tube is not functioning properly. In general, if a chest tube is not functioning properly and the patient is deteriorating, remove the tube and insert another one. Manipulating the tube by pushing it deeper into the chest cavity can lead to an increased risk for infection.

A rare complication of tube thoracostomy is unilateral reexpansion pulmonary edema. The pulmonary edema ranges from mild to severe, but fatalities have been reported.[34] The condition may occur shortly after reexpansion or may be delayed a number of hours. A common factor in these cases seems to be a prolonged period between the development of a pneumothorax and the onset of treatment, but the exact time frame is quite variable. Usually, the pneumothorax has been present for at least 3 to 4 days. Proposed mechanisms include anoxic damage to the alveolar-capillary basement membrane from prolonged pulmonary collapse, loss of surfactant, or rapid fluid shifts. Treatment is supportive, with ventilatory support occasionally being required. Reintroduction of air back into the pleural space and temporary occlusion of the ipsilateral pulmonary artery have been other suggested, but unproved interventions.

References are available at www.expertconsult.com

Cardiac Procedures

CHAPTER 11

Techniques for Supraventricular Tachycardias

Bohdan M. Minczak

INTRODUCTION

Patients in the emergency department frequently complain of palpitations, heart fluttering, or a rapid heart beat, and this is often coupled with weakness, chest pain, or dizziness. The physician must determine the exact rate, rhythm, origin, and cause of the tachycardia and then "gain control" of the heart rate (HR) by slowing or normalizing it or by treating the underlying cause. Determining the cause, origin, and rhythm of the tachycardia is often complicated by the fact that the underlying rate may be very fast (in excess of 150 to 300 beats/min), which makes interpretation of the electrocardiogram more difficult. Furthermore, the sources or pacemakers producing or facilitating the tachyarrhythmia may be from one or multiple locations: in the sinoatrial (SA) node, in one or more ectopic atrial foci, in the atrioventricular (AV) node, or in the ventricular free walls or septum. There may also be an abnormal conduction pathway between the atria and the ventricles. In some conditions, one or more "pacemakers" can be discharging simultaneously. To facilitate the diagnostic process, discrimination between atrial and ventricular electromechanical activity must be attempted. This chapter provides a framework to facilitate the decision-making process with a focus on emergency interventions for various tachydysrhythmias.

Techniques for unmasking, identifying, and treating the various forms of tachyarrhythmias are presented in Box 11-1. This chapter addresses the utility of the vagal reflex in treating and managing various pathophysiologic conditions and the use of medications and cardioversion as they apply to the treatment of various supraventricular tachycardias (SVTs). The major focus is on the evaluation and treatment of SVTs. A more comprehensive discussion regarding the treatment of ventricular tachycardia (VT) is provided in Chapter 12.

OVERVIEW AND SIGNIFICANCE: ANATOMY AND PHYSIOLOGY OF SUPRAVENTRICULAR TACHYCARDIA

Normally, the human heart beats at approximately 80 beats/min (±20 beats/min). If the HR exceeds 100 beats/min, it is called *tachycardia*. If it drops below 60 beats/min, it is called *bradycardia*. The heart's ability to increase the rate of a *normal sinus rhythm* is primarily related to age: *the maximum HR possible with a sinus tachycardia is approximately 220 beats/min minus age*, with normal variations as high as 10 to 20 beats/min. As an example, a 60-year-old man cannot usually mount a sinus tachycardia higher than 160 beats/min in response to sepsis, exercise, fever, anxiety, or adrenergic stimulation. Faster rates would indicate a pathologic cardiac rhythm, not a physiologic response.

There are two general categories or types of tachycardias: SVT and VT. The term *supraventricular tachycardia* describes a rapid HR that has its electrochemical origin either in the atria or in the upper portions of the AV node. *Ventricular tachycardias* originate in the ventricular free walls or interventricular septum (or both). VTs can quickly become unstable and require special consideration (Fig. 11-1F).

SVTs can be further classified as narrow-complex (QRS duration <0.12 second) and wide-complex tachycardias (QRS duration >0.12 second). The rhythms of these dysrhythmias can be regular or irregular. Examples of narrow-complex SVTs are sinus tachycardia (Fig. 11-1A); atrial fibrillation (AF) (Fig. 11-1C); atrial flutter (Fig. 11-1D); AV nodal reentry; atrial tachycardia (Fig. 11-1B), both ectopic and reentrant; multifocal atrial tachycardia (MAT); junctional tachycardia; and accessory pathway-mediated tachycardia. The term *wide-complex tachycardia* describes rhythms such as VT (Fig. 11-1F), SVT with aberrancy (Fig. 11-1E), or a preexcitation tachycardia facilitated by an accessory pathway between the atria and ventricles.

Tachycardias may be benign or can have significant physical effects on the patient. When the HR is 60 beats/min, approximately one cardiac cycle of contraction (systole) and relaxation (diastole) occurs per second. The excitation for cardiac contraction typically originates in the SA node, the intrinsic "pacemaker" of the heart. The pacemaker impulse traverses across and depolarizes the atria, which causes atrial contraction or systole. Subsequently, the depolarization reaches the AV node. On initiating depolarization of the AV node, the conduction velocity of this depolarizing impulse transiently decreases (i.e., undergoes "decremental conduction") so that the ventricles can fill with blood from the

---

BOX 11-1 | **Diagnostic and Therapeutic Approaches to Supraventricular Tachycardias**

VAGAL MANEUVERS

Carotid sinus massage
   Pressure on the carotid sinus
Valsalva technique
   Forced expiration of air against a closed glottis
Apneic facial exposure to cold water ("cold water diving reflex")
   Immersion of the face into cold water
Oculocardiac reflex
   The trigeminovagal reflex initiated by pressure on the eyeball

PHARMACOLOGIC AGENTS

Adenosine
Calcium channel blockers (verapamil, diltiazem)
β-Blockers, including esmolol
Digoxin
Amiodarone
Procainamide

CARDIOVERSION

Administration of a synchronized shock

---

antecedent atrial contraction. *(Remember:* The duration of diastole must be roughly twice the duration of systole to allow adequate ventricular filling.) *The AV node also serves as a gate or selective block to prevent an excessive number of depolarizing impulses from reaching the ventricles when the atrial rate is accelerated.*

Immediately thereafter, this depolarizing wave accelerates as it travels down the bundle of His to the Purkinje fibers and causes ventricular depolarization leading to contraction. Subsequently, the ventricles begin to relax (i.e., enter *diastole* and begin to fill with blood before the next depolarization). This describes the events of one cardiac cycle or heartbeat. The changes in electrochemical voltage during these events are depicted on the electrocardiogram in the usual sequential PQRST (the P wave indicates SA nodal depolarization, the PR interval denotes atrial depolarization followed by activation of the AV node, and the QRS complex summarizes electrical activity during ventricular depolarization) (Fig. 11-2).

The discharge rate of the SA node is usually modulated by a balance of input from the sympathetic and parasympathetic nerves (i.e., the autonomic nervous system). Sympathetic input to the heart is provided by the adrenergic nerves, which innervate the atria and ventricles, and by circulating hormones such as epinephrine and norepinephrine, which are released from the adrenal gland and cause the *HR to increase*. Parasympathetic input to the heart is provided by the vagus nerve (cranial nerve [CN] X) fibers. These nerve fibers innervate the SA and AV nodes. Vagal output to the SA node causes slowing of the HR by decreasing the depolarization rate of the "intrinsic pacemaker," whereas vagal output to the AV node enhances nodal blockade of atrial depolarization impulses to the ventricles. *Hence, vagal stimulation results in slowing of electrical activity, examples being termination of an SVT, slowing of the ventricular rate of AF (via the AV node), or simply producing a sinus bradycardia (via the SA node).* Under normal physiologic circumstances, the HR is modulated to meet the metabolic needs

of the body's peripheral circulation. Changes in AV electrochemical events (i.e., rates and rhythms) are manifested as changes in the electrocardiographic intervals and waveforms.

As noted earlier, SVT rhythms can be either sinus (i.e., originating in the SA node: sinus tachycardia) or ectopic (i.e., originating in atrial myocytes above the ventricles). The rate of discharge of the SA node often varies as a result of various physiologic and pharmacologic stimuli, including fever, hypovolemia, shock, anemia, hypoxia, anxiety, pain, cocaine, and amphetamines. These conditions often require or precipitate increased blood flow and hence cardiac output (CO) to peripheral tissues. This increase in peripheral blood flow or CO is accomplished by an increase in HR (*Remember*: CO = HR × SV [stroke volume]). These are usually normal, benign physiologic responses to various stimuli or triggers. Direct treatment of these rhythms is not generally necessary; however, determining and treating the cause of the sinus tachycardia usually eliminates the fast HR. Nonetheless, when single or multiple ectopic, spontaneously discharging foci develop in the atria or upper portions of the AV node, they can begin to "take over" or "override" the normal pacemaker activity in the heart (i.e., the SA node) and produce a rapid HR exceeding 100 beats/min. These foci may develop as a result of increased irritability or automaticity of atrial myocytes secondary to electrolyte abnormalities, hypoxia, pharmacologic agents, or atrial stretch caused by volumetric overload. If these foci are not treated or suppressed and the atrial depolarization rate proceeds to accelerate to rates greater than 150 beats/min (i.e., the heart is beating in excess of 2 beats/sec) and the impulses get through the AV node to the ventricles, the time for diastolic filling of the ventricles will be compromised and result in a precipitous drop in SV. This will ultimately cause a drop in CO regardless of the increase in HR. Furthermore, as CO begins to drop, mean arterial blood pressure (MABP) will decrease and cause hypoperfusion of the brain and other peripheral tissue (*Remember*: MABP is the product of CO times total peripheral resistance [TPR]—MABP = CO × TRP). Treatment of this tachycardia can be achieved pharmacologically by suppressing the automaticity of myocytes with medications (e.g., calcium channel blockers or β-blockers) and subsequently treating the underlying cause or causes—hypoxia, electrolytes, and the like. Decreasing the hemodynamic consequences of this arrhythmia requires increasing the "blocking" of these impulses from reaching the ventricles via the AV node. This can be done by enhancing vagal input to the AV node or by pharmacologic enhancement of AV blockade. Multiple rapid depolarizations of the atria, which are conducted to the ventricles, can ultimately have a bimodal type of response: a modest increase in HR will cause an increase in CO, whereas a massive increase in the atrial rate with a concomitant increase in the ventricular rate will cause a drop in CO. This can lead to an unstable patient with signs and symptoms such as confusion, altered mental status, or persistent chest pain. When the patient becomes unstable, immediate treatment is indicated.

In addition to areas of increased automaticity that can precipitate SVTs, a condition described as *reentry* can also cause SVTs. Reentry describes a condition whereby a depolarization impulse is being propagated down a pathway in which some of the myocytes are still in the effective refractory period and a "unidirectional block" is present and preventing the impulse from traveling normally down this pathway. However, as the impulse travels around the area of the

Figure 11-1 Tachydysrhythmias. A, Sinus tachycardia. **B,** Supraventricular tachycardia (SVT). **C,** Atrial fibrillation. **D,** Atrial flutter. **E,** SVT with aberrancy. **F,** Ventricular tachycardia.

"unidirectional block," the tissue allows the depolarization front to travel in the opposite (antidromic) direction, back to the initial point of entry into this pathway. This allows the depolarization wavefront to restimulate the myocytes and initiate another propagated depolarization through the same tract (Fig. 11-3). If this condition persists and these impulses stimulate the atria effectively and traverse the AV node, an

SVT may develop as a result of reentry. Suppression of this dysrhythmia can be achieved by terminating the conditions favoring reentry, and the hemodynamic consequences may be attenuated by enhancing AV nodal blockade of the ventricles (e.g., through vagal stimulation, medication), thus slowing the ventricular response to this condition. Termination of reentry can be accomplished by either pharmacologic modification of

ECG AND MEMBRANE POTENTIAL OF VENTRICULAR CELLS

Figure 11-2 Electrocardiographic and membrane potential of ventricular cells.

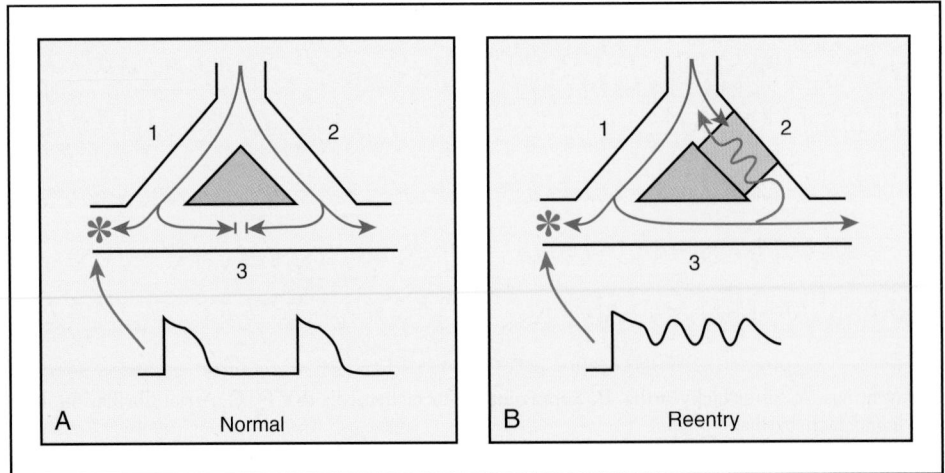

Figure 11-3 Cardiac conduction with supraventricular tachycardia. **A,** Normal depolarization down paths *1* and *2* that will "extinguish" or "cancel out" normal depolarization/repolarization and conductance at point *3*. **B,** Abnormal. *1,* Normal conduction; *2,* delayed/slowed conduction with a unidirectional block; *3,* normal conduction pathway.

the myocytes to render them refractory to depolarization impulses for a longer period in a stable patient or by synchronized cardioversion to uniformly depolarize the myocytes and terminate the conditions favoring the SVT.

Another situation to consider in the development and propagation of SVTs is the presence of preexcitation or an accessory pathway between the atria and the ventricles. Arrhythmias secondary to these causes can be managed with the use of appropriate pharmacologic agents to either suppress conduction through the accessory pathway or block AV nodal transmission without enhancing conduction through the accessory pathway.

To complete this discussion, we must also consider that there may be the possibility of an interventricular conduction delay being present before the development of an SVT. If this is the case, the SVT may appear as a wide-complex tachycardia and can be confused with other dysrhythmias. However, an even more dangerous situation can occur if a wide-complex tachycardia of ventricular origin (VT) is present and is misdiagnosed as an SVT with aberrancy. As a result, the patient could be treated inappropriately, with the intervention causing suppression of ventricular activity and ultimately cardiac arrest. VT with a pulse is considered an unstable rhythm that often requires synchronized cardioversion (discussed in more detail in Chapter 12).

The clinician must have a means of slowing down and sorting out these physiologic events so that appropriate diagnosis and treatment or intervention decisions can be made. With the application of vagal maneuvers, in some cases the activity of the atria and ventricles may be isolated enough to facilitate a correct diagnosis. An understanding of the underlying pathophysiology will guide appropriate treatment.

VAGAL MANEUVERS

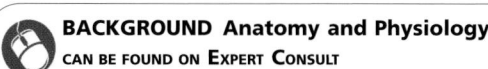

> **BACKGROUND** Anatomy and Physiology
> CAN BE FOUND ON EXPERT CONSULT

Indications for Vagal Maneuvers

Vagal maneuvers are potentially useful in attempting to slow down or break an SVT. They are also indicated in settings in which slowing conduction in the SA or AV node could provide useful information (Box 11-2 and Figs. 11-4*A-E* and 11-5*A-D*). Such settings include patients with wide-complex tachycardia, in whom carotid sinus massage (CSM) aids in the distinction between SVT and VT. CSM can elucidate narrow-complex tachycardia in which the P waves are not visible or aid in detection of suspected rate-related bundle branch block or pacemaker malfunction. After CSM, a wide-complex SVT may be converted to normal sinus rhythm, P waves may be revealed after increased AV node inhibition, or ventricular complexes may narrow as the ventricular rate slows. Because CSM slows atrial and not ventricular activity, AV dissociation may be seen more easily and is indicative of VT (see Fig. 11-4). In rapid AF or atrial flutter with a 2 : 1 block, either P waves or irregular ventricular activity with absent P waves may be revealed (Figs. 11-5*A* and *B*). Sinus tachycardia may also be more apparent once P waves are unmasked by slowing the SA node (see Figs. 11-4*C* and *D*). Adenosine may be used

---

BOX 11-2 **Potential Observations with Vagal Maneuvers in the Management of Tachydysrhythmias**

1. Vagal maneuvers may slow the atrial rate in VT or complete heart block and may therefore demonstrate previously hidden P waves or obvious (AV) dissociation.
2. Abrupt changes in the heart rate without conversion are a result of increasing AV block.
3. Gradual slowing of the ventricular rate suggests the presence of sinus rhythm. Only rarely do vagal maneuvers decrease AV conduction in the presence of a sinus mechanism.
4. The dysrhythmias most likely to convert to sinus rhythm are PAT and paroxysmal nodal tachycardia.
5. Dysrhythmias that are associated with AV conduction defects (PAT with block, atrial flutter, and atrial fibrillation) infrequently convert to a sinus rhythm, but the ventricular rate slows. Rarely, atrial slowing will be sufficient to allow 1 : 1 AV conduction, which may actually increase the ventricular rate (see Fig. 11-6).

AV, atrioventricular; PAT, paroxysmal atrial tachycardia; VT, ventricular tachycardia.

BOX 11-3 **Order of *Decreasing* Frequency of ECG Changes with Vagal Maneuvers**

1. Sinoatrial slowing, which occurs in approximately 75% of cases and leads to sinus arrest approximately 3% of the time
2. Atrial conduction defects, as manifested by an increase in width of the P wave on the electrocardiogram
3. Prolongation of the PR interval and higher degrees of atrioventricular block, which are seen in approximately 10% of cases
4. Nodal escape rhythms
5. Complete asystole, defined as sinus arrest without ventricular escape lasting longer than 3 seconds, which occurs in 4% of cases
6. Premature ventricular contractions

---

for the same diagnostic purpose in these situations as well.[7] In order of decreasing frequency, the electrocardiographic changes seen with CSM and vagal maneuvers are presented in Box 11-3.

Vagal maneuvers, CSM in particular, may also be a useful aid to the diagnosis of syncope in the elderly. Some 14% to 45% of elderly patients referred for syncope are thought to have *carotid sinus syndrome* (CSS).[6,8,9] CSS is defined as an asystolic pause longer than 3 seconds or a reduction in systolic blood pressure greater than 50 mm Hg in response to CSM (Fig. 11-6). Because it shares many characteristics with sick sinus syndrome, it has been suggested that both are manifestations of the same disease. CSS causes cerebral hypoperfusion, which can lead to dizziness and syncope. Analysis of patients with CSS indicates that it results from baroreflex-mediated bradycardia in 29%, hypotension in 37%, or both in 34%.[10,11] Therefore, syncope, chronic near-syncope, or a fall of unclear

Figure 11-4 A, Ventricular tachycardia. Carotid sinus massage (CSM) slows the atria but not the ventricles, thus establishing the presence of atrioventricular (AV) dissociation and supporting the diagnosis of ventricular tachycardia. The QRS interval measures 0.16 sec. Note the atrial rate slowing from 102 to 88 beats/min while the ventricular rate is unaffected. **B,** Paroxysmal atrial tachycardia with variable block. CSM uncovers P waves hidden in the ventricular complex. The upper strip resembles atrial flutter or atrial fibrillation with ventricular ectopic beats. The lower strip shows paroxysmal atrial tachycardia with variable block at an atrial rate of 166 beats/min. **C,** Sinus tachycardia. The sinus P wave is obscured within the descending limb of the T wave. CSM transiently slows the sinus rate and exposes the P wave. The rate then increases. The strips are continuous. **D,** Sinus tachycardia with a high-level block. *Arrows* indicate sinus P waves. Strips are continuous. The basic rhythm is sinus, but a marked first-degree AV block is present. A high-degree (advanced) AV block associated with transient slowing of the sinus rate is produced by CSM. **E,** Paroxysmal atrial tachycardia. CSM abolishes the dysrhythmia and results in a period of sinus suppression with a junctional (*J*) escape beat. Prolonged periods of asystole may produce anxiety in physicians waiting for the resumption of a sinus pacemaker. (*A and B, From Lown B, Levine SA. Carotid sinus—clinical value of its stimulation. Circulation. 1961;23:766. Reproduced by permission; C, from Silverman ME. Recognition and treatment of arrhythmias. In: Schwartz GR, Safar P, Stone JH, et al, eds. Principles and Practice of Emergency Medicine. Vol 2. Philadelphia: Saunders; 1978. Reproduced by permission; D, from Chung EK. Electrocardiography. 2nd ed. New York: Harper & Row; 1980. Reproduced by permission; E, from Silverman ME. Recognition and treatment of arrhythmias. In: Schwartz GR, Safar P, Stone JH, et al, eds. Principles and Practice of Emergency Medicine. Vol 2. Philadelphia: Saunders; 1978. Reproduced by permission.*)

etiology in the elderly is an important indication for diagnostic CSM.[12,13]

Although the use of digoxin has been overshadowed by the use of other potentially less toxic agents such as calcium channel blockers and β-blockers, the clinician can still prospectively simulate the cardioinhibitory effects of digoxin on a patient by performing vagal maneuvers. This can guide use and dosage of the medication before initiating treatment with digoxin. Significant slowing or block with CSM suggests a similar sensitivity to digoxin, and a smaller loading dose should be considered (Table 11-1).

Equipment and Setup

Before the initiation of any clinical intervention such as vagal maneuvers, administration of medication, or cardioversion for

EFFECTS OF CAROTID SINUS MASSAGE ON VARIOUS ARRHYTHMIAS

Figure 11-5 A, Atrial flutter. Carotid sinus massage (CSM) (*downward arrow*) produces marked slowing of the ventricular rate in atrial flutter. Note the obvious flutter waves with an atrial rate of 300 and a long period of ventricular standstill. The strips are continuous. **B,** Atrial fibrillation. CSM slows the ventricular response transiently, and thus the fibrillating baseline is revealed. The ventricular rate subsequently accelerates. **C,** Occult premature ventricular contractions. CSM reveals ventricular extrasystoles, thereby explaining the cause of palpitations in this case. **D,** A run of ventricular tachycardia is seen immediately after a supraventricular dysrhythmia is terminated by CSM. The patient remained asymptomatic, and a normal sinus rhythm was established spontaneously within a few seconds. If asystole is prolonged, ask the patient to cough vigorously (cough-induced cardiopulmonary resuscitation) or apply a precordial thump. (*A, From Chung EK.* Electrocardiography. *2nd ed. New York: Harper & Row; 1980. Reproduced by permission; B, from Silverman ME. Recognition and treatment of arrhythmias. In: Schwartz GR, Safar P, Stone JH, et al, eds.* Principles and Practice of Emergency Medicine. *Vol 2. Philadelphia: Saunders; 1978. Reproduced by permission; C, from Lown B, Levine SA. Carotid sinus—clinical value of its stimulation.* Circulation. *1961;23:766. Reproduced by permission.*)

SVT, place the patient on a cardiac monitor, establish intravenous (IV) access, and infuse a slow, keep-vein-open (KVO; 60 mL/hr saline IV) solution through the IV line. Monitor the patient with a pulse oximeter and blood pressure monitor. Keep numerous antiarrhythmic medications readily available at the bedside. Keep a defibrillator/pacemaker at the bedside in anticipation of a worsening dysrhythmia. Administer oxygen for the procedure, especially if conscious sedation is anticipated. Place the patient in the Trendelenburg position if tolerated. Merely placing the patient in this position may terminate the SVT as a result of increased pressure on the carotids and maximum carotid bulb stimulation. This position may also prevent syncope if there is a significant decrease in blood pressure or HR.

Carotid Sinus Massage

CSM is a bedside vagal maneuver involving digital pressure on the richly innervated carotid sinus (Fig. 11-7). It takes

advantage of the accessible position of this baroreceptor for diagnostic and therapeutic purposes. Its main therapeutic application is for termination of SVTs caused by sudden paroxysmal atrial tachycardia. It also has diagnostic utility in the assessment of tachydysrhythmias and rate-related bundle branch blocks. In addition, it can provide clues to latent digoxin toxicity, as described previously, by potentiating manifestations of the toxicity. It can also be used to sort out the differential diagnosis of syncope. Further information can be found on Expert Consult.

Returning to the use of CSM as a diagnostic technique for assessing digoxin toxicity, the adverse effects and toxicity from digoxin depend more on the response of the host than on the actual digoxin level. In cases of suspected digoxin toxicity, before the digoxin level is available or when it is in the "normal range," CSM may be a useful diagnostic adjunct. Significant inhibition of AV node conduction associated with ventricular ectopy, especially ventricular bigeminy, should lead to suspicion of digoxin toxicity.[1]

Contraindications

CSM is *contraindicated* in the very rare patient likely to suffer neurologic or cardiovascular complications from the procedure. Patients with a *carotid bruit should not undergo CSM* because of the risk for carotid embolization or occlusion. *A recent cerebral infarction is another contraindication* because even a marginal reduction in cerebral blood flow may produce further infarction. Age, by itself, is not a contraindication to CSM. However, the elderly are more likely to have carotid artery disease and may experience transient and, very rarely, permanent neurologic or visual symptoms after CSM. Complications are thought to be due to transient cerebral

Figure 11-6 Hyperreactive carotid sinus reflex. Gentle pressure was applied to the carotid sinus for 3 seconds, which resulted in a pause of approximately 7 seconds in sinus rhythm. This syndrome may be the cause of syncope. *(From Bigger JT Jr. Mechanisms and diagnosis of arrhythmias. In: Braunwald E, ed.* Heart Disease. *Vol 1. Philadelphia: Saunders; 1980. Reproduced by permission.)*

TABLE 11-1 Ventricular Response to Carotid Sinus Massage and Other Vagal Maneuvers

TYPE OF ARRHYTHMIA	ATRIAL RATE (bpm)	RESPONSE TO CAROTID SINUS MASSAGE AND RELEASE
Normal sinus rhythm	60-100	Slowing with return to the former rate on release
Normal sinus bradycardia	<60	Slowing with return to the former rate on release
Normal sinus tachycardia	>100-180	Slowing with return to the former rate on release; appearance of diagnostic P waves
AV nodal reentry	150-250	Termination or no effect
Atrial flutter	250-350	Slowing with return to the former rate on release; increasing AV block; flutter persists
Atrial fibrillation	400-600	Slowing with persistence of a gross irregular rate on release; increasing AV block
Atrial tachycardia with block	150-250	Abrupt slowing with return to a normal sinus rhythm on release; tachycardia often persists
AV junctional rhythm	40-100	None; ± slowing
Reciprocal tachycardia using accessory (WPW) pathways	150-250	Abrupt slowing; termination or no effect; may unmask WPW
Nonparoxysmal AV junctional tachycardia	60-100	None; ± slowing
Ventricular tachycardia	60-100	None; may unmask AV dissociation
Atrial idioventricular rhythm	60-100	None
Ventricular flutter	60-100	None
Ventricular fibrillation	60-100	None
First-degree AV block	60-100	Gradual slowing caused by sinus slowing; return to the former rate on release
Second-degree AV block (I)	60-100	Sinus slows with an increase in block; return to the former rate on release
Second-degree AV block (II)	60-100	Slowing
Third-degree AV block	60-100	None
Right bundle branch block	60-100	Slowing with return to the former rate on release
Left bundle branch block	60-100	Slowing with return to the former rate on release
Digitalis toxicity–induced arrhythmias	Variable	Do not attempt CSM

Adapted from Braunwald E, ed. *Heart Disease: A Textbook of Cardiovascular Medicine.* 6th ed. Philadelphia: Saunders; 2001:642.
AV, atrioventricular; bpm, beats per minute; *CSM,* carotid sinus massage; *WPW,* Wolff-Parkinson-White (syndrome).

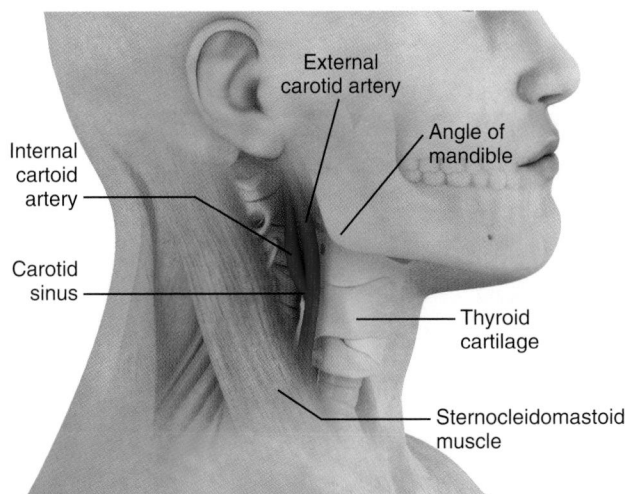

Figure 11-7 The carotid sinus. This baroreceptor is found just below the angle of the mandible at the upper level of the thyroid cartilage, anterior to the sternocleidomastoid muscle.

Labels: External carotid artery; Angle of mandible; Internal cartoid artery; Carotid sinus; Thyroid cartilage; Sternocleidomastoid muscle

ischemia or embolization of plaque, similar to a transient ischemic attack.

The presence of diffuse, advanced coronary atherosclerosis is associated with increased sensitivity of the carotid sinus reflex. This hypersensitivity is further augmented during an anginal attack or acute myocardial infarction. Brown and coworkers[14] found that the degree of carotid sinus hypersensitivity was directly proportional to the severity of coronary artery disease as documented by cardiac catheterization. Patients with acute myocardial ischemia or with recent myocardial infarction are already at higher risk for VT or ventricular fibrillation (VF). A CSM-induced prolonged asystole may further predispose them to these dysrhythmias. Therefore, CSM should be avoided in these patients.

Both digoxin and CSM act through a vagal mechanism to inhibit the AV node. Patients taking digoxin may experience greater inhibition of the AV node with a longer AV block as a result. Patients with apparent manifestations of digoxin toxicity or known digoxin toxicity should not undergo CSM because the AV inhibition may be profound.[15]

Technique

This technique can be performed with or without a concomitant Valsalva maneuver. Alternatively, pressure can be applied to the abdomen by an assistant. Some clinicians prefer to place the patient supine or with the head of the bed tilted downward. Begin CSM on the patient's right carotid bulb because some investigators have found a greater cardioinhibitory effect on this side.[12,16,17] However, scientific agreement on this issue is not unanimous. *Simultaneous bilateral CSM is absolutely contraindicated* because the cerebral circulation may be severely compromised. Before attempting CSM, first auscultate for carotid bruits on both sides of the neck (Fig. 11-8, *step 2*). The presence of a bruit is a contraindication to massage.

Keep the patient relaxed for two reasons. A tense platysma muscle makes palpation of the carotid sinus difficult, and an anxious patient will be less sensitive to CSM as a result of heightened sympathetic tone.

Tilt the patient's head backward and slightly to the opposite side. Palpate the carotid artery just below the angle of the mandible at the upper level of the thyroid cartilage and

anterior to the sternocleidomastoid muscle (see Figs. 11-7 and 11-8, *step 3*). Once the pulsation is identified, use the tips of the fingers to administer CSM for 5 seconds in a posteromedial direction, aiming toward the vertebral column. Although earlier practitioners used a longer duration of massage, a shorter period minimizes the risk for complications and is adequate for diagnostic purposes in the majority of patients.[18] Pressure on the carotid sinus may be steady or undulating in intensity; the force, however, must not occlude the carotid artery. The temporal artery may be simultaneously palpated to ensure that the carotid remains patent throughout the procedure.

If unsuccessful, repeat CSM after 1 minute. If the procedure is still unsuccessful, massage the opposite carotid sinus in a similar fashion. Perform simultaneous Valsalva maneuvers with the patient in the head-down position to enhance carotid sinus sensitivity before the technique is abandoned (Fig. 11-8, *step 4*). *CSM may be repeated once antiarrhythmic medications (e.g., calcium channel blockers and β-blockers) have been given, and often the combination is more effective. However, repetition of CSM after the administration of adenosine is not thought to have any utility.*

Complications

Neurologic complications of CSM are rare and usually transient. In a review of neurologic complications in elderly patients undergoing the procedure, Munro and associates[19] found seven complications in a total of 5000 massage episodes, for an incidence of 0.14%. Reported deficits included weakness in five cases and visual field loss in two others. In one case the visual field loss was permanent. Patients in this study were excluded from CSM if they had a carotid bruit, recent cerebral infarction, recent myocardial infarction, or a history of VT or VF. The duration of massage was 5 seconds. Lown and Levine[1] described one patient with brief facial weakness during several thousand tests. Carotid emboli and hypotension have both been implicated as possible causes of the neurologic deficits. Unintentional occlusion of the carotid artery may also be responsible for some neurologic complications.

Cardiac complications include asystole, VT, or VF. A normal pause of less than 3 seconds is part of the physiologic response to CSM; a longer pause may be diagnostic of CSS (see Fig. 11-6). In a review of reported cases of ventricular tachydysrhythmia, five cases were described.[20] All five patients were receiving digoxin, and in several cases VT or VF followed AV block. Digoxin is associated with more prolonged AV block from CSM, which perhaps leaves these patients more vulnerable.

Valsalva Maneuver

In general, mean changes in bradycardia are greatest with the Valsalva maneuver and the diving response.[2,21,22] During the Valsalva maneuver (i.e., exhaling against a closed glottis or bearing down as though to defecate), intrathoracic pressure increases and leads to increased arterial pressure as a result of increased afterload. This increased pressure is transferred to the peripheral vascular system. Venous return to the heart is decreased, which results in a decrease in the SVT. This is followed by increased venous pressure. All these changes in pressure lead to an initial increase in HR and carotid sinus pressure. As the maneuver is sustained, vagal tone is increased, thereby leading to a compensatory decrease in SA and AV

CAROTID SINUS MASSAGE

Prior to carotid sinus massage, place the patient on a cardiac monitor, initiate an IV line, and have antiarrhythmic medications and a defibrillator ready.

Auscultate for carotid bruits on both sides of the neck. The presence of a bruit is a contraindication to massage.

With the patient's head tilted backward and slightly to the opposite side, palpate the carotid pulse just below the angle of the mandible at the upper level of the thyroid cartilage and anterior to the sternocleidomastoid muscle. Once the pulsation is identified, use the fingertips to administer CSM for 5 seconds in a posteromedial direction, aiming toward the vertebral column.

If the initial massage is unsuccessful, repeat after 1 minute. The opposite side may be massaged in similar fashion.

Simultaneous vagal maneuvers may also be beneficial, such as the Valsalva maneuver depicted here, as might repeated massage after the administration of calcium channel or beta blockers.

Figure 11-8 Carotid sinus massage (CSM). *IV,* intravenous.

conduction. This is the expected or desired diagnostic or therapeutic response.

Contraindications

Patients must be able to cooperate with the clinician's commands. Dyspneic or tachypneic patients may not be able to hold their breath for the period needed to complete the maneuver.

Technique

With the patient supine, monitor in place, IV access secured, antiarrhythmics available, and defibrillation available, have the patient take a deep breath and hold it. Instruct the patient to bear down and try to exhale without allowing air to leave the lungs. The patient should try to hold this position for 10 to 20 seconds.[23,24] An adjunctive method is to have the patient take and hold a deep breath and try to push against the clinician's hand with the abdomen while the clinician gently pushes on the anterior wall of the abdomen.

Apneic Facial Exposure to Cold ("Diving Response," Diving Bradycardia): Technique

This technique can be viewed as a variation on the simple Valsalva maneuver. It has been found to be useful in children who may be unable to cooperate with or may be incapable of performing a Valsalva maneuver. Classically, the technique consists of covering the face with a bag of crushed ice and cold water (0°C to 15°C) for 15 to 30 seconds and then observing the electrocardiogram for a break in the tachycardia. Another variation of this technique is to drip ice water into the nostril of a small child. The procedure is based on the classic diving reflex of bradycardia. Slowing the SVT to unmask the hidden, underlying rhythm is similar to the effects of CSM. Conversion of sudden atrial tachycardia to sinus rhythm should be observed in 15 to 35 seconds. The procedure is convenient and noninvasive and can be self-administered.[25-30]

Berk and colleagues[16] demonstrated in healthy volunteers that immersion of the face in cold water and the Valsalva maneuver can produce a greater vagal response than CSM can. Lim and associates in 1998[31] and Mehta and coworkers in 1988[17] also found that the Valsalva maneuver was more effective than CSM for conversion of induced SVT.

Another technique that was used but has fallen out of favor is direct ocular pressure. There are many contraindications to this technique, such as retinal or lens surgery, glaucoma, thrombotic-related eye conditions, and penetrating or recent blunt trauma to the eye. This procedure is no longer recommended.

SELECTED PHARMACOLOGIC AGENTS

A pharmacologic approach to SVT is preferred in stable patients. In the presence of severe hypotension, chest pain, or other evidence of extremis, cardioversion is the preferred intervention. In unusual circumstances, such as rapid AF in patients with known Wolf-Parkinson-White (WPW) syndrome, certain medications should be used with caution, and cardioversion may be considered the first-line intervention.

Adenosine

The use of vagal maneuvers has been eclipsed in recent years by the use of adenosine, an endogenous, ultrashort-acting, vagal-stimulating purine nucleoside that is ubiquitous in body cells. Its action is to slow conduction time through the AV node and depress the AV node. If vagal maneuvers have been attempted and failed to produce the desired response, use of adenosine is an appropriate subsequent intervention.

Extracellular adenosine is cleared rapidly from the circulation by the erythrocyte and vascular endothelium system that transports adenosine intracellularly. Here, rapid metabolism via a phosphorylation or deamination cycle produces inosine or adenosine monophosphate. Adenosine produces a short-lived pharmaceutical response because it is metabolized rapidly by the described enzymatic degradation. The half-life of adenosine is less than 10 seconds, with the metabolites becoming incorporated into the high-energy phosphate pool.[32-35]

Indications and Contraindications

Most forms of paroxysmal supraventricular tachycardia (PSVT) affect a reentry pathway involving the AV node, and adenosine depresses the AV node and sinus node activity. Adenosine is indicated for the conversion of PSVT associated with or without accessory tract bypass conduction (WPW, Lown-Ganong-Levine [LGL]). The other use of adenosine is for diagnostic slowing of SVT to unmask AF, atrial flutter, or VT. The diagnostic and therapeutic effects of adenosine on tachydysrhythmias are similar to those elicited by vagal maneuvers. Adenosine's safety is derived from its short duration of action—usually about 10 to 12 seconds.

Adenosine should not be used in patients with a known history of second- or third-degree AV block or sick sinus syndrome unless there is a functioning internal pacer. Also, if the patient has a known hypersensitivity to adenosine or a history of severe reactive airway disease or active wheezing, the drug should not be used. In addition, adenosine should not be used in patients with an underlying accessory pathway (WPW, LGL) in the setting of AF. In this circumstance, the HR may increase because the enhanced AV node blockade permits conduction through the bypass tract.

Figure 11-9 Treatment of supraventricular tachycardia (SVT) with adenosine. **A,** Because of its ultrashort half-life (<10 seconds), adenosine must be given rapidly, followed by a 20-mL saline flush. **B,** Adenosine slows conduction through the atrioventricular node, thereby effectively converting supraventricular tachycardia (*left side of the screen*) to sinus rhythm (*right side of the screen*).

Dosage

The initial dose recommended is a 6-mg rapid bolus administered over a period of 1 to 3 seconds. The dose should be followed by a 20-mL saline flush (Fig. 11-9). If no response occurs within 1 to 2 minutes, a 12-mg dose should be administered in the same manner as the initial dose. This second dose should also be followed by a 20-mL saline bolus.

Side effects of adenosine are common and transient. *Many patients experience an unsettling feeling, and this should be explained to the patient before administering the drug.* Common sensations include flushing, dyspnea, and chest pain. Important drug interactions include theophylline or related methylxanthines (caffeine and theobromine), which can block adenosine receptor sites. If these medications are being taken by the patient, administer a larger dose of adenosine. If the patient is taking dipyridamole or carbamazepine, these drugs may block uptake of adenosine and potentiate its effects, so contemplate administering a smaller IV dose of adenosine (e.g., 3 mg).[36] Adenosine is safe and effective in pregnancy.[37] Also, if the patient has a central line or a transplanted heart, try an initial 3-mg dose.

Calcium Channel Blockers

Diltiazem

Diltiazem is a nondihydropyridine calcium channel blocker. It controls the rate of influx of calcium into myocytes during depolarization. This calcium channel blocker slows conduction of impulses through the AV node and prolongs the refractory period of the AV node. As a result, this drug is capable of terminating reentry-based tachycardias that have not converted with the use of adenosine or vagal maneuvers, and it can be used to control the ventricular response rate in a variety of SVTs (AF, atrial flutter). In addition, diltiazem can be used for the treatment of stable, narrow-complex tachycardias that are driven by automaticity (e.g., ectopic, multifocal, or junctional tachycardias).

Its effects on AV nodal tissue are selective in that it reduces AV conduction in tissue responsible for the tachydysrhythmia but spares normal conduction tissue.[34,38-40]

Indications and Contraindications

The beneficial effects of diltiazem are (1) ventricular slowing of rapid AF or atrial flutter without accessory bypass conduction and (2) rapid conversion of narrow-complex PSVT to sinus rhythm.[33,36,38,40,41]

Diltiazem is contraindicated in the following settings: (1) sick sinus syndrome, second-degree block, and third-degree block, except in the presence of an internal pacer; (2) severe hypotension or cardiogenic shock; (3) hypersensitivity to diltiazem; (4) use of IV β-blockade within a few hours of needing to use diltiazem; (5) AF or atrial flutter with coexisting accessory bypass tract conduction (WPW, LGL); and (6) VT.

Dosage

Give an initial dose of 0.25 mg/kg followed by a repeated dose of 0.35 mg/kg. Start a maintenance infusion of 5 to 15 mg/hr.[15,36,38,40] Consider pretreating with calcium IV if the patient is hypotensive (see below).

Verapamil

Verapamil is also a calcium channel blocker. This medication blocks the slow channel for entry of calcium into myocytes. Verapamil blocks not only the calcium channels in the specialized conduction tissue of the myocardium but also the contracting cells of the heart. As a result, verapamil prolongs the effective refractory period within the AV node and slows conduction.[2,39] It also has a modest effect on myocardial contractility.[2]

Indications and Contraindications

Verapamil is effective in (1) converting narrow-complex PSVT to normal sinus rhythm and (2) controlling the ventricular response in AF or atrial flutter if the AF or atrial flutter is not complicated by the presence of an accessory bypass tract (WPW, LGL). With specific regard to WPW syndrome and rapid AF, caution is advised with the use of verapamil. However, verapamil has been reported to be safe in those with overt or concealed accessory conduction pathways.[42]

Verapamil should not be used or be used with caution in the following settings: (1) PSVT with accessory bypass tract conduction, (2) AF or atrial flutter with accessory bypass tract conduction (WPW syndrome), (3) coexistence of sick sinus syndrome or second- or third-degree AV block unless an internal pacer is present, (4) severe left ventricular dysfunction (systolic blood pressure <90 mm Hg) or cardiogenic shock, and (5) patients with known verapamil hypersensitivity.[7,33,34,38-40] Because of its prolonged activity, verapamil should used with caution in patients with congestive heart failure.

In the presence of SVT, hypotension may be caused by the negative inotropic and vasodilating effects of verapamil. Administration of calcium before IV verapamil results in a decreased incidence of hypotension without compromising the effectiveness of channel blockers. The most common adverse effect of IV calcium is flushing. Use of digoxin does

not contraindicate calcium pretreatment. A dose of calcium gluconate, 1 g (ionized calcium, 90 mg) administered over a period of 3 minutes, is recommended for preventing or lessening the hypotensive effect of verapamil without affecting its antiarrhythmic effects.[43]

Dosage

Administer 2.5 to 5 mg IV over a 1- to 2-minute period. It may be repeated every 10 minutes to a maximum of 15 to 20 mg total. Pretreatment with calcium (calcium gluconate, 1 g IV over a period of 2 to 3 minutes) is suggested in hypotensive patients.

β-Adrenergic Blockade

β-Blockers are very useful agents for control of the ventricular response in patients with PSVT, AF or atrial flutter, and atrial tachycardia. No β-blocker offers a distinctive advantage over another because when used clinically, they can all be titrated to a desired effect on dysrhythmias and hypertension. Examples of β-blockers are atenolol, metoprolol, propranolol, and esmolol. What separates the different drugs and their use is the various pharmacologic characteristics that control adverse reactions, speed of onset, dosage regimens, contraindications, and drug interactions.

The electrophysiologic effect of β-blockers results from inhibition of binding of catecholamine at β-receptor sites. These medications reduce the effects of circulating catecholamines, and this is manifested as a decrease in HR, blood pressure, and myocardial contractility. The PR interval may be prolonged, but the QRS and QT intervals are not affected. Their actions are most noted on cells that are most stimulated by adrenergic actions. Typically, these sites are the sinus node, the Purkinje fibers, and ventricular tissue when it is stimulated by catecholamines.[2,33,34,39] These medications also have various cardioprotective effects in patients suffering from acute coronary syndromes. They exert their cardioprotective effects by decreasing myocardial workload, and hence they decrease myocardial oxygen consumption and demand.[2] β-Blockers are useful in the treatment of narrow-complex tachycardias that originate secondary to a reentry phenomenon or an automatic focus (MAT, an ectopic pacemaker, or a junctional rhythm). These drugs can also be used to control rates in patients suffering from AF or atrial flutter, as long as ventricular function is nominal. Some representative doses of these β-blockers are (1) *atenolol* (β_1), 5 mg IV slowly over a period of 5 minutes; if no effect, repeat in 10 minutes; (2) *metoprolol* (β_1), 5 mg IV slowly, may repeat up to 15 mg total; and (3) *propranolol*, 0.1 mg/kg IV by slow push and divided into three equal doses at 2- to 3-minute intervals; the total dose may be repeated in 2 minutes. The administration rate of the drug should not exceed 1 mg/min.

In general, β-blockers should *not* be used in patients with a history that includes diabetes, lung disease, bradycardia, or heart block; use of a calcium channel blocker; hypotension; or the presence of a vasospastic condition. β-Blockers should also not be used in patients with AF in the presence of bypass tracts, as is true for the calcium channel blockers adenosine and amiodarone.

Propranolol

Propranolol is the representative drug of the β-adrenergic blockade agents. It is nonselective and has β_1 and β_2 effects on the heart, which allows it to be used to control rapid ventricular rates. Rate slowing is caused by (1) slowing of impulse formation in the SA node and (2) depression of myocardial contractility. The usual effects on the electrocardiogram are rate reduction and prolongation of the PR interval. The QRS and QT intervals are not affected. Because it is relatively nonselective (has effects on both β_1 and β_2 receptors), its contraindications are somewhat extensive.[33,39,44]

Esmolol

Esmolol is a rapid-, short-acting, β_1-selective (cardioselective) β-blocker. At therapeutic doses it inhibits β_1 receptors in cardiac muscle. At higher doses its selectivity is lost and it affects β_2 receptors in the lung and vascular system. Esmolol is rapidly metabolized in erythrocytes and has a half-life of about 2 to 9 minutes. Its elimination half-life is approximately 9 minutes.[34,38]

Indications and Contraindications

Esmolol is indicated for the rapid conversion of SVT and rapid control of the ventricular rate in patients with non-preexcited AF or atrial flutter. In addition, it can be used to control the rate of noncompensated sinus tachycardia when the clinician believes that the tachycardia requires slowing. It has also been proved to have benefit as adjunctive therapy for the VT of torsades de pointes.[34,36,38,39]

Esmolol should not be used in patients with second- or third-degree heart block or in frank heart failure. Like all β-blockers, exercise care when using this drug in patients with bronchospastic disease and diabetes.

Dosage

Esmolol has a complicated dose regimen. First, give a loading dose of 0.5 mg/kg over the first 1 minute. Follow this with a maintenance infusion of 50 µg/kg/min over a 4-minute period. If this is not successful, administer a second bolus dose of 0.5 mg/kg followed by a maintenance infusion of 100 µg/kg over a 4-minute period. The bolus/maintenance dosing can be repeated up to a maximum infusion rate of 300 µg/kg/min for 4 minutes.[34,38,39] Similar dosing has been recommended for children: a 100- to 200-µg/kg maintenance rate between 100-µg/kg increases in bolus doses.[34]

Procainamide

A time-honored antiarrhythmic, procainamide slows conduction and decreases the automaticity and excitability of atrial, ventricular, and Purkinje tissue. It also increases refractoriness in atrial and ventricular tissue. Procainamide prolongs the QT interval without having much effect on Purkinje fibers or ventricular tissue.[36]

Indications and Contraindications

A long-established clinical application is for management of the rate of SVT, SVT with aberrant conduction (wide-complex SVT), AF or atrial flutter associated with WPW conduction, and VT. The advantage of using procainamide is the ability to convert to the oral form when rate control is achieved.

The dose of procainamide recommended by advanced cardiac life support is usually 15 to 18 mg/min, although in urgent situations up to 50 mg/min can be used. Procainamide is generally used in clinical situations in which time is not a factor in patient care. Long-term management in the emergency department necessitates monitoring of the plasma concentrations of procainamide and its N-acetylprocainamide metabolite. Hypotension and conduction disturbances (torsades de pointes, heart block, and sinus node dysfunction) are often signs of high plasma levels. Use caution in patients with a history of hypokalemia, long QT intervals, and torsades de pointes. Hematologic and rheumatologic disturbances are factors in long-term use. The end point of administration of the drug is when the arrhythmia is suppressed, hypotension occurs, the QT duration increases by 50% over baseline, or a maximum of 17 mg/kg of the drug has been administered (1.2 g in a 70-kg adult).[32]

Digoxin

Digoxin is a time-honored drug used for the treatment of AF and atrial flutter. It is the only antidysrhythmic with inotropic characteristics. Digoxin is less useful for the emergency clinician because of its long delay of onset.

Digoxin is a cardiac glycoside found in a number of plants. It is extracted from the leaves of *Digitalis lanata*. Digoxin increases intracellular Na^+ and K^+ by inhibiting sodium-potassium adenosine triphosphatase, the enzyme that regulates the quantity of Na^+ and K^+ inside the cell. An intracellular increase in Na^+ stimulates Na^+-Ca^+ exchange, which leads to increased intracellular Ca^+. The effects of digoxin are both direct action on cardiac muscle and indirect action on the cardiovascular system. The indirect effects are mediated by the autonomic nervous system. The results of these actions are vagomimetic effects on the SA node and the AV node.

The consequences of these actions are (1) increased force and velocity of myocardial contraction (positive inotropic effect), (2) slowing of HR and AV nodal conduction (vagomimetic effect), and (3) a decrease in symptomatic nervous system effects (neurohormonal-deactivating effect).[32,33,45-48]

Indications and Contraindications

Although its use in controlling the ventricular response rate in chronic AF is well established, it is no longer the mainstay of therapy for narrow-complex tachycardias, for which newer agents have replaced digoxin. Its inotropic character is still widely used in the setting of heart failure.

Use of digoxin should be avoided in the clinical settings of sinus node disease and AV blockade. It may cause complete heart block or severe sinus bradycardia. Do not use digoxin in patients with accessory bypass tract rhythms (WPW or LGL). It may cause a rapid ventricular response or VF. Patients with idiopathic hypertrophic subaortic stenosis, restrictive cardiomyopathy, constrictive pericarditis, or amyloid heart disease are particularly susceptible to digoxin toxicity.[49]

Dosage

Give an IV loading dose of 10 to 15 µg/kg, followed by individual parenteral dosing until the desired rate is achieved.[32-34,36,39,50-53]

Amiodarone

Amiodarone has become one of the workhorses of treatment of dysrhythmia in the emergency department. It is often considered a Vaughan-Williams class III drug because it is a potassium channel blocker. However, this medication also blocks sodium and calcium channels and α- and β-adrenergic

BOX 11-4 Recommendations for Cardioversion

RECOMMENDATIONS FOR PHARMACOLOGIC AND ELECTRICAL CARDIOVERSION OF AF*

1. Immediate electrical cardioversion is advised in patients with paroxysmal AF and a rapid ventricular response who have ECG evidence of acute MI or symptomatic hypotension, angina, or heart failure that does not respond promptly to pharmacologic measures.
2. Cardioversion is suggested in patients without hemodynamic instability when the symptoms of AF are unacceptable.

RECOMMENDATIONS FOR ANTITHROMBOTIC THERAPY TO PREVENT ISCHEMIC STROKE AND SYSTEMIC EMBOLISM IN PATIENTS WITH ATRIAL FIBRILLATION UNDERGOING CARDIOVERSION†

1. For patients with AF lasting 48 hours or longer or of unknown duration for whom pharmacologic or electrical cardioversion is planned, we recommend anticoagulation with an oral vitamin K antagonist (VKA), such as warfarin,‡ to a target INR of 2.5 (range, 2.0 to 3.0) for 3 weeks before elective cardioversion and for at least 4 weeks after sinus rhythm has been maintained.

   Remark: This recommendation applies to all patients with AF, including those whose risk factor status would otherwise indicate a low risk for stroke. Patients with risk factors for thromboembolism should continue anticoagulation beyond 4 weeks unless there is convincing evidence that sinus rhythm is maintained.
2. For patients with AF lasting 48 hours or longer or of unknown duration who are undergoing pharmacologic or electrical cardioversion, we recommend either immediate anticoagulation with IV unfractionated heparin (target PTT, 60 seconds; range, 50 to 70 seconds) or LMWH (at full DVT treatment doses) or at least 5 days of warfarin (target INR, 2.5; range, 2.0 to 3.0) at the time of cardioversion and performance of screening multi-plane TEE). If no thrombus is seen, cardioversion is successful, and sinus rhythm is maintained, we recommend anticoagulation (target INR, 2.5; range, 2.0 to 3.0) for at least 4 weeks. If a thrombus is seen on TEE, cardioversion should be postponed and anticoagulation should be continued indefinitely. We recommend performing TEE again before attempting later cardioversion (all grade 1B addressing the equivalence of TEE-guided versus non–TEE-guided cardioversion).

   Remark: The utility of the conventional and TEE-guided approaches is probably comparable. This recommendation applies to all patients with AF, including those whose risk factor status would otherwise indicate a low risk for stroke. Patients with risk factors for thromboembolism should continue anticoagulation beyond 4 weeks unless there is convincing evidence that sinus rhythm is maintained.
3. For patients with AF of known duration and shorter than 48 hours, we suggest that cardioversion be performed without prolonged anticoagulation. However, in patients without contraindications to anticoagulation, we suggest beginning IV heparin (target PTT, 60 seconds; range, 50 to 70 seconds) or LMWH (at full DVT treatment doses) at initial encounter.

   Remark: In patients with risk factors for stroke, it is particularly important to be confident that the duration of AF is less than 48 hours. In such patients with risk factors, a TEE-guided approach is a reasonable alternative strategy. Postcardioversion anticoagulation is based on whether the patient has experienced more than one episode of AF and on the patient's risk factor status.
4. For emergency cardioversion in a hemodynamically unstable patient, we suggest that IV unfractionated heparin (target PTT, 60 seconds; range, 50 to 70 seconds) or LMWH (at full DVT treatment doses) be started as soon as possible, followed by at least 4 weeks of anticoagulation with an oral VKA, such as warfarin‡ (target INR, 2.5; range, 2.0 to 3.0), if cardioversion is successful and sinus rhythm is maintained.

   Remark: Long-term continuation of anticoagulation is based on whether the patient has experienced more than one episode of AF and on the patient's risk factor status.
5. For cardioversion of patients with atrial flutter, we suggest the use of anticoagulants in the same way as for cardioversion of patients with AF (grade 2C).

ADDITIONAL GUIDELINES§

1. Strict heart rate control in patients with AF is not more beneficial than lenient control.
2. The antiplatelet drug clopidogrel, plus aspirin, might be considered to reduce the risk for major vascular events, including stroke in patients who are poor candidates for the anticoagulant drug warfarin.
3. Catheter ablation is useful to maintain normal sinus rhythm in patients with AF.

AF, *atrial fibrillation*; DVT, *deep venous thrombosis*; ECG, *electrocardiographic*; INR, *international normalized ratio*; IV, *intravenous*; LMWH, *low-molecular-weight heparin*; MI, *myocardial infarction*; PTT, *partial thromboplastin time*; TEE, *transesophageal echocardiography*.
*From Fuster V, Ryden LE, Asinger RE, et al. ACC/AHA/ESC guidelines for the management of atrial fibrillation. Circulation. 2001;104:2118.
†From Singer DE, Albers GW, Dalen JE, et al. Antithrombotic therapy in atrial fibrillation: American College of Chest Physicians evidence based guidelines (8th edition). Chest. 2008;133(6 suppl):546S.
‡Dabigatran is useful as an alternative to warfarin for the prevention of stroke and systemic thromboembolism in patients with paroxysmal to permanent AF and risk factors for stroke or systemic embolization who do not have a prosthetic heart valve or hemodynamically significant valve disease, severe renal failure (creatinine clearance <15 mL/min), or advanced liver disease (impaired baseline clotting function). (Wann S, Curtis AB, Ellenbogen KA et al. 2011 ACCF/AHA/HRS focused update on the management of atrial fibrillation: update of dabigatran. J Am Coll Cardiol. 2011;57:1330.)
§From Wann LS, Curtis AB, January CT, et al. Focused update on the management of atrial fibrillation. Circulation. 2011;123:104.

receptors. As a result of its potassium-blocking properties, amiodarone prolongs the action potential duration and increases refractoriness of the atria and ventricular tissue, the sinus and AV nodal tissue, and Purkinje fibers. Amiodarone also blocks sodium channels in depolarized tissue. It slows depolarization in the SA node and slows conduction through the AV node. Its calcium antagonist effect is minimal.[15,33,34,38]

Indications and Contraindications

Amiodarone is used for the control of narrow-complex supraventricular and ventricular dysrhythmias. It is useful in the management of narrow-complex tachycardias that originate from a reentry rhythm (SVT). It is effective in the conversion of stable wide-complex tachycardias, and it is useful in managing polymorphic VT with a normal QT interval. Amiodarone can be used for wide-complex tachycardias of undetermined origin. This drug can also be used for the management of AF and atrial flutter with aberrancy, SVT with accessory pathway conduction, and the rare adult junctional tachycardia. Another use for this medication is control of the rapid ventricular rate as a result of accessory pathway conduction in preexcited atrial arrhythmias. It is a strong second-line choice with procainamide for hemodynamically stable VT.

Its use can precipitate heart failure, hypotension, and severe bradycardia. When used with β-blockers and calcium channel blockers, amiodarone can have the added risk of hypotension and bradycardia. Torsades de pointes has been reported after the use of amiodarone in conjunction with drugs that have increased the QT interval. Also, amiodarone should be used with great caution, if at all, in the presence of AF with accessory pathways; there are several case reports of patients decompensating after receiving IV amiodarone when it was used for rapid AF plus WPW syndrome.[54-59] In the setting of possible AF with an accessory pathway, procainamide is safer. Finally, note that amiodarone will also prolong the QT interval, so it is best to avoid this drug in patients with a preexistent long QT interval, just like procainamide.

Dosage

The IV dosage is 150 mg administered over 10 minutes. Follow this with a 1-mg/min infusion for 6 hours and then a 0.5-mg/min maintenance infusion over an 18-hour period. If a dysrhythmia is refractory or resistant, 150 mg can be repeated every 10 minutes to a maximum of 2.2 g/24 hr.[54-59] The major adverse effects of amiodarone are bradycardia and hypotension.

ELECTRICAL CARDIOVERSION

In life-threatening or unstable situations, patients in AF are to be immediately cardioverted because the risk for continued AF outweighs the risk for thromboembolism.[38,60-68] Cardioversion is specifically indicated when the patient is unstable; that is, a change in mental status occurs, the patient becomes hypotensive, ischemic chest pain develops, heart failure develops, or the ventricular rate exceeds 140 to 150 beats/min.[39] Urgent

restoration of normal rhythm in patients with symptomatic new-onset AF is best achieved by direct cardioversion with either a monophasic or a biphasic defibrillator. Success rates with biphasic defibrillators are reported to be approximately 94% to 95%.[69-71] The cardioversion procedure is discussed in greater detail in Chapter 12.

Current guidelines for the treatment of symptomatic new-onset AF focus on the length of time that the patient has been in AF or atrial flutter. This is the determining factor for the initiation of anticoagulation when confronted by the need for cardioversion to sinus rhythm. Accordingly, onset within 48 hours or less has been determined to be the time limit that a patient with new-onset AF can undergo cardioversion without the need for anticoagulation. Studies have shown that staying under the 48-hour limit allows cardioversion to occur with the lowest risk for thromboembolism.[38,61,66,72] Patients who have been in AF for longer than 48 hours and are not in need of urgent care need to undergo anticoagulation to an international normalized ratio (INR) of 2.0 to 3.0 for a 3-week duration before cardioversion.[44] If this approach is not clinically acceptable, transesophageal echocardiography (TEE) should be performed in addition to heparinization.

If no clot in the left atrial appendage is visualized on TEE, the heparinized patient should immediately undergo cardioversion and take anticoagulants for the next 4 weeks. If a clot is visualized in left atrial appendage, the patient should first be anticoagulated to an INR or 2.0 to 3.0 for 3 weeks' duration before cardioversion[73-77] (see Box 11-4).

An alternative treatment strategy with a reported success rate of 50% to 70% is ibutilide in a bolus IV infusion. Be cautious when using ibutilide in patients with prolonged QT intervals or severe left ventricular dysfunction. Ibutilide has a 4% risk for ventricular arrhythmia. Pretreatment with ibutilide before electrical cardioversion can increase the chance for successful conversion to nearly 100%.[32,33,39,78-81]

CONCLUSION

The advent of β-blockers, calcium channel blockers, adenosine, amiodarone, and other effective medications to treat tachydysrhythmias—particularly SVT—has diminished the therapeutic use of vagal maneuvers. However, the vagal maneuvers still remain an important diagnostic tool. They are especially important in unmasking the underlying rhythms of narrow-complex tachydysrhythmias and in determining the presence of CSS in patients with syncope.

The advent and availability of medications that quickly and safely control the rate of tachydysrhythmias has given the emergency clinician a more varied and powerful armamentarium to be used in cardioverting these life-threatening dysrhythmias to normal sinus rhythm.

References are available at www.expertconsult.com

CHAPTER 12

Defibrillation and Cardioversion

Bohdan M. Minczak

INTRODUCTION

Defibrillation is an emergency procedure performed to terminate ventricular fibrillation (VF) (Fig. 12-1A). VF is a potentially lethal, but survivable "rhythm" commonly found in victims of sudden cardiac arrest (SCA).[1,2] VF can be caused by myocardial infarction, myocardial ischemia, undiagnosed coronary artery disease, and electrical injuries. Medications such as tricyclic antidepressants, digitalis, quinidine, and other proarrhythmics can cause QT-segment prolongation and changes in the refractory period of the cardiac cycle that are capable of precipitating VF. Furthermore, chest trauma, hypothermia, cardiomyopathy, electrolyte disturbances, and various toxidromes can induce conditions favoring the development of VF. Hypoxia is another culprit that frequently precipitates VF in adults and the pediatric population. Congenital malformations of the heart and great vessels have also been associated with an increased incidence of VF in young children. The most effective treatment of VF in its early phase is defibrillation.[3] It can also be used to terminate pulseless

ventricular tachycardia (VT) (Fig 12-1B). Patients with VF or pulseless VT are unresponsive, pulseless, and apneic. These patients sometimes require appropriate integration of cardiopulmonary resuscitation (CPR) with defibrillation to establish the return of spontaneous circulation (ROSC). Other dysrhythmias may also be encountered in patients with SCA, such as pulseless electrical activity (PEA) and even asystole; however, in this chapter discussion is limited to the treatment of VF and pulseless VT.

Defibrillation entails passing a therapeutic burst of electrical current across the chest wall through the myocardium for the purpose of terminating the chaotic electromechanical activity that is impeding the ventricles from ejecting blood into the circulation (Fig. 12-2). Failure to recognize and terminate VF promptly makes suppression of VF via defibrillation more difficult.[4] For every minute that the heart is in VF without treatment, the potential for the initial defibrillation to be successful and for the victim of SCA to survive decreases by 7% to 10%.[5] However, the integration of CPR with defibrillation, when appropriate, increases the chance for successful defibrillation and survival from SCA.[6]

Cardioversion is performed to suppress dysrhythmias that produce a rapid pulse and cause the patient to become unstable; such dysrhythmias include supraventricular tachycardia (SVT), atrial fibrillation (AF), atrial flutter, and unstable monomorphic VT (Fig. 12-3). These patients do have a pulse, albeit weak, but can rapidly decompensate, become hypotensive, experience chest pain, or have a change in mental status that will require rapid intervention (i.e., cardioversion). CPR is obviously not indicated because these patients have a pulse and their peripheral tissues are being perfused. Cardioversion is very similar to defibrillation; however, the shock is

---

Defibrillation and Cardioversion

Indications

Defibrillation
  Ventricular fibrillation
  Pulseless ventricular tachycardia
Cardioversion (usually reserved for unstable rhythms)
  Ventricular tachycardia with a pulse
  Supraventricular tachycardia
  Atrial fibrillation
  Atrial flutter

Contraindications

Defibrillation
  Presence of a pulse
  Asystole or pulseless electrical activity
  Obvious signs of death
  Valid do-not-resuscitate order
Cardioversion
  Arrhythmias due to digitalis toxicity
  Sinus tachycardia

Complications

Chest wall burns
Shock of a health care worker
Myocardial tissue injury

Equipment

Cardiac monitor/defibrillator
(other supportive equipment not shown)

Review Box 12-1 Defibrillation and cardioversion: indications, contraindications, and equipment.

administered during the refractory period of the cardiac cycle. This is accomplished by setting the defibrillator to the synchronized mode.

The shock is delivered in similar fashion; however, the defibrillator discharges at a particular point in the cardiac cycle. Failure to set the synchronized defibrillator controls properly can result in the conversion of a perfusing rhythm to a nonperfusing rhythm, thereby leaving the patient pulseless.

PRINCIPLES OF RESUSCITATION

The clinical approach to cardiac resuscitation is an evolving and dynamic endeavor, and guidelines frequently change or

A

B

Figure 12-1 Ventricular dysrhythmias. **A,** Ventricular fibrillation. **B,** Ventricular tachycardia.

Figure 12-2 During ventricular fibrillation, chaotic electromechanical activity prevents the ventricle from ejecting blood into the circulation. Defibrillation passes a therapeutic burst of current through the myocardium and terminates this activity.

are altered. Recommendation from the American Heart Association (AHA) are considered the most reasonable guidelines for the clinician, but many of the principles and caveats are based on minimal data, can be contradictory, and are subject to change; more importantly, any guideline is best applied by considering a specific clinical scenario. Most recently, cardiac resuscitation has been reviewed and new AHA guidelines were released in 2010.[7-10] On the basis of the strength of the evidence available, the AHA developed recommendations to support the interventions that showed the most promise. The new algorithms reflect alterations in the sequence of actions to be performed and stress high-quality CPR with compressions of adequate rate and depth that allow complete chest recoil after compressions, minimize interruptions in chest compressions, and avoid excessive overventilation. These modifications stress the interposition of effective CPR (Fig. 12-4) with defibrillation and have been organized in such a way that the time until the first shock is minimized and time to initiation of effective chest compressions is not unnecessarily delayed.

ANATOMY, PHYSIOLOGY, AND PATHOPHYSIOLOGY

The normal human heart rate (HR) is approximately 80 (±20) beats/min. With each beat the heart ejects a stroke volume (SV) of approximately 70 to 80 mL of blood from each ventricle. Multiplying HR by SV produces a value termed cardiac output (CO) (i.e., $HR \times SV = CO$). The product of CO times total peripheral resistance (TPR) produces the value for mean arterial blood pressure (MABP) (i.e., $CO \times TPR = MABP$). When the HR falls to zero or the heart fails to eject an SV (as in VF), MABP drops precipitously. Subsequently, vital organ perfusion is compromised. Hence, blood flow to the brain, the heart, the lungs, and other peripheral organs ceases.

A

B

C

Figure 12-3 Atrial dysrhythmias. **A,** Supraventricular tachycardia. **B,** Atrial fibrillation. **C,** Atrial flutter.

Failure to promptly restore blood flow will lead to significant mortality, morbidity, and SCA. Therefore, any interruption in cardiac contraction must be recognized quickly and corrected promptly. Cardiac contraction occurs as a result of a sequence of electromechanical events occurring in myocytes. The human heart has several unique characteristics that enable it to perform its physiologic role. These myocardial characteristics are automaticity, conductivity, excitability, and contractility. Individual cells have a "variable blend" of these characteristics. Some characteristics are more prominent than others, depending on the anatomic location of the cells in the heart. For example, the "pacemaker cells" have more automaticity, the conduction system has increased conductivity, and ventricular free-wall myocytes have more contractility. The electrical properties of these cells can be assessed by performing regional recordings of the changes in voltage in the tissue with respect to time (i.e., action potentials) (Fig. 12-5). The electrical impulse for myocardial contraction originates spontaneously in the sinoatrial (SA) node and spreads through the atria, which causes it to contract. As the impulse arrives at the atrioventricular (AV) node, it undergoes decremental conduction in which the electrical impulse is slowed down as the atria contract and "preload" the ventricles. Subsequently, the impulse activates the bundle of His and Purkinje fibers, which then causes ventricular contraction via excitation-contraction coupling. The electrical events precede the mechanical events. These events are graphically represented in Figure 12-6, which depicts the change in membrane voltage with respect to time as a result of temporal changes in ion permeability across the myocyte membranes. These sequential changes in ion permeability occur as the membrane potential varies, thereby producing the characteristic cardiac action potential.

As the original impulse from the SA node travels through the atria and into the ventricles, various action potentials are generated regionally. The summation of all these action potentials produces the characteristic electrocardiographic (ECG) tracing PQRST (see Figs. 12-5 and 12-6). The ECG tracing is a graphic representation of the electrical activity that induces the mechanical activity of systole. Systole occurs as a result of excitation-contraction coupling. Calcium ion

Figure 12-4 High-quality cardiopulmonary resuscitation is essential in the resuscitation of victims of sudden cardiac arrest. Push hard and push fast to a depth of 2+ inches at a rate of 100 compressions per minute. Minimize interruptions and avoid overventilating the patient. Allow full recoil of the chest between compressions.

Figure 12-5 Regional action potentials and electrocardiographic correlation. *AV,* atrioventricular; *SA,* sinoartrial. (*Netter illustration from* www.netterimages. com. © *Elsevier Inc. All rights reserved.*)

Relation of Action Potential from the Various Cardiac Regions to the Body Surface ECG

Action potentials

SA node
Atrial muscle
AV node
Common bundle
Bundle branches
Purkinje fibers
Ventricular muscle

P   QRS   T   U

0.2   0.4   0.6

Seconds

levels in the cytoplasm increase and trigger the contractile proteins to interact. As the ion channels reset, the myocytes return to the resting membrane potential (intracellular calcium is resequestered), and diastole occurs. The membrane pumps restore the ion concentrations to normal. This cycle keeps occurring about 80 times per minute. Each "cardiac cycle" lasts approximately 300 msec. During each cardiac cycle there are two periods that need to be addressed: the absolute and relative refractory periods (Fig. 12-7). During the absolute refractory period, the myocytes do not respond to excitatory stimuli because the channels are in full operation. During the relative refractory period, the myocytes can be stimulated with a stimulus that is proportionately larger than usual as more and more ion channels reset. These facts have relevance with regard to cardioversion and will be discussed further later in the chapter.

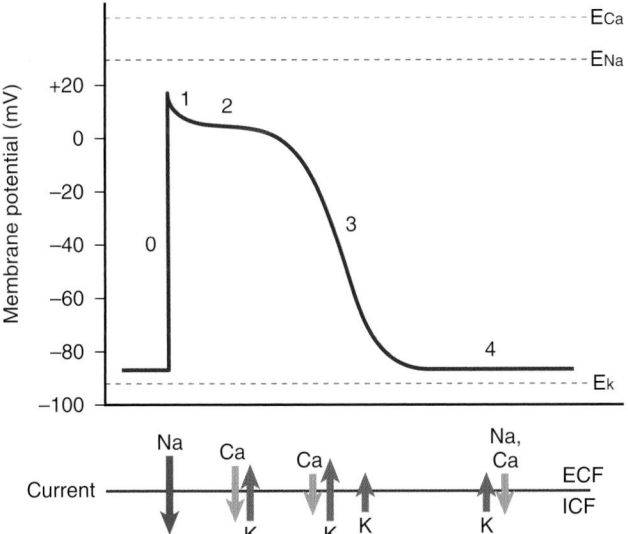

Figure 12-6 The cardiac action potential is a result of ion flux across the cell membrane. *ECF,* extracellular fluid; *ICF,* intracellular fluid. (*Adapted from Costanzo LS: Physiology. 4th ed. Philadelphia: Saunders; 2009, Fig. 4-13.*)

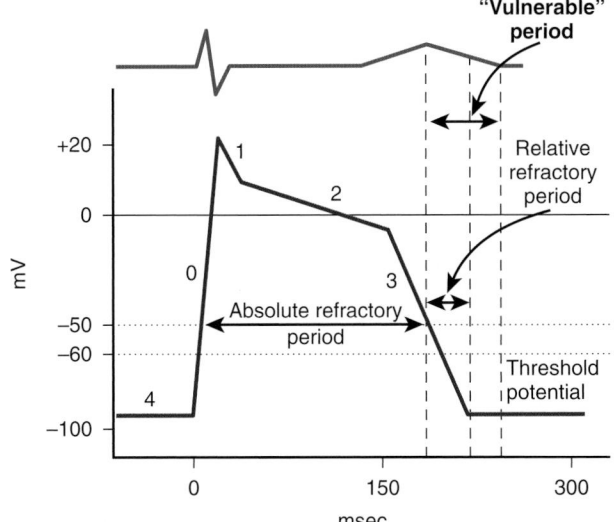

Figure 12-7 Absolute and relative refractory periods.

Mechanisms of Cardiac Dysrhythmias

As is evident from the preceding discussion, normal cardiac activity is a compendium of complex, sequential electrochemical, physiologic, and mechanical events. It includes three mechanisms: enhanced automaticity, triggered activity, and reentry. If alterations in the action potential phases or a modification of the refractory periods occurs and another impulse stimulates the myocyte at a time that it is out of synch with the normal depolarization-repolarization process, the coordinated normal excitation-contraction coupling becomes asynchronous. If conditions favor the development of ectopic foci, individual loci in the ventricular free walls and septum become "pacemakers" and the myocardium begins to contract uncontrollably (see Fig. 12-2) and produce an irregular ECG tracing (see Fig. 12-1A). CO falls to zero, with SCA ensuing. Another proposed mechanism that can precipitate the development of a dysrhythmia is a malfunction in propagation secondary to errors in conductivity and excitability and reentry of already propagated impulses (Fig. 12-8).

Defibrillation and Sudden Cardiac Arrest

When the heart is in VF or pulseless VT, applying a sufficient "burst" of therapeutic current across the myocardium will cause all the membrane channels that are involved in excitation-contraction coupling to be activated and mobilized into the absolute refractory period. As the myocardium enters the relative refractory period and returns to the resting state, the SA node will resume the role of "pacemaker" of the heart and normal AV contraction will resume. HR will increase, the ventricles will resume ejection of a normal SV, and CO will be adjusted to meet tissue needs. Subsequently, ROSC should ensue.

Cardiopulmonary Resuscitation: Ventricular Fibrillation and Pulseless Ventricular Tachycardia

When SCA occurs and the heart is in VF or pulseless VT, ventricular contraction is absent and circulation of blood comes to a standstill. To initiate CPR, mechanically compress the heart between the sternum and vertebral column. This causes pulsatile ejection of blood into the circulation, including the coronary circulation. For these compressions to be effective, perform them quickly and with sufficient displacement of the sternum (i.e., at least 2 inches) to produce adequate flow. Furthermore, keep interruptions in CPR to a minimum so that adequate perfusion pressure is maintained in the vasculature. Although the flow is not at physiologic levels, enough circulation occurs in the tissues, especially the myocardium, that the by-products of VF are "washed out" and the myocardium becomes less refractory to defibrillation.[11] During VF, the myocytes are actually consuming oxygen and adenosine triphosphate at a rate believed to be the same or higher than during normal contraction.[12,13] Several other concerns must be reinforced. During chest compressions, make sure that the chest recoils completely to the resting state so that blood can enter from the vena cava and pass into the right atrium. The rate of compressions should *exceed 100 compressions/min* so that adequate forward flow of blood is produced. Remember that HR × SV = CO.

Figure 12-8 Reentry as a mechanism of cardiac dysrhythmia. **A,** Two pathways are available for conduction of the cardiac impulse. **B,** One pathway has a unidirectional block to excitation (i.e., it can conduct only "backward"), and the other pathway has slowed conduction. **C,** As the impulse travels down the antegrade pathway (*left* in the schematic), it loops around and excites the other limb in a retrograde fashion. **D,** A reentrant circuit has been created, with the original limb now being excited by the impulse propagating up from the other side.

INDICATIONS FOR AND CONTRAINDICATIONS TO DEFIBRILLATION

Prompt electrical defibrillation is the most effective treatment of acute SCA and VF.[3,4] Prompt initiation of CPR in patients with SCA or VF is also critical for successful resuscitation and ROSC. Starting with the onset of collapse, the survival rate for patients with SCA or VF drops 7% to 10% for every minute of downtime without defibrillation.[5] If CPR is initiated, the survival rate declines less rapidly (i.e., 3% to 4% per minute of downtime).[4] If an SCA is witnessed and immediate CPR is provided, coupled with immediate defibrillation, survival from such events has been reported to increase up to fourfold.[4-6] Therefore, *immediate defibrillation is indicated as soon as VF or pulseless VT is diagnosed.* Few absolute specific contraindications to early defibrillation exist other than the presence of a pulse, absence of SCA, medical futility for the procedure, or a valid do-not-resuscitate order.

If a patient is found unresponsive, pulseless, and apneic and the "downtime" is unknown, immediately perform good-quality, effective CPR while preparing for defibrillation. Previous recommendations called for immediate defibrillation in lieu of a short period of CPR. The newest development in the 2010 AHA guidelines for CPR is also a change in the basic life support sequence of steps from the "ABCs" (airway, breathing, chest compressions) to "CAB" (chest compressions, airway, breathing) for adults and pediatric patients (children and infants, excluding newborns). As CPR is performed, prepare for rhythm analysis and initiate defibrillation if indicated. After performing CPR for 2 minutes (*5 cycles at a rate of 30 compressions to 2 ventilations*), perform rhythm analysis. If VF or pulseless VT is diagnosed, promptly perform defibrillation. When the time until the first shock is delayed during prehospital resuscitation (because of prolonged response times), data have demonstrated that the rate of successful defibrillation increases if patients receive bystander CPR before defibrillation.[2-6] A scientific evaluation of this information proposed that CPR enhances the defibrillation threshold

by restoring substrates to myocytes for the facilitation or resumption of normal excitation-contraction coupling. Furthermore, CPR may wash out myocardial depressants that have built up during prolonged VF. Therefore, administration of CPR before defibrillation in patients with suspected, prolonged VF is recommended in the prehospital setting. Data to substantiate this sequence for in-hospital resuscitation have not been presented. Thus, the issue of unknown downtime, though not a definitive contraindication to immediate defibrillation, may be a factor in the clinician's decision-making process regarding the resuscitation sequence.

Victims of SCA as a result of traumatic injuries do not usually survive.[13] The heart, aorta, and pulmonary arteries may have sustained injury that will prevent resumption of normal cardiovascular function. There is a high probability that the underlying hypovolemia and organ damage may preclude successful resuscitation. However, the cause of the trauma may have been SCA with subsequent loss of consciousness. In such cases, if SCA or VF is present in a trauma patient, attempt treatment with CPR and defibrillation; if unsuccessful, search for and treat the underlying cause of the trauma and pursue the SCA. Therefore, *trauma is not a contraindication to defibrillation*, although the resuscitative effort may be futile.

If the victim of VF or pulseless VT is a pregnant female, treatment of the mother is critical. Therefore, prompt defibrillation is indicated as per the same guidelines and sequencing as for nonpregnant patients.[14] No harm to the fetus has been reported as a result of defibrillation, and thus pregnancy is not a contraindication to defibrillation.

Previous recommendations suggested delivering a "stacked" sequence of up to three shocks without interposed chest compressions if the first shock was unsuccessful in terminating VF. This was done to decrease transthoracic impedance with the monophasic damped sinusoidal (MDS) defibrillators in use and to deliver more current to the myocardium. However, this recommendation has been rescinded because of lack of supporting evidence. Now, with the higher first-shock efficacy (90%) in successfully terminating VF (termination of VF for 5 seconds) through the use of biphasic defibrillators,[8] the recommendation to repeat a shock if the first treatment was unsuccessful is harder to justify. Hence, the AHA now recommends a one-shock protocol for VF. Evidence has accumulated that even short interruptions in CPR are harmful. Thus, rescuers should minimize the interval between stopping compressions and delivering shocks and should resume CPR immediately after delivery of a shock.

Defibrillation is also an effective treatment modality for terminating pulseless VT. *If the patient has a pulse, is stable, and has a perfusing rhythm while in VT, defibrillation is contraindicated.* However, if the patient in VT becomes unstable and signs of poor perfusion, a change in mental status, or persistent chest pain with pulmonary edema, hypotension, and subsequent shock develop, *synchronized cardioversion* is recommended. This procedure is addressed later. If the patient becomes unstable as a result of polymorphic VT or becomes *pulseless during the episode of VT, an unsynchronized shock (i.e., defibrillation) is indicated.*

Patients "found down" or who have just become unresponsive can have other "rhythms present" beside VF or pulseless VT (e.g., PEA or asystole). Defibrillation is contraindicated in individuals with PEA. True asystole is not a shockable rhythm, and current evidence suggests that defibrillating patients with "occult" or false asystole is not beneficial and may actually be harmful. Therefore, defibrillation is contraindicated in patients in asystole as long as fine VF has been ruled out (discussion below).

Some patients who succumb to SCA may have various medication-releasing patches (e.g., nitroglycerin, contraceptive hormones, antihypertensive agents, smoking cessation adjuncts) present on their chest. Their presence is not a contraindication to defibrillation. However, modify the placement of the electrodes or paddles used for defibrillation to avoid contact with these patches. If necessary, remove these items before defibrillation to avoid diversion of current from the myocardium, current arcing, sparks, and other problems.

Developments in defibrillation and computer electronics have led to the availability and use of implantable defibrillators (automatic implantable cardiac defibrillators [AICDs], pacemakers) in the chest of patients who have known coronary artery disease. These patients are prone to dysrhythmias and may have episodes of VT and VF that are automatically detected and defibrillated or cardioverted. However, these devices can malfunction, so if these patients have SCA or VF, perform defibrillation as indicated. *The presence of an AICD or pacemaker is not a contraindication to defibrillation.* The only caveat is to avoid placement of the defibrillation paddles over the AICD or pacemaker because the current for defibrillation may be redirected away from the fibrillating myocardium and compromise termination of VF. In addition, because current from the defibrillation could enter the AICD or pacemaker, the device could be prone to future malfunction. These devices should be reevaluated after the patient has been defibrillated.

Current trends in fashion sometimes include piercing of the body in various locations. In addition, certain items of clothing and jewelry may require modification of electrode or paddle placement. The presence of metal in locations proximal to the heart or in locations on the chest should be avoided to minimize the potential for diverting the defibrillating current from the myocardium. Also, if the metal object provides a potential short circuit from the patient or leads to "ground," this object should be removed, if feasible, to avoid diversion of current from the myocardium or arcing and burns across the chest. However, the presence of these materials, such as *jewelry or body piercings, is not a contraindication to defibrillation.*

In this part of the chapter on defibrillation the recommendations are intended for application to an adult (defined as older than 8 years or weighing more than 25 kg [55 lb]) patient with SCA or VF. If the patient is a child (e.g., 1 to 8 years of age or weighing less than 25 kg [55 lb]), modifications in the sequence, defibrillation energy, energy attenuation equipment, and size of the defibrillation paddles are necessary. Pediatric defibrillation details are discussed later in this chapter. If a defibrillator or automatic external defibrillator (AED) and equipment suitable for use in children are not available, the health care provider can resort to using a standard AED or defibrillator. Use of AEDs or defibrillators in infants younger than 1 year has not been studied.

Defibrillation can be an ignition source for explosion if arcing occurs or if there are any stray or aberrant electrical discharges that occur as a result of paddle or electrode discharge. Therefore, in an environment in which volatile explosive material is present, such as the operating room or other areas of critical care, be careful during defibrillation to avoid electrical arcing and to ensure that electrical conductivity through the patient's chest is optimal. Avoid using anesthetic agents and oxygen. A potentially explosive environment is a relative contraindication to defibrillation.[15]

When performing defibrillation, take care to avoid excessive moisture on the chest or around the patient. Although it is unlikely that there will be any significant or dangerous current leaks from the patient onto a wet floor, take care to avoid creating an electrical hazard. Try to ensure that the area is not wet; however, a wet surface is not an absolute contraindication to defibrillation. Defibrillation can be performed on ice and wet pavement.

Finally, defibrillation of an "occult" or "false" asystole or a very fine VF not detectable because of paddle or electrode position may be considered but is *not recommended.*[13] Fine VF can occasionally masquerade as ventricular standstill or asystole. This may be a function of perpendicular electrode orientation with respect to the wavefront of depolarization. When evaluating the rhythm of a patient, if there is any doubt or confusion regarding the type of rhythm present, make sure that several leads are checked and rotate the paddles 90 degrees from their original position to ensure that asystole is indeed present before abandoning the possibility of defibrillation. If fine VF is unmasked, consider providing aggressive CPR before defibrillation. Also, place the controls on the ECG monitor on maximal gain to ensure adequate amplification of weak signals.

CONDUCTIVE MATERIAL

Use of conductive material is important to lower the impedance or resistance to flow of current at the electrode–chest wall interface.[16-18] Multiple factors affect the range of impedance (e.g., body weight, chest size, chest hair, moisture on the skin surface of the patient, paddle size [diameter], paddle contact pressure, phase of respiration, and type of conductive

Figure 12-9 Use of conductive material is essential during defibrillation to lower the impedance to flow of current at the electrode-chest interface. **A,** If standard defibrillation paddles are being used, electrode gel *must* be applied before the procedure. **B,** Self-adhesive pad electrodes have conductive material incorporated into the adhesive. Use of gel with these pads is unnecessary. The use of self-adhesive pads is highly recommended.

material used). High impedance or resistance to flow of current can compromise the amount of current actually delivered to the myocardium and lead to a failed first shock. Inappropriate use of conductive material can result in current bridging or a short circuit and arcing of electrical current secondary to streaking of the material across the chest. This can produce sparks and unnecessary burns on the patient's skin. In addition, arcing of electricity can become a possible explosion hazard, depending on the circumstances. Conductive material needs to be used with the handheld electrodes. Various electrode gels are available on the market and should be kept in the proximity of the defibrillator, on the prearranged cart ready to use (Fig 12-9*A*).

Self-adhesive pad electrodes now have a resistance-reducing, conductive material incorporated into the adhesive, thus rendering the use of a gel or other conductive material unnecessary. Firmly applying the self-adhesive electrode pads to the skin will usually be sufficient to minimize impedance, allow adequate ECG acquisition, and if indicated, defibrillate (see Fig. 12-9*B*).

PROCEDURE

Witnessed Sudden Cardiac Arrest

(Figs. 12-10 and 12-11)

When confronted with a patient who has just become unresponsive, prepare for immediate defibrillation (Fig. 12-12). As soon as the defibrillator is available and the patient is connected to the monitor, assess the rhythm. In the interim, turn on the defibrillation equipment, place the paddles or electrodes on the chest, begin assessment of the patient, and initiate the steps in CPR by applying the CAB principle.[7]

Cardiopulmonary Resuscitation

Perform a pulse check (<10 seconds; see Fig. 12-11, *step 1*). If a pulse is definitely present, provide 1 breath *for 1 second* every 5 to 6 seconds or 8 to 10 breaths/min. The breaths can be delivered with either a bag-valve-mask (BVM) or some type of barrier device. Observe the patient for visible chest wall rise and fall so that the thorax dose not become overinflated. Hyperinflation of the chest can lead to inadvertent pressurization of the esophagus, which can cause lower esophageal sphincter pressure to be exceeded. This can lead to retrograde flow of gastric contents into the esophagus with the potential for subsequent aspiration of acid and debris into the trachea if the airway is not adequately protected. Overventilation of the thorax can also lead to an increase in intrathoracic pressure and impedance of blood flow to and from the heart, which should be avoided. Reassess the patient's pulse every 2 minutes.

If no pulse is present, begin a sequence of 30 chest compressions followed by 2 ventilations/breaths (see Fig. 12-11, *step 2*). Keep your hands on the lower half of the sternum and compress it at least 2 inches (5 cm) at a rate of at least 100 compressions/min. The time allotted for compression should be 50%/50% for compression and relaxation of the chest. Watch for full chest recoil to allow adequate ventricular filling (*do not lean on the chest*) before the next compression. When the defibrillator or AED arrives, continue the 30:2 ratio of compressions to ventilations during CPR, attach the patient to the defibrillator via electrodes, pads, and paddles applied to the patient's chest, and initiate the rhythm check (see Fig. 12-11, *step 3*). Every attempt should be made to minimize interruption of compressions.

Rhythm Assessment

Once the defibrillator is at the bedside, turn on the defibrillator/monitor and place electrodes on the patient's chest in the form of either quick-look paddles or the multifunctional electrode pads that can acquire ECG signals and be used concomitantly to defibrillate the patient. To decrease chest wall impedance, apply a gel or saline pads to the contact surface of the handheld electrode paddles to function as conductive material.

The correct position for placement of either the handheld quick-look paddle electrodes or the self-adhesive pads is illustrated in Figure 12-13. Frequently, the pads are labeled with a diagram as a guide to placing the electrodes on the chest wall. Using the patient's right side for orientation, place the sternal electrode just below the clavicle and just to the right of the sternum. Place the apical electrode in the midaxillary line around the fifth or sixth intercostal space. Once the electrodes or pads are in position, set the selector dial or switch

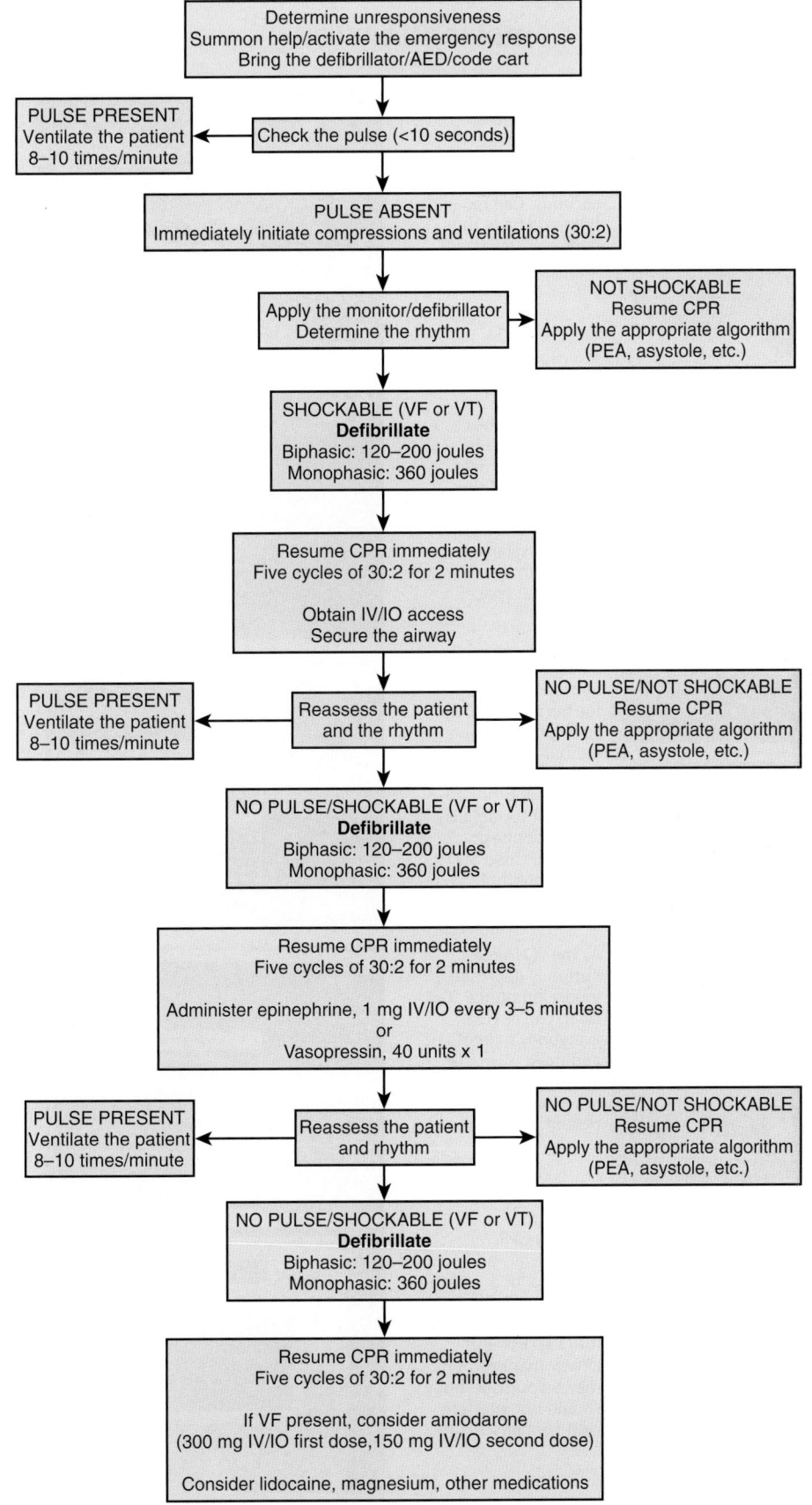

Figure 12-10 Adult defibrillation algorithm. *Note:* The use of epinephrine and its safety and beneficial effects for an improved cardiac arrest outcome has recently been questioned. No ACLS drug has been proved to improve long-term survival. *AED,* automatic external defibrillator; *CPR,* cardiopulmonary resuscitation; *IO,* intraosseous; *IV,* intravenous; *PEA,* pulseless electrical activity; *VF,* ventricular fibrillation; *VT,* ventricular tachycardia.

DEFIBRILLATION

Assess patient responsiveness, breathing, and circulation. Check for a pulse for <10 seconds. Call for help and have the code cart delivered to the bedside.

If there is no pulse, begin CPR at a rate of >100 compressions per minute with a ratio of 30 compressions to 2 ventilations. Avoid interruptions in CPR, and PUSH HARD and PUSH FAST.

Apply the electrodes to the patient's chest. Place the sternal electrode below the clavicle, to the right of the sternum. Place the apical electrode in the midaxillary line at the fifth intercostal space.

Check the rhythm on the monitor. If there is a shockable rhythm (i.e., VF or pulseless VT), prepare for immediate defibrillation.

Select the appropriate energy for the initial shock. For biphasic defibrillators, a default energy of 200 J is appropriate (see text for details). For monophasic machines, use 360 J. Make sure that "SYNC" is turned *off*.

Once the energy has been selected and the decision to defibrillate confirmed, press the "CHARGE" button on the defibrillator.

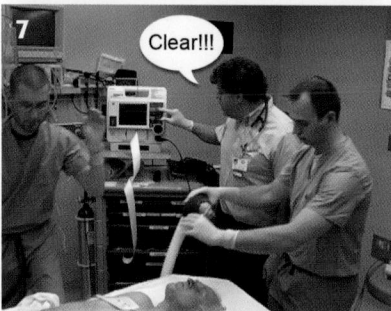

As the "CHARGE" button is depressed, loudly announce "I'm clear, you're clear, everybody's clear!" and make sure that all caregivers are not in contact with the patient.

Check once again to make sure that everyone is clear, and then depress the "SHOCK" button to defibrillate the patient.

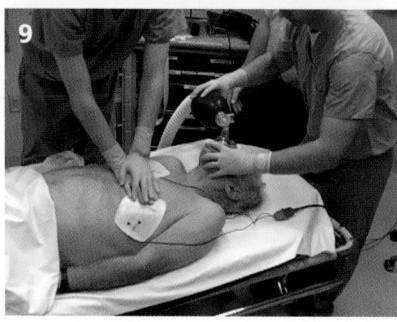

Resume CPR *immediately* and continue for 5 cycles/2 minutes. Additional interventions such as IV/IO access and airway management may be pursued but should not interfere with continuous CPR.

After 2 minutes of CPR, reassess the patient and the rhythm. Refer to the text and algorithms in this chapter for additional information.

Figure 12-11 Defibrillation. *CPR*, cardiopulmonary resuscitation; *IO*, intraosseous; *IV*, intravenous; *VF*, ventricular fibrillation; *VT*, ventricular tachycardia.

Figure 12-12 All resuscitation equipment should be kept on a "code cart" equipped with the monitor/defibrillator, airway supplies, emergency medications, and other essentials.

Figure 12-13 Electrode positioning for defibrillation. Place the sternal electrode just to the right of the sternum, underneath the clavicle. Place the apical electrode in the midaxillary line at the fifth to sixth intercostal space.

on the defibrillator monitor to the appropriate position to acquire the ECG signal from the input source—either the handheld quick-look paddles or the multifunctional electrode pads. Errors sometimes occur when the selector switch is in the position for the patient cable and electrode pads while the operator is attempting to use the handheld paddles. This could lead to misinterpretation of the rhythm, with the operator perceiving that the patient is in asystole, whereas in reality, VF, pulseless VT, or some other rhythm is actually present. Be familiar with the operation of the switches. In addition, adjust the controls for gain of the ECG signal to increase the sensitivity or gain of the ECG amplifier to ensure that fine VF is not interpreted as asystole. As the ECG rhythm appears on the monitor, make a diagnosis of the type of rhythm or lack thereof (see Fig. 12-11, *step 4*). If a shockable rhythm such as VF or pulseless VT is present, defibrillation is indicated. Proceed to select the appropriate energy level for the anticipated defibrillation.

Energy Selection

As noted previously, two major types of defibrillators are available: biphasic and monophasic (Fig. 12-14). Currently, the biphasic defibrillator, which is more likely to be found in the clinical setting, produces either a biphasic rectilinear waveform or a biphasic truncated exponential (BTE) waveform. However, there are still monophasic defibrillators present that usually produce an MDS waveform. Current data do not support one waveform over another, but biphasic defi-

brillators appear to be more efficient in achieving defibrillation with the first shock.

Therefore, the following recommendations are made: in general, a defibrillator using the biphasic rectilinear waveform should be set to an energy level of 120 J. If a BTE defibrillator waveform is being used, energy levels of 150 to 200 J are suggested for the first shock. If the type of waveform of the biphasic defibrillator is unknown or unavailable, a consensus default energy level of 200 J is suggested.

If the defibrillator is an older monophasic model using the MDS waveform, use 360 J for the first shock.

Mode Selection

Before defibrillation, check to make sure that the defibrillator is set to the unsynchronized mode. *Most defibrillators default into the unsynchronized mode between shocks.* Nonetheless, this control should be checked to make sure that it is in the unsynchronized mode; otherwise, the defibrillator may not discharge when the shock buttons are depressed because it is looking for the QRS complex, which is not present in VF. This is discussed in more detail in the "Cardioversion" section later.

Defibrillate

Continue CPR until the defibrillator is charged and ready to defibrillate. Once the energy level has been selected and the decision made to defibrillate, clear the patient for defibrillation by loudly stating "I'm clear, you're clear, everybody's

Figure 12-14 Biphasic and monophasic defibrillator waveforms. Most machines encountered in clinical practice today will be of the biphasic variety.

clear," and then activate the button to charge the defibrillator (see Fig. 12-11, *steps 6* and *7*). Once the defibrillator has been charged and everyone is clear, apply firm pressure to the defibrillation paddles (25 lb) to increase contact and deflate the lungs to the end-expiration state. This will decrease impedance at the paddle–chest wall interface. Subsequently, depress the defibrillation controls and deliver the shock (see Fig. 12-11, *step 8*). This will usually be followed by a perceptible whole-body muscle twitch in the patient. If no obvious response or twitch of the patient is seen, check the defibrillator controls to make sure that it is in the unsynchronized mode and that the paddles are activated. If using the multifunctional pads, no pressure is needed.

Resume Cardiopulmonary Resuscitation

Once the shock has been delivered, resume resuscitation with immediate chest compressions (see Fig. 12-11, *step 9*). Continue chest compressions for approximately 5 cycles of 30 compressions to 2 ventilations, or about 2 minutes of CPR. This facilitates the transition from SCA to ROSC after the heart has been stunned by the defibrillation and may not be functioning at optimal contractility for a few minutes after the shock. If additional monitoring devices are in place such as arterial lines or Swan catheters, modify this step accordingly as dictated by the resuscitation team leader.

Continue CPR for approximately 2 minutes. If the rescuers become fatigued, rotate the compressor and ventilator.

Reassess the Patient: Management of the Airway and Intravenous Access

After 2 minutes of CPR (5 cycles at a 30:2 ratio of compressions to ventilations), check the patient's perfusion status or carotid pulses. If there is no palpable pulse, resume compressions *immediately* and prepare for delivery of a second defibrillatory shock.

As preparation for the second shock begins, other members of the resuscitation team can work on securing the airway via endotracheal intubation, a laryngeal mask airway, or another appropriate device. Proceed with blood drawing and intravenous (IV) line placement or intraosseous (IO) if applicable, but do not interfere with chest compressions. The goal is to maintain uninterrupted chest compressions and to avoid any unnecessary interruptions.

Changes in Cardiopulmonary Resuscitation

Once an advanced airway has been secured, the compression and ventilation cycles are no longer delivered as just described.

Now, the compressor will continue to deliver compressions at a rate higher than 100 compressions/min *continuously*, without pausing for interposition of ventilation. Ask an assistant to deliver the ventilations at a rate of 8 to 10 breaths/min. Be careful to not overinflate the chest or to use too much force during ventilation because this can overpressurize the airways and esophagus, potentiate reflux, and impede venous return to the heart.

Energy and Mode Selection for the Second Shock

The energy for the second shock can be the same as that used before, but a higher energy level can be chosen at the discretion of the resuscitation leader. *Check the mode selector again to be certain that it is in the unsynchronized position.*

Second Defibrillation

Once the energy level has been selected, charge the defibrillator. When the defibrillator is ready to shock, halt CPR, clear the patient as discussed earlier, and deliver the second shock.

Resume CPR immediately after delivering the second shock. This step can be modified at the discretion of the resuscitation team leader, if there is clinical evidence of ROSC, or if devices are being used to monitor circulatory status (e.g., central venous pressure monitor, Swan-Ganz catheter, or direct arterial line).

If the patient does not have a shockable rhythm, proceed to the appropriate algorithm for VT, PEA, or asystole. Regarding airway management, consider using a supraglottic airway or endotracheal intubation without causing any significant interruption in chest compressions. Also, initiate end-tidal carbon dioxide measurements (capnography) to determine the adequacy of CPR and ROSC when applicable.[7]

It is now believed that when SCA occurs in a presumably nonhypoxic heart, there is enough oxygen in the functional residual capacity (FRC) of the lungs (FRC = ERV [expiratory reserve volume] + RV [residual volume]) that with compressions only, blood will be oxygenated in the lungs for a short period. Therefore, airway management is not as urgent as when restoring circulation that has totally ceased. Also, there is no need to overventilate the patient because hyperinflation of the lungs will cause an increase in intrathoracic pressure and compromise venous return to the right side of the heart.

Unwitnessed Arrest

When encountering a patient who is unresponsive and has been down for an unknown amount of time, assess the patient,

Figure 12-15 Automated external defibrillator.

BOX 12-1 **Defibrillation Equipment**

LIST OF MATERIAL FOR DEFIBRILLATION
- Defibrillator/ECG monitor
- Handheld defibrillation electrode "quick-look" paddles
- Patient interface cables; multifunctional for ECG monitoring and defibrillation
- Electrodes and pads for ECG signal acquisition and defibrillation
- Conductive gel (*not* ultrasound gel)

ADDITIONAL "EQUIPMENT" (PERTINENT TO VF/VT)*
ACLS Medications
- Epinephrine
- Vasopressin
- Amiodarone
- Lidocaine
- Magnesium sulfate
- Procainamide
- Atropine

Miscellaneous
- IV access equipment, central line kits, etc.

ACLS, *advanced cardiac life support;* ECG, *electrocardiographic;* VF, *ventricular fibrillation;* VT, *ventricular tachycardia.*
*List of suggested equipment and medications for a code cart.

summon help, and initiate CPR immediately, if indicated. Perform CPR until the defibrillator or AED is brought to the patient's side. As preparations are being made for defibrillation, consider performing 5 cycles of 30 : 2 compressions to ventilations before performing defibrillation.

Automated External Defibrillator Application
The availability of AEDs or semi-automated defibrillators in hospitals has increased, especially in non–critical care areas (Fig. 12-15). Although AEDs are designed for lay public use, application of these devices may also occur in the clinical setting. As in the algorithm, assess the patient, summon help, and apply the AED. Operation of the AED is guided by voice and visual prompts. Turn the device on, apply the patient electrodes in the appropriate positions, analyze the rhythm, and deliver a shock if a shockable rhythm is present. The AED will determine the rhythm and choose the energy level. Integrate CPR with the shocks to enhance the potential outcome of SCA resuscitation.

Medication
As per the 2010 AHA guidelines, there are insufficient data to demonstrate that any drugs or mechanical CPR devices improve long-term outcome after cardiac arrest. There is now some concern that epinephrine, a long-time universally recommended adjunct to CPR, may actually worsen outcomes in patients with SCA. The routine use of medications has been deemphasized, but not abandoned, in the current recommendations for resuscitation of SCA, VF, and pulseless VT (Box 12-1). Whether increased long-term survival from cardiac arrest can be expected with the use of any medications during CPR remains uncertain.

Complications
Complications of defibrillation include soft tissue injury, myocardial injury, and cardiac dysrhythmias. The availability of multifunctional electrode pads and better applicators for electrode gel has decreased the potential for soft tissue injuries such as chest burns.[19] In fact, many clinicians now prefer to use the multifunctional electrode pads for ECG acquisition and for defibrillation.

The development of new, energy-efficient biphasic defibrillation waveforms, such as the BTE and the rectilinear biphasic waveform, has increased first-shock success and decreased the incidence of dysrhythmias after defibrillation.[8] As a result, fewer shocks are needed to defibrillate the myocardium and less current is applied to the myocardium, which results in less electrical damage to myocytes.

Use of AEDs in public access defibrillation programs has not been reported to have produced any significant mishaps or adverse outcomes.[20]

Some older recommendations, such as use of the precordial thump, have been retracted. This procedure has been reported to have caused asystole or complete heart block (or both) when applied.[21]

In addition, the use of procainamide, though not a complication, has fallen out of favor because of long infusion times and mixed results regarding the efficacy of the effects of procainamide during the acute phase of VF and pulseless VT resuscitation.[22]

PEDIATRIC DEFIBRILLATION

Cardiac arrest in infants and children should initially be considered to be secondary to respiratory arrest. SCA, VF, and pulseless VT are much less likely to occur in children than in adults. However, 5% to 15% of pediatric and adolescent SCA events demonstrate VF in the prehospital setting. In in-hospital arrests, a 20% occurrence of VF at some point during the resuscitation is reported. Nonetheless, rapid intervention and defibrillation improve outcomes from SCA. Causes of SCA, VF, and pulseless VT are more diverse in pediatric patients.[22] Cardiac arrest does not usually occur as a result of a primary cardiac cause. Therefore, the approach to resuscitation of a pediatric patient in VF or pulseless VT may differ depending on the cause of the arrest.

Ventricular Fibrillation in Children

VF is much less common in children than in adults. The etiology of VF and SCA in children is most likely to be sudden infant death syndrome, respiratory compromise, sepsis, neurologic disease, or injuries from motor vehicle crashes, burns, accidental firearm discharge, and drowning, which are preventable.[23,24] The most common terminal rhythms reported in children younger than 17 years are PEA, bradycardia, and asystole.[25] The etiology of these pediatric arrhythmias is most often hypoxemia, hypotension, hypoglycemia, and acidemia. In addition, focal electrical ectopy is less likely to initiate VF in a young heart. A significant myocardial mass must be unstable and fibrillating before VF becomes established. In children (from birth to 8 years old) with nontraumatic arrest, only 3% of the dysrhythmias are reported to be VF. In victims aged 8 to 30 years, the number of patients with VF increases by almost sixfold (17%).[23] Several subpopulations of pediatric patients at various ages with cardiomyopathy or myocarditis or who have undergone heart surgery are at increased risk for a primary dysrhythmia.

As noted previously, the incidence of VF in cardiac arrest rhythms of pediatric patients is reported to range from 7% to 20%.[26] Patients with rhythms who have been defibrillated from VF have been reported to have a higher survival-to-discharge rate than do children who sustained asystole or PEA.[27] Therefore, there is a definite indication for early defibrillation in the pediatric population.

Procedure and Technique

The procedure for pediatric defibrillation is similar to the algorithm for adult defibrillation (Fig. 12-16). However, a few differences must be addressed. These guidelines do not apply to children younger than 1 year.

Pediatric Sudden Cardiac Arrest

When cardiac arrest occurs in a child, it is usually a terminal event associated with respiratory compromise or shock. The probability of SCA resulting from a primary cardiac cause is extremely low.[23] Nonetheless, it can and does occur. If resuscitation is prompt, the potential for a positive outcome, including preservation of the patient's neurologic integrity, is quite high. To enhance the outcome of SCA resuscitation, defibrillation and CPR must be effectively integrated. The pediatric resuscitation guidelines incorporated findings from a comprehensive review of the data.[28] Revised steps for the recommended resuscitation sequence are described in the following sections.

Equipment.   To perform pediatric defibrillation, a defibrillator monitor capable of adjustments in energy appropriate for children is needed. If an AED is to be used, it should have an energy attenuator for adjusting the energy to the appropriate level for a child (Fig. 12-17A). In addition, the quick-look electrode paddles (Fig. 12-17B) should have adapters attached to the adult paddles to ensure appropriate contact with the chest wall in a child without causing the electrodes to overlap. If adhesive pads are used, choose the appropriate size that will not overlap (Fig 12-17C). Use gels as in adults while being careful to prevent bridging across the chest wall from streaks of conductive material that may have been carelessly applied to the chest.

Paddle and Pad Application and Use of Conductive Material.   To acquire the electrical rhythm and subsequently administer an effective defibrillatory shock, place the appropriate-sized pads and paddles correctly on the chest. Use of the appropriate size and placement of paddles or pads will ensure that the appropriate current density is delivered across the myocardium to effectively defibrillate the myocytes. Furthermore, appropriate pad or paddle size—the largest surface area possible without direct electrode-to-electrode contact—will decrease transthoracic impedance and enhance defibrillation.[29] To accomplish this, use infant paddles for children weighing less than 10 kg. However, use larger paddles if they do not contact each other. If contact is made between the paddles, an electrical arc or short circuit could occur.[30] In children who weigh more than 10 kg (mean age, 1 year), use adult pads or paddles (8 to 10 cm in diameter).[29] Use a conductive agent to enhance skin contact and decrease transthoracic impedance. Never use dry paddles because the resistance to flow of current will be very large. However, refrain from using saline-soaked pads in children because they may cause arcing as a result of the proximity of the pads on the chest. Remember that electricity will take the path of least resistance and that the current from defibrillation will travel across the chest if there is a saline bridge between the electrodes. In addition, the use of ultrasound gel and alcohol pads is discouraged because of poor electrical conductivity and potentially high impedance.[30]

Apply the paddles or pads firmly to the chest, one to the right of the sternum, just below the clavicle, and the other to the left of the left nipple, over the ribs and the apex of the heart (see Fig. 12-13A). An option when using self-adhesive pads is to place one pad just to the left of the sternum and the other over the back so that they approximate the position of the heart (see Fig. 12-13B).

Procedure in an Unresponsive Child

When confronted with an unresponsive child, immediately summon assistance and start the ABCs of CPR. Bring equipment for resuscitation expediently to the patient's side. If no help is immediately available, first perform about 2 minutes of CPR before leaving the patient's side. Remember that the arrest may have been the result of respiratory compromise and that performance of CPR may ameliorate the condition.

If the victim is unresponsive to verbal and tactile stimuli, begin chest compressions immediately (30:2) at a rate greater than 100/min. Open the airway by using the head-tilt/chin-lift method. If a spinal cord injury is suspected, use the jaw-thrust maneuver without head tilt. The team can initiate other actions. Next, determine breathlessness. If there is no perceivable evidence of breathing, provide two slow rescue breaths (1 breath/sec) that make the chest rise. Do not use excessive force while ventilating because this could cause regurgitation or aspiration, impede venous return to the heart, and decrease coronary blood flow as a result of increased intrathoracic pressure. After interposing the breaths, proceed to assess the circulation by checking for a pulse in either the carotid or femoral artery (<10 seconds). If there is no palpable pulse or a very slow pulse less than 60 beats/min in very young children after 10 seconds of attempting to feel a pulse, initiate

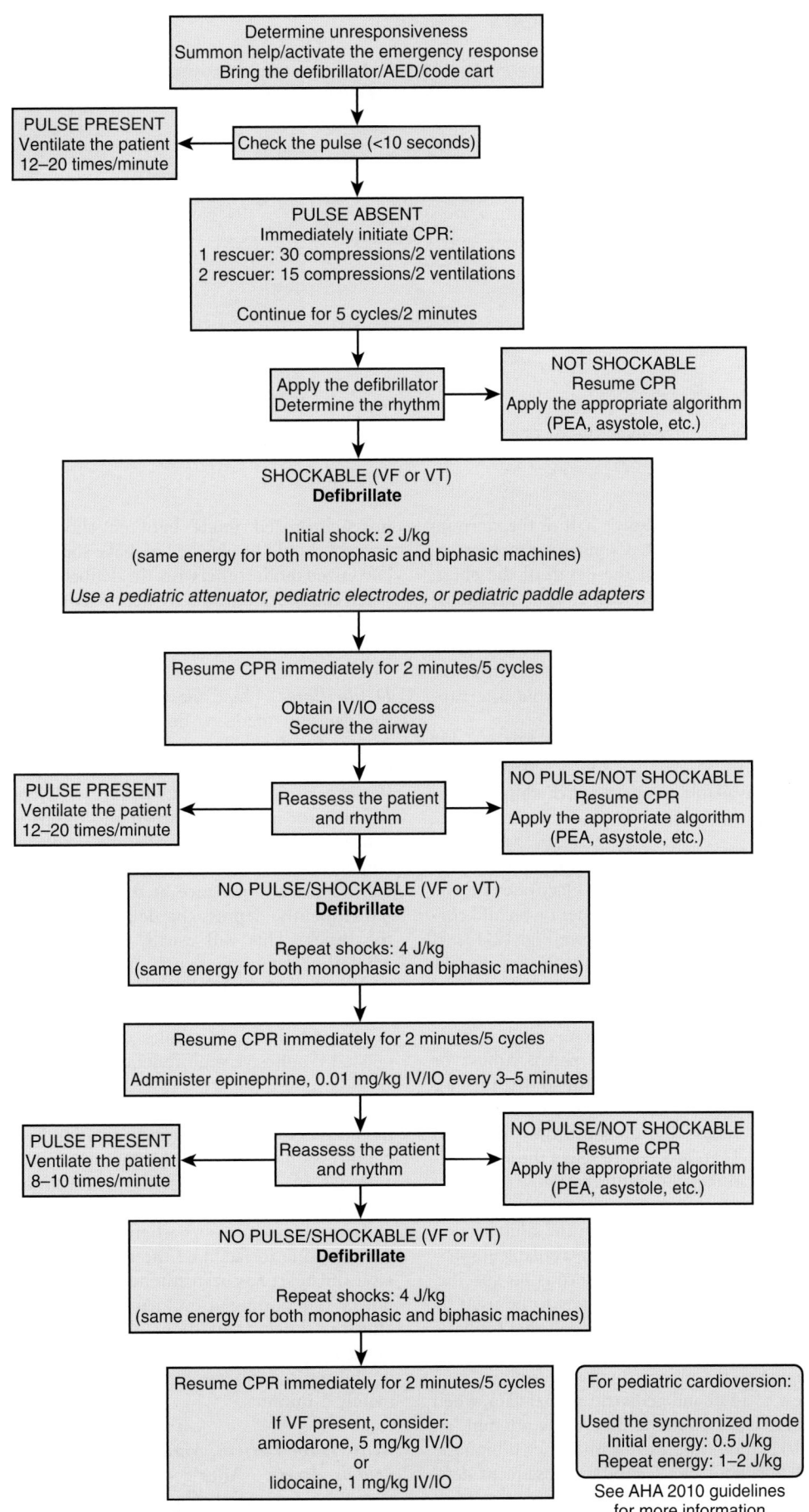

Figure 12-16 Pediatric defibrillation algorithm. *Note:* The use of epinephrine and its safety and beneficial effects for an improved cardiac arrest outcome have recently been questioned. No ACLS drug has been proved to improve long-term survival. *AED*, automatic external defibrillator; *CPR*, cardiopulmonary resuscitation; *IO*, intraosseous; *IV*, intravenous; *PEA*, pulseless electrical activity; *VF*, ventricular fibrillation; *VT*, ventricular tachycardia.

Figure 12-17 Pediatric defibrillation equipment. **A,** Pediatric energy attenuator for the automated external defibrillator. **B,** Pediatric quick-look electrode paddle adapters. **C,** Pediatric adhesive electrode pads.

chest compressions. Compress the lower half of the sternum while avoiding the xiphoid process. Compress the chest to approximately one third to one half the depth of the chest. The rate of compressions should be at least 100 compressions/min. If a single rescuer is performing the compressions and ventilations, the compression-to-ventilation ratio should be 30:2. If two rescuers are available, the compression-to-ventilation ratio should be 15:2. Attempt to avoid interruption of the chest compressions.

If an adequate pulse is present, interpose 12 to 20 breaths/min (1 breath every 3 to 5 seconds). Once a defibrillator monitor or an AED is available, prepare for rhythm analysis and defibrillation.

Rhythm Assessment. Once the defibrillator or monitor is at the patient's side, turn it on and place the electrodes on the patient's chest. The positions of the electrodes on a child correspond to the positions used in an adult (see Fig. 12-13). If quick-look paddles are used, carefully apply the conductive gel to the electrodes' surface. If self-adhesive multifunctional electrode pads are used, there is no need to use conductive gel. Make sure that the input selector switch is reading from the appropriate source (i.e., paddles or pads). Adjust or increase the gain or sensitivity of the monitor so that fine VF is not missed because of low amplitude. As the ECG rhythm appears on the monitor, assess and diagnose the rhythm. If VF or pulseless VT is present, proceed to select the appropriate energy level for the anticipated defibrillation.

Energy Selection. As mentioned earlier in the adult section of the chapter, two types of defibrillators are available: biphasic and monophasic. As of this writing, there is no specific, detailed differentiation between energy levels to be used by either type of defibrillator. However, the caveat that biphasic shocks are at least as effective as monophasic shocks and that they are less damaging to the myocardium still applies.

Based on a review of adult and pediatric animal data, when a manual defibrillator is used for the first shock attempt, an energy level of 2 J/kg should be used with either a biphasic or a monophasic defibrillator. If a second or subsequent defibrillation is indicated, 4 J/kg should be used with either type.[7,27]

Mode Selection. Before defibrillation, check to make sure that the defibrillator is set to the unsynchronized mode for defibrillation. Most defibrillators default into the unsynchronized mode between shocks. Nonetheless, this control should be checked to make sure that it is in the unsynchronized mode; otherwise, the defibrillator may not discharge when the shock buttons are depressed because it is looking for the QRS complex, which is not present in VF (this is discussed in more detail in the later section "Cardioversion").

Defibrillate. Once the energy level has been selected and the decision made to defibrillate, simultaneously clear the patient for defibrillation by loudly stating "I'm clear, you're clear, everybody's clear" while the button is activated to charge the capacitor. *Continue CPR until ready to shock.* Once the defibrillator has been charged and the patient cleared, apply firm pressure to the defibrillation paddles (25 lb) to increase contact and deflate the lungs to the end-expiration state. This will decrease impedance at the paddle–chest wall interface. Subsequently, depress the defibrillation controls and deliver the shock. This will usually be followed by a perceptible whole-body muscle twitch by the patient. If no obvious response or twitch of the patient is seen, check the defibrillator controls to make sure that it is in the unsynchronized mode and that the paddles are activated. No pressure is needed if adhesive multifunctional pads are used.

Resume Cardiopulmonary Resuscitation. Once the shock has been delivered, resume resuscitation with immediate chest compressions. Continue the compressions for approximately 5 cycles of 30 compressions to 2 ventilations or about 2 minutes of CPR. If two rescuers are available, use a 15:2 ratio and switch compressors when the first compressor fatigues. This is done to facilitate the transition from SCA to ROSC after the heart has been stunned by the defibrillation and may not be functioning at optimal contractility for a few minutes after the shock. If additional monitoring devices are in place in the hospital setting, modify this step accordingly as decided by the resuscitation team leader. Continue CPR for approximately 2 minutes.

Reassess the Patient, Manage the Airway, and Gain Intravenous Access. After 2 minutes of CPR, 5 cycles of 30:2, check the patient's perfusion status or carotid pulses. If no pulse is palpable, resume compressions immediately and prepare to deliver a second defibrillatory shock.

While the operator is preparing for the second shock, other members of the resuscitation team can work on securing the airway via endotracheal intubation, a laryngeal mask airway, or another appropriate device. Blood draws and IV line placement (or IO if applicable) should proceed but not interfere with chest compressions. The goal is to maintain uninterrupted chest compressions and avoid any unnecessary interruptions.

Change in Cardiopulmonary Resuscitation. Once an advanced airway has been secured, compression and ventilation cycles are no longer delivered. Now, the compressor will continue to deliver compressions at a rate of 100/min continuously without pausing for interposition of ventilations. When delivering the ventilations, provide 8 to 10 breaths/min, but be careful to not overinflate the chest or use too much force during ventilation to avoid overpressurizing the airways and esophagus and potentiating reflux. Lesser force also decreases the possibility of compromising CO as a result of elevated intrathoracic pressure.

Second Shock: Energy Selection and Mode. The second shock, if indicated, should occur after 2 minutes of CPR. The energy level for the second shock should be 4 J/kg. Be sure to check that the defibrillator or monitor is in the unsynchronized mode.

Immediately after the second shock, resume CPR and continue for about 2 minutes. If assessment of the rhythm and circulatory status shows continued VF or pulseless VT and no ROSC, continue CPR and consider medications such as a vasopressor (e.g., epinephrine).

Medications. The same caveats concerning the lack of proven benefit of any medications to improve long-term survival in adults also applies to children.

Automatic External Defibrillators in Children

As mentioned previously, the incidence of VF and pulseless VT in children is low. Nonetheless, the presence of VF or pulseless VT is an indication for using an AED or defibrillator. The age range for use of an AED or defibrillator is 1 to 8 years. No recommendations for the use of a defibrillator or AED in children younger than 1 year have been provided as of this writing.[31] A pediatric energy dose attenuator (see Fig. 12-17*A*) should be used to prevent the delivery of too much current to the myocardium. If a pediatric dose attenuator is not immediately available, a standard defibrillator should be used at the lowest appropriate setting.

Use of the AED entails bringing the AED to the patient's side, turning the device on, following the voice or visual prompts, and connecting the electrodes to the patient. Once the pads are applied to the patient, the AED will initiate the rhythm analysis automatically or the rescuer will be prompted to press a button to activate the "analyze mode" of the AED. Subsequently, the AED will diagnose the rhythm and advise a shock if indicated. The energy level and mode are all preprogrammed into the AED electronics.

CARDIOVERSION
Introduction and Physiology

Cardioversion is the application of a direct current (DC) "shock" across the chest or directly across the ventricle to normalize the conduction pattern of a rapidly beating heart. This shock is delivered during the absolute refractory period

of the ECG QRS—it is synchronized to the peak of the R wave.

A patient with significant tachycardia may be asymptomatic or may complain of chest pain or discomfort, lightheadedness, or shortness of breath. These symptoms are the result of altered cardiovascular physiology. Rapid cardiac rhythms allow less time for ventricular filling and thereby result in reduced preload and hypotension. The reduced preload, as well as the increased ventricular work caused by the rapid HR, may also result in ventricular ischemia. Pulmonary capillary wedge pressure may also rise despite the shortened filling time because of reduced ventricular compliance secondary to ventricular ischemia. Elevated pulmonary capillary wedge pressure can then lead to pulmonary edema.

Termination of rapid rhythms to alleviate or prevent these symptoms must occur quickly to prevent further deterioration. Persistently poor CO because of a rapid HR results in the development of lactic acidosis, which further compromises cardiac function and makes cessation of the dysrhythmia even more difficult. Unchecked myocardial ischemia may lead to infarction with its attendant sequelae. Drug therapy, rapid cardiac pacing, and cardioversion are the methods available to terminate tachydysrhythmias.

In many cases, DC cardioversion has specific advantages over drug therapy. The speed and simplicity of electrical cardioversion enhance its usefulness in the ED setting. Cardioversion is effective almost immediately, has few side effects, and is often more successful than drug therapy in terminating dysrhythmias. In addition, the effective dose of many antidysrhythmic medications is variable, and there is often a small margin between therapeutic and toxic dosages. Although they can often suppress an undesirable rhythm, drugs may also suppress a normal sinus mechanism or may create toxic manifestations that are more severe than the dysrhythmia being treated.

In the clinical setting of hypotension or acute cardiopulmonary collapse, cardioversion may be lifesaving. Key concepts in the use of this procedure include understanding the indications for its use, the equipment involved, the importance of adequate sedation, and the concerns for health worker safety.

Indications and Contraindications

All decision regarding the need for cardioversion are best made at the bedside by the clinician assessing the given scenario. There are no firm guidelines on exactly what defines an unstable clinical situation, and definitions are relative terms that lend themselves to real-time clinical decision making and clinician interpretation. Cardioversion is often indicated whenever a reentrant tachycardia is causing chest pain, pulmonary edema, lightheadedness, or hypotension. This excludes tachydysrhythmias that are known to be caused by digitalis toxicity, as well as a known sinus tachycardia. It is also indicated in less urgent circumstances when medical therapy has failed. In elderly patients, in whom a prolonged rapid heartbeat can be anticipated to cause complications (e.g., clots, thrombi) related to cardiac ischemia or dysfunction, early intervention with cardioversion may also be beneficial.

A reentrant tachydysrhythmia should be suspected when a sudden change in HR occurs within a few beats. Unless the dysrhythmia is noted while the patient is being monitored, it can be inferred only from the patient's history of a sudden onset of symptoms. In the unusual case of sinus node reentrant tachycardia, rapid onset and offset may be the only clues.[32] Other clues to the presence of a reentrant dysrhythmia are a history of Wolff-Parkinson-White (WPW) syndrome or another known accessory pathway syndrome. Ventricular rates in excess of those predicted for age strongly suggest an accessory pathway.

Dysrhythmias caused by enhanced automaticity *will not* be terminated by uniformly depolarizing myocardial tissue because a homogeneous depolarization state already exists. Enhanced automaticity is the cause of most cases of digitalis toxicity–induced dysrhythmia, sinus tachycardia, and multifocal atrial tachycardia. Although cardioversion will not work in these cases, medications that suppress automaticity, including potassium and magnesium, may be useful.

In digoxin toxicity, not only is cardioversion ineffective, but it is also associated with a higher incidence of post-shock VT and VF.[33] However, in a patient with a therapeutic digoxin level, the risk associated with cardioversion is now thought to be no different from that of other patients. Digoxin is still generally withheld for 24 hours before cardioversion as a precaution against inadvertently elevated levels. Pregnancy at any stage is not a contraindication to cardioversion.[15]

Treatment

Therapy is dictated by the specific wide-complex tachycardia and the patient's clinical findings (Fig. 12-18). The initial approach must always be led—and modified if necessary—by the patient's signs and symptoms and subsequent changes. Synchronized monophasic or biphasic cardioversion is the appropriate first choice of treatment for unstable patients.[11] In patients deemed to be stable, the therapeutic options are more diverse. Stable, wide-complex tachycardia can always be considered VT and treated according to current VT algorithms.[34] A reasonable treatment protocol for stable patients may be the use of adenosine, procainamide, lidocaine, and finally, cardioversion. Amiodarone is effective for most SVTs, and its use for stable unknown wide-complex SVT is both appropriate and safe.[7]

Equipment and Setup

The critical components of preparation for cardioversion are IV access, airway management equipment, drugs for sedation, monitoring, and DC delivery equipment (cardioverter) (Fig. 12-19, *step 1*).

Secure IV access is essential for delivery of sedatives, antidysrhythmics, fluids, and possibly paralytic agents. Although many of these drugs are not used routinely, if they are needed, timing is likely to be critical. A large-bore IV catheter should be inserted and firmly taped to the patient's skin.

A significant and preventable complication of procedures involving sedation is hypoventilation leading to hypoxia. Airway management equipment includes the secure IV catheter discussed previously, working suction with a tonsil-tipped device attached, BVM apparatus, oxygen, and appropriately sized laryngoscope and endotracheal tube. A pulse oximeter is generally recommended for patients undergoing conscious sedation. Another adjunct is continuous monitoring of carbon dioxide pressure (Pco_2). A rising Pco_2 level will be an earlier clue to hypoventilation secondary to sedation because oxygen

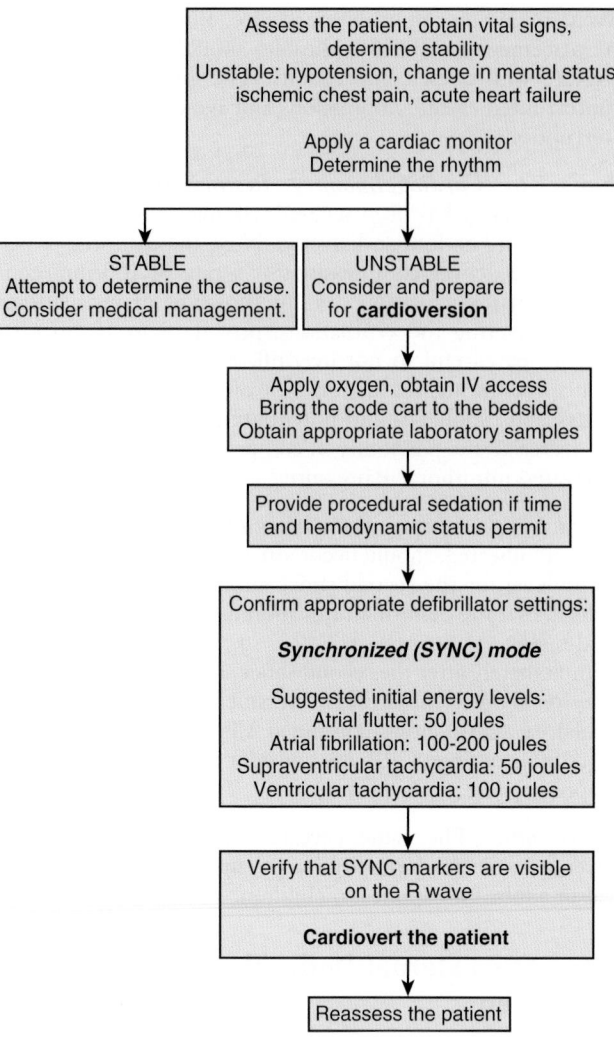

Figure 12-18 Cardioversion algorithm. *IV*, intravenous.

saturation may remain normal for several minutes, especially if the patient has been preoxygenated.

Sedative medications should be ready for use in labeled syringes, along with a prefilled saline syringe for flushing the catheter. Antidysrhythmic medications for ventricular dysrhythmias (e.g., amiodarone, lidocaine) and for unexpected bradycardia (e.g., atropine) should be readily accessible.

Technique

If time permits, metabolic abnormalities such as hypokalemia and hypomagnesemia should be corrected before attempting cardioversion. At a minimum, hypoxia should be corrected with supplemental oxygen. If a patient has metabolic acidosis, compensatory hyperventilation after endotracheal intubation may be indicated before cardioversion. Respiratory acidosis should always be treated before the use of sedative drugs.

Sedation

Cardioversion may be extremely painful or terrifying, and patients must be adequately sedated before its use (see Fig. 12-19, *step 2*). Patients who are not adequately sedated may experience extreme anxiety and fear.[35] Several IV medications

CARDIOVERSION

Obtain IV access, administer oxygen, and place the patient on cardiac, pulse oximetry, and end-tidal CO_2 monitors. Anticipate and prepare sedative and antidysrhythmic medications.

Administer procedural sedation if time and the clinical scenario permit.

Push the "SYNC" button to select the synchronized mode. Check to see that the machine is correctly identifying the R wave of the complexes (*arrow*).

Select the appropriate energy level. This will depend on the rhythm being cardioverted. See text and the cardioversion algorithm for details.

Once the energy has been selected and the decision to cardiovert confirmed, press the "CHARGE" button on the defibrillator.

As the "CHARGE" button is depressed, loudly announce "I'm clear, you're clear, everybody's clear!" and make sure that all caregivers are not in contact with the patient.

Clear!!!

Check once again to make sure that everyone is clear, and then depress the "SHOCK" button to cardiovert the patient.

After delivery of the energy reassess the patient and heart rhythm.

Figure 12-19 Cardioversion.

are available for sedation of patients before cardioversion, including etomidate (0.15 mg/kg), midazolam (0.15 mg/kg), methohexital (1 mg/kg), propofol (0.5-1.0 mg/kg), and thiopental (3 mg/kg). In addition, IV ketamine (1.5 mg/kg), with or without a benzodiazepine or slightly reduced-dose propofol, and IV fentanyl (1.5 μg/kg), a synthetic opioid analgesic, may be administered 3 minutes before induction (Table 12-1).

Midazolam (Versed) is probably the most commonly used agent, with induction occurring approximately 2 minutes after a dose of about 0.15 mg/kg, or at least 5 mg for an average-sized adult. Although induction with midazolam takes slightly longer than with the other medications, it has the advantage that a commercial antagonist, flumazenil, is available for reversal if necessary. Small additional doses of fentanyl (1 to 1.5 μg/kg) may be added for more profound sedation. Fentanyl can cause respiratory depression, but its action can be reversed with naloxone. Methohexital has the advantage of quick onset and a somewhat shorter duration of action than midazolam does, but it has a rare association with laryngospasm. All the drugs except etomidate and ketamine may cause a small drop in blood pressure, and infusion of propofol and etomidate is painful. Ketamine is a reasonable choice in patients with borderline hypotension.

TABLE 12-1 Commonly Available Intravenous Medications Used for Sedation in Cardioversion

DRUG	DOSE	COMMENTS
Midazolam	0.15 mg/kg	Most commonly used Induction occurs in about 2 min Small drop in blood pressure Flumazenil antagonist available
Methohexital	1 mg/kg	Quicker onset than midazolam Shorter duration than midazolam Small drop in blood pressure Rare complication of laryngospasm
Etomidate	0.15 mg/kg	No drop in blood pressure Painful IV infusion
Propofol	1.5 mg/kg	Small drop in blood pressure Painful IV infusion
Thiopental	3 mg/kg	Painful IV infusion
Fentanyl	1.5 μg/kg	An opiate Added for more sedation Can cause respiratory depression
Ketamine	1.5 mg/kg	Will not cause hypotension May be combined with reduced-dose propofol (0.5 mg/kg) or a full-dose benzodiazepine

IV, intravenous.

In elderly patients, the pharmacodynamics and kinetics are altered by coexisting illness and polypharmacy rather than by any intrinsic effect of old age.[36] Drug doses should be reduced in these patients.

Administer the anesthetic agent or agents intravenously over a period of about 30 seconds and wait until the patient is unable to follow simple commands and loss of the eyelash reflex is noted. Administering the agent too quickly may result in hypotension; administering it too slowly may not allow blood levels to reach a therapeutic range if the agent has a rapid rate of metabolism.

Cardioverter Use

Selection of the synchronized or nonsynchronized mode is the next critical step (see Fig. 12-19, *step 3*). In the synchronized mode, the cardioverter searches for a large positive or negative deflection, which it interprets as the R or S wave. It then automatically discharges an electric current that lasts less than 4 msec, thereby avoiding the vulnerable period during repolarization when VF can easily be induced. Once the cardioverter is set to synchronize, a brief delay will occur after

the buttons are pushed for discharge as the machine searches for an R wave. This delay may be disconcerting to an unaware operator.

If concern exists about whether the R wave is large enough to trigger the electrical discharge, the clinician can place the lubricated paddles together and press the discharge button. Firing should occur after a brief delay. When the R- or S-wave deflection is too small to trigger firing, change the lead that the monitor is reading or move the arm leads closer to the chest.

If there is no R or S wave to sense, as in VF, the cardioverter will not fire. Always turn off "synchronization" if VF is noted.

Electrode Position: Same As for Defibrillation

Electrode paddles may be positioned just as they are for defibrillation. Safety is a key concern in the performance of cardioversion. Any staff member acting as a ground for the electrical discharge can be seriously injured. The operator must announce "all clear" and give staff a chance to move away from the bed before discharging the paddles. Care must be taken to clean up spills of saline or water because they may create a conductive path to a staff person at the bedside.

Energy Requirements

The amount of energy required for cardioversion varies with the type of dysrhythmia, the degree of metabolic derangement, and the configuration and thickness of the chest wall (see Fig. 12-19, *step 4*). Obese patients may require a higher energy level for cardioversion, and the anteroposterior paddle position is sometimes more effective in these patients. If patients are shocked while in the expiratory phase of their respiratory cycle, energy requirements may also be lower.

VT in a hemodynamically stable patient should be treated with amiodarone, 150 mg intravenously, and this can be repeated as needed up to a dose of 2.2 g/24 hr. If unsuccessful, cardioversion is then performed. Cardioversion with 10 to 20 J is successful in converting VT in more than 80% of cases. Cardioversion will be accomplished with 50 J in 90% of cases, and conversion should initially be attempted at this energy level.[7] Cardioversion should be synchronized unless the T wave is large and could be misread as the R wave by the cardioverter. If the initial attempts at electrical cardioversion are unsuccessful, the energy level should be doubled—and doubled again if necessary—until a perfusing rhythm is restored. Immediately after conversion of VT, antidysrhythmic medications should be given to prevent recurrence.

Patients with pulseless VT should be initially shocked with 200 J, followed by 300 J if the first shock is not successful. Reentrant SVTs generally respond to low energy levels. Atrial flutter, for example, usually requires less than 50 J for conversion.[7] Cardioversion of atrial flutter in the emergency department (ED) is indicated when the ventricular rate is not slowing in response to pharmacologically enhanced AV node blockade or if the patient is unable to tolerate the aberrant rhythm.

The majority of patients with paroxysmal atrial tachycardia respond to adenosine. If they do not or if urgent conversion is needed because of a high ventricular rate, an electrical countershock should be administered in the synchronized mode at 50 J and doubled if necessary.

In patients with AF, the response to cardioversion is dependent on the duration of the AF and its underlying cause. Most patients with AF do not require cardioversion in the ED unless their ventricular response is high because of a bypass tract, as in WPW syndrome. They may also require cardioversion when sequelae of rapid ventricular contraction are present or anticipated and the ventricular rate is not responding to drug therapy aimed at slowing AV node conduction. Conversion of AF generally requires more energy than reentrant SVTs do ($\approx$100 J in most cases).[7]

Complications

Complications of cardioversion may affect the patient, particularly those with a cardiac pacemaker, as well as health care personnel at the bedside. Injuries to health care personnel during cardioversion or defibrillation include mild shock and burns.

Patient complications are dose related and may involve the airway, heart, or chest wall, or they may be psychological. Hypoxia may develop in patients if sedation is excessive or the airway becomes compromised. With proper preparation and precautions, airway complications can be minimized. Respirations may also be depressed by any of the anesthetic agents, and the adequacy of tidal volume must be continually assessed by either direct observation or end-tidal CO_2 monitoring. If another clinician is available, that clinician should be placed in charge of monitoring the patient's airway. Routine supplemental oxygen is suggested for all patients undergoing sedation.

Chest wall burns resulting from electrical arcing are generally superficial partial-thickness burns, although deep partial-thickness burns have occurred.[37] They are preventable by adequate application of conductive gel and firm pressure on the paddles. Paddles should not be placed over medication patches or ointments, especially those containing nitroglycerin, because electrical discharge may cause ignition and result in chest burns.[38]

Cardiac complications after cardioversion are proportionate to the energy dose delivered. In the moderate energy levels used most commonly, the hemodynamic effects are small. At higher energy levels, however, complications include dysrhythmias, hypotension, and rarely, pulmonary edema, which may occur several hours after the countershock.

The dysrhythmias occurring after high-dose ($\approx$200 J) DC shocks include VT and VF, bradycardia, and AV block, in addition to transient and sustained asystole. Sustained VT or VF was reported following 7 of 99 shocks in a study of patients undergoing electrophysiologic study and requiring cardioversion for VT, VF, or AF. These episodes occurred only in patients with prior VT or VF. Patients with ischemia or known coronary artery disease appear to be at much higher risk for significant post-shock bradycardia, with rate support pacing being required after 13 of 99 shocks in the aforementioned study. Asystole requiring pacing occurred only once in 99 countershocks. Therefore, the proclivity for dysrhythmias is greater with high-dose cardioversion of an ischemic heart.

Conclusion

Cardioversion is a safe and effective method of quickly terminating reentrant tachycardia. Complications related to psychological trauma, respiratory depression, and unintentional shock in health care workers can be avoided with proper precautions. Adequate sedation is essential. Synchronized shock should be administered after close scrutiny of the lead used for sensing to be sure that the R or S wave is significantly larger than the T wave. Be prepared for post-shock VT or VF, and if VF occurs, switch the cardioverter to "nonsynchronized" and defibrillate. Atropine and temporary pacing equipment should be available to treat post-shock bradycardia, especially in patients with myocardial ischemia or infarction.

Pediatric Cardioversion

Pediatric cardioversion is similar to adult cardioversion. As described previously, the purpose of the procedure is to depolarize the myocytes completely at the most opportune time, during the peak of the R wave so that VF is not precipitated, and allow a slower perfusing rhythm to resume. However, the energy levels for pediatric cardioversion are different from those for adults. In the pediatric procedure, the initial recommended energy dose is 0.5 to 1 J/kg with the defibrillator in the synchronized mode. If needed, repeated cardioversion may be attempted at 2 J/kg, again while the defibrillator is in the synchronized mode. Remember to resynchronize the defibrillator after each cardioversion attempt and look for the appropriate markers on the monitor to ensure that the current is delivered at the appropriate phase of the cardiac cycle. If medication is needed, amiodarone at a dose of 5 mg/kg intravenously over a 60-minute period or procainamide at a dose of 15 mg/kg over a 60-minute period can be used (*do not give these drugs together*).

Acknowledgment

The editors and author would like to acknowledge the significant contributions to this chapter in previous editions by Steven Gazak, MD, William Burdick, MD, Jerris R. Hedges, MD, Michael Greenberg, MD, and John Krimm, DO.

References are available at www.expertconsult.com

Assessment of Implantable Devices

James A. Pfaff and Robert T. Gerhardt

Patients with implanted pacemakers or automatic implantable cardioverter-defibrillators (AICDs) are commonly seen in the emergency department (ED). Fortunately, the increased reliability of these devices has prevented a marked increase in patients with true emergencies related to device malfunction, but such patients clearly have serious underlying medical problems that must be considered. Pacemaker complications are not uncommon, with rates ranging from 2.7% to 5%.[1] Many pacemakers fail within the first year.[2] AICD complication rates, including inadvertent shocks, occur in up to 34% of patients with the device.[3] The basic evaluation and treatment of patients with cardiac complaints are not substantially different in patients with pacemakers and AICDs than in those without. However, a general knowledge of the range of problems, complications, and techniques for evaluating or inactivating pacemakers or AICDs is important for emergency clinicians. These devices are complicated, so appropriate consultation may be necessary, depending on the clinical situation.

PACEMAKER CHARACTERISTICS

In essence, a pacemaker consists of an electrical pulse–generating device and a lead system that senses intrinsic cardiac signals and then delivers a pulse. The pulse generator is hermetically sealed with a lithium-based battery device that weighs about 30 g and has an anticipated lifetime of 7 to 12 years. A semiconductor chip serves as the device's central processing unit. The generator is connected to sensing and pacing electrodes that are inserted into various locations in the heart, depending on the configuration of the pacemaker. Newer models are programmable for rate, output, sensitivity, refractory period, and modes of response.[4] They can be reprogrammed radiotelemetrically after implantation.

Pacemakers are classified according to a standard five-letter code developed by the North American Society of Pacing and Electrophysiology/British Pacing and Electrophysiology Group (Table 13-1). Known as the NBG code, it consists of five positions or digits. The first letter designates the chamber that receives the pacing current; the second, the sensing chamber; and the third, the pacemaker's response to sensing. The fourth letter refers to the pacemaker's rate modulation and programmability, and the fifth describes the pacemaker's ability to provide an antitachycardia function. Whereas standard pacemakers generally do not have an antitachycardia function, AICDs do have this capability and overdrive pacing is the device's first response to tachycardia. In normal practice, only the first three letters are used to describe the pacemaker (e.g., VVI or DDD).[5]

Pacemaker wires are embedded in plastic catheters. The terminal electrodes, which may be unipolar or bipolar, travel from the generator unit to the heart via the venous system. In a unipolar system, the lead electrode functions as the negatively charged cathode, and the pulse generator case acts as the positively charged anode into which electrons flow to complete the circuit. The pulse generator casing must remain in contact with tissue and be uninsulated for pacing to occur. In the case of bipolar systems, both electrodes are located within the heart. The cathode is at the tip of the lead, and the anode is a ring electrode roughly 2 cm proximal to the tip. Bipolar leads are thicker, draw more current than unipolar leads, and are commonly preferred because of several advantages, including a decreased likelihood of pacer inhibition as a result of extraneous signals and decreased susceptibility to interference by electromagnetic fields.[6]

The typical entry point for inserting the leads is the central venous system, which is generally accessed via the subclavian or cephalic vein. The terminal electrodes are placed either in the right ventricle or in both the right ventricle and the atrium under fluoroscopic guidance. Proper lead placement and sensing and pacing thresholds are assessed with electrocardiograms (ECGs).[7] The typical radiographic appearance of an implanted pacemaker is shown in Figure 13-1.

The pacemaker is typically programmed to pace at a rate of 60 to 80 beats/min. A significantly different rate usually indicates malfunction. When the battery is low, the rate generally begins to drop and gets slower as the battery fades. Sensing of intracardiac electrical activity is a combination of recognizing the characteristic waveforms of P waves or QRS complexes while discriminating them from T waves or external interfering signals, such as muscle activity or movement. The pacing electrical stimulus is a triphasic wave consisting of an intrinsic deflection, far-field potential, and an injury current, which typically delivers a current of 0.1 to 20.0 mA for 2 msec at 15 V.[8]

Pacemakers have a reed switch that may be closed by placing a magnet over the generator externally on the chest wall; this inactivates the sensing mechanism of the pacemaker, which then reverts to an asynchronous rate termed the *magnet rate*. Essentially, *the magnet turns the demand pacemaker into a fixed-rate pacemaker*. The magnet rate is usually, but not always, the same as the programmed rate.

Several innovations in rate regulation have been incorporated into some pacemakers. When present, the hysteresis feature causes pacing to be triggered at a rate greater than the intrinsic heart rate. When the hysteresis feature is used in a single-chamber ventricular pacemaker, it is designed to maintain atrioventricular (AV) synchrony at rates that are lower than what would be normal for a ventricular-paced rhythm alone. To illustrate, were the hysteresis feature of the pacemaker set at 50 beats/min, an intrinsic rate lower than 50 beats/min would trigger ventricular pacing. Unlike a standard ventricular pacemaker, the hysteresis feature might be set to offer a ventricular pacing rate at 70 beats/min or greater once the pacer is triggered.[9]

Rate modulation by sensor-mediated methods is an additional feature triggered and mediated by a sensed response to various physiologic stimuli.[9] The primary application for this rate modulation feature is in patients with pacemakers who continue to engage in vigorous physical activity. When present, the rate regulation feature is engaged and modulated through motion sensors installed within a pulse generator

TABLE 13-1 North American Society of Pacing and Electrophysiology/British Pacing and Electrophysiology Group Generic Pacemaker Code (NBG Code)

I	II	III	IV	V
Chamber Paced	Chamber Sensed	Response to Sensing	Rate Modulation and Programmability	Antitachycardia Features
0—None A—Atrium V—Ventricle D—Dual	0—None A—Atrium V—Ventricle D—Dual	0—None I—Inhibited T—Triggered D—Dual	0—None I—Inhibited M—Multiple C—Communicating R—Rate modulation	0—None P—Antitachycardiac pacing S—Shock D—Dual

Figure 13-1 A, Various radiographs of an implanted pacemaker and automatic implantable cardioverter-defibrillator showing battery and lead wires. Posteroanterior (PA; **A1**) and lateral (**A2**) chest radiographs demonstrate a biventricular pacing system. There are three leads—the first is positioned in the right atrium, the second is in the right ventricular apex, and the third courses posteriorly in the coronary sinus and into the posterolateral cardiac vein. **B,** PA chest radiographs of a dual-chamber pacemaker. **B1,** The ventricular lead is passing through an atrial septal defect into the left ventricle. **B2,** The lead is repositioned in the right ventricular apex. **C,** A dual-chamber implantable cardioverter-defibrillator with active fixation leads has been implanted via a transvenous approach to place the atrial lead in the systemic venous atrium and the ventricular lead across the baffle into the morphologic left ventricle.

Continued

device, with a corresponding increase or decrease in the pacing rate depending on the degree of motion sensed by the pacemaker device. Other physiologic sensors that may be installed as part of the pacemaker system include those designed to sense minute ventilation, the QT interval, temperature, venous oxygen saturation, and right ventricular contractions. The latter sensors generally require that additional leads be placed.

Characteristics of AICDs

The basic components of an AICD, including sensing electrodes, defibrillation electrodes, and a pulse generator (Fig. 13-2), can be seen on a chest radiograph. Transvenous electrodes have obviated the previous need for surgical placement. They are inserted into the pectoralis muscle. Many transvenous systems consist of a single lead containing a distal sensing electrode and one or more defibrillation electrodes in the right atrium and ventricle.[10] Leads are inserted through the subclavian, axillary, or cephalic vein into the right ventricular apex. The left side is preferred because of a smoother venous route to the heart and a more favorable shocking vector.[11] In an effort to improve the efficiency of defibrillation, an additional defibrillation coil may be used.[11] Various placements of AICDs are demonstrated in Figure 13-3.

The pulse generator is a sealed titanium casing that encloses a lithium–silver–vanadium oxide battery. It has voltage converters and resistors, capacitors to store charge, microprocessors and integrated circuits to control analysis of the rhythm and delivery of therapy, memory chips to store electrographic data, and a telemetry module.[12] Whereas a pacemaker can draw the voltage required for function from

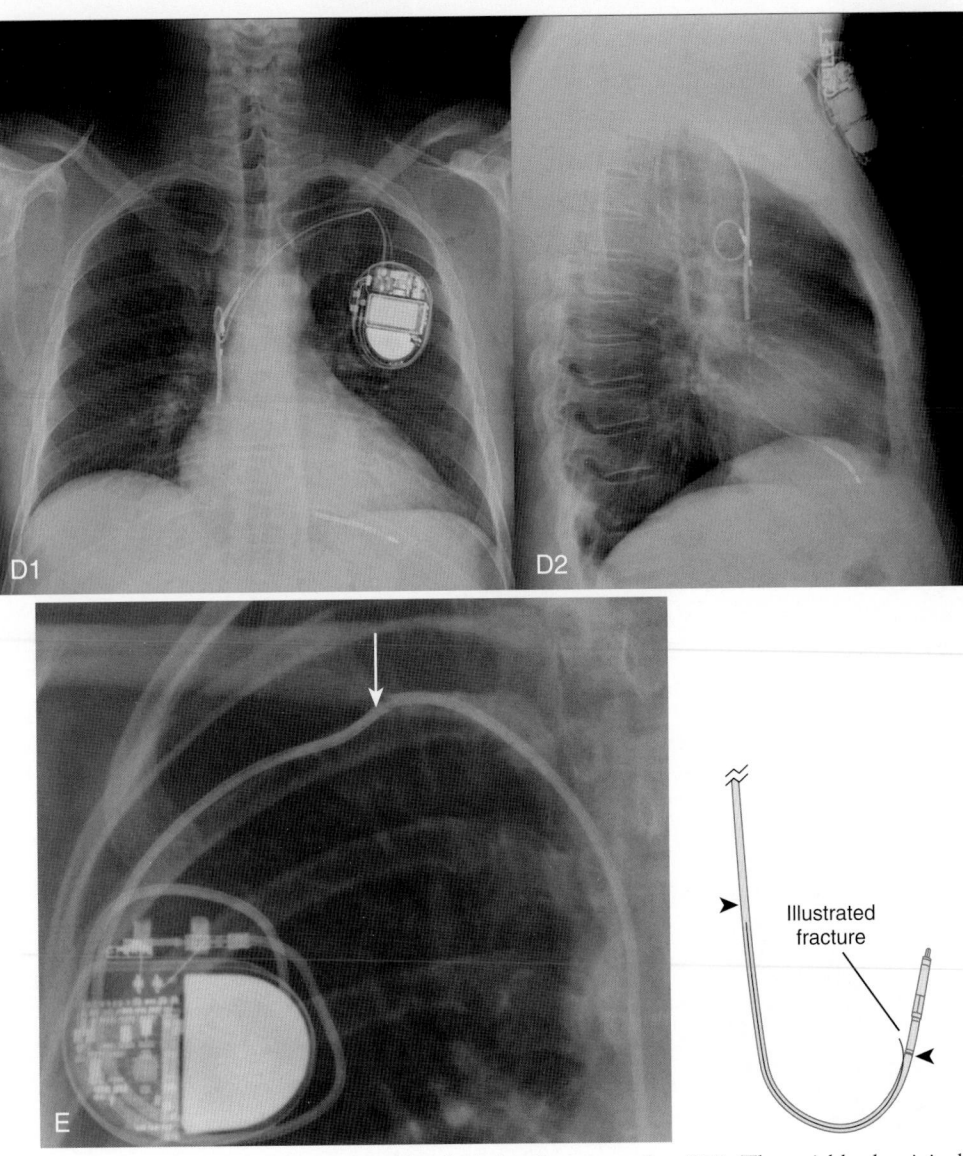

Figure 13-1, cont'd   D, PA chest radiograph of a patient with a dual-chamber pacemaker (**D1**). The atrial lead, originally positioned in the right atrial appendage, is clearly no longer positioned in the right atrial appendage. A lateral view (**D2**) also shows definite dislodgment of the atrial lead. **E,** Close-up view of a portion of the PA chest radiograph of a patient with a single-chamber pacemaker. The lead has fractured (a subtle finding) at the point where it passes below the clavicle (*arrow*). The device showed intermittent ventricular failure to capture and intermittent failure to output on the ventricular lead. Impedance was intermittently measured at more than 9999 Ω. *Inset,* Diagram of the fracture site. (*E inset, Courtesy of Telectronics Pacing Systems, Englewood, CO.*)

its component battery, the energy needed for defibrillation requires a battery that is prohibitively large.[6] To circumvent this problem, an AICD contains a capacitor that maximizes the voltage required by transferring energy from the battery before discharge. To achieve the energy required, AICDs use capacitors that are charged over a period of 3 to 10 seconds by the battery and then release this energy rapidly for defibrillation.[10] The maximal output is 30 J in most units and 45 J in higher-energy units.[6] *This energy is high enough that a discharge is very obvious and often distressing to the patient.*

Most AICDs use a system in which the pulse generator is part of the shocking circuit, often described as a "can" technology, and most of them have a dual-coil lead with a proximal coil in the superior vena cava and a distal coil in the right ventricle.[13] Current flows in a three-dimensional configuration from the distal coil to both the proximal coil and the generator.[14] This dispersion of the electrical field increases the likelihood of depolarizing the entire myocardium at once, thereby leading to successful defibrillation.[14]

AICDs may have the same programming capabilities as pacemakers and can be single chambered, dual chambered, or used with cardiac resynchronization therapy (CRT) .[15] Single-chamber devices have only a right ventricular lead. They often have difficulty identifying atrial arrhythmias, which can result in *inappropriate defibrillation of atrial tachycardias.* Dual-chamber AICDs have right atrial and right ventricular leads and improved ability to discriminate rhythms. In most studies, dual devices have been found to offer improved discrimination between ventricular and supraventricular arrhythmias,

Figure 13-2 A, Automatic implantable cardioverter-defibrillator. **B,** Implantable pacemaker. (*A, SOLETRA device; courtesy of Medtronics, Inc., Minneapolis.*)

thus decreasing inappropriate shocks as a result of rapid supraventricular rhythms or physiologic sinus tachycardia.[16] Approximately 50% of AICDs implanted in the United States are dual-chamber devices.[17] CRT devices add an additional left ventricular lead that is placed in the coronary sinus or epicardium. In patients requiring both AICD and pacemaker functions, both these devices are placed together. The advent of technology has allowed placement of a single device that can perform both pacemaker and defibrillator functions.

AICDs use a combination of antitachycardia pacing, low-energy cardioversion, defibrillation, and bradycardiac pacing in a combination also known as *tiered therapy.* They are programmed with specific algorithms that identify and treat specific rhythms. *Ventricular arrhythmias may initially be converted (or undergo attempts at conversion) with antitachycardiac pacing as opposed to immediate defibrillation.* This *overdrive pacing* may terminate the rhythm without the need for electrical defibrillation in up to 90% of events. It is most successful for terminating monomorphic ventricular tachycardia with a rate of less than 200 beats/min.[1] Overdrive pacing is better tolerated by patients than cardioversion and reduces the risk for inducing atrial fibrillation.[18] These events may be silent, not felt by the patient, and discovered only by interrogating the device.

If unsuccessful, the next intervention may be low-energy cardioversion (<5 J). The device may be programmed to very low levels of electricity that, again, are better tolerated by the patient. This works best for ventricular rates higher than 150 and lower than 240 beats/min.[14] This may be followed by a high-energy defibrillation. Traditionally, the energy level of the first shock is set at least 10 J above the threshold of the last defibrillation measured.[12] If the first shock fails, a backup shock may be required, but this may induce or aggravate ventricular arrhythmias (see the later section "Pacemaker-Mediated Tachycardia"). Unlike the proarrhythmic effects of medication, these arrhythmias are almost never fatal, although they may be associated with increased morbidity.[11] Currently used biphasic waveforms have improved defibrillation thresholds.[12]

This tiered approach obviates the need for unnecessary energy requirements. The devices also have antibradycardiac pacing that allows these patients to have one device instead of separate units. Additional complications associated with AICDs that have antibradycardiac pacing algorithms include a tendency toward oversensing, increased current drain, potential detection problems, and an increased incidence of

Figure 13-3 Diagrammatic demonstration of various automatic implantable cardioverter-defibrillator (AICD) configurations. **A,** Single-chamber AICD. **B,** Dual-chamber AICD. **C,** Biventricular AICD.

hardware and software design problems.[1] At the time of insertion the amount of energy required for various AICD functions, such as the defibrillation threshold, is determined for any given patient, and output and sensing functions can be adjusted by reprogramming as needed.

INDICATIONS FOR PLACEMENT OF IMPLANTABLE PACEMAKERS AND AICDs

The most common indication for placement of a cardiac pacemaker is for the treatment of symptomatic bradyarrhythmias.[19] Roughly 50% of pacemakers are placed in such patients for the treatment of sinus node dysfunction (sick sinus syndrome). Other diagnoses include symptomatic sinus bradycardia, atrial fibrillation with a slow ventricular response, high-grade AV block (including Mobitz type II and third-degree AV block), tachycardia-bradycardia syndrome, chronotropic incompetence, and selected prolonged QT syndromes. Though not classified as absolute indications, pacemakers are sometimes placed for the treatment of severe refractory neurocardiogenic syncope, paroxysmal atrial fibrillation, and hypertrophic or dilated cardiomyopathy.

In recent years, CRT has emerged as a primary approach for patients with severe diastolic dysfunction and a low left ventricular ejection fraction (LVEF).[19] Commonly, such patients manifest low-grade AV blocks and left bundle branch block.[20] The resultant delay in left ventricular conduction often results in corresponding biomechanical delays in ventricular contraction, which in turn causes a further decrement in cardiac output and worsening congestive heart failure. Such prolongation may occur in as many as 33% of patients with advanced heart failure.[20] This electromechanical "dyssynchrony" has been associated with increased risk for sudden cardiac death.[21]

CRT comprises atrial-synchronized, biventricular pacemaking, which overcomes the atrial and ventricular blocks while optimizing both preload and LVEF.[22] Clinical trials and systematic reviews have confirmed the efficacy of CRT, with decrements in mortality of 22% to 30%, as well as improved LVEF and quality of life.[23,24] It is therefore likely that emergency physicians will see the CRT configuration with increasing frequency in patients with implanted pacemakers and AICDs.

The 2008 American Heart Association guidelines for implantation of a cardiac pacemaker are summarized in Box 13-1.[19] AICD technology is used principally for both primary and secondary prevention in patients at risk for sudden death. Primary prevention is an attempt to avoid a potentially malignant ventricular arrhythmia in patients identified as being at high risk.[25] Secondary prevention is for patients who have already had a ventricular arrhythmia and are at risk for further events. In addition, AICDs are implanted for a number of other congenital or familial cardiac conditions. Box 13-2 is a summary of class I indications for the placement of AICDs.[26]

PACEMAKER AND AICD RESPONSE TO MAGNET PLACEMENT

In the clinical setting, placement of a magnet over the pulse generator of a pacemaker is a technique that might be used either diagnostically or therapeutically by the emergency clinician. It is important to note that each pacemaker is programmed to respond in a specific fashion as determined by the manufacturer. The response to magnet placement may vary not only by manufacturer but also by model and by the particular mode in which the pacemaker is currently operating. In most cases, manufacturers set the asynchronous baseline pacing rate in a range approximating 70 beats/min. An indicator of aging of the pacemaker and weakening of the battery is that this asynchronous baseline pacing rate will decrease over time as the battery approaches the point at which replacement is required.

Keeping these provisions in mind, there are standard responses that the provider might expect to see in most circumstances. In the case of single-chamber ventricular pacemakers, the response will most likely be asynchronous pacing (V00). In the case of dual-chamber pacemakers, placement of a magnet usually results in dual-chamber asynchronous pacing (D00). In either case it is important for the clinician to note that placement of a magnet over the pacemaker pulse generator *will not turn the pacemaker off.*

Placing a magnet over any of the currently available AICD models will temporarily *disable tachyarrhythmia intervention* (Fig. 13-4). An ECG should be obtained before and after magnet placement for comparison (Fig. 13-5). Most commercially available pacer magnets are 7 cm in size and can be used with most implantable devices. Each of the present models may have a slightly different response to the magnet. The magnetic field closes a reed switch in the generator circuit that will disable recognition of tachyarrhythmias and subsequent firing of the device. There may be a variety of tones (continuous, intermittent, or silence) during activation or inactivation with the magnet, which are dependent on the manufacturer. Some devices may be programmed to not respond at all.[27] After the desired effect is obtained, the magnet should be secured to maintain inactivation.

Pacemaker and AICD patients should carry an identification card that includes information regarding manufacturer, model type, and lead system, as well as a 24-hour emergency number to allow rapid identification of the model when it is necessary to inactivate the device. In lieu of the availability of a device identification card, the general type, polarity, and number of ventricles involved with the implanted device may be inferred accurately by viewing an overpenetrated anteroposterior chest radiograph.

If a patient with an AICD has a ventricular arrhythmia, the assumption should be made that the device is inoperable and standard advanced cardiac life support (ACLS) protocols should be used to stabilize the patient.

Of further note, in some obese patients or those with heavily developed chest wall musculature, the magnetic field emitted by a single magnet device may not be strong enough to elicit the desired effect on the implanted device. In such cases the clinician may find greater efficacy by using two magnets, one on top of the other.[28]

CLINICAL EVALUATION OF PATIENTS WITH IMPLANTED PACEMAKERS AND AICDs

History

Although patients who go to the ED because of implantable pacemaker–related issues may have one or more of several complaints, those with AICD-related issues are generally seen because their device has discharged. They will often describe

A. PACING FOR BRADYCARDIA CAUSED BY SINUS AND ATRIOVENTRICULAR NODE DYSFUNCTION

1. Sinus nodal dysfunction (SND) with documented symptomatic bradycardia.
2. Sinus bradycardia causing symptomatic chronotropic incompetence.
3. Permanent pacemaker implantation is indicated for symptomatic sinus bradycardia resulting from the drug therapy required for medical conditions.
4. SND with a heart rate lower than 40 beats/min with significant symptoms of bradycardia.
5. Syncope of unexplained origin when clinically significant abnormalities in sinus node function are discovered or provoked in electrophysiologic studies.

B. ACQUIRED ATRIOVENTRICULAR BLOCK IN ADULTS

1. Third-degree and advanced second-degree atrioventricular (AV) block at any anatomic level associated with bradycardia, with symptoms (including heart failure) or ventricular arrhythmias presumed to be due to AV block.
2. Third-degree and advanced second-degree AV block at any anatomic level associated with arrhythmias and other medical conditions that require drug therapy resulting in symptomatic bradycardia.
3. Third-degree and advanced second-degree AV block at any anatomic level in awake, symptom-free patients in sinus rhythm with documented periods of asystole of 3.0 seconds or longer or any escape rate less than 40 beats/min or with an escape rhythm that is below the AV node.
4. Third-degree and advanced second-degree AV block at any anatomic level in awake, symptom-free patients with atrial fibrillation and bradycardia with one or more pauses of at least 5 seconds or longer.
5. Third-degree and advanced second-degree AV block at any anatomic level after catheter ablation of the AV junction.
6. Third-degree and advanced second-degree AV block at any anatomic level associated with postoperative AV block that is not expected to resolve after cardiac surgery.
7. Third-degree and advanced second-degree AV block at any anatomic level associated with neuromuscular diseases with AV block, with or without symptoms.
8. Second-degree AV block with associated symptomatic bradycardia regardless of the type or site of block.
9. Third-degree AV block at any anatomic site with average awake ventricular rates of 40 beats/min or faster if cardiomegaly or left ventricular dysfunction is present or if the site of block is below the AV node. Second- or third-degree AV block during exercise in the absence of myocardial ischemia.

C. CHRONIC BIFASCICULAR BLOCK

1. Permanent pacemaker implantation is indicated for advanced second-degree AV block or intermittent third-degree AV block.
2. Permanent pacemaker implantation is indicated for type II second-degree AV block.
3. Permanent pacemaker implantation is indicated for alternating bundle branch block.

D. PACING FOR ATRIOVENTRICULAR BLOCK ASSOCIATED WITH ACUTE MYOCARDIAL INFARCTION

1. Permanent ventricular pacing is indicated for persistent second-degree AV block in the His-Purkinje system with alternating bundle branch block or third-degree AV block within or below the His-Purkinje system after ST-segment elevation myocardial infarction.
2. Permanent ventricular pacing is indicated for transient advanced second- or third-degree infranodal AV block and associated bundle branch block. If the site of block is uncertain, an electrophysiologic study may be necessary.
3. Permanent ventricular pacing is indicated for persistent and symptomatic second- or third-degree AV block.

E. HYPERSENSITIVE CAROTID SINUS SYNDROME AND NEUROCARDIOGENIC SYNCOPE

Permanent pacing is indicated for recurrent syncope caused by spontaneously occurring carotid sinus stimulation and carotid sinus pressure that induces ventricular asystole lasting longer than 3 seconds.

F. CARDIAC TRANSPLANTATION

Permanent pacing is indicated for persistent inappropriate or symptomatic bradycardia not expected to resolve and for other class I indications for permanent pacing.

G. RECOMMENDATIONS FOR PACING TO PREVENT TACHYCARDIA

Permanent pacing is indicated for sustained pause-dependent ventricular tachycardia, with or without QT prolongation.

H. CARDIAC RESYNCHRONIZATION THERAPY IN PATIENTS WITH SEVERE SYSTOLIC HEART FAILURE

For patients who have a left ventricular ejection fraction of 35% or lower, a QRS duration of 0.12 second or shorter, and sinus rhythm, cardiac resynchronization therapy with or without an implantable cardioverter-defibrillator is indicated for the treatment of New York Heart Association functional class III or ambulatory class IV heart failure symptoms along with optimal recommended medical therapy.

I. OBSTRUCTIVE HYPERTROPHIC CARDIOMYOPATHY

Permanent pacing is indicated for SND or AV block in patients with hypertrophic cardiomyopathy as described previously (see Section 2.1.1, "Sinus Node Dysfunction," and Section 2.1.2, "Acquired Atrioventricular Block in Adults").

J. PACING IN CHILDREN, ADOLESCENTS, AND PATIENTS WITH CONGENITAL HEART DISEASE

1. Permanent pacemaker implantation is indicated for advanced second- or third-degree AV block associated with symptomatic bradycardia, ventricular dysfunction, or low cardiac output.
2. Permanent pacemaker implantation is indicated for SND with correlation of symptoms during age-inappropriate bradycardia. The definition of bradycardia varies with the patient's age and expected heart rate.
3. Permanent pacemaker implantation is indicated for postoperative advanced second- or third-degree AV block that is not expected to resolve or that persists for at least 7 days after cardiac surgery.
4. Permanent pacemaker implantation is indicated for congenital third-degree AV block with a wide QRS escape rhythm, complex ventricular ectopy, or ventricular dysfunction.
5. Permanent pacemaker implantation is indicated for congenital third-degree AV block in infants with a ventricular rate lower than 55 beats/min or with congenital heart disease and a ventricular rate lower than 70 beats/min.

BOX 13-2 American Heart Association Class I Recommendations for Automatic Implantable Cardioverter-Defibrillator Placement

PRIMARY PREVENTION OF SCD IN PATIENTS WHO ARE NEW YORK HEART ASSOCIATION CLASS II OR III

1. Patients with LV dysfunction caused by a previous MI whose MI occurred at least 40 days earlier and who have an LVEF of less than 30% to 40%
2. Patients with nonischemic dilated cardiomyopathy who have an LVEF of less than 30% to 35%

SECONDARY PREVENTION OF SCD

1. Patients who survived VF or hemodynamically unstable VT
2. Patients with VT and syncope who have an LVEF of less than 40%

3. Patients with LV dysfunction as a result of previous MI who have hemodynamically unstable sustained VT to decrease mortality by reducing SCD
4. Patients with nonischemic dilated cardiomyopathy and sustained VT
5. Patients with hypertrophic cardiomyopathy who have sustained VT and/or VF
6. Patients with Brugada's syndrome or prolonged QT syndrome with previous cardiac arrest
7. Patients with congenital heart disease and previous cardiac arrest who have had reversible causes excluded

LV, left ventricular; LVEF, left ventricular ejection fraction; MI, myocardial infarction; SCD, sudden cardiac death; VF, ventricular fibrillation; VT, ventricular tachycardia.

Figure 13-4 A, This patient suffered from 13 discharges of his automatic implantable cardioverter-defibrillator over the course of 1 hour. In the emergency department he was noted to have a discharge while in sinus rhythm, and a magnet (*arrow*) was placed over the device to deactivate it. **B,** An electrophysiology specialist came to the emergency department to interrogate the device. Note that newer devices can communicate wirelessly. **C** and **D,** Interrogation and intracardiac electrocardiograms were consistent with fracture of the right ventricular lead. The device was deactivated and replaced shortly thereafter.

a sensation of being kicked or punched in the chest, and the *sensation is not subtle*. In fact, some patients live in fear of the shock after having experienced it previously, and this is one reason for removal of the device. Ask the patient about the number of discharges and associated symptoms, including chest pain, shortness of breath, lightheadedness, palpitations,

syncope, extremity edema (raising concern for congestive heart failure or lower extremity deep vein thrombosis), or dyspnea on exertion. In addition, elicit general symptoms such as fever, chills, nausea, or vomiting, which could be indicative of infection. Inquire about medication history. Ask about the specific implanted device that they possess. Most pacemaker

A   B

Figure 13-5 A, Electrocardiogram (ECG) of a patient with a nonfiring pacemaker. The intrinsic cardiac rate is 80 beats/min, and no pacemaker activity is seen. **B,** ECG of the same patient with a magnet applied over the pacemaker, which produced a paced rhythm. Pacer spikes are evident (*arrows*), and the magnet rate is 85 beats/min. Note the left bundle branch bundle typical of a pacer lead in the right ventricle.

and AICD patients should have an identification card on their person that will identify the manufacturer, model number, lead system, and a 24-hour emergency contact number. Sophisticated information and the prior electrical events and settings of the device can be ascertained in the ED by simply placing an external interrogating device over the unit.

Physical Examination

First, assess for airway patency, adequate ventilation, and cardiovascular status. The patient's mental status may also be an important clue to the severity of the symptoms. Perform an appropriate physical examination with emphasis on examining the heart and lung to seek murmurs, pericardial friction rubs, and evidence of pulmonary effusion or other abnormalities. Inspect the pacemaker or AICD site for erythema or edema. Palpate the skin for evidence of obvious lead abnormalities. Examine the extremities for evidence of edema or erythema.

Radiography

The imaging modality of choice, at least initially, in a patient with complaints related to an implanted pacemaker or AICD is the plain chest radiograph. If the patient's stability is in question, obtain a portable anteroposterior film. In addition to the standard cardiac, pulmonary, vascular, and skeletal evaluation, this study will probably confirm the location of the pulse generator case, as well as the current location of any leads. Survey the radiograph for evidence of lead fracture or displacement (see Fig. 13-1*E*). Compare with previous chest films. *If the patient does not have a device identification card in immediate possession, take an overpenetrated radiograph to look for a radiopaque marker identifying the model type.*

Electrocardiography

Perform an ECG to seek evidence of pacing, ectopy, and ST-segment or T-wave abnormalities. A comparison ECG may be helpful. If an AICD shock has been delivered, the shock itself can cause transient electrocardiographic changes, and waiting for several minutes to repeat the ECG may identify whether the changes are due to the discharge or an ongoing disease process.[29]

Cardiopulmonary Resuscitation, ACLS Interventions, and External Cardiac Defibrillation in Patients with Implanted Pacemakers or AICDs

In general, ACLS interventions may be performed safely and effectively in patients with pacemakers and AICDs when indicated. Cardiopulmonary resuscitation (CPR) can usually be performed in standard fashion. If an AICD is present, rescuers may notice mild electrical shocks while performing CPR; these shocks are harmless to the rescuer. If the AICD shocks are impeding rescuer performance of CPR or if supraventricular tachycardias are noted during resuscitation, disable the AICD by applying a magnet over the corner of the device from which the leads emerge. This location is generally found easily by palpation but may be located blindly by slowly relocating the magnet until AICD activity ceases.

External cardiac defibrillation may be performed safely in patients with pacemakers and AICDs with the standard expected efficacy; however, it is recommended that external paddles or defibrillator pads be placed at a location approximately 10 cm distant from the pulse generator if possible.[30] A transcutaneous cardiac pacemaker may also be used in similar fashion, again with a recommendation that the pacing pads be placed in anatomically appropriate locations but preferably at a distance of 10 cm from the pulse generator.

Placing the external defibrillation or transcutaneous pacemaker pads in an anteroposterior configuration is advised because this configuration may circumvent energy shunting and shielding.[11] *Every attempt should be made to avoid application of the defibrillators directly over the device.* Use of the lowest possible energy setting for cardioversion or defibrillation is recommended. If available, biphasic cardioverter-defibrillators are further suggested.[30] In the event of successful resuscitation and return of spontaneous circulation, the pacemaker or AICD should be interrogated expeditiously by a cardiologist or electrophysiologist to ensure that no damage was sustained as a result of the resuscitation effort.

Regarding pharmacologic adjuncts, amiodarone has been reported to be more effective for the treatment of potentially lethal arrhythmias in the setting of implanted devices.[31] *Antiarrhythmic medications may be required for a resistant malignant rhythm when the AICD is functioning properly but the arrhythmia persists* (Fig. 13-6*G*).

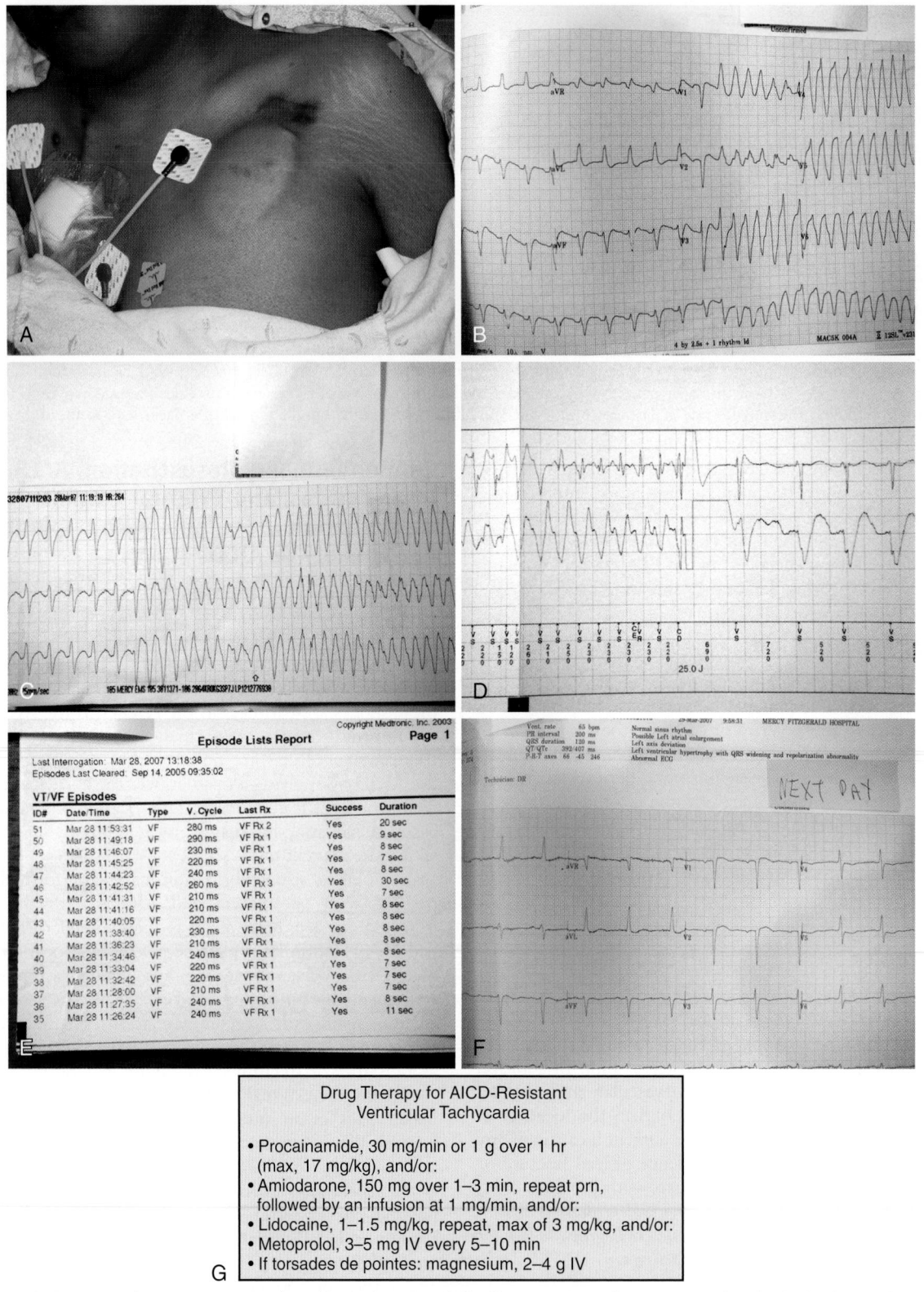

Drug Therapy for AICD-Resistant
Ventricular Tachycardia

• Procainamide, 30 mg/min or 1 g over 1 hr
  (max, 17 mg/kg), and/or:
• Amiodarone, 150 mg over 1–3 min, repeat prn,
  followed by an infusion at 1 mg/min, and/or:
• Lidocaine, 1–1.5 mg/kg, repeat, max of 3 mg/kg, and/or:
• Metoprolol, 3–5 mg IV every 5–10 min
• If torsades de pointes: magnesium, 2–4 g IV

Figure 13-6 A, Patient with an automatic implantable cardioverter-defibrillator (AICD) who experienced multiple discharges from an AICD because of recurrent ventricular tachycardia (VT). **B,** Electrocardiogram (ECG) of VT in the presence of an underlying tachycardia as the possible cause. **C,** A rhythm strip demonstrates persistent polymorphic (torsades de pointes) VT. **D,** After attempts at overdrive pacing failed, the AICD appropriately discharges with temporary termination of VT. **E,** Interrogation of the device uncovers a history of more than 20 episodes of recurrent VT within thirty minutes. *This patient was terrified of a subsequent shock because he could sense the VT and knew of the impending shock. In addition to antiarrhythmic medication, a quiet dark room and aggressive sedation are suggested to reduce catecholamine levels.* **F,** ECG after medical therapy with multiple medications, including magnesium. *Metoprolol seemed to be the deciding factor in terminating the VT in this case.* **G,** Current suggested medical therapy for VT in the presence of an appropriately functioning AICD.

Several additional considerations are unique to the setting of ACLS in patients with a pacemaker or AICD. In cases of acute myocardial infarction involving areas of the myocardium in contact with the pacemaker leads, the implanted pacemaker may experience operative failure. Therefore, maintain a high level of suspicion for the potential requirement for supplemental transcutaneous or transvenous cardiac pacing.

Also, in the postresuscitation setting involving a patient with an implanted pacemaker or AICD, it is important to maintain a higher index of suspicion for device lead fracture or disruption resulting from CPR. Finally, in the postresuscitation phase the clinician should closely watch for the development of pneumothorax, hemothorax, pericardial effusion, or other aforementioned pathophysiologic processes that could adversely affect the function of the implanted device.

COMPLICATIONS AND MALFUNCTION OF IMPLANTED PACEMAKERS

Complications associated with pacemakers are listed in Box 13-3. In addition, patients with previously implanted and otherwise stable pacemakers may experience complications related to direct or indirect trauma affecting the pulse generator or leads. Major complications of pacemaker placement or those caused by subsequent injuries that the emergency clinician might encounter include local or systemic infections resulting from pacemaker placement, thrombophlebitis involving the transvenous route of the pacemaker leads, a venous thromboembolic event, pneumothorax or hemothorax, pericarditis, air embolism, localized hematoma interfering with pacemaker operation or sensing, lead dislodgment,[32] cardiac perforation, hemopericardium with possible progression to cardiac tamponade, and development of the phenomenon known as *pacemaker syndrome*. This condition is often seen in patients with single-chamber ventricular pacemakers who have an underlying component of congestive heart failure. It is believed to be a consequence of the loss of AV synchrony resulting from the ventricular pacing and may be manifested as vertigo, syncope, hypotension, and signs specific to the exacerbation of congestive heart failure.

In addition to the complications associated with initial pacemaker placement, malfunctions of these devices may occur in the short-, intermediate-, and long-term phases of their functional life spans. Most malfunctions result from one or a combination of three primary problems: failure of the pace generator to provide output, failure to capture, or failure to sense the intrinsic cardiac rhythm.

Pacemaker Output Failure

Pacemaker generator output failure is present when no pacing "spike" is noted on the ECG despite an indication for pacing. This condition may result from battery failure, fracture or loss of insulation in the pacer leads, oversensing of extraneous signals resulting in pacer inhibition, disconnection of the leads from the pacer generator, or in the case of a dual-chamber pacer, erroneous sensing of the pacemaker's atrial signal by a ventricular sensor.[33] The latter phenomenon is commonly referred to as *crosstalk*.[34]

Given that the reason for pacemaker implantation in most cases was for the treatment of an underlying bradycardia condition, initial clinical management of patients with some

---

BOX 13-3	**Complications of Permanent Pacemakers**

FAILURE TO PACE (NO PACEMAKER ACTIVITY PRESENT)
Lead fracture
Lead disconnection
Battery depletion
Component failure
Oversensing
External interference

FAILURE TO SENSE (CONSTANT PACEMAKER SPIKES DESPITE ONGOING INTRINSIC CARDIAC ELECTRICAL ACTIVITY)
Lead dislodgment
Lead fracture
Fibrosis around the tip of the lead
Battery depletion
Pacer in asynchronous mode
External interference
Low-amplitude intracardiac signal

FAILURE TO CAPTURE (PACEMAKER SPIKES BUT NO SUBSEQUENT CARDIAC ACTIVITY)
Lead dislodgment, including perforation
Lead fracture
Lead disconnection
Poor lead position
Fibrosis around the tip of the lead
Battery depletion
Metabolic abnormalities
Medications

INAPPROPRIATE PACEMAKER RATE (RUNAWAY PACEMAKER)
Pacemaker reentrant tachycardia
Resetting from external interference
Battery depletion

OTHER
Infections: pocket, wires
Lead displacement: cardiac perforation, tamponade, pericarditis, vascular perforation
Vascular complications: thrombosis, superior vena cava syndrome
Psychiatric: anxiety, panic attacks

---

degree of pacer output failure will usually focus on pharmacologic management aimed at restoring an acceptable intrinsic heart rate. Subsequently, a transcutaneous or transvenous pacemaker may be required to ensure stabilization of the patient. Once stabilization has been accomplished, further ED management should include a thorough secondary survey, 12-lead electrocardiographic and continuous cardiovascular monitoring, portable chest radiograph to assess the condition of the pacemaker leads and identify related pathology, and any other pertinent diagnostic studies. At this point the clinician should seek to identify the type and model of the pacemaker and should consult an available cardiologist or electrophysiologist. Final disposition of the patient depends on the results of the stabilization, diagnostic studies, and cardiology consultation, and admission is often required.

Failure to Capture

In the case of failure to capture, pacemaker spikes are present on the ECG. However, some or all of the spikes are not followed by atrial or ventricular complexes, as appropriate for the pacemaker model in question. Failure to capture may result from deterioration of lead insulation; fracture or dislodgment of the leads; electrolyte disturbances, including hyperkalemia or hypocalcemia; a new condition requiring an elevated pacing threshold; acid-base disturbance; direct damage to the myocardium, which is in contact with the pacer lead's tip (such as myocardial infarction or direct trauma); or dysfunction of the microcircuitry of the pulse generator. In addition, flecainide, a class IC antiarrhythmic medication, has been identified as an acute cause of the rise in ventricular capture thresholds in patients with implanted pacemakers.[32] Likewise, all class I antiarrhythmic agents (sodium channel antagonists) may affect pacer capture thresholds and should therefore be identified as potential etiologic agents in patients suffering failure to capture.

Failure to Sense

Failure of an implanted cardiac pacemaker to sense the patient's intrinsic cardiac rhythm may be subdivided into conditions related to oversensing or undersensing. *Oversensing* is present when the pacemaker erroneously identifies extrinsic electrical signals, such as those from skeletal muscle potentials or electromagnetic interference (EMI), and is inhibited from delivering an appropriate pacemaker pulse. For additional information on extrinsic EMI, refer to "Electromagnetic Interference and Implantable Devices" later in this chapter.

Management of pacemaker failure to sense will be driven largely by the patient's clinical condition. A prudent clinician will order cardiovascular monitoring, intravenous access, and a portable chest radiograph, with additional measures as dictated by the patient's condition. In the event of symptomatic bradycardia, placement of a magnet over the pacemaker pulse generator may be indicated because this maneuver will usually place the pacemaker in an asynchronous ventricular pacing mode and thereby restore a stable and regular paced ventricular rhythm while a consulting cardiologist or electrophysiologist is summoned.

Undersensing is said to occur when the pacemaker fails to identify intrinsic cardiac depolarization and delivers a pacing signal. This condition may result from damage or dislodgment of the pacemaker leads, myocardial infarction, direct cardiac trauma, failure of the pacemaker's power source, and even the application of a magnet. Initial ED management of this condition is similar to that performed in the case of oversensing. Magnet placement may also be appropriate in this setting because it will restore a stable, regular, and normal cardiac rhythm until the pacemaker and its leads may be more thoroughly examined.

Runaway Pacemaker Syndrome

This condition is seen almost exclusively in older pacemaker models, particularly as they approach the end of their battery life or when the pulse generator is damaged by exposure to radiation or direct impact. The hallmark of runaway pacemaker syndrome is uncontrolled tachycardia resulting in ventricular rates approaching 300 to 400 beats/min. In addition to initial attempts at stabilization, magnet placement may be attempted. However, this is often ineffective. If the patient is hemodynamically unstable in the setting of runaway pacemaker syndrome, it may be necessary to disconnect the pulse generator. To do this, identify the location of the pacer leads by physical examination or a portable chest radiograph. Dissect through the skin and subcutaneous tissue and then sever the leads with a wire cutter or similar tool.

Pacemaker-Mediated Tachycardia

In some circumstances, patients with implanted pacemakers or AICDs may be seen in the ED because of symptomatic tachycardias resulting specifically as a complication of their pacemaker devices. This condition, referred to as *pacemaker-mediated tachycardia* and, alternatively, as *pacemaker-induced tachycardia*, most often results from one of three clinical scenarios. In patients with dual-chamber pacemakers, one of the pacemaker leads may function as a pathway for either anterograde or retrograde conduction and result in what is referred to as *endless loop syndrome* and thus a tachycardiac arrhythmia, which may often become hemodynamically unstable. In general, patients suffering from endless loop syndrome will not have a ventricular rate greater than the maximum tracking rate of the pacemaker device. Consequently, this condition will rarely be manifested as hemodynamic instability. One caveat, however, is that patients with underlying coronary artery disease and endless loop syndrome may experience coronary ischemia. In such a case or in a patient who is hemodynamically unstable because of the increased ventricular rate, application of a magnet will terminate the syndrome in most cases. Once stabilized, this condition may be prevented or at least mitigated by reprogramming of the pacemaker's atrial sensor lead by an electrophysiologist.

A second scenario in patients with dual-chamber pacemakers occurs under the circumstance in which the patient experiences an intrinsic atrial tachycardia, at which point the implanted pacemaker begins to continuously discharge at its maximum preprogrammed ventricular rate. This condition may continue until the underlying atrial tachycardia is terminated by intervention.

A third instance of pacemaker-mediated tachycardia occurs in patients with AICD units that have backup antibradycardia pacing capability. It appears that if this pacemaker feature is switched on in such patients and an ectopic ventricular stimulus is delivered after a sudden pause in the intrinsic ventricular depolarization cycle, a ventricular tachyarrhythmia may be triggered.[2,35]

Diagnosis of Acute Myocardial Infarction in the Presence of a Paced Cardiac Rhythm

Patients undergoing active ventricular pacing from an implanted pacemaker device will normally have ECGs that resemble a left bundle branch block pattern. As a result, electrocardiographic diagnosis of acute ischemic changes is equally challenging in both populations. Sgarbossa and coworkers[36] published a series of criteria in 1996 that offer some utility in the interpretation of ECGs in patients with active ventricular pacing in whom acute coronary syndromes are suspected. These criteria are depicted in Table 13-2.[7]

TABLE 13-2 Criteria for Electrocardiographic Diagnosis of Acute Myocardial Infarction in the Setting of a Ventricular Paced Rhythm

ELECTROCARDIOGRAPHIC CRITERION	SENSITIVITY (%)	SENSITIVITY (%)	*P*
Discordant ST-segment elevation >5 mm	53	88	0.025
Concordant ST-segment elevation >1 mm	18	94	NS
ST-segment depression >1 mm in precordial leads V₁-V₃	2	82	NS

NS, not significant.

Automatic Implantable Cardioverter-Defibrillators—Unique Malfunctions

Issues with sensing problems, lead migration, and battery failure are similar to pacemaker complications, and most occur within 3 months after implantation.[37] A potential malfunction unique to AICDs is inappropriate or lack of defibrillation of the device. An analysis of 23,000 Medicare patients with AICDs revealed a complication rate of 11%, with lead dislodgement being the most common problem followed by hematoma or hemorrhage, infection, and pneumothorax.[38]

The AICD may not terminate ventricular arrhythmias, which may or may not be the result of malfunction of the device. AICD malfunction may be a result of battery depletion, component failure, failure-to-sense, or lead malfunction. Failure to cardiovert or defibrillate occurring in the setting of a functioning AICD system may be caused by inappropriate cutoff rates, failure to satisfy multiple detection criteria, completed and exhaustion of therapies, and cross-inhibition by a separate pacemaker.[11] The advent of AV or *dual-chamber AICD* devices has improved the sensitivity of detecting arrhythmias and thus preventing the delivery of inappropriate shocks.

Inappropriate AICD-delivered shocks occur in 20% to 25% of patients[38] and are the most common adverse events observed in AICD patients.[32] The main causes are atrial arrhythmias, sinus tachycardia, nonsustained ventricular tachycardia, lead fracture or EMI, or *electrical storm*.[38] By definition, this phenomenon occurs when three or more shocks are delivered in a 24-hour period, occurs in 10% to 20% of AICD patients,[39] and constitutes a medical emergency.[40] AICD patients who experience this phenomenon may have end-stage cardiac failure and increased long-term mortality.[41] Specific causes of electrical storm are unclear, but it is associated with ventricular tachycardia in the setting of LVEF lower than 30% and occurs more frequently in patients with demonstrated coronary artery disease who have not as yet undergone revascularization procedures. Suggested initial treatment includes the administration of amiodarone and β₂-adrenergic antagonists to pharmacologically suppress the arrhythmias and urgent cardiology consultation for possible pacemaker interrogation, overdrive pacing, or even catheter ablation.[41-43]

The AICD may discharge inappropriately in response to rapid supraventricular rhythms such as atrial fibrillation, supraventricular tachycardia, or even sinus tachycardia. Multiple shocks may be a manifestation of inefficient termination

BOX 13-4 Outcome of Automatic Implantable Cardioverter-Defibrillator Placement: Estimated Events over a 5-Year Period after Placement for Current Criteria*

For every 100 patients in whom an AICD is placed:
   30 patients will die anyway because of underlying disease.
   7-8 patients will be saved by AICD.
   10-20 will have a shock delivered that is not needed.
   5-15 will have an ICD complication.
The rest will not experience the device firing.
Some will ask to have it removed to allow natural death.

Adapted from Stevenson LW, Desai AS. Selecting patients for discussion of the ICD as primary prevention for sudden death in heart failure. J Card Fail. 2006;12:407. AICD, automatic implantable cardioverter-defibrillator; ICD, implantable cardioverter-defibrillator.
**Left ventricular ejection fraction less than 30% to 35% and anticipated survival with good functional capacity beyond 1 year.*

of tachycardia, such as inappropriately low-energy delivery at the first shock, increased defibrillation thresholds, and migration or dislodgment of the defibrillation lead system or failure of the defibrillator system. Shocks that occur every few minutes may suggest that recurring ventricular tachyarrhythmias are being terminated appropriately (see Fig. 13-6).

AICD discharges in the setting of chest pain may be a result of myocardial ischemia–induced tachyarrhythmias.[28] As noted earlier, any electrocardiographic abnormalities noted immediately after shocks should be interpreted with caution because ST elevation or depression can occur immediately after a shock.[29] If the patient receives shocks in association with chest pain, ischemia is suggested, but other causes, including hypokalemia, hypomagnesemia, drug-induced proarrhythmia, or drugs that can prolong the QT interval (such as phenothiazines), should also be considered as underlying causes.[11]

In some settings, the AICD may fail to sense sustained ventricular tachycardia or fibrillation. Such failure may be caused by an intrinsic arrhythmia rate below the programmed detection rate, usually as a result of concurrent pharmacologic therapy. If the patient is hemodynamically stable, it may be advantageous for the cardiologist to interrogate the pacer before initiating further antiarrhythmic therapy. If unsuccessful or if the patient is experiencing a nonperfusing ventricular arrhythmia, other pharmacologic interventions include procainamide[26,44] or amiodarone. Box 13-4 depicts the outcome of AICD placement in a general population.

Use of a Magnet for AICD

A patient who is experiencing *inappropriate* AICD discharges in the ED can be treated by inactivation of the device with a magnet, similar to the approach described earlier for pacemaker patients. *If the patient is experiencing recurrent rhythms that require activation of the AICD, do not inactivate the device because it is functioning as required.*

Technique

The method for inactivating an AICD device is outlined in Box 13-5. The orientation of the device in the abdominal pocket should be determined, with the lead connections normally being cephalad. A ring magnet is then placed over the corner adjacent to the lead connections (usually the upper

---

| BOX 13-5 | Method for Inactivation of an Automatic Implantable Cardioverter-Defibrillator |

1. Determine the orientation of the device in the abdominal pocket radiographically or by palpation.
2. Place a ring magnet over the upper right-hand corner of the device.
3. A beeping tone will sound that corresponds to the sensing of QRS complexes.
4. Leave the magnet in place for at least 30 seconds.
5. When the beeping changes to a continuous tone, the device is inactivated.
6. Remove the magnet.

Adapted from Munter DW, DeLacey WA. Automatic implantable cardioverter-defibrillators. Emerg Med Clin North Am. 1994;12:579. Used with permission.

right-hand corner of the device). A series of beeping tones will sound that correspond to the sensed QRS complexes. In the absence of organized QRS activity, random beeps will sound.[45] When the magnet is left in place for 30 seconds, a continuous beep is heard. This indicates that the AICD is inactivated. The magnet should then be removed, and the AICD will remain inactivated. The AICD may be reactivated by applying the magnet for 30 seconds and removing it when the steady beep changes to intermittent beeping. Note that unlike a pacemaker, in which a magnet will turn a demand pacemaker to a fixed-rate pacemaker, a magnet will not affect the pacing function of an AICD.

"Twiddler's Syndrome"

In some cases, patients with implantable pacemakers choose to "twiddle" with the device: they manipulate the pulse generator case within its physiologic pocket under the skin in the chest. Note that a generator may also be placed in the abdominal wall (Fig. 13-7). This practice of "twiddling" may result in coiling, dislodgment, or disconnection of the pacemaker leads (Fig 13-8). It may even lead to actual displacement of the pulse generator case. At a minimum it may result in physical discomfort and may, in fact, precipitate cardiac arrhythmias or other complications local to the site of pacemaker placement. After initial stabilization of the complaint, these patients may require readjustment or replacement of their pacemaker devices. As part of their care, pacemaker patients should be educated to avoid manipulating their pacemakers.[46]

Mental Health Issues Related to Implanted Pacemakers and AICDs

Patients with these devices may manifest a number of anxiety-related complications, including adjustment disorder, panic attacks, depression, imaginary shock, and defibrillator dependence, abuse, or withdrawal.[47,48] These patients may benefit from psychiatric referral either as an outpatient or as part of the admission evaluation if applicable. The conditions may be severe enough that the device is removed by patient request.

Implantable Pacemaker and AICD Recalls

Since 1990 there have been approximately 29 Food and Drug Administration safety alerts and recalls affecting nearly

Figure 13-7 Pacemakers and automatic implantable cardioverter-defibrillators may be implanted in the abdominal wall, as well as in the more common pectoralis muscle.

Figure 13-8 Twiddler's syndrome. Note the twisting of the pacemaker leads as they exit the device (*arrow*). This twisting is a direct result of the patient "twiddling" with the device and may result in dislodgement or disconnection of the pacemaker leads.

337,000 AICDs.[49] These advisories were issued as a result of unanticipated failure of devices identified after release of the product and widespread clinical use.[49] The decision to remove the devices is complex, and there has been difficulty reaching consensus on the optimal management of patients with these recalled devices. The decision to replace them should be multifactorial and take into consideration the estimated malfunction rate of the device, anticipated consequences of failure of the device, the individual center's procedural risk for complications resulting from generator replacement, and patient preferences and desired level of risk tolerance.[50]

Electromagnetic Interference and Implantable Devices

Given the plethora of new technologies, there is always concern about the interaction of EMI with pacemakers and AICDs. The sources of EMI comprise a significant spectrum and may involve radiated and conducted sources.

The most common response of implanted devices to EMI is inappropriate inhibition or triggering of pacemaker stimuli, reversion to asynchronous pacing, and spurious detection of tachyarrhythmias by the AICD. Reprogramming of operating parameters and permanent damage to the circuitry of the device or the electrode-tissue interface can also occur but are

---

BOX 13-6 | **Sources of Electromagnetic Interference and Their Potential Effects on Implanted Pacemakers and Automatic Implantable Cardioverter-Defibrillators**

GENERALLY THOUGHT TO BE SAFE WITH EMI
Copy machines
Electric blankets
Household appliances (microwaves, washer/dryer)
DVD/CD players, TVs
Personal computers
Remote controls
Heating pads

SOME EVIDENCE OF INTERACTION
Cell phones
Induction ovens

Power toothbrushes
Battery-powered, cordless power tools
Arc welding equipment
Chain saws
Drills
Hedge clippers
Lawn mowers
Leaf blowers
Snow blowers
High-voltage lines
Theft detection systems
Airport scanners/metal detectors

AVOID BECAUSE OF INTERACTION
Electrolysis
MRI
Jackhammers

MEDICAL DEVICES REQUIRING CAUTION
Electrocautery (especially unipolar) equipment
High-energy radiation sources
TENS units
MRI scanners
Body fat–measuring scales
Diathermy equipment

Electrolysis equipment
Spinal cord stimulators
Direct current external cardioversion/defibrillation equipment
Radiofrequency catheter ablation equipment
Lithotripsy equipment

SAFE MEDICAL DEVICES
CT scanners
Dental drills
Diagnostic x-ray machines
Electrocardiography equipment
Ultrasound equipment

Adapted from Cardiosource. Available at www.cardiosource.com. Used with permission.
CT, computed tomography; EMI, electromagnetic interference; MRI, magnetic resonance imaging; TENS, transcutaneous electrical nerve stimulation.

BOX 13-7 | **Follow-Up of Patients with an AICD**

Follow-up assessments of patients with an AICD are made on a routine basis, every 3 to 6 months, and when discharge of the device occurs. Analysis of any previous clinical event and testing of defibrillation function are readily accomplished. Internet-based remote follow-up systems may replace some office follow-up. Follow-up can occur remotely with vendor-specific equipment to interrogate and upload data. Remote follow-up, however, permits only device interrogation and retrieval of diagnostic data, not threshold testing or reprogramming. Device interrogation includes the following:
- Determination of pacing and sensing thresholds.
- Analysis of recorded episodes of arrhythmia detection and AICD activation, including pacing and delivered shocks. Data include the date and time of each episode and a stored electrocardiogram from the event.
- Battery status.

DEFIBRILLATOR DISCHARGE

An appropriate shock is delivered in about 50% of patients by 2 years after implantation. Patients may not sense antitachycardiac

(overdrive) pacing to terminate arrhythmias. Not all episodes of defibrillator discharge require immediate medical evaluation, although many patients go to the ED immediately. Patients with a first shock may be seen on an urgent or elective basis to ascertain the specifics of the event and to determine whether the device is functioning properly. Discharges that are accompanied by changes in cognition (syncope, seizure, or loss of consciousness) require ED evaluation.

Per guidelines, patients who have had a single AICD discharge with immediate return to baseline clinical status and no associated symptoms (e.g., chest pain, shortness of breath, lightheadedness) may have the device interrogated within 1 to 2 days.

Delivery of frequent shocks or clusters of shocks is either appropriate (because of recurrent VT) or inappropriate (because of atrial fibrillation, supraventricular tachycardia, or device malfunction). Such patients generally require emergency evaluation and hospital admission to determine the cause. Additional therapy (such as an antiarrhythmic drug or catheter ablation) may be required.

AICD, automatic implantable cardioverter-defibrillator; ED, emergency department; VT, ventricular tachycardia.

---

much less frequent.[30] Additional adverse effects that may occur include inhibition of bradycardia pacing, inadvertent delivery of a shock, or antitachycardia pacing.

The use of hermetic shielding in metal cases, filtering, interference rejection circuits, and bipolar sensing have helped mitigate most of this interference.[50] Nonetheless, the clinician should be familiar with common sources of EMI that may affect pacemakers and AICDs.

Several caveats will help avoid the deleterious effects of EMI on implantable devices. Cell phones should not be kept in a pocket over the device. When in use, they should be held at least 6 inches away from the device. In the case of hands-free headphones, when used these devices should be placed in the ear opposite the implanted pacemaker or AICD. In

addition, patients should be advised to not linger in theft detection areas or airport metal detectors. Box 13-6 identifies different devices and the corresponding potential EMI that can occur with pacemakers and AICDs.[51,52]

Out-of-Hospital Discharge of AICD

Patients are told to adhere to standard advice defining an appropriate response to out-of-hospital discharges of the AICD (Box 13-7). Many, however, come to the ED for evaluation after every shock. There is no standard ED intervention mandated by historical information, and clinical decisions are made on an individual basis corresponding to the current scenario. Options include prolonged ED observation, consul-

Figure 13-9 Sophisticated bedside interrogation of an automatic implantable cardioverter-defibrillator (AICD) can be accomplished in a few hours by calling the manufacturer. Using a noninvasive AICD-interrogating device, the clinician can determine the patient's name, diagnosis, AICD settings, and surgeon and can view recent and remote information about the heart and AICD activity. This takes away all the guesswork when trying to determine what happened to the patient to prompt an AICD-related ED visit to the emergency department (ED). Such information can also be obtained periodically over the phone in lieu of an ED or office visit.

tation, cardiac monitoring, laboratory testing (such as electrolytes and cardiac enzymes), or interrogation.

Disposition Criteria

In the majority of cases, patients seen in the ED with pacemaker complications or malfunctions will be symptomatic. Accordingly and regardless of the clinical requirement for admission, they will probably require device interrogation and possible recalibration or replacement by a cardiologist. In most cases this will be accomplished during hospital admission.

With regard to AICD malfunctions and disposition, patients who have had a single shock and no other specific complaints or comorbidity can be discharged with follow-up in 24 to 48 hours. Patients with symptoms concerning for ischemia, potentially lethal arrhythmias, or symptomatic illness should be admitted and specialty consultation obtained expeditiously. Patients who have had multiple shocks will need admission for observation and interrogation of their AICD device. Interrogation reveals significant information about the device, such as why it fired, the rhythm history, and an accurate assessment of the underlying problem (Fig. 13-9).

References are available at www.expertconsult.com

CHAPTER 14

Basic Electrocardiographic Techniques

Richard A. Harrigan, Theodore C. Chan, and William J. Brady

The electrocardiogram (ECG) is a graphic recording of the electrical activity of the heart. The standard ECG is obtained by applying electrodes over the chest and limbs to record the electrical activity of the cardiac cycle. Developed 100 years ago, the ECG remains the most important initial diagnostic tool for the assessment of myocardial disease, ischemia, and cardiac dysrhythmias.

Electrocardiography is performed widely throughout the health care field, including ambulances, ambulatory clinics, emergency departments (EDs), and in-patient hospital units. Standard electrocardiography machines are small, self-contained, and portable, thus allowing them to be used in virtually any setting. As a result, clinicians, nurses, and many other health care providers should be familiar with the procedure of standard 12-lead electrocardiography. Emergency clinicians should also be familiar with the alternative leads and other accessory techniques available in electrocardiography, as well as the pitfalls of lead misplacement, misconnection, and tracing artifacts.

BACKGROUND
CAN BE FOUND ON EXPERT CONSULT

INDICATIONS

The most frequent indication for electrocardiography in the ED is the presence of chest pain. Other common indications include abnormal rhythm, palpitations, dyspnea, syncope, and diagnosis-based (e.g., acute coronary syndrome [ACS], suspected pulmonary embolism) and system-related (e.g., "rule out myocardial infarction [MI]" protocol, admission purposes, and operative clearance) indications.[9] The ECG is used to help establish a diagnosis, select appropriate therapy, determine the response to treatment, assist in correct disposition of the patient, and help predict risk for both cardiovascular complication and death.

The initial 12-lead ECG obtained in the ED can be an important tool for determination of cardiovascular risk and, accordingly, the choice of in-hospital admission location. Brush and coworkers[10] classified the initial ECG into high- and low-risk groups. The low-risk electrocardiographic group had normal ECGs, nonspecific ST-T-wave changes, or no change when compared with a previous ECG. High-risk ECGs had significant abnormalities or confounding patterns—such as pathologic Q waves, ischemic ST-segment or T-wave changes, left ventricular hypertrophy, left bundle branch block, or ventricular paced rhythms. Patients with initial ECGs classified as low risk had a 14% incidence of acute myocardial infarction (AMI), a 0.6% incidence of

life-threatening complications, and a 0% mortality rate. Patients with initial ECGs classified as high risk had a 42% incidence of AMI, a 14% incidence of life-threatening complications, and a 10% mortality rate.[10] Another approach to risk prediction involves simple calculation of the number of electrocardiographic leads with ST-segment deviation (elevation or depression)—with an increasing number of leads being associated with higher risk. Along similar lines, the clinician is also able to predict risk with a summation of the total millivolts of ST-segment deviation; once again, higher totals are associated with greater risk.[10]

The limitations of the ECG must be recognized, however. The ECG is widely reported to have a sensitivity for AMI of only approximately 55%; in one study of 1000 patients with ischemic symptoms, sensitivity improved to 68% with serial ECGs and monitoring of ST-segment trends.[11] In another series, the sensitivity of the ECG for AMI ranged from 43% to 65% over a 12-hour period after the onset of ischemic symptom, yet the negative predictive value of a normal ECG (defined as normal or with nonspecific changes or isolated fascicular blocks) for AMI did not improve above 93% during this period.[12] In a large series of more than 10,000 patients, in 889 (8%) of whom AMI was ultimately diagnosed, 19 (2%) were inappropriately discharged from the ED. A nonischemic ECG emerged as one of five risk factors for that inappropriate disposition decision (along with female gender, age <55 years, nonwhite race, and dyspnea as a chief complaint); 2 of those 19 had a normal tracing, whereas the other 17 had nonischemic findings on their ECGs.[13]

BASIC EQUIPMENT

The 12-Lead ECG

Although there is variability depending on the workplace, most ECGs in use today are three-channel recorders with computer memory. Such multichannel systems, which record electrical events in several leads concurrently, offer advantages over the antiquated single-channel recorder systems: capturing transient events on multiple leads simultaneously; banking the data in computer memory for storage, comparison, and transmission; and allowing presentation of data on a single sheet of paper.[14] The electrocardiographic tracing is printed in a standardized manner on standardized paper by the electrocardiograph, which has default settings regarding the speed at which the paper moves through the machine, as well as the amplitude of the deflections to be made on the tracing (Fig. 14-1A). Electrocardiographic paper is divided into a grid with a series of horizontal and vertical lines; the thin lines are 1 mm apart, and the thick lines are separated by 5 mm. At the standard paper speed of 25 mm/sec, each vertical thin line thus represents 0.04 second (or 40 msec), and the thick vertical lines correspond to 0.20 second (or 200 msec). Recordings from each of the 12 leads are typically displayed for 2.5 seconds by default setting; the leads appearing horizontally adjacent to each other are separated by a small vertical hash mark to represent lead change.

The standard ECG includes 12 leads derived from 10 electrodes placed on the patient; each is color-coded and represented by a two-character abbreviation (Table 14-1; see also Fig. 14-1B). Placement of limb leads on the left and right arms (LA and RA, respectively) and the left and right legs (LL and RL, respectively) by color can be recalled with the help

Figure 14-1 A, Standard electrocardiographic (ECG) tracing. By convention, the thick lines are 5 mm apart, and the thin lines (barely visible on this reproduction) are 1 mm apart. At the standard paper speed of 25 mm/sec, each vertical thin line represents 0.04 sec (40 msec) and each vertical thick line represents 0.20 sec (200 msec). (The *inset* represents one "big box," which is outlined by thick lines 5 mm apart.) **B,** Standard 12-lead ECG machine. Note the color coding of the leads.

TABLE 14-1 Conventional Electrodes for the 12-Lead ECG

LOCATION	NOTATION	COLOR
Right arm	RA	White
Left arm	LA	Black
Left leg	LL	Red
Right leg	RL	Green
Precordial leads	V_1	Brown/red
	V_2	Brown/yellow
	V_3	Brown/green
	V_4	Brown/blue
	V_5	Brown/orange
	V_6	Brown/violet

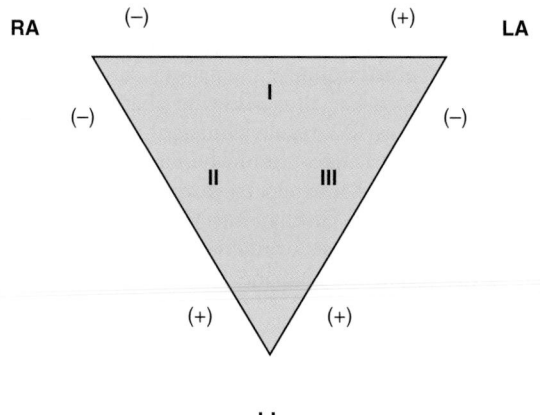

Figure 14-2 Bipolar limb leads. Leads I, II, and III are shown as a triangle, known as *Einthoven's triangle*. Left arm (LA), right arm (RA), and left leg (LL) placement is shown. Orient these bipolar leads so that the positive poles lie inferiorly and to the left (given that the bottom apex of the triangle is directed toward the left leg), as does the major electrical vector of the heart.

of several mnemonics, including the following: "Christmas trees below the knees (the green and red leads are placed on the lower extremities), "white on right and green to go" (the white lead is placed on the RA, the green lead is placed on the leg that controls the gas pedal, and the red lead is correspondingly placed on the leg that is closer to the brake), and "smoke over fire" (the black LA lead is placed over the red LL lead, as with telemetric monitoring pads). Use of these mnemonics may help prevent right/left confusion during electrode placement—and the consequences of limb electrode reversal and misinterpretation of the ECG (see "Electrode Misplacement and Misconnection" later in this chapter).

Standard 12 Leads

The standard 12-lead ECG depicts cardiac electrical activity from 12 points of view, or leads, that can be grouped according to planar orientation. Six leads (I, II, III, aVR, aVL, and aVF) are oriented in the frontal, or coronal, plane and derived from the four limb electrodes. The six precordial leads (V_1, V_2, V_3, V_4, V_5, and V_6) are oriented in the horizontal, or transverse, plane, with each representing cardiac electrical activity from that perspective. Leads I, II, and III are termed *limb leads* and are bipolar in that they record the potential difference between two electrodes (Fig. 14-2). The fourth electrode located on the right leg serves as an electrical ground. The positive poles of these bipolar leads lie to the left and inferior, a position approximating the major vector forces of the normal heart. This early convention was established so that the tracing would feature primarily upright complexes. In contrast, augmented leads aVR, aVL, and aVF are unipolar leads with the positive electrode located at the respective extremities. These augmented leads serve to fill the electrical gaps between leads I, II, and III. Lead aVR stands alone with a polarity and resultant orientation opposite that of the other limb and augmented leads because of the fact that its positive electrode is located in the opposite direction (superior and to the right) of the major vector force of the normal heart (inferior and to the left); thus

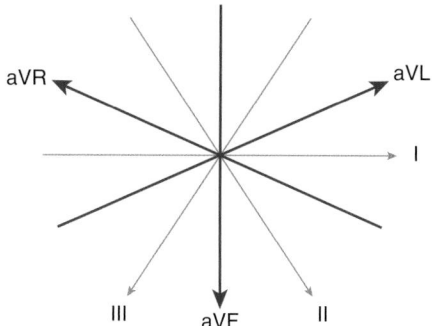

Figure 14-3 Hexaxial system of limb and augmented leads in the frontal plane. Each lead is separated by 30 degrees in this frontal-plane representation of the limb and augmented leads. Augmented leads are shown in boldface. Arrows denote positive polarity. Note that the inferior leads (II, III, aVF) logically lie at the bottom of this figure and the lateral leads (I, aVL) lie on the left side of the figure, where the lateral aspect of the heart is located if this were superimposed on a patient.

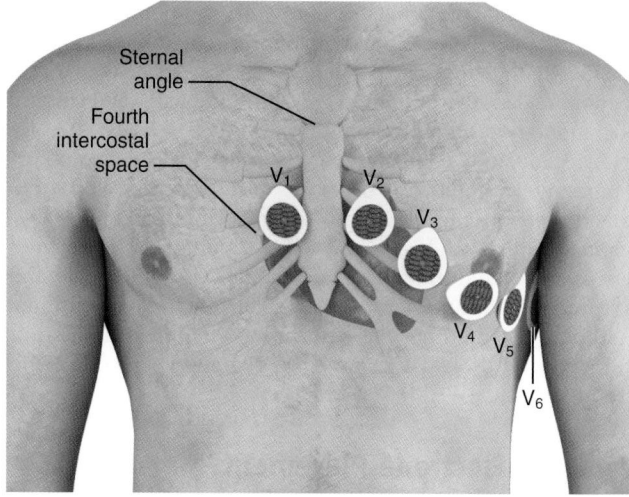

Figure 14-4 Precordial lead placement for the standard 12-lead electrocardiogram. If multiple or repeated electrocardiographic tracings are anticipated, mark the original lead placements on the patient's chest wall or leave stick-on leads in place after the electrocardiographic wires are removed.

its complexes usually appear "opposite" those in most or all of the other leads.

Merging of the vector axes of the limb and augmented leads around a central axis yields a hexaxial system representing cardiac electrical activity in the frontal plane (Fig. 14-3). The six precordial leads, oriented in the horizontal plane, represent six unipolar electrodes with vector positivity oriented toward the chest surface and the central terminal of the hexaxial system serving as a negative pole. In contrast to the frontal-plane leads, the angles between each of the precordial leads in the horizontal plane are not equal. They can vary depending on electrode placement and body habitus.

Electrode Placement

The four limb electrodes are conventionally placed on the extremities as follows: RA on the right wrist, LA on the left wrist, RL on the right ankle, and LL on the left ankle. Electrodes may be affixed more proximally on the limbs if necessary (e.g., amputation, severe injuries), ideally with a notation made on the ECG.[15] Others note that the electrodes may be placed on any part of the arms or legs, provided that they are distal to the shoulders or inguinal/gluteal folds, respectively.[16]

Mason-Likar electrode placement is commonly used by hospital staff and paramedics; this approach does not alter precordial electrode placement but instead moves the limb electrodes to the torso. Originally described in 1966, the Mason-Likar configuration differs from standard electrode placement in that the arm electrodes are relocated to the infraclavicular fossae (medial to the borders of the deltoid muscles and 2 cm below the clavicles) and the leg electrodes are positioned along the anterior axillary lines (halfway between the costal margins and the iliac crests). Actual torso positioning may differ in practice because of individual variation or an attempt to simulate limb electrode placement. A rightward frontal-plane access shift has been described when torso electrode placement is used for the limb electrodes instead of standard positioning on the extremities. Mason-Likar positioning has also been associated with diminution of inferior Q waves, thus making detection of inferior MI more

difficult.[17] An alternative electrode configuration is the Lund system, in which the arm electrodes are placed laterally on the left and right arms at the level of the axillary folds and the leg electrodes are positioned laterally on the major femoral trochanters. The Lund system has been found to more directly approximate the electrocardiographic recordings obtained with conventional positioning than the Mason-Likar configuration does.[18,19]

The precordial electrodes should be placed as follows: V_1—right sternal border, fourth intercostal space; V_2—left sternal border, fourth intercostal space; V_3—midway between V_2 and V_4; V_4—left midclavicular line, fifth intercostal space; V_5—left anterior axillary line, same horizontal level as V_4; and V_6—left midaxillary line, same horizontal level as V_4 and V_5 (Fig. 14-4). Note that V_4 to V_6 are placed at the same horizontal level, not all in the fifth intercostal space. If V_5 and V_6 are situated so that they follow the contour of the intercostal space rather than being on the same horizontal level, they will be superiorly displaced as the ribs curve around the side of the thorax. Minor changes in the position of the precordial leads will alter the ECG tracing, so it is important to keep the adhesive leads in place throughout the ED stay so that lead placement is identical during serial ECG comparisons.

Intercostal space number can be determined by first palpating the sternal angle (angle of Louis), which is the junction of the manubrium and body of the sternum (see Fig. 14-4). This transverse bony ridge is located about 5 cm caudad from the sternal notch in adults. Immediately lateral and inferior to it is the second intercostal space; two spaces farther down lies the fourth intercostal space, where V_1 and V_2 should be placed. Alternatively, one can count down from the medial aspect of the clavicle; beneath the clavicle lies the first rib, below which is the first intercostal space. The precordial electrodes should not be simply "eyeballed" by the technician because as little as 1 to 2 cm of electrode displacement can result in significant morphologic alteration in the precordial QRS complexes.[17,20]

If the patient's anatomy or injury precludes placement of a precordial electrode as just described, it is permissible to attach it within the radius of the width of one interspace of the recommended position, with appropriate notation on the tracing. If the situation demands further displacement, it is recommended that the lead be omitted, with appropriate documentation on the tracing.[15]

A recent study compared conventional 12-lead electrocardiography with the use of disposable, prewired electrodes linked together and placed on the precordium and torso in a manner similar to Mason-Likar positioning. The prewired device saved time (median, 25 seconds, or 20% faster) and featured significantly less artifact than did the conventional method—at four times the cost, however. Only a slight shift in the mean QRS axis was noted (6 degrees when comparing group means).[21]

Pediatric Electrode Placement

In addition to the standard 12-lead tracing, leads V_4R and V_3R should also be recorded; these are mirror images of their left-sided counterparts (see "Additional Leads" later in this chapter). The chest of a tiny infant may not accommodate all the precordial electrodes; in such cases the following array is recommended: V_3R or V_4R, V_1, V_3, and V_6. Limb electrode placement is the same as in adults.[22]

FEATURES OF THE ECG

Interpretation of the ECG is beyond the scope of this chapter. Other features of the procedure itself, including a description of the other data found on the electrocardiographic tracing, are detailed later.

Information Provided by the Computer

In addition to the patient demographic data entered by the operator, the tracing will often feature computations regarding rate, intervals, and axes along the top of the paper. On some tracings a computer-generated "reading" will also be displayed at the top of the tracing. *These interpretations are not infallible.* A sample of nine of these programs was compared

with the readings of eight cardiologists; the "gold standard" in this study was clinical diagnosis made independently of the interpretations of these tracings based on other objective data (e.g., echocardiography, cardiac catheterization). The performance of the programs was good, with correct interpretations in a median of 91% of cases, but the cardiologists were significantly better (median of 96% correct).[23] *The computer programs demonstrated a median sensitivity for anterior and inferior MI of only 77% and 59%, respectively.*[23] Of note, this study did not evaluate interpretation of acute ischemia and cardiac rhythm disturbance—perhaps the most critical issues in electrocardiographic interpretation. Others have found both the computer programs and clinicians to be lacking in their ability to exclude cardiac disease with the ECG, with a negative predictive value for each of between 80% and 85%.[24] When diagnosing atrial fibrillation, both general practitioners (sensitivity, 80%; specificity, 83%) and computer software (sensitivity, 83%; specificity, 99%) are flawed; when combined, diagnostic accuracy improves but is still imperfect (sensitivity, 92%; specificity, 91%).[25]

It is worthwhile to read and consider the computer reading of the ECG, but the emergency clinician should not be beholden to it.

Adjustable Features

Somewhere on the tracing—usually in the left lower corner of the recording—notation of electrocardiographic paper speed (in millimeters per second), calibration (in millimeters per millivolt), and the frequency response (in hertz) will be evident. *Calibration,* or standardization, refers to the amplitude of the waveforms on the tracing. It is usually set at a default value of 10 mm/mV and is graphically depicted by a plateau-shaped waveform that appears at the extreme left side of the tracing, in front of the first complex (Fig. 14-5A). This calibration can be modified by the operator or by the computer itself, as was the case in Figure 14-5B, in which the patient appeared to have acquired voltage criteria for left ventricular hypertrophy when in reality the tracing was unchanged from his baseline (see Fig. 14-5A). Increasing the calibration to 20 mm/mV is helpful when trying to decipher

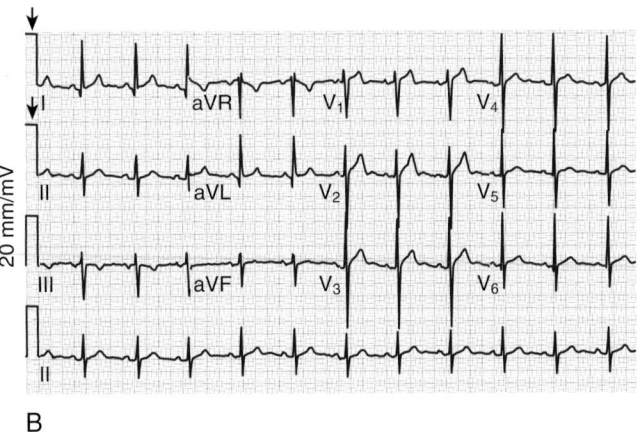

A   B

Figure 14-5 A, Normal 10-mm/mV calibration. Note the box-shaped mark to the left of the complexes (*arrows*); this is a graphic representation of the calibration for the tracing. Routinely note this parameter before interpretation of the electrocardiogram (ECG). Note the change in **B. B,** Abnormal 20-mm/mV calibration. The calibration in this tracing was (inexplicably and unexpectedly) changed to 20 mm/mV by the computer, not by the operator. When compared with a baseline ECG, it appeared that voltage criteria had developed for left ventricular hypertrophy, as well as ST-segment elevation. *A* was recorded minutes later with correction of calibration to the standard 10 mm/mV and was unchanged from baseline tracings.

P-wave morphology. Decreasing the calibration to 5 mm/mV is helpful in cases in which the amplitude of the QRS complex (usually in the precordial leads) is so large that it encroaches on those of adjacent leads. Standardization may not be uniform throughout a given tracing. At times, calibration will be automatically adjusted by the computer based on the waveform amplitudes that it perceives. For example, it is possible to have normal calibration (10 mm/mV) in the limb and augmented leads with half-standard calibration in the precordial leads (5 mm/mV). This may occur in instances of marked left ventricular hypertrophy. In this case the calibration pulse at the left-hand side of the paper will have a downward stairstep appearance.

Paper speed is usually set at a default of 25 mm/sec. It may be manipulated for purposes of deciphering a dysrhythmia, as described later (see "Alteration in Amplitude and Paper Speed"). *It is important that the clinician examine all electrocardiographic tracings for standardization and paper speed parameters before rendering an interpretation.*

ADDITIONAL LEADS

Though not performed routinely and not an ED standard of care, additional electrocardiographic leads may be used in the evaluation of a patient with possible ACS. These leads can be considered in a patient with findings consistent with ACS yet an unrevealing or nondiagnostic 12-lead ECG. These additional, or nontraditional, leads include posterior leads (V_7, V_8, and V_9), right ventricular leads (especially V_4R), and procedural leads (transvenous pacemaker wire placement and pericardiocentesis). Acute posterior and right ventricular MIs are likely to be underdiagnosed because the standard 12-lead ECG does not assess these areas directly. The standard ECG coupled with these additional leads constitutes the 15-lead ECG, the most frequently used extra-lead ECG in clinical practice.

15-Lead ECG

In a study of all ED patients with chest pain, Brady and associates[26] reported that the 15-lead ECG provided a more accurate description of myocardial injury in patients with AMI yet failed to alter rates of diagnosis or use of reperfusion therapies or to change disposition locations. Looking at a more selected population of ED patients, Zalenski and colleagues[27] investigated use of the 15-lead ECG in patients with chest pain and a moderate to high pretest probability of AMI who were already identified as candidates for hospital admission. In this 15-lead ECG study, the authors reported a 12% increase in sensitivity with no loss of specificity (i.e., no increase in false-positive findings) for the diagnosis of ST-segment elevation AMI (STEMI). They concluded that "the findings of ST segment elevation by use of these extra leads can strengthen the ED diagnosis of acute myocardial infarction on the initial tracing and may provide an indication for thrombolytic treatment." They further suggested that in the diagnosis of posterior AMI, leads V_8 and V_9 are superior to reliance on detecting the reciprocal ST-segment depression seen in leads V_1 to V_3. Aqel and colleagues used balloon inflation during coronary angiography for ostial or proximal left circumflex disease to simulate proximal left circumflex STEMI; they found that the posterior leads were significantly better at detecting simulated

STEMI when this vessel was occluded. Interestingly, 11% of their 53 patients had 1-mm or greater ST-segment elevation in a posterior lead with no ST-segment elevation or depression in any other lead.[28]

Possible indications for 15-lead ECGs in patients with suspected acute ischemic heart disease include (1) ST-segment depression in leads V_1 through V_3, (2) all STEMIs involving the inferior or lateral regions, (3) isolated ST-segment elevation in leads V_1 or V_2 (or both), or (4) high clinical suspicion for AMI without electrocardiographic evidence of STEMI on a 12-lead ECG (e.g., to detect occult left circumflex STEMI).

In a novel approach, consideration of the 12 traditional leads plus their vector opposites to render a "24-lead ECG" using only the standard 10 electrodes has been advanced as a means of deriving more data to both increase sensitivity for STEMI and more accurately localize coronary occlusion with the 12-lead ECG. For example, ST-segment elevation in lead III with ST-segment depression in lead aVL is equivalent to ST-segment elevation in two contiguous leads: lead III and lead (–) aVL, which are 30 degrees apart.[29]

Posterior Leads

The posterior electrodes V_8 and V_9 are placed on the patient's back—V_8 at the tip of the left scapula and V_9 in an intermediate position between lead V_8 and the left paraspinal muscles. An additional electrode, V_7, may also be used and is placed on the posterior axillary line equidistant from electrode V_8 (Fig. 14-6). The degree of ST-segment elevation in the posterior leads is often less pronounced than the ST-segment elevation seen in the standard 12 leads in patients with STEMI. This diminution in posterior lead ST-segment elevation results from both the relatively greater distance of these leads from the posterior surface of the heart and the presence of air and soft tissue between the epicardium and the electrocardiographic electrodes. It has been suggested that the threshold criterion for intervention be lowered from the standard 1 mm of ST-segment elevation to 0.5 mm when evaluating the posterior leads for STEMI.[30]

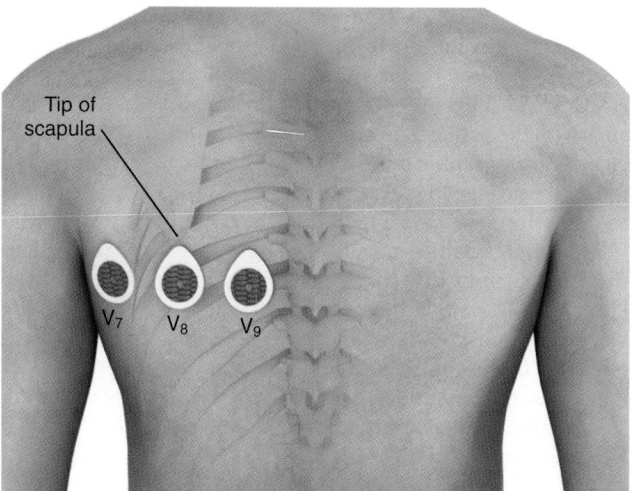

Figure 14-6 Posterior lead placement. Place leads V_7, V_8, and V_9 on the same horizontal plane as V_6, with V_7 at the posterior axillary line, V_8 at the tip of the left scapula, and V_9 near the border of the left paraspinal muscles.

Figure 14-7 Right-sided lead placement. Place right-sided leads V₁R to V₆R on the chest as a mirror image of the standard precordial leads.

Figure 14-8 Right-sided precordial leads. This tracing displays the right-sided precordial leads in an elderly man with chest pain, and they are consistent with acute coronary syndrome. There is ST-segment elevation that is somewhat subtle in the inferior leads (II, III, and aVF), which together with the reciprocal ST-segment depression seen in lead aVL is consistent with a diagnosis of acute inferior myocardial infarction. Leads V_1 to V_6 are in actuality leads V_1R to V_6R—right-sided precordial leads. The convex upward ST-segment elevation seen in leads V_3R to V_6R is indicative of concomitant right ventricular infarction. This patient was found to have a subtotal proximal occlusive lesion of his right coronary artery at cardiac catheterization.

Right-Sided Leads

The right ventricular electrocardiographic electrodes are placed across the right side of the chest in a mirror image of the standard left-sided electrodes and are labeled V_1R to V_6R; alternatively, RV_1 to RV_6 is another commonly used nomenclature for this electrode distribution (Fig. 14-7). Lead V_4R (right fifth intercostal space, midclavicular line) is the most useful lead for detecting ST-segment elevation associated with right ventricular infarction and may be used solely for the evaluation of possible right ventricular infarction. The ST-segment elevation that occurs in association with right ventricular infarction is frequently quite subtle because of the relatively small muscle mass of the right ventricle; at other times the ST-segment elevation is quite prominent, similar in appearance to the ST-segment changes seen with the standard 12 leads (Fig. 14-8).

Invasive Procedural Leads

Patients with severely compromising bradydysrhythmia may require a transvenous pacemaker. In such instances it may be necessary to place the pacing wire without the benefit of fluoroscopy. Advance the wire under electrocardiographic guidance with the patient connected to the limb leads of a grounded electrocardiographic machine and the pacing wire connected to the V lead (see Figs. 15-5 and 15-6). As the electrode enters the superior vena cava and high right atrium, the P wave and QRS complex will be negative. While traversing the atrium, the P wave and QRS complex will become positive, and the latter will become larger as the ventricle is approached. If a balloon-tipped flotation catheter is used, deflate the balloon once it is in the right ventricle. Next, advance it until contact is made with the endocardium and the ventricle is captured. Ventricular wall contact will be indicated by marked ST-segment elevation. Further details regarding emergency cardiac pacing can be found in Chapter 15.

For patients with suspected pericardial effusion who are undergoing urgent pericardiocentesis, an electrocardiographic lead may be placed on the syringe needle. This form of monitoring will assist in correct positioning of the catheter in the pericardial space. Monitor the ST segments while advancing the needle. A sudden appearance of ST-segment elevation indicates that the needle has moved too far internally (i.e., beyond the pericardial space) and has made contact with the epicardium. The emergence of bedside ultrasonography in the ED has made this technique less relevant. Further details regarding pericardiocentesis can be found in Chapter 16.

Body Surface Mapping

An emerging electrocardiographic tool, body surface mapping uses numerous leads to provide a more detailed electrical description of the heart than possible with the 12-lead ECG. The body map ECG that is most commonly used is based on an 80-lead ECG with 64 anterior and 16 posterior leads. This more detailed imaging of the myocardium allows potentially greater diagnostic accuracy in the early detection of STEMI, as well as detection of infarction in more traditionally electrocardiographic "silent" areas of the heart.[31-33]

Clinical information is displayed in three basic formats: a standard 12-lead ECG, an 80-lead ECG (Fig. 14-9), and torso maps (Fig. 14-10). The 80-lead ECG demonstrates a single electrocardiographic P-QRS-T cycle for all 80 leads. In the torso maps, colorimetric imaging is used. Positive structures (i.e., electrocardiographic waveforms located above the baseline) are indicated by red—either a QRS complex with an R wave, an ST segment with elevation, or a prominent upright T wave. Electrocardiographic structures found below the baseline are blue in color—a QRS complex with either prominent Q or S waves, ST-segment depression, or inverted T waves. The color green notes a QRS complex that is isoelectric (i.e., no net positive or negative deflection) and ST segments and T waves that are normal.

The body map ECG should not replace the typical 12-lead ECG in patients with chest pain. It should be used only as a second-tier tool in the evaluation of patients with intermediate to high clinical suspicion for ACS and an unrevealing initial 12-lead ECG. In this instance the clinician is in search of STEMI in electrocardiographically silent areas—namely, the far inferior and lateral walls, the posterior wall, and the right ventricle. Secondary indications include (1) patients with an initially lower suspicion for ACS and a nondiagnostic

Name: William Brady   Patient reference: 99999   Recording Time: October 30, 2006 at 15:53   Analysis BeatView
Age: 29   Gender: Male   Race: White
25 mm/sec   10 mm/mV   0.05–40.0 Hz   60 Hz~

Referring Physician: Brady
Recording Information
  Hospital: UVA
  Department: Emergency
      Department

Analysis Information

Analysed By: AUTO
Date and Time: October 30, 2006 at 15:56
Software Revision: 1.7

Unconfirmed
Signature:
Date:

Heartscape Technologies: PRIME ECG ® Version 1.7:

Figure 14-9 The 80-lead electrocardiogram.

ECG who later demonstrate a significantly positive serum marker and (2) patients with inferior wall STEMI and additional cardiac segment involvement (e.g., inferoposterior STEMI or inferior STEMI with right ventricular infarction). In a recent study, the OCCULT MI (Optimal Cardiovascular Diagnostic Evaluation Enabling Faster Treatment of Myocardial Infarction) study group obtained simultaneous 12-lead and 80-lead ECGs in patients suspected of having ACS. The 80-lead ECG improved the rate of diagnosis of STEMI by an incremental 27.5% when compared with the embedded 12-lead ECG. In this small study, time to percutaneous coronary intervention was markedly longer, however, in the STEMI group evaluated with an 80-lead ECG only (1002 minutes versus 54 minutes, 80 lead versus 12 lead, respectively), although the outcomes were similar.[34]

ALTERNATIVE TECHNIQUES FOR ASSESSMENT OF RHYTHM

Electrocardiographic rhythm assessment depends on a clear signal of both atrial and ventricular electrical activity over a period of time. Although continuous 12-lead electrocardiographic rhythm monitoring has the advantage of recording cardiac activity over multiple leads (thus maximizing atrial and ventricular monitoring), it is often impractical. Moreover, correct identification of the cardiac rhythm on an ECG can be difficult, depending on the clinical setting. Rapid atrial or ventricular rates, especially those above 150 beats/min, often lead to simultaneous or nearly simultaneous deflections that can alter the usual waveforms or cause smaller deflections to be buried within larger ones (such as P waves buried within the QRS complex). In addition, rapid rates result in smaller, narrower waveforms, which makes visual recognition on the ECG challenging. Finally, assessment of atrial activity in general is more difficult because of the smaller electrical impulse and resulting electrocardiographic waveform generated by the atria.

Lead V_1 is generally considered the best lead for detecting the P wave, followed by lead II. In a study of 62 measurements in 28 patients, lead V_1 demonstrated the tallest P wave 53% of the time, followed by lead II (29%), lead I (7%), and lead III (3%).[35] A number of alternative techniques have been developed to improve assessment of rhythm, including

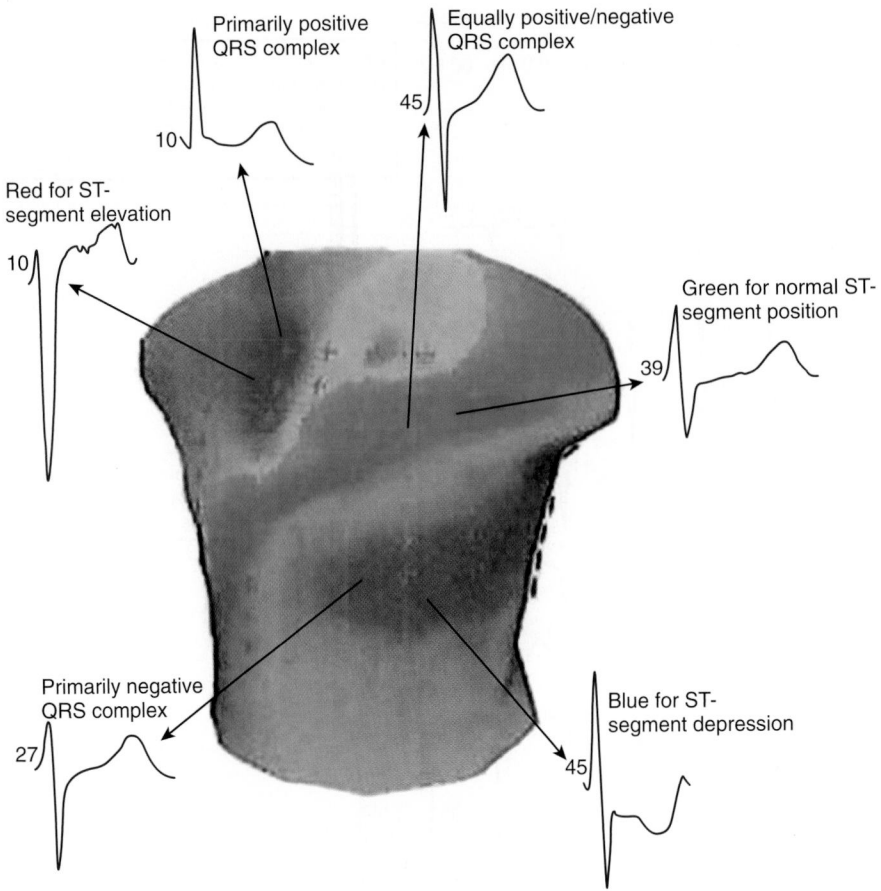

Figure 14-10 Colorimetric interpretation of the torso body map. *Green* indicates either a normal ST segment (i.e., no elevation or depression) or a QRS complex that has a net negative amplitude (neither positive nor negative), *red* shows either ST-segment elevation or a predominantly positive QRS complex, and *blue* shows either ST-segment depression or a predominantly negative QRS complex.

alterations in the standard 12-lead ECG, as well as the addition of nonstandard leads to monitor cardiac and, in particular, atrial rhythm activity.

Alteration in Amplitude and Paper Speed

Most 12-lead electrocardiography machines today allow alteration of both amplitude and paper speed from the basic 10-mm/mV and 25-mm/sec standards, respectively. Increasing the amplitude, most commonly to double the standard, or 20 mm/mV, can increase the prominence of smaller deflections, such as the P wave, and improve recognition of the atrial rhythm (Fig. 14-11). In addition, clinicians have also used photocopy enlargements of the standard ECG to visually enhance smaller deflections.[36]

Increasing the paper speed, again most commonly to double the standard, or 50 mm/sec, has the effect of artificially slowing the rhythm. This technique is most advantageous when assessing patients with marked atrial or ventricular tachycardia. Increasing the paper speed exaggerates any existing irregularity (such as in atrial fibrillation) and can improve recognition of smaller deflections, such as P waves, in the presence of a significant tachycardia. Faster paper speeds also make it possible to measure short electrocardiographic intervals (such as PR or R-R) more accurately (Fig. 14-12).

Accardi and coworkers[37] found that overall diagnostic accuracy improved when clinicians were provided ECGs recorded at the faster 50-mm/sec paper speed, as opposed to

a standard 12-lead ECG, in patients with narrow-complex tachycardia. Moreover, they reported that this improved rhythm assessment probably would have resulted in fewer treatment errors.

Alternative Leads

Assessment of rhythm often requires electrocardiographic monitoring over a longer and continuous period, thus making the standard 12-lead ECG (which requires 10 electrodes) and even unipolar precordial V_1 monitoring (which requires 5 electrodes) not feasible. A number of alternative lead systems requiring fewer electrodes have been described. Many of these systems use the limb bipolar leads (RA, LA, LL) in alternative positions over the chest. Leads I, II, or III are then recorded, depending on the positions of the positive and negative electrodes. *Although various alternative leads provide additional information to the clinician, there are no standard guidelines mandating the use of any alternative leads in the ED. The following leads are rarely used in the ED and are beyond the technical capability of many EDs.*

Lewis Leads
In 1910, Thomas Lewis[38] first described alternative positions for the RA and LL leads to enhance detection of atrial fibrillation. The RA lead was placed over the right second costochondral junction, whereas the LL lead was placed in the right fourth intercostal space 1 inch to the right of the sternum—with the LA and RL leads left in their usual positions. Lewis[38]

Figure 14-11 A, Baseline electrocardiogram (ECG) of a patient before the development of an abnormal rhythm (10 mm/mV). Note the P-wave morphologies, especially in leads I, II, and V_1. **B,** ECG during ectopic atrial tachycardia (10 mm/mV). Note the change in P-wave morphology, especially in lead V_1. **C,** ECG during ectopic atrial tachycardia (20 mm/mV). The P waves are now easier to see in all leads. **D,** ECG after reversion to a normal atrial focus (20 mm/mV). Contrast these accentuated P waves with those in **C.**

Figure 14-12 A, Electrocardiogram (ECG) with tachycardia at normal paper speed (25 mm/sec). Because of the rapid rate, the actual P waves are difficult to discern, thus making determination of the rhythm difficult. The computerized interpretation is sinus tachycardia with a first-degree atrioventricular (AV) block. **B,** ECG with tachycardia at double paper speed (50 mm/sec). With increased paper speed, atrial P-wave activity is accentuated, and atrial flutter with a 2:1 AV block is demonstrated.

TABLE 14-2 Alternative Leads for Assessment of Rhythm

Lead I*	RA = negative electrode	LA = positive electrode
Lead II*	RA = negative electrode	LL = positive electrode
Lead III*	LA = negative electrode	LL = positive electrode
ALTERNATIVE LEAD	**NEGATIVE ELECTRODE POSITION**	**POSITIVE ELECTRODE POSITION**
Lewis†	Right second costochondral junction	Right fourth intercostal space, 1 inch right of the sternum
Drury	Second right costochondral junction Center of the sternum	Seventh right costal cartilage Inferior angle of the scapula 2 inches right of the spine
Schoenwald	Third intercostal space along the right sternal border Third intercostal space along the R sternal border	Left leg Right arm
Lu	1st intercostal space directly above V_1	Approximately 3 inches directly below V_4
Vertical sternal ("Barker leads")	Below the suprasternal notch at the manubrium	Xiphoid process
MCL_1	Left shoulder (1 cm inferior to the left midclavicle)	V_1 (fourth intercostal space, right sternal border)
MCL_6	Left shoulder (1 cm inferior to the left midclavicle)	V_6 (≈sixth rib, midaxillary line)

*First, set the electrocardiographic machine to record the rhythm strip with this lead. If the recording rhythm strip is lead I, the RA wire becomes the negative electrode, which is placed as noted in the table, and the LA wire becomes the positive electrode, which is placed as noted in the table. If lead II or lead III is the lead that is set to record the rhythm strip, the positive and negative electrodes will vary.

†*Example:* One way to record the Lewis lead is to set the electrocardiographic machine to record lead I, use the RA wire as the negative electrode, and place it in the right second costochondral junction. Use the LA wire as the positive electrode and place it in the right fourth intercostal space, 1 inch to the right of the sternum. The Lewis lead may also be recorded on lead II and lead III, but the wires that serve as the positive and negative electrodes will vary.

reported enhancement of atrial activity when the RA served as the negative electrode and LL as the positive electrode (lead II) in this new configuration. Other alternative lead placements to enhance detection of atrial activity have also been described[39-41] (Table 14-2 and Fig. 14-13).

Vertical Sternal "Barker" Leads
In this alternative lead system, the positive electrode is placed at the xiphoid process and the negative electrode is placed just below the suprasternal notch on the manubrium. Herzog and associates[36] reported that vertical sternal leads produce a larger P wave than other systems do, including the Lewis leads. In addition, the vertical sternal leads are placed over bone, which may reduce artifact from muscle activity on recordings (see Fig. 14-13).

Limb-Precordium Leads
A sequential pattern of bipolar leads on the chest, termed *limb-precordium leads*, has been proposed in combination with the original Einthoven limb leads. In this system, standard limb leads are placed on the patient. The RA electrode is then repositioned sequentially at the fourth intercostal space just to the right of the sternum, the fourth intercostal space just to the left of the sternum (low parasternal), the first intercostal space just to the left of the sternum, and the first intercostal space just to the right of the sternum (high parasternal). During this sequential mapping, tracings are recorded for leads I and II until atrial activity is identified. Brenes-Pereira[42] reported that this mapping system allowed the identification of P waves in a majority of patients when none were detected initially on the standard 12-lead ECG.

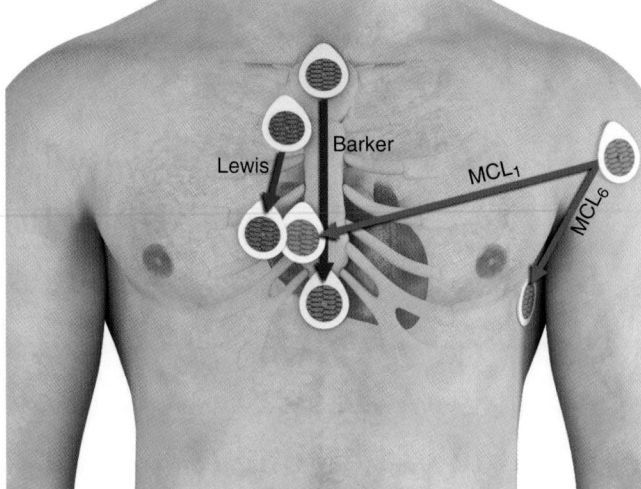

Figure 14-13 Alternative leads. Three of the more commonly used alternative lead strategies for clarification of the atrial rhythm (Lewis leads, vertical sternal or Barker leads, and modified bipolar chest lead 1 [MCL_1]) and monitoring of the ST-T wave (MCL_6) are shown.

Modified Bipolar Chest Leads
Modified bipolar chest leads (MCLs) are the most commonly used leads for monitoring cardiac rhythm. The positive electrode is placed on the chest at a precordial position (V) concordant with the MCL desired (e.g., the V_1 position for MCL_1). The negative electrode is placed on the left shoulder. On standard electrocardiographic machines, the LA electrode is placed at V_1, RA at the left shoulder, LL at V_6, and RL at a remote location on the chest to serve as ground. Lead I

would then reflect MCL$_1$ and lead II, MCL$_6$. MCL$_1$ may be useful in distinguishing atrial activity, MCL$_5$ and MCL$_6$ more commonly in monitoring of the ST-T wave, and both MCL$_1$ and MCL$_6$ in evaluating wide-complex tachycardias[43] (see Fig. 14-13).

Esophageal Leads

The esophageal lead (E) was first described by Brown in the 1930s.[44] Since that time, both unipolar and bipolar esophageal leads have been developed.[45] Because of its posterior location, this lead is often superior in detecting atrial deflections and recording the activity of the posterior surface of the left ventricle. The electrode, which is connected to the ECG by thin wires, is either swallowed or passed through the nares into the esophagus. Once in the esophagus, the location of the electrode is determined either by fluoroscopy or by making a series of low to high esophageal recordings. The position of the electrode in the esophagus is adjusted by slowly pulling the electrode wire out the nares or mouth. In normal adults, leads E$_{15-25}$ (the electrode is located in the esophagus 15 to 25 cm from the nares) generally records atrial activity; E$_{25-35}$, activity of the atrioventricular groove; and E$_{40-50}$, activity of the left ventricular posterior surface. The E lead should be recorded through lead channel I simultaneously with lead channel II and the other surface channels.

Central Venous Catheter Intracardiac Leads

In patients in whom a central venous catheter was placed for vascular access (or for other reasons such as cardiac pacing, hemodialysis, or Swan-Ganz monitoring), that catheter, when filled with saline, can be used as a modified intracardiac electrode for recording of atrial activity. Once filled with saline, a needle was then left in a side access port of the catheter and attached via an alligator clip to lead V$_1$. With this method, the distal port of the saline-filled central venous catheter demonstrated significantly larger P waves than the standard 12-lead ECG and the Lewis lead did.[35]

ELECTRODE MISPLACEMENT AND MISCONNECTION

Limb Electrode Reversal

Although the limb electrodes are not often misplaced, the cables that link them to the ECG are at times improperly connected. This can result in "electrocardiographic changes" that are, in actuality, artifacts. A multitude of possibilities for misconnection of the limb electrodes exists; some of the most probable are summarized here. It is helpful to categorize these possibilities into those that are easily recognizable without comparison to an old ECG versus those that are not. Failure to recognize limb electrode reversal may lead to misattribution of ECG "changes" to a disease that is, in fact, due to technical misadventure. Even though the incidence of electrode reversal in the ED has not been quantified, it has been observed to occur in an intensive care unit setting in 4% to 5% of tracings.[46,47]

Easily Recognizable without an Old ECG

The most common of all misconnections is reversal of the LA and RA electrodes[48] (Fig. 14-14). *The hallmark is a negative P wave and a primarily negative QRS complex in lead I*, which

Figure 14-14 Arm electrode reversal (LA ↔ RA). The most common of limb electrode reversals, the clues lie in leads I and aVR. Lead I features a negative P wave, as well as a principally negative QRS complex and T wave. This could suggest dextrocardia, but the precordial leads demonstrate a normal transition, which is not consistent with dextrocardia. Note also the unusual appearance of aVR in this tracing.

creates a right or extreme axis deviation (depending on the principal vector of the QRS complex in lead aVF). Dextrocardia should also be considered with such findings; the pattern of precordial lead transition will differentiate between dextrocardia and arm electrode reversal, however, with dextrocardia featuring progressive diminution in QRS amplitude as the eye moves from lead V$_1$ (right sided) toward lead V$_6$ (left sided). Moreover, lead aVR is actually aVL in this circumstance, and thus lead aVR may feature both an upright P wave and QRS complex; the former does not occur in normal sinus rhythm, and the latter is clinically unusual—the QRS vectors in leads aVR and V$_6$ are usually opposite unless the heart has a superior frontal-plane axis.[49] A further clue to arm electrode reversal is the resultant discrepancy in the major QRS vectors of leads I and V$_6$. Because the vectors of these two leads are leftward, the QRS complexes are expected to point in similar directions when the ECG is performed properly. These two leads will feature discordant QRS vectors when the arm electrodes are reversed (see Fig. 14-14). Transposition of the RA and LL cables is also easily recognized; all leads are upside down in comparison to the usual patterns, with the exception of aVL, which is unchanged.[48,50]

Anytime that the RL electrode is transposed with another extremity lead, one of the limb leads will appear as virtually a straight line and thus is easily recognized if this finding is not incorrectly ascribed to poor electrode contact or function. The most common is RA/RL reversal,[51] which causes a nearly flat line in lead II (Fig. 14-15). An exception to this rule is if the leg electrodes are reversed (RL ↔ LL), in which case the ECG is virtually identical to one with correct placement of the limb electrodes. Reversal of the leg electrodes is largely insignificant in that the potentials at the left and right legs are essentially the same.[50]

Not Easily Recognizable without an Old ECG

One limb electrode reversal that is not readily recognizable without comparison to a previous tracing is transposition of the LA and LL electrodes. This causes transposition of lead I with lead II on the tracing, as well as lead aVL with aVF. In effect, two inferior leads (II and aVF) have become the lateral leads (I and aVL) and vice versa—thus making this

A   B

Figure 14-15 Right-sided electrode reversal (RA ↔ RL). **A,** In this tracing the nearly flat line in lead II (*arrow*) suggests that the right leg electrode has been switched with the right arm electrode. The trivial voltage in lead II reflects the expected lack of potential difference between the two legs (the right leg electrode is in the right arm position; lead II normally runs from the right arm to the left leg, but now it effectively runs from the right leg to the left leg). **B,** The second tracing was acquired with correct electrode placement.

A   B

Figure 14-16 A, Left-sided limb electrode reversal (LA ↔ LL). A patient with a history consistent with acute coronary syndrome was brought to the emergency department after this electrocardiogram was recorded in a clinic. Leads I and aVL suggest an acute high lateral infarction, but surprisingly, there are no corresponding changes in leads V_5 and V_6. The deep T-wave inversions in III and aVF were at first thought to be inferior ischemia or reciprocal changes (see also **B**). **B,** Correction of electrode reversal (LA ↔ LL). After the electrodes were reconnected, this tracing reveals an acute inferior wall myocardial infarction (MI), as well as deep T-wave inversion in aVL—a harbinger of acute inferior MI. In comparing this tracing with that in *A*, note the following: lead I ↔ lead II, lead aVL ↔ aVF, and lead III is inverted. Thus, inferior changes become lateral, and lateral changes become inferior—the hallmark of LA ↔ LL reversal.

misconnection difficult to detect at times without a baseline ECG for comparison. Furthermore, lead III will be upside down (although a negative QRS complex in lead III is not unusual), and aVR will be unchanged (Fig. 14-16).[50] Suspect LA/LL reversal when comparing two ECGs with changes that do not make clinical sense; if the P-QRS-T–wave morphologies in lead III in the two tracings are mirror opposites, repeat the ECG with close attention to correct electrode connection. Clues to limb electrode reversal are summarized in Table 14-3.

Precordial Electrode Misplacement and Misconnection

Unlike the limb electrodes, the precordial electrodes are more prone to misplacement, especially when variations in body habitus (e.g., obesity, breast tissue, pectus excavatum, chronic lung disease) make proper electrode placement more difficult. This may cause some variability in the amplitude and morphology of the complexes in the precordial leads. However, these changes are not usually grossly abnormal and therefore can be difficult to detect. Variation often becomes evident when comparing the current tracing with an old ECG.[50] In such cases it is useful to go to the bedside and examine where

the electrodes were positioned relative to the recommended placement (see "Electrode Placement" earlier in this chapter). One cannot ensure, however, that the baseline ECG was done with proper electrode placement. When comparing the precordial leads on the current ECG with a baseline tracing, ST-segment and T-wave changes should be viewed in the context of the relative morphologies of the associated QRS complexes. If a marked difference is noted between the two tracings in the amplitude or polarity of the QRS complex in a given precordial lead—the R/S ratio for that QRS complex—the corresponding ST-T-wave changes may be due to variability in electrode placement, although cardiac ischemia cannot be completely excluded as the cause.

Some studies have reported that placement of chest electrodes by more than 20 to 25 mm from the standard positions can be associated with clinically significant changes on the ECG. It has been observed that leads V_1 and V_2 are typically placed too high and that the lateral leads are placed too laterally and too low. McCann and colleagues[52] demonstrated a high degree of variability between experienced clinicians in identifying anatomic landmarks for precordial electrocardiographic electrode placement. There was frequently a large difference in the measured distance from the actual to the "standardized" electrode position that ranged between 0 and

TABLE 14-3 Clues to Improper Limb Electrode Connections

REVERSED LEADS	NEED OLD ECG FOR DETECTION?	KEY FINDINGS
LA ↔ RA	No	P-QRS-T waves upside down in lead I Precordial leads normal (not dextrocardia)
LA ↔ LL	Yes	III upside down from baseline I ↔ II, aVL ↔ aVF, no change in aVR
LA ↔ RL	No	III is a straight line
RA ↔ LL	No	P-QRS-T waves upside down in all leads except aVL
RA ↔ RL	No	II is a straight line
LL ↔ RL	Cannot detect change	Looks like normal electrode placement
LA ↔ LL + RA ↔ RL	No	I is a straight line aVL and aVR are the same polarity and amplitude and II is upside down III

From Surawicz B, Knilans TK. *Chou's Electrocardiography in Clinical Practice*, 5th ed. Philadelphia: Saunders; 2001.
LA, left arm; *LL*, left leg; *RA*, right arm; *RL*, right leg.

A   B

Figure 14-17 A and **B,** Precordial electrode reversal (V₂ ↔ V₃). Note that the usual precordial progression of R-wave growth in leads V₂ and V₃ is disrupted in the tracing displayed in **A. B** shows a return to a normal V₃ transition zone.

105 mm in the vertical direction (mean, 14 mm; median, 10 mm) and between 0 and 120 mm in the horizontal plane (mean, 17 mm; median, 10 mm). Overall, 20.8% of the paired measurements in the vertical direction and 26.6% of those in the horizontal plane differed by more than 25 mm.

Misconnection of the precordial cables is usually easy to detect. The expected progression of P-, QRS-, and T-wave morphologies across the precordium will be disrupted (Fig. 14-17). An abrupt change in wave morphology evolution—followed by a seeming return to normalcy in the next lead—is a good clue to misconnection of the precordial electrodes.[50]

ARTIFACT

Electrocardiographic artifact is commonly encountered yet not always easy to recognize. It can be attributed to either physiologic (internal) or nonphysiologic (external) sources; the former includes muscle activity, patient motion, and poor electrode contact with the skin. Tremors, hiccups, and shivering may produce frequent, narrow spikes on the tracing and simulate atrial and ventricular dysrhythmias[48,53] (Fig. 14-18).

Figure 14-18 Artifact secondary to a physiologic cause. The patient's monitor was alarming because of a perceived heart rate greater than 200 beats/min, and the computerized alert system called this ventricular tachycardia. The patient, who has Parkinson's disease, was without complaint. The electrocardiogram demonstrates a marked artifact that is giving the appearance of atrial flutter in lead V₁.

Figure 14-19 Artifact secondary to rigors. This tracing features a pseudodysrhythmia. The intrinsic RR interval can be traced back through the "dysrhythmia" and reveals an underlying sinus rhythm. The patient was clinically stable and asymptomatic during the event, except for his rigors.

A wandering baseline featuring wide undulations, as well as other "noise" on the ECG, can often be traced to patient movement and high skin impedance, which leads to inadequate contact of the electrode with the skin. Minimizing skin impedance and artifact may be achieved by (1) avoiding electrode placement over bony prominences, major muscles, or pulsating arteries; (2) clipping rather than shaving thick hair at electrode sites; and (3) cleaning and, most importantly, drying the skin surface before reapplying the electrode if the tracing features substantial artifact.[48,54] Nonphysiologic artifact is most often due to 60-Hz electrical interference, which is ascribable to various other sources of alternating current near the patient. This will be manifested as a wide, indistinct isoelectric baseline. Electrocardiographic artifact should be considered when the clinical picture indicates stability and status quo and coincident procedures are in progress (e.g., hemodialysis, blood warmer, bronchoscopy) or devices are in use (e.g., nerve stimulators)—the list of causative equipment is long and varied.[55] Other sources of nonphysiologic artifact include those attributable to the monitoring equipment: loose connections, broken monitor cables, and mechanical issues with the machine (e.g., broken stylus, uneven paper transport). The 60-Hz artifact caused by electrical current interference can be minimized by shutting off nonessential sources of current in the vicinity, as well as by straightening the lead wires so that they are parallel to the patient's body in the long axis.[48,53,56]

Differentiation of artifact from true electrocardiographic abnormality is intuitively important; moreover, clinical consequences have been reported that are directly attributable to confusion of artifact with disease. Unnecessary treatment and procedures—including cardiac catheterization, electrophysiologic testing, and even implantation of a pacemaker and an automatic defibrillator—have been reported.[57] Characteristics that may aid in differentiating artifact from dysrhythmia include the absence of hemodynamic instability during the event (or even absence of any symptoms), normal QRS complexes occurring during the "dysrhythmia," instability of the baseline on the tracing during and immediately after the "dysrhythmic" event, association with body movement, and observance of "notches" amid the complexes of the pseudodysrhythmia that "march out" with the normal QRS complexes that precede and follow the disturbance[58,59] (Fig. 14-19).

References are available at www.expertconsult.com

CHAPTER 15

Emergency Cardiac Pacing

Edward S. Bessman

The purpose of cardiac pacing is to restore or ensure effective cardiac depolarization. Emergency cardiac pacing may be instituted either prophylactically or therapeutically. Prophylactic indications include patients with a high risk for atrioventricular (AV) block. Therapeutic indications include symptomatic bradyarrhythmias and overdrive pacing. Pacing for asystole has very minimal success but has been used for this condition. Several approaches to pacing can be taken, including transcutaneous, transvenous, transthoracic, epicardial, endocardial, and esophageal. Transcutaneous and transvenous are the two techniques most commonly used in the emergency department (ED). Because it can be instituted quickly and noninvasively, transcutaneous pacing is the technique of choice in the ED when time is of the essence. Transvenous pacing should be reserved for patients who require prolonged pacing or have a very high (>30%) risk for heart block. Transcutaneous pacing is generally a temporizing measure that may precede transvenous cardiac pacing. Although it is not an expectation that all emergency clinicians will be adept at placing emergency cardiac pacemakers, many have mastered the techniques and are often the only clinicians available to perform this lifesaving procedure.

EMERGENCY TRANSVENOUS CARDIAC PACING

The transvenous method of endocardial pacing is commonly used and is both safe and effective. In skilled hands, the semifloating transvenous catheter is successfully placed under electrocardiographic (ECG) guidance in 80% of patients.[1] The technique can be performed in less than 20 minutes in 72% of patients and in less than 5 minutes in 30%. However, in some instances, anatomic, logistic, and hemodynamic impediments can prohibit successful pacing by even the most skilled clinician. As with other medical procedures, it should not be performed without a thorough understanding of its indications, contraindications, and complications.[2]

However, because this procedure is essentially performed in a blind manner, sometimes it will not be successful. This may be because the condition is not amenable to pacing (e.g., asystole, drug overdose) or because of technical difficulties inherent with the procedure.

Background

The ability of muscle to be artificially depolarized was recognized as early as the 18th century. Initial efforts focused on the transcutaneous approach (see later in this section). Over the succeeding years several scattered experiments were reported, and in 1951 Callaghan and Bigelow first used the transvenous approach to stimulate asystolic hearts in hypothermic dogs.[3]

Furman and Robinson demonstrated the transvenous endocardial approach in humans in 1958.[4] They treated two patients with complete heart block and Stokes-Adams seizures, thus reconfirming that low-voltage pacing could completely control myocardial depolarization. The catheter remained in the second patient for 96 days without complication. Other early clinical studies also demonstrated the utility of transvenous pacing.[5] Fluoroscopic guidance was used for placement of the pacing catheter in all these studies.

In 1964 Vogel and coworkers demonstrated the use of a flexible catheter passed without fluoroscopic guidance for intracardiac electrocardiography.[6] One year later, Kimball and Killip used this technique to insert endocardial pacemakers at the bedside.[7] They noted technical problems in 20% of their patients, including intermittent capture, difficulty passing the catheter, and catheter knotting. During the same year, Harris and colleagues confirmed the ease and speed with which this procedure could be accomplished.[8]

Before 1965 all intracardiac pacing was done asynchronously, which meant that the pacing catheter could cause electrical stimulation during any phase of the cardiac cycle. Asynchronous pacing frequently resulted in the pacemaker firing during the vulnerable period of an intrinsic depolarization; this occasionally caused ventricular tachycardia or fibrillation. In 1967 a demand pacemaker generator that sensed intrinsic depolarizations and inhibited the pacemaker for a predetermined period was used successfully by Zuckerman and associates in six patients.[9] Since then there has been steady progress in the design and functionality of pacemakers. Table 15-1 summarizes the four-letter code that is used to describe modern pacemakers (there is a fifth letter for combined pacemaker-cardioverter/defibrillators). The most commonly used emergency transvenous pacemaker is represented by the code VVI: the ventricle is paced, the ventricle is sensed, and when a native impulse is sensed, the pacemaker is inhibited. Dual-chamber pacing (DDD or DDDR) is the preferred methodology for permanent pacing but is rarely used on an emergency basis because of the increased complexity of the procedure.

Rosenberg and coworkers introduced an improved pacing catheter known as the Elecath semifloating pacing wire.[1] The Elecath was stiffer than the Flexon steel wire electrode that was in prevailing use. Rosenberg and coworkers[1] achieved pacing in 72% of their patients with an average procedure time of 18 minutes. They also noted that 30% of their patients were paced in 5 minutes or less. In 1970, Swan and Ganz introduced the technique of heart catheterization with a flow-directed balloon-tipped catheter.[10] Schnitzler and colleagues successfully used this method for placement of a right ventricular pacemaker in 15 of 17 patients.[11]

In 1981 Lang and associates compared bedside use of the flow-directed balloon-tipped catheter with insertion of a semirigid electrode catheter in 111 perfusing patients.[12] These researchers found a significantly shorter insertion time (6 minutes 45 seconds versus 13 minutes 30 seconds), a lower incidence of serious arrhythmias (1.5% versus 20.4%), and a lower incidence of catheter displacement (13.4% versus 32%) with the balloon-tipped catheter. They concluded that the balloon-tipped catheter was the method of choice for temporary transvenous pacing (Table 15-2).

Transvenous Cardiac Pacing

Indications

Bradycardias
  Symptomatic sinus node dysfunction
  Second- and third-degree heart block
  Atrial fibrillation with a slow ventricular response
  With myocardial infarction: new left bundle branch block,
    bifasicular block, alternating bundle branch block
  Malfunction of an implanted pacemaker
Tachycardias
  Supraventricular dysrhythmias
  Ventricular dysrhythmias

Contraindications

Prosthetic tricuspid valve
Severe hypothermia

Complications

Inadvertent arterial puncture
Venous thrombosis/thrombophlebitis
Pneumothorax/other anatomic injury
Ventricular arrhythmia
Misplacement of the pacing catheter
Myocardial/pericardial perforation
Entanglement of the pacing catheter

Equipment

The contents of a typical transvenous pacemaker kit are shown here. Additional equipment required for insertion of the sheath introducer is reviewed in Chapter 22. Individual kits may vary by manufacturer; be familiar with the equipment available at your institution before performing the procedure.

Review Box 15-1 Transvenous cardiac pacing: indications, contraindications, complications, and equipment.

TABLE 15-1 Four-Letter Pacemaker Code

FIRST LETTER	SECOND LETTER	THIRD LETTER	FOURTH LETTER
Chamber Paced	Chamber Sensed	Sensing Response	Programmability
A = Atrium	A = Atrium	T = triggered	P = Simple
V = Ventricle	V = Ventricle	I = Inhibited	M = Multiprogrammable
D = Dual	D = Dual	D = Dual (A triggered and V inhibited)	R = Rate adaptive
O = None	O = None	O = None	C = Communicating
			O = None

Birkhahn and coworkers retrospectively compared the experience of emergency physicians with that of cardiologists in placing transvenous pacemakers under ECG guidance.[13] They reported a 13% risk for major complications in both groups of specialists. They concluded that pacemaker placement by emergency physicians under ECG guidance without fluoroscopy had success and complication rates that were comparable to those of their cardiology colleagues.

Indications

The purpose of cardiac pacing is to stimulate effective cardiac depolarization. In most cases the specific indications for cardiac pacing are clear; however, some areas are still controversial. The decision to pace on an emergency basis requires knowledge of the presence or absence of hemodynamic compromise, the cause of the rhythm disturbance, the status of the AV conduction system, and the type of dysrhythmia. *The clinician caring for the patient is in the best position to decide on the value, or nonvalue, of pacing based on nuances of the clinical scenario that are not possible to unravel by any theoretical discussion.* Controversy exists throughout the literature, and this discussion *is not meant to set a standard of care for individual circumstances.*

In general, the indications can be grouped into those that cause either tachycardias or bradycardias (see Review Box 15-1). Transcutaneous cardiac pacing (TCP) has become the mainstay of emergency cardiac pacing and is often used pending placement of a transvenous catheter or to determine whether potentially terminal bradyasystolic rhythms will respond to pacing.

TABLE 15-2	History of Transvenous Pacing	
DATE	**INVESTIGATOR**	**EVENT**
1700	Early investigators	First restimulation studies
1951	Callaghan and Bigelow	First transvenous approach in dogs
1952	Zoll	Transcutaneous cardiac stimulator
1958	Falkmann and Walkins	Implanted pacing wires after surgery
1959	Furman and Robinson	First transvenous pacer in humans
1964	Vogel et al.	Flexible electrocardiographic catheter without fluoroscopy
1965	Kimball and Killip	First bedside transvenous pacing
1966	Goetz et al.	Demand pacemaker developed
1967	Zuckerman et al.	Use of a demand pacemaker clinically
1969	Rosenberg et al.	Semifloating pacing catheter
1973	Schnitzler et al.	Balloon-tipped pacers

Bradycardias
Sinus Node Dysfunction
Sinus node dysfunction may be manifested as sinus arrest, tachybrady (sick sinus) syndrome, or sinus bradycardia. Although symptomatic sinus node dysfunction is a common indication for elective permanent pacing, it is seldom cause for emergency pacemaker insertion.

Seventeen percent of patients with acute myocardial infarction (AMI) will experience sinus bradycardia.[14] It occurs more frequently with inferior than with anterior infarction and has a relatively good prognosis when accompanied by a hemodynamically tolerable escape rhythm. However, sinus bradycardia is not a benign rhythm in this situation; it has a mortality rate of 2% with inferior infarction and 9% with anterior infarction.[15] Sinus node dysfunction frequently responds to medical therapy but requires prompt pacing if such therapy fails.

Asystolic Arrest
Transvenous pacing in an asystolic or bradyasystolic patient has little value and is not recommended.[16] In a study of 13 patients who had suffered cardiac arrest, capture of the myocardium was noted in 4 patients, but there were no survivors.[17] Transvenous pacing alone may also not be effective for post-countershock pulseless bradyarrhythmias.[18] This failure of pacing has likewise been demonstrated with transcutaneous pacemakers, thus suggesting that failure of effective pacing is primarily related to the state of the myocardial tissue.[17] Cardiac pacing may be used as a "last-ditch" effort in bradyasystolic patients but is rarely successful and is not considered standard practice. Early pacing is essential when done for this purpose if success is to be achieved[19] (see later in this section). Most importantly, given the continued emphasis on the importance of maximizing chest compressions during cardiopulmonary resuscitation (CPR), interrupting CPR to institute emergency pacing is not recommended.[20]

AV Block
AV block is the classic indication for pacemaker therapy. In symptomatic patients without myocardial infarction (MI) and in asymptomatic patients with a ventricular rate lower than 40 beats/min, pacemaker therapy is indicated.[21]

In patients with AMI, 15% to 19% progress to heart block: first-degree block develops in approximately 8%, second-degree block in 5%, and third-degree block in 6%.[22] First-degree block progresses to second- or third-degree block 33% of the time, and second-degree block progresses to third-degree block about one third of the time.[23]

AV block occurring during anterior infarction is believed to result from diffuse ischemia in the septum and infranodal conduction tissue. Because these patients tend to progress to high-degree block without warning, a pacemaker is often placed prophylactically. Some patients are prophylactically paced on a temporary basis, even in the absence of hemodynamic compromise.

During inferior infarction, early septal ischemia is the exception and typically block develops sequentially from first-degree to Mobitz type I second-degree and then to third-degree AV block. These conduction abnormalities frequently result in hemodynamically tolerable escape rhythms because of sparing of the bundle branches. A hemodynamically unstable patient who is unresponsive to medical therapy should be paced promptly. Whether and when stable patients should be paced is unclear, but placing a transcutaneous pacer is one option that can be attempted before placing a transvenous pacing catheter.

Trauma
Pacing is not a standard intervention in traumatic cardiac arrest, but in selected cases it may be considered. Several rhythm and conduction disturbances have been documented in patients with nonpenetrating chest trauma. In these patients, traumatic injury to the specialized conduction system may predispose to life-threatening dysrhythmias and blocks that can be treated by cardiac pacing.[24]

Hypovolemia and hypotension can cause ischemia of conduction tissue and cardiac dysfunction.[25] Marked bradyarrhythmias that persist even after vigorous volume replacement may rarely respond to cardiac pacing in patients with such trauma.[26]

Bundle Branch Block and Ischemia
Bundle branch block occurring in AMI is associated with a higher mortality rate and a greater incidence of third-degree heart block than is uncomplicated infarction. Atkins and colleagues noted that 18% of patients with MI had bundle branch block.[27] Of these patients, complete heart block developed in 43% who had right bundle branch block (RBBB) and left axis deviation, in 17% who had left bundle branch block (LBBB), in 19% who had left anterior hemiblock, and in 6% who had no conduction block. The investigators concluded that RBBB with left axis deviation should be paced prophylactically.

TABLE 15-3 Influence of Different Variables on the Risk for High-Degree AVB in Patients with BBB during MI

PATIENTS	PROGRESSING TO HIGH-DEGREE AVB (%)
Infarct location	
Anterior	25
Indeterminate	12
Inferior or posterior	20
PR interval	
>0.20 sec	25
≤0.20 sec	19
Type of BBB	
LBBB	13
RBBB	14
RBBB + LAFB	27
RBBB + LPFB	29
ABBB	44
Onset of BBB	
Definitely old	13
Possibly new	25
Probably new	26
Definitely new	23

From American Heart Association from Hindman MC, Wagner GS, JaRo M, et al. The clinical significance of bundle branch block complicating acute myocardial infarction. 2. Indications of temporary and permanent pacemaker insertion. *Circulation.* 1978;58:690.
ABBB, alternating bundle branch block; *AVB,* atrioventricular block; *BBB,* bundle branch block; *LAFB,* left anterior fascicular hemiblock; *LBBB,* left bundle branch block; *LPFB,* left posterior fascicular hemiblock; *MI,* myocardial infarction; *RBBB,* right bundle branch block.

A study by Hindman and associates confirmed the natural history of bundle branch block during MI.[28] In their study the presence or absence of first-degree AV block, the type of bundle branch block, and the age of the block (new versus old) were used to determine the relative risk for progression to type II second-degree or third-degree block (Table 15-3).

Because of the increased risk, consider pacing for the following conduction blocks: *new-onset* LBBB, RBBB with left axis deviation or other bifascicular block, and alternating bundle-branch block.[28] Though controversial, one authority recommends prophylactic pacing for all new bundle branch blocks when MI is evident.[29]

Whether to place a transvenous pacemaker prophylactically in patients with LBBB before insertion of a flow-directed pulmonary artery catheter (PAC) remains controversial. Some researchers strongly advocate this procedure because of the risk for transient RBBB and life-threatening complete heart block associated with PAC placement.[30] One study noted that this risk is low in patients with previous LBBB but continued to recommend temporary catheter placement for all cases of *new* LBBB.[31] One solution to this problem is to place a transcutaneous pacemaker before catheterization as an emergency measure should heart block develop. In these cases a temporary transvenous pacemaker can be placed in a semi-elective manner when needed.[32] In any event, the trend toward decreased PAC use, particularly outside the critical care setting, makes it unlikely that this will be an issue in the ED.[33]

One final point to bear in mind regarding bradydysrhythmias in the setting of AMI is that most of the studies investigating temporary pacing were done in the era before the use of thrombolytic agents or percutaneous coronary angioplasty. Modern treatment of AMI is substantially different, but more recent studies, particularly those involving prophylactic pacing, are lacking.

Tachycardias

Hemodynamically compromising tachycardias are usually treated by medical means or electrical cardioversion. Since 1980 there has been increasing interest in pacing therapy for symptomatic tachycardias. Supraventricular dysrhythmias, with the exception of atrial fibrillation, respond well to atrial pacing. By "overdrive" pacing the atria at rates 10 to 20 beats/min faster than the underlying rhythm, the atria become entrained, and when the rate is slowed, the rhythm frequently returns to normal sinus. A similar procedure is done for ventricular dysrhythmias.[34] Overdrive pacing is especially useful for arrhythmias with recurrent prolonged QT intervals such as those seen with quinidine toxicity or torsades de pointes.[35] Though an attractive thought, there is no reported experience with these techniques in the ED. Transvenous pacing is also useful in patients with digitalis-induced dysrhythmias, in whom direct current cardioversion may be dangerous, or in patients in whom there is further concern about myocardial depression with drugs.[36]

Cardiac Pacing for Drug-Induced Dysrhythmias

Significant dysrhythmias can be caused by excessive therapeutic medication (often in combination therapy) and overdose of cardioactive medications. Because these drugs have direct effects on cells of the myocardial pacemaker and conduction system, *cardiac pacing is usually of little therapeutic value.* Both bradycardias and tachycardias may result. Tachycardic rhythms from amphetamines, cocaine, anticholinergics, cyclic antidepressants, theophylline, and other drugs do not benefit from cardiac pacing. Drug-induced torsades de pointes may theoretically be overdriven by pacing, but data on this technique are lacking. Any drug that affects the central nervous system (e.g., opiates, sedative-hypnotics, clonidine) may produce bradycardia. Uncommon causes of toxin-induced bradycardia include organophosphate poisoning, various cholinergic drugs, ciguatera poisoning, and rarely, plant toxins. Cardiac pacing is not used for bradycardias from these sources; rather, the underlying central nervous system depression is addressed.

Severe bradycardia and heart block often accompany overdose of digitalis preparations, β-adrenergic blockers, and calcium channel blockers. Although intuitively attractive, *cardiac pacing is not generally effective for serious toxin-induced bradycardias,* even though there have been case reports of success.[37-40] In β-blocker overdose, pacing may increase the heart rate but rarely benefits blood pressure or cardiac output. Worsening of blood pressure may occur as a result of loss of atrial contractions with ventricular pacing. Likewise, calcium channel blocker overdose and digitalis-induced bradycardia and heart block rarely benefit from cardiac pacing. Pharmacologic interventions, such as digoxin-specific Fab, glucagon, calcium, inotropic medications, and vasopressors, remain the mainstay in the treatment of drug-induced dysrhythmias. Given the lack of success of pacing, possible downsides, and the greater effectiveness of specific antidotes, it is not standard to routinely attempt transvenous cardiac pacing in the setting of drug overdose. However, as a last resort, cardiac pacing can be supported.[41]

Contraindications

The presence of a prosthetic tricuspid valve is generally considered to be an absolute contraindication to transvenous cardiac pacing.[42] Also, severe hypothermia will occasionally result in ventricular fibrillation when pacing is attempted. Because ventricular fibrillation under these conditions is difficult to convert, caution is advised when considering pacing severely hypothermic and bradycardiac patients. Rapid and careful rewarming is often recommended first, followed by pacing if the patient's condition does not improve.

Equipment

Several items are required to insert a transvenous pacemaker adequately. Like most special procedures, a prearranged tray is convenient. The usual components required to insert a transvenous cardiac pacemaker are depicted in Review Box 15-1.

Pacing Generator

Many different pacing generators are available, but in general they all have the same basic features. The controls will frequently have a locking feature or cover to prevent the generator from being switched off or reprogrammed inadvertently. An amperage control allows the operator to vary the amount of electrical current delivered to the myocardium, usually 0.1 to 20 mA. *Increasing* the setting *increases* the output and *improves* the likelihood of capture. The pacing control mode is determined by adjusting the gain setting for the sensing function of the generator. By increasing the sensitivity, one can convert the unit from a fixed-rate (asynchronous mode) to a demand (synchronous mode) pacemaker. The typical pacing generator has a sensitivity setting that ranges from about 0.5 to 20 mV. The voltage setting represents the minimum strength of electrical signal that the pacer is able to detect. *Decreasing* the setting *increases* the sensitivity and *improves* the likelihood of sensing myocardial depolarization. In the fixed-rate mode the unit fires despite the underlying intrinsic rhythm; that is, the unit does not sense any intrinsic electrical activity. In the full-demand mode, however, the pacemaker senses the underlying ventricular depolarizations, and the unit does not fire as long as the patient's ventricular rate is equal to or faster than the set rate of the pacing generator. A sensing indicator meter and a rate control knob are also present.

Temporary pacing generators are battery operated, and thus it is always good practice to install a fresh battery whenever pacing is anticipated. An example of a pacing generator is shown in Figure 15-1.

Pacing Catheters and Electrodes

Several sizes and brands of pacing catheters are available. In general, most range from 3 to 5 Fr in size and are approximately 100 cm in length. Lines are marked along the catheter surface at approximately 10-cm intervals and can be used to estimate catheter position during insertion. Pacing catheters differ with respect to their stiffness, electrode configurations, floating characteristics, and other qualities. For emergency pacing, the semifloating bipolar electrode catheter with a

Figure 15-1 Pacemaker energy source: controls and connections.

Figure 15-2 Balloon-tipped pacing catheter.

balloon tip is used most frequently (Fig. 15-2). The balloon holds approximately 1.5 mL of air, and the air injection port has a locking lever to secure balloon expansion. Before insertion, the balloon is checked for leakage of air by inflating and immersing it in sterile water. The presence of an air leak is noted by a stream of bubbles rising to the surface of the water. An inflated balloon helps the catheter "float" into the heart, even in low-flow states, but is obviously not advantageous in the cardiac arrest situation.

For all practical purposes, temporary transvenous pacing is accomplished with a bipolar pacing catheter. The terms *unipolar* and *bipolar* refer to the number of electrodes in contact with the portion of the heart that is to be stimulated. All pacemaker systems must have both a positive (anode) and a negative (cathode) electrode; hence, *all stimulation is bipolar*. In the typical bipolar catheter used for temporary transvenous pacing, the cathode (stimulating electrode) is at the tip of the pacing catheter. The anode is located 1 to 2 cm proximal to the tip, and a balloon or an insulated wire separates the two electrodes. The distinction between unipolar and bipolar pacing catheters is that a bipolar catheter has both electrodes in relatively close proximity on the catheter and both may contact the endocardium. In a bipolar catheter, the electrodes are usually stainless steel or platinum rings that encircle the pacing catheter. When properly positioned, both electrodes will be within the right ventricle so that a field of electrical excitation is set up between the electrodes. With a bipolar catheter, the cathode does not need to be in direct contact with the endocardium for pacing to occur, although it is preferable to have direct contact.

A unipolar system is also effective but is used infrequently for temporary transvenous pacing. In a unipolar system, the cathode is at the tip of the pacing catheter and the anode is located in one of three places: in the pacing generator itself, more proximally on the catheter (outside the ventricle), or on the patient's chest. A bipolar system may be converted to a unipolar system by simply disconnecting the positive proximal connection of the bipolar catheter from the pacing generator and running a new wire from the positive (pacing generator) terminal to the patient's chest wall. Such a conversion may be required in the unlikely event of failure of one lead of the bipolar system.

ECG Machine

An ECG machine can be used to record the heart's inherent electrical activity during insertion of the pacer and to aid in localization of the tip of the catheter without fluoroscopy. The ECG machine must be well grounded to prevent leakage of alternating current, which can cause ventricular fibrillation. Such leakage should be suspected if interference of 50 to 60 cycles per second (Hz) is noted on the ECG tracing.

The ECG machine should be placed in a manner that allows easy visibility of the rhythm during insertion. One method is to place the machine near the level of the patient's midthorax facing the operator, on either side of the patient as logistics and operator preference allow (Fig. 15-3). Note that the operator stands at the head of the patient during passage of the catheter through the internal jugular or subclavian vein and at the midabdomen for insertion through the femoral or brachiocephalic vein. Newer patient monitors may be equipped with suitable ECG connections to allow their use in place of a stand-alone ECG machine. Because these patients will already be attached to a monitor, it may prove convenient to use the same piece of equipment to assist in insertion of the pacemaker.

Introducer Sheath

An introducer set or sheath is required for venous access (see Chapter 22). Some pacing catheters are prepackaged with the appropriate equipment, whereas others require a separate set. The introducer set is used to enhance passage of the pacing catheter through the skin, subcutaneous tissue, and vessel wall. The sheath must be larger than the pacing catheter to allow it to pass. The size of the pacing catheter refers to its outside diameter, whereas the size of the introducer refers to its inside diameter. Thus, a 5-Fr pacing catheter will fit through a 5-Fr introducer. Introducer sheaths are available with a perforated elastic seal covering the opening through which the pacing catheter is passed (pacer port). The seal allows the catheter to be manipulated while preventing blood from escaping or air from entering the vein. A side port allows the sheath to be used for central venous access. A makeshift sheath can be fashioned with an appropriately sized

intravenous (IV) catheter. For a 3-Fr balloon-tipped catheter, a 14-gauge 1.5- to 2-inch IV catheter is suitable. A 4-Fr balloon-tipped catheter will also fit through a 14-gauge catheter or needle. However, without a seal over the hub, blood will leak from the end of the IV catheter.

Overall, the key to success with this procedure is preparation. In a typical ED there are often a variety of vascular access kits and devices, not all of which will work well, if at all, for passing a pacing catheter. It is imperative that one examine all the components of the tray before starting the procedure to ensure that all wires, sheaths, dilators, and syringes fit as expected. Ideally, all the equipment and accessories needed for emergency pacemaker insertion should be kept together in a designated location.

Procedure

A checklist for the preparation and initial setup of a pacing generator is shown in Box 15-1. It may be useful to have a copy of this checklist or a similar list stored with the pacemaker to have on hand in emergency situations.

Patient Preparation

Patient instruction is an extremely important aspect of any procedure. Frequently, there is not enough time to give patients a detailed explanation or to obtain written informed consent. Nonetheless, sufficient information should be provided so that the patient feels at ease. It is always prudent to obtain and document informed consent from the patient, if possible, before any invasive procedure or to document that the circumstances did not allow informed consent. Patients should be assured that they will feel no discomfort after the venipuncture site has been anesthetized and that they will feel better when the catheter is in place and is functional. Continued reassurance is required during the procedure because patients are usually facing away from the operator and their faces are often covered; thus they may be unsure of what is

Figure 15-3 Position of an electrocardiographic device during insertion of a pacemaker catheter through the left subclavian vein.

occurring. Sedation and analgesia should be considered when appropriate.

All operators should wear surgical masks, caps, gloves, and gowns to decrease the risk for infection before catheter placement. Patients should be prepared and draped in the usual sterile fashion. This aseptic precaution should also be explained to the patient.

Site Selection

The four venous channels that provide easy access to the right ventricle are the brachial, subclavian, femoral, and internal

---

BOX 15-1 **Checklist for a Temporary Transvenous Pacing Generator***

- Insert a new battery.
- Turn the pacemaker ON.
- Set the RATE (80 beats/min), OUTPUT (5 mA), and SENSITIVITY (3 mV).[†]
- Connect the patient cable to the pacemaker.
- Open both connector terminals on the patient cable.
- Insert the PROXIMAL (+) pin of the pacing catheter into the POSITIVE (+) connector terminal on the patient cable.
- Tighten the connection firmly.
- Use alligator clips to connect the DISTAL (−) pin of the pacing catheter to lead V_1 of electrocardiographic machine.
- When the catheter is in position, remove the DISTAL (−) pin from V_1 and insert it into the NEGATIVE (−) connector terminal on the patient cable.
- Tighten the connection firmly.

*Adjust pacemaker settings as needed to achieve proper capture and sensitivity (see text).
[†]Guidelines only. Follow the recommendations of the device's manufacturer if different.

---

jugular veins (Table 15-4). The route selected is often one of personal or institutional preference. *The right internal jugular and left subclavian veins have the straightest anatomic pathway to the right ventricle and are generally preferred for temporary transvenous pacing* (Fig. 15-4). In some centers a particular site is preferred for permanent transvenous pacemaker placement, and if possible, this site should be avoided for temporary placement.

The subclavian vein can be accessed through both an infraclavicular and a supraclavicular approach; the infraclavicular approach is most commonly reported for all temporary transvenous pacemaker insertions. This route is preferred because of its easy accessibility, close proximity to the heart, and ease in catheter maintenance and stability. The supraclavicular approach has been described in the literature for several years and has gained popularity among some clinicians.[43,44]

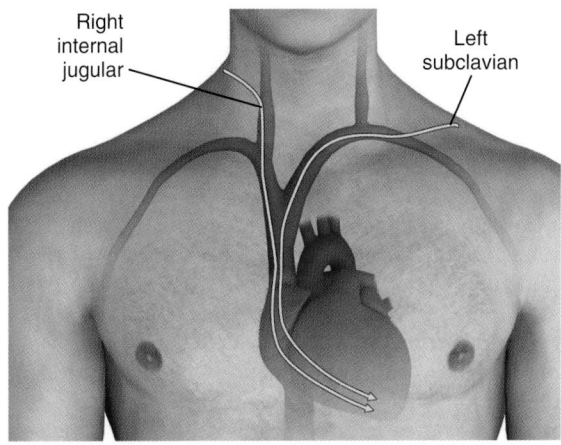

Figure 15-4 The right internal jugular and left subclavian veins have the straightest anatomic pathway to the right ventricle and are generally preferred for temporary transvenous pacing.

TABLE 15-4   Advantages and Disadvantages of Pacemaker Placement Sites

VENOUS CHANNELS	ADVANTAGES	DISADVANTAGES
Brachial	Very safe route Vessel easily accessible, either by cutdown or a percutaneous approach Compressible	Often requires a cutdown Easily displaced and poor patient mobility Not reusable if a cutdown technique is performed The catheter is more difficult to advance than in central or larger vessels
Subclavian	Direct access to the right side of the heart (especially via the left subclavian) Rapid insertion time Good patient mobility	Pneumothorax and other intrathoracic trauma are possible Noncompressible
Femoral	Direct access to the right side of the heart Rapid insertion time Compressible	Increased incidence of thrombophlebitis Can be dislodged by leg movement Poor patient mobility Infection
Internal jugular	Direct access to the right side of the heart (especially via the right internal jugular) Rapid insertion time Compressible	Possible carotid artery puncture Dislodgment with movement of the head Thrombophlebitis

The *left* subclavian vein is preferred because of the less acute angle traversed than with the right-sided approach, but either side may be used.[43,44]

The internal jugular approach may also be used. In this case, the *right* internal jugular vein is preferred because of the direct line to the superior vena cava. Problems with this approach include dislodgment of the pacemaker with movement of the head, puncture of the carotid artery, and thrombophlebitis.

During CPR, use of the right internal jugular vein and the left subclavian vein for pacemaker insertion has been demonstrated to result in the highest rates of proper placement in the right ventricle.[45] The right internal jugular vein is the more direct route of the two and may be the most appropriate site.

Femoral veins, like neck veins, are compressible and easily catheterized. Problems include easy dislodgment, infection, and increased risk for thrombophlebitis.[46,47]

Brachial vein catheterization is easy to perform but results in a high incidence of infection and vessel thrombosis.[48] In addition, the catheter is easily dislodged with arm motion. This approach is seldom used in the emergency setting.

Although the left subclavian and right internal jugular veins are the preferred routes for access, in emergency situations clinicians should use the approach with which they are most experienced to minimize the time spent in cannulating the vein and reduce the potential for complications from the venipuncture.

Skin Preparation and Venous Access

Clean the skin over the venipuncture site twice with an antiseptic solution such as chlorhexidine or povidone-iodine. Prepare a wide area because of the tendency for guidewires and catheters to spring from the hands of an unsuspecting operator. Similarly, drape widely in the standard manner to maintain a sterile field and to allow clear visibility of the venipuncture site.

The infraclavicular approach is used in this chapter to illustrate venous access, although the mechanics is generally the same as for other vascular approaches.

Occasionally, a patient who already has a central venous line in place requires emergency placement of a pacing catheter. An existing central venous pressure (CVP) line can be used to place the pacing catheter if the lumen of the catheter is large enough to accept a guidewire. Withdraw the CVP line 3 to 5 cm to expose an area of sterile tubing. Transect the tubing through a sterile area while holding it firmly at skin level. Pass a guidewire through the tubing, and then withdraw the tubing so that only the wire is left in the vein. Never release the guidewire and the tubing because embolization may result.

With the guidewire in place, pass a dilator and introducer sheath together over the guidewire, as is done in the Seldinger technique. Remove the dilator and guidewire and pass the pacing catheter through the introducer sheath (Fig. 15-5, *step 1*). One key additional step to help preserve sterility while manipulating the pacing catheter is to attach an extensible sleeve on the end of the introducer before inserting the pacing catheter (see Fig. 15-2, *steps 1 and 6*). In this way the pacing catheter can be advanced and withdrawn multiple times without fear of contamination.

Bedside ultrasound (US) can be useful as an aid in securing central venous access, and its use in the setting of emergency transvenous pacing has been reported.[49,50]

Pacemaker Placement
ECG Guidance

Connect the patient to the limb leads of an ECG machine, and turn the indicator to record the chest (V) lead.

With newer ECG machines, the pacemaker may be attached to any of the V leads (usually V_1 or V_5) that are displayed during rhythm monitoring. The *distal* terminal of the pacing catheter (the cathode or lead marked "negative", "−," or "distal") must be connected to the V lead of the ECG machine by a male-to-male connector or by an insulated wire with an alligator clip on each end. Some prepackaged kits contain an alligator clamp that can be connected to the lead with an adapter pin (see Fig. 15-5, *step 2*). The pacing catheter is thus an exploring electrode that creates a unipolar electrode for intracardiac ECG recording. The ECG tracing recorded from the electrode tip *localizes the position of the tip of the pacing electrode*. Because the tracing on the ECG machine may be slightly delayed, advancement of the catheter after initial insertion must be evaluated carefully. If a balloon-tipped catheter is used, inflate the balloon with air *after* the catheter enters the superior vena cava ($\approx$10 to 12 cm for a subclavian or internal jugular insertion) (see Fig. 15-5, *step 3*). The inflation port should be locked and the syringe left attached.

Advance the pacing catheter both quickly and smoothly. Monitor the V lead, and observe the P wave and QRS complex to ascertain the location of the tip of the pacing catheter (see Fig. 15-5, *step 4*). Use of electrocardiography to guide placement of a pacing catheter is based on two concepts. First, the complex will vary in size depending on which chamber is entered. For example, when the tip of the pacing catheter is in the atrium, one will see large P waves, often larger than the corresponding QRS complex. Second, the sum of the electrical forces will be negative if the depolarization is moving away from the catheter tip and positive if the depolarization is moving toward the catheter tip. Therefore, if the tip of the catheter is *above* the atrium, both the P wave and QRS complex will be negative (i.e., the electrical forces of a normally beating heart will be moving away from the catheter tip). As the tip progresses inferiorly in the atrium, the P wave will become isoelectric (biphasic) and will eventually become positive as the wave of atrial depolarization advances toward the tip of the catheter. The ECG tracing resembles an aVR lead initially when in the left subclavian vein (Fig. 15-6A) or the midportion of the superior vena cava (see Fig. 15-6B). At the high right atrial level, both the P wave and QRS complex are negative. The P wave is larger than the QRS complex and is deeply inverted (see Fig. 15-6C and D). As the center of the atrium is approached, the P wave becomes larger and biphasic (see Fig. 15-6E). As the catheter approaches the lower atrium (see Fig. 15-6F), the P wave becomes smaller and upright. The QRS complex is fairly normal. When striking the right atrial wall, an injury pattern with a P-Ta segment is seen (Fig. 15-6G). As the electrode passes through the tricuspid valve, the P wave becomes smaller and the QRS complex becomes larger (see Fig. 15-6H). Placement in the inferior vena cava may be recognized by a change in the morphology of the P wave and a decrease in the amplitude of both the P wave and the QRS complex (see Fig. 15-6I).

Once the pacing catheter is in the desired position, deflate the balloon by unlocking the port, observing that the syringe refills with air spontaneously, and then removing the syringe (Fig. 15-5, *step 5*). One should avoid drawing back on the syringe because this may rupture the balloon. If the syringe

EMERGENCY TRANSVENOUS CARDIAC PACING

1

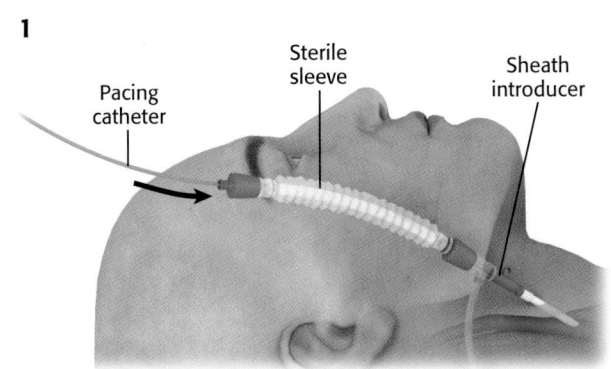

Establish a sheath introducer in the selected vein. Attach the still-compressed sterile sleeve to the introducer hub. Check the balloon for integrity and then advance the catheter into the sleeve. (Full sterile drapes should be used but are not depicted here.)

2

Instruct an assistant to make the following nonsterile connections. Attach the proximal (+) lead to the positive terminal of the connecting cable and the distal (−) lead to the V_1 lead of an ECG machine with an alligator clamp. (Alternatively, an insulated wire with an alligator clip on each end may be used.)

3

Advance the catheter approximately 10 to 12 cm so that the tip lies within the superior vena cava. Then inflate the balloon with 1.5 mL of air. Close the stopcock valve to keep the balloon inflated.

4

Advance the pacing catheter quickly and smoothly. Monitor the V lead on the electrocardiogram to ascertain the location of the tip of the pacing catheter. The P wave and QRS complex will vary in size depending on which chamber the tip is in, and the sum of the electrical forces will be negative if depolarization is moving away from the catheter tip and positive if depolarization is moving toward it. ST-segment elevation will occur when the tip contacts the endocardium.

5

When the pacing catheter is in the desired position, deflate the balloon by unlocking the stopcock and allow the syringe to spontaneously refill with air.

6

Extend the sterile sleeve so that it fully covers the pacing catheter. If your sheath and sleeve have valves, close them by turning clockwise to keep the wire and sleeve in place.

Figure 15-5 Emergency transvenous cardiac pacing. Note that by attaching the pacing catheter to the electrocardiographic (ECG) machine (step 2) and observing the V_1 ECG tracing, the negative lead now becomes an exploring lead that tells the operator the position of the tip of the pacing catheter in the body (see Fig. 15-6).

Continued

EMERGENCY TRANSVENOUS CARDIAC PACING, CONTINUED

7

Rate

Output

Sensitivity

Distal lead attached to the connector cable

Disconnect the catheter's distal (negative) lead from the ECG machine and attach it to the energy soure via the connector cable. Set the rate to 80, the output to 5 mA, and the sensitivity to full-demand mode (most sensitivity), and turn the pacer on.

8

Pacer spike

QRS complex

Assess for *electrical capture* by looking for a QRS complex to follow each pacer spike on the ECG monitor. Assess for *mechanical capture* by checking for a palpable pulse that equals the pacemaker rate. Reposition the catheter if needed.

9

TESTING THRESHOLD
a. Set rate to 80 beats/min.
b. Set output to 5 mA.
c. Set sensitivity to maximum.
d. Reduce output slowly until capture is lost. This output is the threshold.
e. Increase output to 2.5 times the threshold to ensure consistency of capture (usually 2 to 3 mA).

10

TESTING SENSING
a. Set the rate at 10 beats/min greater than intrinsic rhythm.
b. Place the pacemaker in asynchronous mode (minimum sensitivity) and ensure that there is complete capture.
c. Adjust the sensitivity to midposition (approx. 3 mA).
d. Decrease the rate until pacing is suppressed by the intrinsic rhythm.
e. Check that the sensing indicator signals each time that a native beat is sensed.
f. If the pacer fails to sense an intrinsic rhythm, increase the sensitivity.
g. If the pacer oversenses (e.g., triggered by P or T waves or artifact), decrease the sensitivity.
h. Once the sensitivity threshold is determined, set the millivoltage to half that value.

Figure 15-5, cont'd

does not refill spontaneously, the operator should suspect that the balloon might be ruptured. The balloon should not be inflated and the pacing catheter should be withdrawn and the balloon checked for leaks. If a leak is found, a new pacing catheter should be used.

After successful passage of the catheter into the right ventricle, advance the tip until contact is made with the endocardial wall. When this occurs, the QRS segment will show ST-segment elevation (see Fig. 15-6*J*). Ideally, the tip of the catheter should be lodged in the trabeculae at the apex of the right ventricle; however, pacing may also be successful if the catheter is in various other positions within the ventricle or outflow tract.

If the pacer enters the pulmonary artery outflow tract, the P wave again becomes negative, and the QRS amplitude diminishes (see Fig. 15-6*K*). If the catheter is in the pulmonary artery, withdraw the pacing catheter into the right ventricle and readvance it. Sometimes a clockwise or counterclockwise twist of the catheter will redirect its path in a more favorable direction. If catheter-induced ectopy develops, withdraw the catheter slightly until the ectopy stops, and then readvance it. Occasionally, an antidysrhythmic drug such as lidocaine may be needed to desensitize the myocardium. Once ventricular endocardial contact is made, disconnect the catheter from the ECG machine and connect the distal lead to the negative terminal on the

Figure 15-6 As one advances the pacing catheter and records the electrocardiographic complex that is obtained from the distal electrode (the exploring lead), the location of the tip of the pacing wire can be ascertained. With the tip of the pacer in the high right atrium (**D**), above the sinoatrial node, the P waves are large and negative, which indicates that the cardiac forces are moving away from the tip of the catheter. With the exploring electrode in the low right atrium (**F**), the P waves are now positive because the sinus depolarization is now coming toward the tip of the electrode. With the recording electrode tip free in the right ventricle (**H**), positive P waves and large QRS complexes are seen. When lodged against the ventricular wall, the current of injury denotes proper pacer tip placement (**J**). (*A-F and H-K, From Bing OH, McDowell JW, Hantman J, et al. Pacemaker placement by electrocardiographic monitoring. N Engl J Med. 1972;287:651; **G**, from Goldberger E. Treatment of Cardiac Emergencies. 3rd ed. St. Louis: Mosby; 1982:252.*)

pacing generator (see Fig. 15-5, *step* 7). Set the pacing generator at a rate of 80 beats/min or 10 beats/min faster than the underlying ventricular rhythm, whichever is higher. Select the full-demand mode with an output of about 5 mA. The pacing generator is then turned on.

Assess the patient for electrical and mechanical capture. Electrical capture will be manifested on the ECG monitor as a pacer spike followed by a QRS complex (see Fig. 15-5, *step* 8). If a pacer spike is seen but no QRS follows, capture is not occurring. *Mechanical capture* means that a pacer spike with its corresponding QRS triggers a myocardial contraction. This can be assessed by checking that a palpable pulse is present and equal to the rate set on the pacemaker. If complete capture does not occur or if it is intermittent, the pacer will need to be repositioned. When proper capture occurs, assess the pacer for optimal positioning. This is done by testing the thresholds

for pacing and sensing and by physical examination, electrocardiography, and chest radiography.

Catheter Placement in Low-Flow States

If cardiac output is too low to "float" a pacing catheter or if the patient is in extremis, there may not be enough time to advance a pacing catheter via the previously described techniques. Such a situation would be asystole or complete heart block with malignant ventricular escape rhythms (although one can make a case for TCP in such conditions). In such emergency situations, connect the pacing catheter to the energy source, turn the output to the maximum amperage, and select the asynchronous mode. Advance the catheter blindly in the hope that it will enter the right ventricle and pacing will be accomplished. Rotate, advance, withdraw, or otherwise manipulate the pacing catheter according to clinical response. The right internal jugular approach is the most practical access route in this situation.

US Guidance

As bedside US has become more widely available in the ED, new uses have been discovered. One promising technique involves using US to assist in the placement of emergency transvenous pacing catheters.[51,52] US may also help demonstrate whether mechanical capture has been achieved. The advantages of US over fluoroscopy are its safety and ready availability. Further experience will be necessary to confirm its utility (see Ultrasound Box).

Testing Threshold

The threshold is the minimum current necessary to obtain capture. Ideally, it is less than 1.0 mA, and usually it is between 0.3 and 0.7 mA. If the threshold is in this ideal range, good contact with the endocardium can be presumed.

To determine the threshold, set the pacing generator to maximum sensitivity (full-demand mode) at 5-mA output and a rate of approximately 80 beats/min (or at least 10 beats/min greater than the patient's intrinsic rate) (see Fig. 15-5, *step 9*). Reduce the current (output) slowly until capture is lost. This current is the threshold. Carry out this maneuver two or three times to ensure that this value is consistent. Increase the amperage to 2.5 times the threshold to ensure consistency of capture (usually between 2 and 3 mA).

Testing Sensing

Test the sensing function in patients who have underlying rhythms. Set the rate at about 10 beats/min greater than the endogenous rhythm, place the pacemaker in asynchronous mode (*minimum* sensitivity, which is the *maximum* setting on the sensitivity voltage control), and ensure that there is complete capture (see Fig. 15-5, *step 10*). Then adjust the sensitivity control to its midposition or approximately 3 mV, and gradually decrease the rate until pacing is suppressed by the patient's intrinsic rhythm. The sensing indicator on the pacing generator should signal each time that a native beat is sensed and should be in synchrony with each QRS complex on the ECG monitor. If the pacer fails to sense the intrinsic rhythm,

increase the sensitivity (decrease the millivolts) until the pacer is suppressed. Conversely, if the sensing indicator is triggered by P or T waves or by artifact, decrease the sensitivity until only the QRS complex is sensed. Once the sensitivity threshold is determined, set the millivoltage to about half that value.

Securing and Final Assessment

After the pacemaker's position has been tested for electrical accuracy, it must be secured in place. If a sealed introducer sheath was used, the hub should be fixed firmly to the skin with suture (e.g., 4-0 nylon or silk). A fastening suture should be sewn to the skin and the hub tied securely in place. If a plain introducer was used, withdraw it to prevent leakage and suture the catheter in place. In either case, coil the excess pacing catheter and secure it in a sterile manner underneath a large sterile dressing. Assess pacemaker function again, and take a chest film to ensure proper positioning. Ideal positioning of the pacing catheter is at the apex of the right ventricle (Fig. 15-7).

A 12-lead ECG tracing should be obtained after placement of the transvenous pacemaker. If the catheter is within the right ventricle, a left bundle branch pattern with left axis deviation should be evident in paced beats (Fig. 15-8). If an RBBB pattern is noted, coronary sinus placement or left ventricular pacing secondary to septal penetration should be suspected.

With a properly functioning ventricular pacemaker, large cannon waves may be noted on inspection of the venous pulsations at the neck. When the pacemaker achieves ventricular capture, there may be times when the atria contract against a closed tricuspid valve and a cannon wave results. On auscultation of the heart a slight murmur may be evident secondary to tricuspid insufficiency from the catheter interfering with the tricuspid valve apparatus.[53] Following each pacemaker impulse a clicking sound may be heard during expiration that is believed to represent either intercostal or diaphragmatic muscular contractions caused by the pacemaker.[54] Note that this can also be a sign of cardiac perforation.[55] On auscultation of the second heart sound, paradoxical splitting may be noted. This represents a delay in closure of the aortic valve because of delayed left ventricular depolarization.

Figure 15-7 Normal pacemaker position in the apex of the right ventricle on posteroanterior (**A**) and lateral (**B**) chest films.

ULTRASOUND: Transvenous Cardiac Pacing
by Christine Butts, MD

Using ultrasound to guide placement of a transvenous pacemaker (TVPM) gives the physician the advantage of direct visualization of the tip of the pacemaker and the ability to directly maneuver it into the correct position to obtain capture. Although placement of a TVPM is a relatively rare procedure in the emergency department, the use of ultrasound has been described to facilitate the procedure.[1,2] Ultrasound can also be used to evaluate placement in cases in which blind attempts at transvenous pacing are unsuccessful. Additionally, ultrasound is useful in achieving the central venous access used to introduce the pacemaker.

Equipment

A low-frequency (2 to 5 mHz) transducer offers the optimum depth to evaluate the heart. A phased-array or microconvex transducer is ideal for this purpose because its small footprint enables the sonographer to "see" between the patient's ribs. In the absence of a phased-array or micro-convex transducer, a curvilinear transducer may be adequate as well. Although insertion of a TVPM is a sterile procedure, the transducer does not need to be sterile if it is used away from the field. If the transducer will be used near or on the field, it can be placed inside a sterile cover or a sterile glove.

Image Interpretation

The subxiphoid view of the heart is the optimum view for this procedure (Fig. 15-US1). It enables the operator to view all four chambers of the heart at once. The subxiphoid view is obtained by placing the transducer just inferior to the xiphoid process with the indicator pointing toward the patient's right (Fig. 15-US2). A hand should be placed a hand on top of the transducer to enable the sonographer to push downward into the epigastric area. The transducer can then be aimed toward the left side of the chest until the four-chambered view of the heart is seen. In this view the left lobe of the liver is seen at the top of the image. Deep to this is the heart, with the right atrium and ventricle abutting the liver.

Figure 15-US2 Placement of the ultrasound transducer to obtain a subxiphoid image of the heart. *(Image courtesy of Christy Butts, MD.)*

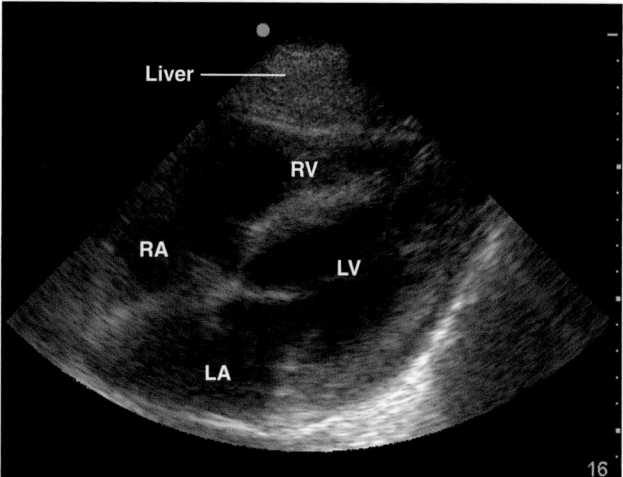

Figure 15-US1 Subxiphoid image of the heart. In this ultrasound image the liver is seen at the top of the image. The heart is seen below, with the right ventricle (RV), right atrium (RA), and left atrium (LA) abutting the left lobe of the liver. The left ventricle (LV) and atria are deep to the right side at the bottom of the image.

Figure 15-US3 Pacing wire within the right ventricle (*arrows*). **A,** Sonographic image. **B,** Schematic representation. The right ventricle is seen through the subxiphoid window, which provides excellent views of the heart without interfering with placement of the pacemaker line. The pacemaker wire is seen as a brightly echogenic structure within the right ventricle.

Continued

ULTRASOUND: Transvenous Cardiac Pacing—cont'd

Procedure and Technique

To guide placement of the pacemaker, the procedure should begin in the usual fashion (as described above). Once the pacer wire has been inserted, the sonographer should begin observing the right atrium. The wire will appear as a hyperechoic (white) linear echo as it enters the right atrium and can be seen to advance in real time (Fig. 15-US3). The wire should be followed as it enters the right ventricle. This can be observed simultaneously with the electrical readings on the monitor. Capture of the pacemaker can be confirmed by visualization of coordinated, rhythmic contractions of the myocardium at the set rate. The monitor can also be evaluated for signs of electrical capture.

REFERENCES:

1. Aguilera P, Durham B, Riley D. Emergency transvenous cardiac pacing placement using ultrasound guidance. *Ann Emerg Med.* 2000;36:224-227.
2. Macedo W, Sturmann K, Kim JM, et al. Ultrasonographic guidance of transvenous pacemaker insertion in the emergency department. *J Emerg Med.* 1999;17:491-496.

Figure 15-8 Electrocardiographic pattern of a right ventricular pacemaker.

As in any procedure, assess the patient for improvement in clinical status. Evaluate vital signs, mentation, congestive symptoms, and urinary output. In addition, look for complications secondary to the procedure and treat as needed.

Complications

The complications associated with emergency transvenous cardiac pacing are numerous and represent a compendium of those related to central venous catheterization,[13,56] those related to right-sided heart catheterization, and those unique to the pacing catheter itself (Table 15-5).

Problems Related to Central Venous Catheterization

Inadvertent arterial puncture is a well-known complication of the percutaneous approach to the venous system.[60] This problem is usually recognized quickly because of the rapid return of arterial blood. Firm compression over the puncture site will almost always result in hemostasis in 5 minutes or less.

Venous thrombosis and thrombophlebitis are also potential problems with central venous catheterization. Thrombophlebitis, which occurs early after insertion, is an uncommon complication. Thrombosis of the innominate vein is also a rare problem, with pulmonary embolism being an even more uncommon event.[61] Femoral vein thrombosis, however, appears to be a much more common event associated with femoral vein catheterization.[46,59] Studies using noninvasive techniques have shown a 37% incidence of femoral vein thrombosis, with 55% of these patients having evidence of pulmonary embolism on ventilation-perfusion scans.[59] At least one study suggests that the use of low-dose enoxaparin is safe and effective in reducing pacemaker-related femoral vein thrombosis.[62]

TABLE 15-5 Complications of Transvenous Cardiac Pacing

YEAR	REFERENCE	PATIENTS (N)	CATHETER	ROUTE	RESULT
1969	Rosenberg et al.[1]	111	Flexon steel wire vs. unipolar semifloating (ECG)	96 Subclavian 5 Basilic 1 External jugular	12 with inconsistent pacing, 3 local infections, 2 pneumothoraces, 1 subclavian artery puncture; 16% complication rate
1973	Schnitzler et al.[11]	17	3-Fr bipolar semifloating balloon (ECG)	Antecubital vein	2 PVCs, stable pacing, no thrombophlebitis
1973	Weinstein et al.[47]	100	6-Fr bipolar (fluoroscopy)	Femoral	2 ventricular tachycardias, 2 perforations, 2 required repositioning, 1 with questionable thrombophlebitis and pulmonary embolism, 1 local infection
1973	Lumia and Rios[57]	142 insertions in 113 patients	Bipolar (fluoroscopy)	61 Brachial 81 Femoral	12 ventricular tachycardias and fibrillation in 9 patients, 3 perforations in 2 patients; local hematoma, abscess, and bleeding in 30%; 16.9% complication rate
1980	Pandian et al.[58]	20	5-Fr bipolar (fluoroscopy)	Femoral	25% with deep vein thrombosis
1980	Nolewajka et al.[59]	29	6-Fr Cordis (fluoroscopy)	Femoral	34% with venous thrombosis by venography, 60% of these with pulmonary embolism by V̇/Q̇ scan
1981	Lang et al.[12]	111	Balloon, semifloating vs. semirigid	Subclavian	Serious dysrhythmia: 1.5% with balloon tipped, 20.4% with semirigid Catheter displacement: 13.6% ± 4.4% days balloon tipped; 32% ± 1.9% days semirigid
1982	Austin et al.[46]	113 insertions in 100 patients	4- to 7-Fr bipolar (fluoroscopy)	Brachial Femoral	Failure to sense or pace in 37%; repositioning of brachial insertions in 37%; repositioning of femoral insertions in 9%; fever, sepsis, local infection only with femoral insertions; 20% complication rate

ECG, electrocardiogram; PVC, premature ventricular contraction; V̇/Q̇, ventilation-perfusion.

Pneumothorax is consistently a problem with the various approaches to the veins at the base of the neck. The decision to place a chest tube in patients with this complication depends on the extent of the air leak and the clinical status of the patient. In addition, laceration of the subclavian vein with hemothorax,[63] laceration of the thoracic duct with chylothorax, air embolism, wound infections, pneumomediastinum, hydromediastinum, hemomediastinum,[64] phrenic nerve injury,[65] and fracture of the guidewire with embolization[66,67] are all potential complications.[35,63]

Complications of Right-Sided Heart Catheterization

A frequent complication of the pacing catheter is dysrhythmia, with premature ventricular contractions being a common occurrence. One study noted a 1.5% incidence of serious dysrhythmias with a balloon-tipped catheter inserted under ECG guidance as opposed to a 32% incidence with insertion of a semirigid catheter under fluoroscopic guidance, thus suggesting that the balloon catheter was the preferred type of catheter.[12] Another study noted a 6% incidence of ventricular tachycardia during insertion.[46] An ischemic heart is

I	aVR	V₁	V₄
II	aVL	V₂	V₅
III	aVF	V₃	V₆

Figure 15-9 Coronary sinus pacing. Note the paced right bundle branch block pattern.

more prone than a nonischemic heart to dysrhythmias.[68] Therapy for catheter-induced ectopy during insertion involves repositioning the catheter in the ventricle. This usually stops the ectopy; however, if after repeated attempts it is found that the catheter cannot be passed without ectopy, myocardial suppressant therapy may be used to desensitize the myocardium.

Misplacement of the pacing catheter has been well studied. Passage of the catheter into the pulmonary artery can be diagnosed electrocardiographically by observing the return of an inverted P wave and a decrease in the voltage of the QRS complex. Misplacement in the coronary sinus may occur and should be suspected in patients in whom a paced RBBB pattern on the electrocardiogram is seen with right ventricular pacing (Fig. 15-9). Rarely, an RBBB pattern can be seen with a normal right ventricular position; therefore, all RBBB patterns do not represent coronary sinus pacing.[69] Further evidence of coronary sinus location can be obtained by viewing the lateral chest film. Normally, the tip of the catheter should point anteriorly toward the apex of the heart; however, with placement in the coronary sinus, the tip of the catheter is displaced posteriorly and several centimeters away from the sternum (Fig. 15-10). Other potential forms of misplacement include left ventricular pacing through an atrial septal defect or a ventricular septal defect, septal puncture, extraluminal insertion, and arterial insertion.[70]

Perforation of the ventricle is a well-described complication that can result in loss of capture,[71] hemopericardium, and tamponade.[72,73] Reported symptoms and signs of this problem include chest pain, pericardial friction rub, and diaphragmatic or chest wall muscular pacing.[74] At least one case of a postpericardiotomy-like syndrome and two cases of endocardial friction rub have been reported without perforation.[75,76]

Figure 15-10 Coronary sinus position. **A,** Posteroanterior view. **B,** Lateral view. Normally, the tip of the catheter should point anteriorly toward the apex of the heart. With coronary sinus placement, the tip is displaced posteriorly and several centimeters from the sternum. (*A and B, From Goldberger E. Treatment of Cardiac Emergencies. 3rd ed. St. Louis: Mosby; 1982.*)

Pericardial perforation is suggested radiographically when the pacing catheter is outside or abuts the cardiac silhouette and is not in proper position within the right ventricular cavity (Fig. 15-11).[77] ECG clues include a change in the QRS complex and T-wave axis or failure to properly sense. In suspected cases, a two-dimensional echocardiogram usually demonstrates the catheter's extracardiac position. Simply pulling the catheter back and repositioning it in the right ventricle can usually treat uncomplicated perforation.

During insertion of a temporary pacing catheter when a nonfunctioning permanent catheter is in place, there is a small risk of entanglement or knotting.[78] This potential also exists with other central lines and PACs. Even without the presence of other lines, the pacing catheter can become knotted.[79]

Frequently, these lines can be untangled under fluoroscopy with the use of specialized catheters.

Local and systemic infection,[48] balloon rupture, pulmonary infarction,[80] phrenic nerve pacing,[81] and rupture of the chordae tendineae are also potential complications.

Complications of the Pacing Electrode

Complications related to the pacing electrode can be separated into three groups: mechanical, organic, and electrical.

Mechanical failures include displacement, fracture of the catheter, and loose leads. Displacement can result in intermittent or complete loss of capture or improper sensing, malignant dysrhythmias, diaphragmatic pacing, or perforation.

Figure 15-11 A pacing catheter tip (*arrow*) that is outside or abuts the cardiac silhouette and is not properly positioned within the right ventricular cavity suggests myocardial perforation. (*From Tarver RD, Gillespie KR. The misplaced tube. Emerg Med Clin North Am. 1988;20:97.*)

Displacement should be suspected with changes in amplitude, with changes of greater than 90 degrees in vector, or with a change in threshold.[82] Frequently, catheter fractures may be detected by careful review of the chest film or may be suspected because of a change in the sensing threshold. As with displacement, catheter fractures may result in intermittent or complete loss of capture.

Organic causes of pacemaker failure result in changes in the threshold or sensing function.[83] Progressive inflammation, fibrosis, and thrombosis may result in more than doubling of the original threshold.[84] However, this process takes several weeks and is of no concern in the setting of pacemaker placement in the ED.

Electrical problems with pacing in the past have included failure of the pacemaker generator, dysrhythmias, and outside interference. Modern devices are extremely reliable and resistant to outside interference. Although ventricular tachycardia and ventricular fibrillation have been reported to result from pacemakers, these dysrhythmias are rare. Therefore, patients with such dysrhythmias should be evaluated for a non–pacemaker-induced cause.[85] Defibrillation and cardioversion are safe in patients who have temporary pacemakers.

EMERGENCY TRANSCUTANEOUS CARDIAC PACING

TCP is a rapid, minimally invasive method of emergency cardiac pacing that may temporarily substitute for transvenous pacing. Electrodes are applied to the skin of the anterior and posterior chest walls, and pacing is initiated with a portable pulse generator. In an emergency setting, this pacing technique is faster and easier to initiate than transvenous pacing. Pulse generators are sufficiently portable to be used in EDs, hospital wards, intensive care units, and mobile paramedic vehicles.

In 1872, Duchenne de Boulogne reported successful resuscitation of a child by attaching one electrode to a limb while

Transcutaneous Cardiac Pacing

Indications
General indications are identical to those for transvenous pacing (see Review Box 15-1)
Initial stabilization of patients requiring pacing while arrangements for transvenous pacing are being made
Pacing in various environments (prehospital, hospital ward, etc.)
Pacing in patients treated with thrombolytics or other anticoagulants

Contraindications
No absolute contraindications

Complications
Failure to recognize the presence of underlying treatable ventricular fibrillation
Induction of ventricular fibrillation (rare)
Soft tissue discomfort

Equipment

Review Box 15-2 Transcutaneous cardiac pacing: indications, contraindications, complications, and equipment.

a second electrode was rhythmically touched to the precordium of the thorax.[86] Successful overdrive pacing of the human heart with a precordial electrode was reported by VonZiemssen in 1882.[87]

In 1952, Zoll introduced the first practical means of TCP. Using a ground electrode attached to the skin and a subcutaneous needle electrode over the precordium, he reported successful resuscitation of two patients in ventricular standstill.[88] One patient was paced for 5 days and subsequently discharged from the hospital. Zoll later introduced a machine that delivered impulses lasting 2 msec through metal paddles 3 cm in diameter pressed firmly against the anterior chest wall. This device was the first commercial transcutaneous cardiac pacemaker. During the 1950s, Zoll and coworkers and Leatham and colleagues demonstrated the effectiveness of TCP in patients with bradycardia and asystole.[89-92] Leatham and colleagues used larger electrodes (4 × 6 cm) and a longer pulse duration (20 msec) to successfully pace two patients with bradydysrhythmias.[92]

Until the late 1950s, TCP was the only clinically accepted method of cardiac pacing. The original technique involving bare metal electrodes had adverse effects, including local tissue burns, muscle contraction, and severe pain.[88,92] With the development of the first implantable pacemakers from 1958 through 1960 and the improvement in transvenous electrodes during the early 1960s, TCP was rapidly discarded.[93]

Refinements in electrode size and pulse characteristics led to the reintroduction of TCP into clinical practice.[94,95] Increasing the pulse duration from 2 to 20 msec or longer was found to decrease the current output required for cardiac capture.[96,97] Longer impulse durations also make induction of ventricular fibrillation less likely.[96] Electrodes with a larger surface area (80 to 100 cm^2) decrease the current density at the underlying skin and therefore decrease pain and the possibility of tissue burns.[94]

Indications and Contraindications

General indications for cardiac pacing were discussed earlier. TCP is the fastest and easiest method of emergency pacing. This technique is useful for initial stabilization of patients in the ED who require emergency pacing while arrangements or decisions about transvenous pacemaker insertion are being made. The equipment is readily mastered, the procedure is fast, and it is minimally invasive.[95,98] Refinements in equipment have made TCP the emergency pacing procedure of choice. TCP is also widely used in the prehospital environment, as well as in the hospital in the cardiac catheterization laboratory, operating room, and intensive care units and on general medical floors.[99-101] The technique may be preferable to transvenous pacing in patients who have received thrombolytic agents or other anticoagulants. No central venous puncture, with the attendant risk of hemorrhage, is required. Limited experience suggests that TCP may also be useful in the treatment of refractory tachydysrhythmias by overdrive pacing.[102-107] Although small pediatric electrodes for TCP have been developed, experience with pediatric TCP has been limited.[108-110]

TCP is indicated for the treatment of hemodynamically significant bradydysrhythmias that have not responded to medical therapy. *Hemodynamically significant* implies hypotension, anginal chest pain, pulmonary edema, or evidence of decreased cerebral perfusion. This technique is *temporary* and is indicated for short intervals as a bridge until transvenous pacing can be initiated or the underlying cause of the bradydysrhythmia (e.g., hyperkalemia,[98] drug overdose) can be reversed.[111] Though generally unsuccessful, TCP may be attempted for the treatment of asystolic cardiac arrest. In this setting the technique is efficacious only if used early after the onset of arrest (usually within 10 minutes).[112,113] TCP is not indicated for the treatment of prolonged arrest victims with a final morbid rhythm of asystole.[109,114-116]

Delay from the onset of arrest to the initiation of pacing is a major problem that limits the usefulness of TCP in prehospital care. Hedges and associates reported that the everyday availability of pacing increased the number of patients who underwent pacing within 10 minutes of hemodynamic decompensation and increased long-term patient survival as well.[113] Prehospital pacing may be most useful in the treatment of patients with a hemodynamically significant bradycardia who have not yet progressed to cardiac arrest (e.g., heart block in the setting of AMI) or in patients who arrest after the arrival of prehospital providers.[112,113]

In conscious patients with hemodynamically stable bradycardia, TCP may not be necessary. It is reasonable to attach electrodes to such patients and to leave the pacemaker in standby mode against the possibility of hemodynamic deterioration while further efforts at treatment of the patient's underlying disorder are being made. This approach has been used successfully in patients with new heart block in the setting of cardiac ischemia.[117] Generally, when a transvenous pacemaker becomes available, it is preferred because of better patient tolerance.

Equipment

Since their reintroduction, transcutaneous pacemakers have undergone rapid evolution and are now standard equipment in most EDs, as well as in other hospital settings and the prehospital environment. The pacemakers introduced in the early 1980s tended to be asynchronous devices with a limited selection of rate and output parameters. Units introduced more recently have demand mode pacing and more output options and are often combined with a defibrillator in a single unit. Combined defibrillator-pacers offer advantages in cost, ease, and rapidity of use when compared with stand-alone devices. An example of a combined unit is shown in Review Box 15-2.

All transcutaneous pacemakers have similar basic features. Most allow operation in either a fixed rate (asynchronous) or a demand mode (VVI). Most allow rate selection in a range from 30 to 200 beats/min. Current output is usually adjustable from 0 to 200 mA. If an ECG monitor is not an integral part of the unit, *an output adapter to a separate monitor is required* to "blank" the large electrical spike from the pacemaker impulse and allow interpretation of the much smaller ECG complex. Without blanking protection, the standard ECG machine is swamped by the pacemaker spike and uninterpretable. This could be disastrous because the large pacing artifacts *can mask treatable ventricular fibrillation* (Fig. 15-12). Pulse durations on available units vary from 20 to 40 msec and are not adjustable by the operator.

Two sets of patient electrodes are usually required for operation of the device. One set of standard ECG electrodes is used for monitoring. The much larger pacing electrodes deliver electrical impulses for pacing. Newer combined

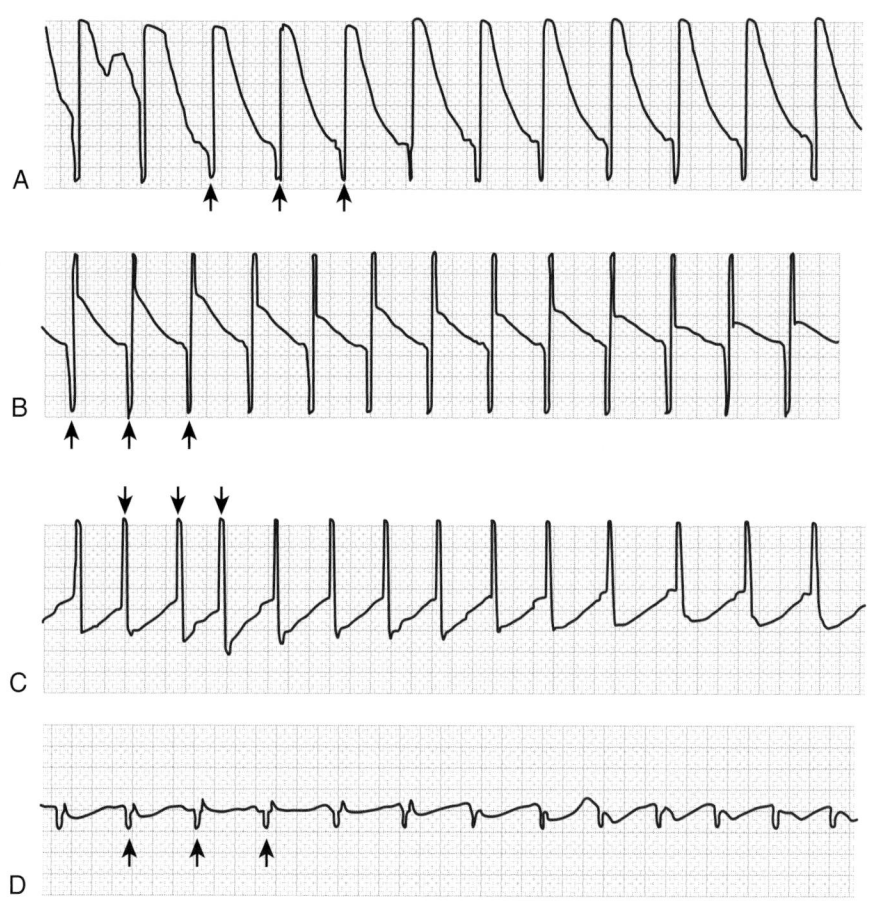

Figure 15-12 A-C, The top three rhythm strips are taken from a standard wall-mounted electrocardiographic monitor. They all demonstrate large pacer spikes without capture (*arrows*). The underlying rhythm cannot be determined and could be treatable ventricular fibrillation. **D,** The bottom rhythm strip demonstrates a tracing on the same patient with the external pacer monitor (special dampening). Note that the pacing spikes are much smaller, and it is easy to see that the underlying rhythm is asystole, without pacer capture. The presence of a T wave after the QRS complex is a good indicator of ventricular capture.

defibrillator-pacemakers can use a single set of electrodes for ECG monitoring, pacing, and defibrillation. This approach makes the device simpler to use, although the ECG waveform and analysis may be suboptimal. Provisions are generally made for separate ECG monitoring electrodes for use as desired by the operator.

Along with the widespread use of TCP come problems arising from lack of standardization of equipment. Pacing electrodes placed on a patient before arrival at the hospital may be incompatible with the transcutaneous pacemaker used in the ED, and likewise, the equipment in the ED may differ from inpatient units. Efforts should be made to establish a single standard for pacing electrode connectors within an institution and out to the prehospital environment if possible.

To facilitate rapid setup, the pacing electrodes should be connected to the pacemaker at all times. With conventional packaging the leads are inside the packet with the pads, which means that the packet must be opened to allow connection to the pacing unit. However, exposure to air causes the electrodes to dry out and lose their conductivity, thus requiring continual replacement of the unused electrodes. Newer packaging leaves the connectors outside the packet, thus allowing connection to the pacemaker while preserving the shelf life of the pacing electrodes.

Technique

Pad Placement

The pacing electrodes are self-adhesive. Position them as shown in Figure 15-13. Take care to avoid placing the electrodes over an implanted pacemaker or defibrillator. Remove any transdermal drug delivery patches if they are in the way. Remove excessive hair if time permits. Place the anterior electrode (cathode or negative electrode) as close as possible to the point of maximal impulse on the left anterior chest wall. Place the second electrode directly posterior to the anterior electrode (Fig.15-13A and B). The posterior electrode serves as the ground. An alternative arrangement for the pacing electrodes is shown in Figure 15-13C. On females, place the electrode beneath the breast and against the chest wall. Because data regarding optimum electrode placement are scarce, selection can be based on the clinician's preference and the patient's habitus.[118,119] Nonetheless, suboptimal capture as a result of poor electrode placement may be rectified with a small change in electrode position. Although the polarity of the electrodes does not appear to be important for defibrillation, at least one study has indicated that it may important be for pacing.[120] The electrodes are labeled by the manufacturer to indicate which should be placed over the precordium, and it is prudent to observe this recommendation. ECG electrodes (if used) are placed on the chest wall or limbs, or both, as required and connected to the instrument cable. Some clinicians prophylactically apply pacing electrodes to all critically ill patients with bradycardia to facilitate immediate TCP should decompensation occur.

There is little risk for electrical injury to health care providers during TCP. The power delivered during each impulse is less than $\frac{1}{1000}$ of that delivered during defibrillation.[121] Chest compressions (CPR) can be administered directly over the insulated electrodes while pacing.[122]

Figure 15-13 Correct placement of transcutaneous pacemaker electrodes. **A** and **B**, Anteroposterior positions. **C**, Anterolateral positions (see text).

Inadvertent contact with the active pacing surface results in only a mild shock.

Pacing Bradycardiac Rhythms

To initiate TCP, apply the pacing electrodes and activate the device (Fig. 15-14, *steps 1 and 2*). Slowly increase the output from minimal settings until capture is achieved. (Fig. 15-14, *step 4*) Rate and current (output) selections are adjustable. Generally, a heart rate of 60 to 70 beats/min will maintain adequate blood pressure (by blood pressure cuff or arterial catheter) and cerebral perfusion.

Assess electrical capture by monitoring the ECG tracing on the filtered monitor of the pacing unit (see Fig. 15-14, *steps 5 and 6*). Assess mechanical capture by palpating the pulse as for transvenous pacing. Because of muscular contractions triggered by the pacer, carotid pulses may be difficult to assess, so palpating the femoral pulse may be easier. Additionally, bedside US may prove useful in determining ventricular capture.[123,124] Ideally, continue pacing at an output level just above the threshold of initial electrical capture to minimize discomfort. One study involving 16 normal male volunteers who were paced without sedation noted cardiac capture at a mean current of 54 mA (range, 42 to 60 mA).[125] Most subjects could tolerate pacing at their capture threshold; only one subject required discontinuation of pacing at 60 mA because of intolerable pain. Heller and coworkers compared subjective pain perception and capture thresholds in 10 volunteers paced with five different transcutaneous pacers.[126] Capture rates (40% to 80%), thresholds (66.5 to 104 mA), and subjective discomfort varied from pacemaker to pacemaker.

Failure to capture with TCP may be related to electrode placement or patient size. Patients with barrel-shaped chests and large amounts of intrathoracic air conduct electricity poorly and may prove refractory to capture. In one study, the scarring associated with thoracotomy was found to nearly double the pacing threshold.[127] A large pericardial effusion or tamponade will also increase the output required for capture.[128] Failure to electrically capture with a transcutaneous device in these settings is an indication to consider immediate placement of a transvenous pacer.

Patients who are conscious or who regain consciousness during TCP will experience discomfort because of muscle contraction.[117,125,126] Analgesia with incremental doses of an opioid agent, sedation with a benzodiazepine compound, or both, will make this discomfort tolerable until transvenous pacing can be instituted.

Overdrive Pacing

Overdrive pacing of ventricular tachycardia or paroxysmal supraventricular tachycardia is performed in patients who are stable enough to tolerate the brief delay associated with the preparation needed for this technique.[102-107] Few data exist on the efficacy or use of this procedure in the ED. Sedate the patient as explained earlier, place pacing and monitoring electrode pads in the standard positions as detailed earlier, and initiate brief trains (6 to 10 beats) of asynchronous pacing. Set the pacer rate at approximately 20 to 60 pulses/min greater than the dysrhythmia rate.[129] Generally, an impulse rate of 200 pulses/min is used for ventricular tachycardias (the rate is usually 150 to 180 beats/min), and a rate of 240 to 280 pulses/min is used for paroxysmal supraventricular tachycardias (the rate is commonly 200 to 250 beats/min).

Because rhythm acceleration is possible during overdrive pacing, it is essential to keep resuscitation equipment, including a defibrillator, at the bedside.

Complications

The major potential complication of TCP is *failure to recognize the presence of underlying treatable ventricular fibrillation.* This complication is primarily due to the size of the pacing artifact on the ECG screen, a technical problem inherent in systems without appropriate dampening circuitry.

A rare complication of TCP is induction of ventricular fibrillation. Studies of fibrillation thresholds using large precordial electrodes have shown that the longer impulse durations used in modern devices seem to decrease the chance of inducing ventricular fibrillation with TCP. Nonetheless, asynchronous TCP for tachydysrhythmias has been associated with acceleration in rhythm and the development of ventricular fibrillation.[105]

Studies looking at prolonged TCP in humans have not been extensive. Zoll and colleagues reported 25 humans paced for up to 108 hours with impulses of 20-msec duration.[91] Pacer-induced dysrhythmias did not occur. Leatham and colleagues paced one patient for 68 hours with impulses 20 msec in duration.[92] The patient died 2 days after pacing was discontinued. Pathologic examination revealed no evidence of

EMERGENCY TRANSCUTANEOUS CARDIAC PACING

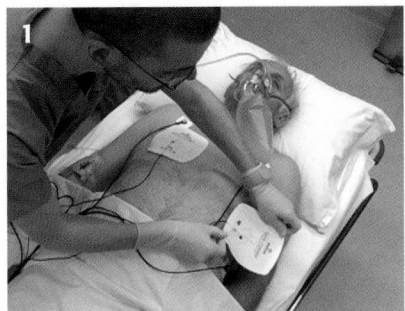

Apply the pacing pads in either the anteroposterior or the anterolateral positions.

Excessive hair may be removed if time permits.

Turn the pacemaker on (*long arrow*), and check to make sure that the pacemaker is sensing the intrinsic rhythm (*short arrows*).

Select the pacing rate by using the Rate button.

Generally, a rate of 60 to 70 beats/min will maintain adequate blood pressure and cerebral perfusion.

Slowly increase the current output from minimal settings until capture is achieved.

Note the presence of pacer spikes (*arrows*) and the absence of subsequent QRS complexes.

Electrical capture has not been achieved and the current needs to be increased.

With higher current electrical capture has been achieved (QRS after every pacer spike, *arrows*).

Check for mechanical capture by palpating for a pulse.

Figure 15-14 Emergency transcutaneous cardiac pacing.

pacer-induced myocardial damage. Madsen and colleagues paced 10 healthy volunteers at threshold for 30 minutes and found no enzyme or echocardiographic abnormalities.[130] TCP appears unlikely to produce cardiac injury with short-term use in the ED.

Soft tissue discomfort with the potential for injury may still occur with current transcutaneous pacemakers. Most patients are able to tolerate the discomfort, especially after sedation and analgesia. Nonetheless, prolonged use may still induce local cutaneous injury, particularly in pediatric patients because of the use of smaller electrodes.[131,132] Patients who cannot tolerate TCP or who will need long-term pacing are candidates for transvenous pacing.

References are available at www.expertconsult.com

CHAPTER 16

Pericardiocentesis

Haney A. Mallemat and Semhar Z. Tewelde

DEFINITION

Pericardial effusion, the presence of fluid within the pericardial space, has a number of causes. As fluid accumulates, a critical point is reached at which pericardial pressure negatively affects cardiac filling and causes circulatory insufficiency. This is called pericardial tamponade. Once compensatory mechanisms begin to fail, obstructive shock ensues and failure to restore hemodynamics leads to cardiac arrest. Only removal of fluid can stabilize hemodynamics at this point.

ANATOMY AND PHYSIOLOGY

Pericardium and Pericardial Space

The pericardium is a two-layered fibroelastic sac surrounding the heart.[1] The pericardium is avascular but well innervated, so inflammation induces severe pain. The visceral pericardium is a single-cell layer that adheres to the epicardium. The outer parietal pericardium consists mostly of collagen with some elastin. These two layers create the pericardial space, which normally contains 15 to 50 mL of serous fluid.[2] Pericardial fluid provides lubrication for cardiac contractility and acts as a "shock absorber" for deceleration forces.

The pericardium is a tense structure, but it also has some elasticity. These properties limit the amount of cardiac dilation that is possible during diastole and enhance mechanical interactions between the atria and ventricles during systole.[3] This semi-elastic property can also tolerate an acute (i.e., over a period of hours to days) accumulation of pericardial fluid (80 to 120 mL) without significantly increasing intrapericardial pressure, which is the flat portion of the pressure-volume curve for pericardial pressure (Fig. 16-1).[4,5] Once a critical volume is reached, adding as little as 20 to 40 mL can double intrapericardial pressure (the steep portion of the pressure-volume curve [see Fig. 16-1]) and cause clinical decompensation (cardiac tamponade). Cardiac tamponade typically occurs with an intrapericardial pressure of 15 to 20 mm Hg.[6]

Slow and chronic accumulation of pericardial fluid (over a period of weeks to months) causes the pericardium to expand circumferentially, and it can accommodate several liters of fluid with minimal alteration in intrapericardial pressure. Patients with this condition may be asymptomatic despite large effusions. No specific pericardial volume predicts the hemodynamic consequences of an effusion. Such consequences depend on the acuity of accumulation of the fluid.

Pericardiocentesis

Indications

Diagnostic
  Determining the cause of pericardial effusion
Therapeutic
  Hemodynamic instability
  Cardiac arrest, pulseless electrical activity

Contraindications

Absolute
  None (if hypotension or hypoperfusion is evident
  or if the patient is in cardiac arrest)
Relative
  Coagulopathy
  Prosthetic heart valve
  Pacemakers and cardiac devices
  Lack of direct visualization (e.g., ultrasound) during the procedure
  Traumatic pericardium (thoracotomy preferred)

Complications

Dysrhythmias   Fluid reaccumulation
Air embolism   Intercostal vessel injury
Coronary artery puncture   Suppurative pericarditis
Hemothorax pneumothorax   Costochondritis
Pneumopericardium   Left ventricular injury
Intraabdominal injury   Internal mammary artery injury

Equipment

Chlorhexidine
Sterile drape
Lidocaine
10-mL syringe/25-gauge needle
60-mL syringe
Ultrasound
18-gauge spinal needle
J-tipped guidewire
Dilator
8-Fr pigtail catheter
3-way stopcock
ECG wire with alligator clips

Review Box 16-1 Pericardiocentesis: indications, contraindications, complications, and equipment.

Pathophysiology of Pericardial Tamponade

To generate an effective stroke volume, the left ventricle (LV) must be filled, and this process relies primarily on adequate filling of the right ventricle (RV). Normal inspiration promotes RV filling. Negative intrathoracic pressure increases venous return to the right side of the heart. This reduces wall tension in the RV, which causes dilation and more filling of the chamber.

Elevated intrapericardial pressure (i.e., early tamponade) results in abnormal RV filling and then abnormal LV filling. In this situation, the free wall of the RV cannot expand against the pericardial fluid during inspiration. To accommodate the filling, the interventricular septum bows abnormally into the LV, which reduces its volume. LV filling, stroke volume, and ultimately cardiac output are reduced.[7] This phenomenon is responsible for pulsus paradoxus (PP, described later in this chapter), which is sometimes observed with tamponade.[8] LV filling is also reduced by the collapse of right-sided structures. After a critical volume is reached on the pressure-volume curve (see Fig. 16-1), the intrapericardial pressure is transmitted to the inferior vena cava (IVC) and right atrium. These thin-walled structures then become compressed and reduce filling of the RV.

The atria and pulmonary circulation are at much lower pressure than systemic arterial pressure and are also vulnerable to rising intrapericardial pressure (Fig. 16-2). Late in tamponade a "pressure plateau" occurs in which right atrial pressure, RV diastolic pressure, pulmonary artery diastolic pressure, and pulmonary capillary wedge pressure are virtually identical. This equalization of chamber pressure leads to a reduction in venous return and the echocardiographic hallmark of tamponade: diastolic collapse of the RV. At this point, hemodynamic collapse is imminent, with severe hypotension, bradycardia, and potentially pulseless electrical activity (PEA) developing. Unless intrapericardial pressure is decreased immediately, cardiac arrest will ensue.[9]

Compensatory Mechanisms and Pericardiocentesis

To maintain physiologic cardiac output, the sympathetic nervous system increases the heart rate, arterial vasoconstriction (to maintain mean arterial blood pressure), and venoconstriction (to maintain normal venous-atrial and atrioventricular filling gradients). Early in tamponade, these compensatory mechanisms are usually effective in maintaining adequate cardiac output.

Compensatory mechanisms also preserve normal cardiac contractility and myocardial perfusion.[7,10,11] However, when pericardial pressure overwhelms the compensatory mechanisms, coronary perfusion pressure is reduced, which leads to myocardial ischemia. Experimental induction of severe tamponade demonstrated microscopic ischemic cardiac injury.[12] Lactic acidosis (resulting from reduced cardiac output and systemic hypoperfusion) may directly cause cardiac depression and thereby reduce cardiac contractility and, ultimately, cardiac output.[9]

Removal of pericardial fluid (i.e., pericardiocentesis) reverses the pathophysiologic processes just described by

Figure 16-1 Production of cardiac tamponade by injection of saline into the pericardial sac. The pericardial space can accommodate the acute introduction of 80 to 120 mL of fluid without a significant increase in pericardial pressure, but with about 200 mL of saline, pressure increases steeply and blood pressure (BP) drops. Once critical volumes are reached, very small increases cause significant hemodynamic compromise. (*From Fowler NO. Physiology of cardiac tamponade and pulsus paradoxus. II: physiological, circulatory, and pharmacological responses in cardiac tamponade. Mod Concepts Cardiovasc Dis. 1978;47:116. Reproduced by permission of the American Heart Association, Inc.*)

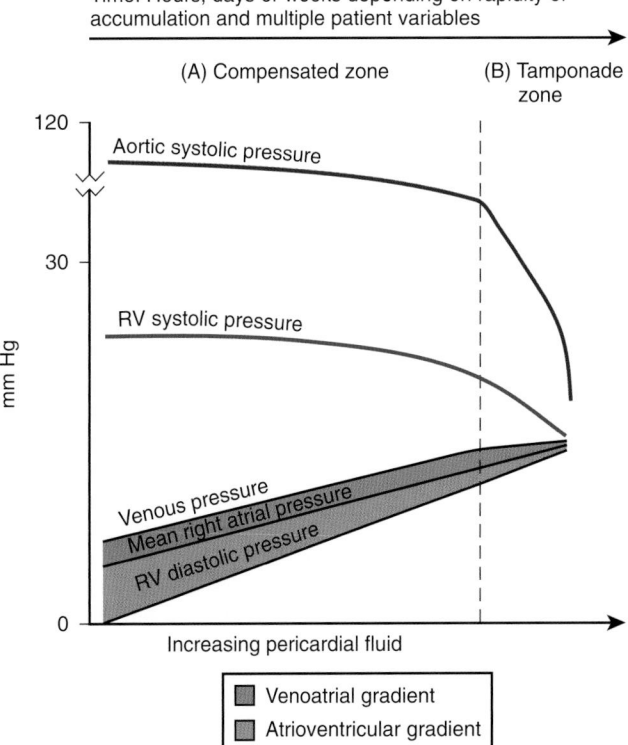

Figure 16-2 Summary of physiologic changes in tamponade. *RV,* right ventricular. (*From Shoemaker WC, Carey JS, Yao ST, et al. Hemodynamic monitoring for physiologic evaluation, diagnosis, and therapy of acute hemopericardial tamponade from penetrating wounds. J Trauma. 1973;13:363; and Spodick D. Acute cardiac tamponade: pathologic physiology, diagnosis, and management. Prog Cardiovasc Dis. 1967;10:65. Reproduced by permission.*)

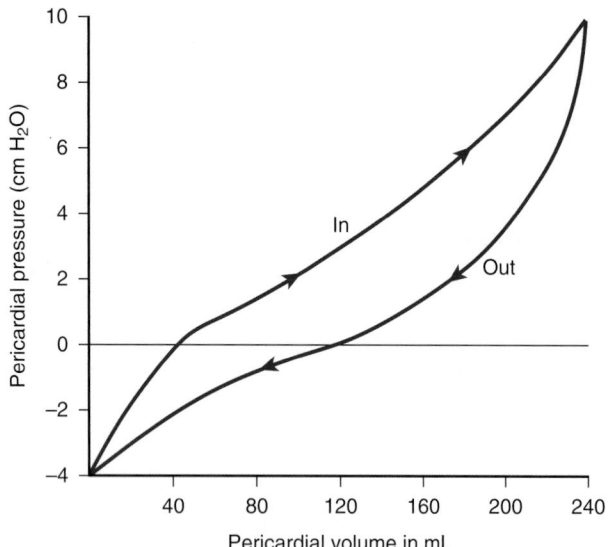

Figure 16-3 Relationship of intrapericardial pressure to volume of pericardial fluid. Pressure drops rapidly when a small amount of fluid is removed. *(From Pories W, Gaudiani V. Cardiac tamponade. Surg Clin North Am. 1975;55:573. Reproduced by permission.)*

improving cardiac filling and output. Interestingly, the pressure-volume relationship of the pericardial space demonstrates hysteresis; that is, withdrawing a certain quantity of fluid reduces intrapericardial pressure more than addition of the same amount of fluid increases intrapericardial pressure. This effect, however, is not universal and may vary among patients and in various disease states (Fig. 16-3).[2]

Special Considerations in Patients with Pericardial Effusion and Tamponade

Under normal circumstances, positive pressure ventilation (e.g., mechanical ventilation) reduces venous return to the right side of the heart by increasing intrathoracic pressure. This could be detrimental for patients with tamponade because right-sided filling is already compromised and further reductions can lead to severe hemodynamic instability.[13] Therefore, *positive pressure ventilation should be avoided in patients with known or suspected tamponade unless it is absolutely necessary.*

Low-pressure pericardial tamponade is defined as a hemodynamically significant effusion with lower than expected intrapericardial pressure.[14] This category of tamponade occurs in certain hypovolemic patients with subacute or chronic effusions (e.g., associated with long-term diuretic use, dehydration, excessive dialysis).[15] The diagnosis may be challenging because the classic symptoms and findings on physical examination (e.g., distended neck veins) may be absent.[16] Fluid boluses may temporize the hemodynamic compromise while pericardial decompression is being arranged.

EPIDEMIOLOGY

The major categories of pericardial effusion include infection, malignancy, trauma, and metabolic abnormalities. Effusion may also be associated with aortic disease, connective tissue disease, or idiopathic causes. It is often difficult to report the exact incidence of each type of pericardial effusion because of variations in patient populations, local epidemiology, and the diagnostic protocols used during evaluation. The prevalence of a chronic effusion is also difficult to ascertain because it is often asymptomatic and underreported. General autopsy studies demonstrate an overall prevalence of 3.4%.[17]

CAUSES OF PERICARDIAL EFFUSION
(Box 16-1)

Acute Hemopericardium

Acute hemopericardium, or rapid accumulation of blood in the pericardial space, can have a traumatic or nontraumatic etiology. It is one of the most feared causes of tamponade because the semi-elastic pericardium cannot accommodate acute increases in pericardial fluid and clinical deterioration can be rapid. This diagnosis can be challenging to make because there may be little or no evidence during the initial evaluation (e.g., pericardial size might be normal on a chest radiograph).

Traumatic Hemopericardium
Penetrating Trauma

Penetrating cardiac trauma can cause acute hemopericardium by either external forces (e.g., a stab wound to the heart) or internal forces (e.g., iatrogenic injury during placement of a pacemaker). Cardiac perforation can lead to rapid clinical deterioration and PEA.

External cardiac puncture is associated with stab wounds or projectile injuries (e.g., gunshot wounds). Tamponade develops in 80% to 90% of patients with cardiac stab wounds as opposed to 20% of those with gunshot wounds.[18,19] Stab wounds cause tamponade more frequently because if the pericardial injury is small, it can reseal and trap blood within the pericardial space.[20] On the other hand, a gunshot typically produces large pericardial wounds that allow continuous drainage into the pleural space.[21] Clinical deterioration is usually secondary to hypovolemia.[21] Any penetrating injury to the chest, back, or upper part of the abdomen may injure the pericardium and cause tamponade.

Internal penetrating trauma is typically caused by invasive diagnostic or therapeutic procedures. The procedures most often associated with this injury are pacemaker insertion and cardiac catheterization (angioplasty or valvuloplasty).[22-24] Hemopericardium results from puncturing the cardiac chamber, a coronary artery, or a great vessel (e.g., the superior vena cava). Ironically, pericardiocentesis itself (treatment of a pericardial effusion) can cause hemopericardium if coronary vessels or the myocardium is injured during the procedure.[25,26]

Internal jugular and subclavian venous catheters (e.g., central venous or hemodialysis catheters) are commonly inserted in the emergency department (ED). During such procedures, hemopericardium results from perforation of the superior vena cava, right atrium, or RV. Hemopericardium can occur immediately or can be delayed up to 2 days subsequent to erosion of the catheter through myocardial or vascular tissue.[27,28] Although this complication seldom occurs, it should always be considered when a patient experiences sudden hemodynamic deterioration following an invasive procedure.

BOX 16-1 Causes of Pericardial Effusion

NEOPLASM
Mesothelioma
Lung
Breast
Melanoma
Lymphoma

PERICARDITIS
Radiation related (especially
    after Hodgkin's disease)
Viral
Bacterial
    Staphylococcus
    Pneumococcus
    Haemophilus
Fungal
Tuberculosis
Amebiasis

Toxoplasmosis
Idiopathic

CONNECTIVE TISSUE DISEASE
Systemic lupus erythematosus
Scleroderma
Rheumatoid arthritis
Acute rheumatic fever

METABOLIC DISORDERS
Myxedema
Uremia
Cholesterol pericarditis
Bleeding diatheses

CARDIAC DISEASE
Acute myocardial infarction
Dissecting aortic aneurysm

Congestive heart failure
Coronary aneurysm

DRUGS
Hydralazine
Phenytoin
Anticoagulants
Procainamide
Minoxidil

TRAUMA
Blunt
    Major trauma
    Closed-chest cardiopulmo-
        nary resuscitation
Penetrating
    Major penetrating trauma
Intracardiac injections

Transthoracic and transvenous
    pacing wires
Pericardiocentesis
Cardiac catheterization
Central venous pressure
    catheter

MISCELLANEOUS
Serum sickness
Chylous effusion
Löffler's syndrome
Reiter's syndrome
Behçet's syndrome
Pancreatitis
Postpericardiotomy
Amyloidosis
Ascites

Data from Guberman BA, Fowler NO, Engel PJ, et al. Cardiac tamponade in medical patients. Circulation. 1981;64:633; and Pories WJ, Caudiani VA. Cardiac tamponade. Surg Clin North Am. 1975;55:573.

Blunt Trauma

Major blunt chest trauma can cause hemopericardium with or without obvious signs of injury.[29] Myocardial rupture can be uncontained or contained.[30,31] Patients with uncontained rupture do not typically survive long enough to reach the hospital.[32] Contained rupture may be found soon after injury or may be a late finding (in some cases up to 12 days later).[33] Tamponade can also be caused by a deceleration mechanism of injury that induces either aortic or vena caval disruption.[34] In one case series the incidence of tamponade following deceleration injury was found to be 2.3% (1 in 43 patients).[35]

Miscellaneous Trauma

Chest compressions during cardiopulmonary resuscitation (CPR) can also cause hemopericardium from broken ribs, bleeding intercostal vessels, or penetrating injury (e.g., intracardiac injection of medication, which is rarely performed today).[36] Hemopericardium following CPR has been described in case reports[37,38] but is unlikely to be significant, much less to cause tamponade.

Atraumatic Hemopericardium

Atraumatic hemopericardium is difficult to diagnose. Diagnosis is often delayed because it occurs spontaneously and the clinical findings can be less obvious than those of hemopericardium from traumatic causes. Maintain a high index of suspicion for this condition in patients with risk factors, such as recent myocardial infarction (MI). Common causes of atraumatic hemopericardium are discussed below.

Bleeding diathesis is an important cause of spontaneous hemopericardium and may be associated with the use of anticoagulants (reported incidence of 2.5% to 11%)[22] or thrombolytic therapy (incidence <1%).[39] Patients who have undergone cardiac surgery are at increased risk because of the anticoagulative effects of the cardiopulmonary bypass machine and medications started postoperatively (e.g.,

clopidogrel, warfarin).[40] Fortunately, tamponade has a low incidence and is generally detected in the postoperative period before discharge.[41,42] This complication is usually prevented by the intraoperative placement of mediastinal or pericardial drains.[22,43]

Hemopericardium can develop following MI. Early after a transmural MI (1 to 3 days), the necrotic myocardium causes inflammation of the overlying pericardium and then effusions can form. Late-developing effusions (weeks after an MI) are caused by an autoimmune pericarditis called Dressler's syndrome.[1] Improved reperfusion techniques have reduced the incidence of post-MI pericarditis and effusion.[44]

Ascending aortic dissection causes rapid and usually fatal hemopericardium. The dissection may expand in a retrograde fashion by extending to the base of the aorta and into the pericardial sac. Risk factors for aortic dissection include hypertension, atherosclerosis, vasculitis (e.g., giant cell arteritis, syphilis), collagen vascular disease (e.g., Marfan's syndrome), and the use of sympathomimetics (e.g., cocaine).[45-47]

Ventricular free-wall rupture is a rapidly fatal cause of acute hemopericardium that can occur after MI. This complication is less common today than in the past (<1%)[39] secondary to improved revascularization techniques, better therapeutic medications, and faster intervention times (shorter door-to-balloon times) for coronary ischemia. Despite a reduction in its overall incidence, 7% of all deaths related to MI are caused by this complication.[48,49] Survival is possible with prompt recognition and treatment, but the prognosis is grim once tamponade occurs.[50,51]

Nonhemorrhagic Effusions

Nonhemorrhagic pericardial effusions usually accumulate slower than acute hemopericardium does (over a period of weeks to months). Chronic fluid accumulation allows the pericardium to stretch circumferentially and accommodate up to 2000 mL of fluid without any hemodynamic compromise.[52] Effusions that grow slowly allow the circulatory system to adapt to the intrapericardial pressure, thereby further maintaining hemodynamic stability. Thus, asymptomatic patients with moderate to large effusions may not need emergency pericardiocentesis, in contrast to patients with acute hemopericardium.[53,54]

Nonhemorrhagic effusions have several causes (see Box 16-1), and the exact one may not be obvious during the initial evaluation without diagnostic pericardiocentesis. Common causes of nonhemorrhagic effusions are discussed in the following sections.

Idiopathic Effusions

Most idiopathic effusions are believed to be viral in origin and most commonly caused by infection with coxsackievirus, echovirus, or enterovirus. Idiopathic pericardial effusions may be asymptomatic or have an associated component of pericarditis (e.g., positional pain or diffuse ST-segment changes on the electrocardiogram [ECG]).[55] These effusions are often labeled "idiopathic" because the diagnosis cannot be made noninvasively (i.e., based on the history, physical examination, or serum testing) and the risk associated with diagnostic pericardiocentesis outweighs the risk of observation in asymptomatic adults who appear to be well.[56] Diagnostic pericardiocentesis may be recommended for idiopathic effusions that are persistent or symptomatic without a known cause.[57]

Neoplastic Effusion

Tumors of the pericardium or myocardium may cause nonhemorrhagic effusions.[54,58] Primary cardiac tumors are less common (0.001% to 0.003%) than metastases from another site (2% to 18%), but either may cause a malignant effusion.[59] Although no malignancy preferentially metastasizes to the heart, certain tumors commonly involve the heart when they metastasize; frequently implicated are lung cancer, breast cancer, mediastinal tumors, malignant melanoma, leukemia, and lymphoma.[46]

Cardiac metastasis is usually a late finding in cancer; other foci are generally evident first.[47] The classic signs and symptoms of tamponade (e.g., chest pain and dyspnea) may not be obvious with malignant tamponade. When present, they may be mistakenly attributed to the underlying malignancy.[46] Thus, in the relevant clinical scenario, consider screening patients with malignancy for pericardial effusion (e.g., ultrasound) before the clinical findings of tamponade appear.

Congestive Heart Failure

Congestive heart failure (CHF) is a cause of pericardial effusion. Diagnosis may be difficult because of overlapping signs and symptoms with exacerbations of CHF (e.g., chest pain or dyspnea). Adding to the diagnostic complexity is that 12% to 20% of patients with CHF have a coexisting pericardial effusion.[60] Fortunately, treatment of CHF-associated pericardial effusion does not differ from that for an effusion from other causes: treat the underlying cause unless the patient has evidence of hemodynamic compromise.

Radiation

Pericardial effusions (secondary to radiation-induced pericarditis) can develop acutely during radiation therapy or nay be delayed for years. Risk factors include the radiation dose, duration of exposure, and age of the patient. Patients treated with radiation for Hodgkin's disease have the highest association of radiation-induced pericarditis and subsequent effusions.[22] These effusions can be serous, hemorrhagic, or fibrinous.[57]

HIV-Associated Effusions

Human immunodeficiency virus (HIV) can cause nonhemorrhagic pericardial effusion and tamponade (see Review Box 16-1).[61,62] The incidence has been reported to be approximately 11% in patients with HIV infection or acquired immunodeficiency syndrome (AIDS), and 13% of cases are classified as moderate to severe. It is unclear whether antiretroviral therapy has affected these data.[17]

HIV-related effusions have been attributed to bacterial (e.g., *Staphylococcus aureus*), viral (e.g., cytomegalovirus), fungal (*Cryptococcus neoformans*), and mycobacterial causes (e.g., tuberculosis, which is the most common cause of HIV-related effusions worldwide).[63] Kaposi's sarcoma and lymphoma can cause noninfectious pericardial effusions in HIV patients.[64,65]

Renal Failure and Uremia

Pericardial effusion develops in approximately 15% to 20% of dialysis patients, and tamponade may eventually occur in as many as 35% of that group.[66,67] Up to 7% of chronic dialysis patients have effusions with volumes of 1000 mL or greater.[68] In many cases, effusions secondary to renal failure can be managed solely with aggressive dialysis without pericardiocentesis. Any sign of hemodynamic compromise, however, warrants strong consideration of pericardiocentesis.

Hypothyroidism

Hypothyroid patients are at risk for pericardial effusions (up to 30%), but the fluid accumulates gradually, so tamponade develops in only a few patients.[54] If pericardial effusions are present, other areas of the body usually demonstrate serositis (e.g., pleural effusions). Treating the underlying hypothyroidism often reverses the effusion without the need for pericardiocentesis.

Special Considerations in Pericardial Disease

Pericardial tamponade is classically described as being secondary to circumferential effusion, which causes a generalized increase in pericardial pressure and compression of multiple cardiac chambers. Loculated effusions (caused by a local hematoma or an infectious process) or pericardial adhesions (from previous inflammation) can compress one or two cardiac chambers and thus reduce both cardiac filling and cardiac output.[69,70]

Constrictive pericarditis occurs following chronic pericardial inflammation, infection, or mediastinal irradiation. These processes cause scarring, fibrosis, or calcification, and the pericardium eventually becomes a nonelastic and "constrictive" sac around the heart. Myocardial relaxation and cardiac filling are impaired, and diastolic dysfunction ensues. Without echocardiography, constrictive pericarditis can be difficult to distinguish from pericardial tamponade.[1]

Effusive-constrictive pericarditis is defined by the presence of both pericardial effusion and pericardial constriction. It may be quite difficult to differentiate between effusive-constrictive pericarditis and pericardial tamponade in stable patients because both are associated with effusions.[71] Fortunately, distinguishing between these diagnoses is less important in hemodynamically unstable patients because they are treated identically (i.e., with pericardiocentesis).[72]

Pneumopericardium is an interesting, though rare cause of cardiac tamponade. It is most commonly associated with pneumothorax caused by barotrauma (e.g., mechanical ventilation).[73] It also occurs spontaneously during acute asthma exacerbations,[74] and it can follow blunt chest injury.[75,76] Although typically benign, tension pneumopericardium has been reported as a cause of life-threatening tamponade after blunt[77,78] and penetrating chest trauma.[79,80]

DIAGNOSING CARDIAC TAMPONADE

Diagnosis of pericardial effusions requires integration of the patient's history, findings on physical examination, and diagnostic testing. Unfortunately, even experienced clinicians may not initially consider pericardial effusion because the clinical findings are often vague and nonspecific. Nonspecific symptoms, such as chest pain and dyspnea, can be ascribed to more common conditions (e.g., CHF or pulmonary pathology), so the diagnosis might be delayed until diagnostic testing is performed (e.g., computed tomography [CT] of the chest for pulmonary embolism)[81] or until hypotension develops and bedside ultrasound is performed.[82]

Acute pericardial tamponade (e.g., secondary to blunt chest wall trauma) is usually challenging to diagnose because the findings on physical examination may resemble those of other life-threatening conditions (e.g., tension pneumothorax, hemothorax, hypovolemia, pulmonary edema, severe contusion of the RV, aortic dissection, or pulmonary embolism).[67] In hemodynamically unstable patients, diagnostic (e.g., bedside ultrasound) and therapeutic (e.g., pericardiocentesis) interventions must be performed even with a paucity of findings on physical examination because rapid clinical deterioration and cardiac arrest can occur before a definitive diagnosis can be made.

Once a pericardial effusion is suspected (or diagnosed), the next step is to determine its size and hemodynamic significance and presence of underlying or associated diseases.[83] Specific therapy will hinge on this information and is discussed in the following sections.

History: Patient Profile and Symptoms

The historical features of pericardial effusions are nonspecific and the diagnosis may be overlooked initially. However, an astute clinician might be suspicious based on comorbid conditions (e.g., warfarin therapy or a history of myxedema) and the time course of the symptoms (e.g., free-wall rupture several days after MI, dyspnea in a patient with uremic pericarditis). Box 16-2 lists important details to be ascertained from the history when pericardial effusion is suspected.[84]

BOX 16-2 Information to Obtain from Patients When Pericardial Effusion Is Suspected

ONSET AND DURATION OF SYMPTOMS

Acute

Trauma
Recent cardiac surgery
Recent myocardial infarction
Acute aortic dissection
Recent diagnostic or therapeutic intervention (e.g., catheterization)
Recent upper thoracic vascular procedure (e.g., hemodialysis catheter, central line, peripherally inserted central catheter line, Mediport)
Recent placement of a pacemaker or automatic implantable cardioverter-defibrillator

Subacute/Chronic

Metabolic (e.g., uremia)
Endocrine (e.g., hypothyroidism)
Infectious
- Viral (e.g., human immunodeficiency virus)
- Bacterial (e.g., *Staphylococcus*)
- Fungal (e.g., *Aspergillus*)
Neoplastic
- Primary cardiac
- Metastatic
Autoimmune disorders (e.g., lupus)
Inflammatory
- Vasculitis

MEDICAL/SURGICAL HISTORY

Autoimmune disorders
- Lupus
- Mixed connective tissue disease
- Vasculitis
Endocrine disease
- Hypothyroidism
- Ovarian hyperstimulation syndrome
Metabolic diseases
- End-stage renal disease
- Uremia
- Coagulopathies
Artificial cardiac valves
- Anticoagulation medications
- Risk for myocarditis
Cardiac disease
- Anticoagulation medications
- Pericarditis
- Aneurysm
Recent placement of a vascular catheter
Recent cardiac surgery
Recent cardiac intervention
Recent thoracic radiation

MEDICATIONS

Anticoagulants
- Aspirin
- Warfarin
- Clopidogrel

Antiarrhythmic
- Procainamide (drug-induced lupus)
Tuberculosis therapy
- Isoniazid (drug-induced lupus)

COMMON SYMPTOMS

Altered mental status, confusion
Fatigue
Dizziness, lightheadedness
Orthostatic changes
Exercise intolerance
Hoarseness
Hiccups
Fever
Chills
Chest pain
- Substernal
- Pleuritic
- Scapula (phrenic nerve irritation)
- Palpitations
- Cough
- Dyspnea
- Myalgia
- Arthralgia

BOX 16-3 Physical Examination Findings Suggestive of Pericardial Effusion or Tamponade

VITAL SIGNS
Normal vital signs
Tachycardia (tamponade)
Hypotension (tamponade)
Narrow pulse pressure
Pulsus paradoxus
Fever (if the cause is infectious or neoplastic)

APPEARANCE
Normal appearance
Anxiety
Sense of impending doom
Diaphoresis
Cold and clammy

Pallor
Altered mental status, confusion

NECK
Supraclavicular retractions
Distended neck veins (may be flat with hypotension)

CARDIOVASCULAR
Normal findings on examination
Tachycardia
Increased pain with a supine position, relieved by leaning forward

Muted, distant heart sounds
Pericardial friction rub (inflammatory pericarditis)
Displaced point of maximal impulse
Increased cardiac borders with percussion
Distended neck veins
Auscultatory dullness along the left scapular area

PULMONARY
Telegraphic speech
Respiratory distress
Supraclavicular retractions
Cough

Hoarseness
Clear breath sounds (may distinguish tamponade from congestive heart failure)

ABDOMINAL
Hepatomegaly
Splenomegaly

SKIN
Cool extremities
Clammy extremities
Dilated head and scalp veins
Peripheral edema
Anasarca

TABLE 16-1 Shoemaker System of Grading Cardiac Tamponade

GRADE	PERICARDIAL VOLUME (mL)	CARDIAC INDEX	STROKE INDEX	MEAN ARTERIAL PRESSURE	CENTRAL VENOUS PRESSURE	HEART RATE	BECK'S TRIAD
I	<200	Normal or ↑	Normal or ↓	Normal	↑	↑	Venous distention, hypotension, muffled heart sounds usually not present
II	≥200	↓	↓	Normal or ↓	↑ (≤12 cm H₂O)	↑	May or may not be present
III	>200	↓↓	↓↓	↓↓	↑↑ (30-40 cm H₂O)	↑	Usually present

From Shoemaker WC, Carey SJ, Yao ST, et al. Hemodynamic monitoring for physiologic evaluation, diagnosis, and therapy of acute hemopericardial tamponade from penetrating wounds. *J Trauma.* 1973;13:36.

Physical Examination

Physical examination of patients with pericardial effusion (e.g., displaced point of maximal impulse, muffled heart sounds) lacks sensitivity and specificity. If the history suggests pericardial effusion, the physical examination should focus on determining the underlying cause (e.g., stigmata of hypothyroidism) to guide definitive diagnostic testing (e.g., echocardiography). Ironically, many pericardial effusions are not diagnosed from the history or findings on physical examination but are found incidentally during the evaluation for other diseases.

In 1935, Beck characterized the physical manifestations of tamponade with two triads—one for chronic and one for acute tamponade.[85] Beck's "chronic" triad consists of increased central venous pressure (CVP) (i.e., distended neck veins), ascites, and a small, quiet heart. "Beck's triad" is a classic description of acute cardiac compression, which includes increased CVP, decreased arterial pressure, and muffled heart sounds. Almost 90% of patients have one or more of these "acute" signs,[86] *but only about 33% demonstrate the complete triad.*[9,87] The utility of this triad is further limited because all three signs are usually observed shortly before cardiac arrest.

It would be clinically desirable to identify patients in early tamponade, before hemodynamic collapse. Unfortunately, findings on physical examination in early tamponade are nonspecific and may be indistinguishable from those of other critical diseases (e.g., septic shock, right heart failure).[57] Patients initially seen in late tamponade also have nonspecific findings. They may be agitated, panic-stricken, confused, uncooperative, restless, cyanotic, diaphoretic, acutely dyspneic, or hemodynamically unstable. Such patients should undergo a brief and focused physical examination because the time between initial evaluation and full arrest may be brief.

Some of the findings on physical examination associated with tamponade are described below. A more comprehensive list is presented in Box 16-3.

Vital Sign Abnormalities

The three stages occur sequentially and reflect the natural history of acute tamponade (Table 16-1).[88] The time course within each stage varies from patient to patient. Some patients are stable within a given stage for hours, whereas others proceed through all three stages and cardiac arrest within minutes.[9,88] Grade I tamponade is characterized by normal blood pressure and cardiac output with an increase in the heart rate and CVP (measured invasively with a central venous catheter). Grade II tamponade is defined by normal or slightly reduced blood pressure; CVP and the heart rate remain increased. Grade III tamponade is identified on the basis of Beck's triad: hypotension, tachycardia, and elevated CVP.

Nearly all patients with tamponade have sinus tachycardia, although its specificity is low.[89] The physiologic purpose of tachycardia is to maintain normal cardiac output despite reductions in stroke volume from worsening tamponade. Exceptions to the pairing of tachycardia with tamponade usually relate to the underlying cause of the effusion (e.g., myxedema) or the concomitant use of certain medications (e.g., β-blockers).

Adding to the diagnostic complexity, not all patients in tamponade have a reduction in blood pressure. In fact, Brown and coworkers[90] described several tamponade patients with elevated blood pressure. These patients were previously hypertensive and paradoxically had reduced systolic blood pressure following pericardiocentesis.

Pulsus Paradoxus

PP is an exaggerated decrease in systolic blood pressure (>12 mm Hg) during inspiration secondary to reduced stroke volume (Fig. 16-4*A*).[30,91,92] Patients with moderate to severe tamponade typically demonstrate PP greater than 20 mm Hg.[9,86,93] Unfortunately, PP is not pathognomonic for tamponade. It is observed in other conditions, such as hypotension associated with labored breathing (secondary to extreme reductions in intrathoracic pressure [Fig. 16-4*B*]), severe emphysema, severe asthma, obesity, cardiac failure, constrictive pericarditis, pulmonary embolism, and cardiogenic shock.[9,86,93]

The absence of PP does not rule out tamponade because it can occur with several conditions: atrial septal defects, aortic insufficiency, positive pressure ventilation, loculated pericardial effusions, and elevated left ventricular diastolic pressure (e.g., poor left ventricular compliance secondary to chronic hypertension).[14] Finally, PP should be interpreted with caution in patients with traumatic tamponade because it can be unreliable.[94-96] In a study of 197 patients with traumatic tamponade, only 8.6% had PP.[97]

Measuring PP is useful only occasionally because it is difficult, time-consuming, and not specific or sensitive for tamponade. Its description here is for historical value and for use in hemodynamically stable patients. When managing unstable patients, especially those in extremis, assessment for PP should not replace more definitive testing such as bedside ultrasound.

Neck Vein Distention and Elevated CVP

Neck vein distention (a surrogate for measuring CVP) occurs late in tamponade, when right-sided chambers (e.g., the RV) collapse. Neck vein distention may be obvious on examination (Fig. 16-5*A*), but visualization of such distention is less accurate than measuring CVP by central venous catheter or evaluation with ultrasound (Table 16-2). Patients with significant tamponade typically have a CVP of 12 cm H_2O or higher.[95] Finally, although initial CVP readings are useful and diagnostic when grossly elevated (e.g., 20 to 30 cm H_2O),[95,98] upward CVP trends can be a more sensitive diagnostic tool.[95]

Overreliance on increased CVP and venous distention should be avoided because they do not always indicate tamponade. For example, increased intrathoracic pressure (as induced by positive pressure ventilation or Valsalva maneuvers) increases CVP and causes neck vein distention even without pericardial effusion. Conversely, hypovolemic patients

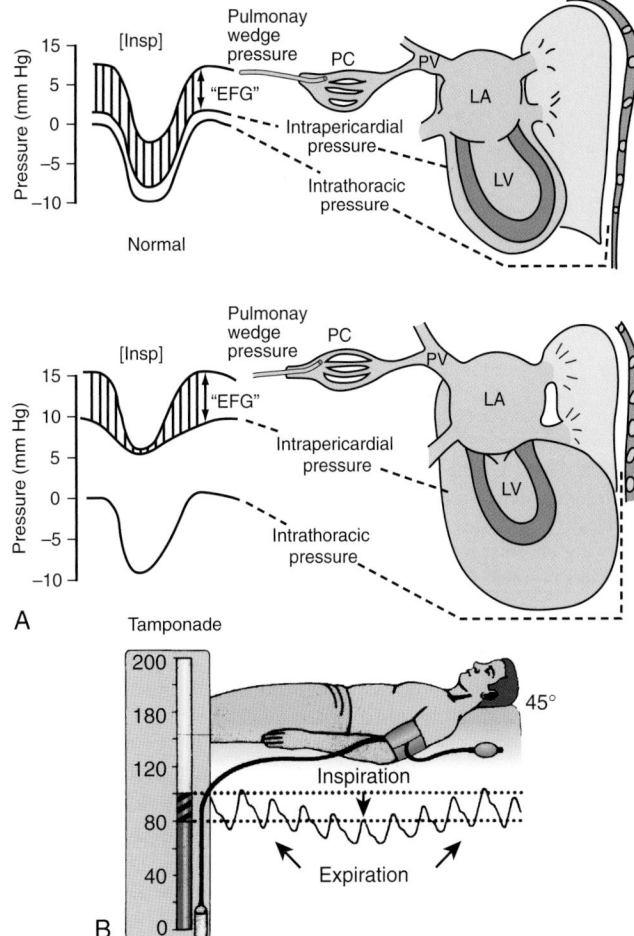

Figure 16-4 Pulsus paradoxus. **A,** *Top,* The normal situation in which changes in intrathoracic pressure are transmitted to both the pericardial sac and the pulmonary veins. The effective filling gradient (EFG) changes only slightly during respiration. *Bottom,* Cardiac tamponade in which changes in intrathoracic pressure are transmitted to the pulmonary veins but not to the pericardial sac. The EFG falls during inspiration (Insp). *LA,* left atrium; *LV,* left ventricle; *PC,* pulmonary capillaries; *PV,* pulmonary veins. **B,** Normally, systolic blood pressure drops slightly during inspiration. To assess for pulsus paradoxus, have the patient breathe normally while lying at a 45-degree angle. Inflate the blood pressure cuff well above systolic pressure and slowly deflate it. When the pulse is first heard only during expiration, this is the upper value. Deflate the cuff until the pulse is heard during both inspiration and expiration; this is the lower value. A difference of more than 12 mm Hg between the two values indicates pulsus paradoxus. (*A, Adapted from Sharp JT, Bunnell IL, Holand JF, et al. Hemodynamics during induced cardiac tamponade in man. Am J Med. 1960;25:640.*)

may have reduced CVP and no neck vein distention despite having clinical tamponade. The absence of distended neck veins may also result from severe venoconstriction secondary to intrinsic sympathetic discharge, vasopressor use, or severe hypovolemia.[9,88,93,95]

Diagnostic Testing

Diagnostic testing should be initiated when pericardial effusion or tamponade is suspected. Definitive diagnosis requires imaging such as CT or, preferably, cardiac ultrasound (Fig.

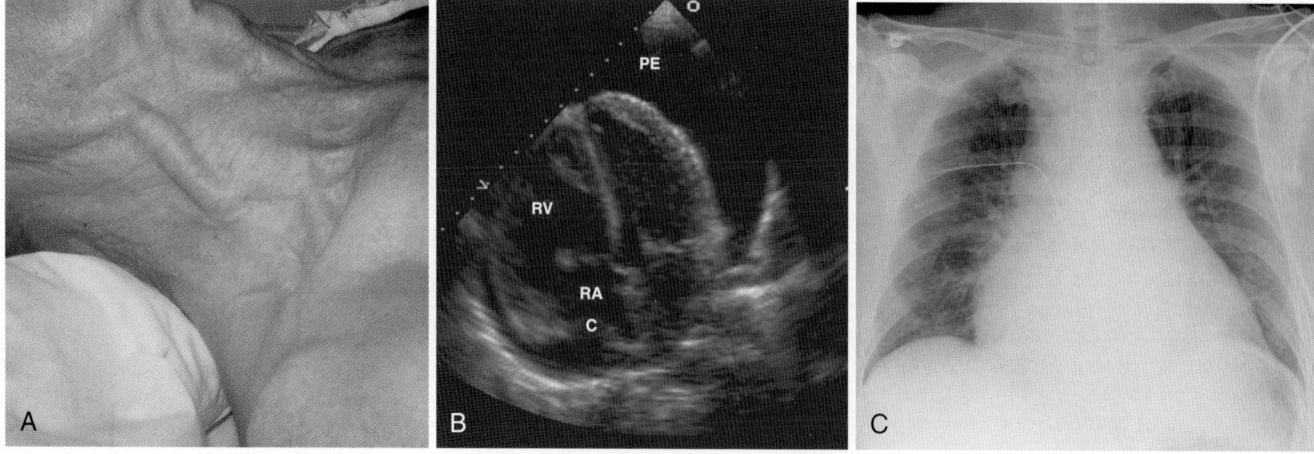

Figure 16-5 A, The neck veins might be markedly distended with cardiac tamponade, but this finding is not universal, especially in patients with hypovolemic trauma. **B,** Ultrasound. An apical view of a large pericardial effusion in early ventricular diastole reveals marked right atrial collapse. *C,* collapsed segment of the right atrial wall; *PE,* pericardial effusion; *RA,* right atrium; *RV,* right ventricle. **C,** Chest radiograph showing an enlarged, globular cardiac silhouette (water-bottle heart) in a patient with tamponade caused by a malignant effusion. The chest film has minimal value in diagnosing tamponade but is usually abnormal when significant *chronic* effusions are present.

TABLE 16-2 Noninvasive Estimation of Right Atrial Pressure with Ultrasound

DIAMETER (cm) OF INFERIOR VENA CAVA	CHANGE IN DIAMETER WITH RESPIRATION	ESTIMATED RIGHT ATRIAL PRESSURE (mm Hg)
Normal (<2.1)	Decrease >50%	~3 (normal, 0-5)
Dilated (<2.1)	Decrease <50%	~8 (normal, 5-10)
Dilated (>2.1)	Decrease >50%	~8 (normal, 10-15)
Dilated (>2.1)	Decrease <50%	>15

Based on Rudski LG, Lai WW, Afilalo J, et al. Guidelines for the echocardiographic assessment of the right heart in adults: a report from the American Society of Echocardiography endorsed by the European Association of Echocardiography, a registered branch of the European Society of Cardiology, and the Canadian Society of Echocardiography. *J Am Soc Echocardiogr.* 2010;23:685.

16-5*B*). Bedside ultrasound is the fastest and most reliable diagnostic tool because it is noninvasive, does not emit radiation, and can be performed at the bedside without transporting unstable patients outside the ED.

As discussed previously, pericardial effusions are occasionally discovered incidentally during evaluation for other disorders. For example, the chest film and ECG of a patient being assessed for acute coronary syndrome (ACS) may suggest tamponade. If the clinical context supports pericardial effusion as the primary diagnosis rather than ACS, further workup for the effusion (e.g., an echocardiogram) should be ordered. If neither diagnosis is more likely than the other, dual workups may be necessary.

Chest Radiography

Chest radiographs are not diagnostically useful in patients with acute traumatic tamponade because the pericardium does not have sufficient time to change size or shape (see "Pathophysiology of Pericardial Tamponade"). Radiographs, however, may reveal other associated findings such as

hemothorax, bullets in the thorax, or even pneumopericardium. Chest radiography may also be helpful when other diagnoses (e.g., CHF) have clinical findings similar to those of pericardial effusion. For example, a dyspneic patient with a clear chest film is less likely to have decompensated CHF than tamponade.

In patients with chronic pericardial effusions, chest films often demonstrate an enlarged, saclike, "water-bottle" cardiac shadow or pleural effusion (Fig. 16-5*C*). Unfortunately, it is difficult to differentiate a large effusion from myocardial enlargement (e.g., dilated cardiomyopathy) because radiographs demonstrate only the cardiac silhouette and do not reveal the physiologic differences between these two diagnoses.

Electrocardiography

Pericardial effusion secondary to acute pericarditis is suspected on the basis of typical changes on the ECG. Pericarditis has four stages: (1) diffuse ST-segment elevation with PR depression, (2) ST- and PR-segment normalization, (3) diffuse T-wave inversion, and (4) normalization of T waves.[99]

Electrocardiography has acceptable specificity but poor sensitivity[93,100,101] in diagnosing pericardial effusion and tamponade. In a study of patients with pericardial effusion, electrocardiography had an overall sensitivity of 1% to 17% and a specificity of 89% to 100%.[93] Therefore, an ECG may suggest but should never be the only means of diagnosing a pericardial effusion (Fig. 16-6). Furthermore, electrocardiography cannot reliably differentiate tamponade from effusion.[102]

The three most commonly described electrocardiographic findings in pericardial effusion are PR depression, low-voltage QRS complexes, and electrical alternans. PR-segment depression is the most common finding and is defined as depression of 1 mV or greater in at least one lead other than aVR. Low-voltage QRS complexes (most frequently associated with moderate to large effusions) are defined by a QRS complex with an amplitude of 5 mV or less across all limb leads. Alternatively, low-voltage QRS complexes can be identified by a sum of 30 mV or less for all limb lead QRS amplitudes.

ELECTRICAL ALTERNANS IN PERICARDIAL TAMPONADE

Figure 16-6 Electrical alternans may develop in patients with pericardial effusion and cardiac tamponade. Notice the beat-to-beat alternation in the P-QRs-T axis; this is caused by the periodic swinging motion of the heart in a large pericardial effusion. Relatively low QRS voltage and sinus tachycardia are also present. Overall, the electrocardiogram has low sensitivity for pericardial effusion and tamponade. Note that electrical alternans may be more evident in the V leads.

Figure 16-7 Areas of the chest to obtain basic echocardiographic windows: *A,* subxiphoid (subcostal) view; *B,* parasternal view; *C,* apical four-chamber view.

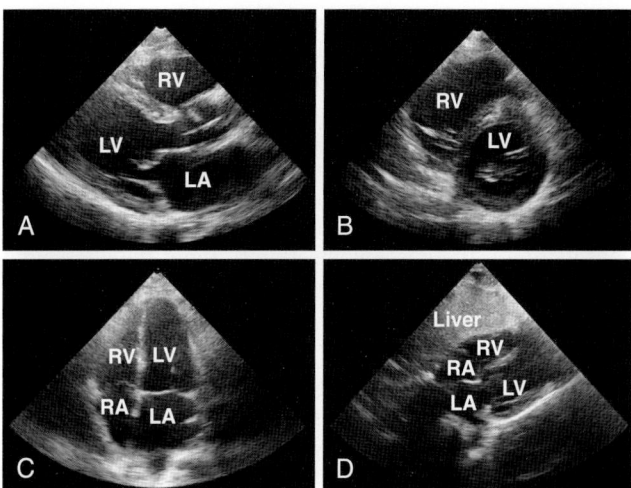

Figure 16-8 Normal echocardiographic views: **A,** Parasternal long-axis view. **B,** Parasternal short-axis view. **C,** Apical four-chamber view. **D,** Subxiphoid (subcostal) view. *LA,* left atrium; *LV,* left ventricle; *RA,* right atrium; *RV,* right ventricle.

Figure 16-9 Examples of pericardial effusion. **A,** Small pericardial effusion (parasternal long-axis view). **B,** Moderate pericardial effusion (parasternal long-axis view). **C,** Large pericardial effusion (apical four-chamber view). **D,** Large pericardial effusion (subcostal/subxiphoid view). *LA,* left atrium; *LV,* left ventricle; *PE,* pericardial effusion; *PL,* pleural effusion; *RA,* right atrium. *RV,* right ventricle.

Electrical alternans is a beat-to-beat alternation in QRS amplitude caused by the pendulum motion of the heart within the fluid-filled pericardial sac.[103] Alternans has been observed in 22% of medical patients with tamponade[104] and in 5% of patients with tamponade secondary to cancer.[105] Electrical alternans of P waves and QRS complexes (i.e., total electrical alternans) is a rare finding but, when seen, is pathognomonic of tamponade (see Fig. 16-6).[93,106]

Echocardiography
Echocardiography is the best tool for diagnosing pericardial effusion or tamponade (see Figs. 16-7 to 16-9 and the Ultrasound Box). It not only demonstrates the presence of a pericardial effusion but also detects hemodynamic abnormalities. Ultrasonography (used interchangeably with *echocardiography* from here on) has the advantage that it is noninvasive and portable for use at the bedside and involves no ionizing

radiation.[9] Echocardiography is a very sensitive and specific tool for the diagnosis of pericardial effusion and tamponade,[57,87,89] and its use in diagnosing pericardial effusions has been endorsed by several academic societies.[107-110]

Diagnosing Pericardial Effusions and Tamponade
Fluid within the pericardial space is not always pathologic—the pericardial space normally holds 15 to 50 mL of fluid. Small effusions may be clinically insignificant. The sonographer/clinician should exercise caution to not overread an effusion, particularly when the patient is hemodynamically stable.[111]

Once a pericardial effusion is discovered, evaluate the patient for evidence of hemodynamic compromise. Echocardiographic signs include (1) diastolic collapse of the right atrium (highly specific and sensitive for tamponade, especially when the collapse occurs for more than a third of the cardiac cycle)[112]; (2) early diastolic collapse of the right ventricular free wall (less sensitive than right atrial collapse but specific for tamponade)[113]; (3) left atrial collapse (a very specific sign of tamponade)[114]; (4) a small, slitlike, hyperkinetic left ventricle; (5) dilation of the hepatic veins and IVC; and (6) swinging of the heart to and fro within the pericardial sac.[115] The presence of any of these signs should alert the clinician to the possibility of hemodynamic instability. Obtain expert consultation if there is any uncertainty about the ultrasound findings.

Limitations of Ultrasound

Ultrasound is the best diagnostic tool for pericardial effusion and tamponade, but great care must be taken when it is used as the only diagnostic modality. In a postoperative series of cardiac surgery patients, 60% of loculated effusions causing tamponade were missed on transthoracic echocardiography but were visualized with transesophageal echocardiography.[116]

Many ultrasound findings that suggest pericardial effusion are actually false positives. Examples include pericardial thickening, large pleural effusions, atelectasis, and mediastinal lesions.[17] Epicardial (or anterior) fat pads can also be misinterpreted as pericardial effusions, although several details help distinguish between the two entities. First, epicardial fat pads tend to occur anteriorly, unlike circumferential effusions, which occur posteriorly. If a fat pad is suspected, multiple ultrasound views should be obtained to rule out a posterior effusion. Second, the echocardiographic appearance of an epicardial fat pad is isoechoic and homogeneous. This differs from blood in the pericardial space, which may look like fronds of clot waving within an anechoic (black) pericardial space. Third, an epicardial fat pad does not alter hemodynamics like tamponade does—it should not cause diastolic collapse of the right ventricular free wall, dilation of the IVC, or any signs indicating hemodynamic compromise. After careful examination, if doubt still exists regarding the presence of an effusion, hemodynamically stable patients should have a formal echocardiogram or CT scan.

CT Scan

CT may be the only diagnostic option at institutions where ultrasound or formal echocardiography is not available in the ED. CT can demonstrate dilated hepatic veins, a plethoric IVC, and interventricular septal bowing.[117] This modality is less desirable than bedside ultrasound because it requires patients to be transported to the radiology suite. Thus, patient safety and cardiopulmonary stability must be considered before the decision is made to transport the patient. Unstable patients should never be transported until they are fully stabilized.

For stable patients, CT is effective in defining the presence, severity, and extent of pericardial effusions (i.e., circumferential versus loculated). In certain circumstances it even provides a more definitive diagnosis than echocardiography does because it may reveal the type of pericardial fluid (by differences in tissue density) and pericardial disease (e.g., constrictive pericarditis).[118] In one series, eight equivocal echocardiograms were evaluated by follow-up CT.[119] Two patients thought to have pericardial effusion by ultrasonography were found to have pleural effusions. Another patient in whom a pericardial effusion was diagnosed on ultrasonography was found by CT to have an epicardial lipoma. CT defined three

loculated pericardial effusions not identified by ultrasonography. Finally, two patients had hemopericardium visualized by CT but not by ultrasonography.

Treating Pericardial Effusions and Tamponade

Treatment of pericardial effusions in the ED depends on the degree of hemodynamic compromise. Patients with stable effusions should be treated supportively while the underlying cause (known or suspected) is addressed. For example, stable patients with pericardial effusions secondary to uremia may best be treated with dialysis, observation, and serial echocardiograms.[120] Even when the diagnosis is unknown there may be no need to perform emergency pericardiocentesis if the effusion is small to moderate.[121] Deferring diagnostic pericardiocentesis to the inpatient setting may be preferred because the cardiac catheterization laboratory or operating room is a more sterile and controlled environment than the ED.[57]

Patients with evidence of tamponade need urgent pericardiocentesis (discussed in the next section). Even those with early tamponade who are stable can decompensate quickly with little warning. Fluid boluses may improve hemodynamics temporarily, especially in patients with concomitant hypovolemia.[89] Administration of vasopressors and an inotrope is a temporizing measure and should be initiated while preparing for emergency pericardiocentesis. Finally, positive pressure ventilation (e.g., mechanical ventilation) should be avoided if possible because as discussed in the section on physiology, it can lead to hemodynamic collapse secondary to changes in intrathoracic pressure.

INDICATIONS FOR PERICARDIOCENTESIS

There are two indications for pericardiocentesis: (1) to diagnose the cause or presence of a pericardial effusion (diagnostic pericardiocentesis) and (2) to relieve tamponade (therapeutic pericardiocentesis). Diagnostic pericardiocentesis is an elective procedure. It is ideally performed under visual guidance (e.g., ultrasound). Therapeutic pericardiocentesis can be done semi-electively with ultrasound guidance or on an emergency basis (with electrocardiographic assistance).

Diagnostic Pericardiocentesis

Use of pericardiocentesis to determine the cause of nonhemorrhagic effusions is common practice, even though opinions on its utility vary.[52,122,123] Recovery of neoplastic cells, blood, bacteria, and viruses from pericardial fluid can be valuable in making the diagnosis. Measurement of pericardial fluid pH can also be helpful because inflammatory fluid is significantly more acidotic than noninflammatory fluid.[124] When a specific cause is suspected, additional diagnostic testing may be useful (e.g., adenosine deaminase in patients with tuberculosis and carcinoembryonic antigen in those with suspected malignancy).[125]

The diagnostic accuracy of pericardiocentesis is variable, and certain diagnoses are unlikely to be made from pericardial fluid. In one large series, fluid samples were obtained in 90% of aspirations, but the specific cause was determined from only 24% of those specimens.[126] Another series demonstrated false-negative cytologic results in certain cases of lymphoma and mesothelioma.[126] In some HIV patients, effusions secondary to Kaposi's sarcoma and cytomegalovirus infection have been diagnosed by pericardial biopsy following nondiagnostic fluid analysis.[127,128]

The most helpful clinical predictors of diagnosis before pericardiocentesis are the size of the effusion (larger effusions and tamponade are more likely to yield a diagnosis) and signs of inflammation (e.g., fever, pericardial friction rub, ST-segment elevation).[58] Unfortunately, the only definitive methods of diagnosis are pericardial fluid aspiration and analysis and pericardial biopsy.

Subxiphoid pericardiotomy can also be used in stable patients with pericardial effusion. This technique collects both pericardial fluid and a pericardial biopsy specimen, and because a tissue sample is obtained, a definitive diagnosis is more likely.[129] This procedure can be performed safely in the operating suite without general anesthesia.[130] In a prospective series of 57 patients who underwent subxiphoid pericardiotomy, a definitive diagnosis was obtained in 36%, a probable diagnosis in 40%, a possible diagnosis in 16%, and no diagnosis in 7%. It is uncertain whether this technique is safer than ultrasound-guided pericardiocentesis, but published reports show low rates of complications in experienced hands.[58]

Diagnostic pericardiocentesis has limited utility for hemopericardium secondary to traumatic causes. When used diagnostically after trauma to assess for the presence of pericardial bleeding, the procedure has a false-negative rate (i.e., no blood aspirated) of between 20% and 40%.[95,131-133] The high false-negative rate is due to the fact that posttraumatic blood tends to clot within the pericardial space and therefore cannot be aspirated.[19] Furthermore, pericardiocentesis should not delay emergency thoracotomy if cardiac tamponade is suspected.[134] If there is uncertainty about the presence of tamponade, the focused abdominal sonography in trauma (FAST) examination rapidly and noninvasively identifies pericardial fluid.[135-137]

Therapeutic Pericardiocentesis

The ultrasonographic finding of a large pericardial effusion in a stable patient should lead to early cardiology or cardiothoracic surgery consultation for percutaneous drainage or placement of a pericardial window. Patients with a pericardial effusion who remain hypotensive despite fluid resuscitation require emergency therapeutic drainage. The decision to wait for consultants is best made by the emergency physician at the bedside and should be based on clinical judgment. For patients in extremis, pericardiocentesis should be performed immediately even if consultation is unavailable. The clinician who performs the procedure should be the one who is most experienced in both sonography and pericardial fluid aspiration.

Tamponade of Uncertain Cause: Pulseless Electrical Activity

A major indication for emergency pericardiocentesis is a patient in cardiac arrest with PEA. Always consider cardiac tamponade in the differential diagnosis for PEA, especially if jugular venous pressure is elevated or a pericardial effusion is demonstrated on ultrasound. In a series of 20 patients with PEA, 3 had tamponade and another 5 had some degree of

pericardial effusion.[138] In this setting, blind (i.e., landmark method), ECG-guided, or ultrasound-guided pericardiocentesis can be lifesaving.

Tamponade Caused by Nonhemorrhagic Effusions

Most nonhemorrhagic effusions are liquid. They can be drained by pericardiocentesis with a small needle or by a catheter left in the pericardial space. Removal of even a small amount of fluid can cause immediate and dramatic improvement in blood pressure and cardiac output. Pericardiocentesis relieves tamponade caused by nonhemorrhagic effusions in 60% to 90% of cases.[54,126,139]

If small-needle pericardiocentesis fails, the patient might have a purulent, malignant, or well-organized effusion. Placement of a pericardial catheter may be more useful in the long-term management of these patients. In Krikorian and Hancock's series,[126] 24% of patients were managed successfully with a single pericardiocentesis procedure, but 37% needed multiple aspirations or an indwelling catheter (39% required surgical drainage and 55% of these patients had traumatic hemopericardium). Therefore, if time and patient stability permit, consider pericardiocentesis with a catheter to reduce the necessity for repeated aspirations.

Patients with renal failure and tamponade require urgent pericardiocentesis. Without signs of tamponade, however, these patients may be better managed by dialysis. In one series, 63% of renal failure patients were managed successfully with only dialysis.[126] There is some evidence that needle pericardiocentesis is a poor choice in patients who need pericardial drainage; in one series, 9 of 10 patients had serious complications following this procedure.[66] Consultation with specialists is advised when there is no evidence of hemodynamic collapse but pericardial drainage is still being considered.

An algorithm for the urgent management of nonhemorrhagic cardiac tamponade is presented in Figure 16-10.

Pericardiocentesis in Patients with Hemorrhagic Tamponade

For hemorrhagic tamponade, pericardiocentesis is never the definitive treatment because this strategy has several drawbacks.[140,141] Aspiration of a small quantity of fluid may cause a dramatic improvement in hemodynamics, but pericardial clots can prevent adequate drainage, so blood usually reaccumulates.[93,106] Patients with traumatic pericardial hemorrhage ultimately require thoracotomy to explore and repair the cardiac injury. Pericardiocentesis simply delays this definitive procedure. A study investigating traumatic cardiac injury found that all patients who underwent surgery within 2 hours of the injury survived but the mortality rate was higher in patients who experienced longer operating room delays.[140]

Sugg and associates documented a 43% mortality rate when pericardiocentesis was the sole treatment of traumatic tamponade as compared with 16% in those who also underwent surgical intervention.[132] All patients managed by pericardiocentesis had repairable wounds at autopsy, thus suggesting that in this population, operative repair is preferable. The number of deaths from stab wounds has been decreasing over time in response to a shift in trauma philosophy in which early thoracotomy is supported rather than repeated pericardiocentesis.[95,133,141,142]

Pericardiocentesis may improve a trauma patient's hemodynamics temporarily, and benefit may be derived from this

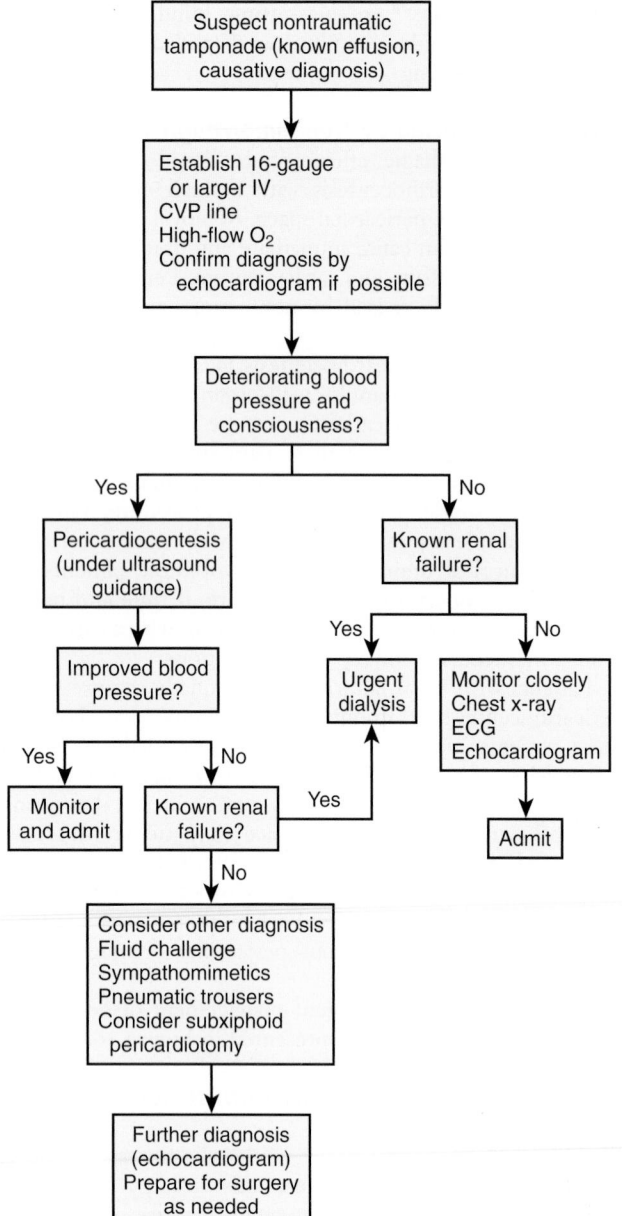

Figure 16-10 Management of nontraumatic cardiac tamponade. *CVP*, central venous pressure; *ECG*, electrocardiogram; *IV*, intravenous line.

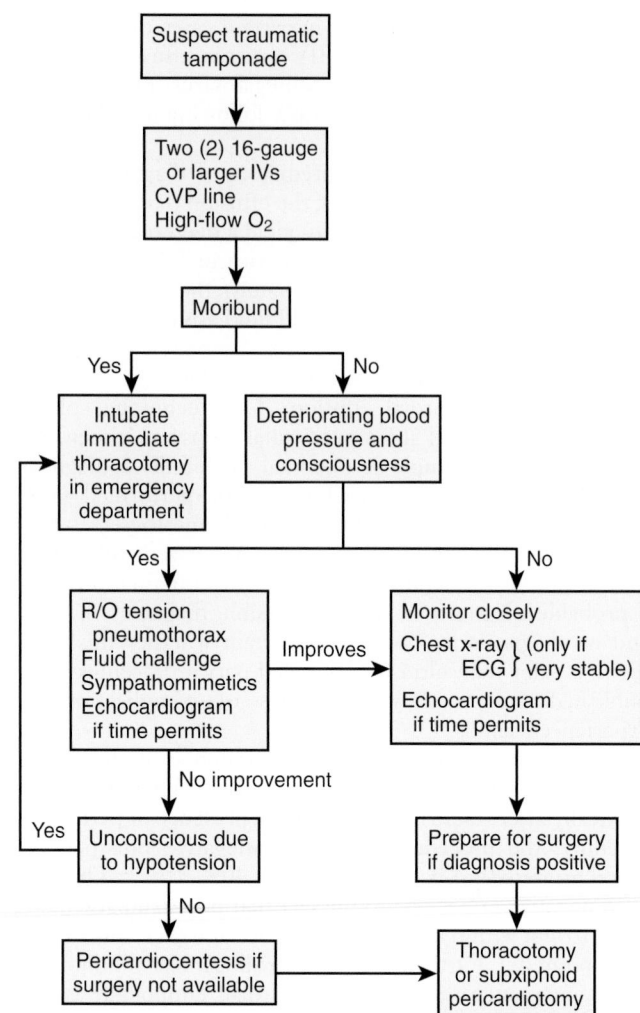

Figure 16-11 Management of traumatic cardiac tamponade. *CVP*, central venous pressure; *ECG*, electrocardiogram; *IVs*, intravenous lines; *R/O*, rule out.

approach, but only when definitive surgical treatment is being arranged (Fig. 16-11). A study of penetrating trauma patients with tamponade found that preoperative pericardiocentesis decreased the mortality rate from 25% to 11%.[143]

CONTRAINDICATIONS

There are no absolute contraindications to pericardiocentesis in hemodynamically unstable patients. Relative contraindications to pericardiocentesis include coagulopathy; previous thoracoabdominal surgery; the presence of prosthetic heart valves, pacemakers, or cardiac devices; inability to visualize the effusion with ultrasound during the procedure; and situations in which better treatment modalities are immediately available (e.g., thoracotomy for trauma patients).

Ideally, pericardiocentesis is performed in the cardiac catheterization laboratory under fluoroscopic or echocardiographic guidance. With the advent of bedside ultrasound and immediate visualization of large pericardial effusions, pericardiocentesis is being performed in the ED more frequently. Ultrasound can accurately identify the area of the heart with the greatest fluid accumulation and clarify its relationship to the body wall.[40,144,145] This allows the physician to choose an entry site and angle of penetration with the greatest likelihood of obtaining fluid while avoiding vital structures.

OVERVIEW OF TECHNIQUES AND EQUIPMENT

In an urgent situation (e.g., PEA arrest) with no adjunctive equipment available, pericardiocentesis can be performed with minimal equipment. Use a long 18-gauge spinal needle attached to a 10-mL syringe to withdraw fluid from the pericardial sac. Although the procedure can be done with these two simple devices, access to several others would be beneficial during the procedure. Of all the components, the most essential is an ultrasound machine, which first is used to determine whether a pericardial effusion is present and then assists

Figure 16-12 For emergency pericardiocentesis, a long 18-gauge spinal needle is connected to a V lead of an electrocardiographic machine via a cable with alligator clips.

in accurate needle placement. Ideally, use a probe with a small-footprint and a frequency of 2 to 4 MHz. If this type of probe is not available, use a 2- to 3.5-MHz curvilinear probe in the subxiphoid view, which will also provide excellent images of the heart.

Before the introduction of real-time sonography to guide needle placement, electrocardiographic monitoring was used to indicate appropriate needle placement. This was done by connecting the electrocardiographic machine to one of the precordial leads (e.g., V_1). That precordial lead was then attached to the distal end of a spinal needle with an alligator clamp (Fig. 16-12). The precordial lead was used as a rhythm strip to monitor the needle tip continuously.

Other tools that are desirable for urgent pericardiocentesis can be found easily in the ED or in a pericardiocentesis kit (see Review Box 16-1): a finder needle; Seldinger wire; dilator; flexible catheter guide; 6- to 8-Fr pigtail catheter; plastic drainage tube; extra syringes; sterile hat, gown, gloves, and drape; and local anesthetic.

PROCEDURE

Temporizing Measures

Cardiac tamponade is an emergency that requires urgent therapy. Therapy typically consists of either pericardial drainage by needle aspiration or placement of a pericardial window. These procedures cannot be readily performed in an ED, so temporizing methods are the mainstay of therapy unless the patient is unstable (e.g., in PEA arrest). The most common therapeutic procedures used as temporizing measures in the setting of tamponade are intravascular volume expansion and administration of vasopressors.[5,14,146] Although most textbooks and protocols encourage the use of these temporizing methods, they are backed by only sparse scientific evidence.[147,148] Studies in animals have shown an increase in cardiac output and improvement in blood pressure with expansion of central blood volume; the validity of this in humans with cardiac tamponade is uncertain. Fluid resuscitation in a trauma patient with penetrating cardiac injury might cause deterioration. Animal experiments indicate that the response depends on whether fluid boluses produce recurrent bleeding from the cardiac wound.[149] Despite the lack of

evidence, judicious volume expansion with or without an adjunctive vasopressor before definitive therapy may be the only option for patients with tamponade.

Norepinephrine, isoproterenol, dopamine, and dobutamine have all been evaluated as the vasopressor of choice in patients with cardiac tamponade. Norepinephrine and isoproterenol increased cardiac output in animal models of tamponade but failed to increase it in humans.[150,151] Dopamine and dobutamine increased cardiac output and improved hemodynamics in the setting of tamponade.[33,148] Either of these agents may be helpful as a temporizing agent, but theoretically, dobutamine might be preferable because of its greater β-adrenergic activity.[151]

Preparation

Before preparing for pericardiocentesis, place all resuscitation equipment at the bedside in anticipation of clinical deterioration. Most patients undergoing pericardiocentesis in the ED have already experienced hemodynamic collapse and are lying supine. If the patient is able to cooperate, elevate the chest 30 to 45 degrees to bring the heart closer to the chest wall. Sedation of stuporous patients is typically forgone because of the risk for further hemodynamic collapse. If the patient is awake and undergoing the procedure without obvious hemodynamic compromise, short-acting medications (e.g., midazolam or fentanyl) are preferred.

Every effort should be made to ensure aseptic technique. Prepare the chest and upper part of the abdomen with a chlorhexidine-based solution. Drape the patient and ensure that all care providers involved in the procedure are wearing a sterile hat, mask, gown, and gloves. If the patient is awake, anesthetize the skin and the proposed route with 1% lidocaine (see Review Box 16-1). Because the pericardium is extremely sensitive, it should be anesthetized.[152]

The approach to pericardiocentesis depends on the clinical status of the patient, the availability of ultrasound, and the distribution of pericardial fluid. Pericardial fluid is not always distributed circumferentially in the pericardial sac, so ultrasound can quickly identify the maximal effusion pocket and demarcate the appropriate site for needle placement. Pericardiocentesis with ultrasound guidance is currently the safest and most reliable method for the diagnosis and treatment of pericardial effusion and tamponade.[153] Studies of echocardiography-directed pericardiocentesis have found that the apical approach is the best site for puncture.[145,154,155] Cadaver studies have corroborated this finding and demonstrated greater safety with an apical approach. However, these studies also revealed that an apical approach is associated with a greater incidence of pneumothorax than a traditional subcostal approach is. Before the advent of ultrasound guidance, the subxiphoid approach (discussed later in this chapter) was the preferred method of pericardiocentesis. It is still used frequently during cardiac arrest and when ultrasound is not readily available.

ECG Monitoring

If ultrasound is not readily available to guide needle placement, electrocardiographic monitoring can serve as a useful adjunct. Electrocardiographic monitoring is used to prevent puncture of the ventricle. When using this method, an assistant is essential to ensure sterile technique, observe for

Figure 16-13 Current of injury. There is an obvious change in the electrocardiogram when the pericardiocentesis needle touches the epicardium. Following slight withdrawal (*arrow*), the ST-segment elevation diminishes. This is best seen when the needle is directly attached to the electrocardiographic V lead.

dysrhythmias, and make sure that the electrocardiographic machine is functioning properly.

After all equipment is sterile, attach an alligator clip from one of the precordial leads (e.g., V_1) to the distal end of the spinal needle. Record a rhythm strip of this lead (the "exploring electrode") continuously. Advance the needle through the skin while remembering that any contact with the epicardium will cause a current-of-injury pattern that can be seen on the ECG. Typically, this is represented as a wide-complex premature ventricular contraction with an elevated ST segment (Fig. 16-13). When a current-of-injury pattern is seen, the needle is probably touching the epicardium. Withdraw it several millimeters to prevent laceration of the myocardium or coronary vessels. After slight withdrawal, the needle should be within the pericardial space. Aspirate any fluid, but watch for any changes on the ECG. Electrocardiographic monitoring is not infallible: if the patient has an abnormal myocardium from conditions such as a previous MI or the formation of scar tissue, no current-of-injury pattern will be generated on the rhythm strip.

Ultrasound-Guided Pericardiocentesis

Pericardiocentesis has traditionally been performed blindly. This approach was associated with a low success rate and a high rate of complications, such as inadvertent puncture of the lung, ventricle, or epicardial vessels. Using ultrasound to both diagnose and guide pericardiocentesis has resulted in increased success rates, as well as a lower rate of complications. The techniques are described in the Ultrasound Box.

Subxiphoid/Subcostal Approach

As mentioned earlier, the traditional blind subxiphoid approach can still be used for pericardiocentesis in the ED (e.g., for patients in cardiac arrest and when ultrasound is not available). The technique is performed as follows: introduce the needle 1 cm inferior to the left xiphocostal angle at a 30-degree angle to the skin (Fig. 16-14). Because the heart is an anterior structure, angles greater than 45 degrees may lacerate the liver or stomach. Aim toward the left shoulder and advance the needle slowly while continuously maintaining negative pressure on the syringe to aspirate any fluid. Aspirate with an "in-and-out" vector only, not "side to side," which may lacerate tissue. If no fluid is aspirated, withdraw the needle completely and redirect it in a deeper posterior trajectory. If no fluid is aspirated after redirecting the needle, withdraw the needle and redirect it, working from the patient's left to right, until it is aimed at the right shoulder.

Recommendations regarding needle trajectory vary widely, including toward the right shoulder, sternal notch, and left shoulder.[146,152]

Apical Approach

The apical approach is sometimes used as an alternative to the subcostal approach to drain a pericardial effusion when ultrasound is available. Use ultrasound to identify the largest area of the apical effusion (Fig. 16-15*A*) or simply feel for the apex. If the apex cannot be palpated, it typically lies within the area of cardiac dullness, often between the fifth, sixth, or seventh intercostal space, between the midclavicular and midaxillary lines. Introduce the needle 1 cm lateral to and into the intercostal space below the apical heartbeat. Advance the needle over the cephalad border of the rib and aim it toward the right shoulder to avoid the neurovascular bundle located caudal to the rib space. This area is close to the lingula and the left pleural space, thus making pneumothorax a frequent complication. Theoretically, this technique is used because the coronary vessels are small at the apex; therefore, if a ventricle is entered, it is the thick-walled LV, which is more likely to seal off after ventricular injury. With echocardiographic guidance, the apical approach is used more commonly.[156]

Parasternal Approach

The parasternal approach is an alternative approach to the previously described techniques. First, identity the largest area of the parasternal effusion on ultrasound if possible. If ultrasound is not available or if the effusion is not clearly identified on the ultrasound image, proceed by introducing the needle 1 cm lateral to the sternal border at the left fifth or sixth intercostal interspace. Advance the needle over the cephalad border of the rib to avoid the neurovascular bundle on the caudal aspect of the rib. Avoid going too far laterally from the sternal border because of potential injury to the internal mammary artery.[157] Occasionally, a right parasternal approach may be used when ultrasound predicts superior access to an effusion from this direction.

Tsang and coworkers[158] described this technique for ultrasound-guided pericardiocentesis in 1998. The ideal site for skin puncture is where the largest area of fluid accumulation is closest to the skin surface. On ultrasound, this is indicated by a large anechoic (black) area at the top of the screen, usually corresponding to the left anterior chest wall (rather than the subcostal region). This approach also avoids injury to the liver (common with the subcostal approach). Inadvertent puncture of the lung is also prevented with this approach because air in the lung will not conduct sound waves and will prevent visualization of the heart when located immediately beneath the probe. Avoid choosing a site that could puncture the internal mammary artery, which lies 3 to 5 cm from either parasternal border, or the neurovascular bundle, which is located at the inferior border of the rib. Mark the best site with a sterile pen.

Procedure and Technique

Confirm the trajectory and depth of the needle before puncturing the skin. Be aware that repositioning the patient alters the position of the heart and pericardial sac within the chest, so reassessment will be necessary. Prepare the skin

PERICARDIOCENTESIS (SUBXIPHOID APPROACH)

1 Examine the patient and identify the xiphoid process and the costal margin.

Prepare the area with antiseptic and administer local anesthetic.

2 Introduce the needle 1 cm inferior to the left xiphocostal angle at a 30-degree angle to the skin.

Aim toward the left shoulder.

3 Aspirate during needle advancement and monitor for fluid return.

Stop advancing once fluid is returned.

4 ST segment elevation   Needle withdrawn ST segment returns to normal

If using electrocardiographic monitoring, observe for current of injury during needle advancement, which indicates epicardial contact. If this occurs, withdraw the needle slightly.

5 Advance a J-tipped guidewire through the needle and into the pericardium.

6 Remove the needle, while leaving the guidewire in place in the pericardium.

7 Advance a 6- to 8-Fr dilator over the wire and then remove the dilator.

8 Advance a 6- to 8-Fr pigtail catheter over the wire and into the pericardium.

9 Remove the wire and drain the pericardial fluid.

Figure 16-14 Pericardiocentesis (subxiphoid approach). *(From Custalow CB. Color Atlas of Emergency Department Procedures. Philadelphia: Saunders; 2005:123.)*

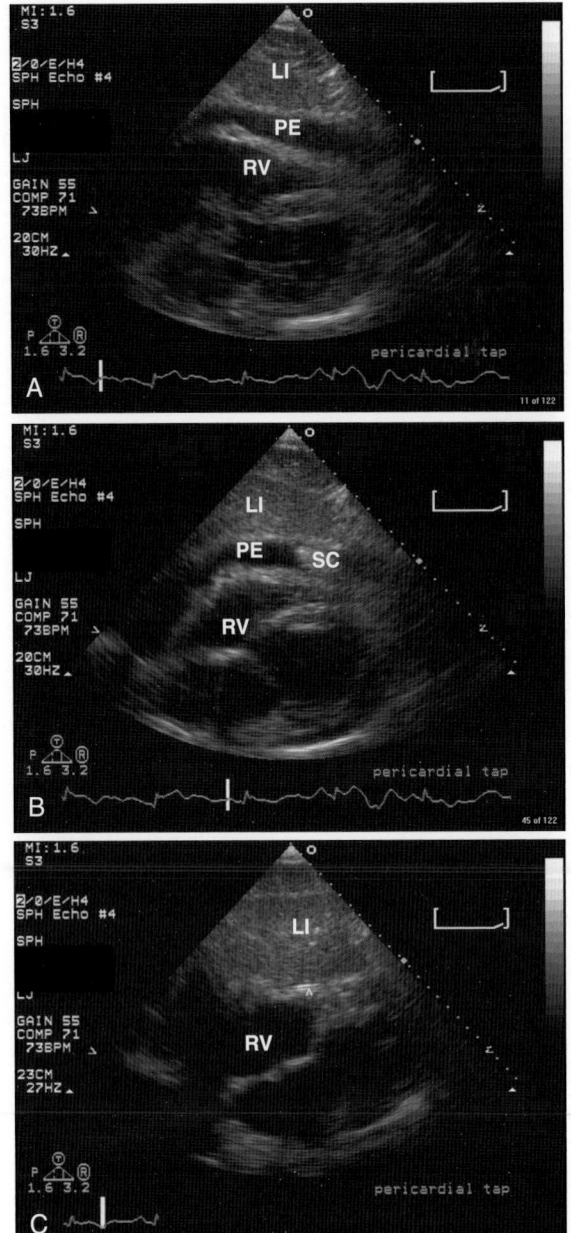

Figure 16-15 Placement of a pigtail catheter in the pericardial space under ultrasound assistance: subcostal view of a small but hemodynamically significant pericardial effusion during pericardiocentesis. **A,** The effusion. **B,** After the injection of approximately 0.1 mL of agitated saline through the pericardiocentesis needle to confirm its position in the pericardial space. **C,** The shaft of the pigtail catheter (arrowhead, two discrete parallel echogenic lines reflect the catheter walls; the echo-free area represents the catheter lumen) lying in the pericardial space after the majority of fluid has been drained. *LI,* liver; *PE,* pericardial effusion; *RV,* right ventricle; *SC,* saline contrast.

antiseptically and place a sterile cover over the ultrasound probe. If time permits, anesthetize the selected area with 1% lidocaine, with the superior border of the adjacent rib being used as a landmark. Select an 18-gauge spinal needle. Ideally, the needle should have a sheath that allows it to be withdrawn after the pericardial space is entered. This helps avoid injury to the heart and other vital structures. Attach a saline-filled syringe to the needle, and gently aspirate while slowly advanc-

ing the needle. Keep the ultrasound probe on the chest wall, immediately adjacent to the aspiration site.

Once the pericardial space is entered, inject agitated saline to confirm needle placement, particularly if the pericardial fluid is grossly bloody or if there is any question about needle position (see Fig. 16-15*B*). Prepare a saline echocardiographic contrast medium by using two 5-mL syringes, one with saline and the other with air. Connect them via a three-way stopcock to the needle and catheter. Rapidly inject saline between the syringes and then inject it into the sheath. Monitor the entrance of the agitated saline into the pericardial space sonographically—it appears as a brightly echogenic stream. If the use of agitated saline proves to be inconclusive or suboptimal, use an echocardiographic contrast agent (e.g., Definity) as a safe and successful alternative.[159,160] Contrast agents contain gas microbubbles, which markedly enhance the fluid echo by introducing multiple liquid-gas interfaces. Inject this solution as a bolus. If the contrast material clears immediately after administration (as occurs with agitated saline) or persists temporarily within the cardiac chambers, an intracardiac location is suggested.

Fluid Aspiration and Evaluation

Removal of even a small amount of pericardial fluid (e.g., 30 to 50 mL) usually results in either return of spontaneous circulation or hemodynamic improvement. After any approach used for pericardiocentesis, place a temporary drain not only to ensure rapid access into the pericardial sac but also to allow more fluid to be removed quickly if hemodynamic collapse recurs. After needle placement is confirmed, a temporary drain can be placed by the Seldinger technique, described in Chapter 22.

Remove the syringe from the needle, advance a guidewire through the needle, and then remove the needle. Position a dilator (6- to 8-Fr Cordis) over the wire. If a dilator is not used, particularly with the subxiphoid approach, the pigtail catheter tip may get caught in the subcutaneous tissue and make placement of the catheter difficult. Remove the dilator and slide an introducer sheath dilator (6- to 8-Fr Cordis) over the wire. Remove the wire and the dilator while leaving the introducer sheath in place. Insert the pigtail angiocatheter through the introducer sheath, and aspirate fluid to confirm placement.[154,158] After the catheter is advanced into place, it should be secured with a suture to ensure that it does not migrate after the procedure; an appropriate catheter dressing should be applied. The catheter should be attached to a three-way stopcock and connected to a water seal to drain by gravity. The pigtail catheter allows prolonged drainage and safe access into the pericardial sac without requiring the introduction of another needle.[161,162] If drainage of pericardial fluid becomes sluggish, flush the catheter with a heparinized saline solution to ensure patency of the lumen.[152]

Aspiration of blood during pericardiocentesis raises the possibility of cardiac puncture. Blood retrieved from the ventricle usually clots faster than bloody fluid aspirated from the pericardium. In general, hemorrhagic pericardial effusions have local fibrinolytic activity, which prevents clot formation. If the bleeding is brisk enough, however, blood may still clot and does not necessarily point toward ventricular puncture. The hematocrit of pericardial fluid should always be lower than that of a sample from the systemic vascular system, except in patients with aortic dissection or acute myocardial rupture. These circumstances aside, a hematocrit value similar to that for systemic blood should raise concern for an intracardiac needle location. Several other simple laboratory tests can differentiate normal from abnormal pericardial fluid, but they require the availability of a centrifuge system and time. Under normal conditions, pericardial fluid is less than 50 mL in volume and clear to pale yellow in color with no red or white blood cells, inflammatory markers, bacteria, or cancer cells and with a glucose concentration similar to that of blood.

Immediately following the procedure, obtain a chest film to ensure the absence of pneumothorax and free air under the diaphragm. Place the patient on continuous cardiac monitoring for 24 hours and watch for signs of reaccumulating fluid or iatrogenic complications. Repeating the ultrasound examination in 24 hours is recommended. Diagnostic evaluation of nonhemorrhagic fluid is similar to that for pleural fluid (see Chapter 9).

Suture the pigtail catheter to the skin, but be careful to not occlude the catheter by tying it too tightly. Wrap the catheter in gauze at the skin and cover it with a sterile dressing. Attach the catheter to suction tubing and a drainage system.

COMPLICATIONS

Emergency physicians often perform pericardiocentesis under duress on a patient in PEA arrest. Many also perform the technique blindly because they have little or no time to gather adjunctive assistance or tools. It is critical for the emergency physician to be aware of both the traditional and contemporary methods of performing the procedure and the complications that can be associated with these methods (see Review Box 16-1).

With the advent of ultrasound- and CT-guided pericardiocentesis, the complication rate has been greatly reduced. Complication rates as low as 4% have been reported in large observational studies. Earlier studies of blind pericardiocentesis documented morbidity rates of 20% to 40% and mortality rates as high as 6%.[163] Because pericardiocentesis is performed in moribund patients, the likelihood of cardiac arrest and death is high. However, they are not usually a direct complication of pericardiocentesis but of poor cardiopulmonary reserve. Cardiac arrest and death are rarely associated with echocardiographically guided pericardiocentesis. When blind or electrocardiographically guided pericardiocentesis is performed, the patient is usually already in full arrest and attributing the cause of death to the procedure is nearly impossible. In a series of 52 patients the only death occurred in a patient in cardiogenic shock in whom pericardiocentesis was nonproductive and who was found to have severe arteriosclerotic heart disease, not tamponade, on postmortem examination.[164] In a series of 352 fluoroscopically guided pericardiocenteses, two deaths were documented.[165] Ultrasonographic or CT confirmation of effusion was used in all but 15 cases. The two deaths occurred during or after the procedure, but whether they could be attributed to the procedure is unclear. One patient with aortic rupture that penetrated into the pericardial space died of cardiac arrest immediately after the puncture. The other death, in a post-MI patient with a left ventricular aneurysm, was caused by ventricular fibrillation that occurred about 15 minutes after the procedure.

Figure 16-16 Air-fluid level (*arrow*) in the pericardial space immediately after pericardiocentesis. A minor pneumopericardium is inconsequential; a larger collection may cause tamponade.

One of the most frequent complications is a "dry tap," especially when a blind approach is used. A "dry tap" is often caused by blockage of the needle with clotted blood or a skin plug. With the parasternal approach, the needle can become blocked by vigorous probing of the anterior costal cartilage. The problem can be solved by repositioning or irrigating the needle, which allows the effusion to be aspirated unless it is loculated.

Preventricular contractions are frequently noted after the needle enters the pericardial sac; however, no serious dysrhythmias resulting in hemodynamic compromise have been mentioned in the literature. Several case series report no dysrhythmias.[54,67,154] Krikorian and Hancock[126] reported one episode of ventricular tachycardia and several "hypotensive vasovagal reactions" that were associated with bradycardia and responded to atropine and fluid loading. Duvernoy and associates[165] reported 1 case of ventricular tachycardia and 1 case of atrial fibrillation in 352 procedures. Maggiolini and coworkers reported transient third-degree heart block in a single patient.[166] The traditional subxiphoid approach carries a risk for liver laceration. Fortunately, inadvertent needle passage into the liver has not been reported to cause significant hemorrhage or death.[167]

The parasternal and apical approaches have been documented as causing pneumothorax and pneumopericardium in several case series, but without any clinical consequence (Fig. 16-16). The pneumothoraces were treated with 100% oxygen or thoracostomy. There have also been infrequent reports of pneumopericardium after removal of a pericardiocentesis catheter. The cause of the pneumopericardium is thought to be the formation of a bronchopericardial fistula, but the exact mechanism is unclear. The mortality rate associated with tension pneumopericardium is about 50%, so consider pneumopericardium when patients complain of dyspnea and hypotension after removal of their catheter.[168-170]

Very few studies have reported ventricular or coronary vessel laceration during pericardiocentesis. These complications occur more frequently during blind or electrocardiographically guided procedures. Most cardiac perforations occur in the RV, but punctures in the LV and atria have also been reported.[25] When these perforations occur, they tend to

ULTRASOUND: Pericardiocentesis

by Christine Butts, MD

Pericardiocentesis has traditionally been performed blindly. This approach was associated with a low success rate and a high rate of complications, such as inadvertent puncture of the lung, ventricle, or epicardial vessels.[1] Using ultrasound to both diagnose and guide pericardiocentesis has resulted in increased success rates, as well as a lower rate of complications.[2,3]

Bedside ultrasound may additionally allow the emergency physician to make a rapid diagnosis of pericardial effusion. Evidence of impending cardiac tamponade, including right ventricular collapse and distention of the inferior vena cava, can also be identified.

Equipment

The pericardium should be imaged with a low-frequency (2 to 4 mHz) transducer to achieve adequate depth. A phased-array or microconvex transducer is preferred for its smaller footprint, which enables the sonographer to image between the ribs. However, a curvilinear transducer may be used if that is what is available.

Image Interpretation

The initial step in the procedure is to evaluate the pericardium in multiple windows. This will allow identification and characterization of the effusion, as well as planning of the best approach for drainage. This chapter focuses primarily on the views most commonly used in this procedure, the subxiphoid and parasternal.

The subxiphoid view is best known to most emergency physicians as part of the focused abdominal sonography in trauma (FAST) examination. This view provides a four-chamber view of the heart and uses the left lobe of the liver as an acoustic window. To obtain this view, the transducer is placed just inferior to the xiphoid process in the midline. The indicator faces the patient's right side (Fig. 15-US1). To obtain the best image possible it is best to place the hand over the transducer and press down into the epigastric area. The transducer can then be aimed toward the left side of the chest until the heart comes into view. The depth may need to be adjusted to view all four chambers of the heart, as well as the pericardium.

In this view the left lobe of the liver can be seen at the top of the image. Deep to the liver, a four-chambered view of the heart should be seen, surrounded by the brightly echogenic (white) border of the pericardium (Fig. 15-US2). The right ventricle will abut the liver, with the left ventricle located deeper into the body. A pericardial effusion can be identified as an anechoic (black) or hypoechoic (dark gray) collection

between the heart and pericardium (Fig. 15-US3). Although fluid will typically collect at the most gravity-dependent area, loculated collections may not follow this rule.

The parasternal view is obtained by placing the transducer to the left of the patient's sternum in the fourth to fifth intercostal space. The indicator should be pointing toward the patient's right shoulder (Fig. 15-US4). Slight adjustments in angle may be needed to obtain the best image of the heart. If the patient's hemodynamic status allows, placing the patient in a left lateral decubitus position may improve this view by moving the heart closer to the anterior chest wall and displacing the air-filled lungs.

The parasternal view will demonstrate the left atrium, left ventricle, and a small portion of the right ventricle (Fig. 15-US5). The pericardium can be seen as an echogenic (white) border surrounding the heart. As in the subxiphoid view, an effusion will appear as an anechoic (black) or hypoechoic (dark gray) collection between the heart and pericardium (Fig. 15-US6).

Procedure and Technique

Once the views have been evaluated and an effusion has been identified, the pericardium should be evaluated in multiple views to determine the

Figure 16-US2 Normal subxiphoid view of the heart seen with ultrasound. The pericardium (arrow) can be identified as a bright white (hyperechoic) outline, typically best seen at the inferior aspect of the heart. The pericardium should directly abut the heart, as seen in this image.

Figure 16-US3 Subxiphoid view demonstrating a pericardial effusion. When comparing this image with the normal view, a black (anechoic) fluid collection (arrow) can be seen between the pericardium and the left ventricle.

Figure 16-US1 Placement of the ultrasound transducer to obtain a subxiphoid image of the heart.

ULTRASOUND: Pericardiocentesis, cont'd

Figure 16-US4 Placement of the ultrasound transducer to obtain a parasternal long-axis view of the heart.

Figure 16-US5 Normal parasternal long-axis view of the heart. The pericardium can be seen as a bright white (hyperechoic) outline surrounding the heart (arrow). As with the subxiphoid image, the pericardium should directly abut the heart with no intervening fluid.

Figure 16-US6 Parasternal long-axis view demonstrating a pericardial effusion. An anechoic (black) fluid collection can be seen on the right of the image (arrow), between the left ventricle and the pericardium. The right ventricle, at the top of the image (arrowhead), can be seen to "bow" inward from the pressure exerted by the effusion. This finding, right ventricular collapse, indicates that the effusion is causing hemodynamic compromise.

be advanced in the predetermined location along the predetermined trajectory. This can be done blindly or can be guided directly by the transducer. Gentle continuous pressure should be applied to the syringe until the pericardial space is entered and fluid is obtained.

If there is any question of whether the needle tip is in the pericardial space, agitated saline can be injected through the catheter under direct ultrasound guidance. This will allow analysis of the location of the needle tip. Prepare saline echocardiographic contrast medium by using two 5-mL syringes, one with saline and the other air, connected via a three-way stopcock to the needle catheter sheath. Saline in one syringe is rapidly injected between the syringes and then injected into the sheath once it is agitated. Entrance of the agitated saline into the pericardial space will appear sonographically as a brightly echogenic area.

Complications

Complications may occur when a pericardial effusion is misdiagnosed. The most common factor causing misdiagnosis is the presence of a fat pad anterior to the heart. Unless the effusion is loculated, it should lie within the most dependent portion of the heart and should be circumferential, depending on its size. Considering these factors and evaluating the pericardium in multiple views will aid in decreasing this misdiagnosis. Additionally, care should be taken in performing pericardiocentesis in stable patients, particularly when the effusion is small. Smaller effusions may be more difficult to access and thereby lead to increased complications.

REFERENCES

1. Salem K, Mulji A, Lonn E. Echocardiographically guided pericardiocentesis—the gold standard for the management of pericardial effusion and cardiac tamponade. *Can J Cardiol.* 1999;15:1251-1255.
2. Tsang TS, El-Najdawi EK, Seward JB, et al. Percutaneous echocardiographically guided pericardiocentesis in pediatric patients: evaluation of safety and efficacy. *J Am Soc Echocardiogr.* 1998;11:1072-1077.
3. Vayre F, Lardoux H, Pezzano M, et al. Subxiphoid pericardiocentesis guided by contrast two-dimensional echocardiography in cardiac tamponade: experience of 110 consecutive patients. *Eur J Echocardiogr.* 2000;1:66-71.
4. Tsang T, Freeman WK, Sinak LJ, et al. Echocardiographically guided pericardiocentesis: evolution and state-of-the-art technique. *Mayo Clin Proc.* 1998;73:647-652.

best area to attempt pericardiocentesis. Tsang and colleagues described the procedure for echocardiographically guided pericardiocentesis in detail in 1998.[4] Ideally, the procedure should be attempted at the site at which the largest fluid collection is closest to the skin surface. Typically, the anterior chest wall is preferred because of its proximity to the pericardium and the absence of vital interfering structures such as the liver. The air-filled lung creates a scatter artifact that does not allow the ultrasound beam to pass. Therefore, if the heart and pericardium can be viewed clearly, avoidance of the lung can be ensured. The sonographer should also attempt to approximate and avoid the location of the internal mammary artery, which lies 3 to 5 cm lateral to the sternum. Once the optimum site is identified, the practitioner should note the trajectory of the ultrasound beam. This is the trajectory that should be followed by the needle.

The field should be sterilized and the area to be traversed should be adequately anesthetized with local anesthetic. The ultrasound transducer should also be placed in a sterile covering. Care should be taken to not reposition the patient after initial assessment because this will alter the position and trajectory. A 16-gauge catheter with a retractable needle should be used to minimize potential injury to the underlying structures. After the field is prepared, the catheter with an attached syringe should be silent and result in hemopericardium and death. In patients taking anticoagulants, it is important to check coagulation factors and monitor them closely after a seemingly insignificant pericardiocentesis because hemopericardium could develop just from the procedure itself.

In the series compiled by Krikorian and Hancock,[126] hemopericardium developed in 13 of 123 patients as a result of pericardiocentesis, 1 as a result of a lacerated coronary artery. One patient died of a punctured ventricle. Surgical control was necessary in four patients in whom tamponade developed, whereas it did not develop in eight patients with hemopericardium, and they were managed conservatively. Guberman and colleagues[54] reported three lacerations of the RV in 46 patients; one was fatal. Wong and colleagues[164] found five punctures of the RV, four in patients with nonproductive pericardiocentesis, but none caused any adverse sequelae. In their series of 352 procedures, Duvernoy and associates[165] reported 23 penetrations. In two cases both the RV and LV had been perforated, and in all other cases the RV had been entered.

Researchers differ in their opinions regarding the adverse effects of ventricular puncture. Most ventricular punctures involve the lower aspect of the RV. The wall of the RV is thin and therefore vulnerable to laceration. However, pressure in the RV is low,[2] so a puncture should cause little bleeding. In a series of patients who underwent ultrasound-directed pericardiocentesis, ventricular puncture occurred in 1.5% but was without consequence.[154] In another study, laceration of the RV occurred in 1 patient despite the use of echocardiography; it resulted in tamponade and necessitated emergency surgery.[123] Of the 23 perforations in the series by Duvernoy and associates, 3 were considered major complications (two patients required thoracotomy). Left ventricular pseudoaneurysm typically occurs as a complication of MI. It is rarely seen after surgery, trauma, or infection. Rare cases of severe left ventricular pseudoaneurysm after pericardiocentesis have been reported recently.[171,172]

Even when pericardiocentesis has induced no physical injury, adverse events have been documented. Most have to do with the fact that during pericardiocentesis the stroke volume of the previously collapsed RV increases 75% after the first 200 mL of fluid is removed.[7] In general, this increase in stroke volume is greater initially than that demonstrated by the LV. This imbalance can cause significant consequences for both right and left ventricular function. Three of six patients in whom large effusions were removed by pericardiocentesis experienced right ventricular dilation and overload, abnormal septal motion, and either no increase or a decrease in the right ventricular ejection fraction.[173] These patients subsequently and slowly returned to normal hemodynamic status.

Pulmonary edema following pericardiocentesis has also been reported, presumably caused by a sudden increase in venous return to the LV when peripheral vascular resistance is still high from compensatory catecholamine secretion.[174-178] Supporting evidence for this explanation is that right ventricular stroke volume increases more than left ventricular stroke volume after relief of tamponade.[10] Circulatory collapse with persistently low arterial blood pressure has been reported in a patient from whom 700 mL of clear fluid was drained at a rate of 100 mL/min.[179] Thus, many authors recommend that the pericardial drainage rate not exceed 50 mL/min.

Acknowledgment

The editors and authors acknowledge the contributions of Richard J. Harper to this chapter in previous editions. Linda J. Kesselring, MS, ELS, from the Department of Emergency Medicine at the University of Maryland School of Medicine, copyedited the manuscript for the sixth edition.

(References are available at www.expertconsult.com)

CHAPTER 17

Artificial Perfusion during Cardiac Arrest

Benjamin S. Abella, Mariana R. Gonzalez, and Lance B. Becker

Cardiopulmonary resuscitation (CPR) can be lifesaving for a patient in cardiac arrest, particularly in conjunction with other therapies such as defibrillation or delivery of medications. In several large clinical studies, data have shown that prompt delivery of CPR serves as an important predictor of successful outcome and increases the chance of survival by up to twofold. Each minute without treatment, on the other hand, is associated with a 10% to 15% decrease in the probability of survival.[1,2]

The quality of CPR is an important technical issue and has a direct effect on patient outcome. For example, shallow chest compressions have an adverse impact on the success of defibrillation.[3] Because of these and related data, emphasis has recently been placed on improving the quality of CPR, and such priority has been codified in consensus CPR guidelines promulgated by the American Heart Association. These guidelines are formulated through a formalized data evaluation process and are updated every 5 years.[4]

Worrisome data have shown that the quality of CPR during actual resuscitation is endemically poor.[5,6] Specifically, chest compressions are often administered too slowly with inadequate depth. In addition, pauses in chest compressions are too long, and hyperventilation of arrest patients is common. These deficiencies may be due to a variety of factors, including infrequent training, lack of awareness of the quality of CPR during resuscitation, and inadequate team leadership during resuscitation efforts.[7]

CONVENTIONAL CPR

Although CPR is widely taught to health care personnel and reassessed periodically, the importance of high-quality CPR cannot be stressed enough. High-quality CPR immediately before defibrillation increases the chance of successful restoration of circulation.[3,8] Although another recent multicenter investigation of out-of-hospital arrest did not support this claim,[9] it is generally believed that for unwitnessed arrest or arrest events with a long downtime, early CPR and defibrillation have a significant impact on patient survival and recovery.[10,11] Quality chest compression also increases the efficacy of drugs administered during resuscitation, whereas inadequate circulation leads to minimal effects from peripherally delivered drugs.[12] Hyperventilation is also widely prevalent and dramatically compromises hemodynamics. In animal studies, hyperventilation leads to reduced survival from arrest. In this section we review the key procedural aspects of manual CPR.

Compressions

The 2010 resuscitation guidelines emphasize the importance of quality chest compression[4] by recommending that clinicians focus on maintaining proper chest compression depth and rate. Compress the sternum to a depth of at least 2 inches with a rate of at least 100 compressions/min. Box 17-1 provides a summary of procedural recommendations for CPR. If possible, place a backboard under the victim to ensure appropriate thoracic compression. In addition, adjust the height of the bed or have the rescuer stand on top of a step-stool so that the entire weight of the rescuer above the waist is directed onto the patient's sternum (Fig. 17-1A). This enhances the depth of compressions and helps prevent leaning on the patient's chest between compressions, which is another key deficiency that has been widely observed. Extend the arms fully and place them perpendicular to the patient's chest while making sure to pull away from the chest sufficiently between compressions to allow full chest recoil. Rotate rescuers aggressively (approximately every 2 to 3 minutes) to avoid deteriorating quality of compressions because of exhaustion. Properly delivered compressions are highly fatiguing, and rescuer bravado often interferes with the realization of declining CPR quality over time.

Minimize pauses in chest compressions because even short pauses have profound effects on coronary perfusion pressure and outcomes.[13] As stated earlier, long pauses in chest compressions before delivery of a shock are associated with failure of defibrillation.[3] Do not stop CPR to deliver medications because the drugs can be administered at the same time as the compressions. Keep pauses in chest compressions to a minimum (e.g., for procedures such as intubation or pulse checks).

Ventilations

Deliver ventilations at a rate of 8 to 10 breaths/min (see Fig. 17-1B). Hyperventilation (e.g., ventilation rates greater than 30/min) is common during resuscitation. To prevent unwittingly hyperventilating the patient, ask the rescuer who is providing ventilations to remove his or her hand completely off the bag-valve-mask apparatus between ventilations. The team leader should be vigilant in the observation of delivery of ventilations and should be ready to verbally prompt rescuers to ventilate the patient at the appropriate rate if hyperventilation is performed.

Pulse Checks

Pulse checks are generally performed too frequently during resuscitation efforts and take too much time. If a pulse cannot be readily felt within seconds, return to chest compressions as soon as possible. No studies have suggested that CPR is harmful to a patient with a very weak pulse, so use of a Doppler ultrasound device to detect the pulse is discouraged. If rescuers need ultrasound to find a pulse, the patient is at the very least markedly hypotensive and should probably be receiving CPR. Attempt pulse detection at the location of the carotid or femoral artery because peripheral pulse checks during profound shock or cardiac arrest states are notoriously unreliable. Frequently, a "pulse" can be detected during CPR itself; this phenomenon is often due to venous backpressure during compressions and does not indicate that compressions should be stopped, nor does it necessarily suggest that the compressions are of adequate quality.

Monitoring end-tidal CO_2 pressure (P_{ETCO_2}) also affords an opportunity to detect a pulse during CPR. During ongoing

COMPRESSIONS

At least 100 compressions/min
Depth of at least 2 inches/compression
Allow full chest recoil between compressions
Minimize pauses in compressions

VENTILATIONS

8-10 ventilations/min (avoid hyperventilation)
Minimize pauses in chest compression for intubation
Use of continuous capnography recommended for intubated
    patients

CPR, *cardiopulmonary resuscitation.*

Figure 17-1 Conventional cardiopulmonary resuscitation (CPR). *Note*: No alternative technique or device in routine use has consistently been shown to be superior to conventional CPR. **A,** Compress the sternum to a depth of at least 2 inches at a rate of 100 compressions/min. Better CPR can be achieved by having the rescuer stand on a stepstool during compressions, rotating rescuers every 2 to 3 minutes, and minimizing pauses. **B,** Deliver ventilations at a rate of 8 to 10 breaths/min. Avoid hyperventilation during resuscitation.

resuscitation of a pulseless patient, capnography will generally remain low (often less than 20 mm Hg), which is indicative of low blood flow. If the patient achieves return of spontaneous circulation (ROSC), a sharp increase in the PETCO$_2$ value (usually greater than 25 to 30 mm Hg) is consistent with return of adequate perfusion.[14]

Leadership and Teamwork

Cardiac arrest resuscitations are often crowded, chaotic events filled with stress and anxiety. To maximize calm and efficiency and to ensure quality of care, establish a team protocol. Designate someone to be the leader of the resuscitation, and make sure that all participants are clearly aware of this designation. The designated team leader should be responsible for monitoring the rhythm, for giving orders to initiate and terminate chest compressions, and for delivery of drugs and other therapies. The team leader should be situated either at the head of the bed or at a place where you can direct the resuscitation. As the team leader, it is important that you do not actually perform compressions, ventilations, or other specific procedures unless absolutely necessary because you may quickly lose control of the resuscitation. Since most rescuers are unable to detect when their own quality of compressions is diminishing, observe CPR closely and order rescuer rotations throughout the duration of the resuscitation.[15]

New Directions: CC-CPR

Chest compression–only cardiopulmonary resuscitation (CC-CPR) has been shown in a number of investigations to be as effective as standard CPR in resuscitation efforts initiated by members of the lay public.[16,17] Give compressions at a rate of at least 100/min.

Because of its simplicity, CC-CPR minimizes pauses in chest compressions while maintaining proper rate and depth. Lay rescuers in the community may be less experienced with standard CPR and uncomfortable with the performance of mouth-to-mouth resuscitation. The simplicity of CC-CPR makes it relatively easy for first responders to initiate resuscitation efforts and for emergency medical dispatchers to guide lay rescuers remotely. The American Heart Association's 2010 guidelines have shifted emphasis from "ABC" ("airway, breathing, compressions") to "CAB" ("compressions, airway, breathing") for lay rescuers. Their endorsement of

"hands-only CPR" (a synonym for CC-CPR) educational programs reflects additional evidence that a focus on chest compressions during CPR may lead to an increase in bystander CPR, as well as improvements in patient outcomes.[18] Recent investigations have shown that CC-CPR is associated with improved survival of patients with out-of-hospital cardiac arrest when performed by lay bystanders. A period of CC-CPR before intubation and rhythm evaluation also improves outcomes when used by emergency medical service (EMS) personnel.[19,20] The EMS community is likely to see more widespread adoption and use of CC-CPR by lay public educational programs in the upcoming years.

ADJUNCTS TO IMPROVE THE QUALITY OF CPR

Numerous techniques and adjunctive devices have been investigated in attempts to improve long-term survival rates with CPR. Data are conflicting and contrary, and as of this writing, no alternative technique or device in routine use has consistently been shown to be superior to conventional CPR. Unless breakthrough technology or new information on the parameters affecting the outcome of CPR emerge, this admonition will probably endure. Nonetheless, a variety of technologies have been developed to improve the quality of CPR. Some of these tools directly improve chest compressions, whereas others are less direct and aim to improve human performance or enhance hemodynamics during the delivery of chest compressions. This section describes some of these promising, intuitively useful, yet still unproven techniques.

ACD-CPR

Active compression-decompression cardiopulmonary resuscitation (ACD-CPR) is a variant of CPR in which the passive relaxation phase of CPR is converted into an active phase by means of a handheld or mechanical suction device, which can theoretically improve both myocardial and cerebral circulation when compared with traditional CPR.[21,22] However, data on these devices are mixed; there have been studies on out-of-hospital cardiac arrest using this technique that did not find any improvements in either initial outcome or survival to discharge, and as with many devices, there are instances when its application is impractical.[23,24]

ITD

The impedance threshold device (ITD) optimizes chest compression hemodynamics via manipulation of intrathoracic pressure. From a practical standpoint, the ITD is a relatively simple device that is placed between the endotracheal tube and the bag-valve apparatus, much like a colorimetric $PETCO_2$ detector, which is familiar to most ED clinicians (Fig. 17-2). The ITD contains a valve that prevents air from flowing through the device that is less than 10 cm H_2O in pressure. During resuscitation, the ITD prevents air from entering the thorax during recoil of the chest wall after each compression by generating a small but hemodynamically significant negative pressure within the chest. In laboratory studies this negative pressure enhances venous return to the heart and results in increased cardiac output with each subsequent chest compression.

The ITD can be used during resuscitation either with mask ventilation or via an endotracheal tube and is therefore appropriate for both basic life support care in the field and ED resuscitation. Apply the device and administer ventilations at a rate of 8 to 10 breaths/min as per standard resuscitation guidelines. The Res-Q-Pod ITD has a flashing light timed to prompt the appropriate ventilatory rate as well. When using it with a face mask, it is important to continuously maintain a tight seal between the patient's face and the mask during CPR to maintain efficacy of the ITD. This is best accomplished with a two-person ventilation technique in which one person holds the face mask and the second person squeezes the bag. If a pulse is restored, remove the ITD from the respiratory circuit.

Current data are conflicting on whether ITDs improve clinical outcomes when used as an adjunct to resuscitation efforts. Numerous studies and clinical trials using one particular model of ITD (Res-Q-Pod, Advanced Circulatory Systems, Inc., Eden Prairie, MN) have demonstrated improved hemodynamics during CPR and have suggested that use of an ITD during resuscitation efforts may lead to improved survival and patient outcomes.[25-27] However, the

Figure 17-2 Impedance threshold device (ITD). The ITD is placed in-line between the mask or endotracheal tube and the bag-valve apparatus. This is the Res-Q-Pod; the flashing light indicator is used to time the respiratory rate. (*Courtesy of Advanced Circulatory, Roseville, MN.*)

findings from recent randomized controlled trials of ITD use in patients suffering out-of-hospital cardiac arrest have offered opposing data, thus suggesting that there is not a significant improvement in patient outcomes when these devices have been used.[28]

Monitoring and Feedback Devices

Emphasis on CPR quality and minimizing interruptions has spurred the development of devices to monitor the quality of chest compressions and ventilations and then provide audio or visual prompts to improve performance. These devices aim to improve human delivery of CPR and, unlike ACD-CPR or the ITD, do not enhance hemodynamics or patient physiology directly.

One method of monitoring chest compressions involves placing a relatively small external device on the patient's sternum and performing chest compressions on top of the device (Fig. 17-3). The device measures the quality of compressions via a force detector or accelerometer (or both) that determines the rate and depth of chest compressions. Different versions of these CPR quality–monitoring and feedback devices are on the market. Some are incorporated into defibrillators (MRx-QCPR, Philips Healthcare, Andover, MA; R series with Real CPR Help, Zoll Medical Corp, Chelmsford, MA), whereas others are stand-alone devices applied to the chest. In recent trials, use of such a defibrillator with CPR monitoring and feedback improved CPR performance and, in one out-of-hospital trial, improved the rate of initial resuscitation.[29] Further research will be required to assess the magnitude of improvement in survival that these devices can offer and what training mechanisms can maximize team responses to feedback messages.

Figure 17-3 Cardiopulmonary resuscitation–sensing defibrillator. The chest compression pad with force detector and accelerometer is indicated (*arrow*). Several such devices are currently marketed; this is the MRx-QCPR (Philips Healthcare, Andover, MA).

Figure 17-4 The LUCAS-2 mechanical cardiopulmonary resuscitation device (Jolife Corp., Lund, Sweden).

Mechanical CPR Devices

The adjuncts described previously all rely on human performance of CPR. Another general approach to improve CPR quality is to provide compressions via a mechanical device that is independent of human fatigue or vagaries in performance. Such tools have been introduced in previous decades but fell out of favor because of unwieldy design and other practical considerations.

A newer generation of devices has brought the notion of mechanical CPR back to active consideration. One such device uses a "load-distributing compression band" (Autopulse, Zoll Corp., Chelmsford, MA). The Autopulse device works via a wide band that is attached to a backboard and battery-powered motor and placed across the torso. Through cycles of constriction and relaxation, the band compresses the chest in a circumferential manner at a fixed rate and "depth" consistent with resuscitation guidelines. In this fashion, pauses are also minimized by eliminating rescuer switching. Such devices have a unique role in out-of-hospital arrest because compressions can be delivered while transporting a patient down stairs or into an ambulance.

Recent studies to determine the efficacy of the Autopulse have had mixed results. Although initial smaller investigations appeared promising, a large multicenter randomized trial was stopped early because patients in the manual CPR arm had survival equivalent to those receiving care via the Autopulse, with a trend toward worse outcomes in the Autopulse group.[30]

A separate nonrandomized trial showed a marked improvement in survival when using the device.[31] A recent randomized trial in Europe has demonstrated the utility and feasibility of automated compression devices (in this case the Autopulse) in the resuscitation of out-of-hospital cardiac arrest patients.[32] The survival benefit of such devices may very much depend on the specifics of how they are applied and used; an upcoming large clinical trial (the Circulation Improving Resuscitation Care [CIRC] Trial) seeks to examine the effectiveness of the Autopulse device, improve EMS education and proper use of automated compression devices, and minimize confounders that may have affected previous investigations.[33]

Another mechanical CPR device has been developed in Europe (LUCAS, Jolife Corp., Lund, Sweden) and is currently being evaluated in clinical trials outside the United States (Fig. 17-4). This device, in contrast to the band mechanism of the Autopulse, uses a piston/suction cup to compress the anterior aspect of the chest, much like during manual CPR, with the suction cup providing some degree of active compression-decompression, as described earlier in this chapter. A pilot study found no difference in survival to discharge between patients who received manual chest compressions and those who were resuscitated using the LUCAS device.[34] A larger clinical trial involving the LUCAS device is currently under way and will provide additional information on the clinical impact of this particular mechanical CPR device.[35]

To highlight an intriguing opportunity available with mechanical CPR devices, there has been much discussion about the potential utility of these tools in clinical situations in which coronary angiography might be performed *concurrently* with ongoing resuscitation efforts. If clinical evidence suggests a major coronary event as the cause of the arrest, mechanical devices could be used to perform high-quality, continuous chest compressions as percutaneous coronary intervention is being performed. Case studies have demonstrated the feasibility of using the LUCAS device during intra-arrest coronary angiography with good patient outcomes,[36,37] but additional data will be necessary to draw more clear conclusions about clinical practices and patient outcomes in these situations.

Emergency Cardiac Bypass

Extracorporeal cardiopulmonary resuscitation (E-CPR) is an emergency technique that has been investigated as a "last resort" for cardiac arrest patients who have failed to achieve ROSC despite ongoing resuscitation efforts. Several clinical studies have demonstrated successful outcomes for patients in whom E-CPR was used (and thus indicate that E-CPR could be a feasible addition to resuscitation efforts).[35-37] One prospective trial in Japan, which identified patients who failed to respond to other traditional resuscitation efforts, demonstrated a favorable neurologic outcome in patients who were able to undergo both emergency cardiac bypass and therapeutic hypothermia treatment; rapid initiation of E-CPR and attainment of the target temperature were associated with positive neurologic outcomes in this cohort.[38] The specialized training necessary to perform the procedure, as well as significant logistic issues surrounding rapid establishment of extracorporeal membrane oxygenation in the emergency department (ED) setting, raises concern about the widespread applicability of this intervention. Other investigations have highlighted the potential complications related to E-CPR in these critically ill patients.[39,40] Additional research is needed on this topic, and more information will be necessary to clearly identify patients who are likely to benefit from E-CPR, examine the cost of such an intervention, and determine the impact of E-CPR on the survival of cardiac arrest victims.[41]

MONITORING DURING CPR

Overview of CPR

Despite extensive research and attempts to alter the outcome of cardiac arrest, it is discouraging to realize that at present, there are no reliable clinical criteria that clinicians can use to assess the efficacy of CPR. Although P_{ETCO_2} serves as an indicator of the cardiac output produced by chest compressions and may indicate ROSC, there is little other technology available to provide real-time feedback on the effectiveness of CPR. Pulse oximetry is not helpful during arrest. Early defibrillation has been linked to better survival rates, but no medications have been shown to improve neurologically intact survival from cardiac arrest. Despite the widespread use of epinephrine and several studies of vasopressin, no placebo-controlled study has shown that any medication or vasopressor given routinely during human cardiac arrest (for any initial arrest rhythm) increases the rate of long-term survival after cardiac arrest.

Arterial blood gas monitoring during cardiac arrest is not a reliable indicator of the severity of tissue hypoxemia, hypercapnia (and therefore the adequacy of ventilation during CPR), or tissue acidosis. Current evidence in patients with ventricular fibrillation neither supports nor refutes the routine use of intravenous fluids. There is no evidence that any antiarrhythmic drug given routinely during human cardiac arrest increases survival to hospital discharge. There is insufficient evidence to recommend for or against the routine use of fibrinolysis for cardiac arrest.

No blood testing is considered routine or standard during the initial stages of cardiopulmonary arrest, although early serum potassium and blood glucose monitoring is prudent if resuscitation is successful.[14]

Capnography

Capnography measures respiratory CO_2, which is delivered to the lungs and expelled during exhalation (Fig. 17-5). The highest CO_2 levels occur at the end of each exhalation, called P_{ETCO_2}. During cardiac arrest, P_{ETCO_2} falls abruptly at the onset of cardiac arrest, increases during the delivery of effective CPR, and returns to physiologic levels after ROSC. P_{ETCO_2} correlates with cardiac output under low-flow states such as CPR.[42] Because of this relationship with cardiac output, P_{ETCO_2} has been regarded as a probable indicator of the quality of CPR. During effective CPR in animal trials,

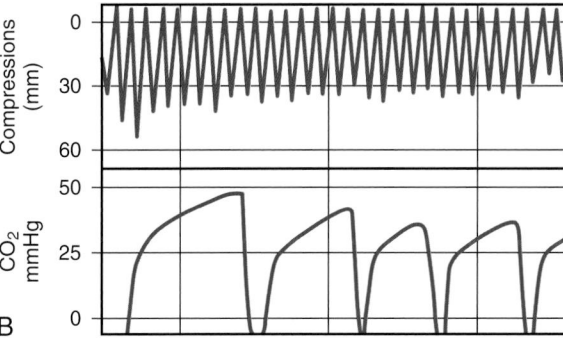

Figure 17-5 Waveform capnography during cardiac arrest. **A,** P_{ETCO_2}: diagram showing a typical ventilation cycle and CO_2 waveform. The point that represents P_{ETCO_2} is marked with an arrow. **B,** P_{ETCO_2} recording during cardiopulmonary resuscitation. This image demonstrates the use of capnography during ongoing resuscitation. The chest compression waveform is shown in red (*panel top*), and the P_{ETCO_2} waveform is shown in blue (*panel bottom*).

P_{ETCO_2} positively correlates with cardiac output, coronary perfusion pressure, efficacy of cardiac compression, ROSC, and even survival. Research is currently being done to further understand the use of P_{ETCO_2} during CPR. At the other end of the spectrum, P_{ETCO_2} could be useful in determining when to terminate resuscitation efforts.[43]

Although capnography is a common method of confirming correct endotracheal tube placement, it has also been regarded as a potential method of measuring hemodynamics and perfusion during cardiac arrest, as well as for determining the outcome of resuscitation efforts (specifically, detection of ROSC). The 2010 resuscitation guidelines recommend continuous waveform capnography for all intubated patients during resuscitation efforts.[14]

Ultrasound Monitoring

With advances in ultrasound equipment, properly trained users can portably and accurately monitor cardiac function in real time. Preliminary studies have demonstrated that trained physicians can assess cardiac function and obtain adequate images rapidly by using a subcostal approach to standard echocardiography in the cardiac arrest setting.[44] If you are adequately trained in this technology, use it during resuscitation efforts to clinically diagnose conditions such as pulseless electrical activity (PEA) and to make a global assessment of cardiac motion during CPR and pulse restoration.

Use ultrasound during arrest to rapidly diagnose and treat conditions such as cardiac tamponade. Get the ED ultrasound machine ready to use when preparing for an incoming cardiac arrest. Remember, however, that ultrasound is only a secondary diagnostic adjunct and should not interfere with the performance of high-quality CPR. Minimize interruptions to perform ultrasound and use it only during resuscitation for specific purposes (e.g., diagnosis of PEA versus hypotensive sinus rhythm). In most cases of arrest, ultrasound is probably of little value. Finally, there is ongoing research on the use of transcranial Doppler ultrasound to determine the prognosis after cardiac arrest. One preliminary study concluded that patients with severely disabling or fatal outcomes could be identified within the first 24 hours with this method.[45]

CONCLUSION

Physicians and other health care workers have been performing CPR for more than 50 years, but only since the 1990s has the full importance of the quality of CPR become apparent through an evidence-based approach. Chest compressions and ventilations appear to be deceptively easy to the newly trained, but in fact they are highly complex skills and are difficult to perform well under stress. New technologies have been developed to assist in delivery of CPR, and use of these tools may improve the ability to save lives from cardiac arrest in the coming years.

References are available at www.expertconsult.com

CHAPTER 18

Resuscitative Thoracotomy

Russell F. Jones and Emanuel P. Rivers

In the United States, trauma is the leading cause of death in people aged 1 through 44.[1] Blunt trauma accounts for the majority of trauma mortality overall, but in urban settings, penetrating trauma, including firearm-related injuries, accounts for an increased proportion of trauma deaths. In 2007, more than 31,000 firearm-related deaths occurred in the United States,[2] with many victims arriving at the emergency department (ED) in extremis.

Penetrating cardiac injuries are associated with a very high mortality rate. On rare occasions, however, an aggressive approach involving the use of emergency department thoracotomy (EDT) leads to survival in patients with impending or recent traumatic arrest. EDT is a dramatic, heroic intervention performed outside the operating room and often in the absence of trained cardiothoracic or trauma surgeons. *Though supported as a potential lifesaving procedure, EDT is not a mandated standard of care nor a procedure that is expected to be*

Resuscitative Thoracotomy

Indications
Penetrating trauma patient in cardiac arrest
Blunt trauma patient with vital signs in the field
Nontraumatic hypothermic cardiac arrest

Contraindications
Blunt trauma arrest patients without vital signs in the field
Trauma patients with open cranial wounds
Initial rhythm of asystole
Cardiopulmonary resuscitation ongoing >15 minutes

Complications
Phrenic nerve injury
Coronary artery injury
Infection
Injury/disease transmission to health care worker

Equipment

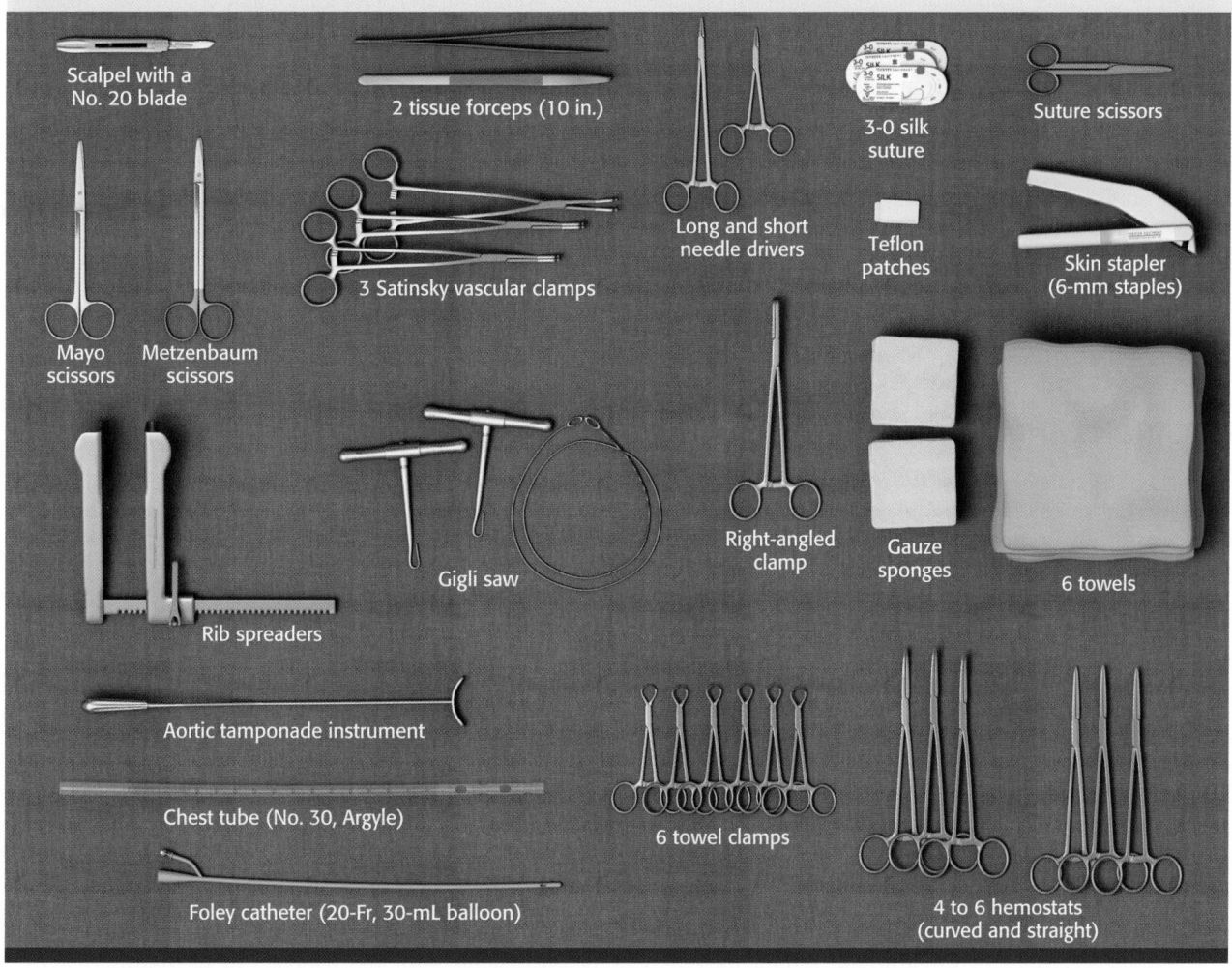

Scalpel with a No. 20 blade
2 tissue forceps (10 in.)
3-0 silk suture
Suture scissors
Mayo scissors
Metzenbaum scissors
3 Satinsky vascular clamps
Long and short needle drivers
Teflon patches
Skin stapler (6-mm staples)
Gigli saw
Right-angled clamp
Gauze sponges
6 towels
Rib spreaders
Aortic tamponade instrument
Chest tube (No. 30, Argyle)
6 towel clamps
Foley catheter (20-Fr, 30-mL balloon)
4 to 6 hemostats (curved and straight)

Review Box 18-1 Resuscitative thoracotomy: indications, contraindications, equipment, and complications.

performed in most EDs. The first successful thoracotomy was reported more than 100 years ago, and the first EDT was reported in 1966.[3] Since then, multiple studies have reported outcomes, indications, techniques, and risks associated with the procedure. In 2003, the National Association of EMS Physicians Standards and Clinical Practice Committee and the American College of Surgeons Committee on Trauma (ACSCOT) proposed specific guidelines for EDT.[4] However, despite the guidelines, EDT remains a procedure done on a case-by-case basis with controversial evidence regarding the ideal indications.

Given the circumstances surrounding the procedure and the associated injuries, few patients survive. The poor overall survival rates, however, should not discourage performance of the procedure in the correct setting and when appropriate surgical backup is available for definitive care.

EDT is not a simple procedure. Identifying specific structures within a chest cavity filled with blood, coupled with a collapsed lung and an injured heart and major vessels, can be formidable. Localizing the injuries that can be reversed quickly and safely is even more difficult.

This chapter focuses on three major objectives: (1) identifying the indications for and contraindications to EDT, (2) describing the technical aspects of the procedure and adjunctive maneuvers to repair specific injuries, and (3) recognizing the associated risks and complications.

Every institution should have guidelines for the appropriate use of resuscitative thoracotomy. An institutional plan for chest wound management and postprocedural care should also be established with the service that will provide backup when members of the surgical team cannot be on site at the time of resuscitation. Debate regarding who should perform EDT is not necessary because everyone who is licensed to perform resuscitative thoracotomy should be trained, competent, and prepared for the technical and initial critical care aspects of patient management. Patient care needs in the event of successful resuscitation should be considered in advance and the surgical and intensive care teams notified so that they can mobilize the appropriate supplies, equipment, and personnel.

INDICATIONS AND CONTRAINDICATIONS

In the ED, the vast majority of thoracotomies are performed on penetrating trauma patients in cardiac arrest. Beall and coworkers initially proposed EDT for the treatment of penetrating cardiac injuries in 1966.[3] Since then, it has been expanded to include extrathoracic injuries, blunt trauma, and nontraumatic pathology. Studies show wide variation in survival rates and outcomes. Taking 40 years of collective EDT data into account, the survival rate of patients undergoing EDT for blunt trauma is nearly 2%, whereas that for penetrating trauma is nearly 16%,[4] but these survival rates depend on many variables and are not applicable to every situation. There are a paucity of data concerning survival rates in patients with EDT performed for nontraumatic causes, and it is not recommended that this procedure be regularly used in these settings.

Make the decision to perform EDT quickly based on whether the patient is likely to benefit from the procedure, has a reasonable chance of survival, and cannot tolerate a delay in operative intervention. Also consider the risks

BOX 18-1 Factors Used to Determine Which Patients May Benefit From EDT

Mechanism of injury
Location of injury
Initial cardiac rhythm
Resuscitation (cardiopulmonary) time
Signs of life

associated with performing the procedure. Trauma researchers have identified several factors that are considered crucial when determining who will benefit from EDT (Box 18-1).

The first assessment is made in the prehospital setting, where determination of the mechanism of injury and the presence or absence of a pulse is critical. Recommendations from the ACSCOT guidelines state that EDT has no role in blunt trauma victims who are apneic and pulseless and lack an organized rhythm.[4] Such patients do not survive, regardless of the intervention. In one of the largest EDT series to date, Branney and coworkers[5] reviewed 868 consecutive patients over a 23-year period. They found that no blunt trauma patients survived EDT when they had no vital signs in the field but that 2.5% of blunt trauma patients survived EDT when vital signs were present in the field. Rhee and colleagues[6] examined 4620 cases of EDT from 24 studies over a 25-year period. The overall survival rate after blunt trauma was just 1.4%, which led to EDT falling out of favor for this indication. Recent articles, however, have challenged the idea of limiting EDT to those in cardiac arrest from penetrating injury only.[7-9] Moore and associates recommended considering EDT in blunt trauma victims who have received less than 5 minutes of cardiopulmonary resuscitation (CPR) and possess signs of life.[7] The survival rate of pulseless trauma patients sustaining penetrating injury is significantly higher than that of blunt trauma patients. EDT should only rarely be used in patients with blunt trauma mechanisms. Several penetrating injury subtypes have been studied: firearm injuries, stab wounds, and penetrating explosive injuries. Thoracic stab wounds consistently show the highest rates of survival after EDT.[5,10-12] This is theoretically due to the decreased amount of tissue damage related to the weapon and the ability to quickly identify anatomic structures and injuries. Penetrating firearm injuries are more likely to result in death because of increased tissue damage from the missile and concussive surrounding forces. Patients with firearm injuries are more likely to have multiple wounds, and the depth of penetration is increased in comparison to stab wounds. One published cohort of combat casualties from explosive penetrating injuries reported similar survival rates as those after firearm-related penetrating injuries.[12]

The location of the penetrating injury helps determine the futility of EDT. A trend toward increased survival rates in patients with thoracic injuries was found in historical data.[4,12-21] Isolated cardiac wounds have the highest survival rate after EDT, with approximately 19% of patients surviving the procedure.[8] Penetrating abdominal injuries have beneficial outcomes when EDT is performed to cross-clamp the aorta, with survival rates in the mid-teens.[5,12,22,23] Extremity injuries rarely require EDT because the use of a tourniquet can control the hemorrhaging until the patient can be transported to the operating room. When EDT is used for traumatic extremity exsanguination, though, survival rates range from 10% to 25%.[12] Patients in cardiac arrest associated with head injuries, especially those with open cranial wounds, have dismal survival rates and are considered poor candidates for further resuscitative efforts, including EDT.[7]

The type of cardiac electrical activity is helpful in determining who may benefit from EDT. Battistella and colleagues[24] reviewed 604 patients undergoing CPR for traumatic cardiopulmonary arrest and found that of the 212 patients who were in asystole, none survived. Fulton and associates[25] found that of patients in traumatic arrest, survival was improved when the patients exhibited ventricular fibrillation, ventricular tachycardia, or pulseless electrical activity rather than asystole or an idioventricular rhythm. In another study of EDT for traumatic arrest, asystole, idioventricular rhythm, or severe bradycardia was indicative of poor outcomes or an unsalvageable patient.[4] In fact, most emergency medical service providers will not transport trauma patients who are in asystole regardless of the mechanism.[26]

The duration of resuscitation before EDT can also be used as a decision point. With traumatic injury, survival rates diminish as the duration of CPR increases. The consensus recommendation based on multiple studies is that any trauma patient who has undergone CPR for longer than 15 minutes has an exceedingly dismal survival rate and further resuscitation should be considered futile.[4,10,11,25-28] Penetrating trauma patients with signs of life and CPR times of less than 15 minutes are candidates for EDT. In fact, penetrating trauma patients who suffer arrest in the ED have acceptable rates of survival and good neurologic outcomes if EDT is performed promptly.[14-17,20,27,29] EDT can be considered in victims of blunt trauma cardiac arrest if CPR has been ongoing for less than 5 minutes.[7] This practice is controversial, however, and each institution should address this situation both in their trauma protocol and on an individual basis before arrival of the patient in the ED.

Perhaps the most critical determinant of the appropriateness of EDT is whether the patient demonstrates "signs of life." Signs of life are objective physiologic parameters that are present in patients who survive EDT. They include pupillary response, extremity movement, cardiac electrical activity, measurable or palpable blood pressure, spontaneous ventilation, or the presence of a carotid pulse. The presence of one or more of these indicators has been associated with good neurologic outcomes and increased rates of survival.[3-9,30]

Although survival remains the ultimate gauge of the effectiveness of EDT, it is essential to consider quality of life also, especially neurologic function of the patient. It is somewhat surprising that survivors of EDT generally have good neurologic outcomes. Rhee and colleagues[6] reported that 280 of 303 (92.4%) patients discharged after EDT were neurologically intact. It is not possible to accurately predict which patients are likely to survive intact, but the study by Branney and coworkers[5] demonstrated that all survivors with full neurologic recovery had respiratory effort at the scene and 75% still had respiratory effort on arrival at the ED. The presence or absence of a palpable pulse was not an absolute prognostic indicator in this study. Sixty-six percent of long-term survivors (11 patients with penetrating trauma and 1 with blunt trauma) had no detectable pulse on arrival at the ED.[9] The first 24 hours after EDT rapidly demonstrates which patients are likely to become long-term survivors. Baker and associates[14] showed that with 168 emergency thoracotomies for mixed trauma, most patients with fatal injuries died within 24 hours. Of patients surviving the first 24 hours, 80% (33 of 41) lived and were discharged from the hospital. Full neurologic recovery occurred in 90% of these survivors. Overall, only 2.4% (4 of 168) remained severely disabled or in a persistent vegetative state. Of these 4 patients, only 1 (0.6%) lived beyond 2 months.

Cardiac Injuries—Penetrating

Sixty percent to 80% of cardiac stab wounds result in pericardial effusion regardless of the presence of shock.[31] Depending on which chamber is involved, tamponade can occur if the wound is smaller than 1 cm in size. Wounds larger than 1 cm usually continue to bleed regardless of which chamber is involved. Low-pressure atrial wounds generally form a thrombus before tamponade develops. The thicker-walled left ventricle may spontaneously seal stab wounds up to 1 cm in length. As little as 60 to 100 mL of blood acutely filling the pericardium will impede diastolic filling, reduce stroke volume, decrease cardiac output, and increase release of catecholamine. Catecholamine release may mask the severity of illness because it maintains blood pressure through an increase in peripheral vascular resistance. In penetrating cardiac injury, the right ventricle is the chamber most likely to be involved because of its anterior location, followed by the left ventricle and the atria.[32,33]

The progression from compensated cardiac function to uncompensated tamponade can be sudden and profound. Although one may suspect tamponade based on well-described signs, clinical diagnosis of pericardial tamponade in an unstable trauma patient is difficult because of the combined effect of hemorrhagic and cardiogenic shock. The classic signs of Beck's triad (distended neck veins, hypotension, and muffled heart sounds) described in 1926[34] have limited diagnostic value for acute penetrating cardiac trauma.[35] The most reliable signs of tamponade are elevated central venous pressure, hypotension, and tachycardia.

The advent of ultrasound and the focused assessment with sonography in trauma (FAST) examination has improved the diagnosis of pericardial effusion and tamponade. Findings indicative of tamponade include the presence of pericardial fluid with right atrial or ventricular collapse during diastole (Fig. 18-1). FAST is a rapid bedside screening examination used to detect hemopericardium and hemoperitoneum and is now important in the evaluation of unstable trauma patients.[36,37] From data collected in 1540 patients, Rozycki and associates[38] reported 100% sensitivity and specificity in detecting pericardial and peritoneal fluid in a hypotensive, unstable trauma patient. Ultrasound can have rare false-negative results when pericardial fluid from a cardiac injury decompresses into the thoracic cavity through a wound in the pericardium.[39]

After EDT for penetrating cardiac wounds, survival is also related to the mechanism of injury. Patients with stab wounds fare better than do patients with gunshot wounds. Rhee and colleagues[6] noted that 16.8% of patients with stab wounds survived to hospital discharge after EDT. Branney and coworkers[5] reported a 29% survival rate in stab wound patients with tamponade and a 15% survival rate in those without tamponade.

In contrast, gunshot wounds are often large injuries unable to seal themselves; tamponade occurs in only 20%. Patients

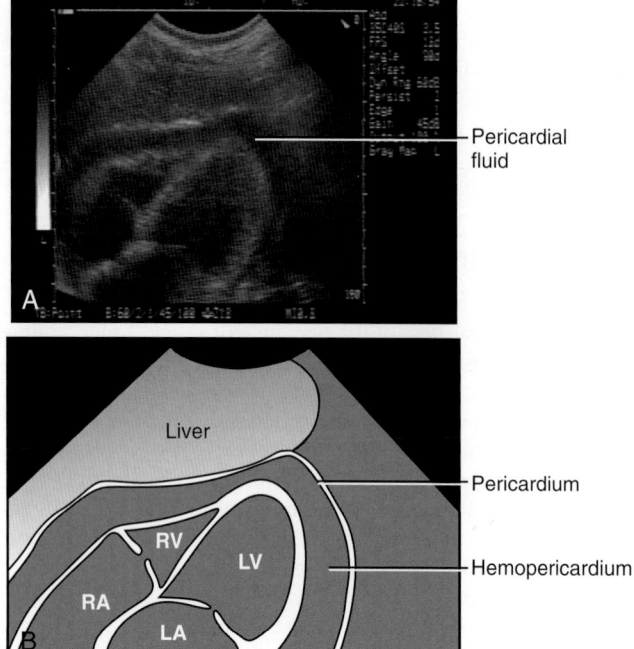

Figure 18-1 A, Bedside ultrasound demonstrating the hemopericardium. **B,** Artist's drawing of the chambers of the heart, the pericardium, and the hemopericardium as seen on ultrasound. *LA,* left atrium; *LV,* left ventricle; *RA,* right atrium; *RV,* right ventricle.

with penetrating cardiac injuries from gunshot wounds are more likely to initially be seen with profoundly compromised hemodynamics. In addition, the increasing popularity of larger-caliber weapons has made it more difficult to resuscitate patients with gunshot wounds to the chest. Of 112 patients with gunshot wounds to the heart,[5] only 2% survived neurologically intact.

Cardiac Injuries—Blunt

Blunt trauma to the heart can range from minor contusion to cardiac rupture. The most common cause of death after non-penetrating cardiac injuries is myocardial rupture, and in approximately 25% of such patients the ascending aorta is ruptured simultaneously.[31] Branney and coworkers[5] observed a 2% survival rate in blunt trauma patients resuscitated with EDT. Those who survived had vital signs present in the field. The poor outcomes associated with this type of injury are a result of the poor cardiac function caused by myocardial contusion, even if the hemorrhage has been treated.

Pulmonary Injuries

Pulmonary injuries can be divided into three types: parenchymal, tracheobronchial, and large vessel. Parenchymal and tracheobronchial injuries rarely require EDT because they are either rapidly fatal or treated initially by tube thoracostomy. Tracheobronchial injury is more common in blunt than in penetrating trauma. Bertelson and Howitz[40] reviewed 1128 patients at autopsy and found only 3 to have this injury. The airway is usually maintained, even with complete transection. The stiff tracheobronchial cartilage tends to hold the lumen open, and the paratracheal and parabronchial fasciae preserve the relationship of the proximal to distal bronchi. Ninety

percent of tracheobronchial tears occur within 2.5 cm of the carina, and most commonly involve the main stem bronchi. Complete division of the trachea is extremely rare. Depending on the size and location of the injury, patients may have massive hemoptysis, airway obstruction, pneumomediastinum, pneumothorax, or tension pneumothorax. Massive subcutaneous emphysema and pneumomediastinum are usually seen, although up to 10% of patients with this injury have no abnormal findings on the initial radiograph.[41] If hemorrhage is profuse or if the site of the injury can be determined, use of a bifid endotracheal tube or unilateral intubation of a main stem bronchus will help secure the airway.

Lacerations of the lung parenchyma that are not accompanied by injury to major vessels generally respond to tube thoracostomy. If the initial chest tube drainage is more than 1500 mL or if there is persistent hypotension or cardiac arrest, consider immediate thoracotomy. For pulmonary injuries, survival after EDT is also related to the mechanism of injury. Branney and coworkers[5] reported a 17% survival rate after pulmonary stab wounds, 3% after gunshot wounds, and 5% after blunt trauma.

AIR EMBOLISM

Air embolism is a complication of pulmonary parenchymal injuries that may require immediate thoracotomy if the patient is hemodynamically unstable. The development of air embolism after penetrating injuries of the lung is often insidious, and the diagnosis is usually made at the time of thoracotomy.[42] Preoperative and postmortem diagnosis of air embolism is difficult, and it is likely that most air emboli are not detected. Air embolism is confirmed at thoracotomy by needle aspiration of a foamy air-blood mixture from the left or right ventricle or by visualization of air within the coronary arteries.

Air embolism may appear in either the right or the left side of the circulatory system. Involvement of the right side of the circulation is referred to as *venous* or *pulmonary* air embolism. Generally, venous air is well tolerated, but death can occur when the volume of air reaches 5 to 8 mL/kg. The rate at which air moves into the circulation and the body's position are important determinants of the volume that can be tolerated. If the body's position allows dispersion of air into the peripheral circulation, more air can be tolerated, although the damage to peripheral structures and end-organs can be extensive. Rapid death usually results from obstruction of the right ventricle or the pulmonary outflow tract. Injuries to the vena cava or the right ventricle can also create portals of entry into the right circulatory system.

Air embolism involving the left side of the circulatory system is referred to as *arterial* or *systemic* air embolism. The lethal volume depends on the organs to which it is distributed. As little as 0.5 mL of air in the left anterior descending coronary artery can lead to ventricular fibrillation. Two milliliters of air injected into the cerebral circulation can be fatal. The formation of traumatic bronchovenous fistulas creates potential entry points for air to move into the left side of the circulatory system. The only requirement is the formation of an air-blood gradient conducive to the inward movement of air. Although lowered intravascular pressure from hemorrhage is a risk factor, the most important element in all reports of air embolism has been the use of positive pressure ventilation.[43]

In a review of 447 cases of major thoracic trauma, Yee and coworkers[44] found adequate chart data to suggest the diagnosis of air embolism in 61 patients. About 25% of patients with air embolism have blunt trauma with associated lung injury secondary to multiple rib fractures or hilar disruption. The overall mortality is higher than 50%.

The diagnosis of air embolism is easily overlooked because the signs and symptoms are similar to those of hypovolemic shock. Two valuable signs that are present in 36% of patients are hemoptysis and the occurrence of cardiac arrest *after intubation and ventilation.* The development of focal neurologic changes, seizures, or central nervous system dysfunction in the absence of head injury is also suggestive of the diagnosis.[45] Overall, the diagnosis is subtle and must be considered when there is no evidence of the more common causes of extremis in a trauma patient.

Blunt and Penetrating Abdominal Injury

In the setting of penetrating abdominal injury, thoracotomy with cross-clamping of the thoracic aorta has been advocated as a means of controlling hemorrhage, redistributing blood flow to the brain and heart, and reducing blood loss below the diaphragm. Unfortunately, aortic cross-clamping can also have detrimental effects. Kralovich and colleagues[46] studied the hemodynamic consequences of aortic occlusion in a swine model of hemorrhagic arrest. There was no difference between groups in return of spontaneous circulation; however, the occluded aorta group experienced statistically greater impairments in left ventricular function and systemic oxygen utilization in the postresuscitation period. Branney and coworkers[5] found that 8 of 76 patients undergoing EDT for *penetrating abdominal injury* survived neurologically intact. More recently, Seamon and colleagues[23] achieved a 16% survival rate with good neurologic outcomes (8 of 50 patients) when EDT was used before laparotomy for abdominal exsanguination from trauma. Of note, none of the survivors in this study were in cardiac arrest at the time of EDT, but they did have severe hemorrhagic shock, and six of the eight had unmeasurable blood pressure. Current recommendations suggest that EDT be performed judiciously in patients with abdominal trauma as an adjunct to definitive repair of the abdominal injury.

Open-Chest Resuscitation for Nontraumatic Arrest

At present, less than 6% of CPR attempts conducted outside hospital special care units result in survival.[47] The first case of a human survivor of open-chest cardiac massage (OCCM) was reported in 1901. In 1960, Kouwenhoven and associates[48] published favorable survival rates with closed-chest CPR as opposed to OCCM. After further refinement by Pearson and Redding, closed-chest CPR gradually became the preferred method of cardiac compression.[49]

The goal of CPR is to restore coronary perfusion pressure (CPP), which is the prime determinant for return of spontaneous circulation as established in animal models. Paradis and associates[50] found that humans need a minimal CPP of 15 mm Hg to achieve return of spontaneous circulation. Although a CPP of 15 mm Hg does not guarantee return of spontaneous circulation, there is 100% failure of resuscitation if CPP is below this level. Despite the limited number of

human studies on OCCM, its hemodynamic superiority over closed-chest CPR is compelling. Del Guercio and coworkers[51] measured cardiac output during both closed-chest CPR and OCCM in in-hospital cardiac arrest patients. OCCM produced a mean cardiac index of 1.31 L/min/m^2 as opposed to 0.6 L/min/m^2 during closed-chest CPR. Boczar and colleagues[52] further examined 10 patients who were unresponsive to closed-chest CPR and measured CPP during closed-chest CPR followed by OCCM. Mean CPP in the closed-chest group was 7.3 mm Hg versus 32.6 mm Hg in the open-chest group. All patients achieved a CPP of at least 20 mm Hg at some time during their OCCM phase. This easily surpassed the minimal CPP required for return of spontaneous circulation. Outcomes after OCCM have not been well established. Animal models suggest not only improved hemodynamic parameters but also a possible increase in 24-hour survival rates.[53] Neurologic outcomes, however, are unknown, and the American Heart Association guidelines for CPR do not promote the regular use of OCCM in patients with out-of-hospital cardiac arrest.[47]

At present, the precise indications for open-chest resuscitation after nontraumatic arrest are not well defined, and the procedure is not considered the standard of care. Despite demonstrated hemodynamic superiority in both animal and human models of open-chest versus closed-chest CPR, outcome benefit is lacking. There are a paucity of human data evaluating the window of time during which this treatment can be effective. Consider performing OCCM in patients with witnessed in-hospital cardiac arrest who do not have any significant underlying comorbid conditions, who have mechanical lesions, or for whom closed-chest CPR may be ineffective. A prehospital cardiac arrest patient who remains without a perfusing rhythm after the initial defibrillation has a poor prognosis with conventional treatment. Whether OCCM has a role in the management of these patients has yet to be established.

Nontraumatic Hypothermic Cardiac Arrest

In the setting of cardiac arrest from hypothermia, consider the use of EDT and OCCM. Cardiopulmonary or venovenous bypass is the most rapid method of core rewarming, but it is rarely available immediately. Open thoracotomy with mediastinal irrigation has been used successfully in cases of severe hypothermia with cardiac arrest. Brunette and McVaney[54] reported 11 patients with hypothermic cardiac arrest, 7 of whom underwent EDT with OCCM and mediastinal rewarming. Five patients survived, and all had positive neurologic outcomes despite cardiac arrest times of between 10 and 90 minutes (although one patient died of gastrointestinal hemorrhage and sepsis following resuscitation, the other four patients survived with full neurologic recovery). The other four patients who did not undergo EDT did not survive despite being taken promptly to the operating room for cardiopulmonary bypass rewarming. Although the number of cases is limited, this study is evidence that OCCM can provide prolonged hemodynamic support and good neurologic outcomes. It should be noted that similar case reports also exist in which closed-chest CPR was maintained for prolonged periods and resulted in successful hypothermic resuscitation.[55] EDT with mediastinal irrigation can produce core rewarming rates as fast as 8°C/hr, with the heart and lungs preferentially being rewarmed first.[54] Mediastinal irrigation involves heating sterile saline in a microwave oven to 40°C and then pouring it slowly over the heart and into the thorax. Performing a thoracotomy for hypothermic arrest does not preclude the use of cardiac bypass inasmuch as it was subsequently used after EDT in three of the survivors from the Brunette and McVaney study.[54]

EQUIPMENT

Carefully select the instruments to be included in the EDT equipment tray. See Review Box 18-1 for a complete list.

PROCEDURE
Preliminary Considerations

All trauma patients arriving at the ED with hypotension must be assumed to be hypovolemic and be treated accordingly. Rapidly exclude other causes as well, including tension pneumothorax, cardiac tamponade, air embolism, and neurogenic or cardiogenic shock. A useful algorithmic overview of the approach to chest trauma is presented in Figure 18-2. The use of autotransfusion, if available, has several benefits, but its use is not widespread or considered standard.[56]

Airway Control

Intubate the patient orotracheally, if possible, but be aware that access to the thoracic organs, surgical repairs, or surgical procedures may be hampered by frequent inflations of the left lung. If necessary, *selectively intubate the right lung by blindly advancing a standard single-lumen endotracheal tube to a depth of 30 cm (measured from the corner of the mouth) in adult patients.*[57] Although the left lung and the right upper lobe are not ventilated with the tracheal tube in this position, animal studies and data from humans suggest that selective right lung ventilation provides adequate oxygenation and ventilation for at least 60 minutes.[57] With the left lung deflated one can expedite thoracotomy by maximizing space in the left thoracic cavity. Keep in mind that extending the thoracotomy into the right thoracic cavity may necessitate switching to bilateral lung ventilation or left lung ventilation to allow maximum right thoracic exposure.

Anesthesia and Amnesia

Comatose patients undergoing resuscitation may regain consciousness during successful EDT, but this awareness may not be apparent if they are still pharmacologically paralyzed. Anticipate and recognize this phenomenon and administer adequate analgesic, amnestic, and muscle-relaxing agents to a ventilated patient who may also be in shock. No specific regimen has been studied, but ketamine appears an ideal agent to use in the ED. It is prudent to administer anesthetic agents routinely if a paralyzed patient demonstrates perfusion during resuscitation. This is not only humane but decreases systemic oxygen consumption.

Anterolateral Thoracotomy Incision

Manually ventilate the patient during the procedure. Ask an assistant to pass a nasogastric tube, which helps differentiate the esophagus from the aorta, but do not allow this procedure

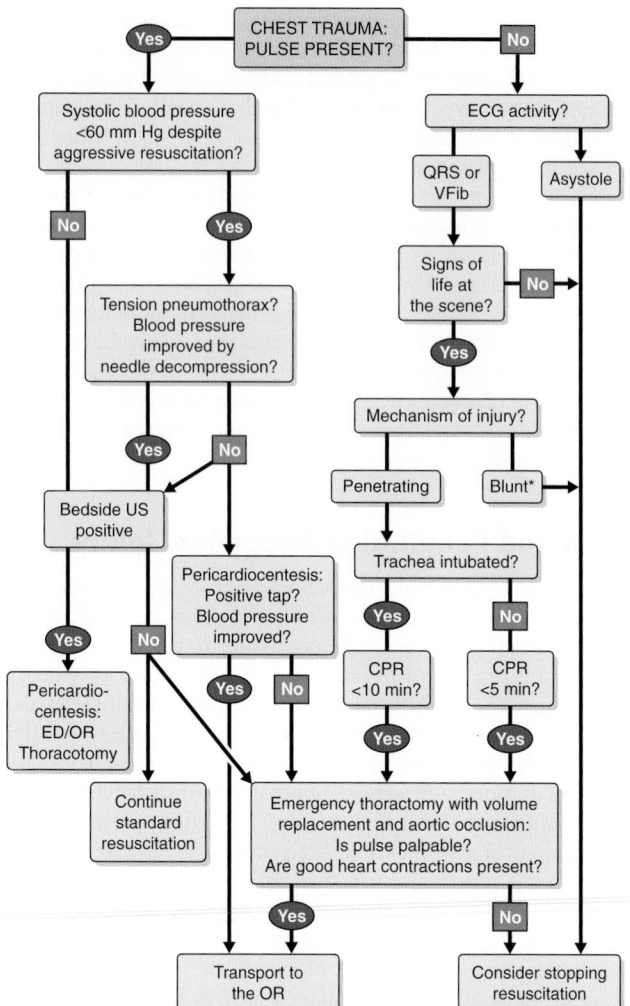

Figure 18-2 An algorithmic approach to chest trauma. *CPR,* cardiopulmonary resuscitation; *ECG,* electrocardiographic; *ED,* emergency department; *OR,* operating room; *QRS,* organized electrical activity; tap, pericardial tap yielding blood; *US,* ultrasonography; *VFib,* ventricular fibrillation. *Pulseless blunt trauma management is controversial, with some data supporting stopping resuscitation immediately[4] and recent data recommending emergency department thoracotomy if CPR has been ongoing for less than 5 minutes.[7]

to delay thoracotomy. If CPR is being performed, ask an assistant to continue closed-chest compressions up to the point of making the initial incision. Take universal precautions to avoid blood exposure and use a suction catheter to minimize contact with blood. Sterile gloves (consider double-glove protection), gown, mask with an eye shield, and an operative surgical cap are recommended for the procedure.

Prepare the skin of the left anterior aspect of the chest with antiseptic if readily available. Wedge towels or sheets under the left posterior part of the chest and place the patient's left arm above the head (Fig. 18-3A). On the left side of the chest, make an anterolateral incision at the fourth to fifth intercostal space with a scalpel with a No. 20 blade (Fig. 18-4, *step 1*). Do not take the time to count ribs; simply estimate the location to be just beneath the nipple in males and at the inframammary fold in females (see Fig. 18-3). It is important to establish wide exposure by beginning the incision on the right

Figure 18-3 Left anterolateral thoracotomy. **A,** Place several towels or sandbags under the left scapula and raise the arm above the head. The patient should be intubated. Insert a nasogastric (NG) tube to differentiate the esophagus from the aorta. Make a left anterolateral submammary incision. **B,** *Dashes* indicate the incision site in the inframammary fold in women. *ET,* endotracheal.

RESUSCITATIVE THORACOTOMY GENERAL TECHNIQUE

1 Make an anterolateral incision at the 4th to 5th intercostal space.

Begin at the right side of the sternum and extend the incision past the posterior axillary line.

2 Cut the intercostal muscles with scissors.

Incise along the top of the rib to avoid the intercostal artery.

3 Use scissors to incise the parietal pleura and gain entry into the thoracic cavity.

4 Use your hands to spread the ribs.

5 Place a rib spreader between the ribs with the handle and ratchet bar facing downward.

Carefully spread the ribs open.

6 PERICARDIOTOMY
Lift the pericardial sac with forceps, and cut pericardium with scissors.

Incise in a caudal-to-cephalad direction; stay anterior and parallel to the phrenic nerve.

7 AORTIC CROSS-CLAMPING
Bluntly dissect the surrounding fascia and temporarily apply an aortic clamp.

Additional injury-specific procedures are depicted elsewhere in this chapter.

Figure 18-4 Resuscitative thoracotomy, general technique. *(From Custalow CB.* Color Atlas of Emergency Department Procedures. *Philadelphia: Saunders; 2005.)*

side of the sternum and extending the skin incision past the posterior axillary line. Beginning here will save time if the right side of the chest needs to be opened as well. Inadequate exposure, rib fractures, and additional delays occur when the skin incision is too limited. *With the first sweep of the scalpel,* separate skin, subcutaneous fat, and the superficial portions of the pectoralis and serratus muscles.

Cut the intercostal muscles with scissors to expose the thoracic cavity (Fig. 18-4, *step 2*). Use scissors to divide the intercostal muscles because the risk for lung laceration is greater when a scalpel is used. Make the incision just over the top of the rib to avoid the intercostal neurovascular bundle. Just before opening the pleura, stop ventilations momentarily. This will allow the lung to collapse away from the chest wall. Should the internal mammary artery be transected during the procedure, hemorrhage is generally minimal until after perfusion is reestablished, at which time bleeding may be profuse. If actively bleeding, the internal mammary artery should be ligated or clamped. Do not forget to address the internal mammary artery if perfusion is reestablished because this can be a source of significant bleeding.[30]

After entering the pleural cavity, gain good exposure. Karmy-Jones and associates[58] found that 20% of their patients undergoing EDT via the anterolateral approach needed to have the initial incision extended. To gain better exposure, first use your hands to open the chest cavity. Then place a Finochietto retractor (rib spreader) between the ribs with the handle and the ratchet bar directed downward toward the axilla (Fig. 18-4, *step 5*). If the retractor were to be placed with the handle up, the ratchet bar would prevent extension of the incision into the right side of the chest. Ribs may be broken during spreading, so be careful to not get cut on the sharp bone edges. If massive hemothorax is encountered, remove the clots manually, suction out the blood, and use towels to absorb any blood spilling from the chest. If the site of injury is to the right of the heart and cannot be reached, extend the incision into the right side of the chest with a Gigli saw, Liebsche knife, sternal osteotome, or standard trauma shears. Before performing EDT it would be prudent to familiarize oneself with the instruments included in the EDT tray, but do not take the time for this during an actual case.

Pericardiotomy

In a patient in cardiac arrest, if there is no other obvious injury in the chest and the myocardium cannot be visualized, open the pericardium. *It may be difficult to definitively rule out pericardial tamponade by visual inspection alone. If in doubt, use forceps to elevate a portion of pericardium and carefully incise it to assess for hemopericardium.*

If you are confident that there is no pericardial tamponade, leave the pericardial sac closed while you address other life-threatening injuries. Opening the pericardium increases the risk for complications such as delay in the onset of cardiac compressions, damage to the myocardium or coronary vessels, or cutting of the left phrenic nerve. Previous pericardial disease may also have caused adhesions, and if you attempt to separate these adhesions rapidly, you can tear the atria or right ventricular wall. The incidence of traumatic rupture of the atria or the right ventricle during massage is greater when the pericardium is open. Furthermore, with an intact pericardium, pressure is distributed over a larger area and the

pericardial fluid seldom allows compressing fingers to remain in one spot for a prolonged period.

Perform pericardiotomy if tamponade is present or suspected. This procedure is performed *anterior and parallel to the left phrenic nerve* (Fig. 18-4, *step 6*). Begin the incision near the diaphragm to avoid injury to the coronary arteries. *Lift the pericardial sac with toothed forceps*, and use scissors to make a small hole. Extend the incision with scissors in a cephalad direction along the anterior aspect of the pericardium. Extend the incision so that it reaches from the apex of the heart to the root of the aorta. When the pericardium is under tension, it may be difficult to grasp the pericardium with forceps. In this case, use sharp, straight Mayo scissors to divide the pericardium by layers. If the heart is in arrest, speed is important, so use sharp scissors to "catch" the pericardium and start the pericardiotomy. To do this, hold the point of the scissors almost parallel to the surface of the heart and use enough pressure to create a wrinkle in the pericardium to puncture it as the scissors move forward. Apply moderate pressure to puncture the fibrous pericardium. Be cautious because if the point of the scissors is unnecessarily angled toward the heart, the sudden "give" that occurs when you open the pericardium may result in laceration of the myocardium. Remove clots of blood from the pericardial sac with a sweeping motion with your gloved hand, sterile lap sponges, or gauze pads. If cardiac repair or cardiac compressions are needed, deliver the heart from the pericardial sac. To do this, place your right hand through the pericardial incision and encircle the heart, pull it into the left side of the chest, and place the pericardial sac behind the heart.

Internal Cardiac Defibrillation

It is not uncommon to encounter cardiac dysrhythmias during EDT resuscitative efforts. Recommendations for internal defibrillation are the same as those for external defibrillation: ventricular fibrillation and tachycardia without pulses are immediate indications for defibrillation. With an chest open, internal defibrillation is the procedure of choice.

To perform internal defibrillation, place the *internal paddles* on the anterior and posterior aspects of the heart. The current is delivered through the circular tips of the paddles onto the surface of the heart. There is decreased electrical impedance with direct myocardial contact, and as a result less energy is needed than with standard defibrillation (typically 10 to 50 J). If internal paddles are not available, perform defibrillation in the usual manner with external paddles or electrodes.

Direct Cardiac Compressions

Three techniques for cardiac compression have been described: one-handed compression, one-handed sternal compression, and two-handed (bimanual) compression (Fig. 18-5). To perform the one-handed compression method, place your thumb over the left ventricle, the opposing fingers over the right ventricle, and your palm over the apex of the heart. To perform one-handed sternal compression, hold your fingers flat. Keep the fingers tightly together to form a flat surface over the left ventricle and compress the heart up against the sternum with your fingers. To perform two-handed compression, cup the left hand and place it over the right ventricle. Hold the fingers of the right hand tightly together to form a flat surface supporting the left ventricle. Push the flat surface of your right-hand fingers to compress the heart

Figure 18-5 Two-handed method of cardiac massage. Compress the ventricles toward the interventricular septum. Note how the hands flank the left anterior descending artery, which overlies the septum. Avoid using excessive fingertip pressure or lifting the heart, which slows ventricular filling by distorting the soft atrial-caval junction. *NG*, nasogastric.

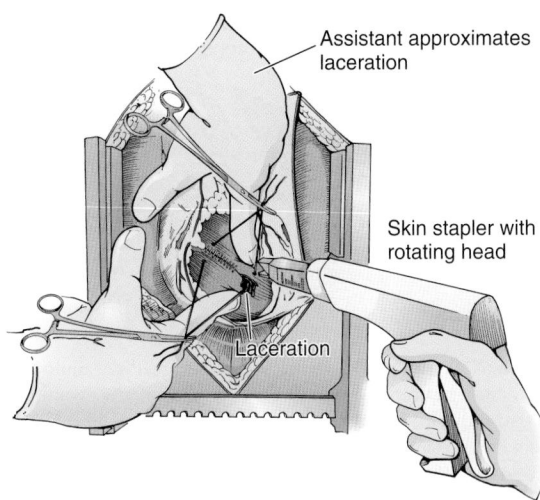

Figure 18-6 Technique of cardiac stapling to temporarily control hemorrhage. Ask an assistant to approximate the tissues with fingertip pressure, or as illustrated, use two half-horizontal sutures to approximate the wound edges and reduce bleeding. Use a skin stapler with wide (6-mm) staples and place them 5 mm apart. This technique may be used for atrial and ventricular lacerations. After stabilizing the patient's condition, revise the wound in the operating room.

against the cupped surface of the left hand. The bimanual technique has been shown to be consistently superior.[59]

A difference of opinion exists regarding the optimal rate at which the heart should be compressed. Some recommend a rate of 50 to 60 compressions/min; however, no physiologic data support such a recommendation. Recent American Heart Association guidelines for closed-chest CPR recommend a rate of at least 100 compressions/min.[47] It is conceivable that this would also apply to OCCM.

It is important to remember the following points while performing cardiac compression:

1. Use the entire palmar surface of the fingers. Avoid fingertip pressure.
2. For each method, adjust the force of compression so that it is perpendicular to the plane of the septum. The anterior descending coronary artery is located over the interventricular septum, so this is a helpful landmark to orient your hand properly.
3. Position your fingers so that the coronary arteries will not be occluded.
4. Venous filling of the heart is especially sensitive to changes in position. Maintain a relatively normal anatomic position of the heart to prevent kinking of the vena cava and pulmonary veins. Do not angle the heart more than 30 degrees into the left side of the chest.
5. It is essential to completely relax the heart between compressions to allow it to refill completely.

Control of Hemorrhagic Cardiac Wounds

To partially control active bleeding from a ventricular wound, place one finger over the wound and use the other hand to

stabilize the beating heart. This maneuver buys time while you begin to repair the injury and continue with resuscitation. If the heart is not beating, you may perform closure of the injury before resuscitation and defibrillation, although this is controversial. If you elect to repair the injury before attempting to restart the heart, perform intermittent cardiac massage. Surgical staples can be used to close a ventricular wound and are an extremely rapid method for controlling hemorrhage (Fig. 18-6).[60] This technique is particularly useful with large or multiple lacerations. Another advantage is that stapling does not expose the operator to the risk associated with needlestick. Macho and coworkers[61] reported a 93% success rate in temporarily controlling hemorrhage in 28 patients (33 lacerations) with penetrating injuries to both the atria and ventricles by using a standard skin stapler with wide (6-mm) staples placed at 5-mm intervals (Auto-Suture 35W, U.S. Surgical Corp., Norwalk, CT). The rotating long neck of the Ethicon Proximate Quantum Skin Stapler (Model PQW-35, Ethicon, Inc., Somerville, NJ) is helpful in obtaining proper orientation of the staples during placement. The staples can be left in place and reinforced or replaced on further exploration in the operating room.

Alternatively, repair the wound by placing several horizontal mattress sutures under the tamponading finger (Fig. 18-7). Polypropylene 2-0 or 3-0 monofilament (Prolene) suture is recommended for cardiac repair, but nonabsorbable silk can also be used. Avoid smaller sutures and nylon sutures. *If multiple sutures are needed, lay them all in place before they are tied.* This allows you to attain equal distribution of wound tension, which prevents tearing of the myocardium.[62] Alternatively, pass the suture underneath, over, and through Teflon pledgets to prevent the suture from cutting through the myocardium. Pledgets are especially important for reinforcement when the myocardium has been weakened by the blast effect of a bullet[63] or when suturing the thinner-walled atria or right ventricle. An alternative to Teflon pledgets is to use small rectangles of pericardial tissue cut from the opened pericardium.

Figure 18-7 Technique of cardiac suture repair. Place multiple horizontal mattress sutures 6 mm from the edge of the wound before tying. Close the wound just enough to stop the bleeding. Use Teflon pledgets on the cardiac surface, and pass all surface sutures through these reinforcements. Sutures come from underneath, lie over, then pass back through the pledgets. Closure without pledgets incurs the risk of sutures ripping through the contracting myocardium. Similarly, the use of simple vertical sutures should be discouraged because of the risk for suture dissection through the myocardium. For repairs near a coronary artery, take care to pass the suture under the artery. Note that rectangles of pericardial tissue may be substituted for ready-made Teflon pledgets.

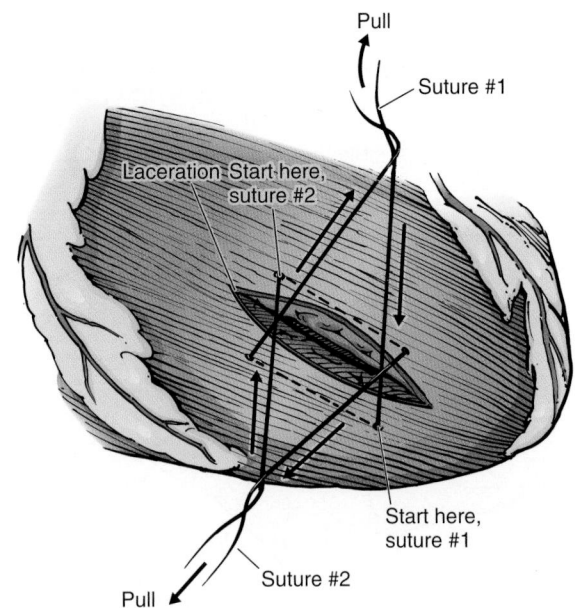

Figure 18-8 Control of hemorrhage with two widely placed incomplete mattress sutures. Ask an assistant to cross two half-horizontal sutures to bring the wound edges into apposition. By controlling the hemorrhage in this manner, the assistant's hands are outside the operative field and the edges of the wound are fully exposed. This facilitates more orderly closure of the wound. After the wound is repaired, the sutures may be either removed or tied to each other.

For large wounds that cannot be controlled with pressure, place an incomplete horizontal mattress suture on either side of the wound (Fig. 18-8). Cross the free ends to stop the bleeding. Then the actual reparative sutures can be placed accurately. It must be stressed that suturing the myocardium requires good technique. Excessive tension may tear the myocardium and aggravate the situation. Keys to success include using appropriately sized suture, obtaining a generous "bite" with the needle, and applying only enough tension to control the bleeding.

If exsanguinating hemorrhage is not controlled by the aforementioned methods, temporarily occlude inflow to the heart. Apply inflow occlusion intermittently for 60 to 90 seconds. During occlusion, the heart shrinks, hemorrhage is controlled, and you can place sutures in a decompressed injury. Two techniques that are useful are vascular clamping of the superior and inferior vena cava for partial inflow occlusion[64] and the Sauerbruch grip (Fig. 18-9).[65] The Sauerbruch grip can be performed quickly with the added advantage of cradling and stabilizing the heart while you repair the wounds over either the ventricle or the left atrium. It involves occlusion of the vena cava between the ring and middle fingers of the left hand to create partial occlusion of inflow. The Sauerbruch grip will interfere only with the repair of wounds involving the right atrium.

Another technique for temporarily controlling hemorrhage is to insert a Foley catheter (20 Fr with a 30-mL balloon) through a wound.[66] After inserting the catheter, inflate the balloon, clamp the catheter to prevent air embolism, and *apply gentle traction* (Fig. 18-10). Apply enough traction to slow the bleeding and provide an acceptable level to visualize and repair the wound. Excessive traction can pull the catheter out and enlarge the wound. The balloon will effectively occlude the wound internally. A purse-string suture is then used to close the wound. When repairing the wound, be careful with the suture needle because it can easily rupture the balloon. Temporarily pushing the balloon into the

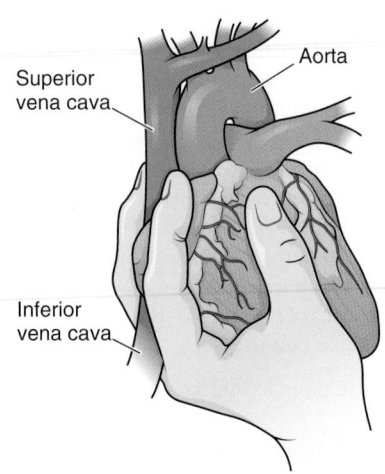

Figure 18-9 The Sauerbruch maneuver is the method of choice for reducing heavy bleeding from cardiac wounds. Occlusion of venous inflow is achieved by using the first and second or second and third fingers as a clamp.

ventricular lumen during passage of the needle can be done to avoid this complication. Use normal saline when inflating the balloon because using air could result in air embolism if the suture needle ruptures the balloon.

Foley catheters have several advantages over other methods for controlling cardiac wounds. With the digital method, your fingertip will often slip if there is a strong heartbeat, you cannot visualize the wound during repair, and digital pressure significantly interferes with cardiac massage. Intermittent total venous inflow occlusion is an effective method of controlling bleeding and decompressing the heart, but such

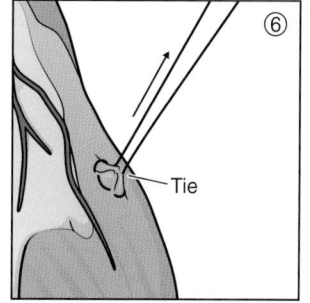

A

Figure 18-10 A, Serial illustration. Gentle traction on an inflated Foley catheter may control hemorrhage and allow repair. Inflate the balloon with saline while taking care to not rupture the balloon with the suture needle. This technique is particularly useful for injuries to the inferior cavoatrial junction, for posterior wounds, and during cardiac massage. Volume loading can be achieved by infusion of blood or crystalloid solution through the lumen of the catheter. Take care to avoid an air embolus through the lumen of the catheter during placement. **B,** Foley catheter in an atrial stab wound. Keep gentle traction on an inflated balloon and *inject saline directly into the heart via the catheter. Note how difficult it is to identify structures in the chest cavity.* The heart is collapsed and not beating, which makes even this organ hard to find. The aorta could not be isolated before stopping resuscitation efforts.

B

control will be at the expense of poor cardiac output. Attempting to elevate the heart for control and repair of posterior cardiac wounds often results in cardiac arrest by reducing both venous and arterial flow. With posterior injuries, use of a Foley catheter does not require continued viewing after initial placement. If bleeding can be controlled, repairs in this location should await full-volume expansion or cardiopulmonary bypass.[67] Regardless of location, the most valuable feature of the Foley catheter is that you can control hemorrhage without interfering with cardiac compression. Also, the catheter can be used for infusion of fluids (Fig. 18-10*B*).[68]

To initially manage wounds of the atria, use partial-occlusion clamps (Fig. 18-11). Because of the thin structure and instability of the atrial wall, you will not be able to effectively stop bleeding with digital pressure. Injuries near the caval-atrial junction are not amenable to clamping; in this location, use a Foley catheter to tamponade the wound.[66] Be careful to not obstruct atrial filling with the inflated balloon. Skin staples may also be used for closure of atrial wounds.[61]

Wounds of the septa, valves, and coronary arteries require definitive repair in the operating suite. Hemorrhage from a

Figure 18-11 Use a partial-occlusion clamp in different locations for control of bleeding and subsequent repair.

Figure 18-12 Cross-clamping for control of subclavian bleeding is difficult and time-consuming. Compression with laparotomy pads in the apical pleura from below and the supraclavicular fossa from above will control hemorrhage while the patient's condition is stabilized and the patient is transported to the operating room. *NG*, nasogastric.

Figure 18-13 Manual cardiac massage and cross-clamping of the aorta can be used to increase coronary and cerebral perfusion selectively. *IVC*, inferior vena cava.

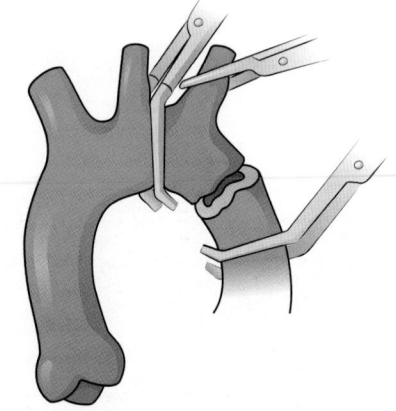

Figure 18-14 Traumatic rupture of the aorta is *usually a fatal injury*. Three clamps are required for control. Backbleeding will occur if fewer than three clamps are used.

coronary artery can generally be controlled with digital pressure. Avoid ligation of a coronary artery whenever possible.

Control of Hemorrhagic Great-Vessel Wounds

Wounds of the great vessels can be controlled with digital pressure or partial-occlusion clamps. If desired, close small aortic wounds with 3-0 Prolene suture.[69] To prevent exsanguinating hemorrhage from the left subclavian artery, try to cross-clamp the intrathoracic portion of the artery. Cross-clamping of the right subclavian artery is very difficult. For injuries to this vessel, use laparotomy pads for compression in the apex of the pleura from below and the supraclavicular fossa from above (Fig. 18-12) to prevent further bleeding as the patient is stabilized and moved to the operating suite.[60]

Aortic Cross-Clamping

For persistent hypotension (systolic blood pressure <70 mm Hg) after thoracotomy and pericardiotomy, perform temporary occlusion of the descending thoracic aorta. This maneuver can maintain myocardial and cerebral perfusion (Fig. 18-13; also see Fig. 18-4, *step* 7), although Kravolich and colleagues[46] suggested that the benefit of significant improvement in CPP may be overstated. When the aorta has been injured by blunt trauma, selective clamping is necessary (Fig. 18-14). Aortic occlusion has a limited role in controlling hemorrhage below the diaphragm. In patients with a tense

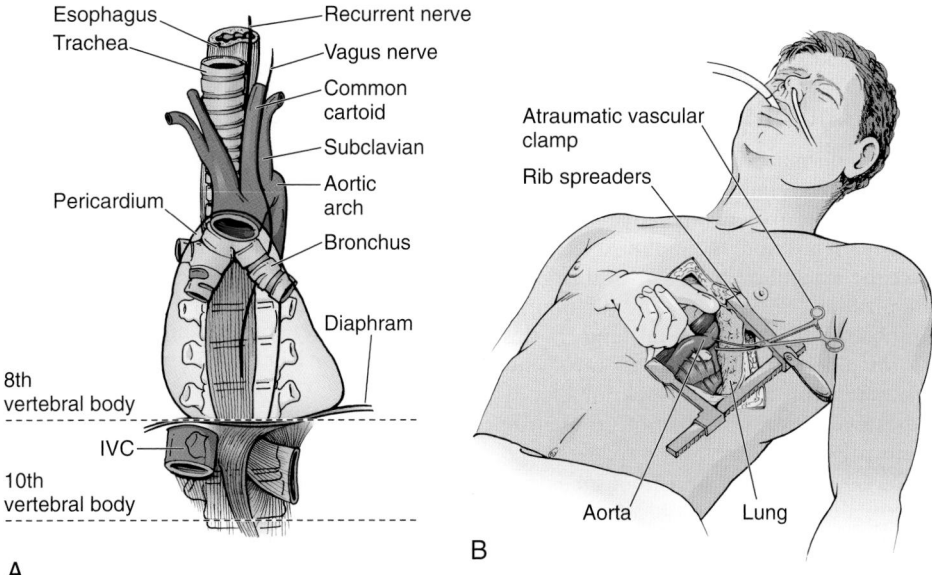

Esophagus
Trachea
Recurrent nerve
Vagus nerve
Common cartoid
Subclavian
Aortic arch
Pericardium
Bronchus
Diaphram
8th vertebral body
IVC
10th vertebral body
A

Atraumatic vascular clamp
Rib spreaders
Aorta
Lung
B

Figure 18-15 A, *Identification of the aorta is very difficult during emergency department thoracotomy.* If possible, first pass a nasogastric tube to help identify the esophagus. The aorta is in the posterior mediastinum, directly anterior to the vertebral bodies. The esophagus is anterior and slightly medial to the aorta. In the lower part of the thorax, both are covered on the anterolateral surface by the mediastinal pleura, which must be dissected before isolating the aorta for cross-clamping. **B,** Aortic cross-clamping. Using blunt dissection, spread the pleura above and below the aorta. Fully mobilize the vessel and clearly separate the esophagus before clamping. The aorta is the more posterior structure and is in contact with the vertebral bodies.

abdomen and massive hemoperitoneum, aortic cross-clamping is beneficial when applied just before laparotomy.[23]

The aorta can be very difficult to identify in an ED, especially when collapsed as a result of exsanguination. It is situated immediately anterior to the vertebrae and actually lies on the vertebral bodies themselves. The esophagus lies anterior and slightly medial to the aorta. Passing a nasogastric tube from above may help in identifying the esophagus. To expose the descending aorta, ask an assistant to retract the left lung in a superomedial direction. To achieve adequate exposure it is sometimes necessary to divide the inferior pulmonary ligament (be careful to not injure the inferior pulmonary vein). Identify the aorta by advancing the fingers of the left hand along the thoracic cage toward the vertebral column. Open the mediastinal pleura and bluntly dissect the aorta away from the esophagus anteriorly and the prevertebral fascia posteriorly before clamping. To locate the aorta, use a DeBakey aortic clamp or a curved Kelly clamp for blunt dissection and spread the pleura open above and below the aorta (Fig. 18-15). Alternatively, if excessive hemorrhage limits direct visualization, bluntly dissect with the thumb and fingertips. Separate the aorta from the esophagus, which lies medially and slightly anteriorly. It may be difficult to separate the esophagus from the aorta by feel in a hypotensive or cardiac arrest situation. When the aorta is completely isolated, use the index finger of the left hand to flex around the vessel and apply a large Satinsky or DeBakey vascular clamp with the right hand. Check brachial blood pressure immediately after the occlusion. If systolic pressure is higher than 120 mm Hg, slowly release the clamp and adjust it to maintain a systolic pressure of less than 120 mm Hg.[22]

Given the need for timely intervention, the simplest and most desirable approach to aortic occlusion is to have an assistant digitally compress it or use the aortic tamponade instrument (Fig. 18-16). The aortic tamponade instrument,

Figure 18-16 Use of a Conn aortic compressor is an excellent method for aortic occlusion because it is fast, does not interfere with the operative field, and is associated with minimal risk for injury. Alternatively, direct digital occlusion can be used, but this technique is more awkward.

however, may be applied blindly to the vertebral column and permits safe, quick, and complete aortic occlusion.[70] This technique may be most prudent when isolation of the aorta is difficult. The instrument's unique shape allows it to remain in place and to provide atraumatic occlusion with little interference in the operative field when compared with digital compression. The degree of occlusion can be varied by the amount of pressure exerted by the operator.

Potential complications of aortic cross-clamping include ischemia of the spinal cord, liver, bowel, and kidneys. In addition, iatrogenic injury to the aorta and the esophagus may occur. Fortunately, these complications are infrequent. The metabolic penalty of aortic cross-clamping becomes exponential when occlusion time exceeds 30 minutes.[71] Whenever possible, unclamp the aorta for 30 to 60 seconds every 10 minutes to increase distal perfusion. Perform final release of the aorta gradually.

Management of Air Embolism

In those at risk for air embolism, spontaneous ventilation is preferred. It is essential that the source of the air embolism be controlled rapidly. Place the patient immediately in the Trendelenburg (head-down) position to minimize cerebral involvement and direct the air emboli to less critical organs. If the chest injury is unilateral, consider isolating the injured lung by selectively intubating the contralateral lung. If this is unsuccessful, perform a left anterolateral thoracotomy. *Flood the exposed thorax with sterile saline* and look for bloody froth created during positive pressure ventilation to identify peripheral bronchovenous fistulas. Carry out a quick search for hilar injuries. If the source of the air embolism is not readily apparent, perform a contralateral thoracotomy. Once the bronchovenous communication is controlled, use a needle to aspirate the residual air that commonly remains in the left ventricle and the aorta. If the patient is hypotensive, consider cross-clamping the aorta. Be aware, though, that cross-clamping the aorta before controlling bronchovenous fistulas and removing residual air may result in further dissemination of air to the heart and brain.

Air emboli traverse capillary beds if the blood pressure is high enough. After controlling the bronchovenous fistula, produce a brief period of proximal aortic hypertension by cross-clamping the descending aorta. Maintain systemic arterial pressure with adequate fluid resuscitation. Vasopressors such as dopamine, epinephrine, or norepinephrine may be required to increase systemic pressure and facilitate the passage of air bubbles from left to right.[72]

Maintain left atrial pressure at a high level. Keep the ventilator inspiratory pressure as low as possible, and use 100% oxygen to facilitate diffusion of nitrogen from emboli. Consider high-frequency ventilation, which allows the use of small volumes and has been used successfully in individual patients. The most important adjunctive therapy is hyperbaric oxygen. Although it is best to begin treatment within 6 hours of the traumatic insult, there are cases of success and improvement when hyperbaric oxygen has been started even 36 hours after injury.[73]

INTERPRETATION AND HEMODYNAMIC MONITORING

Use systolic blood pressure after the first 30 minutes of resuscitation as a decision point for further treatment. A report of EDT for blunt and penetrating trauma demonstrated a relationship between blood pressure at 30 minutes and the eventual outcome.[74] Of the 146 cases reviewed, 45 patients (31%) were transferred to the operating room after initial resuscitation and aortic cross-clamping when necessary. For patients who survived with full neurologic recovery, the average systolic blood pressure after the first 30 minutes of resuscitation was 110 mm Hg. In those who were long-term survivors but had significant brain damage, the average systolic blood pressure was 85 mm Hg. No survivals were recorded when mean systolic blood pressure was lower than 70 mm Hg. *Transfer of these patients to the operating room for definitive repair of these mortal wounds would be futile.*

EDT IN CHILDREN

Trauma is the leading cause of death and morbidity in children older than 1 year.[1] Just as in adults, improved transportation of injured children to the hospital has resulted in the survival of more patients who would have been pronounced dead at the scene. Although the role of EDT has been reviewed extensively in the adult population, experience and data in the pediatric population are limited. Overall survival rates in children undergoing EDT for penetrating thoracic trauma are approximately 11% to 12% and, for blunt trauma, 1% to 2%.[4] General consensus from the practice management guidelines for EDT is to use the same parameters as used for adults.[4]

COMPLICATIONS

A variety of significant complications occur in patients surviving EDT, but most of them are related to the primary injury rather than the thoracotomy. Techniques to avoid iatrogenic complications include noting the position of the left phrenic nerve and coronary arteries during EDT. Surprisingly, serious infections are uncommon. Patients receiving antibiotics during or immediately after the procedure have a low rate of infectious complications. Standard antibiotic regimens targeting skin flora are recommended but should not delay the procedure.[75] As a general rule, excessive attention to antiseptic skin preparation should be avoided because it may delay performance of the procedure.[76]

Another potentially serious complication of EDT is injury or transmission of disease to health care workers. In an emotionally charged environment in which many clinicians are attempting to perform a lifesaving procedure under difficult conditions, it is easy for a needle, scalpel, or scissors to cause injury. Sharp ribs can cut clinicians quite easily (Fig. 18-17). The seroprevalence of human immunodeficiency virus (HIV)

Figure 18-17 Note the sharp edges of this rib (indicated by the circled clamp), which was fractured during unsuccessful emergency department thoracotomy. The incidence of blood-borne diseases (e.g., human immunodeficiency virus, hepatitis) in trauma patients may be high and transmission to a health care worker may occur if sharp bone fragments puncture the gloves and skin.

in U.S. EDs is estimated to range from 2% to 6% or 9% in urban areas.[77] Tardiff and colleagues[77] noted an HIV-positive rate of 7.2% in a study of trauma patients taken to their urban ED. Occupational exposure to both hepatitis B and hepatitis C virus is of concern to health care workers as well. Sloan and associates[78] found a 3.1% incidence of hepatitis B in trauma patients brought to their inner-city ED. Hepatitis C is now the most common viral hepatitis seen in health care workers since advent of the hepatitis B vaccine. Approximately 2200 health care workers per year seroconvert after occupational exposure. The risk for seroconversion after occupational exposure to HIV is estimated to be 0.3% for needlestick and as high as 4.5% for deep injury.[79] Hepatitis C seroconversion rates after occupational exposure are estimated to be between 1.8% and 10%.[79] Keep the risk for exposure to staff in mind, and rigorously follow universal precautions. Although EDT must be performed rapidly to be of value to the patient, excessive haste is not warranted if it threatens the health of members of the medical team.

Acknowledgment

The editors and authors wish to acknowledge the contributions of Robert L. Bartlett, MD, and Michael E. Boczar, MD, to this chapter in previous editions.

References are available at www.expertconsult.com

Vascular Techniques and Volume Support

CHAPTER 19

Pediatric Vascular Access and Blood Sampling Techniques

Genevieve Santillanes and Ilene Claudius

Obtaining vascular access and blood samples in an infant or child can challenge and frustrate even the most skilled emergency clinician. Vascular access can be especially challenging in children who are dehydrated or in shock. This chapter reviews the basic principles and techniques of blood sampling, as well as placement of peripheral and central intravenous (IV) and intraarterial catheters in infants and children, including the use of umbilical catheters in newborns. Also reviewed are hydration techniques for dehydrated children. For critically ill and injured children, intraosseous (IO) access is the preferred technique if peripheral vascular access cannot be secured rapidly (see Chapter 25). Though rarely required, emergency cutdown is occasionally lifesaving, and a section of this chapter is devoted to cutdown techniques.

PATIENT PREPARATION AND RESTRAINT

Fear and anticipation of pain associated with procedures or injections make the hospital experience traumatic for children. Before beginning any painful procedure in a child, explain the procedure to the parents, as well as the reasons that it needs to be done. For children capable of understanding, explain the procedure in developmentally appropriate language before starting and before each successive step. Avoid using deceptive phrases such as "this won't hurt." A gentle, honest explanation that the procedure will hurt a bit and a statement such as "it is okay to cry, but not to move" will provide realistic expectations for the child and set limits as well. Depending on the situation, most parents wish to remain with their child during the procedure.[1] Others will not. The potential for parents to faint at the sight of blood or needles should always be addressed, and it is preferable that they sit down during the procedure. If present, the parent's

role should be to provide comfort to the child but not to assist in any potentially painful procedure. If possible, distract the child with simple conversation regarding school, friends, hobbies, pets, or TV shows to help decrease the child's anxiety.

The success of blood sampling or obtaining vascular access depends on proper positioning and restraint of the patient. In most cases, this requires the assistance of at least one other staff person and restraint of the extremity a joint above and below the intended insertion site. A significant amount of time may be required to perform venipuncture or vessel cannulation in neonates or young infants. Consequently, they may become hypothermic if disrobed and exposed for a prolonged period, especially if perfusion is compromised because of sepsis or hypovolemic shock. Use overhead lights, warm blankets, or other warming modalities to prevent accidental hypothermia in vulnerable patients.

Anesthesia

Many products are available to decrease the pain associated with vascular access. Do not delay attempts at access in critically ill or injured children to use these medications or devices, but consider using them in stable patients. These medications and products are discussed in more detail in Chapter 29. Options include vapocoolants, topical anesthetics such as lidocaine-prilocaine (EMLA), 4% liposomal lidocaine (LMX-4), and injection of lidocaine via a needleless jet injector (J-tip). Orally administered sucrose solution (Sweet-Ease) has been demonstrated to decrease the pain response in young infants during procedures.[2,3] Procedural sedation is commonly used during central venous and arterial cannulation in children (Chapter 33).

BLOOD SAMPLING TECHNIQUES
Capillary Blood Sampling
Indications and Contraindications

Capillary blood sampling is frequently used to obtain blood samples from young infants. In infants, the heel is the most common location for capillary blood sampling, whereas in older children and adults, blood samples are more commonly obtained from the finger, toe, or earlobe. This technique is useful when repeated measurements such as blood glucose or serial hemoglobin are needed. It is also an option for obtaining "arterialized" blood for blood gas analysis when arterial access is unavailable, such as in chronically ill neonates and young infants or when the clinician is not comfortable obtaining a percutaneous arterial blood sample. If a sufficient volume is obtained, blood from a capillary sample can also be sent for other routine laboratory studies. Do not send this type of specimen for blood culture because of the risk for contamination. Heel sticks are more painful than venipuncture but are useful in the event of difficult access or when arterialized samples are needed.[4]

Avoid sampling from an area of local inflammation or hematoma. Avoid repetitive sampling from the same site because it may induce inflammation and subsequent scarring. In general, heel stick sampling is not ideal for blood gas analysis when the infant is hypotensive, the heel is markedly bruised, or there is evidence of peripheral vasoconstriction.

Equipment and Setup (Box 19-1)
Use a 3-mm lancet (Becton-Dickinson, Rutherford, NJ) or an automated disposable incision device (e.g., Tenderfoot, Surgicutt) to perform this procedure. Perform blood collection with either heparinized capillary tubes or 1-mL Microtainer tubes with a collector attachment (Becton-Dickinson, Rutherford, NJ).

Technique
The heel stick method of capillary blood sampling will be described, but capillary blood samples can also be obtained from a finger, toe, or earlobe (Fig. 19-1). To avoid penetration of the calcaneus and the risk for osteochondritis, puncture only the most medial and lateral portions of the plantar surface of the heel.[5] Some research suggests that when using automated lancets, any site on the heel can be safely punctured in a term neonate.[6] Prewarm the foot for 5 minutes to produce hyperemia and enhance blood flow. Immobilize the foot in a dependent position with one hand. First cleanse the heel with antiseptic solution and allow it to dry. Next, puncture the skin with the lancet. Allow the alcohol to dry to avoid false elevations in the glucose level. Avoid squeezing the foot because it may inhibit capillary filling and actually decrease the flow of blood. Furthermore, squeezing may lead to hemolysis and make analysis less accurate. If blood does not flow freely, another puncture may be required.

Wipe away the first small drop of blood with gauze and allow a second drop to form. Place a heparinized capillary tube in the drop of blood and invert the proximal end of the tube to allow it to fill by capillary action. Fill the capillary tube until blood reaches the demarcation line on the tube. Overfilling or underfilling may result in clotting or erroneous test results. If 1-mL Microtainer tubes are used, hold the tube at an angle of 30 to 45 degrees from the surface of the puncture site. Touch the collector end of the tube to the drop of blood and allow the blood to drain into

the tube. Gently tap the tube to facilitate flow to the bottom. Once filled, seal the tube with the accompanying cap. After an adequate specimen is obtained, apply a dry dressing to the puncture site.

When a heel stick is performed for an arterialized blood sample, use a technique that is similar to that discussed previously for routine blood sampling, with the following differences. Wrap the infant's foot in a warm towel for a few minutes and discard the first drop of blood while allowing the remaining blood to flow freely into a heparinized capillary tube. Place the tip of the tube as near the puncture site as possible to minimize exposure of the blood to environmental oxygen. Fill the tube as completely as possible. Avoid collecting air in the tube and excessive squeezing of the foot because this may artificially lower Po_2. When the tube is full, occlude the free end with the gloved finger to prevent the entry of air, and cap both ends.

Complications
When performed properly, heel sticks are associated with a low incidence of complications. Use a proper incision device to prevent lacerations. Rare complications include infection, scarring, and calcified nodules.[7]

Interpretation
Multiple studies have demonstrated a good correlation between arterial and capillary specimens for determining pH and Pco_2 in hemodynamically stable patients.[8,9] However, determination of Po_2 is not reliable when performed on blood obtained by capillary sampling.

Venipuncture
Indications and Contraindications
Although many laboratory tests for small infants may be performed on blood obtained by heel stick, larger volumes of blood may be required, which makes heel sticks impractical. Use venipuncture to obtain larger quantities of blood from infants and children and to obtain blood for culture. When collecting blood for culture, prepare the area of venipuncture with an appropriate antiseptic solution and allow the skin to dry. The blood culture collection bottle will probably indicate a desired volume of sample for optimal results, but 1 mL of blood is generally acceptable for a small infant. Wash off the cleanser promptly after blood has been collected because iodine solutions and other detergents can irritate infant skin.

Equipment and Setup (Box 19-2)
A small-gauge butterfly needle and syringe are usually preferred over a needle and syringe for obtaining blood from infants and young children. It is easier to control the

---

BOX 19-1 Equipment for Capillary Blood Sampling

Warm wet towel or diaper
Alcohol pads
Lancets or automated disposable incision devices
Blood collection tubes (capillary tubes or Microtainers)
Clay sealer (if using capillary tubes without accompanying caps)

BOX 19-2 Equipment for Venous Blood Sampling in Infants and Children

Alcohol pads (or povidone-iodine swabs if blood cultures are needed)
Tourniquet (rubber band for scalp veins and small infants)
21- or 23-gauge butterfly needle
3-, 5-, or 10-mL syringe
Evacuated blood tubes

CAPILLARY BLOOD SAMPLING

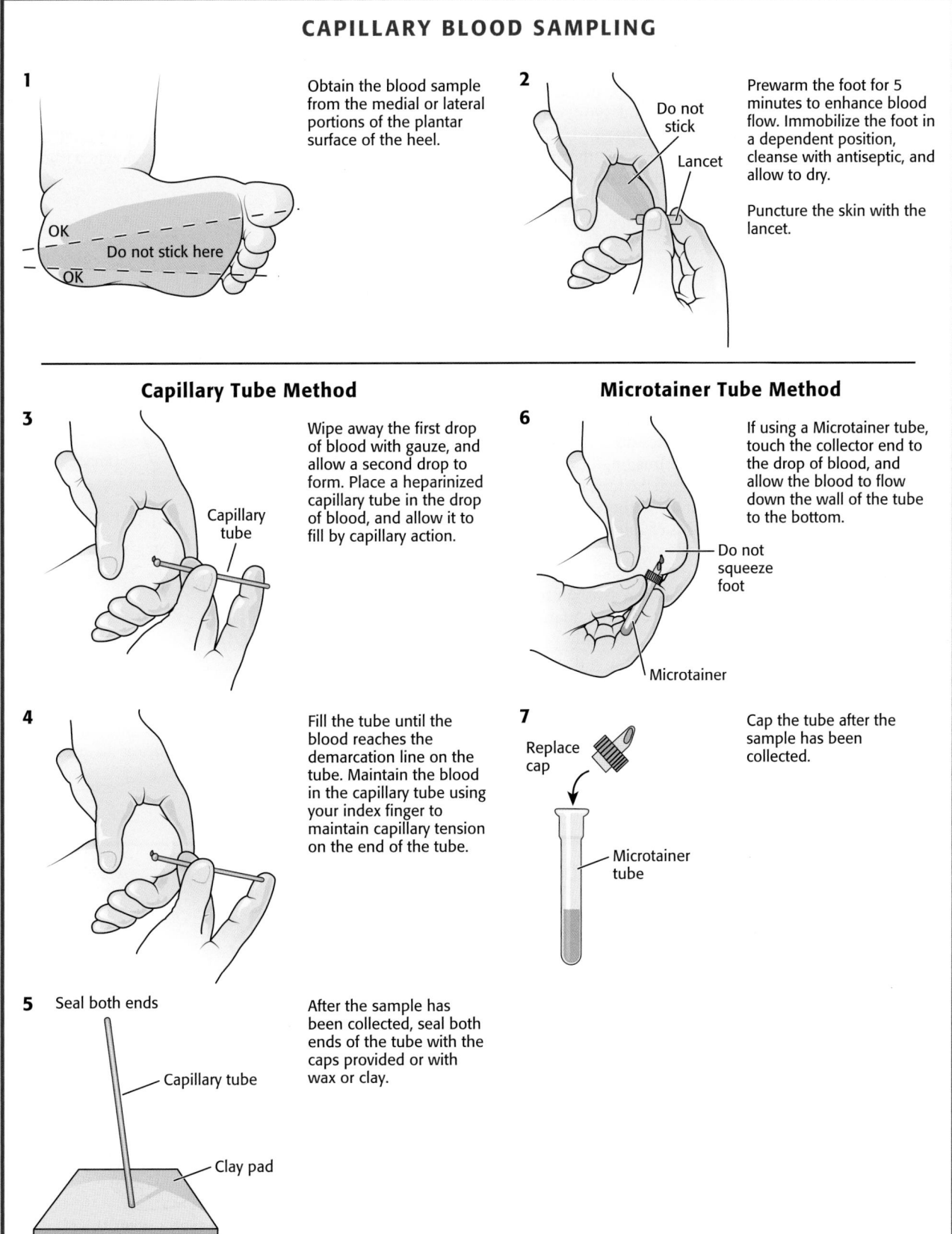

1 Obtain the blood sample from the medial or lateral portions of the plantar surface of the heel.

OK
Do not stick here
OK

2 Prewarm the foot for 5 minutes to enhance blood flow. Immobilize the foot in a dependent position, cleanse with antiseptic, and allow to dry.

Puncture the skin with the lancet.

Do not stick
Lancet

Capillary Tube Method

3 Wipe away the first drop of blood with gauze, and allow a second drop to form. Place a heparinized capillary tube in the drop of blood, and allow it to fill by capillary action.

Capillary tube

4 Fill the tube until the blood reaches the demarcation line on the tube. Maintain the blood in the capillary tube using your index finger to maintain capillary tension on the end of the tube.

5 Seal both ends

Capillary tube

Clay pad

After the sample has been collected, seal both ends of the tube with the caps provided or with wax or clay.

Microtainer Tube Method

6 If using a Microtainer tube, touch the collector end to the drop of blood, and allow the blood to flow down the wall of the tube to the bottom.

Do not squeeze foot

Microtainer

7 Replace cap

Microtainer tube

Cap the tube after the sample has been collected.

Figure 19-1 Capillary blood sampling: capillary tube and Microtainer tube methods.

position and to suction with a butterfly needle and syringe. If other access is not available, the butterfly needle may also serve as an infusion line after an adequate amount of blood is obtained. A 23-gauge butterfly needle will generally suffice for venipuncture, regardless of the age group. In older children and adolescents, a straight needle and syringe or the Vacutainer system (Becton-Dickinson, Rutherford, NJ) can be used more easily than in infants. However, the negative pressure within the evacuated blood tube may be sufficient to collapse the punctured vein. Use a 3- or 5-mL syringe because it is less likely than a 10-mL syringe to cause vein collapse in small children.

Technique

As in adults, the usual site for venipuncture in infants and children is the antecubital fossa. However, any reasonably accessible or easily visible peripheral vein may be used, such as those on the hands, feet, or scalp for very small infants (Fig. 19-2). Veins on the dorsum of the hand can be used, provided that they will not be needed for IV cannulation. The external jugular and femoral veins or arterial sites are rarely needed for routine samples in a stable patient. Imaging devices (e.g., ultrasound, transillumination, or infrared devices) may also be used to locate and identify veins for IV catheter placement. These devices are discussed later in this chapter (see "Vascular Line Placement: Venous and Arterial").

Assemble all necessary equipment and make sure that everything is ready for immediate use. Ask an assistant to help immobilize the patient when drawing blood from infants and small children. Assemble the equipment, especially needles, out of sight of the child. If an extremity vein is to be used, apply a tourniquet proximal to the selected vein. In small infants, a rubber band can be used as a tourniquet. Be sure that the tourniquet is not so tight that it impedes arterial filling. It is absolutely essential that the tourniquet be removed after the procedure.

Cleanse the area surrounding the chosen site of skin penetration with antiseptic solution and allow it to dry. Apply slight distal traction to the skin to immobilize the vein. Insert the needle quickly through the skin and advance it slowly into the vein at an angle of approximately 30 degrees with the bevel facing up (Fig. 19-3, *step 1*). Successful vessel penetration is heralded by a flashback, or flow, of blood into the butterfly tubing. Apply gentle suction by slowly withdrawing

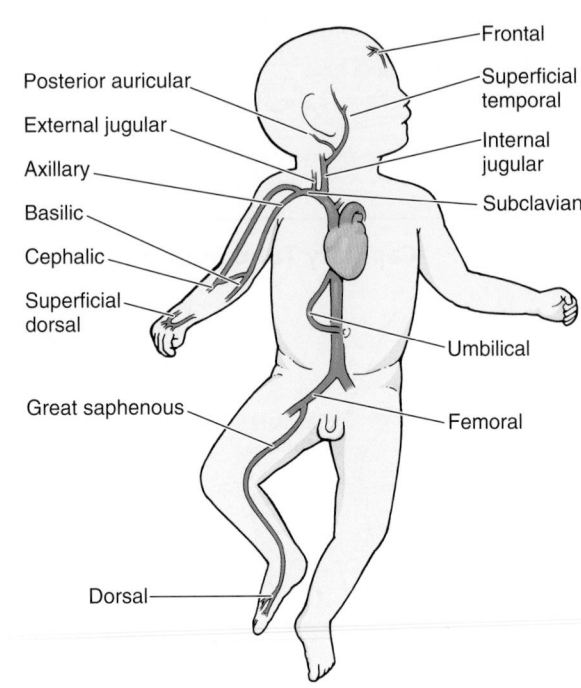

Figure 19-2 Venous access sites in neonates and young infants. If venous access is unavailable, arterial blood may be used for most laboratory tests, including blood cultures.

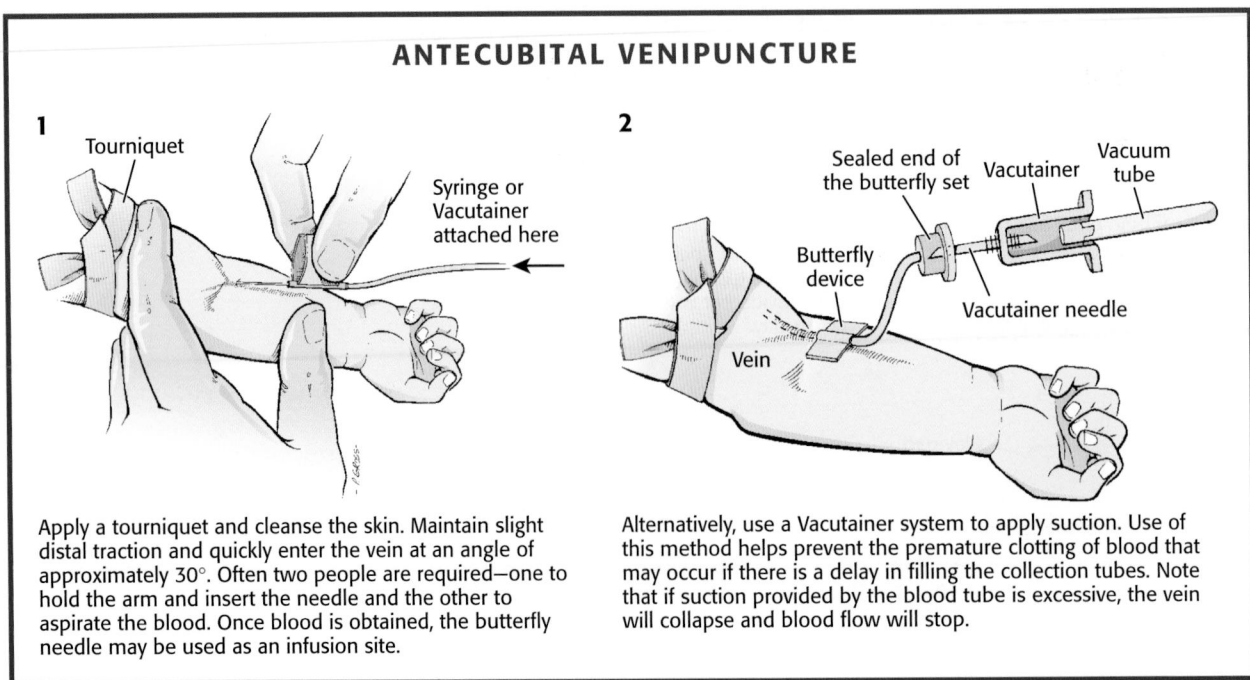

ANTECUBITAL VENIPUNCTURE

Apply a tourniquet and cleanse the skin. Maintain slight distal traction and quickly enter the vein at an angle of approximately 30°. Often two people are required—one to hold the arm and insert the needle and the other to aspirate the blood. Once blood is obtained, the butterfly needle may be used as an infusion site.

Alternatively, use a Vacutainer system to apply suction. Use of this method helps prevent the premature clotting of blood that may occur if there is a delay in filling the collection tubes. Note that if suction provided by the blood tube is excessive, the vein will collapse and blood flow will stop.

Figure 19-3 Antecubital venipuncture.

the plunger of the syringe. If the required amount of blood is greater than the capacity of the attached syringe, pinch off the tubing, remove the filled syringe, attach a new syringe, and apply gentle suction again after releasing the pinched tubing. After the required amount of blood is withdrawn, remove the needle and apply a sterile dressing and direct pressure to the puncture site.

Apply suction with a Vacutainer system in which the needle punctures the sealed end of the butterfly device (see Fig. 19-3, *step 2*). There are also butterfly systems available with a second needle that is occluded by a rubber shield located at the opposite end of the butterfly tubing. Once the vein has been entered, the needle at the opposite end of the butterfly tubing is pushed through the top of the vacuum-sealed tube. In either case, if the suction is excessive, the vein will collapse and blood flow will stop.

Although peripheral sites for venous blood sampling are preferable in infants, the external jugular and femoral veins may also be used for venipuncture during resuscitation or when peripheral sites are inadequate. The external jugular vein lies in a line from the angle of the jaw to the middle of the clavicle and is usually visible on the surface of the skin (Fig. 19-4). When the infant is crying, this vein is more prominent. Ask an assistant to restrain the infant in a supine position with the head and neck extended over the edge of the bed. Alternatively, place a towel roll or pillow under the child's shoulders. Turn the head approximately 40 to 70 degrees from the midline. Cleanse the skin surrounding the area to be punctured with alcohol or another antiseptic solution. Apply finger pressure just above the clavicle to help distend the jugular vein. Use a 21- to 25-gauge straight needle or a 21- to 25-gauge butterfly needle attached to a syringe. Puncture the skin and then advance the needle slowly until the jugular vein is entered and a flashback of blood is observed. Keep the syringe connected to the needle at all times to maintain constant negative pressure and avoid air embolism. After the appropriate amount of blood is obtained, withdraw the needle and apply slight pressure to the vessel. Place the infant in an upright position after the needle is removed, and hold pressure over the puncture site for 3 to 5 minutes. Observe the puncture site closely afterward to identify persistent bleeding.

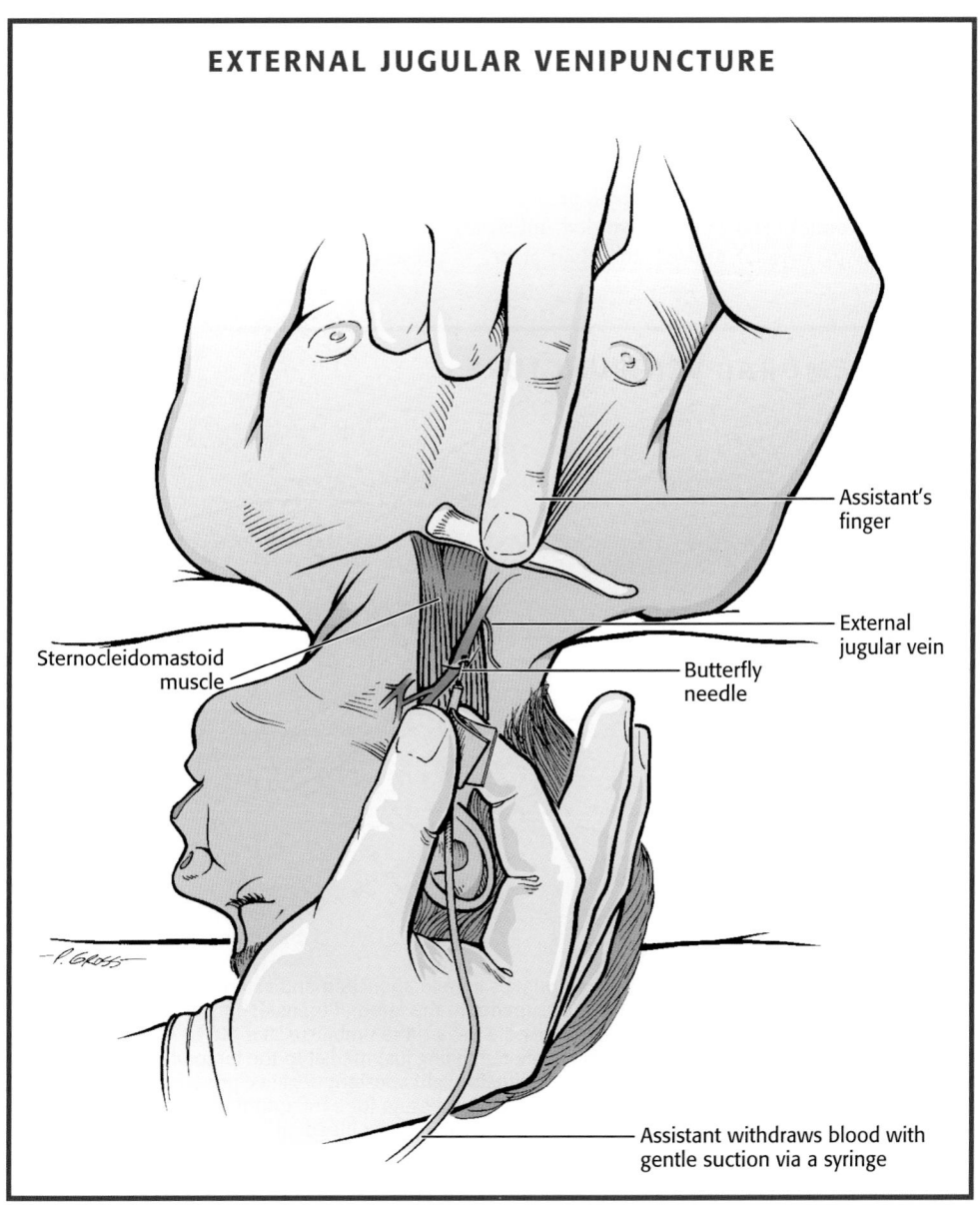

EXTERNAL JUGULAR VENIPUNCTURE

Assistant's finger

External jugular vein

Butterfly needle

Sternocleidomastoid muscle

Assistant withdraws blood with gentle suction via a syringe

Figure 19-4 External jugular venipuncture. A syringe or a butterfly needle may be used. Venous distention is aided when an assistant's finger occludes the vein or when the infant cries. The neck is extended, either over the side of the bed or by placing a rolled towel under the shoulders. This procedure requires two people.

In most patients, the femoral vein lies medial to the femoral artery and inferior to the inguinal ligament (Fig. 19-5*A*). Ask an assistant to position the patient's hips in mild abduction and extension while you palpate the artery. Identify its location by placing a mark on the skin just superior to the femoral triangle. If available, use ultrasound to assess the position of the femoral vessels. Prepare the femoral triangle with alcohol or another antiseptic agent. Use a povidone-iodine or chlorhexidine scrub when obtaining blood for culture. Use a technique of needle insertion that is similar to that for external jugular venipuncture (see Fig. 19-4). Puncture the skin and then direct the needle or catheter toward the umbilicus at a 30- to 45-degree angle to the skin and just medial to the pulsation of the femoral artery (see Fig. 19-5*B*). Apply slight negative pressure constantly throughout insertion. After the needle enters the femoral vein, withdraw the desired blood samples. Afterward, remove the needle or catheter unless an IV catheter for venous access is desired in this location. Apply pressure over the puncture site in the femoral triangle for a minimum of 5 minutes. Observe closely for recurrent bleeding.

Scalp veins can be very useful for venous sampling in small infants when other options are not possible or readily available.[10] The anatomic considerations and technique are discussed later (see "Peripheral Venous Catheterization: Percutaneous" and "Peripheral Venous Catheterization: Venous Cutdown").

Complications
Complications of venipuncture include hematoma formation, local infection, injury to adjacent structures (e.g., vessels), and phlebitis. These complications are all uncommon. Use special care when attempting to puncture the external jugular or femoral vein. Inadvertent deep puncture in the neck can injure the carotid artery, the vagus nerve, the phrenic nerve, or the apex of the lung. The femoral artery or nerve can be injured during puncture of the area around the femoral triangle. Fortunately, these injuries are unlikely when proper technique is used.

Arterial Blood Sampling

Indications and Contraindications
Arterial blood gas analysis provides useful and important information for evaluating the respiratory status and acid-base equilibrium in infants or children with respiratory distress or metabolic derangements. Use arterial blood for routine laboratory analysis or blood culture if venous blood is difficult to obtain. Potential sites for arterial blood sampling include the radial, brachial, dorsalis pedis, posterior tibial, and, in newborn infants, the umbilical arteries.

The radial artery has several advantages that make it the most commonly used artery for blood sampling. First, its location makes it easy to palpate and puncture (Fig. 19-6*A*). The ulnar artery is more difficult to locate. Second, no vein or nerve is immediately adjacent to the radial artery, which minimizes the risk of obtaining venous blood or damaging a nerve. Another advantage of the radial artery is the presence of good collateral circulation from the ulnar artery. The brachial artery has little collateral circulation and should be avoided unless no other options are available.[11] Limit use of the ulnar artery to preserve collateral circulation to the hand.

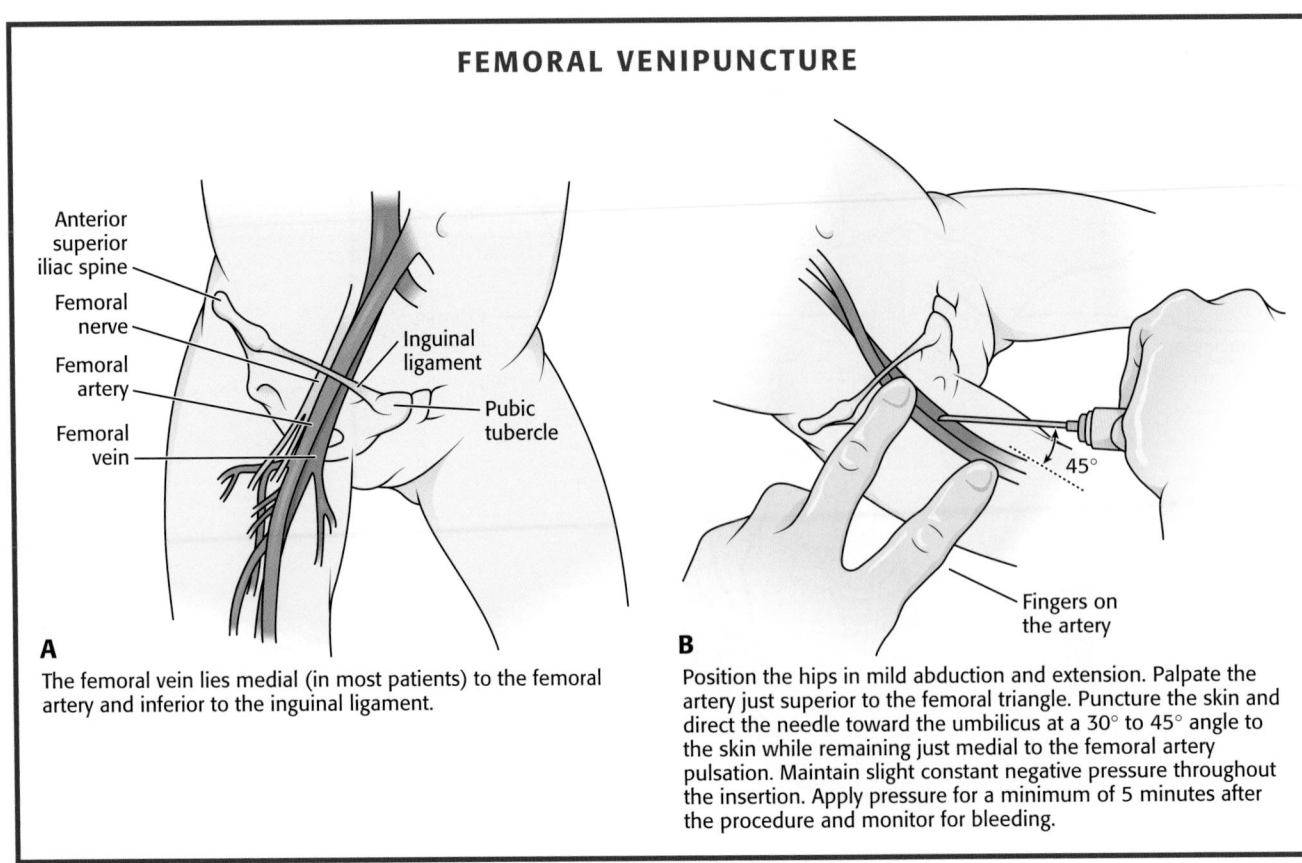

FEMORAL VENIPUNCTURE

Anterior superior iliac spine
Femoral nerve
Femoral artery
Femoral vein
Inguinal ligament
Pubic tubercle

45°

Fingers on the artery

A
The femoral vein lies medial (in most patients) to the femoral artery and inferior to the inguinal ligament.

B
Position the hips in mild abduction and extension. Palpate the artery just superior to the femoral triangle. Puncture the skin and direct the needle toward the umbilicus at a 30° to 45° angle to the skin while remaining just medial to the femoral artery pulsation. Maintain slight constant negative pressure throughout the insertion. Apply pressure for a minimum of 5 minutes after the procedure and monitor for bleeding.

Figure 19-5 Femoral venipuncture. **A,** Anatomy. **B,** Technique.

As a general rule, do not use the femoral artery for obtaining routine blood samples.

Avoid puncture of an artery if the overlying skin is infected, burned, or otherwise damaged. Also, consider the presence of adequate collateral circulation and any potential coagulation disorders.

Equipment and Setup (Box 19-3)

For arterial puncture in infants and children, a small-gauge butterfly needle is preferable to a needle and syringe. As for venipuncture, a 23-gauge butterfly needle is used most often, although a 25-gauge butterfly needle may be better in newborns. Some clinicians prefer to use a 25-gauge needle connected to a syringe, but a butterfly allows better control of the needle while an assistant aspirates the syringe. This technique may also permit a larger volume of blood to be withdrawn.

Technique

The radial artery is the one most frequently used vessels to obtain intermittent arterial samples, so the technique for arterial puncture at this site will be described. (See also Chapter 20 for a discussion of the Allen test and the effect of heparin on arterial blood sampling.)

Hold the infant's wrist and hand in your nondominant hand (see Fig. 19-6B). Hold the hand fully supinated with the wrist slightly extended (i.e., dorsiflexed). Palpate the arterial pulsation just proximal to the transverse wrist creases. Do not overextend the wrist because this can cause loss of the arterial pulse during palpation. Make a small indentation in the skin with a fingernail to mark the insertion site. Cleanse the area with antiseptic and allow the skin to dry. The topical anesthetic options discussed previously may be used if the clinical situation permits. Penetrate the skin at a 30- to 45-degree angle. While the plunger of the syringe is gently withdrawn by an assistant, advance the needle slowly until the radial artery is punctured or resistance (bone) is met (Fig. 19-7). In contrast to performing the procedure in adults, provide continuous, but gentle suction with the plunger of the syringe in infants. Pulsating or rapidly flowing blood that appears in the hub of the needle is a good indication that the radial artery has been punctured. Some clinicians prefer to attach the syringe to the butterfly needle only after blood return is noted. Suction can be applied afterward.

BOX 19-3 | **Equipment for Arterial Blood Sampling in Infants and Children**

Alcohol pads
Povidone-iodine solution
Heparin solution for coating the syringe or a prepackaged heparinized syringe if obtaining a sample for blood gas analysis
1- or 3-mL syringe
23- or 25-gauge butterfly needle
Ice-filled container (bag or cup)

RADIAL ARTERIAL BLOOD SAMPLING

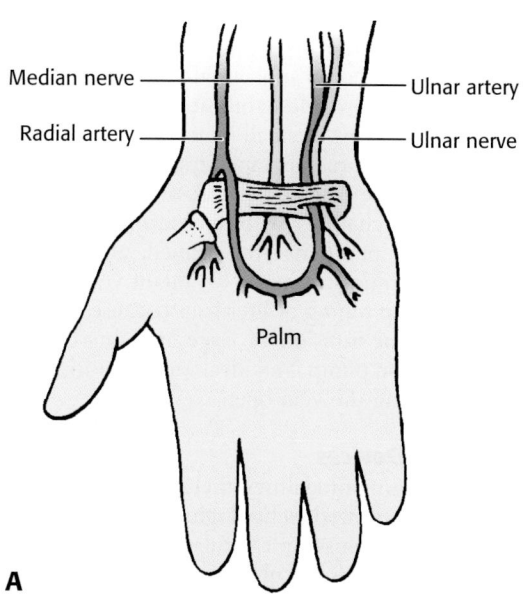

A The radial artery is preferred for sampling procedures. Its superficial location is easy to palpate and puncture, and there are no immediately adjacent nerves or veins that may be injured or accidentally punctured.

B Hold the wrist in a position of supination and slight extension. Insert the needle at a 30° to 45° angle while applying continuous, gentle suction with the plunger. Advance the needle until the radial artery is punctured and blood is returned or until resistance is met (see Fig. 19–7).

Figure 19-6 Radial arterial blood sampling. **A,** Anatomy. **B,** Technique.

Figure 19-7 Resistance met during passage of the blood gas needle usually indicates contact with bone. The needle should be withdrawn slowly. If the needle has traversed both walls of the artery, blood will be obtained as the needle is slowly withdrawn into the arterial lumen.

If resistance is met while pushing the needle deeper, withdraw the needle slowly since both walls of the artery may have been punctured but the tip may reenter the lumen on withdrawal. If no blood returns, withdraw the needle slowly to the point at which only the distal tip of the needle remains beneath the skin. Repeat the procedure after checking the location of the pulse. Reorient the needle slightly more laterally or medially if necessary. After the desired amount of blood is obtained, remove the needle and apply pressure for 5 minutes or longer to control the bleeding.

Complications

Complications of radial artery puncture include infection, hematoma formation, arterial spasm, tendon injury, and nerve damage.[12,13] With proper technique, however, the complication rate is extremely low. If the infant starts to cry before blood is obtained, the Po_2 and Pco_2 values may not reflect the infant's true steady state.

VASCULAR LINE PLACEMENT: VENOUS AND ARTERIAL

Intravascular lines are indicated when access to the venous or arterial circulation is necessary. Techniques to secure access to these intravascular spaces are discussed in the following sections. Remember to consider using topical or intradermal anesthetics or procedural sedation if the clinical situation permits.

Peripheral Venous Catheterization: Percutaneous

Indications and Contraindications

In general, peripheral IV lines are indicated when the patient is unable to attain medical and nutritional goals with enteral therapy. These lines provide fluids for resuscitation and maintenance and access for the administration of medications.

Equipment and Setup (Box 19-4)

Over-the-needle catheters such as the Angiocath, Medicut, or Quikcath are the mainstay of peripheral venous catheterization. These thin-walled, flexible catheters range in size from 14 to 24 gauge. Select the appropriate gauge and length of the catheter based on the size of the child and the clinical situation. Larger-diameter catheters allow more rapid administration of fluids in emergency situations, but large catheters may decrease the success of cannulation in young children with small veins. In general, use the smallest-gauge catheter that is appropriate for the clinical situation. For infants, a 22- to 24-gauge catheter is generally appropriate.

Use a T-connector extension tubing connected to the catheter after insertion to facilitate withdrawal of blood for specimen collection. This device makes flushing the catheter and maintaining patency easier (especially while taping and securing the IV line). It also allows dressing changes without disturbing the IV insertion site. In recent years, traditional catheters have been replaced with similar over-the-needle catheters that have a protective cap into which the needle is retracted after cannulation to reduce needlestick injuries.

Use either a homemade or commercially available device to protect the IV site from a child's attempts to remove the line. An arm or leg board appropriate for the size of the child should be handy to provide stabilization of the extremity after insertion. In newborns or small infants, fashion an arm board from two tongue depressors taped together and covered with a 4- × 4-inch piece of gauze to provide the length needed. Keep an IV fluid chamber with microdrip tubing and a continuous infusion pump nearby, primed, and ready to use. Monitor fluid administration in an infant very carefully. Do not use macrodrip tubing or liter bags because they can result in the inadvertent infusion of large amounts of fluid in an infant. An infusion pump is an ideal way of limiting fluid infusion while keeping the vein open.

Vein Imaging Devices

A variety of imaging modalities, including ultrasound, transillumination, and infrared technologies, have been used to help locate peripheral veins for cannulation. In adults there are data supporting the use of ultrasound to facilitate peripheral vein cannulation in those with difficult access.[14,15] However, the use of ultrasound to aid in the placement of peripheral IV lines in pediatric patients is not common practice. One recently published study demonstrated that ultrasound could be used to detect peripheral veins in young children that were not "clinically apparent" (nonvisible and nonpalpable).[16] The study also found that lack of ultrasound visualization increased the chance of unsuccessful placement.[16] Other small studies have shown mixed results, and further research is needed.[17-19]

Some emergency departments (EDs) use transillumination devices commonly found in neonatal intensive care units to assist in finding veins in infants.[20,21] The Venoscope II (Venoscope LLC, Lafayatte, LA) and the Neonatal Transilluminator (Graykon Scientific, Victoria, Australia) are two such devices that work by projecting a high-intensity light into the patient's subcutaneous tissue. The light causes the veins to contrast with the surrounding tissue, which makes them easier to locate.[22]

A newer vein imaging technology, VeinViewer (Luminetx Corp., Memphis, TN) uses near-infrared technology to project an enhanced image of the subcutaneous veins onto the patient's skin. Theoretically, knowledge of the location of the venous valves and the course of the vessel can assist the clinician in selecting the best area to be cannulated.[23] Early small studies have not demonstrated improved overall success rates in obtaining IV access, but the technology may be useful in patients with difficult IV access.[24-26]

Technique

A number of IV sites are available for placement of a peripheral IV line in an infant (see Fig. 19-2). The most common sites chosen for IV insertion in infants and children are the superficial veins of the dorsum of the hand, the antecubital fossa, the dorsum of the foot, and the scalp (in newborns and small infants). The veins of the dorsum of the hand are the vessels most frequently used. Because these veins are relatively straight and lie flat on the metacarpals, they are easily stabilized. If the hand is chosen, take the child's age and hand preference into consideration. Avoid placing an IV line in a hand used for thumb sucking whenever possible. Veins in the antecubital fossa (cephalic and basilic veins) are easily accessible; however, the angulation across the fossa makes advancement of the catheter difficult. These veins may not be easily visible and yet may be palpable. Select the most distal vein that is large enough to accommodate the catheter and leave the larger, more proximal veins in case the initial attempts are unsuccessful or if prolonged IV therapy is needed and percutaneous central venous catheter placement (e.g., a peripherally inserted central catheter line) is being contemplated. Tributaries of the dorsal venous arch on the dorsum of the foot, like those on the dorsum of the hand, are relatively straight, and the extremity is easily immobilized after insertion. Because indwelling catheters in this location prevent mobility, consider using this site only in preambulatory patients or after attempts at other sites have been unsuccessful. The scalp veins are easy to cannulate, but their use is primarily limited to very small infants. If a peripheral vein on the hands, feet, or antecubital fossa is being used, immobilize the extremity first by taping it to an arm board, a padded splint, or a commercially available immobilization device. The particular site is a matter of preference, so choose the vein that appears to be the easiest to cannulate.

With few exceptions, the same techniques used for IV insertion in adults may be used in infants and children, especially in the veins of the distal ends of the extremities. If the peripheral end of an extremity is used, place a tourniquet proximal to the planned site of entry. Warm the extremity to induce vasodilation in the surface veins, which makes them easier to cannulate. Flush the tubing of the T-extension set before venipuncture with a sterile IV solution, such as normal saline (NS), to prevent air embolism. Direct the IV catheter through the skin at a 10- to 20-degree angle and slowly advance it until blood return is noted (Fig. 19-8, *step 1*). Next, advance the catheter over the needle and into the vein. Retract the needle and connect the IV line to the hub of the catheter by means of a T-extension set (see Fig. 19-8, *step 2*). After 1 mL of saline has been flushed through the line, inspect the site for signs of infiltration, such as hematoma or local swelling.

Fix the catheter to the skin with a 0.5-inch piece of tape passed over the catheter hub and skin. Place a second piece of tape adhesive side up and slip it under the catheter hub. Cross it over the catheter hub in a V shape (Fig. 19-8, *step 2*). After securing the catheter with tape, cover the entire area with a transparent sterile dressing such as Tegaderm (3M, St. Paul, MN) or OP Site (Smith and Nephew Medical, Massillon, OH). Loop back the tubing of the T-extension set, place a piece of tape midway over the tubing, and secure it to the skin. This ensures that the IV tubing will not be accidentally dislodged if is suddenly pulled. Securely tape the hand and forearm to an arm board for immobilization (see Fig. 19-8, *step 3*). Occasionally, the flow rate of the infusion may depend on the position of the catheter, especially if the catheter spans a joint or the tip abuts a venous valve. Adjust the hand position or catheter with strategically placed sterile gauze or withdraw the catheter slightly to remedy the problem.

Obtain blood specimens just after IV insertion. If the IV line has been flushed, the initial blood draw will be diluted. To prevent dilution, withdraw 5 mL of blood from the catheter before collecting the samples. This 5 mL of "waste" can be either discarded or reinstilled into the patient. Next, remove the syringe. Connect the T-extension tubing to the IV infusion tubing, and set the infusion pump at the desired rate. Send blood for culture only if the skin was cleaned with an appropriate antiseptic before insertion of the IV catheter.

If the scalp veins are used, trim the hair in the surrounding area to expose the vessels. To differentiate between arteries and veins on the scalp, arteries are usually more tortuous than veins.[10] If an artery is entered during placement of the needle and fluid is infused, blanching will occur in the area. If this happens, remove the IV catheter, maintain slight pressure for 5 minutes, and repeat the procedure at another site. A rubber band may be used as a tourniquet around the scalp to produce venous dilation, but it is rarely required. Place a piece of tape on the rubber band before placement on the scalp to facilitate lifting the rubber band away from the scalp.

If a scalp vein butterfly infusion set is used, grasp the wings of the butterfly between the thumb and forefinger and introduce the needle beneath the skin approximately 0.5 cm distal to the anticipated site of vein entrance (Fig. 19-9, *step 1*). Advance the needle slowly toward the vessel until blood appears in the tubing, which indicates that the vessel has been entered. Next, remove the tourniquet. Flush the needle with 0.5 to 2 mL of IV fluid, such as NS, to ensure that the needle is properly in place within the vein. If infiltration occurs, as noted by a subcutaneous bump, remove the IV line and repeat the process at another site.

After the wings are secured, tape the tubing of the butterfly set in a loop on the scalp so that it is not pulled inadvertently. Place a wisp of cotton under the wings of the butterfly if the flow rate of the infusion is affected by the position of the catheter. Tape a small medication cup over the wings and the needle to protect the IV line (see Fig. 19-9, *step 2*).

PERIPHERAL INTRAVENOUS CATHETERIZATION

Direct the catheter at a 10° to 20° angle toward the insertion site and advance until blood return is seen in the catheter and hub. Advance the catheter over the needle and into the vein.

Remove the needle, and attach the T-extension set to the catheter hub. Flush with saline, and secure the catheter to the skin with tape.

Secure the hand and forearm to an arm board.

Cover the insertion site with the plastic wrapper from the extension set for additional protection.

Figure 19-8 Pediatric peripheral intravenous catheterization. (See Figure 21-6 for additional details on proper intravenous technique.)

Connect the tubing of the butterfly set to the tubing from the IV system. It is generally preferable to use standard over-the-needle IV catheters whenever possible, whether for extremity or scalp IV lines, because they are less likely to infiltrate and will last longer. However, a small butterfly needle that can be inserted temporarily until additional access is possible is sometimes the only option short of IO access.

External Jugular Venous Catheterization
The external jugular vein is superficial and easily visible. It can be used when other attempts at peripheral IV access have been unsuccessful. The external jugular vein is undesirable as a primary catheterization site during resuscitative efforts because manipulation of the head and neck may compromise management of the airway. Moreover, it is not a suitable site for central venous catheterization because of the acute angle of entry of the external jugular vein into the subclavian vein.[27]

Technique. Because central venous access is not the goal of this approach, the external jugular vein is most often entered with a standard over-the-needle IV catheter. The external jugular vein lies in a line from the angle of the jaw to the middle of the clavicle and is usually visible on the surface of the skin. The vein is more prominent when the child is crying. Ask an assistant to restrain the patient in a supine position with the head and neck extended over the edge of the bed. Alternatively, place a towel roll or pillow under the shoulders. Turn the head approximately 40 to 70 degrees from the midline (see Fig. 19-4). Cleanse the skin surrounding the area to be punctured with alcohol (or another antiseptic solution). Cover the area with a sterile drape, and infiltrate 1% lidocaine into the skin. Place a finger just above the clavicle to distend the jugular vein.

Attach an 18- to 22-gauge over-the-needle catheter to a syringe. Align it parallel to the vein, and puncture the skin

Figure 19-9 Scalp vein intravenous catheterization.

approximately one half to two thirds of the distance from the angle of the jaw to the clavicle. Advance the catheter slowly until the jugular vein is entered. Keep the syringe connected to the catheter at all times and maintain constant negative pressure to avoid air embolism. After the appropriate amount of blood is obtained, advance the catheter and secure it in place. Apply a sterile occlusive dressing.

Complications

Complications of peripheral IV lines and IV fluid therapy include infection, phlebitis, inadvertent arterial puncture, injection of sclerosing agents into the subcutaneous space with resultant necrosis and sloughing of the skin (especially in small infants), air embolism, and administration of inappropriate volumes of fluid. Because the life span of an IV needle or catheter is usually fairly short (<72 hours) in a small infant, the decision concerning elective removal and replacement of the IV system is not usually a problem. Of course, it is important to pay meticulous attention to antiseptic procedures during insertion and maintenance of the IV system to decrease the risk for infection.

Peripheral Venous Catheterization: Venous Cutdown

Indications and Contraindications

With the development of small IV catheters and the rapidity and safety of IO needle placement for emergency access (Chapter 25), peripheral venous cutdown is rarely performed in the ED. Even in experienced hands a saphenous vein cutdown may take more than 10 minutes and is associated with a higher rate of infection than other routes of vascular access are.[28] Nevertheless, if peripheral venous, central venous, or IO access cannot be obtained, venous cutdown may provide an alternative means of emergency venous access. For the purpose of illustration, exposure and cannulation of the saphenous vein will be discussed (Fig. 19-10). The same principles apply when cutdown is performed on most peripheral veins.

Equipment and Setup (Box 19-5)

Successful venous catheterization via cutdown in infants and small children requires sterile instruments, an assistant, good lighting, and a selection of catheters. Silastic catheters, which can be obtained in 2-, 3-, and 4-Fr sizes (Dow Chemical Company, Midland, MI), seem to remain patent longer and can be sterilized with the instruments to make a "cutdown tray." Standard 18- to 22-gauge IV catheters are also useful.

Technique

Begin with complete immobilization of the thigh, leg, ankle, and foot by taping them to a padded leg board. Attach this board in turn to the table or bed where the procedure is being performed (Fig. 19-10, *step 1*). Prepare the area around the medial malleolus with antiseptic solution and drape it with sterile towels. Perform local anesthesia (intradermal 1% lidocaine) in an area about 1 cm proximal and 1 cm anterior to the medial malleolus. No major nerves or tendons accompany the vein in this location.

Place a tourniquet proximally on the leg and make a transverse skin incision (usually about 2 cm in length) in the anesthetized area. Insert a small mosquito hemostat into the wound with the concavity of the clamp upward. Advance the tip of the hemostat to the bone in one corner of the wound, and "scoop up" all tissue lying against the bone and in the subcutaneous region with the hemostat (see Fig. 19-10, *step 2*). This will invariably lift the vein out of the wound along with the surrounding tissue. Use fine forceps or a mosquito hemostat to separate and remove all nonvenous structures so

VENOUS CUTDOWN

1 Immobilize the ankle and the site of skin incision.

Incision

Saphenous vein

Tibia

Medial malleolus

2 Use a curved hemostat to scoop up the vein. Keep the point of the hemostat against the bone.

Curved hemostat

Anterior aspect

Saphenous vein

Medial malleolus

Posterior aspect

3 Dissect the vein free with the curved hemostat.

4 Place silk sutures around the distal and proximal end of the exposed vein. Tie *only* the distal suture. Make a small venotomy with a scalpel or fine scissors.

5 Grasp the catheter (prefilled with saline) with a hemostat.

6 Advance the catheter into the vein.

7 Use a vein dilator or forceps to hold the ventomy incision open.

Vein lifter

Cannula or catheter

Traction on distal end of vein

8 Advance the catheter 2–3 cm into the vein.

Vein lifter

Vein

9 Close the incision with 4–0 nylon sutures. Place a sterile dressing over the wound, and secure the ankle to the foot board.

Figure 19-10 Venous cutdown (saphenous vein). (*From Suratt PM, Gibson RS. Manual of Medical Procedures. St. Louis: Mosby; 1982. Reproduced by permission.*)

Equipment for Peripheral Venous Cutdown in Infants and Children

Padded leg board	Fine forceps
Antiseptic solution and sterile drapes	4-0 silk sutures
	Fine scissors or scalpel
Local anesthetic	Vein dilator or lifter
Tourniquet	Silastic catheter
Mosquito hemostat	

Figure 19-11 The mini-cutdown procedure using a standard intravenous catheter-over-the-needle system is technically easier than a full cutdown and may be preferred in an emergency.

that only the saphenous vein is left tented over the hemostat (see Fig. 19-10, *step 3*). To avoid injury to the vein during dissection, spread the ends of the hemostat parallel to the direction of the vein, never transversely.

Pass two 4-0 silk sutures under the vein. Pull one distally to stabilize the vein, and pull the other proximal to the site of venipuncture. The distal suture may be tied, but if left untied it can still be used for stabilization of the vein and to occlude blood flow by applying gentle traction. Removing the untied distal suture after cannulation of the vein may allow subsequent recannulation after eventual catheter removal. Use fine scissors or a scalpel blade to make an oblique or V-shaped incision (venotomy) in the anterior wall of the vein between the sutures (see Fig. 19-10, *step 4*).

Grasp the Silastic catheter (prefilled with saline solution) with forceps and advance it into the vein for a distance of 2 to 3 cm (see Fig. 19-10, *steps 5 and 6*). This is usually the most difficult and time-consuming portion of the procedure. Use a vein dilator, L-shaped lifter, or forceps to hold the venotomy incision open (see Fig. 19-10, *steps 7 and 8*). Pull downward on the distal tie to provide countertraction and stabilize the vein during advancement of the catheter. Remove the tourniquet and tie the proximal suture around the vein with the catheter inside while taking care to not occlude the catheter by tying the suture too tightly. If the distal suture was tied, the free ends of the suture can be tied around the catheter to provide additional stability. If the distal suture was not tied, remove it at this point. Tie the proximal suture to secure the catheter, but leave the ends long enough so that the suture can be removed to allow recannulation once the infusion is removed.

Continued infusion of saline through the catheter from an attached syringe will ensure patency. Orient the catheter into either corner of the incision and close the incision with interrupted 4-0 nylon suture. Wrap the skin suture nearest the catheter around it and tie it to hold the catheter in place. Control bleeding with direct pressure. Place antibiotic ointment over the wound, and apply a sterile occlusive dressing. Connect the IV tubing and tape it securely to the foot board to prevent inadvertent removal of the catheter (see Fig. 19-10, *step 9*).

Change the dressing carefully every day with sterile technique and reapply antibiotic ointment. When cared for properly, catheters can remain in place for as long as 7 to 10 days. Generally, though, it is best to replace the catheter and insert it into another site after 3 to 4 days. At the first sign of infiltration or infection, remove the catheter. Unfortunately, once the vein has been used for cutdown, it is usually rendered useless for future venous cannulation.

Mini-Cutdown

Cannulation of a small vein with a catheter or tube may be difficult and very time-consuming if one is not experienced in the technique. As an alternative, use the mini-cutdown procedure. For this technique, once the vein is exposed through a skin incision and subcutaneous dissection, cannulate it directly with a standard IV catheter (e.g., Medicut, Angiocath, Quikcath) rather than nicking it with a scalpel (Fig. 19-11). Place a silk suture or hemostat under the vein to immobilize it during the puncture, but do not tie off the vein after cannulation. Although the catheter will not be as secure with this modification, the technique is useful when time is critical. Moreover, the vein is not destroyed by this technique. In essence, a mini-cutdown uses the percutaneous technique of cannulation, except that venipuncture is performed through a skin incision under direct visualization (see Chapter 23).

Complications

In addition to the problems with percutaneous catheter placement that were discussed previously, venous cutdown can result in wound infection and phlebitis. Adjacent structures may be injured during the incision and subsequent blunt dissection. When using the mini-cutdown technique without ligatures, extravasation of infusate may result. Light pressure on the closed wound will generally prevent continued extravasation.

Central Venous Catheterization: Percutaneous

Percutaneous placement of central venous lines has become the technique of choice for many clinicians to secure central venous access in neonates and young infants. This technique has nearly supplanted the technique of cutdown for central venous catheterization, which is seldom performed in the ED. Both percutaneous and venous cutdown catheterizations require central venous catheters, which can be purchased separately or within self-contained kits (e.g., Arrow International, Inc., Reading, PA; Gesco International, San Antonio, TX).

Indications and Contraindications

Central venous cannulation is indicated in the ED when peripheral venous access is limited or impossible and when precise hemodynamic monitoring is needed in a critically ill or injured child. Contraindications to percutaneous placement of central venous catheters include an uncorrected coagulopathy; local infection or burns at the insertion site; malformations or deformations that may distort the vascular anatomy; vascular insufficiency of an extremity; or obstruction or compression of the access veins by tumor, abnormal vessels, hematoma, thrombus, abscess, or malformation. Peripheral venous or IO access is preferred over central access during cardiac arrest to minimize complications and interruptions in cardiopulmonary resuscitation (CPR), but if a central line is in place, medications should be given centrally rather than peripherally.[29]

Equipment and Setup (Box 19-6)
Percutaneous central venous catheterization in infants and children can be performed with any number of sterile over-the-needle catheters ranging in size from 22 to 16 gauge (the choice depends on the age of the patient) and equipment similar to that used for percutaneous peripheral venous catheterization. If insertion of a larger indwelling catheter is desired, commercially available kits are convenient because they contain most of the items needed for the procedure (Gesco International, Inc., San Antonio, TX; Arrow International, Inc., Reading, PA; Cook, Inc., Bloomington, IN). The catheters in these kits are typically made of a silicone elastomer, polyvinyl chloride, or polyethylene; some are available with an antimicrobial coating, which may reduce infection rates. Catheter length is variable, and one- to three-lumen catheters are available. Rapid volume replacement, as in the case of severe dehydration or acute blood loss from trauma, is best achieved by inserting a short, large-bore catheter for the initial resuscitation and stabilization.

Other equipment necessary includes antiseptic solution, gauze pads, sterile drapes, gowns, sterile gloves, caps, masks, syringes (3, 5, and 10 mL), sterile transparent skin coverings (e.g., Tegaderm, 3M Company, St. Paul, MN; OP Site, Smith and Nephew Medical, Massillon, OH), Luer-Lok three-way stopcocks, 0.25% to 1.0% lidocaine, flush solution (1 to 2 U heparin/mL NS), and IV tubing with a T-connector extension. Depending on the vein to be accessed, restraint of the extremity, pelvis, or head may require a padded support, an assistant, or both.

Techniques
Percutaneous placement of central venous catheters can be accomplished with either a guidewire (Seldinger) technique

---

BOX 19-6 **Equipment for Central Venous Catheterization**

Antiseptic solution and sterile drapes
Local anesthetic
Syringes (3, 5, and 10 mL)
Introducer needle or over-the-needle catheter (16 to 22 gauge, depending on the age of the patient)
Guidewire
Scalpel with a No. 11 blade
Dilator
Central venous catheter
Intravenous tubing
Saline flush
Sterile skin dressing

---

or an over-the-needle catheter. Details of the femoral, internal jugular, and subclavian approaches follow. In the last several years, experience in using real-time ultrasound to facilitate placement of central venous lines in adults has prompted a number of organizations to recommend it for widespread use.[30,31] The use of ultrasound to guide placement of central venous catheters in children has been studied, but the body of literature remains small.[32] Pediatric studies have focused primarily on localization of the internal jugular and have shown mixed results when comparing ultrasound-guided cannulation with a landmark-based technique. One study looked specifically at femoral vein catheterization and found no difference in success rates with the use of ultrasound but a significantly lower complication rate when ultrasound was used.[33]

Femoral Catheterization
The safety and efficacy of percutaneous femoral venous catheterization have been demonstrated.[34,35] Femoral venous catheterization is the central venous access route most commonly used in infants and children in emergency situations (Fig 19-12). The femoral anatomy is easily learned and the arterial pulse provides a landmark for insertion of the catheter. In the event of inadvertent arterial puncture or venous laceration, hemostasis can be achieved by the application of direct pressure. In addition, femoral catheterization is less likely to interfere with emergency procedures in the region of the head, neck, and chest during medical or trauma resuscitation. Femoral vein catheterization may be associated with a higher risk for infection than subclavian catheterization but has a higher success rate in children and does not carry any risk for hemothorax, pneumothorax, or puncture of the subclavian artery.[36-39]

Technique. Restrain the child adequately to permit exposure of the inguinal region. In some situations, sedation may be appropriate to facilitate successful catheterization (see Chapter 33). Use the introducer needle supplied with the kit with or without a syringe to enter the femoral vein. Palpate the femoral artery with one finger, and place the needle in the skin just medial to the artery. Enter the skin at a 30- to 45-degree angle approximately 1 cm below the inguinal ligament. Direct the general course of the needle in a line toward the umbilicus. When blood return is noted, gently pass the wire through the needle into the proximal end of the vein. If a syringe has been attached to the introducer needle, apply continuous, gentle suction while inserting the needle. When the syringe is removed to insert the wire, place a sterile gloved finger over the open hub of the needle to prevent air embolism or blood loss. The wire should not meet resistance when introduced gently. Make sure that the proximal end is always visibly protruding from the hub of the needle. If resistance to passage of the wire is encountered, remove it to assess the needle's position within the vessel. If resistance to removal of the wire is encountered, withdraw the needle and the wire together to prevent shearing off the end of the wire.[40] An alternative method that may be useful when placing the 4-Fr double-lumen Arrow catheter is to remove the tubing from a 21-gauge butterfly needle (Abbott Hospitals, Inc., North Chicago, IL) and use the needle to enter the vein (Fig. 19-12, *step 1*). The butterfly needle is very easy to hold in a stable position and is also shorter than the needles supplied with the preassembled kits. When blood return is obtained, pass the wire through the butterfly needle into the proximal end of the vein.

Make a small incision (1 to 2 mm) in the skin at the wire's entry point to allow passage of the dilator (see Fig. 19-12, *step 2*) or the catheter itself. The incision is generally made with a No. 11 scalpel blade with the sharp edge of the blade pointed away from the wire. Advance the dilator gently over the wire and then remove it. Advance the catheter over the wire into the vein and remove the wire (see Fig. 19-12, *step 3*). Occasionally, it is useful to gently rotate and advance the dilator (or catheter) simultaneously as it enters the vein. Withdraw blood from the catheter ports, and then flush them with a sterile saline solution. Secure the catheter with silk or nylon sutures (see Fig. 19-12, *step 4*). Place a sterile transparent skin covering over the exit site for use as an impermeable dressing.

This technique is useful in children as small as 1000 g. When placing femoral venous catheters in children smaller than 1500 g, use a smaller single-lumen catheter (3 Fr or 24 gauge) because a larger catheter may occlude blood flow through the femoral vein.

Note that during CPR, palpable pulsations or Doppler tones in the femoral *vein* may be detected. Hence, if the vein is not found medial to the pulsations, consider catheterization of the pulsating vessel during CPR as a last resort when other options for vascular access or drug delivery are unavailable. Prepare both sides of the groin with antiseptic solution in the event that the initial attempt is unsuccessful.

Internal Jugular Venous Catheterization
The internal jugular veins lie within the carotid sheath containing the carotid artery and vagus nerve. The lower part of the vein lies within the triangle formed by the sternal and clavicular heads of the sternocleidomastoid muscle and becomes more lateral and anterior to the artery as it joins the subclavian vein. The right internal jugular vein is preferred over the left because the internal jugular, the innominate vein, and the superior vena cava form a nearly straight line into the right atrium. This decreases the chance for pneumothorax or injury to the thoracic duct.

Technique.   Three approaches to internal jugular catheterization are possible (including the anterior, median or central, and posterior approaches, as discussed in Chapter 22). The

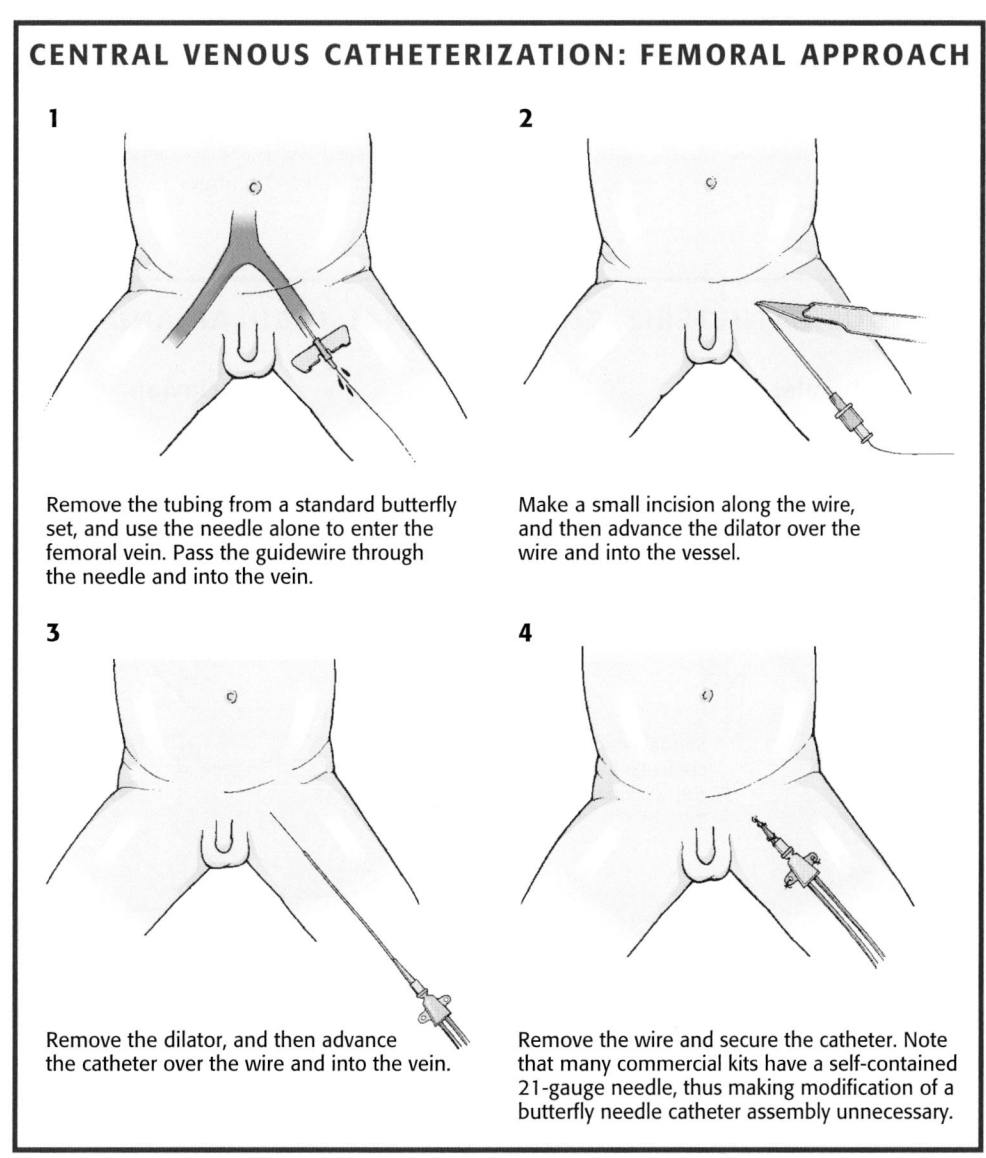

CENTRAL VENOUS CATHETERIZATION: FEMORAL APPROACH

1

Remove the tubing from a standard butterfly set, and use the needle alone to enter the femoral vein. Pass the guidewire through the needle and into the vein.

2

Make a small incision along the wire, and then advance the dilator over the wire and into the vessel.

3

Remove the dilator, and then advance the catheter over the wire and into the vein.

4

Remove the wire and secure the catheter. Note that many commercial kits have a self-contained 21-gauge needle, thus making modification of a butterfly needle catheter assembly unnecessary.

Figure 19-12 Central venous catheterization: femoral approach.

median or central approach is recommended in pediatric patients and is described here. Use of ultrasound to guide elective cannulization of the internal jugular vein in infants has been described and appears to improve success rates (see Chapter 66).[41-43] Position the child in the same fashion as that described for external jugular venous catheterization. For the medial or central approach, use the apex of the angle formed by the sternal and clavicular heads of the sternocleidomastoid muscle as the puncture site. If one could imagine a line from the mastoid process to the sternal notch, the apex of the angle formed by the two muscular heads would fall approximately along the middle third of that line.[40] Cleanse the skin surrounding the area to be punctured with antiseptic solution. Cover the area with a sterile drape, and infiltrate the skin with 1% lidocaine. Introduce an 18- to 22-gauge needle attached to a syringe at the apex of the triangle at an angle of 30 degrees downward relative to the coronal plane and direct it caudad toward the ipsilateral nipple (Fig. 19-13). Advance the needle slowly until the jugular vein is entered. Keep the syringe connected to the needle at all times to maintain constant negative pressure and avoid air embolism. After blood flow is obtained, remove the syringe and place a finger over the hub of the needle. Insert a guidewire during a positive pressure breath or exhalation. Remove the needle and introduce a catheter via the Seldinger technique. Pass the catheter far enough to reach the junction of the superior vena cava and right atrium. Check the catheter for blood return, secure the line with sutures, and apply a sterile occlusive dressing. Obtain a chest radiograph to assess the proper location of the catheter, as well as to rule out pneumothorax.

Subclavian Venous Catheterization

The subclavian vein is a popular site for central venous access in adult patients but is used far less frequently in children (see Fig. 19-13). The technique is more difficult in children because of the smaller size of the vessel, as well as a more cephalad location under the clavicles. In addition, there is a risk for pneumothorax and hemothorax, especially in younger patients and when performed during emergencies. Subclavian venous access may interfere with resuscitative efforts or be unavailable because of placement of cervical spine immobilization devices in a trauma patient.

Technique. The technique for subclavian venous catheterization differs from that for adults in that the approach to the vein is more lateral in children. The infraclavicular approach is described. The equipment needed is the same as that used for femoral catheterization. Turn the patient's head away from the side to be punctured and place a towel roll under the shoulders. The right side is preferred because the dome of the lung is more cephalad on the left side. The needle insertion site is at the distal third of the clavicle in the depression created between the deltoid and the pectoralis major muscles. Prepare the skin with antiseptic solution. Cover the area with a sterile drape, and infiltrate the skin with 1% lidocaine.

Introduce the finder needle bevel up and advance it slowly while applying negative pressure with the attached syringe. Keep the syringe and needle parallel to the frontal plane. Direct the needle medially and slightly cephalad, beneath the clavicle toward the posterior aspect of the sternal end of the clavicle (i.e., toward a fingertip placed in the sternal notch).

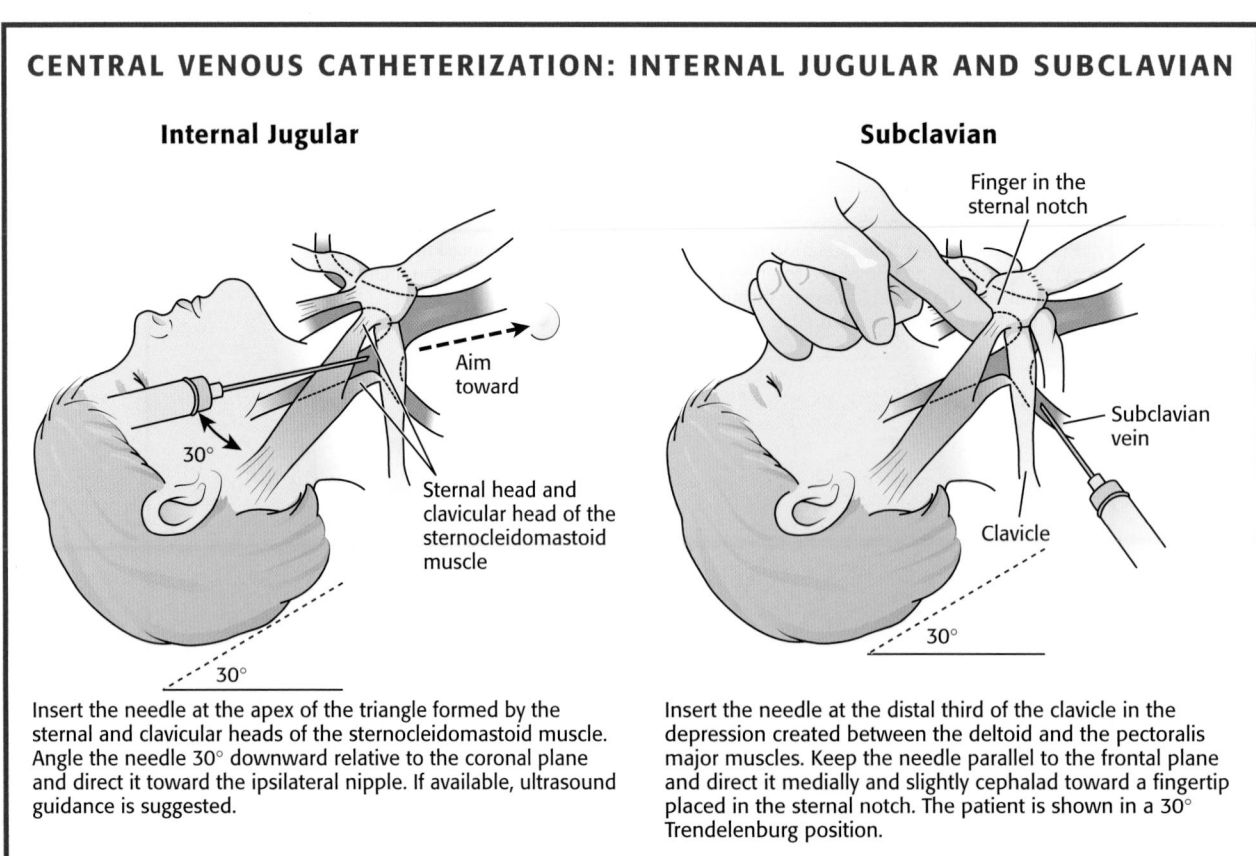

CENTRAL VENOUS CATHETERIZATION: INTERNAL JUGULAR AND SUBCLAVIAN

Internal Jugular

Aim toward

30°

Sternal head and clavicular head of the sternocleidomastoid muscle

30°

Insert the needle at the apex of the triangle formed by the sternal and clavicular heads of the sternocleidomastoid muscle. Angle the needle 30° downward relative to the coronal plane and direct it toward the ipsilateral nipple. If available, ultrasound guidance is suggested.

Subclavian

Finger in the sternal notch

Subclavian vein

Clavicle

30°

Insert the needle at the distal third of the clavicle in the depression created between the deltoid and the pectoralis major muscles. Keep the needle parallel to the frontal plane and direct it medially and slightly cephalad toward a fingertip placed in the sternal notch. The patient is shown in a 30° Trendelenburg position.

Figure 19-13 Central venous catheterization: internal jugular and subclavian approaches.

Advance the needle until blood return is obtained. Turn the syringe so that the bevel of the needle points caudad to direct the guidewire to the superior vena cava. Remove the syringe from the needle and insert the wire during a positive pressure breath or natural exhalation. Remove the needle and introduce the catheter over the wire via the Seldinger technique as previously described for femoral catheterization. As in adults, the cardiac monitor may show a rhythm disturbance if the wire is advanced too far. Perform auscultation of bilateral breath sounds and obtain a chest radiograph to confirm proper positioning of the catheter in the superior vena cava and to rule out procedural complications such as pneumothorax or hemothorax. Secure the catheter in place with sutures, and apply a sterile, occlusive dressing.

Complications

Infection and thrombosis are the major risks associated with central venous catheters.[38,44] Subclavian and internal jugular catheters additionally carry serious risks for pneumothorax and hemothorax. Other complications include arterial puncture, accidental displacement, phlebitis, hemorrhage, hematoma, dysrhythmia, air embolism, vascular obstruction or perforation, right atrial perforation, and localized edema. Perform blood sampling from indwelling central venous lines with caution because the risk for contamination increases each time that the system is opened. Remove catheters as soon as they are no longer needed to minimize the risk for these complications.

Emergency Vascular Access

Vascular access is a key component of any resuscitation to allow the administration of fluid and medications and to obtain blood samples. However, achieving venous access during pediatric resuscitation can challenge even the most seasoned clinician.[45,46] In a review of pediatric resuscitations by Rossetti and colleagues, IV access required 10 or more minutes in 24% of cases.[45] The average time required for a cutdown was 24 minutes. Children who were successfully resuscitated had vascular access achieved significantly sooner than did those who were not resuscitated. Emergency IV access was most prolonged in children younger than 2 years. This last finding is important because the majority of cardiopulmonary arrests in children occur in this younger age group.

For these reasons, clinicians should obtain IO access in critical patients if IV access is not established quickly rather than delay treatment with attempts to place peripheral or central venous catheters (see Chapter 25).[29] IO lines are underused in many EDs.[47] If no IV or IO line is available, give certain drugs via the endotracheal tube (see Chapter 26) while attempts at venous access are initiated. However, endotracheal drug administration has been shown to be less efficacious than IV administration in adults, and this route of administration should be used only when no alternatives are available.[48,49] Central venous access may be desirable in critical patients. In pediatric resuscitation, the femoral vein is generally chosen because its consistent anatomic location and large size make it the safest and easiest central vein to catheterize. The femoral vein can also be accessed with minimal interference with resuscitative efforts. However, central venous access in children takes significantly longer than IO line placement. Generally, placement of a central line in children should occur after initial stabilization through a peripheral IV or an IO line.

Umbilical Vein Catheterization

Indications and Contraindications

The major indication for umbilical vein catheterization is the need to access the vascular system for emergency resuscitation and stabilization of neonates. It may also be used for exchange transfusions and short-term central venous access in newborns. The umbilical vein may remain patent for up to 2 weeks after birth.[50] In neonates who require emergency access in the ED, a peripheral vein would be preferable, but attempting to cannulate one of the umbilical vessels could be lifesaving. Moreover, umbilical vein catheterization is technically easier than umbilical artery cannulation.

Equipment and Setup

See Box 19-7 for the supplies and equipment necessary for catheterization. Place the infant beneath a radiant warmer because keeping the infant warm during the procedure is critical. Restrain the extremities. Wear a mask, cap, gown, and sterile gloves. Assess the length of catheter needed before the procedure. Methods to estimate the best length for both umbilical vein and artery lines are discussed below.

Technique

Hold the umbilical stump upright and scrub the cord with a bactericidal solution. Avoid pooling of liquid at the infant's side because this may be associated with blistering of the skin under a radiant warmer. Drape the umbilical area in sterile fashion with the infant's head left exposed for observation.

Place a loop of umbilical tape or a purse-string suture at the junction of the skin and the cord to provide hemostasis and to anchor the line after placement (Fig. 19-14, *step 1*). Cut the cord with a scalpel about 1 cm from the skin (often less in infants who are not newly born), and identify the vessels. The vein is usually located at 12 o'clock and has a thin wall and large lumen. It may continue to bleed after cutting. The two arteries have thicker walls and smaller lumens. Constriction reduces bleeding after the vessels are cut. Occasionally, a persistent urachus may be mistaken for the umbilical vein, but the presence of urine in the urachus may help correctly identify that structure.

Flush the catheter (3.5 Fr [preterm infants] to 5.0 Fr [term infants]) with heparinized saline and attach it to a three-way

---

BOX 19-7 Equipment for Umbilical Vein and Artery Catheterization

Sterile drapes
3-0 silk suture on a curved needle
Small clamps, forceps, scissors, and needle holder
Curved iris forceps without teeth
Umbilical artery catheter (3.5 to 5 Fr)
Fluid chamber, intravenous tubing, infusion pump, filter (0.22 μm), short length of intravenous IV tubing, and three-way stopcock
10 mL of heparinized solution for flushing (1 to 2 units heparin per milliliter of fluid)
Infusion solution (usually 5% to 10% dextrose in water with electrolytes. Some clinicians also add 1 unit heparin per milliliter of fluid to prevent clotting in the catheter)

UMBILICAL VEIN CATHETERIZATION

1

Umbilical vein

Umbilical arteries

Purse-string suture or loosely tied umbilical tape

Hold the umbilical stump up and scrub it with bactericidal solution. Place a loop of umbilical tape or a purse-string suture at the junction of the skin and the cord. Cut the cord with a scalpel 1 cm from the skin and identify the vessels. The single vein is thin walled, has a large lumen, and may continue to bleed after cutting. The two arteries have thicker walls and smaller lumens and do not usually bleed.

2

Advance a preflushed catheter into the vein and gently advance it.

For emergency use, advance only 1–2 cm beyond the point at which good blood return is obtained. This is usually only 4–5 cm for a term-sized infant.

For longer-term use, the catheter may be passed into the inferior vena cava. (See text for details.)

Umbilical vein

Umbilical arteries

Figure 19-14 Umbilical vein catheterization. *(From Zaoutis L, Chiang V. Comprehensive Pediatric Hospital Medicine. Philadelphia: Elsevier; 2007.)*

stopcock. Place the catheter into the lumen of the umbilical vein and advance it gently (see Fig. 19-14, *step 2*). An umbilical vein line can be placed in a fashion that is intended either for emergency use or for more chronic use. In an emergency case, advance the catheter only 1 to 2 cm beyond the point at which good blood return is obtained. This is usually only 4 to 5 cm in a term-sized infant. If the catheter is pushed farther than this distance, it may enter the ductus venosus and then move into the inferior vena cava, or it may enter a branch of the portal vein within the liver (as evidenced by resistance at 5 to 10 cm). Infusion of medications into a catheter in this location can result in liver necrosis.

The inferior vena cava site may be a desirable location in some newborn infants in whom peripheral vascular access is limited and for whom longer-term central venous access is desired. It is also useful for monitoring central venous pressure or infusion of medications, high concentrations of glucose (>10%), IV fluids, and hyperalimentation solutions. The catheter must be inserted approximately 10 to 12 cm in a term-sized infant to reach the inferior vena cava. Radiographs are required in this case to identify and prevent accidental entry into the portal vein, thereby limiting utility in an emergency situation. Note that an umbilical venous catheter will proceed directly cephalad (without making a downward loop) until it passes through the ductus venosus (Fig. 19-15).

Some practitioners use standardized graphs to estimate the length of insertion. Such graphs are based on the shoulder-to-umbilicus length (Fig. 19-16A) and are useful if stored in the drawers of the warming beds used to resuscitate newborns and small infants, along with the catheters and other equipment. Shoulder-to-umbilicus length is the perpendicular line measured from the tip of the shoulder to the horizontal level of the umbilicus. If the graph is not available, the

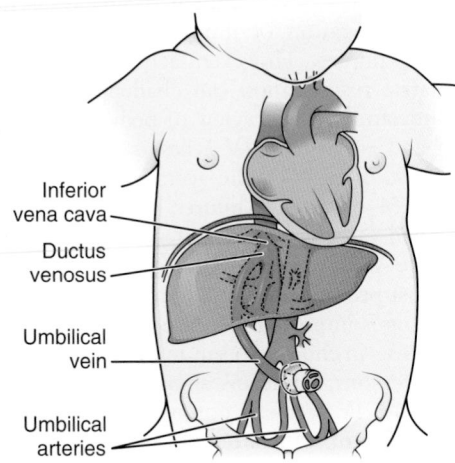

Inferior vena cava

Ductus venosus

Umbilical vein

Umbilical arteries

Figure 19-15 An umbilical venous catheter will proceed directly cephalad (without making a downward loop) until it passes through the ductus venosus.

shoulder-to-umbilicus length multiplied by 0.6 gives an approximate insertion length that will result in the tip of the catheter being above the diaphragm but below the right atrium in the inferior vena cava.[50] Formulas based on birth weight are also used to estimate catheter length.[51]

Air embolism may occur at the time of catheter removal if the infant generates sufficient negative intrathoracic pressure (as during crying) to cause air to be drawn into the patent umbilical vein. Therefore, caution must be used during removal of the catheter to ensure that the vein is promptly occluded (by tightening a purse-string suture or applying pressure on or just cephalad to the umbilicus).

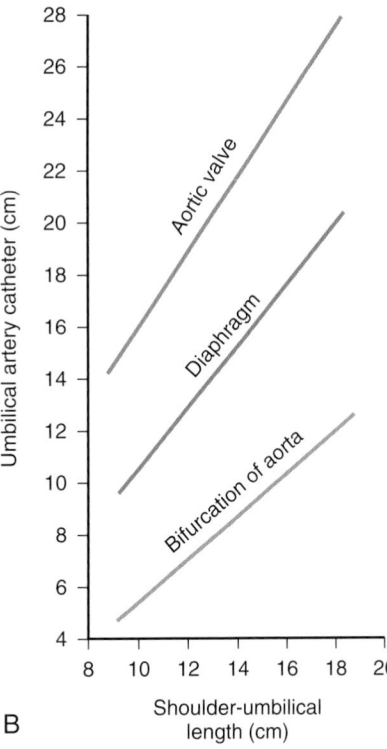

Figure 19-16 After measuring the shoulder-to-umbilicus length, a standardized graph can be used to determine the appropriate length of the umbilical venous catheter (**A**) or umbilical arterial catheter (**B**). The venous catheter should be inserted into the inferior vena cava below the level of the right atrium. The appropriate length of the arterial catheter depends on whether a "high" or "low" line is desired (see text for explanation). (*A and B, From The Johns Hopkins Hospital, Nechyba C, Gunn VL. The Harriet Lane Handbook: A Manual for Pediatric Home Officers. 16th ed. St. Louis: Mosby; 2002.*)

Complications

Complications of umbilical venous catheters include hemorrhage, infection, injection of sclerosing substances into the liver (resulting in hepatic necrosis), air embolism, catheter tip embolism, and vessel perforation.[52,53] Follow careful technique during insertion and maintenance of catheters to minimize such complications.

Umbilical Artery Catheterization

Indications and Contraindications

Umbilical artery catheterization is a useful procedure in the care of newborn infants who require frequent monitoring of arterial blood gases and arterial blood pressure, fluid and medication administration, and exchange transfusions.[53] Either one of the two umbilical arteries may be cannulated for resuscitation purposes, but an umbilical vein is generally technically easier to cannulate and may be preferred in an emergency. Complications are discussed later, but one should avoid cannulating the arteries if omphalitis, peritonitis, necrotizing enterocolitis, or intestinal hypoperfusion is present.

Equipment and Setup

The equipment required for umbilical artery catheterization is identical to that used for umbilical venous catheterization (see Box 19-7). Additional equipment needed for continuous arterial pressure monitoring and infusion should be readily available. Estimate the catheter length needed before starting the procedure. Do this by using a standard graph (see Fig. 19-16B) or a birth weight regression formula.

Technique

The technique of umbilical artery catheterization is similar to that described for umbilical vein catheterization in the preceding section. After the umbilical arteries have been located

(Fig. 19-17, *step 1*), grasp the cord with a curved hemostat near the selected artery. Ask an assistant to use two hemostats to grasp each side of the cord and slightly evert the edges to aid in exposure of the arteries. Using curved iris forceps without teeth, gently dilate the artery (see Fig. 19-17, *step 2*). Sometimes, repeated passes of the forceps are required because the umbilical artery can spasm and make the procedure difficult. Attach a 3.5- to 5-Fr catheter to a three-way stopcock and flush it with a sterile heparinized solution. Introduce the catheter into the dilated artery (see Fig. 19-17, *step 3*). Use a 3.5- to 4-Fr catheter for infants weighing less than 2 kg and a 5-Fr catheter for those weighing 2 kg or more.

When the catheter is being inserted, place gentle tension on the cord in a cephalad direction, and advance the catheter with slow, constant pressure toward the feet. Resistance is occasionally felt at 1 to 2 cm. Overcome this with gentle, sustained pressure. On the other hand, if the catheter passes 4 to 5 cm and then meets resistance, this generally indicates that a "false passage" through the vessel wall has occurred. Occasionally, one may bypass the perforation by reattempting catheterization with a larger catheter.

Acceptable positions of umbilical arterial catheters are between T6 and T9 ("high line") and between L3 and L5, just above the aortic bifurcation ("low line"). High lines are associated with a lower incidence of thrombotic complications.[54] Use graphs and formulas to estimate the proper catheter length for insertion at both the high and low positions (see Fig. 19-16B), but confirm placement with a radiograph. These formulas may not be as accurate in babies at the extremes of weight. Once sterile technique is broken, do not advance the line. It is therefore preferable to position the catheter too high and to withdraw it as necessary according to postinsertion radiographs. This will show the catheter proceeding from the umbilicus down toward the pelvis, making an acute turn into the internal iliac artery, continuing toward

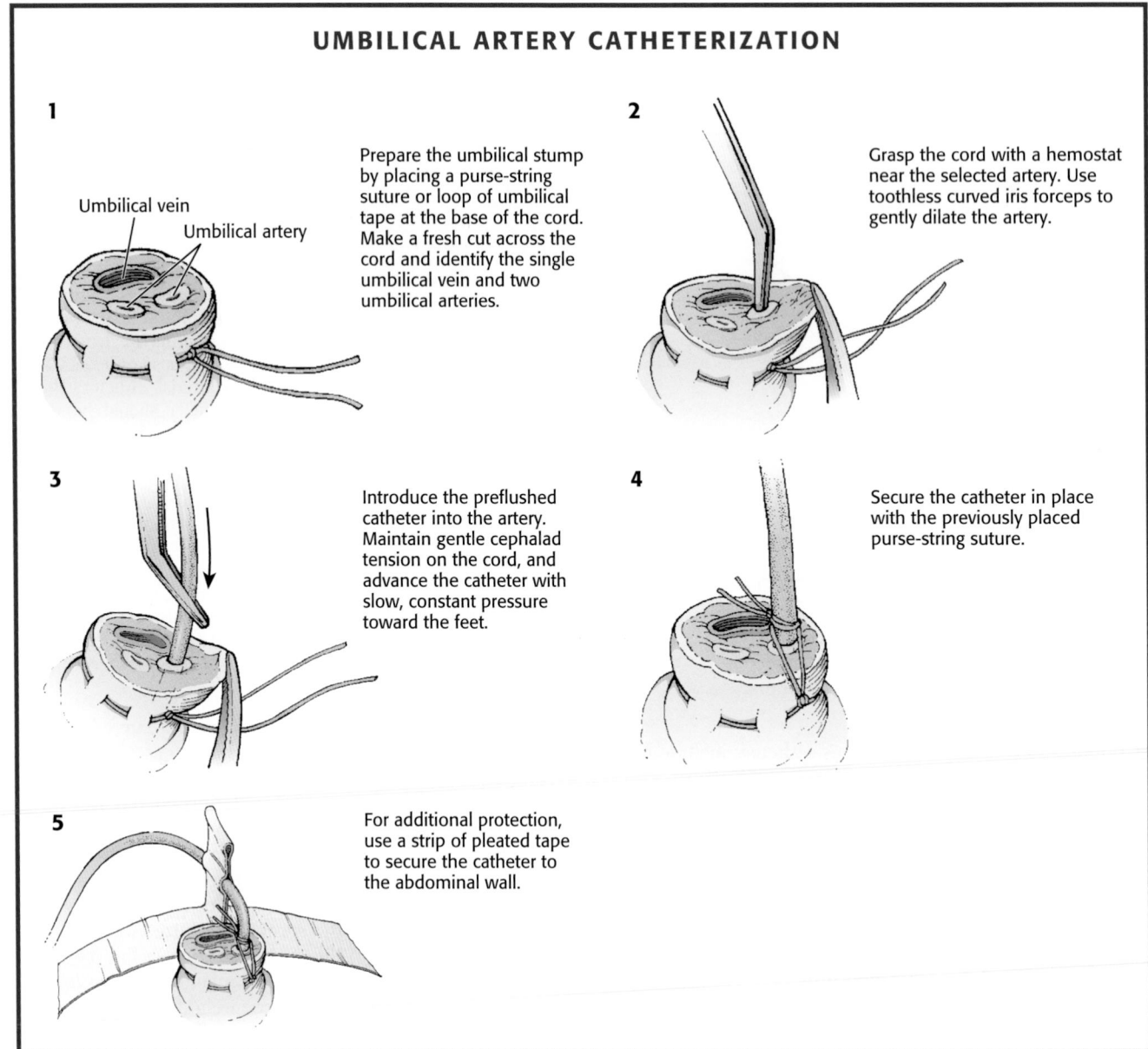

UMBILICAL ARTERY CATHETERIZATION

1 Prepare the umbilical stump by placing a purse-string suture or loop of umbilical tape at the base of the cord. Make a fresh cut across the cord and identify the single umbilical vein and two umbilical arteries.

Umbilical vein
Umbilical artery

2 Grasp the cord with a hemostat near the selected artery. Use toothless curved iris forceps to gently dilate the artery.

3 Introduce the preflushed catheter into the artery. Maintain gentle cephalad tension on the cord, and advance the catheter with slow, constant pressure toward the feet.

4 Secure the catheter in place with the previously placed purse-string suture.

5 For additional protection, use a strip of pleated tape to secure the catheter to the abdominal wall.

Figure 19-17 Umbilical artery catheterization.

the head into the bifurcation of the aorta, and then moving up the aorta slightly to the left of the vertebral column (Fig. 19-18). After it has been properly positioned, tie the catheter with the previously placed suture and tape it to the abdominal wall (see Fig. 19-17, *steps 4 and 5*).

Most unsuccessful umbilical artery catheterization attempts fail because the catheter perforates the arterial wall approximately 1 cm below the umbilical stump, where the umbilical artery begins curving toward the feet. In this instance, the catheter is advanced in the extraluminal space, and resistance is encountered at 4 to 6 cm.

Complications

Complications of umbilical artery catheterization include hemorrhage, infection, thromboembolic phenomena (especially involving the kidneys, gastrointestinal tract, and lower extremities), aortic thrombosis, aortic aneurysm, vasospasm,

air embolism, vessel perforation, peritoneal perforation, and hypertension.[53]

If the catheter becomes plugged or fails to function properly or if there is blanching or discoloration of the buttocks, the heels, or the toes, remove the catheter at once. Umbilical arteries are most easily cannulated in the first few hours of life but may provide a viable vascular route as late as 5 to 7 days of age.

Percutaneous Arterial Catheterization

Indications and Contraindications

Despite the growing use of noninvasive devices for monitoring transcutaneous oxygen and carbon dioxide, percutaneous peripheral arterial catheterization is indicated when there is a need for frequent blood gas sampling, cotinuous monitoring of arterial blood pressure, or both. Arteries used for peripheral

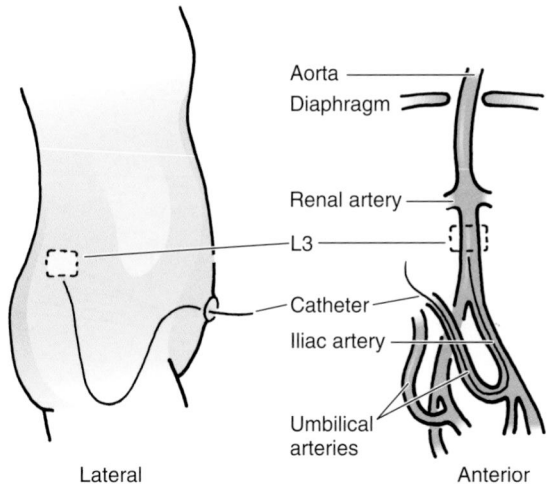

Figure 19-18 The umbilical artery catheter makes a loop downward before heading cephalad (schematic drawing of a radiograph interpretation).

catheters in infants and children include the radial, ulnar,[55] femoral,[56] dorsalis pedis, and posterior tibial arteries. This procedure is rarely performed in the ED.

Percutaneous radial artery catheterization has become widely accepted and has been shown to be safe in infants and children. The catheter allows preductal blood gas determinations if placed in the right radial artery. Only the procedure for radial artery catheterization is described here, but catheterization of other vessels is similar.

Peripheral arterial catheterization is contraindicated when (1) adequate peripheral arterial samples can be obtained by percutaneous puncture, (2) the circulation of the extremity to be catheterized is compromised, (3) occlusion of the vessel to be catheterized compromises perfusion of the extremity, (4) there is an ongoing bleeding diathesis, (5) localized infection or inflammation overlies the artery to be cannulated, or (6) intensive monitoring of line function is not available.

Equipment and Setup
The equipment needed for arterial catheterization is essentially the same as that required for percutaneous peripheral venous catheterization (see Box 19-4). Some centers use commercially available arterial line kits, which come with all the necessary supplies and equipment. Alternatively, standard 22- or 24-gauge over-the-needle IV catheters, a T-piece connector, and a three-way stopcock will work fine. Connect the T-piece and the stopcock and then fill them with NS solution. Prepare an infusion pump with heparinized saline.[57]

Technique
Perform the procedure with good lighting and an adequate work area and monitor the infant's heart rate and respiratory rate closely. Palpate the radial artery proximal to the transverse wrist crease on the palmar surface of the wrist, medial to the styloid process of the radius. Before the procedure, compress the artery and observe the hand and fingers for change in color. If blanching or cyanosis is noted (indicating poor collateral circulation), do not perform catheterization. If locating the artery by palpation is difficult, a transillumination device,[58] Doppler probe, or ultrasound may be helpful.[59-61]

Secure the infant's or child's hand and lower part of the forearm to an arm board with the wrist dorsiflexed 45 to 60 degrees by placing a roll of gauze underneath it. Take care to leave the fingers exposed to allow assessment of the peripheral circulation. Palpate the radial artery at the point of maximal impulse and mark it by making a gentle indentation with a gloved fingernail. Prepare the area over the radial artery with povidone-iodine or another antiseptic solution and wash it with alcohol. Use a topical or local anesthetic (such as 1% lidocaine without epinephrine), or both, at the planned insertion site. Insert the catheter with the needle through the skin just proximal to the transverse wrist crease at a 10- to 20-degree angle (Fig. 19-19A). Advance the catheter with the needle slowly until blood appears in the catheter hub, which signifies puncture of the anterior arterial wall. Slowly advance the catheter until blood appears in the needle and then carefully lower the angle of the needle to approximately 10 degrees. Slowly advance the catheter over the needle and into the lumen of the artery. Remove the needle. Attach the stopcock and T-piece connector to the catheter hub. Open the stopcock to the syringe to confirm return of pulsatile blood. Flush it with 0.5 mL of heparinized solution very gently to clear the catheter while observing the fingers and the hand for evidence of blanching or cyanosis.

Fix the catheter to the skin with a thin piece of tape placed adhesive side up under the catheter hub and cross it over the catheter in a V shape. Pass a second piece of tape around and over the catheter hub to fix it to the wrist (Fig. 19-19B). Add a transparent sterile dressing such as Tegaderm (3M, St. Paul, MN) or OP Site (Smith and Nephew Medical, Massillon, OH) for an additional layer of security and protection. Use a small piece of tape to attach the T-piece connector to the wrist area or to the splint. Be sure that the fingers are easily visible.

Use only heparinized NS or half-normal saline for infusion. Do not infuse medications, blood, blood products, amino acid solutions, IV fat solutions, or hypertonic solutions through the catheter. Remove the catheter if there is evidence of blanching or cyanosis, if it is impossible to withdraw blood from the catheter, or if it becomes difficult to flush the catheter.

Complications
Complications, which have been reported with every type of arterial catheter, include hemorrhage, thrombosis, spasm, infection, scars, air embolism, retrograde blood flow, transient elevation in blood pressure with rapid (<1 second) infusion, and nerve damage. Thrombosis or spasm may result in blanching or cyanosis of the extremity or skin.[53] There is the potential for loss of digits, an entire extremity, or large areas of skin. However, complications from ED-placed arterial lines are uncommon and generally minor.[12]

Arterial Cutdown Catheterization

Indications and Contraindications
Arterial catheterization by cutdown of the posterior tibial artery or radial artery may be indicated when frequent monitoring of arterial blood gases or blood pressure is needed and percutaneous access is not possible. Contraindications to arterial cutdown are similar to those cited for percutaneous arterial catheterization. Because of their experience with a wide variety of percutaneous vascular access techniques, emergency

RADIAL ARTERY CATHETERIZATION

A Introduce the catheter assembly into the radial artery through the skin at a 10°- to 20°-angle. This is a smaller angle than that used for simple arterial puncture.

B One technique of taping the arterial catheter. The arm board should be well padded and secured.

Figure 19-19 Radial artery catheterization. (See Figure 20-5 for additional details on this technique.)

clinicians may find that percutaneous arterial catheterization is easier and likely to be more successful than performing an arterial cutdown.[62]

Equipment and Setup (Box 19-8)
Successful arterial cutdown catheterization in a small infant requires sterile instruments, an assistant, good lighting, and a selection of catheters. The equipment required can be found on a cutdown tray, which is available in most EDs. Also needed are a 22- or 24-gauge over-the-needle catheter, T-extension connector tubing, a stopcock, a 5- or 10-mL syringe filled with flush solution (NS with 1 to 5 U heparin/mL), and silk suture ties. The operator prepares for the procedure by scrubbing and donning a mask, cap, gown, and sterile gloves.

Technique
The anatomy (Fig. 19-20) and technique for posterior tibial arterial cutdown are described in detail (Fig. 19-21). The same technique is applicable for the radial artery. Stabilize the foot in a neutral position by taping the externally rotated lower part of the leg to a splint. Localize the posterior tibial artery with Doppler ultrasound just posterior to the medial malleolus. Prepare the skin of the foot with a povidone-iodine or other antiseptic solution.

After subcutaneous injection of 1% lidocaine, make a 5- to 7-mm transverse incision in the skin over the artery posterior to and at the midlevel of the medial malleolus (see Fig. 19-21, step 1). Using blunt dissection in a vertical direction (parallel to the vessels), separate the tissue with a pair of small, curved forceps. Identify the artery, which courses with the vein just anterior and superficial to the nerve and is usually pulsatile. Isolate the artery by sliding small, curved forceps beneath it and gently elevating the vessel (see Fig. 19-21, step 2). Excessive manipulation of the artery can cause spasm; if this occurs, apply a few drops of 1% lidocaine locally to induce dilation.

BOX 19-8 **Equipment for Arterial Cutdown Catheterization**

Padded arm or foot board
Antiseptic solution
Sterile drapes
Local anesthetic
Scalpel
Small curved forceps
Silk ties
22- or 24-gauge over-the-needle catheter
Preflushed connector tubing
Infusion tubing

Place a silk tie (without a needle) beneath the artery to stabilize it during cannulation (see Fig. 19-21, step 3).

At a 10-degree angle, insert a 22- or 24-gauge over-the-needle catheter (bevel downward) into the artery over the surface of the forceps. When blood return is seen, advance the catheter over the stylet to its full length (see Fig. 19-21, steps 4 and 5). Remove the needle stylet and connect the catheter to the T-connector tubing and a three-way stopcock that has been prefilled with heparinized flush solution. Check for patency by observing blood return with pulsations. Flush the catheter slowly and gently. Remove the silk suture and secure the skin incision with sutures. Suture the catheter to the skin over the heel. Secure the catheter and connector to the heel with tape (see Fig. 19-21, step 6). Connect the stopcock to the infusion line.

Complications
The complications of arterial cutdown are similar to those with percutaneous arterial catheterization and include hemor-

Figure 19-20 Anatomy of the posterior tibial artery and surrounding structures.

ARTERIAL CUTDOWN CATHETERIZATION (POSTERIOR TIBIAL)

1

Medial malleolus

Make a 5- to 7-mm incision posterior to and at the midline level of the medial malleolus.

2

Isolate the artery by sliding small curved forceps beneath it and gently elevate the vessel.

3

Place a silk tie under the vessel to stabilize it during cannulation. Insert a 22- or 24-gauge over-the-needle catheter into the vessel, bevel down, over the surface of the forceps.

4

When blood return is seen, advance the catheter over the needle.

5

Remove the needle after the catheter has been fully advanced, and connect to a preflushed connector tubing assembly.

6

Suture the skin incision, and secure the catheter and connector to the patient with sutures and/or tape. Use a padded leg board for extra protection.

Figure 19-21 Arterial cutdown catheterization (posterior tibial).

TABLE 19-1 Estimating Dehydration

DEHYDRATION	SYMPTOMS	SIGNS	FLUID LOST IN INFANTS	FLUID LOST IN OLDER CHILDREN	TREATMENT
Mild	Thirsty	Slightly dry mucous membranes	50 mL/kg	3-5% total fluid	ORS, 50-100 mL/kg over a 2-to 4-hr period Consider other methods if not tolerated No laboratory studies
Moderate	Decreased urine output Absent tears	Tachycardia Capillary refill >2 sec Dry mucous membranes Weak pulse Abnormal respirations Sunken eyes	100 mL/kg	6-9% total fluid	ORS, 50-100 mL/kg over a 2-to 4-hr period Consider other methods if not tolerated No laboratory studies
Severe	Abnormal mental status, lethargy	Abnormal skin turgor Sunken fontanelle Hypotension	150 mL/kg	>9% total fluid	20-60 mL/kg of NS by IV bolus Serum chemistries

IV, intravenous; *NS,* normal saline; *ORS,* oral rehydration solution

rhage, thrombosis, or spasm resulting in loss of tissue; infections; permanent scars; and nerve damage. These complications have been reported with all types of arterial cutdowns.

REHYDRATION TECHNIQUES IN INFANTS AND CHILDREN

Approach to Dehydration

Assessing whether a child with acute gastroenteritis is dehydrated and to what degree is complicated by inconsistency in the literature. Parental report of symptoms and signs associated with dehydration (emesis, diarrhea, poor fluid intake, decreased urine output, weak cry, sunken fontanelle, sunken eyes, decreased tears, dry mouth, and cool extremities) has 73% to 100% sensitivity in predicting moderate or great dehydration but poor specificity.[63] Table 19-1 presents a more thorough list of the signs, symptoms, and definitions of mild, moderate, and severe dehydration.

Oral Rehydration

Oral rehydration therapy (ORT) has been shown to be equivalent to IV therapy in children with acute gastroenteritis in terms of rehydration, subsequent diarrheal episodes, and the development of sodium abnormalities.[64] Failure rates are 4.9% as compared with 1.3% for IV therapy, and use of ORT can avoid the need for IV hydration in 24 of every 25 patients.[65] This is the modality of choice for rehydration of a mildly to moderately dehydrated infant or child 1 month or older. Oral rehydration solutions come in a number of commercial forms (World Health Organization rehydration salts, Enfalyte, Pedialyte, Rehydralyte, CeraLyte). A solution can be made at home with 5 cups of water, 8 teaspoons of sugar, and 1 teaspoon of salt. The target volume is 50 to 100 mL/kg over a period of 2 to 4 hours. Typically, this is

Figure 19-22 Oral rehydration with a syringe. The parent is instructed on the technique in the emergency department.

started with a spoon, cup, or syringe delivering 5 mL to children younger than 2 years and 10 mL to children older than 2 years every 5 minutes and then increasing volumes slowly as tolerated (Fig. 19-22). Vomiting is not a contraindication to attempting ORT since children can typically tolerate these small volumes. Some practitioners fear accompanying electrolyte abnormalities; however, hypernatremic dehydration responds well to ORT.

Oral rehydration can be facilitated with the use of an antiemetic. Ondansetron has been shown to decrease ED vomiting with a number needed to treat (NNT) of 5, decrease the need for IV hydration (NNT = 5), and decrease need for admission (NNT = 14).[66] Ondansetron is administered at a dose of 0.15 mg/kg in the form of syrup or oral dissolving tablets. An alternative, simplified dosing regimen is to give 2 mg for children 8 to 15 kg, 4 mg for children 15 to 30 kg, and 8 mg for children greater than 30 kg.[67] Most oral ondansetron studies include children 6 months and older, but several studies using IV ondansetron have included infants as young as 1 month. Concern has been raised regarding the possibility of the use of ondansetron delaying the identification of more pathologic diagnoses. A metaanalysis has shown no difference in return visit rates in those who do not receive antiemetic therapy, and it has been shown to not mask alternative diagnoses.[4,68] Outpatient prescriptions for ondansetron do not affect recidivism or readmission rates. Ondansetron has recently received attention for its ability to prolong the QT interval. In children, it lengthens the duration of the QT interval by 10 to 17 msec, an amount unlikely to be induce torsades de pointes in an otherwise healthy child.[69] Other antiemetics and antimotility agents are not recommended by the American Academy of Pediatrics for use in children younger than 5 years, and they have a high incidence of side effects.[70] There is a Food and Drug Administration "boxed warning" against the use of promethazine in children younger than 2 years and a strong recommendation against its use even in older children.

Laboratory Tests

The American Academy of Pediatrics recommends electrolyte testing in patients with severe dehydration, those who need IV rehydration, or children with moderate dehydration and findings on the history or physical examination inconsistent with straightforward diarrheal episodes.[8] A prospective study of patients 2 months to 9 years of age deemed to require parenteral rehydration on clinical grounds demonstrated a 48% rate of laboratory abnormalities, 10.4% of which changed management. More than 9% of their patients had hypoglycemia, so obtaining a glucose level urgently, as well as electrolytes when feasible in patients who require IV rehydration, is recommended.[71] It is difficult to provide recommendations regarding the management of low bicarbonate because the level has been found to correlate poorly with clinical signs of dehydration. One study found a bicarbonate level of less than 16 mmol/L in 35% of patients with no dehydration and a level greater than 20 mmol/L in 15% of patients with moderate dehydration, thus indicating that it may be a poor determinant of management.[72] Urine specific gravity tends to lag behind the child's hydration status and is particularly unreliable in infants younger than 1 year.[73]

Parenteral Rehydration

Obtaining IV access is covered elsewhere in this section. If parenteral administration of fluids is deemed appropriate, standard therapy involves 20-mL/kg boluses of NS or lactated Ringer's solution infused over a 60-minute period each until normalization of pulse, perfusion, and mental status occurs. Recent literature has demonstrated comparable safety and efficacy of rapid rehydration protocols involving the administration of 50 to 60 mL/kg over a 60-minute period in otherwise healthy children.[74-76] Fourteen percent of children rapidly rehydrated required a return ED visit, which did not differ significantly from the proportion of children returning after a standard rehydration protocol.[12]

Children who have received parenteral fluids and subsequently tolerated oral fluids can typically be discharged home from the ED. If the child requires admission for continuance of maintenance fluids, isotonic saline is recommended because of a documented 17% to 45% risk for hyponatremia with the use of hypotonic fluid.[77-79] The amount of maintenance fluid is calculated as 100 mL/kg for the first 10 kg of body weight, 50 mL/kg for 10 to 20 kg of body weight, and 20 mL/kg for the remaining body weight in a 24-hour period. For example, a 50-kg child would require (100 mL × 10 kg) + (50 mL × 10 kg) + (20 mL × 30 kg) divided evenly over 24 hours.

If parenteral fluid administration is required and IV access is not readily achieved, IO access has recently been made faster and easier to achieve with use of the intraosseous drill (EZ-IO) (see Chapter 25).[80] Available sites are the same as those with standard insertion, with the flat area of the proximal end of the tibia two fingerbreadths below and 1 to 2 cm medial to the tibial tuberosity being widely accepted as the preferred site in children. Skin overlying the site is prepared and anesthetized, and the appropriate needle is connected to the drill. Needle options for the EZ-IO include pink 15-mm (3 to 39 kg), blue 25-mm (>40 kg), and yellow 45-mm (>40 kg with excess subcutaneous tissue) needles. The needle and drill are placed at a 90-degree angle to the bone, and the drill trigger is depressed while applying gentle pressure. A sudden "give" or "pop" is felt when the intramedullary space is reached. At this point the drill is removed from the embedded needle, and a connector is attached to the hub of the needle. A bolus of 5 to 10 mL of NS while feeling the posterior surface of the calf for evidence of extravasation will confirm appropriate placement. Pain associated with the infusion is minimized by the administration of 0.5 mg/kg of 1% preservative-free lidocaine (cardiac lidocaine is most readily available at most centers) to an adult maximum of 20 to 50 mg through the IO line.[81] IV tubing is connected and the infusion initiated. Pushing fluid via a syringe or the use of a pressure bag is recommended to allow an acceptable rate of delivery.[18] Securing an IO line is difficult, but a simple solution is to surround the needle and proximal tubing with a small inverted paper cup with the bottom removed and the cup taped to the leg (Fig. 19-23). Success rates are high and adverse events minimal. However, if the initial attempt is unsuccessful

Figure 19-23 Intraosseous line protected by a paper cup.

because of extravasation, the contralateral tibia or another site must be selected.

Nasogastric Tube Rehydration

Nasogastric rehydration is a potentially effective technique in children who refuse to take fluids orally in the quantity required for rehydration. When compared with IV hydration, the cost is 18% less,[82] and it is an option in children in whom IV access cannot be established easily. Several studies have demonstrated its safety and efficacy in mildly to moderately dehydrated patients.[83,84] Studies in developing nations have found this technique effective for severe dehydration as well.[85-87] Nasogastric rehydration is accomplished by placement of a nasogastric tube, with a 5-Fr feeding tube typically being adequate for children younger than 3 years. Use of topical anesthetic or nebulized lidocaine (5 mg/kg diluted in NS) before insertion is recommended for comfort. A bolus of 50 mL/kg of electrolyte solution (e.g., Pedialyte) is administered by continuous infusion via an enteral feeding pump over a 3-hour period. Twenty-four-hour rehydration regimens (50 to 100 mL/kg for the first 10 kg of body weight and then 25 to 50 mL/kg for the remaining body weight) have also been proposed but seem to have equivalent outcomes to more rapid rehydration protocols.[88] In one study, 18% of patients nasogastrically rehydrated required a return visit to the ED, which was not significantly different from those who received IV rehydration.[21] No study has evaluated the use of frequent, small boluses; however, experience with ORT would indicate that 5- to 10-mL parent-administered syringe boluses to equal 50 mL/kg would be an option in the event that a pump for continuous administration is unavailable.

Subcutaneous Rehydration

Subcutaneous rehydration therapy, also known as hypodermoclysis, is an option in children with mild to moderate dehydration in whom IV or IO access is not available or feasible. Its utility as a bridge to facilitating commencement of IV hydration in severely dehydrated children has been postulated, but not studied. Although the potential has been recognized since the early 1900s, the hyaluronan-containing intercellular matrix of subcutaneous tissue prevents easy delivery and absorption of large quantities of fluid, and the previous preparations of hyaluronidase (enzymes that hydrolyze hyaluronan) were animal based and allergenic. More recently, a recombinant formulation of human hyaluronidase, HuPH20 (Hylenex), has become available, thus making this technique more accessible. Its primary utility has been in geriatric and hospice patients requiring hydration, but several studies have substantiated its safety and efficacy in pediatric patients as young as 2 months.[89]

After sterile preparation, a 22- or 24-gauge angiocatheter or 25-gauge butterfly needle is inserted at a 30- to 45-degree angle to the hub into subcutaneous tissue. After placement of a small piece of gauze under the hub of the catheter to maintain the angle, it is secured with a sterile occlusive dressing. Although the interscapular area is often used, the thigh, abdomen (left iliac fossa), chest, and upper part of the arm are also options.[90] If possible, an area with a pinchable fat fold of 1 inch should be selected. The catheter should be aspirated for *absence* of blood return. A 150-unit dose of hyaluronidase is injected through the catheter, and the fluid infusion is

Figure 19-24 Subcutaneous rehydration with normal swelling 5 minutes after beginning the infusion. *(Courtesy of Dr. Corburn Allen; reproduced with permission from Pediatrics)*

TABLE 19-2 Troubleshooting Subcutaneous Rehydration Complications

The catheter becomes dislodged.	Restart in the same area without an additional dose of hyaluronidase[90]
The infusion pump indicates occlusion.	Slow the infusion rate by 10 mL/hr.
The area becomes firm, indurated, and painful.	Administer an additional dose of hyaluronidase.
The child fails outpatient therapy.	Continue infusion of fluid through the catheter for 48 hours as maintenance.

started. Typically, isotonic fluids such as 0.9% NS are used. Mean fluid infusion rates are highly variable in adults and range in children from 18.9 mL/kg over the first hour to 38.4 mL/kg for a 4-hour infusion.[89] An eventual infusion rate around 20 mL/kg/hour should be selected and titrated down if the infusion pump indicates occlusion. Because the hyaluronidase requires about 15 minutes to take full effect, some providers prefer to start more slowly and titrate upward.[91] Initially, an erythematous swelling may appear at the infusion site (Fig. 19-24), but it will decrease in size after 5 minutes and disappear 1 to 2 hours after cessation of the fluid infusion. Some pain may occur at infusion site. Suggestions for troubleshooting subcutaneous infusion problems can be found in Table 19-2. Maximal diffusion of fluid into the IV compartment occurs in 1 hour.[92] An injection of hyaluronidase allows subcutaneous infiltration for 48 hours, and maintenance fluids, including those containing dextrose and potassium, can be infused through the catheter after the bolus if required. No special care is required following removal of the catheter.

Subcutaneous rehydration is not recommended in patients with signs of shock, coagulation deficits, gross edema, significant electrolyte abnormalities (sodium >150 or <130 mEq/L), or no intact skin sites (e.g., massive burns).[30,93] The most common adverse events reported are redness, swelling, or

TABLE 19-3 Discharge Instructions for Mild to Moderate Dehydration

Oral recommendations for acute rehydration*	ORS, 50-100 mL/kg over a 3- to 4-hr period
Diet recommendations following correction of dehydration	Continue breastfeeding or formula Resume a normal unrestricted diet
Oral intake to avoid	Juices, sodas, sports drinks (osmotic diarrhea), foods high in simple sugar
Fluid requirements <10 kg for ongoing losses	60-120 mL per diarrheal stool or emesis episode
Fluid requirements >10 kg for ongoing losses	120-240 mL per diarrheal stool or emesis episode
Return precautions	Bloody stool, signs of dehydration, altered mental status

ORS, oral rehydration solution.

*Typically, the acute rehydration phase takes place in the emergency department. These recommendations apply to a child who is doing well and leaves to finish acute rehydration at home.

bruising at the infusion site.[94] Allergic reactions have not been reported with the newer formulation of hyaluronidase, and skin infections are rare. In one study, this technique facilitated discharge home in 84% of patients and allowed definitive rehydration in 94% of patients, with no return visits requiring admission.[29]

Discharge

Commonly held beliefs include avoidance of dairy products, need for formula change or overdilution of formula with water, gut rest for 24 hours or longer, and the BRAT diet (bananas, rice, applesauce, toast). These beliefs are not supported by the literature in most cases. Once rehydration has been achieved, return to a normal diet is suggested as soon as possible. Advice for discharge instructions is listed in Table 19-3.[95]

Most children seen in the ED with acute dehydration will be corrected and discharged home. Admission criteria include inadequate care at home or inability to follow return precautions, inability to take or failure of rehydration with ORT, concern for more serious pathology, severe dehydration, and neonatal dehydration.[34]

References are available at www.expertconsult.com

Arterial Puncture and Cannulation

Hyung T. Kim

Arterial puncture is the most accurate blood sampling technique for true arterial blood gas (ABG) and acid-base determination. The absence of arterial blood pressure defines cardiac arrest and serves as a definitive end point for resuscitative efforts. Intraarterial cannulation with continuous blood pressure measurement remains an accepted standard in critically ill patients. Intraarterial monitoring of blood pressure better reflects the force of systemic perfusion and is one of the most important determinants of cardiac work. In recent years, noninvasive technologies have achieved an accuracy that is nearly equal to that of invasive monitoring, but these techniques also have limitations.[1,2] Invasive modalities require specific expertise and support to perform.[3]

HISTORICAL PERSPECTIVE

Hippocrates suggested that the blood and arteries deliver life-giving energy to the body. Building on these ideas, the ancient Greek physician Galen first noted that arteries carry blood from the heart although he wrongly asserted that the heart constantly produced new blood. The concept of circulating blood volume generating pulse and pressure was not recognized until the Age of Enlightenment. The Spanish physician Severetus was among the first to accurately describe the circulation in 1580, but most of his writings were destroyed when he was executed for his teachings. Soon thereafter in 1616, William Harvey described a circulatory system with a finite amount of blood and the heart at its center. Stephen Hales first recorded blood pressure measurement in 1733 using a brass pipe. He inserted a pipe into a horse's artery and connected it to a glass conduit in which he observed blood rising and falling.[1,4]

The first measurement of human blood pressure was accomplished in 1847 with the kymograph. It was developed by the German physiologist Carl Ludwig and involved the insertion of catheters directly into the artery. In 1949, Peterson and colleagues illustrated continuous recording of pulse waves and blood pressure with a catheter percutaneously inserted into the brachial artery. Soon thereafter,

Arterial Puncture And Cannulation

Indications
Blood gas sampling
Continuous pressure monitoring
Need for frequent blood sampling
Inotropic support (use of continuous infusion of vasoactive agents)
Majory surgery involving fluid shifts/blood loss
Hypothermia (induced or environmental)
Diagnostic angiography
Therapeutic embolization

Contraindications

Strict	Relative
Inadequate circulation	Previous surgery in the area
Raynaud's syndrome	Anticoagulation/coagulopathy
Buerger's disease	Skin infection at the site
Full-thickness burns	Atherosclerosis
	Inadequate collateral flow
	Partial-thickness burns

Complications
Hematoma formation
Infection
Bleeding
Ischemia
Thrombosis/embolism
Arteriovenous fistula formation
Pseudoaneurysm formation

Equipment
Arterial Puncture

Arterial Cannulation

(Not shown: bag of normal saline, pressure infuser)

Review Box 20-1 Arterial puncture and cannulation: indications, contraindications, complications, and equipment.

percutaneous femoral artery cannulation with a polyethylene catheter through a large-bore needle was described by Peirce. Barr described radial artery cannulation with a Teflon catheter in 1961.[5]

An important accomplishment in vascular access occurred in 1953 when Seldinger presented a technique in which percutaneous catheterization could be achieved over a guidewire.[5,6] In the 1960s, the introduction of electrical monitoring of arterial pressure with transducers and recorders allowed mathematical waveform analysis in addition to visual analysis. More recent advances have included continuous, invasive monitoring of ABG values.[7] Currently, there are a growing number of noninvasive devices and methods for accurate monitoring of arterial blood pressure; however, none match the proven accuracy of intraarterial monitoring.

A growing acceptance of using venous blood gas measurements instead of arterial gases in many clinical settings has reduced the frequency of arterial puncture. With ongoing improvements in noninvasive monitoring devices, it is possible that invasive monitoring may become less common.

INDICATIONS AND CONTRAINDICATIONS

Indications for and contraindications to arterial puncture and cannulation are listed in Review Box 20-1. The use of arterial lines for continuous monitoring is generally reserved for the intensive care setting; however, arterial cannulation may be initiated in the emergency department (ED). The indications for placement of an arterial catheter fall into three major categories[8,9]:

1. *Repetitive and direct arterial blood sampling.* Catheter access removes the need for multiple arterial punctures and allows either repeated sampling or placement of sensors for continuous monitoring of blood gas and other chemistry values.
2. *Continuous real-time monitoring of blood pressure.* Catheter access allows superior monitoring and moment-to-moment detection of changes. Intraoperative and intensive care unit (ICU) management is often facilitated by placement of an arterial line.
3. *Failure or inability to use indirect blood pressure monitoring.* Some patients such as those with severe burns, dialysis grafts or shunts, or morbid obesity may need ongoing monitoring of perfusion, which can best be accomplished by arterial catheterization.

Although acute respiratory decompensation and metabolic emergencies are the most common reasons for ABG sampling, all blood tests performed on venous blood are also possible on an arterial sample. Cultures performed on blood obtained from an indwelling arterial line have a sensitivity and specificity similar to that of cultures performed on blood obtained from a venipuncture site.[10,11] Patients with moderate respiratory decompensation may be managed without arterial puncture by using continuous, noninvasive pulse oximetry, end-tidal or transcutaneous carbon dioxide monitoring, carboxyhemoglobin and methemoglobin monitoring, or any combination thereof.[12] Nonetheless, a role still exists for arterial blood sampling. The initial correlation between noninvasive values and acid-base status via arterial sampling is often important in critical illness to set a baseline or verify a trend. Some authors use ABG sampling in the initial evaluation of

critically ill trauma patients.[13] Vasoactive drugs (e.g., nitroprusside and norepinephrine) are best administered with continuous monitoring of arterial pressure to guide titration. The response of trauma and post-cardiac arrest patients to acute resuscitative efforts may also be more easily monitored with the use of arterial catheterization.

Few contraindications to arterial puncture exist; none are absolute. For example, after thrombolysis, arterial cannulation should be performed only if it will provide essential data that cannot be obtained by any other method. If absolutely necessary, a single arterial puncture of the readily compressible radial artery is preferred. Arterial puncture can be performed safely in patients who are anticoagulated or who have other coagulopathies, but it should be undertaken with extreme caution in patients with severe disseminated coagulopathies.

There are reports of patients with bleeding complications who require transfusion. Some patients have suffered compression neuropathies secondary to hematomas at the puncture site.[14] Repeated arterial sampling in such patients should be accomplished by insertion of an indwelling cannula to minimize trauma to the arterial wall.

The presence of severe arteriosclerosis, with or without diminution in flow, is a relative contraindication to arterial puncture. In hemodynamically unstable patients with advanced cardiovascular disease, the benefits of invasive monitoring may nonetheless outweigh its risks.[9] Consider an alternative site if an isolated, decreased palpable pulse or bruit is felt over the site selected. Consider an alternative site if there is evidence of decreased or absent collateral flow in areas where flow normally exists, such as in Raynaud's syndrome or an abnormal result on the modified Allen test (discussed later in the section "Techniques"). Avoid puncturing a specific arterial site when infection, burn, or other damage to cutaneous defenses exists in the overlying skin. In addition, avoid performing an arterial puncture through or distal to a surgical shunt.

Arterial versus Venous Analysis

Arterial sampling has been the traditional approach to evaluating acid-base abnormalities in critically ill patients, especially those being maintained on a ventilator. In most ED settings, however, venous blood gas analysis may suffice. Studies have demonstrated that analysis of venous blood (especially central venous blood) for pH, bicarbonate, lactate, base excess, and carbon dioxide pressure (Pco_2) are within 95% limits of agreement with arterial sampling and can safely supplant it.[15-17] On the other hand, arterial blood sampling is still required for accurate analysis of oxygen pressure (Po_2).[18-20]

EQUIPMENT: ARTERIAL PUNCTURE

Arterial Puncture with a Needle/Syringe

To obtain a single sample of arterial blood by the percutaneous method, attach a 3-mL syringe (preferred and most common) to a needle. Base the needle size on puncture location and patient size and age. For an adult, use a 20-gauge, 2.5-inch needle for a femoral sample and a 22 gauge, 1.25 inch needle for a radial artery puncture. For pediatric arterial sampling, use a needle with a slightly shorter length in the range of 22 to 24 gauge at the same sites as in adults.

Figure 20-1 Arterial blood gas syringe. This device is precoated with dry lithium heparin. Additionally, the plunger is vented, which allows air in the syringe to escape through the plunger as the sample is collected. To use this type of syringe, pull back the plunger to the desired volume before arterial puncture. When the needle enters the artery, blood will fill the syringe spontaneously—there is no need to pull back on the plunger.

Precoated blood gas plastic syringes (with dry lithium heparin) are commonly used and allow a longer shelf life and ready use (Fig. 20-1). Such devices are designed to minimize sampling error as a result of heparin.[21] If necessary, prepare a regular syringe with 1 or 2 mL of a heparinized saline solution (1000 IU/mL) drawn into the syringe to coat the barrel and needle. Fully eject the heparin through the needle immediately before skin puncture to minimize heparin-related errors. Although the syringe may appear devoid of heparin, enough heparin remains in the needle and syringe to provide anticoagulation. Even dry heparin may produce abnormalities in ABG results because of a heparin-induced dilutional effect.

The latest blood gas and chemistry analyzers require only 0.2 mL of whole blood for accuracy, and some point-of-care devices can perform analyses on single drops of blood. However, sample sizes of less than 1.0 mL of blood aspirated into heparin-coated syringes may result in a heparin-related error on ABG values.

Stored heparin solution has higher Po_2 and lower Pco_2 values than blood does.[22] A dilutional effect from heparin would mean that the addition of 0.4 mL of heparin solution to a 2-mL sample of blood (dilution of 20%) will lower Pco_2 by 16%.[21] Proper technique with dry lithium heparin-prefilled syringes or full ejection of excess heparin will prevent such problems if more than 2 mL of blood is collected. A falsely low Pco_2 is the most clinically significant change caused by excess heparin.[21,22] Neither Po_2 nor pH levels are significantly altered by the addition of heparin in most instances, although a slight increase in Po_2 and a minimal decrease in pH may occur if high concentrations of heparin (25,000 IU/mL) are used.[23] If 2 to 3 mL of blood is collected, heparin-related effects are likely to be clinically inconsequential.

Continuous Monitoring via Arterial Catheter

The fluid-filled recording systems used with arterial cannulation have a great influence on the accuracy of pressure measurements. The frequency responses of tubing, transducers, and other components of the monitoring system influence the accuracy of systolic and diastolic pressure measurement. Failure to recognize recording system artifacts will lead to errors in interpretation of the pressure.[3]

Various catheter types have demonstrated similar frequency-response characteristics, but some studies have

found different complication rates. Teflon catheters may carry an increased rate of thrombosis.[24,25] Another contributing element leading to thrombosis is catheter diameter; the incidence of thrombosis is inversely related to the ratio of vessel lumen to catheter diameter.[26,27] Thus, the risk for thrombosis increases as the diameter of the catheter decreases. The incidence of thrombosis also increases with increased duration of catheter placement. In contrast, a higher risk for thrombosis was seen in the femoral artery than in the radial artery in a study involving a pediatric population.[28] Catheters coated with a combination of chlorhexidine and silver sulfadiazine have produced lower infection rates.[29]

Preparation for Arterial Cannulation

Box 20-1 lists the usual equipment for arterial cannulation, although the majority of prepackaged kits contain the supplies most needed (see Review Box 20-1). Shorter catheters are ideal for peripheral artery cannulation, whereas use of a longer catheter and the Seldinger technique is preferable for the femoral artery.

For arterial cannulation in adults, use a 16- to 18-gauge catheter for the femoral artery and a 20-gauge catheter for the radial artery (Fig. 20-2). Small children and infants require a 22- to 24-gauge catheter, which may need to be inserted percutaneously via the Seldinger technique or through a femoral cutdown. Based on patient size, older pediatric patients usually require 20- to 22-gauge catheters.

The tubing that connects the catheter to the pressure transducer has a significant effect on accuracy of the monitoring system. The higher the frequency response of the entire

Figure 20-2 Catheters for arterial cannulation. **A,** Standard intravenous catheter. Use 20 gauge for the radial artery and 16 or 18 gauge for the femoral artery. **B,** Arrow Arterial Catheterization Kit. This device has a self-enclosed guidewire that is advanced into the artery by moving the actuating lever forward. When the lever reaches the reference mark on the barrel of the device, the tip of the guidewire is at the opening of the needle lumen. (*Arrow International, Reading PA.*)

Figure 20-3 Arterial pressure monitoring systems. **A,** System for continuous flushing. A 1-L bag of normal saline is pressurized to 250 to 300 mm Hg with a metered blood pump (not shown). The continuous flush device is set to deliver 3 mL/hr of saline. A mechanical pressure transducer is depicted. The transducer device is a sterile, inexpensive, fully assembled monitor that can be used during patient transfer. Alternatively, the electronic transducer depicted in **B** may be used. **B,** System for manual flush. A saline flush solution can be injected manually through a syringe at the proximal or distal port. The transducer dome should be maintained at the level of the patient's heart. (*From Beal JM, ed.* Critical Care for Surgical Patients. *New York: Macmillan; 1982. Reproduced by permission.*)

system, the more accurate the determination of systolic and diastolic pressure; however, artifact also becomes more of a problem.[8,30] Use stiff, low-capacitance plastic tubing for arterial catheterization and monitoring. Place the electronic pressure transducer connection as close as possible to the patient and zero it appropriately because the frequency response of a tube is inversely related to its length.[30-32]

The pressure wave produced with each contraction is transmitted from the artery through the catheter and connecting tubing to a measuring device. The arterial fluid wave is received by an electromechanical transducer that changes the mechanical pressure wave into an electrical signal that can be displayed on the monitor. The most basic technique for obtaining blood pressure values involves the use of a simple manometer.[33] This system can be assembled quickly if the material is available.

A continuous method of flushing the pressure tubing is required to maintain patency of the catheter lumen during intraarterial pressure monitoring. A three-way stopcock through which the tubing is intermittently flushed (a minimum of every 15 to 30 minutes) with saline is a simple, effective method. Continuous flush devices push a set amount of fluid (usually 2 to 3 mL/hr) through the line.[9] A typical monitoring system that includes this device is shown in Figure 20-3. The pressure transducer must be mounted at the level of the patient's heart. Current pressure-monitoring setups include not only built-in stopcocks but also in-line flushing plungers to facilitate clearance of blood after sampling.

Intravascular transducers were initially seen as an improvement over the external electromechanical transducers in use since the mid-1970s. Many of the numerous brands are fragile, temperature sensitive, of variable quality, and much more difficult to place in vessels than catheters are. Despite anecdotal reports of fibrin deposition on these devices, no increased incidence of thrombus formation has been noted. The most important advantages of intravascular transducers are the ability to continuously monitor ABG values and elimination of the potential error induced by catheters, stopcocks, and connecting tubing.[34,35]

SITE SELECTION

The radial, brachial, and femoral arteries are the sites usually punctured for blood gas sampling in adults. Pediatric sites commonly used for arterial puncture include arteries in the foot and the umbilical artery in newborns.

When an artery is cannulated for longer-term use, consider the potential consequence of complete loss of blood flow through a vessel as a result of intraluminal thrombosis. This is important when choosing a site for arterial puncture. Because the most frequent complication of arterial catheterization is bleeding, the ability to control hemorrhage must also be considered. For these reasons, the radial and femoral arteries are favored because of their good collateral blood flow and ease of compression in case of hemorrhage. Patient comfort and nursing care concerns should also be considered during selection of the site.

TECHNIQUES
Arterial Puncture

Palpate the arterial pulse to ascertain the location of the vessel and prepare the overlying skin with an antiseptic solution (Fig. 20-4, *step 1*). Anesthetize the patient's skin with a wheal

ARTERIAL PUNCTURE (RADIAL ARTERY)

1

Position the wrist in slight dorsiflexion, cleanse the skin with antiseptic solution, and palpate the radial pulse.

2

Optionally, place a small wheal of local anesthetic (e.g., 1% lidocaine without epinephrine) over the entry site. Avoid placing too large of a wheal, which may obscure the artery.

3

Hold the syringe in your hand like a dart, with the bevel up. Palpate the artery with the index and middle fingers of your other hand. Puncture the skin distal to your finger, and slowly advance the needle at a 30° angle toward the pulsating vessel.

4

As soon as blood flows, stop advancing the needle. Allow the syringe to fill on its own. If bone is encountered, withdraw slowly because both vessel walls may have been penetrated and the lumen may be entered as the needle is withdrawn.

5

Remove the needle from the artery after the syringe has filled. Apply a bandage and firm pressure to the puncture site for a minimum of 3 to 5 minutes.

6

End cap

Remove all air from the syringe by holding it upward, gently tapping it, and depressing the plunger. Attach the end cap to the syringe to maintain anaerobic conditions, and submit the sample to the laboratory.

Figure 20-4 Arterial puncture (radial artery).

TABLE 20-1 Parameters That Affect Interpretation of Arterial Blood Gases

PARAMETER	HEPARIN*	AIR BUBBLE IN SAMPLE	DELAYED ANALYSIS†
Po_2	No significant change‡	Elevated	Variable†
Pco_2	Lowered§	No significant changes‖	Elevated¶
pH	Unchanged§	No significant changes‖	Lowered¶

*Use only a 1000-IU/mL concentration. Fill the dead space of the needle and syringe only and collect 3 mL of blood.
†Changes unpredictable at 20 minutes regardless of the storage method.
‡There are reports of slight increases in Po_2 with excessive heparin.
§The falsely lowered Pco_2 that occurs with added heparin is the most clinically significant change noted. pH may be decreased if a large volume of concentrated heparin (25,000 IU/mL) is used.
‖If stored at 4°C for 20 minutes. Anaerobic storage at room temperature for 20 minutes results in no significant change.
¶Minimal changes up to 2 hours if stored at 4°C.

of local anesthetic (e.g., 1% lidocaine without epinephrine) through a small needle (25 or 27 gauge) (see Fig. 20-4, *step 2*). If local anesthesia is to be performed, take care to use only a small amount of local anesthetic because a large wheal may obscure the pulse. One study found no significant alterations in Pco_2 or pH from the pain or anxiety of an unanesthetized arterial puncture (Table 20-1).[36] If the patient is in extremis or unresponsive to pain in the area to be punctured, the anesthetic infiltration step may be omitted.

Isolate the arterial pulsation with the index and middle fingers of the gloved, nondominant hand and identify the course of the vessel. Puncture the skin through the anesthetic wheal, immediately distal to the palpated pulse under the index finger (Fig. 20-4, *step 3*). The older technique of placing the needle between the index and middle finger risks self-puncture and is no longer advised. Hold the syringe like a dart with the bevel up and the syringe kept in view so that blood flow can be seen immediately. Advance the needle slowly toward the pulsating vessel at an approximately 30-degree angle. A larger angle is required to puncture the deeper femoral artery. Once the needle enters the arterial lumen, allow the syringe plunger to rise with the arterial pressure on its own to discriminate between arterial and venous sampling (see Fig. 20-4, *step 4*). As soon as blood flows, stop advancing the needle and allow the syringe to fill. If no blood flow is obtained or if bone has been hit, withdraw the needle slowly because both walls of the vessel may have been punctured and the lumen may be entered as the needle is withdrawn. Redirect the needle only when the needle has been retracted to a location just deep to the dermis. After at least 1 to 2 mL of blood has been obtained, remove the needle from the artery. Apply firm pressure at the puncture site for a minimum of 3 to 5 minutes (see Fig. 20-4, *step 5*). If the patient is anticoagulated or has a coagulopathy, 10 to 15 minutes of pressure is required.

Use of ultrasound is rapidly becoming a standard in procedures involving central vascular access. The same ultrasound-guided techniques are also being applied to arterial cannulation (see Ultrasound Box.)

In their review of the current literature, Shiloh and colleagues reported 71% improvement in the likelihood of success at the first attempt when using ultrasound guidance.[37] Vascular Doppler can also be used to improve success rates. Hold the probe over the artery just proximal to the puncture site. An important indication of vessel identification is the loss of audible pulsations with compression.

Proper handling of the sample and rapid analysis are very important. When the needle is withdrawn, expel any air bubbles present in the syringe to avoid a false elevation in Po_2.[38] Remove the air neatly and easily by tapping the inverted syringe (needle pointing upward) to force any air to the top; then carefully and slowly depress the syringe plunger to push out the remaining air (see Fig. 20-4, *step 6*). A gauze pad or alcohol wipe may be used to collect any excess blood expelled with the syringe held upright and the plunger side down. Remove the needle and cap the syringe to ensure anaerobic conditions. Alternatively, many of the commercially available arterial blood gas kits come with an air bubble removal device (Filter-Pro) that allows the clinician to expel air bubbles from the sample and reduce potential exposure from the blood product.

Air in the sample will significantly increase Po_2 (mean increase, 11 mm Hg) after 20 minutes of storage, even if kept at 4°C. pH and Pco_2 are not significantly altered by air bubbles if the blood is stored at 4°C for 20 minutes and no significant deterioration has occurred.[23,38] If blood is stored at room temperature for longer than 20 minutes, Pco_2 will increase and the pH will decrease, probably as a result of leukocyte metabolism. In a stored sample, Po_2 varies to such an extent that the change is unpredictable for chemical interpretation at 30 minutes, regardless of the storage method. High leukocyte or platelet counts, such as those seen in leukemic patients, may shorten acceptable storage intervals.[39,40]

Thus, ABG samples should always be kept on ice and analyzed within 15 to 20 minutes. Samples that cannot be analyzed within this time frame should be considered unreliable.

PERCUTANEOUS TECHNIQUE FOR ARTERIAL CANNULATION

Direct Over-the-Needle Catheter Cannulation

Placement of an angiocatheter directly into an arterial lumen in a manner similar to placement of an intravenous catheter is the most practiced and simplest method, but it is not always successful because of technical difficulties. The only routine site for this technique is the radial artery. Use of a catheter over a guidewire as per the Seldinger technique is strongly advised at most other sites.

Take time to ensure proper alignment of the desired site. Delays, complications, and inability to successfully cannulate an artery often occur as a result of failure to properly prepare the desired site and involved limb. An important preparatory step is to ensure that the target limb is secured flat and not rotated; any rotation could result in the desired artery being shifted from the expected anatomic position and make it more difficult to cannulate. For example, to adequately prepare the radial artery, immobilize the wrist and hand in mild dorsiflexion with some padding for support underneath the wrist (Fig. 20-5, *step 1*). Prepare the skin with sterile technique. Inject local anesthetic with a 25-gauge or smaller needle and achieve

ULTRASOUND: Arterial Puncture

by Christine Butts, MD

Much as ultrasound can be used with great success in the placement of peripheral and central intravenous lines, it can also be used for the placement of arterial catheters.

The target vessel should first be identified with ultrasound. A high-frequency transducer (10 to 12 mHz) should be used to ensure proper resolution. The target vessel is typically easiest to identify in the transverse plane (with the indicator pointing toward the patient's right side) (Fig. 20-US1). Arteries usually appear as rounded structures with thick walls, as opposed to veins. Depending on the size of the vessel, pulsations may be noted. Application of color flow Doppler to a suspected artery will frequently demonstrate a pattern of pulsatile flow (Fig. 20-US2). Although arteries are usually thought to resist collapse from outside pressure (such as from applying pressure to the overlying transducer), smaller arteries in the periphery may show a degree of collapse. When seeking to identify the target vessel, multiple means of identification should be used before an attempt at cannulation.

Once the vessel has been identified, ultrasound can also be used to directly guide cannulation. Sterile technique should be maintained, particularly when accessing central arteries such as the femoral artery. A full description of the technique of ultrasound-guided venous access can be found in both the general ultrasound chapter (Chapter 66) and the central venous access chapter (Chapter 22) in this textbook. The principles of these procedures also apply to arterial cannulation, although a few points should be emphasized. When guiding access to the radial artery, a transverse approach is typically used because the vessel is small and difficult to visualize in the longitudinal approach. Additionally, it may be difficult to keep the image of the longitudinal vessel centered on the screen, especially when one physician is directing both the ultrasound and the needle.

Figure 20-US1 Placement of the transducer over the distal end of the arm in the transverse plane to localize the radial artery.

Figure 20-US2 Image of the radial artery with color flow. Applying color flow will enable the operator to correctly identify the artery.

sufficient infiltration to ensure a painless procedure. Subcutaneous infiltration of lidocaine or a similar anesthetic may also reduce vessel spasm at the time of arterial puncture.

Check the catheter assembly for proper movement and function. Alternatively, a 3-mL syringe with the plunger removed can be used as a blood reservoir. Advance the catheter toward the palpated artery at a comfortable angle for the operator, generally 30 to 45 degrees from the skin (see Fig. 20-5, *step 2*). Make a small incision with a No. 11 scalpel blade or a larger-bore needle to eliminate the problem of damage to the catheter from kinking on the skin. The tip of the needle is often perceived to pierce the artery, but successful puncture is confirmed by identifying a "flash" of arterial blood flow into the needle hub and reservoir. As the needle-catheter assembly advances through the skin toward the artery, the initial flash of arterial blood is obtained by the needle alone, which protrudes beyond the catheter. For this reason, the needle-catheter assembly should be lowered and advanced 2 mm forward to ensure that the tip of the catheter has cannulated the vessel, along with the needle (see Fig. 20-5, *step 3*). The position of the catheter within the vessel lumen is confirmed by continuous return of arterial blood. The catheter alone can

now be advanced with care over the needle into the artery (see Fig. 20-5, *step 4*). If the catheter fails to thread, it has not properly entered the vessel lumen and should not be forced to advance without confirmation of placement by active blood return.

When blood flow into the needle-catheter assembly has ceased, it may have pierced the backside of the arterial wall. This double-puncture method is useful for cannulating small vessels, yet it is not recommended as a routine procedure for inexperienced clinicians.[5] If double puncture has occurred and blood has ceased to flow into the collection reservoir, do not remove the entire needle-catheter assembly. Instead, simply retract the needle slightly to determine whether blood flow into the catheter can be reestablished. If blood flow occurs, gently advance the catheter. If not, slowly withdraw the catheter until pulsatile blood flow reappears and then advance the catheter into the artery. It is important for the clinician to be aware of whether the tip of the needle or the catheter is the leading edge within the vessel.[8]

Once the catheter is fully advanced into the vessel lumen, maintain occlusive pressure on the proximal end of the artery to limit blood loss, and then remove the needle (see Fig. 20-5,

ARTERIAL CANNULATION: OVER-THE-NEEDLE CATHETER TECHNIQUE

1

Immobilize the hand and wrist in mild dorsiflexion on a padded arm board. Prepare the skin with antiseptic, anesthetize, and apply a sterile drape.

2

Advance the needle into the artery at a 30° to 45° angle to the skin. Confirm arterial puncture by observing a flash into the needle hub.

3

Lower the angiocatheter and advance it 2 mm forward to ensure that the tip has cannulated the vessel. Confirm proper placement by observing continuous arterial blood return.

4

Carefully advance the catheter over the needle and into the artery. Do not force the catheter; if it fails to easily thread, it has not properly entered the vessel lumen. (See text for troubleshooting tips.)

5

Tamponade over the artery proximal to the tip of the catheter (to prevent blood loss), and remove the needle.

6

Attach the tubing from the pressure transducer to the catheter. Suture the catheter hub to the skin and cover with a sterile dressing, such as Tegaderm.

Figure 20-5 Arterial cannulation: over-the-needle catheter technique. Note that in this example the angiocatheter *does not have a safety mechanism* such as a retracting needle. This allows a syringe to be attached to the back of the hub as a blood reservoir. Such angiocatheters may be difficult to find in some institutions.

step 5). Next attach narrow-bore, low-compliance pressure tubing to the catheter (see Fig. 20-5, *step 6*). Apply an appropriate sterile dressing after the apparatus has been securely sutured to the wrist.

Occasionally, one will encounter difficulty advancing the catheter into the lumen. The "liquid stylet" method may aid further passage of the catheter.[41] Fill a 10-mL syringe with about 5-mL of sterile normal saline. Attach the syringe to the catheter hub, and aspirate 1 to 2 mL of blood to confirm intraluminal position. Then slowly inject the fluid from the syringe and advance the catheter behind the fluid wave.

Ultrasound guidance is now routinely used for both peripheral and central venous access and can also assist in arterial cannulation (see Ultrasound Box). When compared with the palpation technique, ultrasound-guided arterial cannulation significantly improves the likelihood of success on the first attempt.[42] With B-mode ultrasound, the targeted artery can be visualized in real-time by using a 7.5- to 10-MHz linear-array transducer. Differentiate the target artery from the adjacent vessel by its pulsatility and noncompressibility with mild pressure by the transducer. Use color Doppler to further assist in distinguishing between arteries and veins. Either transverse or longitudinal views can be applied during arterial cannulation, but the transverse view is often more useful in smaller arteries. Once the catheter has entered the artery and it is confirmed by blood flow, place the ultrasound transducer on the field to free up the nondominant hand.[42,43]

The number of attempts with additional arterial punctures increases the size of the developing hematoma and the real risk for vessel wall damage, thrombosis, and even loss of arterial flow through the vessel. Despite the added trauma, there is no reported increase in complications when both walls, rather than one, are punctured in a single cannulation attempt.[44-46]

Guidewire Techniques for Arterial Cannulation

A modified Seldinger technique can often rescue a failed direct cannulation attempt with an over-the-needle catheter (Fig. 20-6). If the catheter has been placed in the arterial

ARTERIAL CANNULATION: GUIDEWIRE TECHNIQUE

Prepare the wrist and insert the needle as described in Figure 20–5. Look for pulsatile blood return in the flash chamber.

Hold the catheter in place and remove the needle. Pulsatile blood should flow from the catheter. If not present, slowly back the catheter out, and observe for blood return.

Insert the guidewire through the catheter. It should advance freely and easily into the vessel. Do not force it.

Advance the catheter over the wire and into the artery. Remove the wire, attach the catheter hub to the transducer tubing, and secure it to the skin.

Figure 20-6 Arterial cannulation: guidewire technique.

lumen with blood return, pass a properly sized guidewire through the catheter into the artery. Advance the catheter fully into the vessel over the guidewire. The clinician is cautioned that stiffer guidewires, unlike most prepackaged ones, do not have a softer, more flexible end tip and that the vessel wall may be damaged or even perforated with excessive force. Alternatively, catheter sets are available with an attachable, catheter-contained, wire stylet that permits a modified Seldinger technique for placement of the catheter. The over-the-needle catheter follows the self-contained guidewire during cannulation. Numerous commercially available sets feature styles of guidewire and reservoir attachments that are different from an over-the-needle catheter assembly. Most resemble the Arrow Arterial Catheterization Kit (Arrow International, Inc., Reading, PA) (Fig. 20-7; also see Fig. 20-2). These kits are extremely practical for smaller vessels, especially the radial, brachial, and axillary arteries, and have excellent success rates for first-time placement. Although some authors have suggested that guidewire-based techniques will improve arterial cannulation success rates in certain patients,[47] it appears that success is more a function of operator experience and personal preference.[48]

Seldinger Technique

The Seldinger technique[6] for venipuncture is described in detail in Chapter 22. Overall success rates with the Seldinger, guidewire-directed technique are superior to those with direct arterial cannulation.[48] A few available kits are designed specifically for cannulation of larger arteries, but single-lumen venous catheters with guidewires may be used if catheter size and length are appropriate for specific arteries (see the following section for guidelines). The guidewire technique should be used initially for critical patients.

Place the needle percutaneously into the arterial lumen, as described previously. Then place a guidewire through the needle into the vessel lumen, and remove the needle. Thread the catheter over the wire, and pull the wire out. Although

ARTERIAL CANNULATION: ARROW ARTERIAL CATHETERIZATION KIT

Ensure that the actuating lever is fully retracted, and then insert the needle into the artery. Monitor for blood flashback in the hub of the needle to confirm intraarterial placement.

Stabilize the needle and advance the guidewire into the vessel by using the actuating lever. When the lever reaches the reference mark (*black arrow*) on the device, the wire begins to exit the needle.

After the wire is fully inserted, advance the entire assembly 1–2 mm farther into the vessel. Firmly hold the needle in position, and advance the catheter over the wire and into the vessel. A slight rotating motion may be helpful.

Remove the needle and guidewire assembly and attach the transducer tubing to the catheter hub. Use the wing clip (*arrow*) to suture the catheter to the skin, and then cover with a sterile dressing.

Figure 20-7 Arterial cannulation: Arrow Arterial Catheterization Kit.

most kits have vessel dilators, especially with larger catheter sizes, caution is advised. Dilate the tract only and not the artery to avoid unnecessary blood loss and excessive arterial injury.

Cutdown Technique for Arterial Cannulation

The cutdown technique is rarely used, but in certain circumstances it may be performed to obtain arterial access. With the increasing use of ultrasound-assisted catheter placement, this technique should seldom be required. Perform cannulation after direct visualization of the vessel. A cutdown can be performed on any artery but is most commonly reserved for distal lower limb arteries and, rarely, the brachial artery. After a site has been selected, prepare the overlying skin with an antiseptic solution. Using sterile technique, inject local anesthetic solution subcutaneously in a horizontal line 2 to 3 cm long and perpendicular to the artery. Omit this step if the patient is unconscious or otherwise anesthetized at the cutdown site.

Use a No. 10 or 15 scalpel blade to incise the skin along the anesthetic wheal. Spread the underlying tissues parallel to the artery with a mosquito hemostat. Palpate the pulse repeatedly throughout the procedure to ensure proper positioning. Once the surrounding soft tissue has been retracted and after exposing approximately 1 cm of the artery, isolate the artery by passing two silk sutures underneath it with the hemostat. Strip away only enough perivascular tissue to expose the artery. Perivascular tissue will help limit bleeding at the time of catheter removal. Introduce an over-the-needle catheter device, such as the kind used in the percutaneous method, and introduce it through the skin just distal to the incision. Advance it into the surgical site (Fig. 20-8).[41] Alternatively, use a modified Seldinger guidewire setup to catheterize the artery. Puncture the arterial wall with the tip of the needle, and thread the catheter into the vessel lumen. When this has been accomplished, remove the two silk sutures, which have been used only to control the vessel, and close the skin incision. Do not tie off the artery the way that a vein is tied off during a venous cutdown. Apply firm pressure, as used after arterial puncture, over the cutdown site. Separation of the soft tissues during the procedure may allow considerable hemorrhage into the tissue if pressure is not applied.

Local Puncture Site and Catheter Care

Once the catheter has been placed successfully, advance it until the hub is in contact with the skin. Secure the catheter by fastening it to the skin with suture material. Silk (2-0) or nylon (4-0) sutures provide the best anchoring. To accomplish this, take a moderate bite of skin with the needle, and tie a knot in the suture while leaving both tails of the suture long. Care should be taken to avoid pinching the skin too tightly. Tie the loose ends of the suture around the catheter at its hub. Then, after laying two ties, place a second set of knots on the back portion without occluding the lumen by constriction (Fig. 20-9).

Another option to secure these lines is to apply commercially available sutureless securement devices. According to one study, sutured lines are associated with a 10% rate of catheter-related bloodstream infection. In comparison, lines that were secured with a sutureless method had an infection rate of less than 1% and eliminated the potential for accidental needlestick from suturing.[49]

After tying the catheter in place, apply a drop of antibiotic ointment to the puncture site[50] and a self-adhesive dressing over the area. Further secure the catheter and its connecting tubing with sterile sponges and adhesive tape. Make sure that all tubing connections are tight and secure. If the tubing becomes disconnected inadvertently, the patient can exsanguinate rapidly.

Fluid-Pressurized Systems

When successful arterial cannulation has been performed, attach the catheter to a pressurized fluid-filled system. A three-way stopcock can be interposed between the patient and the transducer for blood gas sampling and to allow flushing of the system. Flushing can be periodic or continuous at a rate of 3 to 4 mL/hr through a continuous-flow device. Most institutions use normal saline in place of heparinized solution to maintain patency. Use of a heparinized flush solution in pressurized arterial lines may result in greater long-term accuracy of pressure monitoring, but no real difference in catheter blockage has been reported, and this approach avoids heparin-related complications such as drug incompatibility, thrombosis, local tissue damage, and hemorrhage.[51-55] For short-term setups as in the ED, saline is sufficient.

Blood samples are obtained easily from the arterial catheter system. Attach a syringe to the three-way stopcock and aspirate and discard the blood to clear the line. Studies examining the necessary discard volume of flushed blood solution have found considerable variation, depending on the volume of the system.[56,57] Short lengths of tubing between the catheter and the aspiration port minimize the necessary discard volume. For a tubing length of 91 cm (36 inches), aspirate 4

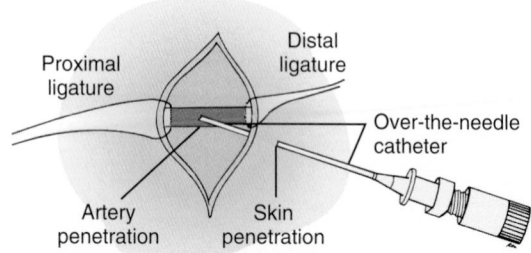

Figure 20-8 Placement of an arterial line using the cutdown technique. Note that the catheter enters the surgical wound percutaneously to minimize entry of bacteria into the healing wound and permit better stabilization of the catheter. Entry of the catheter into the vessel is more parallel to the vessel than illustrated. Ligatures are used only to *temporarily* isolate the artery and to control bleeding. *The artery should not be tied off.* The catheter is secured by suturing the hub to the skin.

Figure 20-9 A technique for securing a vascular catheter to adjacent skin.

to 5 mL[57]; for a tubing length of 213 cm (84 inches), aspirate 8 mL.[56] Attach a second syringe that has been heparinized, and aspirate 3 mL of blood to send for ABG analysis. If the blood is to be used for other tests, the second syringe does not need to be heparinized. Self-contained, nondetachable, blood sample–withdrawing systems allow less blood wasting for sampling. Flush the stopcock and line to avoid clotting.

SELECTION OF ARTERIES FOR CANNULATION

Radial and Ulnar

The radial artery is most frequently used for prolonged cannulation. Widespread collateral flow is present in the wrist because of two major palmar anastomoses known as arches (Fig. 20-10). The superficial palmar arch lies between the aponeurosis palmaris and the tendons of the flexor digitorum sublimis. The arch is formed mainly by the terminal ulnar artery and the superficial palmar branch of the radial artery. The other major communication of these two vessels, the deep palmar arch, is formed by connections of the terminal radial artery with the deep palmar branches of the ulnar artery.[58] Some collateral flow is almost always present at the wrist, with the deep arch alone being complete in 97% of 650 hand dissections at autopsy.[59] Despite these findings, Friedman[60] noted the absence of palpable ulnar pulses in 10 of 290 (3.4%) healthy children and young adults. Interestingly, this was always a bilateral finding. Radial pulses were present in all subjects, however.

Before attempting radial artery cannulation, one may assess the adequacy of collateral flow to the hand by performing a bedside examination. This examination was originally described by E. V. Allen in 1929[61] and is used to assess arterial stenosis in the hands of patients with thromboangiitis obliterans. The Allen test identifies patients at increased risk for ischemic complications from radial artery catheterization.

The procedure has seen many modifications[62,63] since originally being described in a cooperative patient. The modified Allen test is performed as follows: occlude both the radial and ulnar arteries with digital pressure and then ask the patient to tightly clench the fist repeatedly to exsanguinate the hand. Then open the hand and release the occlusion of the ulnar artery (Fig. 20-11). After 2 minutes, repeat the test in the same manner with release of the radial artery. Rubor should return rapidly to the hand following the release of pressure from either vessel.

An abnormal (positive) Allen test result, suggestive of inadequate collateralization, is defined as the continued presence of pallor 5 to 15 seconds after release of the artery.[6,26,63,64] If return of color takes longer than 5 to 10 seconds, do not

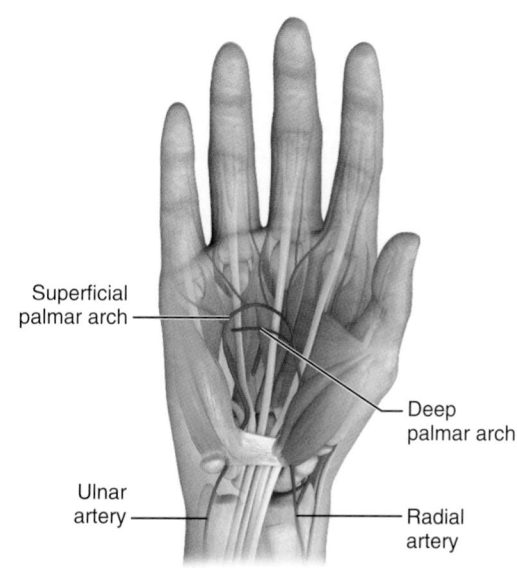

Figure 20-10 Arterial anatomy of the hand and wrist.

THE ALLEN TEST

1 Radial artery   Ulnar artery

Compress both the radial and ulnar arteries to occlude arterial flow, and instruct the patient to repeatedly make a tight fist to squeeze venous blood out of the hand. Alternatively, the hand may be squeezed first and then the arteries occluded.

2

Instruct the patient to relax the hand and extend the fingers. Carefully observe the hand—it should be blanched.

3

Release the ulnar artery and observe the hand for return of rubor, which signifies good flow in the ulnar artery. If filling does not occur within 5 to 10 seconds, radial artery cannulation should not be done. If brisk filling occurs, repeat the test with release of the radial artery to assess radial artery patency. If both the radial and ulnar arteries demonstrate patency, the wrist may be used for arterial cannulation.

Figure 20-11 Allen test. Before puncturing the radial artery for cannulation, it is important to identify a competent ulnar artery should injury to the radial artery occur. This is not generally required, nor standard, for a single arterial puncture. *(Adapted from Schwartz GR, ed.* Principles and Practice of Emergency Medicine. *Philadelphia: Saunders; 1978:354. Reproduced by permission.)*

perform radial artery puncture. Be careful to avoid overextension of the hand with wide separation of the digits, which may compress the palmar arches between fascial planes and yield a false-positive result.[65] Time permitting, performance of some variation of the Allen test is desirable before ulnar or radial puncture for prolonged cannulation. This test is not considered mandatory or standard for one-time radial artery puncture for blood gas sampling. Moreover, the utility of the Allen test is still questioned because of numerous reports of permanent ischemic sequelae after cannulation even after a normal Allen test result.[63,66,67] Notably, other studies have found no ischemic complications following radial artery catheterization and abnormal results on the Allen test.[45,68] Although there are no guarantees against digital ischemia after radial artery cannulation,[69] the finding of an abnormal Allen test result should be documented and lead one to search for an alternative site for the procedure.

At the wrist, the radial artery rests on the flexor digitorum superficialis, flexor pollicis longus, and pronator quadratus and against the radius.[59] Isolate the pulsation of the artery on the palmar surface of the wrist. The radial artery is more superficial as it moves closer to the wrist. In this location it provides a more consistent site for cannulation because of its fixation and decreased mobility. Dorsiflexing the wrist at about a 60-degree angle over a towel or sandbag and preferably fixing the wrist to an arm board will also considerably help isolate the artery. This degree of preparation should be considered standard when time for setup permits (see Fig. 20-5, step 1).[44,45]

Antegrade radial artery cannulation may be accomplished in infants and children when the radial arteries are obstructed and retrograde blood flow is observed during a failed cutdown attempt at standard retrograde arterial cannulation.[70] In addition, displacement of perivascular interstitial fluid in neonates and bright light make the course of the artery visible so that under direct vision, cannulation of the artery becomes as easy as venous cannulation.[71] Doppler ultrasound on selected patients with poor peripheral pulses may facilitate percutaneous radial artery cannulation and minimize the number of punctures needed for placement.[72]

The ulnar artery is seldom used because its smaller size makes it more difficult to puncture than the radial artery. At the wrist, the ulnar artery runs along the palmar margin of the flexor carpi ulnaris in the space between it and the flexor digitorum sublimis.[59] Use caution because the artery runs next to the ulnar nerve as both pass into the hand just radial to the pisiform bone. Minimize any potential injury by approaching the ulnar artery from the radial side.[73] Make the ulnar artery more accessible with dorsiflexion of the wrist.

Brachial

Although it appears safe for arterial puncture, the brachial artery does not have the anatomic benefit of the collateral circulation that is found in the wrist. The brachial artery begins as the continuation of the axillary artery and ends at the head of the radius, where it splits into the ulnar and radial arteries. The preferred puncture site of the brachial artery is in or just proximal to the antecubital fossa. In this region the artery lies on top of the brachialis muscle and enters the fossa underneath the bicipital aponeurosis with the median nerve on the medial side of the artery (Fig. 20-12). Both the radial and the axillary arteries are preferred over the brachial artery

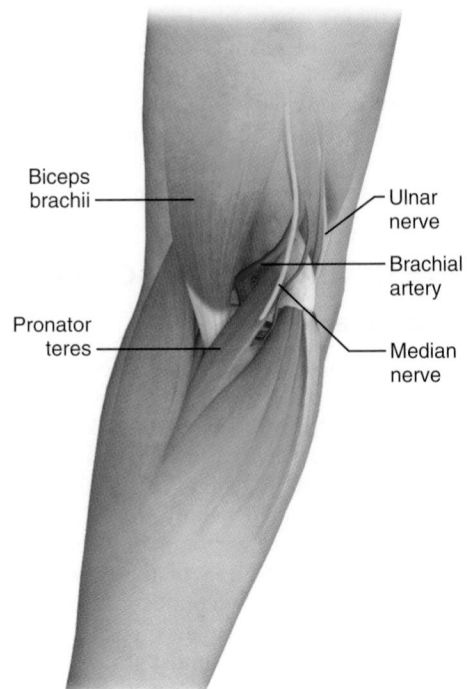

Figure 20-12 Brachial artery anatomy.

in the upper extremity. There is increased risk for ischemic complications from the reduced collateral circulation, as well as the need to maintain the arm in extension for puncture and for prolonged cannulation. Nonetheless, safe cannulation of the brachial artery has been demonstrated by some investigators.[74] Bazaral and coworkers[75] found only one minor thrombotic occurrence in more than 3000 brachial artery catheterizations over a 3-year period in cardiac surgery patients. A longer catheter (10 cm) is required for the brachial artery so that sufficient length is available to traverse the elbow joint.

Dorsalis Pedis

The dorsalis pedis artery continues from the anterior tibial artery and runs from approximately midway between the malleoli to the posterior end of the first metatarsal space, where it forms the dorsal metatarsal and deep plantar arteries. The lateral plantar artery, a branch of the posterior tibial artery, passes obliquely across the foot to the base of the fifth metatarsal. The plantar arch is completed at the point where the lateral plantar artery joins the deep plantar artery between the first and second metatarsals. On the dorsum of the foot, the dorsalis pedis artery lies in the subcutaneous tissue parallel to the extensor hallucis longus tendon and between it and the extensor digitorum longus (Fig. 20-13).[76]

Cannulate the artery in the midfoot region. Although this vessel is amenable to cutdown, the vascular anatomy of the foot is quite variable. This is of no consequence if a pulse can be palpated, but Huber,[77] in his dissection of 200 feet, noted that the dorsalis pedis artery was absent in 12% of patients. In 16% of patients the dorsalis pedis artery provides the main blood supply to the toes.[78] Although the dorsal pedis and posterior tibial arteries form similar collateral foot circulation as in the hand, the nature of advancing vascular disease makes

Figure 20-13 Dorsalis pedis artery anatomy.

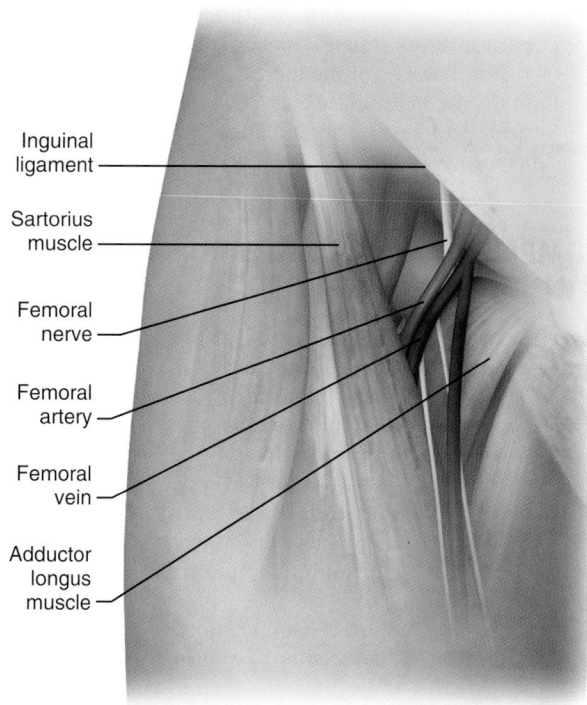

Figure 20-14 Femoral artery anatomy.

this a more difficult cannulation, with higher complication rates than in the wrist. This site has its major utility in pediatric monitoring cases. Attempts to predetermine collateral flow with a modified Allen test using the posterior tibial and dorsalis pedis arteries is not as easily performed in the foot as in the hand, nor are there good data to prove its validity. Monitoring problems also exist with this artery. The pressure wave obtained with an electronic transducer attached to the dorsalis pedis artery will be 5 to 20 mm Hg higher than that of the radial artery and, in addition, will be delayed by 0.1 to 0.2 second.[76]

Femoral

The femoral artery is the second most commonly used vessel for arterial cannulation. Based on its ease of cannulation and low record of complications, it has been called the vessel of choice for arterial access.[79-81] Along with the axillary artery, the femoral artery more closely resembles aortic pressure waveforms than those from any other peripheral site.[7] The femoral artery is the direct continuation of the iliac artery and enters the thigh after passing below the inguinal ligament. Arterial puncture must always occur distal to the ligament to prevent uncontrolled hemorrhage into the pelvis or peritoneum.[82] The artery may be palpable easily midway between the public symphysis and the anterior superior iliac spine. The advantage of cannulating the artery at a site just distal to the inguinal ligament is that the artery can be compressed against the femoral head. Cannulation becomes more difficult the more distal the puncture site is from the inguinal ligament because the femoral artery splits into the superficial femoral and the deep femoral arteries. These arteries, especially the deep femoral, can be challenging to compress if bleeding needs to be controlled. One method of locating an appropriate arterial puncture site is to place the thumb and fifth finger on the pubis symphysis and the anterior iliac spine and locate the artery underneath the middle knuckle. When puncturing this vessel, be careful to avoid the femoral nerve and vein, which form the lateral and medial borders, respectively (Fig. 20-14).

A longer, larger-diameter catheter is required for accurate monitoring of the femoral artery because of the relatively greater depth at which it lies and its size. Only the Seldinger technique is recommended for this site, which enables placement of a 15- to 20-cm plastic catheter for prolonged monitoring. Avoid using catheter-through-the-needle or over-the-needle catheter devices because of the vessel's distance beneath the skin. Leakage around the catheter can occur with catheter-through-the-needle or over-the-needle catheter devices as a result of the high arterial pressure and the loose fit of the cannula in the hole in the vessel wall. Regardless of the device used, enter the skin with the needle at an angle of about 45 degrees instead of the usual 15 to 20 degrees.

The extremely large ratio of arterial diameter to catheter diameter is thought to reduce the incidence of thrombosis, particularly total occlusion. However, occlusion has been reported with femoral cannulation for monitoring purposes.[83] A commonly perceived disadvantage of this site is the increased possibility of bacterial contamination because of its proximity to the warm, moist groin and perineum; however, no studies have confirmed this hypothesis.[84] The femoral area is inconvenient for any patient who is awake and mobile or for a patient who is able to sit in a chair. If the patient is that mobile, reconsider the risk-benefit ratio of invasive monitoring. Despite theoretical difficulties, some hospitals use femoral arterial lines almost exclusively, and the ICU nursing staff is often more comfortable caring for these lines than those at other sites.

Umbilical and Temporal

In neonates, arterial access can be accomplished for a short time through the umbilical artery (see Chapter 19). After this artery closes, the temporal artery provides a safe alternative. Prian described use of the temporal artery and noted its accessibility and lack of clinical sequelae if it undergoes thrombosis.[85] Use the cutdown method with a 22-gauge catheter after the artery's course has been traced with an ultrasonic flow detector. Because of the increasing accuracy of ear oximeters and the use of capillary blood gas samples for determination of pH, prolonged arterial cannulation will become less frequent during infant care.

COMPLICATIONS OF ARTERIAL CANNULATION

Arterial cannulation is safe if care is taken to avoid complications. Most can be avoided by adhering to a few simple principles. Reported clinical sequelae of arterial puncture and cannulation range from simple hematomas to life-threatening infections and exsanguination. In addition, ischemia, arteriovenous fistula, and pseudoaneurysm formation are possible. The incidence of complications varies with the site selected, the method of cannulation, and the clinician's level of skill and experience. Early detection of complications is greatly aided by enhanced vigilance.

It is difficult to compare complication rates at various sites because most published studies have primarily used only the radial artery. No studies have compared the approach and complication rates of arterial catheters in the ED with those placed in the ICU or operating room. In a large study spanning 24 months, 2119 ICU patients had arterial catheters placed at admission: 52% at the radial site and 45% at the femoral site. The most common complication was vascular insufficiency (4%), followed by bleeding (2.1%) and infection (0.6%). No difference was reported in infection rates at femoral versus radial sites.[86] There are reports of complications from arterial puncture for procedures unrelated to cannulation, such as arteriography or simple puncture for blood sampling as routinely performed in the ED. In a study of 2400 consecutive cardiac catheterizations over a 12-month period, complications occurred in 1.6% of patients, including 17 needing vascular repair and 28 requiring transfusion.[87]

Hematoma formation at the puncture site is common. Zorab reported this complication in 50% of all catheterizations.[88] Bruising was of minimal clinical significance in this report, but leakage can be dangerous when it occurs around the catheter or from the puncture site after the catheter is removed (Fig. 20-15). Compression neuropathies requiring surgical decompression have been reported after arterial puncture secondary to hematoma formation.[14,89,90] The large amount of soft tissue surrounding the femoral artery makes bleeding in this area difficult to control. Large hematomas are not uncommon after femoral artery catheterization; indeed, Soderstrom and colleagues[80] reported two cases of bleeding that required transfusion after femoral puncture. Though uncommon, a clinician should be aware of the potential development of a retroperitoneal hematoma, a morbid complication, following femoral artery cannulation. Suspect this complication in patients in whom hypovolemic shock with a falling hematocrit develops following the procedure.[91,92] Another serious complication is the formation of a pseudoaneurysm as the walls of the punctured artery fail to seal properly. Although most pseudoaneurysms can be managed conservatively, they are susceptible to both rupture and infection. Several treatment options are now available, and identification of a pseudoaneurysm should prompt referral to a vascular surgeon.[93,94] More commonly, hematomas are painful,

Figure 20-15 Right groin hemorrhage with resulting hematoma. The injury resulted from a failed attempt to place a right femoral artery catheter via the Seldinger technique. A large femoral hematoma is pictured here 3 days after iatrogenic injury.

slow to resolve, and prone to infection. Multiple-site punctures and inadequate pressure applied for insufficient time account for most hematomas. Multiple punctures can be avoided in most instances by experienced operators and the use ultrasound-aided techniques.

Thrombotic occlusion after radial arterial cannulation occurs in nearly 50% of infants and small children; however, ischemia from occlusion is rare because of collateral blood supply from the ulnar artery.[95] Insertion sites closest to the bend of the wrist increase the chance of maintaining patency. Nonpatency is four times more likely with insertion at sites 3 cm or more proximal to the bend in the wrist.[96] Slogoff and associates[68] described 1700 cardiovascular surgery patients who underwent radial artery cannulation without any long-term ischemic complications despite evidence of radial artery occlusion after decannulation in more than 25% of the patients. Serious complications after radial artery cannulation are extremely rare in the absence of contributing factors such as preexisting vasospastic arterial disease, previous arterial injury, protracted shock, high-dose vasopressor administration, prolonged cannulation, or infection.[67,97]

Prevention of bleeding complications can be accomplished with frequent careful inspection of the puncture site and the use of prolonged compression after removal of the catheter or needle. Maintain firm pressure for 10 minutes or longer after removing a peripheral artery catheter and longer after femoral cannulation or if the patient has received anticoagulants. Five minutes of pressure is sufficient after puncture for a blood gas sample in an individual with normal coagulation. Exsanguination may occur if the arterial line apparatus becomes disconnected. This is more common in an obtunded or combative patient, and restraints are often required for patients with indwelling arterial cannulas. Exsanguination should not occur if tight connections are maintained throughout the system and if frequent, careful inspections of both the circuit and the patient are made.

Meticulous attention to aseptic technique is necessary during insertion and catheter maintenance to minimize the risk for catheter-related infections.[98,99] Serious infections rarely complicate arterial cannulation. Simple interventions can reduce the risk for serious catheter-related infection. Evidence supports the use of full-barrier precautions during catheter insertion, specialized nursing care, and newer-generation catheters with antiseptic hubs or antimicrobial agent–impregnated catheters.[98] The incidence of catheter-related infections increases with prolonged cannulation.[84] Catheters placed via sterile technique have an extremely low rate of infection in the first 96 hours after placement. Catheters changed over a guidewire every 96 hours have an infection rate of about 10% at the radial and femoral sites.[81]

Most infections begin locally at the puncture site and remain localized, although systemic sepsis has been reported.[97] The radial and femoral sites have a similar incidence of complications, but axillary cannulation seems to have a much higher incidence of infection (although no large studies of cannulation at this site exist).[85,100] Arterial cannulas are more prone than other vascular catheters to infectious complications. Many mechanisms have been proposed for this increased incidence.[99,101] The arterial pressure–monitoring system usually consists of a long column of fairly stagnant fluid and is subject to frequent manipulation. Stamm and coworkers[100] found that patients were at greater risk for systemic infection if they had an arterial line and required frequent blood gas determinations than if they had the cannula alone. The sampling stopcock is a site of frequent bacterial contamination.

The risk for infection also increases as the duration of cannulation is prolonged. Older studies recommend that catheters be changed after 4 days if continued monitoring is necessary.[100,101] In addition, Makai and Hassemer[101] recommended changing the entire fluid-filled system, including the transducer chamber domes and continuous flow devices, every 48 hours. However, the risk for noninfectious complications increases with more frequent catheter and site changes. Therefore, daily evaluation of the site is advised, and catheter change should not be mandatory until 7 to 8 days if the site remains clean.

Shinozaki and colleagues[102] demonstrated a marked reduction in equipment contamination when the continuous flush device was located just distal to the transducer, as opposed to closer to the three-way stopcock used for sampling. This setup reduces the length of the static column of fluid between the sampling stopcock and the transducer. As mentioned previously, a drop of iodophor or antibiotic ointment applied to the puncture site decreases the incidence of local wound infection.[51] This technique has drawn a great deal of criticism, however. The current standard is a clean, nonocclusive, dry dressing. An antibiotic- or silver-impregnated catheter is recommended for long-term placement.

Thrombosis of the vessel in which the cannula is placed is another frequently encountered problem. The incidence of thrombosis varies with the method used to determine the presence of clots. Bedford and Wollman[25] found a greater than 40% occlusion rate when radial artery catheters were left in place for longer than 20 hours. All these occluded vessels eventually recanalized. Angiographic studies show deposition of fibrin on 100% of catheters left in place for longer than 1 day, although clinical evidence of ischemia secondary to occlusion by such thrombi is seen in less than 1% of cases in most studies.[103] Most reports of nonangiographic catheterization involve the radial artery. Therefore, it is difficult to compare the incidence of thrombosis at other sites, although during the 176 femoral catheterizations reported by Soderstrom and colleagues[80] and Ersoz and associates,[104] dorsalis

pedis pulses were decreased in only two patients and no clinical signs of ischemia were noted. Larger catheter sizes, trauma during cannulation, and the presence of atherosclerosis have all been postulated to increase the incidence of thrombosis; however, conflicting studies abound.

Arterial spasm after puncture (usually following multiple attempts) can predispose to thrombus formation and can even lead to ischemic changes without fibrin deposition. Successful reversal of spasm with intraarterial lidocaine, reserpine, and phentolamine has been reported, but no reliable studies of their efficacy in this clinical situation have been published.[105]

Thrombosis can be minimized by decreasing the duration of catheterization and proper flushing. Surgical embolectomy or thrombectomy is rarely required because the smaller vessels that are most likely to occlude usually have good collateral circulation. The larger femoral artery, which has poor collateralization, rarely occludes with catheterization when used for monitoring purposes.

Thrombosis can result in occlusion of the catheter. Time until occlusion of radial and femoral artery catheters has been compared. Radial cannulas became occluded at an average of 3.8 days, whereas femoral cannulas became occluded after 7.3 days.[81] The importance of this comparison is minimal if the clinician follows infection prophylaxis guidelines and changes arterial catheters after 4 days.

A few less common complications are easily prevented. One that occurs only with the percutaneous catheter-through-the-needle method is catheter embolization. Once the catheter has been placed through the needle, it should never be pulled back because the end of the catheter may be sheared off by the sharp needle bevel. If this complication occurs, surgical removal of the tip of the catheter is necessary.

Skin necrosis is a complication of radial artery cannulation that involves an area of the volar surface of the forearm proximal to the cannula.[106,107] Wyatt and colleagues[108] believed this to be secondary to the poor blood supply in this area and thought that proper technique would decrease the incidence of necrosis.

One feared complication of indwelling radial and brachial arterial catheters is the occurrence of a cerebrovascular accident secondary to embolization from flushing of the catheters.[27,106] As little as 3 to 12 mL of flush solution has been shown to reflux to the junction of the subclavian and vertebral arteries.[80] A fatality caused by air embolism from a radial artery catheter has been reported and was re-created in a primate model.[109] Although these animals were much smaller (7 kg) than an adult human, as little as 2.5 mL of air introduced at a relatively low flush rate was found to embolize in retrograde fashion to the brain. Cerebral embolization can be prevented with the use of continuous flush systems (3 mL/hr) and by ensuring the integrity of the tubing and transducer systems to prevent entry of air. In addition, small volumes (<2 mL) of intermittent flush solution should be used.

Complication rates also vary according to the method of arterial cannulation. Mortensen[110] studied the three main techniques (discussed earlier in "Techniques"), but unfortunately, most of his arterial cannulations were for angiographic purposes. The complications associated with prolonged cannulation time are therefore underrepresented. In Mortensen's series,[110] cutdown arteriotomy exhibited the lowest incidence of complications (7.7%), whereas the Seldinger technique had a 17.7% incidence of complications. The complication rate with percutaneous cannulation was 11.3%. False passage of the guidewire, the catheter, or both was associated with increased intimal damage and complications. It is imperative that the wire or catheter be advanced only if no resistance is met.

Once the monitoring system is set up, manipulate it as little as possible. Perform any handling with aseptic technique. Change the tubing and other fluid-filled devices every 48 hours, and insert catheters into a vessel that provides the largest vessel-to-catheter ratio as possible.

If these principles are followed and the patient and system are carefully inspected at frequent intervals, complications of arterial puncture and cannulation can be minimized.

INTERPRETATION

An indwelling arterial catheter provides continuous blood pressure monitoring. The trend of a patient's pressure facilitates assessment of the effect of various therapeutic interventions. The absolute systolic and diastolic pressure measured will vary at different catheter sites, with higher peak systolic pressure measured at the periphery. The pressure will also be higher when measured at the distal end of the lower limb.[30,80] A wide variance between direct arterial pressure and the pressure measured with a standard pneumatic cuff will always exist in some patients. Oscillometric blood pressure measurement can significantly underestimate arterial blood pressure.[111] For this reason, regularly compare a cuff pressure with that obtained via invasive monitoring. Moreover, a change in their relationship may be the first indication of difficulty with the direct measuring system.

Waveform analysis may also provide an early indication of thrombosis in the arterial catheter. Many variables affect the waveform, including cardiac valvular disease and arteriosclerosis.[112] Waveforms may vary tremendously among patients, but after an adequate monitoring system has been established, a change in an individual's pressure wave is usually indicative of thrombosis or a malfunction in the monitoring system. A change in waveform may also indicate a change in the patient's cardiovascular status, such as a papillary muscle rupture. Before making a therapeutic decision based on an electronically generated number, recheck the patient's blood pressure with a pneumatic cuff. This device is less fallible than the electromechanical system.

Radial systolic arterial pressure poorly estimates the actual ascending aortic pressure, with more than 50% of cases reporting a difference in values of 10 to 35 mm Hg. Mean arterial pressure and diastolic pressure, in contrast, are highly accurate with greater than 90% of the values being within 3 mm Hg of aortic values.[113] Longer catheters have also been used successfully from radial sites to more accurately reflect central aortic pressure for cardiac surgery patients.[114]

An indwelling arterial cannula can provide valuable information about the hemodynamic status of a patient (through continuous pressure monitoring) and about the patient's respiratory and metabolic status (through intermittent sampling for ABG analysis and other blood tests). The Pco_2 and pH of the blood can be used to define four major groups of metabolic derangement: respiratory acidosis or alkalosis and metabolic acidosis or alkalosis. Rarely will a disorder be strictly classified into one of these groups; however, a simple chart such as that provided in the Appendix helps determine the relative effects of metabolic and respiratory influence on blood pH. (See also discussion in Appendix 1.)

Adequacy of blood oxygenation can be determined from the measured Po_2 of arterial blood and the known concentration of oxygen that the patient is inspiring. To avoid iatrogenic complications of intensive care, one must be absolutely certain that the data are from an arterial sample that has been properly analyzed before basing one's treatment decisions on the numbers obtained. Not uncommonly, a venous sample is interpreted as though it were arterial. Furthermore, false readings may result if the sample is not free of air bubbles, not promptly chilled, or not analyzed within 20 to 30 minutes. Though still controversial, blood gas values that are not corrected for body temperature appear to be more appropriate for guiding therapy in hypothermic patients.[115,116]

CONCLUSION

As intensive care knowledge and technology grow and develop, cannulation of the arterial system may decrease in frequency. Oximeters can determine the quality of blood oxygenation transcutaneously and are becoming more accurate and sophisticated. Electronic sphygmomanometers are being refined for continuous indirect blood pressure monitoring. As these devices improve and noninvasive sampling methods for clinically relevant electrolytes and physiologic markers are refined, the indwelling arterial cannula may in time become considered overly invasive. Despite improvements in noninvasive monitoring devices, the current need for frequent blood sampling for chemical and hematologic analysis remains an indication for its use in selected critically ill patients. Overzealous blood gas analysis may lead to iatrogenic anemia in the ICU. Multiple reports have documented the advantages of limiting frequent blood sampling.[117-119]

Arterial puncture and cannulation are invaluable aids to the emergency and critical care clinician. Long-term catheterization is a safe procedure when the catheter is placed, maintained, and removed with care. The radial artery is the most favored location for puncture, but as more experience is gained and reported with femoral artery catheterization, the latter may become a more frequently used site. Selection of either site is associated with a low complication rate and should be determined by the skill of the clinician, the nursing team, and the relative convenience and comfort of the patient. Ultrasound guidance for arterial catheter placement is rapidly becoming the standard and should be considered in every instance to reduce the need for multiple puncture attempts.

Acknowledgment

The author would like to acknowledge the work of Drs. Dave Milzman and Tim Janchar, who were the authors of this chapter in the previous edition.

References are available at www.expertconsult.com

CHAPTER 21

Peripheral Intravenous Access

Shan W. Liu and Richard D. Zane

INTRODUCTION

Intravenous (IV) access is a mainstay of modern medicine. IV cannulation is a procedure performed by a wide array of health care professionals, including physicians, nurses, physician assistants, phlebotomists, and emergency medical technicians. In the emergency department (ED), uncomplicated peripheral venous access is usually secured by a nurse or technician. In the United States, more than 25 million patients have peripheral IV catheters placed each year as vascular access for the administration of medications and fluids and sampling of blood for analysis. IV access can usually be accomplished in less than 5 minutes.[1-4] Despite their growing number, dedicated IV teams are very costly and not always cost-effective.[5,6] Moreover, in the ED setting multiple providers may be called on to obtain IV access, thus making it an essential skill for both emergency physicians and nurses to master. Subtleties in technique are important and can be improved with practice; this is why some providers are able to place IV lines in even the most challenging situations.

HISTORICAL PERSPECTIVE

Bloodletting, or bleeding, dates to the time of Hippocrates. The ancient technique consisted of tying a bandage around the arm to distend the forearm veins, opening a vein with a sharp knife, and collecting the blood into a basin. In the Middle Ages this was performed by barber-surgeons. In 1656, Sir Christopher Wren injected opium into dogs intravenously with a quill and bladder, thereby becoming the father of modern IV therapy.[7] Blood transfusions also date back to the mid-1600s. The French physician Jean Denis is credited with the first successful transfusion by giving lamb's blood to a 15-year-old boy.[8,9]

Originally, 16- to 18-gauge indwelling steel needles were used for IV infusions. In the 1950s the Rochester needle was introduced, which was a resinous catheter on the outside of a steel introducer needle. Because of increased comfort and mobility, plastic catheters have replaced indwelling metal needles and are now almost universal.[7,10]

INDICATIONS AND CONTRAINDICATIONS

Obtaining timely and adequate vascular access is a major priority during any resuscitation. In patients with normal perfusion, differences in delivery times for injections centrally versus peripherally are minimal—within seconds.[11] During cardiopulmonary resuscitation (CPR), however, medications have been shown to reach the central circulation faster with central access than with peripheral venous access.[12] A change in outcome, though, has not been demonstrated with the central administration of advanced cardiac life support drugs;

Peripheral Intravenous Access

Indications	Contraindications	Complications	
Venous blood sampling	Extremity with significant edema, burns, sclerosis, phlebitis, or thrombosis	*Early*	*Late*
Intravenous fluid infusion		Bruising	Phlebitis
Intravenous medication infusion	Ipsilateral radical mastectomy or fistula	Infiltration	Infection
Blood transfusion	Overlying cellulitis	Air embolism	Nerve damage
Intravenous contrast infusion			Thrombosis

Equipment

Review Box 21-1 Peripheral intravenous access: indications, contraindications, complications, and equipment.

hence, peripheral IV cannulation is the procedure of choice even during CPR because of the speed, ease, and safety with which it can be accomplished. In less critically ill patients, the role of IV therapy is more often debated and access is ultimately unnecessary in a large proportion of patients in whom it is obtained.[13] In broad terms, IV access or therapy is needed in patients for whom IV medications are required or when oral therapy is *inadequate* (e.g., severe shock states), *contraindicated* (e.g., surgical emergencies), or *impossible* (e.g., intractable vomiting).

Saline or heparin locks are preferable when IV medications are needed and there are limited foreseeable fluid requirements. Saline locks cost less than a full IV fluid and tubing assembly and are especially helpful when vascular access is needed suddenly.[14,15] Access to the catheter requires irrigation with a separate syringe and flush.

A peripheral IV central catheter (PICC) shares the attributes of both central and peripheral venous IV lines (see Chapter 24). A PICC is composed of a thin tube of biocompatible material with an attachment hub. It is inserted percutaneously, under ultrasound guidance by a dedicated PICC team, into a peripheral vein and then advanced into a large central vein, followed by radiographic confirmation of placement. PICCs are suitable for long-term vascular access for blood sampling, infusion of antibiotics and hyperosmolar solutions such as total parenteral nutrition, and infusion of certain chemotherapeutic agents. Insert a PICC line as soon as long-term access is anticipated.[3]

Peripheral IV lines should not be placed in extremities with massive edema, burns, sclerosis, phlebitis, or thrombosis due to risk for extravasation or suboptimal volume flow. When practical, avoid placing an IV line in extremities on the same side as radical mastectomies, though they can be used when an urgent condition exists and other peripheral access is not possible. When feasible, cannulation at infected sites, such as through an area of cellulitis, as well on extremities with shunts or fistulas, should be avoided because it may cause bacteremia or thrombosis. If possible, do not cannulate a vein over or distal to a recent fracture site on an extremity (Fig. 21-1). Veins that drain from an area affected by trauma or major vascular disruption (e.g., distal to a ruptured aorta) are also suboptimal because fluid or medications may not be delivered to the circulatory system.

Figure 21-1 Do not place peripheral intravenous (IV) access (*long arrow*) near or distal to a fracture in an extremity (*short arrow*). In this case an IV line for pain medication was placed before obtaining the radiograph. The scaphoid fracture was not suspected and the opposite arm had difficult access.

Blood samples for laboratory analysis are usually drawn before IV cannulation to avoid contamination with IV fluid or medication. However, studies have shown that accurate basic electrolyte and hematologic values can be obtained with peripheral IV lines when infusions are shut off for at least 2 minutes, at least 5 mL of blood is wasted, and all tubes are filled to avoid inaccurate bicarbonate readings.[16-18] By adopting this technique, one can reduce the number of peripheral needlesticks, minimize trauma or sclerosis of the vein, and improve patient satisfaction.

ULTRASOUND GUIDANCE AND TRANSILLUMINATION

Though more commonly used with central venous access, ultrasound can also assist in the placement of peripheral lines. For IV placements that have been designated "difficult" after a certain number of attempts by nursing staff, use of ultrasound guidance increases the success rate and decreases the number of attempts necessary for successful cannulation in both adult and pediatric patients.[19-22] One recent prospective randomized control study, however, did not show a benefit; conflicting evidence may ultimately stem from differences in the experience of ultrasound operators.[23] The caliber of the vein identified on ultrasound is predictive of its ability to be cannulated. If no vessel is identified, cannulation is not usually possible.[24,25] An additional issue with ultrasound-guided peripheral IV lines is their longevity. One study has brought attention to the high premature failure rate of ultrasound-guided peripheral lines.[26] This is probably related to the depth of the veins being cannulated, the length and type of catheter used, and the angle of the catheter through soft tissue.

Other devices transilluminate the veins to increase their visibility, especially in infants. Although little evidence is available to evaluate their utility, such devices, though not routinely available, can be useful, especially in departments with a large pediatric population. As emergency providers become more comfortable with these advancing technologies, ultrasound-guided or illumination-assisted insertion of peripheral lines will probably increase.

ANATOMY

The success of cannulation depends on familiarity with the vascular anatomy of the extremities. In the upper extremity, the veins of the hands are drained by the metacarpal and dorsal veins, which connect to form the dorsal venous arch (Fig. 21-2). These sites are excellent for IV therapy and comfortably accommodate 22- and 20-gauge catheters. The venous supply of the wrist and forearm consists of the basilic vein, which courses along the ulnar portion of the posterior aspect of the forearm. It is often ignored because of its location but can easily be accessed if the patient's forearm is flexed and the clinician stands at the head of the patient.[27] On the radial side of the forearm, the cephalic is best known as the "intern vein." Readily accessible, this vein can accommodate 22- to 16-gauge catheters. The median veins of the forearm course through the middle of the forearm, and the accessory cephalic veins on the radial aspect of the forearm are easily stabilized and accessible.

The antecubital veins consist of the medial cubital, basilic, and cephalic veins, and these veins are often selected for

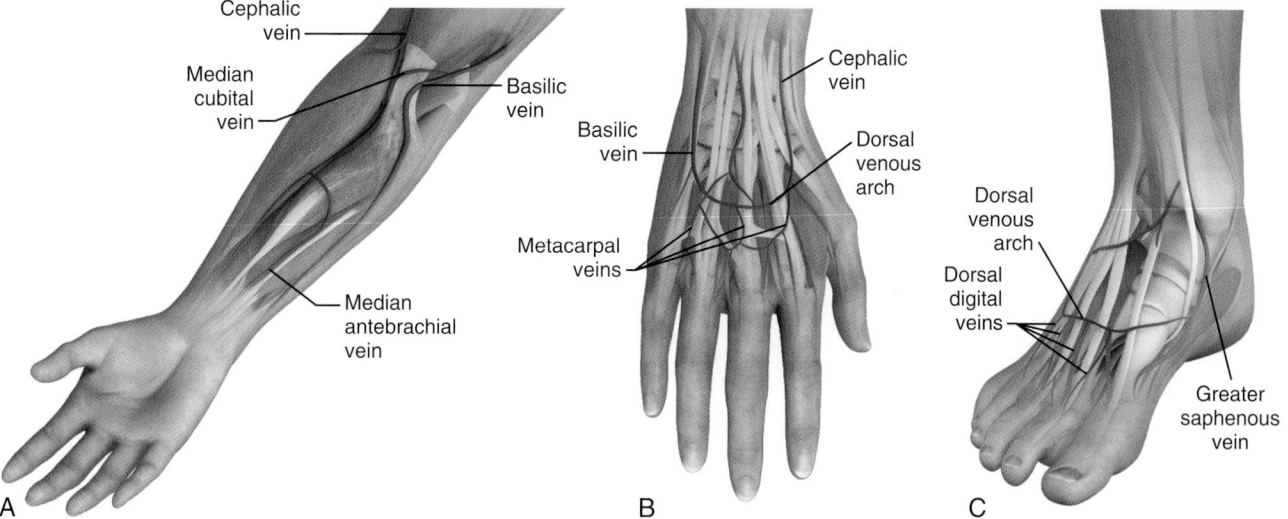

Figure 21-2 Anatomy of extremity veins for peripheral intravenous cannulation.

catheters or blood drawing. IV placement here is easy, but mobility of the arm is restricted once the catheter is in place. The larger veins above the antecubital space, the cephalic and basilic veins, are often more difficult to see but can be accessed without difficulty if necessary.

The relevant lower extremity venous anatomy starts with the dorsal digital veins, which become the dorsal metatarsal veins and form the dorsal venous arch. The arch ultimately splits into the great saphenous vein, which travels up the medial aspect of the ankle, and the small saphenous vein, which courses laterally up the opposite side. These are the vascular structures most easily accessible for IV therapy.

The external jugular vein is formed below the ear and behind the angle of the mandible (Fig. 21-3). It then passes downward and obliquely across the sternocleidomastoid and under the middle of the clavicle to join the subclavian vein. It is important to note the presence of valves in the external jugular, usually about 4 cm above the clavicle, because they can significantly impede IV function.[28]

PREPARATION

Safety

Universal precautions must be applied to all patients, especially in emergency care settings, in which the risk for exposure to blood is increased and the infection status of patients is largely unknown.[29] One study showed that 11% of all hospital IV catheter injuries to health care workers occurred in the ED.[30] Newer catheter devices have emerged that prevent inadvertent needle injuries (Fig. 21-4). The Protectiv IV Catheter Safety System has a protective sleeve that encases the sharp stylet as it is retracted from the catheter. The needle of the Insyte Autoguard Shielded IV Catheter is instantly encased inside a tamper-resistant safety barrel by pressing an activation button. The Saf-T-Intima IV catheter, Punctur-Guard Safety Winged Set, Vacutainer Safety-Lok, Shamrock safety winged needle, and Angel Wing Safety Needle systems are all types of winged safety devices with shields that advance over the needle to prevent exposure of the needle.[7]

Figure 21-3 External jugular anatomy. *SCM*, sternocleidomastoid.

Figure 21-4 Intravenous catheter safety device. When the activation button is depressed (*arrow*), the spring is released and the needle is retracted into the safety barrel.

Figure 21-5 Various gauges of intravenous catheters. Needles are sized according to gauge, from large to small (14 to 24 gauge).

Choosing the Catheter Gauge

The specific gauge of catheter to use depends on the clinical scenario (Fig. 21-5). The narrowest catheter typically used in adults is a 22 gauge, which is sufficient for the routine administration of maintenance fluids and antibiotics. A 20 or 18 gauge is necessary for the administration of blood products, and a 16-gauge needle is preferred in resuscitation settings when large amounts of fluid must be given quickly.[27] A second IV line at a different location allows additional IV therapy and also acts as a backup line in critical resuscitations. An 18-gauge catheter in the antecubital fossa is the standard device for IV contrast–enhanced computed tomography (CT) studies such as pulmonary CT angiogram.

Appropriate Site

Site selection depends largely on the expected duration of IV therapy, the patient's activity level, and the condition of the extremities. When choosing a location to initiate IV access, the best place to start is the hand and then advance cephalad as necessary. Hand veins are appropriate for 22-gauge catheters. Cephalic, accessory, or basilic veins are ideal for larger-bore IV lines. Avoid veins that are not resilient and feel hard or cordlike because they are often thrombosed.[7] Deep, percutaneous antecubital venipuncture and external jugular vein cannulation are also options in patients with difficult veins or those who may need IV access quickly.[7] The lower extremities veins can also be useful locations, especially in pediatric patients. In patients who have undergone radical mastectomy, avoid the arm on the same side as the surgery because circulation may be impaired, flow may be affected, and edema and other complications such as thrombosis could result.[7,22] Scalp veins are commonly used in neonates.[3,31]

Adjuncts for Finding a Vein

Patients often have nonvisible and nonpalpable veins. A common method of increasing venous distention is to ask patients to open and close their fist. Lowering the arm below the level of the heart can also increase venous distention. Light tapping can likewise be effective, although heavy tapping may cause the vein to spasm. If these methods are inadequate, heat packs can be applied for 10 to 20 minutes to increase venous engorgement. This is particularly useful in the pediatric population.[7]

Nitroglycerin ointment applied to the hands of patients with small-caliber veins has been shown to increase the diameter of the vein by two to six times and increase the rate of successful first-attempt cannulation. Once the tourniquet is applied to the wrist, a quarter inch of 2% nitroglycerin is applied to a 2.5-cm^2 area, left on for 2 minutes, and then rubbed off.[32] Nitroglycerin has been found to be useful and safe in the pediatric population as well.[33] This technique is contraindicated in hypotensive patients.

In the late 1980s, several small studies demonstrated the potential use of a venous distention device—a cardboard mailing tube that was placed over the forearm with a sealed bulb at one end that would cause a vacuum within the tube. Of the patients predetermined to be difficult to access, 90% were cannulated when this device was used. Reported complications were few and included petechiae and discomfort.[34,35]

Anesthesia

Though somewhat time-consuming, local anesthesia at the site should be considered part of routine care. Local anesthesia significantly decreases pain before cannulation.[36-38] Anesthetics such as lidocaine or bupivacaine may be instilled just beneath the skin at the site of planned cannulation through a tuberculin (1-mL) syringe equipped with a 27- or smaller-gauge needle. Adding bicarbonate (e.g., buffered lidocaine), warming the solution to room temperature, instilling the solution slowly, and distracting the patient during injection all contribute to reducing pain.[39] In the pediatric population, 2.5 g of EMLA (eutectic mixture of local anesthetics) can be applied topically over the site.[7,40] Its main disadvantage is slow onset, with as long as an hour needed for induction of anesthesia before cannulation.[41] Other options include ethyl chloride topical spray,[42] which temporarily numbs the skin, and oral sucrose in infants.[43]

IV Assembly

Review Box 21-1 itemizes the materials necessary for IV cannulation. The procedure is detailed in Figure 21-6. The first step is to prepare the IV fluids and tubing. Remove the cap from the IV tubing and the tab from the IV bag. Clamp the IV tubing shut and insert the spiked end into the IV fluid bag. Pinch the drip chamber and fill it halfway. Open the clamp slightly to flush the IV tubing. If saline locks are being used, flush them similarly before cannulation. To do this, attach the lock to a saline-filled syringe and push saline through it.

Inspection and Positioning

After collecting and preparing the equipment and supplies, palpate the veins. Position the patient comfortably on a flat surface. Place a 1-inch-wide tourniquet on the upper part of the patient's arm or forearm and pull it sufficiently tight to impede venous flow but not tight enough to compromise arterial flow. Place the tourniquet under the arm. Fold both ends of it above the arm and cross the ends. Pull the overlying end taut and tuck the middle portion below the underlying end to create a loop. After placement of the tourniquet, palpate the veins with the index and middle finger of one's nondominant hand. The veins are soft, elastic, resilient, and pulseless.[27]

BOX 21-1 Medications and Solutions That May Cause Tissue Injury When Extravasation Occurs in a Peripheral Vein*

Aminophylline	Metaraminol
Calcium chloride 10%	Mithramycin
Carmustine	Mitomycin
Chlordiazepoxide	Nafcillin
Colchicine	Neo-Synephrine
Crystalline amino acids 4.25%/ dextrose 10%	Nitroglycerin
	Norepinephrine
Crystalline amino acids 4.25%/ dextrose 25%	Parenteral nutrition solutions
	Phenytoin[†]
Dactinomycin	Potassium solutions
Daunorubicin	Propylene glycol
Dextrose 10%	Renografin-60
Dextrose 50% in water	Sodium bicarbonate 8.4%
Diazepam	Sodium thiopental
Dobutamine	Tetracycline
Dopamine	Vasopressin
Doxorubicin	Vinblastine
Epinephrine	Vincristine
Ethyl alcohol	Vindesine
Mechlorethamine	

*Many medications and intravenous solutions will cause pain and occasionally skin sloughing if significant amounts extravasate into soft tissues. Thus any complaint of pain during infusion or signs of tissue swelling should prompt an investigation for extravasation. Most extravasations have no specific therapy, so prevention is the only option. Phentolamine, injected subcutaneously to reverse vasoconstriction, is the most common technique, but its efficacy has not been well studied.
[†]Use a maximum concentration of 2 mg/mL of saline or fosphenytoin solution to minimize this risk.

Cannulation

Wash your hands, don gloves (nonsterile is adequate), and clean the injection site with iodine, alcohol, or both. Iodine is a better antiseptic than alcohol and results in fewer infections.[44] If using alcohol, allow it to dry on the surface of the skin. Stabilize the vein without contaminating the prepared site. One method is to position one's thumb alongside the vein and pull down while the index finger is positioned more cephalad and pulls upward. Take the angiocatheter between the thumb and forefinger of the dominant hand. With the bevel up, angle the angiocatheter 10 to 30 degrees between the catheter and the vein and parallel to the vein. Puncture the vein. Once a flash of blood is seen, advance the catheter several millimeters more to ensure that the catheter has entered the vein and not just the wall. Avoid advancing too far and puncturing the posterior wall. Loosen the stylet and advance only the catheter. Use the fingers that were anchoring the vein to occlude the vein at the tip of the catheter to prevent extravasation of blood from the angiocatheter. Remove the needle; connect the saline lock, IV lining, or syringe for phlebotomy; and release the tourniquet.[27]

Cannulation of the external jugular vein deserves a special note (Fig. 21-7). In patients with otherwise limited peripheral access, it can be cannulated as follows. Place patient in the Trendelenburg position to fill the external jugular vein. Rotate the head to the opposite side and prepare the area as above. Take the cannula and align it in the direction of the vein with the point aiming toward the ipsilateral shoulder. Puncture midway between the angle of the jaw and the midclavicular line while lightly compressing the vein with the free finger above the clavicle. Proceed as described previously for cannulation.

Anchoring the Device

After the IV cannula has been connected to the saline lock or IV tubing, anchor the device (see Fig. 21-6). Use a half-inch-wide strip of tape, adhesive side up, under the hub of the catheter and fold it over in a bow-shaped manner. This will secure the catheter and prevent lateral movement. Clear polyurethane dressings can also be used with or instead of tape. Saline locks can be connected to needleless hubs to prevent accidental needle injury. Then secure the loose saline lock or IV tubing with tape to prevent accidental dislodgement. Connect the IV tubing to the angiocatheter and anchor it. Alternatively, use a commercially available securing device. Sign and date the dressings to ensure timely dressing changes.[7] As an option, topical antibiotics or iodophor ointment may be applied to the insertion site to prevent infection, though the efficacy of doing so is unproven.[45]

Maintaining Patency

An important component of IV care is maintaining patency with frequent flushing. Until recently, heparin solutions were used to flush catheters and maintain patency, but heparin can cause problems such as hemorrhage. Saline flushes are as effective as heparin in maintaining patency and preventing phlebitis but do not carry the risks of bleeding or heparin-induced thrombocytopenia.[46-48]

Dressing

It is not cost-effective to continually re-dress peripheral venous catheters at periodic intervals. Sterile gauze or transparent, semipermeable, polyurethane dressings can be left in place until removal of the catheter without increasing infection rates, as long as the site is regularly evaluated.[49] Securing techniques that use proprietary devices, such as the StatLock IV, a sterile, adhesive-backed anchor, and distal male Luer-tip extensions, may reduce complications by decreasing mobility and risk of dislodgement.[50] Commonly used topical antimicrobial ointments have not been consistently proved to reduce the rate of peripheral catheter–related infection but have been associated with increased rates of antimicrobial resistance and *Candida* colonization. Such ointments are not harmful in the ED, but their routine use is not supported.

Percutaneous Brachial Vein Cannulation

Brachial vein cannulation is an option when attempts at peripheral IV access have failed or are contraindicated and may obviate the need for central venous access or surgical cutdown. Complications include brachial artery puncture, hematoma, and transitory paresthesias.

To cannulate the brachial vein, palpate the brachial artery in the antecubital fossa. Prepare the site in the usual manner and apply a tourniquet above the antecubital space. At a point immediately medial or lateral to the pulse, insert an angiocatheter with an attached syringe and advance it at a 45-degree angle while maintaining suction on the syringe. After entrance into the vein, continue 2 to 3 mm further to ensure

PERIPHERAL INTRAVENOUS ACCESS

1

Pull the plug from the IV bag.

2

Insert the spiked end of the IV tubing into the bag.

3

Pinch the drip chamber to fill the bulb halfway before infusing fluid.

4

Flush the IV tubing.

5

Flush the saline lock.

6

Apply a tourniquet 3 to 4 cm proximal to the insertion site.

7

Cross the tourniquet ends and apply tension.

8

Tuck the middle portion of one end under opposite end to make a loop.

Figure 21-6 Peripheral intravenous (IV) access. IV lines placed in the dorsum of the hand are associated with the lowest infection rates from venous cannulation.

PERIPHERAL INTRAVENOUS ACCESS, CONT'D

Leave the distal portion of the tucked end free for one-hand tourniquet release.

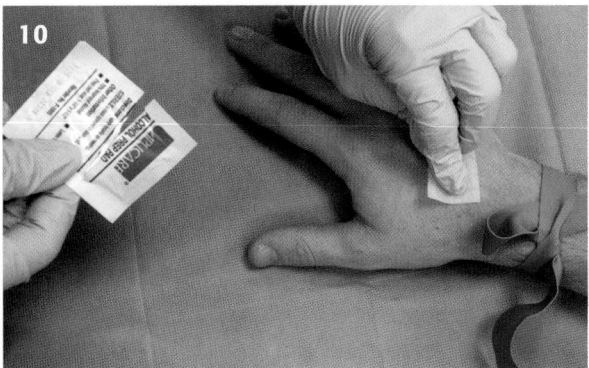

Prepare the insertion site with an alcohol pad.

Grasp the skin and apply linear traction along the course of the vein.

Insert the IV catheter with the bevel facing upward.

Advance the needle until a flash of blood is seen.

Advance the catheter over the needle until flush with the skin.

Remove the needle. Apply pressure at the tip of the catheter (*X*) to stop backbleeding.

Attach the preflushed saline lock.

Figure 21-6, cont'd

Continued

PERIPHERAL INTRAVENOUS ACCESS, CONT'D

Attach the catheter to skin with tape.

Cover the insertion site with Tegaderm (or similar) dressing.

Secure the distal end of the saline lock with tape.

Attach IV tubing to the saline lock for IV fluid administration.

Figure 21-6, cont'd

cannulation. Advance the catheter and remove the needle as usual.[26,42]

COMPLICATIONS

Although IV placement is a common procedure, it is not without complications. Fortunately, morbidity is rarely severe. Phlebitis, infiltration, infection, nerve damage, air embolism, bruising, and thrombosis are the most common complications and rarely cause significant morbidity or fatality.

Phlebitis is a common complication after IV cannulation and is described as the presence of a palpable cord accompanied by warmth, erythema, tenderness, and induration over the involved vein (Fig. 21-8). Phlebitis necessitates removal of the catheter and replacement on another extremity. Avoiding IV placement in the lower extremities (where there is more often stagnant blood flow) and across joints (where motion traumatizes the venous wall) minimizes the incidence of IV catheter–related phlebitis.[7] Other causes of phlebitis include IV infusion of potassium chloride, certain antibiotics (vancomycin, erythromycin), many cytotoxic chemotherapy agents, phenytoin, and any hyperosmolar solution (e.g., 50% dextrose solution).[51,52] The role of in-line filters to prevent phlebitis is controversial. Particulates from reconstituted medications, degradation products, precipitates, glass from vials, and other foreign debris may all play a part in postinfusion phlebitis. In-line filters may therefore play a role in preventing phlebitis, but given their cost, risk of clogging, and paucity of evidence that they improve outcomes, these filters have not become routine.[53]

Even with the most pristine technique, there is about a 0.5% incidence of catheter-related bloodstream infection with peripheral IV catheters. IV devices facilitate infection by damaging epithelial barriers and thereby providing microorganisms direct access to the bloodstream.[54] The risk for infection with peripheral venous catheters is higher in the lower extremity than in the upper extremity and higher in the wrist or upper part of the arm than in the hand. The most common infectious complication of peripheral IV access is self-limited cellulitis.[55] The safety of maintaining peripheral IV lines for up to 72 hours before they are relocated has been established in a large, prospective study.[49] With rates of clinically significant bacteremia lower than 0.5%, some argue that routine replacement of catheters is now no longer needed.[56] Nonetheless, infection can be a costly and potentially devastating complication of IV therapy. Suppurative thrombophlebitis is extremely rare. It most frequently occurs in patients with thermal injury and long-term or lower extremity cannulation.[54] Local signs of inflammation or suppuration are often absent and can occur 2 to 10 days after removal of the catheter.[57] Treatment is immediate surgical excision of the entire length of the involved vein and tributaries. Though rare with peripheral IV catheters, intravascular device–related bloodstream infection may be an unrecognized cause of nosocomial infection. Peripheral IV catheters are most

Figure 21-7 External jugular cannulation. **A,** Note that traction on the vein is applied with the thumb of the nondominant hand while the index finger tamponades the vessel (*arrow*) (essentially serving as a tourniquet) near the clavicle. Flow is dependent on neck position. **B,** Intravenous catheters may be sutured in place for stability. The Trendelenburg position and a Valsalva maneuver can facilitate cannulation.

Figure 21-8 A, Suppurative phlebitis from a peripheral intravenous line. **B,** After incising and cleaning the infected subcutaneous tract, a gauze pack was placed for 24 hours and oral antibiotics were given with good results.

often associated with staphylococcal and candidal species.[58] Infectious complications can be reduced significantly by hand washing, wearing gloves, preparing the site with iodine, and monitoring the site for signs of infection.[7]

Bruising is a common complication of IV therapy. Contrary to popular belief, flexing of the elbow after venipuncture does not prevent bruising in the antecubital site.[59] Applying direct pressure immediately after decannulation is the most useful technique to prevent bruising.

Tissue or interstitial infiltration occurs when the catheter is dislodged from the vein during infusion. It is a common and usually relatively minor complication of IV therapy. Extravasation of certain infusions, such as hypertonic solutions, vasopressors, or chemotherapeutic agents, however, poses a significant risk for necrosis and skin sloughing when infiltration and extravasation occur. In extreme cases, skin grafting may be required.[7] For extravasation of dopamine or epinephrine, local injection of antidotes such as phentolamine may be used to reverse the tissue damage.[60]

Nerve injury is rare after IV cannulation. Any peripheral nerve is potentially vulnerable to a needle-induced injury, and sequelae can range from a minor motor or sensory abnormality to complete paralysis. Nerve damage may be due to direct injury by the needle, intraneural microvascular damage from hematomas, or toxic effects of the agent injected.[61] The first symptoms are usually pain, numbness, or paresthesia. Pain may persist for years and can be debilitating. Fortunately, most simple procedures do not result in nerve injury because

nerves tend to roll or slide away from a needle. Like all procedures, knowledge of the relevant anatomy is essential. Should a patient complain of numbness or severe pain after a needle puncture, stop the injection immediately.[62,63]

Thrombosis and subsequent pulmonary embolism (PE) are commonly associated with centrally placed IV catheters.[7] Though rare, thrombosis followed by clinically significant PE may occur in patients with peripheral IV lines if saline locks are not flushed or IV fluids run dry. Should this occur, aspirate the line. If the return fluid appears bloody, discard the syringe and then gently flush the saline lock and resume the infusion. If there is no bloody aspirate, use 2 to 3 mL of saline to gently flush the line. If resistance is encountered, stop flushing immediately because there is a risk for development of an embolism. Attempt IV insertion at another site.[64]

Venous air embolism is another significant, though exceedingly rare complication of peripheral IV access. Symptoms include chest pain, shortness of breath, sudden vascular collapse, cyanosis, and hypotension. If air embolism is suspected, place the patient in the left lateral decubitus Trendelenburg position. Invasive maneuvers include aspiration of air through a central venous catheter and even thoracotomy with direct aspiration from the heart (see Chapter 18). This complication can be prevented by eliminating air from the IV tubing before initiating therapy and not allowing IV lines to run dry.[7] If air bubbles are present in an IV line, tap the tubing while holding it taut to allow the air to escape to the top. Similarly, curl the tubing around a pen or syringe to accomplish the same goal. If the air is near a Y connector, one can use a needle and syringe to directly remove it. If all else fails and there is air between the Y connector and the patient, disconnect the tubing and flush it.[65]

Recommendations of the Centers for Disease Control and Prevention for IV catheter care to prevent complications are as follows:

1. Record and date the time of catheter insertion in an obvious location near the insertion site.
2. Do not palpate the insertion site after the skin has been cleansed with antiseptic.
3. Palpate the insertion site for tenderness daily through an intact dressing.
4. Visually inspect the site if the patient reports tenderness.
5. Wash hands before and after palpating, inserting, replacing, or dressing any intravascular access site.
6. Replace dressings when they are damp, loose, or soiled.[55]

EXTRAVASATION OF MEDICATIONS AND VASOPRESSORS

Usually, infiltration of a vein is a relatively minor and common complication of IV therapy if only sterile fluid extravasates, even in large amounts. This often occurs when the catheter is dislodged from the vein during infusion. However, if the infusions consist of hypertonic substances, vasopressors, or chemotherapeutics, there is a significant risk for skin sloughing if infiltration and extravasation occur (see Box 21-1). Pain at the infusion site or the alarm sounding on an infusion pump device requires inspection of the infusion site for extravasation. In extreme cases, grafting may be required for skin sloughing (Fig. 21-9).[5] If dopamine, phenylephrine (Neo-Synephrine), or norepinephrine extravasate, phentolamine may be used as an antidote to prevent ischemia locally; its use is encouraged as soon as extravasation is identified. Reversal of ischemia with phentolamine is a common technique, but its ability to totally reverse or prevent skin sloughing is not guaranteed. However, if infiltration of these vasopressors occurs, the authors suggest that it be used routinely. There are few downsides to this intervention, although hypotension is a theoretical side effect because phentolamine is an α-adrenergic antagonist. To inject phentolamine, place 5 mg in a vial and dilute with equal parts of saline (final form: 5 mg in 2 mL). For large areas, use two vials with the contents of each vial injected 10 minutes apart through a 25- to 27-gauge needle or a tuberculin syringe. If the IV line is still in place, inject about 1 mL of phentolamine through the catheter before it is removed; however, the IV line is often removed before this can be done.

The entire area of skin blanching—or suspected area of extravasation—is injected with multiple small aliquots of the solution, about 0.25 to 0.5 mL each. The procedure may be repeated in 2 to 4 hours. Hyaluronidase is probably benign and has been suggested in the past to ameliorate some effects of extravasation of other solutions. Though it has been a common suggestion, its efficacy has not been well established, and the product is not readily available. Ice and heat have varying effects in counteracting fluid extravasation. Extravasation of IV contrast material is discussed in Chapter 36.

Figure 21-9 A, Infiltration of calcium chloride in an infant. Once this occurs, there is no treatment except débridement and possible skin grafting. Calcium gluconate will not cause such a reaction. Extravasation of hypertonic dextrose, phenytoin, and vasoconstrictors or vasopressors will cause similar necrosis. **B,** Full-thickness tissue injury from doxorubicin extravasation, not obvious until 7 to10 days after the infusion.

TABLE 21-1   Possible Antidotes for Extravasated Chemotherapeutic Agents*

CHEMOTHERAPEUTIC AGENT	ANTIDOTE	DOSE
Anthracycline	Dexrazoxane hydrochloride[†]	First dose, inject the equivalent of 500 mg dexrazoxane intravenously over 1-2 hr, second dose at 24 hr, and third dose at 48 hr
Mechlorethamine	Sodium thiosulfate	Multiple subcutaneous injections in and around the area of extravasation with a 25-gauge needle: 4 mL of 10% sodium thiosulfate + 6 mL water
Vinca alkaloids (vincristine, vinblastine, and vinorelbine)	Hyaluronidase	Inject subcutaneously in and around the area of extravasation with a 25-gauge needle: 150 units (1 mL) For vinca alkaloids, apply local hot compresses
Doxorubicin	Granulocyte-macrophage colony-stimulating factor[‡]	Inject subcutaneously in and around the area of extravasation with a 25-gauge needle
Doxorubicin, daunorubicin, and mitomycin	Dimethyl sulfoxide (free radical scavenger)	Apply a 50-70% solution topically qid for 14 days. Leave uncovered
Mitomycin	Pyridoxine[‡]	Inject subcutaneously in and around the area of extravasation with a 25-gauge needle
Nonspecific	Saline	Inject subcutaneously in and around the area of extravasation with a 25-gauge needle
Nonspecific	Corticosteroids[§]	Inject subcutaneously in and around the area of extravasation with a 25-gauge needle: hydrocortisone, 500 mg diluted in 500 mL saline

*Many of these interventions are anecdotal and none are guaranteed to reverse or ameliorate tissue injury. Controversy surrounds the actual benefit, and no randomized prospective trials have been conducted for many of the suggested regimens. Also consider elevation and surgical débridement when necessary.
[†]Approved by U.S. Food and Drug Administration for this indication.
[‡]Not well studied, theoretical benefit.
[§]Results are variable; injury is not an inflammatory reaction.

Extravasation of chemotherapy solutions is particularly common and can produce full-thickness tissue sloughing. The patient may complain of pain and burning at the time of infusion, but skin sloughing may be delayed for many days. Table 21-1 lists possible antidotes and dosages for chemotherapy-induced extravasation injury. Results of these interventions vary.

Injury from extravasation of phenytoin can be minimized or avoided by using dilute solutions, no more than a 2-mg/ mL concentration (1 g in 500 mL saline), or by using fosphenytoin instead of phenytoin. When possible, use calcium gluconate, not calcium chloride, in a peripheral IV line.

The bottom line is that most extravasated chemotherapy and other agents have no specific antidote or reversal agents to alter the final outcome. At most extravasation sites it may be best to avoid the empirical use of suggested treatments such as sodium bicarbonate, sodium thiosulfate, heparin,

ULTRASOUND: Peripheral Intravenous Access   *by Christine Butts, MD*

Ultrasound-guided access is indicated when standard placement is difficult. This may include patients with no palpable or visible peripheral veins, history of intravenous drug use or multiple previous peripheral lines causing scarring or thrombosis, obesity, or previous surgeries causing distortion of the anatomy. Use of ultrasound to achieve peripheral intravenous access has been found to increase the rate of success, decrease both the time to placement and the number of attempts, and increase overall patient satisfaction.[1] Nursing use of ultrasound to guide peripheral intravenous access has also shown promise in improving success and decreasing complications.[2]

There are two methods by which the ultrasound may be used to access peripheral veins. In the first method, ultrasound is used to simply evaluate the underlying anatomy. Frequently, veins are present superficially but cannot be seen or palpated from the surface of the skin. Apply the transducer to rapidly locate an ideal vein and cannulate it "blindly" in the typical fashion. The second method calls for ultrasound to be used to directly guide venous access. This method may be most practical when the veins are deeper within the tissues or adjacent to other more important structures.

Use a high-frequency (7.5- to 10-mHz) transducer to obtain the necessary resolution for evaluating the anatomy. Typically, for peripheral venous access, a sterile field is not necessary. However, it is important to clean the area with alcohol or chlorhexidine solution before the procedure. Use universal precautions. Apply a tourniquet when appropriate to assist in distending the veins and to make them easier to identify.

Multiple peripheral vessels are available for ultrasound-guided access. The basilic vein lies on the ulnar aspect of the forearm and the cephalic vein can be found on the radial aspect (Fig. 21-US1). The larger median cubital vein represents the junction of these two veins and lies in the antecubital fossa (Fig. 21-US2). The deep brachial vein is found on the median aspect of the distal end of the arm in the bicipital groove (Fig.

21-US3). The external jugular vein is found superficially in the neck and runs diagonally across the sternocleidomastoid muscle.

Distinguishing the artery from the vein may prove more challenging than with central vessels. Peripheral veins and arteries are smaller, and even arteries may collapse with pressure. Evaluate the veins before application of the tourniquet. Veins should collapse easily and in fact may collapse from only the pressure of applying the transducer to the skin. Placing the heel of the operator's hand on the patient's arm and then applying the transducer may decrease this effect. Arteries can be further identified by evaluating the Doppler flow pattern of the vessel. Even small arteries will have a biphasic, pulsatile flow pattern versus the

Figure 21-US2 Ultrasound image of the median cubital vein (*arrow*).

Figure 21-US3 Ultrasound image of the deep brachial vein (*large arrow*). Another smaller vein can be seen more superficially to the right of the image (*small arrow*).

Figure 21-US1 Ultrasound image of the basilic vein (*arrow*).

Continued

ULTRASOUND: Peripheral Intravenous Access, cont'd

Figure 21-US4 Demonstration of venous augmentation. **A,** Ultrasound view of a suspected vein (*arrow*). **B,** Once the wrist is lightly squeezed, adding color Doppler flow to the area will demonstrate a "flush" of color within the vessel (*arrow*).

steady low-amplitude venous pattern. Finally, venous augmentation can be used for confirmation. Color flow imaging is used over the vessel in question. Squeezing the arm distal to the area should cause a temporary flush of flow in the vein (Fig. 21-US4). The artery should not show any change in its typical pulsatile flow.

Once a location for cannulation has been chosen, scan the relevant area to locate the desired vessel. Once the vein has been identified, the cannulation procedure is identical for all peripheral veins. A transverse, or short-axis, approach is universally used because of the small size of the peripheral veins. Center the transducer over the target vessel. The depth of the image on-screen should be decreased as much as possible so the best possible image is obtained. A blunt object (e.g., a fingertip) is applied over the center of the transducer to ensure that the vessel in question is centered. Then introduce the needle at a 45-degree angle slightly back from the transducer (Fig. 21-US5). Once the tip of the needle is identified on-screen, advance it toward the vessel. Watch the catheter closely for a flash of blood. Once the flash is obtained, set the ultrasound aside and continue the procedure in the typical fashion.

A pitfall that may frustrate the sonographer is kinking or difficulty threading or advancing the catheter once a flash has been obtained. This frequently occurs in deeper vessels, such as the deep brachial. Using a longer, stiffer catheter (e.g., 1¾-inch Arrow twin catheter or the longer catheter from the Arrow arterial line kit) may help reduce this problem.

Figure 21-US5 A, Introduce the needle at a 45-degree angle, slightly back from the transducer. **B,** Identify the tip of the needle on-screen. **C,** Advance the tip of the needle (*arrow*) toward the vessel.

REFERENCES:

1. Costantino T, Parikh A, Satz WA, et al. Ultrasonography-guided peripheral intravenous access versus traditional approaches in patients with difficult intravenous access. *Ann Emerg Med.* 2005;46:456-461.
2. Brannam L, Blaivas M, Lyon M, et al. Emergency nurses' utilization of ultrasound guidance for placement of peripheral intravenous lines in difficult-access patients. *Acad Emerg Med.* 2004;11:1361-1363.

calcium gluconate, magnesium sulfate, lidocaine, cimetidine, diphenhydramine, and other chemical substances that are believed to inactivate drugs and reduce toxic effects on cells. In some experimental settings these substances have made the necrosis and ulceration worse.[53-56]

References are available at www.expertconsult.com

CHAPTER 22

Central Venous Catheterization and Central Venous Pressure Monitoring

Christopher R. McNeil, Salim R. Rezaie, and Bruce D. Adams

Central venous access remains a cornerstone of resuscitation and critical care in both the emergency department (ED) and intensive care unit. Advanced hemodynamic monitoring, rapid infusion of fluid, placement of transvenous pacemakers, and administration of selected medications all require reliable central venous access. Central venous catheterization has also gained acceptance in the resuscitation and treatment of critically ill children (see Chapter 19). Traditionally, the subclavian vein (SV), internal jugular (IJ) vein, and femoral vein have provided reliable and easily obtainable vascular access through the use of identifiable anatomic landmarks. Over the past decade, the increased availability of, training in, and provider competence in bedside ultrasonography have had a significant impact on the standard approach to both peripheral and central venous catheterization. Ultrasound-guided central venous catheterization has improved success rates, reduced complication rates, decreased the time required to perform the procedure, and resulted in overall cost savings.

The various techniques described in this chapter each have inherent advantages and disadvantages, but all have a place in the practice of emergency medicine. Frequently, a clinician's previous experience with a particular technique determines the preferred approach, but clinicians responsible for acute resuscitation of the ill and injured should master several of these techniques.

HISTORICAL PERSPECTIVE

In 1667, the first known central venous catheter (CVC) was placed into a human IJ vein by Lower for a blood transfusion into the carotid artery of a sheep.[1] Modern central venous catheterization heralds back to at least 1928 when Werner Forssmann, a 25-year-old German surgeon, performed a venous cutdown on his own left antecubital vein, inserted a ureteral catheter to a distance of 65 cm, and then climbed several flights of stairs to the radiology suite to confirm that it terminated in the right atrium. Although the hospital fired Dr. Forssmann for not obtaining permission, he went on to win the 1956 Nobel Prize for his pioneering efforts.[1,2]

Duffy reported a large series of femoral, jugular, and antecubital vein catheterizations in 1949.[3] Aubaniac developed subclavian venipuncture while working on French Army casualties between 1942 and 1952.[4] His infraclavicular SV approach was refined by Keeri-Szanto in 1956, and the supraclavicular approach to the vein was first described by Yoffa in 1965.[5,6] Aside from Duffy's earlier work, Hermosura (1966) and English (1969) are generally credited with scientific development of the percutaneous IJ approach.[7]

The most important advancement in modern CVC came in 1953 when the Swedish radiologist Sven Seldinger had the idea of advancing large catheters over a flexible wire that was inserted through a percutaneous needle.[8,9] The role of central venous pressure (CVP) monitoring in the maintenance of optimal blood volume helped popularize central catheterization in the United States.[10] This was accelerated by the advent of the pulmonary artery catheter, which was developed by Jeremy Swan and William Ganz in 1968.[11] Swan, who was inspired by his observations of a sailing boat during a picnic with his children, developed a flow-directed balloon that allowed measurement of pulmonary artery pressure.[12]

ANATOMY

SV System

The SV begins as a continuation of the axillary vein at the outer edge of the first rib. It joins the IJ vein to become the innominate (sometimes referred to as the brachiocephalic) vein 3 to 4 cm proximally. The SV has a diameter of 10 to 20 mm, is approximately 3 to 4 cm long, and is valveless. After crossing over the first rib, the vein lies posterior to the medial third of the clavicle. It is only in this area that there is an intimate association between the clavicle and the SV. The costoclavicular ligament lies anterior and inferior to the SV, and the fascia contiguous to this ligament invests the vessel. Posterior to the vein and separating it from the subclavian artery is the anterior scalene muscle, which has a thickness of 10 to 15 mm. The phrenic nerve passes over the anterior surface of the scalene muscle laterally and runs immediately behind the junction of the SV and the IJ vein. The larger thoracic duct (on the left) and the smaller lymphatic duct (on the right) pass over the anterior scalene muscle and enter the SV near its junction with the IJ vein. Superior and posterior to the subclavian artery lies the brachial plexus. The dome of the left lung may extend above the first rib, but the right lung rarely extends this high (Fig. 22-1).

IJ Vein

The IJ vein begins just medial to the mastoid process in the jugular foramen at the base of the skull and is formed by the inferior petrosal sinus and the sigmoid sinus. It runs inferiorly and passes under the sternal end of the clavicle to join the SV and form the innominate or brachiocephalic vein. At the level of the thyroid cartilage, the IJ vein, the internal carotid artery, and the vagus nerve course together in the carotid sheath just deep to the sternocleidomastoid (SCM) muscle. Within the carotid sheath, the IJ vein typically occupies the anterior lateral position and the carotid artery lies medial and slightly posterior to the vein. This relationship is relatively constant, but studies have found that the carotid artery may overlap the IJ. Note that normally the IJ vein migrates medially as it nears the clavicle, where it may lie directly over the carotid artery. When using the most common (central) approach, the IJ tends to be more lateral than expected.[13,14] Furthermore, in 5.5% of those studied, the IJ vein may even be medial to the carotid artery.[14-17] The relationship between the IJ vein and the carotid artery also depends on head position. Excessive head rotation can cause the carotid artery to rotate over the IJ vein.[18,19]

Anatomic landmarks for locating the vein include the sternal notch, the medial third of the clavicle, and the SCM.

Central Venous Catheterization

Indications

Central venous pressure monitoring
High-volume/flow resuscitation
Emergency venous access
Inability to obtain peripheral venous access
Repetitive blood sampling
Administering hyperalimentation, caustic
  agents, or other concentrated fluids
Insertion of transvenous cardiac pacemakers
Hemodialysis or plasmapheresis
Insertion of pulmonary artery catheters

Complications

Arterial puncture and hematoma
Pneumothorax (subclavian and internal jugular approach)
Hemothorax (subclavian and internal jugular approach)
Vessel injury
Air embolism
Cardiac dysrhythmia
Nerve injury
Infection
Thrombosis
Catheter misplacement

Contraindications

Infection over the placement site
Distortion of landmarks by trauma or congenital anomalies
Coagulopathies, including anticoagulation and thrombolytic therapy
Pathologic conditions, including superior vena cava syndrome
Current venous thrombosis in the target vessel
Prior vessel injury or procedures
Morbid obesity
Uncooperative patients

Equipment (contents of a typical central venous catheterization kit)

1% lidocaine
without epinephrine

5-mL syringe
(for venipuncture)

5-mL syringe
(for anesthetic)

18-gauge needle
(for venipuncture)

25- and 22-gauge needles
(for anesthetic)

Dilator

Chlorhexidene

Scalpel with a No.11 blade

Sterile drape

Triple-lumen catheter

Guidewire

Catheter clamp

Silk suture

Review Box 22-1 Central venous catheterization: indications, contraindications, complications, and equipment.

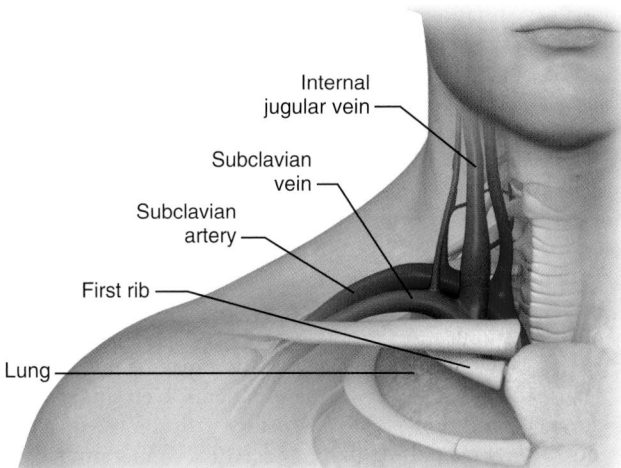

Figure 22-1 Subclavian vein anatomy. The subclavian vein runs parallel to the clavicle and anterior to the subclavian artery. The cupula of the lung lies just caudad to these structures. If the introducer needle is kept almost parallel to the clavicle, the artery and lung should not be encountered.

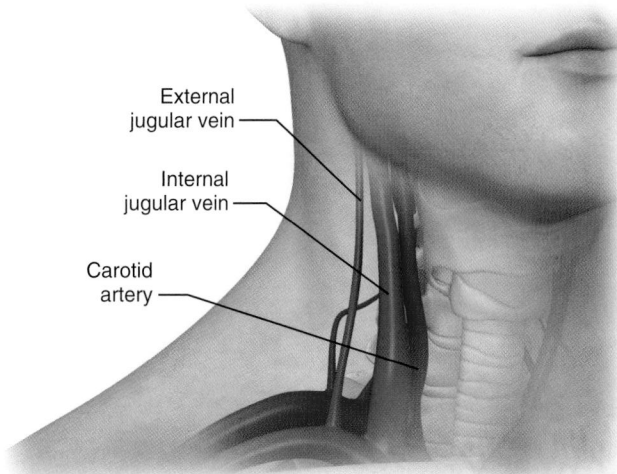

Figure 22-2 Internal jugular anatomy. The internal jugular vein runs parallel and lateral to the carotid artery but lies almost directly above the carotid artery at the level of the clavicle.

The two heads of the SCM and the clavicle form a triangle that is key to understanding the underlying vascular anatomy. The IJ vein can be located at the apex of the triangle as it courses along the medial head of the SCM and occupies a position in the middle of the triangle at the level of the clavicle before it joins the SV and forms the innominate vein. At the level of the thyroid cartilage, the IJ vein can be found just deep to the SCM.

Generally, the right IJ is bigger than the left IJ because of its connection to the SV and the right atrium. The IJ vein can be pulsatile, but in contrast to the aorta, these pulsations are not palpable. When visualized, however, the presence of venous pulsations can give an indication of patency of the IJ vein to the right atrium. The IJ vein also changes size with respiration. Because of the negative intrathoracic pressure at end-inspiration, blood in the IJ vein is actually drawn into the right atrium and the diameter of the IJ vein shrinks. In contrast, at end-expiration the increased intrathoracic pressure will limit return of blood to the right atrium and the diameter of the IJ vein will increase. Another unique characteristic of the IJ vein is its distensibility. The IJ vein will enlarge when pressure in the vein is increased, such as when flow of blood back to the right atrium is obstructed, as with thrombosis. This distensibility can be advantageous for the placement of central venous access. Use of a head-down (Trendelenburg) position or a Valsalva maneuver will increase the diameter of the IJ vein and thereby increase the likelihood of successful puncture (Fig. 22-2).

Femoral Vein

The femoral anatomy is less complex than that of the neck and shoulder and contains fewer vital structures. The femoral vein is most easily cannulated percutaneously in patients with a palpable femoral pulse. The femoral vein begins at the adductor canal (also known as Hunter's canal) and ends at the inferior margin of the inguinal ligament, where it becomes the external iliac vein. It is contained within the femoral triangle (inguinal ligament, medial border of the adductor longus, and lateral border of the sartorius muscle). Medially,

the femoral vein abuts a robust system of lymphatics. Laterally, the vein is intimately associated with the femoral artery. The femoral nerve courses down into the leg just lateral to the femoral artery. These relationships from lateral to medial can be remembered with the mnemonic NAVEL (nerve, artery, vein, empty space, lymphatics). Note that as the femoral artery and vein course down the leg within the femoral sheath, their side-by-side relationship frequently rotates such that the femoral artery may lie on top of the vein. Therefore, to avoid arterial puncture, keep cannulation attempts just under the inguinal ligament. When cannulating this vessel distal to the inguinal ligament, ultrasound guidance can be helpful to avoid arterial puncture (Fig. 22-3).

INDICATIONS

Central venous access has several clinical indications (see Review Box 22-1). If necessary, any central venous approach could be used for each of these situations. However, certain approaches offer advantages over others in specific clinical settings. The clinical indications are discussed in detail in the following sections.[20-22]

CVP Monitoring and Oximetry

For a period, pulmonary artery catheterization somewhat supplanted CVP monitoring; however, there is little evidence that this practice has any benefit with regard to patient mortality or quality of life. In the specific setting of resuscitation of patients in septic shock, CVP monitoring has reemerged as an important component of "early goal-directed therapy."[23,24] Continuous or episodic measurements of central venous O_2 saturation play a prominent role in current protocols for the aggressive treatment of septic shock.[23,24]

Central venous catheterization is widely used as a vehicle for rapid volume resuscitation. Notwithstanding, short large-caliber peripheral catheters can be as effective as central access because of the properties of Poiseuille's law, which states that the rate of flow is proportional to the radius of the catheter and inversely proportional to its length.[3] To illustrate, the

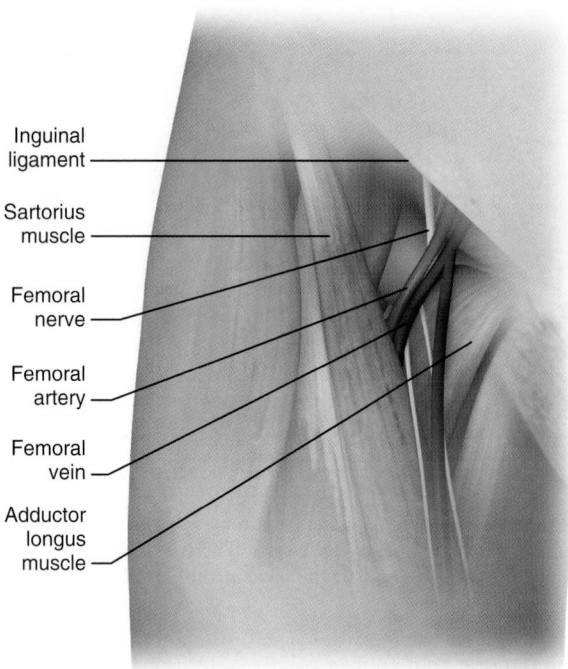

Inguinal ligament

Sartorius muscle

Femoral nerve

Femoral artery

Femoral vein

Adductor longus muscle

Figure 22-3 Femoral vein anatomy. The femoral vital structures are located in the femoral triangle: inguinal ligament superiorly, sartorius muscle laterally, and adductor longus muscle medially. The triangle can be remembered by the mnemonic "SAIL" (*s*artorius, *a*dductor longus, and *i*nguinal *l*igament). Note the femoral structures from lateral to medial: *n*erve, *a*rtery, *v*ein, *e*mpty canal, and *l*ymphatics (mnemonic—NAVEL). The femoral vein lies medial to the femoral artery. *Important anatomic note:* At sites more distal from the inguinal ligament, the vein lies directly above the artery.

gravity flow rate of saline through a peripheral 5-cm, 14-gauge catheter is roughly twice that through a 20-cm, 16-gauge CVC. Consequently, placement of large-bore peripheral catheters is generally the fastest method of volume loading.

Delivery of High-Flow Fluid Boluses and Blood Products

The advent of thermoregulating high-volume rapid infusers affords the advantage of using central venous catheterization in the setting of severe hemorrhagic shock or hypothermia. The available systems can infuse blood warmed to 37°C through an 8.5-Fr introducer sheath 25% more rapidly than through a 14-gauge peripheral intravenous (IV) line and up to 50% faster than through an 18-gauge peripheral IV line.[25] The Level 1 Rapid Infuser and the Belmont FMS 2000 are examples of modern systems with infusion rates as high as 1500 mL/min.[25] Massive air embolism was a concern with early rapid infusers, but safety precautions have now been engineered to prevent this. Still, if the catheter is misplaced, fluid or blood can be rapidly infused into the thorax, mediastinum, or peritoneum with serious consequences.

Emergency Venous Access and Inability to Achieve Peripheral Access

The predictable anatomic locations of the subclavian and femoral veins and the speed with which they can be cannulated have prompted their use in cardiac arrest and other emergency situations. The need for a central line during cardiopulmonary resuscitation (CPR) is controversial.[26-28] When achieved easily, central venous cannulation, especially via the IJ or SV route, is preferred over peripheral venous access because it provides a rapid and reliable route for the administration of drugs to the central circulation of patients in cardiac arrest. With resuscitation for aortic catastrophes or thoracoabdominal trauma, two CVCs, "one above and one below" the diaphragm, are often used.

Patients with a history of IV drug use, major burns, chronic disease, dehydration, or morbid obesity and those who require long-term access may have inadequate peripheral IV sites. Central venous cannulation may be indicated as a means of venous access in these patients even under non-emergency conditions.[29] More recently with the use of ultrasound, deep brachial, axillary, and basilic vein cannulation may be attempted before central venous catheterization. This approach avoids the complications that can be associated with central venous access.

Routine Serial Blood Drawing

The potential complications of CVCs make them inappropriate solely for routine blood sampling. However, lines already in place may be used for this purpose if they are properly cleared of IV fluid. A 20-cm, 16-gauge catheter contains 0.3 mL of fluid, so at least this much must be withdrawn to avoid dilution of blood samples. Moreover, to avoid aspiration of crystalloid-diluted blood from the peripheral vein, it is advised that the IV line be turned off for at least 2 to 3 minutes before using the catheter for a blood draw. Because of the increased risk for infectious complications, air embolism, and venous backbleeding, the IV tubing should not be repeatedly disconnected from the catheter hub. Interposition of a three-way stopcock in the IV tubing simplifies access and is an acceptable method for sampling blood in the intensive care setting, regardless of the IV site. The oxygen level in blood from the SV can be determined for guidance in early goal-directed therapy for sepsis if one chooses not to place a continuous oximetric monitor.

Additionally, serial lactate levels may help guide early goal-directed resuscitation. With an imbalance in oxygen supply (Do_2) and consumption (Vo_2), tissue hypoperfusion and hypoxia lead to anaerobic metabolism. The final product of this process is lactate. Arterial lactate levels would best represent overall perfusion since such samples contain blood coming from the pulmonary veins, superior vena cava (SVC), and inferior vena cava (IVC). Peripheral lactate preferentially reflects perfusion and metabolism in the compartment from which the blood was drawn, but not overall perfusion. Arterial and central venous lactate correlate closely more than 96% of the time, whereas peripheral venous lactate and arterial lactate correlate only 87% of the time.[30]

Infusion of Hyperalimentation and Other Concentrated Solutions

Central venous hyperalimentation is safe and reliable. Use of the infraclavicular subclavian technique frees the patient's extremities and neck; this procedure is therefore well suited for long-term applications. Hyperosmolar or irritating solutions with the potential to cause thrombophlebitis if given through small peripheral vessels are frequently infused

TABLE 22-1 Advantages and Disadvantages of Central Venous Access Techniques

TECHNIQUE	ADVANTAGES	DISADVANTAGES
IJ	Good external landmarks Improved success with ultrasound Less risk for pneumothorax than with SV access Can recognize and control bleeding Malposition of the catheter is rare Almost a straight course to the superior vena cava on the right side Carotid artery easily identified	More difficult and inconvenient to secure Possibly higher infectious risk than with SV access Possibly higher risk for thrombosis than with SV access
Femoral	Good external landmarks Useful alternative with coagulopathy	Difficult to secure in ambulatory patients Not reliable for CVP measurement Highest risk for infection Higher risk for thrombus
SV, infraclavicular	Good external landmarks	Unable to compress bleeding vessels "Blind" procedure Should not be attempted in children younger than 2 yr
SV, supraclavicular	Good external landmarks Practical method of inserting a central line in cardiorespiratory arrest	"Blind" procedure Unable to compress bleeding vessels

CVP, central venous pressure; *IJ,* internal jugular; *SV,* subclavian vein.

through central veins. Examples are potassium chloride (>40 mmol/L), hyperosmolar saline, 10% calcium chloride (but not calcium gluconate, which can safely be given peripherally), 10% dextrose infusions, chemotherapeutic agents, and acidifying solutions such as ammonium chloride. Vasoactive substances (e.g., dopamine, norepinephrine) are best administered through a CVC because they may cause soft tissue necrosis if extravasation occurs in peripheral sites.

Central catheters, though safer than peripheral IV lines, are not immune to extravasation; indeed, fatal cases have been reported if the catheter becomes wedged up against the vessel wall, valves, or endocardium.[31] Strategies to avoid this complication include delivering vesicant drugs only through the distal ports or reconfirming that the proximal port is safely in the vein by aspirating blood through it.[31]

Other Indications

Other indications for central venous access include insertion of a pulmonary artery catheter or transvenous pacemaker, cardiac catheterization, pulmonary angiography, and hemodialysis. A pulmonary artery catheter can be valuable for determining fluid and hemodynamic status in the critically ill. Its widespread use in the 1980s and 1990s drew heavy criticism because data showing a benefit in patient-oriented outcomes were lacking. Pulmonary artery catheters have subsequently lost popularity and should be used only when the diagnostic benefits outweigh the potential risks.[32,33] Catheters such as the Uldall and Quinton devices can be inserted within minutes, thereby permitting emergency or short-term hemodialysis. However, these catheters are very large and relatively stiff and have been known to perforate the vena cava or atrial walls, with fatal outcomes.[34,35] Extra caution should be applied during their insertion, possibly under ultrasound or fluoroscopic guidance.

CONTRAINDICATIONS

General contraindications to the various techniques of central venous access are presented in Review Box 22-1. Table 22-1 lists the general advantages and disadvantages with each approach. Most contraindications listed are relative and should be viewed in the context of the patient's overall condition, urgency of need, and availability of alternative options for vascular access. Perhaps the only true absolute contraindication is insertion of catheters impregnated with antibiotics (most commonly tetracycline, rifampin, or chlorhexidine) if the patient has a serious allergy to the drug.[36,37] Local cellulitis and distorted local anatomy or landmarks are relative contraindications to any access route. Each technique is contraindicated in patients with distorted local anatomy or landmarks preventing safe insertion. Insertion of catheters through freshly burned regions, though somewhat challenging, is not associated with a higher incidence of infection until approximately 3 days after the burn, when bacterial colonization accelerates.[38,39] One of the more commonly encountered impediments to CVC placement is morbid obesity.[40] Surface landmarks in the neck are often obscured, and an abdominal pannus can block the femoral access site and consequently require deeper insertions and steeper angles. An ultrasound-guided IJ approach is safer under these circumstances.[40] Insertion of another catheter on the same side as a preexisting one risks the complication of entrapment.[41] Combativeness is an important factor in the decision to place a CVC because the risk for mechanical complications greatly increases in uncooperative patients. Sometimes it is best to sedate and intubate critically ill patients before attempting central venous catheterization. Other relative contraindications include conditions predisposing to sclerosis or thrombosis of the central veins, such as vasculitis, previous long-term cannulation, or illicit IV drug use via any of the deep venous systems.

Coagulopathy is a frequent concern surrounding insertion of a CVC, with the overall risk for clinically significant hemorrhage in these patients approximating 2%.[42] A transfusion of fresh frozen plasma is commonly used to correct any existing coagulopathy. However, a recent review concluded that if good technique is used, correction of coagulopathy is not generally required before or during the procedure.[43] Mumtaz and coworkers found that even in thrombocytopenic patients (platelet count <50 × 10⁹/L), bleeding complications occurred about 3% of the time and were limited to bleeding at the insertion site[44]; these complications were managed with additional sutures. Although the occasional patient may require a blood transfusion or replacement of clotting factors if a hemorrhagic complication arises, prophylactic correction of an abnormal international normalized ratio or platelet count before the procedure is not routinely necessary.[43-45] Risk can be further reduced in coagulopathic patients with the use of ultrasound-guided placement techniques.[14,46-49]

Subclavian Approach

SV access is contraindicated in patients who have previously undergone surgery or sustained trauma involving the clavicle, the first rib, or the subclavian vessels; those with previous radiation therapy involving the clavicular area; those with significant chest wall deformities; and those with marked cachexia or obesity. Patients with unilateral deformities not associated with pneumothorax (e.g., fractured clavicle) should be catheterized on the opposite side. Subclavian venipuncture is not contraindicated in patients with penetrating thoracic wounds unless the injuries are known or suspected to involve the subclavian vessels or SVC. Generally, cannulate the vein on the same side as the chest wound to avoid the possibility of bilateral pneumothoraces. When (preexisting) SV injury is suspected, cannulate on the opposite side. Exercise greater caution when placing a CVC in the SV in coagulopathic patients because this vessel is not compressible. Formerly, subclavian venipuncture was not recommended for use in small children, but in experienced hands it has been demonstrated to be safe.[50-52]

IJ Approach

Cervical trauma with swelling or anatomic distortion at the intended site of IJ venipuncture is the most important contraindication to the IJ approach. Likewise, the presence of a cervical collar is problematic. Although bleeding disorders are relative contraindications to central venous cannulation, the ultrasound-guided IJ approach is preferred over the SV route because the IJ site is compressible. However, prolonged compression of the artery to control bleeding could impair the cerebral circulation if collateral blood flow is compromised. In a study by Oguzkurt and colleagues, only minor bleeding complications occurred in less than 2% of patients after ultrasound-guided IJ catheterization.[47] In the setting of severe bleeding diatheses, the ultrasound-guided femoral approach is an acceptable alternative. Ultrasound-guided IJ placement is preferred in patients with abnormal anatomy from previous IJ trauma, small IJ vessels, and morbid obesity. Historically, carotid artery disease (obstruction or atherosclerotic plaque) is a relative contraindication to IJ cannulation because inadvertent puncture or manipulation of the artery could dislodge

a plaque. If a preceding SV catheterization has been unsuccessful, the ipsilateral IJ route is generally preferred for a subsequent attempt. In this manner, bilateral iatrogenic complications can be avoided.

Femoral Approach

Contraindications to femoral cannulation include known or suspected intraabdominal hemorrhage or injury to the pelvis, groin, iliac vessels, or IVC. Additionally, avoid the femoral approach when known or suspected deep venous thrombosis is present. Palpation for femoral pulsations during CPR is difficult, and the pulsations are often venous rather than arterial.[28,53] Ultrasound-guided catheterization of the femoral vein during CPR is more successful and less likely than the standard landmark-oriented approach to incur inadvertent arterial puncture.[28]

PROCEDURE

The most commonly used method for central venous cannulation is the Seldinger (guidewire) technique, in which a thin-walled needle is used to introduce a guidewire into the vessel lumen. Seldinger originally described this technique in 1953 as a method of placing a catheter for percutaneous arteriography.[17] The Seldinger technique is illustrated in Figure 22-9. To obtain vascular access, insert a small needle into the intended vessel. Once the introducer needle is positioned within the lumen of the vessel, thread a wire through the needle and then remove the needle. The wire, now within the vessel, serves as a guide over which the catheter is inserted. Although the Seldinger technique involves several steps, it can be performed quickly once mastered. More importantly, this technique broadens the application of central venous cannulation by permitting the insertion of standard infusion catheters, multilumen catheters, large-bore rapid infusion systems, introducer devices, hemodialysis devices, and even peripheral cardiopulmonary bypass cannulas. Given this flexibility, the use of Seldinger-type systems is advantageous despite their greater cost.

Ultrasound guidance has revolutionized the cannulation of central veins. As with all anatomic structures in the human body, veins are highly variable in their location. Not surprisingly, research has demonstrated that the ability to see the internal structure's location and proximity to other structures greatly increases the safety and success rate while decreasing the time required to perform the procedure.[46-49,54-56] These advantages have been recognized by national organizations. In a report from the Agency for Healthcare Research and Quality (AHRQ), use of ultrasound guidance was listed as one of the top 10 ways to reduce morbidity and mortality.[57] Many hospitals now require the use of ultrasound guidance for the placement of all CVCs.

The basic materials required for central venous cannulation are shown in Review Box 22-1 and are discussed in further detail below. The catheter may be a component in a guidewire system or may be of the over-the-needle variety (the other widely used method for catheter placement). Several types of CVC Seldinger-type prepackaged kits are commercially available, and the variations in each kit are discussed in the next section.

EQUIPMENT

Preparation and organization of equipment ahead of time are imperative for a successful procedure. Most catheters now come from the manufacturer in convenient sterile kits. We strongly recommend stocking all additional equipment such as sterile gowns, gloves, and drapes in a dedicated "central line cart." This is a fundamental part of the "bundling" practice that has been shown to reduce the search for supplies, improve compliance with full-barrier technique, and subsequently decrease catheter-related infections.[58-63] Sterile barrier precautions with cap, face mask, sterile gown, and gloves should be used at all times during insertion of CVCs.[61,64,65]

Ultrasound

Historically, many clinicians preferred to first locate the position of a central vein with a small exploratory or "finder" needle rather than directly cannulating the vein with a larger needle to accommodate a guidewire or catheter. This practice is less practical for the SV approach and has largely been replaced with the use of bedside ultrasound. Ultrasound-guided CVC placement allows the provider to survey the anatomy before the procedure, guide insertion of the needle into the correct vessel, and confirm placement of the catheter in the vessel.[14,47-49] See the Ultrasound Box.

Needle

Virtually any needle or catheter can be used to introduce a guidewire into a vessel, but there are advantages to using needles specifically designed for passage of a guidewire. These needles must be large enough to accommodate the desired wire yet be as small as possible to minimize bleeding complications. The introducer needles provided with CVCs or introducer devices are usually thin walled to maximize lumen size relative to the overall needle diameter. If a needle that is not thin walled is used, choose a size that is 1 gauge smaller (larger bore) than that listed in Table 22-2. If unsure, simply test the equipment first to ensure compatibility.

Standard needles may have a uniformly straight-bore lumen throughout their length. A wire passing into a straight needle may encounter an obstacle at the proximal end. The proximal end of a Seldinger needle incorporates a funnel-shaped taper that guides the wire directly into the needle (Fig. 22-4). It is advisable to use a non–Luer-Lok or slip-tip type of syringe because the added twisting that is required to remove a Luer-Lok syringe from the introducer needle may dislodge a tenuously placed needle. Safety syringe systems exist that permit passage of the wire without removal of the aspirating syringe by using a central tunnel in the barrel. This device incorporates a hollow syringe through which the guidewire can pass directly into the introducing needle without detachment. It also reduces the risk for air embolism, which can occur when the needle is open to air. It is not uncommon for the wire to become snagged at the junction of the safety syringe and the needle hub. In this case, simply remove the syringe and insert the wire directly.

Guidewire

Two basic types of guidewires are used: straight and J shaped. Straight wires are for use in vessels with a linear configuration,

TABLE 22-2 Needle Sizes for Venous and Arterial Catheters*

STANDARD FULL-LENGTH COIL GUIDEWIRE CATHETER SIZE (Fr)	NEEDLE GAUGE†
3	21
4-4.5	20
5-6.0	20-19
6-8.5	19-18

*Any size of catheter from 3.0 to 8.5 Fr may be introduced with a 22-gauge needle if a solid wire (e.g., Cor-Flex, Cook Critical Care) is used.
†All needle gauges are for thin-walled needles only, the type supplied in central line kits.

Figure 22-4 Introducing needles. **A,** Ordinary needle with a straight-bore lumen. **B,** Seldinger needle with a tapered lumen, which allows easy entry of the guidewire.

Figure 22-5 J-wire. **A,** Plastic sleeve in the retracted position demonstrating the J-tip. **B,** Plastic sleeve advanced to straighten the curve for easy introduction into the needle hub. **C,** Plastic sleeve inserted into needle hub. In an emergency, take care to not misplace or throw the sleeve away. Without it, placing the J-wire into the hub of the needle is very difficult. Some wires may have a "soft-tipped" straight end on the opposite end of the wire. These wires are engineered to be flexible (to avoid vessel injury) and may be used if there is difficulty passing the J end.

whereas J-wires are for use in tortuous vessels. Both wires have essentially the same internal design (Fig. 22-5). The flexibility of the wire is the result of a stainless steel coil or helix that forms the bulk of the guidewire. Within the central lumen of the helix is a straight central core wire, called a mandrel, that adds rigidity to the steel coil. The mandrel is usually fixed at one end of the helix and terminates 0.5 and 3.0 cm from the other end to create a flexible or floppy tip. Wires are also available with two flexible ends, one straight and the other J shaped. The flexible end of the guidewire allows the wire to flex on contact with the wall of a vessel. If the contact is tangential, as with an infraclavicular approach to the SV, a straight wire is generally preferred. If the angle is more acute, as with an external jugular approach to the SV, or if the vessel is particularly tortuous or valves must be traversed, a J-shaped wire may be used. The more rounded leading edge of the J-wire provides a broader surface to manipulate within the vessel and decreases the risk for perforation. This is especially advantageous when attempting to thread a wire through a vessel with valves. Many guidewires also contain a straight safety wire that runs parallel to the mandrel to keep the wire from kinking or shearing.

The standard size for guidewires is 0.025 to 0.035 inch (0.064 to 0.089 cm) in diameter, which permits introduction through an 18-gauge thin-walled needle. A modification of this standard wire uses a bare mandrel with the flexible coil soldered to its end. This construction provides a wire with a diameter of just 0.018 inch (0.047 cm) but with the same rigidity as the larger wires. The manufacturer states that such a wire can be introduced through a 22-gauge thin-walled needle yet still guide an 8.5-Fr catheter (Micropuncture Introducer Sets and Trays with Cor-Flex Wire Guides, Cook Critical Care, Inc., Bloomington, IN).

It is important to emphasize that guidewires are delicate and may bend, kink, or unwind. A force of 4 to 6 lb may cause a wire to rupture. Wires should thread easily and smoothly and never be forced; the worst complications of CVC placement are associated with the application of excessive force across parts of the apparatus that are not threading smoothly.[66] If a wire is not passing easily, withdraw the wire and the introducer needle as a single unit. Embolization of portions of the guidewire is possible, and sharp defects in the wire may perforate vessel walls (Fig. 22-6). If one encounters a good flash of blood but cannot readily manipulate the wire, this may indicate that the outer wire coils are entrapped against the proximal sharp edge of the needle bevel. The J can be straightened remotely by applying gentle force on the wire in each direction, which may allow retrieval of the wire.[55] Wires should be inspected for small defects such as kinks, sharp ends, or spurs before use and especially after a failed attempt. Wires may be threaded into the introducer needle hub more easily by using the plastic sleeve attached to the wire as shown in Figure 22-5C.

Catheters

A number of different catheter and introducer devices have been developed, and the method of passage into the vessel varies accordingly. The functions of catheters have become more sophisticated as well, most notably for continuous monitoring of central venous oxygen saturation and cardiac output. Generally, one can place single-, double-, and triple-lumen catheters by sliding the catheter directly over a guidewire into the intended vessel (Fig. 22-7A). Catheter insertion lengths are listed in Table 22-3. Larger catheters or devices without lumens can be introduced with a sheath-introducer system. Over-the-needle catheters can be introduced once intravascular placement is attained.

The Desilets-Hoffman–type sheath introducer became available in 1965 to aid in arteriography procedures that require many catheter changes. This device is commonly but incorrectly termed a "Cordis," which is a proprietary trade

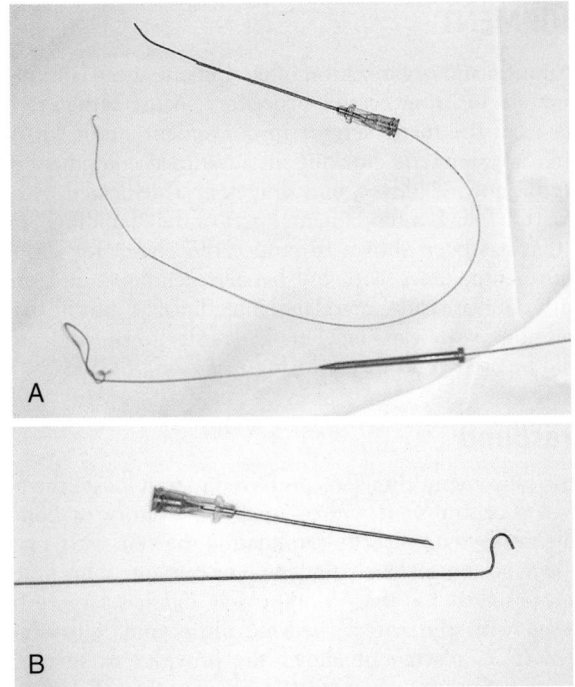

Figure 22-6 A and **B,** Although newer guidewires are more resistant to shearing, if a guidewire will not advance, *withdraw both the needle and the wire in one motion.* These pictures demonstrate a permanently deformed guidewire that could not be advanced. Withdrawing the wire with the indwelling introducer needle in place within a vessel may shear off a portion of the wire and result in systemic embolization.

name. The sheath-introducer unit includes two parts, an inner dilator and an outer sheath as shown in Figure 22-7B. The dilator is rigid with a narrow lumen to accommodate the guidewire. It is longer and thinner than its sheath and has a tapered end that dilates the subcutaneous tissue and vessel defect created by the needle. The sheath (or introducer catheter when used as a cannula for inserting Swan-Ganz catheters, transvenous pacemakers, or other devices) has a blunt end and is simply a large-diameter catheter.

Many modifications of the sheath exist, such as side arms and diaphragms to aid in the placement of devices without lumens. Care must be taken when using side-arm sets for rapid administration of fluid because some catheters are 8.5 Fr in diameter but have only a 5-Fr side arm. Some sets have a "single-lumen infusion catheter," which performs the same function but is more easily secured to the sheath introducer. Selection of the appropriate diameter of introducer catheter should correspond to the indication for placement of a CVC. Generally, an 8.5-Fr catheter is used to facilitate placement of a Swan-Ganz catheter and a 6.0-Fr catheter is used to facilitate transvenous placement of a pacemaker. If the introducer catheter is larger than required to support the intraluminal device, a leak may develop at the diaphragm insertion point.

Special catheters have been developed to prevent bacterial contamination and line sepsis.[37,67,68] These catheters are impregnated with either antiseptics (silver sulfadiazine and chlorhexidine) or antibiotics (minocycline, rifampin, or cefazolin) to reduce bacterial colonization and microbial growth. Also, heparin-coated catheters are available that prevent fibronectin binding, thereby inhibiting the formation

A

B

Figure 22-7 A, Triple-lumen catheter. The catheter ports are used for infusion of fluids, administration of medications, and monitoring of central venous pressure and are typically labeled as proximal, medial, and distal. The distal or brown port, typically 16 gauge, facilitates passage of the guidewire. Note that the end cap of the distal port (arrow) must be removed before insertion to allow passage of the guidewire. **B,** Sheath introducer. This large-bore device (8.5 Fr) is used as an introduction catheter for devices such as Swan-Ganz catheters and transvenous pacemakers. Note that the dilator must be placed through the catheter *before* the device is inserted into the patient.

TABLE 22-3 Formulas for Catheter Insertion Length Based on Patient Height and Approach

SITE	FORMULA	IN SVC (%)	IN RA (%)
RSC	(Ht/10) − 2 cm	96	4
LSC	(Ht/10) + 2 cm	97	2
RIJ	Ht/10	90	10
LIJ	(Ht/10) + 4 cm	94	5

From Czepizak C, O'Callaghan JM, Venus B. Evaluation of formulas for optimal positioning of central venous catheters. *Chest.* 1995;107:1662. Reproduced by permission.

Ht, patient height (in cm); *LIJ,* left internal jugular; *LSC,* left subclavian; *RA,* right atrium; *RIJ,* right internal jugular; *RSC,* right subclavian; *SVC,* superior vena cava.

of bacterial biofilm on the catheter's surface. These catheters can decrease catheter-associated infection (CAI) significantly and are cost-effective when the prevalence of CAI is greater than 2%.[42] They should be avoided in patients with a history of heparin-induced thrombocytopenia.[69] Minocycline- and rifampin-impregnated catheters are currently considered to be the most effective.[37,67] Other interventions that decrease

central line infections include the use of full sterile barrier precautions,[61,65] skin preparation with chlorhexidine solution,[61-63,70] and placement by experienced physicians.[65,71-73]

Many different catheters are currently manufactured. Although this leads to great flexibility in choice and cost, it often results in confusion when a clinician is handed an unfamiliar catheter during an emergency. It is best to use one brand routinely and to ensure that all medical personnel are thoroughly familiar with its use.[74]

TECHNIQUE

Preprocedure Preparation

When possible, discuss the procedure with the patient and obtain written informed consent. Place the patient and yourself in an appropriate position for the specific vessel being accessed. If available, perform an ultrasound survey to identify the patient's anatomy, ensure vessel patency, and confirm the puncture site (Fig. 22-8). Ultrasound-guided CVC placement has been shown to decrease procedure times, as well as complication rates.[46-49] Additionally, compliance with a central line bundling policy has been shown to significantly decrease central line–associated bloodstream infections.[60-63] Prepare and drape the puncture site while maintaining sterile technique, and observe universal precautions throughout the procedure (Fig. 22-9, *steps 1 and 2*). A gown, surgical cap, mask, eye protection, and sterile gloves should be worn throughout the procedure when possible. When performing ultrasound-guided placement of a CVC, ensure that a sterile transducer sheath and sterile transducer gel are used during the procedure (see Fig. 22-9, *step 3*). Using an assistant will prove valuable in patient preparation, maintenance of sterility, and handling of the equipment.

Guidewire Placement with the Seldinger Technique

When performing ultrasound-guided placement of a CVC, begin with an ultrasound survey of the target vein, surrounding structures, and venipuncture location, as shown in Figure 22-8. Veins can easily be distinguished from the nearby artery by applying external pressure with the transducer. Veins collapse completely with pressure, whereas arteries may deform but do not usually collapse. Occasionally, the vein does not collapse with pressure. If this occurs, a thrombus may be present in the vein or the structure has been misidentified. If a suspected vein does not collapse with pressure, it is not an appropriate vessel for cannulation. If available, Doppler functions may also be helpful in the differentiation of veins and arteries. Select a venipuncture location where branching of the vein will allow the shortest path of the needle, will not obstruct passage of the catheter, and will not allow inadvertent puncture of other vital anatomic structures. (See Chapter 66 for additional information and descriptions of the ultrasound technique.)

Prepare the catheter for insertion by flushing each lumen with sterile normal saline. Anesthetize the insertion site with lidocaine or bupivacaine (see Fig. 22-9, *step 5*). Attach a small syringe to an introducing needle that is large enough to accommodate the guidewire. Insert the needle and syringe together. Slowly advance the needle into the vein and apply steady negative pressure on the syringe (see Fig. 22-9, *step*

Figure 22-8 A, Ultrasound survey. Perform an ultrasound survey to identify the anatomy before beginning the procedure. **B,** Cross-sectional view of the artery (*left*) and noncompressed vein (*right*). **C,** Cross-sectional view of the artery (*left*) and compressed vein (*right*).

6). When performing ultrasound-guided CVC placement, follow the needle trajectory in the soft tissue and observe penetration of the vessel. If the tip of the needle is not visualized at all times with ultrasound, the needle may be passed into structures other than the vein. The key concept in using ultrasound guidance for venous access is to visualize the tip of the needle at all times during cannulation (Fig. 22-10). Once the tip of the needle enters the vessel lumen, blood will be aspirated freely. Stabilize the needle hub to prevent movement of the needle and displacement of the tip from the vessel, and remove the syringe. The need to disconnect the syringe can be eliminated by use of the Arrow Safety Syringe. After removing the syringe, cap the needle hub with your thumb before passing the guidewire to minimize the potential for air embolism.

Confirm that the blood flow is nonpulsatile. Bright red pulsatile blood is very suggestive of arterial puncture. Be aware that in shock states or marked arterial desaturation, dark, nonpulsatile blood does not rule out arterial cannulation. If there are concerns about possible arterial puncture, either remove the introducer needle and draw a sample for blood gas analysis from the needle to compare with an arterial blood gas sample or insert an 18-gauge single-lumen catheter over the wire and into the vessel because this step does not require the use of a dilator. The catheter can then be connected to a pressure transducer to confirm the presence of venous waveforms and venous pressure.

Introduce the flexible end of the guidewire into the hub of the needle (see Fig. 22-9, *step* 7). It may be easier to introduce the J-wire by advancing the plastic sleeve contained in the kit onto the floppy end of the wire to straighten the J shape. This straightened end is then introduced into the needle hub. The guidewire should thread smoothly through the needle into the vessel without resistance. Do not force the wire if resistance

is encountered, but remove it from the needle and reattach the syringe to aspirate blood and reconfirm intravascular needle placement. It is important for the wire to slip easily from the needle during removal. If resistance to removal of the wire is felt, the wire and needle should be removed as a single unit to prevent shearing of the wire and resultant wire embolism. It has been recommended by some that no wire should ever be withdrawn through the introducing needle.[75] Although there are no clinical data to support this recommendation and newer wires are stronger and more resistant to shearing, it represents the safest course of action. The recommendation to remove the needle and wire as a unit is sometimes disregarded because of reluctance to abandon a potentially successful venipuncture. The clinician performing the procedure must use both caution and good judgment to determine the best course of action but should not withdraw the guidewire against resistance. Manipulation of the wire within an introducer needle should be done only with standard coil guidewires. Solid wires (such as Cor-Flex Wire Guides from Cook Critical Care) have a small lip at the point at which the flexible coil is soldered to the wire. This lip can become caught on the edge of the tip of the needle and shear off the coil portion of the wire. Solid wires must thread freely on the first attempt or the entire wire and needle assembly must be removed. Keep backup wires on hand.

Occasionally, a wire must be teased into the vessel; rotating the wire or needle often helps in difficult placements. If the wire does not thread easily, pull back slightly on the needle itself just before advancing the wire. This helps if the opening of the needle is abutting the vessel's inner wall and blocking entry of the wire or if the vein is compressed by introduction of the needle. Changing wire tips from a straight wire to a J-wire or vice versa may also solve an advancement problem. If the inner lumen of a vessel is smaller than the

CENTRAL VENOUS CATHETERIZATION (INTERNAL JUGULAR APPROACH)

Prepare the area with chlorhexidine solution. A gown, surgical cap, mask, eye protection, and sterile gloves should be worn throughout the procedure.

Apply a full-body, sterile drape. Meticulous attention must be paid to sterile technique to avoid iatrogenic infection.

Insert the ultrasound probe into a sterile sheath, and use sterile ultrasound gel during the procedure. Enlist the help of an assistant in patient preparation and maintenance of sterility.

Identify the anatomic structures with ultrasound. The internal jugular vein (*IJ*) and carotid artery (*CA*) must be clearly distinguished from each other (see text for more details).

Anesthetize the tissues overlying the vein with local anesthetic. Here, the operator is using ultrasound guidance to ensure a proper entry site.

Insert the needle and syringe while slowly advancing and applying negative pressure to the plunger. Follow the needle trajectory with ultrasound until the vein is entered and blood enters the syringe (*arrow*).

Remove the syringe and advance the guidewire through the needle. Use the straightener (*arrow*) to facilitate entry of the J-wire into the hub. NEVER FORCE THE WIRE!

Once the wire has been inserted to the appropriate depth (see text for details), remove the needle (*arrow*). It is *essential* to *always* maintain a grip on the wire throughout the procedure (!).

Figure 22-9 Ultrasound-guided internal jugular central venous catheterization.

Continued

CENTRAL VENOUS CATHETERIZATION (INTERNAL JUGULAR APPROACH)

Make an incision at the site of the wire to facilitate dilator and catheter passage. Make the incision the width of the catheter and extend it completely through the dermis.

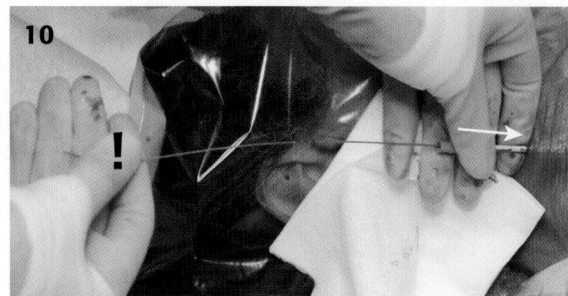

Thread the dilator over the guidewire. The wire must *always* be protruding from the end of the dilator and firmly in your grasp (!). Advance the dilator several cm into the vessel and then remove.

Advance the catheter over the wire. It can be difficult to align the two pieces; hold the very end of the catheter and the wire to make this step easier.

Advance the catheter into the vessel. The guidewire will emerge from the distal port. It is essential that the guidewire protrudes from the hub and is grasped before catheter advancement (!).

Remove the wire. Cover the open port with your thumb (*arrow*) until the end-cap is screwed on.

Flush all ports with saline.

Suture the catheter into place using non-absorbable silk sutures. Several knots should be made to secure the line. Avoid making knots that place excessive pressure on the skin.

Clean the area around the catheter insertion site with chlorhexidine. Place a simple dressing, avoiding excessive amounts of gauze and tape.

Figure 22-9, cont'd

Figure 22-10 A, Ultrasound-guided insertion of the introducer needle. **B,** Cross-sectional ultrasound image of the needle (*arrow*) within the vessel.

diameter of the J, the wire will be prevented from returning its natural shape and the spring in the coil will generate resistance. Any advantages of a J-wire will be negated if the wire fails to regain its intended shape. In this instance, a straight tip should be able to be introduced without a problem. Alternatively, if the angle of entry of the needle into the vessel is more acute than was suspected, a straight wire may not be able to bend appropriately as it encounters the vessel's far wall. A J-tipped wire may be used and threaded in such a manner that the wire resumes its J shape away from the far wall. All these maneuvers are performed with gentle free motions of the wire within the needle. If at any time the wire cannot be advanced freely, suspect improper placement and reevaluate the attempt.

If threading easily, advance the guidewire until at least one quarter of the wire is within the vessel. The further into the vessel the wire extends, the more stable its location when the catheter is introduced. However, advancing the guidewire too far may result in ventricular ectopy secondary to endocardial irritation, myocardial puncture leading to tamponade, or entanglement in a previously placed pacemaker, internal defibrillator, or IVC filter. In both the left and right IJ vein and infraclavicular SV approaches, fluoroscopic study during passage of the guidewire has determined the mean distance from skin to the SVC-atrial junction to be 18 cm.[75] This distance has been recommended as the greatest depth of guidewire insertion for these approaches. It should be noted that 18 cm is not necessarily the appropriate final depth for the catheter being placed (see discussion below).

Cardiac monitoring may be helpful during the insertion of central lines. Any increase in premature ventricular contractions or a new ventricular dysrhythmia should be interpreted as evidence that the guidewire is inserted too far and should be remedied by withdrawing the wire until the rhythm reverts to baseline. Usually, the procedure can be continued after a moment, with care taken to not readvance the wire. Persistent ventricular dysrhythmias require standard advanced cardiac life support treatment and consideration of a new vascular approach.

Occasionally, a wire threads easily past the tip of the needle and then suddenly will not advance farther. If the introducer needle demonstrated free return of blood at the time of wire entry and the initial advancement of the wire met no resistance, the two options are to halt the procedure or seek confirmation of wire position. The guidewire within the lumen of the vessel can be visualized and confirmed via cross-sectional and longitudinal views on ultrasound. Alternatively, the needle may be removed, the wire fixed in place with a

Figure 22-11 Cross-sectional (**A**) and longitudinal (**B**) ultrasound images demonstrating a guidewire (*arrows*) in the lumen of the targeted vein.

sterile hemostat, and a radiograph taken to confirm the position of the wire.[75,76] A freely advancing wire may suddenly stop once it is well within a vessel if the vessel makes an unsuspected bend or is being compressed or deviated by another structure, such as a rib or muscle. This seems especially common with the infraclavicular approach to the SV and can sometimes be remedied by a more lateral approach.

Sheath Unit and Catheter Placement

Once the wire is placed into the vessel, remove the needle in preparation for passage of the catheter (see Fig. 22-9, *step 8*). Proper positioning of the guidewire within the vessel lumen can be confirmed by cross-sectional and longitudinal ultrasound imaging (Fig. 22-11).[76] This can be done at any point while inserting the wire to ensure that the correct vessel has been cannulated and that puncture of the posterior wall has not occurred. This technique can be quite useful when resistance is encountered while feeding the guidewire. A small skin incision is required at the site of the wire to widen the opening (see Fig. 22-9, *step 9*). Make the incision approximately the width of the catheter to be introduced and extend it completely through the dermis.

When placing soft multiple-lumen catheters, the tissue must be dilated from the skin to the vessel before placement of the catheter. Thread the guidewire through the distal opening of the rigid dilator until it extends through the proximal end of the dilator (see Fig. 22-9, *step 10*). The wire must always be visibly protruding from the end of the dilator or catheter during insertion to avoid inadvertent advancement of the wire into the circulation and potential loss of the wire. While maintaining control of the guidewire proximally, thread the dilator over the wire into the skin with a twisting motion. Advance the rigid dilator only a few centimeters into the vessel, and then remove it. Once the dilator is removed, thread the soft catheter into position over the wire. Placement of multiple-lumen catheters requires identification of the distal lumen and its corresponding hub. Find the distal lumen at the very tip of the catheter. The corresponding hub is usually labeled "distal" by the manufacturer. If there is any confusion, inject a small amount of sterile saline through each hub until it is observed exiting the distal lumen. Once the distal hub is identified, remove its cover cap to allow passage of the guidewire. Place the catheter by threading the guidewire into the distal lumen and advancing it until it protrudes from the identified hub (see Fig. 22-9, *step 11*). It is imperative that the guidewire protrude from the catheter hub and that it be firmly grasped as the wire and catheter are advanced. If the wire does not protrude from the proximal end of the catheter, withdraw the wire at the skin entry point until it protrudes enough to be grasped. While maintaining control of the guidewire proximally, advance the catheter into the vessel to the desired catheter insertion length (see Fig. 22-9, *step 12*). Ultrasonography can be used to verify proper catheter placement. After insertion of the catheter the wire must be removed (see Fig. 22-9, *step 13*) and the catheter must be anchored to the skin with sutures. When removing the wire from a catheter it must slip out easily. If any resistance is met, remove both the wire and the catheter as a single unit and reattempt the procedure. A common cause of a "stuck wire" is a small piece of adipose tissue wedged between the wire and the lumen of the catheter. Avoid this problem by creating a deep enough skin nick and adequate dilation of the tract before inserting the catheter.

When placing a single-lumen, Desilets-Hoffman sheath-introducer system, the dilator and larger single-lumen catheter are inserted simultaneously as a dilator-sheath unit. The dilator-sheath unit must first be assembled by inserting the dilator through the catheter's diaphragm (Fig. 22-12, *step 2*). When assembled correctly, the dilator "snaps" into place within the lumen of the sheath and protrudes several centimeters from the distal end of the catheter.

After successful guidewire placement and after the skin incision is made, thread the dilator-sheath assembly over the wire (see Fig. 22-12, *step 3*). It is imperative that the guidewire protrude from the proximal end of the dilator-sheath assembly and that it be firmly grasped as the wire and unit is advanced. If the wire does not protrude from the proximal end of the assembly, withdraw the wire at the skin entry point until it protrudes enough to be grasped. While maintaining

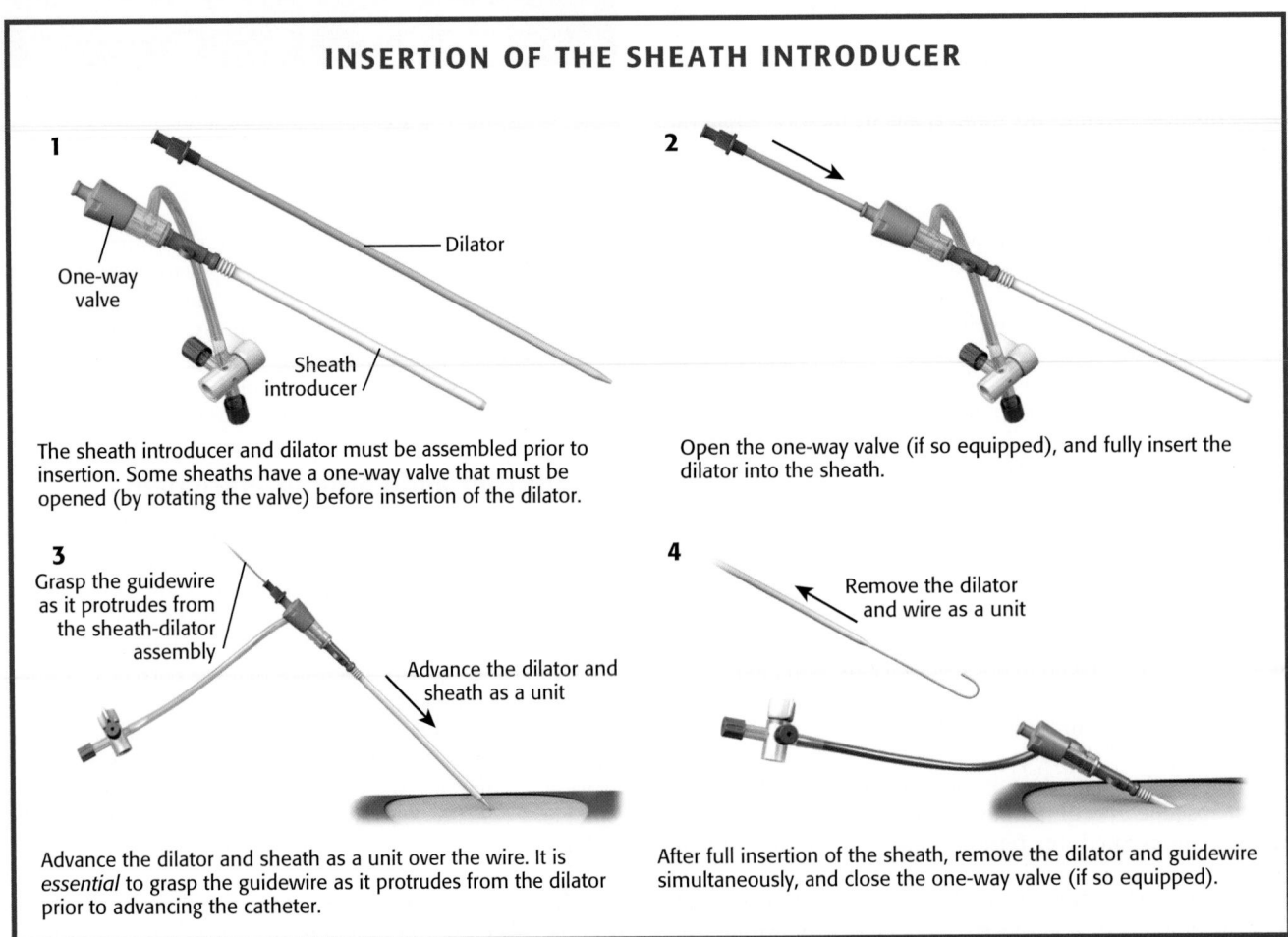

Figure 22-12 Insertion of the sheath introducer. Insertion of a sheath introducer varies slightly from that for a triple-lumen catheter—the dilator and the catheter are inserted simultaneously as depicted. The remainder of the steps are analogous to those in Figure 22-9. Once inserted, sheath introducers facilitate the placement of devices such as pulmonary artery catheters and transvenous pacemakers.

control of the guidewire proximally, advance the assembly through the skin with a twisting motion until it is within the vessel. Grasp the unit at the junction of the sheath and dilator. This prevents the thinner sheath from kinking or bending at the tip or from bunching up at the coupler end. Keep the assembly intact and advance it through the skin to the hub. Once the catheter is placed, remove the wire and dilator from the sheath simultaneously (see Fig. 22-12, *step 4*). When removing the wire and dilator, the dilator must "unsnap" from the sheath unit, and the wire must slip out easily. Once the single-lumen sheath-introducer catheter is placed correctly, it may be used to facilitate the placement of additional intralu-minal devices such as a pulmonary artery catheter, trans-venous cardiac pacemaker, or additional multiple-lumen catheter. At times, critically ill patients who require initial large-volume resuscitation will later require multiple medica-tions and therapies that dictate the need for a multiple-lumen catheter. An alternative method of placing a multiple-lumen catheter is to thread the catheter through a standard Desilets-Hoffman sheath-introducer system.

It is important to consider the depth of insertion of the catheter (see Table 22-3). The proper depth of catheter inser-tion is site specific (see below). After successful CVC place-ment, the catheter should be anchored to the skin with sutures (see Fig. 22-9, *step 15*). Each port should be immediately capped and flushed with a saline solution (see Fig. 22-9, *step 14*). The catheter insertion site should be dressed appropri-ately and all sharp implements disposed of in appropriate receptacles (see Fig. 22-9, *step 16*).

Replacement of Existing Catheters

In addition to placing new catheters, clinicians may use the guidewire technique to change existing catheters. Many patients with CVCs are seriously ill and will require subse-quent monitoring of pulmonary artery wedge pressure, place-ment of a transvenous pacemaker, or insertion of a different catheter. The CVC that is initially inserted should have a lumen large enough to accept a guidewire and facilitate con-version to a different catheter. Clinicians may use the guide-wire technique to change a single-lumen CVC to a triple-lumen catheter or a sheath-introducer set. Not all commercially available CVCs will accept a guidewire.

Replacement of an existing catheter begins with selecting a guidewire longer than either of the devices to be exchanged. Use meticulous aseptic technique.[70] Insert the guidewire into the existing CVC until a few centimeters of wire is protruding from the proximal end. With one hand holding the wire securely, remove the catheter and wire as a single unit until the tip of the catheter just clears the patient's skin. Grasp the wire at the point where it exits the skin and only then release the wire at the other end. Then slide the catheter off the wire and insert the new device in the normal fashion. Exercise caution with this technique because catheter embolization can occur, especially if a catheter is cut to allow use of a shorter guidewire for the exchange. In patients without evidence of line sepsis, exchanging the guidewire does not increase the incidence of CAI if performed properly.[70]

Over-the-Needle Technique

An optional method for cannulation is to place an over-the-needle catheter percutaneously. Over-the-needle devices

(such as the Angiocath) use a tapered plastic catheter that passes through the vessel wall into the lumen, with the tip of the needle being used as a guide. There are advantages with this system. The catheter does not pass through a sharp needle and there is less risk of shearing and resultant catheter embolization. Also, the hole made by the needle in the vessel wall is smaller than the catheter, thus producing a tighter seal. The IJ vein and SV via the supraclavicular approach are the most popular and appropriate approaches for this technique. These devices may be useful when rapid central venous access is required (e.g., in cardiac arrest). These catheters are not suitable for high-volume fluid resuscitation, and they are too small for passage of a pacemaker lead. Once the clinical situ-ation stabilizes, exchange this device for a larger central cath-eter via the Seldinger technique.

Prepare the skin with chlorhexidine solution. Use a longer peripheral-type catheter (such as a 16-gauge, $5\frac{1}{4}$-inch angio-catheter) in an adult. Smaller-diameter devices, such as 20-gauge catheters, may be easier to pass but provide slower infusion rates. Attach the needle to a syringe, and slowly advance it into the vein with steady negative pressure applied to the syringe. This may be difficult because of the longer length of the needle relative to the catheter. When using bedside ultrasound, follow the trajectory of the needle into the soft tissues and visualize penetration of the vessel. With over-the-needle catheters, the needle extends a few millime-ters past the tip of the catheter. Return of blood will be obtained when the tip of the needle is in the vein, although the catheter may actually be outside the lumen. If the needle is withdrawn before the catheter is advanced, the tip of the catheter will remain outside the vein. It is therefore important to advance the needle a few millimeters after the venous flash is seen and then hold it steadily while advancing the catheter into the vein. Secure the catheter and verify its placement as detailed later in this chapter.

SITE SELECTION

Subclavian Approaches

Subclavian venipuncture is the most frequently used means of achieving central venous access. The infraclavicular SV approach was the first popular means of central venous access and has been used widely for nearly half a century. It is useful in many clinical situations and relatively easy to learn. It is often the best approach in trauma because a cervical collar can interfere with the IJ technique. The supraclavicular SV approach may be preferable during CPR because it minimizes physical interference in chest compressions and airway man-agement. In addition, the supraclavicular SV technique has been performed in the sitting position in patients with severe orthopnea. Finally, the left SV provides a more direct route to the SVC and is the preferred site for pacemaker placement and CVP monitoring.

IJ Approach

The IJ vein provides an excellent site for placement of a CVC. However, there is a 5% to 10% risk for complications, with serious complications occurring in about 1% of patients.[46] Failure rates have been found to be 19.4% for landmark-placed IJ catheterization by a junior practitioner and 5% to 10% by a clinician with extensive experience.[77] Despite its potential complications, the IJ vein is in many cases preferred over other options for central venous access. In contrast to the SV, arterial punctures are easier to control because direct pressure can be used, and the incidence of pneumothorax is lower. Hematoma formation is easier to diagnose because of the close proximity of the IJ vein to the skin. In addition, the right IJ vein provides a straight anatomic path to the SVC and right atrium. This is advantageous for passage of catheters or internal pacemaker wires to the heart. Disadvantages of IJ vein cannulation over other sites include a relatively high carotid artery puncture rate and poor landmarks in obese or edematous patients.[40,46]

The IJ technique is useful for routine central venous access and for emergency venous access during CPR because the site is removed from the area of chest compressions. The differences in morbidity between the SV and the IJ vein approach have probably been overstated.[20,73,78,79] Catheter malposition is more frequent in the SV, but the risk for infection is probably slightly higher with IJ sites.[20,22,42,65] The rate of arterial puncture is higher with IJ attempts, but the SV is not a compressible site.[20,42] Though counterintuitive, the evidence available does not support a significant difference in the rate of pneumothorax and hemothorax.[20,42] Although there may be a slight difference in complications between the two routes, in the absence of specific contraindications clinicians should use the technique with which they are most familiar. The rapid development of real-time ultrasound guidance may tip the scales toward the IJ as the preferred site.[14,47-49,80,81]

Femoral Approach

Cannulation of the femoral vein for central venous access has become increasingly popular, especially for venous access, infusion ports, passage of transvenous pacemakers, and placement of pressure measurement catheters in critically ill patients.[81] The relatively simple and superficial anatomy surrounding the femoral vein affords a rapid approach to the central venous system and avoids many of the more significant complications associated with cannulation of the IJ vein and SV. These benefits are tempered somewhat by several long-term disadvantages, including higher infection rates and an increased risk for venous thrombosis. Other indications for ED femoral cannulation include emergency cardiopulmonary bypass for resuscitation purposes, charcoal hemoperfusion for severe drug overdoses, and dialysis access. The femoral area is less congested than the head and neck area with monitoring and airway equipment, and conscious patients who are still bedridden may turn their head and use their arms more freely without moving the central line. The femoral site is contraindicated in ambulatory patients who require central access.

SPECIFIC VESSEL ACCESS TECHNIQUES

If SV or IJ vein approaches are planned, prepare the skin in the area, including puncture sites for both the infraclavicular and supraclavicular SV and IJ vein approaches. This permits the clinician to change the site after an unsuccessful attempt without repeating the preparation or having to obtain an interval chest radiograph. Prepare the area, including the ipsilateral anterior aspect of the neck, the supraclavicular fossa,

and the anterior chest wall 3 to 5 cm past the midline and the same distance above the nipple line. Prepare for femoral access by trimming groin hairs and applying chlorhexidine to cover an area the breadth of and extending 10 cm above and below the inguinal ligament.

Each approach to central venous cannulation is described separately below. As with any invasive procedure, briefly describe the procedure to awake patients, and restate each step as it is about to be performed. After descriptions of the common approaches to the central veins, puncture site care, verification of placement, and other adjuncts to the procedure are summarized.

Infraclavicular Subclavian Approach

Descriptions of subclavian venipuncture often focus unduly on angles and landmarks. Indeed, recent studies have demonstrated that some traditional positioning maneuvers may actually hinder successful cannulation efforts.

Positioning

Place the patient supine on the stretcher with the head in a neutral position and the arm adducted at the side. Some authors have advocated various shoulder-, back-, head-, and arm-positioning maneuvers, but they take extra time and the help of an assistant and are often not helpful.[82-92]

We believe that the best position for almost all infraclavicular SV attempts is the neutral shoulder position with the arm adducted.[82-93] Turning the head away may be helpful but is certainly not required if cervical injuries are suspected.[83,85,90] Interestingly, Jung and colleagues found that in children, tilting the head toward the catheterization site improved catheter malposition rates.[94] This technique has not been studied in adults.

In difficult cases, placing a small towel roll under the ipsilateral shoulder[90] or having an assistant place caudal traction of about 5 cm on the extremity may also be helpful.[93] Placing the patient in a moderate Trendelenburg position (10 to 20 degrees) decreases the risk for air embolism.[85,95] The claim that this position distends the vein is controversial, but it may do so to a small favorable degree.[83,85,87] If the Trendelenburg position is impractical, the SV approach is probably less affected than the IJ approach when resorting to a neutral or even an upright position.[83,85,87]

Placing a pillow under the back is commonly recommended to make the clavicle more prominent, but as the shoulder falls backward, the space between the clavicle and the first rib narrows, thus making the SV less accessible.[92] Significant compression of the subclavian vessels between these bony structures occurs as the shoulders retract, which can cause a "pinch off" of the catheter as it slides through the SV between the clavicle and the first rib.[92,96]

Venipuncture Site

The right SV is usually selected first because of the lower pleural dome on the right and the need to avoid the left-sided thoracic duct. The more direct route between the left SV and the SVC is a theoretical advantage of left-sided subclavian venipuncture; however, there is no higher incidence of catheter malposition when the right infraclavicular SV approach is used. In conscious patients, anesthetize the point of needle entry with 1% lidocaine. If possible, infiltrate the periosteum of the clavicle to make the procedure less painful. Opinions vary regarding the best point of needle entry, more so than for the IJ or femoral approaches. With nonobese patients, look for the "deltopectoral triangle," which is bounded by the clavicle superiorly, the pectoralis major medially, and the deltoid muscle laterally.[88,97] The junction of the middle and medial thirds of the clavicle lies just medial to this triangle. Further medially, the vein lies just posterior to the clavicle and above the first rib, which acts as a barrier to penetration of the pleura. This protective effect is theoretically diminished when a more lateral location is chosen. However, when approaching the vein more medially, some clinicians have difficulty puncturing the SV, dilating the tissues, and passing the J-wire. Other recommended sites of approach include lateral and inferior to the junction of the clavicle and the first rib, with the needle aimed at this junction, and entry at the site of a small tubercle in the medial aspect of the deltopectoral groove. We recommend puncturing the skin at the lateral portion of the deltopectoral triangle via a shallow angle of attack.[88]

Needle Orientation

Orient the bevel of the needle inferomedially to direct the wire toward the innominate vein rather than toward the opposite vessel wall or up into the IJ vein. Align the bevel of the needle with the markings on the barrel of the syringe to permit awareness of bevel orientation after skin puncture.

Before inserting the needle, place your left index finger in the suprasternal notch and your thumb at the costoclavicular junction (Fig. 22-13). These landmarks serve as reference points for the direction that the needle should travel. Aim the needle immediately above and posterior to your index finger. Watch for vessel entry, signaled by flashback of dark venous blood, which usually occurs at a depth of 3 to 4 cm. If the tip of the needle is truly intraluminal, there will be free-flowing blood. Return of pulsatile flow signifies arterial puncture, and the needle should be withdrawn immediately. A single arterial puncture without laceration rarely causes serious harm. Using this technique eliminates the need to measure angles, to

Figure 22-13 Infraclavicular subclavian approach. Place your index finger in the suprasternal notch and your thumb at the costoclavicular junction; these landmarks will serve as reference points for the direction that the needle should travel. Orient the bevel of the needle inferomedially, and aim the needle above and posterior to your index finger.

"walk" the clavicle, or to concentrate excessively on maintaining the needle parallel to the chest wall. Avoid using sweeping motions of the tip of the needle to prevent unseen injuries.

Unsuccessful Attempts

Cannulation of the SV may not succeed on the first attempt. It is reasonable to try again, but after three or four unsuccessful attempts, it is wise to move to a different anatomic approach or to allow a colleague to attempt the procedure. Use a new setup each time that blood is obtained because clots and tissue will clog the needle and mislead the clinician even if the vein has been entered successfully on subsequent attempts. If several attempts are made, inform the admitting clinician or anesthesiologist so that proper precautions are taken to identify subsequent complications. It is advisable to obtain radiographs of the chest even after unsuccessful attempts. If the initial puncture site was placed properly, use the same needle hole for subsequent attempts if possible for aesthetic reasons. If the SV route is unsuccessful on one side, attempt IJ vein catheterization on the same side rather than SV cannulation on the opposite side to avoid bilateral complications.

Supraclavicular Subclavian Approach

Positioning

The goal of the supraclavicular SV technique is to puncture the SV in its superior aspect as it joins the IJ vein. Insert the needle above and behind the clavicle, lateral to the clavicular head of the SCM muscle. Advance it in an avascular plane while directing it away from the subclavian artery and the dome of the pleura (Fig. 22-14). The right side is preferred because of the lower pleural dome, its more direct route to the SVC, and location of the thoracic duct on the left side. The patient's head may be turned to the opposite side to help identify the landmarks.

Needle Orientation

After the area of the supraclavicular fossa has been prepared and draped, identify a point 1 cm lateral to the clavicular head of the SCM and 1 cm posterior to the clavicle. Alternatively, use the junction of the middle and medial thirds of the clavicle as the landmark for needle entry. Anesthetize the area with 1% lidocaine. If a 3-cm-long needle is used for anesthesia, it may also be used to locate the vessel in a relatively atraumatic manner. The SV can almost always be located with this needle because of its superficial location and the absence of bony structures in the path of the needle. Advance a 14-gauge needle (or 18-gauge thin-walled needle) along the path of the scout needle. Apply gentle negative pressure with an attached syringe.

When seeking the SV, aim the needle so that it bisects the clavicosternomastoid angle and the tip points just caudal to the contralateral nipple. Orient the bevel medially to prevent the catheter from getting trapped against the inferior vessel wall. Point the tip of the needle 10 degrees above the horizontal. Successful vessel puncture generally occurs at a depth of 2 to 3 cm.

Subclavian Ultrasound Technique

Typically, puncture of the SV occurs at the point where the vein is coursing deep to the clavicle. However, with ultrasound, visualization of the SV can be difficult at this location because of interference with the overlying bone. Fortunately,

Figure 22-14 Supraclavicular subclavian approach. **A,** Anatomy. As the subclavian vein passes over the first rib, it is separated from the subclavian artery by the anterior scalene muscle. The dome of the pleura is posterolateral to the confluence of the great veins. *Arrow,* needle target; *ASM,* anterior scalene muscle; *IJ,* internal jugular vein; *SA,* subclavian artery; *SCM,* sternocleidomastoid muscle, sternal head; *SV,* subclavian vein. **B,** Approach. Insert the needle 1 cm posterior to the clavicle and 1 cm lateral to the clavicular head of the SCM such that the angle made by the clavicle and lateral border of the muscle is bisected. The needle traverses an avascular plane and punctures the junction of the subclavian and IJ veins behind the sternoclavicular joint. The right side is preferred because of a direct route to the superior vena cava and absence of the thoracic duct. The needle is directed 45 degrees from the sagittal plane and 10 to 15 degrees upward from the horizontal plane and aimed toward the contralateral nipple. Note that the vein is just posterior to the clavicle at this juncture.

more distally the vein lies farther away from the clavicle and chest wall. Hence, access to the SV typically occurs lateral to the curve of the clavicle bone, in the proximal axillary vein. As the vein moves laterally, the mean depth from the skin increases from 1.9 to 3.1 cm while the distance from the rib cage to the vein increases from 1 to 2 cm. The arteriovenous distance also increases from 0.3 to 0.8 cm, and there is less overlap of the artery and vein.[98] Because the vein is not in close proximity to the clavicle, if a hematoma develops, manual pressure can be used to stop the bleeding. Furthermore, the axillary vein is farther from the chest wall and pleural surface, thus decreasing the possibility of pleural injury and subsequent pneumothorax. In clinical studies, ultrasound-guided axillary vein access had a first–needle pass

success rate of 76% with successful placement in 96% of cases. Despite the use of ultrasound, however, the catheter malposition rate was unchanged at approximately 15%.[99]

IJ Approach

Positioning
Position is critical for maximizing the success of blind (landmark technique) cannulation of the IJ vein. Place the patient in a supine position with the head down and turned about 15 to 30 degrees away from the IJ vein to be cannulated. Rotate the head slightly away from the site of insertion. Rotating the head more than 40 degrees has been shown to increase the risk for overlapping the carotid artery over the IJ vein.[19] Occasionally, placing a towel roll under the scapula helps extend the neck and accentuate the landmarks. Stand at the head of the bed with all equipment within easy reach. This may involve moving the bed to the center of the room to allow a table or work surface to be placed at the head of the bed.

Ask the patient to perform a Valsalva maneuver just before inserting the needle to increase the diameter of the IJ vein. Alternatively, the patient can be asked to hum. Trendelenburg positioning, the Valsalva maneuver, and humming all increase the area of the vessel by about 30% to 40%.[100] If the patient is unable to cooperate, coordinate the insertion with respiration because the IJ vein is at its largest diameter just before inspiration. In intubated patients, this relationship is reversed because mechanical ventilation increases intrathoracic pressure at end-inspiration. External abdominal compression also helps distend the IJ vein.

Venipuncture Site
The right IJ vein provides a more direct route to the right atrium for transvenous pacing. The left IJ vein is often more tortuous and catheters must negotiate two 90-degree turns at the junction of the left IJ vein with the SV and at the junction of the SV with the SVC. However, if the right IJ vein is obstructed or scarred by previous access, the left IJ vein may be accessed with the same technique. Of note, the right IJ vein has been observed to be twice the size of the left IJ vein in 34% of normal adults.[101]

Aspirate before injecting anesthetic so that it is not injected into the carotid artery or IJ vein. Once infiltration is completed, use the needle to locate the IJ vein by aspirating blood into the syringe. Note the depth and angle of needle entry and use this as a mental guide to finding the IJ vein with the introducer needle. Typically, an 18-gauge 2.5-cm introducer needle attached to a syringe is used initially to puncture the IJ vein. However, needle selection may vary depending on the central line kit used. The operator may choose from three approaches: central, posterior and anterior (Fig. 22-15).

Central Route
This approach is favored by some who believe that the incidence of cannulation of the carotid artery is decreased and the cupula of the lung is avoided.[101] First, palpate and identify the triangle formed by the clavicle and the sternal and clavicular heads of the SCM. Use a marking pen or a local anesthetic skin wheal to mark the lateral border of the carotid pulse, and perform all subsequent needle punctures lateral to this point.

When using the scout needle technique, attach a 22-gauge, 3-cm needle to a 5- to 10-mL syringe. Insert the needle near the apex of the triangle and direct it caudally at an angle

ANTERIOR APPROACH

Insert needle along the medial edge of the sternocleidomastoid, 2–3 fingerbreadths above the clavicle.

Entry angle = 30° to 45°.

Aim towards the ipsilateral nipple.

Note: Palpate the carotid artery during venipuncture. The artery may be slightly retracted medially.

CENTRAL APPROACH

Insert needle at the apex of the triangle formed by the heads of the sternocleidomastoid muscle and the clavicle.

Entry angle = 30°.

Aim towards the ipsilateral nipple.

Note: Estimate the course of the IJ vein by placing three fingers lightly over the carotid artery as it runs parallel to the vein. The vein lies just lateral to the artery, albeit often minimally so.

POSTERIOR APPROACH

Insert needle at the posterior (lateral) edge of the sternocleidomastoid, midway between the mastoid process and the clavicle.

Entry angle = 45°.

Aim towards the suprasternal notch.

Note: Avoid the external jugular vein, which crosses the posterior SCM border. During needle advancement, apply pressure to the SCM to lift the body of the muscle. The vein is usually reached at a depth of 7 cm.

Figure 22-15 Approaches to the internal jugular (IJ) vein. *SCM,* sternocleidomastoid.

of 30 to 40 degrees to the skin. Direct the needle initially parallel and slightly lateral to the course of the carotid artery. Estimate the course of the IJ vein by placing three fingers lightly over the course of the carotid artery as it runs parallel to the vein. The vein consistently lies just lateral to the carotid artery, albeit often minimally so. Prolonged deep palpation of the carotid artery may decrease the size of the vein, so use the three-finger technique lightly to identify the course of the artery.

Posterior and Anterior Routes

In the posterior approach, make the puncture at the posterior (lateral) edge of the SCM approximately midway between its origin at the mastoid process and its insertion at the clavicle. The external jugular vein courses in this area and can be used as a landmark, with the puncture occurring where the external jugular vein crosses the posterolateral border of the SCM. Be careful to not strike the external jugular vein. Advance the needle toward the suprasternal notch, just under the belly of the SCM, at an angle of approximately 45 degrees to the transverse plane. During advancement of the needle, apply pressure to the SCM in an effort to lift the body of the muscle. The vein is usually reached at a depth of 7 cm in an average-sized adult. Because the posterior approach occurs higher in the neck, there is less risk for hemothorax, pneumothorax, or carotid puncture.[102] The benefits of the posterior approach are more dramatic in obese patients, with carotid puncture occurring in 3% of patients versus up to 17% with the anterior approach.[103]

In the anterior approach, needle puncture occurs along the anterior or medial edge of the SCM about two to three fingerbreadths above the clavicle. Insert the needle at an angle of 30 to 45 degrees toward the ipsilateral nipple, away from the carotid pulse. If cannulation is unsuccessful, withdraw the needle to the skin and redirect it slightly toward the carotid artery.

Once the approach is chosen, slowly advance the needle toward the IJ vein. Create gentle negative pressure with the syringe while advancing the needle. Once blood is seen, stop advancing the syringe. Remove the syringe from the needle to determine whether the vessel is pulsatile. Be careful to not allow negative intrapleural pressure to draw air into the venous system through the open needle. Because the tip of the introducer needle is beveled, lateral motions of the needle tip may cause lacerations of the deep structures of the neck. It is therefore very important to remove the needle from the neck completely before any redirection of the needle.

Once cannulation of the IJ vein has been confirmed, remove the syringe from the needle and place a gloved digit over the needle hub to prevent air embolism. Insert a guidewire through the needle into the IJ vein and place the catheter using the Seldinger technique. Once the wire is inserted into the IJ vein, reduce the angle to the skin to make the needle nearly parallel to the vein. This allows a greater chance of directing the wire toward the heart. Do not let the guidewire extend into the right atrium. The average distance from the insertion site to the junction of the SVC and right atrium is 16 ± 2 cm for the right IJ vein and 19 ± 2 cm for the left IJ vein. The spring wires supplied in kits are often much longer, up to 60 cm in length. If the full length of the wire is inserted, the wire could enter the right atrium or ventricle and cause myocardial irritability and subsequent dysrhythmias. Monitor cardiac rhythm during insertion of the spring wire to detect cardiac irritability. The distance that the catheter is introduced depends on the distance from the site of introduction to the junction of the SVC and right atrium. This distance will be shorter with the right IJ vein than with the left IJ vein.

IJ Ultrasound Technique

Cannulation of the IJ vein is an optimal location for the use of ultrasound guidance. Whereas the landmark approach is associated with a complication rate of between 5% and 10% irrespective of the technique used or experience of the operator, with the use of ultrasound, the complication rate is significantly reduced.[101] Even with novice users of ultrasound for IJ vein cannulation, first-attempt success is significantly increased when compared the blind landmark technique, 43% versus 26%.[104] With experience, however, the first-attempt success rate improves to more than 75%.[16,17,105] Use of ultrasound for placement of central lines in the IJ vein has also been shown to decrease overall catheter placement failures by 64%, reduce complications by 78%, and decrease the need for multiple catheter placement attempts by 40% in comparison to the standard landmark placement technique.[106,107] The primary reason for the increased success rate is the variation in anatomy of the IJ vein relative to the carotid artery. The anatomy of the IJ vein has been shown to be aberrant in 9% to 19% of cases.[101,104,107] Furthermore, the IJ vein may be unusually small (i.e., <0.5 cm) in up to 14% of patients. In some patient populations the IJ vein is thrombosed in up to 2.5%.[104]

With the use of ultrasound there is no need for reliance on normal anatomy for cannulation. Therefore, the IJ vein may be cannulated despite abnormal anatomy. Hence, cannulation may occur at the apex of the triangle, near the base at the junction with the innominate vein, or anywhere in between.

Femoral Approach

Positioning and Needle Orientation

Place the patient in the supine position for the femoral vein approach. This approach does not require any special positioning or tilting of the bed. Fully expose and thoroughly cleanse the area with a soapy washcloth or surgical scrub brush to remove obvious soiling, which may be more common at this site. Next, prepare the skin at the site broadly with chlorhexidine, including the anterior superior iliac spine laterally and superiorly, extending to the midline, and continuing 10 to 15 cm below the inguinal ligament. Tape a urethral catheter to the contralateral leg. In an obese patient, have an assistant retract the abdominal pannus manually or secure it with wide tape.

After the instillation of local anesthetic, introduce the needle at a 45-degree angle in a cephalic direction approximately 1 cm medial to this point and toward the umbilicus (Fig. 22-16). Palpate the femoral pulse two fingerbreadths beneath the inguinal ligament. Note that while palpating the artery, pressure from the operator's fingers can compress the adjacent vein and impede cannulation. Avoid this anatomic distortion by releasing digital pressure while keeping the fingers on the skin to serve as a visual reference to the underlying anatomy. The depth of the needle required to reach the vein varies with body habitus, but in thin adults, the vein is quite superficial and is usually reached at a depth of approximately 2 to 3 cm. Return of dark, nonpulsatile blood signals successful venous penetration.

Although using the femoral arterial pulse as a guide is ideal, it may not be palpable in an obese or hypotensive patient. A more detailed understanding of the femoral landmarks can be used to guide cannulation attempts. On all but the most

Inguinal ligament

Figure 22-16 Femoral approach. Palpate the femoral artery two fingerbreadths beneath the inguinal ligament. Introduce the needle at a 45-degree in a cephalic direction 1 cm medial to this point and toward the umbilicus. Importantly, more distally the *vein lies over the artery*, so place the catheter near the inguinal ligament, or use ultrasound guidance.

severely injured trauma patients with a disrupted pelvis (in which case a femoral approach would be contraindicated), the anterior superior iliac spine and the midpoint of the pubic symphysis are easily palpated. The line between these two bony references describes the inguinal ligament. When this line is divided into thirds, the femoral artery should underlie the junction of the medial and middle thirds. The femoral vein will lie approximately one fingerbreadth medial to this point. Alternatively, the vascular anatomy of the region can be evaluated and the line placed via ultrasound guidance.

Venipuncture

During advancement of the needle, maintain gentle negative pressure on the syringe at all times while the needle is under the skin. Direct the needle posteriorly and advance it until the vein is entered, as identified by a flash of dark, nonpulsatile blood. If the vessel is penetrated when the syringe is not being aspirated, the flash of blood may be seen only as the needle is being withdrawn. The femoral vein lies just medial to the femoral artery at the level of the inguinal ligament. It is closer to the artery than many clinicians appreciate. As the vein progresses distally in the leg, it runs closer to and almost behind the femoral artery.

Femoral, Ultrasound Technique

Cannulation of the femoral vein under ultrasound guidance is very similar to that for the IJ vein. Using ultrasound, the common femoral vein, its junction with the saphenous vein, and the branches of the common femoral vein—the superficial and deep femoral veins—are easily identified. Typically, placement of the catheter should occur proximal to the bifurcation of the common femoral vein and preferably proximal to the junction with the saphenous vein.

AFTERCARE

Anchoring the Central Line

After the central venous catheter is placed, it will need to be anchored in place by one of three techniques: StatLock, suture, or staple (Fig. 22-17). The StatLock may not hold well in patients with oily skin but is excellent for older patients with thin skin. For suturing, one will need the sterile, nonabsorbable suture material (usually 2-0 silk) provided in the CVC kit. The straight suture needles found in many sets are awkward for many clinicians, so a curved needle with a driver may be helpful. To avoid a needlestick with

---

ULTRASOUND: Central Venous Catheterization   *by Christine Butts, MD*

IJ Vein

When evaluating the internal jugular (IJ) vein, the transducer (7.5 to 20 MHz) should be initially placed over the right or left side of the neck to evaluate the anatomy. An ideal initial location to begin is at the apex of the triangle formed by the two heads of the subclavian muscle (Fig. 22-US1). Placing the transducer over this area in the transverse orientation will enable the vessels to be located in cross section, where they can best be evaluated. The internal carotid artery and IJ vein will be seen as paired structures with anechoic central areas (Fig. 22-US2). The position of one relative to the other can be variable, but typically the IJ lies lateral and superficial to the carotid. Several characteristics of the IJ serve to distinguish it from the carotid. The IJ is typically more oval in shape (versus the rounded shape of the carotid), is thinner walled, and will

compress with gentle pressure. Additionally, the size of the IJ will change with respiration and should be seen to increase in size with a Valsalva maneuver.

Complications can be reduced by several methods. First is to ensure that the target vessel is indeed the vein and not the artery. Variant anatomy or variations in volume status (either depletion or overload) may make the vessels difficult to distinguish from one another. Confirmation should be attempted by noting multiple characteristics of the vessel (compressibility, shape, anatomic location, etc). Once the vessel has

Figure 22-US2 Transverse image of the carotid artery (CA) and internal jugular (IJ) vein. The IJ can be recognized by its oval or triangular shape, its thinner walls, and collapse with light pressure. Although both are rounded and contain anechoic (*black*) fluid, the IJ is slightly larger and more oval in shape. Though not evident in this image, slight pressure will cause collapse of the IJ.

Figure 22-US1 Placement of the ultrasound transducer at the apex of the triangle formed by the heads of the sternocleidomastoid.

Continued

ULTRASOUND: Central Venous Catheterization, cont'd

been confirmed as the vein, the operator must take great care to ensure that the position of the tip of the needle is apparent at all times. Most complications occur when the tip of the needle is deeper or more medial than the operator realizes, thus placing it in proximity to other structures (e.g., lung, carotid artery). An extensive discussion of each approach can be found in the basic ultrasound chapter (see Chapter 66), and each approach has its drawbacks in determining position. In the transverse method, the angle of approach can be difficult to ascertain and cause the tip of the needle to be deeper than the operator realizes. Additionally, the tip of the needle may be difficult to follow. In the longitudinal approach, the medial to lateral orientation of the needle can be difficult to appreciate. Additionally, slight movements of the transducer may result in loss of the appropriate image. A combination of these two, or an oblique approach, may minimize these difficulties.

Femoral Vein

The femoral artery and vein lie together with the femoral nerve within a common sheath. They can be found at the level of the inguinal crease on the medial aspect of the thigh. Palpating the femoral pulse will also aid in localizing the vascular bundle. The transducer (7.5 to 10 MHz) should be placed in a transverse or slightly oblique orientation overlying this area. Slightly externally rotating the thigh may facilitate this step. Classically, the artery is described to lie lateral to the vein. However, this is often not the case and multiple variations may be noted. The femoral artery and vein will appear as rounded anechoic structures (Fig. 22-US3). The femoral vein can be recognized by its thinner walls, slightly more oval shape, and collapse with gentle pressure. It will also typically increase in size when the lower part of the leg is squeezed. The vascular bundle may need to be followed inferiorly or superiorly to determine the most optimal location for puncture.

Complications can be reduced by several methods. First is to ensure that the target vessel is indeed the vein and not the artery. Variant anatomy or variations in volume status (either depletion or overload) may make the vessels difficult to distinguish from one another. Confirmation should be attempted by noting multiple characteristics of the vessel (compressibility, shape, anatomic location, etc). Once the vessel has

been confirmed as the vein, the operator must take great care to ensure that the position of the tip of the needle is apparent at all times. The tip of the needle may be difficult to follow in the transverse approach and result in an inadvertent puncture of the posterior wall of the vessel. When the artery lies deep to the vein, arterial puncture or cannulation may result. In the longitudinal approach, the medial to lateral position of the needle may be difficult to appreciate and result in accidental arterial puncture. The oblique approach may minimize these difficulties.

Subclavian Vein

The subclavian vessels can be imaged from either a supraclavicular or an infraclavicular approach. For the supraclavicular approach, the transducer (7.5 to 10 MHz) is placed along the long axis of the clavicle on the superior aspect (Fig. 22-US4). It should be angled downward. In this view the vessels should be seen in their long axis (Fig. 22-US5). The vein can be identified by its variation with respiration and change in size

Figure 22-US4 Placement of the ultrasound transducer superior to the clavicle to enable visualization of the subclavian vessels in the long axis.

Figure 22-US3 Transverse image of the femoral artery (FA) and femoral vein (FV). Similar to vessels in the neck, the femoral vein is more oval or triangular in shape. Though not evident in this image, slight pressure will cause collapse of the vessel.

Figure 22-US5 Long-axis view of the subclavian vein. The subclavian artery, not seen in this image, will be seen as a similar-appearing vessel deep to the vein. Color flow and Doppler can be used to distinguish between the two vessels.

ULTRASOUND: Central Venous Catheterization, cont'd

with the Valsalva maneuver. The vein can also be followed to identify the junction with the IJ vein, thereby offering further confirmation. In the infraclavicular approach, the transducer is placed beneath the clavicle at its most lateral aspect, in a sagittal or slightly oblique orientation, following the position of the clavicle (Fig. 22-US6). In this view the vessels will be seen in cross section or a slightly oblique plane (Fig. 22-US7). The pleura may also be seen deep to the vessels as an echogenic vertical line that slides back and forth with respiration.

A longitudinal approach should be used in which the needle is introduced from the end of the transducer in either the infraclavicular or the supraclavicular approaches. This will enable a shallow angle to be used and thereby minimize the chance of damaging deeper structures such as the lung. Once a flash of blood has been obtained, the ultrasound transducer can be set aside and the procedure continued as described above.

The subclavian artery and vein lie in close opposition to the pleura, so pneumothorax is a more common complication. Using a long-axis approach (in which the needle is introduced from the end of the transducer rather than from the middle) offers the advantage of visualizing the entirety of the needle in its course toward the vein. A shallow angle can be used, and the relationship of the needle to the pleura can also be appreciated.

Figure 22-US6 Placement of the ultrasound transducer inferior to the clavicle to enable visualization of the subclavian vessels in short axis. A sagittal (shown) or slightly oblique orientation should be used.

Figure 22-US7 Short-axis view of the subclavian artery (*arrowhead*) and vein (*arrow*) as seen from the inferior aspect of the clavicle.

the straight needle, pass the blunt end of the needle through the anchoring devices and pull the suture forward manually. Place the suture in the skin approximately a half centimeter from the catheter to anchor the central line in place. Several knots should be made to secure the line. Avoid making knots that place excessive pressure on the skin because this can lead to difficulty removing the knots and necrosis. Loose knots can lead to migration of the catheter and loss of access. Stapling a central line into place can be just as effective as suturing; however, the staples tend to fall out after a few days.

Dressing

Clean the area around the catheter insertion site with chlorhexidine, and then use a clear dressing (such as Tegaderm) to cover up the insertion site of the catheter once secured (see Fig. 22-9, *step 16*). Apply a chlorhexidine patch (Biopatch) at the site where the catheter enters the skin (see Fig. 22-17*E* and *F*). Because dressings are inspected and changed periodically, place a simple dressing and avoid excessive amounts of gauze and tape. Take care to protect the skin against maceration.

Assessing Line Placement

Check all tubing and connections for tightness to prevent air embolism, loss of fluid, or bleeding. Before infusing IV fluids, lower the IV fluid reservoir to below the level of the patient's right atrium and check the line for backflow of blood. Free backflow of blood is suggestive but not diagnostic of intravascular placement. Backflow could occur from a hematoma or hemothorax if the catheter is free in the pleural space. A pulsatile blood column may be noted if the catheter has been inadvertently placed in an artery. Less pronounced pulsations might also occur if the catheter is advanced too far and reaches the right atrium or ventricle. In addition, pulsations may be noted with changes in intrathoracic pressure as a result of respirations, although these pulsations should occur at a much slower rate than the arterial pulse. A final method of checking intravascular placement is to attach a syringe directly to the catheter hub and aspirate venous blood. It is also advisable to ensure that the catheter is easily flushed with a saline solution. This carries the additional benefit of removing air from the system. Radiographs are also always indicated to verify catheter location and assess for potential complications, except after routine femoral line placements. In an awake

SECURING A CENTRAL VENOUS CATHETER

A white rubber clamp is provided to secure the catheter when the full length is not needed. Twist open the pliable clamp and place it over the catheter at a site a few centimeters from the insertion site.

The rubber clamp is covered with a blue plastic fastener, and both the clamp and fastener are sutured to the skin to secure the catheter. The hub of the catheter is also sutured to the skin.

To avoid a needlestick, the blunt end of the needle is used to pass the suture through the holes of the fastening devices.

Alternatively, skin staples may be used. Tent the skin and pass the staples through the anchoring eyes.

This Biopatch is a chlorhexidine-containing hydrophilic covering placed at the site where the catheter enters the skin to deliver local antisepsis for 7 days.

A simple Tegaderm clear covering is then applied.

Figure 22-17 Methods to secure a central venous triple-lumen catheter.

patient, infusing fluids via a catheter tip positioned in the IJ vein may produce an audible gurgling or flowing sound in the patient's ear.[108]

Radiographs

Following placement of lines involving puncture of the neck or thorax, listen to the lungs to detect any inequality of lung sounds suggestive of a pneumothorax or hemothorax. Obtain a chest film as soon as possible to check for hemothorax,

pneumothorax, and the position of the tip of the catheter (Fig. 22-18). Because small amounts of fluid or air may layer out parallel to the radiographic plate with the patient in the supine position, take the film in the upright or semi-upright position whenever possible. In ill patients, a rotated or oblique projection on a chest radiograph may be obtained, and the clinician may be confused about the proper position of the catheter. In such cases, repeat the radiograph. A misplaced catheter tip is usually obvious on a properly positioned standard posteroanterior chest radiograph (Fig. 22-19), but

Figure 22-18 Chest radiographs obtained after placement of right internal jugular (**A**) and left subclavian (**B**) central venous catheters. The tips of the catheters are appropriately placed in the superior vena cava (*arrows*). The tip should not lie within the right atrium or the right ventricle.

Figure 22-19 Chest radiograph obtained after left internal jugular catheterization. Note that the course of the catheter (*small arrows*) does not cross the midline and that the tip (*large arrow*) projects to the left of the midline near the aortic arch. Although the catheter may have been located intravascularly in a venous anatomic variant, it was decided to remove this line and replace it with a new catheter.

occasionally, injection of contrast material may be required. For example, a catheter in one of the internal thoracic veins may simply appear more lateral than expected, but because of the close proximity of these veins and the SVC, malposition may not be appreciated by this subtle finding. Misplaced catheters should be repositioned or replaced.

Attention should also be given to the possibility of a retained guidewire. Although this complication is rare, if not specifically considered it can be overlooked by both clinicians and radiologists.[109,110]

Postprocedure radiographs are not always necessary for routine replacement of catheters over guidewires. If such patients are stable and being hemodynamically monitored, radiography may be deferred safely in the absence of apparent complications or clinical suspicion of malposition.[111,112]

Redirection of Misplaced Catheters

Improper catheter tip position occurs commonly. It has been reported that only 71% of SV catheters are located in the

SVC on the initial chest film. Complications of improper positioning include hydrothorax, hemothorax, ascites, chest wall abscess, embolization to the pleural space, and chest pain. More commonly, improper location yields inaccurate measurements of CVP or is associated with poor flow caused by kinking. An unusual complication attributable to improper tip position is cerebral infarction, which can occur following inadvertent cannulation of the subclavian artery.

Misdirection or inappropriate positioning of the tip of a CVC, when promptly recognized and corrected, is an inconsequential complication. Loop formation, lodging in small neck veins, tips directed caudally, and innominate vein position are common problems. Reposition misplaced catheters as soon as logistically possible. If the catheter is being used for fluid resuscitation, the malposition may be tolerated for some time. If vasopressors or medications are infused, proper positioning of the tip of the catheter is more critical. A number of options are available to remedy malpositioning. One strategy is to insert a 2-Fr Fogarty catheter through the lumen of the central line and advance it 3 cm beyond the tip. Withdraw the entire assembly until only the Fogarty catheter is in the SV. Inject 1 mL of air into the balloon, and advance the Fogarty catheter. It is hoped that blood flow will direct the assembly into the SVC. Deflate the balloon and advance the central line over the Fogarty catheter, which is then withdrawn.

Another anecdotal strategy is to withdraw the catheter until only the distal tip remains in the cannulated vessel. This measurement is best appreciated by comparing the length of the indwelling catheter with another unused catheter. The clinician then simply readvances the catheter in the hope that it becomes properly positioned. Other manipulations with guidewires have been suggested, but reinsertion with another puncture is often required for the misplaced catheter to be positioned properly. This approach also decreases the risk for infection by avoiding the introduction of bacteria into the vessel from any nonsterile segment of the CVC.

SPECIAL CONSIDERATIONS FOR OTHER VESSELS

External Jugular Vein Approach

Central venous catheterization via the external jugular vein is time-consuming and often difficult. The difficulty in converting an external jugular catheter into a CVC frequently renders it a lower-yield clinical procedure. Use of the external jugular vein for achieving central venous access requires that a guidewire be used. After cannulation of the vein and intraluminal placement of the guidewire, advance the guidewire into the thorax by rotating and manipulating the tip into the central venous circulation. Advancement of the guidewire is the most difficult and time-consuming portion of the procedure, and the time requirement limits the usefulness of this technique in an emergency. A small-radius J-tipped wire, a distended vessel lumen, and exaggeration of patient head tilt, coupled with skin traction, may facilitate successful passage of the guidewire. Partially withdrawing the wire and twisting it 180 degrees before readvancing the tip may also be helpful.

Basilic and Cephalic Approaches

Passing a catheter into the central circulation is difficult via the basilic and cephalic routes, and failure is common. Insertion of a peripheral IV central catheter through these routes is often performed by specialized teams and is less suitable for emergency indications. The cephalic vein may terminate inches above the antecubital fossa or bifurcate before entering the axillary vein and send a branch to the external jugular vein. The cephalic vein may also enter the axillary vein at a right angle, thereby defeating any attempt to pass the catheter centrally. Furthermore, both the basilic and the cephalic systems contain valves that may impede catheterization. Abduction of the shoulder may help advance the catheter if resistance near the axillary vein is encountered. The incidence of failure to place the catheter in the SVC ranges from a high of 40% to a low of 2%.[44,113] The greatest success rate (98%) reported was obtained with slow catheter advancement and the patient in a 45- to 90-degree upright position.[44] A flexible catheter was introduced into the basilic vein until the tip was judged to be proximal to the junction of the cephalic and basilic veins and distal to the junction of the IJ vein with the innominate vein. The wire stylet was withdrawn 18 cm, and the catheter was advanced slowly 1 cm at a time, with 2 seconds allowed between each 1-cm insertion. The natural flexibility of Bard catheters contributed to negotiation into the SVC when the patient was upright. This time-consuming technique is contraindicated when the patient cannot tolerate an upright position.

The basilic and cephalic venous systems are entered through the large veins in the antecubital fossa. Placement of a tourniquet aids venous distention and initial venous puncture. When veins are not visible, they may be identified with bedside ultrasound (as described in Chapter 66). The basilic vein, located on the medial aspect of the antecubital fossa, is generally larger than the radially located cephalic vein. Furthermore, the basilic vein usually provides a more direct route for passage into the axillary vein, SV, and SVC.

Vascular Access in Cardiac Arrest

Immediate vascular access is required for resuscitation during cardiac arrest. Femoral CVCs are often used in this setting. The infraclavicular SV approach is also commonly used during cardiac arrest if logistics permit. The intuitive rationale for femoral CVC placement has been that much of the resuscitation activity, including chest compressions, occurs on the thorax, thus limiting the clinician's ability to safely place

a higher line. During cardiac arrest, the availability of drugs delivered to the central circulation may be slower via the femoral route than via supraclavicular SV or IJ vein infusions.[113,114] Additionally, pulsations felt in the groin during CPR may be venous instead of arterial,[28] and there is a high rate of unrecognized catheter malposition and arterial injury.[28,115] To place a femoral catheter blindly (without ultrasound guidance or clear identification of the arterial pulse), divide the distance from the anterior superior iliac spine to the symphysis pubis into thirds. The artery typically lies at the junction of the medial and middle thirds and the vein 1 cm medial to this location. Blind femoral central line insertions during arrest are less than optimal. The increasingly available intraosseous placement systems and bedside ultrasonography are beginning to supplant such "blind" CVC placements during cardiac arrest and other emergencies that require immediate vascular access.

CVP MONITORING

CVP Measurement

Although described by Forssman in 1931, it was not until the early 1960s that measurement of CVP became commonplace as a means of assessing cardiac performance and guiding fluid therapy.[10] CVP measurements are most frequently used as a guide for determination of a patient's volume status and fluid requirements and for investigation of tamponade.[116] CVP monitoring has often been criticized as ineffective, outmoded, and unreliable,[117] but in the last few years a resurgence in its use has occurred.[118] Astute clinicians can maximize the usefulness of this diagnostic tool by understanding its basic principles, indications, and limitations.[119-121]

Physiology

Simply stated, CVP is the pressure exerted by blood against the walls of the intrathoracic venae cavae. Because pressure in the great veins of the thorax is generally within 1 mm Hg of right atrial pressure, CVP reflects the amount of blood or pressure at which blood is returning to the heart. Pressure in the central veins has two significant hemodynamic effects. First, the pressure promotes filling of the heart during diastole, a factor that helps determine right ventricular end-diastolic volume (preload). Second, CVP is also the backpressure of the systemic circulation and opposes return of blood from peripheral blood vessels into the heart. CVP is therefore a measure of both the ability of the heart to pump blood (cardiac function) and the tendency for blood to flow from the peripheral veins (venous return to the heart). The CVP reading is determined by a complex interaction of intravascular volume, right atrial and ventricular function, venomotor tone, and intrathoracic pressure.[116,117,119,120]

To measure CVP, place the tip of a pressure-monitoring catheter into any of the great systemic veins of the thorax or into the right atrium.[119,121] You can also use the femoral vein for measurement as long as there is no evidence of increased abdominal pressure.[10,122] The catheter is connected to a simple manometer or to an electronic pressure transducer interfaced with a monitoring system, at the level of the right atrium, that is capable of calculating a mean pressure value and displaying pressure waveforms.[119,121] The waveforms produced correlate with the cardiac cycle and create a typical wave pattern.

Central Venous Pressure Measurement

Indications
Acute circulatory failure
Anticipated massive blood transfusion or fluid
  replacement therapy
Cautious fluid replacement in patients with
  compromised cardiovascular status
Suspected cardiac tamponade
Fluid resuscitation during goal-directed therapy
  for severe sepsis

Contraindications
Other resuscitative interventions that take priority over
  central venous access and central venous pressure setup
Large vegetations on the tricuspid valve
Superior vena cava syndrome
Right atrial tumor or thrombus

Complications
Faulty central venous pressure readings:
  Increased intrathoracic pressure (ventilator, straining, coughing)
  Failure to calibrate or zero the transducer
  Malposition of the tip of the catheter
  Obstruction of the catheter
  Air bubbles in the circuit
  Readings during the wrong phase of ventilation
  Vasopressors (presumed)

Equipment

Review Box 22-2 Central venous pressure measurement: indications, contraindications, complications, and equipment.

Indications for and Contraindications to CVP Measurement

The five traditional major indications for monitoring CVP are:

1. Acute circulatory failure
2. Anticipated massive blood transfusion or fluid replacement therapy
3. Cautious fluid replacement in patients with compromised cardiovascular status
4. Suspected cardiac tamponade
5. Fluid resuscitation during goal-directed therapy in patients with severe sepsis

The procedure is contraindicated when other resuscitative therapeutic and diagnostic interventions take priority over central venous access and CVP transducer setup and calibration or in the setting of large vegetations on the tricuspid valve, SVC syndrome, or tumors or thrombus in the right atrium.

A common misconception is that CVP consistently reflects pressure in the left side of the heart. The measurement that best reflects changes in left ventricular pressure and reserve is left atrial pressure or the nearly equivalent pulmonary capillary wedge pressure (PCWP). Development of the flow-directed pulmonary artery catheter has allowed repeated measurements of PCWP, thus permitting reliable estimation of left atrial pressure.[121]

CVP monitoring is most helpful in patients without significant preexisting cardiopulmonary disease. Numerous studies highlight the unreliability of right-sided hemodynamic monitoring in patients with underlying cardiac or pulmonary disease.[111,115] Ultimately, however, the differences noted are not a failure of CVP monitoring to reflect central hemodynamics. Rather, the disagreements noted by previous authors simply highlight the complexity of the relationship between ventricular and vascular compliance, blood volume, and filling pressure in various disease states. As with pulmonary artery occlusion pressure measurements, the clinician is cautioned to be aware of the assumptions involved and to recognize the scenarios in which these assumptions do not hold true.

Procedure

Although CVP may be determined with a manometry column assembled at the bedside (Fig. 22-20), the most common technique in practice is measurement with an electronic transducer interfaced to a monitoring system (Fig. 22-21). Typical transducers include a nipple valve attached to a pressurized bag of saline to allow easy flushing of the system. To use these manometers, attach the transducer to the patient's central line with a length of flexible, yet fairly rigid-walled tubing filled with saline. Place a three-way stopcock between the patient and the transducer to simplify line flushing and calibration.

Flush all air bubbles from the system by opening the stopcock to air and flushing saline through the line. Do not flush air bubbles into the patient. Even tiny bubbles left in the tubing will dampen the CVP wave and potentially cause underestimation of venous pressure.

MEASUREMENT OF CENTRAL VENOUS PRESSURE: MANOMETRY

1

Manometer

Flow

Assemble the manometer as depicted above. When the stopcock is turned to direct flow of fluid to the patient, the manometer is bypassed. This is the position that is maintained to keep the catheter patent. Remember to always flush all tubing before connecting it to the patient's central catheter.

2

Flow

To measure central venous pressure, first turn the stopcock to fill the manometer to 25 cm H_2O.

3

Flow

Patient reference point

Next, open the stopcock to the patient and the manometer. Allow the column of water in the manometer to fall and stabilize before a reading is taken. Note that the zero mark must be horizontally aligned with the tricuspid valve (which is estimated as the midaxillary line in a supine patient).

Figure 22-20 Measurement of central venous pressure with a manual manometer.

After the system has been flushed, place the stopcock (with the transducer still open to air) at the level of the patient's right atrium. Zero (calibrate) the monitor detecting the transducer's signal with the transducer at the level of the right atrium, which can be approximated on the skin surface as a point at the midaxillary line and the fourth intercostal space.[119,121] Finally, set the stopcock so that the transducer is in continuity with the patient's venous catheter.

In spontaneously breathing patients, take readings at the end of a normal inspiration. If the patient is receiving positive pressure ventilation, the changes in CVP during the respiratory cycle are reversed: it rises with inspiration and decreases with expiration. In these patients, take readings near the end of expiration.[121] Thus, during both normal and mechanical ventilation, the lowest reading is a useful estimate of mean CVP.

MEASUREMENT OF CENTRAL VENOUS PRESSURE: TRANSDUCER

Insert a bag of normal saline into a pressure bag and inflate to the recommended pressure (usually 300 mm Hg).

Flush all air bubbles from the system by opening the stopcock and running saline through the line. Any air left in the system will cause erroneous CVP readings. Take care to not flush air into the patient.

Connect the flushed transducer tubing to the patient's central line.

Transducer at level of right atrium

Mount the transducer at the level of the patient's right atrium. This level can be approximated on the skin surface as a point at the midaxillary line and fourth intercostal space.

Adjust the stopcock so that the transducer is open to air, and zero the system. The exact process for the zeroing procedure will vary by the equipment manufacturer.

Finally, set the stopcock so that it is open to the transducer and the central venous catheter. Observe for a venous waveform and CVP reading on the monitor (*arrow*).

Figure 22-21 Measurement of central venous pressure (CVP) with an electronic transducer.

Take a reading after accurate placement of the tip of the catheter has been established. To ensure optimal measurement, place the patient in the supine position. Whenever the patient is repositioned, take care to ensure that the transducer has been recalibrated to reflect the new position of the patient.

Errors in CVP Measurement

A number of extrinsic factors may alter the accuracy of the CVP reading (Box 22-1).[116,119,121] In addition to the position of the patient, such factors include changes in intrathoracic pressure, malposition of the tip of the catheter, obstruction of the catheter, and failure to calibrate or zero the line. Activities that increase intrathoracic pressure, such as coughing or straining, may cause spuriously high measurements. Make sure that the patient is relaxed at the time of measurement and breathing normally. In mechanically ventilated patients, CVP will be elevated to an extent directly proportional to the ventilatory pressure being delivered and inversely proportional to the mechanical compliance of the lung. Care should be exercised in interpreting filling pressure in this circumstance because ventilator-induced elevations in CVP are not

---

BOX 22-1 Reasons for Faulty CVP Readings

Increased intrathoracic pressure (ventilator, straining, coughing)
Failure to calibrate or zero the transducer
Malposition of the tip of the catheter
Obstruction of catheter
Air bubbles in the circuit
Readings during the wrong phase of ventilation
Vasopressors (presumed)

CVP, central venous pressure.

---

artifactual but represent changes in the hemodynamic physiology of the patient. As in spontaneously breathing patients, CVP measurements are meaningful only in relaxed, sedated, or paralyzed subjects.

Another reason for faulty readings is malposition of the tip of the catheter. If the catheter tip has not passed far enough into the central venous system, peripheral venous spasm or venous valves may yield pressure readings that are inconsistent with the true CVP.

If the tip of the catheter has passed into the right ventricle, a falsely elevated CVP measurement is obtained. Recognition of a characteristic right ventricular pressure waveform on the patient's monitor should hopefully preclude this error. Such fluctuations may also occasionally be seen in appropriately positioned CVP lines when significant tricuspid regurgitation or atrioventricular dissociation (a cannon "a" wave) is present.[117] Inaccurate low venous pressure readings are seen when a valvelike obstruction at the tip of the catheter occurs as a result of either clot formation or contact against a vein wall. Wave damping secondary to air bubbles in the transducer or tubing also leads to faulty readings. Using poorly zeroed lines may result in inaccurate measurements that may be interpreted as a change in the patient's status when none has actually taken place. The transducer should be zeroed to the same level for every measurement.

Interpretation of CVP Measurement

Normal CVP values are as follows:

Low: <6 cm H_2O
Normal: 6 to 12 cm H_2O
High: >12 cm H_2O

In the late stages of pregnancy (30 to 42 weeks), CVP is physiologically elevated, and normal readings are 5 to 8 cm H_2O higher. A CVP reading of less than 6 cm H_2O is consistent with low right atrial pressure and reflects a decrease in the return of blood volume to the right heart. This may indicate that the patient requires additional fluid or blood. A low CVP reading is also obtained when vasomotor tone is decreased, as with sepsis, spinal cord injury, or other forms of sympathetic interruption.

A CVP reading falling within a normal range is viewed in relation to the clinical scenario. A reading higher than 12 cm H_2O indicates that the heart is not effectively circulating the volume presented to it. This may occur in a normovolemic patient with underlying cardiac disease such as left ventricular hypertrophy (with associated poor ventricular compliance) or in a patient with a normal heart who is volume-overloaded. High CVP can also be related to variables other than pump failure, such as pericardial tamponade, restrictive pericarditis, pulmonary stenosis, tricuspid regurgitation, pulmonary hypertension, and pulmonary embolism.[123]

Changes in blood volume, vessel tone, and cardiac function may occur alone or in combination with one another; therefore, it is possible to have a normal or elevated CVP in the presence of normovolemia, hypovolemia, and hypervolemia.[123] Interpret the specific CVP values with respect to the entire clinical picture. The response of CVP to an infusion is more important than the initial reading.

Fluid Challenge

Monitoring CVP may be helpful as a practical guide to fluid therapy.[116,118-121] Serial CVP measurements provide a fairly reliable indication of the capability of the right side of the heart to accept an additional fluid load. Although PCWP is a more sensitive index of left heart fluid needs (and in some clinical situations measurement of PCWP is essential), serial measurement of CVP can nonetheless provide useful information.

A fluid challenge can help assess both volume deficits and pump failure.[120] Although a fluid challenge can be used with either PCWP monitoring or CVP monitoring, only the fluid challenge for CVP monitoring is discussed here. Slight variations in the methodology of fluid challenge are reported in the literature. Generally, fluid boluses of 250 to 500 mL of crystalloid are administered sequentially and CVP is measured 10 minutes after each bolus. Repeat the fluid challenge until measurements indicate that adequate volume expansion has occurred. Discontinue the fluid challenge as soon as hemodynamic signs of shock are reversed or signs of cardiac incompetence are evident.

Cardiac Tamponade

In cardiac tamponade, pericardial pressure rises to equal right ventricular end-diastolic pressure. The pericardial pressure encountered in pericardial tamponade characteristically produces an elevated CVP.[123] The degree of elevation in CVP is variable, and one must interpret measurements cautiously; CVP readings in the range of 16 to 18 cm H_2O are typically seen with acute tamponade, but elevations of up to 30 cm H_2O may be encountered. The precise CVP reading is often lower than one might intuitively expect, and it is not uncommon to encounter tamponade with a CVP of 10 to 12 cm H_2O. A normal or even low CVP reading may be seen if the tamponade is associated with significant hypovolemia. An excessive rise in CVP after fluid challenge may be more important than a single reading in the diagnosis of pericardial tamponade.

Excessive straining, positive pressure ventilation, agitation, inflation of pneumatic antishock garments, and tension pneumothorax may all increase intrathoracic pressure, produce a high CVP reading, and erroneously suggest the diagnosis of pericardial tamponade. Increases in vascular tone, as seen with the use of dopamine or other vasopressors, may also elevate CVP and thus mimic tamponade and complicate estimations of volume.

COMPLICATIONS

The medical literature is replete with reports of CVC complications. Understanding the pathophysiology surrounding CVC complications helps clinicians anticipate, recognize, and manage complications should they arise and better educate patients and their families during the informed consent process.

More than 15% of patients who receive CVCs experience some type of complication, and complications occur despite pristine technique.[42,73] This percentage is not surprising in view of the close proximity of vital structures, the complexity of patients' medical conditions, and the emergency circumstances under which many of these procedures are often performed. The number of complications increases, especially those involving thrombosis and infection, with longer durations of catheterization and increasing severity of illness.[25] Although clinicians strive to limit complications, their occurrence cannot naïvely be viewed as evidence of faulty technique or substandard care. Common complications with the different approaches are summarized in Box 22-2 and Table 22-4 and can generally be categorized as mechanical, infectious, and thrombotic. Key complications and injuries by approach are discussed below.

The number of lumens does not directly affect the rate of catheter-related complications.[42,73] One 3-year retrospective

BOX 22-2 Complications of Central Venous Access

GENERAL

Mechanical

Puncture of an adjacent artery
Hematoma formation
Air embolus
Pneumothorax
Pericardial tamponade
Catheter embolus
Arteriovenous fistula
Mural thrombus formation
Large-vein obstruction
Dysrhythmias
Catheter knotting
Catheter malposition

Infectious

Bloodstream infection
Generalized sepsis
Septic arthritis
Osteomyelitis
Cellulitis at the insertion site

Thrombotic

Pulmonary embolism
Venous thrombosis

SV AND IJ APPROACHES

Pulmonary

Pneumothorax
Hemothorax
Hydrothorax
Chylothorax
Neck hematoma and tracheal obstruction
Endotracheal cuff perforation
Tracheal perforation

Neurologic

Phrenic nerve injury
Brachial plexus injury
Cerebral infarct

FEMORAL APPROACH

Intraabdominal

Bowel perforation
Psoas abscess
Bladder perforation

IJ, *internal jugular;* SV, *subclavian vein.*

TABLE 22-4 Anatomic Structures That Can Be Injured by Central Venous Cannulation

STRUCTURE	ANATOMIC RELATIONSHIP TO VEIN	ERROR IN PROCEDURE	INJURY
Subclavian Vein Cannulation			
Subclavian artery	Posterior and slightly superior, separated by the scalenus anterior—10-15 mm in adults, 5-8 mm in children	Insertion too deep or lateral	Hemorrhage, hematoma, possible hemothorax
Brachial plexus	Posterior to and separated from the subclavian vein by the scalenus anterior and the subclavian artery (20 mm)	Same as with the subclavian artery	Possible motor or sensory deficits in the hand, arm, or shoulder
Parietal pleura	Contact with the posteroinferior side of the subclavian vein, medial to the attachment of the anterior scalenus muscle to the first rib	Needle penetrates beneath or through both walls of the subclavian vein	Pneumothorax
Phrenic nerve	Same as with the parietal pleura	Placement of the needle above or behind the vein or penetration of both its walls	Paralysis of the ipsilateral hemidiaphragm
Thoracic duct	Crosses the scalenus anterior and enters the superior margin of the subclavian vein near the internal jugular junction	Same as with the phrenic nerve	Soft tissue lymphedema or chylothorax on the left
Internal Jugular Vein Cannulation			
Carotid artery	Passes with the jugular vein in the carotid sheath, consistently medial and deep to the vein	Insertion site too medial or the course of the needle not directed at the ipsilateral nipple	Hematoma, possible cerebral thromboembolism or airway obstruction
Phrenic nerve	Passes along the anterior surface of the scalenus anterior, behind the vein	Insertion too deep	Paralysis of the ipsilateral hemidiaphragm
Brachial plexus	Separated from the internal jugular by the scalenus anterior	Insertion too deep or too lateral	Possible motor or sensory deficits in the hand, arm, or shoulder
Femoral Vein Cannulation			
Femoral artery	Lies lateral to the vein in the femoral triangle	Needle passed too laterally	Hematoma
Psoas muscle	Directly posterior to the artery and vein	Needle passed too deep	Hematoma, psoas abscess
Bowel	Proximal and deep to the femoral vein	Needle passed too deep and above the inguinal ligament	Enterotomy, peritonitis
Synovial capsule of the hip	Deep to the psoas muscle	Needle passed too deep, particularly in small children	Arthritis, septic joint

From Knopp R, Dailey RH. Central venous cannulation and pressure monitoring. *JACEP.* 1977;6:358.

review of all central catheters placed in the ED (supraclavicular SV, IJ, and femoral lines) reported a mechanical complication rate of 3.4%, or 22 of 643 lines placed.[124] Complications were defined as pneumothorax, hematoma, line misplacement, hemothorax, or any issue with the CVC (excluding infection or thrombosis) that required an inpatient consultation. In general, failure and complication rates increase as the number of percutaneous punctures increase. Historically, operator skill and experience have reliably predicted complication or success rates.[42,73] It has previously been reported that clinicians who have placed more than 50 CVCs have less than half the complication rates of those who have fewer than 50 attempts.[73]

Published complication rates vary in the literature and can now be classified according to whether ultrasound guidance was used during the procedure (Table 22-5).[42,47] Recent studies have demonstrated that ultrasound-guided CVC placement techniques have improved success rates, reduced complication rates, and decreased time needed to perform the procedure.[46-49] As a result, ultrasound guidance for CVC placement is recommended by the U.S. Department of Health and Human Services. Reports by the AHRQ list ultrasound guidance for central vein cannulation as one of its most highly rated safety practices.[57,125]

Mechanical Complications

The most commonly reported mechanical complications are arterial puncture, hematoma, and pneumothorax. Inadvertent arterial puncture and hematoma formation are usually easily recognized and controlled with simple compression. Rarely, an artery is lacerated to such an extent that bleeding is significant and operative repair is necessary. In cardiac arrest, low-flow, or shock states, arterial puncture may not be obvious, and arterial cannulation and intraarterial administration of medications have occurred. This can lead to the subsequent development of ischemia or thrombosis of the artery and limb. When systolic blood pressure rises, arterial pulsations become more obvious. In critically ill patients, however, this complication may escape detection for some time. It has been reported that ultrasound-guided placement of IJ CVCs decreases the rate of arterial puncture to 1.4%.[47]

Though poorly studied, patients with a coagulopathy may experience significant bleeding from CVC placement, especially if arterial puncture or laceration has occurred. Mumtaz and coworkers cited a 3% bleeding rate in coagulopathic patients who experienced only minor bleeding that could be controlled with digital pressure.[44] Although central venous access may be performed safely in patients with underlying disorders in hemostasis without correction of the coagulopathy, caution is nevertheless urged. Areas amenable to arterial compression are preferred in these patients.[44]

Pneumothorax occurs in up to 6% of subclavian venipunctures and can also occur with the IJ approach[42,73,126] (Fig. 22-22A). Initially, the importance of this complication was minimized, but reports of fatalities caused by tension pneumothorax, bilateral pneumothorax, and combined hemopneumothorax followed.[55] One would expect a higher incidence of pneumothorax if the procedure is performed during CPR or positive pressure ventilation. A small pneumothorax can quickly become a life-threatening tension pneumothorax with positive pressure ventilation. Treatment of a catheter-induced pneumothorax is controversial, but not all patients will require formal tube thoracostomy. Some authors have reported that many stable outpatients exhibiting a pneumothorax after insertion of a CVC can be managed successfully by observation alone (60% in one series) or catheter (pigtail/Heimlich valve) aspiration, with large tube thoracostomy being reserved for refractory cases or emergency settings.[126,127] Critically ill patients or those undergoing mechanical ventilation are more likely to require invasive treatment of a catheter-induced pneumothorax.

Hemothorax may occur after laceration of the SV or subclavian artery, puncture of the pulmonary artery, or intrathoracic infusion of blood (Fig. 22-22B). Hydrothorax occurs as a result of infusion of IV fluid into the pleural space. Hydromediastinum is also possible. These are rarely serious complications, but fatalities have been reported. Surgical repair is occasionally required. Arteriovenous fistula formation has also been reported.[128] Additional pulmonary complications include tracheal and endotracheal cuff perforation.

Air embolism is a very rare, but potentially life-threatening complication of central venous cannulation. Undoubtedly, minor and clinically inconsequential amounts of air enter the

TABLE 22-5 Frequency of Complications without and with Ultrasound Guidance

COMPLICATION	WITHOUT ULTRASOUND			WITH ULTRASOUND
	IJ	SV	Femoral	IJ
Arterial puncture	6.3-9.4%	3.1-4.9%	9.0-15.0%	1.8%
Hematoma	<0.1-2.2%	1.2-2.1%	3.8-4.4%	0.4%
Hemothorax	0%	0.4-0.6%	NA	0%
Pneumothorax	<0.1-0.2%	1.5-3.1%	NA	0%
Infection (rate per 1000 catheter-days)	8.6	4	15.3	NA
Thrombosis (rate per 1000 catheter-days)	1.2-3	0-13	8-34	NA

Data from References 47, 78, 129.
IJ, internal jugular; *NA*, not applicable; *SC*, subclavian vein.

Figure 22-22 Pneumothorax and hemothorax. A chest radiograph should be taken routinely to assess the position of a central venous catheter introduced via the subclavian or internal jugular route. This confirms placement of the catheter. Chest radiography can also show potential complications of the procedure. **A,** Large right pneumothorax after right internal jugular catheterization. The catheter is still in place (*large arrow*), and the absence of lung markings on the right and the pleural reflection (*small arrows*) are readily apparent. **B,** Left hydropneumothorax after left subclavian venipuncture (the catheter was removed before this radiograph). Note the straight line of fluid (air-fluid level) and no meniscus, a finding indicating that a *pneumothorax must also be present.* The edge of the partially collapsed lung is difficult to appreciate. No clinician can place central venous catheters and fail to have at least some complications that are inherent to the procedure, regardless of even flawless technique.

venous circulation during many cannulation procedures. Maintaining constant occlusion (with the operator's finger) on all needles that are located in central veins can minimize this occurrence. A 14-gauge needle can transmit 100 mL of air per second with a 5-cm H_2O pressure difference across the needle.[95] Air embolism may occur if the line is open to air during catheterization or if it subsequently becomes disconnected. The recommended treatment is to place the patient in the left lateral decubitus position to relieve air bubble occlusion of the right ventricular outflow tract.[95] If this is unsuccessful, aspiration with the catheter advanced into the right ventricle has been advocated.[95] Emergency thoracotomy

to aspirate air (see Chapter 18) and cardiothoracic surgical consultation may also be warranted.

Catheter or wire embolization resulting from shearing of a through-the-needle catheter by the tip of the needle is a serious and generally avoidable complication. Embolization can occur when the catheter or wire is withdrawn through the needle or if the guard is not properly secured. Adverse events after embolization include arrhythmias, venous thrombosis, endocarditis, myocardial perforation, and pulmonary embolism.[75] The mortality rate in patients who did not have these catheters removed has been reported to be as high as 60%.[75] Transvenous retrieval techniques by interventional radiology are usually attempted, followed by open surgery if they are unsuccessful.[75] Entire guidewires may also embolize to the general circulation if the tip is not constantly secured by the operator throughout the procedure. Although the precise incidence of retained or "lost" guidewires is unknown, it is rarely reported in the literature. Initiatives by national safety bodies such as the National Quality Forum in the United States have focused on reducing the incidence of retained wires by classifying them as "never" events that require mandatory reporting in many states.

Delayed perforation of the myocardium is a rare, but generally fatal complication of central venous catheterization by any route.[129] The presumed mechanism is prolonged contact of the rigid catheter with the beating myocardium. The catheter perforates the myocardial wall and causes tamponade either by bleeding from the involved chamber or by infusion of IV fluid into the pericardium. The right atrium is involved more commonly than the right ventricle.[95] All clinicians who insert such catheters or care for such patients should be aware of this deadly complication, which results in profound deterioration with hypotension, shortness of breath, and shock. Emergency echocardiography, pericardiocentesis, and operative intervention by a thoracic surgeon may all be required for salvage of the patient. This can also occur with misplacement of the CVC in the pericardiophrenic vein.[130,131] Fortunately, this complication is preventable by using a postinsertion chest film to confirm the position of the tip of the catheter and repositioning any catheter if the tip is within the cardiac silhouette.

Catheter knotting or kinking may occur if the catheter is forced or repositioned or if an excessively long catheter is used.[130-132] The most common result of kinking is poor flow of IV fluids, although rare complications as severe as SVC obstruction have been seen.[130-132]

Thoracic duct laceration is a frequently discussed complication of left-sided subclavian venipuncture; however, it is extremely uncommon and has been reported only as a complication of IJ, not SV cannulation.

Neurologic complications are extremely rare and presumably caused by direct trauma from the needle during venipuncture. Brachial plexus palsy and phrenic nerve injury with paralysis of the hemidiaphragm have been reported.[133,134] Infusing hypertonic medications into the IJ vein via a malpositioned catheter may result in a variety of neurologic complications from retrograde perfusion of intracranial vessels.[135]

Infectious Complications

Infectious complications include local cellulitis, thrombophlebitis, generalized septicemia, osteomyelitis, and septic arthritis.[54] The incidence of septic complications varies from 0% to 25%.[70,136] The frequency with which infectious complications occur is directly related to the attention given to aseptic technique during insertion and aftercare of the catheter. Femoral venous catheterization carries a greater risk for infection than subclavian catheterization does. Merrer and associates reported the overall infectious complication rate from femoral and subclavian catheters to be 19.8% and 4.5%, respectively.[129] Ultrasound-guided IJ CVC placement has resulted in a decrease in the rates of central line–associated bloodstream infections (CLABSIs).[49] The exact mechanism by which ultrasound-guided CVC placement results in a lower risk for infection is unclear; it may be related to a reduced number of skin punctures. Organisms most commonly recovered from colonized femoral catheters are coagulase-negative staphylococci, Enterobacteriaceae, *Enterococcus* species, and *Pseudomonas aeruginosa*.[129]

CVCs cause an estimated 80,000 CLABSIs and are implicated in up to 28,000 deaths per year in patients in the intensive care unit.[60-62] The average cost has been estimated at $45,000 per patient with a CLABSI, with an cumulative cost of $2.3 billion annually.[60-62] Recently, the Centers for Disease Control and Prevention has recommended that central line bundling policies be implemented to significantly decrease the incidence of CLABSI.[61,62] This bundling policy includes five evidence-based interventions: (1) hand washing, (2) maximal barrier precautions, (3) chlorhexidine skin antisepsis, (4) optimal catheter site selection with avoidance of the femoral vein if possible, and (5) daily review of the necessity for the line and prompt removal of unnecessary lines.[63]

Thrombotic Complications

Thrombosis and thrombophlebitis are significant risks associate with placement of a CVC. The risk for catheter-related thrombosis is directly related to the site of access. In one trial, catheter-related thrombosis was reported in up to 21.5% of patients with femoral CVCs and in 1.9% of patients with SV CVCs. For SV and IJ CVCs, it is important to determine that the tip of the catheter rests in the SVC, especially during the infusion of irritating or hypertonic solutions.[129] Thrombi may form secondary to prolonged contact of the catheter against the vascular endothelium. One autopsy study found a 29% incidence of mural thrombi in the innominate vein, SVC, and right ventricle of patients who had central lines in place an average of 8 days before death.[65] The clinical importance of these thrombi remains unclear; however, any thrombosis has the potential to embolize. Moreover, catheter-related thrombosis is a cause of SVC obstruction syndrome.[137]

Subclavian Approaches

Although both approaches to the SV are relatively safe, the infraclavicular SV approach is more likely to be associated with complications. In a randomized, prospective comparison of supraclavicular SV and infraclavicular SV puncture in 500 ED patients, complication rates were 2.0% and 5.1%, respectively.[138] The most significant complications are pneumothorax and puncture of the subclavian artery; the highest reported incidence of pneumothorax is 2.4%.[18,66,138] Adherence to the techniques recommended for supraclavicular SV puncture decreases the risk for these complications because the needle is directed away from the pleural dome and subclavian artery. The relatively superficial location of the vein when approached from above the clavicle (1.5 to 3.5 cm) lessens the risk for puncture or laceration of deep structures.

IJ Approach

Many complications of IJ cannulation are similar to those of SV access. The incidence of complications appears to be higher with use of the left IJ vein than with the right.[16] One common complication unique to the IJ approach is a localized hematoma in the neck.[139] With the IJ approach, pressure can easily be maintained on the area of swelling, and most hematomas will resolve spontaneously. If puncture of the carotid artery is recognized and treated with compression, it rarely causes significant morbidity in the absence of marked atherosclerotic disease, although arteriovenous fistulas may occur after IJ puncture.[128] Several neurologic complications unique to the IJ site of venipuncture have also been reported as a result of hematomas or direct injury. Such complications include damage to the phrenic nerves, iatrogenic Horner's syndrome, trauma to the brachial plexus, and even passage of a catheter into the thecal space of the spinal canal.[135] If the carotid artery is punctured, one may again attempt IJ or SV cannulation on the same side after appropriate, prolonged (15- to 20-minute) compression. The IJ vein valve is frequently damaged when cannulated, which often results in incompetence of the valve. The clinical significance of this, if any, is unknown.[140]

Femoral Approach

Because vital structures in the neck and chest are not at risk, complications of femoral vein cannulation are generally less severe than those of other routes for central venous access. The most common immediate complications involve bleeding from damage to either the femoral artery or the femoral vein (Fig. 22-23). This can usually be managed with 10 to 15 minutes of direct pressure. Extra care should be taken in anticoagulated patients or after the administration of thrombolytic agents. In extreme cases when hemostasis cannot be achieved through direct pressure, a vascular surgeon should be consulted.

The peritoneum can also be violated with resultant perforation of the bowel. Bowel penetration is especially likely if the patient has a femoral hernia. Injury to the bowel is usually minimal and unlikely to require specific treatment. Nonetheless, the potential bacterial contamination of the femoral puncture site can pose a significant problem. Aspiration of air during placement of a femoral line necessitates removal of the catheter and reinsertion at another site. Other complications include muscular abscesses, infection of the hip joint, damage to the femoral nerve, and puncture of the bladder. Risk for these outcomes can be mitigated by strict aseptic technique, thorough assessment of landmarks, careful control of the needle's depth, and the use of bedside ultrasound.

Two more complications merit special mention. The first is the increased risk for catheter infection. Presumably caused by anatomic association with the anogenital region, many studies have found that femoral lines become infected at significantly higher rates than IJ or supraclavicular SV lines do.[61,62,65,129] Of note, some studies have failed to find a

Figure 22-23 A femoral vein catheter is more prone to deep vein thrombosis and infection than a subclavian or internal jugular line is, but it is a standard access route in the emergency department. Strict attention to sterile technique and limiting use to a few days will negate most of the negatives of this approach. **A,** Significant hemorrhage can occur after puncture of the femoral artery, but this area is readily compressed. The femoral route may be the approach of choice in a patient with an inadvertently placed arterial catheter who requires a central line. **B,** Bleeding from an inadvertently placed arterial catheter that was removed without adequate pressure in an anticoagulated patient.

statistical difference, and it is unclear how much of the effect is due to the actual location of the line versus how it is placed and managed.

The majority of studies show that the incidence of deep vein thrombosis is also increased in lines placed via the femoral route,[129,141] although the clinical significance of these clots has not been definitively addressed.

TRAINING AND SIMULATION

CVC placement and ultrasound guidance techniques have a relatively steep learning curve. Simulation is recommended by the AHQR to teach these techniques.[57,125] Simulation training is independently associated with higher rates of correct needle insertion on the first attempt, as well as with higher successful CVC placement rates.[125,142,143] There are many simulation models that can be used. Kendall and Faragher described a phantom model as an easy, inexpensive method for ultrasound-guided CVC placement training.[144]

References are available at www.expertconsult.com

CHAPTER 23

Venous Cutdown

Veronica Vasquez and Pablo F. Aguilera

Management of critically ill or injured patients requires immediate and adequate vascular access, especially during trauma resuscitation, when rapid infusion of crystalloid or blood products may be necessary. Venous cutdown, a time-honored surgical technique, has largely been replaced by alternative methods of obtaining venous access, including intraosseous lines, the Seldinger technique, and ultrasound-guided central venous cannulation.[1] Nonetheless, venous cutdown still has a role as an emergency method of achieving vascular access when other techniques and equipment are unavailable, particularly in settings outside the United States.

First described by Keeley in 1940 and Kirkham in 1945,[2,3] venous cutdown offered an alternative to venipuncture in patients with shock. Though no longer taught as a mandatory procedure in the Advanced Trauma Life Support course, venous cutdown is considered optional and continues to be taught at the discretion of the instructor.[4] Realistically,

percutaneous vascular access may be infeasible in a pulseless, hypovolemic, or anatomically scarred patient. With a thorough understanding of the anatomy, the procedure, and its potential complications, this mechanically simple procedure can be performed quickly and effectively.[5]

INDICATIONS

Venous cutdown may be used as an alternative to venipuncture for critical patients in need of vascular access when less invasive options have been exhausted or are not available. Patients with severe shock, asystole, or pulseless electrical activity will lack palpable femoral pulses, thus making percutaneous femoral vein catheterization more difficult. Surface landmarks may be obscured and veins may be unusable in intravenous (IV) drug users, the extensively injured, or severely burned patients. Attempts at percutaneous venous cannulation may be complicated or even impossible in such patients. Venous cutdown and interosseous routes (see Chapter 25) are both viable options in such scenarios.

Children

Venipuncture in small children poses a challenge in even the healthiest of patients, let alone those in extremis, whose veins may be poorly visualized. Central vein catheterization, intraosseous line placement, or venous cutdown should be considered as alternative means of emergency vascular access when other peripheral sites have been exhausted. The distal

---

Venous Cutdown

Indications

As an alternative to venipuncture in critically ill patients in need of vascular access and in whom venipuncture may be difficult:

Shock

Asystole or pulseless electrical activity

Sclerosed veins of intravenous drug abusers

Extensive burn or other injury

Small children

Contraindications

Absolute:

When less invasive options exist for venous access

Major blunt or penetrating trauma at proposed cutdown site

Relative:

Overlying soft tissue infection

Bleeding diasthesis

Immunocompromise

Extremity injuries proximal to the site

Complications

Transection of the vein	Phlebitis
Transection of the artery	Sepsis
Bleeding	Thrombus formation
Hematoma	Injury to surrounding structures

Equipment

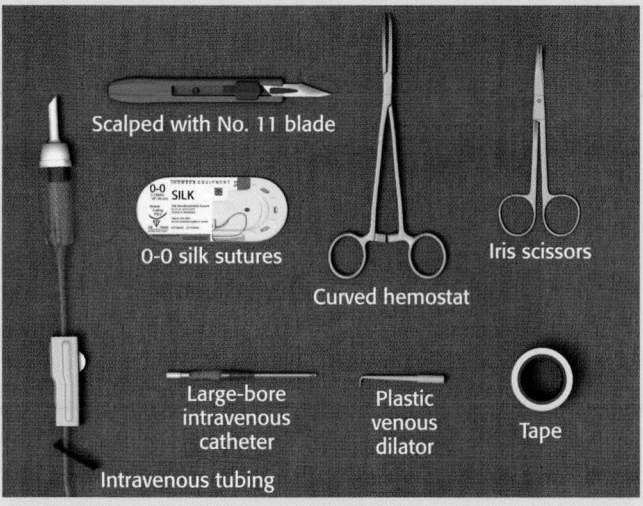

Scalped with No. 11 blade

0-0 silk sutures

Curved hemostat

Iris scissors

Large-bore intravenous catheter

Plastic venous dilator

Tape

Intravenous tubing

Review Box 23-1 Venous cutdown: indications, contraindications, complications, and equipment.

saphenous vein at the ankle is often recommended for venous cutdown in children given its large diameter and anatomic predictability at this location.[6,7]

Hypovolemic Shock

Initially popularized during the Vietnam War for rapid transfusion, venous cutdown has since been used for resuscitation of patients with profound hypovolemia.[8,9] The flow rate of saline through a standard IV extension set cut to a length of 28 cm (12 inches) and inserted directly into the vein is 15% to 30% greater than through a 5-cm, 14-gauge catheter. This difference is larger if pressure is applied to the system. Moreover, the improvement in flow rate through large-bore lines is greater for blood than for crystalloid solutions because the viscous characteristics of blood impede its passage through small-bore tubing.[9] A unit of blood can be transfused in as little as 3 minutes through IV extension tubing inserted directly into the vein. Consequently, large-bore lines placed by venous cutdown are an excellent mechanism for the treatment of severe hypovolemia.

CONTRAINDICATIONS

Venous cutdown is contraindicated when less invasive alternatives exist and when performing the procedure would cause excessive delay.[10] Highly skilled clinicians may perform a cutdown in less than 60 seconds.[11] However, multiple studies by Westfall,[12] Rhee,[13] Iserson,[14] and their colleagues have indicated that on average, the procedure takes at least 5 to 6 minutes to complete. Use of the modified Seldinger technique described both by Shockley and Butzier and by Klofas has been shown to decrease that time by 22%.[15,16] In general, the use of percutaneously inserted central venous catheters in either the subclavian, internal jugular, or femoral vein is preferable to a cutdown.

Absolute contraindications include major blunt or penetrating trauma involving the extremity on which the procedure is to be performed.[17] Relative contraindications include vascular injury proximal to the cutdown site, overlying soft tissue infection, coagulopathies, compromised host defense mechanisms, and impaired wound healing. Other considerations include any previous saphenous vein harvest for coronary artery bypass or other vascular surgery proximal to the anticipated cutdown site.[18] The indications for venous cutdown should be weighed against the potential complications.

ANATOMY AND SELECTION OF THE SITE

Knowledge of the relevant anatomy is imperative for success. Veins in both the upper and lower extremities may be used. The size and accessibility of the target vessel along with the clinician's experience and training are the principal factors in selection of the site. There are four primary locations at which venous cutdown is performed: the great saphenous vein distally at the ankle and proximally at the thigh, the basilic vein above the elbow, and the cephalic vein below it. Brachial vein cutdown is no longer recommended as an emergency venous access route because of its time-consuming dissection and risk for neurovascular injury. The anatomy of individual vessels

and their relative merits as cutdown sites are described in the following sections.

The Great Saphenous Vein

The great saphenous vein is the longest vein in the body, and it runs subcutaneously throughout much of its course (Fig. 23-1). It is most easily accessible at the ankle but may also be cannulated below the knee and below the femoral triangle. The great saphenous vein begins just anterior to the medial malleolus, where it is a continuation of the medial marginal vein of the foot. The vein crosses 1 cm anterior to the medial malleolus and, together with the saphenous nerve, ascends along the anteromedial aspect of the leg.[19,20] The saphenous nerve at this level is of relatively little clinical significance in that, if transected, it causes sensory loss in only a small area along the medial aspect of the foot. At the ankle, the vessel can be exposed with minimal blunt dissection. The vein's superficial, predictable, and isolated location has made the distal saphenous vein the traditional pediatric cutdown site.[19]

At the knee, the saphenous vein lies superficially and medially. A cutdown performed 1 to 4 cm below the knee and immediately posterior to the tibia has been described in the pediatric literature.[6] This site is seldom used, however, because of its many disadvantages, including kinking of the line as the knee is flexed and risk for injury to the saphenous branch of the genicular artery and the saphenous nerve.[21] Of note, the

Femoral artery
Femoral vein

Great (long) saphenous vein

Saphenous vein

Medial malleolus

Figure 23-1 Superficial veins of the lower limb.

Figure 23-2 Subcutaneous dissection in the proximal part of the thigh. The saphenous vein is easily distinguished from surrounding fat with blunt dissection. *(Courtesy of Pablo Aguilera, MD. Hospital Dr. Sótero del Río, Santiago, Chile.)*

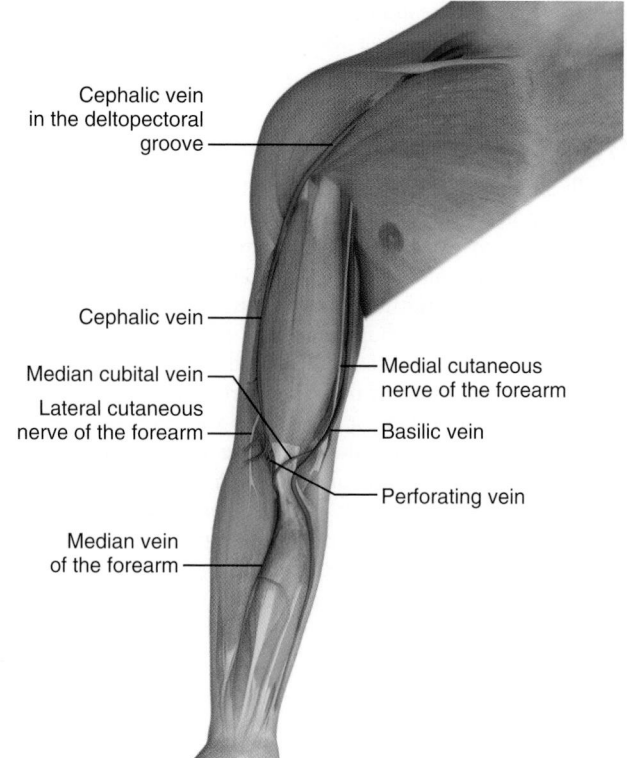

Figure 23-3 Veins of the upper limb.

great saphenous vein is duplicated in the calf in 25% of the population and may be present on exploration.[22]

In the thigh, the saphenous vein begins on the medial aspect of the knee and crosses anterolaterally as it ascends toward the femoral triangle. Approximately 4 cm below the inguinal ligament and 3 cm lateral to the pubic tubercle, the saphenous vein dips through the fossa ovalis, where it penetrates the femoral sheath and joins the femoral vein. The saphenous vein is easily isolated from the surrounding fat at this site because of its large caliber (4 to 5 mm in outside diameter) and superficial relationship to the femoral sheath (Fig. 23-2). Also lying anteromedially in the thigh is the lateral femoral cutaneous vein, which has a smaller diameter and lies lateral to the great saphenous vein.[20] The saphenous vein at the thigh is a preferred site for cutdown given its large diameter and ease of accessibility. An 8.5-Fr catheter is easily introduced at this level and is ideal for rapid infusion of crystalloid or blood during resuscitation.[17]

The Basilic Vein

The basilic vein is a preferred site for venous cutdown in the upper extremity because of its predictable anatomic location. The size of this vein enables it to be located easily, even in hypotensive or hypovolemic patients. Superficially at this level there are no important associated structures, but the brachial artery and the median nerve are found deep to the basilic vein.

Veins of the dorsal venous network of the hand unite to form the cephalic and basilic veins, which travel along the radial and ulnar sides of the forearm, respectively (Fig. 23-3). At the midforearm level, the basilic vein crosses anterolaterally and then courses ventrally at the medial epicondyle. The median cubital vein crosses over from the radial side of the arm to join the basilic vein just above the medial epicondyle. The basilic vein then continues proximally, where it occupies a superficial position between the biceps and pronator teres muscles. In this segment it lies in close proximity to the medial cutaneous nerve, which supplies sensation to the ulnar

side of the forearm. At approximately midway in the upper part of the arm, the basilic vein perforates the deep fascia, where it joins the brachial vein and continues on into the axillary vein.[20]

The basilic vein is consistently found at the antecubital fossa 2 cm above and 2 to 3 cm lateral to the medial epicondyle on the anterior surface of the upper part of the arm. It is exposed through a transverse incision on the medial aspect of the proximal antecubital fossa. It is this predictability in anatomic location that makes the basilic vein an ideal site for venous cutdown in the upper extremity.

A more proximal cutdown site had previously been recommended to avoid the network of interconnecting veins at the level of the antecubital fossa.[23] However, a closer association between the basilic vein and the medial cutaneous nerve in this segment may result in transection of the nerve and subsequent sensory loss on the ulnar side of the forearm.

The Cephalic Vein

This cephalic vein begins on the radial aspect of the wrist, crosses anteromedially, and ascends toward the antecubital fossa. In the forearm, it lies in close association with the lateral cutaneous nerve, which supplies sensory innervation to the radial aspect of the forearm (see Fig. 23-3). In the antecubital fossa, it lies subcutaneously and just lateral to the midline. It is at this level where the median cubital vein connects to the cephalic and basilic veins. The cephalic vein then ascends in the upper part of the arm over the lateral aspect of the biceps muscle and through the deltopectoral groove. Just below the clavicle, it pierces the clavipectoral fascia, becomes a deep structure, and enters the axillary vein.[20]

Venous cutdown is easily performed on the cephalic vein because of its large diameter and superficial location. In the forearm, it is important to avoid the lateral cutaneous nerve. A preferred location is in the antecubital fossa at the distal flexor crease. Cutdown on the cephalic vein at the wrist has also been reported, but the thin skin overlying the vein at this level usually permits simple percutaneous cannulation when the vein is available for cannulation.[24] The cephalic vein may also be entered in the deltopectoral groove. However, the slightly deeper position and possible interference with the performance of other procedures make this approach more difficult.

EQUIPMENT

The material required to perform a formal venous cutdown is shown in Review Box 23-1. Perhaps the most important piece of equipment and the most difficult to find is the vein dilator/lifter, a plastic device with a 90-degree angle that is used to facilitate entrance of a catheter into the cut vein. For pediatric patients, use a warming table or radiant warmer and a padded extremity board as well.

Choose a catheter based on the desired function of the venous line. When central venous pressure (CVP) needs to be monitored, choose a catheter long enough to reach the superior vena cava. Approximate this distance by aligning the catheter over the chest with the tip at the level of the manubrial-sternal junction. The average distance from the antecubital fossa to the superior vena cava is 54 cm in adult men. Lumen size is relatively unimportant when the line is inserted for monitoring CVP or to infuse drugs, but it is a critical factor in the treatment of hypovolemia. Short, large-bore catheters are preferred when fluid must be delivered rapidly. Silastic catheters, IV plastic tubing, or 5- or 8-Fr pediatric feeding tubes may be used as infusion catheters in older children and adults.

Tables 23-1, 23-2, and 23-3 list the flow rates of various fluids through some commonly used catheter systems. It is essential to know the relative flow rates if maximal benefit is to be obtained from the time spent performing the cutdown. Excellent flow rates can be achieved by threading IV tubing directly into the vein or by using a 5-cm, 10-gauge IV catheter. Cut sterile tubing to the appropriate length and leave a slight bevel on the end to facilitate cannulation of the opened vein.[11,25]

TABLE 23-1 Comparative Average Flow Rates (mL/min) for Tap Water CAN BE FOUND ON EXPERT CONSULT

TABLE 23-2 Comparative Average Flow Rates (mL/min, 200–mm Hg Pressure) for Red Blood Cells CAN BE FOUND ON EXPERT CONSULT

TABLE 23-3 Comparative Average Flow Rates (mL/min) CAN BE FOUND ON EXPERT CONSULT

TECHNIQUE

The technique of venous cutdown is essentially the same regardless of the vessel cannulated (Fig. 23-4). Prepare the skin around the incisional area with an antiseptic solution and then cover it with sterile drapes. Place a tourniquet proximal to the cutdown site to help visualize the vein. For children, immobilize the lower part of the leg or elbow (depending on the cutdown site) on a padded board before beginning the procedure.

In conscious patients, apply a local anesthetic before the procedure. Make a skin incision perpendicular to the course of the vein. A longitudinal incision, even though it decreases the risk of transecting neurovascular structures, may not provide sufficient exposure. Incise the skin through all its layers until subcutaneous fat bulges through the incision. Very carefully dissect the subcutaneous tissues bluntly by spreading them gently with a curved hemostat parallel to the course of the vein and with the tips pointed downward. This is the most difficult and delicate portion of the procedure and may damage the vein and render it unable to be cannulated. Bleeding, however, is usually minimal unless the vein is nicked. Use a tissue spreader or a self-retaining retractor, if needed, to provide a wider field. Isolate the vein from the adjacent tissue and mobilize it for 1 to 3 cm.

For the standard venous cutdown technique, after mobilizing the vein, use a hemostat to pass proximal and distal silk ties under the vein for stabilization (Fig. 23-5).

Tie the distal ligature after initial placement, but leave the ends long for maneuvering the vein. As an option, use traction on the distal suture to control the vein, but do not tie it off. If the distal suture is tied, the vein will be sacrificed for future use. Leave the proximal ligature untied to maneuver the vein for insertion of the catheter or tubing and control of back-bleeding (by lifting the sutures). Elevate the vein with a hemostat and stretch it flat. This provides good visualization, controls the vessel, and limits bleeding when the vessel is incised. Alternatively, place gentle traction on the proximal tie to control oozing around the puncture site. Using a No. 11 scalpel blade or a pair of iris scissors, incise through one third to one half the diameter of the vein at a 45-degree angle. If the incision is too small, the catheter may pass into a false channel in the adventitia. Conversely, if the incision is too large, the vein may tear completely and retract from the field buried within tissue.[26] If desired, make a longitudinal incision in the vein to avoid transecting the vessel, but realize that this technique makes it more difficult to identify the lumen. Also be aware that some bleeding will normally occur after the vein has merely been nicked on the surface. To perform a mini-cutdown at this point, puncture the vein with an IV catheter and introducer needle and do not make an incision in the vein.

Before introducing the cannula into the vein, make a bevel in the cannula at a 45-degree angle. This is unnecessary if the cannula has a tapered tip. Make the bevel short, but be careful to not make it sharp to avoid piercing the posterior wall or otherwise damaging the vein. If using the rounded tip of a feeding tube, it may be more difficult to introduce but can be advanced less traumatically. If using an IV cannula, introduce it directly through the skin incision or through a separate stab incision.

Threading the catheter into the vein is often the most difficult and time-consuming portion of the procedure. Difficulty threading has several causes. The lumen may have been

VENOUS CUTDOWN

1 After applying a tourniquet and cleansing the skin, make a skin incision perpendicular to the course of the vein.

2 Bluntly dissect, isolate, and mobilize the vein.

3 Use a hemostat to isolate the vein and pass silk ties under it, proximal and distal to the proposed cannulation site.

4 Tie the distal suture only. Optionally, you can apply traction on the distal *untied* suture to control bleeding and remove it after cannulation.

5 Incise the vein while retracting the proximal ligature. Lift the proximal untied suture to control backbleeding.

6 Use the venous dilator to lift the flap and then advance the catheter into the vein. Attach intravenous tubing to the catheter.

7 Tie the proximal silk suture around the vein and catheter. Remove the proximal suture and suture the skin. If the distal suture has not been tied, remove it before suturing the skin.

Figure 23-4 Venous cutdown. *(Adapted from Custalow CB. Color Atlas of Emergency Department Procedures. Philadelphia: Saunders; 2005.)*

Figure 23-5 With the assistance of a hemostat, proximal and distal silk ties may be placed under the vein for stabilization. Above, a distal tie is placed under the great saphenous vein at the thigh to aid in stabilizing the vein during cannulation. Traction on this suture will occlude blood flow and minimize bleeding during catheterization of the vein. Traction on the proximal suture will also control backbleeding (proximal suture not shown here). Note that a small incision has been made in the vein to accept a catheter, but traction on the distal suture prevents bleeding. Once the catheter is in place, the distal suture is usually tied. *(Courtesy of Pablo Aguilera, MD. Hospital Dr. Sótero del Río, Santiago, Chile.)*

Figure 23-6 Advancement of the standard intravenous catheter under direct vision through the great saphenous vein at the thigh. The distal suture is tied, thereby sacrificing the vein for further use. The proximal suture is not yet secured around the catheter. *(Courtesy of Pablo Aguilera, MD. Hospital Dr. Sótero del Río, Santiago, Chile.)*

incorrectly identified, or a false passage into the adventitia may have been created. This can be difficult to recognize because a catheter can easily pass between layers of the vessel wall and never reach the lumen of the vein. Other causes include penetrating the posterior vessel wall, getting stuck in a valve, or using a catheter that is too large to cannulate the vein.

Use of a plastic venous dilator can help identify and elevate the vessel lumen. Thread the small, pointed tip of the dilator into the vein to expose the lumen before advancing the tip of the catheter. Alternatively, bend a sterile 20-gauge needle at a 90-degree angle to serve as a venous dilator or elevator. A vein dilator is useful for very small veins, such as in pediatric cutdowns, but is generally unnecessary in adults. To thread large catheters in adults, grasp the proximal edge of the vessel with small forceps or a mosquito hemostat. Apply counter-traction and advance the catheter. Never force a catheter that will not advance easily (Fig. 23-6).

Once the catheter is advanced into the lumen, backbleed any air from the cannula and connect it to IV tubing. Tie the proximal ligature around both the vessel and the cannula (Fig. 23-7). If the distal suture has not been tied, remove it. If it has been tied, cut the ends of the suture near the knot. Remove the tourniquet, affix the catheter to the skin, and close the incision. Apply antibiotic ointment at the point where the catheter passes through the skin, and dress the wound. In an emergency situation one may delay skin closure if necessary and simply wrap the wound with sterile dressing. Loop the IV tubing under the outer layers of the dressing to minimize the risk of pulling the cannula out if the external IV line is inadvertently tugged.

Figure 23-7 Once the catheter is inserted into the lumen of the vein, tie the proximal ligature around both the vessel and the cannula. *(Courtesy of Pablo Aguilera, MD. Hospital Dr. Sótero del Río, Santiago, Chile.)*

Mini-Cutdown

The mini-cutdown is an alternative method designed to preserve the vein and bypass the time-consuming step of inserting a catheter into the vein.[27] It is preferred if time is limited. Basically, a deep vein is cannulated through an incision under direct vision with a standard peripheral IV catheter. Use a skin incision and blunt dissection to locate the vessel. Once identified, puncture the vein under direct vision with a percutaneous venous catheter. Introduce the needle through either the skin incision or a separate stab incision. If an over-the-needle device (e.g., Angiocath, Medicut) is used, withdraw the needle and discard it. With a through-the-needle device, thread the cannula into the vein and withdraw the needle to the surface of the skin (Fig. 23-8). Place a guard on the tip of the needle, fix the catheter device to the skin, and close the incision. This method eliminates the need for tying or cutting the vein, thereby permitting repeated catheterization. Venipuncture is easier and uses the same equipment as percutaneous venous cannulation. A simple skin incision may also permit direct visualization of veins in an obese patient and facilitate standard percutaneous venipuncture.

Hansbrough and associates described a mini-cutdown procedure with a 10-gauge IV catheter (Deseret 10-gauge Angiocath).[25] Flow rates of blood and saline with this catheter are equal to those obtained when IV extension tubing is placed in a vein via the more time-consuming standard venous cutdown technique. This catheter allows one to infuse a unit of whole blood in 2 to 3 minutes if high pressure and oversized IV tubing are used.

Modified Cutdown Technique

Shockley and Butzier described a further modification in which a guidewire, dilator, and sheath system is inserted after standard cutdown and venotomy.[15] To perform this modification, set up the guidewire, dilator, and sheath system before making the skin incision. Once the vein has been incised, insert the end of the guidewire followed by the dilator and sheath. Remove the wire and dilator while leaving the sheath. Ligatures are not usually needed with this technique. These authors found that when performed by novices, this technique saved more than 2 minutes in comparison to the standard technique. Moreover, in the event of a transection, there was an increased vein salvage rate. Klofas used a similar technique at the distal saphenous vein.[16] He also developed a model for teaching the modified technique with wood, gauze, cast padding, and tape.

To remove catheters inserted by cutdown, cut the skin stitches holding the catheter in place and then withdraw the catheter. Control backbleeding from the proximal venous end by applying a simple pressure dressing.

COMPLICATIONS

Complications of venous cutdown include local hematoma, infection, sepsis, phlebitis, embolization, wound dehiscence, and injury to associated structures. An indirect but significant complication is deterioration of an unstable patient during a time-consuming attempt at cutdown. Documentation of complications and their frequency in the literature has been sparse. Bogen reported a 15% complication rate in 234 cases.[28] Infection and phlebitis each occurred at a rate of 4%. Infectious complications may result from the introduction of pathogens during placement of the line, transcutaneous invasion along the course of the cannula, or deposition of blood-borne organisms on the tip of the catheter.[29] A clear correlation exists between the incidence of infectious complications and the length of time that a catheter is left in place. Moran and colleagues found that the infection rate rose from 50% to 78% when a catheter was left in place for more than 48 hours.[30] Druskin and Siegel,[29] studying a mixed population of patients who had undergone cutdown and others who had catheters inserted percutaneously, found that the incidence of culture-positive catheter tips rose from 0% to 52% after 48 hours.[29] In the study by Moran and coworkers,[30] *Staphylococcus albus* was the predominant organism that was isolated, but organisms more commonly thought of as pathogenic (*Staphylococcus aureus*, *Enterococcus* spp., and *Proteus* spp.) were isolated with greater frequency from cutdowns that had been in place for long periods. Rhee and coauthors reported a 1.4%

Blood flow

1

2

3

4

Figure 23-8 The mini-cutdown technique is an alternative to the venous cutdown method. The vein is cannulated under direct vision with standard percutaneous catheters. A separate entry site (shown) may be used, or the vein can be cannulated through the skin incision. Note that the vein is not tied off with this technique. A standard Angiocath intravenous set may also be used instead of the through-the-needle catheter shown here.

infection rate and one episode of cellulitis after 73 cutdown attempts.[13] All catheters were removed within 24 hours.

Some evidence indicates that the rate of infectious complications decreases when a broad-spectrum topical antibiotic ointment is applied to the cutdown site. Moran and colleagues found an infectious complication rate of 18% when topical polymyxin B–neomycin-bacitracin (Neosporin) was used as opposed to a 78% rate in a placebo-treated group.[30] In this study, topical antibiotic use resulted in only a moderate decrease (from 53% to 37%) in the incidence of phlebitis but a significant decrease (from 86% to 14%) in the incidence of phlebitis associated with positive cultures. This suggests that phlebitis is often a chemical or an irritative process rather than the result of infection. Whatever the cause, the incidence of phlebitis is clearly related to the duration of catheterization.[8,28,31] Early catheter removal is a key factor in the prevention of both phlebitis and the infectious complications of venous cutdown. This is especially true of lines inserted during emergency resuscitative treatment. Such lines should be removed as soon as the patient's condition permits and alternative access routes are in place.[9,10]

Proper attention to details of the surgical technique will limit the occurrence of minor complications such as local hematoma, abscess, and wound dehiscence. One can avoid injury to associated structures by selecting a site at which the vein is well isolated and the physician feels most comfortable performing the procedure.

Acknowledgment

The authors and editors wish to sincerely thank Patricia Lanter and Justin Williams for their contributions to this chapter in prior editions.

References are available at www.expertconsult.com

CHAPTER 24

Indwelling Vascular Devices: Emergency Access and Management

Scott H. Witt and Diann M. Krywko

Indwelling vascular lines provide routes for short- and long-term infusion of antibiotics, antifungal agents, hyperalimentation fluids, chemotherapeutic agents, blood products, analgesics, and anesthetic agents. In addition, they provide access for lifesaving procedures such as hemodialysis (HD) and plasmapheresis. As of 2008, nearly 382,000 patients were receiving HD therapy, with 3 to 5 million central venous catheters being placed yearly in patients in the United States.[1,2] For the purpose of this chapter, all implanted devices and intermediate- to long-term catheters for vascular access are considered vascular access devices (VADs). Arteriovenous (AV) fistulas and AV grafts are included because of their similarities to VADs.

HISTORICAL PERSPECTIVE

A major advance that ultimately led to the development of several types of indwelling catheters was the introduction of Silastic (polymerized silicone rubber) in 1948 by the Dow Corning Corporation. This biocompatible material is an ideal substrate for intravenous (IV) catheters because it is chemically inert, antithrombogenic, rigid at room temperature, and pliable at body temperature. In 1973, Broviac and coworkers used this material to develop a 90-cm × 0.22-mm indwelling right atrial (RA) catheter for total parenteral nutrition (TPN).[3] In 1979, Hickman and colleagues reported their experience with a 0.32-mm catheter that could be used for blood products and drug therapy in bone marrow transplant recipients.[4] A totally implantable vascular access device (TIVAD) was described by Fortner and Pahnke in 1976.[5] Since that time, TIVADs have become a mainstay of treatment in oncology patients. TIVADs allow less painful IV access and improve quality of life by permitting unrestricted mobility.

Temporary access for HD via an external AV shunt was pioneered by both Quinton and Scribner and their coworkers in 1960.[6,7] This original shunt was composed of a loop of tubing lying on the volar aspect of the forearm that connected the radial artery to a wrist vein. Although it provided effective dialysis, it was associated with a high rate of infection, thrombosis, and restriction of patient activity. Brescia and colleagues then introduced the peripheral subcutaneous autogenous AV fistula in 1966.[8] This Brescia-Cimino internal fistula used a side-to-side anastomosis (the current procedure of choice for long-term HD) to connect the radial artery to the cephalic vein in the nondominant hand. Erben and associates described the routine use of percutaneous cannulation of the subclavian vein for HD in 1969.[9] In 1979, Uldall and coworkers reported the development of a single-needle, subclavian HD catheter.[10]

INDWELLING VADs

VADs are typically chosen based on the least invasive, smallest catheter with the lowest risk for complications that will last as long as the length of therapy that is anticipated.[11] Length of therapy is often the major consideration when choosing a device. Long-term VADs consist of cuffed, tunneled RA catheters and implantable ports. Medium-term VADs include midline catheters (lasting weeks), peripherally inserted central catheter (PICC) lines (lasting months), and Silastic subclavian or jugular catheters (percutaneous multilumen catheters). Short-term devices (see Chapter 21) include short peripheral IV, subcutaneous (butterfly), subclavian, and jugular catheters. Additional VADs include those used for dialysis, as well as AV fistulas and grafts.

Cuffed, Tunneled RA Catheters (Broviac, Hickman, Hemocath, Leonard, Raaf)

Several cuffed, tunneled RA catheters are available, each with differences tailored to specific applications (Fig. 24-1*A*). The *Broviac* is an all-Silastic single-lumen catheter with a 1.0-mm internal diameter (ID). It is 90 cm long with a thin intravascular segment (55 cm). The *Hickman*, also a Silastic catheter, has a 1.6-mm ID. It allows more frequent blood sampling without jeopardizing luminal patency.[12] Single-, double- and triple-lumen variations exist. *Hemocath/Permacath* has the largest bore of the RA catheters, 2.2 mm ID. *Quinton* Instrument Company manufactures these catheters for HD, plasmapheresis, long-term nutritional support, and pain control. The main advantage of a cuffed catheter is that it can be used immediately, but it is not recommended for long-term access in patients undergoing dialysis if an AV fistula or graft is possible. Long-term dialysis with tunneled catheters has been associated with an increased risk for death, a 5- to 10-fold increase in the risk for infection, and a decreased likelihood of adequate dialysis.[13] Ideally, these catheters should be used only as a bridge to longer-term devices.[14]

Nonemergency insertion of RA catheters is typically done in an operating room or interventional radiology suite. The device is introduced via the upper anterior chest wall and tunneled subcutaneously to enter the superior vena cava (SVC) system via the cephalic, subclavian, internal, or external jugular vein (Fig. 24-2). The distal tip of the flexible catheter is advanced to the distal SVC or into the mid-RA area. The subcutaneous tunnel isolates the venous puncture site from the skin and decreases the potential for bacterial contamination. Dacron cuffs (one near the venous entrance site and one near the skin exit site) anchor the catheter and are believed to inhibit colonization of the SVC by skin organisms.[15] However, no study has been able to support this belief. Advantages of an RA catheter include ease of insertion and use, minimal interference with patient activity, low incidence of major complications or unintended dislodgment, ease of removal, and potential repair via a kit. Disadvantages include the need for regular maintenance and the potential for unacceptable cosmesis.

Figure 24-1 A, Broviac Pediatric 4.2-French Single-Lumen CV Catheter with SureCuff Tissue Ingrowth Cuff and VitaCuff Antimicrobial Cuff. **B,** The Groshong catheter has a valve to prevent backbleeding.

Groshong Catheter

In contrast to the Broviac and Hickman catheters, the *Groshong* catheter has slitlike openings just proximal to the end of the intravascular portion of the catheter (see Fig. 24-1*B*). This functions as a one-way valve to stop backbleeding and prevent air entry and embolism from the negative intrathoracic pressure. This feature obviates the need to use a heparin lock (saline may be used). In addition, external catheter clamping is not necessary. Disadvantages are its high cost and requirement for pressurized infusion systems.[16]

TIVADs/Ports (Port-A-Cath, Proport, Infuse-A-Port, Mediport)

Since 1983, implanted ports have become the mainstay for long-term cancer therapy. TIVADs are tunneled RA catheters, but they differ from Broviac and Hickman catheters in that they have a subcutaneous titanium or plastic portal with a self-sealing septum (Fig. 24-3) that may be accessed by puncturing a specially designed needle (90-degree angled Huber needle) through intact skin (Fig. 24-4). Cosmetically, they are superior to external tunneled catheters, require less maintenance, and afford patients greater freedom of movement and activities such as swimming or bathing.

TIVADs may be inserted on an outpatient basis under local anesthesia via a subcutaneous tunnel or open cutdown. The cutdown technique offers potential speed (mean placement time, 15 minutes), safety (negligible risk for pneumothorax),

Figure 24-2 A, Subclavian-placed catheter with a subcutaneous tunnel. **B,** Quinton dialysis catheter in the right internal jugular vein, often used for emergency dialysis or as a bridge until a dialysis fistula or graft is ready for use (i.e., when it matures).

along with avoidance of early and late complications.[17] Placement is typically in the nondominant arm with the portal in the upper part of the arm or chest unless a vein is occluded or radiation therapy is planned on that side.

Disadvantages of this type of device include increased cost, the need for a specific noncoring Huber access needle, and the small gauge (20 to 22) of the access needle, which limits fluid infusion rates.[16]

PICC (Nontunneled, Noncuffed)

PICC lines are centrally placed lines that were first described in the 1970s and originally developed for the neonatal population. Subsequently, their use expanded into the adult arena for prolonged antibiotic therapy, IV fluids, chemotherapy,

C   Infuse-a-Port

Figure 24-3 A, Port-a-Cath double-lumen port (for chest placement). **B,** Port-A-Cath single-lumen port (for upper extremity placement). The Port-A-Cath system is accessed by inserting a Huber needle through the skin into the portal septum. **C,** The Infuse-A-Port is similar to the Port-A-Cath.

A

B

Figure 24-4 A, Porta-A-Cath system (Deltec, Inc., St. Paul, MN). This device is subcutaneous and accessed with a Huber needle introduced through the skin into the portal septum. **B,** The Huber needle is used to access the septum. Always use sterile technique.

Figure 24-5 The double-lumen percutaneously inserted central catheter (5.0 Fr, 18 gauge) is placed in the arm with the tip of the catheter in the superior vena cava. Shorter 20-cm versions (not shown) look similar but terminate in the axillary vein and are termed midline peripheral catheters.

TPN, and delivery of medications that are irritating to peripheral vessels. PICCs (Fig. 24-5) are made of two substances, either polyurethane (Intracath) or silicone (Intrasil), are radiopaque, and measure 50 to 60 cm in length with an outside diameter of 2 to 7 Fr. The catheter may have a single- or double-lumen configuration and can be open or closed ended or valved (e.g., Groshong). An open-ended PICC cannot prevent feedback of blood into the catheter and therefore must be flushed one or more times daily with heparinized saline. The Groshong valve reduces backup of blood into the catheter and therefore requires flushing as infrequently as once a week. The most common type of PICC line in use today is the 5-Fr, double-lumen, closed-ended catheter.

Selection of the device should be based on the number of lumens necessary for therapy. Selection of the access site depends on many factors, including the suitability of target vessels, body habitus, handedness, ability to manage self-care, comorbid conditions, desired infusion rate, number and compatibility of concurrent infusions, infusate characteristics, and the estimated duration of therapy. Infusate that is hyperosmolar (e.g., TPN) or vesicant requires rapid dilution. Accordingly, the tip must be in the SVC, where the estimated flow rate is 2000 mL/min. PICC lines are most frequently placed in the superficial veins proximal to the antecubital fossa (usually the basilic or cephalic vein) (Fig. 24-6). However, they may also be placed via a transhepatic or translumbar approach when the SVC is thrombosed or occluded.[18]

Advantages of PICC lines include usefulness in a wide variety of clinical situations, ease of placement, and ease of use and maintenance. They do not require surgical insertion and may be placed in an outpatient setting. A PICC line is an excellent vehicle for medium- to long-term IV therapy. With proper care, PICCs can remain in place for long periods, even months to years.[19] To remove a PICC line, simply withdraw it from the vein and apply pressure and a sterile bandage.

Midline Peripheral Catheters

Midline catheters are often confused with PICC lines. They are also placed peripherally in the superficial veins of the antecubital fossa or upper part of the forearm. They differ from PICCs in that they are peripheral, not central catheters.

Figure 24-6 A, Percutaneously inserted central catheter (PICC) line placement in the upper extremity with the internal catheter tip at the superior vena cava (SVC). **B,** Most PICC lines are used for outpatient therapy, such as prolonged antibiotic therapy, so proper aseptic technique at the catheter site is essential.

Midlines are typically shorter (20 cm), with the tip terminating near the axillary vein. Placement above the axillary vein results in a higher risk for thrombosis. They are designed for short- to medium-term use, a shorter period than with a PICC. Because midline catheters do not enter the central circulation with high flow, delivery of medication and infusion types are limited, and routine blood withdrawal is not recommended. Differentiating between these two catheters in situ may be difficult because their outward appearance is similar. Obtaining an x-ray film for visualization of tip placement will help in determining catheter type.

Figure 24-7 Mahurkar 11.5-Fr. × 16-cm Double-Lumen Catheter for temporary hemodialysis, apheresis, and infusion.

HD VADs

Vascular access, which is often referred to as the Achilles heel of renal patients, remains problematic. From the moment that the first access is created, an ongoing process is started that will end with loss of all access sites if the patient survives long enough.[20] Clinical practice guidelines of the National Kidney Foundation—Disease Outcomes Quality Initiative (NKF-DOQI) recommend early construction of an AV fistula and avoidance of catheters for permanent or prolonged vascular access,[17,21] with less than 10% of permanent access being in the form of catheters.[22] However, one study demonstrated that more than half the patients began dialysis with a central catheter because a well-developed AV fistula was not available.[23] The risk of requiring three or more vascular access sites is almost double in patients who start HD with a central catheter.

Temporary Dialysis Catheters (Quinton, Mahurkar, Tessio, Vascath, Uldall)

Temporary vascular access catheters (Fig. 24-7) are used for emergency HD or for temporary HD access if a more permanent dialysis route (AV fistula or graft) is not available or has recently been placed and has not matured yet. The advantage of tunneled catheters is the ability to provide immediate access or temporary access while a more permanent structure matures, but this carries a long-term risk for infection, dysfunction, and central venous stenosis. The majority of bacteremia episodes in patients undergoing HD are caused by HD catheters, with an approximate 20% to 25% risk over the average duration of use.

These large-bore catheters allow the necessary blood flow rate of 300 mL/min for dialysis. The *Quinton* catheter has two ports, one to deliver the patient's blood to the dialysis machine and another to return the blood to the patient's circulation (see Fig. 24-2B). These catheters are placed in a central vein, either the internal jugular, subclavian, or femoral. The right internal jugular approach is preferred, even if permanent access is to be created on the right side, because it has the lowest thrombosis rate. The NKF-DOQI recommends avoiding the subclavian vein unless no other options exist or the ipsilateral arm has no more permanent access sites. For patient comfort, a special 180-degree catheter can be used (Fig. 24-8). There are two avenues to place this catheter: percutaneously or surgically. Emergency percutaneous placement may be performed by the emergency clinician at the bedside. Using sterile technique and after injection of a local anesthetic, insert the catheter by following the same procedure for placing a central line into one of the central veins.

The second technique uses a slightly larger catheter (Quinton, Hickman) and is performed in the operating room

Figure 24-8 MedComp Duo-Flow Internal Jugular Vascular Catheter (11.5 Fr × 15 cm). The angle of the catheter makes it more comfortable for the patient.

under local anesthesia with or without general sedation. This catheter is placed in much the same fashion as the tunneled RA catheters described previously. Surgically implanted catheters are preferred if more than temporary use is anticipated because the risk for infection is decreased and they can be used for a longer time.

Chronic HD Vascular Access

The goal of chronic HD vascular access is to provide safe, effective, and repeated easy access to the circulation. The three principal types of access are native AV fistulas, synthetic grafts, and double-lumen tunneled cuffed catheters (described above). The access types differ in failure rates, patency, complications, and other morbidity. In general, fistulas are preferred over grafts because of superior long-term patency and lower complication rates. However, fistulas are more likely than grafts to experience primary failure, defined as being unable to provide reliable access. Both fistulas and grafts must mature before they can be used for HD, a process that may take several weeks to several months. HD is often performed via a Quinton catheter during this hiatus, so a patient in the emergency department (ED) with both a catheter and a shunt either has a nonfunctioning fistula or graft or the access site is still immature. Grafts can usually be cannulated earlier than fistulas, often within weeks of placement. The minimum time for fistula maturation is at least 1 month. Complications common to both grafts and fistulas are thrombosis, infection, steal syndrome, aneurysms, venous hypertension, seromas, and local bleeding (Fig. 24-9). Overall, grafts are more likely to experience infection and thrombosis requiring thrombectomy or require other types of access intervention. The risk for infection with HD grafts is about 10% over prolonged use and 1% to 2% with HD fistulas. Graft infection requires complete excision to eradicate an infection of the foreign material, whereas fistula infections may resolve with IV antibiotic use.

It may be difficult to distinguish a fistula from a graft by gross inspection alone. Grafts are rarely placed in the forearm, which is the preferred site for fistulas. Fistulas tend to be more tortuous and serpentine, whereas synthetic grafts are straighter or C shaped. Both grafts and fistulas are subject to vascular perturbation and integrity issues from the high flow rates and repeated access. Grafts are subject to pseudoaneurysms when there is a breach in the integrity of the graft and are more likely to rupture. Fistulas are also subject to bulging of the vessel walls to form a true aneurysm. Dilated veins in a fistula can simulate an aneurysm. Both types of vascular deformities can rupture. Multiple defects may require a replacement access.

Side of artery to side of vein

End of vein to side of artery

End of artery to side of vein

End-to-end spatulated artery and vein

Figure 24-9 A, Various possible anastomotic configurations between the artery and vein for autogenous fistula formation. A thrill should be palpated if this fistula is functioning. **B,** Older dialysis fistula. Fistulas can develop multiple aneurysms (*arrows*) from multiple time use. It may be difficult to distinguish a fistula from a graft by merely looking at the site. (*A, Adapted from Ozeran RS. Construction and care of external arteriovenous shunts. In: Wilson SE, Owens ML, eds.* Vascular Access Surgery. *Chicago: Year Book Medical; 1980.*)

Edema of the arm, breasts, neck, or face can result from complications of HD access. Causes include venous outflow obstruction in various areas, thrombosis, or infection.

AV Fistulas

An AV fistula is a *direct subcutaneous anastomosis of an artery and vein without prosthetic material* and is the preferred means of

Figure 24-11 Three possible graft configurations for jump grafts in which standard sites have been used. Note the typical C shape of the graft. (*Redrawn from Tilney NL, Lazarus JM, eds.* Surgical Care of the Patient with Renal Failure. *Philadelphia: Saunders; 1982; as shown in Haisch CE. Chronic vascular and peritoneal access. In: Davis JH, Sheldon GF, eds.* Clinical Surgery. *St. Louis: Mosby; 1995.)*

Figure 24-10 Arteriovenous fistula. **A,** Brescia-Cimino (radial-cephalic) fistula performed at the level of the wrist. **B,** Brachial-cephalic fistula performed proximal to the antecubital fossa. **C,** Multiple asymptomatic *pseudoaneurysms* resulting several years after creation of an autogenous wrist (Brescia-Cimino) arteriovenous fistula. (*B, Adapted from Rutherford RB, ed.* Vascular Surgery. *5th ed. Philadelphia: Saunders; 2001.)*

vascular access for HD (see Fig. 24-9). Historically, the percentage of patients with AV fistulas fell well below the recommended goal, with most patients receiving AV grafts or long-term vascular access catheters. The most recent data from the Dialysis Outcomes and Practice Patterns Study (DOPPS) show that from 1996 to 2007, AV fistula use in the United States almost doubled (24% to 47%) and AV graft use fell by 50%.[24] Use of an autogenous fistula is associated with the longest period of patency with relative freedom from thrombotic and infectious complications. Once a fistula matures, long-term patency is high (48% of AV fistulas versus 14% of AV grafts at 5 years), with low infection rates relative to grafts.[25]

An autogenous AV fistula is constructed by anastomosing an artery to a vein (see Fig. 24-9), preferably a nearby one. Various configurations are possible, but AV fistulas are typically an end-to-side vein-to-artery anastomosis. The radial-cephalic (*Brescia-Cimino forearm*) fistula in the forearm is the most frequently used (Fig. 24-10), with the brachial-cephalic, brachial-basilic, and rarely the proximal part of the thigh being alternatives. Over time, the venous portion of the shunt is subjected to high pressure, and flow becomes arterialized (hypertrophied and dilated), which renders it suitable for repeated vascular access. Full epithelialization of the shunt does not occur for 3 to 6 months, thus necessitating anticipatory placement as renal function worsens.

AV Grafts

If a forearm radiocephalic fistula cannot be constructed or has failed, an AV bridge graft using a donor vein or synthetic material is a well-accepted alternative. Several synthetic materials are used for grafts. Polytetrafluoroethylene (PTFE) is the

most commonly used but takes 3 weeks to mature. An available polyurethane graft (Vectra) has the ability to be accessed within 24 hours. A standard graft is 6 to 8 mm in diameter and usually positioned in a U-shaped subcutaneous tunnel in the forearm. The graft is attached by end-to-side anastomoses to the brachial artery and antecubital vein. If no suitable antecubital vein is available, a straight bridge graft between the brachial artery and either the axillary or the basilic vein is often used. Multiple configurations are possible (Fig. 24-11). The characteristic C shape of the graft can aid in differentiating a graft from a more tortuous fistula. A jump graft between opposite extremities with creation of a loop across the chest or anastomosis of the axillary artery to the iliac vein is a possibility if all other sites have been exhausted. When compared with AV fistulas, AV grafts have a significantly higher incidence of thrombosis, infection, pseudoaneurysm formation, and limb loss. PTFE grafts have a low primary patency rate (29% at 1 year according to one study).[26] However, they have a low incidence of aneurysm formation and are comparatively easy to revise. The estimated life span of a PTFE graft in clinical practice is often less than 2 years.

ACCESSING VADs IN THE ED

When IV access is required in patients with VADs, standard methods of peripheral access should be attempted first to preserve the life span of the VAD and avoid complications. However, VADs, AV fistulas, and shunts may be accessed in emergency situations for phlebotomy and infusion of medications and fluids. Because of the complications of infection and catheter malfunction, dislodgment, and fracture, only personnel with the requisite knowledge and skill should access VADs if feasible. When VADs are accessed, ensure antisepsis throughout the procedure.

The emergency need to administer parenteral medications to patients lacking other means of vascular access is the most common reason to access a VAD in the ED. Assuming that proper access methods are used to prevent infection, the greatest risk is sludging in the catheter with resultant occlusion. After administering medications, follow with a saline flush to clear the catheter and ensure that the medications reach the circulation. Do not administer medications concurrently that are known to be incompatible when mixed (e.g., calcium and bicarbonate), even through separate ports of multilumen catheters. Blood specimens, including samples for culture, can also be obtained via VADs. For phlebotomy specimens, stop the infusion, use appropriate catheter antisepsis, remove fluid occupying dead space in the catheter, and follow the blood draw with a flush of heparinized saline.[27]

Accessing Long-Term Venous Access Catheters

To access the catheter (with the exception of Groshong catheters, which have backflow valve protection), first clamp it to prevent air embolism. Patients usually carry their own clamps, but if not available, use a hemostat without teeth. A hemostat with teeth will suffice in an emergency, in which case wrap sterile tape or tubing around the teeth of the hemostat. Remove the cap of the catheter and withdraw any mobile clots with a syringe. Remove about 3 to 5 mL of blood and then attach a 10-mL syringe to a single-dose vial of normal saline. Smaller syringes generate greater amounts of pressure for infusion, which can lead to increased intraluminal pressure and rupture of the catheter. Inject 3 to 5 mL of solution and then again withdraw it to ensure patency. Flush again with saline. More pronounced infusion might be necessary to ensure the patency of Groshong catheters.

To accomplish phlebotomy, withdraw the dead space solution, reclamp it, and use a separate syringe to remove the desired amount of blood.[28] If clots are withdrawn, continue withdrawing blood until it is clot free. Inject bolus medications and infuse IV solutions through the catheter, and clamp it whenever it is unattached. Deliver a 5-mL normal saline flush between medications through a 10-mL syringe. On completion of either blood withdrawal or medication infusion, inject 3 to 4 mL of saline to flush it and then inject 3 to 5 mL of heparin (1000 U/mL). Clamp the line and reposition the cap.[28] Note that 1000 U/mL of heparin should be used; less concentrated solutions may promote clotting. Do not inject larger amounts because it can heparinize the patient systemically. Groshong catheters need not be flushed with heparin but instead may be flushed briskly with 5 to 10 mL of saline. Multilumen central catheters have one port for each lumen, so access each one in the same manner. After antiseptic preparation, gain access either by inserting a needle or a syringe into the protective cap or by removing the cap entirely. Flush with 5-mL normal saline or sterile water, and verify backflow before all subsequent procedures. Perform phlebotomy through the proximal lumen to prevent mixing with medications being delivered through the other ports. Deliver IV infusions in similar fashion, and inject a normal saline flush between medications. Terminate the procedure by flushing 3 to 5 mL of heparin (1000 U/mL) through each port.

Accessing TIVADs

The procedure for accessing TIVADs is unique because these devices are not external. Instead, a circular reservoir (cylinder) lies subcutaneously on the anterior chest wall. First, palpate the cylinder and then prepare the overlying skin with povidone-iodine solution. Fill a 10-mL syringe with normal saline and attach it to connecting tubing. Attach this to a

19- to 22-gauge, 90-degree tapered (Huber) needle. The Huber needle is a specialized needle designed for use with TIVADs to prevent damage to the portal septum. It has a 90-degree bend with a slightly curved tip and the opening on the side rather than on the end. Most importantly, the Huber is a noncoring needle. This avoids damage to the Silastic septum and allows up to 2000 punctures. Do not access the TIVAD with a standard needle unless an arrest is in progress and a Huber needle is not immediately available. Apply a clamp to the connecting tubing whenever the system is open. Expel the air and insert the Huber needle through the septum of the reservoir. Insert the needle slowly and steadily through the diaphragm until it contacts the back of the reservoir. Be aware that although incomplete perforation of the septum will block flow, substantial pressure may also damage the back of the device and bend the tip of the needle. Remove the clamp slowly, and inject 5 mL of solution to ensure patency. If patency is not easily demonstrated, consider using alteplase (recombinant tissue plasminogen activator) as a fibrinolytic agent for catheter occlusion.[29]

Once the solution has been injected, apply gentle negative pressure to demonstrate backflow of blood. Stabilize the Huber needle by building a 4- × 4-inch gauze pad about the needle and further reinforce it with 2.54-cm (1-inch) silk tape. First, remove 8 to 9 mL of blood with a separate syringe and waste it, and then perform phlebotomy through the extension tubing. If necessary, deliver IV solutions through extension tubing, but remember that the rate of flow will be limited by the smaller radius of the Huber needle. Deliver a 5-mL normal saline flush between medications. Complete the procedure with a 3- to 5-mL heparin (1000 U/mL) flush, and remove the Huber needle.[28]

Accessing AV Fistulas, Shunts, and HD Catheters

AV fistulas, shunts, and temporary dialysis catheters are placed in patients who require HD, and they represent the sole access for that purpose. Consequently, routine use of these sites for phlebotomy and fluid administration is strongly discouraged. In fact, venipuncture in the same extremity as a patent AV fistula is not recommended, except for the veins in the dorsum of the ipsilateral hand. When standard IV access cannot be obtained under emergency circumstances, however, fistulas, shunts, and catheters may all be used to administer IV solutions and medications (Fig. 24-12). Though avoided whenever possible, the option to access these sites is based on clinical judgement by the clinician. If possible, ascertain patency of the fistula by noting a bruit and palpable thrill, although these signs may not be appreciable if the patient is in extremis.

Prepare the area overlying the fistula with antiseptic solution and access the fistula with the smallest-gauge needle that is appropriate.[30] Puncture 1 to 2 cm from the end of the anastomosis nearest the venous side, and avoid aneurysmal sites.[30] Access AV shunts similarly by placing the smallest needle possible in the catheter and bridging the arterial and venous circulations. Apply local pressure for at least 5 minutes after the procedure is completed and monitor subsequently for hemorrhage. Access the Uldall and Mahurkar catheters in much the same way that multilumen central catheters are accessed. Remove or inject through the retaining cap on each arm. Up to 5000 units of heparin is present within the two

Figure 24-12 For resuscitation or delivery of advanced cardiac life support drugs, a venous catheter may be used to access a shunt, but otherwise avoid this whenever possible.

BOX 24-1 Complications of Indwelling Vascular Access Devices

INFECTION
Skin/exit site
Reservoir/pocket
Tunnel
Catheter tip/lumen
Sepsis

MALFUNCTION
Occlusion
Failure of delivery of
   medication
Failure to infuse/withdraw
Pinch-off syndrome
Steal syndrome
Malposition
False aneurysms
Catheter dislodgement

HEMORRHAGE/COAGULATION
Bleeding
Local puncture site
Arterial bleeding
Excess heparinization
Thrombosis
Phlebitis
Deep venous thrombosis
Fibrin sheath

MISCELLANEOUS
Embolism
   Air
   Thrombus
   Catheter fragment
Arrhythmias
Cutaneous Dacron cuff erosion
High output cardiac failure
Precipitants

---

lumens, and so it is imperative to aspirate before administering fluid or medications. After use, flush each catheter arm with 10 mL of normal saline and instill 1.5 mL of heparin solution (1000 U/mL) into each one.

COMPLICATIONS OF VADs

VADs are now sufficiently commonplace that patients with these devices are seen in the ED on a regular basis. Given a complication rate of 4% to 10%,[31] it is essential that emergency clinicians be aware of these complications and their management. The risk for complications associated with a VAD is dependent on several factors, including the type of catheter, underlying patient pathology and anatomy, the site chosen for placement, and the experience of health care workers obtaining access and caring for the device.[32]

Complications of VADs include (1) infection, (2) hemorrhage and coagulation abnormalities, (3) malfunction, and (4) miscellaneous problems (Box 24-1).

Infection

Infection is the most common complication leading to removal of VADs and potentially the most serious. Infection can also result in shunt thrombosis, rupture, or massive hemorrhage. An estimated 250,000 to 500,000 cases of nosocomial VAD-related bacteremia occur annually in the United States with an associated 10% mortality rate.[33] Infectious complications include endocarditis, septic arthritis, pulmonary emboli, osteomyelitis, and spinal epidural abscess. The definitions of VAD-related infections are not uniform, which makes it difficult to compare the results of various investigations. However, it is generally agreed that risk factors for infection include the site of insertion, hospital size, duration of catheter placement, type of catheter, and patient factors. Most studies show a lower incidence of infection for TIVADs than for external systems, presumably because of lack of direct access by cutaneous organisms. Rates of VAD infection tend to be highest in the first 3 months after insertion, with skin flora

---

BOX 24-2 Microorganisms Causing Indwelling Catheter Infection

BACTERIAL
Gram-Positive Cocci
Staphylococcus aureus, Staphylococcus epidermidis, Streptococcus faecalis, Streptococcus bovis, group C streptococci, *Streptococcus viridans*

Gram-Negative Bacilli
Pseudomonas aeruginosa, Klebsiella spp., *Acinetobacter* spp., *Serratia* spp.

Gram-Positive Bacilli
Bacillus cereus, Bacillus laterosporus, Corynebacterium spp.

ATYPICAL
Mycobacterium neoaurum, Mycobacterium fortuitum, Mycobacterium chelonae

MYCOTIC
Malassezia furfur, Malassezia pachydermatis, Aspergillus fumigatus, Aspergillus flavus, Candida albicans

---

being most common.[31,34] The rate of infection decreases significantly and reaches a plateau after 5 to 6 months.[34] The most common infecting organisms are listed in Box 24-2.

Clinical findings are unreliable in the diagnosis of infection secondary to VADs. Fever, rigors, and an elevated white blood cell count are nonspecific, whereas purulent drainage at the insertion site is specific but not sensitive. Therefore, evaluation beyond physical examination alone is essential when infection is suspected, including Gram stain of purulent material at the site, blood cultures, and culture of catheter segments. In addition, transesophageal echocardiography is indicated if valvular vegetations are suspected by blood cultures positive for *Staphylococcus aureus*, persistent bacteremia or fungemia after removal of the catheter, or lack of clinical improvement.

Draw two sets of blood for culture, with one set through the catheter itself and one from a peripheral site. Positive blood cultures for *S. aureus*, coagulase-negative staphylococci, or *Candida* species, in the appropriate patient setting and in the absence of another identifiable source of infection, should increase suspicion for catheter-related bloodstream infection.[31] In most studies, blood obtained from a VAD yielding a colony count at least 5- to 10-fold greater than that for blood obtained from a peripheral site suggests a catheter-related source of infection.[35] Similarly, catheter infection should be assumed if cultures of peripherally derived blood are negative and the VAD-derived cultures are positive.[34] Not only is blood drawn from the catheter more likely to yield a positive culture, but it may also occur earlier in the course of infection. One study demonstrated high sensitivity and specificity for diagnosing a VAD-related infection if cultures of blood drawn from the access device became positive 2 or more hours before cultures of peripherally drawn blood.[36]

Infusate-related bloodstream infection is uncommon and defined as isolation of the same organism from both the infusate and separate percutaneous blood cultures, along with no other source of infection. When this diagnosis is suggested, cultures of the infusate should be performed in addition to catheter and peripheral blood cultures.[31]

When a catheter-related infection is suspected, an important management decision is required to determine whether to remove the catheter. Removal is recommended in patients who have a catheter placed solely for short-term use. In patients with long-term catheters, remove the catheter in the setting of severe sepsis, suppurative thrombophlebitis, endocarditis, or persistent positive blood cultures (longer than 72 hours) while on appropriate antibiotics. Also, remove the catheter if the infection is due to *S. aureus*, *Pseudomonas aeruginosa*, fungi, or mycobacteria. For patients who require long-term vascular access for survival or have no other vascular access options, salvage of the catheter may be attempted if the infecting agent is not *Bacillus*, *Micrococcus*, or propionibacteria, in addition to the previously listed organisms. If the catheter is left in place, obtain blood for repeated cultures and remove the catheter promptly if they remain positive following 72 hours of appropriate antibiotic therapy.[37]

If a VAD is removed, culture it to determine the offending organism. Place the catheter in a sterile tube (red top) and send it to the laboratory for culturing. The most widely used laboratory technique for the clinical diagnosis of catheter-related infection is the semiquantitative method, in which a segment of the catheter is rolled across the surface of an agar plate and colony-forming units (CFUs) are counted after incubation overnight. Quantitative culture of the catheter segment requires either flushing the segment with broth or vortexing in broth, followed by serial dilutions and surface plating on blood agar. A yield of 15 CFUs or more from a catheter by semiquantitative culture or a yield of 10^2 or more from a catheter by quantitative culture with accompanying signs of local or systemic infection is indicative of a catheter-related infection.[31]

HD catheters deserve special consideration. The process of HD requires several connections to the graft, thereby increasing the risk for infection. The rate of bacteremia in HD patients attributed to the graft varies from 48% to 73%. The incidence is highest when central venous dialysis catheters are used. Native AV fistulas carry the lowest risk for infection. Unfortunately, AV grafts are more commonly used in the United States.[38] As with other VADs, initiate empirical antibiotic therapy based on epidemiologic and patient factors, followed by narrowed-spectrum therapy after isolation and determination of sensitivities. The most common infecting organism is *S. aureus*. There has been an association between nasal carriage of *S. aureus* in HD patients and catheter infection. Reducing carriage rates has resulted in a decreased incidence of bloodstream infections.[31]

Antimicrobial Therapy

Pending the results of culture, the initial choice of an antibiotic is empirical and depends on the clinical setting, site of infection, type of device, host factors (e.g., immunocompromised state), severity of illness, and whether the device has been removed. If a VAD-related bloodstream infection is suspected, vancomycin should be initiated empirically because coagulase-negative *Staphylococcus* is the most common infectious organism and the prevalence of methicillin-resistant *S. aureus* continues to increase.[39] This should be followed by a semisynthetic penicillin or other appropriate antibiotics as guided by sensitivity studies. If the patient is severely ill, septic, or in an immunocompromised state or has a femoral catheter in place, additional coverage for gram-negative bacilli should be initiated.[39] Institute a third-generation cephalosporin unless the organism is extended-spectrum β-lactamase positive, in which case a carbapenem is more appropriate.[40] If there is concern for *P. aeruginosa*, initiate therapy with a fourth-generation cephalosporin (e.g., cefepime) or carbapenem, with or without an aminoglycoside. In addition to bacterial pathogens, fungemia should be suspected in septic patients who are receiving TPN, those with prolonged use of antibiotics, or those with a history of a hematologic malignancy or a bone marrow or solid organ transplant or if a femoral catheter is in place.[39] If fungemia is suspected or confirmed, initiate an antifungal medication and remove the catheter. An echinocandin medication (e.g., micafungin, caspofungin) is the recommended empirical treatment of suspected fungal infection.[40] Although there are no compelling data to specify a duration of antibiotic therapy, expert recommendation is to treat *S. aureus* infection for 14 days, gram-negative bacilli for 7 to 14 days, and candidal infection with antifungal therapy for 14 days after the first negative blood culture. Complicated infections (e.g., those with suppurative thrombophlebitis, endocarditis, or other similar infections) require 4 to 6 weeks of antibiotic treatment.[40]

Recommendations vary regarding exit site or tunnel or pocket infections. Jones recommended using aggressive local care in the early stages and a topical antibiotic ointment for short-term treatment.[34] Long-term treatment should be avoided because of the risk for *Candida* colonization.[34] Mermel and colleagues,[31] however, recommended that in patients with complicated infections, such as tunnel infection or port abscess, the catheter be removed and antibiotics initiated for 7 to 10 days.

If the VAD is retained, consider antibiotic lock therapy (ALT). ALT is a therapeutic option if the goal is to salvage the catheter. Most infections in tunneled catheters originate in the hub and spread to the catheter lumen. A biofilm can form and make eradication of the organism difficult because systemic antibiotics cannot achieve therapeutic levels there. ALT involves filling the catheter hub and lumen with a higher concentration of antibiotics and leaving them in place for extended periods. It is recommended that dwell times not exceed 48 hours before reinstilling the antibiotic solution.[40,41] If it is a femoral catheter, dwell time should not exceed 24 hours. ALT should always be used in conjunction with systemic antibiotics, and the recommended duration of treatment is 7 to 14 days.[40]

Prophylactic Measures
Antibiotic Prophylaxis during Initial Line Insertion
Prophylaxis with vancomycin or teicoplanin during central line insertion has not consistently demonstrated a reduced incidence of catheter-related bloodstream infection. Based on the limited data available, Centers for Disease Control and Prevention (CDC) guidelines currently recommend against giving vancomycin prophylactically because it is an independent risk factor for the acquisition of vancomycin-resistant enterococci and staphylococci with reduced susceptibility to glycopeptides.[42] Rather than using antibiotic prophylaxis, focus efforts on interventions designed to discourage the emergence of antimicrobial resistance, such as maximal barrier precautions.[43]

Impregnated Catheters
Using antimicrobial- or antiseptic-impregnated catheters or silver-impregnated collagen cuffs may be an effective intervention to reduce VAD-related bloodstream infection. A recent metaanalysis favored impregnated catheters in reducing central line–associated bloodstream infections (CLABSIs), but it was acknowledged that the overall methodology of the studies included was poor.[44] Nonetheless, the CDC currently recommends the use of these devices if the catheter is anticipated to remain in place for more than 5 days and if the institution's CLABSI rate is not decreasing after implementation of a comprehensive strategy to reduce catheter-associated infections.[41]

Routine Line Changing
Despite the incidence of infection and the potential complications, routine changing of VADs is not recommended.[41] Cobb and coworkers found that replacement of VADs every 3 days did not prevent infection and that doing so over a guidewire actually increased the risk for bloodstream infection.[45]

Thrombus Formation

It has been estimated that 2% to 42% of VADs are associated with deep venous thrombosis (DVT).[46] Risk factors for catheter-related DVT include the composition, diameter, and position of the VAD; elevated intraluminal pressure; turbulent blood flow; vascular calcification; endothelial injury; and increased levels of fibronectin.[46,47] Polyurethane and silicone catheters have a lower rate of VAD-related DVT than do polyethylene or Teflon-coated catheters. A catheter with an external diameter of less than 2.8 mm has a lower incidence of DVT. Incorrect placement of the VAD in the SVC, as opposed to the junction of the SVC and right atrium, results in a higher incidence of catheter-related DVT.[46]

DVTs may be asymptomatic and not recognized because of the underlying condition of the patient. The incidence of central venous catheter–related DVT, as assessed by

venography, has been found to range from 27% to 66%. The majority of these thromboses are asymptomatic. The incidence of clinically overt DVT has been found to range from 0.3% to 28.3%, with most studies finding the incidence to be less than 5%. The first 6 weeks after catheter insertion presents the greatest risk for thromboembolic complications.[48]

Most HD access failures (80%) are related to thrombosis, with greater than 90% of these thromboses associated with venous outflow stenosis.[14] Histologically, hyperplasia of the endothelium and fibromuscular vessel wall occurs. Over time, fibrin deposits build up on the tip of the VAD. This may continue to the point of complete occlusion and prevent infusion or aspiration from the VAD. Early detection may be enhanced by maintaining a high index of suspicion and noting prolonged bleeding after withdrawal of the cannula or a change in the bruit over the device, or both. Prompt consultation with a nephrologist and vascular surgeon is indicated. Heparin or local thrombolytic agents, such as alteplase, may be tried (see the next section).

Catheter Occlusion

Occlusion of the catheter or low flow can be caused by improper positioning, kinking, or compression of the catheter; intraluminal thrombi; extraluminal thrombi; fibrin deposits at the tip of the catheter; or intraluminal precipitation of infusate. *Pinch-off syndrome* occurs when the line (most often a PICC) is compressed between the clavicle and the first rib. It is manifested clinically as difficulty injecting that is posturally related.[16] Overzealous withdrawal of the syringe will collapse the catheter and cause occlusion. Chest radiographs may reveal scalloping of the catheter. Maneuvers to facilitate flow include the Valsalva maneuver, the reverse Trendelenburg position, slight tension on the catheter, placement of the catheter more laterally, IV hydration, and extension of the arms above the head.[28,49]

If these measures are unsuccessful, the occlusion may be caused by clot formation. The clinician should be familiar with local institutional recommendations for thrombolysis in the setting of recent VAD occlusion attributed to a fibrin plug. Admission and consultation are usually required, and maneuvers to address clotted or occluded catheters are not a standard ED procedure but may be performed under proper circumstances and according to local guidelines. Alteplase has been shown to be both effective and safe in treating central venous catheter occlusions caused by clot.[50] If attempted, first withdraw any mobile clot by aspiration with a syringe. Instill 2 mL of alteplase (1 mg/mL) and allow it to dwell for up to 120 minutes. If it remains occluded, the dose may be repeated once.

Embolization

A serious but uncommon complication of VAD use is embolization with air, a catheter fragment, or thrombotic emboli.[51-54] Air emboli develop when the lumen of the catheter is left open to air or the catheter is fractured, perforated, or cut. The one-way valve in the Groshong catheter prevents this complication. Be careful to maintain a closed system by clamping the catheter appropriately to prevent delivery of air into the venous circulation. Should the externalized portion of a catheter be damaged, immediately place an appropriate clamp between the damaged portion and the skin.[28] Be suspicious for air embolism if an open or damaged catheter is found in association with tachypnea and hypotension.[51] Place the patient in a left lateral decubitus and Trendelenburg position to reduce ventricular outflow obstruction by air pockets. Initiate supportive measures, including high-flow oxygen. If this is unsuccessful, attempt aspiration with the catheter advanced into the right ventricle, if possible. Emergency thoracotomy to aspirate air (see Chapter 18) and cardiothoracic surgical consultation may also be warranted.

Embolization of a catheter fragment is a potentially life-threatening complication that can cause acute dyspnea, palpitations, atypical chest pain, hypoxia, and atrial fibrillation. As with any foreign-body embolus, sequelae include sepsis, lung abscess, dysrhythmias, vascular or cardiac perforation, and sudden death. Catheter fragments may be identified radiographically or potentially by ultrasonography and may be removed either surgically or by intravascular retrieval methods.[52]

Embolization of thrombi with potentially lethal sequelae may occur during routine flushing and injection of solutions through the catheter. Anderson and coworkers prospectively evaluated the size and frequency of catheter thrombi in 43 patients by aspirating after a urokinase flush.[53] Clots were noted in 40 of 43 subjects and in 153 of 508 total specimens. Thrombi varied in size from small fragments to 5 cm in length. Burns and McLaren reported one case of a hemodynamically significant pulmonary embolus associated with PICC placement in a 77-year-old man.[54]

Hemorrhagic Complications

Bleeding may be seen with any indwelling VAD or AV fistula but more commonly occurs with nontunneled VADs or temporary dialysis catheters. It is often related to mechanical trauma, transient or preexisting thrombocytopenia, uremia- or drug-induced platelet dysfunction, and infection. Repeated cannulation of the fistula or graft weakens the wall of the device. Many fistulas will develop aneurysms from repeated use; synthetic grafts can develop pseudoaneurysms from frequent punctures (Fig. 24-13). Severe life-threatening hemorrhage from this high-pressure system may occur and necessitates rapid control. The primary goal should be to control bleeding and prevent exsanguination; however, take care to minimize damage to the VAD that would prevent future use. Use full universal precautions because there is an increased risk for communicable disease in this patient population (2.4% for hepatitis B virus and 7.4% for hepatitis C virus in the United States).[55] When the bleeding stops, observe the patient for 2 hours for evidence of rebleeding and to detect graft thrombosis. Treatment can be divided into mechanical modalities and correction of coagulopathy.

Mechanical

Literature addressing acute hemorrhage in patients with VADs is clearly lacking. Many of the techniques discussed are anecdotal examples used by emergency clinicians, nephrologists, and vascular surgeons informally polled at our institutions. Individual institutional guidelines, techniques, and preferences may vary; therefore, consultation with these providers is recommended when possible.

Approach to Bleeding Complications

It is important to identify the specific bleeding site, which is challenging when hemorrhage is massive (Fig. 24-14). This is

Figure 24-13 Because of repeated access and high venous pressure, the integrity of the shunt vessel can be compromised. Pseudoaneurysms form in a synthetic graft and are covered with skin. True aneurysms form in a fistula from bulging of the entire vessel. Both can rupture. A tortuous vein under pressure can mimic an aneurysm.

most easily accomplished by digital pressure over the feeding and draining vessels of the shunt above and below the bleeding site. The most easily controlled bleeding is that occurring immediately after dialysis, when simple measures are often effective. Spontaneous bleeding between dialysis treatments often signifies more serious problems, such as infection or mechanical problems with the access site. High pressure from venous stenosis secondary to long-term dialysis complicates the control of bleeding (Fig 24-15).

Direct Pressure

Begin management of bleeding with direct pressure. Always use sterile technique to lessen the chance of infecting a bleeding shunt. With gloved hands, apply direct pressure with fingers and a sterile gauze bandage. For bleeding AV fistulas and shunts secondary to cannulation, apply pressure focally over the site of cannulation. For tunneled catheters, apply pressure over the site of vascular entry of the catheter, not the subcutaneous exit site. Note that this is not possible with subclavian VADs. Hold the pressure for a minimum of 5 minutes and then reevaluate for hemostasis. Holding direct pressure for extended periods or maintaining more diffuse pressure may cause thrombosis and ultimate graft failure, which is a known and unfortunate risk. Wrapping the site with an elastic bandage for a few minutes is acceptable, but longer application in this broad manner may lead to the entire graft clotting.

Dialysis Clamps

Special self-retaining dialysis clamps may be applied over a specific bleeding site (Fig. 24-16). Be careful that the clamp does not slip off the bleeding site because the surface area of the clamp is small. Place sterile gauze or topical thrombin-impregnated gauze under the clamp. Ten to 15 minutes may be required to stop the bleeding, but it is best to avoid frequent checks during the first 5 to 8 minutes to avoid disrupting hemostasis.

Suture

To adequately visualize the bleeding site, (1) apply concomitant digital pressure to the proximal and distal ends of the shunt or fistula (Fig 24-17), or (2) apply a pneumatic blood pressure cuff or tourniquet *distal to* the fistula or graft to

Figure 24-14 A, Spontaneous rupture of this fistula resulted in massive hemorrhage and hypovolemic shock. Failure to put direct pressure over the bleeding site, as indicated in **B,** exacerbated the blood loss. **B,** This infected pseudoaneurysm (*arrowhead*) precipitated the spontaneous massive hemorrhage seen in **A.** The actual graft is exposed. Note that control of bleeding to identify the compromised site is achieved by firm digital pressure on the vessels on both sides of the rupture (*arrows*). Infected grafts must be replaced. Infected fistulas may be salvaged with antibiotics. Bleeding of a shunt can also signal thrombosis of a major vein.

Figure 24-15 Edema of the hand and breast occurred as a result of the high venous pressure of chronic venous stenosis secondary to long-term hemodialysis. **A,** Obstruction of the innominate vein or superior vena cava may cause breast and face swelling, and sometimes headaches because of intracranial hypertension. This may be difficult to differentiate from thrombosis. Anticoagulation will not help this unfortunate patient. Surgical revision to divert blood flow into a patent vein is sometimes possible to restore unobstructed flow. **B,** Arm edema may also be a sign of shunt infection.

impede distal-to-proximal arterial flow, unless it is a loop graft, in which case it is applied above (*proximal to*) the device. Inject the bleeding site subcutaneously with lidocaine with epinephrine. Place a figure-of-eight or horizontal mattress suture of 4-0 nonabsorbable polypropylene or nylon (noncutting needle) at the site of bleeding. Be careful to suture as superficially as possible to prevent damage to the underlying graft or fistula. The patient may require a venogram for evaluation of VAD patency before use. Remove the suture in a few days.

Thrombogenic Agents

If major bleeding has been controlled and oozing is minimal, oxidized cellulose hemostatic agents (Oxycel, Surgicel) may be used to achieve hemostasis. Apply these agents directly over the site of bleeding and hold them in place with gloved hands and a gauze bandage or clamp. The disadvantage of this approach is that the agents are costly and a potential nidus for infection.

Vasoconstrictive Agents

Subcutaneous injection of 2 to 4 mL of lidocaine (2%) with epinephrine to form a wheel around the site may decrease

bleeding by both vasoconstriction and local pressure. This may be used in conjunction with chemical cautery.

Chemical Cautery

Silver nitrate ($AgNO_3$), a mildly caustic and hemostatic agent, may stop residual bleeding. The agent needs to be protected from light until just before use. When ready, remove the wooden stick from the container and black plastic wrap and gently apply the gray-tipped end directly on the site. Do not apply it aggressively because this can result in dissolution or dislodgment of the formed clot.

Once the bleeding is controlled, rebleeding is infrequent. It is prudent to observe the patient for 30 to 45 minutes and have the patient walk around and use the arm gently to ensure that bleeding will not recur when discharged. If no bleeding recurs, discharge is appropriate unless precluded by other conditions.

Coagulopathy

Control of hemorrhage may require treatment of an underlying coagulopathy. HD patients are generally considered to be

Figure 24-16 Bleeding from a dialysis graft or fistula can be massive because of the high pressure. This dialysis graft clamp with sterile gauze (option: impregnate the gauze with topical thrombin) is kept in place for about 10 minutes. Other options for a bleeding graft are discussed in text. Bleeding after dialysis is related to needle size and the degree of anticoagulation, but prolonged bleeding may signal outflow stenosis, infection, or skin atrophy and the need for evaluation of the shunt.

Figure 24-17 To suture a bleeding dialysis shunt, instruct an assistant to apply proximal and distal pressure to stem the flow of blood and then inject the site with lidocaine with epinephrine. Place a figure-of-eight (shown) or horizontal mattress suture as superficially as possible to prevent damage to the underlying graft or fistula.

at increased risk for bleeding because of uremic platelet dysfunction. The incidence of major bleeding in these patients is increased with the concomitant use of anticoagulant medications.[56] Perform laboratory testing for evaluation: complete blood count, blood urea nitrogen, prothrombin time, international normalized ratio (INR), partial thromboplastin time, and other tests depending on the patient's medical history or signs. Consult nephrology, vascular surgery, or both if possible before reversing therapeutic anticoagulation given the potential for graft thrombosis and the need for close follow-up.

Uremic Platelet Dysfunction

If platelet dysfunction is suspected because of uremia, administer desmopressin (DDAVP) or cryoprecipitate to control the hemorrhage.[30] Adult dosing of DDAVP to control uremic bleeding is 0.3 µg/kg intravenously as a single dose or every 12 hours. Onset occurs in 1 to 2 hours, and its duration is 6 to 8 hours after a single dose. Disadvantages include high cost and adverse reactions, including anaphylaxis, water intoxication or hyponatremia, and thrombotic events (rare). Use of DDAVP may be most appropriate if the platelet count and standard coagulation profile is otherwise normal.

Heparin-Associated Coagulopathy

Heparin administration is not routine during dialysis, and if it is used, small doses are infused (3000 to 5000 units). Heparin is usually stopped about 1 hour before the end of dialysis, and hence heparin-related bleeding is unusual in the ED. If uncontrollable bleeding occurs in the context of recent heparin use, reversal of heparin's effect with protamine sulfate may be necessary. Administering 1 mg of protamine sulfate will effectively reverse the anticoagulant effect of 100 units of unfractionated heparin. Protamine is less efficacious in the reversal of low molecular weight heparins. Nonetheless, current recommendations are to administer 1 mg of protamine for every 1 mg of low-molecular-weight heparin that the patient received.[57]

Warfarin-Associated Coagulopathy

The use of warfarin predisposes patients to potentially serious bleeding complications. In an actively bleeding patient with an elevated INR, immediate reversal of the medication's effect can be achieved with fresh frozen plasma or prothrombin complex concentrates (PCCs). PCCs have the advantage of requiring less total volume to achieve reversal of anticoagulation and therefore less risk for volume overload.[57] Vitamin K should also be administered to the patient (10 mg by slow IV infusion).

Catheter Displacement, Migration, or Malposition

Catheter displacement may occur accidentally secondary to patient movement, iatrogenically, or both. The catheter should be firmly secured with sutures, sterile tape strips (with care taken to avoid direct contact with the catheter itself), and premanufactured devices.[19] Even with these measures, migration may still occur. With regard to TIVADs, malposition of the intravascular portion may occur as a result of incorrect initial positioning or secondarily from forceful flushing, neck flexion, obesity, severe coughing, emesis, or upper extremity movement. Malposition of the port body may occur intentionally or by unintentional manipulation of the port (twiddler's syndrome). Obtain a computed tomography scan of the chest to diagnosis this condition. Surgical intervention is usually necessary.[58]

Catheter Fracture

Fracture of a VAD can occur either subcutaneously or in the externalized portion.[59] It may take place with certain physical activities that involve repetitive and excessive motion, such as golfing, swimming, and weight lifting. Subcutaneous fractures cause pain and swelling and require removal of the line. Fractures in the externalized portion may be repaired with commercially available kits and do not always have to be replaced.

Steal Syndrome

Vascular steal syndrome is an uncommon (1% to 3% incidence) but serious complication of AV fistulas that is difficult to predict and often leads to access failure. It occurs because of preferential flow through the low-resistance fistula at the expense of the distal circulation. The syndrome is manifested by classic arterial insufficiency symptoms with exacerbation during dialysis: pain, pallor, numbness, motor weakness, and diminished or absent pulses distal to the fistula.[60] Steal syndrome must be differentiated from diabetic or uremic neuropathy because it may lead to the development of irreversible neuromuscular dysfunction and tissue necrosis. Prompt recognition and correction of hand ischemia lead to increased salvage and use of functioning fistulas. Steal syndrome usually requires ligation or removal of the VAD with placement of a new access device in the opposite extremity.

AFTERCARE INSTRUCTIONS

Before release from the ED, instruct the patient regarding proper catheter care to prolong the device's lifetime and to decrease morbidity and mortality.[28] Patients may bathe and swim normally after maturation of the site; they should avoid direct pressure on the reservoir and report bruising or bleeding immediately. Long-term venous access catheters and multilumen catheters should be dressed in sterile fashion and observed daily for bleeding and signs of infection, including fever, pain, redness, swelling, and purulent drainage. VADs should be gently flushed on a routine basis.[28] Heparin flushes are essential to prevent thrombosis (Table 24-1; see p. 454). Tunneled (e.g., Hickman) and nontunneled (e.g., PICC) catheters require flushing twice weekly with 5 mL of heparin (10 U/mL). TIVADs require flushing with heparin every 4 weeks and after use. Generally, Groshong catheters are flushed with 5 mL of saline once weekly. Mahurkar and Uldall catheters are "flushed" during dialysis. Mahurkar catheters are also used for apheresis, in which case they are treated three times a week with normal saline and heparin, as outlined earlier. Patients should not allow phlebotomy or infusion into an extremity with a VAD or have blood pressure measured in that extremity. Signs of infection and any inability to flush an indwelling catheter should be reported immediately to a clinician.

Acknowledgment

Cemal B. Sozener, MD, and Pino Colone, MD, coauthored the chapter in previous editions of this text. The authors acknowledge the value of their contributions to the current chapter.

References are available at www.expertconsult.com

TABLE 24-1 Standard Intravenous Catheter Flushes*

LINE	FLUSH SOLUTION	HEPARIN STRENGTH	AMOUNT PER FLUSH	INDICATION
Peripheral	NSS	—	1 mL saline only	1. If a running IV line in place—no flush necessary 2. If used intermittently—flush after each use

Central lines
CVP line
  Single lumen
  Double lumen
  Triple lumen
	NSS	—	2 mL in each lumen	If used intermittently; use a 10-mL syringe:
				1. Flush with 3 mL NSS before administering any agent
				2. Flush with 5 mL NSS after medication or blood draws
				3. Each port not being used must be flushed with 3 mL NSS every 8 hr

For all PICCs				
PICC	A. Blood draw must be specifically ordered by the attending physician B. Never use a Vacutainer for PICC blood draw C. After blood is drawn or medication infused, flush as per the protocol below			
Open-ended PICCs—placed in interventional radiology—single lumen and double lumen (white PICC)	NSS	NO HEPARIN When using positive pressure caps	20 mL after blood draw or TPN 5-mL routine flush every 12 hr	Interventional radiology PICCs (open ended) If used intermittently or with a running IV line; use 10-mL syringes: 1. Must use POSITIVE PRESSURE CAPS 2. Flush with 20 mL NSS using two 10-mL syringes for each lumen 3. Pulsatile flush recommended
Closed-ended PICC with valves—placed by an IV team—also known as a Groshong PICC (blue PICC)	NSS	NO HEPARIN	20 mL after blood draw or TPN 5-mL routine flush every 12 hr	IV team PICCs: No heparin needed for a Groshong PICC 1. Using two 10-mL syringes, flush each lumen with 20 mL NSS 2. Pulsatile flush recommended

Implanted port
  Single lumen
  Double lumen
  Chest AND arm ports
	Heparin	100 U/mL
		400 units heparin per lumen
			4 mL per lumen	A. If used intermittently; use 10-mL syringes:
				  1. Flush with 20 mL NSS after medication, TPN, or blood draw
				  2. Followed by 4 mL heparinized saline (100 U/mL)
				B. When not in use, flush frequency = 1/mo
				  1. Draw off the heparin lock until blood is visualized in the syringe (discard the syringe)
				  2. Flush with 20 mL NSS
				  3. Flush with 4 mL heparinized saline (100 U/mL)
				C. Before deaccessing an implanted port:
				  1. Flush with 20 mL NSS
				  2. Flush with 4 mL heparinized saline (100 U/mL)

Tunneled catheter (very rarely used/seen)
A. Groshong
  Single lumen
  Double lumen
B. Hickman, Broviac
	NSS
	Heparin
		—
		100 U/mL
		250 units heparin per lumen
			2.5 mL per lumen	A. If used intermittently; use 10-mL syringes:
				  1. Flush with 10 mL NSS after medication and 20 mL NSS after TPN or blood draw
				  2. The frequency of flushing each port is every 8 hr
				B. When not in use, flush frequency = 1/wk
				  1. Draw off heparin until blood is seen in the syringe (discard the syringe). Do this for each
				  2. Flush each lumen with 20 mL NSS
				  3. Flush each lumen with 2.5 mL heparinized saline (100 U/mL)

From Blackburn P, Kokotis K. BARD access systems: vascular access device selection, insertion, and management. In: Weinstein SM, ed. *Plumers' Principles and Practice of Intravenous Therapy*. 9th ed. Baltimore: Lippincott; 2001; Infusion Nurses Society. *Infusion Therapy in Clinical Practice*. 2nd ed. Philadelphia: Saunders; 2001.
CVP, central venous pressure; *IV*, intravenous; *NSS*, normal saline solution; *PICC*, peripherally inserted central catheter; *TPN*, total parenteral nutrition.
*If an indwelling catheter is used or manipulated in the emergency department, a flush solution is instilled to maintain patency of the catheter.

Intraosseous Infusion

Kenneth Deitch

Establishing vascular access in critically ill and injured patients is central to the practice of emergency medicine. Moreover, placing an intravenous (IV) catheter in an acutely ill child can be one of the most challenging and frustrating procedures that a clinician can be called on to perform. Children have small peripheral vessels that collapse during shock, and their higher proportion of body fat makes visualization and palpation of peripheral vessels difficult. These factors often result in prolonged attempts and high failure rates.

In a review of vascular access success rates in children in cardiac arrest, the average time needed to establish percutaneous peripheral IV access was 7.9 ± 4.2 minutes, with only a 17% success rate.[1] Some authors advocate the use of central venous lines in children, but such lines are also difficult to place and are associated with risk for arterial injury, infection, and pneumothorax. Alternative routes of drug administration, such as the endotracheal and rectal routes, are not reliable in patients in shock or cardiac arrest.[2]

Peripheral IV access can also be difficult in adults, including those who are obese, have burn injuries, are volume-depleted, or are in shock.[3] This difficulty is compounded in the prehospital or military setting, where environmental factors and the need for rapid transport can challenge even the most skilled practitioners.[4]

Intraosseous (IO) access can provide rapid, lifesaving intravascular access in challenging environments and in both pediatric and adult patients. The American Heart Association, the American Academy of Pediatrics, and the American College of Surgeons all recommend IO access in children in emergency situations when IV access is not immediately possible.[5,6] The latest edition of the advanced trauma life support course of the American College of Surgeons also notes that IO access using specially designed equipment is an important option in adult trauma patients.[5] IO access is often faster than IV access, and the success rate after failed IV attempts is high. In a retrospective study of pediatric cardiac arrest patients, time to IO access was significantly shorter than time to IV access.[7] In a similar review of intravascular access during pediatric cardiac arrest, Brunette and Fischer[2] noted that when compared with central venous access and venous cutdown, IO access and IV access were faster, and the success rate for IO access was 83% versus 17% for IV access. IO access can also be a rapid and successful technique in adults.[8] Because of their success under difficult battlefield conditions, the U.S. military has adopted the use of IO infusion devices.[5]

IO access is not always successful. In a 5-year review of prehospital IO needle placement, success rates were higher in children younger than 3 years (85%) than in older children or adults (50%).[7] The main causes of failure were errors in identification of landmarks and bending of the needles. Better needle design and new devices have helped overcome problems with bone penetration (see "Equipment and Setup," later).

HISTORICAL PERSPECTIVE

One of the earliest references describing the IO route is attributed to Drinker and colleagues,[9] who in 1922 examined

Intraosseus Infusion

Indications
Emergency intravascular access when other methods have failed
Cardiac arrest in infants and young children
Military applications
Obtaining blood for laboratory evaluation

Contraindications
Osteoporosis and osteogenesis imperfecta
Fractured bone
Prior use of same bone for IO infusion
Cellulitis or burn overlaying insertion site

Complications

Technical difficulties	Soft tissue and bony complications
Over-penetration	Infection
Incomplete penetration	Bony inflammatory reaction
Needle obstruction	Skin sloughing
Fluid extravasation	Compartment syndrome
	Epiphyseal injury
	Fat embolism
	Pain with infusion

Equipment

Intravenous tubing

Antiseptic

10-mL syringe

Intraosseus needle/device

Review Box 25-1 Intraosseous infusion: indications, contraindications, complications, and equipment.

the circulation of the sternum and suggested it as a site for transfusion. The route was not used clinically until 1934, when Josefson,[10] a Swedish clinician, injected liver concentrate into the sternum of 12 adult patients with pernicious anemia and reported that all 12 improved. Subsequently, the technique became widespread in Scandinavian countries. In 1944, British physician Hamilton Bailey[11] described the utility of sternal IO access in blackout conditions in London during World War II.

In 1940, the technique was introduced to American clinicians by Tocantins and associates,[12-14] who described a series of animal and clinical studies demonstrating that fluid is rapidly transported from the medullary cavity of long bones to the heart. They recommended using the manubrium in older children and adults and the upper part of the tibia or lower part of the femur in children 3 years or younger. Over the next 2 decades, thousands of cases of IO infusion of blood, crystalloid substances, and drugs were reported.[15-19] The procedure was more commonly used in children because of the difficulty in achieving other forms of IV access. Nevertheless, during the 1940s, IO infusion was also used extensively in adults, and a sternal puncture kit for bone marrow infusion was a common component of emergency medical supplies during World War II.[4,20] This resulted in more than 4000 reported cases of successful IO access in wounded soldiers.[19] During this time, relatively few complications were reported despite the fact that the needles were often left in place for 24 to 48 hours. Heinild and coworkers in 1947[17] reviewed 982 cases of IO infusion and reported only 18 failures and 5 cases of osteomyelitis. None of the cases of osteomyelitis occurred in patients who received isotonic solutions.

With the introduction of plastic catheters and improved cannulation techniques, the need for IO infusion as an alternative route for IV access diminished, and the technique was all but abandoned. In the mid-1980s, James Orlowski brought about a renaissance in the use of IO access for pediatric resuscitation. While traveling through India during a cholera epidemic, he observed emergency health care workers using IO access to deliver fluids and medications. In 1984 he wrote an editorial, "My Kingdom for an Intravenous Line,"[20] in which he advocated the use of IO access during pediatric resuscitation. After Orlowski's editorial, others began promoting the use of IO access to allow rapid drug delivery during cardiopulmonary resuscitation (CPR) in children.[1,21,22] In 1988, IO techniques were adopted by the American Heart Association and included in the pediatric advance life support guidelines.[6] Since then, the technique has become widespread throughout the United States and is recognized as an accepted alternative to IV access in pediatric emergencies and, increasingly, in neonatal and adult emergencies. In addition, the safety, ease, and effectiveness of the technique have led to its use in prehospital emergency care.[7,23-26]

ANATOMY AND PHYSIOLOGY

Long bones are richly vascular structures with a dynamic circulation. They are capable of accepting large volumes of fluid and rapidly transporting fluid or drugs to the central circulation. The bone, like most organs, is supplied by a major artery (nutrient artery). The artery pierces the cortex and divides into ascending and descending branches, which further subdivide into arterioles that pierce the endosteal surface of

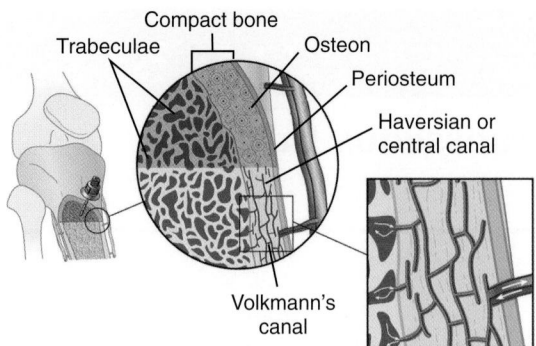

Figure 25-1 Schematic diagram illustrating the vascular anatomy of a long bone with an intraosseous needle in place.

the stratum compactum to become capillaries. The capillaries drain into medullary venous sinusoids throughout the medullary space, which in turn drain into a central venous channel (Fig. 25-1). The medullary sinusoids accept fluid and drugs during IO infusion and serve as a route for transport to the central venous channel, which exits the bone as nutrient and emissary veins.[27] The medullary cavity thus functions as a rigid, noncollapsible vein, even in the presence of profound shock or cardiopulmonary arrest.[28] Radiographic studies have demonstrated that radiopaque dye spreads only a few centimeters in the medullary space before being transported to the venous system.[29]

Almost every drug and fluid commonly used during resuscitation has been reported upon in clinical and preclinical IO studies. Medications and fluids that have been administered through IO infusion are listed in Box 25-1. Crystalloid infusion studies in animals have demonstrated that infusion rates of 10 to 17 mL/min may be achieved with gravity infusion and rates as high as 42 mL/min with pressure infusion.[30-32] In a swine model of hemorrhagic shock, Neufeld and colleagues[31] found that the IO delivery rate of crystalloid was similar to that with both peripheral and central venous administration. IO crystalloid infusions have also been shown to produce a significant increase in blood pressure in a hemorrhagic shock model in rabbits.[32] In small animals (7 to 8 kg), the size of the marrow cavity is the rate-limiting factor, whereas in larger animals (12 to 15 kg), the size of the needle determines the flow.[33,34] Blood under pressure can be infused approximately two thirds as fast as crystalloid fluids.[33] However, in a swine model evaluating IO infusion for mild therapeutic hypothermia, IO infusion of ice-cold saline was not as efficacious as intravenous infusion.[35]

Comparisons of IO and IV infusion of drugs have demonstrated that the drugs reach the central circulation by both routes in similar concentrations and at the same time (Fig. 25-2).[14,36] This holds true even during CPR, during which sodium bicarbonate has been shown to provide greater buffering capacity when administered by the IO route than by the peripheral IV route.[37] Early IO access and infusion of epinephrine improved 24-hour survival in a swine model of ventricular fibrillation versus delayed IV administration.[38] IO infusion of iodinated computed tomographic contrast material has also been reported as being successful,[39] as has scorpion antivenin.[40]

Voelckel and associates[36] demonstrated that bone marrow blood flow responds to both the physiologic stress of hemorrhagic shock and vasopressors given during resuscitation after

| BOX 25-1 | Medications and Fluids That Can Be Administered Intraosseously |

MEDICATIONS

Adenosine
Antibiotics
Antitoxins
Anesthetic agents
Atracurium besylate
Atropine
Calcium chloride
Calcium gluconate
Contrast media
Dexamethasone
Diazepam
Diazoxide
Digoxin
Dobutamine
Dopamine
Ephedrine
Epinephrine
Heparin
Insulin
Levarterenol
Lidocaine
Lorazepam

Mannitol
Morphine
Naloxone
Pancuronium
Phenobarbital
Phenytoin
Propranolol
Sodium bicarbonate
Succinylcholine
Thiopental
Vecuronium

FLUIDS
Crystalloids

Dextrose solutions
Sodium chloride solutions
Lactated Ringer's solution

Colloids

Blood and blood products
Packed red blood cells
Plasma

Data from Getschman SJ, Dietrich AM, Franklin WH, et al. Intraosseous adenosine. As effective as peripheral or central venous administration? Arch Pediatr Adolesc Med. 1994;148:616; and Sawyer RW, Bodai BI, Blaisdell FW, et al. The current status of intraosseous infusion. J Am Coll Surg. 1994;179:353.

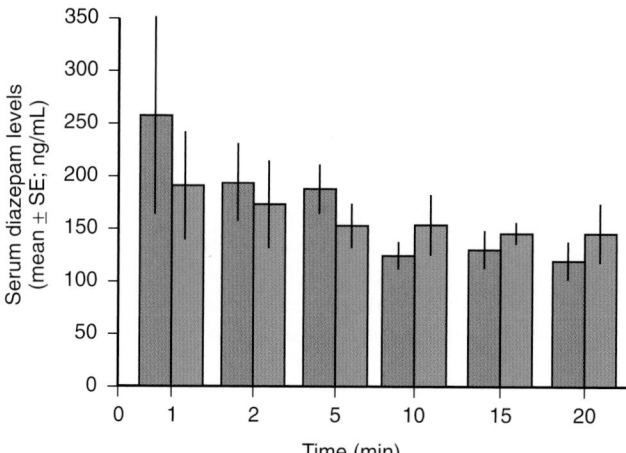

Figure 25-2 Serum diazepam levels graphed for the intraosseous (*blue*) and intravenous (*purple*) groups as a function of time when injected during normal perfusion. Initially, the intravenous drug level is slightly higher, but overall the difference between the two routes of administration is not significant.

hypovolemic cardiac arrest in dogs. After successful resuscitation, bone marrow blood flow decreased after high-dose epinephrine but was maintained after high-dose vasopressin. These findings in animal models suggest the need for pressurized IO infusion techniques during hemorrhagic shock and certain drug therapies.

INDICATIONS

When children or adults need immediate resuscitation and IV access cannot be achieved quickly or reliably, the IO route provides a rapid and effective means of administering drugs, fluid, and blood. Once the patient has been stabilized, percutaneous peripheral or central intravascular access may be achieved.

Obtaining venous access can be a difficult task even under the best circumstances. This difficulty is compounded during high-stress situations or low-flow states such as cardiac arrest. Studies have shown that IO devices provide a rapid and effective means of fluid and drug administration during pediatric CPR.[1] This is also true during resuscitation of critically injured infants and children, in whom IO infusion of blood, colloids, or crystalloids (or any combination thereof) may be lifesaving. IO infusion is also beneficial in the management of children with other medical conditions, including those with respiratory distress, neurologic insults, dehydration and sepsis.[42-44] The widespread use of IO devices has led to improved prehospital vascular access and a marked reduction in critical transport with failed vascular access.[45]

IO access is not commonly used in infants, but it is recommended as an alternative for medication and crystalloid administration when venous access is not readily obtained.[46] IO infusion has been used with success in both premature and term infants.[47-49] In one study, 30 IO lines were placed in 20 preterm and 7 full-term neonates with a variety of illnesses (e.g., respiratory distress syndrome, perinatal asphyxia, congenital cardiac anomalies) in whom conventional venous access had failed.[48] All survived resuscitation with no long-term effects from IO line placement. Gestational age ranged from 32 to 41 weeks and birth weight ranged from 515 to 4050 g.[48] In 2000, Abe and coworkers[49] reported on the speed and ease of establishing newborn emergency vascular access by using turkey bones and plastic infant legs to simulate IO access and fresh umbilical cord to simulate umbilical venous catheterization. They demonstrated that for individuals who do not perform newborn resuscitation frequently, IO placement was easier and quicker than umbilical venous catheterization. A comparison of umbilical venous versus IO access in a simulated model of neonatal resuscitation showed that IO access was faster with no difference in error rate or perceived difference in ease of use.[50]

IO infusion is also indicated for adult patients in whom attempts at peripheral or central venous access have been unsuccessful. This may include adult patients with burns, trauma, shock, dehydration, or status epilepticus.[51] Multiple sites, including the iliac crest, femur, proximal and distal ends of the tibia, radius, clavicle, and calcaneus may be used.[52-55] Of these, the tibia may be less desirable because red marrow is replaced by less vascular yellow marrow or fat by the fifth year of life. In contrast, the sternum has been advocated as the best site to establish IO access in adults because it is large and flat and can readily be located.[56] In addition, the sternum's cortical bone is thin (1 to 2 mm) and the marrow space relatively uniform (6 to 11 mm).[57]

There has also been renewed interest in IO access by the U.S. military. In addition to logistic constraints that limit the volume of isotonic crystalloid fluids available to resuscitate injured soldiers, hypotension, environmental and tactical conditions, and the presence of mass casualties can lead to excessive delay in obtaining vascular access.[4] The Army Institute for

Research has compared several IO infusion devices, including the FAST-1 Intraosseous Infusion System (PYNG Medical Corporation, Richmond, British Columbia, Canada), the Bone Injection Gun (BIG; Waismed, Yokenam, Israel), the Sur-Fast Hand-Driven Threaded-Needle (Cook Critical Care, Bloomington, IL), and the Jamshidi Straight-Needle (Allegence Health Care, McGaw Park, IL).[56] Success rates with these devices were similar (94% to 97%), and all were inserted in less than 2 minutes. The participants rated no individual device as being significantly better than the others. It was concluded that each device was easy to master and could be used appropriately during special operations when IV access could not be accomplished.[56] A recent randomized controlled trial (RCT) of the BIG device versus the EZ-IO showed no significant differences in success rates or overall ease of use. Of 40 adults in the prehospital setting, vascular access was successfully achieved on the first attempt in 80% to 90% of patients within 2 minutes.[58] Another recent RCT showed that a Jamshidi 15-gauge needle could be placed significantly faster than the FAST-1 device but had similar success and complication rates, as well as perceived ease of use.[59]

In addition to serving as a route for fluid administration, the IO needle may be used to obtain blood for typing, cross-matching, and determining blood chemistry in the marrow cavity. Serum electrolyte, blood urea nitrogen, creatinine, glucose, and calcium levels are very similar to those in samples obtained from an IO aspirate.[60,61] Blood gas values obtained from the IO site were similar to those obtained from central venous sites during steady and low-flow states in one animal model.[62] Brickman and colleagues[63] demonstrated that bone marrow aspirates obtained from an IO needle in the iliac crest could be used reliably to type and screen blood for transfusion. A complete blood cell count may not be reliable because it reflects the marrow cell count rather than the cell count in the peripheral circulation. Furthermore, the aspirated blood usually clots within seconds, even if placed in a tube that contains heparin.

CONTRAINDICATIONS

Relatively few contraindications to IO infusion exist. Osteoporosis and osteogenesis imperfecta are associated with a high potential for fracture; therefore, unless absolutely necessary, the procedure should be avoided when these diagnoses are known. A fractured bone should be avoided because as fluid is infused, it increases intramedullary pressure and forces fluid to extravasate at the fracture site. This may slow the healing process, cause nonunion of the bone, or lead to a compartment syndrome. Similar extravasation of fluid can occur through recent IO puncture sites placed in the same bone. Hence, recent previous use of the same bone for IO infusion represents a relative contraindication to IO line placement. Needle insertion through areas of cellulitis, infection, or burns should also be avoided. Patients with right-to-left intracardiac shunts (e.g., tetralogy of Fallot, pulmonary atresia) may be at higher risk for fat or bone marrow embolization.[64,65]

EQUIPMENT AND SETUP

The following is a review of products currently available for IO infusion. Information regarding the use of these products is limited, and few prospective studies have compared IO needles or devices in clinical practice. Until more information becomes available, practitioners are encouraged to review the products available and choose those that best meet their needs.

IO Needles (Fig. 25-3)

Needles used for IO access range in size from 13 to 20 gauge and must be sturdy enough to penetrate bone without bending or breaking. They must also be long enough to reach the marrow cavity. *Standard needles for drawing blood or administering medications are not adequate for IO infusions;* they are not sturdy enough to penetrate bone and do not have a stylet to prevent bone from plugging the lumen. A cadaver study of IO puncture suggested that nonstyleted needles (2.5-cm, 18-gauge phlebotomy needles and 7.6-cm, 14-gauge IV needles) enter the marrow space successfully only about half the time.[66] In the past, an 18-gauge spinal needle was commonly used in children younger than 12 to 18 months. This needle, though readily available in most EDs, often bends, is too long for rapid infusion of fluid, and has a greater risk for occlusion from clotted blood.[67] Very small "butterfly" needles have been used with success in preterm infants.[68]

Bone Marrow Aspiration Needle

Bone marrow aspiration needles can be used if needles specifically designed for IO access are not available. These needles are large enough (16 gauge) to be used in older children and adults and are suitable for rapid administration of fluid.

Jamshidi Bone Marrow
Aspiration Needle

Illinois Sternal/Iliac
Aspiration Needle

Jamshidi Disposable
Sternal/Iliac Aspiration Needle

Cook IO Needle

Sur-Fast Needle

Figure 25-3 Various intraosseous needles.

Illinois Sternal/Iliac Aspiration Needle

The Illinois Sternal/Iliac Aspiration Needle (Monojet, Division of Sherwood Medical, St. Lonis, MO) was designed for bone marrow aspiration but can be used for IO infusion. The needle is available in both 16 and 18 gauge. It has an adjustable plastic sleeve to prevent the needle from penetrating through the opposite bony cortex. However, its long shaft and poorly designed handle make it prone to dislodgment during transport and other procedures.

Jamshidi Disposable Sternal/Iliac Aspiration Needle

Like the Illinois Sternal/Iliac Aspiration Needle, the Jamshidi Disposable Sternal/Iliac Aspiration Needle (Cardinal Health, Dublin, OH) was designed for bone marrow aspiration, but it has a shorter shaft and smaller handle, which makes it easier to use. It comes in either 15 or 18 gauge and also features an adjustable plastic sleeve to prevent overpenetration. Once inserted, the needle protrudes approximately 2 inches from the skin, which increases the risk for accidental dislodgment. In a study using a turkey bone model, participants rated the Jamshidi needle easier to use than the Cook IO needle.[69]

Cook IO Needle

The Cook IO Needle (Cook Critical Care, Bloomington, IN) is specifically designed for IO insertion and infusion. It comes in a variety of sizes from 18 to 14 gauge and can be inserted to a depth of 3 to 4 cm. It has a detachable handle, which reduces the risk of it being dislodged, and a depth marker to help ensure proper placement.

Sur-Fast Needle

The Sur-Fast Needle (Cook Critical Care, Bloomington, IN) is also specifically designed for IO insertion and infusion. It has a threaded shaft that helps secure the needle in the bone and a detachable handle that may be reused with multiple needles. In a study by Jun and associates,[70] the Sur-Fast IO needle had a success rate similar to that of a standard bone marrow aspiration needle.

IO Devices

FAST-1 Intraosseous Infusion System (Fig. 25-4)

The FAST-1 Intraosseous Infusion System (PYNG Medical, Richmond, British Columbia, Canada) uses an impact-driven device designed for sternal placement only. The FAST-1 has been used successfully by both military and prehospital care providers.[56,71] In one prehospital study, flow rates of 80 and 150 mL/min were obtained by using gravity and a pressure bag, respectively.[72] In a prospective prehospital evaluation, the mean time to successful placement was 67 seconds.[73] The device has a series of stabilizing probes that help maintain good contact with the sternum and serve as the depth control mechanism for insertion of the needle. These probes use the surface of the manubrium rather than the patient's skin to ensure the proper depth of insertion. Once the device is positioned against the sternum, additional pressure triggers the release of a hollow needle into the medullary space. The needle comes preconnected to IV tubing. The handle is automatically released from the stylet and infusion tubing once the needle has met its preset depth. Removal of the needle requires a threaded tool provided with the device. The FAST-1 is larger and heavier than other IO devices and, once triggered, cannot be reused.

Bone Injection Gun—BIG (Fig. 25-5)

The BIG (Waismed, Yokenam, Israel) is another spring-loaded, impact-driven device that comes in both pediatric and adult sizes. Like the FAST-1 system, this device is designed for single use only. An advantage of the BIG is the ability to adjust the depth of insertion, which allows it to be used at different sites (e.g., tibia, humerus). However, if the device is not carefully stabilized before and during insertion, incorrect placement can easily occur. In addition, there is the potential for operator and patient injury if the device is accidentally triggered or mistargeted.[71] In a prospective, prehospital setting the BIG device was shown to have a 71% success rate in children and a 73% success rate in adults.[74] In another prehospital study, 91% of 181 patients had successful insertion on the first attempt.[75]

EZ-IO Device (Fig. 25-6)

The EZ-IO Device (Vida-Care, San Antonio, TX) handheld, battery-powered device that drills an IO needle to the appropriate depth in the IO space. The EZ-IO device allows the operator to control the pressure or force used during insertion.[76] Placement can be achieved in less than 10 seconds in the vast majority of patients, with first-time successful insertion rates ranging from 77% to 97%.[77-80]

TIAX Reusable IO Infusion Device (Fig. 25-7)

The TIAX Reusable IO Infusion Device (TIAX LLC, Cambridge, MA) has developed a compact, portable, and reusable

Figure 25-4 FAST-1 Intraosseous Infusion System. (*Courtesy of PYNG Medical Corporation, Richmond, British Columbia, Canada.*)

Figure 25-5 Bone Injection Gun. (*Courtesy of BIG, Waismed, Yokenam, Israel.*)

IO infusion device for quick vascular access through the sternum of soldiers wounded in combat. The device is lightweight (217 g), can be operated with one hand, and has a reusable driver/depth control system to insert single-use IO needles. The device is currently in phase II trials.

Figure 25-6 EZ-IO Device.

Figure 25-7 TIAX Reusable IO Infusion Device. *(Courtesy of TIAX LLC, Cambridge, MA.)*

PROCEDURE

Sites for IO Needle Placement

The patient's age and size are the two most important factors when choosing the best site for needle penetration. In infants and children younger than 6 years, the proximal end of the tibia is the preferred site, followed by the distal ends of the tibia and femur. Other sites such as the clavicle and humerus have been used, but neither has gained popularity. In adults, the distal part of the tibia has been the most common site for IO access. However, with the introduction of spring-loaded and drill devices, IO locations once reserved only for children are now potential sites in adults as well. In addition, the FAST-1 System makes the sternum a simple and effective location for IO access in adults.[78]

Proximal Tibia

The tibia is a large bone with a thin layer of overlying subcutaneous tissue that allows landmarks to readily be palpated. Insertion here does not interfere with airway management or CPR. This is one of the most common infusion sites. On the proximal end of the tibia, the broad, flat, anteromedial surface is used and the tibial tuberosity serves as a landmark. The site of IO cannulation is approximately 1 to 3 cm (2 finger widths) below the tuberosity (Fig. 25-8*A*). This location is far enough away from the growth plate to prevent damage, but it is in an area where the bone is still soft enough to allow easy penetration with the needle. In adults, penetrating the thick bone in the proximal end of the tibia is much more difficult and requires a 13- to 16-gauge needle. A spring-loaded device such as the BIG or a battery-powered drill such as the EZ-IO can make penetration much easier and allows the use of smaller-gauge needles. In a comparison of first-attempt success between tibial and humeral IO insertion during out-of-hospital cardiac arrest, tibial placement was significantly more successful (90%) than humeral placement (60%) with a lower rate of needle dislodgement.[81]

Figure 25-8 Intraosseous (IO) insertion sites. **A,** Proximal tibia. The IO needle is inserted 1 to 3 cm distal to the tibial tuberosity and over the medial aspect of the tibia. The bevel of the needle is directed away from the joint space. **B,** Distal tibia. The IO needle is inserted on the medial surface of the distal end of the tibia at the junction of the medial malleolus and the shaft of the tibia, posterior to the greater saphenous vein. The needle is directed cephalad, away from the growth plate. **C,** Distal femur. The IO needle is inserted 2 to 3 cm above the femoral condyles in the midline and directed cephalad away from the growth plate.

Distal Tibia

The distal end of the tibia, though a preferred site in adults, may be used in children as well.[67,82] The cortex of the bone and the overlying tissue are both thin. The site of needle insertion is the medial surface at the junction of the medial malleolus and the shaft of the tibia, posterior to the greater saphenous vein (see Fig. 25-8B). The needle is inserted perpendicular to the long axis of the bone or 10 to 15 degrees cephalad to avoid the growth plate.[83]

Sternum

The sternum has several advantages over peripheral bones but is rarely used in the ED. Its advantages include a large, relatively flat body that can be readily located; retention of a high proportion of red marrow, which allows rapid transfer of infused fluids and drugs to the central circulation; and thinner, more uniform cortical bone overlying a relatively uniform marrow space. In addition, the sternum is less likely to be fractured in major trauma.[72] Introduction of the FAST-1 System, which allows safe and effective penetration of the sternum, has led to increased use and popularity of sternal IO insertion in adults.

Humerus

The proximal end of the humerus is a relatively new option for IO access, but it is well tolerated and easily accessed. The close proximity of the greater tubercle of the humerus to the heart provides rapid infusion of medication and fluid into the general circulation. The humerus has been shown to be an effective site relative to peripheral or central access in a prospective resuscitation model.[84,85]

Other Sites

The distal portion of the femur is occasionally used as an alternative site in children, but because of thick overlying muscle and soft tissue, it is more difficult to palpate bony landmarks (Fig. 25-8C). If chosen, the needle should be inserted 2 to 3 cm above the femoral condyles in the midline and directed cephalad at an angle of 10 to 15 degrees from the vertical.[85] Other sites, including the clavicle and calcaneus, can be used as alternatives, but these sites are less popular.

Site Preparation

To prepare the proximal end of the tibia or distal end of the femur for IO insertion, a small support such as a towel roll should be placed behind the knee. All insertion sites should be cleansed with chlorhexidine, povidone-iodine, or an alcohol-based antibacterial solution. If the patient is conscious, the skin and periosteum should be anesthetized.

Manual Needle Insertion (Fig. 25-9)

Before insertion, stabilize the site with the free hand (i.e., the hand not holding the IO needle) and use it to identify the landmarks. For example, during proximal tibial insertion, stabilize the proximal end of the tibia with the thumb and index finger of the free hand and use them to palpate the tibial tuberosity (the main bony landmark for proximal tibial insertion). During insertion, avoid injury to this hand by keeping it out of the plane of insertion and clear of the puncture site. Direct the IO needle perpendicular (90 degrees) to the bone's long axis and slightly caudad (60 to 75 degrees). Directing the

needle slightly caudad helps avoid penetration of the growth plate. Advance the needle with a twisting or rotating motion (but not a rocking motion) to drive it into the bone and to puncture the cortex. Once the cortex has been penetrated, there will be a sudden decrease in bony resistance and a "crunchy" feeling as the needle enters the marrow cavity. Penetration of the inner cortex usually occurs at a depth of approximately 1 cm. Aspirate for blood or marrow contents (or both) to confirm correct placement. Other signs of correct placement include the needle's ability to remain upright without support and to have free-flowing fluid without signs of extravasation into surrounding tissue.[86,87]

Once proper placement is confirmed, secure the needle and tubing with tape. Fastening the leg to an appropriately sized leg board helps further stabilize a lower extremity insertion site in infants and small children. Protect the needle from accidental dislodgment by cutting the bottom out of a plastic cup and taping and bandaging the cup in place over the device. Commercially made shields are also available for this purpose. Remove the IO needle as soon as IV access has been secured, and apply a sterile dressing over the site. Control excessive bleeding by applying direct pressure over the site for 5 minutes.[88]

USE OF SPECIFIC IO DEVICES

FAST-1 (Fig. 25-10)

The FAST-1 device was designed specifically to penetrate the sternum.[56,89] It is prepackaged with alcohol and iodine and comes with a protective dressing to hold the device in place. It also includes a threaded tip remover for easy removal of the metal tip and infusion tubing.

After disinfecting the skin site over the sternum, place the target patch over the midline of the manubrium with the hole in the middle of the target approximately 1.5 cm below the sternal notch. Next, place the FAST-1 introducer in the center of the target zone. The introducer has a "bone cluster" of needles that form a circle. These needles "sense" the cortex of the sternum and help ensure proper needle depth. Once the introducer is in position over the target zone, apply pressure to the handle to release an inner needle located in the center of the bone cluster. This needle has a small metal tip that is preconnected to plastic infusion tubing. After release, the central IO needle advances 5 mm beyond the circular cluster of needles, stops at the bony cortex, and positions the metal tip at the cortex-medullary junction. At this point, withdraw the handle so that only the plastic infusion tube is left protruding from the insertion site. Marrow aspiration and rapid flow of fluid help verify the appropriate position. Attach the plastic dome to the target patch via Velcro fasteners and secure the tubing in place. Removal of the infusion tube requires the use of a threaded-tip remover, which is included. The tube can also be removed by directly pulling it; however, the metal tip is sometimes left behind and must be extracted through a small incision.[56]

BIG (Fig. 25-11)

The BIG incorporates a loaded spring to facilitate penetration of the bone. To adjust the depth of insertion, remove the safety pin from one end and turn the other end clockwise or counterclockwise to reduce or increase needle depth,

MANUAL INTRAOSSEOUS NEEDLE INSERTION

Cleanse the skin with antiseptic.

Stabilize the leg and identify the tibial tuberosity with your free hand. Insert the needle perpendicular or slightly caudad with a twisting or rotating motion.

Remove the stylet once the cortex is penetrated (feel for a decrease in resistance and a "crunchy" feeling).

Aspirate blood and/or marrow to confirm the correct position. If the patient is awake, very slowly infuse 2–5 mL of 2% lidocaine a few minutes prior to infusion. Flush the needle with 10 mL of saline to prime the infusion.

Connect the IV tubing to the needle.

Secure the IO needle in place with tape.

Protect the needle from dislodgment with a plastic cup in which the bottom has been cut out, and then tape and bandage if in place over the needle.

Figure 25-9 Manual interosseus (IO) needle insertion. *IV,* intravenous.

FAST-1 INTRAOSSEOUS DEVICE

Cleanse the overlying skin with antiseptic and then place the adhesive target patch over the midline of the manubrium; the target hole should be approximately 1.5 cm below the sternal notch.

Place the introducer in the center of the target zone. Apply pressure to the handle to release the needle. The central IO needle will advance to the cortex-medullary junction.

Attach the plastic dome to the target patch to secure the tube in place.

Figure 25-10 Insertion of the FAST-1 Intraosseous Device.

respectively. Place the BIG firmly against the skin perpendicular or slightly caudad to the long axis of the bone. Fire the gun by applying palmar force on the back of the unit and pulling on the flanges with the middle and ring fingers. Confirm placement by aspirating marrow, flushing with the same syringe, and observing flow through the IV tubing. Slide the slotted safety pin into the needle to maintain stability. To remove the needle, rotate it back and forth with the small clamps provided with the unit. Dress the site in a manner determined by the care provider.

EZ-IO Needle (Figs. 25-12 and 25-13)

This battery-operated "drill" can drive the IO needle through thick bone with relative ease. The EZ-IO kit comes with a battery-operated drill and an IO needle with a stylet; the EZ-IO AD comes with a 15-gauge, 25-mm IO needle for use in patients heavier than 40 kg; and the EZ-IO PD comes with a 15-gauge, 15-mm needle for use in patients lighter than

39 kg. To operate the drill, insert the needle into the driver tip and make sure that it is securely seated onto the drill. Remove the safety cap from the needle and position the drill perpendicular (or slightly caudad) to the insertion site. Squeeze the trigger while applying gentle pressure to penetrate the skin. When the tip of the needle comes in contact with the bone, at least 5 mm of the IO catheter should be visible. If not, the overlying soft tissue may be too deep for the needle to enter the marrow cavity. To penetrate the bone, continue to squeeze the trigger while applying steady downward pressure until a sudden "give" or "pop" occurs, which signals entry into the medullary space. Too much pressure on the device can cause the drill to stall and prevent the needle from penetrating the cortex.

After entry into the marrow cavity, attach the EZ-Connect extension set provided with the EZ-IO kit and aspirate blood and bone marrow contents to confirm correct placement. Once catheter placement has been checked, fluids or medications can be infused. Avoid attaching syringes and IV tubing directly to

THE BONE INJECTION GUN (BIG)

1 Hold the bottom part of the device firmly, perpendicular to the leg.

2 Squeeze and pull out the safety latch.

3 While holding firmly at the bottom part, press down with the palm of your hand.

4 Pull up the Bone Injection Gun (BIG) slowly.

5 Remove the trocar needle.

6 Secure with the safety latch.

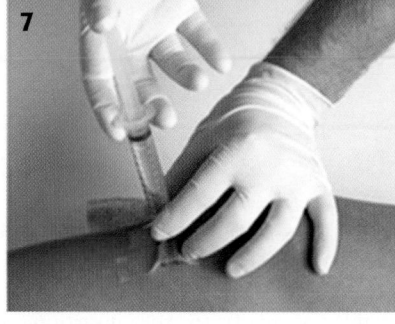
7 Flush with 10–20 mL of normal saline.

Figure 25-11 Use of the Bone Injection Gun (BIG).

the IO needle because this can enlarge the hole in the cortex and result in extravasation of fluid. Secure the tubing with tape and cover the area with appropriate dressing.

COMPLICATIONS
Technical Difficulties

Technical difficulties are the most common complications, but they decrease as familiarity with the technique increases

(Fig. 25-14). The most common mistake is to place excessive pressure on the needle during insertion and force it entirely through the bone and out the other side (Fig. 25-15). Minimize this risk by using appropriate landmarks and keeping the needle perpendicular to the long axis of the bone. In addition, hold the needle with the index finger approximately 1 cm from the bevel. When this finger touches the skin, the needle should be in the marrow cavity and no further pressure needs to be applied. Some IO needles have a mark 1 cm from the bevel (e.g., Cook IO Needle), whereas others have a special

EZ-IO INTRAOSSEOUS DEVICE

1

Chlorhexidine

Cleanse the site with an antiseptic agent per institutional protocol.

2

Connect the appropriate needle set to the driver (pink 15 mm = patients 3–39 kg; blue 25 mm = patients >40 kg; yellow 45 mm = proximal humerus, patients with excessive tissue over the site).

3

Position the driver at the insertion site with the needle at a 90-degree angle to the surface of the bone. Gently pierce the skin with the needle set and advance needle *without using the trigger yet*, until the needle set tip touches the bone.

4

Gentle downward pressure

Squeeze trigger

Penetrate the bone cortex by now squeezing the driver's trigger and applying gentle, consistent, steady downward pressure. Allow the driver to do the work.

5

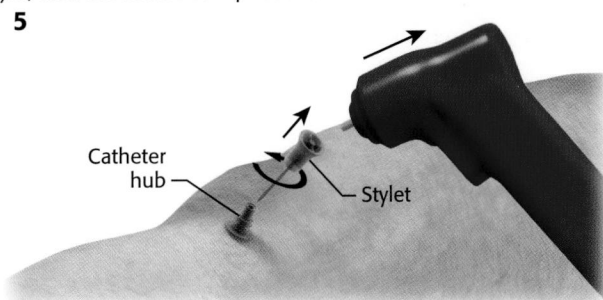

Catheter hub

Stylet

Remove the power driver from the needle set while stabilizing the catheter hub, and then remove the stylet by turning it counterclockwise.

6

EZ-Connect tubing

Attach the EZ-Connect tubing to the Luer-lok adapter on the catheter hub. Confirm placement by aspirating blood and/or marrow contents.

7

If the patient is responsive to pain, consider *slowly* administering plain 2% lidocaine for anesthetic effect *before* flushing with 10 mL of saline. Begin the infusion with a pressure bag.

8

Remove the device within 24 hours. Connect a sterile Luer-lok syringe to the catheter hub, and rotate clockwise while pulling straight up. Avoid rocking the needle on removal.

Figure 25-12 Use of the EZ-IO Device.

EZ-IO PROXIMAL HUMERUS INSERTION

1

Acromion
Greater tubercle
Surgical neck of humerus
Deltoid
Bicipital groove

Position the patient with the arm adducted and the hand over the umbilicus. This results in internal rotation of the humerus and shifts the greater tubercle to a more anterior position. Identify the greater tubercle of the humerus (firm pressure may be required because of overlying structures such as the deltoid). Identify the surgical neck of the humerus by palpating up the humerus until a "notch" or "groove" is felt.

2

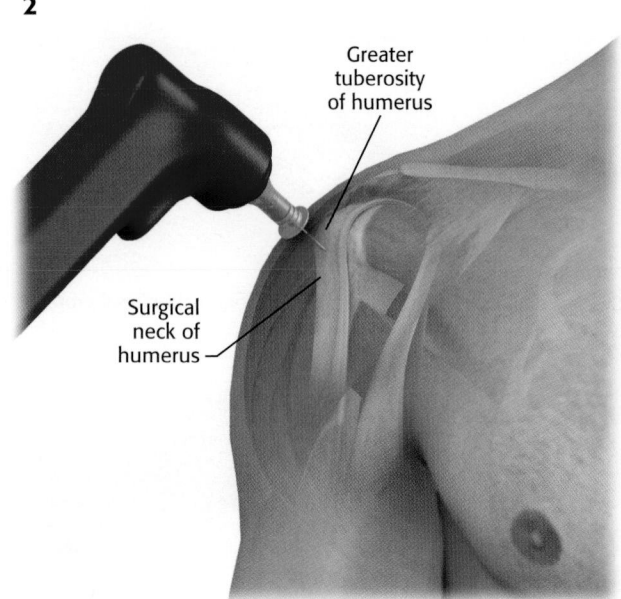

Greater tuberosity of humerus
Surgical neck of humerus

The appropriate insertion site is 1 cm superior to the surgical neck for most adults. Use the yellow 45-mm needle set. The process of EZ-IO insertion and removal at the humerus site is identical to that described in Figure 25–12.

Figure 25-13 EZ-IO proximal humeral insertion.

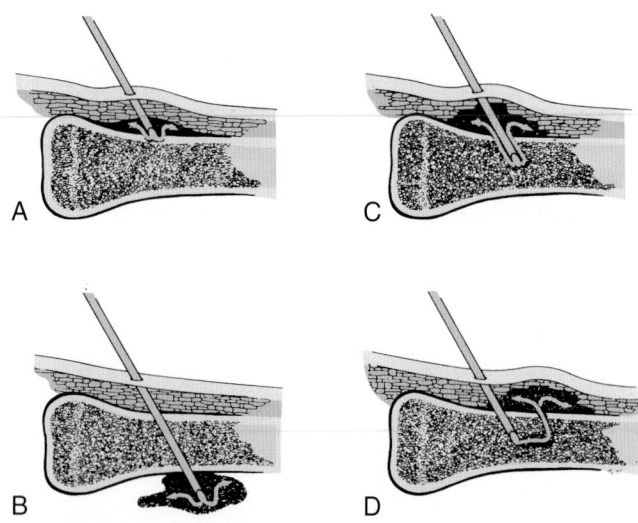

A

B

C

D

Figure 25-14 Schematic diagram of possible problems encountered with intraosseous infusion. **A,** Incomplete penetration of the bony cortex. **B,** Penetration of the posterior cortex. **C,** Fluid escaping around the needle through the puncture site. **D,** Fluid leaking through a nearby previous cortical puncture site.

Figure 25-15 Radiograph of bilaterally misplaced intraosseous needles with penetration through the posterior tibial cortices.

guide or mechanism to ensure proper insertion and depth of penetration (e.g., Illinois Sternal/Iliac Aspiration Needle). If available, use of these adjuncts will also help prevent overpenetration.

At times, the needle appears to be in the marrow cavity, but blood or bone marrow cannot be aspirated and fluids do not flow freely. This may follow incomplete penetration of the bone or overpenetration into the opposite cortex. Incomplete penetration usually results in extravasation of fluids and can be corrected by replacing the stylet and slowly advancing the needle until successful aspiration of marrow contents and free flow of fluids occur. Penetration into the opposite cortex generally results in little or no flow. If overpenetration is suspected, pull the needle back 1 to 2 mm and check for free flow of fluids.

To ensure flow, rapidly inject 10 mL of saline into the marrow. This is a painful procedure in awake patients, but failure to initially flush the compartment is a common reason for inadequate flow. A pressurized bag system is suggested if large volumes of fluid are administered. Flush each dose of medication with 3 to 5 mL of saline. Fluids that initially flowed freely may stop flowing if the needle becomes clogged by blood clots or bone spicules. Flush the needle frequently with 3 to 5 mL of saline to help avoid this problem. If none of these maneuvers results in free flow of fluid, remove the needle and reinsert it in the opposite extremity or another site. This helps avoid fluid extravasation through the hole that is left after removing the needle.

Extravasation of fluid is less common but may be associated with a number of adverse events.[90,91] Extravasation may be caused by fluids being infused under excessive pressure and with prolonged use of an IO site.[92] As noted previously, extravasation may also result from incomplete needle penetration or penetration through the opposite cortex. Even when an IO needle has been positioned properly, fluid can leak out through holes made by previous IO attempts or through an insertion site made too large from "rocking" during insertion or from an improperly secured needle that becomes loose with movement.[91-93] Interestingly, the type of needle used does not appear to influence extravasation rates.[94] Regardless of the cause, if extravasation occurs, remove the needle quickly and apply pressure to the site. If left unchecked, extravasation can lead to a number of adverse events (see "Soft Tissue and Bony Complications" below). In addition, though not directly harmful, extravasation of fluid through multiple cortical defects from previous IO attempts has been associated with lower serum levels of infused drugs.[95]

Soft Tissue and Bony Complications

Infection
In the past, concerns about infection have led clinicians to shy away from using the IO route. Although the potential for infection is real, its actual incidence is low. A literature review of more than 4000 cases from 1942 to 1977 found a 0.6% infection rate.[3] Although most of the affected access sites were not placed under emergency conditions, the needles were often left in place for 1 to 2 days, thus increasing the likelihood of infection. A survey of more than 1000 U.S. and foreign medical schools found that the incidence of infection for IO needles placed in emergency conditions was less than 3%.[96] The most common infection is cellulitis at the puncture site, which usually responds well to antibiotics. Osteomyelitis

Figure 25-16 Radiograph (**A**) and bone scan (**B**) of the tibia demonstrating an inflammatory reaction 4 days after the patient received intraosseous phenytoin and phenobarbital. The periosteum is elevated along the length of the bone and is mimicking osteomyelitis on the plain film and the bone scan. Diagnosis of osteomyelitis requires either clinical evidence of infectious toxicity or positive cultures (blood or periosteal aspirate).

is less common but also usually responds well to antibiotics. Heinild and coworkers[17] reported three cases of osteomyelitis in 25 patients who received infusions of undiluted 50% dextrose in water. More recently, Platt and coworkers[97] reported a case of fungal osteomyelitis and sepsis secondary to an IO infusion device. A case of tibial osteomyelitis with IO abscess was also recently reported.[98]

In addition to infection, inflammatory reactions of the bone may be seen. Such reactions are most common when hypertonic or sclerosing agents are used and may produce an elevation of the periosteum on plain radiographs or a positive bone scan (Fig. 25-16). Unlike patients with osteomyelitis from bacteria, a child with a sterile inflammatory reaction should not appear ill. One hypertonic sclerosing drug that may be used during cardiac arrest is sodium bicarbonate. Heinild and coworkers[17] reported 78 cases of bicarbonate infusion with no complications. Animal studies have reported a decrease in cellularity with edema and destruction of some cells, but these changes are temporary and resolve completely in a few weeks.[99-102] A case of systemic fibrinolysis through IO vascular access in a patient with ST-elevation myocardial infarction has recently been reported.[103]

Skin Sloughing
Skin sloughing and myonecrosis have been reported secondary to extravasation of infused fluids and medications.[102] This occurs if fluid or drugs extravasate from the puncture site into the surrounding tissue. When drugs such as calcium chloride, epinephrine, and sodium bicarbonate are infused, care should be taken to prevent dislodgment of the needle and extravasation into tissue. In addition, it is best to infuse such drugs only by gravity because infusion under pressure increases the risk for extravasation.

Compartment Syndrome

Compartment syndrome may occur when fluids leak out of the bone into a closed compartment such as the anterior or deep posterior compartment of the lower leg.[104-107] The risk for compartment syndrome can be reduced by carefully placing and securing the IO needle, limiting the number of attempts in the same bone, and removing the needle once IV access has been obtained. In addition, it is prudent to check the insertion site frequently, especially when fluids are being infused under pressure.

Epiphyseal Injuries

Injury to the growth plate and subsequent developmental abnormalities of the bone are ongoing concerns with the IO route. Regardless, these fears are largely unsupported in the available literature. In fact, there have been no reports of growth plate damage or permanent abnormalities of the bone. Two animal studies specifically examined damage to the epiphysis. Sodium bicarbonate was injected directly into the epiphysis and no radiologic evidence of epiphyseal injury was found.[108,109] In addition, two prospective radiologic analyses failed to identify any growth abnormalities 1 year after tibial IO insertion.[110,111] By pointing the needle away from the joint space and using the previously mentioned landmarks for insertion, the risk for epiphyseal injury is remote.

Whereas growth plate abnormalities appear to be very rare, tibial fractures have been reported after IO placement.[112] Hence, it is appropriate to take follow-up radiographs of patients who have undergone IO needle attempts or placement. Cortical defects may be seen on radiographs for up to 40 days after injection.[113]

Fat Embolism

Fat embolism is another potential complication of IO insertion.[3,67] This condition is rare, however, and has been reported only in adult patients.[64] Animal studies have found no changes in blood gases during IO infusion and limited evidence of fat globule collections in the lungs.[64,65] In a swine cardiac arrest model, there was no difference in the risk for fat emboli in pigs that had an IO line inserted versus those receiving IV medications.[114,115] Because the marrow in infants and children is primarily hematopoietic, this potential complication is unlikely to occur in this population.

Pain with Infusion

Most patients undergoing IO infusion will not be in a condition to sense pain, but infusion into bone marrow can be quite painful. Infusing 2 to 5 mL of 2% lidocaine before infusion has been suggested to relieve pain in awake patients. Medications intended to remain in the medullary space, such as local anesthetics, *must be injected very slowly until the desired anesthetic effect if achieved.* A recent study suggests that lidocaine is efficacious in attenuating the pain related to IO infusion.[116]

TRAINING

Procedural training can be performed on simulation models, animal bones (e.g., chicken or turkey legs), or cadavers. IO insertion techniques are part of the curriculum of the pediatric advanced life support, advanced pediatric life support, and advanced trauma life support courses. Training typically consists of an hour of didactics followed by a hands-on session. Novice users have achieved success rates of 93% to 97% for manual and battery-powered IO placement in a variety of simulated settings.* Battery-powered IO placement has also been shown to have high success rates after training.

Acknowledgment

The author would like to sincerely thank Rachael Stanley, MD, for her contribution to this chapter in previous editions.

> References are available at www.expertconsult.com

*References 5, 22, 49, 56, 80, 117, 118.

CHAPTER 26

Alternative Methods of Drug Administration

Steven J. Bauer and Carl R. Chudnofsky

The rapid administration of lifesaving, pain-relieving, and sedative medications lies at the core of the practice of emergency medicine. The intravenous (IV) route is usually the delivery method of choice. However, there are circumstances in which vascular access is either not available or contraindicated. Thus, emergency providers need to have a working knowledge of alternative routes of drug administration. This chapter describes the endotracheal (ET), intranasal, and rectal routes. Intraosseous (IO) access is covered in Chapter 25.

ET ADMINISTRATION OF MEDICATION

Certain drugs can be delivered simply, rapidly, and effectively to the central circulation by way of the ET tube. This method is best reserved for situations in which a patient's condition warrants immediate pharmacologic intervention but more conventional means of drug delivery, such as IV and IO, are not readily available. Such circumstances frequently arise in the prehospital or cardiac arrest scenario. Knowledge of the appropriate drugs and dosages that can be delivered effectively by this route may prove to be lifesaving.

Historical Perspective

ET drug administration dates back to 1857, when Bernard[1] demonstrated that the lung could rapidly absorb a solution of curare. In this historical experiment he instilled a fatal solution into the upper respiratory tract of dogs by way of a tracheostomy. Over the following decades, other investigators expanded this work and demonstrated that solutions containing salicylates, atropine, potassium iodide, strychnine, and chloral hydrate were also rapidly absorbed from the lung and excreted in urine after injecting aqueous solutions into the tracheas of experimental animals.[2] The use of intrapulmonary medication for the treatment of lung disease gained further acceptance when studies demonstrated that inhaling epinephrine mist dramatically relieved the symptoms of asthma.[3]

In the late 1930s and 1940s, several important observations were made concerning ET drug therapy: (1) penicillin delivered by the ET route demonstrated a depot effect, which resulted in therapeutic blood levels that lasted twice as long as those with intramuscular injection[4]; (2) various diluents mixed with penicillin affected both the rate and the degree of absorption from the lungs[5]; and (3) higher serum drug levels were attained with direct ET drug administration than with aerosolized administration.[5] In the 1950s it was noted that drugs delivered endotracheally were absorbed much more rapidly than those applied to the posterior part of the pharynx. Drugs applied locally to the larynx and trachea were absorbed rapidly and even resulted in blood levels significant enough to cause adverse anesthetic reactions.[6]

In 1967, Redding and coworkers[7] studied the use of ET administration as a route of drug delivery in a canine model of cardiopulmonary arrest. They administered epinephrine by the IV, intracardiac, and intratracheal routes to resuscitate dogs that had undergone both respiratory and circulatory arrest secondary to hypoxia. They then evaluated the effectiveness of the epinephrine after administration of the drug by all three of these routes. Their study revealed that all three

Endotracheal Medication Administration

Indications
Cardiac arrest with no peripheral or intraosseous access

Contraindications
Peripheral or intraosseous access

Complications
Depot effect of drug
Transient hypoxemia
Loss of catheter or needle down endotracheal tube

Equipment

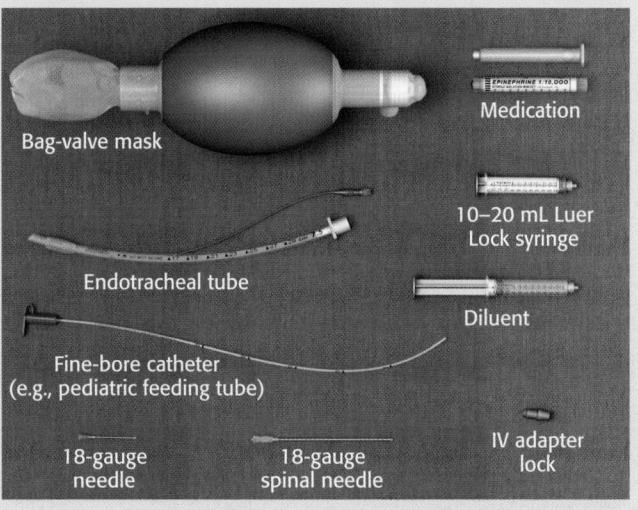

Bag-valve mask

Medication

10–20 mL Luer Lock syringe

Endotracheal tube

Diluent

Fine-bore catheter (e.g., pediatric feeding tube)

18-gauge needle

18-gauge spinal needle

IV adapter lock

Review Box 26-1 Endotracheal medication administration: indications, contraindications, complications, and equipment.

routes of drug administration were equally effective in restoring the circulation of dogs in hypoxia-induced cardiac arrest, again demonstrating that the ET route of drug delivery provides effective access to the systemic circulation.

In the late 1970s, Roberts, Greenberg, and colleagues[8-11] studied ET drug delivery in a series of laboratory experiments and clinical applications of ET epinephrine. Since that time, a number of important animal and human studies, as well as case reports, have been published in which the various aspects of ET drug administration were investigated. These studies have addressed (1) the appropriate dose of drug to administer; (2) the effect of the drug solution's volume; (3) the effect of different diluent solutions; (4) the role of different ET drug delivery techniques; and (5) the effects of hypoxia, hypotension, shock, and cardiopulmonary arrest on the absorption, distribution, and efficacy of endotracheally administered drugs.

Recommendations For ET Drug Delivery

It is imperative to remember that ET drug delivery is not the delivery method of choice. The American Heart Association (AHA) recommends that if IV access is not available, IO access should be obtained.[12] Although the AHA makes specific recommendations regarding the use of ET drug delivery for cardiac resuscitation (Table 26-1),[12-14] much of the existing literature is controversial and contradictory at times. It is therefore possible that some of these issues will continue to be the subject of future investigations.

Appropriate Dose

All investigators agree that the ET dose of a medication should be at least equal to the IV dose of the same drug when given for the same indication, but most studies indicate that higher doses are needed when administering drugs endotracheally. For advanced cardiac life support (ACLS) medications in adults, the AHA recommends a dose that is 2.0 to 2.5 times the usual IV dose when administered endotracheally.[12] This would be 2.0 to 2.5 mg (twice the standard IV dose of 1.0 mg). This recommendation is supported by the results of a study of epinephrine administered immediately after intubation in the out-of-hospital setting.[15] Other studies of

endotracheally administered lidocaine indicate that a 3-mg/kg dose (twice the standard IV dose of 1.5 mg/kg of lidocaine) was needed to obtain therapeutic serum levels.[16,17]

Some animal studies[18] and case reports[10] have reported conflicting results, with positive effects or recovery from cardiovascular collapse when epinephrine was used in doses equal to the recommended IV doses. In other animal[19] and human[20] studies, however, epinephrine administered endotracheally at doses of approximately 0.01 and 0.02 mg/kg, respectively, were shown to be unreliable in producing a physiologic response. In addition, studies using both normotensive and cardiac arrest canine models have shown that epinephrine doses of 0.01 mg/kg administered endotracheally produce serum levels approximately a 10th of that produced when the same dose is given intravenously.[9,21,22] These studies recommend increasing the ET epinephrine dose to 0.1 mg/kg and are the basis for the 2010 AHA recommendation to use a 10-fold increased dose when administering ET epinephrine to pediatric patients.[13] Some studies have shown that ET epinephrine at all doses causes a significant decrease in diastolic blood pressure immediately after instillation and that a dose of 0.3 mg/kg increases diastolic blood pressure after 1 minute. This may be due to β-adrenergic blockade at lower doses.[23,24]

ET drug delivery is associated with a depot effect, with ET drugs being "stored" and released slowly over time, similar to a continuous IV drip. This presumably occurs as a result of local vasoconstriction and lymphatic storage of the drug[8] or pooling in lung tissue because of poor lung perfusion.[25] With epinephrine use, the depot effect can produce postresuscitative dysrhythmias, hypertension, and tachycardia together with resultant increased myocardial oxygen demand. Given these conflicting data, it seems reasonable in adults to start with a dose 2.0 to 2.5 times the usual IV dose. If this is ineffective, higher doses may be used subsequently.

Volume for a Single Dose

For ET drugs, the AHA recommends a total volume of 10 mL in adults,[12] 5 mL in pediatric patients,[13] and 1 mL in neonates.[14] In studies involving dogs, Mace[26] compared undiluted lidocaine with diluted lidocaine (volume ≈6.5 mL) and found significantly higher plasma lidocaine levels in the animals

---

TABLE 26-1 American Heart Association Guidelines for Endotracheal Drug Administration

GUIDELINE	ADULT*	PEDIATRIC†	NEONATAL‡
Medication dose	2-2.5 times the recommended intravenous dose	Epinephrine, 0.1 mg/kg (10 times the recommended intravenous dose) Atropine, 0.04-0.06 mg/kg Lidocaine, 2-3 mg/kg	Epinephrine (1 : 10,000) Consider ≤0.1 mg/kg (class indeterminate)
Total volume to instill	10 mL	5 mL	1 mL
Diluent	Normal saline or distilled water	Normal saline	Normal saline

*Adult data from American Heart Association. Guidelines 2010 for cardiopulmonary resuscitation and emergency cardiovascular care, part 8: advanced cardiac life support. *Circulation*. 2010;122:S729.
†Pediatric data from American Heart Association. Guidelines 2010 for cardiopulmonary resuscitation and emergency cardiovascular care, part 14: Pediatric advanced life support. *Circulation*. 2010;122:S876.
‡Neonatal data from American Heart Association. 2010 American Heart Association guidelines for cardiopulmonary resuscitation and emergency cardiovascular care: neonatal resuscitation. *Circulation*. 2010;122:S909.

receiving diluted lidocaine. There were no changes in arterial blood gas values before or after ET drug administration. In another animal study, lidocaine diluted with normal saline to volumes of up to 25 mL produced no changes in arterial blood gases or the clinical condition and no change in the gross anatomy or histology of the lung.[27] In contrast, a study comparing normal saline with distilled water revealed decreased arterial oxygen partial pressure (Pao_2) with both solutions (water producing the greatest effect), but this study used large volumes (2 mL/kg) of solution.[28]

Studies of endotracheally administered lidocaine in human subjects reveal that dilution with distilled water to a total volume of 10 mL results in higher plasma lidocaine levels but also produces a decrease in Pao_2 of approximately 40 mm Hg that persists for longer than 1 hour.[29] A total volume of 5 mL yields lower plasma levels and a shorter period of hypoxemia. Data and volume recommendations in the setting of multiple doses of the drug are lacking.

It may be difficult or impossible to limit the total volume of the drug solution to 10 mL when using prefilled syringes. Prefilled syringes of epinephrine contain 1 mg in 10 mL (1 : 10,000). Giving 2.5 times the IV/IO dose requires the administration of 20 to 25 mL. It is possible to obtain epinephrine 1 : 1000 (1 mg/mL) and dilute it to a total volume of 5 to 10 mL, but the higher concentration of epinephrine may not be readily available during a cardiac arrest code. Likewise, prefilled syringes of atropine contain 1 mg in 10 mL (0.1 mg/mL). Prefilled syringes of lidocaine contain 20 mg/mL (100 mg/5 mL). A dose of 2 to 2.5 times the IV/IO dose could easily amount to 20 mL or more total volume in an obese patient.

Appropriate Diluent

Both normal saline and distilled water may be used as diluents for ET drug administration, but it remains unclear which is preferred. In one study, intubated dogs were administered epinephrine via ET tube, and peak serum epinephrine levels were 13 times higher when distilled water was used as a diluent instead of normal saline.[30] In addition, mean arterial blood pressure increased significantly only in dogs that were administered epinephrine diluted with distilled water. Greenberg and coworkers,[28] however, reported that normal saline administered via the ET route produced fewer detrimental effects on arterial blood gases than distilled water did. Another study found no changes in pulmonary status (arterial blood gas, oxygen saturation, gross anatomy, or histology) in dogs given lidocaine diluted with normal saline in total volumes ranging between 6 and 25 mL.[27] Still another study found no difference in arterial blood gases after the delivery of either diluent solution.[31] Hence, the optimal diluent is controversial; saline may produce less pulmonary dysfunction, but distilled water appears to deliver a greater amount of drug.

Technique for ET Drug Delivery

Techniques for ET drug administration include direct instillation into the proximal end of the ET tube, administration via a catheter that extends just beyond the distal tip of the ET tube, deep endobronchial administration using a longer catheter, administration via ET tube monitoring ports, administration with equipment developed specifically for ET atomized drugs, and injection through the side of the ET tube with a needle. Several studies have indicated that the use of a catheter or feeding tube may not be needed to enhance the drug's

effectiveness. Greenberg and Spivey[32] instilled radiopaque contrast material directly into the proximal end of the ET tube and compared its distribution with that of contrast material instilled via a catheter extending out the distal end of the tube. Both techniques were equally effective in distributing the contrast agent to the peripheral lung fields as long as five rapid manual ventilations followed the instillation. In addition, using a porcine cardiopulmonary arrest model, Jasani and colleagues[33] showed no difference in resuscitation rates or physiologic responses between epinephrine administered by direct injection into the ET tube, via a catheter extending out the distal end of the ET tube, or via a monitoring lumen built into the side wall of the ET tube. Rehan and associates[34] demonstrated that there was no difference in the amount of drug delivered via catheter versus direct instillation in neonates. In studies of patients with normal perfusion, some support "deep bronchial" ET drug administration, whereas others do not.[35-37]

Some studies have suggested that drug absorption with direct instillation into the ET tube is inconsistent during cardiopulmonary arrest.[17,20] To address one specific question, one study found no difference in plasma epinephrine levels when epinephrine was instilled during apnea versus instillation during the ventilator inspiratory cycle.[38]

Given these conflicting studies, use of a catheter to enhance deep pulmonary delivery seems reasonable. However, if a catheter is not readily available, direct injection into the ET tube appears to be justified.

Effects of Hypoxia, Hypotension, and Cardiopulmonary Arrest

Despite concerns that medications might not be absorbed in states of hypoxia or low blood flow, the data available reveal the opposite to be true. In a hemorrhagic shock model, Mace[39] demonstrated that higher plasma lidocaine levels were obtained via the ET route during shock than during nonshock states. In a lamb model, when epinephrine was administered endotracheally, higher plasma epinephrine levels were achieved during hypoxia-induced low pulmonary blood flow than during baseline, normal pulmonary blood flow.[40] Finally, plasma lidocaine levels rose earlier when lidocaine was administered endotracheally to dogs that were hypoxemic than to dogs that were not.[41]

Significant questions remain regarding the efficacy of endotracheally administered medications.[17,19,20,42-44] The 2010 guidelines for neonatal resuscitation[14] discourage the routine use of ET epinephrine. More importantly, these studies serve to emphasize that ET drug administration should not be used in lieu of attempts to obtain definitive access to the systemic circulation. ET drug administration should not be performed when more direct means of accessing the central circulation are available.

Indications

ET drug therapy is indicated when emergency pharmacologic intervention is needed and other access, either IV or IO, is not available. This most frequently occurs during cardiovascular collapse. Though intuitively and experimentally attractive, randomized, controlled trials of the efficacy of ET drug therapy are lacking.[45] Niemann and colleagues, in a retrospective cohort study, examined the outcomes of 596 cardiac arrest patients who received IV or ET medications. There were no

BOX 26-1 **Endotracheally Administered Drugs Shown to Be Effective Experimentally and Clinically**

BOX 26-1 Endotracheally Administered Drugs Shown to Be Effective Experimentally and Clinically

Atropine
Diazepam*
Epinephrine
Lidocaine
Naloxone†

*See text—effective but produced pneumonitis in one animal model.[46]
†See text—not recommended in neonates.[14]

BOX 26-2 Endotracheally Administered Drugs Shown to Be Effective Experimentally but Not Proven Clinically

Flumazenil
Metaraminol
Midazolam
Propranolol
Vasopressin

survivors to hospital discharge in the 101 patients who received ET medications versus a 5% survival rate in patients who received IV medications. However, more patients in the ET group were asystolic, a sign that these patients were already in much worse condition.[45]

Specific indications for the delivery of a drug endotracheally are the same as those for IV and IO administration. However, only a limited number of emergency drugs can be given safely by the ET route (Boxes 26-1 and 26-2). Medications that are appropriate for ET administration based on animal and human studies include epinephrine,[8,10,47] atropine,[48-50] lidocaine,[36,39,41,51] and naloxone.[52,53] ET naloxone is not currently recommended in neonates.[14]

Diazepam has also been shown to be effective.[54,55] However, in one animal model, diazepam produced pneumonitis when 0.5 mg/kg was administered via the ET route.[46] Because diazepam is sparingly soluble in water, it is available only in a solution of propylene glycol, ethanol, and benzyl alcohol. It is unknown whether the reported pneumonitis was due to the direct effect of diazepam or the diluent. The AHA has removed diazepam from its list of medications that can be given safely via the ET route; other routes may be more appropriate for this drug.[13,56,57]

Experimental studies of vasopressin,[58,59] midazolam,[60] flumazenil,[61] propranolol,[48] and metaraminol[62] in animal models suggest that these medications may also be effective when administered endotracheally, but no clinical studies in humans have been conducted to verify these findings. Efrati and coworkers' study[59] demonstrated that ET vasopressin had greater effects on diastolic blood pressure than did ET epinephrine with little effect on the heart rate, but no clinical trials have evaluated its efficacy. Based on a study by Wenzel and colleagues,[58] the 2010 ACLS guidelines added vasopressin to the list of cardiac resuscitation drugs that can

be administered via the ET route (in addition to lidocaine, epinephrine, atropine).[12] It is interesting to note that in the study of midazolam, no pathologic changes were seen in lung sections after the administration of midazolam.[60] In addition, midazolam is available commercially in aqueous solution and could therefore be diluted with normal saline or distilled water for ET administration. However, given that midazolam is approved for intramuscular use, it seems unlikely that ET administration would ever be necessary. Palmer and associates[61] demonstrated that therapeutic blood levels of flumazenil were obtained within a minute after ET delivery of 1 mg of the drug diluted in 10 mL of saline. This is 10 times the recommended IV dose of 0.1- to 0.2-mg aliquots. The role of flumazenil by ET administration remains to be determined.

Contraindications

At present, the only true contraindication to the ET delivery of an appropriate drug is the presence of another form of access to the systemic circulation through which the needed drug can be delivered rapidly and effectively. A complete list of drugs that are *contraindicated* for ET delivery is not available, but specific medications that have been shown to be ineffective or unsafe when given via the ET route include sodium bicarbonate, amiodarone, isoproterenol, and bretylium. In dogs, sodium bicarbonate was shown to inactivate lung surfactant.[63] Isoproterenol, even when given in doses 10 times the IV dose, failed to produce significant changes in arterial blood pressure or heart rate.[49] Studies of bretylium also indicate low serum levels after ET administration, even when administered at doses of 20 mg/kg.[64] Amiodarone induces pneumonitis and pulmonary fibrosis in animals and is therefore not recommended for ET administration.[65]

Equipment

The patient must first be intubated endotracheally. It should be noted that in studies in which the recommended ET tube doses of medications were administered by Combitube (Kendall-Sheridan, Argyle, NY) or laryngeal mask airway (LMA North America, San Diego, CA), absorption of drugs was found to be subtherapeutic.[66-68] A Combitube, when placed in the esophagus (requiring medications to travel out the side holes to reach the trachea), needs 10 times more epinephrine than that used with an ET tube to obtain the same serum concentration and hemodynamic effects.[66] Presumably, a Combitube that enters the trachea directly would function equivalently to an ET tube, but no studies have been done to support this assumption.

The equipment listed here is that required to perform any of the four different techniques described. This equipment is suggested for the ideal situation; at no time should drug delivery be delayed while searching for the "perfect" piece of equipment.

1. Manual bag ventilation device capable of delivering a fraction of inspiratory oxygen (F_{IO_2}) of at least 50%. When ET drug delivery is indicated, the patient's condition almost always warrants supplemental oxygen. Although the technique may not result in any significant deterioration in respiratory function, it is still advisable to administer additional oxygen after drug delivery. Use the bag

ventilation device to also deliver several rapid insufflations immediately after drug delivery to assist in delivery of the drug distally, where it may be absorbed more rapidly and effectively.[32] It should be noted, however, that the priorities of drug administration via the ET route must be balanced against the potential deleterious effects that such rapid insufflation might have on hemodynamics and cerebral perfusion. Excessive hyperventilation of victims of out-of-hospital cardiac arrest is common and associated with poor outcomes.[69]

2. A fine-bore catheter or special ET tube designed to deliver the drug at or beyond the distal end of the ET tube. For adults, select a catheter that is at least 8 Fr in size and 35 cm (14 inches) in length. It should be long enough to protrude past the distal end of the ET tube. The diameter of the catheter should be large enough to allow rapid delivery of 10 mL of solution. Several different types of tubes and catheters commonly available in the emergency department (ED) can be used for this purpose:

   a. A 16-gauge central venous pressure or cutdown catheter. Because most are only 30 cm in length, the proximal end of the ET tube should be shortened so that the catheter can protrude past the end.

   b. An 8- or 10-Fr polyethylene pediatric feeding tube (e.g., Argyle, St. Louis). These tubes are much longer than needed, so cut them to reduce dead space. Luer-Lok ends fit onto the proximal end of the tube. For neonates, use a 5-Fr feeding tube with a syringe and an IV adapter.

   c. An 8-Fr (or larger) pediatric pulmonary suction catheter without the control port. Because this catheter is designed to extend past the tip of the ET tube, it is an ideal length. However, with some brands it is difficult to attach a syringe or IV adapter lock after the suction control port is removed.

   Alternatively, some ET tubes are made with built-in ports that allow the instillation of drugs without removing the bag ventilation device.

3. An IV adapter lock. This can be placed as needed onto the proximal end of the irrigation lumen of the Hi-Lo Jet Tracheal Tube or on the catheters described previously to convert them for use with prefilled syringes. This adapter is generally unnecessary if a standard syringe is used.

4. A 10- to 20-mL syringe, preferably a Luer-Lok type, large enough to deliver the desired volume of drug solution plus an additional 5 mL of air. Most of the medications now prescribed for emergency situations come in prefilled syringes. This type of apparatus does not usually allow one to draw up diluent or an additional volume of air to empty the syringe of solution. In addition, depending on the manufacturer and model, some prefilled syringes have either needles or a needleless system that may require an IV adapter lock to use them for ET injection.

5. Diluent solution. Keep an adequate volume of diluent available, such as normal saline or distilled water.

6. Medications to be instilled (see Box 26-1).

7. An 18- or 19-gauge needle to draw up the medication and inject it. Use an 18-gauge, 8.9-cm (3.5-inch) spinal needle for direct instillation of medications into the proximal end of the ET tube.

8. Alcohol wipes to clean the vials and injection ports.

9. Gloves, mask, and eye protection. After instillation, the solution often refluxes out of the ET tube, which makes blood and body fluid precautions critical.

Procedure

The procedure of choice is one that will deliver the medication to the patient in the least amount of time. Secure the ET tube before instilling medications endotracheally to prevent the tube from being expelled if the patient coughs. Inflate the cuff of the tube, if present.

Direct Instillation into the ET Tube

While the patient is being ventilated, draw up the desired drug into a syringe (or use a prefilled syringe) (Fig. 26-1, *step 1*). Dilute the drug to a final volume of 10 mL (adults), 5 mL (children), or 1 mL (neonates) with normal saline or distilled water. Attach an 18- or 19-gauge needle. Some authors recommend using an 8.9-cm (3.5-inch) spinal needle. If using a prefilled syringe, draw up an appropriate volume of diluent in a second syringe so that the total instillation volume (drug plus diluent) equals 10 mL (adults), 5 mL (children), or 1 mL (neonates). Attach an 18- or 19-gauge needle, which will be used to flush the ET tube after instillation of the drug.

Interrupt the connection between the proximal end of the ET tube and the bag ventilation device. Insert the needle of the syringe into the proximal opening of the ET tube (see Fig. 26-1, *step 2*). Hold the proximal end of the needle with one hand to prevent loss of the needle into the tube. Inject the drug solution rapidly and forcefully. If using a prefilled syringe, flush the tube immediately with the diluent in a second syringe. If the patient makes an effort to cough, place a thumb over the opening of the ET tube to prevent expulsion of the solution. Reattach the bag ventilation device and deliver five rapid insufflations.

Use of a Catheter

Draw the plunger back to add 5 mL of air to the liquid in the syringe. If the drug to be delivered is in a prefilled syringe, place an IV adapter lock on the catheter if necessary to accommodate the syringe needle or needleless tip. Attach the syringe to the catheter at this time or once the catheter has been placed within the ET tube. In addition, draw up the appropriate volume of diluent (normal saline or distilled water) plus 5 mL air into a second syringe to flush the catheter after instillation of the drug from the prefilled syringe. The air flush presumably forces out any medication adhering to the walls of the catheter's lumen. Rehan and colleagues[34] determined that when using a catheter in a neonatal model, more medication was delivered with an additional air flush than without an air flush.

Disconnect the proximal end of the ET tube from the bag ventilation device. Place the catheter into the lumen of the ET tube in such a manner that the distal end of the catheter extends approximately 1 cm beyond the distal end of the ET tube (see Fig. 26-1, *step 3*). For the catheter to reach deep enough, the proximal end of the ET tube may need to be cut to a shorter length. Hold the proximal ends of the catheter and ET tube at all times during the procedure. If it has not already been done, attach the syringe to the catheter. Inject the drug solution rapidly and forcefully through the catheter into the trachea followed by the 5 mL of air needed to flush the catheter of any remaining drug solution (see Fig. 26-1, *step 4*). If using a prefilled syringe, use the second syringe to promptly flush with the diluent and air. Immediately remove the syringe and catheter from the ET tube. Reconnect the bag ventilation device with supplemental oxygen to the ET tube and deliver five rapid ventilations.

ENDOTRACHEAL MEDICATION ADMINISTRATION

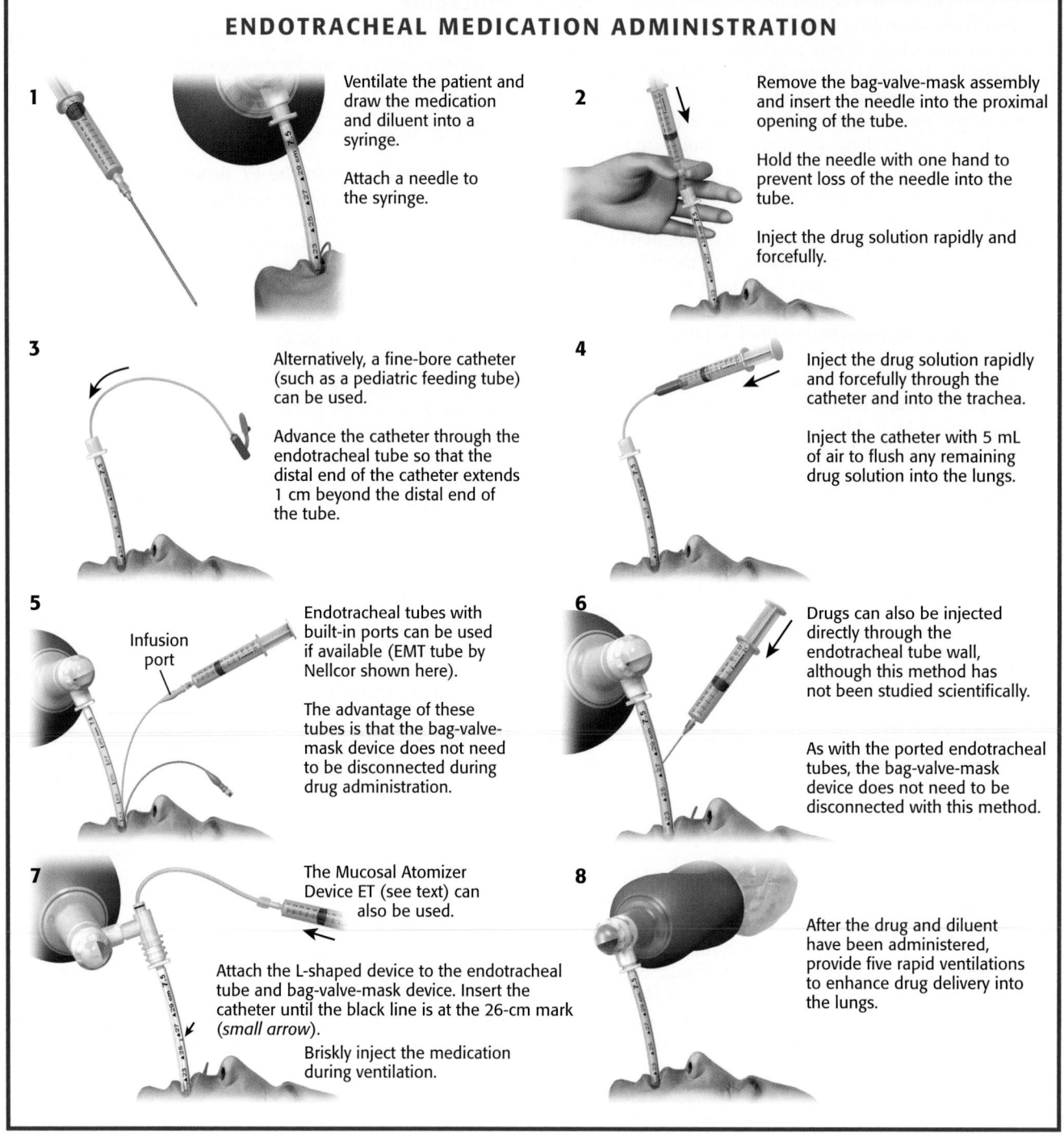

1 Ventilate the patient and draw the medication and diluent into a syringe.

Attach a needle to the syringe.

2 Remove the bag-valve-mask assembly and insert the needle into the proximal opening of the tube.

Hold the needle with one hand to prevent loss of the needle into the tube.

Inject the drug solution rapidly and forcefully.

3 Alternatively, a fine-bore catheter (such as a pediatric feeding tube) can be used.

Advance the catheter through the endotracheal tube so that the distal end of the catheter extends 1 cm beyond the distal end of the tube.

4 Inject the drug solution rapidly and forcefully through the catheter and into the trachea.

Inject the catheter with 5 mL of air to flush any remaining drug solution into the lungs.

5 Infusion port

Endotracheal tubes with built-in ports can be used if available (EMT tube by Nellcor shown here).

The advantage of these tubes is that the bag-valve-mask device does not need to be disconnected during drug administration.

6 Drugs can also be injected directly through the endotracheal tube wall, although this method has not been studied scientifically.

As with the ported endotracheal tubes, the bag-valve-mask device does not need to be disconnected with this method.

7 The Mucosal Atomizer Device ET (see text) can also be used.

Attach the L-shaped device to the endotracheal tube and bag-valve-mask device. Insert the catheter until the black line is at the 26-cm mark (*small arrow*).

Briskly inject the medication during ventilation.

8 After the drug and diluent have been administered, provide five rapid ventilations to enhance drug delivery into the lungs.

Figure 26-1 Endotracheal administration of medication.

Use of ET Tubes with Irrigation and Drug Delivery Lumens

The following tubes have built-in ports:

1. ET tubes designed for bronchoscopy (e.g., Hi-Lo Jet Tracheal Tube; Nellcor, Pleasanton, CA) (Fig. 26-2*A*). These tubes have two additional ports, one for monitoring or irrigation (opaque lumen) and one for jet ventilation (transparent lumen). They are available in only uncuffed sizes. In a porcine cardiopulmonary arrest model, successful resuscitation with this tube was comparable to resuscitation with other forms of ET drug administration.[33]

The major disadvantage of this ET tube is the need to be familiar with the specific ports before use. If one has never seen the tube previously, determining which port is used for irrigation could prove to be time-consuming. In addition, the port requires placement of an IV adapter lock or Luer-Lok to use a prefilled syringe.

2. ET tube with a side port (ETSP; e.g., EMT Emergency Medicine Tube, Nellcor, Pleasanton, CA) (see Figs. 26-1, *step 5*, and 26-2*B*). This tube is designed specifically for ET drug administration but is available in cuffed sizes only. The instillation lumen opens into the tube at Murphy's eye, approximately 1 cm from the end of the tube. The

Figure 26-2 Specialty endotracheal tubes with irrigation/drug delivery lumens. **A,** Hi-Lo Jet Tracheal Tube (Nellcor, Pleasanton, CA). This tube is designed for bronchoscopy and has two additional ports, one for jet ventilation and one for irrigation. This is an uncuffed tube and does not have a balloon inflation port. **B,** EMT Emergency Medicine Tube (Nellcor, Pleasanton, CA). This tube is designed specifically for endotracheal drug administration and has two ports: one for balloon inflation and one for drug instillation.

Figure 26-3 The Mucosal Atomizer Device-Endotracheal Tube (MADett, LMA North America, San Diego, CA). The L-shaped port attaches to both the bag-valve-mask device (BVM) and endotracheal tube (ETT) and allows uninterrupted ventilation during drug administration. The catheter should be inserted until the black depth marker is at the 26-cm mark on the ETT.

injection port has an IV adapter lock, which makes it amenable to use with prefilled syringes. The ETSP is not available in pediatric sizes. In addition, in one study comparing the administration of lidocaine via the ETSP with administration through the proximal end of the standard ET tube, serum lidocaine measurements never reached therapeutic levels in the ETSP group, in contrast to the ET group and IV control group.[70]

3. Uncuffed tracheal tube with a monitoring lumen (Nellcor, Pleasanton, CA). This tube contains a separate monitoring lumen in the wall of the tube that opens inside the distal tip. A three-way stopcock with a Luer-Lok adapter provides access to the monitoring lumen. The major disadvantage of this ET tube is the need to be familiar with the additional port.

The advantage of these specialized ET tubes is that they eliminate the need to disconnect the bag ventilation device and the ET tube.

Injection through the Wall of the ET Tube

This method of drug delivery has not yet been evaluated scientifically but has been used clinically.[71,72] As with ET tubes with drug delivery lumens, this technique requires no interruption of the connection between the bag ventilation device and the ET tube (see Fig. 26-1, *step 6*). In addition, placing an IV adapter lock on the needle allows it to be left inserted in the ET tube for use with additional medications.[72]

Use of the ET Atomizer

The Mucosal Atomizer Device-Endotracheal Tube (MADett, LMA North America, San Diego, CA) is an L-shaped port that attaches to both the ventilator bag and the ET tube (Fig. 26-3; also see Fig. 26-1, *step 7*). A catheter is inserted into the adapter and a mark is aligned at the 26-cm line of the ET

tube. The catheter is then locked into place in the adapter. The L shape allows ventilation of the patient to be uninterrupted while medication is administered via the catheter and atomized into the patient's lung mucosa at the distal tip that protrudes from the end of the ET tube. This device can be used only with ET tubes 7.0 or larger and longer than 28 cm.

Complications

Reported complications of ET drug therapy are rare, in part because of the infrequent use of this technique. Since most patients who receive ET drug therapy are in cardiopulmonary arrest or are otherwise critically ill, it is difficult to ascertain whether an adverse outcome is the result of the therapy.

With regard to the techniques of ET drug administration, no serious complications have been reported. A theoretical complication is loss of a needle or catheter down the ET tube, which can be prevented by holding the catheter or needle while instilling the drug.

After ET drug administration, the well-described systemic effects of drugs administered in emergency situations may produce adverse effects. Administration of epinephrine during cardiopulmonary resuscitation has been noted in case reports to produce prolonged hypertension, tachycardia, and arrhythmias after the return of a perfusing rhythm.[10,21] It appears that these side effects are related to the depot effect, in which larger doses of drugs administered endotracheally are released slowly over time. In addition to epinephrine, atropine and lidocaine also exhibit a depot effect when administered endotracheally.[63] No serious long-term sequelae, however, have been reported to result from this effect.

A potential concern with ET drug therapy is a transient decrease in arterial oxygen content during or after drug delivery. If total volumes are maintained between 5 and 10 mL in adults, the effect on pulmonary function appears to be minimal. Supplemental oxygen should always be administered in an effort to improve oxygenation and offset any transient drop in arterial oxygen content that might develop.

INTRANASAL ADMINISTRATION OF MEDICATION

Anatomy and Physiology

The human nasal cavity is a convenient and readily available site to deliver medications. It has been used for centuries and has recently been introduced into the ED. It has a volume of 15 to 20 mL and a total surface area of approximately 150 cm[2].[2,73] The nasal cavity is divided into two mostly symmetric halves by the nasal septum. Each half consists of four anatomically and histologically distinct regions: the vestibule, atrium, and respiratory and olfactory regions (Fig. 26-4). The respiratory and olfactory regions are areas of high vascularity and good permeability. The respiratory region has the largest surface area at approximately 130 cm[2].[2,74] Blood flow in the nasal mucosa is higher, per cubic centimeter, than in muscle, brain, or liver tissue.[75]

The olfactory mucosa has been theorized to have a direct connection to the brain and bypasses the first-pass metabolism of orally administered medications.[76-78] Drugs that can be delivered via the nasal mucosa are generally small in molecular weight, stabile, and dissolvable in the watery mucus of the nasal passages.[79]

Indications and Contraindications

The intranasal route may be very useful in circumstances where placing an IV line is not possible or practical. This is especially true in patients at the extremes of age. Thus, knowledge of this painless, needleless route of drug administration is important for practicing emergency physicians. Intranasal administration of medication has been shown for more than 30 years to be effective.[80] Many medications are routinely administered nasally in the outpatient setting for both local and systemic delivery,[79] but the majority of these medications have little clinical application in the ED. Drugs used routinely in the ED that have been studied intranasally include the opioid antagonist naloxone, the benzodiazepine midazolam, the sedative-hypnotic ketamine, and the opioids fentanyl and sufentanil. Most of these studies have focused on the pediatric patient population as an alternative to IV medication.

Narcotic Overdose

Intranasal naloxone at a dose of 2 mg was shown to be as effective as IV naloxone in patients with known or suspected opioid overdose.[81] Patients receiving intranasal naloxone had an increase in the respiratory rate that was statistically equivalent to that with IV naloxone. Intranasal naloxone was shown to reduce the need to initiate an IV line in narcotic overdose patients.[82] This could help reduce the risk for needlestick injuries in the prehospital setting in this high-risk patient population. Similarly, *nebulized* naloxone has also been used to treat opioid intoxication in the *non-apneic patient*.

Seizures

Bhattacharyya and colleagues studied intranasal midazolam versus rectal diazepam in pediatric seizure patients. Midazolam, 0.2 mg/kg delivered intranasally, was found to have a significantly more rapid onset of seizure cessation with

Figure 26-4 Regions of the nasal cavity. *(Netter illustration from www.netterimages.com. © Elsevier Inc. All rights reserved.)*

Intranasal Medication Administration

Indications
Pain relief
Anxiolysis/sedation
Seizure control
Narcotic overdose

Contraindications
Abnormal nasal anatomy
Nasal trauma

Complications
Side effects of the specific medication
Local nasal irritation

Equipment

Mucosal atomizing device

Medication

1-mL syringe

Review Box 26-2 Intranasal medication administration: indications, contraindications, complications, and equipment.

minimal effect on respiration and oxygen saturation.[83] The authors suggested that this route could be used in both the prehospital setting and the ED to deliver antiepileptic medication until an IV line can be initiated.

Sedation

Klein and coworkers studied intranasal, buccal, and oral administration of midazolam for pediatric procedural sedation.[84] They demonstrated that 0.3 mg/kg of midazolam administered intranasally exhibited a faster onset of sedation, achieved adequate sedation in a greater proportion of patients, and resulted in more parents of pediatric patients stating that they would chose the same regimen again. However, more patients complained of local irritation of the nasal mucosa. This is probably due to the acidity of midazolam. Local irritation has been noted especially when drops are used to instill the midazolam.[85] Premedication with intranasal lidocaine may decrease the local irritation associated with midazolam.[86]

Ketamine has been studied in the pediatric population both as a stand-alone sedative and in combination with midazolam.[87,88] Ketamine, 3 mg/kg, was found to be very safe and effective when administered intranasally and had good sedation scores and no significant adverse events. Ketamine, 5 mg/kg, in combination with midazolam, 0.3 mg/kg, was administered intranasally as an anesthesia preinduction agent and had rapid onset of sedation. However, this study used a higher dose of ketamine, which could result in prolonged sedation or sedation deeper than desired.

Pain Management

Fentanyl is widely used for the management of acute pain. Intranasal fentanyl has been shown to have desirable pharmacokinetics and high bioavailability in the treatment of acute pain.[89,90] Foster, Upton, and colleagues demonstrated that intranasal fentanyl (75 to 200 μg) had only a slight, nonstatistically significant lag in the onset of analgesia but equivalent pain reduction.[89]

Intranasal fentanyl at 1.7 μg/kg concentrated to 150 μg/mL was compared with IV morphine in pediatric patients with long-bone fractures.[91] Intranasal fentanyl was shown to be as effective as IV morphine and had a similar side effect profile. Intranasal fentanyl can be used to commence pain control in these patients before initiating an IV line or as a noninvasive alternative to IV or intramuscular injection.

Contraindications

There are no absolute contraindications to the intranasal administration of medication with the exception of medication allergy. Abnormal nasal anatomy or increased mucus production may reduce absorption and necessitate repeated dosing.[79]

Notes on Medication Dosing

The medications noted previously have not been studied extensively for appropriate dosing. The doses used correlate with the standard IV or intramuscular doses. It is recommended that the lowest dose possible be used and to repeat the dose if necessary.

Equipment

The only equipment necessary is the desired medication, a needle to draw the medication from the vial, a 1-mL syringe, and an atomizing device if available (Review Box 26-2).

Procedure

Two methods to deliver drugs to the nasal mucosa can be used: drops or aerosol. Nasal drops require a cooperative patient and correct positioning to enhance drug delivery.[92,93] Some authors have noted that much of the drug is lost to the environment by dripping out the nose or into the throat and then swallowed.[92,93] This can result in metabolism of the drug in the liver through first-pass metabolism. Nasal atomization has been found to be the optimal method of enhancing mucosal coverage and increasing plasma concentrations of intranasal medications.[92-94] Regardless of the method, the relatively small volume of the nasal cavity limits the volume of medication to approximately 1 mL per naris. If the volume is greater than 1 mL, split the dose and instill half into each naris. Use concentrated forms of medications to decrease the overall volume.[79]

Nasal Drops

Draw up the appropriate dose and volume of medication. Position the patient properly to enhance delivery to the mucosa and prevent runoff or swallowing. Instill the drops slowly to prevent runoff.

One position is to place the patient on the back with the head down and nose pointing up. Slowly instill the drops into each naris along the nasal septum and allow the medication to flow into the turbinates[92,93] (Fig. 26-5A).

A second position is the lateral decubitus position with the head angled downward[92,93] (see Fig. 26-5B). Use pillows or towels to elevate the body at the shoulders if necessary. Instill the drops into the naris that is "up" so that the medication runs along the nasal septum and turbinates.

An alternative, though more uncomfortable position is to place the patient on the knees with the head down and the vertex parallel to the bed, essentially in a position similar to starting a forward roll[92,93] (see Fig. 26-5C). Instill the medication against the septum and let it flow to the turbinates.

Nasal Atomization

Many commercial devices are available for home and outpatient use to deliver medications intranasally. The Mucosal Atomization Device (LMA North America, San Diego, CA) is small, easy to use, and attaches to nearly any syringe (Fig. 26-6). Atomization of midazolam was found to achieve higher plasma concentrations than nebulized midazolam.[95] Atomization results in very fine particles that distribute over the surface and can be absorbed more readily.

Draw up an appropriate volume of medication into a syringe with an additional amount to accommodate for the dead space of the device (0.1 mL). Insert the device approximately ¼ to ½ inch into the vestibule. Rapidly depress the plunger. If the total volume is greater than 1 mL, repeat this in the other naris (Fig. 26-7).

An obvious advantage to use of an atomizer is that proper positioning is not necessary and the medication is instilled rapidly. This can result in less runoff and requires less cooperation from the patient.

Complications

Aside from the side effects of the medications (allergy, nausea, apnea, etc.), there are few to no complications when using intranasal medications. As mentioned previously, midazolam has been noted to cause short-term local irritation. A single

Figure 26-5 Patient positioning for intranasal administration of medication. **A,** Head down, nose pointing up. **B,** Lateral decubitus position with the head angled down. **C,** "Somersault" position.

Figure 26-6 Mucosal Atomization Device (LMA North America, San Diego, CA).

Figure 26-7 Insert the device approximately 1 cm into the vestibule and rapidly depress the plunger. If the total volume is greater than 1 mL, repeat in the other naris.

case of anosmia following long-term use of intranasal ketamine has been reported.[96]

Nebulized Naloxone

Naloxone has been administered via nebulization, as an alternative to more traditional routes, to reverse opioid

intoxication.[97] The proposed benefit of nebulized naloxone is that intravenous access is not required, the reversal effect may be prolonged or continued as long as the nebulizer is used, and there may be a more gradual, but often not complete, reversal of opioid intoxication, reversing opioid effects without producing acute withdrawal. Most reports are anecdotal experience or case reports, and there are little data on the specific use. The procedure may be applicable to *nonapneic* patients and can be used by both prehospital and ED clinicians. Rescue intramuscular or IV naloxone should be available for those not responding appropriately. Empirical dosing is 2 to 4 mg of naloxone in 3 mL of saline, delivered by an oxygen driven nebulizer, such as those used to deliver aerosolized beta-agonists to asthmatics.

Weber et al[98] reported success with nebulized naloxone in approximately 80% of spontaneously breathing patients with suspected opioid intoxication when the medication was administered by paramedics. Nebulized naloxone is a reasonable option for nonapneic patients with suspected opioid-induced depressed mental status or respiratory depression; however, intravenous or intramuscular naloxone must be used if the desired reversal is not accomplished.

Rectal Administration Of Medication

Indications

Drug administration when more desirable routes are unavailable or impractical:

 Children frightened of intravenous catheterization
 Patients who refuse patenteral drug administration
 Patients with nausea/vomiting or inability to swallow

Contraindications

Immunosuppression
Severe thrombocytopenia or coagulopathy
Active gastrointestinal bleeding
Diarrhea
Chronic anorectal problems (fissures, hemorrhoids, fistulas. etc.)

Complications

Erractic absorption
 Delayed, prolonged, or unusually rapid
Local trauma
Pain

Equipment

Syringe with medication

16- or 18-gauge intravenous catheter

Lubricating jelly

Medication suppository

6- or 8-French pediatric feeding tube

Review Box 26-3 Rectal medication administration: indications, contraindications, complications, and equipment.

RECTAL ADMINISTRATION OF MEDICATION

Medications may be administered rectally when other more preferable routes are not available. This most often occurs when IV access is impractical or impossible, the medication is not suitable for intramuscular administration, or other non-parenteral routes are unavailable or less desirable. In these situations, rectal administration may offer a simple and easy method of drug delivery. The major drawback to rectal drug administration is the unpredictable and often erratic drug absorption.

Drug absorption from the rectum is a simple diffusion process across the lipid membrane. In general, the rate of absorption rises with increasing lipid solubility of the drug and, when applicable, with increased rate of drug release from its carrier (e.g., time to liquefaction of suppository preparations). Other factors affecting transmucosal rectal absorption include the volume of liquid, concentration of the drug, length of the rectal catheter (i.e., site of rectal drug delivery), presence of stool in the rectal vault, pH of the rectal contents, rectal retention of the drug or drugs administered, and differences in venous drainage within the rectosigmoid region.[99]

Anatomy and Physiology

The rectum is the terminal portion of the large intestine; it begins at the confluence of the three taeniae coli of the sigmoid colon and ends at the anal canal. In adults, the anal canal is about 5 cm in length and the rectum is approximately 10 to 15 cm in length. In children, the size of the rectum varies with age (see Table 26-2).

The rectum has two main routes of venous drainage (Fig. 26-8). The superior rectal vein drains into the portal circulation (by way of the inferior mesenteric vein), whereas the middle and inferior rectal veins drain into the caval system (by way of the inferior iliac vein). This pattern of venous drainage has a significant impact on the peak serum

TABLE 26-2 Age-Related Changes in Rectal Dimensions			
AGE	DIAMETER (cm)	LENGTH (cm)	VOLUME (mL)	LENGTH TO INSERT CATHETHER (cm)
1 mo	1.5	3	7	1.5
3 mo	3.0	6	42	3
1 yr	3.5	7	67	3.5
2 yr	4.0	8	100	4
6 yr	4.5	9	143	4.5
10 yr	5.0	12	235	6

From Smith S, Sharkey I, Campbell D. Guidelines for rectal administration of anticonvulsant medication in children. *Pediatr Perinatal Drug Ther.* 2001;4:140–147.

concentrations achieved by rectally administered drugs. Drugs administered high in the rectum (the area drained by the superior rectal vein) are carried directly to the liver via the portal vein and are subject to first-pass metabolism. In contrast, drugs administered low in the rectum are delivered systemically into the inferior vena cava, thereby avoiding first-pass elimination in the liver.

Indications and Contraindications

Rectal drug administration is indicated when more desirable routes are unavailable or impractical. For example, IV access in small children may be very difficult to obtain and frightening to the child. In these situations, the ease of rectal administration may outweigh the benefits of IV drug delivery. Patients who refuse parenteral drug administration may also benefit from rectal delivery, as will those with nausea and vomiting or an inability to swallow.

Vascular Supply of the Anus and Rectum

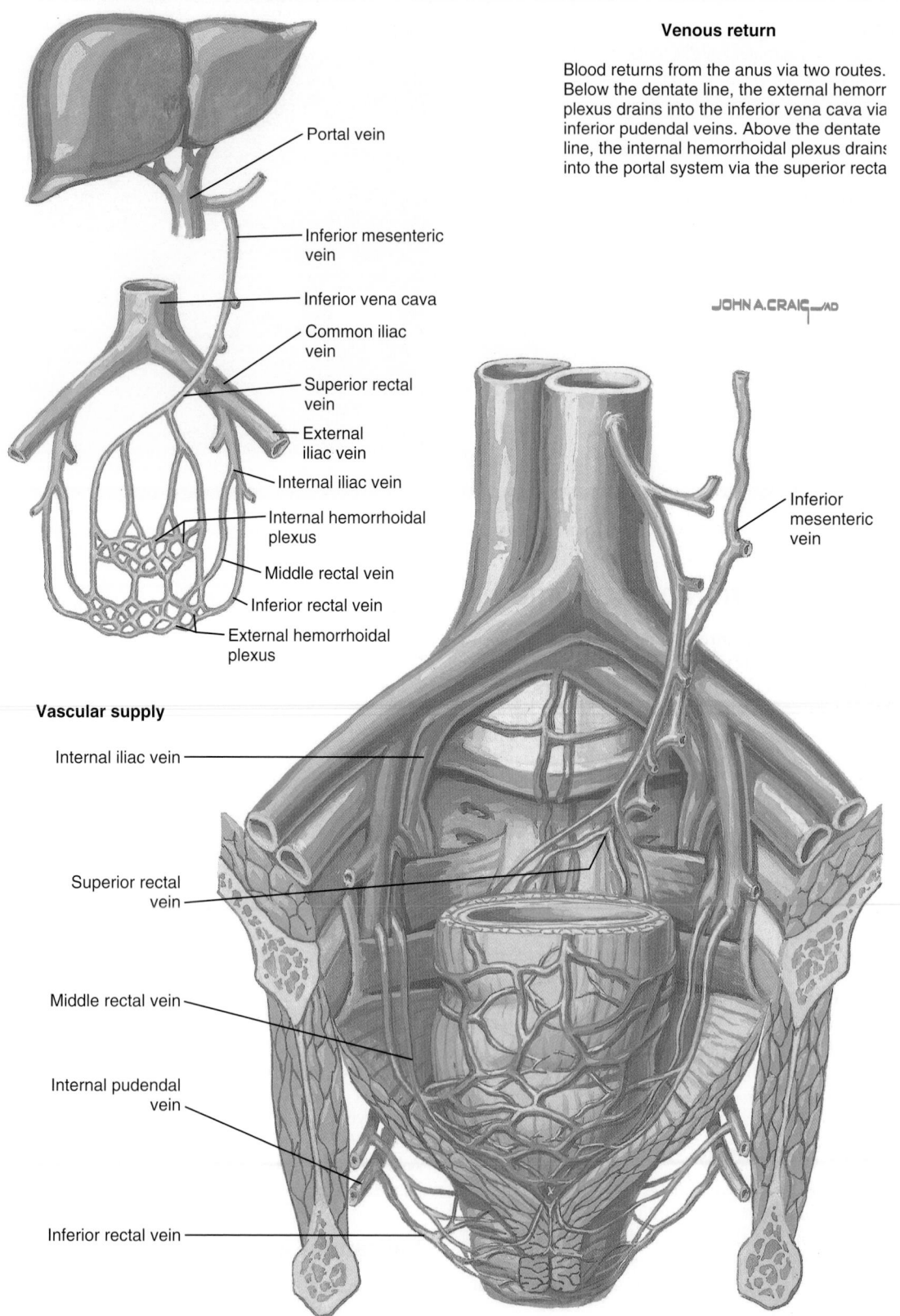

Venous return

Blood returns from the anus via two routes. Below the dentate line, the external hemorr plexus drains into the inferior vena cava via inferior pudendal veins. Above the dentate line, the internal hemorrhoidal plexus drains into the portal system via the superior recta

Portal vein

Inferior mesenteric vein

Inferior vena cava

Common iliac vein

Superior rectal vein

External iliac vein

Internal iliac vein

Internal hemorrhoidal plexus

Middle rectal vein

Inferior rectal vein

External hemorrhoidal plexus

JOHN A.CRAIG AD

Inferior mesenteric vein

Vascular supply

Internal iliac vein

Superior rectal vein

Middle rectal vein

Internal pudendal vein

Inferior rectal vein

Figure 26-8 Venous drainage of the rectum. *(Netter illustration from* www.netterimages.com. *© Elsevier Inc. All rights reserved.)*

There are few, if any absolute contraindications to rectal drug administration. Rectal administration should be avoided in immunosuppressed patients, in whom even minimal trauma could lead to abscess formation, and in patients with severe thrombocytopenia or coagulopathy to avoid difficult-to-control bleeding.[99,100] Patients with active lower gastrointestinal bleeding and those with severe diarrhea are not generally good candidates for rectal drug administration. Finally, patients with a variety of acute or chronic anorectal problems such as fissures, hemorrhoids, or perianal abscesses or fistulas may not tolerate rectal drug administration.

Equipment

In general, no special equipment is required for rectal drug administration. For medications in suppository form, a water-soluble lubricant (e.g., Surgilube) will reduce the discomfort associated with insertion. For liquid and gel formulations, use an appropriately sized syringe attached to a small (e.g., 6- or 8-Fr) rubber feeding tube or an 18- or 16-gauge plastic IV catheter with the needle removed.

Procedure

Suppositories

Place adults and large children in a lateral recumbent position with the upper part of the leg flexed at the knee and hip and the lower part of the leg extended. Infants, because of their small size, can be placed in almost any position. Place the lubricated suppository at the rectal opening and gently push it into the rectum toward the umbilicus until the gloved index finger has been inserted approximately 7.5 cm in adults, 3.5 cm in children, or 1.5 cm in infants (see Table 26-2). To help prevent expulsion of the suppository, do not allow the patient to get up for approximately 10 to 15 minutes after insertion.

Most suppositories have an apex at one end (pointed end) and taper to a blunt base at the other end. For ease of insertion, manufacturers recommend inserting the tapered end first. However, in 1991, Abd-El-Maeboud and colleagues found that inserting suppositories blunt end first resulted in greater retention within the rectum and a lower expulsion rate.[101] Nonetheless, these findings have not been corroborated and have been challenged by nursing educators as insufficient evidence on which to base clinical practice.[102]

Liquids and Gels

Position the patient as described for insertion of a suppository. Draw up the desired dose of medication into an appropriately sized syringe attached to an 6- or 8-Fr rubber feeding tube (adults and large children) or an 18- or 16-guage IV catheter (infants and small children) with the needle removed (Fig. 26-9). The goal is to deposit the drug in the low to midportion of the rectum to avoid first-pass elimination by the liver. For adults, insert the rubber feeding tube approximately 7.5 to 10.0 cm and slowly inject the drug. In children, catheter depth varies with age (see Table 26-2). When administering rectal medication to infants and young children, be sure to squeeze the buttock cheeks closed after withdrawing the catheter to prevent expulsion of the medication. A 3-inch piece of tape placed across the buttocks also works well and frees the clinician to perform other duties.

Figure 26-9 Pediatric rectal administration of medication via a pediatric feeding tube.

Medications

A variety of medications can be administered rectally. In emergency medicine practice the most common medications given rectally are analgesics and antipyretics, sedative-hypnotic agents, anticonvulsants, antiemetics, and cation exchange resins (e.g., Kayexalate).

Analgesics and Antipyretics

Acetaminophen is frequently administered rectally in children for both fever and pain. Common reasons for rectal administration include refusal to take the medication orally, vomiting, and altered mental status. Acetaminophen is commercially available in suppository form and is easy to obtain and administer. Studies comparing oral and rectal administration of acetaminophen have demonstrated equal antipyretic effectiveness.[103,104] Rectal dosing of acetaminophen is the same as oral dosing (Table 26-3).

Though not commonly administered rectally, aspirin, non-steroidal antiinflammatory drugs (NSAIDs), including indomethacin and diclofenac (diclofenac suppositories are not available in the United States), and morphine also come in rectal formulations and can be very useful in a variety of ED encounters. For example, aspirin is commonly administered rectally to adults with symptoms of a transient ischemic attack, an acute stroke, or an acute coronary syndrome who may have an impaired swallowing mechanism or are too unstable to take medication orally. Like acetaminophen, the oral and rectal doses of aspirin are similar (see Table 26-3). Rectal NSAIDs and morphine may be an alternative for patients discharged from the ED who require ongoing analgesia but cannot tolerate oral medications.[105-109] Rectal doses of indomethacin and morphine are provided in Table 26-3.

Sedative-Hypnotic Agents

Sedative-hypnotic agents, including midazolam, methohexital, and thiopental, may be administered rectally in children requiring sedation in the ED.[110-113] This occurs most often in pediatric patients in whom IV access may be problematic or for procedures that may require only minimal sedation in conjunction with the use of local anesthetics (see Chapter 33 for a detailed discussion of sedation and analgesia in children). Rectal administration of methohexital and thiopental is

TABLE 26-3 Drugs Commonly Administered Rectally in the ED

CLASS	RECTAL DOSE/FREQUENCY	ONSET*	DURATION	COMMENTS
Analgesics/Antipyretics				
Acetaminophen	Adults: 325-650 mg q4-6h or 1000 mg q6-8h (max, 4 g/day) Children: 10-15 mg/kg q4-6h (max, 2.6 g/day)	<1 hr	4-6 hr	Studies have demonstrated equal antipyretic efficacy with rectal and oral administration of acetaminophen
Aspirin	Adults: 300-600 mg q4-6h (max, 4 g/day) Children: 10-15 mg/kg q4-6h (max, 4 g/day)	<1 hr	4-6 hr	Contraindications are the same as for oral administration (e.g., children with chickenpox or recent flulike symptoms)
Indomethacin	Adults: 25-50 mg/kg/dose q8-12h (max, 200 mg/day) Children ≥2 yr: 1-2 mg/kg/day q6-12h (max, 4 mg/kg/day) Children >14 yr: see adult dosing	≈30 min	4-6 hr	Indocin suppositories only come in 50-mg doses, which is too high
Diclofenac	N/A			Not available in a rectal formulation in the United States
Morphine	Adults: 10-20 mg q3-4h Children (≥6 mo and <50 kg): 0.15-0.2 mg/kg q3-4h	≈30 min	3-4 hr	Rectal absorption may vary widely; close observation for respiratory depression is mandatory in infants and children
Sedative Hypnotics				
Midazolam	Adults: seldom given rectally Children: 0.25-0.5 mg/kg	10-30 min	60-90 min	Because these drugs cannot be titrated when given rectally, close monitoring for oversedation is mandatory
Methohexital	Adults: seldom given rectally Children: 25 mg/kg	5-15 min	60 min	Prepare a solution of methohexital for rectal administration by adding 5 mL of sterile water or saline to a 500-mg vial and mix well
Thiopental	Adults: 3-4 g/dose Children: 5-10 mg/kg/dose	5-15 min	60 min	
Anticonvulsants				
Diazepam	Adults: 10 mg; may repeat once Children: 0.5 mg/kg; then 0.25 mg/kg in 10 minutes (max, 20 mg)	2-10 min	30 min	Dosing guidelines are for status epilepticus; the adult rectal delivery system contains 4 mL (20 mg) of diazepam gel with a 6-cm tip; the pediatric rectal delivery system contains 2 mL (10 mg) of gel with a 4.4-cm tip (see text for details)
Antiemetics				
Prochlorperazine	Adults: 25 mg Children >9 kg: 0.4 mg/kg/day q6-8h (not recommended in children <10 kg)	≈60 min	12 hr	Central nervous system effects similar to those with other routes of administration for both prochlorperazine and promethazine
Promethazine	Adults: 12.5-25 mg q4-6h Children >2 yr: 0.25-1 mg/kg/day q4-6h (max, 25 mg/dose)	≈30 min	4-6 hr (up to 12 hr)	
Cation Exchange Resin				
Sodium polystyrene sulfonate (Kayexalate)	Adults: 30-50 g q6h Older children: 1 g/kg/dose q2-6h Young children/infants: calculate the dose (1 mEq K^+/g of resin)	2-24 hr	6 hr	Avoid solutions containing sorbitol; see text for details regarding rectal administration

ED, emergency department.

*The onset of action of rectally administered medications may vary widely because of erratic absorption and first-pass elimination in the liver.

particularly useful for sedating children before advanced imaging studies.[111,113] The major drawback of rectal administration is an inability to titrate these medications to the desired level of sedation.

Midazolam, methohexital, and thiopental are administered rectally using the IV formulations of each agent as described previously. The rectal doses of midazolam, methohexital, and thiopental in children are 0.25 to 0.5 mg/kg, 25 mg/kg, and 5 to 10 mg/kg, respectively (see Table 26-3). To prepare a solution of methohexital for rectal administration, add 5 mL of sterile water or saline to a 500-mg vial of methohexital and mix well; this provides a methohexital solution of 100 mg/mL.

Anticonvulsants

Anticonvulsants are generally administered orally or intravenously in the ED. However, there may be situations, such as in actively seizing patients, in which oral or IV administration is impossible or unlikely to be accomplished in a reasonable period. In these cases, rectal administration may be an effective alternative.[114] Studies have demonstrated that diazepam, because of its high lipid solubility, is rapidly absorbed from the rectum and can quickly halt seizures.[114,115] Lorazepam has much lower lipid solubility and is not recommended for rectal use.

Diazepam is commercially available in a gel formulation that is preloaded in a rectal delivery system (Diastat AcuDial). However, the undiluted parenteral formulation can also be used. The preloaded rectal delivery system is available for both pediatric and adult use. The adult device contains 4 mL (20 mg) of diazepam gel and has a 6-cm tip for rectal administration. This device is designed to deliver set doses of 10, 12.5, 15, 17.5, and 20 mg of diazepam. Two pediatric devices are available: one contains 0.5 mL of a 5-mg/mL gel, and the other contains 2 mL of a 5-mg/mL gel. The latter is designed to deliver set doses of 5, 7.5, and 10 mg of diazepam. Both pediatric devices have a 4.4-cm tip for rectal administration. The recommended dose of diazepam rectal gel for treating actively seizing children and those in status epilepticus is 0.5 mg/kg, followed by 0.25 mg/kg in 10 minutes if needed (maximum dose, 20 mg); the adult dose is 10 mg, which may be repeated once (see Table 26-3).

Antiemetics

Antiemetics are frequently used in the ED for patients with nausea and vomiting. In most cases, these medications are given intravenously. However, for patients with mild symptoms who do not otherwise require IV access and for discharged patients expected to have ongoing nausea and vomiting (e.g., patients with a viral gastroenteritis), rectal administration is a reasonable alternative. Rectal administration may also be used as the initial treatment of ED patients with active vomiting in whom IV access will be delayed, such as those requiring central venous access.

The two most common antiemetics administered rectally in the ED are prochlorperazine and promethazine. Both come in suppository formulations, which makes rectal administration easy. Prochlorperazine requires a higher dose when given rectally, whereas promethazine dosing is the same regardless of the route of administration (see Table 26-3).

Cation Exchange Resin

The most commonly available cation exchange resin is sodium polystyrene sulfonate (Kayexalate). In the gut, sodium polystyrene sulfonate absorbs potassium and releases sodium. Each gram of resin may bind as much as 1 mEq of potassium and release 1 to 2 mEq of sodium. In the ED, Kayexalate is frequently given to patients with hyperkalemia as a temporizing measure before dialysis.

Sodium polystyrene sulfonate may be given orally or rectally as a retention enema. Oral dosing is more effective if intestinal motility is not impaired. Common reasons for rectal administration include an inability or refusal to swallow (the oral solution is not very palatable), vomiting, and altered mental status. The resin comes in two forms: a powder that must be reconstituted and a premixed suspension containing sorbitol. The latter should be avoided whenever possible because it has been linked to the development of intestinal necrosis.[116,117] Nevertheless, sodium polystyrene sulfonate in sorbitol remains the most frequently used preparation in the ED.[118]

Before drug administration, perform a cleansing enema with warm tap water. Prepare a sodium polystyrene sulfonate enema by dissolving 50 g of the resin in 100 to 150 mL of tap water warmed to body temperature. In adults, administer the resin emulsion via a 6- or 8-Fr rubber feeding tube placed about 20 cm from the rectum with the tip well into the sigmoid colon. Retain the enema in the colon for at least 30 to 60 minutes and for several hours if possible. Once retention is complete, irrigate the colon with 50 to 100 mL of a non-sodium-containing fluid. The recommended dose of sodium polystyrene sulfonate for rectal administration in adults is 30 to 50 g every 6 hours. For older children, the dose is 1 g/kg per dose every 2 to 6 hours. Use lower doses in small children and infants. To calculate this dose, use the exchange ratio of 1 mEq K^+/g of resin (see Table 26-3).

Complications

In general, systemic complications of rectally administered medications are the same as for other routes of administration. Complications specific to rectal administration include erratic absorption and local trauma.

Absorption of a rectally administered drug may be delayed or prolonged, or uptake may be almost as rapid as though the agent were administered intravenously.[99] Unusually rapid absorption has resulted in the death of a $7\frac{1}{2}$-month-old child receiving rectal morphine for postoperative pain.[119] In addition to erratic absorption, peak serum concentrations may vary considerably depending on how much of the drug undergoes first-pass elimination in the liver. These factors make rectal drug administration less desirable in most cases when parenteral administration is possible.

Insertion of a suppository or catheter into the rectum may cause mild pain and mucosal irritation, which is usually well tolerated by most patients. Similarly, bleeding from local trauma is usually of no clinical consequence, except in patients with a clinically significant coagulopathy or severe thrombocytopenia.[100] Development of a perianal or perirectal abscess is a theoretical concern in neutropenic patients, and thus rectal drug administration is best avoided in such patients.

References are available at www.expertconsult.com

CHAPTER 27

Autotransfusion

Mark J. Neavyn, Margarita E. Pena, and Charlene Irvin Babcock

INTRODUCTION

Autologous blood transfusion, or autotransfusion, is the collection and reinfusion of a patient's own blood for volume replacement.[1] Preoperative blood banking and intraoperative cell salvage techniques have increased in a multitude of surgical specialties.[2-7] Autotransfusion in the emergency department (ED) is usually limited to patients with severe, traumatic hemothorax and clinically significant blood loss.

Autotransfusion is usually performed in trauma centers or in EDs with high trauma volume. Though not a uniform standard of care, it is applicable to any ED. Since the procedure requires familiarity with the equipment, continuing education, and quality control, it may be counterproductive to institute it in a hospital that has a low trauma census or in a setting in which it will be used infrequently enough that staff education issues are problematic. Clinicians practicing in more austere environments with a paucity of clinical resources, such as combat and disaster zones, may find that the procedure's benefits outweigh its risks.[8-10]

BACKGROUND

Reports of autotransfusion can be found as early as 1818 when Blundell, an English practitioner, reinfused shed blood after witnessing a woman exsanguinate from uterine hemorrhage.[11] In 1886, Duncan published the first known human account of autotransfusion in which he reinfused shed blood in a patient with a traumatic amputation without any notable ill effects.[12] In 1917, Elmendorf published a description of the first case of autotransfusion in a patient with traumatic hemothorax.[13]

The discovery of ABO blood typing at the turn of the century and the institution of blood banks in the 1930s led to the almost exclusive use of allogeneic (homologous) blood up to and following World War II. During the 1960s and 1970s,

Autotransfusion

Indications

Hemothorax containing >1500 mL
Hemothorax with an immediate need for transfusion and insufficient allogeneic blood available
Hemothorax with an urgent need for blood and the patient's religious beliefs prohibit the use of banked blood

Contraindications

Coagulopathy or disseminated intravascular cougulation
Possibility of malignant cells in the salvaged blood
Active infection
Gross contamination of pleural blood from gastrointestinal contents

Complications

Hematologic

Decreased platelet count
Decreased fibrinogen level
Increased fibrin split products
Prolonged prothrombin time
Prolonged partial thromboplastin time
Red blood cell hemolysis
Elevated plasma free hemoglobin
Decreased hematocrit

Nonhematologic

Bacteremia
Sepsis
Microembolism
Air embolism
Renal insufficiency

Equipment

Chest drainage and autotransfusion system.
*(Atrium Ocean ATS shown above,
Atrium Medical Corporation, Hudson, NH)*

Review Box 27-1 Autotransfusion: indications, contraindications, complications, and equipment.

cardiopulmonary bypass surgery and combat trauma experience during the Vietnam War generated extensive data regarding intraoperative retrieval of large quantities of blood for reinfusion.[14-17] This revitalized interest, coupled with increased experience in surgical, trauma, and combat situations, has thus initiated a new era in autotransfusion.

ANATOMY

Hemothorax refers to a collection of blood within the pleural space. Severe hemorrhage is more often associated with laceration of vessels on the inside of the chest wall, such as the internal mammary and intercostal arteries. Blunt trauma and penetrating trauma are by far the most common causes of hemothorax. Spontaneous hemothorax can occur secondary to intrathoracic malignancy,[18] pulmonary infarction, bullous emphysema, virulent pulmonary or mediastinal infection, vascular malformation, and endometriosis of the pleura (catamenial).[19]

PATHOPHYSIOLOGY

The pathophysiologic sequelae of hemothorax include both hemodynamic instability and respiratory compromise. The pleural cavity can accommodate more than 50% of the total blood volume, so clinically significant intrathoracic blood loss can occur with minimal external signs of bleeding. The clinician should suspect hemothorax in the setting of chest trauma with clinical signs of hypovolemia. Physical examination may demonstrate decreased breath sounds and reduced tactile fremitus. Imaging during the initial resuscitation period is usually limited to supine chest radiographs, which may show haziness in the affected lung field as blood layers in the posterior pleural space (Fig. 27-1). Ultrasound is also useful in the initial evaluation of hemothorax (Fig. 27-2).[20] Tube thoracostomy is the treatment of choice for acute hemothorax, with thoracotomy and video-assisted thoracic surgery performed as indicated for severe or ongoing hemorrhage.

ADVANTAGES

Shed blood from traumatic hemothorax is immediately available for rapid transfusion. The blood is normothermic and compatible, which avoids the risk of allergic reaction or infection from transfusion transmissible diseases. There are numerous transfusion transmissible diseases, including viruses such as human immunodeficiency virus and hepatitis, bacteria, parasites, and most recently reported, variant Creutzfeldt-Jakob disease.[21,22] Although the risk for transfusion transmissible diseases has decreased dramatically in developed countries, it is still very problematic worldwide.[23] Immunologic transfusion reactions and posttransfusion sepsis continue to be risks as well.[24] In trauma patients, allogeneic transfusions have been shown to be an independent risk factor for infection,[25-28] which may be dose dependent and independently associated with increased morbidity and mortality.[28-30] In patients whose religious convictions (e.g., Jehovah's Witness) prohibit transfusions with homologous blood, reinfusion of autologous blood that does not involve blood storage may be an acceptable alternative.[31]

Autologous blood provides societal benefits by preserving the limited stores of banked blood and reducing the cost of medical care.[32-34] Adias and colleagues compared the direct cost of banked blood with the cost of autologous blood transfusion and found substantial savings with autotransfusion.[35] Box 27-1 summarizes the advantages of autotransfusion.

INDICATIONS

In general, all victims of severe trauma, whether blunt or penetrating, should be considered potential candidates for autotransfusion. Several categories of patients for whom emergency autotransfusion is suitable have been described and are summarized in Review Box 27-1. Reul and associates described the ideal autotransfusion candidate as a blunt or penetrating trauma victim with hemothorax consisting of 1500 mL or more of blood.[41] Other patients who may benefit include those with an immediate need for transfusion for whom insufficient homologous blood is available (because of a shortage or a difficult crossmatch) and those whose religious convictions prohibit homologous transfusion.[36,39,40]

Figure 27-1 Hemothorax secondary to a gunshot wound. Note the haziness over the right hemithorax with the bullet seen in the right upper lobe. In this supine radiograph the volume of the hemothorax may not be fully appreciated. *(From JA Marx. Rosen's Emergency Medicine. 7th ed. St. Louis: Mosby; 2009.)*

Figure 27-2 Ultrasonographic appearance of hemothorax. Blood in the pleural cavity appears anechoic (*arrow*) and is easily seen interspersed between the collapsed lung and diaphragm.

BOX 27-1   Advantages of Autotransfusion

1. Immediately available—no delay in crossmatching and no storage required
2. Blood compatibility and allergic reaction not an issue
3. Autologous blood usually normothermic
4. No risk for transfusion transmissible disease
5. No risk for hypocalcemia or hyperkalemia[36,37]
6. Decreased risk for acute respiratory distress syndrome
7. Higher levels of 2,3-diphosphoglycerate than in banked red blood cells[38]
8. Decreased use of banked blood; more available for subsequent patients in need[34]
9. Decreased cost of medical care[32-34]
10. May be acceptable to religions opposed to homologous blood transfusions[36,39,40]
11. May be a valuable alternative to banked blood in developing countries where infected donor blood is a problem

---

CONTRAINDICATIONS

In some situations emergency autotransfusion may pose more risk than benefit. Coagulopathy and disseminated intravascular coagulation (DIC) are important contraindications.[8,42] Others include active infection, gross contamination, and the possibility of malignant cells in the salvaged blood.[43] With direct autotransfusion of pleural blood through a microfilter, the risk of reinfusing tumor cells is unknown. However, recent work using perioperative cell salvage suggests that the risk for dissemination of malignant disease is minimal.[44] Concerns regarding gross contamination from concomitant gastrointestinal tract injury have also been disputed.[45] An early study of autotransfusion before cell washing was implemented found that despite reinfusion of massively contaminated blood, 17 of 25 patients survived without evidence of septic complications.[46]

Recent work on contamination involving cell salvage systems incorporates a cell-washing step.[47,48] Several investigators believe that reinfusion of limited amounts of contaminated blood from the peritoneal cavity may now be accomplished with acceptable risk. Nonetheless, the current consensus is that exsanguinating hemorrhage without available homologous blood is the only acceptable indication for autotransfusion when there is recognized intestinal contamination.[49-51] Concurrent use of systemic antibiotics is advised.[8,9,47,48,51,52]

Autotransfusion should be performed within 4 to 6 hours from the time of injury,[37,53] although it has been performed after this period in combat situations without significant complications.[8,48]

EQUIPMENT AND MATERIAL
Blood Filters

In-line filtration is used routinely during reinfusion of blood products to reduce the danger of microembolization and resultant pulmonary insufficiency.[1,37,53] The relationship between the presence of microaggregates and the development of acute respiratory distress syndrome is controversial.[1] However, most investigators advise the use of a micropore filter with pore size recommendations ranging from 20 to

170 μm.[54-56] The majority of investigators believe that a pore size of 40 μm minimizes the risk for microembolization without undue elevation in filtration pressure.[41,57,58] The manufacturers of the commercial devices discussed in this chapter also recommend at least a 40-μm filter size.

Vacuum Suction

The level of vacuum suction should be limited to minimize hemolysis of red blood cells.[58] The precise level at which clinically significant hemolysis occurs is uncertain, and there is wide variation (5 to 100 mm Hg) in recommendations.[14,41,55,59-61] Several commercial products recommend a starting vacuum pressure of 20 mm Hg.[62]

Anticoagulation

Blood retrieved from the pleural and abdominal cavities frequently will not clot because it is devoid of fibrinogen.[63] This is believed to be due to the fact that moderate rates of bleeding allow time for defibrination by contact with the serosal surfaces and by mechanical agitation from respiratory and cardiac movement. For this reason, some recommend simple reinfusion through a filter without any anticoagulant.[17,54,60,64] However, wounds of the great vessels may bleed at a rate that allows coagulable blood to enter the collection reservoir and clot the entire system.[52,60,61] In the ED setting where autotransfusion is indicated for rapid blood loss, anticoagulation is recommended.

The use of heparin as an anticoagulant in trauma patients is not recommended by the manufacturers of autotransfusion devices.[62] Heparin anticoagulation is possible; however, local heparinization of the tubing and reservoir may lead to the formation of platelet microaggregates on the filter and in the line, as well as increase the risk for systemic heparinization.[41,65]

Citrate compounds, an alternative to heparin, are frequently recommended for autotransfusion.[42] Citrates bind with the calcium ion and prevent conversion of protein fibrinogen into insoluble fibrin, which would cause the blood to clot. Because citrate binds only with calcium, it anticoagulates just the blood in which it is dissolved. Once the anticoagulated blood is infused, citrate is rapidly metabolized by the liver. Early studies used acid citrate dextrose (ACD).[37] More recently, citrate phosphate dextrose (CPD) has been used because it necessitates less volume as an anticoagulant and results in less acidosis than ACD.[41,66,67] Rarely, excessive use of CPD can cause cardiac dysrhythmias.[41] Moreover, use of insufficient or outdated CPD may result in clotting of collected blood. Baldan and colleagues described the use of simple autotransfusion in more than 200 patients with penetrating chest injuries and recommended using half-dose citrate phosphate dextrose adenine (CPDA) solution.[9] Although anticoagulant therapy and dosage recommendations are at the discretion of the physician, commercially available devices do offer some general guidelines (Table 27-1).

Historical Techniques Using Standard ED Equipment

Before purpose-built systems were available, autotransfusion was possible by using common items available in most EDs. These techniques have not been as widely tested and are more appropriate for use in dire situations, such as may occur in a disaster or on the battlefield.[9]

Symbas described a simplified collecting system involving a standard chest tube bottle.[68] More than 400 patients were autotransfused via this method with no adverse effects attributable to the procedure. After insertion of a chest tube, blood was collected into a standard bottle containing 400 mL of normal saline, with suction maintained at 12 to 16 mm Hg. The blood collected in the chest bottle can be reinfused in one of two possible ways as shown in Figure 27-3. Improvements on his historical technique, such as the addition of anticoagulation and blood filters, should be considered.

Autotransfusion Units

All the commercially available autotransfusion systems (ATSs) are based on the same three-stage system (called the "three-bottle system") for collection of pleural fluid (Fig. 27-4). Currently used devices incorporate the three-bottle system into one unit. Stage 1 is the collection of pleural fluid (blood). Stage 2 is the water seal stage, in which water acts as a one-way valve (water seal) that allows air to be sucked out of the pleural space but not leak back in. Stage 3 is the suction control stage, which is essentially a safety stage so that if the degree of suction suddenly increases beyond the set point, the system will pull air from the atmosphere instead of inappropriately increasing suction in the pleural cavity. Historically, water was (and still frequently is) used in the suction control stage.

The disadvantage of using water in stages 2 or 3 is that if the device is knocked over, loss of the water seal and spillage of water from the suction control stage can occur. Newer designs have solved this problem, and two systems currently available do not use water (Atrium Express and Pleur-evac Sahara). These newer devices use a one-way valve instead of a water seal in stage 2 and a pressure regulator instead of water in the suction control stage (stage 3). Table 27-2 describes features of several of the more commonly used devices.

To collect blood for autotransfusion, a collection bag can be connected beforehand in series with the chest drainage system. With this arrangement, blood goes from the patient to the blood collection bag to the chest drainage system. When the

TABLE 27-1 ACD-A and CPD Dosage Recommendations

BLOOD VOLUME EXPECTED	FOR 1:7, ADD THIS AMOUNT OF ACD-A	FOR 1:20, ADD THIS AMOUNT OF ACD-A
ACD-A DOSAGE RECOMMENDATIONS* (RATIO OF ACD-A TO BLOOD)		
Low = 140-250 mL	20-35 mL	7-12 mL
Incremental volume over 250 mL	1 mL for each 100 mL of collected blood	5 mL for each 100 mL of blood collected
Medium = 250-500 mL	40-70 mL	12.5-25 mL
High = 500-1000 mL	70-140 mL	25-50 mL
CPD DOSAGE RECOMMENDATIONS		
Anticoagulant CPD solution can be added at the discretion of the physician at a control dosage of 14 mL of CPD solution to 100 mL of blood collected (70 mL CPD/500 mL blood)		

From *A Personal Guide to Managing Chest Drainage Autotransfusion.* Atrium Medical Corporation, pp 26, 27; available at http://www.atriummed.com/PDF/Red%20Handbook.pdf.
ACD-A, Acid Citrate Dextrose anticoagulant; *CPD,* citrate phosphate dextrose.
*Dosage ratios are approximate. Note that 35 mL of ACD-A provides a 1:7 ratio of ACD-A to blood for low volume and a 1:20 ratio for high-volume blood and may be a good starting point if it is unclear how much blood will accumulate.

Figure 27-3 Historical technique of autotransfusion for traumatic hemothorax. **A,** Blood is collected into a sterile blood collection bottle with 400 mL of normal saline. **B,** After blood is collected, the chest tube is disconnected from the collection bottle. **C,** Blood is infused directly from the blood collection bottle while a new chest tube drainage bottle is connected to the chest tube, or **D,** blood collected from the chest tube is transferred into a sterile blood bag. **E,** Blood transferred into the blood bag is infused into the patient. (*From Symbas PN. Extraoperative autotransfusion from hemothorax. Surgery. 1978;84:722.*)

blood bag is filled, it is removed and replaced with a new blood collection bag. If the bag overfills, the fluid will spill into the usual chest fluid collection system. Eventually, when no more blood needs to be autotransfused, the blood collection bag is taken out of the series and the chest tube drainage system

functions as usual. Because blood goes directly into the blood collection bag, anticoagulant needs to be added to the blood collection bag before the blood flows into it.

Blood may also be drawn directly from a chest drainage system. Some devices have an additional port at the bottom called an ATS access line. This is referred to as a self-filling ATS. Not all devices permit withdrawal of blood directly from the chest drainage system. In devices without this option, any blood that goes into the chest drainage system is not available for transfusion. The advantage of the ATS access line is that autotransfusion need not be anticipated before the chest tube collection system is connected to the chest tube. Because blood first goes to the collection chamber of the chest drainage device, anticoagulant needs to be added to the collection chamber before blood enters it.

Some models allow these chest drainage systems to be connected directly to the patient to provide continuous autotransfusion. In this setup, a blood filter with intravenous (IV) blood tubing is hooked up to an IV infusion pump. The blood can then be continuously reinfused as it collects in the chest drainage system; it goes from the blood collection chamber out the ATS access line and is pumped into the patient with an IV infusion pump in a closed system (Fig. 27-5). Other models offer continuous infusion directly from a blood collection bag and not the chest drainage device. The blood simply goes from the chest tube into the blood collection bag, and a port on the bag is accessed to return the blood back to the patient.

Figure 27-4 Three-bottle chest drainage system. *A,* From the patient's chest tube. *B,* Connection to a water seal bottle (stage 2). *C,* Connection to the suction control bottle. *D,* Connection to suction. *E,* Vent tube for suction control.

TABLE 27-2	Chest Drainage Devices for Autotransfusion					
	OCEAN 2000 SERIES	**OASIS 3600 SERIES**	**EXPRESS 4000 SERIES**	**A-7000, A-8000 SERIES**	**A-6000**	**SAHARA S-1100**
Designer	Atrium	Atrium	Atrium	Pleur-evac	Pleur-evac	Pleur-evac
Company	Atrium*	Atrium*	Atrium*	Teleflex[†]	Teleflex[†]	Teleflex[†]
Water seal stage	Water based	Water based	Dry one-way valve	Water based	Water based	Dry one-way valve
Suction control seal	Water based	Dry one-way valve	Dry one- way valve	Water based	Dry regulator valve	Dry regulator valve
If tipped over	Loss of water seal, spillage of water into the suction control chamber	Loss of water seal	No problem	Loss of water seal, spillage of water into the suction control chamber	Loss of water seal	No problem
Blood for reinfusion can be withdrawn directly from the chest drainage system	Yes, Model 2050	Yes, Model 3650	Yes, Model 4050	No	No	No
Comments	24/7 help by telephone*	24/7 help by phone*	24/7 help by phone*	8 AM-7 PM EST by telephone[†]	8 AM-7 PM EST by telephone[†]	8 AM-7 PM EST by telephone[†]
Continuous transfusion capability	Yes, Model 2050—directly from the unit to the patient	Yes, Model 3650—directly from the unit to the patient	Yes, Model 4050—directly from the unit to the patient	No	Yes, Model A9250—from the blood collection bag to the patient	Yes, Models S1150 and S1152—from the blood collection bag to the patient

*Atrium: (800) 528-7486; www.atriummed.com.
[†]Teleflex: (919) 544-8000; http://www.teleflexmedical.com.

Figure 27-5 Continuous autotransfusion. Blood is continuously reinfused into the patient as it collects in the chest drainage system. *ATS,* autotransfusion system. *(Courtesy of Atrium Medical Corporation, Hudson, NH.)*

Pleur-evac® A-7000/A-8000
A Carrying handle
B High-negativity relief valve
C High-negativity float valve
  and relief chamber
D Collection chamber
E Patient air leak meter
  (A-7000 only)
F Calibrated water seal
G Self-sealing diaphragm in
  water seal chamber
H Suction control chamber
I Positive pressure relief valve

Pleur-evac® A-6000
A Carrying handle
B High-negativity relief valve
C High-negativity float valve
  and relief chamber
D Collection chamber
E Patient air leak meter
F Calibrated water seal
G Self-sealing diaphragm
H Suction control dial
I Suction control indicator
  window with fluorescent float
J Positive pressure relief valve

Pleur-evac® Sahara
A-1 Suction dial
A-2 Suction indicator
A-3 Negative pressure indicator
B-1 Air leak diagnostics
B-2 Needleless injection site
B-3 Positive pressure relief valve
B-4 Filtered high-negativity relief valve
C-1 Collection chamber.

Figure 27-6 Pleur-evac chest drainage systems. *(Courtesy of Teleflex Medical, Research Triangle Park, NC.)*

PROCEDURE FOR AUTOTRANSFUSION

Whether in-line, self-filling, or continuous techniques are chosen depends on the chest tube drainage system used. Some systems allow more than one technique to collect blood for autotransfusion. The specific port locations and connections may vary slightly among the different designs, but the general concepts are relatively universal. See Figures 27-6 and 27-7 for a description of several different systems from Atrium and Pleur-evac.

A. Atrium Ocean water seal chest drain

B. Atrium Oasis dry suction chest drain

C. Atrium Express chest drain

D. Atrium ATS continuous autotransfusion system

Figure 27-7 Atrium chest drainage systems. *ATS,* autotransfusion system. *(Courtesy of Atrium Medical Corporation, Hudson, NH.)*

ATRIUM IN-LINE AUTOTRANSFUSION: BLOOD COLLECTION

1

Chest tube connector
Chest tube clamp
Protective caps
Drainage system connector
Autotransfusion blood bag
Bag clamps

Hang the autotransfusion blood bag on the chest drain. Close both autotransfusion blood bag clamps and remove the protective caps. Close the patient chest tube clamp.

2

Move the clamp next to the connector. Close before separation of the connector.

Chest tube connector
Drainage system connector

Depress the connector lock and pull the tube up to separate the connector.

Separate the connectors between the patient's chest tube connector and the Ocean chest drainage system by depressing the connector lock.

3

Drainage system connector
Male bag connector
Chest tube connector
Female bag connector

Insert the male chest tube connector into the female bag connector, and the male bag connector into the female drainage system connector. Open the clamps in the 1-2-3 sequence depicted above. Blood will then flow from the chest tube into the blood bag. Once the bag is full (600 mL), close the patient chest tube clamp and both bag clamps.

4

Connect the blood bag connectors to each other.
Reconnect the chest tube connector to the drainage system and then open the clamp.
Keep the blood bag clamps closed.

First disconnect the blood bag from the drainage system and then disconnect the blood bag from the chest tube connector. Attach the chest tube connector to the drainage system, and attach the blood bag connectors to each other. Open the chest tube clamp so that drainage resumes into the drainage system.

Refer to text for instructions on how to infuse the collected blood.

Figure 27-8 Atrium in-line autotransfusion: blood collection. *(Courtesy of Atrium Medical Corporation, Hudson, NH.)*

Atrium Chest Drainage Devices

The procedure described here is for the Ocean model; however, all Atrium models have similar connectors.

In-Line Autotransfusion Blood Collection and Infusion Procedure (Fig. 27-8)

1. Place the autotransfusion blood bag onto the chest drain via the attached flexible hanger.

2. Close both autotransfusion blood bag clamps and remove the protective caps over the autotransfusion bag connectors.

3. Close the patient's chest tube clamp.

4. Separate the connectors between the patient's chest tube and the Ocean chest drain by depressing the connector lock.

5. Insert the male patient chest tube connector into the female autotransfusion bag connector.

6. Insert the male autotransfusion bag connector into the female Ocean chest drain connector.
7. Open the clamps in the following order:
   a. Open the autotransfusion bag clamp going to the Ocean chest drain.
   b. Open the autotransfusion bag clamp going to the patient's chest tube.
   c. Open the patient's chest tube clamp to resume drainage. (Blood will then flow from the patient's chest tube into the autotransfusion blood bag.)
8. When the blood bag is filled (600 mL maximum), close the patient's chest tube clamp and both autotransfusion blood bag clamps.
9. Disconnect the autotransfusion blood bag connection with the Ocean chest drain connection first.
10. Disconnect the autotransfusion blood bag from the patient's chest tube connector.
11. Insert the male patient chest tube connector into the female Ocean chest drain connector.
12. Open the patient's chest tube clamp so that drainage may resume into the Ocean chest drain device.
13. Connect the male and female autotransfusion bag connectors to each other.
14. Connect and pre-prime the blood filter and the IV blood tubing with sterile saline (spike the blood tubing into the filter).
15. Invert the autotransfusion bag so that the spike port at the bottom points upward.
16. Remove the tethered cap with sterile technique.
17. Insert the saline-primed filter spike into the autotransfusion bag spike port with a firm twisting motion.
18. Return the autotransfusion bag to an upright position and place it on a standard IV pole.
19. Open the filtered air vent located on top of the autotransfusion bag first, and then open the IV tubing clamp.
20. Evacuate all the remaining air from the IV line and attach it to the patient to begin the infusion.
21. For gravity infusion, leave the air vent at the top of the autotransfusion bag open.
22. For pressure infuser application, the filtered air vent must remain closed (the maximum ATS bag infuser pressure is 150 mm Hg).

Self-Filling Autotransfusion Blood Collection and Infusion Procedure

1. Identify the chest drain ATS access line (at the bottom of the collection chamber of the Ocean chest drain), and close the ATS access line clamp (Fig. 27-9).
2. Remove the spike port cap of the ATS access line and insert the autotransfusion bag spike into the Ocean ATS access line spike port with a firm twisting motion.
3. Position the autotransfusion bag at least 2 to 4 inches below the base of the Ocean chest drain.
4. Open the clamps to the autotransfusion blood bag (on the ATS access line and on the autotransfusion blood bag).
5. Activate the autotransfusion bag spring-generated vacuum by gently bending the autotransfusion bag upward where indicated to initiate transfer of blood. A "pop" will be heard and the bag will expand when properly activated. The self-filling autotransfusion bag will begin to fill and expand as blood enters from the chest drain. Do not

Figure 27-9 The chest drain autotransfusion system (ATS) access line is found at the bottom of the drainage system. *(Courtesy of Atrium Medical Corporation, Hudson, NH.)*

Figure 27-10 Activation of the self-filling Atrium autotransfusion bag. *(Courtesy of Atrium Medical Corporation, Hudson, NH.)*

activate the autotransfusion bag before connecting it to the chest drain (Fig. 27-10).
6. Displace any air in the autotransfusion bag by gently squeezing the autotransfusion bag as necessary.
7. When the autotransfusion blood bag is filled (700-mL capacity), close both the ATS access line clamp and the autotransfusion blood bag clamp and cap the end of the ATS access line.
8. Remove the autotransfusion blood bag spike from the ATS access line spike port and place the spike back into the original bag port. Position the ATS access line in the holder on top of the Ocean chest drain. Keep the ATS access line clamp fully closed at all times when not in use.

9. Connect the filter to the IV blood infusion set (spike the filter with the blood tubing spike) and pre-prime the blood filter and IV blood tubing with sterile saline.
10. Invert the autotransfusion bag so that the spike port at the bottom of the autotransfusion bag points upward.
11. Remove the tethered cap via sterile technique.
12. Insert the saline-primed filter spike into the autotransfusion bag spike port with a firm twisting motion.
13. Return the autotransfusion bag to an upright position and place it on a standard IV pole.
14. Open the filtered air vent located at the top of the autotransfusion bag first, and then open the IV line clamp.
15. Evacuate all the remaining air from the IV line and attach it to the patient to begin infusion.
16. For gravity infusion, leave the air vent at the top of the ATS bag open.
17. For pressure infuser application, the filtered air vent must remain closed (the maximum ATS bag infuser pressure is 150 mm Hg).

Continuous Autotransfusion (Fig. 27-11)

For direct reinfusion of shed autologous blood via a blood-compatible infusion pump, a microemboli blood filter and nonvented, blood-compatible IV administration set must be used.

1. Spike the blood IV tubing set into the filter and prime it with sterile saline.
2. Identify the chest drain ATS access line at the bottom of the Ocean chest drain and close the ATS access line clamp (see Fig. 27-9).
3. Drape the ATS access line around the hanger or the patient's line so that the terminal end of the ATS access line is facing the floor.
4. Remove the spike port cap on the ATS access line and insert the blood filter spike into the ATS access line.
5. Turn the filter to a "spike down" position.
6. Unclamp the ATS access line and IV tubing.
7. Use a 60-mL syringe to aspirate blood through the filter and into the drip chamber of the IV tubing set.
8. When the drip chamber is ¼ full, turn the filter to the "spike up" position and continue purging air from the line.
9. When purging is complete, insert the IV cassette into the pump.
10. Purge all air before connection to the patient.
11. Set the pump to the desired volume and rate (mL/hr) to be infused.
12. Watch the infusion carefully and make sure that the infusion pump is programmed to stop before all the blood in the Ocean chest drain is empty to prevent air embolism.

Pleur-evac Chest Drainage Devices

All Pleur-evac models have similar designs. The method described here is for the Sahara design.[69]

In-Line Blood Collection and Autotransfusion Procedure

1. Close the two clamps on the top of the autotransfusion bag (Fig 27-12).
2. Attach the autotransfusion bag to the side of the chest drain device by aligning the bottom leg and the lever of

Figure 27-11 Infusion pump setup for continuous autotransfusion. Note the intravenous (IV) tubing with the microemboli blood filter in the "spike up" position. *A,* Autotransfusion system (ATS) access line. *B,* End of the ATS access line. *C,* Blood filter. *D,* IV tubing with the spike port in the upward position. *E,* Blood-compatible IV infusion pump. *G,* Patient IV access. *(Courtesy of Atrium Medical Corporation, Hudson, NH.)*

Figure 27-12 Pleur-evac Sahara in-line autotransfusion setup. *(Courtesy of Teleflex Medical, Research Triangle Park, NC.)*

the adapter with their mating receptacles on the chest drain system. Insert with a downward motion until the lever "clicks" into position. The autotransfusion bag should be firmly attached to the chest drain device (Fig. 27-13).
3. Close the clamp on the patient's chest tube and disconnect the red and blue connectors separating the patient's chest tube from the chest drainage device.
4. Remove the red protective cap from the autotransfusion bag tube and connect this end to the patient's chest tube.
5. Remove the blue protective cap from the autotransfusion collection bag tube and connect this end to the chest drainage device (red connected to red and blue connected to blue).
6. Open all the clamps. The autotransfusion blood bag will begin to fill.

Pleur-evac SAHARA system
with attached autotransfusion bag

Figure 27-13 Pleur-evac Sahara in-line autotransfusion setup with the autotransfusion bag attached to the chest drain device. *(Courtesy of Teleflex Medical, Research Triangle Park, NC.)*

7. To discontinue autotransfusion, first reduce excessive negative pressure with the high-negativity relief valve on the Sahara chest drain.
8. Close the clamp on the patient's chest tube, and then close both clamps on the autotransfusion bag.
9. Separate the red connectors going to the patient's chest tube and the blue connectors going to the Sahara chest drain.
10. Connect the red and blue connectors on the autotransfusion bag.
11. Join the patient's chest tube red connector to the Sahara chest drain blue connector.
12. Open the clamp on the patient's chest tube so that drainage from the patient to the Sahara chest drain may resume.
13. Remove the autotransfusion bag from the Sahara chest drain by depressing the lever and lifting the autotransfusion bag up.
14. Remove the adaptor bracket from the wire frame of the autotransfusion bag by twisting it slightly to disengage the bottom and then unhook the top.
15. Slide the autotransfusion bag off the wire support frame. Make sure that the red and blue connectors on the top of the autotransfusion bag are secure and that the clamps on the autotransfusion bag are closed.
16. Connect the filter and IV blood tubing (spike the filter with the IV blood tubing spike).
17. Invert the autotransfusion bag so that the spike port points upward and then remove the protective cap.
18. Insert the filter (use the spike end of the filter) into the spike port on the autotransfusion bag.
19. Evacuate residual air from the autotransfusion bag by opening the IV infusion set clamp, keep the autotransfusion bag inverted, and carefully squeeze all the air from the autotransfusion bag through the filter and IV line.
20. Continue to squeeze the autotransfusion bag to allow blood to slowly prime the filter. Continue squeezing until the filter is saturated with blood and the drip chamber on the IV tubing is half full.
21. Close the IV clamp.

22. Invert the autotransfusion bag and suspend it from an IV pole.
23. Open the IV infusion line clamp to carefully flush all the blood tubing of any remaining air.
24. Attach the distal end of the infusion set to the patient's IV line and begin infusion.

Continuous Infusion

1. Set up a blood-compatible IV pump.
2. Connect the filter to the IV blood tubing (spike the blood tubing into the filter), and then connect it to a bag of saline (spike the filter into the saline bag). Prime the filter, drip chamber, and IV blood tubing with the sterile saline bag. Remove the bag of saline used to prime it.
3. Remove the blue protective cap from the autotransfusion bag and spike the autotransfusion bag with the blood filter spike.
4. Use an IV pump to prime the filter, drip chamber, and infusion line with blood.
5. If needed, depress the high-negativity relief valve on the top of the Sahara chest drain to relieve excessive negative pressure.
6. Make sure that the infusion line is filled with blood and contains no air, and then attach it to the patient's IV catheter.
7. Make sure that all the connections are secure.
8. Set the infusion rate on the IV pump.
9. Attach the Sahara drain and the autotransfusion bag to the bed rail with hangers.

COMPLICATIONS

In general, complications from autotransfusion are clinically insignificant if proper technique is followed. Complications may be categorized as hematologic and nonhematologic (Review Box 27-1).

Hematologic Complications

The degree to which autotransfusion contributes to the development or exacerbation of coagulopathy in an actively bleeding patient has still not been conclusively determined.[70]

Broadie and coworkers found that blood collected from trauma victims during thoracotomy or laparotomy had markedly elevated prothrombin, partial thromboplastin, and thrombin times, as well as absent fibrinogen.[63] The dilemma is that severely injured trauma patients who are candidates for autotransfusion are more likely to have other independent risk factors for coagulopathy, such as hypothermia and acidosis. Horst and colleagues studied 154 trauma patients who underwent intraoperative autotransfusion and found that patients who received more than 15 units of autologous blood or more than 50 units of combined autologous and banked blood were coagulopathic but also more severely injured, hypothermic, and acidotic.[71] Although coagulation test abnormalities following the infusion of salvaged blood have been interpreted as evidence of DIC, these changes are probably the result of infusion of fibrin degradation products and do not represent consumptive coagulopathy.[72] In general, even though coagulopathy should be anticipated, it has not proved to be clinically important when volumes of autotransfused blood remain below 1500 to 2000 mL in adult patients.[73,74] When reinfused

---

BOX 27-2 **General Autotransfusion Information**

1. Use each liner bag only once.
2. Insert a new filter for each autotransfusion bag used.
3. To minimize risk for bacterial overgrowth, blood collected must be reinfused within 6 hours from the time of injury.*
4. After reinfusing a total of 3500 mL (about 7 units) of autologous blood, it has been suggested that 1 unit of fresh frozen plasma be given for every 2 units (about 1000 mL) of autotransfused blood.[41]
5. If some or all of the collected blood becomes clotted in the liner bag, the blood should be discarded.
6. To reduce the risk for air embolism, remove all the air from the bag with the collected blood before hanging it for reinfusion.[76]

The American Association of Blood Banks suggests no more than a 6-hour shelf life between collection and reinfusion.[53] The age of blood collected should be calculated from time of injury. Blood reinfused after this time should be considered hazardous.

---

volumes exceed 3500 mL, laboratory evidence of dilutional coagulopathy may become evident.[56] When volumes of autotransfused blood are greater that the patient's total blood volume, animal studies suggest that the risk for a true consumptive coagulopathy is increased.[38]

Recommendations regarding the volume of autologous blood that should trigger the infusion of plasma or platelets range from 25% of the total blood volume (about 1250 mL in a 70-kg adult) to 3500 mL[56,75] (Box 27-2). Others advise reliance on laboratory tests and clinical findings rather than a volume-based protocol.[38] Prudent clinical judgment dictates application of the more liberal guidelines for replacement therapy in patients with extensive hepatic injury, intractable shock, or ongoing loss requiring immediate surgical intervention.

Hemolysis occurs with autotransfusion, in part because of prolonged exposure of cells to the serosa of the traumatized body cavities.[76] Hemolysis also results from mechanical damage during collection and reinfusion or from excessive exposure to air-fluid interfaces.[41] The hematocrit falls in direct proportion to the quantity of blood transfused, with the average decline being 10% to 20%.[41,50,68] However, nontraumatized red blood cell survival has been reported to be normal in all cases studied.[17,56,77]

Nonhematologic Complications

The theoretical risk for sepsis after the administration of potentially contaminated blood always exists within the nonsterile environment of the typical ED. Experience has shown this risk to be minimal after autotransfusion from an isolated hemothorax, and there is no evidence suggesting that routine prophylaxis with systemic antibiotics is beneficial.[15,37] Collected blood is generally transfused as soon as the collection bag is full. The American Association of Blood Banks

guidelines allow a 6-hour interval between collection and reinfusion.[53] The age of collected blood, however, should be calculated from the time of injury (see Box 27-2). Blood reinfused after this 6-hour period should be considered potentially hazardous.

The risk for microemboli secondary to platelet aggregation and fat emboli has largely been eliminated by the use of micropore filters.[50,56,59] During reinfusion of collected blood there is usually a mild increase in screen filtration pressure, indicative of the formation of microemboli trapped by the filter.[59] There has been no clinical evidence of pulmonary insufficiency or elevation of the alveolar-arterial oxygen gradient that might be attributed to the passage of microemboli beyond micropore filter systems.[41]

As with all IV infusions, improper technique, such as applying pressure to air-containing systems, may lead to air embolism. This uncommon but potentially fatal complication has been associated with autotransfusion systems that use automated roller pump units in which the aspirate reservoir was inadvertently allowed to run dry.[37,78-80] Air embolism with gravity or with a manually assisted technique is rare.

Infusion of large quantities of unwashed blood that contains hemolyzed red blood cells may contribute to renal failure, particularly in patients with preexisting renal insufficiency.[43] Elevated plasma free hemoglobin is a consistent finding in patients who have undergone autotransfusion.[41,65,68] In the past it was believed that elevated levels of free hemoglobin following hemolytic transfusion reactions caused renal failure by its precipitation and obstruction of renal tubules. However, more recent evidence suggests that the mechanism in this setting is independent of free hemoglobin but rather is the result of an antigen-antibody–induced intravascular coagulation that when compounded by vasoconstriction and hypotension, leads to renal ischemia.[81] Even though renal failure as a direct consequence of autotransfusion has not been reported, transient elevations in serum creatinine do occur. In the presence of shock and systemic acidosis, acute tubular necrosis remains a potential complication.[28,36,82] The clinician must weigh the urgency of blood transfusion against the timely availability of an alternative source.

RESOURCES

Brief educational videos are available online for Atrium products at http://www.atriummed.com/EN/Chest_Drainage/edu-files/ATS-video1.asp (accessed July 2012) and show in detail the step-by-step processes to initiate autotransfusion with their devices. They also have a 24-hour help line to assist with any questions during the setup or use of their devices (800-528-7486). Pleur-evac has some limited information available online (www.teleflexmedical.com) and can be contacted during regular business hours (919-544-8000, 8 AM to 7 PM EST) to answer questions.

References are available at www.expertconsult.com

Transfusion Therapy: Blood and Blood Products

Diane L. Gorgas and Colin G. Kaide

Transfusion of blood components (red cells, white cells, platelets, whole plasma, or plasma fractions) is commonplace in the emergency department (ED). Annually in the United States, 15 million blood donations take place and 14 million units of red blood cells (RBCs) are transfused.[1] Although acute hemorrhage is the most common emergency indication for blood transfusion, more nonemergency transfusions and blood component therapy now occur in the ED as a result of the general migration of health care away from inpatient settings. Technical advances have made component therapy directed at specific acute and chronic pathologic conditions practical, safe, and affordable.

BACKGROUND

RBC Antigens and Antibodies

The first documented transfusion took place in the early 1600s, and sporadic advancement in transfusion medicine occurred over the next 3 centuries, mainly dabbling in cross-species whole blood transfusions. It was not until the early 1900s that the Austrian Karl Landsteiner found that an individual's serum reacted with the red cells of some but not all other individuals, thereby discovering the red cell antigen-antibody system.

RBC membranes contain a series of glycoprotein moieties, or antigens, that give the cell an individual identity. Two different genetically determined antigens, type A and type B, occur on the cell surface. Any individual may have one, both, or neither of these antigens. Because the type A and type B antigens on the surface of the cell make the RBC susceptible to agglutination, these antigens are termed agglutinogens. The presence or absence of agglutinogens is the basis for the ABO blood group classification, and the blood types are named accordingly as A, B, or AB. Blood type O contains neither the A nor the B agglutinogen. These blood type antigens are represented in Figure 28-1. The relative frequencies of the different blood groups are listed in Table 28-1.

Within the first year of life, antibodies begin to form against the standard red cell agglutinogens not present in the individual patient. These agglutinins are γ-globulins of the IgM and IgG types and are probably produced by exposure to agglutinogens in food, bacteria, or exogenous substances other than blood transfusions. In the absence of type A agglutinogens (blood types B and O), anti-A antibodies, or agglutinins, spontaneously develop in the plasma. Similarly, in the absence of type B agglutinogens (blood types A and O), anti-B antibodies develop. When both A and B agglutinogens are present (blood type AB), no agglutinins are formed. Blood

groups and their genotypes and constituent agglutinogens and agglutinins are shown in Figure 28-1.

The reaction between red cell antigens and the corresponding agglutinins results in red cell destruction when noncompatible blood types are mixed. As many as 300 different red cell antigens have been identified, but clinically the A and B antigens are most important; with the first transfusion of ABO-incompatible blood, severe, potentially fatal agglutination can occur. The Rh system is likewise very important because there is a chance that transfusion of Rh-positive blood to an Rh-negative patient will result in the formation of Rh antibodies. These antibodies are capable of causing severe hemolysis following a second exposure to the Rh antigen. Of the 40 antigens in the Rh system, D is the most antigenic, but others can also stimulate the production of antibodies in recipients lacking the antigen and thus complicate future transfusions. Other antigen systems in which antibodies could potentially cause hemolytic reactions are the Kell (K and k alleles), Duffy (Fy^a and Fy^b), Kidd (Jk^a and Jk^b), and MNS (M and N and closely linked S and s) systems. Other antigen systems are rarely of clinical importance in transfusion therapy, except in certain patient populations who may require repeated transfusions, such as those with sickle cell anemia.

Crossmatching

Compatibility testing, or crossmatching, involves mixing the donor's RBCs and serum with the serum and RBCs of the recipient to identify the potential for a transfusion reaction. The end point of all crossmatches is the presence of RBC agglutination (either gross or microscopic) or hemolysis. Testing is performed immediately after mixing, after incubation at 37°C for varying times, and with and without an antiglobulin reagent to identify surface immunoglobulin or complement. Each unit of blood product, when properly crossmatched, can be administered with the expectation of safety. Full crossmatching takes approximately 45 minutes to complete.

Types of RBC Preparations

Whole Blood

The normal blood volume of a healthy adult and healthy child is approximately 70 and 80 mL/kg, respectively. Though intuitively an ideal transfusion agent, whole blood is seldom used except for autologous transfusions (e.g., autotransfusion) and for exchange transfusions. Whole blood is not indicated for the treatment of hypovolemic shock, which can be treated effectively with a combination of crystalloids (e.g., lactated Ringer's [LR] solution, 0.9% sodium chloride), colloids (e.g., plasma protein, albumin), and packed red blood cells (PRBCs). It is also not indicated for the correction of thrombocytopenia, replacement of coagulation factors, or treatment of anemia.[2] The incidence of transfusion reactions following transfusion with whole blood is approximately 2.5 times greater than that with PRBCs.[3] Whole blood contains antigenic leukocytes and serum proteins, which carry higher risk (approximately 1%) for an allergic reaction. Nevertheless, warm fresh whole blood has seen increased popularity in military settings and has been proposed as an alternative to component therapy for civilian use in massive transfusion protocols.[4]

Figure 28-1 Blood group types and their associated antibodies and antigens. *(From Abbas AK. Cellular and Molecular Immunology. 7th ed. Philadelphia: Saunders; 2011.)*

TABLE 28-1   Frequency of Blood Groups in the U.S. General Population

BLOOD GROUPS	FREQUENCY (%)
Type	
O	44
A	42
B	10
AB	4
Rh factor	
Rh⁻	15
Rh⁺	85

From Guyton AC, ed. *Textbook of Medical Physiology.* 6th ed. Philadelphia: Saunders; 1981.

PRBCs

PRBCs are prepared by centrifugation and removal of most of the plasma from citrated whole blood. One unit of PRBCs contains the same red cell mass as 1 unit of whole blood at approximately half the volume and twice the hematocrit (55%

to 80%) in 250 mL of volume.[5] *One unit of PRBCs raises the hematocrit approximately 3% in an adult or increases the hemoglobin level of a 70-kg individual by 1 g/dL.* In children, there is an approximate rise in hematocrit of 1% for each 1 mL/kg of packed cells. For example, if 5 mL/kg of PRBCs is transfused, the hematocrit will rise by approximately 5%. Actual changes depend on the state of hydration and the rate of bleeding. Because most of the plasma has been removed, PRBCs cause fewer transfusion and allergic reactions than whole blood does.

PRBCs contain less sodium, potassium, ammonia, citrate, hydrogen ions, and antigenic protein than whole blood does. This may offer advantages in patients with reduced cardiovascular, renal, or hepatic function. The rate of urticaria is still relatively high at 1% to 3% of transfusions, but the incidence of adverse reactions to packed cells is approximately one third of that noted with whole blood. The benefit of increased hemoglobin must be weighed against the potential for volume, electrolyte, and acid-base imbalances following PRBC administration. In cases of massive transfusion (>10 units), there is a significant risk for metabolic and respiratory acidosis, as well as hypocalcemia, which can reach life-threatening levels. Although underlying illness or injury obviously plays a major role in the cause of death, the overall mortality of patients requiring massive PRBC transfusions is approximately 60%.[6,7]

| BOX 28-1 | **Indications for the Use of Specialty RBCs for Transfusion** |

IRRADIATED

Neonates
Patients with hematologic malignancies
Stem cell transplant patients
Directed donations from family members
HLA-matched platelets
Patients with cellular immune deficiency

WASHED

Recipients with a history of severe allergic transfusion reactions
IgA-deficient patients
Paroxysmal nocturnal hemoglobinuria

LEUKOCYTE REDUCED

Multiply transfused patients
Multiparous females
Cancer patients undergoing chemotherapy

CMV AND EBV SERONEGATIVE

Seronegative patients who are currently pregnant
Premature or low-birth-weight infants
Bone marrow or organ transplant recipients
Immunosuppressed patients

Abstracted from Williamson LM, Warwick RM. Transfusion-associated graft-versus-host disease and its prevention. Blood Rev. 1995;9:251-261; and Cushing MM, Ness PM. Principles of red blood cell transfusion. In: Hoffman R, Benz EJ, Shattil S, et al, eds. Hematology: Basic Principles and Practice. 5th ed. Philadelphia: 2009:2210-2216
CMV, *cytomegalovirus*; EBV, *Epstein-Barr virus*; RBCs, *red blood cells.*

Transfusion of PRBCs is indicated to provide additional oxygen-carrying capacity and expansion of volume. Packed cells are most commonly used to treat acute hemorrhage and anemia not amenable to nutritional correction. When treating acute hemorrhage, PRBCs are usually given (1) if the hemoglobin level falls below established critical levels for that particular given patient population (see the section "Transfusion Thresholds"), (2) after rapid crystalloid infusion fails to restore normal vital signs, or (3) concurrently with crystalloid infusion in the treatment of obvious life-threatening blood loss.

Specially prepared or screened types of red cells are listed in the following sections. Their indications for use are presented in Box 28-1.

Washed RBCs

After centrifugation, red cells can be washed to further remove leukocytes, platelets, microaggregates, and plasma proteins. Washing reduces the titer of anti-A and anti-B, thereby permitting safer transfusion of type O PRBCs into non-O recipients.

Leukocyte-Reduced RBCs

Leukocyte-reduced blood products contain less than 5×10^6 leukocytes/unit, whereas standard RBC units contain 1 to 3 $\times 10^9$ leukocytes. Reduction can be performed at the time of collection, in the transfusion laboratory, or at the bedside during transfusion. Leukocyte-reduced products are used to decrease the likelihood of febrile reactions, immunization to leukocytes, and transmission of disease. Currently, about 60% to 75% of the U.S. blood supply is leukoreduced.[8] Several groups advocate the use of 100% leukocyte-reduced blood products because of the many adverse transfusion reactions that are associated with leukocytes. Non–leukocyte-reduced products are virtually the exclusive method of transmission of several viruses, including human T-lymphotropic virus 1 and 2, Epstein-Barr virus (EBV), and cytomegalovirus (CMV). Additionally, they help reactivate and disseminate CMV and human immunodeficiency virus (HIV). Moreover, increased rates of bacterial contamination and postoperative and line infections have been associated with the use of non–leukocyte-reduced products. Furthermore, leukocytes lead to HLA alloimmunization, which results in increased graft rejection and platelet refractoriness.[9]

Irradiated RBCs

Blood products can be irradiated to reduce the risk for graft-versus-host disease (GVHD) in susceptible patients. Irradiation destroys the donor lymphocytes' ability to respond to host foreign antigens. Box 28-1 lists the indications for use of irradiated PRBCs.

Infectious Complications of Transfusions

Though relatively uncommon, transmission of infectious diseases is the transfusion-related complication most feared by the lay public. Transmission of a wide variety of infectious diseases has been reported, but modern screening methods have sharply reduced the frequency of transmission. Viral illnesses remain the most problematic.

Between 1985 and 1999, 694 deaths associated with transfusion were reported to the Food and Drug Administration (FDA). Seventy-seven (11.1%) of these deaths were caused by bacterial contamination. However, sepsis is an uncommon occurrence because both the citrate preservative and refrigeration kill most bacteria. Concern over sepsis is responsible for the practice of completing transfusions within 4 hours and returning unused blood products to the blood bank refrigerator for future use only if they have been unrefrigerated for less than 30 minutes. Both gram-negative and gram-positive organisms are transmitted, with gram-negative virulence being more commonly associated with mortality. A prospective observational study found that the rate of nosocomial infections was significantly higher in patients receiving blood transfusion. Leukoreduction did not significantly reduce the rate of infection.[10] A recent multicenter study by the Centers for Disease Control and Prevention further evaluated the risk for bacterial contamination in the blood pool. The results showed the rate of bacterial sepsis to be much lower than previously thought. Only 0.21 cases and 0.13 deaths per million red cell transfusions occurred. The rate was slightly higher for platelet transfusions, with 10 cases and 2 deaths per million transfusions.[11] Mandatory screening of platelets for bacterial contamination began in 2004 and has further reduced the rate of reported death.

Syphilis may theoretically be transmitted by transfusion, but both refrigeration and citrate markedly reduce the survival of *Treponema pallidum*. Thus, only fresh blood or platelet transfusions are of concern for its transmission. The incubation period for syphilis transmitted by transfusion is 4 weeks to 4 months, and the initial clinical manifestation is commonly a rash. No cases of transfusion-transmitted syphilis have been recognized for many years.[12,13]

The risk for parasitic infection via transfusion is exceedingly low (<1 per 1,000,000), although prospective blood product donors who have been to an endemic region within 12 months or treated with malarial prophylaxis within 3 years are prohibited from blood donation. Those with a history of babesiosis or Chagas' disease are permanently barred. Donors with a history of Lyme disease may donate if they are symptom free and have undergone a complete course of treatment.

Viruses are the organisms most likely to be transmitted by transfusion and the agents with the greatest potential to cause serious disease. They include CMV, EBV, HIV, West Nile virus (WNV), and the hepatitis viruses.

Most blood products have the potential to transmit hepatitis. Routine testing of blood donors for hepatitis C virus (HCV) has occurred since 1991, but the initial screening tests were relatively inaccurate. Since April 1999, the use of nucleic acid amplification testing (NAAT) to detect HCV RNA has been mandatory. This test has essentially eliminated false positives and has a sensitivity of greater than 99%.[14,15] The American Association of Blood Banks reported the risk for transmission of HCV to be less than 1 per 1,000,000 transfusions. The incubation period for HCV is 2 to 12 weeks following parenteral infusion. The reported risk for transmission of hepatitis B virus (HBV) is higher at 1 per 137,000 transfusions.

Both CMV and EBV may cause a mononucleosis-like syndrome 2 to 6 weeks after a transfusion. Indications for CMV- and EBV-negative preparations are listed in Box 28-1. Alternatively, leukocyte-reduced products can help protect against CMV and EBV.

The acquired immunodeficiency syndrome (AIDS) epidemic has affected transfusion therapy profoundly. In the United States, 3% of AIDS cases have been linked to blood products. The estimated likelihood of transmitting HIV through transfusion is 1 in 1,900,000. Currently, NAAT is used to detect HIV in blood. Because the test detects genetic material in lieu of antibody to the virus, it has significantly reduced the window period during which infection is undetected. Other methods of reducing transmission, including techniques to kill the virus in collected samples (viral inactivation) and the use of blood component substitutes, are being investigated.

Efforts to reduce the risk for transmission of HIV to the general population receiving blood products began early in the course of the epidemic and have had considerable success. Voluntary deferment of blood donation by high-risk groups was encouraged beginning in 1983, and formal screening of all blood products commenced in 1985.

Transmission of WNV by blood transfusion was first documented in the United States in 2002.[16,17] Since 2003, universal screening for WNV by investigational NAAT occurs on all blood donations. From 2003 to 2005, 1400 potentially infectious donations were removed from the blood pool. Since that time, however, multiple cases of transfusion-associated transmission of WNV have been confirmed. This residual risk for transmission is due to blood units with low levels of viremia. Public health authorities continue to look for ways to eliminate this risk from the blood pool.[17,18]

Emerging infectious risks to the blood supply are always under investigation. Blood-transmitted infections under current surveillance include parvovirus B19, dengue virus, and the prions that cause Creutzfeldt-Jacob disease. Although a viremic phase of human herpesvirus-8, avian flu (H5N1), H1N1, and Lyme disease has been well documented, no cases of transmission through transfusion have been noted.[18,19]

A summary of infections risks associated with red cell transfusion is presented in Table 28-2.

Transfusion Reactions

Transfusion reactions can be divided into two phases, acute and chronic. The vast majority of transfusion reactions occur proximate to or concurrently with the administration of red cells. If the ED is the site for a nonemergency transfusion and

TABLE 28-2 Estimated Risks of Transfusion per Unit PRBCs in the United States

RISK	RATE
Major allergic reactions	1/100
Anaphylaxis	1/20,000-50,000
Anaphylactic shock	1/500,000
Hemolytic reaction (minor)	1/6000
Hemolytic reaction (fatal)	1/100,000 allergic reactions
Death from sepsis (RBC)	1/5 million
Death from sepsis (platelets)	1/500,000
Parasitic infections (Lyme, malaria, Chagas)	<1/million—data lacking
Hepatitis C	<1/million
Hepatitis B	1/140,000
Parvovirus, Creutzfeldt-Jacob disease	Extremely rare—data lacking
HTLV 1/2 infection	1/200,000
HIV infection	1/2 million
West Nile virus	Extremely rare—data lacking
CMV/Epstein-Barr	Rare—data lacking
Acute lung injury	1/500,000
Graft-versus-host disease	Extremely rare—data lacking
Immunosuppression	Unknown
Syphilis[‡]	No cases reported currently

CMV, cytomegalovirus; *HIV*, human immunodeficiency virus; *HTLV*, human T-cell lymphotropic virus; *PRBCs*, packed RBCs; *RBC*, red blood cell.

the patient is otherwise stable enough for discharge, it is a common practice for the patient to be released shortly after the transfusion is completed.

Acute Reactions
Allergic
The most common manifestation of a minor allergic transfusion reaction is urticaria; however, wheezing and angioedema can also be observed. The allergic response is due to the presence of atopic substances that interact with antibodies in the donor or recipient plasma, but the severity is not dose related.[5] Whenever a transfusion reaction is suspected, the first step in management is to stop the transfusion. Treatment is the same as for other allergic reactions and includes antihistamines, steroids, and epinephrine if needed. For mild reactions (e.g., those limited to skin findings), the transfusion can be resumed once treatment has been given.

Anaphylactic
The reported incidence of transfusion-associated anaphylaxis is 1 in 20,000 to 50,000. Anaphylaxis occurs most commonly in IgA-deficient patients who have IgA-specific antibodies of the IgE class.[20] Manifestations of an anaphylactic transfusion reaction include shock, hypotension, angioedema, dyspnea, bronchospasm, and laryngospasm. The symptoms are typically rapid in onset and begin within seconds to minutes of starting the transfusion. If this type of reaction occurs, the transfusion must be stopped immediately. Treatment includes airway management as necessary, epinephrine, fluids, and steroids, followed by appropriate supportive care and continued close observation. If a transfusion is still required, the patient needs to be pretreated with steroids and antihistamines 30 to 60 minutes before the transfusion. Alternatively or in addition, washed cellular products can be used.

Febrile (Nonhemolytic)
A febrile, nonhemolytic reaction is defined as an increase in temperature of 1°C or higher during or within 6 hours of the transfusion. The mechanism for this type of reaction is most commonly attributed to an interaction between recipient antibodies and donor leukocytes.[21,22] This stimulates the release of cytokines such as interleukin-1, which ultimately produces a febrile response. Although this type of reaction is not life-threatening, it is difficult to distinguish from more serious transfusion reactions. Accordingly, all patients with a fever attributable to a transfusion must have the transfusion stopped. Symptoms can be treated with acetaminophen or nonsteroidal antiinflammatory drugs. There is no role for antihistamines in the treatment of this type of reaction. Although controversy exists, premedication with antipyretics and antihistamines may prevent these transfusion reactions.[23]

Acute Hemolytic
An acute hemolytic reaction is usually the result of donor-recipient major ABO incompatibility. This in turn is most commonly the result of blood product misassignment related to clerical error. Hemolytic transfusion reactions are estimated to occur once per every 6000 blood units transfused, with a fatality rate of 1 per every 100,000 units transfused.

When incompatible blood is given, the result may range widely from no effect to death. If the recipient does not have antibodies (naturally occurring or acquired) directed against the foreign RBC antigen received, there will be no immediate reaction, but antibodies to the infused blood may develop within weeks, thus limiting the safety of subsequent transfusions from the same donor or same antigenic type. If the recipient's serum has preformed antibodies directed against the donor RBCs (e.g., an incompatibility in the major cross-match), the recipient will begin to hemolyze the donor cells within seconds or minutes. In most cases of major crossmatch reactions, RBCs of the donor blood are agglutinated and hemolyzed. It is rare for transfused blood to produce agglutination of the recipient's cells because the plasma portion of the donor blood becomes diluted by the plasma of the recipient. This reduces the titer of the infused agglutinins to a level too low to cause significant agglutination. Because the recipient's plasma is not diluted to any significant degree, the recipient's agglutinins can react with donor cells. The end result of antigen-antibody incompatibility is red cell hemolysis. Occasionally this occurs immediately, but more often the cells first agglutinate. They are then trapped in small vessels and become phagocytized over a period of hours to days and release hemoglobin into the circulatory system.[24] Clinical manifestations of acute hemolysis include chills, fever, tachycardia, abdominal pain, back pain, hypotension, fainting, and a feeling of "impending doom." Derived from the liberation of intracellular material associated with hemolysis, vasoactive substances may cause hypotension and shock; other substances may precipitate disseminated intravascular coagulation and high-output cardiac failure. Acute renal failure may also result. The presence of hemoglobinemia and hemoglobinuria is essential in making the diagnosis. A decrease in hematocrit and haptoglobin or an increase in lactate dehydrogenase (LDH) may also be seen.

Treatment of an acute hemolytic reaction begins with immediate cessation of the transfusion. The blood bank should be alerted immediately because a second patient is now at risk for receiving the wrong product. Resuscitation and supportive care along with close monitoring of laboratory values are essential. A sample of blood from the recipient needs to be obtained for a direct antiglobulin test, plasma-free hemoglobin, and repeated type and crossmatch. Urine can also be tested for free hemoglobin. Renal function and electrolytes should be monitored for evidence of renal failure and hyperkalemia. Dialysis is occasionally required.[24,25] Fluid resuscitation and diuresis with normal saline are recommended to maintain urine output above 100 to 200 mL/hr. LR solution should be avoided because calcium can precipitate clotting.

Drug-Induced Hemolysis
Drug-induced hemolysis is not a transfusion reaction per se; however, it can be indistinguishable from an acute hemolytic reaction in patients receiving blood transfusions. In this case, both autologous and transfused cells are affected. A patient's serum can react with red cells in the presence of certain drugs. Two examples of drugs that can cause this type of reaction are cefotetan and ceftriaxone.

TRALI
Transfusion-related acute lung injury (TRALI) refers to noncardiogenic pulmonary edema occurring during or shortly after the transfusion of blood products. A leading cause of transfusion-related mortality and morbidity, TRALI has been reported to occur in as many as 3% of patients receiving transfusions.[26,27] TRALI appears to be associated with

components from female plasma; preferential distribution of male plasma by the American Red Cross has recently decreased its incidence.[28]

The potential for TRALI is one reason why some authorities are reluctant to transfuse high ratios of plasma to PRBCs in massive transfusion protocols. TRALI is thought to result from the activation of recipient neutrophils in the lung and the production of vasoactive mediators, which leads to increased pulmonary capillary permeability and leakage. Initial symptoms include respiratory distress, hypoxia, hypotension, fever, and bilateral pulmonary edema; however, the spectrum of TRALI can also include much milder reactions.[29,30]

Treatment of TRALI is supportive and includes supplemental oxygen, endotracheal intubation, and cardiovascular support as necessary. Diuresis and corticosteroids are not effective.[31,32]

Delayed
Delayed Hemolytic

Even when major and minor crossmatches indicate compatibility, delayed hemolytic transfusion reactions can occur days to weeks after transfusion. This is due to antibody production by either the donor or recipient B cells in response to exposure to antigens on red cells. Usually seen in multiply transfused patients or in multigravida women, these reactions may be unavoidable without complete RBC antigen typing, a procedure occasionally indicated for recipients of repeated transfusions. An incompatibility in the minor crossmatch does not usually result in a serious reaction, although the recipient's red cells can be hemolyzed if the titer of the antibody is sufficiently large. Fortunately, 90% of transfusions are now given as PRBCs, which contain a very small volume of plasma, thus minimizing the chance of a transfusion reaction occurring as a result of donor sensitization.

The signs and symptoms of a delayed hemolytic reaction include low-grade fever, a decrease in hemoglobin, mild jaundice, a positive direct antiglobulin test, and elevation of LDH.

Treatment of a delayed hemolytic reaction is not needed unless there is evidence of brisk hemolysis. In the case of brisk hemolysis, treatment consists of fluids, antigen-negative (type O) blood transfusions, or red cell exchange.

GVHD

GVHD is a transfusion complication most commonly associated with allogeneic hematopoietic cell transfusions. However, it can occur whenever immunologically competent lymphocytes are transfused, especially in immunocompromised hosts. Donor lymphocytes engraft in the recipient and then attack host tissue. Symptoms are typically observed 7 to 14 days after the transfusion and include fever, rash, and diarrhea. Hepatitis and marrow aplasia also occur. GVHD is often fatal; failure of the host's marrow leads to overwhelming infection or bleeding. The use of gamma-irradiated cellular components prevents this complication by making the donor lymphocytes incapable of proliferating.[21,29]

Posttransfusion Purpura

In rare cases, profound thrombocytopenia can develop 1 to 3 weeks after a transfusion associated with an antibody response to a platelet antigen. A probable pathophysiologic mechanism for this is the production of low-affinity antibodies that cross-react with autologous platelets. Eventually, as the immune response matures, the low-affinity antibody is eliminated and the thrombocytopenia resolves spontaneously. Only patients at risk for bleeding or hemorrhage need to be treated. Treatment consists of high-dose immune globulin, plasmapheresis, or platelet transfusion.

Miscellaneous Transfusion Issues

Transfusion Thresholds

PRBCs are a precious commodity. Guidelines to limit transfusions to those that are absolutely necessary have set transfusion thresholds or "triggers." A liberal transfusion trigger is approximately 10 g/dL of hemoglobin, whereas restrictive thresholds are set at 7 to 8 g/dL. The limits for restrictive thresholds stem from the finding that aerobic metabolism can still occur at hemoglobin concentrations as low as 5 g/dL.[33,34] Clinically, however, almost all patients show signs of physiologic stress at hemoglobin concentrations of less than 6 g/dL.[34,35] It is at this level that patients will begin to reliably demonstrate the symptoms and signs of anemia: dyspnea on exertion or even at rest; pallor, particularly of the palms and mucous membranes (Fig. 28-2); and resting tachycardia.

The Transfusion Requirements in Critical Care study compared a strategy of restrictive transfusion triggers with conventional, more liberal triggers.[36] The authors concluded that a *restrictive strategy appears to be at least as effective as a more liberal strategy*, with the possible exception of patients with coronary insufficiency. In trauma patients, more liberal use of blood has also been questioned.[37] One of the risks associated with restrictive transfusion thresholds is an increased incidence of infection.[37] Nonetheless, mortality, cardiac events,

Figure 28-2 Physical finding of anemia. Marked pallor of the palmar creases (*above*) is apparent when compared with a patient with a normal hemoglobin level (*below*). This anemic patient had a hemoglobin level of 4.5 g/dL.

and length of hospital and intensive care unit (ICU) stay appear to be unaffected by more restrictive thresholds.[38]

No single criterion should be used as an indication for red cell component therapy. Multiple factors related to the patient's clinical status and oxygen delivery needs should be considered. Current practice focuses on the needs of the individual patient. Particularly close attention should be paid to the subset of patients at risk for coronary ischemia, with more liberal triggers possibly being applied to these patients. Wu and colleagues,[39] in a U.S.-based study of Medicare patients with acute myocardial infarction, found RBC transfusions to be beneficial in elderly patients when hematocrit values were lower than 33%. In the setting of severe sepsis, a more conservative threshold of 10 g/dL may also be appropriate.[40] In contrast, new data from pediatric ICU settings suggest that adopting a threshold of 7 g/dL imparts no worse clinical outcome and may result in benefits in long-term mortality and morbidity.[41] Similar findings were documented in pediatric postsurgical patients.[42]

In addition to cost and transmitted infections, there is a risk for systemic inflammatory response syndrome with transfusion. This syndrome is closely associated with diminished organ function and mortality in critically ill adult patients and its incidence increases with the administration of more than 4 units of PRBCs.[43,44] Red cell administration is also associated with an increased risk for life-threatening acute respiratory distress syndrome[45] and multiple-organ failure.[46,47] This has been linked to immunologic alterations and their effects on plasma cytokine and cytokine receptor concentrations. In patients receiving more than 15 units of PRBCs, levels of both interleukin and soluble tumor necrosis factor were elevated.[31,46] It remains unclear whether the use of leukocyte-reduced PRBCs can mitigate the expected inflammatory response.

The judicious and restricted administration of PRBCs appears to be clinically founded in the majority of patients. By implementing a restrictive transfusion strategy, the probability of a patient requiring blood can be decreased by 42% and the volume of PRBCs transfused can be decreased by 0.93 units per patient.[38,48,49]

Another area of study focuses on the projected need for administration of PRBCs in any given patient. Knowing which patients will probably need blood based on their initial findings can be helpful in resource allocation and determination of the need for crossmatching. Studies have correlated the base deficit (BD) with the need for transfusion by using a cutoff of −6 mEq/L. Patients with a BD larger than −6 mEq/L have a 72% chance of requiring blood, whereas those with BDs smaller than −6 have only an 18% of requiring PRBCs. More elaborate scales have been proposed based on easily assessable parameters. The emergency transfusion score is a point system based on systolic blood pressure, the presence of free fluid on focused assessment with sonography for trauma (FAST), an unstable pelvic ring fracture, advanced patient age, admission from the scene, motor vehicle collision, or a fall as being predictors of future transfusion requirements.[50]

In summary, it is impossible to define strict PRBC transfusion recommendations in the ED setting. Such decisions must be made in real time after factoring in multiple factors, some of which may not be known at the time. In summary, *definitive data are lacking at this time and no dogmatic recommendations can possibly apply to all ED scenarios. As a general concept, however, the likelihood of a transfusion being of benefit is high when the patient's hemoglobin level is less than 6 to 7 g/dL and low when it* *is greater than 10 g/dL. The correct strategy is unclear when the hemoglobin level is between 7 and 10 g/dL. Continued blood loss of varying degrees renders transfusion strategies even more obscure. The elderly and those with cardiovascular or respiratory disease may not tolerate anemia as well as those without these parameters.*

Massive Transfusion

Massive transfusion is loosely defined. In the 1970s it was considered to be the transfusion of more than 10 units of blood to an adult, equivalent to 1 blood volume, within 24 hours. Historically, massive transfusion was associated with dismal survival rates (<10%).[51,52] As blood banking technology and storage methods have improved, the mortality associated with massive transfusions has decreased significantly. There is no clear physiologic threshold to define a massive transfusion. Mortality in patients receiving fewer than 5 units is currently around 10%, in those receiving 6 to 9 units it is approximately 20%, and in those receiving 10 or more units it is greater than 50%.[53] Some sources have recently narrowed the definition of massive transfusion to include only patients who receive more than 50 units of PRBCs within the first 24 hours of resuscitation. Alternative triggers for initiation of a massive transfusion protocol are now being proposed, including elevation of the international normalized ratio (INR) and BD, in addition to hemoglobin. Despite the challenges of treating the expected posttransfusion inflammatory and immunologic complications, patients requiring massive transfusions can have good outcomes.

Transfusion Coagulopathy

Pathologic hemostasis occurs following massive blood transfusions.[52,54-57] Coagulopathy and subsequent uncontrolled bleeding are major contributors to trauma-related deaths.[58,59] Although such abnormalities rarely develop within the time frame of the initial resuscitation in the ED, an understanding of the problem can lead to a more thoughtful approach to transfusion practices and the anticipation of potential problems. Significant alterations in blood and blood products occur during storage. Moreover, in patients who are given a transfusion equal to 2 blood volumes, only approximately 10% of the original elements remain. The development of transfusion coagulopathy is multifactorial; important factors include tissue injury, acidosis, the duration of shock, and hypothermia, in addition to activation, consumption, and dilution of coagulation factors.[60-62]

Transfusion coagulopathy is also related in part to dilution of the recipient's platelets by transfused blood devoid of functioning platelets. Dilutional thrombocytopenia is a well-recognized complication of massive transfusion, and a platelet count should be obtained routinely if more than 5 units of blood are transfused.

Disseminated intravascular coagulation (from a hemolytic reaction) may play a secondary role in posttransfusion bleeding. Factors V and VIII are labile in stored blood and absent in packed cells. Fibrinogen is relatively stable in stored blood but is absent in packed cells. A deficiency of most clotting factors, especially factors V and VIII and fibrinogen, occurs with massive transfusions. This deficiency probably occurs on a "washout" (i.e., dilutional) basis, although the dynamics are poorly understood. Replacement of these factors may be required. Specific assays for the individual factors are available, but it is more practical to measure the prothrombin time (PT), partial thromboplastin time (PTT), and fibrinogen levels. Plasma has been used to correct clotting factor abnormalities secondary to dilution from massive transfusions, but its effectiveness has not been firmly established. Cryoprecipitate has also been used to replace factor VIII and fibrinogen, but it is rarely required because plasma contains some fibrinogen. Fresh frozen plasma (FFP) should be infused to correct the coagulopathy as indicated by clotting studies. Cryoprecipitate may be required if fibrinogen levels fall below 100 mg/dL despite the use of plasma. Although blood component therapy can be based on measured coagulopathy parameters, as a general guide, 1 to 2 units of plasma for each 5 to 6 units of blood may be given empirically.[63,64]

Numerous massive transfusion protocols exist. Traditionally, transfusion-related coagulopathies have been evaluated and treated as per laboratory indicators, but rapid or massive transfusions do not allow equilibration or timely laboratory analysis. Although this approach is quite acceptable in most patients, the aim of transfusion protocols is to prevent transfusion-related coagulopathy before it occurs. Obviously, one cannot simply continue to transfuse only PRBCs to patients experiencing significant blood loss, and some combination or ratio of plasma to PRBCs to platelets should be adopted. The ideal combination is, however, not known with certainly, and it is largely dependent on the underlying need for transfusion and specific patient characteristics. Most protocols recommend a plasma-to-PRBC ratio of 1:1.5 or 1:1.8.[65] Other protocols also include empirical platelet administration and use ratios of RBCs to platelets to FFP of 1:1:1.[66] At this time, however, no specific transfusion ratio has been proved superior. Strict adherence to any protocol must be balanced against the risk for multisystem organ failure and infection associated with high doses of platelets and plasma. All protocols recommend warming of blood and blood products because hypothermia occurs quickly during massive transfusions and can contribute to further coagulopathy.

Severe Trauma and Coagulopathy

A transfusion coagulopathy often develops in individuals injured during military combat who received transfusions because of widespread tissue trauma. The U.S. military has advocated an approach to transfusion therapy that includes prompt initiation of 1:1:1 resuscitation ratios with RBCs, pre-thawed universal-donor AB plasma, and apheresis platelets, with conversion to fresh whole blood as soon as it can be obtained. This ratio has not been universally adopted by civilian hospitals.

Emergency Transfusions

In an emergency, three alternatives to fully crossmatched blood exist. The preferred substitute is type-specific blood with an abbreviated crossmatch. The abbreviated crossmatch includes ABO and Rh compatibility. In addition, the recipient's serum is screened for unexpected antibodies, and an immediate "spin" crossmatch is performed at room temperature. This abbreviated crossmatch requires approximately 30 minutes. Many institutions are now using this procedure as their standard crossmatch for most patients. The safety and utility of the type-specific abbreviated crossmatch have been demonstrated repeatedly, with transfusion reactions occurring only rarely.[67,68] Brickman and coworkers demonstrated that bone marrow aspirates obtained with an intraosseous needle can also be used for crossmatching.[69]

The second preference for an alternative to fully crossmatched blood is type-specific blood that is only ABO and Rh compatible, without screen or immediate spin crossmatch. The patient's ABO group and Rh factor can be determined within 2 minutes, and in an emergency, typing of the blood group and the Rh factor is all that is necessary before transfusion. Type-specific blood that has not been crossmatched has been used in numerous military and civilian series without serious consequences. While the type-specific blood is being transfused, the antibody screen and crossmatch are carried out in the laboratory. The transfusion should be stopped if an incompatibility is found.

A third alternative to fully crossmatched blood is group O blood, although type-specific blood is generally preferable.[5,70] Commonly, this is available at the point of care and has the advantage of being immediately available in cases of severe shock with ongoing bleeding. Thus, despite the theoretical preference for type-specific blood in emergency situations, type O is often a reasonable and practical alternative.

One may transfuse both Rh-positive and Rh-negative group O packed cells into patients who are in critical condition. It is a common misconception that patients who are Rh negative will have an immediate transfusion reaction if given Rh-positive blood. There is no particular advantage in determining the Rh factor because preformed, naturally occurring anti-Rh antibodies do not exist. Theoretically, individuals who are Rh negative may become sensitized either through pregnancy or by previous transfusions, and a delayed hemolytic transfusion reaction will result if Rh-positive blood is transfused. However, this scenario is very rare and is of little significance when compared with life-threatening blood loss. Sensitization to the Rh factor is most problematic for Rh-negative women of reproductive age.[71,72] Any sensitized patient may experience a transfusion reaction if exposed again to Rh-incompatible blood. However, significant subsequent transfusion reactions with Rh-incompatible blood in men sensitized to the Rh factor are very rare. Many advise routine use of the more widely available type O Rh-positive packed cells in all patients in whom the Rh factor has not been determined, except in females of childbearing age, for whom future Rh sensitization may be an important consideration. Once resuscitated with Rh-positive packed cells, patients may receive their own type without a problem. Because individuals with type O Rh-negative blood represent only 15% of the population and the blood may be in short supply, it is reasonable to save type O Rh-negative blood for Rh-negative females of childbearing potential and to use type O Rh-positive packed cells routinely as the first choice for emergency transfusions. In a study of emergency blood needs, Schmidt and colleagues reported 601 units of blood into 262 untyped patients, including 8 Rh-negative women, before the blood type was determined.[71] No acute hemolytic reactions occurred, and no women were sensitized. A non–emergency-based study found the rate of Rh sensitization in Rh-negative recipients receiving Rh-positive blood to be about 8%, and this figure may be reduced if Rh immune globulin is given after transfusion.[73,74] Thus, prophylaxis with Rh immune globulin is recommended only for Rh-negative women of childbearing potential receiving Rh-positive blood.

Rh immune prophylaxis with $Rh_0(D)$ human immune globulin (RhoGAM) is also indicated for Rh-negative pregnant women who may be bearing Rh-positive children and may have fetomaternal transplacental hemorrhage, including bleeding in early pregnancy, such as spontaneous or elective abortion, ectopic pregnancy, and other potential causes of antepartum hemorrhage such as trauma. RhoGAM suppresses the immune response of Rh-negative women to Rh-positive RBCs and is effective when given up to 72 hours after exposure to fetal erythrocytes. Standard doses are 50 µg for women up to 12 weeks of pregnancy and 300 µg in the second and third trimester. In the setting of fetal-maternal transfusion greater than 15 mL (usually only in the third trimester when fetal blood volume becomes more substantial), higher doses may be necessary. In such circumstances, the correct dose may be calculated by quantitative testing for fetal erythrocytes in the mother's blood (Kleihauer-Betke test).[75]

If non-crossmatched blood is transfused, the laboratory should receive a plain (e.g., without a serum separator) red-topped tube of venous blood as soon as possible to begin a formal crossmatch procedure. Whenever possible, this sample should be drawn before any blood is transfused.

Metabolic Disturbances

RBCs undergo metabolic, biochemical, and molecular changes during storage that are collectively known as the erythrocyte "storage lesion."[76,77] These changes are generally subtle but can be measured: a decrease in levels of 2,3-diphosphoglycerate (2,3-DPG), pH, and intracellular potassium and a concomitant increase in supernatant potassium.

Theoretically, citrate salts, which are the usual anticoagulants in donor blood, may combine with ionized calcium in plasma and produce hypocalcemia and rarely hypocalcemic-related cardiovascular depression. In clinical practice, the hemodynamic consequences of citrate-induced hypocalcemia are minimal, although the QT interval may be prolonged on the electrocardiogram with citrate infusion. Supplemental calcium administration is not usually necessary even during massive blood replacement, as long as circulating volume is maintained, because the liver is able to remove citrate from the blood within a few minutes. Alterations in this recommendation may be necessary in patients with severe liver disease. If calcium replacement is deemed necessary by clinical judgment, 10 to 20 mL of calcium gluconate may be given intravenously, via a different vein, for each 500 mL of blood transfused. If calcium chloride is used, only 2 to 5 mL per 500 mL of blood should be given. Calcium chloride may be preferable in patients with abnormal liver function, such as those with bleeding esophageal varices, since citrate metabolism is decreased, which results in slower release of ionized calcium. Care must be taken to avoid administering too much calcium and inducing hypercalcemia, ideally by monitoring the ionized calcium concentration.

Directed and Autologous Donations

The system of "directed donations" by which friends or family members may donate blood for a specific individual has been proposed in response to concerns about the transmission of infectious disease. At this time, directed donation systems are in place in some institutions but the practice has not been widely supported. Directed donations probably do not decrease the risk for infectious disease transmission and may disrupt the normal anonymous blood donor system and thus leave fewer units available for other needy patients.[78,79]

Though of limited clinical applicability in emergencies, autologous donations are commonplace in elective surgery. It

has been suggested that up to 10% of the blood supply could be provided through this mechanism. However, current studies show that at its peak, autologous donations represented less than 2% of the total blood collections, and this number is declining.[80] Applications at this time include elective cardiac, gynecologic, orthopedic, and vascular surgery. Benefits include avoidance of exogenous blood-borne disease and sensitization. An individual can donate 1 unit of blood weekly until 3 days before surgery. Because blood can be stored up to 35 days, donations usually begin 5 weeks before needed. The blood donor will require iron supplements and must maintain a hemoglobin level higher than 11 g/dL.

RBC Substitutes

Concerns over infection, availability, storage difficulties, and risk for transfusion reactions have fueled interest in the development of blood substitutes. The ideal blood substitute should (1) deliver oxygen efficiently, (2) require no compatibility testing, (3) cause few or no side effects, (4) have prolonged storage qualities, (5) persist in the circulation, and (6) be affordable.[81] Blood substitutes can be categorized as synthetic emulsions and hemoglobin-based oxygen carriers (HBOCs) or "stromal-free" hemoglobin solutions.

HBOCs can be derived either from humans (typically from outdated human PRBCs) or from animals, notably bovine. HBOCs are created by lysing red cells, extracting the hemoglobin, and then chemically cross-linking single hemoglobin molecules to create a larger molecule, one less likely to cause impairment in renal function by obstruction of the renal tubules.[82] Early HBOCs had a propensity to cause renal injury, but this has markedly improved in subsequent generations. Advantages of HBOCs over packed red cells include a much longer shelf life (1 to 4 years) and no need for crossmatching.[83] An important disadvantage is a much shorter circulating half-life (1 day versus 31 days).[5]

Perfluorocarbons are carbon-fluorine compounds that have high oxygen- and carbon dioxide–dissolving capacity.[84] They are not miscible with water and must therefore be emulsified for administration. Perfluorocarbons are totally synthetic, essentially limitless in supply, chemically stable, and harbor no risk for infection.[85] However, they are limited by a short half-life, with degradation occurring within 48 hours of administration. Trials to date have focused mainly on their adjunctive use with standard transfusion therapy.

Other potential blood analogues in the investigation phase include biodegradable micelles and hemerythrin, an oligomeric protein responsible for transport of oxygen in the marine invertebrate.[48] Alternative sources for red cell therapy include stem cells[86] and placental umbilical cord blood[87] as another stem cell analogue to create greater supplies of transfusion-safe blood.

OTHER BLOOD PRODUCTS

When it has been decided that a patient needs a transfusion and the patient's condition is stable enough, ask the patient or relatives about any previous transfusion reactions and whether the patient abides by any religious prohibitions to transfusion. Blood should be drawn from the patient (≈2 mL for every unit of blood product to be crossmatched) and put into a red-topped, nonanticoagulated tube (Fig. 28-3, *step 1*).

BLOOD TRANSFUSION

Collect a blood sample in a red-topped nonanticoagulated tube *(without serum separator gel)*. The tube must be signed by the individual who drew the blood sample according to institutional policy.

Initiate an intravenous line with a 14- to 16-gauge catheter if possible. Flush the system with a solution of normal saline before administering the blood. Do not use any intravenous fluids other than saline, and do not infuse any medications through the line.

Prior to transfusion, carefully check patient and blood unit identities according to institutional protocol. Many centers use a two-nurse mandate for checking and double-checking blood before it is administered.

Connect the blood to a tubing set with an appropriate filter. Here, the blood is being transfused through a standard blood administration tubing set.

Begin the blood transfusion. One unit of whole blood can be safely administered to a hypotensive patient at a rate of at least 20 mL/kg/hr. In the setting of hypovolemic shock and continued hemorrhage, there is no limit to the transfusion rate. In a stable patient, infuse 1 unit of whole blood or packed red blood cells over approximately a 2-hour period.

Carefully monitor the patient for evidence of a transfusion reaction. Look for hives, chills, diarrhea, fever, pruritus, flushing, abdominal or back pain, tightness in the throat, and respiratory distress. Stop the transfusion immediately if there is an increase in the pulse rate, decrease in blood pressure, respiratory symptoms, chest or abdominal discomfort, or a sensation of impending doom.

Figure 28-3 Blood transfusion steps.

The tube must not contain a serum separator gel. The label should be signed by the individual drawing the blood sample. This identifying signature will be used in the blood bank's crossmatching procedures. The individual blood components are discussed in the following sections. A summary of the dosages and characteristics of each component is provided in Table 28-3.

Platelet Concentrates

Platelet concentrates are prepared by rapid centrifugation of platelet-rich plasma. Platelets are obtained by single-donor apheresis or from pooled random-donor whole blood units. Platelets obtained by single-donor apheresis have the advantage of exposing the recipient to only one donor. This reduces the risk for exposure to many different donors and confers a lower risk for transfusion-transmitted disease and other complications. HLA-matched platelets may be used when HLA antibodies develop as a result of repeated random-donor platelet transfusions. Platelet concentrates contain most of the platelets from 1 unit of blood in 30 to 50 mL of plasma.

Confusion sometimes arises about how to order platelets. Platelets are typically ordered by the "pack." Many institutions use a "6-pack" composed of 6 individual units of platelets. Some institutions use a 4-pack. A 4- to 6-pack of random-donor units delivers about the same amount of platelets as a single-donor apheresis unit. Unfortunately, some hospitals also refer to the "4- or 6-pack" as a unit. It is important to become familiar with the blood bank terminology at your hospital. For this discussion, the term "unit" is used to describe individual units and not a 4- or 6-pack.

One individual unit of random-donor platelet concentrate raises the platelet count by 5000 to 10,000/mm³. The usual adult dose is 1 random-donor unit for every 10 kg of body weight. In an average adult, this works out to approximately 6 to 8 units of platelet concentrate. Assuming a zero platelet level, 6 units (or one 6-pack) or one single-donor apheresis unit given to a normal-sized adult should increase the platelet count to around 50,000/mm³. If there is no evidence of platelet consumption, this transfusion should be adequate for 3 to 5 days. In cases of severe platelet consumption, transfusion may be required every 6 to 24 hours. Some hospital blood banks prepare platelet concentrates regularly; in some cities, a central blood bank service, such as the American Red Cross, prepares platelet concentrates regularly and delivers units on an as-needed basis within 1 to 2 hours of

TABLE 28-3	Summary and Dosage of Blood Products		
BLOOD COMPONENT	**DOSE**	**NOTES**	**EXPECTED RESULTS**
Platelets	≈1 unit/10 kg 1 apheresis pack or a 6-pack of pooled platelets	ABO and Rh compatible is preferred but in an emergency is not necessary 30-50 mL/U ≈ 180-300 mL/6-pack Available in 5-15 min 3× the usual dose to reverse clopidogrel and ASA The duration of platelet life is severely diminished with ITP	Each unit should raise the platelet count by 5000-10,000, so a 6-pack or 1 apheresis unit should raise the count by 30,000-60,000
Fresh frozen plasma	15 mL/kg or ≈1000 mL or 4 units in a 70-kg patient	ABO compatibility is desirable but not required in an emergency, and Rh compatibility is never required 200-250 mL/bag Available in 45-60 min Should begin with 4 units minimum to correct an elevated INR Not possible to get an INR <1.5 with FFP	Each unit raises all coagulation factors by 2-3% in average-sized adults
Cryoprecipitate	10-20 bags, depending on the indication	ABO compatibility is desirable but not required in an emergency, and Rh compatibility is never required Hypofibrinogenemia <100 mg/dL: give 10 bags, 15-20 mL/bag Fibrinolytic-induced bleeding: give 10-12 bags Factor VIII deficiency when specific factor therapy is not available: 1 bag/5 kg Available in 20 min	With fibrinolytic-induced bleeding, recommended doses may help correct bleeding In factor VIII deficiency, the recommended dose will raise factor VIII to 50% of normal

ASA, acetylsalicylic acid; *FFP,* fresh frozen plasma; *INR,* international normalized ratio; *ITP,* idiopathic thrombocytopenic purpura.

the request. Platelet concentrates are viable for 5 days when kept at room temperature and gently agitated at intermittent periods or when kept in motion. They should not be refrigerated.

The issue of prophylactic platelet transfusion remains controversial. Spontaneous bleeding rarely occurs if the platelet count is greater than 10,000 to 20,000/mm^3. Even in the event of surgery or trauma, excessive bleeding is uncommon in patients whose platelet count exceeds 50,000/mm^3. It is generally recommended that active hemorrhage be treated by platelet transfusion if the platelet count is lower than 50,000/mm^3, but prophylactic transfusion may be withheld safely until the count is lower than 20,000/mm^3, and more recent data suggest that this threshold can be lowered to less than 10,000 or even 5000/mm^3.[88,89]

Patients with idiopathic thrombocytopenic purpura (ITP) may be severely thrombocytopenic. Despite low platelet counts in ITP, it is uncommon to see spontaneous bleeding. Because of the presence of antiplatelet antibodies in these patients, transfused platelets may last only a short time (minutes to hours) before being removed from the circulation. Nonetheless, patients with ITP and life-threatening bleeding or severe head trauma should be given platelets at two to three times the normal dose.[90]

Platelet transfusion should be avoided in patients with thrombotic thrombocytopenic purpura (TTP), a rare microangiopathic hemolytic anemia, because platelets will result in further microemboli. TTP may be suspected in patients with both anemia and thrombocytopenia but not leukopenia. Clinical features often include fluctuating neurologic symptoms and signs, jaundice, renal dysfunction, and fever. Laboratory confirmation includes the identification of intravascular hemolysis on a peripheral blood smear (e.g., schistocytes), as well as other laboratory evidence of hemolysis. Treatment consists of plasma exchange, although emergency treatment may begin with an infusion of FFP.[91]

In patients with traumatic intracranial hemorrhage (ICH) who are taking platelet inhibitors such as aspirin and clopidogrel, limited retrospective studies suggest an increase in morbidity and possibly increased mortality in comparison to controls not taking antiplatelet agents.[92] One ex vivo study involving 11 healthy volunteers found that complete normalization of platelet function could be obtained in patients taking platelet inhibitors by giving 10 to 15 random-donor units (two to three 4- or 6-packs) or 2 to 3 single-donor apheresis units.[93] Given the devastating nature of ICH in patients taking antiplatelet agents, the benefits of large-volume platelet transfusions may outweigh the risks; however, this is still unclear.

Crossmatching is unnecessary for platelet transfusion, but the donor and the recipient should be ABO and Rh compatible. Note that platelet concentrates contain enough RBCs to sensitize an Rh-negative individual. In an emergency situation, if ABO-compatible platelets are not available, unmatched platelets can be transfused. This will reduce the number of platelets available from the transfusion but otherwise does not cause the same reaction that is expected with an incompatible red cell transfusion. Most institutions have a policy that limits the amount of incompatible platelets that can be given.[94] There may be a diluting effect of the platelet count that results in thrombocytopenia with massive blood transfusions. When more than 10 units of blood is transfused, the platelet count must be routinely evaluated

and platelets must be replaced accordingly. Clinically significant platelet depletion rarely occurs if less than 15 units of blood (or 1.5 to 2 times the blood volume) has been transfused.[95]

Each 4 to 6 units of platelets contains 250 to 350 mL of plasma ($\approx$1 unit of FFP), which includes coagulation factors and may reduce the requirement for FFP. Platelets may be infused rapidly (1 unit/10 min) with the use of specialized platelet filters.

FFP

FFP is prepared by separating plasma from the cellular components of single-donor whole blood, followed by rapid freezing and storage at 18°C or lower. Freezing preserves the soluble coagulation factors of the contact activation (intrinsic) and tissue factor (extrinsic) clotting systems, including the labile factors V and VIII. FFP also contains fibrinogen, though not as much as cryoprecipitate does. Plasma stored for 3 months retains approximately 60% of the normal factor VIII activity and has a shelf life of up to 1 year. Thawed solvent- or detergent-treated plasma stored at 4°C for 6 days still contains sufficient coagulant activity of factors II, V, VII, VIII, IX, XI, and XII, fibrinogen, antithrombin, protein C, and von Willebrand factor (vWF) antigen and can be safely administered.[96] Ideally, transfused plasma should be compatible with the recipient's ABO group. Rh compatibility is not considered essential.[97] Each unit of FFP has a volume of approximately 200 to 250 mL. The INR of a unit of FFP is about 1.5. Transfusion of even very large amounts of FFP into a patient with an elevated INR will not correct the INR to below 1.5. It is not clinically useful to give FFP to patients with an INR lower than 1.7.[98]

Because each unit of FFP increases levels of all coagulation factors by 2% to 3% in an average-sized adult, it is useful in clinical scenarios involving depletion of clotting factors. FFP may also be valuable in patients with hereditary or acquired clotting abnormalities, such as a deficiency of factor II, V, VII, X, XI, or XIII; von Willebrand syndrome; hemophilia A (factor VIII deficiency); hemophilia B (factor IX deficiency); or hypofibrinogenemia. However, its effectiveness is limited in these inherited diseases with severe clotting abnormalities because of the large volume that is generally required. Specific factor replacement, when available, is always preferred over FFP.

FFP is also indicated for clotting factor deficiencies resulting from massive blood replacement. However, pathologic hemorrhage after massive transfusions is often caused by thrombocytopenia rather than by a depletion of clotting factors. More aggressive FFP replacement formulas are becoming commonplace, rather than the accepted 1 unit of FFP for every 5 to 6 units of PRBCs (see "Massive Transfusions," earlier).

FFP can be used for rapid reversal of serious acute bleeding from warfarin anticoagulants or for prophylaxis before surgery or an invasive procedure. Timing of FFP administration is key. In a study on warfarin-related ICH, each 30-minute delay in administering the first dose of FFP translated into a 20% lower chance of reversing the patient's coagulopathy within the first 24 hours (a significant predictor of mortality).[99] In an emergency situation, 5 to 10 mL/kg of FFP will effect a rapid reversal of the vitamin K-dependent factors II, VII, IX, and X. In life-threatening hemorrhage from warfarin excess, factor IX concentrate (Konyne 80, Proplex, Mononine) may be used, but such therapy carries a higher risk for hepatitis and thromboembolic disease.[100] It is appropriate to use FFP to treat the acquired deficiency of multiple factors, such as seen in patients with severe liver disease, disseminated intravascular coagulation, or vitamin K depletion, and for plasma exchange in those with TTP or hemolytic-uremic syndrome. It is not appropriate for volume expansion or enhancement of wound healing.

Reactions to FFP include fever, chills, and allergic responses, and recipients have a risk for HIV infection and hepatitis similar to the risk with whole blood. FFP should be infused rapidly after thawing because the clotting factors are labile and rapidly lost.

One less common but very serious complication of the administration of blood products containing plasma (FFP and platelets) is TRALI. It is believed to be an immune-mediated process and can occur in up to 1 in 5000 transfusions containing plasma. It carries a mortality of 6% to 9%. Although it is more common with plasma products, it can also occur with RBC transfusions because of the small amount of residual plasma in PRBCs.[101,102] It was described earlier in the section "Transfusion Reactions."

Start by giving 4 units of FFP if the PT is greater than 1.5 to 1.7 times normal or the activated PTT is greater than 1.5 times the top normal value.[103] Each 5 to 6 units of platelets contain the equivalent of 1 unit of FFP, so concomitant platelet infusions may lower the requirements for FFP. In critically ill patients with acute hemorrhage and suspected coagulopathy (e.g., end-stage liver disease), it is appropriate to begin empirical treatment before the laboratory values are known.

Cryoprecipitate

Cryoprecipitate is prepared from single-donor plasma by gradual thawing of rapidly frozen plasma. This process causes precipitation of proteins rich in fibrinogen, as well as factor VIII. Each unit of cryoprecipitate typically yields 100 to 250 mg of fibrinogen, 80 to 100 units of factor VIII, and 50 to 60 mg of fibronectin.[104] Cryoprecipitate is a plasma product and therefore requires ABO compatibility (see earlier discussion in the section "Fresh Frozen Plasma"). The volume of each bag unit is about 15 to 18 mL.

Cryoprecipitate is indicated for the treatment of patients with fibrinogen deficiency, congenital afibrinogenemia, dysfibrinogenemia, and factor XIII deficiency and in some patients with hemophilia A or von Willebrand's disease.[105,106] It can also be used as a second-line treatment to correct a deficiency in coagulation factor VIII (in hemophilia A) when factor VIII concentrates are not readily available. Because cryoprecipitate contains no factor IX, it is of no value in the treatment of factor IX deficiency (hemophilia B).

Mild deficiencies in factor VIII are defined as 10% to 30% of normal activity and severe deficiencies as less than 3% of normal activity. When treating bleeding, the goal depends on the site and severity of hemorrhage, but in general, one should aim for at least 50% of normal factor VIII activity. For life-threatening hemorrhage, aim for 100% activity. The amount of cryoprecipitate required to correct coagulation defects ranges from 10 to 20 U/kg for minor bleeding, such as hemarthrosis, to 50 U/kg for control of bleeding in surgery or trauma. Guide specific replacement by laboratory assay of

factor VIII activity. The half-life of factor VIII in plasma is 8 to 12 hours.

One bag of cryoprecipitate per 5 kg of body weight will raise the recipient's factor VIII level to approximately 50% of normal. In a 70-kg patient, this equals 14 bags. The large number of units that must be given increases the chance of exposure to blood-borne diseases. Factor VIII concentrate is a better choice because of improved methods of viral inactivation and the availability of factor VIII prepared with recombinant DNA technology.

The vWF in cryoprecipitate degrades during storage, thus leading to variable amounts in each bag. It can be used for life-threatening bleeding in patients with von Willebrand's disease but only when the proper preparations of concentrated vWF (Humate-P) are not available.

Cryoprecipitate may be required to correct significant hypofibrinogenemia (<100 mg/dL). A typical adult dose of around 10 bags of cryoprecipitate raises the fibrinogen level by up to 1 g/L (60 to 100 mg/dL). In cases of severe bleeding after the use of a fibrinolytic agent such as tissue plasminogen activator, cryoprecipitate can be used to help control the bleeding. A consensus on dosing has not been reached, but many sources recommend between 10 and 12 bags.[107]

Specific Factor Therapy

A summation of the dosages and characteristics of each factor appears in Table 28-4.

Factor VII

Activated recombinant factor VII (rFVIIa) is a recombinant DNA product that has been approved by the FDA for the control of bleeding in patients with hemophilia A or B who have inhibitors to factors VIII and IX. It works by binding to the surface of activated platelets, which then activate factor X by using the tissue factor pathway (formerly known as the extrinsic pathway). This obviates the need for either factor VIII or IX. Activated factor X then complexes with factor Va, which leads to thrombin burst and clot formation. Factor VII has a half-life of 2.7 hours. A thromboembolic rate of 1% to 2% has been reported.[108] A large metaanalysis of 35 randomized trials showed that arterial clots were more common than venous clots and the risk appeared to increase with age.[109]

Increasingly, activated factor VII is being used to control bleeding in patients who are not hemophiliacs.[110] One multicenter study found that of 701 patients receiving factor VII, 92% were for off-label uses.[111] Several randomized, controlled trials have investigated the use of rFVIIa in specific settings, including ICH, gastrointestinal bleeding, and trauma. Dosing has varied markedly from 5 to 400 μg/kg. A significant consideration when contemplating the use of factor VII is cost. At an average cost per dose of $5000 (80 μg/kg), this can be a limiting factor, especially when some studies use protocols consisting of eight sequential doses.[112]

ICH

ICH is a predictor of poor survivability and neurologic function in a patient who has undergone an acute stroke. The risk for hemorrhage expansion within the first 24 hours is between 20% and 40% in these patients, and thus goal-directed therapy to minimize this risk is critical.[113] In 2005, Mayer and associates[114] published a double-blind, placebo-controlled trial that evaluated the use of rFVIIa for acute ICH. They

TABLE 28-4   Comparison of Correction of the INR in Warfarin-Anticoagulated Patients with PCC, rFVIIa, and FFP

REVERSAL AGENTS	ADVANTAGES	DISADVANTAGES
PCC United States: Profilnine	1. Onset within 10 min 2. Low risk for viral contamination	1. The Bebulin VH product (but not Profilnine) contains heparin—this would not be appropriate when heparin-induced thrombocytopenia is suspected 2. Clotting events have been reported 3. *Duration of 12-24 hr may be an advantage or disadvantage* 4. Cost: ≈0.59 per unit (Profilnine); at 35 U/kg, ≈$1445.50 in a 70-kg patient
rFVIIa	1. A recombinant product does not carry risks associated with blood products 2. Onset within 10 min 3. Storage at room temperature	1. Newer data suggest that although the INR may be reversed in warfarin anticoagulation, clinical bleeding may not be significantly affected 2. Some clotting events have been reported, especially at doses above 1 mg 3. Cost: approximately $1200 for a 1-mg dose: 90 µg/kg in a 70-kg patient, ≈$7560 4. Short duration of 6 hr may be an advantage or disadvantage—multiple doses may be required
FFP	Cost: about $65/unit 15ml/kg with 250ml/unit in a 70-kg adult = $273. Clinician familiarity Available everywhere	1. High volume of fluid may be undesirable for heart failure 2. Slow onset 3. Frozen—must be thawed over a 30-min period 4. Risk for TRALI

FFP, fresh frozen plasma; *INR*, international normalized ratio; *PCC*, prothrombin complex concentrate; *rFVIIa*, recombinant factor VIIa; *TRALI*, transfusion-related acute lung injury.

randomized 399 patients to placebo or to 40, 80, or 160 µg/kg of rFVIIa within 1 hour of a baseline computed tomography (CT) scan of the head. CT was repeated in 24 hours. The primary outcome measured was the percent change in volume of ICH from the initial to the repeat scan. The study showed a 29% increase in the volume of ICH in the placebo group versus 16%, 14%, and 11% in the treatment groups, respectively. Ninety-day outcomes were also evaluated and showed a 69% rate of death or severe disability in patients in the placebo group and 55%, 49%, and 54% in the rFVIIa groups, respectively. When looking at mortality alone, the rate was 29% in the placebo group and 18% in the rFVIIa groups combined. A subsequent study of 841 patients by the same investigators also showed a reduction in growth of the hematoma with rFVIIa, but in contrast to the initial study, no improvement in mortality or functional outcome occurred.[115] Studies of traumatic ICH have yielded similar findings. In a retrospective study by Stein and coworkers[116] of 63 patients with severe traumatic brain injury and coagulopathy at admission, 29 who received rFVIIa were compared with 34 who received FFP. Time to surgical intervention was less in the rFVIIa group; however, there was no difference between the groups at discharge with respect to neurologic outcome or mortality. In a prospective, dose escalation study of factor VII in patients with traumatic ICH, Narayan and colleagues[117] found no differences in mortality rates or ICH volume in the placebo and rFVIIa groups.

Trauma
Several investigators have examined the use of factor VII in the setting of trauma. A study by Bofford and coworkers[118] in 2005 enrolled 301 ED patients with major trauma who

required at least 8 units of PRBCs. The treatment group received three doses of rFVIIa immediately after the eighth unit of blood had been given. The doses were repeated at hours 1 and 3. The primary outcome measured was the total transfusion requirement, and subgroup analysis was performed for blunt and penetrating trauma. For blunt trauma, there was a small decrease in the transfusion requirement (7.0 units in the treatment group versus 7.5 in the placebo group) and a decrease in the number of patients needing massive transfusion (14% of the treatment group versus 33% of the placebo group). In the penetrating trauma group the differences were not statistically significant. In the entire cohort, no differences were found in mortality at 48 hours or 30 days in comparison to placebo. Thromboembolic events were uncommon (4%) and did not differ between the treatment and placebo groups. Raobaikady and colleagues[119] evaluated a group of 48 patients with traumatic pelvic fracture who were scheduled for surgical repair. Patients were randomized to a dose of 90 µg/kg of rFVIIa or placebo at the time of first incision. No significant difference was found in the primary outcome measure of transfusion requirement. Other groups have found that the administration of factor VII can favorably affect the subsequent need for other blood products, specifically PRBCs, cryoprecipitate, and platelets; however, mortality is not significantly affected.[120,121] A 2008 Cochrane review of seven trials involving 1214 subjects (687 patients receiving rFVIIa) concluded that there is *no advantage or disadvantage of rFVIIa over placebo in any of the studied outcomes.*[122] Although rFVIIa has a well-defined role in patients with hemophilia, its use as a more general hemostatic drug remains unproven, and use outside its current approved indications and clinical investigations should be avoided.

Factor VIII Concentrate

Human Antihemophilic Factor

Factor VIII extracted from pooled human plasma produces a concentrated stable product with a shelf life of up to 2 years. Significantly more concentrated than cryoprecipitate and available for home use, factor VIII concentrate was a major breakthrough in the treatment of hemophilia. Unfortunately, the presence of viruses in the donor pool contributed to the high prevalence of hepatitis and HIV infection in hemophiliacs who used earlier versions of this product. Newer products (Alphanate, Hemofil, Humate-P, Koate-DVI, Monarc-M, Monoclate-P) are produced with one or more methods to reduce viral contamination. These methods have markedly reduced the risk for viral transmission, especially lipid-encapsulated viruses (HIV, HBV, HCV). To date, there have been no reports of transmission of these viruses with the newer preparations.

Recombinant Antihemophilic Factor

Since the gene for production of factor VIII was discovered in 1984, research into recombinant genetics has aimed to provide a safer product that will theoretically be more readily available and less expensive to produce. Two recombinant DNA-derived factor VIII preparations (Recombinate, Kogenate) were approved by the FDA in 1993. More recent introductions include Bioclate, Helixate, Helixate FS, and Kogenate FS. These genetically engineered products have hemostatic activity equivalent to that of plasma-derived factor VIII and minimal risk for viral contamination. Because some of these products are prepared from human albumin and other animal proteins, there is a potential for transmission of viruses. Products such as Helixate FS and Kogenate FS are prepared without human albumin, which should eliminate the possibility of viral contamination. Though costlier, they are a better choice for young patients with a newly diagnosed condition who have not already been exposed to hepatitis or HIV.[123]

Factor VIII Concentrate

Administration of 1 unit of factor VIII concentrate per kilogram of body weight should increase factor VIII activity by 2%. The dosage should be individualized according to the severity of bleeding, the known deficiency of factor VIII activity, and the presence of factor VIII antibodies. Factor VIII levels should be increased to 20% to 40% of normal for minor bleeding (e.g., small joint), 40% to 60% for moderate bleeding (e.g., large joint, neck, oral cavity), and 60% to 100% for life-threatening bleeding (e.g., intracranial, intraabdominal, pharyngeal).

Antibodies develop in up to 15% of factor VIII recipients. Administration of massive doses of factor VIII has proved beneficial in overwhelming the endogenous antibody response. In addition, immunoadsorbent techniques to remove the antibody have met with some success. The general use of immunosuppressives and plasmapheresis has also had limited success.

FEIBA

Factor VIII inhibitor–bypassing activity (FEIBA) is a product derived from pooled human plasma that contains factors II, VII, IX, and X. It promotes coagulation by bypassing the need for factors VIII and IX. FEIBA is vapor-heated to achieve greater than 10 logs of reduction in all target viruses, and its safety profile is favorable.[124] FEIBA is used to treat bleeding episodes in hemophilic patients with antibodies to factor VIII

and is generally efficacious in this role.[106] Adverse reactions include headache, fever, chills, flushing, nausea, vomiting, and an occasional allergic reaction. The risk for thrombotic complications exists, especially in patients with liver and heart disease or those who are pregnant or breastfeeding.

DDAVP

A synthetic analogue of pituitary vasopressin, 1-deamino-(8-D-arginine)-vasopressin (DDAVP) has been found to stimulate the endogenous production of factor VIII in a subset of mild hemophiliacs. The exact mechanism is unknown, but treatment with 0.3 mg/kg intravenously over a 15-minute period has been recommended when avoidance of the inherent risks of the factor VIII concentrate is desired.

Factor VII in the Hemophiliac Population

Although factor VII is being used increasingly in nonhemophiliac patients, its original indication was for hemophiliacs in whom factor VIII inhibitors had developed and who were having acute bleeding events. Study dosages in these patients were generally higher than for off-label use (100 to 300 μg), but the drug was effective in controlling bleeding episodes with an acceptably low rate of thromboembolic events.[125,126]

Factor IX Concentrate

Factor IX is prepared from pooled human plasma and is available as a lyophilized powder (AlphaNine, Mononine). Factor IX is also available in recombinant technology as BeneFix.

Historically, the use of factor IX concentrate has carried a very high risk for transmission of viral hepatitis. However, improved donor screening and new methods of viral reduction have substantially reduced the risk for transmission of viruses. As with factor VIII concentrate, the risk for transmission of HIV and hepatitis is very low with current human-derived products. Recombinant factor IX is not derived from human products and carries no risk for viral transmission.

Factor IX is indicated for the treatment of bleeding episodes in hemophilia B patients with a severe deficiency of factor IX. Administration of 1 U/kg body weight will increase the factor IX concentration by approximately 1%. High levels of factor IX are not required to control bleeding. Levels should be increased to 15% to 25% of normal for mild to moderate bleeding and to 25% to 50% of normal for more serious bleeding or before major surgery.

PCC, FFP, and Reversal of Warfarin

Prothrombin complex concentrate (PCC) is a plasma-derived concentrate of nonactivated clotting factors II, VII, IX, and X. These preparations undergo a process of viral inactivation to reduce the risk for viral transmission. PCCs are divided into two groups: three-factor preparations and four-factor preparations. This nomenclature can be confusing because both preparations contain four factors; however, the three-factor preparations have very low amounts of factor VII, whereas the four-factor preparations contain clinically relevant amounts. Some PCC products also contain protein C and protein S. These are added to balance the procoagulant effect of the concentrated clotting factors. At the time of publication, only the three-factor preparations were available in the United States for use outside study protocols. The two most commonly available products are Profilnine SD (Grifols) and Bebulin VH (Baxter). Clinical trials in the United States are under way for four-factor preparations such as Octaplex

(Octapharma) and Beriplex P (CSL Behring). Four-factor preparations have been used in Europe for many years.

In the ED, PCCs can play a very important role in the reversal of anticoagulation from warfarin (see below). PCCs and activated PCCs (FEIBA) may also be effective in reversing some of the newer anticoagulants such as the oral factor X inhibitors (rivaroxaban [Xarelto]) and the factor II inhibitors (dabigatran [Pradaxa]). One concern with these preparations is a possible prothrombotic effect. A recent systematic review of 14 studies (460 patients) found only seven thrombotic complications: three strokes, two myocardial infarctions, and two deep venous thromboses. This translates to a 1.5% risk for inappropriate clotting with PCC administration.[127]

Dosing ranges for PCCs have varied. One study suggested a standard absolute dose for patients with an elevated INR (500 units for INR <5 and 1000 units for INR >5).[128] This study used four-factor preparations only available outside the United States; the same authors found suboptimal reversal effects with three-factor preparations in this fixed-dosing regimen. Other studies have suggested unit/kg dosing, with the amount varying according to the degree of INR elevation.[129,130]

Elevated INRs may be encountered fortuitously or in patients with trauma or serious medical conditions. Guides to approaching and treating such patients are found in Table 28-5. Reflex reversal of an elevated INR should be avoided, especially in the absence of bleeding. Even minor bleeding can be tolerated in lieu of losing the beneficial effects of anticoagulation in selected patients (e.g., those with mechanical heart valves, left ventricular assist devices, or active clots). In the presence of significant trauma or serious hemorrhage, however, any warfarin effect should be reversed.

Warfarin works as a vitamin K antagonist by inhibiting synthesis of the active forms of the vitamin K–dependent coagulation factors II, VII, IX, and X. The first step in the reversal of warfarin is to administer vitamin K according to the recommended dosing and route guidelines outlined in Table 28-5. Vitamin K can be given either orally or intravenously (Fig. 28-4). Oral use is universally safe and should be used when possible. Although intravenous (IV) administration has been implicated in anaphylactoid-like systemic reactions, the incidence of these reactions is very small and should not preclude its use when the oral route is unavailable. Because of erratic absorption patterns, subcutaneous administration of vitamin K is no longer recommended.[131] Reduction in the INR begins within 2 hours, and correction to within the normal range is generally achieved within 24 hours if hepatic function is normal and a sufficiently large dose is given.[132]

The next step in the rapid correction of an elevated INR is to replace the missing clotting factors (II, VII, XI and X). Traditionally, FFP has been used for this purpose. FFP is effective but requires a significant volume and takes time to thaw and prepare for administration. PCCs have been used in Europe and other parts of the world for many years to reverse undesirable warfarin effects. Studies have demonstrated the effectiveness of PCCs in normalizing elevated INRs within 15 minutes after administration without the complication of excessive volume or a delay in time to administration.[130,133,134] A comparison of FFP, PCC, and factor VII is provided in Table 28-4. Another strategy to reverse warfarin-related coagulopathy is to bypass the need for the missing factors by

---

TABLE 28-5 Managing Elevated INRs

CONDITION	ACTION
INR above the therapeutic range but <5.0 *AND* No bleeding	Lower or omit the dose, monitor more frequently, and resume at a lower dose when the INR is therapeutic; if only minimally above the therapeutic range, no dose reduction may be required.
INR ≥5.0 but ≤9.0 *AND* No significant bleeding	Omit the next 1 or 2 doses, monitor more frequently, and resume at a lower dose when the INR is in a therapeutic range. Alternatively, omit the dose and give vitamin K, 1-2.5 mg orally, particularly if at increased risk for bleeding. If more rapid reversal is required because the patient needs urgent surgery, vitamin K$_1$ (2-4 mg orally) can be given with the expectation that a reduction in the INR will occur in 24 hr. If the INR is still high, additional vitamin K (1-2 mg orally) can be given.
INR >9.0 *AND* No significant bleeding	Hold warfarin therapy and give a higher dose of vitamin K (5-10 mg orally) with the expectation that the INR will be reduced substantially in 24-48 hr. Monitor more frequently and use additional vitamin K if necessary. Resume therapy at a lower dose when the INR is therapeutic.
Serious or life-threatening bleeding at any elevation of INR	Hold warfarin therapy and give vitamin K (10 mg by slow intravenous infusion), supplemented with fresh frozen plasma or prothrombin complex concentrate, depending on the urgency of the situation; recombinant factor VIIa may be considered an alternative to prothrombin complex concentrate; vitamin K can be repeated every 12 hr.

Adapted from Ansell, J, Hirsh, J, Hylek, E, et al. Pharmacology and management of the vitamin K antagonists: American College of Chest Physicians Evidence-Based Clinical Practice Guidelines (8th Edition). *Chest.* 2008;133(6 suppl):160S-198S.
INR, international normalized ratio.

Figure 28-4 Vitamin K administered by the intravenous (IV) route has been implicated in serious systemic reactions and, rarely, fatalities. The oral route is universally safe and should be used when possible. If the IV route is mandated, use a dilute solution (such as 5 to 10 mg in 100 mL), begin at a slow rate, and be on the lookout for systemic reactions. The best remedy for a systemic reaction, probably an idiosyncratic reaction, is unknown, but general supportive measures for anaphylactoid reactions seem to work well. Vitamin K_1 can be used to reverse warfarin-induced coagulopathy, but selective use is encouraged. The IV preparation can be given orally to titrate small amounts. Tablets are available in only 5-mg strength.

creating a very large thrombin burst (e.g., by directly activating factor X). rFVIIa has been used off-label for this purpose. Although rapid normalization of the INR is achieved, sustaining the correction requires additional doses because of the short half-life of rFVIIa. Although the INR can be corrected rapidly, some studies have called into question the effects of rFVIIa on actual clinical reversal of bleeding.[135,136]

Reversal of Other Agents

With the introduction of new anticoagulants, direct factor Xa inhibitors (rivaroxaban [Xarelto]) and direct factor II inhibitors (dabigatran [Pradaxa]), there are now concerns about reversal during acute bleeding. Because these inhibitors act at key points in the coagulation cascade, they are theoretically difficult, if not currently impossible to reverse. As of this writing there is no proven way to reverse the anticoagulation of dabigatran. Although the drug is removed by dialysis, such intervention is rarely practical in an acutely bleeding patient. Current recommendations are largely based on case reports, animal models, and human volunteer studies, and no reversal agents have been approved specifically for these direct inhibitors or have proved to be clinically efficacious (Table 28-6). However, in one recent study, PCC (50 IU/kg of Cofact, not available in the United States) immediately and completely reversed the anticoagulant effect of rivaroxaban in healthy subjects. It had no influence on the anticoagulant action of dabigatran at the dose used in this study (http://www.ncbi.nlm.nih.gov/pubmed/21900088). See the footnote in Table 28-6. In cases of life-threatening bleeding in patients receiving direct factor X or factor II inhibitors, the off-label use of PCC, activated PCC (FEIBA), or activated factor VIIa (or any combination) have all been used but none is proven.

COLLECTION AND STORAGE OF BLOOD PRODUCTS

Table 28-7 lists some characteristics of blood for transfusion. Whole blood is collected from donors into 500-mL plastic bags containing 63 mL of citrate-phosphate-dextrose (CPD) with a resultant hematocrit of 35% to 40%. Immediately after collection, sophisticated techniques permit separation of the whole blood into various components and fractions. Blood components such as FFP, PRBCs, granulocytes, and platelets are prepared from a single donor, separated, and transfused as single units. Minor blood fractions, including albumin, γ-globulin, cryoprecipitate, and fibrinogen, are often pooled from multiple donors. Within 24 hours, blood is essentially devoid of normally functioning platelets and some clotting factors, especially the labile factors V and VIII. Separation into individual components permits specialized storage and transfusion techniques designed to optimize the survival and availability of each component.

As is true of whole blood, PRBCs can be stored up to 21 days, although newer preservatives such as ADSOL (adenine, dextrose, saline, mannitol, and water) may allow 49-day storage. Red cell viability decreases approximately 1% per day. Storage of blood contributes to a variety of other derangements or "storage lesions." Cell metabolism continues during storage and causes a mild acidosis. This acidosis is buffered effectively by the bicarbonate derived from the metabolism of citrate, assuming normal hepatic function. Even with massive transfusions, acidosis is more often the result of disruption of normal physiologic function than the storage of blood products themselves. Levels of 2,3-DPG decrease during storage, thereby shifting the oxygen-hemoglobin dissociation curve to the left. This shift is of small clinical significance because 2,3-DPG levels are usually normal in transfusion recipients within 24 hours of infusion. Potassium commonly leaks from red cells during storage because of a less efficient sodium-potassium adenosine triphosphatase (ATPase)-dependent pump. Most of the potassium is either absorbed by the remaining blood cells, excreted by the kidneys, or shifted back into the cells as a result of the alkalosis produced by metabolism of citrate in the preservative. Hyperkalemia may be of particular importance in newborns and patients with renal impairment.

ORDERING OF BLOOD

Ordering a type and crossmatch procedure on a blood product implies that the decision has already been made to administer a transfusion. Blood should be drawn from the patient (≈2 mL for every unit of blood product to be cross-matched) and put into a red-topped, nonanticoagulated tube (see Fig. 28-3, *step 1*). The tube must not contain a serum separator gel. The label should be signed by the individual drawing the blood sample. This identifying signature will be used in the blood bank's cross-matching procedures. The individual blood components are discussed in the following sections. A summary of the dosages and characteristics of each component is provided in Table 28-3. A "type and hold" or "type and screen" (no crossmatch) request alerts the blood bank to the possibility that a blood product will be required for the patient so that appropriate units can be acquired and kept on hand. A type and crossmatch procedure takes 45 minutes and restricts

TABLE 28-6   Summary and Dosage of Reversal Agents*

AGENT	DOSE	NOTES
Vitamin K	1-10 mg PO or IV	SC delivery is no longer used Vitamin K will begin to work in about 2 hr but takes 24 hr to provide adequate reversal
DDAVP	0.3 µg/kg IV	Promotes platelet adherence Consider for bleeding with platelet inhibitor use Consider in mild vWD
Prothrombin complex concentrate[†] Profilnine)	INR 2-4: 25 IU/kg by IV push INR 4-6: 35 IU/kg by IV push INR >6: 50 IU/kg by IV push Alternative strategy: INR <5: 500 units; INR >5: 1000 units	Multiple dosing strategies INR-based dosing is most effective with 3-factor preparations
aPCC (Feiba)	INR <5: 500 units; INR >5: 1000 units In factor II and X inhibitor bleeding: 50 U/kg	May be more thrombogenic than PCC May be effective in reversing factor II (dabigatran) and factor X (rivaroxaban) inhibitor bleeding
rFVIIa (NovoSeven)	No specific dose has been proved 90 µg/kg is often used	Doses between 5 and 400 µg/kg have been used. Most uses are off-label and doses vary widely May not actually reverse clinical bleeding from warfarin May be useful for bleeding resulting from factor X inhibitors (both direct [rivaroxaban] and indirect [fondaparinux])

aPCC, activated prothromin complex concentrate; *DDAVP*, desmopressin; *INR*, international normalized ratio; *rFVIIa*, recombinant activated factor VII; *vWF*, von Willebrand factor.
*Most of the dosing is off-label and is derived from various studies using these agents for unapproved conditions. Other dosing regimens may exist.
[†]Recent reports suggest that PCCs may reverse the anticoagulant effect of rivaroxaban but not that of dabigatran, but the investigation is ongoing and the issue is currently unsettled (Eerenberg ES, Kamphuisen PW, Sijpkens MK, et al. Reversal of rivaroxaban and dabigatran by prothrombin complex concentrate: a randomized, placebo-controlled, crossover study in healthy subjects. *Circulation.* 2011;124:1573-1579).

TABLE 28-7   Transfusion of Blood Products

BLOOD PRODUCT*	WAITING TIME UNTIL RECEIPT IN THE ED	VOLUME	HEMATOCRIT (%)
Un-crossmatched Rh⁺ or Rh⁻ PRBCs	0-5 min	250 mL	70
Un-crossmatched type-specific whole blood	15 min	450 mL	35-40
Typed and screened whole blood	25 min	450 mL	35-40
Crossmatched whole blood	90 min	450 mL	35-40
PRBCs	90 min	250 mL	70
Frozen RBCs	4-6 hr (if not prepared in house)	250 mL	70

ED, emergency department; *PRBCs*, packed red blood cells.
*Approximate rise of 1 g/dL hemoglobin per unit PRBC transfused. Each unit of PRBCs raises the hematocrit 2% to 3%. In children, each 1 mL/kg of PRBCs raises the hematocrit by 1%.

a unit of blood to a specific patient. In the ED, a crossmatch procedure should be considered for a blood product only if the adult patient (1) manifests shock, (2) has symptomatic anemia (usually associated with a hemoglobin level <10 g/dL) in the ED, (3) has a documented loss of 1000 mL of blood, or (4) requires a blood-losing operation immediately (e.g., thoracotomy).[137] A type and hold can safely be requested for all other situations in which a blood transfusion is considered possible during the patient's care; a desirable ratio of units crossmatched to units transfused can thus be achieved. Hooker and colleagues[138] found that the empirical trigger of prehospital hypotension (systolic blood pressure <100 mm Hg) was a useful discriminator for ordering early crossmatched blood.

The number of units requested for a crossmatch procedure is determined by the size of the patient, the response of the patient to the injury and subsequent emergency treatment, and the presence of ongoing blood loss (e.g., arterial or massive gastrointestinal bleeding). Table 28-7 provides specific guidelines for administering blood components.

Red cell preparations for transfusion are not routinely tested for the presence of sickle hemoglobin. Donors with sickle trait are not excluded, and blood with sickle trait can be safely given to almost every patient because occlusion of blood flow caused by intravascular sickling would occur only in extreme conditions of acidity, hypoxia, or hypothermia, which are unlikely to be compatible with life. Nonetheless, when a transfusion is being performed in infants and patients with known sickle cell anemia, the blood bank should be alerted, and a "sickle preparation" should be requested for donor blood to avoid the infusion of blood with sickle trait into such patients. Patients receiving multiple transfusions for sickle cell disease are at increased risk for alloimmunization. Directed donation may be helpful to decrease this risk.[139,140]

Blood Request Forms

Proper identification of the patient and the intended unit of blood is critical. Transfusion of an incorrect unit is a potentially fatal error. Most transfusion reactions are attributable to clerical error, and the vast majority of such errors occur at the bedside (e.g., not in the blood bank).[141] Just before administering the blood, the nurse or clinician (or both) must check the identity of the numbered labels. In addition, the blood bank laboratory slip must identify the patient by name and number and contain the identification number of the unit of blood.

Usual procedures require a separate blood bank request form for each unit of RBCs or whole blood ordered. A number of units of FFP, cryoprecipitate, and platelet concentrates may be ordered on one form with proper identification (depending on individual blood bank procedures).

Blood Products for Jehovah's Witnesses

There are approximately 1.2 million Jehovah's Witnesses in the United States. Based on the religious belief that the Bible prohibits blood or blood product transfusion (Acts 15:28-29), devout Jehovah's Witnesses do not accept transfusions of whole blood, packed cells, white blood cells, platelets, plasma, or autologous blood.[142] Since 1961, willing acceptance of a blood transfusion by an unrepentant member has been grounds for expulsion from the religion.[143,144] An individual's decision to abandon the teachings of the church and accept blood products can lead to congregational disciplinary actions, including "disfellowshipping," a term for formal expulsion and shunning. Some members may permit the infusion of albumin, clotting factor solutions, plasma expanders, or intraoperative autotransfusion.[145] Although no guidelines for the administration of blood products to Jehovah's Witnesses are absolute, certain recommendations can be made. Even though a transfusion may be necessary to save a patient's life and would otherwise be considered standard care, administration of blood or blood products in the face of refusal can legally be considered battery. In an awake and otherwise competent adult, courts have ruled that clinicians cannot be held liable if they comply with a patient's directive and withhold lifesaving blood administration after refusal of transfusion when

specific and detailed information of the consequences of such an omission in treatment are provided. The issue becomes clouded when patients are incompetent, unconscious (most Jehovah's Witnesses carry cards informing medical personnel of their religious beliefs), or minors.

In the absence of specific directives to the contrary, it is prudent to administer blood products to patients who are unconscious, judged to be incompetent adults, or minors.[146] Explicit documentation of the intent of the clinician to preserve life coupled with an accurate description of discussion of the issue with the patient or the family and clarification of the patient's mental capacity is mandatory. Furthermore, emergency legal assistance (e.g., court orders, appointment of a temporary guardian) should be sought immediately with rapid judicial resolution.[147] Various clinical techniques to maximize oxygen delivery and minimize oxygen consumption should be used. Examples include limited blood drawing, the use of high-dose erythropoietin and nutritional support with aggressive iron supplementation, hypothermia, volume expansion, sedation, oxygen, and the use of synthetic hemoglobin substitutes.[148,149] Hyperbaric oxygen therapy (HBO) can dissolve sufficient oxygen to sustain life in the absence of hemoglobin and may be another option when blood cannot be used.[150-152] HBO can be used in a pulsed fashion (3 to 4 hr/day) to reduce the oxygen debt until hemoglobin can rise to adequate levels.

ADMINISTRATION OF BLOOD PRODUCTS

IV Transfusions

Do not open a unit of blood unless a free-flowing IV access line has been established in a large-bore vein. Use a 14- to 16-gauge IV catheter if possible, both to minimize hemolysis and to ensure rapid infusion of fluid for the treatment of hypovolemia or hypotension. When a large quantity of blood must be given rapidly, administer it by means of a high-flow infusion system if possible. The purpose of a large-bore infusion line is defeated if blood is piggybacked with an 18- to 20-gauge needle through a side port in the infusion tubing. For an elective transfusion, however, blood may be given through a smaller lumen. Combining hemodilution (250 mL of saline with 1 unit of PRBCs) and pressurization can safely increase the flow rate through 20- and 22-gauge catheters severalfold.[153] No significant hemolysis occurs when small (21-, 23-, 25-, and 27-gauge) short needles are used for the transfusion of fresh blood or packed cells in infants and children and when the maximum rate of infusion is less than 100 mL/hr.[154] For rapid infusion, however, connect the blood administration tubing directly to the infusion catheter. Monitor the infusion site for infiltration, infection, or local reactions.

If the patient already has a suitable IV line in place, flush the system with a solution of normal saline before administering the blood (see Fig. 28-3, *step 2*). Do not use other IV fluids because of the risk for hemolysis or aggregation (e.g., with 5% dextrose in water).[155,156] Do not place any medications in the unit of blood or infusion line for the same reasons.

Errors associated with blood transfusions have serious consequences and frequently result in severe transfusion reactions and death. The Joint Commission on Accreditation of Healthcare Organizations (JCAHO) has set forth guidelines in an attempt to reduce these errors, including the following:

- Training personnel in procedures and recognition of reactions
- Revising staffing models
- Redesigning methods to identify patients, attain patient and blood verification, gain consent, and process multiple samples. It was strongly suggested that room numbers be discontinued as a method of identifying patients and use of a unique identification band be considered for patients receiving blood
- Enhancing technical and computer support of the process
- Discontinuing the use of refrigerators for multiple blood units

Many EDs have moved to a two-nurse mandate for checking patient and blood unit identities before administration (see Fig. 28-3, *step 3*). As the risk for infectious complications associated with transfusion medicine gradually declines, medical errors have supplanted them as the most serious cause of transfusion mishaps.[157]

IO Transfusions

Although IV administration is by far the most common route of blood and blood component therapy, intraosseous (IO) administration appears to be safe and effective. Administration rates via an IO route are generally slower (on average 21 versus 35 mL/min by the IV route) but appear to be metabolically and hemodynamically equivalent.[158] In animal models, no evidence of fat embolism and lung or kidney inflammation was noted after IO PRBC infusion. Administration of IO liposome-encapsulated hemoglobin (one of the forms of HBOC therapy) is also effective and may have additional advantages over the IV route.[159] Similarly, limited studies on the administration of other blood products via the IO route have been promising.[160]

Filters

Infuse all blood and blood products through an appropriate filter, such as those supplied in-line in blood administration tubing sets (see Fig. 28-3, *step 4*). In the past, filtration was required merely to keep the IV line from becoming blocked by clots. Adverse consequences from infusing unfiltered blood products have since been recognized. Debris consisting of clots and aggregates of fibrin, white blood cells, platelets, and intertwined RBCs (ranging in size from 15 to 200 μm) accumulates progressively during the storage of blood. The usual filter, made of a single layer of plastic with multiple 170-μm pores, traps larger particles yet allows the rapid infusion of 2 to 3 units of blood before flow is obstructed. Purified components of blood plasma can be safely administered through a filter with pores as fine as 5 μm.

It has been suggested that microaggregates of debris that can pass through a 170-μm filter may in part contribute to the syndrome of "shock lung" seen after the transfusion of many blood units in patients suffering from severe trauma and hemorrhage. Some clinicians therefore recommend using a microaggregate blood infusion filter with a mesh pore size of 40 μm when multiple units of blood are administered to trauma victims, patients with compromised pulmonary function, and neonates. Microaggregate filters tend to become blocked, impede the rate of infusion more quickly, and are not commonly required in the emergency setting.[161] A significant

number of platelets are removed by microaggregate filters, and some advise against using these filters when platelet packs are infused. Others believe that although platelets are removed with the microaggregate filters, the trapped platelets can be removed with a saline flush without any significant loss.[162]

Replace standard filters after 2 to 3 units of blood product have been administered. Change microaggregate filters after each unit.

Rate of Infusion

One unit of whole blood can be safely administered to a hypotensive patient at a rate of at least 20 mL/kg/hr (see Fig. 28-3, *step 5*). In the setting of hypovolemic shock and continued hemorrhage, there is no limit to the transfusion rate. Multiple units may be transfused simultaneously, even under pressure. Use of a rapid transfuser device can assist in the rapid administration and warming of blood (Fig. 28-5). In stable patients, administer 1 unit of whole blood (500 mL) over approximately a 2-hour period (3 to 4 mL/kg/hr). After this time, RBCs begin to lose metabolic activity. In addition, the unit of blood, which is an excellent culture medium, is likely to become contaminated if bacteria and fungi are allowed to grow at room temperature. Give packed cells at approximately the same rate. Give plasma products more rapidly; in a patient without cardiovascular compromise, administer FFP at a rate faster than 15 to 20 min/unit because the coagulant activity begins to deteriorate rapidly after thawing. In patients with severe anemia and congestive heart failure, administer a rapidly acting diuretic, such as furosemide, at the onset of transfusion to prevent circulatory overload.

Figure 28-5 Use of a rapid transfuser allows transfusion rates up to 300 mL/min via a 14-gauge peripheral intravenous line. All fluids administered via the rapid transfuser will be warmed to approximately 37°C.

If a transfusion of blood must be interrupted or delayed for any reason, return the remainder of the blood unit to the blood bank. Refrigerators in the ED or on the hospital unit should not be used to store blood products unless they are specifically equipped and authorized to do so.

For patients in hemorrhagic shock, administer blood through two large-bore catheters at different sites if necessary. Usually, gravity provides a sufficient pressure gradient if the unit is raised above the patient to increase the rate of infusion when the clamps are wide open. Using a pressure pump makes the infusion quicker.[163] Do not use a standard sphygmomanometer cuff wrapped around a unit of blood to create increased infusion pressure because the nonuniform application of pressure could burst the plastic bag containing the blood component.

If desired, dilute PRBCs with normal saline (0.9% without dextrose) before infusion simply by opening the clamps on the upper tubes of the Y infusion set and leaving the lower (recipient end) clamps closed. Although it is generally agreed that LR solution should not be mixed with blood because of possible clot formation, multiple studies have challenged this belief and results have shown that small amounts of LR solution (up to 150 mL) are safe in the clinical setting.[164,165] Furthermore, larger volumes of LR solution have not been found to produce microaggregate clots in laboratory settings when using AS-3–preserved PRBCs, a typical additive nutritive solution containing sodium chloride, sodium citrate, sodium phosphate, citric acid, dextrose, and adenine.[166]

Diluting blood, while increasing its volume, will allow more rapid infusion by decreasing blood viscosity, which is dependent on hematocrit. Alternatively, add approximately 200 mL of normal saline directly to the bag of PRBCs to bring the hematocrit in the blood bag to approximately 45%.

Rewarming

Blood is stored at approximately 4°C to maintain cellular integrity and prevent the growth of microorganisms. Blood products usually passively warm to 10°C by the time that they are administered to the patient unless administered under pressure. The adverse effects of hypothermia on cardiac conduction and flow rates are evident when rapid administration of a large volume of blood is performed without prewarming.

Various mechanisms have been used to warm blood to 35°C to 37°C. An ideal blood warmer should allow liberal flow rates while preventing thermal hemolysis of blood cells. Commonly used devices include those with bath coils that allow a plastic tube to reside in a closely regulated warm water bath and dry heat devices that allow blood to circulate through flat, thin bags sandwiched between aluminum blocks that contain electric heating elements. Both devices have relatively low flow rates and suboptimal thermal clearance.[5] Immersion of blood bags in warm water baths is safe but is considered imprecise and slow. Despite some evidence of their safety, the use of microwave heating devices is not recommended by the Association of Blood Banks because of concerns of hemolysis.[167] Herron and colleagues[168] advocated keeping PRBC temperature below 50°C because they noted significant hemolysis beginning at 51°C to 53°C.

Rapid admixture warming is a promising alternative technique.[169] Mix the unit of whole blood with an equal amount of normal saline that has been preheated to 60°C to 70°C.

Once mixed, administer the product to the patient, which has a resultant delivery temperature of approximately 35°C. This technique combines dilution of blood product and warming into one step. Regardless of the rewarming technique used, warming refrigerated blood to body temperature decreases its viscosity twofold to threefold and avoids venous spasm, thus facilitating transfusion.

Monitoring

During the first part of the transfusion of any blood product, carefully monitor the patient for evidence of a transfusion reaction (see Fig. 28-3, *step 6*). Look for signs and symptoms such as hives, chills, diarrhea, fever, pruritus, flushing, abdominal or back pain, tightness in the chest or throat, and respiratory distress. A potentially life-threatening acute hemolytic transfusion reaction in a patient who has previously received transfusions may differ clinically from a minor allergic reaction only by its effects on the patient's pulse and blood pressure. Treat an allergic reaction (hives, itching) to leukocytes or plasma proteins by administering an antihistamine (but not in the blood infusion line), and stop the transfusion.

Stop the transfusion immediately when the following signs are encountered: an increase in pulse rate, a decrease in blood pressure, respiratory symptoms, chest or abdominal discomfort, or a sensation of "impending doom." Administer normal saline to maintain blood pressure and urine output. Send samples of urine and blood to the laboratory to verify the presence of free hemoglobin. Also send the blood bank a clotted sample of blood to reassess for the presence of an immune reaction. If the blood bank concludes that the reaction is a nonhemolytic allergic response, premedicate with antihistamines (diphenhydramine or hydroxyzine) and antipyretics before the next transfusion. Alternatively, use washed cells.

If a hemolytic transfusion reaction is suspected, treat the patient vigorously and promptly.[170] Most morbidity and mortality are due to hypotension and shock with subsequent cardiovascular instability, renal insufficiency, respiratory manifestations, or hemorrhagic complications of disseminated intravascular coagulation. Infuse crystalloid or vasopressors to treat the hypotension directly, if required. Determine the volume and rate of infusion by blood pressure response. Treat symptomatically with acetaminophen, a warming blanket, antihistamines, and inhaled or subcutaneous β-agonists for bronchospasm or subglottic edema.

If an acute hemolytic transfusion reaction occurs, alkalinize the urine with IV sodium bicarbonate to prevent the precipitation of free hemoglobin. Force diuresis with mannitol to maintain urine output at 50 to 100 mL/hr. The benefit of alkalization and diuresis in preventing acute renal failure is uncertain, although the use of these techniques is commonly advocated.[171] After shock is controlled, assess hemostasis, respiratory function, renal function, and cardiac function to help direct therapy for complications; disseminated intravascular coagulation may require the administration of plasma, platelets, or fibrinogen, and acute tubular necrosis may complicate fluid management.

Delayed, or "late," hemolytic transfusion reactions may occur days or even weeks after the transfusion of RBCs. Such reactions are characterized by falling hemoglobin levels, jaundice, hemoglobinemia, and indirect hyperbilirubinemia.[172] This complication is usually self-limited and is not

BOX 28-2 Caveats Regarding Transfusion of Blood Products in the Setting of Acute Blood Loss

The total volume of blood circulating in the body is about 7% of ideal body weight in adults and 8% to 9% in children. A 70-kg adult, therefore, has a total blood volume of about 5 L.

DEFINITION OF MASSIVE BLOOD LOSS

Loss of total blood volume (10 units in a 70-kg adult) in 24 hours or loss of 50% of total blood volume over a 3-hour period.

GENERALIZED GUIDE TO TRANSFUSION OF RBCS*

Rarely transfuse if the hemoglobin level is higher than 10 g/dL; usually transfuse if the level is lower than 6 g/dL. In general, the aim is to keep the hemoglobin level at about 7 to 8 g/dL and the hematocrit about 30% to 35% to sustain hemostasis and oxygen delivery.[†]

In critically ill patients, a restrictive transfusion policy of administering RBCs if the hemoglobin level drops below 7 g/dL and maintaining levels in the 7- to 9-g/dL range is at least as beneficial as more liberal criteria, except perhaps for patients with acute coronary ischemia.

GENERAL GUIDE TO PLATELET TRANSFUSION

Aim for a platelet count of $50,000/mL^3$ or higher in actively bleeding patients,[‡] but lower thresholds may be safe, especially in the absence of bleeding.

FFP

Fibrinogen levels may fall to a critical level (<1 g/dL) after 150% loss of blood volume; therefore, consider FFP after 1 blood volume

has been lost. Other labile clotting factors fall to 25% activity after about 200% blood loss. Transfusing 1 unit of FFP per every 5 to 6 units of RBCs has been traditional teaching, but decisions are best based on coagulation profiles. Preliminary evidence indicates that an FFP/RBC ratio of 1:1 may be more beneficial in patients with exsanguinating hemorrhage.

CRYOPRECIPITATE[§]

If FFP does not raise fibrinogen levels to more than 1 g/dL, consider cryoprecipitate. Use in the ED is supported, but not mandated.

PROTHROMBIN COMPLEX CONCENTRATES[§]

Autoplex T, Proplex, and Feiba VH are all products contain that factor VII but no fibrinogen. Reversal of the INR to normal is the goal. Concomitant vitamin K is used to initiate production of clotting factors that have been blocked by warfarin. Use in the ED is supported but not mandated.

RECOMBINANT FACTOR VIIA[§]

No strict guidelines or proven benefits exist. May consider if
1. No heparin/warfarin effect remains.
2. Surgical control of bleeding is not possible.
3. Bleeding continues despite adequate replacement of other coagulation factors (FFP, platelets, cryoprecipitate).
4. Acidosis is corrected.

Use in the ED is supported but not mandated.

Adapted from Stainsby D, MacLennan D, Thomas J, et al. Guidelines on the management of massive blood loss. Br J Haematol. 2006;135:634; and Hébert PC, Wells G, Blajchman MA, et al. A multicenter, randomized, controlled clinical trial of transfusion requirements in critical care. N Engl J Med. 1999;340:409.
ED, emergency department; FFP, fresh frozen plasma; INR, international normalized ratio; RBCs, red blood cells.
Depends on the rate of blood loss and underlying medical condition. RBC transfusion is probably required with 30% to 40% blood volume loss.
[†]*RBCs can contribute to hemostasis by their effect on platelet margination and function.*
[‡]*This level can be anticipated by the time that the patient has received 2 blood volumes of fluid or RBC transfusions, but substantial variations exist.*
[§]*Use in the ED is supported but not mandated; it is usually administered under the advice of a consultant.*

life-threatening. Therapy is symptomatic, but future attempts at crossmatching for transfusions may be difficult because of the presence of RBC antibodies. Individuals thus affected should wear identification tags or bracelets to alert medical personnel that previous transfusion reactions have occurred.

On completion of a transfusion, make an entry in the patient's record to indicate the type and volume of the transfusion and the presence or absence of any reaction. The progress note, the transfusion record sheet, or the transfusion laboratory slip can be used for this purpose and should be signed and dated by the clinician, in accordance with hospital policies.

Emphasize to the patient and family how critically important any blood transfusion is to the patient's care. Suggest that

the family consider arranging for replacement donations of units of blood to afford future patients the luxury of an ample, available supply of blood products.

CONCLUSION

Some general guidelines and caveats regarding the transfusion of blood products in the setting of acute blood loss are outlined in Box 28-2.

References are available at www.expertconsult.com.

Anesthetic and Analgesic Techniques

CHAPTER 29

Local and Topical Anesthesia

Douglas L. McGee

Local anesthetic agents are important tools used in the everyday practice of emergency medicine. This chapter describes the mechanism of action, the nuances of clinical use, and the adverse reactions to anesthetics that are commonly used in the emergency department (ED). Detailed technical guidance for the performance of topical and infiltrative local anesthesia is provided.

BACKGROUND

The first local anesthetic was cocaine, an alkaloid in the leaves of the *Erythroxylon coca* shrub from the Andes Mountains. Early Incan society used cocaine for invasive procedures, including cranial trephination. In 1884, Koller[1] used topical cocaine in the eye and was credited with the introduction of local anesthesia into clinical practice. In the same year, Zenfel used a topical solution of alcohol and cocaine to anesthetize the eardrum, and Hall[2] introduced the drug into dentistry. In 1885 Halsted[3] demonstrated that cocaine blocked nerve transmission, thereby laying the foundation for nerve block anesthesia. The search for alternatives to cocaine led to synthesis of the benzoic acid ester derivatives and the amide anesthetics used today. It was not until the 1960s that detailed understanding of the physiochemical properties, mechanism of action, pharmacokinetics, and toxicity of these agents emerged.

PHARMACOLOGY AND PHYSIOLOGY
Chemical Structure and Physiochemical Properties

Most useful local anesthetic agents share a basic chemical structure:

Aromatic segment—Intermediate chain—Hydrophilic segment

Subtle variations in this basic structure determine each agent's main physiochemical properties: the negative log of dissociation constant (pK_a), the partition coefficient (a measurement of lipid solubility), and the degree of protein binding. Each of these properties determines the drug's potency, onset, and duration of action. However, physiochemical properties are not the sole determinant of clinical activity; other factors influence the drug's effect. The intermediate chain between the aromatic and the hydrophilic segments is either an amino-ester or an amino-amide; these chemical structures form the basis for the two main classifications of local anesthetics. Common ester-type agents include procaine, chloroprocaine, cocaine, and tetracaine. Common amide-type agents include articaine, lidocaine, mepivacaine, prilocaine, bupivacaine, and etidocaine. Different biochemical pathways metabolize each class. Esters are hydrolyzed by plasma pseudocholinesterase. Cocaine, an ester, is also partly metabolized by N-demethylation and nonenzymatic hydrolysis. Individuals with pseudocholinesterase deficiency may have a greater potential for cocaine toxicity if large doses are used, although this has not been an issue when cocaine is used clinically as an anesthetic. Amides are metabolized in the liver by enzymatic degradation. Local anesthetics are poorly soluble weak bases combined with hydrogen chloride to produce the salt of a weak acid. In solution, the salt exists both as uncharged molecules (nonionized) and as positively charged cations (ionized). The nonionized form is lipid soluble, which enables it to diffuse through tissues and across nerve membranes. The ratio of nonionized to ionized forms depends on the pH of the medium (vial solution or tissue milieu) and on the pK_a of the specific agent. The pK_a is the pH in which 50% of the solution is in the uncharged form and 50% is in the charged form. When the pH of the solution or tissue is less than the pK_a, more of the drug is ionized. When the pH increases, more of the drug is in the nonionized form. Because the nonionized form of drug can diffuse through tissues and nerves, manipulating the pH of the solution can alter a drug's diffusion properties.

Local anesthetics are available in single-dose vials or ampules and in multidose vials, with and without epinephrine. Most solutions have a pH higher than 5. Multidose vials contain methylparaben, an antibacterial preservative. Local anesthetics premixed with epinephrine also contain an antioxidant (sodium bisulfite or sodium metabisulfite) to prevent deactivation of the vasoconstrictor. These solutions must be adjusted to a more acidic pH, approximately 3.5 to 4.0, to maintain the stability of epinephrine and its antioxidant. These properties as they relate to the amide group are depicted in Table 29-1.

TABLE 29-1 pH and Additives of Amide Local Anesthetics

SOLUTION CONTENT	pH (RANGE)	PRESERVATIVE (METHYLPARABEN)	ANTIOXIDANT
Plain, single dose	4.5-6.5	–	–
Plain, multidose	4.5-6.5	+	–
Commercial epinephrine, single dose	3.5-4.0	–	+
Commercial epinephrine, multidose	3.5-4.0	+	+
Prepared epinephrine, single dose	4.5-6.5	–	–

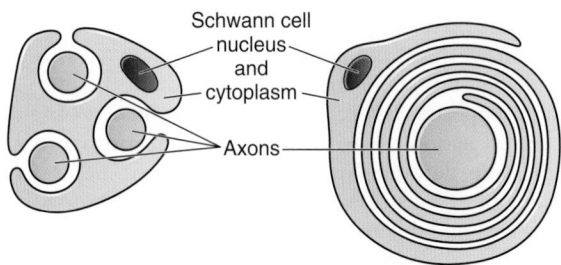

Figure 29-1 Schwann cell sheath of unmyelinated (left) and myelinated (*right*) nerve fibers. (*From Wildsmith JAW. Peripheral nerve and local anesthetic drugs.* Br J Anaesth. *1986;58:692. Reproduced by permission.*)

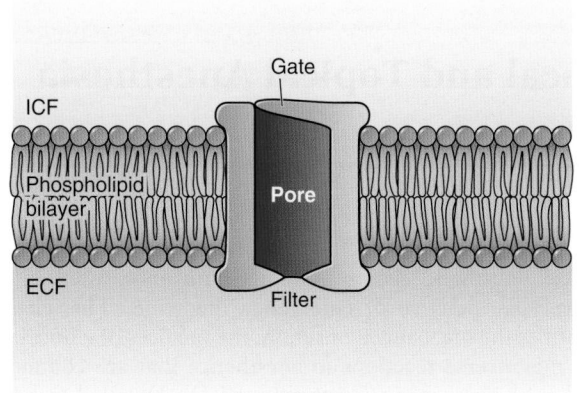

Figure 29-2 Axon membrane. *ECF,* extracellular fluid; *ICF,* intracellular fluid. (*From Wildsmith JAW. Peripheral nerve and local anesthetic drugs.* Br J Anaesth. *1986;58:692. Reproduced by permission.*)

Nerve Structure and Impulse Transmission

Functional and Structural Components of a Peripheral Nerve

The functional nerve unit includes the nerve axon and its surrounding Schwann cell sheath. The Schwann cell (Fig. 29-1) may surround several unmyelinated axons or a single myelinated nerve fiber and form a myelin sheath. Junctions between sheaths along the axon called *nodes of Ranvier* contain sodium channels necessary for depolarization. As myelin sheath thickness increases from autonomic to sensory to motor fibers, the nodes of Ranvier are spaced farther apart. The most important structure affecting transmission of nerve impulses is the axon membrane (Fig. 29-2). The membrane consists of a double layer of phospholipids into which are embedded protein molecules that serve as channels containing pores for the movement of ions in and out of the cell. Most pores have a filter, or gate, that controls ion-specific movement and a sensory mechanism that opens or closes the gate. Bundles of nerve fibers (Fig. 29-3) are embedded in the endoneurium, which is made of collagen fibrils, and they are surrounded by a cellular layer, the perineurium. The perineurium functions as a diffusion barrier and maintains the composition of extracellular fluid around the nerve fibers. Surrounding the entire structure is the outer layer of a peripheral nerve, the epineurium, which is composed of areolar connective tissue.

The Nerve Impulse and Transmission

The inside of a nerve fiber, or axoplasm, is negative (–70 mV) at rest in comparison to the outside. This resting potential is the net result of the differences in ionic concentration on each side of the axonal membrane and the forces that tend to

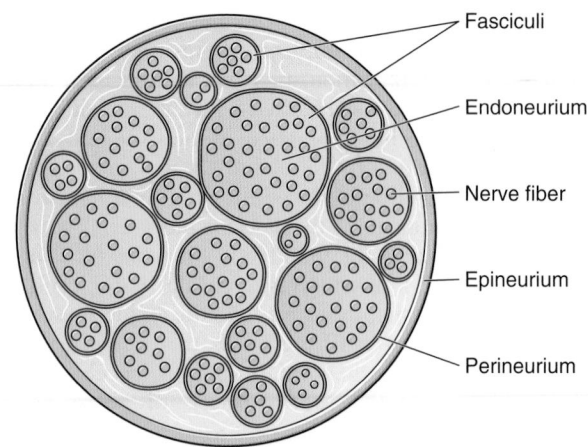

Figure 29-3 Cross-section of a peripheral nerve. (*From Wildsmith JAW. Peripheral nerve and local anesthetic drugs.* Br J Anaesth. *1986;58:692. Reproduced by permission.*)

maintain that difference. Specifically, there is a surplus of sodium extracellularly and potassium intracellularly. The sodium channel is closed, thereby preventing these ions from moving along their concentration gradient (out → in). Although potassium can leave the cell to follow its concentration gradient (in → out), the need to maintain electrical neutrality inside the cell prevents it from completely doing so. Potassium is in equilibrium between the concentration gradient and the electrochemical gradient, thus creating the negative resting potential.

The sodium channel opens when a nerve is stimulated. Sodium ions enter slowly at first until a critical threshold is reached. They then enter the cell rapidly, along the electrochemical and concentration gradients, and cause depolarization. The influx of sodium is halted when the membrane potential reaches +20 mV, but potassium continues to move out of the cell and repolarizes it until the resting potential is reached. When the excitation process has been completed and the nerve cell is electrically quiet, the relative excess of sodium inside the cell and potassium outside the cell is readjusted by the adenosine triphosphate-dependent sodium-potassium pump.

Depolarization of a portion of the nerve causes a current to flow along the adjacent nerve fiber. This current makes the membrane potential less negative and actuates the sensor to open the next sodium channel. The action potential cycle is repeated, thereby propagating the impulse. Nerve conduction is essentially unidirectional because the sodium channel is not only closed but inactivated as well and delayed closure of specific potassium channels prevents the critical threshold from being reached in the segment just depolarized. An impulse spreads continuously down the axon in unmyelinated nerve fibers. In myelinated fibers, current flows from node to node and depolarizes intervening segments at once. This saltatory conduction causes a faster rate of impulse transmission in myelinated fibers.

Mechanism of Action

How local anesthetic agents block nerve conduction depends on the active form of the agent and the specific physiologic and cellular activity.

The Active Form
Anesthetic solutions contain uncharged and charged forms. The concentration of the uncharged form increases in more alkaline milieus. Only this uncharged lipid-soluble form can cross tissue and membrane barriers. Once the uncharged drug is through a barrier, it reequilibrates into uncharged and charged forms in a proportion dependent on the prevailing pH. Because local anesthetics are more effective in alkaline solutions, it was originally thought that the uncharged form was responsible for conduction blockade. Alkaline solutions are currently believed to be more effective because of increased penetration through tissue barriers. The cationic charged form is responsible for the actual neuronal blockade.

The Physiologic and Cellular Basis for Neuronal Blockade
Prevention of sodium influx across the nerve membrane forms the physiologic basis for conduction blockade. Local anesthetics slow sodium influx, thereby decreasing the rate of rise and amplitude of depolarization. If sufficient anesthetic is present and the firing threshold is not reached, the action potential is not formed. With no action potential, no impulse is transmitted and conduction is blocked, which results in local anesthesia.

How anesthetic agents prevent sodium influx is still not completely understood. It is believed that the cationic charged

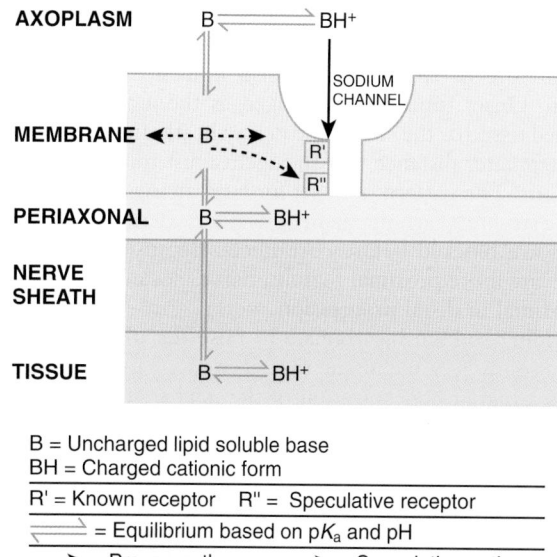

Figure 29-4 Mechanism of action of local anesthetic agents (see text for details). (*Modified from Ritchie JM. Mechanism of action of local anesthetic agents and biotoxins.* Br J Anaesth. *1975;47:196. Reproduced by permission.*)

form blocks the action potential from inside the membrane; the agent enters the sodium channel from the axoplasmic side and binds to a receptor.[4,5] This "specific receptor" theory is well accepted and is considered the predominant mechanism in preventing influx of sodium. However, this theory cannot account for the action of benzocaine and other neutral compounds or the uncharged base forms of the common local anesthetics.

In summary (Fig. 29-4), when a local anesthetic (other than benzocaine) surrounds the perineurium, it equilibrates into its uncharged and charged forms based on tissue pH and pK_a. In a more alkaline environment, a greater proportion of the uncharged form is present. The uncharged lipid-soluble form penetrates tissue, nerve sheath, and nerve membrane to gain access to the axoplasm and reequilibrates into both charged and uncharged forms. The charged form enters the sodium channel, decreases movement of sodium into the cell, and halts nerve transmission. The uncharged base is also involved in sodium channel blockade, but the exact nature of this mechanism is unknown.

Activity Profile during Neuronal Blockade

A local anesthetic's onset, potency, duration, and ability to produce a differential blockade in mixed nerves are a function of its physiochemical properties, the physiologic environment, and to some extent, manipulation by the clinician.

Onset of Action
The pK_a of an anesthetic is the primary physiochemical factor that determines its onset of action. Increased tissue penetration and a shortened onset of action are found in drugs with a lower pK_a because more of the lipid-soluble uncharged form is present (Tables 29-2 and 29-3). Although in isolated nerve fibers the onset of action directly parallels pK_a, other physiochemical factors also influence drug activity. For example, prilocaine and lidocaine have the same pK_a, but lidocaine's

onset is faster because of its enhanced ability to penetrate through nonnerve tissue.

The site of administration also influences the onset of action. Onset times are prolonged as the amount of interspersed tissue or the size of the nerve sheath increases because of the greater distance that the agent must travel to reach its receptor. The pattern of onset for large nerves is determined by the structural arrangement of its fibers. Peripheral (mantle) fibers are blocked before core fibers. Because mantle fibers innervate more proximal regions, nerve blockade proceeds in a proximal to distal progression.

Adding sodium bicarbonate to raise the pH of the anesthetic solution (a technique that decreases pain on injection) yields a higher concentration of the uncharged lipid-soluble form and decreases onset time. Increasing the total dose by using a higher concentration of the same volume or a greater volume of the same concentration also shortens onset time. For most procedures performed in the ED, the time of onset of most agents is short enough that manipulation to achieve shorter times is unnecessary.

Potency

The lipid solubility of an anesthetic is a primary physicochemical factor determining potency. The drug's partition coefficient, not the concentration of the lipid-soluble form determined by the pK_a or pH, confers its lipid solubility. Because the nerve membrane is lipid, lipophilic anesthetics pass more easily into the cell and few molecules are needed to block conduction (see Tables 29-2 and 29-3).

The degree of vasodilation produced by the anesthetic also affects potency because vasodilation promotes vascular absorption, thereby reducing the amount of locally available drug. Lidocaine is more lipid soluble than prilocaine or mepivacaine, but it produces more vasodilation. Although lidocaine is twice as potent as prilocaine or mepivacaine in vitro, it is equipotent in vivo. Though not a primary reason for its use, epinephrine, by producing vasoconstriction and making more molecules available to the nerve, increases the depth of anesthesia. Drugs more readily absorbed by fat have reduced potency. Increased concentration also increases potency. Choosing an anesthetic for its potency is not usually necessary for any given site because the commercially available concentration of an agent may be manipulated to make most drugs equianesthetic. For example, lidocaine, being one fourth as potent as bupivacaine, is usually used at four times the concentration (1% to 2% versus 0.25% to 0.5%, respectively). For different sites and techniques, different concentrations and volumes of a given agent are needed to produce adequate blockade.

Duration

The degree of protein binding of an anesthetic primarily determines its duration of action. Agents that bind more tightly to the protein receptor remain in the sodium channel longer (see Tables 29-2 and 29-3). Like potency, the duration of action is reduced by the vasodilation produced by local anesthetics. Prilocaine, which is less protein bound than lidocaine, has a longer duration of action because of its lesser degree of vasodilation. The duration of action also varies with the mode of administration. It is shorter when agents are applied topically.

The duration of action may be prolonged by several methods. Increasing the dose, usually by increasing the

---

TABLE 29-2   Activity Profile with a Primary Physiochemical Determinant

AGENT	ONSET: pK_a	POTENCY:LIPID SOLUBILITY	DURATION: PROTEIN BINDING
Tetracaine	Slow	8	Long
Procaine	Slow	1	Short
Chloroprocaine	Fast	1	Short
Lidocaine	Fast	2	Moderate
Mepivacaine	Fast	2	Moderate
Prilocaine	Fast	2	Moderate
Bupivacaine	Moderate	8	Long
Etidocaine	Fast	4-6	Long

TABLE 29-3   Physiochemical Properties of Selected Local Anesthetics

AGENT	TYPE	SITE OF METABOLISM	pK_a	LIPID SOLUBILITY (PARTITION COEFFICIENT)	PROTEIN BINDING (%)
Tetracaine	Ester	Plasma	8.5	High (4.1)	76
Procaine	Ester	Plasma	8.9	Low (0.02)	6
Chloroprocaine	Ester	Plasma	8.7	Low (0.14)	—
Lidocaine	Amide	Liver	7.9	Medium (2.9)	64
Mepivacaine	Amide	Liver	7.6	Medium (0.8)	78
Prilocaine	Amide	Liver	7.9	Medium (0.9)	55
Bupivacaine	Amide	Liver	8.1	High (27.5)	95
Etidocaine	Amide	Liver	7.7	High (141.0)	94

Note: A common way to remember the class of anesthetic (amide versus ester) is that all amides have the letter "i" appearing twice in the generic name. The others are esters. Cocaine, not listed in this table, is also an ester.

concentration, prolongs the duration to limits imposed by toxic effects. Raising the pH of the anesthetic solution has also been shown to prolong duration.[6,7] The most practical way to increase duration is to use solutions that contain epinephrine.[8] Epinephrine causes vasoconstriction, decreases systemic absorption, and allows more drug to reach the nerve. The effect of epinephrine varies according to the agent. Anesthetics that intrinsically produce more vasodilation (e.g., procaine, lidocaine, mepivacaine) benefit more from epinephrine's vasoconstrictive action. The long-acting, highly lipid-soluble agents (e.g., bupivacaine, etidocaine) are less affected because they are substantially taken up by extradural fat and released slowly. In fact, lidocaine with epinephrine may be effective for as long as bupivacaine without epinephrine. Generally, most ED procedures can be accomplished quickly before the anesthesia wears off regardless of which drug is selected. Choose agents with a long duration of action when the procedure is lengthy or if postoperative analgesia is desired.

TOPICAL ANESTHESIA

Local anesthetic agents may be applied topically to mucous membranes, intact skin, and lacerations. There are sufficient differences among these sites to merit a separate discussion of each one. Topical anesthesia of the eye is discussed in Chapter 62.

Mucous Membranes

Agents and Uses

Effective anesthesia of the intact mucous membranes (not intact skin) of the nose, mouth, throat, tracheobronchial tree, esophagus, and genitourinary tract may be provided by several anesthetics (Box 29-1). Tetracaine, lidocaine, and cocaine are the most effective commonly used agents (Table 29-4 and Box 29-1). Benzocaine (14% to 20%) is commonly used for intraoral or pharyngeal anesthesia (Fig. 29-5). The anesthesia produced is superficial and does not relieve pain that originates from submucosal structures. The onset of action may be slow, which limits its usefulness in urgent situations (such as passing a nasogastric tube). Agents applied topically can be absorbed systemically, and concentrated topical agents can cause toxicity.

Tetracaine solution is an effective and potent topical agent with a relatively long duration of action. It is used in concentrations from 0.25% to 1% with a recommended maximum

adult dose of 50 mg. In overdose, it has the disadvantage of severe cardiovascular toxicity without any preceding central nervous system (CNS) stimulatory phase.

Lidocaine is also an effective topical agent that is marketed in a variety of forms (solutions, jellies, and ointments) and concentrations (2% to 10%). The 10% form is most effective, and minimal topical anesthesia is achieved with less potent concentrations. Lidocaine is commonly used as the 2% viscous solution prescribed for inflamed or irritated mucous membranes of the mouth and pharynx. Patient misuse of viscous lidocaine, by repeated self-administration, can lead to serious toxicity. Topical lidocaine provides an adequate duration for most procedures, with the maximum safe dose being 250 to 300 mg.

Cocaine is an effective, but potentially toxic topical agent that is applied to the mucous membranes of the upper respiratory tract. Although it is an ester, hepatic metabolism occurs,

---

BOX 29-1 **Common Local and Topical Anesthetics Used in the ED**

- Benzocaine spray will produce transient anesthesia of the mucous membranes. Rarely, it can precipitate methemoglobinemia in standard doses. Anbesol is a popular over-the-counter benzocaine anesthetic for dental problems, such as teething. See Figure 30-3 for a description of an excellent topical combination of lidocaine, prilocaine, and tetracaine (preferred by editors).
- EMLA cream (lidocaine and prilocaine) will produce anesthesia of intact skin, but it must be in place for about 60 minutes to provide significant benefit. ELA-Max is another topical lidocaine preparation with a more rapid onset of action.
- "Magic mouthwash" contains equal parts of diphenhydramine elixir, Maalox, and 2% viscous lidocaine. Each 5-mL teaspoon contains less than 50 mg of lidocaine. It is swished, held in the mouth for 1 to 2 minutes, and expectorated.
- Lidocaine (2%) may be used intraorally, but repeated use may produce systemic toxicity, especially in children. Each 5-mL teaspoon contains 100 mg of lidocaine. It should not be swallowed but, instead, expectorated after holding it in the mouth for a few minutes. Viscous lidocaine is not useful for acute pharyngitis. Systemic narcotics are preferred if the pain is severe.

ED, emergency department; EMLA, eutectic mixture of local anesthetics.

TABLE 29-4 Practical Agents for ED Use: Mucosal Application

AGENT	USUAL CONCENTRATION (%)	MAXIMUM DOSAGE* Adult (mg)	MAXIMUM DOSAGE* Pediatric (mg/kg)	ONSET (min)	DURATION (min)
Tetracaine	0.5	50	0.75	3-8	30-60
Lidocaine	2-10	250-300[†]	3-4[†]	2-5	15-45
Cocaine[‡]	4	200	2-3[†]	2-5	30-45

ED, emergency department.
*These are conservative figures; see text for explanations.
[†]The lower dosage should be used for a maximum safe dose when feasible.
[‡]The 10% cocaine solution is best avoided because of minimal additional clinical benefit and the potential for coronary vasoconstriction in patients with coronary artery disease.

Figure 29-5 Topical anesthetics can provide effective anesthesia of intact mucous membranes. Here, Hurricaine spray (benzocaine 20%) is used before incision and drainage of a peritonsillar abscess. A rare side effect of topical benzocaine is methemoglobinemia.

Figure 29-6 Peak blood levels of lidocaine. *(Modified from Raj [ed]. Textbook of Regional Anesthesia. New York: Churchill Livingstone; 2002.)*

as does hydrolysis by plasma pseudocholinesterase. Absorption is enhanced in the presence of inflammation. Cocaine is the only anesthetic that produces vasoconstriction at clinically useful concentrations, hence its popularity for treating epistaxis. This major advantage is offset by its susceptibility to abuse and toxic potential. The toxic effects are due to direction stimulation of the CNS and blockade of norepinephrine reuptake in the peripheral nervous system. *Cocaine should not be administered to patients who are sensitive to exogenous catecholamines or who are taking monoamine oxidase (MAO) inhibitor antidepressants.* Clinical manifestations of toxicity include CNS excitement, seizures, and hyperthermia. Central and peripheral effects of hypertension, tachycardia, and ventricular arrhythmias may also be seen. Acute myocardial infarction has been reported after topical application.[9] Cocaine is commonly used as a 4% solution with a maximum safe dose of 200 mg (2 to 3 mg/kg). A 10% solution is available, but this concentration adds little to the topical effect while enhancing the potential for toxicity. Coronary vasoconstriction may occur with doses as low as 2 mg/kg applied to the nasal mucosa. Although the clinical effect of this vasoconstriction is usually benign and without electrocardiographic changes, topical cocaine should be used cautiously in patients with known or suspected coronary artery disease. *Dyclonine* offers advantages over other topical anesthetic agents. It is a ketone derivative without an ester or amide linkage and may be used in patients who are allergic to the common anesthetics. Extensive experience with the topical preparation has shown it to be effective and safe.[10] Dyclonine is marketed in 0.5% and 1% solutions, often in sore throat preparations, with a maximum adult recommended dose of 300 mg.

Benzocaine is an ester that is marketed in its neutral form in 14% to 20% preparations (Cetacaine, Americaine, Hurricaine) (see Fig. 29-5). Its low water solubility prevents significant penetration of the mucous membranes, thus reducing systemic toxicity if applied to intact mucosa. However, it is not a potent anesthetic and has a brief duration of action. It is more allergenic than other topical agents. Benzocaine is usually dispensed in an admixture with other therapeutic ingredients and is clinically effective only at relatively high

(>14%) concentrations. Benzocaine is available as a nonprescription gel and liquid (6.3% to 20% Anbesol, for example) and is used for a variety of maladies, including ear pain, mouth pain, and teething. It is commonly used by dentists to produce mucosal anesthesia before intraoral nerve blocks (see Chapter 30). Adriani and Zepernick[10] recommended this agent for lubricating catheters, airways, endotracheal tubes, and laryngoscopes and reported only one adverse reaction (methemoglobinemia) in their experience with approximately 150,000 patients. Methemoglobinemia occurs rarely after mucosal absorption of benzocaine used repeatedly for teething infants and after standard doses of benzocaine sprays used in endoscopic procedures.[11]

An excellent topical preparation is a combination of lidocaine, prilocaine, and tetracaine, especially useful for dental mucosa anesthesia (see Fig. 30-3). Topical gel mixtures of 2.5% lidocaine and 2.5% prilocaine (eutectic mixture of local anesthetics [EMLA]) are commonly used on intact skin but have also been used on mucous membranes. EMLA is more effective than 20% benzocaine when applied to the oral mucosa before needle injection for dental anesthesia. One study demonstrated that pain was reduced more quickly with EMLA than with benzocaine when applied to the buccal mucosa.[12]

As with infiltrated anesthesia, toxic reactions to topically applied anesthetics correlate with the peak blood levels achieved and not necessarily with the dose administered. Systemic absorption of a topical agent is more rapid, with a higher level being achieved than with the same dose given by infiltration (Fig. 29-6). *The total dose of a topical anesthetic should be considerably less than that used for infiltration at a given site.* Fractionating the total dose into three portions administered over a period of several minutes effectively reduces peak blood levels. Inadvertent suppression of the gag reflex, combined with difficulty swallowing, may lead to aspiration, an important potential adverse reaction to topical anesthesia of the nose, mouth, and pharynx. Infections from drug solutions in multidose vials for topical anesthesia of the larynx and trachea have not been substantiated.

Technique and Precautions

A commonly used "magic mouthwash" for the topical treatment of painful gingivostomatitis in children is often prescribed by emergency clinicians and pediatricians. There has been little scientific study of the preparation and it is not available commercially, but it has been used safely for decades. It consists of equal parts viscous lidocaine (2%), Maalox as a binder, and diphenhydramine elixir. Corticosteroids or nystatin is often added when the mixture is used to treat chemotherapy-induced mucositis.[13] However, a recent review found no evidence that magic mouthwash is effective in treating this condition.[14] The creamy mixture is swished around the mouth and expectorated or painted on specific lesions with a cotton swab. Packing an area with a cotton ball soaked with this mixture is one option. Repeated doses or swallowing of the elixir can produce systemic toxicity, so careful instruction should be given to limit use of the solution to every few hours. This combination would be theoretically less toxic than simply using topical lidocaine.

Emergency clinicians often prescribe 2% viscous lidocaine (20 mg/mL) for patients with pharyngitis, stomatitis, dental pain, or other inflammatory or irritative lesions in the oropharynx. Although this intervention is widely used and generally safe, the common misconception that topical anesthesia is totally innocuous may result in poor patient instructions and serious consequences. Topical lidocaine is helpful for painful mouth lesions but is of little practical value for acute pharyngitis, for which systemic analgesics are usually a better option. Seizures and death from topical lidocaine have been reported when excessive repeated doses have been administered.[15,16] Toxic blood levels may occur because the anesthetic effect of viscous lidocaine lasts for only 30 to 60 minutes and patients with recurrent pain may either ignore or be ignorant of the safe dosing interval of 3 hours and medicate themselves more frequently. Patients tend to increase each dose to obtain greater relief, and inflammation may increase systemic absorption. In addition, painful oral lesions may last for several days.

Children are at higher risk for the rare toxicity of oral lidocaine. When compared with adults, children may exhibit increased lidocaine absorption, decreased clearance, and a longer half-life.[17] Continued medication use allows lidocaine and its major metabolites monoethylglycinexylidide (MEGX) and glycinexylidide (GX) to accumulate. Both MEGX and GX are produced from the hepatic metabolism of lidocaine and are excreted in urine. They possess anesthetic and antiarrhythmic activity and have the potential for CNS toxicity. Although these metabolites are less potent than lidocaine, their elimination half-lives are considerably longer. Several investigators regard MEGX and GX to be the cause of CNS toxicity with prolonged topical use of lidocaine.[16] The length of time that viscous lidocaine is retained in the mouth and whether the excess is expectorated or swallowed also affect the blood level produced. Expectorating the medication after swishing it in the mouth produces much lower blood levels than when it is swallowed. It seems logical that the most hazardous mode of administration would be to retain the solution in the mouth "until absorbed."

Clearly explain the proper way to use viscous lidocaine and inform patients *not to dose themselves ad libitum*. Note that a 2% solution contains 20 mg/mL, or 100 mg per standard teaspoon (5 mL). The recommended maximum adult dose is 300 mg (15 mL of a 2% solution) no more frequently than every 3 hours. When possible, instruct the patient to decrease the dose by using direct cotton swab application. When gargled or swished in the mouth, limit application time to 1 to 2 minutes, and instruct the patient to expectorate excess solution. Limit use to 2 or 3 days, especially if swallowing the solution is necessary to obtain relief. Prescribe lower doses for patients at risk for decreased clearance (see "Systemic Toxic Reactions" later in this chapter). Doses for children are prescribed at 3 mg/kg. Because infants cannot expectorate well, do not use viscous lidocaine for minor oral irritation and teething. Recommend that no food be eaten for 1 hour after application because anesthesia of the oropharynx can interfere with swallowing and cause aspiration. Special note should be made of the over-the-counter availability of benzocaine, commonly used for toothaches and teething. A gel or liquid (Anbesol) is available in 6.3% to 20% formulations. When used repeatedly in the oral cavity on irritated tissue, systemic toxicity, including methemoglobinemia, may occur.

Lidocaine 4% solution can be atomized with a standard nebulizer device commonly used for delivering asthma medications and inhaled by the patient before insertion of a nasogastric tube. This method effectively anesthetizes the nasopharyngeal and oropharyngeal tissues, thereby easing the pain with tube insertion.[18,19]

Intact Skin

Agents and Uses

The stratum corneum provides a cutaneous barrier that prevents the commonly marketed aqueous solutions (acid salts) from producing anesthesia, but saturated solutions of the bases of local anesthetics are effective on intact skin. When applied topically to abraded skin, most anesthetic agents result in peak blood levels similar to those resulting from infiltration in 6 to 10 minutes.

Lidocaine Cream

Lubens and coworkers[20] used 30% lidocaine cream, saturated on a gauze pad and adherent to an elastic patch, for a myriad of procedures. Despite its effectiveness, safety, and painless application, the practicality of its use in an emergency setting is limited. In 1974, Lubens and coworkers[20] reported an impressive list of uses, including minor operative procedures (e.g., excision of lesions, incision and drainage of abscesses), lumbar puncture, venipuncture, and allergy testing. Lidocaine remains one of the most commonly used topical compounds.

EMLA Cream, ELA-Max, and Tetracaine Base Patch

Various topical anesthetics have been suggested to decrease the pain of venipuncture or injections and to provide topical anesthesia for painful skin abrasions and lesions. These agents have been studied extensively and are safe, but they are not practical in many ED settings because of their slow onset of action and inadequate efficacy. However, their activity profiles make them more applicable than 30% lidocaine cream to emergency medicine. Tetracaine base is available as a solution, a gel, and a patch preparation. It is effective in crossing the lipid-rich barrier of the stratum corneum because it is highly lipophilic. EMLA was approved in the United States in 1992. It contains 2.5% lidocaine and 2.5% prilocaine in a unique oil-and-water emulsion yielding 5% EMLA. The mild lipophilic and hydrophilic properties of the component drugs are greatly increased when mixed together, thereby allowing absorption through intact skin. ELA-Max and ELA-Max5 are topical lidocaine anesthetic creams with a more rapid onset of action than EMLA cream. ELA-Max is a 4% concentration, and 5% ELA-Max is marketed as an anorectal cream that may benefit patients undergoing painful rectal procedures. Neither product has prilocaine, as is found in EMLA cream, and neither has U.S. Food and Drug Administration approval for pain relief before painful injections or intravenous (IV) insertion, but both have such potential.[21]

Tetracaine base seems to offer the advantage of being able to achieve effective anesthesia with a shorter application time and a longer duration.[22] For tetracaine and EMLA preparations, onset, depth of anesthesia, duration, and blood levels vary directly with application time, use on thinner or inflamed skin, and larger doses.[23] These preparations exhibit a reservoir effect.[24] The drug is deposited in the stratum corneum and continues to diffuse along its concentration gradient, even after it is removed from the skin.

Tetracaine base, lidocaine cream, and EMLA can be useful in the ED for providing anesthesia for many procedures: venous cannulation, venipuncture, or any needle insertion, including preinfiltration anesthesia and lumbar puncture; a variety of minor surgical procedures; and anesthetizing the tympanic membrane and external auditory canal. EMLA has also been used effectively for débridement of ulcers.[25]

EMLA and 5% lidocaine cream are equally effective in reducing the pain of IV insertion.[26] Luhmann and colleagues[27] demonstrated that 5% lidocaine cream applied for 30 minutes under an occlusive dressing was as effective as infiltrated buffered lidocaine before IV catheter insertion in children. Obviously, infiltrative administration of buffered lidocaine requires skin puncture, but its onset of anesthesia is almost immediate. When time is not an issue, topical creams may be an acceptable alternative to infiltrated anesthesia or no anesthesia at all. About a 60-minute interval after application is required for these preparations to provide optimal topical analgesia to the intact skin for such procedures as venipuncture. Early cutaneous placement of these agents (e.g., over common IV sites while the patient is being triaged) is important for practical ED use.

Ethyl Chloride and Trichloromonofluoromethane and Dichlorodifluoromethane (Fluori-Methane) Sprays

These topical agents are often used for limited skin incisions (e.g., drainage of small abscesses), trigger point injections, joint aspiration, or injection of bursitis or tendonitis. These agents evaporate quickly from the skin and cool it to the point of freezing. Anesthesia is effective and immediate, but drawbacks include its short duration (only up to 1 minute), potential pain on thawing, and possibly lowered resistance to infection and delayed healing. Highly volatile ethyl chloride spray is flammable. Ethyl chloride has been studied in children to reduce the pain of venipuncture, but the results are mixed.[28,29] Given their short duration of action and the time needed to perform pediatric venipuncture, these preparations have limited use for this purpose.

Technique
Lidocaine Cream

This 30% cream is saturated on a gauze pad that is adherent to an elastic patch and placed over the area to be injected or incised.[20] The high concentration of anesthetic and an occlusive patch are needed to achieve effective skin penetration. The duration of action varies with the application time. A 45-minute application time is needed for most procedures. To achieve a topical anesthetic duration of 30 minutes, a 2-hour application is necessary.

Tetracaine Base Patch and EMLA Cream

Because both agents demonstrate a reservoir effect, anesthesia may increase or begin many minutes after removal of the drug. A precise description of application times and duration is not possible. Tetracaine base requires a minimum of 20 to 30 minutes of application time to produce several hours of anesthesia. EMLA requires an application time of 1 to 2 hours for a reported duration of 30 minutes to several hours. Occlusive dressings seem to increase penetration of EMLA whenever the cream is used. Patches are more convenient and cause no loss of effectiveness.

EMLA dosing is based on the amount of cream applied, not on the amount of anesthetic. Each gram of EMLA cream contains 25 mg of lidocaine and 25 mg of prilocaine. Dosages are given in grams of cream, not milligrams of anesthetic. In general, apply EMLA as a thick layer over intact skin under an occlusive dressing for about 1 hour before a procedure. Application of a thick layer approximates to 1 to 2 $g/10$ cm^2. For minor procedures such as needle insertions, apply 2.5 g of EMLA over 20 to 25 cm^2 for at least 1 hour. For more painful procedures, apply about 2 g of cream per 10 cm^2 for at least 2 hours. The maximum application area (MAA) determines the appropriate total dose applied. Base the MAA on the patient's weight as follows: up to 10 kg, MAA = 100 cm^2; 10 to 20 kg, MAA = 600 cm^2; more than 20 kg, MAA = 2000 cm^2.

Ethyl Chloride and Fluori-Methane Sprays

Collect all the equipment required and make all preparations needed to immediately perform the desired procedure. Invert the bottle 25 cm from the skin and spray a stream along the proposed incision site until the area turns white and hard. Make the incision or local anesthetic injection immediately or during actual spraying of the agent for optimal results because the effect is fleeting. Some clinicians use these vapocoolant sprays to decrease the pain of injection of a more traditional local anesthetic such as lidocaine.

Iontophoresis

Anesthetic agents may be drawn into the skin without needles by electrical current applied through electrodes in a process called *iontophoresis*. Lidocaine with epinephrine administered via iontophoresis provides adequate anesthesia before venipuncture in pediatric patients and is superior to EMLA in providing cutaneous anesthesia.[30-33] Iontophoresis is not widely used in emergency medicine but may be another alternative to applied anesthetic agents.

Microneedle Pretreatment

Recently developed technology known as microneedle pretreatment may improve the efficacy of cutaneously applied topical anesthetics. A functional microarray of fine needles painlessly perforates the stratum corneum to facilitate the penetration of applied medications without using traditional needle injections. A recent study demonstrated that perforation of the skin of healthy volunteers with a microneedle to which dyclonine was applied resulted in decreased time to anesthesia and a greater degree of pain reduction than did application of dyclonine to nonperforated skin.[34] This emerging technology may improve the practical application of anesthetics to intact skin in the ED.

Jet Injection

Jet injection of anesthetic through intact skin may overcome some of the limitations imposed by the cutaneous application of anesthetics without needle infiltration. A jet injector is a device containing carbon dioxide gas that rapidly forces a plunger to expel drug through a small orifice applied over intact skin. Medication penetrates the epidermis to a depth of 5 to 8 mm in 0.2 second and causes the drug to be rapidly dispersed through the skin. Safety is improved because no needles are used to penetrate the skin. Several studies have demonstrated that jet injection of anesthetics provides more rapid anesthesia than does topical application of anesthetic agents and is preferred by patients over no anesthesia at all for painful procedures such as IV insertion and arterial blood gas sampling.[35-37]

Complications

General adverse reactions to anesthetic agents are discussed in the "Complications" section later in this chapter.

Tetracaine base is quite safe, with a low blood concentration after proper use. In one study, cutaneous erythema developed at the site of application in approximately 25% of patients.[24] This vasodilatory effect may actually be an advantage when starting IV lines or performing venipuncture. EMLA is also quite safe. Although it has a high rate of local skin reactions, they are mild and transient, with disappearance 1 to 2 hours after removal of the cream. Despite the reported successful use of EMLA cream on skin ulcers, Hansson and associates[25] and Powell and coworkers[38] described an increase in bacterial growth, infection, and inflammation when used in experimental wounds. Methemoglobinemia resulting from the metabolites of prilocaine may occur with EMLA.[23] The risk for clinically significant methemoglobinemia seems remote when EMLA is used properly. It is contraindicated in any infant younger than 3 months and in infants between 3 and 12 months of age who are currently taking methemoglobinemia-inducing drugs (nitrites, sulfonamides, antimalarials, phenobarbital, and acetaminophen). The risk for adverse effects is increased in patients with anemia, respiratory or cardiovascular disease, and deficiencies in glucose-6-phosphate dehydrogenase or methemoglobin reductase. Prolonged inhalation of ethyl chloride spray may produce general anesthesia, coma, or cardiorespiratory arrest. Ethyl chloride is also flammable, thus precluding its use with electrocautery.

Topically applied anesthetics are often covered with an occlusive dressing to contain the medication. Covering the medication with an occlusive dressing may dramatically increase drug absorption and the amount of metabolites. Oni and associates demonstrated that 4% lidocaine cream applied to volunteers with an occlusive dressing resulted in three times the level of serum lidocaine and double the level of MEGX when the same dose was applied to volunteers without occlusion.[39] Use caution when occluding topical anesthetics over intact skin because markedly elevated serum level of drug may be reached.

Lacerations

Background

In 1980, Pryor and colleagues[40] reported their experience with a topical anesthetic solution (tetracaine-adrenaline-cocaine [TAC]) for wound repair. The original formula, used in most subsequent studies, consists of a solution of 0.5% tetracaine, 1:2,000 epinephrine (adrenaline), and 11.8% cocaine. Traditionally, anesthesia is produced by firmly applying a solution-saturated gauze pad or cotton ball directly to the laceration for 10 minutes. The resulting loss of cutaneous sensation is centered about the area of application. Gel formulations of topical wound anesthesia (TWA) with alternative mixtures of agents promise to improve the ease and safety of topical anesthetic solutions for wound repair in the ED. Advantages of TWA include painless application, no distortion of wound margins, good hemostasis, and good patient and parental acceptance in the pediatric age group.

Indications and Contraindications

Use of TWA is generally restricted to young children with wounds less than 5 cm in length in whom the delay in application of an anesthetic is acceptable and proper application can be ensured (Fig. 29-7). TWA containing vasoconstricting agents is not generally used in structures without a collateral blood supply (e.g., digits, tip of the nose, pinna of the ear, penis), although there is no evidence that this is unsafe. When some wound preparation is desired before anesthesia, remove large debris and clotted blood to allow the appropriate application of TWA and then finish wound preparation once the wound is properly anesthetized.

TWA appears to be less effective on the trunk and extremities than on the face and scalp and less effective than lidocaine infiltration in these areas. The 10- to 20-minute onset time may be unacceptable in a busy ED.[41] Two other often mentioned drawbacks may be more theoretical than real. Vasoconstrictor-induced higher infection rates (see "Complications" later in this chapter) have not been clearly demonstrated. The argument that the necessary 10-minute application period is time-consuming and takes valuable nursing time is partially offset by using the child's caretaker or adhesive paper tape alone to hold the solution in place. It is not necessary for anyone to "hold" the medicine in place when gel is used.

Some EDs still stock topical anesthetic gels that contain cocaine. Cocaine use is complex because of cost and federal regulations requiring storage in a locked cabinet and maintenance of separate written records of its use. In view of the evidence that mixtures without cocaine are efficacious, avoid the potential complications related to cocaine, and do not have the potential for abuse that cocaine does, the practicality of cocaine-containing TWA has been questioned.[42]

Agents and Effectiveness
TAC and Related Mixtures

Three clinical trials directly compared TAC with infiltrated lidocaine. Without specifying wound location, Pryor's group[40] found equal anesthetic effect. Complete anesthesia with TAC was achieved in 82% to 86% of patients as compared with

Figure 29-7 Topical wound anesthesia. **A,** The topical anesthetic (in this case, lidocaine-epinephrine-tetracaine gel) is applied to a cotton ball or gauze pad. **B,** The anesthetic is held in place with an occlusive dressing such as Tegaderm. **C,** After a 30-minute application period, vasoconstriction of local tissue can be readily observed (*arrow*), and effective anesthesia has been achieved. **D,** Local wound repair, including additional infiltrative anesthesia if necessary, can proceed with little if any patient discomfort.

83% to 92% for subcutaneous lidocaine. The remaining patients obtained partial anesthesia. Hegenbarth and associates[43] and Anderson and coworkers[44] demonstrated results similar to those of Pryor's group.[40] Hegenbarth and associates found TAC to be equal to lidocaine only on the face and scalp and inferior to it at other locations. In contrast, other studies have confirmed excellent rates of effectiveness, especially on the face and scalp.[45-49] TAC is more effective than its component drugs alone. On the face and scalp, TAC was found to be superior to tetracaine alone, although on nonfacial areas, both produced equally poor results.[45] TAC was found to be more effective than cocaine alone and more effective than a tetracaine-epinephrine solution in the same dosage ratio.[47,50]

In 1990, Bonadio and Wagner[48] showed that an epinephrine-cocaine solution (1:2,000 epinephrine and 11.8% cocaine) was equal to TAC in effectiveness. Bonadio and Wagner[46] also found that half-strength TAC (0.25% tetracaine, 1:4000 epinephrine, 5.9% cocaine) achieved excellent results in patients with dermal lacerations of the face, lip, and scalp. Smith and Barry[51] compared three strengths of TAC and found equal effectiveness among them; they recommended the lowest-strength cocaine formulation (1% tetracaine, 1:4000 epinephrine, 4% cocaine). Ernst and colleagues[52] found similar effectiveness to TAC when a slightly different lidocaine-epinephrine-tetracaine (LET) solution (4% lidocaine, 1:2000 epinephrine, 1% tetracaine) was used.

TAC has also been compared with EMLA when placed in a wound for 60 minutes before wound repair. In a study of 32 wounds, supplemental anesthesia was required less often with EMLA.[53] The non–cocaine-containing formulations are generally considered less toxic and have advantages in terms of reduced cost and avoidance of controlled substance precautions during storage.

LET and Related Solutions

Many variations of mixtures that do not contain cocaine have been studied; these include variations LET, lidocaine-epinephrine, tetracaine-phenylephrine, tetracaine-lidocaine-phenylephrine, bupivacaine-norepinephrine, and prilocaine-phenylephrine. Schilling and associates[54] found that a LET solution (4% lidocaine, 1:1000 epinephrine, 0.5% tetracaine) was as effective as TAC. LET gel preparations are at least as effective as LET solutions.[55] Singer and Stark[56] determined that EMLA or LET gel placed in a wound on initial evaluation and before infiltration with lidocaine reduced the pain of infiltration, thereby allowing essentially painless injection of lidocaine.

Technique and Dosage

Because the topical mixtures noted earlier (especially TAC) are not innocuous anesthetics, pay close attention to the technique of application and the recommended maximum dose. There is no uniformly accepted application technique, composition of components, or concentration of components.

Generally, apply topical solutions such as TWA to the wound in a gravity-dependent position and carefully fill the wound cavity. After 3 minutes, place a single 2- × 2-cm gauze pad or cotton ball saturated with TWA on the wound. Tape or hold the pad firmly in place for 15 to 20 minutes. The person holding the gauze should wear latex examination gloves to minimize the risk for cutaneous absorption of the solution. The average dose of TWA mixture for most wounds is 2 mL.

Gaufberg and coauthors[57] described "sequential layer application" (SLA) of topical lidocaine with epinephrine (TLE) to deeper wounds that might not typically be amenable to the use of TWA. Cotton soaked with TLE was applied to the wound surface and 2 mm of surrounding skin for 10 to 15 minutes and then removed. A second similarly soaked piece of cotton was packed deeper into the wound for 10 to 15 minutes. Deep wounds were treated with a third piece of TLE-soaked cotton placed deeper into the wound. Anesthesia was presumed when 3 mm or more of pallor was seen on all wound margins. The group receiving lidocaine by SLA was compared with a group receiving infiltrated 2% buffered lidocaine with epinephrine. Both groups experienced a similar degree of anesthesia during suturing. Mean time to anesthesia with SLA was 29 minutes versus 5 minutes for the infiltration group. Despite the longer time in the SLA group, the authors argued that the additional time is worthwhile because the painful injection, risk for hollow-bore needle injury, and tissue distortion with infiltration were eliminated. If time permits, the SLA technique may be useful for wounds that would have otherwise required infiltrated anesthesia.

Hegenbarth and associates[43] estimated the maximum safe dose of full-strength TAC to be 0.09 mL/kg based on the known maximal safe dose of infiltrated tetracaine, the mucosal application of cocaine, and an estimate of absorption of solution onto the applicator. The key to safety is to avoid TAC on mucosal surfaces or areas in which sniffing or swallowing may accidentally occur. Topical mucosal anesthesia is discussed elsewhere in this chapter.

Prepare an epinephrine-cocaine gel by adding 0.15 g of methylcellulose to 1.5 mL of epinephrine-cocaine solution. Stir the mixture thoroughly for a minute or two until a gel consistency is obtained. After sterile preparation, place the wound in a gravity-dependent position and apply the gel with a cotton-tipped swab to coat the entire wound cavity and margins. Allow the wound to stand for 15 to 20 minutes and thoroughly wash the wound cavity to remove the gel. In Bonadio and Wagner's study,[49] the average dose used was 0.35 mL of gel containing only 40 mg of cocaine. Again, other agents are equally efficacious and safer; select these over cocaine-containing mixtures whenever possible.

Complications

Most adverse events associated with TWA occur with mixtures that contain cocaine. Lidocaine toxicity is a well-recognized adverse event when higher doses are used (see "Systemic Toxic Reactions" later in this chapter), but lidocaine toxicity has not been reported with TWA mixtures.

Mucosal application may rarely lead to significant systemic toxicity; fatalities have been reported after application. Even after nonmucosal TAC use, cocaine levels appear in the blood and cocaine metabolites appear in the urine in the majority of patients,[58,59] but tetracaine does not. Gel formulations of TAC tend to stay in the wound and thus reduce the risk of solution runoff onto mucosal surfaces. There is no need to use a gauze pad to apply the medication in a gel formulation or to hold it in place. Because the entire applied dose will stay in the wound, a lower dose can be used. Gel also provides more uniform application to tissues, which improves the anesthetic effect. In tissues containing end-arteries, ischemia caused by vasoconstrictors may occur. Avoid TAC on the digits, the tip of the nose, the penis, and the pinna of the ear. Use TAC with caution on patients with coronary artery disease, uncontrolled hypertension, seizures, or peripheral vascular disease. Patients with decreased plasma cholinesterase levels are theoretically at increased risk for systemic toxic effects, but this potential risk is of little clinical concern.

INFILTRATION ANESTHESIA

Background

Injection of an anesthetic agent directly into tissue before surgical manipulation is known as *infiltration anesthesia* (Fig.

Figure 29-8 Infiltration anesthesia for incision and drainage of a pilonidal abscess. Minimize pain by using a small needle (ideally 30 gauge if injecting through intact skin or 25 to 27 gauge if going through the cut edges of a wound), buffering the anesthetic with sodium bicarbonate, warming the anesthetic to body temperature, and injecting slowly in the subdermal plane.

29-8). Field block anesthesia is also considered a form of infiltration anesthesia, particularly since the agents, concentrations, and recommended maximum dosages are the same. To create a field block, inject a field of anesthetic around the operative site. Make the injection proximal to or surrounding the area that you plan to manipulate. Combine infiltrative anesthesia with procedural sedation (see Chapter 33) to reduce anxiety or motion.

Indications and Contraindications

Infiltration anesthesia is indicated when good operative conditions can be obtained with this technique. It may be used for the majority of minor surgical procedures such as excision of skin lesions and suturing of wounds. Infiltration anesthesia is considered quicker and safer than nerve block and general anesthesia. Local infiltration can provide hemostasis, both by direct distention of tissue and by the concurrent use of epinephrine.

A disadvantage of local infiltration over nerve blocks is that a relatively large dose of the drug is needed to anesthetize a relatively small area. For extensive wounds, the amount of anesthetic required may risk systemic toxicity. The maximum allowable volume can be increased by adding epinephrine, using a lower concentration of the anesthetic agent, or both (Table 29-5). When large volumes are anticipated and a nerve block is anatomically feasible, the nerve block is preferred. Avoid using infiltration for large procedures in small children and in apprehensive patients, especially those with previous adverse reactions to the medications (whether vasovagal or otherwise). Local infiltration distorts the tissues that will be incised or repaired, which makes it undesirable in areas requiring precise anatomic alignment (e.g., some lip repairs).

Choice of Agent

The local anesthetic agents most frequently used for infiltration are 0.5% to 1% lidocaine, 0.5% to 1% procaine, and 0.25% bupivacaine (Table 29-6). Higher concentrations are of no additional benefit. Lidocaine is most commonly used because of its excellent activity profile, low allergenicity, low toxicity, user familiarity, and ready availability. Procaine is useful for patients who are allergic to amide anesthetics. Some clinicians prefer bupivacaine because of its prolonged duration. Bupivacaine may also be preferred when postoperative analgesia is desired, for prolonged procedures, for dental anesthesia, or even for short procedures that may be interrupted in a busy ED.

A comparison of equianesthetic doses of lidocaine and bupivacaine for infiltration anesthesia (Table 29-7) revealed that the duration of action is the major difference between the two agents. For the majority of ED procedures it is not necessary to extend the duration of anesthesia beyond 1 hour; which makes plain lidocaine a logical anesthetic choice. Patients experience a moderate amount of pain after repair of a laceration when the lidocaine wears off in about 1 hour.[60] Bupivacaine reduces the pain after repair of lacerations for at least 6 hours. This benefit of a prolonged duration of anesthesia must be weighed against the hazards of injury to the mucous membranes or an unprotected limb or the annoyance of prolonged numbness in patients who have undergone simple surgical procedures.

A prolonged duration of anesthesia can also be achieved by adding epinephrine, sodium bicarbonate, or both to lidocaine.

TABLE 29-5 Maximum Allowable Volume (Adults)

AGENT	CONCENTRATION (%)	MAXIMUM* SAFE DOSE (mg)	MAXIMUM VOLUME (mL)
Lidocaine	0.5	300	60
	1	300	30
Bupivacaine†	0.25	175	70
Lidocaine-epinephrine	0.5	500	100
	1	500	50
Bupivacaine-epinephrine	0.25	225	90

*These are quite conservative figures for infiltration anesthesia; see text for explanation.
†Some physicians recommend 400 mg as the maximum safe dose for bupivacaine.

TABLE 29-6 Practical Agents for ED Use: Local Infiltration

AGENT	CONCENTRATION (%)	MAXIMUM DOSE*†		ONSET (min)	DURATION‡
		Adult (mg)	Pediatric (mg/kg)		
Procaine	0.5-1.0	500§ (600)	7 (9)	2-5	15-45 min
Lidocaine	0.5-1.0	300 (500)	4.5 (7)‖	2-5	1-2 hr
Bupivacaine	0.25	175 (225)	2 (3)¶	2-5	4-8 hr

ED, emergency department.
*These are quite conservative figures; see text for explanation.
†The higher maximum dose for solutions containing epinephrine appears in parentheses.
‡These values are for the agent alone; they can be extended considerably with the addition of epinephrine.
§Some authorities recommend up to 1000 mg or 14 mg/kg for procaine.
‖Some authorities recommend up to 7 mg/kg for plain lidocaine in children older than 1 year.
¶Because of lack of clinical trial experience, drug companies do not recommend the use of bupivacaine in children younger than 12 years, but bupivacaine is commonly used without problems in children.

TABLE 29-7 Comparison of 1% Lidocaine and 0.25% Bupivacaine: Infiltration Anesthesia

	LIDOCAINE	BUPIVACAINE	ADVANTAGE
Onset	2-5 min	2-5 min	Equal
Effectiveness (equianesthetic dose)	Excellent	Excellent	Equal
Duration	1-2 hr	4-6 hr	B
Infection potential	No	No	Equal
Administration pain	Less	More	L
Maximum volume*—plain lidocaine	Less	More	B
Maximum volume—epinephrine	Less	More	B
Toxic potential	Less cardiotoxic; equal CNS	More cardiotoxic; equal CNS	L

B, bupivacaine; *CNS*, central nervous system; *L*, lidocaine.
*See Table 29-6 for volume and concentration comparison.

ADVANTAGES

1. Prolongs the duration
2. Provides hemostasis
3. Slows absorption:
   Decreases the agent's toxic potential
   Allows an increased dose
4. Increases the level of blockade

DISADVANTAGES

1. Impairs host defenses—increases the incidence of infection*
2. Delays wound healing*
3. Do not use for
   Areas supplied by end-arteries
   Patients "sensitive" to catecholamines
4. Toxicity—catecholamine reaction†

Based on laboratory studies and of unknown clinical importance.
†*For example, in patients taking monoamine oxidase inhibitors.*

Epinephrine provides excellent wound hemostasis and slows systemic absorption. This latter property decreases the peak blood level, reduces the potential for a toxic reaction, and allows a greater volume of agent to be used for extensive lacerations. The major disadvantage of epinephrine is theoretical damage to host defenses, but it is generally clinically inconsequential (Box 29-2). Bicarbonate added to the anesthetic just before injection decreases the pain of administration. Bupivacaine, if used with due caution, is safe and easy to use. The deciding factors are many, but some logical choices are as follows:

- For a wound with excessive bleeding, use lidocaine with epinephrine and sodium bicarbonate.
- For an apprehensive patient, use lidocaine with sodium bicarbonate.
- For anticipated prolonged postprocedure pain, use bupivacaine.

Equipment

The pain of injection is reduced with the use of small-gauge needles. Ideally, a 30-gauge needle is used if the injection is made through skin. If the injection is made through the cut edges of the wound, a 25- to 27-gauge needle suffices. A small-gauge needle slows the rate of injection and reduces the rate and pain of tissue distention. A 10-mL syringe is recommended both for its ease of handling and for the relatively slow rate of injection that it allows.

Technique

Once an agent has been chosen, proper administration technique minimizes pain, prevents spread of bacteria, and avoids intravascular injection. Buffering, temperature manipulation, and careful infiltration also reduce the pain of injection.

Buffering

Raising the pH of an anesthetic by adding sodium bicarbonate decreases pain dramatically, whereas lowering the pH by adding epinephrine increases pain. Buffering is probably the best way to reduce the pain of local anesthetic injections, and its routine use is highly recommend. It is probable that pH is not the sole factor in producing pain because the pain produced by various agents does not correlate strictly with the pH. Sodium bicarbonate probably works by increasing the ratio of nonionized to ionized molecules, which either renders the pain receptors less sensitive or causes more rapid diffusion of solution into the nerve and a shorter time to the onset of anesthesia.

To alkalinize lidocaine, add 1 mL of sodium bicarbonate (8.4%, 1 mmol/mL) to every 10 mL of anesthetic solution. As the pH of the solution is raised, the anesthetic becomes unstable and has a decreased shelf life. It was initially recommended that buffered lidocaine be prepared just before use to avoid precipitation and degradation, but buffered lidocaine retains its effectiveness for 1 week and refrigeration may further increase its shelf life.[61,62] Bicarbonate may be combined with plain lidocaine for both infiltrative anesthesia[63,64] and digital nerve blocks.[65] In one volunteer study, sodium bicarbonate was effectively combined with lidocaine and epinephrine.[62]

Sodium bicarbonate can be added to bupivacaine, but the solution tends to precipitate as the pH rises. The clinical effect of such precipitation is unclear, but if it occurs, it is probably prudent to use another solution prepared with less buffer. Precipitation varies directly with the concentration of bupivacaine and the time since mixture.[66] Cheney and coworkers[67] showed that 0.05 mL of 8.4% sodium bicarbonate (measured in a tuberculin syringe) could be mixed with 10 mL of 0.5% bupivacaine without precipitation. The goal of using bupivacaine is to prolong the duration of anesthesia; this effect can also be accomplished somewhat by using buffered lidocaine (plain or with epinephrine).

In view of the amount of published literature demonstrating that adding sodium bicarbonate to lidocaine before infiltrative anesthesia reduces the pain of injection without adverse effects, lidocaine should almost always be buffered when infiltrated in the ED; there is no practical reason to avoid the addition of bicarbonate.

Temperature Manipulation

Warming an anesthetic to body temperature (37°C to 42°C) reduces the pain of infiltration,[68,69] but warming may not reduce injection pain as much as buffering with sodium bicarbonate does. Bartfield and colleagues[70] found that lidocaine warmed to 38.9°C was more painful than room-temperature buffered lidocaine during intradermal injection. Brogan and associates,[71] using lidocaine warmed to 37°C, found the warmed lidocaine and room-temperature buffered lidocaine to be equivalent during wound infiltration. Neither study found a synergistic effect with combined warming and buffering. Martin and coworkers[72] found that warmed (37°C) lidocaine was no less painful than buffered lidocaine. Anesthetic solutions can be warmed in a baby food warmer with thermostat temperature control or in an IV solution warmer. Warming is not believed to adversely affect the shelf life of the local anesthetic.

Locally cooling the area to be infiltrated may provide additional pain relief. Leff and colleagues[73] demonstrated that patients receiving local infiltrative anesthesia for repair of an inguinal hernia had less pain when the incision area was cooled before infiltration. Patients were randomized to two groups and had a 1000-mL bag of saline placed over the

Figure 29-9 A, Except in the setting of gross contamination, wounds should be anesthetized by inserting the needle *through the cut edges, not through the intact skin*. Patients often will not feel a 25-gauge or smaller needle passed into subcutaneous tissue when it is advanced slowly through the cut edge. However, pain generally occurs with distention of tissue by the anesthetic, and hence injection should be slow and deliberate. **B,** If a wound is grossly contaminated, the anesthetic may be introduced through the intact skin. The operator should limit the number of needlesticks. The needle is first introduced at a point in line with the wound and beyond the wound edge (*1*), and while the anesthetic is slowly injected, the needle is advanced to include one entire side of the wound (if possible) to a point well past the opposite end of the wound. The other side may be anesthetized by passing the needle through the area already infiltrated by the first injection (*3*) to make the skin puncture painless. A 3.8-cm (1.5-inch) 27-gauge needle is a good choice. If the needle is not long enough to encompass the entire wound, the skin is painlessly punctured at a midway point that has already been anesthetized (*2*). **C,** Inject local anesthetic *through subcutaneous tissue, not intact skin.*

inguinal area for 5 minutes. One group used saline bags at room temperature; the other group used saline bags cooled to 4°C. A significant decrease in pain perception was found in the group in which the inguinal area was cooled before lidocaine infiltration. Cooling of wounds in the ED before infiltration has not been studied.

Injection

The pain from injection of local anesthetics is primarily a result of skin puncture (which can be minimized with small-gauge needles) and subcutaneous injection. Although patients fear the needle, there is little perceived pain merely from the needle's presence in subcutaneous tissue. Place the injection in *subdermal* tissue to minimize needle puncture pain and the tissue distention that occurs with *intradermal* placement. Place the needle "up to the hub" and inject while withdrawing along the just-created subdermal tunnel to minimize tissue distention. After an initial injection, instead of totally withdrawing the needle from the tissue, *redirect it along another path to lessen the number of skin punctures.* Slowly inject the smallest volume necessary to reduce pain.

Because the patient barely feels a needle placed subcutaneously and skin puncture is often quite painful, *make all wound injections through the wound edge and not through the skin* (Fig. 29-9).[74,75] Spread of infection beyond the wound margin has not been demonstrated clinically with this technique. Some clinicians choose to inject the anesthetic through intact skin in patients with a grossly contaminated wound. Bierman[76] described a technique of patient distraction by applying light pressure to alternate sides of the wound with one's fingers and repeated ambiguous questioning about feeling the

light pressure rather than the ongoing wound injection. Ask school-aged children to count backward or to say the "ABCs" to distract them during injection. Inject 1% lidocaine through intact skin with the needle bevel facing upward because this is less painful than injecting with the needle bevel facing downward.[77]

To prevent a systemic toxic reaction, avoid giving an intravascular injection. For infiltration anesthesia with a small-gauge needle, however, aspiration is usually unnecessary unless the injection is deeper than the subcutaneous area or the area to be injected contains many large vessels.

SPECIAL CONSIDERATIONS

Hematoma Block

Hematoma block has been used for many years to provide anesthesia for fracture reduction, particularly of the distal end of the forearm and hand (Fig. 29-10). Its popularity has waned somewhat because of the fear (unproven and theoretical) of introducing infection at the fracture site and its limited efficacy. Although several studies have shown hematoma block to be safe, the anesthesia that it provides is not as good as that provided by a Bier block (see Chapter 32). Nevertheless, there are several reasons to consider this technique.[78,79] The procedure is simple and quick to perform and does not require additional personnel. There is no need to wait for an anesthesiologist. A lower dose of the anesthetic agent is required for a hematoma block than for a Bier block (see Chapter 32). A hematoma block is particularly useful when a Bier block and general anesthesia are contraindicated.

Figure 29-10 Hematoma block. This technique is useful for reducing fractures of the distal end of the forearm and hand. Here it is being used before reduction of a distal radius (Colles) fracture. To perform the block, slowly inject 5 to 15 mL of plain 1% lidocaine into the fracture cavity and around the adjacent periosteum.

Prepare the skin over the fracture site with antiseptic solution and insert the needle into the hematoma, as confirmed by aspirating blood. Slowly inject 5 to 15 mL of plain 1% lidocaine or 5 to 10 mL of plain 2% lidocaine into the fracture cavity and around the adjacent periosteum. Larger fractures require larger volumes of local anesthetic. Adequate anesthesia occurs in about 5 to 10 minutes and may last for several hours. A common error is to attempt the procedure too soon after injection. Do not perform this procedure through dirty skin or with open fractures.

Intraarticular Anesthesia and Analgesia

Findings from the history and physical examination of an acutely traumatized joint, such as the knee, often underestimate the severity of the injury. Instillation of 5 mL of 1% lidocaine after joint aspiration may help relieve pain and facilitate an examination, but its use is not routinely recommended.[80] Since spasm and apprehension are often not relieved by local anesthesia, the information gained from this maneuver does usually not influence the ED treatment plan. Intraarticular anesthesia of the knee has no effect on gait pattern or joint proprioception.[81] Postprocedure weight bearing may be allowed without fear of producing or increasing injury if otherwise indicated. Intraarticular anesthesia may enhance elbow use after aspiration of a hemarthrosis associated with a radial head fracture.[82] The technique of administration is analogous to arthrocentesis (see Chapter 53). Intraarticular lidocaine has been effective in facilitating reduction of a shoulder dislocation. Animal experiments have demonstrated chondrotoxicity when local anesthetics are continuously infused into a joint.[83,84] Although continuous joint infusion of anesthetic may be harmful when used in a postoperative setting, there is no evidence that a single injection of intraarticular anesthetic in the ED is harmful.

Morphine may be injected directly into joints for postoperative pain relief and potentially provide prolonged analgesia after reduction of fractures. Theoretically, there are local opioid receptors in joints that are capable of being stimulated by rather small doses of morphine to provide relief for up to 24 hours with a single dose. There may also be some systemic absorption of the intraarticular morphine that contributes to analgesia, but adverse systemic opioid effects are not seen with this technique. Data are sparse on the exact mechanism and optimal doses. Three to 6 hours may be required for analgesia to reach it maximum effect. In a systematic review, Gupta and colleagues concluded that postoperative intraarticular morphine injected into the knee joint at doses of 2 to 4 mg provides analgesia for up to 24 hours.[84a] There is a wide variability in efficacy, which may be dose related. Though studied primarily for postoperative use after knee surgery, a similar concept may be intuitively applied to traumatic joint pain, but this has not been studied adequately.

Intrapleural Anesthesia

Indications
Intrapleural anesthesia introduces a local anesthetic into the pleural space (i.e., between the parietal and visceral pleura) through an epidural catheter. The anesthetic can be introduced through a previously placed chest tube. The technique can provide relief for several conditions, primarily postthoracotomy pain, postcholecystectomy pain, and most importantly for emergency clinicians, posttraumatic chest pain (e.g., rib fractures, pneumothorax, hemothorax). This procedure is not only useful for pain relief but also facilitates turning, coughing, and deep breathing. Several studies have demonstrated improved respiratory mechanics when intrapleural anesthesia is used.[85,86] Though not unanimous, most studies show that intrapleural anesthesia is effective in providing analgesia.[87,88] Concern has been raised that intrapleural anesthesia may create a level of anesthesia below the umbilicus and make posttraumatic abdominal examinations unreliable. Until this issue is clarified, it seems prudent to rule out intraabdominal injury before intrapleural anesthesia is used.[89]

Technique
If a chest tube is in place, it is preferable to inject anesthetic into the pleural space through the chest tube. Clamp the tube for 10 to 15 minutes to allow the anesthetic to diffuse. When the tube cannot be taken off suction or if no tube is present, inject the local anesthetic percutaneously.[90] With the patient in the lateral position (with the affected side up), place a 16-gauge Tuohy needle 8 to 10 cm from the posterior midline in the eighth intercostal space. Angle the needle 30 to 40 degrees with respect to the skin and aim medially, with the bevel up and directed just above the rib. After perforating the posterior intercostal membrane (felt as a distinct resistance), remove the stylet and attach a well-wetted, air-filled glass syringe to the Tuohy needle. Advance the needle until it enters the pleural space, which is denoted by the plunger being drawn down the syringe as a result of the negative pressure created during inspiration. Remove the syringe and introduce an epidural catheter 5 to 6 cm into the pleural space. Remove the Tuohy needle, obtain a chest radiograph to confirm proper position, and secure the catheter.

The most commonly used anesthetic and dose is 20 mL (0.3 mL/kg) of 0.5% bupivacaine. A dose repeated every 8 hours is safe and effective.[91] Alternatively, infuse 0.25% bupivacaine at 0.1 to 0.2 mL/kg/hr after a bolus has been administered.[85] The solution presumably diffuses from the pleural space "back" through the parietal pleura and the intercostal muscle to reach the intercostal spaces, where it blocks the intercostal nerves. The level of anesthesia can extend from T2 to T12 and involve the skin, chest, abdominal wall, and potentially the viscera if the visceral afferent fibers are blocked at the sympathetic chain in the paravertebral gutter.

Though not yet a consistently proven or a completely standardized technique, intrapleural anesthesia offers promise for patients and is a valuable procedure for the emergency clinician to master.

COMPLICATIONS

Local Anesthetic Effect on Wounds

Wound Healing

Local anesthetics produce cytotoxic effects on cell structure and function in a dose- and time-related manner. These effects, at doses well below those used clinically, involve fibroblasts more than nervous tissue. Local anesthetics impair mitochondrial function and fibroblast proliferation and hasten apoptosis in vitro; the clinical relevance of these effects to the ED use of local anesthetics is likely to be minimal.[92,93] Collagen synthesis is inhibited by lidocaine and bupivacaine.[94] Morris and Tracey[95] found that lidocaine in increasing concentrations progressively reduces the tensile strength of wounds. Epinephrine added to 1% and 2% concentrations of lidocaine further reduced tensile strength, but when epinephrine was added to distilled water or to 0.5% lidocaine, it had little effect. Several conclusions may be clinically relevant. Although it may delay the onset of anesthesia, 0.5% lidocaine solution, without epinephrine, may be best for maintaining wound strength.

Eriksson and associates[96] found that lidocaine reduces the inflammatory response in wounds by decreasing the number of white cells and their metabolic activity. Although an inflammatory response may be beneficial in a contaminated wound, it can be detrimental in a sterile wound because of tissue toxicity created by the release of superoxide anions, lysosomal enzymes, thromboxanes, leukotrienes, and interleukins. The clinical relevance of this is unknown. None of the concerns mentioned earlier should prohibit the use of standard anesthetics or epinephrine when their use is otherwise indicated.

Wound Infection

Though not generally appreciated, it has long been known that local anesthetics possess antimicrobial activity in vitro. Lidocaine and procaine demonstrate concentration-dependent inhibition of culture growth of most gram-negative organisms.[97-99] Gram-positive isolates are also significantly affected by lidocaine and, to a lesser extent, by procaine. Lidocaine inhibits the growth of common nosocomial pathogens, including *Enterococcus faecalis*, *Escherichia coli*, *Pseudomonas aeruginosa*, and several strains of methicillin-resistant *Staphylococcus aureus* and vancomycin-resistant enterococci.[99] Administering anesthetics before obtaining material for culture, including injecting a joint before arthrocentesis, may give false-negative culture results. To avoid this problem, if possible inject the skin at the injection site and along the needle tract but not into the actual joint space until after a synovial fluid specimen has been obtained for culture. Berg and coworkers[100] demonstrated that lidocaine administered before tissue biopsy of chronic wounds did not affect the

culture results when the exposure time before culture was less than 2 hours. This effect is also significant when anesthetic ointments are applied before culture. EMLA cream applied before culture demonstrates powerful antimicrobial properties.[100] Furthermore, it has been shown that adding sodium bicarbonate to lidocaine greatly enhances its inhibitory effect on bacteria.[101] Although local anesthetics can interfere with culture testing, several studies have shown that local anesthetics, by themselves, do not appear to alter the incidence of wound infection.[102,103]

Epinephrine appears to exert a deleterious effect on host defenses, at least in animal models. Studies of infiltrated and topically applied epinephrine solutions in contaminated animal wounds show an increased potential for infection.[102,103] Epinephrine-induced vasoconstriction may contribute to tissue hypoxia, retard the killing of *S. aureus* by leukocytes, and reduce leukocyte migration into the tissue.[104] Most clinical studies using topical anesthetics with vasoconstrictor properties (e.g., TAC mixtures) do not demonstrate a significant rise in infection rates.[40,43,44,49] The concerns mentioned earlier should not prohibit the use of epinephrine for wound preparation when its use is otherwise appropriate.

Local Injuries

Injury may result from the direct application of an anesthetic agent to a nerve or from passage of a needle through soft tissue structures. Factors implicated in transient or persistent neuropathy include acidic solutions, additives, the agent itself, needle trauma, compression from hematomas, and inadvertent injection of neurolytic agents. Born[105] described a series of 49 wrist and metacarpal blocks with bupivacaine in which significant neuropathy developed in eight patients. He postulated that damage occurred from trapping of the drug in a confined space and recommended that whenever bupivacaine is used in this situation, it should be low in concentration and volume. Infection, hematomas, and broken needles are other local problems that can be avoided by using proper technique. Erroneous needle placement can also produce complications such as pneumothorax during a brachial plexus or intercostal block.

Use of Epinephrine with Local Anesthetics

Epinephrine in conjunction with local anesthetics prolongs the duration of anesthesia and produces a temporary hemostatic effect, but its inclusion in digital block solutions has traditionally been discouraged because of the belief that it can lead to ischemia and necrosis. Areas of special concern include the digits, penis, tip of the nose, and earlobe. Although tissue ischemia and sloughing have been reported with concentrations of 1:20,000, current practice involves concentrations in the range of 1:100,000 to 1:200,000 and the use of submaximal doses. Several authors suggest that epinephrine-containing solutions can be safely injected into the fingers without adverse sequelae.[106-109]

A study of more that 3000 cases of elective injection of low-dose epinephrine (≤1:100,000) into the hand and fingers failed to identify a single case of digital tissue loss, and phentolamine was not required to reverse vasoconstriction.[106] Of 1111 procedures reported by Chowdhry and coauthors[110] involving digital blocks with 1% lidocaine plus epinephrine (1:100,000) at a dose ranging between 0.5 and 10 mL (average, 4.3 mL), no patient in the epinephrine group exhibited digital

TABLE 29-8   Differentiating Systemic Adverse Reactions

FINDINGS	TOXIC REACTIONS	ALLERGY	VASOVAGAL	EXCESS CATECHOLAMINES, ANXIETY* (ENDOGENOUS), VASOCONSTRICTOR (EXOGENOUS)
Relatively specific signs and symptoms	Metallic taste Tongue numbness Drowsiness Nystagmus Slurred speech Seizures[†] Coma Respiratory arrest[†]	Acute rhinitis Pruritus[†] Dermatitis Urticaria[†] Facial swelling Laryngospasm Bronchospasm[†]	Syncope[†,‡]	Headache Hypertension[†] Palpitations Apprehension[†,§]
Overlapping signs and symptoms	Paresthesia Light-headedness Tinnitus Tremor Tachypnea Tachycardia (early) Bradycardia[†] Hypotension[†] Cardiac arrest	Light-headedness Tachycardia[†] Hypotension[†] Cardiac arrest Nausea and vomiting Dyspnea	Light-headedness Tinnitus Tachypnea Tachycardia (early) Bradycardia[†] Hypotension[†] Diaphoresis	Paresthesia[†] Light-headedness[†] Tremor Tachypnea[†] Tachycardia[†] Nausea and vomiting Dyspnea Diaphoresis

*Anxiety reaction, including hyperventilation syndrome.
[†]Denotes common and significant reactions.
[‡]Vasovagal syncope occurs with the patient upright; any loss of consciousness in the recumbent position implies a severe toxic or anaphylactic reaction.
[§]Although apprehension is classically associated with anxiety and vasoconstrictor reactions, milder toxic and allergic reactions may cause patient apprehension.

ischemia or experienced nerve injuries or unusually delayed wound healing. Current data support the use of epinephrine, when correctly applied, for the performance of digital blocks of the fingers and toes.

The use of phentolamine (Regitine), which produces postsynaptic α-adrenergic blockade, is recommended for clinically significant vasoconstrictor-induced tissue ischemia. This medication is usually given by local infiltration, in the area where epinephrine has been injected, at a dose of 0.5 to 5.0 mg diluted 1:1 with saline. If local infiltration is ineffective because of tension within a tissue compartment or if the area of vasoconstriction is large, give phentolamine by the intraarterial route.[111]

Systemic Toxic Reactions

Although systemic toxic reactions occur in only 0.1% to 0.4% patients after the administration of local anesthetics, they are the most frequent serious adverse reactions encountered (Table 29-8).[112] After the administration of a local anesthetic, some of the drug reaches its intended target and some is absorbed quickly into the systemic circulation. Peak blood levels are generally produced within 30 minutes. Many vagal reactions, nonspecific anxiety reactions, and sensitivity to preservatives have been attributed to "allergies" or to systemic toxicity to local anesthetics. Patients may also demonstrate systemic reactions to hidden allergens that may mimic a systemic reaction, such as anaphylactic reactions to the latex in surgical gloves.

High Blood Levels
Systemic toxic reactions result from high blood levels of local anesthetic. Several factors are important in producing high

blood levels, including the site and mode of administration, rate, dose and concentration, addition of epinephrine, specific drug, clearance, maximum safe dosage, and inadvertent intravascular injection.

Site and Mode of Administration
In comparing the routes of administration for a given dose, the intravascular route produces the highest levels, followed by topical mucosal application and then infiltration (see Fig. 29-6). The more vascular the site, the more systemic absorption that occurs and the higher the level obtained. The following blocks are arranged in decreasing order of systemic absorption: intercostal, caudal, epidural, brachial plexus, and subcutaneous. It follows that the site of administration is an important variable in determining the safe dose of an anesthetic. For example, 400 mg of lidocaine may produce a nontoxic blood level with subcutaneous abdominal wall infiltration but produce a toxic level when used for an intercostal nerve block.

Rate
A more rapid IV injection will produce a higher blood level than a slower injection. A single topical application leads to a higher level than a dose that is fractionated over time.

Dose and Concentration
The larger the total dose, the higher the peak blood level. It is uncertain whether increasing the concentration while maintaining the total dose by decreasing the volume affects the serum level.

Addition of Epinephrine
Epinephrine produces vasoconstriction and reduces systemic absorption, thereby resulting in lower peak blood levels. Occasionally, the apprehension, tachycardia, or palpitations

induced by epinephrine can be incorrectly interpreted by both the clinician and patient as an "allergic" reaction.

Specific Drug. The more potent agents are more toxic on a milligram-to-milligram basis. Because anesthetics are used in equipotent doses (e.g., 1 mg of bupivacaine versus 4 mg of lidocaine), they are approximately equitoxic. The blood levels achieved by a particular agent depend on the agent's absorption, distribution, and clearance from the circulation. Agents with high lipid solubility and lower protein binding (etidocaine > bupivacaine > lidocaine > mepivacaine) tend to become sequestered in tissue and have slower absorption and lower blood levels. Agents with a greater volume of distribution or faster clearance (etidocaine > lidocaine > mepivacaine > bupivacaine) also produce lower blood levels. Together, these effects produce margins of safety for each anesthetic, with etidocaine having the greatest safety margin, followed by bupivacaine, which is equal to or better than lidocaine.

Esters are difficult to measure in blood because of their rapid hydrolysis by pseudocholinesterase. As a group, toxicity is inversely proportional to the rate of hydrolysis. Tetracaine is slowly hydrolyzed and is most toxic. Chloroprocaine is quickly hydrolyzed and is the least toxic. Procaine falls between the two.

Clearance

The liver metabolizes amides, with the clearance rate being a function of hepatic blood flow and the extraction capacity of the liver. Decreased hepatic blood flow, produced by norepinephrine, propranolol, or general anesthesia, slows clearance and potentially raises drug blood levels. Decreased drug extraction, associated with congestive heart failure, cirrhosis, or hypothermia, may produce a higher blood level. Hypovolemia, which decreases hepatic flow, does not raise blood levels because it causes an offsetting decrease in absorption.

Decreased clearance of esters and an increased risk for toxicity occur in patients with either low levels or an atypical form of pseudocholinesterase. Low levels occur in various disease states, including severe liver disease and renal failure, and in pregnancy. Atypical pseudocholinesterase is an inherited trait, and its presence reduces the hydrolysis rate of procaine to a greater extent than low levels do.

There are significant differences between pediatric and adult drug distribution and metabolism. Neonates exhibit both reduced levels of pseudocholinesterase and reduced hepatic metabolism, thus increasing the risk for toxicity. In older children, the effects of increased hepatic metabolism and a relatively larger volume of distribution increase their tolerance for higher doses.

Because lidocaine is metabolized in the liver by cytochrome P-450 enzymes, drugs that inhibit these enzymes may slow lidocaine clearance and increase the risk for lidocaine toxicity. Although the effect of ciprofloxacin and erythromycin on infiltrated lidocaine has not been studied, these drugs decrease the metabolism of lidocaine and increase the concentration of its major metabolites when lidocaine is injected intravenously.[113-115] The clinical effect of this previously discussed phenomenon is unknown and probably of little consequence in ED wound care.

Maximum Safe Dosage

The *maximum safe dose* of a drug may be defined as the dose that produces a blood level of the drug just below the toxic level (Table 29-9). One maximum dose of an anesthetic agent

TABLE 29-9 Calculation of Anesthetic Doses

Anesthetic solutions are marketed with the drug concentration expressed as a percentage (e.g., bupivacaine 0.25%, lidocaine 1%). To ascertain the strength of a solution in milligrams per milliliter, consider the following:

A 1% solution is prepared by dissolving 1 g of drug in 100 mL of solution.

Therefore, 1 g/100 mL = 1000 mg/100 mL = 10 mg/mL.

To calculate the strength from the percentage quickly, simply move the decimal point one place to the right, as follows:

0.25% = 2.5 mg/mL	e.g., bupivacaine
0.5% = 5 mg/mL	e.g., tetracaine
1% = 10 mg/mL	e.g., lidocaine
2% = 20 mg/mL	e.g., viscous lidocaine
4% = 40 mg/mL	e.g., cocaine
5% = 50 mg/mL	e.g., lidocaine ointment
20% = 200 mg/mL	e.g., benzocaine

When combined in an anesthetic solution, epinephrine is usually in a 1:100,000 or a 1:200,000 dilution.

1 mL of 1:1000 epinephrine = 1 mg.

0.1 mL of 1:1000 epinephrine in 10 mL of anesthetic solution = 1:100,000 dilution = 0.010 mg/mL.

0.1 mL of 1:1000 epinephrine in 20 mL of anesthetic solution = 1:200,000 dilution = 0.005 mg/mL.

Some examples detailing epinephrine content:

	1:100,000	**1:200,000**
5 mL	0.050 mg	0.025 mg
10 mL	0.100 mg	0.050 mg
20 mL	0.200 mg	0.100 mg

Therefore, 50 mL of 1% lidocaine with epinephrine 1:200,000 contains 500 mg of lidocaine and 0.25 mg of epinephrine.

appropriate for all patients and all conditions cannot be stated. A maximum safe dose cannot be based solely on the weight of a patient. In an adult, peak blood levels do not correlate well with weight because the volume of drug distribution is relatively constant.[116,117] As an approximation, Arthur and McNicol[118] recommended that maximum dosages for children be based on weight. Plain lidocaine may be used in doses of up to 4.5 mg/kg, and the addition of epinephrine allows a maximum dose of 7 mg/kg. Bupivacaine is not recommended for children younger than 12 years, although it is commonly used without adverse consequences. Furthermore, the dose should be modified according to the site and mode of administration.

Maximum safe doses as stated on package inserts should be used only as guidelines because most of them are derived from animal experiments and are based on absorption data only. Levels vary with the site of administration, use of a vasoconstrictor, and to some extent, the health of the patient.

Levels can often be exceeded safely when the drug is administered accurately. Drugs may be toxic even within the "safe range" when inadvertently injected intravenously.

Inadvertent Intravascular Injection

Most toxic reactions are caused by inadvertent intravascular injection of anesthetics whose doses were calculated for their intended extravascular sites. For example, lidocaine, 300 mg, is a safely infiltrated dose that would probably cause toxicity if directly injected into the bloodstream.

Anesthetics that are injected intravascularly must pass through the lungs before they reach other organs. Lung tissue sequesters a significant amount of drug, which lowers the arterial blood concentration. Anesthetics that bypass the lungs, in cases of inadvertent injection into the carotid or vertebral arteries or in patients with intracardiac right-to-left shunts, can produce CNS toxicity at low doses. Intraarterial injections into subcutaneous end-arteries about the head or neck are capable of retrograde flow into the cerebral circulation if the injection pressure exceeds arterial pressure. Because the blood volume in the brain is only about 30 mL at any given moment, even 1 mg of lidocaine injected into the carotid artery can theoretically produce toxic concentrations. Patients with low cardiac output or hypovolemia and preferential cerebral blood flow may suffer enhanced CNS toxicity.

Host Factors

Four factors tend to lower the body's systemic tolerance to local anesthetic agents: hypoxia, acid-base status, protein binding, and concomitant drug use.

Hypoxia

It was initially thought that an overdose of a local anesthetic produces CNS stimulation and subsequent intracellular hypoxia, which then became the key precipitant for all toxic manifestations of the drug. It is now known that hypoxia may enhance anesthetic toxicity but is not the primary factor.

Acid-Base Status

Although studies of metabolic alkalosis have produced conflicting results, acidosis, particularly respiratory acidosis, can increase toxicity. The elevated CO_2 produced by respiratory acidosis crosses the blood-brain barrier, where it may act directly on the receptor and indirectly by lowering intracellular pH. The lower pH causes more drug to ionize, thereby furthering the block in the sodium channel and increasing the potential for toxicity.

Protein Binding

The of concentration unbound drug relates more closely to toxic effects than does the total drug concentration (bound plus unbound) as measured in the blood. The amount of α-acid glycoprotein (AAG), the major plasma protein responsible for binding local anesthetics, is considerably decreased in neonates in comparison to adults. Arthur and McNicol[118] implied that the low AAG levels in neonates are responsible for the increased toxic potential. Tucker and colleagues[119] listed several disease states that alter AAG levels and protein binding but question whether they lead to changes in free drug concentration in vivo.

Concomitant Drugs. For years, barbiturates were used to prevent and treat local anesthesia-induced seizures. Barbiturates were found to worsen anesthetic-induced apnea and cardiovascular depression. CNS depressants are used with caution when concern exists for local anesthetic toxicity. CNS stimulants have been shown to increase anesthetic-induced excitability and are avoided. Mixtures of local anesthetics have an additive effect on toxicity. If two drugs are used at half strength, they produce the same degree of toxicity as though each were used alone at normal strength. As discussed previously, drugs that slow metabolism by inhibiting hepatic enzymes may increase the risk for toxicity.

Recognition of CNS Toxicity

The earliest manifestation of systemic toxicity is CNS stimulation resulting from blockade of inhibitory synapses. CNS depression follows and is produced by direct depression of the medulla, although hypoxia may play a role. The signs and symptoms are dose related. Potential signs and symptoms of CNS toxicity, in progressing order, are numbness of the tongue, light-headedness, tinnitus, visual disturbances, muscle twitching, convulsions, coma, and apnea. Drowsiness, commonly seen with lower doses of lidocaine, is not associated with bupivacaine or etidocaine. Tetracaine may produce apnea or cardiovascular toxicity without CNS manifestations.

Recognition of Cardiovascular Toxicity

Moderate blood concentrations of local anesthetics produce slight increases in cardiac output, heart rate, and arterial pressure because of the effects of direct peripheral vasodilation and CNS stimulation. At concentrations generally well above CNS toxicity levels, local anesthetics cause direct myocardial depression, hypotension, and bradycardia, perhaps leading to cardiovascular collapse. These agents also slow electrical conduction and lead to reentry phenomena and various supraventricular and potentially lethal ventricular dysrhythmias, especially with bupivacaine and etidocaine.

Prevention of Toxicity

Knowledge of factors contributing to toxicity guides preventive measures. Avoid esters in patients with an atypical form or a quantitative deficiency of pseudocholinesterase. Use amides with caution in patients with severe liver disease or congestive heart failure. Pay attention to maximum safe dosages based on the site, technique, use of epinephrine, and patient status. Add epinephrine when possible to decrease the rate of drug absorption at vascular sites. Reduce the drug concentration by saline dilution to increase the volume for administration when a large area must be infiltrated. Frequently aspirate in areas of high vascularity, even though a negative aspiration may not prevent IV administration.[120] Slow infiltration is advised for safety and is also associated with less pain.

Treatment of Systemic Toxicity

Local anesthetics should not be administered without the ability to recognize and treat a toxic reaction, including having all necessary equipment and drugs readily available and being knowledgeable in their use. Despite taking all possible precautions, toxic reactions still occur, and close observation of the patient allows early detection and treatment.

Providing proper oxygenation and ventilation at the earliest sign of a reaction is the cornerstone of treatment. Encourage patients who are alert to moderately hyperventilate to lower the pressure of carbon dioxide (Pco_2) and raise the seizure threshold. Intubation with high-flow oxygen and hyperventilation is performed for patients who cannot adequately ventilate. Initiate IV access and monitor vital signs and cardiac rhythm closely.

Seizures are generally self-limited but are treated if they persist or prevent adequate ventilation. Because respiratory depression secondary to toxicity may follow, low-dose lorazepam or an ultrashort-acting barbiturate (thiopental or sodium methohexital) is preferred. Intubate the patient to ensure an effective airway and prevent further lactic acidosis if the seizures persist. If toxicity is caused by an ester, especially if there is an associated pseudocholinesterase problem, succinylcholine will compete with the anesthetic for the pseudocholinesterase and may increase the toxicity of both compounds.

Treat hypotension and bradycardia with fluids, leg elevation, α- and β-agonists (epinephrine, ephedrine, or dopamine), or atropine as the need dictates. Although lidocaine (with diazepam pretreatment) has been shown to be effective for bupivacaine-induced ventricular dysrhythmias, strong theoretical and experimental evidence indicates that bretylium is more effective.[121,122] However, until bretylium becomes available again, amiodarone is a reasonable alternative. High doses of atropine and epinephrine can be successful in correcting pulseless idioventricular rhythm. Cardiopulmonary resuscitation is instituted when necessary.

Intravenous Lipid Emulsion

Animal studies, case reports/small series, and personal opinion have advocated the use of 20% lipid emulsion intravenously as a remarkable antidote to resuscitate bupivacaine- and mepivacaine-related cardiac arrest, a situation that is usually fatal (see http://lipidrescue.com). Rosenblatt and associates[123] described the IV injection of 100 mL of 20% Intralipid (Baxter formulation used for hyperalimentation) followed by an infusion (0.5 mL/kg/min over a 2-hour period) and related this intervention to successful resuscitation in a scenario that appeared hopeless. Picard[124] considers lipid emulsion a "crucial antidote" that should be available when local anesthetics are used for peripheral nerve blocks. It is unclear whether this intervention will prove useful for local anesthetic–related cardiac arrest, but the initial data are encouraging. Lipid emulsion therapy in otherwise hopeless situations of cardiac arrest secondary to local anesthetic overdose is supported (Box 29-3). *It appears prudent and intuitive to initiate this antidote before cardiac arrest when significant local anesthetic toxicity is identified.*

Allergic Reactions

Allergenic Agents

True allergic reactions are rare and account for only 1% to 2% of all adverse reactions, but they are important to recognize because of their serious potential. Ester solutions (procaine, tetracaine) that produce the metabolite paraaminobenzoic acid (PABA) account for the majority of these reactions. Amide solutions (lidocaine, bupivacaine) are rarely involved, and usually the preservative methylparaben (MPB), which is structurally similar to PABA, is responsible. Although pure esters and pure amides do not cross-react, amides may appear to do so if multidose vials containing MPB are used. Patients may manifest an allergic response on first contact with a local anesthetic because of previous sensitization to these agents. MPB is found in creams, ointments, and various cosmetics, and PABA is an ingredient in many sunscreen

---

BOX 29-3 Preliminary Strategies for Lipid Emulsion Rescue Therapy in Patients with Severe Local Anesthetic Toxicity*

Intravenous lipid emulsion (ILE) is available as Liposyn II (20%) or Intralipid (20%).

Protocol: Infuse 20% ILE intravenously. Administer a bolus injection of 1.5 mL/kg[†] over a period of 1 to 2 minutes. It may be repeated 1 to 3 times every 5 minutes. Follow with a continuous infusion at 0.25 mL/kg/min for 30 to 120 minutes.

Increase the rate of infusion to 0.5 mL/kg/min in patients with declining blood pressure.

From Brent J: Poisoned patients are different—sometimes fat is a good thing. Crit Care Med. 2009;37:1157; and http:// lipidrescue.com.
*Can be extrapolated to other toxins. Continue other resuscitative efforts, including cardiopulmonary resuscitation.
†For the initial dose, withdraw 100 mL from a 500-mL bag/bottle and inject with a syringe. Then attach to an infusion pump.

---

preparations. Patients who are latex sensitive may have an allergic reaction incorrectly attributed to the local anesthetic.

Cell-mediated delayed reactions manifested as dermatitis are rare; it is immediate hypersensitivity that most concerns the emergency clinician. A spectrum of signs and symptoms may occur, from rhinitis and mild urticaria to bronchospasm, upper airway edema, or anaphylactic shock. Onset may be immediate and occur even during administration of the agent. Treat anaphylaxis in the usual manner.

The more frequent problem facing emergency clinicians is a patient who claims to have a past history of allergy to local anesthetics. Most patients assume that any adverse reaction to a local anesthetic procedure is an allergy. Because allergy is rarely the cause, a careful history and a review of previous records, if available, are crucial in evaluating these patients. Procaine, trade name Novocaine, was commonly used in dentistry, and many patients who experienced many types of reactions in the dentist's office, rarely true allergy, state they are allergic to Novocaine. Procaine is no longer used in dental practice, but procaine is the local anesthetic in intramuscular penicillin preparations (procaine penicillin G).

Attempts to uncover the actual cause of the past reaction and the specific agent involved are often fruitless. Ask about the exact signs and symptoms, technique of administration, amount of drug used, and how the patient was treated. If an allergic reaction cannot be ruled out and the drug previously used is known, use an agent from the other class (whether amide or ester). Lidocaine from a dental cartridge does not contain MPB, and if this were the allergenic source, an ester agent could be used. However, if lidocaine from a multidose vial is implicated, do not use an ester because MPB may cross-react with PABA. In this case it may be safer to use an amide without MPB or to choose an alternative (see later). In most cases the allergen is an ester, and the patient can safely be given an amide without MPB. Single-dose ampules of 1% lidocaine without MPB, readily obtainable from a resuscitation cart, can be used for this purpose.

Uncertainty often exists regarding the specific agent involved, and the clinician must choose an alternative approach to local anesthesia. If the wounds are extensive and the risk is acceptable, procedural sedation (see Chapter 33) or general anesthesia may be used. Conversely, if minimal pain is expected and the procedure is short (e.g., one or two sutures or staples in the scalp), no anesthesia may be required. These methods may be useful, but the degree of anesthesia produced is frequently not sufficient. Antihistamines injected into a wound have been used successfully for many years and represent a good alternative. Local anesthetic efficacy is found in varying degrees with all antihistamines. Ketamine anesthesia may be a useful alternative in some situations and is commonly used in children.

Diphenhydramine and Benzyl Alcohol
Several studies have demonstrated that 1% diphenhydramine (Benadryl) is as effective as 1% lidocaine for infiltrative anesthesia.[125-127] As long as diphenhydramine is not used at concentrations greater than 1%, potential problems of skin necrosis or significant sedation are rare. Dilute the standard 5% parenteral form to a 1% concentration for subcutaneous injection (1 mL of drug to 4 mL of saline). The duration of action of diphenhydramine is shorter than that of lidocaine but appears to be adequate for most procedures. The injection pain of diphenhydramine exceeds that of lidocaine but can be diminished by reducing the concentration to 0.5%. At this lower concentration, the effectiveness of this agent on facial wounds is lost.[128] The addition of epinephrine to 0.5% diphenhydramine results in a more painful solution with a shorter duration of action than a standard buffered lidocaine with epinephrine solution.[129] Benzyl alcohol (0.9%) with epinephrine (1:100,000) compares favorably with diphenhydramine as an effective local anesthetic. This appears to be a useful alternative to diphenhydramine when lidocaine cannot be used but is of shorter duration than diphenhydramine.[130-132]

Skin Testing
Skin testing and progressive subcutaneous challenge doses deserve special mention because they appear to be logical and well-studied approaches. However, intradermal skin testing with local anesthetics is controversial and often of no practical benefit in the ED. False-positive results are frequently produced by local release of histamine in response to needle trauma, tissue distention, or preservatives in the solution.[133] In addition, a high incidence of false-negative results can occur. It is questionable whether these low-molecular-weight drugs or their allergenic metabolites are ever capable of eliciting positive responses.[134] Other disadvantages of skin testing include its time-consuming nature and potential hazard when even minute traces of an allergen may precipitate a serious reaction. Subcutaneous challenge testing in graduating doses has been advocated and may well eliminate many false responses, but it does not eliminate the problems of time and hazard. Swanson,[135] recognizing that allergy to pure lidocaine is extremely rare, recommended 0.1 mL as a single intradermal skin test. Although his approach eliminates the time disadvantage, intradermal placement can still produce false responses. It would seem more reasonable to give this test dose subcutaneously while exercising due caution in the unlikely event that a patient exhibits a serious reaction.

Summary of Anesthetic "Allergy" Management
Generally speaking, the optimal approach to a patient with a presumed anesthetic allergy is to determine the specific anesthetic agent associated with a presumed allergic reaction and then use a preservative-free agent from the other class (see earlier discussion). If the agent is unknown, use an antihistamine or give 0.1 mL of preservative-free lidocaine as a subcutaneous test dose and proceed with the full dose if no reaction occurs within 30 minutes. Given the studies mentioned earlier, prudent choices would seem to be diphenhydramine (Benadryl) or benzyl alcohol. Epinephrine (1:100,000) can be added to both these drugs to prolong the duration of action. Ketamine anesthesia is also an alternative.

Catecholamine Reactions
Anxiety and vasoconstrictor (epinephrine) reactions are discussed together because each produces similar manifestations caused by elevated catecholamine levels. These relatively common disorders are difficult to distinguish from each other and are not generally serious.

Excess catecholamine levels produce tachycardia, palpitations, hypertension, apprehension, tremulousness, diaphoresis, tachypnea, pallor, and on occasion, anginal chest pain. Thus, catecholamine excess may resemble the CNS stimulation phase of local anesthetic toxicity.

Catecholamine reactions are not usually caused solely by exogenous epinephrine because if it is used in its optimal concentration (1:200,000), the maximum safe dose (0.25 mg) is rarely exceeded. However, many patients produce significant endogenous catecholamines because of anxiety about the anesthetic approach or upcoming procedure. In this case, even the addition of small amounts of epinephrine could trigger a catecholamine reaction. Therefore, patient preparation includes proper explanation and reassurance to decrease anxiety. Exercise caution with patients who have hyperthyroidism, hypertension, or atherosclerotic cardiovascular disease, although these conditions do not contraindicate the judicious use of epinephrine-containing anesthetics. Do not give epinephrine-containing anesthetics to patients taking MAO inhibitors.

Treatment of a catecholamine reaction includes stopping further drug administration, observing the patient closely, and administering α- or β-antagonists or benzodiazepine agents, if necessary, to combat severe reactions.

Vasovagal Reactions
It is not standard to monitor patients (cardiac, pulse oximetry) during routine local anesthesia procedures. Vasovagal reactions are, however, common, especially in dental procedures (reported incidence, 2% to 3%), during which the patient is generally in an upright position. To limit vasovagal reactions related to local anesthesia in the ED, do not draw up medication in a syringe in front of the patient, and inject only when the patient is supine (Figs. 29-11 and 29-12). The patient initially experiences anxiety when a triggering event, commonly the sight or sensation of needle insertion, causes loss of sympathetic tone and an increase in vagal tone. The resultant hypotension and bradycardia may lead to syncope. Address the patient's anxiety and administer the injections with the patient recumbent as useful preventive measures. Cardiac monitoring may help identify the onset of vagally induced bradycardia when suggested by the past history. Lay the patient supine and elevate the legs. Rarely, atropine is required. Should a patient lose consciousness while in a recumbent position, consider diagnoses other than vasovagal syncope, although significant bradycardia and even complete

Figure 29-11 Drawing up local anesthetic with a syringe and needle in front of the patient may lead to anxiety and a vasovagal reaction. Avoid this potential complication by simply performing this task out of view of the patient.

heart block may accompany a vagal reaction in a supine patient.

SUMMARY

Emergency medicine cannot be practiced without the use of local anesthetic agents. Their effectiveness when applied topically or by infiltration makes them extremely adaptable to many clinical circumstances. A working knowledge of commonly used agents is necessary to ensure the safe administration of these medications. Aim specific efforts at maximizing the drugs' anesthetic effects while minimizing the pain of administration and risk for toxicity.

References are available at www.expertconsult.com

Figure 29-12 A, What's wrong in this picture? Almost everything! The patient is sitting upright and directly observing the procedure. This may lead to a vasovagal event, and should he fall from the bed, significant injury may occur. Additional problems include improper positioning of the overhead light (behind the physician's back), lack of privacy (open curtain and door), equipment tray placed too far away, and a hunched-over posture of the physician. **B,** A much better approach. Note that the patient is supine, the bed is raised, the light and equipment tray are in better position, the curtain is closed, and a family member is present (but sitting to avoid a "bystander vagal event") to distract the patient during the procedure. The clinician could also be seated for comfort.

CHAPTER 30

Regional Anesthesia of the Head and Neck

James T. Amsterdam and Kevin P. Kilgore

Intraoral and extraoral regional anesthesia is simple and convenient for everyday use in the emergency department (ED).[1] Nerve blocks provide anesthesia to broad areas of distribution on the face with a minimal amount of anesthetic and tissue distortion. Local anesthetic blocks are effective for closing facial lacerations, especially those of the lips, forehead, midface, and ears, places where the swelling caused by local infiltration may be undesirable. Local anesthetic blocks are also effective for the relief of pain, for anesthesia during facial débridement, and for diagnostic purposes.

Regional blocks are also therapeutic for procedural anesthesia and for control of pain in dental emergencies such as toothaches and dry sockets (see Chapter 64). Patients with dental pain who do not obtain relief with a regional dental block most likely do not have pain of dental origin. In cases in which the patient is thought to be seeking drugs, a dental anesthetic block is frequently the treatment of choice as an alternative to narcotics.

Topical anesthetic solutions such as tetracaine-adrenaline-cocaine (TAC) solution are useful for small lacerations of the scalp and face because of the vascularity of these areas. TAC is not to be used on or near the mucous membranes or the eye (see Chapter 29). More extensive discussion of the general complications of local anesthetics and regional anesthesia is provided in Chapters 29 and 32, respectively. Ophthalmologic anesthesia is discussed in Chapter 62, and blocks about the ears and nasal anesthesia are discussed in Chapter 63.

The procedures and techniques described here generally carry low morbidity. The supraperiosteal, mental nerve, and more sophisticated blocks (e.g., inferior alveolar block) are best learned under the instruction of an experienced clinician, a dentist, or an oral and maxillofacial surgeon.

ANATOMY OF THE FIFTH CRANIAL (TRIGEMINAL) NERVE

The fifth cranial nerve, known as the trigeminal nerve, is the sensory nerve to the face (Fig. 30-1A) and the largest of the cranial nerves. It takes its origin from the midbrain and enlarges into the gasserian, or semilunar, ganglion. Each gasserian ganglion supplies one side of the face. The gasserian ganglion is a flat, crescent-shaped structure approximately 10 mm long and 20 mm wide that divides into three branches: the ophthalmic, maxillary, and mandibular nerves (Fig. 30-1B).

Ophthalmic Nerve

The first division, the *ophthalmic nerve* (V_1), is the smallest branch of the gasserian ganglion. It leaves the cranium through the superior orbital fissure and has five cutaneous branches:

1. The medial and lateral branches of the supraorbital nerve, which emerge on the face through the supraorbital notch.

Regional Anesthesia of The Head and Neck

Indications
Anesthesia of the teeth for dental pain
Anesthesia of the soft tissues of the face

Contraindications
Lack of patient cooperation
Inability to perform the procedure without passing through an infected area
Anticoagulated patients (e.g., warfarin)

Complications
Local anesthetic toxicity if maximum amounts are exceeded
Failure to obtain anesthesia
Allergy to local anesthetic
Infection extending to the deep spaces of the head and neck because of injecting through an infected area
Hematoma
Failure to aspirate blood
Intravascular injection of epinephrine
Needle breakage (rare)
Needlestick of the operator

Equipment

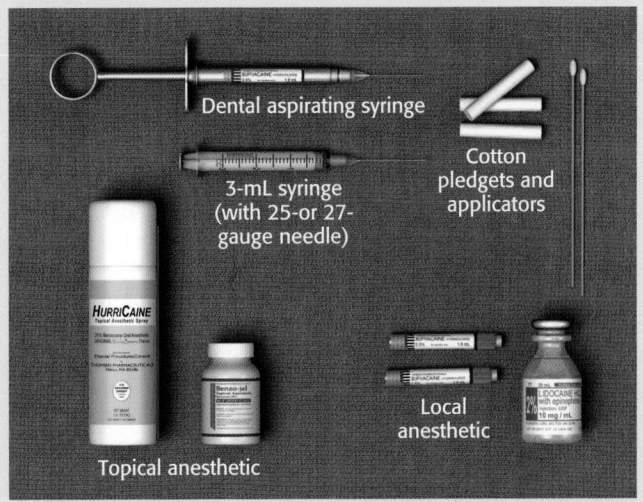

Dental aspirating syringe

3-mL syringe (with 25-or 27-gauge needle)

Cotton pledgets and applicators

Topical anesthetic

Local anesthetic

Review Box 30-1 Regional anesthesia of the head and neck: indications, contraindications, complications, and equipment.

Figure 30-1 A, Cutaneous distribution of the trigeminal nerve (cranial nerve V). Note that the supraorbital, infraorbital, and mental foramina are all in line just medial to the pupil when the person looks straight ahead. **B,** Branches of the trigeminal nerve. (*Adapted from Eriksson E, ed.* Illustrated Handbook in Local Anesthesia. *Philadelphia: Saunders; 1980.*)

These two sensory nerves pierce the frontalis muscle and extend to the lambdoid suture on the back of the skull.

2. The supratrochlear nerve, which provides sensation to the medial aspect of the forehead just above the glabella.
3. The infratrochlear nerve.
4. The lacrimal nerve.
5. The external nasal nerve.

Branches of the ophthalmic nerve provide sensation to the forehead, cornea, upper eyelid, structures in the orbit, and the frontal sinuses.

Maxillary Nerve

The second division, the *maxillary nerve* (V_2), provides sensation to the maxilla and associated structures, including the teeth, periosteum, mucous membranes of the maxillary sinus, nasal cavity, soft and hard palate, lower eyelids, upper lip, and side of the nose. The second division exits the cranium from the foramen rotundum and ultimately enters the face through the infraorbital canal. It terminates as the infraorbital nerve. The infraorbital nerve gives off sensory branches to the lower eyelids, the side of the nose, and the upper lip.

The anatomy of the maxillary nerve is rather complicated because of its numerous branches. The first branch comprises two short sphenopalatine nerves to the pterygopalatine ganglion, also called the *Meckel ganglion* or the *sphenopalatine ganglion*. The next two branches of clinical importance are the nasopalatine and the greater (anterior) palatine nerves. The nasopalatine nerve arises from the pterygopalatine ganglion, courses down along the nasal septum, and is transmitted through the anterior portion of the hard palate by way of the anterior palatine canal. This canal is located in the midline approximately 10 mm palatal to the maxillary central teeth and immediately behind the incisors. The nasopalatine nerve provides sensation to the most anterior portion of the hard

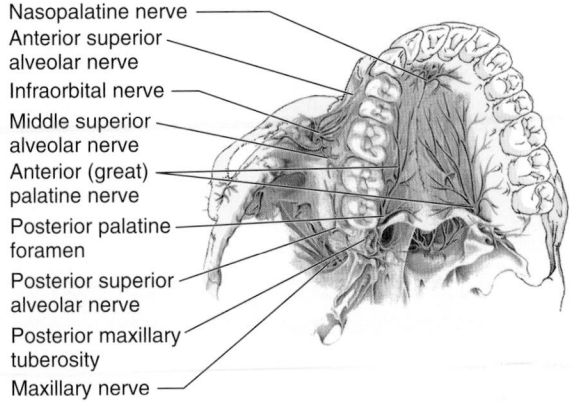

Figure 30-2 The anterior third of the palate, from canine to canine, is anesthetized by a local injection near the anterior palatine canal. There may be some overlapping branches of the anterior palatine nerve. Anesthesia of the posterior two thirds of the palate is obtained by a local injection in the area of the posterior palatine foramen. *Note:* Do not enter the foramen itself because the anesthetic may reach the middle palatine nerve, produce anesthesia of the soft palate, and result in gagging. (*Adapted from Eriksson E, ed.* Illustrated Handbook in Local Anesthesia. *Philadelphia: Saunders; 1980.*)

palate and the adjacent gum margins of the upper incisors. This nerve is rarely blocked in clinical practice, except in dental operations, because it is quite painful as a result of the tightly bound tissues (Fig. 30-2).

The anterior, or greater, palatine nerve arises from the pterygopalatine ganglion and passes down through the posterior palatine foramen. The posterior palatine foramen is located 10 mm palatal to the third molar and the bicuspid teeth and intermingles with the nasopalatine nerve opposite the cuspid tooth. The greater palatine nerve provides sensation to most of the hard palate, as well as the palatal aspect of the gingiva. It is rarely blocked in the ED (see Fig. 30-2).

The next branch consists of the posterior superior alveolar (PSA) nerve, which courses down the posterior surface of the maxilla for approximately 20 mm, at which point it enters one or several small posterosuperior dental foramina (see Fig. 30-2). This nerve supplies all the roots of the third and second molar teeth and two roots of the first molar tooth. A third branch consists of the middle superior alveolar (MSA) nerve, which branches off about midway within the infraorbital canal and then courses downward in the outer wall of the maxillary sinus (see Fig. 30-2). This nerve supplies the maxillary first and second bicuspid teeth and the mesiobuccal root of the first molar. The last branch consists of the anterior superior alveolar (ASA) nerve, which branches off into the infraorbital canal approximately 5 mm behind the infraorbital foramen, just before the terminal branches of the infraorbital nerve emerge (Fig. 30-2). This nerve descends in the anterior wall of the maxilla to supply the maxillary central, lateral, and cuspid teeth; the labial mucous membrane; the periosteum; and the alveoli on one side of the median line. There is intercommunication among the ASA, MSA, and PSA nerves.

Mandibular Nerve

The third division, the *mandibular nerve* (V_3), is the largest branch of the trigeminal nerve. It exits from the cranium through the foramen ovale and divides into three principal branches:

1. The long buccal nerve branches off just outside the foramen ovale. It passes between the two heads of the external pterygoid muscle and crosses in front of the ramus to enter the cheek through the buccinator muscle, buccal to the maxillary third molar. The buccal nerve supplies sensory branches to the buccal mucous membrane and the mucoperiosteum over the maxillary and mandibular teeth. The cutaneous branch provides sensation to the cheek.
2. The lingual nerve courses forward toward the midline. It runs downward superficially to the internal pterygoid muscle and passes lingual to the apex of the mandibular third molar. It enters the base of the tongue at this point through the floor of the mouth and supplies the anterior two thirds of the tongue, the lingual mucous membrane, and the mucoperiosteum.
3. The largest of the V_3 branches is the inferior alveolar nerve. It provides sensation to all the lower teeth, although the central incisors, lateral incisors, and buccal aspect of the molar teeth may receive additional sensory innervation. The nerve descends, covered by the external pterygoid muscle, and passes between the ramus of the mandible and the sphenomandibular ligament to enter the mandibular canal. It is accompanied by the inferior alveolar artery and vein, proceeds along the mandibular canal, and innervates the teeth. At the mental foramen the nerve bifurcates into an incisive branch, which continues forward to supply the anterior teeth. It gives off a side branch, the mental nerve, which exits from the mental foramen to supply the skin. The mental foramen is located approximately between the apices of the lower first and second bicuspids, or premolar teeth. This is a useful site at which to perform a nerve block because the mental nerve provides sensation to the skin of the chin and the mucous membrane of the lower lip.

Figure 30-3 A, Local anesthesia—basic setup for intraoral application using an aspirating dental syringe. **B,** Topical mucosal anesthesia can *make the injection nearly painless*. Swab the *gauze-dried mucosa* with the topical agent or have the patient hold cotton swabs soaked in the agent, and wait for 1 to 3 minutes. Benzocaine can be used as a topical anesthetic (shown here). However, excellent topical anesthesia of mucous membranes can be obtained after 2 minutes by applying a gel mixture of a topical anesthetic consisting of 10% lidocaine, 10% prilocaine, and 4% tetracaine. (*Profound, Steven's Pharmacy, Costa Mesa, CA. Available at* www.stevensrx.com).

EQUIPMENT FOR DENTAL AND CRANIAL NERVE BLOCKS

Extraoral injections can be done easily with a 3-mL Luer-Lok syringe and a $1\frac{1}{2}$-inch, 25- to 27-gauge needle. A needle no smaller than 27 gauge is recommended for deep block techniques because of the inability to perform aspiration. Generally, a long needle is used for nerve blocks and a short needle is used for infiltration. Intraoral local anesthesia can also be conveniently administered with a dental aspirating syringe, which uses a Carpule cartridge of anesthetic along with a disposable needle (Fig. 30-3A). Dental aspirating syringes are not mandatory for intraoral local anesthesia but they make the procedure simpler, particularly when aspirating. Other adjuncts that are helpful in the administration of intraoral anesthesia include topical mucosal anesthetic agents such as gels or sprays because they can *make the injection nearly painless* (Fig. 30-3B). First swab the *gauze-dried mucosa* with a topical agent or have the patient hold cotton swabs soaked in the agent to the anticipated injection site, and wait for 1 to 3 minutes. Excellent topical anesthesia of the mucous membranes can be achieved after 2 minutes by applying a gel mixture of a topical anesthetic consisting of 10% lidocaine, 10% prilocaine and 4% tetracaine (Profound, Steven's Pharmacy, Costa Mesa, CA; www.stevensrx.com).

The anesthetic agent most frequently used is 2% lidocaine with a vasoconstrictor such as epinephrine at a concentration of 1 : 100,000. Many other anesthetic agents, such as mepivacaine (Carbocaine) and Cetacaine (a combination of benzocaine, tetracaine, butamben, and benzalkonium), with or without vasoconstrictor agents, are also available. Bupivacaine (Marcaine 0.5%) with or without epinephrine (1 : 100,000) is a longer-acting anesthetic that is often ideal for procedures performed in the ED. Bupivacaine with epinephrine is theoretically the best choice in the ED because of its longer duration of action. As a result of the rich vascularity of the oral cavity, vasoconstrictors are important in sustaining the duration of anesthesia and should be used whenever possible in the absence of medical contraindications.

GENERAL RECOMMENDATIONS

Use needles no smaller than 27 gauge for block techniques because a higher-gauge needle makes aspiration difficult and can thus result in inadvertent intravascular injection. Intravascular epinephrine, though used in small doses, may produce systemic symptoms (anxiety, tachycardia), as well as painful vasospasm if injected intraarterially, but the amount of local anesthetic is generally inconsequential.[2]

When an intraoral block is performed, the needle should not be inserted to its full length at the hub. Should inadvertent breakage occur in such a situation, retrieval of the needle may be difficult. Furthermore, the direction of the needle should not be changed while the needle is deep in the tissue. Always aspirate before injection, and inject slowly to minimize pain.

A warmed anesthetic solution is also more comfortable for the patient. Place topical anesthetics on mucous membranes before all dental blocks to make the needle puncture less painful. This adjunctive measure is greatly appreciated by the patient and suggested whenever possible.

An important caveat for intraoral local anesthesia is that an injection should not be made into or through an infected area. This is especially important with inferior alveolar nerve blocks, in which extension of an infection can be serious and difficult to treat. Trismus with inadequate oral access or direct extension of infection to the parapharyngeal spaces can result. Therefore, local anesthesia should be only superficial before incision and drainage, unless a block can be performed far proximal to the site of infections.

TECHNIQUE
Topical Anesthesia

Most patients fear dental blocks greatly, and the anxiety and pain may be lessened considerably with the use of topical anesthetics applied to the mucous membranes before injection (Fig 30-4, *step 3*). It is important to *dry the injection site thoroughly with gauze before the injection* (see Fig 30-4, *step 2*) because copious saliva will wash the anesthetic away prematurely. Coat a cotton-tipped applicator generously with 20% benzocaine (Hurricaine, Beutlich, Inc., Niles, IL) or 5% to 10% lidocaine so that the area of injection is completely covered. Allow the patient to hold the cotton swab in place. The area will be anesthetized in 2 to 3 minutes. Use concentrated topical anesthetics because poor results are obtained with weaker preparations such as 2% viscous lidocaine. Cocaine (4%) is another acceptable topical anesthetic.

HEAD AND NECK REGIONAL ANESTHESIA: GENERAL TECHNIQUE

Confirm relevant local anatomy (in this example, the infraorbital nerve block is depicted).

Retract the lip and dry the mucous membranes with gauze or a cotton pledget.

Apply a topical anesthetic, such as Benzo-Jel, on a cotton-tipped applicator (shown here), or use Hurricaine spray (not depicted).

Insert the needle, aspirate the syringe to exclude intravascular placement and then inject the appropriate amount of local anesthetic (usually about 2 mL).

Figure 30-4 Head and neck regional anesthesia—general technique.

Supraperiosteal Infiltration

The most common technique for intraoral local anesthesia of individual teeth is supraperiosteal infiltration (Fig. 30-5). This technique can provide complete relief of a toothache. Select the area to be anesthetized and dry it with gauze. Apply a topical anesthetic, such as 20% benzocaine or 5% lidocaine ointment, as described. Ask the patient to close the jaw slightly and relax the facial musculature. Grasp the mucous membrane of the area with a piece of gauze. Pull the gauze outward and downward in the maxilla and outward and upward in the mandible to extend the mucosa fully and to delineate the mucobuccal fold. Puncture the mucobuccal fold with the bevel of the needle facing the tooth. Aspirate the area and deposit approximately 1 to 2 mL of local anesthetic (2% lidocaine should be used here) at the apex (area of the root tip) of the involved tooth (see Fig. 30-5). It is helpful to place a finger against the *outer* aspect of the lip overlying the injection site. Apply firm and steady pressure against the lip and *slowly inject* the local anesthetic into the supraperiosteal site. This helps prevent ballooning of the lip.

The purpose of the injection is to deposit the anesthetic near the bone that supports the tooth. The anesthetic must penetrate the cortex of bone to reach the nerve of the individual tooth, so the injection may fail if the solution is deposited too far from the periosteum, if the needle is passed too far above the roots of the teeth, or if the bone in the area is unusually thick or dense. If anesthesia is unsuccessful, inject the palatal side. It may take 5 to 10 minutes to achieve full anesthesia with this technique, however, and the procedure may not be as effective for the posterior molars. Infiltration of the area around the maxillary canine and the first premolars will anesthetize the MSA and ASA nerves; lacerations of the upper lip can be treated by bilateral injection in the canine fossa areas.

Posterior or Superior Alveolar Nerve Block

Anatomy

Use the PSA block to anesthetize the maxillary molar teeth (Fig. 30-6). On occasion, the maxillary first molar is not completely anesthetized by this technique alone and may require

Figure 30-5 Supraperiosteal nerve block. **A,** Anatomy and distribution. **B,** Technique. Deposit the anesthetic next to the periosteum at the level of the apex (area of the root tip) of the desired tooth. The palatal side of the tooth may also be injected.

Figure 30-6 Posterior superior alveolar nerve block. **A,** Anatomy and distribution. **B,** Technique. Insert the needle at the upper second molar and direct it toward the maxillary tuberosity to a depth of 2 to 2.5 cm.

an additional block (discussed subsequently). The landmarks for this technique are the posterior-lateral portion of the maxillary tuberosity and the second molar.

Intraoral Approach

For the intraoral approach, apply a topical anesthetic on a cotton-tipped swab to the gauze-dried mucosa for 60 to 90 seconds before introducing the needle for the nerve block.[2] With the patient's mouth half-open and the jaw facing the operator, retract the cheek laterally. Make the puncture in the mucosal reflection just distal to the distal buccal root of the upper second molar (Fig. 30-6B). Direct the needle toward the maxillary tuberosity (i.e., upward, backward, and inward) and then along the curvature of the maxillary tuberosity to a depth of approximately 2 to 2.5 cm. On reaching this depth, aspirate with the needle and inject 2 to 3 mL of anesthetic solution.

Complications

Complications include puncture of the pterygoid plexus and hematoma formation should the syringe not be aspirated before injection. Also, if the needle were advanced too far posteriorly, a division 2 block of cranial nerve V will result.

MSA Nerve Block

Anatomy

Use the MSA block to anesthetize the mesiobuccal root of the maxillary first molar, which will provide complete anesthesia of the tooth (Fig. 30-7). The landmark for this procedure is the junction between the second premolar and first molar.

Intraoral Approach

Apply a topical anesthetic on a cotton-tipped swab to gauze-dried mucosa for 60 to 90 seconds before introducing the needle for the nerve block. Retract the cheek laterally and make a puncture in the mucosal reflection adjacent to the mesiobuccal root area of the first molar (the space between the second premolar and the first molar). Direct the needle at a 45-degree angle (see Fig. 30-7A). When the correct location has been determined and aspiration has been performed, inject 2 to 3 mL of anesthetic solution. Massage the tissue for 10 to 15 seconds after the injection to hasten the onset of anesthesia.

ASA Nerve Block

Anatomy

The landmark for this technique is the apex of the canine tooth (Fig. 30-8).

Intraoral Approach

For the intraoral approach, apply a topical anesthetic on a cotton-tipped swab to gauze-dried mucosa for 60 seconds before introducing the needle for the nerve block. Ask the patient to close the jaw slightly to relax the upper lip. Retract the lip anteriorly and make the puncture in the mucosal reflection at the apex of the canine tooth while directing the needle at a 45-degree angle (see Fig. 30-8B). When the correct location has been determined and aspiration has been performed, inject 2 mL of anesthetic solution. Massage the tissue for 10 to 15 seconds after the injection to hasten the onset of anesthesia.

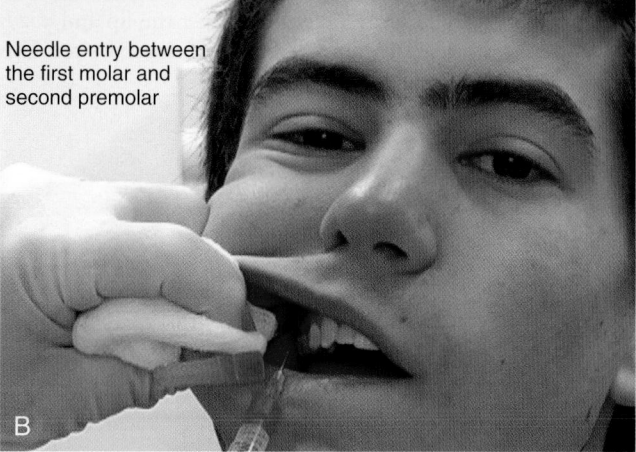

Figure 30-7 Middle superior alveolar nerve block. **A,** Anatomy and distribution. **B,** Technique. Insert the needle between the second premolar and first molar directed at a 45-degree angle.

Infraorbital Nerve Block

Anatomy

An infraorbital nerve block can be used to anesthetize the midface region (Fig. 30-9A). A solution of local anesthetic deposited adjacent to the infraorbital foramen anesthetizes not only the middle and superior alveolar nerves but also the main trunk of the infraorbital nerve, which innervates the skin of the upper lip, the skin of the nose, and the lower eyelid. The nasal mucosa is not anesthetized with this technique.

The infraorbital foramen is difficult to palpate extraorally and almost impossible to feel in the presence of facial swelling. It is found on the inferior border of the infraorbital ridge on a vertical (sagittal) line with the pupil when the patient stares straight ahead. Although one volunteer study found similar patient pain scale scores and overall preference in subjects undergoing both intraoral and extraoral approaches, the intraoral approach seemed to provide nearly twice the duration of anesthesia.[3]

Intraoral Approach

Apply a topical anesthetic on a cotton-tipped swab to gauze-dried mucosa for 60 to 90 seconds before introducing the needle for the nerve block. When performing the intraoral approach, keep the palpating finger in place over the inferior

Anterior Superior Alveolar

Figure 30-8 Anterior superior alveolar nerve block. **A,** Anatomy and distribution. **B,** Technique. Insert the needle at the apex of the canine tooth directed at a 45-degree angle.

Infraorbital—Intraoral Approach

Figure 30-9 Infraorbital nerve block. **A,** Distribution. **B,** Anatomy. **C,** Technique. Needle entry occurs at the upper second bicuspid (premolar); advance the needle parallel to the tooth to a depth of 2.5 cm.

border on the infraorbital rim. Retract the cheek as for the supraperiosteal injection, and make the puncture in the mucosa opposite the upper second bicuspid (premolar tooth) approximately 0.5 cm from the buccal surface (Fig. 30-9*B*). Direct the needle parallel to the long axis of the second bicuspid until it is palpated near the foramen, at a depth of approximately 2.5 cm. If the entry is too acute, one may encounter the malar eminence before approaching the infraorbital foramen. In addition, if the needle is extended too far posteriorly and superiorly, the orbit may be entered. Halt the procedure if you are unsure of the location of the needle or if the patient is not cooperating.

When the proper needle location has been determined and aspiration has been performed, inject 2 to 3 mL of solution *adjacent to, but not within the foramen.* Hold a finger firmly on the inferior orbital rim to avoid ballooning of the lower eyelid with anesthetic solution. If you are not certain of the exact location of the infraorbital foramen, perform a field block to obtain anesthesia. For the latter technique, infiltrate 5 mL of the anesthetic solution in a fanlike distribution in the upper buccal fold. This technique is not as precise as a discrete nerve block but usually produces the same effect. Massage the tissue for 10 to 15 seconds after the injection to hasten the onset of anesthesia.

Extraoral Approach

The infraorbital foramen can also be approached from an extraoral route (Fig. 30-10). The extraoral approach requires external preparation of the skin. With the extraoral approach use similar landmarks to locate the infraorbital foramen. The

Infraorbital—External Approach

Figure 30-10 Infraorbital nerve block, external approach. While injecting, place a finger under the eyelid to minimize lid swelling.

Inferior Alveolar

Figure 30-11 Inferior alveolar nerve block. **A,** Anatomy and distribution. Identify the anterior border of the mandibular ramus (coronoid notch) with the thumb. **B,** Approach. **C,** Technique.

needle can be felt as it passes through the skin, the subcutaneous tissue, and the quadratus labii superioris muscle. After injection, firmly massage the infiltrated tissue for 10 to 15 seconds. It is usually visibly swollen. Place a finger under the eye to limit eye edema.

Be careful to not anesthetize the facial artery and vein because these vessels may lie on either side of the needle. Do not use vasoconstrictors to avoid vasoconstriction of the facial artery. If severe blanching of the face occurs, warm compresses should be applied to the face immediately. Local phentolamine may also be injected into the blanched area to reverse the ischemia.

Inferior Alveolar Nerve Block

In the setting of extreme dental pain, the emergency clinician may find the inferior alveolar nerve block and the lingual nerve block useful. This injection is somewhat more difficult than the other techniques described, and the emergency clinician is advised to view demonstrations of this procedure before attempting it. The inferior alveolar nerve block provides anesthesia to all the teeth on that side of the mandible and desensitizes the lower lip and chin via blockade of the mental nerve. This technique is primarily useful for anesthetizing patients who have sustained severe dentoalveolar trauma; those with complaints of postextraction pain, a dry socket, or pulpitis (toothache); or those with a periapical abscess.

Anatomy

First review the anatomy of the region (Fig. 30-11*A*). The patient can be seated either in a dental chair or upright with the occiput firmly against the back of the stretcher so that when the mouth is opened, the body of the mandible is parallel to the floor. Despite the use of topical anesthesia, be ready for an unexpected quick jerk of the head when an anxious patient first feels the needle. Stand on the side *opposite* the one being injected.

The technique first involves *palpation of the retromolar fossa with the index finger or thumb*. With this maneuver, the greatest

depth of the anterior border of the ramus of the mandible (the coronoid notch) may be identified (Fig. 30-11*A*). With the thumb in the mouth resting in the retromolar fossa and the index finger placed externally behind the ramus at the same height as the thumb (Fig 30-12), the tissues are retracted toward the buccal (cheek) side, and the pterygomandibular

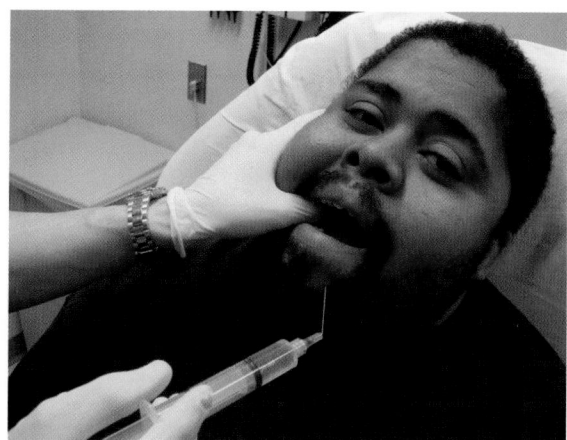

Figure 30-12 To compensate for difficulty obtaining the correct approach with a straight needle for the inferior aveolar nerve block, a 25-gauge 1½ -inch needle is bent 30 degrees with the needle guard.

triangle is visualized (Fig. 30-11*C*). This technique also moves the operator's finger safely away from the tip of the needle.

Approach
Coat the gauze-dried mucosa over the area to be injected with a topical anesthetic, as described previously. When topical anesthesia has been achieved, hold the syringe parallel to the occlusal surfaces of the teeth and angled so that the barrel of the syringe lies between the first and second premolars on the opposite side of the mandible (Fig. 30-11*B*). Failing to appreciate this required angle is the most common reason for failure of this nerve block. If a large-barrel syringe is used, the corner of the mouth may hamper efforts to obtain the proper angle. Facilitate the angle by carefully bending the 25-gauge needle about 30 degrees (see Fig. 30-12). Puncture inside the triangle at a point *1 cm above the occlusal surface of the molars*. If the needle enters too low (e.g., at the level of the teeth), the anesthetic will be deposited over the bony canal and prominence (lingula) that house the mandibular nerve and not over the nerve itself.

The needle can be felt as it passes through the ligaments and the muscles covering the internal surface of the mandible. Stop when the needle has reached bone, which signifies contact with the posterior wall of the mandibular sulcus; bone *must* be felt with the needle. Failure to do so generally results from directing the needle toward the parotid gland (too far posteriorly) rather than toward the inner aspect of the mandible. This will anesthetize portions of the facial nerve. Withdraw the needle slightly and aspirate. Deposit approximately 1 to 2 mL of solution. Three to 4 mL may be required if needle positioning is suboptimal. In children, the angulation is not parallel to the occlusal surfaces of the teeth. Instead, hold the barrel of the syringe slightly higher because the mandibular foramen is lower.

One may anesthetize the *lingual nerve* by placing several drops of anesthetic solution while slowly withdrawing the syringe and needle. The anterior two thirds of the tongue can thus be anesthetized. In actual practice, the lingual nerve is consistently blocked with this procedure because of the close proximity of both nerves. Anesthetize the *long buccal nerve* by injecting 0.2 mL of local anesthetic just distal and buccal to the last mandibular molar. Supplementing the inferior alveolar block with both lingual and buccal nerve blocks helps

anesthetize any aberrant fibers that may also be innervating the teeth. Shortly after a successful injection, the patient will report tingling in the lower lip; however, 3 to 5 minutes is usually required to achieve complete anesthesia.

Complications
Complications include inadvertent administration of anesthetic posteriorly in the region of the parotid gland, which will anesthetize the facial nerve. This is an annoying but relatively benign complication that will cause temporary facial paralysis (similar to Bell's palsy). It will affect the orbicularis oculi muscle and cause an inability to close the eyelid. Should this occur, protect the eye with an eye patch or tape until the local anesthetic has worn off (≈2 to 3 hours). Reassure the patient. Anesthesia with bupivacaine (Marcaine) presents a more significant problem if this complication occurs because bupivacaine anesthesia lasts from 3 to 6 hours (perhaps longer in some patients if epinephrine is used).

Gow-Gates Block
Anatomy
The inferior alveolar nerve block may be unsuccessful because of deposition of anesthetic in a plane medial to the lingula. In addition, the traditional technique involves depositing additional anesthetic for the long buccal nerve. First introduced in the 1970s, the Gow-Gates mandibular block is also an acceptable technique for achieving mandibular anesthesia, especially if traditional approaches fail (Fig. 30-13). The Gow-Gates approach involves the deposition of anesthetic at the lateral aspect of the anterior condylar head below the insertion of the lateral pterygoid muscle, and it uses extraoral landmarks (tragus of the ear and corner of the mouth).[4] The area is much less vascular than the area near the lingula. For this reason, epinephrine mixed with the local anesthetic is not necessary.

Approach
Ask the patient to open the mouth widely (Fig. 30-13*C*). Place a finger inferior to the tragus of the ear as the landmark for the lateral aspect of the anterior condyle (which is now sitting at the eminence). Insert the needle opposite the second molar with the barrel of the syringe between the opposite lower premolars and the corner of the mouth (similar to the inferior alveolar approach). With this plane maintained, advance the needle until it reaches the condylar neck. Withdraw the needle, aspirate, and inject 1 to 2 mL of anesthetic.[4,5]

Complications
The positive vascular aspiration rate with the Gow-Gates procedure is reported to be 1.6%, as compared with a range of positive aspiration with the conventional inferior alveolar technique of 3.5% to 22%.[6] If the needle is directed more toward the medial aspect of the anterior condylar process, the needle is then in the proximity of the pterygoid plexus of veins and the sympathetic plexus of the internal carotid artery. If the sympathetic plexus is anesthetized, Horner's syndrome will temporarily develop.

Mental Nerve Block
Block the mental nerve by infiltrating local anesthetic about the nerve where it exits its bony foramen. Avoid inserting the

Gow-Gates Block

Condylar head
Buccal nerve
Inferior alveolar nerve
Lingual nerve
Second premolar

Figure 30-13 Gow-Gates block. **A,** Distribution. **B,** Anatomy and approach. Angle the needle from the opposite premolars toward the condylar head. **C,** Technique. (*Adapted from Norton NS. Mandibular injections. In:* Netter's Head and Neck Anatomy for Dentistry. *Philadelphia: Saunders; 2007:572-574. Copyright 2007 Elsevier Inc.*)

needle into the mental nerve foramen because the needle or injection of liquid into the foramen can produce neurovascular damage. Infiltrate around the foramen to provide anesthesia of the lower lip. For lacerations over the midline of the lips, administer anesthetic about the mental nerve on each

Figure 30-14 A mental nerve block is ideal for a complicated lower lip laceration because it will not distort tissue.

side of the face. This practice anesthetizes crossover fibers. Use a 1.3-cm (½-inch), 25- or 27-gauge needle on a 3-mL syringe.

Anatomy

The mental nerve is a continuation of the inferior alveolar nerve and innervates the mucosa and skin of the lower lip on the ipsilateral side of the mandible, with limited crossover of midline fibers. The nerve emerges from the mental foramen below the second premolar. Lacerations of the lower lip can be repaired with this block (Fig. 30-14).

Approaches

Like the infraorbital nerve, block the mental nerve via an intraoral or extraoral approach. Syverud and colleagues found that volunteers who received intraoral topical anesthetic followed by an intraoral injection considered the technique to be less painful than the extraoral approach.[7] Before using either approach, identify the mental foramen by palpation about 1 cm inferior and anterior to the second premolar. It is usually best to locate the foramen with a gloved finger placed in the labial area over the mandible. Generally, the foramen will be just medial to the pupil of the eye (while the patient stares straight ahead) along a sagittal plane. The intraoral approach is demonstrated in Figure 30-15.

With the *intraoral* approach it is best to use topical anesthesia before infiltration. Anesthetize the lower labial fold adjacent to the first or second premolar. Approach the mental foramen at about a 45-degree angle, and infiltrate the area adjacent to the foramen with 1 to 2 mL of local anesthetic. Massage as described previously.

Scalp Block

Scalp blocks provide surgical anesthesia for repair of scalp lacerations, drainage of superficial scalp abscesses, and exploration and débridement of scalp wounds.

Anatomy

As shown in Figure 30-16, the scalp receives its nerve supply from branches of the trigeminal nerve (fifth cranial nerve) and the cervical plexus. The forehead is supplied by the supraorbital and supratrochlear nerves. Both nerves are branches of the ophthalmic division of the trigeminal nerve. The temporal

Mental

A

Second premolar

First premolar

Mental foramen

Mental nerve

B

C

Figure 30-15 Mental nerve block. **A,** Distribution. **B,** Anatomy and approach. The mental foramen is found below the second premolar. **C,** Technique.

Supraorbital nerve

Supratrochlear nerve

Zygomatical-temporal nerve

Auriculo-temporal nerve

Greater occipital nerve

Third occipital nerve

Lesser occipital nerve

Great auricular nerve

Figure 30-16 Sources of sensory nerve supply to the scalp. Nerves above the blue line become superficial and converge toward the vertex of the scalp.

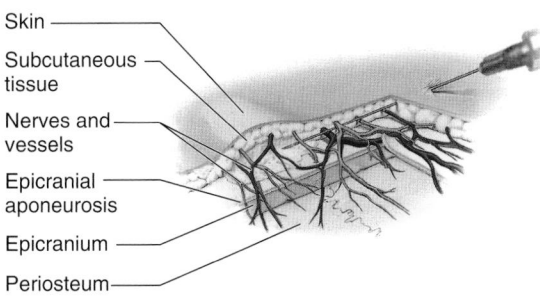

Skin

Subcutaneous tissue

Nerves and vessels

Epicranial aponeurosis

Epicranium

Periosteum

Figure 30-17 Topographic anatomy of the scalp taken above a line drawn from the upper border of the external ear to the occiput and the eyebrows. Generously infiltrating this area in a fanlike motion will block multiple sensory nerves. (*Adapted from Eriksson E, ed.* Illustrated Handbook in Local Anesthesia. *Philadelphia: Saunders; 1980.*)

Topographically, the nerves and vessels of the scalp are located in subcutaneous tissue above the epicranial aponeurosis. From this level they divide into small branches that extend to the deeper layers (epicranium and periosteum) (Fig. 30-17).[8,9]

Approaches

A scalp block can be accomplished by individually blocking each nerve that supplies the scalp, but this approach is time-consuming, difficult, and cumbersome. Because the nerves on the scalp are located superficially, a scalp block can easily be performed by injecting local anesthetic agents into the subcutaneous tissue circumferentially around the area to be blocked. Injection of local anesthetic to deeper levels is necessary only if bone is to be removed. Note that injection of local anesthetic agents only in the deeper layers without subcutaneous infiltration results in an unsuccessful block and a greater amount of bleeding during surgical intervention.

In preparation for the block, clip a band of hair (some clinicians prefer to shave the head, but this procedure is of unproven benefit). A band 1 cm wide and 3 cm away from the wound can be clipped circumferentially. Inject local anesthetic in the clipped area.

region receives its nerve supply from the zygomaticotemporal (a V₂ branch nerve), temporomandibular, and auriculotemporal nerves (V₃ branch nerves).

The posterior aspect of the scalp is innervated by the great auricular and the greater, lesser, and least (third) occipital nerves. The nerves that supply the posterior aspect of the scalp originate from the cervical plexus. All the nerves become superficial above a line drawn from the upper border of the external ear to the occiput and the eyebrows and converge toward the vertex of the scalp (see Fig. 30-16).

Prepare the skin with an antiseptic solution, and raise a skin wheal at any point along the clipped skin with a 1.3-cm ($\frac{1}{2}$-inch), 25-gauge needle. Insert a 7.6-cm (3-inch), 22-gauge needle through the skin wheal and into subcutaneous tissue. Advance it along the scalp circumferentially following the previously clipped area. Inject 0.5% to 1% lidocaine or 0.125% to 0.25% bupivacaine with epinephrine (1 : 200,000). Add epinephrine to the local anesthetic agent to provide vasoconstriction and prevent excessive blood loss and absorption of local anesthetic. The total dose of the local anesthetic agents should not exceed the recommended dose for that particular agent (see Chapter 29). Inject some local anesthetic solution into the temporalis muscle to prevent contraction of the muscle during the primary procedure if necessary.

Colley and Heavner demonstrated that when bupivacaine is used, peak plasma local anesthetic concentrations occur within 10 to 15 minutes after injection.[10] Thus, the first 10- to 15-minute period after the injection is the most critical period to monitor for local anesthetic toxicity. Colley and Heavner also found that despite the scalp's high vascularity, absorption of local anesthetics from the scalp is not excessive.[10] Because that the toxic plasma threshold for bupivacaine is 4 μg/mL, these concentrations suggest that a scalp block using bupivacaine has a wide margin of safety, even without the use of epinephrine. When epinephrine is used with bupivacaine, its effect on absorption becomes more pronounced with concentrations of 0.125% than with 0.25%. This is probably because at low concentrations (0.125%), bupivacaine has a vasoconstrictor property.[11]

Greater and Lesser Occipital Nerve Block

This relatively simple block may be useful in the ED for treating occipital neuralgia and tension headaches. For occipital neuritis, a long-acting corticosteroid such as methylprednisolone (20 to 40 mg) may be combined with the local anesthetic (see Chapter 52).[12]

Anatomy

The posterior aspect of the head is supplied by the posterior rami of the cervical nerves. Two important branches of these nerves are the greater and lesser occipital nerves. The greater occipital nerve becomes superficial on each side at the inferior border of the obliquus capitis inferior muscle and runs superiorly toward the vertex over this muscle. The nerve is located medial to the occipital artery. The lesser occipital nerve is located approximately 2.5 to 3.5 cm lateral and 1 to 2 cm caudal to the greater occipital nerve (see Fig. 30-16).

Approach

It is not usually necessary to shave or clip the scalp before performing greater and lesser occipital nerve blocks. The greater occipital nerve can best be blocked at the nuchal line, which extends from the middle of the external occipital protuberance to the mastoid process. The nuchal line is located between the insertion sites of the trapezius muscle and the semispinalis muscles. At this site the greater occipital nerve is just medial to the occipital artery.

First, palpate the occipital artery. Next, attach a 3.8-cm, 23- to 25-gauge needle to a syringe containing 5 mL of local anesthetic. Insert the needle into the skin (Fig. 30-18*A*). After obtaining paresthesia at the vertex, inject 5 mL of local

Figure 30-18 Occipital nerve blocks. **A,** Block the greater occipital nerve on a line 3 cm lateral to the external occipital protuberance and the base of the occipital bone. **B,** Block the lesser occipital nerve by injection of 2 to 3 mL of anesthetic solution along the posterior border of the mastoid process of the temporal bone.

anesthetic solution. Block the lesser occipital nerve with a fanlike injection of a local anesthetic solution, 2.5 to 3.5 cm lateral and 1 cm caudal to the point described for the greater occipital nerve (Fig. 30-18*B*).

This procedure is not usually associated with any complications; however, intraarterial injections should be avoided by careful aspiration.

Ophthalmic (V₁) Nerve Block

The lateral and medial branches of the supraorbital, supratrochlear, and infratrochlear nerves may be blocked by percutaneous local injection at the point where they emerge from the superior aspect of the orbit. Anesthesia of the forehead and scalp is achieved as far posteriorly as the lambdoid suture. Although anesthesia for suturing lacerations of the forehead and scalp is easily achieved, the nerve block may also be used for débridement or topical treatment of burns or abrasions and for delicate lacerations of the upper eyelid (Fig. 30-19). Such anesthesia is ideal for removing small pieces of glass embedded in the forehead from a windshield injury.

Anatomy

The subtle supraorbital notch, which is in line with the pupil (when the patient is staring straight ahead), can be palpated

Figure 30-19 An ophthalmic (V₁) nerve block would be ideal for this patient with extensive forehead and eyelid lacerations. Additionally, an infraorbital (V₂) block could be used to provide anesthesia for repair of the maxillary laceration.

along the superior orbital rim (Fig. 30-20*B*). This landmark is the site of injection for blockade of the supraorbital nerves. The supratrochlear nerve is found 0.5 to 1.0 cm medial to the notch. The infratrochlear nerve is not usually blocked but is found in the most medial aspect of the superior orbital rim. If the anesthetic is placed on the forehead proper, this block may not produce complete anesthesia of the skin of the upper eyelid if the sensory branches to the eyelid are given off before the supraorbital nerve traverses the forehead.

Approach
With the patient in the supine position, raise a skin wheal. Paresthesias in the form of an electric shock sensation over the forehead will ensure a successful nerve block. Inject 1 to 3 mL of anesthetic in the area of the supraorbital notch (Fig. 30-20*C*). Hold a finger or a roll of gauze firmly under the orbital rim to avoid ballooning of anesthetic into the upper eyelid.

If paresthesias cannot be elicited or if the nerve block is unsuccessful, place a line of anesthetic solution along the orbital rim laterally to medially to ensure a block of all of the branches of the ophthalmic nerve.

Complications
Hematoma formation or swelling of the eyelid may occur but requires only local pressure. Occasionally, ecchymosis of the periorbital region will appear the next day, and the patient should be warned of this possibility.

Although this block is used infrequently, it is easily performed and not associated with serious side effects. Its use should be considered when anesthesia of the forehead or the anterior aspect of the scalp is desired.

CONCLUSION

Nerve blocks about the head and neck are relatively painless when done carefully and slowly after topical mucosal

Supraorbital

The supraorbital notch is in line with the pupil when the patient looks straight ahead

Supraorbital nerve

Supraorbital notch

Subtrochlear nerve

Figure 30-20 Supraorbital nerve block. **A,** Distribution. **B,** Anatomy and approach. **C,** Technique. A finger may be placed just below the margin of the superior orbital rim to avoid swelling of the eyelid.

anesthesia (for intraoral approaches) or local skin anesthesia (for extraoral blocks and approaches). Patients who appear anxious may benefit from sedation before attempting these blocks (see Chapter 33). These blocks should not be attempted on an uncooperative patient.

References are available at www.expertconsult.com

CHAPTER 31

Nerve Blocks of the Thorax and Extremities

Mark Spektor and John J. Kelly

Virtually every peripheral nerve can be blocked at some point along its course from the spine to the periphery, but digital nerve blocks (e.g., fingers and toes) are more commonly used than proximal blocks. Other common applications include femoral blocks for fractures of the femur, ankle blocks for foot injuries and infections, intercostal blocks for rib fractures, and wrist blocks for injuries to the palm.

The preparation, technique, choice of anesthetic, precautions, and complications are similar for all nerve blocks and are described in general in the following sections. The clinician is encouraged to use the same basic techniques and precautions for all nerve blocks. Specific precautions unique to a particular nerve block are included with the description of that block. Obvious precautions, such as aspiration before injection when the needle is in close proximity to a vascular structure, are not restated to avoid redundancy.

GENERAL CONCEPTS

Indications

For most lacerations and injuries seen in the emergency department (ED), local infiltrative anesthesia is adequate and more efficient than using a nerve block (see Chapter 29). Patients who require extensive repair and anesthesia of the entire extremity are often referred to a specialist, who may prefer to examine an unanesthetized limb. A nerve block is indicated when it will provide advantages over other techniques. Scenarios in which this requirement is met include the following:

- When distortion from local infiltration hampers closure (e.g., facial wounds) or compromises blood flow (e.g., fingertip)
- When anesthesia is required over a large area and multiple injections would be painful or when the large amount of anesthetic needed for local infiltration exceeds the recommended dose
- When a nerve block is the most efficacious form of treatment, such as an intercostal block for treating a rib fracture or a patient with chronic obstructive pulmonary disease
- When local infiltration of the wound would be more painful than a regional nerve block, such as in the plantar surface of the foot or the palm of the hand
- When the block is performed to decrease pain during finger or toe dislocation or reduction
- When extensive limb surgery or manipulation is required (e.g., extensive tendon repair) and other options are not available

Preparation

A brief history, including drug allergies (particularly to local anesthetics), medications, and systemic illnesses, should be taken from the patient. Peripheral vascular, heart, and liver disease may increase the risk for severe complications. Therefore, information about the existence of these diseases should also be sought.

Instructions

Explain the procedure to the patient—including the pain of needle insertion, paresthesias, and possible complications that may occur. Also discuss the potential need for additional anesthetic or alternative procedures if the nerve block fails. Be sure that the patient understands that the additional administration of an anesthetic is part of the normal procedure rather than an attempt to correct an improperly performed nerve block. It is not standard to obtain written informed consent for the nerve blocks performed in the ED.

Equipment

For most nerve blocks performed in the ED, the following equipment is required: latex gloves, an antiseptic solution (e.g., Betadine), a 10-mL syringe, an 18-gauge needle for drawing the anesthetic from the vial, and a 3.75-cm, 25- or 27-gauge needle for the nerve block. Note that the needle sizes given in text are general recommendations, but for the majority of blocks, a 25-gauge needle is ideal. In addition, keep standard resuscitation equipment for advanced cardiac life support readily available any time that local anesthetic agents are given.

Choice of Anesthetic

Factors influencing the choice of anesthetic agent for nerve blocks are similar to those for local infiltration (see Chapter 29 for extensive discussion). In general, most nerve blocks are done for the repair of painful traumatic injuries that are likely to cause pain long after the repair is completed. In such cases, select the anesthetic with the longest duration of action to maximize the patient's analgesia. For most of the blocks described in this chapter, 0.25% bupivacaine is suggested as the anesthetic of choice, but equal volumes of 1% lidocaine with epinephrine can be substituted. The use of epinephrine on end-organ areas has traditionally been discouraged (e.g., tip of the nose, peripheral ear pinna, distal end of the penis), although the theoretical risk is unsubstantiated in clinical practice. Recent literature describes the use and confirms the safety of lidocaine with epinephrine (1:100,000 concentration) for digital blocks.[1] It would be prudent to avoid epinephrine-containing anesthetics in injuries involving vascular compromise or for those with obvious peripheral artery disease. Higher concentrations of lidocaine (≤2%) or bupivacaine (0.5%) are commonly used for large nerves. Ropivacaine is a relatively new amide anesthetic with a rapid onset and a long duration of action (several hours). It has been reported to have fewer cardiotoxic and central nervous system effects than bupivacaine does.[2,3] Take care to avoid exceeding the recommended dosages of the anesthetic chosen. Buffering the anesthetic is strongly encouraged to lessen the pain of infiltration (see Chapter 29).

Positioning the Patient

When possible, perform nerve blocks with the patient in the supine position to minimize the vasovagal syncope that may occur when the patient is in an upright position. When drawing up the anesthetic from the vial, hide this anxiety- and fear-inducing portion of the procedure from the patient.

Preparation of the Area to Be Blocked

To limit the incidence of infection, prepare the field in aseptic fashion before needle puncture. Allow the antiseptic solution to dry fully to achieve its maximal antibacterial effect. Sterile drapes and gloves are not routinely required but may be considered in addition to aseptic skin preparation for the initiation of blocks that (1) are close to large joints, vessels, and nerves; (2) are located in inherently contaminated areas of the body (e.g., groin, perineum); or (3) require simultaneous palpation of the underlying structures while injecting.

Choosing the Nerves to Block

Successful anesthesia requires appropriate knowledge of the relevant anatomy. Most areas to be anesthetized have overlapping sensory innervation and therefore require two or more nerves to be blocked. In addition, the cutaneous distribution of the various peripheral nerves differs slightly from patient to patient. Use a liberal margin of error when determining which nerves supply the desired area of anesthesia.

Locating the Nerve

When locating a nerve to be blocked, approach it from a site with easily identifiable anatomic landmarks. The best sites are those with good structural landmarks (e.g., prominent bones or tendons) immediately next to the nerve. For example, the four digital nerves are reliably found at the 2-, 4-, 8-, and 10-o'clock positions around and just superficial to the proximal phalanx, whereas the median nerve lies between the palpable palmaris longus and flexor carpi radialis tendons at the proximal wrist crease. Nerves that course adjacent to easily palpable arteries, such as in the axilla and groin, are also easy to locate and are good sites for performing nerve blocks. Nerves that do not have adjacent structural or vascular landmarks are much more difficult to block.

Blocking nerves with good structural or vascular landmarks is straightforward: palpate the landmarks and follow the course of the nerve in relation to these landmarks. After visualizing the anatomy in the mind's eye, insert the needle in close proximity to the nerve.

Blocking nerves with poor landmarks, such as the radial nerve at the elbow, requires skill, practice, and some degree of luck. To increase the likelihood of successfully blocking these nerves, consider using a nerve stimulator.

Nerve Stimulator

A nerve stimulator is commonly used by anesthesiologists but has never gained popularity among emergency clinicians. Nevertheless, it helps locate nerves that do not have adjacent structural or vascular landmarks, which greatly increases the chances of successfully blocking these nerves.

Ultrasound

Use of ultrasound to identify injection sites for peripheral nerve blocks has been gaining popularity. Ultrasound guidance has been used successfully to locate and block nerves in the neck (e.g., interscalene and phrenic nerve blocks), lower extremity (e.g., femoral and saphenous nerve blocks), upper extremity (e.g., radial, ulnar, and median nerve blocks at the

elbow), and the lumbar plexus.[4-7] Ultrasonographic guidance negates the effects of anatomic variability, provides real-time needle guidance, and allows the operator to visualize the "spread" of local anesthetic.

Paresthesia

A common technique to ensure that the tip of the needle is in close proximity to the nerve is to elicit a paresthesia. Touching and mechanically stimulating the nerve with movement of the needle tip produces a tingling sensation or jolt known as a *paresthesia*, and it is felt along the distribution of the nerve. In practice, the jolt of a true paresthesia is often difficult to distinguish from the "ouch" of a pain-sensitive structure. When blocking proximal nerves at the elbow or axilla, the paresthesia travels far enough away from the injection site that it can be reliably distinguished from locally induced pain. Paresthesias at the level of the hand and wrist are more difficult to distinguish from pain. In both cases, paresthesia is a subjective feeling that requires intelligent and cooperative patients to understand what they are expected to feel and to remain relaxed and attentive so that they can distinguish an "ouch" from a jolt. Before the procedure, a simple explanation of what the patient should or may feel will facilitate cooperation. While eliciting paresthesias is generally reliable in demonstrating that the needle is close to its target, some authors believe that it may theoretically increase the rate of complications as a result of mechanical trauma or intraneural injection.[8-10] Once the paresthesia is elicited, it is important to withdraw the needle 1 to 2 mm before injecting the anesthetic. *If a paresthesia persists, stop the injection and reposition the needle.*

Injecting the Anesthetic

Strive to ensure that the anesthetic agent is not inadvertently injected into a vessel or nerve bundle. In practice, a misplaced intravascular injection is usually of minimal consequence, but small amounts of epinephrine may cause systemic symptoms such as tachycardia or anxiety. Intraarterial injection, theoretically, is more dangerous than intravenous injection. Either way, aspirate the syringe to check for blood before injection. If no blood is aspirated, inject the anesthetic while observing the extremity for blanching, which suggests intravascular injection. If blanching occurs, reposition the needle before further injection.

Nerve bundle injection has the potential to cause nonspecific nerve injury. Severe pain or paresthesia during injection or resistance to depressing the plunger suggests the possibility of intraneural placement of the needle. If any of these problems occur, immediately stop injecting and reposition the needle.

The onset and duration of anesthesia are both greatly influenced by how close the injected anesthetic is to the nerve. Onset occurs within a few minutes if the anesthetic is in immediate proximity to the nerve. Onset takes longer or may not occur at all if the anesthetic must diffuse more than 2 to 3 mm, which underscores the importance of locating the nerve before the injection.

More anesthetic is required if it must diffuse a long distance to the nerve. A range of suggested volumes of anesthetic is given with each nerve block description. For blocks in which a definite paresthesia is elicited or a nerve stimulator or ultrasound is used, the minimal recommended amount of anesthetic suffices. For blocks of smaller nerves, paresthesias are often not easily elicited, and the anesthetic must be injected in the general vicinity of the nerve. For these blocks or when doubt exists about the proximity of the needle to the nerve, larger amounts of anesthetic are recommended. This point cannot be emphasized strongly enough. *The difference between a successful and an unsuccessful block may be merely an additional 2 mL of anesthetic.* When in doubt, err on the high side of the recommended dosage. For blocks of large nerve, many clinicians also opt for 2% lidocaine rather than the 1% solution.

With most blocks the onset of anesthesia occurs in 2 to 15 minutes, depending on the distance that the anesthetic must diffuse to the nerve and the type of anesthetic used. Wait 30 minutes before deciding that a block is unsuccessful.

Complications and Precautions

Complications may result from peripheral nerve blocks but are rare in clinical practice. Most cannot be prevented by even perfect technique. General precautions include measures to minimize nerve injury, intravascular injection, and systemic toxicity. No actual statistics exist on the complication rate from nerve blocks performed by emergency clinicians, but they are extremely rare in clinical practice. Theoretically, infrequently performed blocks, blocks that require high doses of anesthetic, and blocks close to major vascular structures are more likely to have complications.

Nerve Injury

Nerve injury is rare but can occur secondary to (1) chemical irritation from the anesthetic, (2) direct trauma from the needle, or (3) ischemia as a result of intraneural injection. Overall, the incidence of serious neuronal injury is rare and occurs in 1.9 per 10,000 blocks.[11] Given that placement of a nerve block is a blind procedure, nerve injuries do not necessarily represent an error in technique.

Chemical neuritis from the anesthetic is the most common nerve injury.[9,10] The patient may complain of pain and varying degrees of nerve dysfunction, including paresthesia or motor or sensory deficit. Most cases are transient and resolve completely. Supportive care and close follow-up are the mainstays of treatment. Emergency clinicians should not exceed the recommended doses and concentrations of anesthetic (Table 31-1). In general, lidocaine 1% or 2% or bupivacaine 0.25% or 0.5% is safe for nerve blocks performed in the ED.

Direct nerve damage can be minimized by proper needle style, positioning, and manipulation. Use a short, beveled needle and keep the bevel parallel to the longitudinal axis of the nerve. Sharp pain or paresthesia indicates that the needle is close to or in the nerve. Avoid excessive needle movement when the tip of the needle is in contact with the nerve. If a 25-gauge needle is used, physical damage to a nerve should be minimal, even when directly touched by the tip of the needle. A 27-gauge needle is theoretically attractive, but its small size may limit aspiration testing and it may bend or break when attempting to block deep nerves.

Intraneural injection may rarely cause nerve ischemia and injury. Elicitation of a paresthesia or severe pain suggests that the needle has made contact with the nerve. *When a paresthesia is elicited, withdraw the needle 1 to 2 mm before injecting the anesthetic. If the paresthesia occurs during injection, stop the injection and reposition the needle.* Most neurons are surrounded by a strong perineural sheath through which the nutrient arteries

TABLE 31-1 Recommended Volumes of Anesthetic for Various Nerve Blocks

NERVE	VOLUME (mL)
Axillary	40-50*
Elbow	
Ulnar	5-10*
Radial	5-15*
Median	5-15*
Wrist	
Ulnar	5-15*
Radial	5-15*
Median	3-5*
Hip	
Femoral	10-20*
Three-in-one	25-30*
Knee	
Tibial	5-15*
Peroneal	5-10*
Saphenous	5-10*
Ankle	
Posterior tibial	5-10*
Deep peroneal	3-5*
Saphenous, sural, and superficial peroneal	4-10*
Intercostal	5-15*
Hand	
Metacarpal and web space	2-4†
Finger	1-2†
Foot	
Metatarsal	10-15†
Web space	3-5†
Toe	2-5†

*Anesthetic: 1% lidocaine or 0.25% bupivacaine (both with epinephrine).
†Anesthetic: 1% lidocaine or 0.25% bupivacaine (both without epinephrine).

run lengthwise. Injection directly into a nerve sheath may increase pressure within the nerve and compress the nutrient artery. Impaired blood flow results in nerve ischemia and subsequent paralysis. Intraneural injection is often heralded by severe pain, which worsens with further injection and may radiate along the course of innervation. The operator may notice difficulty depressing the plunger of the syringe. If the tip of the needle is in proper position, slow injection of the anesthetic should be minimally painful, and the anesthetic should go in without resistance.

Intravascular Injection

Intravascular injection may rarely result in both systemic and limb toxicity. Inadvertent intravascular injection produces high blood levels of the anesthetic. Exercise care when administering large amounts of anesthetic in close proximity to large blood vessels.

Intraarterial injection of anesthetics with epinephrine may cause peripheral vasospasm and further compromise injured tissue. Intravascular anesthetic is not toxic to the limb itself, although it may produce transient blanching of the skin by displacing blood from the vascular tree. Epinephrine, however, can cause prolonged vasospasm and subsequent ischemia if it is injected into an artery. This is especially worrisome when anesthetizing areas with little collateral circulation, such as the toes, fingers, penis, and tip of the nose. Severe epinephrine-induced tissue blanching or vasospasm may be reversed with local or intravascular injection of phentolamine (see extensive discussion in Chapter 29).

Vasospasm associated with the epinephrine in anesthetic solutions is rare, but experience in related clinical situations can help guide therapy. Roberts and Krisanda used a total of 5 mg of phentolamine infused intraarterially to reverse arm ischemia following 3 mg of epinephrine inadvertently administered into the brachial artery during cardiac resuscitation.[12] Digital ischemia from inadvertent epinephrine autoinjection (Epi-Pen) has been treated both by proximal "digital block" with 2 mg of phentolamine and by local infiltration at the ischemic site with 1.5 mg of phentolamine.[13,14]

The route of phentolamine administration should be guided by the clinical situation. Phentolamine must reach the site of vasospasm. Local infiltration may be effective for ischemia in a single toe or finger, whereas arterial injection has the advantage of delivering the medication directly to the arteries exhibiting spasm. For larger areas of involvement or in instances in which local infiltration is ineffective, use intraarterial injection. A dose of 1.5 to 5 mg appears to be effective in most cases,[12-14] although a total of 10 mg may be used for local infiltration. Phentolamine, 5 mg, can be mixed with 5 to 10 mL of either normal saline or lidocaine. The small volume of the distal pulp space may limit the volume of the infiltration dose to 0.5 to 1.5 mL in the fingertip. Larger volumes and dosages can be used with proximal infiltrations. For intraarterial infusion of the radial artery at the wrist or the dorsalis pedis at the ankle, dosages of 1.5 to 5 mg of phentolamine are suitable. Slow infusion or graded dosages of 1 mg may provide enough phentolamine to reverse the ischemia without excessive systemic effects such as hypotension.

Hematoma
Hematoma formation may result from arterial puncture, particularly during blocks in which a major blood vessel is being used as a landmark to locate the nerve (e.g., axillary or femoral artery). Direct pressure for 5 to 10 minutes usually controls further bleeding. Use of small-gauge needles (e.g., 25- to 27-gauge) also helps minimize bleeding from a punctured artery. A minor coagulopathy is not a contraindication to a nerve block.

Infection
Infection is rare and can be minimized by following aseptic technique and using the lowest possible concentration of epinephrine. Injection should be made through noninfected skin that has been antiseptically prepared. Injection through a site of infection may spread the infection to adjacent tissues, fascial planes, and joints.

Systemic Toxicity
The incidence of systemic toxicity with local anesthetics has diminished significantly in the past 30 years. Interestingly, peripheral nerve blocks have been reported to have the highest incidence of systemic toxicity.[11] Allergic reactions account for only 1% of untoward reactions (see Chapter 29).[15]

Limb Injury
Injury to the anesthetized limb can result if the patient is permitted to use the limb, is advised to use heat or cold application, or performs wound care before the anesthesia has worn off. With major nerve blocks, do not release the patient from the ED until sensation and function have returned.

With minor blocks, the patient may be sent home but should be properly cautioned. Advise the patient to avoid ischemia-producing compression dressings (e.g., elastic bandages) because the anesthetized area may not sense impending problems.

SPECIFIC NERVE BLOCKS
Intercostal Nerve Block
Blocking the intercostal nerves produces anesthesia over an area of their cutaneous distribution (Fig. 31-1) and provides considerable pain relief for patients with rib contusions or fractures. Rib fractures are typically quite painful and cause the patient to try to splint respirations to avoid excessive movement of the injured site. The resulting hypoventilation, atelectasis, and poor expectoration from splinting respirations may cause hypoxia or lead to pneumonia. This is particularly true in patients with preexisting pulmonary disease and minimal respiratory reserve, in whom further impairment of function may cause significant respiratory compromise.

Theoretically, anesthetizing injured ribs eases pain and facilitates deep breathing and coughing. Unfortunately, no controlled studies have compared intercostal blocks and oral analgesics in patients with the types of rib fractures that are commonly managed on an outpatient basis. However, studies do suggest that intercostal blocks may be superior to analgesics in patients who have undergone thoracotomy.[16-18] In these studies, those receiving intercostal nerve blocks had better results on pulmonary function tests, greater oxygenation, and earlier ambulation and discharge than did those receiving opioid analgesics.

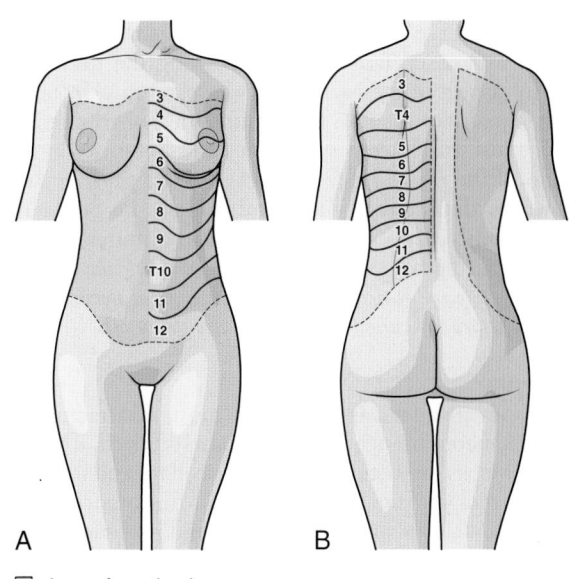

☐ Area of anethesia

Figure 31-1 A and **B,** Intercostal nerve block: area of anesthesia and cutaneous distribution of the intercostal nerves.

There are several arguments against the routine use of intercostal nerve blocks in the ED. First, rib fractures are often tolerated well by young patients, who usually require minimal oral analgesics. Second, these blocks have a relatively short duration of action. The typical duration of action of a long-acting anesthetic with epinephrine is 8 to 12 hours. However, it should be noted that patients often experience partial analgesia for up to 3 days, a period that cannot be attributed to direct action of the anesthetic on the nerve. Perhaps the anesthesia reduces muscle spasm and the associated cycle of pain.

Finally, a wrongly perceived high incidence of pneumothorax and unsuccessful blocks deters many clinicians from performing intercostal nerve blocks in the ED. The true incidence of pneumothorax after intercostal nerve blocks is very low and not significant enough to prohibit the procedure. Moore reported that in more than 10,000 individual rib blocks performed, the incidence of pneumothorax was less than 0.1%.[19] However, Shanti and associates reported that the incidence of pneumothorax was 1.4% for each individual intercostal nerve blocked.[20] If more than one nerve requires blockade, the incidence of pneumothorax may be greater. The suggested approach to discussing intercostal blocks is to give patients the facts with regard to the duration of analgesia and possible complications and then allow them to decide on the method for themselves. Frequently, they prefer oral analgesics initially but may return for further relief of pain, at which time they are more amenable to a nerve block.

Anatomy

Each thoracic nerve exits the spine through the intervertebral foramen, which lies midway between adjacent ribs (Fig. 31-2A). It immediately gives off the posterior cutaneous branch, which supplies the skin and muscles of the paraspinal area. The intercostal nerve then continues around the chest wall and gives off lateral cutaneous branches at the midaxillary line. These branches are the sensory supply to the anterior and posterior lateral chest wall.

The intercostal nerve runs with the vein and artery in the subcostal groove. The vein and artery lie *above the nerve* and are somewhat protected by the rib during a nerve block. Posteriorly, the nerve is separated from the pleura and lungs by the thin intercostal fascia. When blocking the nerve in the posterior aspect of the back, particular care must be taken to avoid puncture of the thin fascia and underlying lung. Fortunately, most rib fractures occur in the anterior or lateral portion of the rib and can be blocked *in the posterior axillary line*, where the internal intercostal muscles lie between the nerve and the lung's pleura and provide a buffer for minor errors in needle placement. *Note that blocking the nerve here will anesthetize the entire course of the intercostal nerve because it is blocked before the cutaneous branches are given off.*

Technique

To achieve adequate analgesia for most rib fractures, the lateral cutaneous branch needs to be anesthetized. Therefore, perform blocks between the posterior axillary and midaxillary line at a point proximal to the origin of this branch (see Fig. 31-2A, arrow). Explain the procedure and its benefits and its risks, including potential pneumothorax, systemic toxicity, and ineffective block, before proceeding.

Use a 10-mL syringe with a 3.75-cm, 25-gauge needle. Prepare the area to be injected in the usual aseptic manner.

Use the index finger of the nondominant hand to retract the skin at the lower edge of the rib cephalad and pull it up and over the rib (see Fig. 31-2B). With the syringe in the opposite hand, puncture the skin close to the tip of the finger that is retracting the skin over the rib. Keep the syringe at an 80-degree angle to the chest wall with the needle pointing cephalad, and rest the hand holding the syringe on the chest wall for stability. In this position, the depth of needle penetration is well controlled. Slowly advance the needle until it comes to rest on the lower border of the rib. *The bone should be felt through the tip of the needle.*

At this point, release the skin retracted over the rib. As the skin returns to its natural position, the shaft of the needle will become perpendicular to the chest wall and the tip of the needle will be at the inferior margin of the rib. Shift the syringe from the dominant hand to the index finger and thumb of the nondominant hand. Rest the middle finger of the same hand against the shaft of the needle and exert gentle pressure on the shaft to "walk" the needle off the lower edge of the rib. Again, keep the palm of the hand planted firmly on the chest wall to ensure control of the needle. With the help of the dominant hand, slowly advance the needle 3 mm. Aspirate to be sure that the needle has not penetrated a blood vessel, and then inject 2 to 4 mL of anesthetic while carefully moving the needle in and out 1 mm to ensure that the compartment containing the nerve between the internal and external intercostal muscles is penetrated. This may also serve to minimize intravascular injection. Repeat the procedure on the *two ribs above and below* to ensure that the overlapping innervation from adjacent nerves is blocked.

Although the procedure just discussed seems extensive, it takes 1 to 2 minutes to perform once the operator is familiar with the technique, and three to five intercostals can be blocked in 10 minutes' total time.

Precautions

Initially place the needle at the lower edge of the rib. If it contacts the rib above this point, it cannot be walked off the lower edge of the rib at the proper angle. If it is inserted too low, over the intercostal space, it may be advanced through the pleura and into the lung before the operator realizes that it is too deep. Before inserting the needle it is always prudent to estimate the depth of the bone. If the bone is not encountered by this depth of insertion, reevaluate the position of the needle. Even after the needle has been properly walked off the edge of the rib, take care to not puncture the pleura and lung. The depth of the intercostal groove in which the nerve runs is 0.6 cm posteriorly and diminishes to 0.4 cm anteriorly.

Because the incidence of pneumothorax is low, a chest radiograph is not routinely required after this procedure. Observe asymptomatic patients for 15 to 30 minutes and instruct them to return if problems arise. If the patient has symptoms of pneumothorax (e.g., cough, a change in nature of the pleuritic pain, or shortness of breath), obtain a chest film before discharge.

If the clinician inadvertently causes a pneumothorax, treatment depends on its size. Many pneumothoraces from this procedure are small and require no specific intervention. Those smaller than 20% may be observed for 6 hours.[21] During this time, administer a high concentration of oxygen to help decrease the size of the pneumothorax. If the pneumothorax does not enlarge, the patient may be released home

INTERCOSTAL NERVE BLOCK

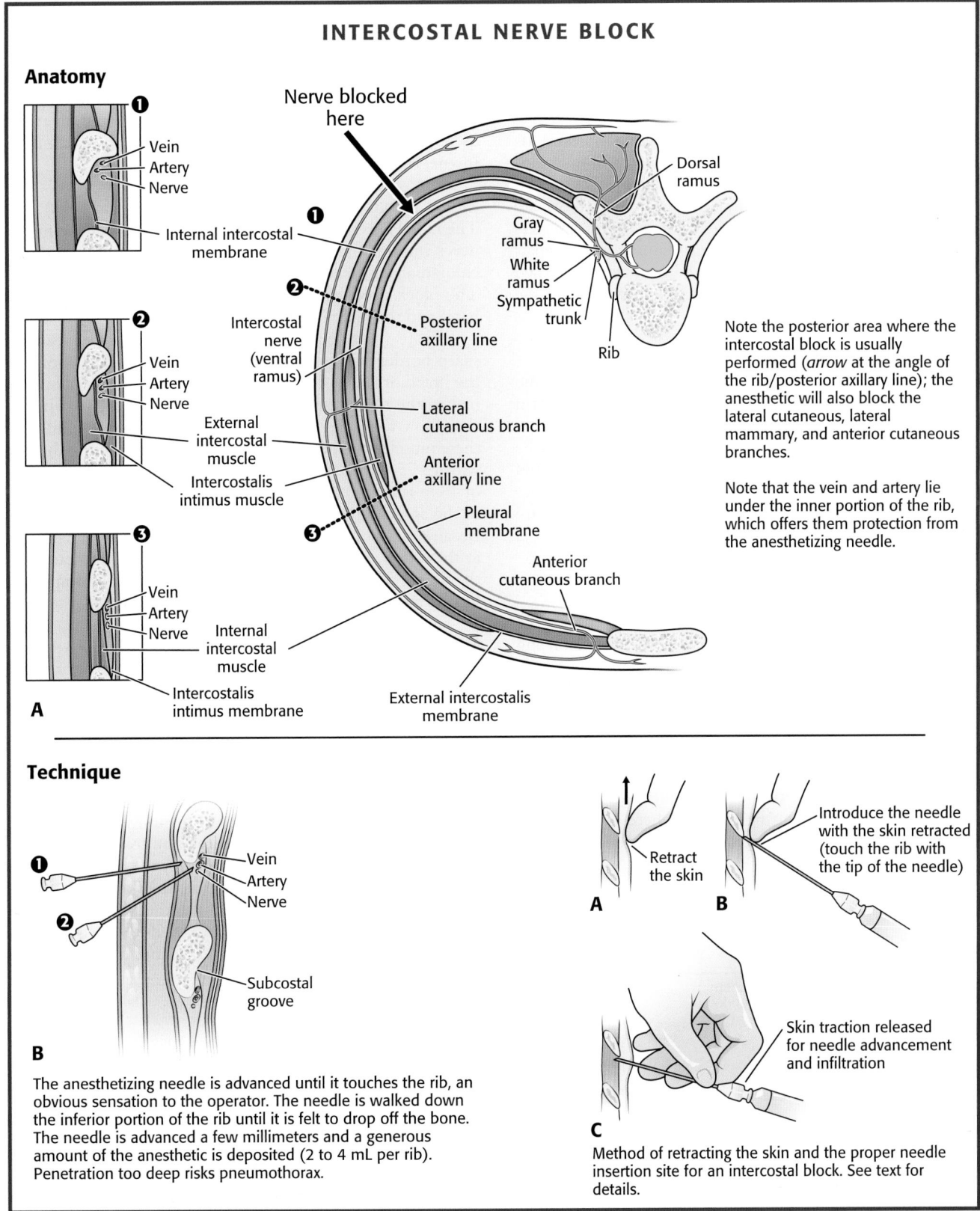

Anatomy

Nerve blocked here

① Vein / Artery / Nerve

Internal intercostal membrane

② Vein / Artery / Nerve

External intercostal muscle

Intercostalis intimus muscle

③ Vein / Artery / Nerve

Internal intercostal muscle

Intercostalis intimus membrane

Dorsal ramus

Gray ramus

White ramus

Sympathetic trunk

Rib

Intercostal nerve (ventral ramus)

Posterior axillary line

Lateral cutaneous branch

Anterior axillary line

Pleural membrane

Anterior cutaneous branch

External intercostalis membrane

Note the posterior area where the intercostal block is usually performed (*arrow* at the angle of the rib/posterior axillary line); the anesthetic will also block the lateral cutaneous, lateral mammary, and anterior cutaneous branches.

Note that the vein and artery lie under the inner portion of the rib, which offers them protection from the anesthetizing needle.

A

Technique

① Vein / Artery / Nerve

② Subcostal groove

B

The anesthetizing needle is advanced until it touches the rib, an obvious sensation to the operator. The needle is walked down the inferior portion of the rib until it is felt to drop off the bone. The needle is advanced a few millimeters and a generous amount of the anesthetic is deposited (2 to 4 mL per rib). Penetration too deep risks pneumothorax.

A Retract the skin

B Introduce the needle with the skin retracted (touch the rib with the tip of the needle)

C Skin traction released for needle advancement and infiltration

Method of retracting the skin and the proper needle insertion site for an intercostal block. See text for details.

Figure 31-2 Intercostal nerve block: anatomy and technique. (*Adapted from Chung J. Thoracic pain. In: Sinatra RS, Hord AH, Ginsberg G, et al, eds.* Acute Pain. *St. Louis: Mosby; 1991.*)

with arrangements for close follow-up. Needle or catheter aspiration of larger pneumothoraces may be all that is needed. A chest tube is necessary if this method fails (see Chapter 10).

Nerve Blocks of the Upper Extremity

The upper extremity is supplied by the brachial plexus. Its branches—primarily the median, radial, ulnar, and musculocutaneous nerves—can be blocked at the axilla, elbow, wrist, hand, or fingers. Nerve blocks at the axilla and elbow are seldom used in the ED. Nerve blocks of the wrist are performed occasionally before painful procedures or for repair of injuries to the hand. Metacarpal and digital blocks are used frequently to treat fractures, lacerations, and infections of the fingers.

Nerve Blocks at the Elbow

The median, ulnar, and radial nerves can be blocked at the elbow to provide anesthesia to the distal end of the forearm and hand (Fig. 31-3). For most injuries extensive enough to require a nerve block at the elbow, all three nerves must be blocked for successful anesthesia because of the variable and overlapping innervation of the forearm. Furthermore, injuries to the proximal and middle aspects of the forearm may require additional circumferential subcutaneous field blocks of the lateral, medial, and posterior cutaneous nerves.

Ulnar Nerve: Anatomy and Technique (Fig. 31-4*A*)

The ulnar nerve can be palpated in the ulnar groove on the posteromedial aspect of the elbow between the olecranon and the medial condyle of the humerus. This nerve supplies innervation to the small finger, the ulnar half of the ring finger, and the ulnar aspect of the hand.

With the elbow flexed, insert a 3.75-cm, 25-gauge needle 1 to 2 cm proximal to the ulnar groove and advance the needle parallel to the course of the nerve. The tip of the needle should come to rest close to the proximal end of the groove. Do not block the nerve in the groove, where it is prone to damage. For similar reasons, a paresthesia may be elicited but

is not vigorously sought. *If a paresthesia occurs during injection, slightly reposition the needle to avoid intraneural injection.* Although an elbow ulnar nerve block is common, many clinicians prefer to block the ulnar nerve at the wrist to limit the risk for injury. Once the tip of the needle is positioned properly, deposit 5 to 10 mL of anesthetic. If a nerve stimulator is used, flexion of the small and ring fingers signals proximity to the nerve.

Radial Nerve: Anatomy and Technique (Fig. 31-4*B*)

The radial nerve and sensory branch of the musculocutaneous nerve run together in the sulcus between the biceps and brachioradialis muscles on the anterolateral aspect of the elbow. The block produces anesthesia of the lateral dorsum of the hand and the lateral aspect of the forearm.

Palpate the sulcus in which the nerve runs between the sharp border of the biceps muscle and the medial border of the brachioradialis muscle in the antecubital fossa just proximal to the skin crease of the elbow. Having the patient flex the elbow to 90 degrees and isometrically contract and relax these muscles will help define their borders. Puncture the skin with a 3.75-cm, 25-gauge needle halfway between the muscles, or 1 cm lateral to the biceps tendon, at a point 1 cm proximal to the antecubital crease and inject 5 to 15 mL of anesthetic. Because of poor landmarks and the depth of the radial nerve at the elbow, a nerve stimulator greatly facilitates search for the nerve, which when stimulated, produces extension of the fingers and wrist.

Median Nerve: Anatomy and Technique (Fig. 31-4*C*)

The median nerve runs medial to the brachial artery in the anteromedial aspect of the elbow. Block of this nerve anesthetizes the index, middle, and radial portion of the ring finger and the palmar aspect of the thumb and lateral part of the palm.

Palpate the brachial artery in the flexed arm at the elbow just proximal to the antecubital crease and medial to the prominent biceps tendon. Once the anatomy is defined and marked in the flexed arm, extend the arm to 30 degrees and insert a 3.75-cm, 25-gauge needle slightly medial to the artery and perpendicular to the skin to the depth of the artery, about 2 to 3 cm, and inject 5 to 15 mL of anesthetic. Again, a nerve stimulator facilitates the process and produces flexion of the wrist and index finger. Most commonly, median nerve blocks are performed at the wrist.

Nerve Blocks at the Wrist

The median, ulnar, and radial nerves may be blocked at the wrist to provide anesthesia to the hand. Most extensive injuries and procedures for which a wrist nerve block could be used can also be managed by local infiltration or a digital block. When compared with direct infiltration, wrist block anesthesia may have a slow and unreliable onset and can require more time to take effect if all three nerves are to be blocked. There are several circumstances, however, in which wrist nerve blocks are more advantageous than other types of blocks or anesthesia.

Diffuse lesions that may be difficult to anesthetize with local infiltration can easily be anesthetized with a wrist block. Deep abrasions with embedded debris, commonly the result of "road burn" from bicycle and motorcycle crashes, can be cleaned and débrided painlessly after a nerve block at the wrist. Hydrofluoric acid burns, which require treatment with

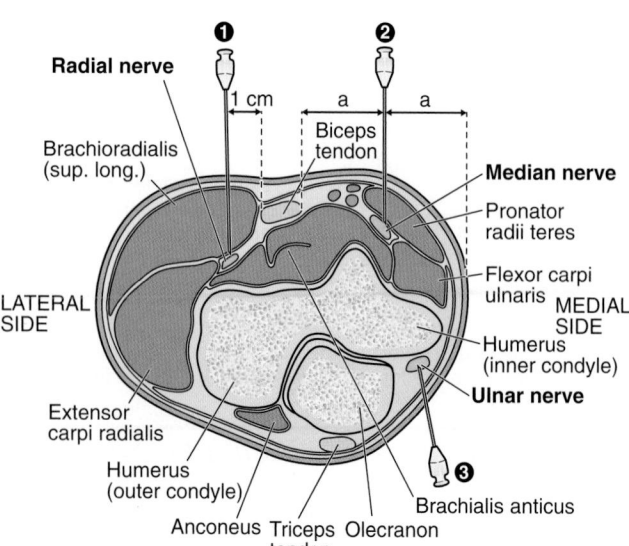

Figure 31-3 Cross section of the elbow looking cephalad, right arm. The radial nerve (*1*), median nerve (*2*), and ulnar nerve (*3*) are demonstrated.

NERVE BLOCKS AT THE ELBOW

Ulnar Nerve

Distribution

A

Anatomy and Technique

With the elbow flexed, insert the needle 1 to 2 cm proximal to ulnar groove, and advance toward groove parallel to the course of the nerve. Deposit 5 to 10 mL of anesthetic.

Radial Nerve

Distribution

B

Anatomy and Technique

Insert the needle on the volar surface of the elbow, 1 cm proximal to the antecubital crease, midway between the brachioradialis and biceps muscles. Deposit 5 to 15 mL of anesthetic.

Median Nerve

Distribution

C

Anatomy and Technique

Palpate the brachial artery in the flexed arm, proximal to the antecubital crease and medial to the biceps tendon. Then with arm flexed at 30 degrees, inject 5 to 15 mL of anesthetic slightly medial to the artery.

Figure 31-4 Nerve blocks at the elbow.

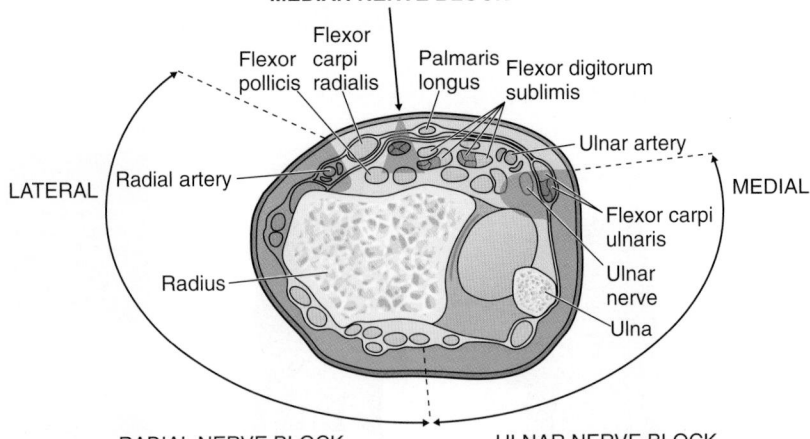

Figure 31-5 Cross section of the wrist looking cephalad, right wrist. The *arrow* points to the (covered) median nerve. The shaded triangle depicts the area infiltrated with anesthetic. Note the relatively superficial position of the median nerve, just radial to the palmaris longus.

numerous subcutaneous injections of calcium gluconate, and thermal burns that require extensive débridement are better tolerated after a wrist nerve block. Wrist blocks are also advantageous in a severely swollen and contused hand, in which small amounts of anesthetic injected locally may increase tissue pressure and produce further pain. Finally, deep lacerations of the palm are very painful to anesthetize with local infiltration and will also benefit from a wrist block.

When compared with nerves in the axilla and elbow, the nerves in the wrist are more easily located anatomically and can be blocked more reliably. All three nerves lie in the volar aspect of the wrist near easily palpated tendons. A nerve stimulator is not necessary but may be useful in locating the nerves, particularly when one is learning how to perform these blocks.

The anatomy and technique for blocking each nerve follow. Note that the median nerve lies in the midline and deep to the fascia and the ulnar and radial nerves lie on their respective sides and have branches that wrap around dorsally. Blocking all three nerves at the wrist requires a block that when viewed end-on, roughly resembles a horseshoe straddling a horseshoe stake (Fig. 31-5).

Median Nerve: Anatomy and Technique (Fig. 31-6A)
In the wrist, the median nerve lies just below the palmaris longus tendon or slightly radial to it between the palmaris longus and flexor carpi radialis tendons. Both tendons are easily palpated, but the palmaris longus may be absent in up to 20% of patients, in which case the nerve is found about 1 cm in the ulnar direction from the flexor carpi radialis tendon. The nerve lies deep to the fascia of the flexor retinaculum, but at a depth of 1 cm or less from the skin. The superficial position of the median nerve at the wrist is emphasized because *a major cause of failure of this block is to instill the anesthetic too deep.*

The palmaris longus tendon is located by having the patient make a fist with the wrist flexed against resistance (Fig. 31-7). Insert a 3.75-cm, 25-gauge needle perpendicular to the skin on the radial border of the palmaris longus tendon just proximal to the proximal wrist crease. Advance the needle slowly until a slight "pop" is felt as the needle penetrates the retinaculum and a paresthesia is produced. If no paresthesia ensues, it may be elicited in a more ulnar direction under the palmaris longus tendon. If a paresthesia is still not elicited, deposit 3 to 5 mL of anesthetic in the proximity of the nerve

at a depth of 1 cm under the tendon. Although the nerve is surprisingly close to the skin, it is better to err slightly on the deep side of the retinaculum and continue depositing anesthetic as the needle is withdrawn because the retinaculum is an effective barrier to a successful nerve block from superficially injected anesthetic.

Radial Nerve: Anatomy and Technique (Fig. 31-6B)
The radial nerve follows the radial artery into the wrist but *gives off sensory nerve branches proximal to the wrist*. These branches wrap around the wrist and fan out to supply the dorsal and radial aspect of the hand.

Nerve block here requires an injection in close proximity to the artery and a field block that extends around the dorsal aspect of the wrist. Insert a 3.75-cm, 25-gauge needle immediately lateral to the palpable artery at the level of the proximal palmar crease. At the depth of the artery, inject 2 to 5 mL of anesthetic. Distribute an additional 5 to 6 mL of anesthetic subcutaneously from the initial point of injection to the dorsal midline. Withdraw the needle and reposition it to complete the block. Withdrawing the needle and repositioning it to a site that has already been anesthetized help decrease the discomfort of numerous needlesticks.

Ulnar Nerve: Anatomy and Technique (Fig. 31-6C)
The ulnar nerve follows the ulnar artery into the wrist, where they both lie deep to the flexor carpi ulnaris tendon. The flexor carpi ulnaris tendon is easily palpated just proximal to the prominent pisiform bone by having the patient flex the wrist against resistance. At the level of the proximal palmar crease, the artery and nerve lie just off the radial border of the flexor carpi ulnaris tendon; however, the nerve lies between the tendon and the artery and deep to the artery, which makes it difficult to approach the nerve from the volar aspect of the wrist without involving the artery.

A nerve block of the ulnar nerve can be carried out by two different approaches: lateral and volar. The lateral approach may be easier because of the reason stated previously. For the lateral approach, insert a 3.75-cm, 25-gauge needle on the ulnar aspect of the wrist at the proximal palmar crease and deposit a wheal of anesthetic horizontally under the flexor carpi ulnaris tendon. Then direct the needle toward the ulnar bone at a point deep to the flexor carpi ulnaris tendon and inject 3 to 5 mL of anesthetic solution as the needle is withdrawn. Like the radial nerve, cutaneous nerves branch off the

NERVE BLOCKS AT THE WRIST

Median Nerve

Distribution

A

Anatomy and Technique

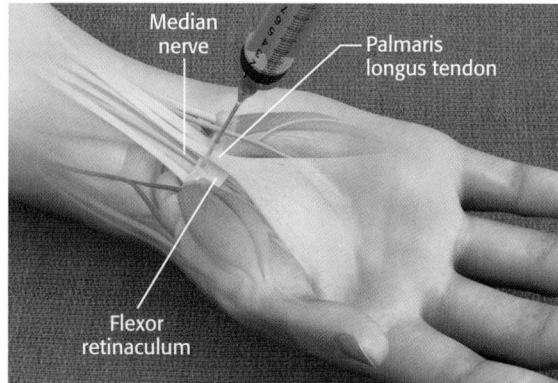

Locate the palmaris longus tendon (see Fig. 31-7). Insert the needle on the radial side of the tendon just proximal to the volar wrist crease. Feel for a "pop" as the needle penetrates the retinaculum, and inject 3 to 5 mL of anesthetic.

Radial Nerve

Distribution

B

Anatomy and Technique

First inject 2 to 5 mL of anesthetic immediately lateral to the radial artery at the level of the proximal palmar crease (not shown). Then inject another 5 to 6 mL from the initial injection point to the dorsal midline.

Ulnar Nerve

Distribution

C

Anatomy and Technique

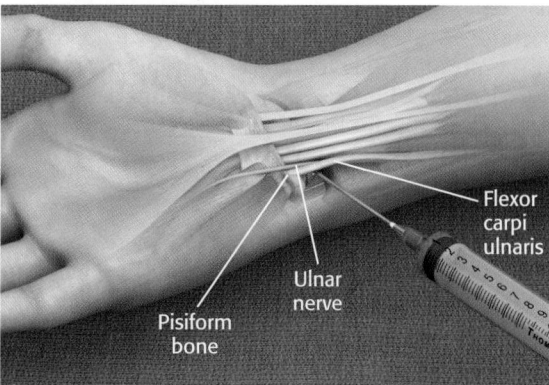

Insert the needle on the ulnar aspect of the wrist at the proximal palmar crease, under the flexor carpi ulnaris tendon. Inject 3 to 5 mL of anesthetic. Next, deposit 5 to 6 mL of anesthetic from the lateral border of the flexor carpi ulnaris to the dorsal midline (not shown).

Figure 31-6 Nerve blocks at the wrist.

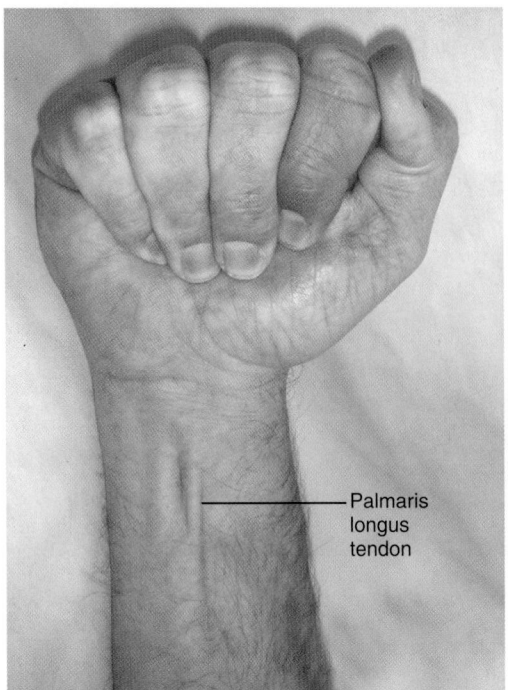

Figure 31-7 The palmaris longus tendon is found by having the patient make a tight fist and flex the wrist. This tendon may be absent in some patients.

Figure 31-8 Schematic cross section of the phalanx demonstrating the relationship of the nerves to the bone. Note that each finger has four digital nerves and that the digital artery and vein run parallel to and near the palmar branches.

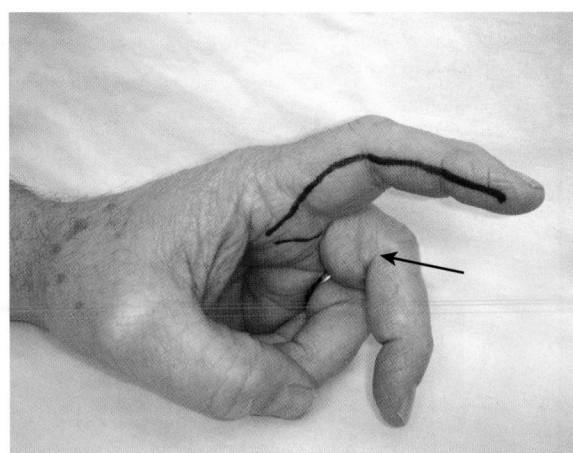

Figure 31-9 Each finger has four digital nerves: two palmar and two dorsal. The palmar nerves travel in a line connecting the top of the skin creases made by flexing the proximal interphalangeal and distal interphalangeal joints (*black line*). The nerves are more palmar than is often appreciated and are almost adjacent to the flexor tendon, so injecting the true lateral portion of the finger may miss the nerve. If the anesthesia needle is inserted at the tip of the skin creases (*arrow*). the nerve will be blocked.

ulnar nerve, wrap around the wrist, and supply the dorsum of the hand. Block these branches by subcutaneously injecting 5 to 6 mL of anesthetic from the lateral border of the flexor carpi ulnaris tendon to the dorsal midline. Another advantage of the lateral approach is that the dorsal branches can be blocked from the same injection site.

Nerve Blocks of the Digits

The digital nerve block is one of the most useful and most used blocks in the ED. Indications for choosing it include repair of finger lacerations and amputations, reduction of fractures and dislocations, drainage of infections, removal of fingernails, and relief of pain (e.g., from a fracture or burn). A digital block is superior to local infiltration in most circumstances. Wound infiltration may be a problem in a finger that has tight skin and can accept only a limited volume of anesthetic. Injection of anesthetic into this restricted space increases tissue pressure, thereby impairing capillary blood flow and causing pain. Fibrous septa in the fingertip also restrict the space available for the injected substance and even limit the spread of small amounts of anesthetic.

Anatomy

Each finger is supplied by two sets of nerves. These nerves, the dorsal and palmar digital nerves, run alongside the phalanx at the 2- and 10-o'clock positions and the 4- and 8-o'clock positions, respectively (Fig. 31-8).

The principal nerves supplying the finger are the palmar digital nerves, also called the common digital nerves. These nerves originate from the deep volar branches of the ulnar and median nerves, where they branch in the wrist. The palmar digital nerves follow the artery along the volar lateral aspect of the bone, one on each side, and supply sensation to the volar skin and interphalangeal joints of all five digits (Fig.

31-9). In the middle three fingers, these nerves also supply the dorsal distal aspect of the finger, including the fingertip and nail bed. Although many clinicians routinely block both sets of digital nerves, in the presence of normal anatomy, only the volar (palmar) branches must be blocked to obtain adequate anesthesia of the middle three fingers distal to the distal interphalangeal joint.

The dorsal digital nerves originate from the radial and ulnar nerves, which wrap around to the dorsum of the hand. They supply the nail beds of the thumb and small finger and the dorsal aspect of all five digits up to the distal interphalangeal joints. Unlike the middle three fingers, which require blocking of only the two volar (palmar) digital nerves, all four nerves are usually blocked in the thumb and fifth finger, particularly to obtain anesthesia of the fingertip and nail bed (Fig. 31-10).

■ Volar digital nerve
innervation

■ Dorsal digital nerve
innervation

Figure 31-10 For the index, middle, and ring fingers, the volar digital nerves provide sensation not only to the volar surface of the fingers but also to the dorsal surface distal to the distal interphalangeal joints. Thus, to obtain anesthesia of the distal portion of these three fingers, only the volar nerves need be blocked. Note that for the thumb and little finger, *both* the dorsal and volar nerves need to be blocked to obtain distal anesthesia.

Technique

The digital nerves can be blocked anywhere in their course, including sites in the finger, in the web space between the fingers, and between the metacarpals in the hand. There are a variety of approaches to the nerves, including the dorsal and palmar approaches and the web space approach. Each has its merits., and the technique is similar at each level.

The dorsal approach has the advantage of thinner, less pain-sensitive skin than encountered with volar approaches. The hand can be held firmly and flat on the table to prevent withdrawal. The disadvantage is that two injections are needed with this approach to block both volar digital nerves.

The dorsal approach can be used in the dorsum of the hand at the metacarpals, just proximal to the finger webs at the proximal end of the proximal phalanx or distal to the web space. Clinical situations may dictate which site to use; however, given equal circumstances, the preferred site is just proximal to the finger web. Here, the nerve's location is more consistent than in the hand, and there is more soft tissue space to accommodate the volume of injected anesthetic than there is in the distal end of the finger. Digital block at the web space is more efficacious in onset and requires less time to achieve anesthesia than does a metacarpal block done proximal to the metacarpophalangeal joint.[22]

A digital block requires aseptic injection technique, and usually only alcohol pad preparation is performed. Sterile gloves and drapes are not necessary, although examination gloves are recommended. The onset of anesthesia occurs in 1 to 15 minutes and it lasts for 20 minutes to 6 hours, depending on the anesthetic agent used.

The clinician must first decide whether two or four digital nerves require blocking (see earlier discussion). As noted previously, the authors recommend performing the block from the dorsal surface where the skin is thinner, easier to penetrate, and less sensitive than skin on the volar surface. Insert a 3.75-cm, 25- or 27-gauge needle at the web space, just distal to the knuckle at the lateral edge of the bone (Fig. 31-11*A*). Once the tip of the needle is subdermal, it usually contacts

the bone. At this point, create a skin wheal by injecting 0.5 to 1 mL of anesthetic without epinephrine. This serves to block the dorsal digital nerve and provide anesthesia at the injection site. Pass the needle lateral to the bone and toward the palmar surface until the palmar skin starts to tent slightly. Withdraw the needle 1 mm and inject 0.5 to 1.5 mL of anesthetic. This procedure is repeated on the opposite side of the finger. The result is a circumferential band of anesthetic at the base of the finger. Firm massage of the injected area for 15 to 30 seconds enhances diffusion of the anesthetic through the tissue to the nerves.

A variation of the dorsal approach is performed as follows. After injecting one side of the finger, pull the needle back slightly (without removing it) and redirect it *across the top of the digit* to anesthetize the skin on the opposite side (see Fig. 31-11*B*). Completely withdraw the needle and reinsert it *at the site that was just anesthetized*, and continue the block as described earlier. The presumed advantage of this method is that it minimizes the pain of the second skin puncture. However, because this technique requires the needle to be placed across the dorsal aspect of the finger, it increases the risk for extensor tendon puncture and trauma.

The palmar and web space approaches can be used most successfully for the middle three fingers when only a single puncture is required to block both volar nerves. This technique takes advantage of the anatomic fact that only the volar digital nerves must be blocked to obtain anesthesia of the total finger (except the proximal dorsal surface). If the thumb or fifth finger must be anesthetized, the dorsal branches must also be blocked to obtain anesthesia of the fingertip and fingernail area (see Fig. 31-10).

The palmar approach requires an injection in the palm, which is more painful than an injection in the dorsal skin. Insert the needle directly over the center of the metacarpal head and slowly inject the anesthetic as the needle is advanced to the bone (see Fig. 31-11*C*). At this point, withdraw the needle 3 to 4 mm and redirect it slightly to the left and right of center to block both digital nerves without withdrawing the needle. To be successful, a palpable soft tissue fullness should be appreciated. The technique requires 4 to 5 mL of anesthetic.

With the web space approach, hold the patient's hand with your thumb and index finger over the dorsal and volar surface of the metacarpal head, respectively. Use your third finger to separate the patient's fingers to expose the web space while your fourth and fifth fingers support the patient's finger being anesthetized (Fig. 31-11*D*). Insert the needle into the web space and inject 1 mL of anesthetic. Slowly advance the needle until it is next to the lateral volar surface of the metacarpal head and inject additional anesthetic. Withdraw the needle slightly and redirect it across the midline of the metacarpal head to the opposite digital nerve. Use the index finger to palpate "a fullness" as the anesthetic is injected. Again, firm massage of the injected area for 15 to 30 seconds enhances diffusion of the anesthetic through the tissue to the nerves. When needed, redirect the needle to the adjacent finger without withdrawing it to block both fingers with a single puncture (Fig. 31-12).

Alternative Techniques
Jet Injection Technique
Jet injection for a digital nerve block can be used effectively and is less painful than standard needle techniques.[23] The

technique described by Ellis and Owens uses 0.15 mL of 1% lidocaine delivered by a jet injector at 2600 psi.[23] Make three injections in the lateral aspect of the proximal phalanx: the first, midway between the volar and dorsal surfaces; the second, dorsal to this; and the third, volar. Administer a combined total of 0.45 mL to each side of the phalanx at the 2-, 3-, and 4-o'clock positions and the 8-, 9-, and 10-o'clock positions in relation to the bone.

Advantages of jet injection are a less painful injection and avoidance of "needle phobia," particularly in children. Potential disadvantages include lacerations, which may occur with tangential injection. Holding the injector perpendicular to the skin avoids this problem. Thick skin associated with older age, manual labor, and male gender may require larger volumes of anesthetic.

Transthecal Digital Block Technique

A transthecal block is performed by making a single injection into the flexor tendon sheath, which produces rapid and complete finger anesthesia. It was first described by Chiu in 1990, who noted rapid finger anesthesia after injection treatment of a trigger finger.[24] Cadaver studies suggest that the injected fluid diffuses out of the tendon sheath and around the phalanx and all four digital nerves.

DIGITAL NERVE BLOCKS

Dorsal Approach

1. Insert the needle at the web space, just distal to the knuckle at the edge of the bone. Once the needle tip is subdermal, inject 0.5 to 1 mL of anesthetic to block the dorsal digital nerve.

2. Advance the needle along the bone toward the palmar surface until the palmar skin begins to tent. Inject another 0.5 to 1 mL of anesthetic to block the volar digital nerve.

3. Repeat steps 1 and 2 on the opposite side of the finger. The result is a circumferential band of anesthetic around the base of the finger. Firmly massage the area for 30 seconds to enhance diffusion of the anesthetic.

A

Dorsal Approach—Alternative Method

1. Block both the dorsal and volar digital nerves on one side of the finger as described above. *Do not* fully remove the needle after blocking the volar nerve.

2. *Without removing the needle*, redirect it across the top of the finger to anesthetize the skin on the opposite side. After injecting the opposite side, remove the needle.

3. Insert the needle at the site that was anesthetized in step 2, and block the other side of the finger. The presumed benefit of this technique is that it minimizes pain at the second skin puncture site.

B

Figure 31-11 Digital nerve blocks.

DIGITAL NERVE BLOCKS, CONT'D

Palmar Approach

1. Insert the needle directly over the center of the metacarpal head and slowly inject anesthetic while advancing the needle to the bone.

C

2. Withdraw the needle 3 to 4 mm (without completely removing it) and slightly angle it to the right or left of center to block one of the volar digital nerves.

3. Repeat on the other side of the digit. To be successful, a palpable soft tissue fullness should be appreciated. Usually 4 to 5 mL of anesthetic is required.

Web-Space Approach

1. Hold the patient's hand with your thumb and index finger over the metacarpal, and spread the fingers to expose the web space.

D

2. Insert the needle into the web space and inject 1 mL of anesthetic. Slowly advance the needle until it is next to the volar surface of the metacarpal head and inject additional anesthetic.

3. Withdraw the needle slightly and redirect it across the midline of the metacarpal head to the opposite digital nerve. Inject additional anesthetic at this location. You will be able to feel the tissue distention by the anesthetic with your thumb, but be careful to avoid passing the needle through the skin and puncturing your thumb.

Figure 31-11, cont'd

Palpate the flexor tendon in the palm proximal to the metacarpophalangeal joint. Introduce a 25-gauge needle attached to a 3-mL syringe at a 45-degree angle and advance it toward the tendon sheath while maintaining constant slight pressure on the plunger of the syringe (Fig. 31-13). When the sheath has been entered, the anesthetic should flow freely. If it does not, it is presumed that the tendon has been entered. If this happens, withdraw the syringe slowly (while keeping slight pressure on the plunger) until anesthetic flows smoothly and easily. Inject a total of 2 mL of anesthetic solution (smaller volumes should be used in children). After the needle is removed, apply pressure over the tendon proximally to facilitate distal spread. The average onset of anesthesia is 3 minutes.[25]

The advantage of this technique is a single injection. However, Hill and colleagues found the technique to be "clinically equal" to traditional digital blocks.[26] Other authors have stated that the traditional digital block is easier to perform and produces less pain during and after injection.[27] Theoretically, the technique may increase risk for injury to the tendon.

Complications and Precautions

The injection should go in smoothly, without resistance during injection. Although the finger is forgiving of transient

Figure 31-12 Web space block techniques. **A,** For a metacarpal head block from the palmar surface, bending the needle 30 to 45 degrees allows easier access to the digital nerves without the syringe getting in the way. **B,** Adjacent fingers can be blocked with one needle puncture in the web space. After blocking the middle finger, withdraw the needle slightly, and without exiting the skin, redirect it to the metacarpal head of the index finger (*arrow*).

Figure 31-13 Transthecal block. The flexor tendon sheath is entered volarly just proximal to the metacarpophalangeal joint. With the use of a 25-gauge needle on a 3-mL syringe, the fluid should flow easily. Inject 2 to 3 mL of anesthetic and apply pressure to the proximal end of the tendon sheath.

pressure from excessive anesthetic, if the injection site becomes excessively tense, digital perfusion may be compromised. Even if epinephrine-containing solutions are used for a digital block in otherwise healthy individuals without peripheral vascular disease, it is unlikely that serious ischemic injury will occur.[28] Significant vasoconstriction generally lasts less than 60 minutes, within the time interval for which an ischemic tourniquet can safely be used in the same area.[29] However, if the entire digit remains blanched for more than 15 minutes, it is prudent to reverse the α-agonism of epinephrine with phentolamine (see Chapter 29). Using a pulse oximeter on the affected finger may help quantitate the degree of ischemia.[30]

The small size of the digital arteries and nerves makes intravascular or intraneural injection less likely. Inadvertent intravascular injection may cause digital ischemia from vasospasm or displacement of blood out of the capillary bed by the anesthetic. Blanching of the finger as the anesthetic is injected suggests intravascular injection. If this is observed, immediately discontinue the injection. Usually, the ischemia is transient and self-resolving, and serious complications are rare. Massage or topical application of nitroglycerin paste may be attempted if the ischemia persists.[31]

Commonly, the digital nerve is lacerated or damaged by the initial injury to the finger. Careful evaluation using two-point discrimination should be performed to determine the extent of nerve injury before blocking the nerve. Even if nerve injury is questionable, it should be documented in the chart, and the patient should be advised of the injury before the nerve block. Careful evaluation and patient education should prevent misconceptions about the cause of the nerve injury. Although most isolated digital nerve injuries are not debilitating, they heal slowly and can be annoying to the patient. Digital nerve injury proximal to the distal interphalangeal joint may be repaired surgically. Nerve repair may be undertaken immediately when specialty consultation is available or be delayed after initial simple closure.

Nerve Blocks of the Lower Extremity

In the lower extremities, nerve blocks can be performed in the groin (e.g., femoral nerve block), ankles, metatarsals, and toes. Femoral nerve block is the least often performed but is an effective method for providing analgesia to ED patients with femoral neck fractures. Ankle, metatarsal, and digital blocks are used frequently to treat ingrown toenails, foreign bodies, fractures, and lacerations of the forefoot and toes.

Femoral Nerve Block (Three-In-One Block)

A femoral nerve block provides significant analgesia to the proximal end of the femur and complete analgesia to the femoral shaft. It has been used to supplement anesthesia for a variety of surgical procedures on the anterior aspect of the thigh and knee and to provide postoperative analgesia after hip surgery.[32] In the ED, this block is primarily used to provide analgesia for patients with hip fractures. It can be especially helpful in the management of elderly patients and those with respiratory compromise or poor pulmonary reserve, in whom high doses of opiate analgesics may be problematic.

The three-in-one nerve block may be used to block the femoral, obturator, and lateral femoral cutaneous nerves with a single injection. The femoral nerve runs down the thigh in a fascial sheath that is continuous with the nerve sheath that contains all three nerves more proximally. If a large amount of local anesthetic is injected into this sheath, it will track proximally, medially, and laterally and thereby block all three nerves and provide more complete analgesia of the femoral neck and hip joint. The technique for performing both a femoral and three-in-one nerve block is identical except that the three-in-one block requires a larger volume of local anesthetic (25 to 30 mL versus 20 mL).

Because the femoral and three-in-one nerve blocks are technically similar and associated with the same potential complications, the fact that the three-in-one nerve block provides better analgesia of the femoral neck and hip joint would seem to make it the logical choice. In clinical practice, however, the lateral femoral cutaneous nerve is less likely to be blocked than the femoral nerve, and the obturator nerve is frequently left unblocked despite proper technique.[33] Nevertheless, because of potentially better analgesia obtained with the three-in-one nerve block and no clinically significant downside in comparison to a femoral nerve block, the remainder of the section will focus on performing the three-in-one nerve block.

Anatomy (Fig. 31-14*A*)

The femoral nerve is formed from the posterior branches of L2-L4 and is the largest branch of the lumbar plexus. The nerve emerges from the psoas muscle and descends between the psoas and iliacus muscles. It passes under the inguinal ligament in the groove formed by these muscles lateral to the femoral artery and divides into anterior and posterior branches. The anterior branches innervate the anterior aspect of the thigh, and the posterior branches innervate the quadriceps muscle and continue below the knee as the saphenous nerve to provide sensory innervation from the medial side of the calf to the medial malleolus.

The lateral femoral cutaneous nerve arises from the second and third lumbar nerve roots. The nerve emerges from the lateral border of the psoas muscle and travels under the iliac fascia, across the iliac muscle, and under the inguinal ligament 1 to 2 cm medial to the anterior superior iliac spine. It branches into anterior and posterior branches 7 to 10 cm below the anterior superior iliac spine. The anterior branch innervates the skin over the anterolateral aspect of the thigh to the knee, whereas the posterior branch of the nerve innervates the lateral part of the thigh from the greater trochanter to the middle of the thigh.

The obturator nerve arises from the anterior divisions of L2-L4. It descends through the fibers of the psoas muscle and emerges from its medial border near the brim of the pelvis. It then passes behind the common iliac arteries and runs along the lateral wall of the lesser pelvis, above and in front of the obturator vessels to the upper part of the obturator foramen. Here, it enters the thigh through the obturator canal and divides into an anterior and a posterior branch. The obturator nerve is responsible for sensory innervation of the skin of the medial aspect of the thigh and motor innervation of the abductor muscles of the lower extremity.

Technique (Fig. 31-14*B*)

Place the patient in a supine position and prepare the skin overlying the femoral triangle in the usual fashion. Palpate the femoral artery 1 to 2 cm distal to the inguinal ligament and inject a subcutaneous wheal of local anesthetic 1 to 2 cm lateral to this point. Keep the nondominant hand on the femoral artery throughout the remainder of the procedure.

Insert a 3.75-cm 25- to 22-gauge needle just lateral to the artery at a 45- to 60-degree angle to the skin. Slowly advance the needle cephalad until one of the following occurs: a "pop" with sudden loss of resistance (signifying penetration into the femoral nerve sheath) is felt, a paresthesia is elicited, or the needle pulsates laterally, which signifies a position adjacent to the femoral artery. Inject 25 to 30 mL of anesthetic. The block usually takes 15 minutes to take effect. If proximity to the nerve is uncertain (e.g., a pop is not appreciated, a paresthesia is not elicited, or the needle does not move with pulsation of the femoral artery), inject the anesthetic in a fanlike distribution lateral to the femoral artery in an attempt to anesthetize the nerve.

Some experts recommend applying finger pressure 2 to 4 cm below the injection site to help spread the local anesthetic proximally to the obturator and lateral femoral cutaneous nerves. However, an imaging study suggested that blockade occurs through lateral (lateral femoral cutaneous nerve) and medial (obturator nerve) spread of injected anesthetic.[34]

Nerve Blocks of the Ankle

Nerve block of the five nerves of the ankle—the deep peroneal (anterior tibial), posterior tibial, saphenous, superficial peroneal (musculocutaneous), and sural nerves—provides anesthesia to the foot. Of all the nerve block techniques described, these are the most technically difficult and most prone to failure. Depending on the desired area of anesthesia, one or more of the five nerves are blocked. These blocks can be used during operative procedures and repair of injuries to the foot. They are particularly useful in providing anesthesia to the sole of the foot for repair of lacerations and removal of foreign bodies.

A nerve block of the foot is better tolerated by the patient than local infiltration in all but the most minor procedures; it is the method of choice for treating injuries (e.g., lacerations, foreign bodies) of the sole. The skin of the sole is thicker and more tightly bound to the underlying fascia by connective tissue septa than is skin in other parts of the body. Puncturing this skin can be difficult and is always quite painful. The fibrous septa can limit the amount and spread of anesthetic. If large amounts of anesthetic are injected, the volume of injected substance quickly exceeds the space available, which can lead to painful distention of the tissue and circulatory compromise of the microvasculature. Local infiltrative anesthesia is adequate for treating minor injuries to the dorsum of the foot in which only small amounts of anesthetic are needed. However, for more extensive procedures such incision and drainage, extensive wound care, and foreign body removal, an ankle block is better tolerated.

Anatomy

The foot is supplied by the five nerve branches of the principal nerve trunks. Three nerves are located anteriorly and supply the dorsal aspect of the foot. Two nerves are located posteriorly and supply the volar aspect.

The anteriorly located nerves are the superficial peroneal, deep peroneal, and saphenous nerves (Fig. 31-15*A*). The superficial peroneal nerve (also called the dorsal cutaneous or musculocutaneous nerve) actually consists of multiple branches that supply a large portion of the dorsal aspect of the foot. These nerves are located superficially between the lateral malleolus and the extensor hallucis longus tendon,

FEMORAL NERVE/"THREE-IN-ONE" BLOCK

Anatomy

Psoas muscle

Lateral femoral cutaneous nerve

Femoral nerve

Obturator nerve

L2
L3
L4
L5

A

The lumbar plexus lies in the psoas compartment between the psoas major and quadratus lumborum muscles. The femoral nerve is formed from the posterior branches of L2-L4 and is the largest branch of the lumbar plexus. The lateral femoral cutaneous and obturator nerves arise from L2-L3 and L2-L4, respectively.

Technique

Inguinal ligament

Femoral artery

Femoral nerve

B

Palpate the femoral artery 2 cm distal to the inguinal ligament. Inject a wheal of lidocaine 1 to 2 cm lateral to this point. Advance the needle at a 45° to 60° angle to the skin until (1) a "pop" and sudden loss of resistance are felt, (2) parasthesia is elicited, or (3) the needle pulsates laterally. Inject 25 to 30 mL of anesthetic. If proximity to the nerve is uncertain, inject in a fanlike distribution lateral to the femoral artery.

Figure 31-14 The femoral nerve/"three-in-one" block.

Saphenous nerve

Superficial peroneal nerve

Deep peroneal nerve

Sural nerve

Posterior tibial nerve

A

B

Figure 31-15 Anatomy and distribution of the sensory nerves of the lower part of the leg and foot.

which is easily palpated by having the patient dorsiflex the big toe. The deep peroneal nerve (also called the anterior tibial nerve) supplies the web space between the big and second toes. In the ankle it lies under the extensor hallucis longus tendon. The saphenous nerve runs superficially with the saphenous vein between the medial malleolus and the tibialis anterior tendon, which is prominent when the patient dorsiflexes the foot. The saphenous nerve supplies the medial aspect of the foot near the arch.

The posteriorly located nerves are the posterior tibial and sural nerves (see Fig. 31-15B). The sural nerve runs subcutaneously between the lateral malleolus and the Achilles tendon

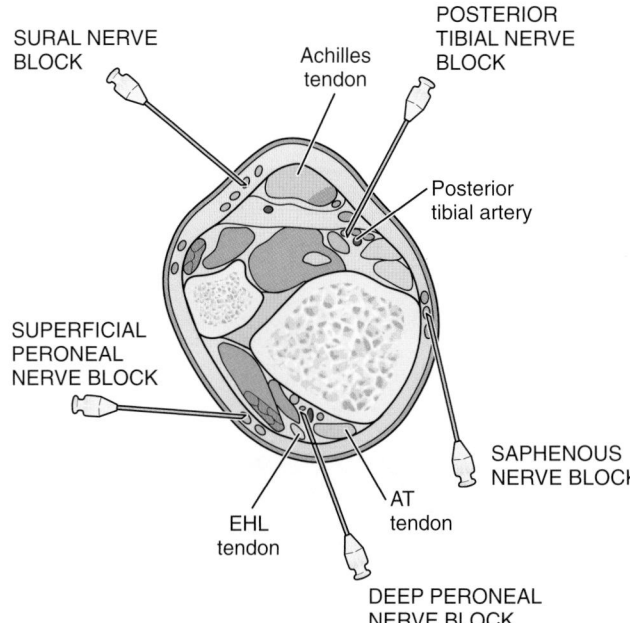

Figure 31-16 A complete nerve block of the foot requires blocking three superficial nerves (sural, saphenous, and superficial peroneal) and two deep nerves (posterior tibial and deep peroneal). *AT,* anterior tibial; *EHL,* extensor hallucis longus.

and supplies the lateral border, both volar and dorsal, of the foot. The posterior tibial nerve runs with the posterior tibial artery, which can be palpated between the medial malleolus and the Achilles tendon. It lies slightly deep and posterior to the artery.

The posterior tibial nerve is one of the major nerve branches to the foot. After passing through the ankle, it branches into the medial and lateral plantar nerves, which supply sensation to most of the volar aspect of the foot and toes and motor innervation to the intrinsic muscles of the foot.

Technique
A complete nerve block of the foot requires blocking three subcutaneous nerves and two deeper nerves (Fig. 31-16). Once familiar with the anatomy, an experienced clinician can anesthetize all five nerves quickly by placing subcutaneous band blocks around 75% of the ankle circumference and two deep injections: one next to the palpable posterior tibial artery and the other under the extensor tendon of the big toe.

The five nerves of the foot are commonly blocked in combinations of two or more. Small procedures clearly within the distribution of one nerve may require only a single nerve block. However, overlap of the nerves' sensory distribution frequently necessitates blocking a number of nerves for adequate anesthesia. Nerve block of the sural and posterior tibial nerves together anesthetizes the bottom of the foot and is the most useful combination.

Posterior Tibial Nerve (Fig. 31-17*A*)
Block the posterior tibial nerve in the medial aspect of the ankle between the medial malleolus and the Achilles tendon. Palpate the tibial artery just posterior to the medial malleolus. The injection site is 0.5 to 1.0 cm superior to

this point. If the artery is not palpable, use a point 1 cm above the medial malleolus and just anterior to the Achilles tendon.

Insert a 3.75 cm, 25-gauge needle at a 45-degree angle to the mediolateral plane (the needle is almost perpendicular to the skin), just posterior to the artery. At the estimated depth of the artery (approximately 0.5 to 1.0 cm deep), wiggle the needle slightly to produce a paresthesia. If a paresthesia is elicited, inject 3 to 5 mL of anesthetic. If no paresthesia is produced, advance the needle inward, again at a 45-degree angle, until it hits the posterior aspect of the tibia. Withdraw the needle about 1 mm and inject 5 to 7 mL of anesthetic while slowing withdrawing the needle another 1 cm. A rise in temperature of the foot, because of vasodilation from loss of sympathetic tone, may herald a successful block.

Sural Nerve (Fig. 31-17*B*)
Block the sural nerve on the lateral aspect of the ankle between the Achilles tendon and the lateral malleolus. Inject 3 to 5 mL of anesthetic subcutaneously in a band about 1 cm above the lateral malleolus between the Achilles tendon and the lateral malleolus.

Superficial Peroneal Nerves (Fig. 31-17*C*)
Block the superficial peroneal nerves on the anterior aspect of the ankle between the extensor hallucis longus tendon and the lateral malleolus by subcutaneously injecting 4 to 10 mL of anesthetic in a band between these landmarks.

Deep Peroneal Nerve (Fig. 31-17*D*)
Block the deep peroneal nerve anteriorly beneath the extensor hallucis longus tendon. The injection site is 1 cm above the base of the medial malleolus between the extensor hallucis longus and anterior tibial tendons. Palpate the tendons by having the patient dorsiflex the big toe and foot, respectively. Create a lidocaine wheel at the injection site. Direct the needle about 30 degrees laterally and under the extensor hallucis longus tendon until it strikes the tibia (at a depth of <1 cm). Withdraw the needle 1 mm and inject 3 to 5 mL of anesthetic.

Saphenous Nerve (Fig. 31-17*E*)
Block the saphenous nerve anteriorly between the medial malleolus and the anterior tibial tendon by injecting 3 to 5 mL of anesthetic subcutaneously between these landmarks.

Nerve Blocks of the Metatarsals and Toes
Like nerve blocks in the hand and fingers, nerve blocks in the foot and toes are commonly used in the ED. Indications for using these blocks include repair of lacerations, drainage of infections, removal of toenails, manipulation of fractures and dislocations, and otherwise painful procedures requiring anesthesia of the forefoot and toes.

Digital nerve blocks in the foot and toes are superior to local infiltration anesthesia for all but the most minor procedures. In the toes, the limited subcutaneous space does not accommodate enough injected material for adequate infiltrative anesthesia. Furthermore, the fibrous septa, which attach the volar skin to the underlying fascia and bone, limit the spread and volume of injected solutions. On the plantar surface, even small amounts of local infiltrate can cause painful distention and local ischemia of the tissues.

NERVE BLOCKS AT THE ANKLE

Posterior Tibial

Distribution

A

Anatomy and Technique

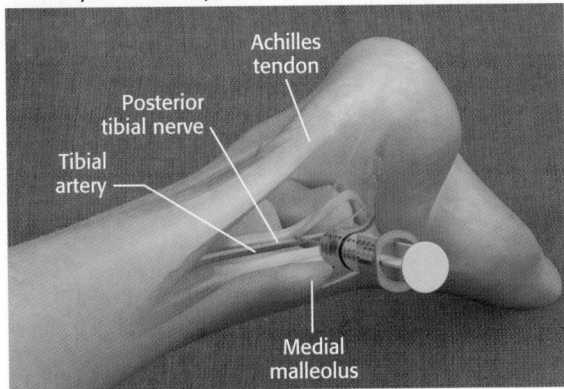

Palpate the tibial artery posterior to the medial malleolus. Insert the needle 1 cm superior to this point, perpendicular to the skin. At a depth of 1 cm, inject 3 to 5 mL of anesthetic. See text for additional details.

Sural Nerve

Distribution

B

Anatomy and Technique

Palpate the Achilles tendon and lateral malleolus. Inject 3 to 5 mL of anesthetic subcutaneously in a band between the Achilles tendon and lateral malleolus, about 1 cm superior to the malleolus.

Superficial Peroneal

Distribution

C

Anatomy and Technique

Palpate the extensor hallucis longus tendon and the lateral malleolus. Inject 4 to 10 mL of anesthetic subcutaneously in a band between the tendon and the malleolus.

Figure 31-17 Nerve blocks at the ankle.

NERVE BLOCKS AT THE ANKLE, CONT'D

Deep Peroneal

Distribution

D

Anatomy and Technique

Palpate the extensor hallucis longus and anterior tibial tendons while the patient dorsiflexes the foot and big toe. Insert the needle at a level 1 cm superior to the medial malleolus, and direct it laterally under the EHL tendon until it strikes the tibia. Inject 3 to 5 mL of anesthetic.

Saphenous

Distribution

E

Anatomy and Technique

First, inject 2 to 5 mL of anesthetic immediately lateral to the radial artery at the level of the proximal palmar crease (not shown). Then inject another 5 to 6 mL from the initial injection point to the dorsal midline.

Figure 31-17, cont'd

Anatomy

Each toe is supplied by two dorsal and two volar nerves, which are branches of the major nerves of the ankle. The dorsal digital nerves are the terminal branches of the deep and superficial peroneal nerves. The volar nerves are branches of the posterior tibial and sural nerves.

The location of the nerves in relation to the bones varies with the site of the foot. In the toes, the nerves lie at the 2-, 4-, 8-, and 10-o'clock positions in close relationship to the bone. In the proximal part of the foot, the nerves run with the tendons and are not in close relationship with the bones (Fig. 31-18).

Technique

The digital nerves can be blocked at the metatarsals, interdigital web spaces, or toes. The bones of the foot can be palpated easily from the dorsum and are used as the landmarks for estimating the location of the nerves. Proximally, the nerves' relationship to the bones is less consistent, which makes definitive needle placement and successful block less reliable. In the toes, the position of the nerves is more consistent; however, minimal subcutaneous tissue space is available for the injected solution. At the web space, the nerves are located in close relationship to the bone, and ample space is available for injecting the anesthetic; hence, for most procedures the web space is the preferred site for a digital nerve block.

The technique for toe and metatarsal blocks is similar (Fig. 31-19). All four nerves supplying each toe are usually blocked because of their sensory overlap. Perform the block from the dorsal surface, where the skin is thinner and less sensitive. Start by placing a 1-mL skin wheal dorsally between the metatarsal bones. Advance the needle until the volar skin tents slightly, and inject 2 mL of anesthetic as the needle

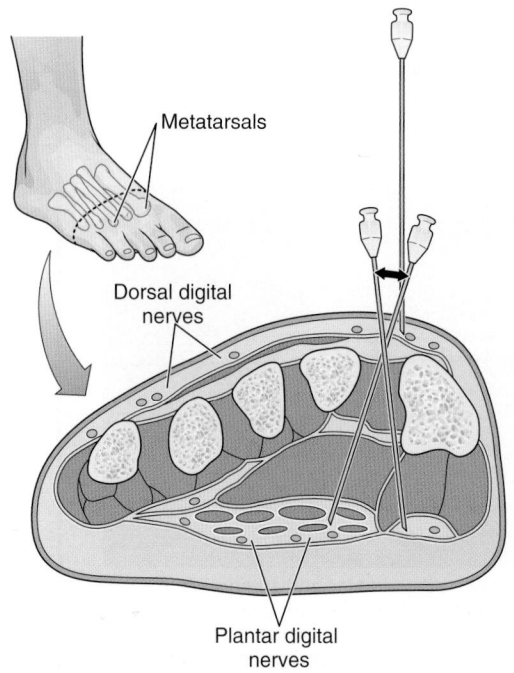

Figure 31-18 Anatomy and technique for a digital nerve block at the metatarsals.

is withdrawn. Without removing it, redirect the needle in a different volar direction, and repeat the procedure. Deposit a total of 5 mL of anesthetic in a fanlike pattern in each metatarsal space. Again, because of sensory overlap, two or more spaces need to be anesthetized for each toe to be blocked.

For a web space block, select a site on the dorsum just proximal to the base of the toe. Insert a 3.75-cm, 27-gauge needle attached to a 10-mL syringe at the lateral edge of the bone and place a subcutaneous wheal between the skin and the bone with 0.5 to 1.0 mL of anesthetic. This serves to block the dorsal nerve and minimize pain at the needle insertion site. Advance the needle just lateral to the bone toward the sole until the needle tents the volar skin slightly. Withdraw the needle 1 mm and inject 0.5 to 1.0 mL of anesthetic. As the needle is withdrawn, inject another 0.5 mL to ensure a successful block. Repeat the procedure on the opposite side of the toe. In this manner, two columns of anesthetic are placed on each side of the toe in the area through which the four digital nerves run. A total of 2 to 4 mL of anesthetic is used. For blocks done in the toe itself, the procedure is the same, but smaller amounts of anesthetic (e.g., <2 mL) are used because of the limited subcutaneous space and fear of vascular compression. Alternative techniques using a single injection site, as described for the finger, can be performed.

Text continued on p. 579

NERVE BLOCKS OF THE TOES

Web Space Block

1. Insert the needle on the dorsum just proximal to the base of the toe. Advance to the edge of the bone and inject 0.5 to 1 mL of anesthetic to block the dorsal nerve.
A

2. Advance the needle along the bone toward the sole until the needle slightly tents the volar skin. Withdraw the needle 1 mm and inject 0.5 to 1 mL of anesthetic.

3. Repeat on the other side of the toe. A total of 2 to 4 mL of anesthetic is typically used.

Alternative Technique

1. Block the dorsal and volar nerves on one side of the toe as described above. *Do not completely remove the needle after anesthetizing the volar nerve!*
B

2. Redirect the needle (without completely removing it) across the dorsal surface of the toe. Inject anesthetic on the dorsal surface of the opposite side of the toe, and then remove the needle.

3. Insert the needle through the newly anesthetized region, and block the dorsal and volar nerves on this side of the toe. This method minimizes pain felt at the second injection site.

Figure 31-19 Nerve blocks of the toes.

ULTRASOUND: Nerve Blocks of the Thorax and Extremities   *by Christine Butts, MD*

Regional nerve blocks are typically performed by identifying anatomic landmarks and blindly injecting anesthetic agents. Nerve stimulators may be used to identify larger nerves and ensure proper placement of anesthetics. However, these techniques are not infallible and improper placement of anesthetic may result. Additionally, some nerve blocks, such as the scalene block, may be avoided because of concern regarding adjacent anatomic structures. Use of ultrasound allows the clinician to identify the nerve in question, as well as to directly guide the application of anesthetic. Furthermore, nearby structures such as arteries or veins can be identified and avoided, thereby offering the operator greater confidence in performing more advanced blocks. Despite a limited number of randomized controlled trials, preliminary evidence seems to support the use of ultrasound, especially with regard to patient safety.[1]

Although each nerve block will require a slightly different approach, similar principles apply. A high-frequency transducer (10 to 12 MHz or higher) should be used to ensure the proper resolution to identify the structures in question (Fig. 31-US1). Equipment should be gathered as described earlier in this chapter. Sterile technique is not typically required for peripheral nerve blocks but should be used when accessing larger, more central structures such as the femoral nerve.

Peripheral nerves have a characteristic appearance when viewed by ultrasound and are usually easily identified, especially in the transverse orientation. They are hyperechoic (white) in appearance and are generally round or oval, although some may also appear more triangular (Fig. 31-US2). In larger nerves, the individual fascicles may be visible, especially when viewed with higher frequency. Nerve trunks (such as those used for scalene blocks) appear as rounded objects with a hypoechoic (darker gray) center (Fig. 31-US3). They may resemble blood vessels and thus care must be taken to ensure that they are distinguished. This can be done by applying color flow Doppler and noting the absence of blood flow.

Once the nerve has been visualized, the "in-plane" technique is often the most useful to guide the needle to the selected area. The transducer is placed in the transverse or slightly oblique plane relative to the nerve. The transducer should be adjusted so that the nerve is further away from the entry point of the needle (Fig. 31-US4). This will ensure that when the needle is inserted under ultrasound guidance, it can be "followed"

Figure 31-US1 High-frequency transducer.

Figure 31-US2 Ultrasound image of a peripheral nerve (*arrow*), in this case the median nerve. Peripheral nerves are characterized by a brightly echogenic (*white*) texture and appear slightly fibrillar.

Figure 31-US3 Ultrasound image of a nerve trunk (*arrow*), in this case a brachial plexus trunk. Nerve trunks appear similar to vascular structures, with a hypoechoic (*light gray*) area surrounded by a hyperechoic (*white*) wall. Applying color flow will aid in distinguishing the two.

Figure 31-US4 Ultrasound image demonstrating movement of the transducer to place the target nerve away from the anticipated entry point of the needle. The path of the needle is approximated by the *arrow*.

Continued

ULTRASOUND: Nerve Blocks of the Thorax and Extremities, cont'd

Figure 31-US5 Introducing the needle along the long axis of the transducer. Use of this technique will allow the sonographer to directly follow the course of the needle as it travels toward the nerve.

Figure 31-US6 Placement of the ultrasound transducer at the level of the thyroid cartilage.

as it advances toward the nerve in question. Once the image has been obtained, the needle is introduced from the end of transducer (Fig. 31-US5). Again, the entry point should be away from the nerve. Once the needle tip or needle is seen on screen, it should be advanced toward the nerve. Once the tip of the needle is seen adjacent to the nerve, anesthetic can be injected under direct ultrasound guidance. The best results are usually obtained by injecting anesthetic in a pattern that surrounds the nerve in a concentric manner. This can be achieved by injecting under ultrasound guidance and then repositioning the tip of the needle under ultrasound guidance until the nerve has been surrounded. The needle can also be inserted from the midpoint of the transducer, although this technique may cause more difficulty in following the tip of the needle.

Detailed descriptions of the anatomy and technique of the individual nerve blocks can be found throughout this chapter. However, it is important to touch on the nerve blocks typically performed under ultrasound guidance because the landmarks differ slightly.

Interscalene Block

The interscalene nerve blocks focuses on the trunks of the brachial plexus, specifically C5, C6, and C7. Blocking these trunks will provide anesthesia to most of the shoulder and upper extremity and spare the medial aspects of the arm and hand (these are innervated by the C8 and T1 nerve roots). This block is ideal for shoulder dislocations or complex lacerations of the upper extremity.

The trunks can be found grouped together in the neck and are typically easily identified with ultrasound. Because a number of critical structures are located near these trunks, using ultrasound to guide the injection will offer the physician increased confidence in the procedure, as well as increased success in the block. Several methods are described in the literature for localizing the nerve trunks. One of the most straightforward is to use the surrounding anatomy. Begin by placing the transducer, in the transverse orientation, lateral to the trachea at the level of the thyroid cartilage (Fig. 31-US6). Move the transducer laterally until the internal jugular vein and carotid artery are visualized (Fig. 31-US7). Once these vessels are seen, continue moving the transducer slightly laterally

Figure 31-US7 Ultrasound at the level of the thyroid cartilage. The internal jugular (IJ) vein is seen as the large vascular structure. Lying just beneath it is the carotid artery (CA).

until the muscle bellies of the anterior and middle scalenes are visible. The border between the muscles may be subtle; however, shifting the transducer to a slightly oblique plane may help better distinguish the anatomy. The trunks of the brachial plexus will be seen as rounded structures lying between the muscle bellies (Fig. 31-US8). They typically have an echogenic (white) border with a hypoechoic (dark gray) to anechoic (black) center. As noted above, the nerve trunks can resemble blood vessels, and thus care should be taken to evaluate the target structures before insertion of the needle.

Once the nerve trunks have been identified, needle insertion can proceed as described above. Typically, 10 to 20 mL of anesthetic is sufficient to achieve blockade, provided that it is injected directly adjacent to the nerve trunks (in the potential space between the trunks and the anterior and middle scalenes) (Fig. 31-US9). Injecting relatively small volumes of anesthetic into this potential space will prevent "overflow"

ULTRASOUND: Nerve Blocks of the Thorax and Extremities, cont'd

Figure 31-US8 A, Ultrasound at the level of the thyroid cartilage. The vascular structures are seen on the right of the image. **B,** The anterior and middle scalenes can be seen with the brachial plexus trunks lying between them (highlighted in the *second image*).

Figure 31-US9 Image of the brachial plexus trunks again highlighted in red. In this image the potential space in the sheath around the trunks is highlighted in *blue*. Placement of an anesthetic agent in this potential space ensures the intended effect on the nerve trunks with minimal spread to adjacent structures.

Figure 31-US10 Placement of the transducer over the middle of the forearm to localize the median nerve. The transducer can then be shifted slightly to the right or left to locate the ulnar and radial nerves.

Figure 31-US11 Ultrasound image of the median nerve. Although the median nerve does not travel with an associated artery, it is easily located in the middle of the forearm and is characterized by its triangular appearance. Its hyperechoic (*white*) structure is highlighted by the *arrow* in this image.

into the potential space anterior to the anterior scalene, where the phrenic nerve is found.

Forearm Nerve Blocks

Although blockade of the nerves that innervate the hand and wrist is typically performed at the wrist by using anatomic landmarks, it can also be performed under direct ultrasound guidance in the forearm. The median, radial, and ulnar nerves are easily identified with ultrasound, and direct visualized injection of anesthetic produces excellent results. Placing the transducer on the middle of the forearm in the transverse orientation will allow rapid identification (Fig. 31-US10). The median nerve is found in the center of the forearm, surrounded by the muscle belly. It is brightly echogenic (white) and usually has an oval or slightly triangular appearance (Fig. 31-US11). The radial nerve can be found toward the radial

ULTRASOUND: Nerve Blocks of the Thorax and Extremities, cont'd

Figure 31-US12 Ultrasound image of the radial nerve with its accompanying vascular structures. In contrast to the median nerve, the radial nerve is smaller but can easily be identified by first locating the radial artery (*arrowhead*). The nerve can be identified as the echogenic (*white*) slightly triangular structure (*arrow*) beside the artery.

Figure 31-US13 Ultrasound image of the ulnar nerve with its accompanying vascular structures. In contrast to the median nerve, the ulnar nerve is smaller but can be easily identified by first locating the ulnar artery (*arrowhead*). The nerve can be identified as the echogenic (*white*) slightly triangular structure (*arrow*) beside the artery.

aspect of the forearm, adjacent to the radial artery and vein (Fig. 31-US12). The ulnar nerve is similarly found on the ulnar aspect of the forearm, adjacent to the ulnar artery and vein (Fig. 31-US13). The radial and ulnar nerves may appear smaller but have a similar echogenic, slightly triangular shape. Once the nerves have been visualized, the block can proceed as described above.

Lower Extremity Blocks

The tibial and common peroneal nerves can be blocked in the popliteal fossa to provide anesthesia to the distal part of the calf, ankle, and foot.

Figure 31-US14 Placement of the ultrasound transducer in the transverse plane in the popliteal fossa to enable visualization of the tibial and peroneal nerves.

Figure 31-US15 Ultrasound image of the tibial nerve (*arrow*) viewed in transverse orientation. The popliteal vein can be seen just below the nerve and serves as a landmark for locating the nerve.

Both are easily identified in the popliteal fossa, where they exist as separate structures. The transducer should be placed transversely in the popliteal fossa, and the popliteal artery should be sought (Fig. 31-US14). It is easily identified as a pulsatile, rounded, anechoic structure. Once the artery has been identified, the tibial nerve can be found slightly superficial ("high and outside") to the artery (Fig. 31-US15). As with other peripheral nerves, the tibial nerve appears as an echogenic, rounded structure. Once the tibial nerve has been found, it should be followed slightly proximally until the common peroneal nerve is identified. It is similar in appearance to the tibial nerve but is seen more superficially (Fig. 31-US16). Once both nerves have been identified, anesthetic can be applied under direct ultrasound guidance as described above.

ULTRASOUND: Nerve Blocks of the Thorax and Extremities, cont'd

Figure 31-US16 Ultrasound image of the tibial and peroneal nerves. The peroneal nerve (*arrow*) is typically slightly more superficial than the tibial nerve (*arrowhead*).

REFERENCE:
1. Liu S, Ngeow JE, Yadeau JT. Ultrasound-guided regional anesthesia and analgesia: a qualitative systematic review. *Reg Anesth Pain Med.* 2009;34:47-59.

Complications and Precautions

Complications of lower extremity nerve blocks are similar to those associated with nerve blocks performed in the upper extremity and include intravascular injection, local anesthetic toxicity, nerve trauma, hematoma formation, and failure of the block.

The precautions that apply to the hand and fingers apply to the foot and toes. Ischemic complications can be avoided by paying attention to changes in the skin during the injection. Blanching heralds possible intravascular injection or vascular compression. If the skin blanches, halt the procedure and reevaluate the position of the needle and the amount and content of the injected solution. The total volume of anesthesia should not exceed the recommended amount. The literature suggests that epinephrine-containing anesthetics are safe for digital nerve blocks,[30] but some clinicians opt for epinephrine-free alternatives because of the theoretical risk for ischemic complications (see the "Complications and Precautions" subsection and Chapter 29).

As with upper extremity nerve blocks, note any neural or vascular injuries before the injection. The close proximity of these structures to the skin and bones means that they are frequently injured. Deficits, even if questionable, should be documented in the record and brought to the attention of the patient before performance of the nerve block.

References are available at www.expertconsult.com

CHAPTER 32

Intravenous Regional Anesthesia*

James R. Roberts and Sharon K. Carney

Clinical use of intravenous regional anesthesia (IVRA) has been well established as a safe,[1-3] quick, and effective alternative to general anesthesia in selected cases requiring surgical manipulation of the upper and lower extremities. Though historically relegated to the operating room, the procedure is readily applicable to outpatient use. Because of its reliability, safety, and ease of use, it is now commonly used in the emergency department (ED) and clinic. In the ED, the technique provides quick and complete anesthesia, muscle relaxation, and a bloodless operating field. The procedure is free from the troublesome side effects associated with other regional blocks, such as the axillary block. The procedure is easily mastered and has a very low failure rate; consistently good results can be expected. Although not a standard requirement of ED personnel, this technique can be safely used by trained ED clinicians, including physician's assistants and nurse practitioners, and does not have to be administered by an anesthesiologist.[3] The first practical use of analgesia associated with the intravenous (IV) injection of a local anesthetic agent

---

*This chapter is modified with permission from Roberts JR. Intravenous regional anesthesia. *JACEP*. 1977;6:261.

was described by August Gustav Bier in 1908.[4] Colbern has since proposed the eponym *Bier block*.[5] Although the procedure has been in existence for many years, the need for special equipment and a safe anesthetic agent limited its use. However, the Bier block has now gained wide acceptance as a safe and effective procedure, and several papers extol its virtues.[6-9] Even though complications do exist, no reported fatalities directly attributable to use of the Bier block *with lidocaine* have been reported. In this chapter the techniques and complications are discussed according to their application in the ED.

INDICATIONS AND CONTRAINDICATIONS

Indications for IVRA include any procedure on the arm or leg that requires operating anesthesia, muscle relaxation, or a bloodless field, such as reduction of fractures and dislocations, repair of major lacerations, removal of foreign bodies, débridement of burns, and drainage of infection (Fig. 32-1). IVRA is commonly used for extremity surgery, such as carpal tunnel surgery or tendon repair. The procedure may be carried out on any patient of any age who is able to cooperate with the clinician.

The only absolute contraindications are allergy to the anesthetic agent and, possibly, uncontrolled hypertension. Relative contraindications include severe Raynaud's disease, Buerger's disease, or a crushed or already hypoxic extremity in which further transient ischemia would be detrimental. Homozygous sickle cell disease is a theoretical contraindication, but few data exist on the treatment of patients with this condition. IVRA is best used for procedures requiring no more than 60 to 90 minutes of tourniquet time. Continuous cardiac or blood pressure monitoring is not standard and not required unless extenuating circumstances prognosticate potential cardiovascular problems. An uncooperative patient

Intravenous Regional Anesthesia

Indications

Procedures of the arm or leg that require operating anesthesia, muscle relaxation, or a bloodless field:

Reduction of fractures and dislocations
Repair of major lacerations
Removal of foreign bodies
Débridement of burns
Drainage of infection

Contraindications

Absolute
Allergy to anesthetic agent
Uncontrolled hypertension

Relative
Severe Raynaud's disease
Buerger's disease
Crushed or hypoxic extremity
Procedures taking >90 minutes

Complications

Lidocaine allergy (rare)
Lidocaine toxicity
Thrombophlebitis
Tissue extravasation of anesthetic agent

Equipment

22-gauge IV catheter or 21-gauge butterfly needle

60-mL syringe

1% lidocaine without epinephrine

Esmarch (elastic) bandage

Sterile saline diluent

Pneumatic tourniquet

Review Box 32-1 Intravenous regional anesthesia: indications, contraindications, complications, and equipment. A double cuff tourniquet is shown. Not shown is a device required to provide continuous cuff pressure (see Fig. 32-2). *Do not use a standard blood pressure cuff.*

Figure 32-1 Intravenous regional anesthesia can be used in the emergency department for any procedure on an extremity that requires anesthesia, muscle relaxation, or control of hemorrhage, such as closed reduction of a displaced distal radius fracture as depicted here.

may delay the procedure rather than contraindicate it. The judicious use of standard ED sedation may facilitate the use of IVRA in an anxious or transiently uncooperative patient.

EQUIPMENT

The equipment required for IVRA consists of the following:
- 1% lidocaine (Xylocaine),* *without epinephrine*, to be diluted to a 0.5% solution (note: 1% lidocaine = 10 mg/mL; hence 1 mL of 1% lidocaine = 10 mg)
- Clonidine, a parenteral opioid such as fentanyl, or ketorolac if used as additives
- Sterile saline solution as a diluent
- 50-mL syringe/18-gauge needle
- Pneumatic tourniquet (single or double cuff) such as the Zimmer A.T.S. 2000 Automatic Tourniquet System (Fig. 32-2) (Note: *Do not use a standard blood pressure cuff.*)
- IV catheters (20 or 22 gauge) or a 21-gauge butterfly needle
- Elastic bandage/Webril padding
- 500 mL of 5% dextrose in water (D₅W) and IV extension tubing (optional)

PROCEDURE

The procedure should be explained to the patient in advance. Premedication with midazolam (Versed), diazepam (Valium), or an opioid (e.g., morphine, fentanyl) may be helpful but need not be used routinely. The only painful portions of the procedure are establishment of the infusion catheter and exsanguination. The procedure should not be done on patients who are persistently uncooperative, intoxicated, or obtunded or who have had a previous reaction to a local anesthetic.

*Commercial preparations with preservatives are commonly used. Lidocaine 0.5% is also available.

Figure 32-2 A digital-controlled double-cuff system by Zimmer (A.T.S. 2000, Zimmer, Inc., Bloomfield, CN) allows safe intravenous regional anesthesia and the ability to lessen pain from the arterial tourniquet.

The patient need not be free of oral intake for a specific period before the procedure, but it is prudent to delay the procedure if the patient has just eaten a large meal. As a precaution, a suggested option is a large-bore catheter and an IV line with D₅W in the unaffected extremity. General resuscitation equipment, including suction, anticonvulsant drugs, bag-valve-mask apparatus, and oxygen, should be available. Continuous cardiac and blood pressure monitoring is not routine but may be used as an option depending on the clinician's assessment of the potential for cardiovascular events.

While the patient is being prepared, keep the lidocaine solution ready, but *withhold it until the injured extremity is exsanguinated and the cuff is in place and inflated*, as discussed later. The standard dose of lidocaine for the arm is 3 mg/kg. Inject it as a 0.5% solution (1% lidocaine mixed with equal parts sterile saline in a 50-mL syringe). Hence, for a 70-kg patient, infuse 210 mg of lidocaine (21 mL of 1% lidocaine) mixed with 21 mL of saline for a total volume in the infusing syringe of 42 mL of 0.5% lidocaine. Farrell and coworkers described a procedure termed the *minidose Bier block* in which 1.5 mg/kg of lidocaine is used and reported a 95% success rate.[10] This lower dose may decrease the incidence of central nervous system side effects and is more desirable in the ED setting. Additional lidocaine may be infused if the initial dose is inadequate. *Lidocaine with epinephrine should not be used.* Plain lidocaine is also available as a 0.5% solution and can therefore be used directly to avoid diluting the stronger solution. Some prefer preservative-free lidocaine, but most clinicians use standard lidocaine with preservatives.

A pneumatic tourniquet with cotton padding (to prevent ecchymosis) under the cuff is applied proximal to the pathology. *It is strongly advised that one not use a regular blood pressure cuff* because these cuffs often leak or rupture and are not designed to withstand high pressure for any length of time. A specially designed portable double-cuff pneumatic system, such as that marketed by Zimmer Corporation, is ideal and preferred by the author.

Premix the anesthetic and saline solution in the syringe. Inflate the tourniquet and place a plastic catheter or a metal butterfly needle in a superficial vein as close to the pathologic site as possible, and securely tape it in place (Fig. 32-3, *step 1*). It is usually desirable to use a vein on the dorsum of the hand, but importantly, the injection site should be at least 10 cm distal to the tourniquet to avoid injection of anesthetic proximal to or under the tourniquet. Keep the hub on the catheter to avoid backbleeding, or attach the syringe to the butterfly tubing. This catheter will be the route of injection of the anesthetic agent. Anesthesia from a fingertip-to-elbow direction seems to occur irrespective of the site of infusion of the anesthetic, but selecting an injection location near the site of pathology may provide more rapid anesthesia at a lower dosage.

Deflate the tourniquet used to obtain IV access, and exsanguinate the extremity so that when the anesthetic agent is injected, it will fill the drained vascular system. Exsanguination may be accomplished by either of two methods. Simple elevation of the extremity for a few minutes may be adequate, but wrapping the extremity in a distal-to-proximal direction with an elastic or Esmarch bandage, while being careful to not dislodge the infusion needle, significantly enhances exsanguination (see Fig. 32-3, *step 2*). Wrapping may be painful, so this step can be eliminated if it causes too much anxiety for the patient. If the wrapping procedure is not done, the extremity should be elevated for at least 3 minutes. During the wrapping procedure, care must be taken to not dislodge or infiltrate the infusion catheter.

With the extremity still elevated or wrapped, the tourniquet is inflated to 250 mm Hg (or 100 mm Hg above systolic pressure), the arm is placed by the patient's side, and the elastic exsanguination bandage is removed (see Fig. 32-3, *steps 3 to 5*). In a child the tourniquet is inflated to 50 mm Hg above systolic pressure. In elderly obese patients with calcified peripheral vessels, arterial occlusion may not be achieved safely.[11] In the leg, cuff pressure of 300 mm Hg or approximately twice the systolic pressure measured in the arms is suggested.

With the tourniquet now inflated, slowly inject the 0.5% lidocaine solution into the infusion catheter at the calculated dose (see Fig. 32-3, *step 6*). Note that the solution is placed *in the arm in which the circulation is blocked, not in the precautionary keep-open IV line on the unaffected side*. At this point, blotchy areas of erythema may appear on the skin. This is not an adverse reaction to the anesthetic agent but merely the result of residual blood being displaced from the vascular compartment, and it heralds success of the procedure.

In 3 to 5 minutes, the patient will experience paresthesia or warmth beginning in the fingertips and traveling proximally, with final anesthesia occurring above the elbow, to the level of the tourniquet. Complete anesthesia ensues in 10 to 20 minutes, followed by muscle relaxation. Note that adequate analgesia may exist even if the patient can still sense touch and position and has some motor function. If the "minidose" technique (initial dose of 1.5 mg/kg of lidocaine) does not provide adequate anesthesia, infuse an additional 0.5 to 1 mg/kg of diluted lidocaine at this time. As an example, for a 70-kg patient, an additional 0.5 mg/kg of lidocaine equals

35 mg lidocaine (3.5 mL of 1% lidocaine), and when the 1% lidocaine is diluted equally with saline, the final volume of the additional 0.5% lidocaine is 7 mL. Additional lidocaine was required in 7% of cases in one series in which the minidose regimen was used.[10] The clinician should be patient, however, and wait a full 15 minutes before infusing additional lidocaine. Alternatively, if analgesia is slow or inadequate, an extra 10 to 20 mL of *saline* solution may be injected to supplement the total volume of solution to enhance the effect. *Do not exceed a 3-mg/kg total dose of lidocaine*. For obese patients, a maximum of 300 mg of lidocaine is suggested for the arm and no more than 400 mg for the leg. Data for very obese patients do not exist. Next, withdraw the infusing needle and tightly tape the puncture site to prevent extravasation of the anesthetic agent. Perform the surgical procedure or manipulation, including postreduction x-ray films and casting or bandaging (see Fig. 32-3, *step 7*).

On completion of the procedure, deflation of the tourniquet may be *cycled* to prevent a bolus effect of any lidocaine that may remain in the intravascular compartment. Deflate the cuff for 5 seconds and reinflate it for 1 to 2 minutes. *Repeat this action two or three times*. This is probably required only if the cuff has been inflated for less than 30 minutes. A single deflation is often performed if the cuff has been inflated for longer than this time.

If the tourniquet has been in place for less than 30 minutes, an increase in transient lidocaine-related side effects may be seen if cycled deflation has not been used because adequate tissue fixation of the lidocaine has probably not occurred. This may result in a higher peak plasma lidocaine level, with increased side effects. If the surgical procedure is completed rapidly and the 3-mg/kg limit of lidocaine has been infused, the tourniquet should remain inflated until 20 to 30 minutes has elapsed, and only then should it be deflated via the cycling technique. It is reasonable to use a 20-minute cutoff if the minidose technique is used or a total of 200 mg or less of lidocaine has been administered because this dose is equal to a commonly administered antiarrhythmic IV bolus.

Sensation returns quickly when the tourniquet is removed, and in 5 to 10 minutes the extremity returns to its preanesthetic level of sensation and function. Many patients describe a transient intense tingling sensation after cuff deflation. If the procedure takes longer than 20 or 30 minutes, many patients complain of pain from the tourniquet because it is not inflated over an anesthetized area. Use of a double-cuff tourniquet may alleviate the problem of pain under the cuff. A wide tourniquet cuff (14 cm) is less painful than a narrow tourniquet (7 cm) when the cuff is inflated 10 mm Hg above loss the of arterial pulse.[12] The reason for pain under the tourniquet is unknown, but this can be a limiting factor because most patients begin to feel significant discomfort after 30 minutes if only a single cuff is used. Tourniquet pain can be significantly reduced and tourniquet time extended by adding ketorolac to the lidocaine anesthetic (see later).

In the *preferred* double-cuff system, two separate tourniquets are placed side by side on the extremity. One is termed the *proximal cuff* and the other the *distal cuff*. The proximal cuff is inflated at the beginning of the procedure, and anesthesia is obtained under the deflated distal cuff. When the patient begins to feel pain under the proximal cuff, the *distal cuff is first inflated over an already anesthetized area, and the pain-producing proximal cuff is then deflated*. One must be certain to inflate the distal cuff before the proximal cuff is released;

INTRAVENOUS REGIONAL ANESTHESIA

1

Place an IV catheter or butterfly needle as close to the pathologic site as possible. The site should be at least 10 cm distal to the tourniquet. A dorsal hand vein is ideal.

2

Exsanguinate the extremity by elevating and wrapping it in a distal-to-proximal fashion. Here, an Esmarch bandage is being used.

3

Apply the tourniquet to the patient's arm.

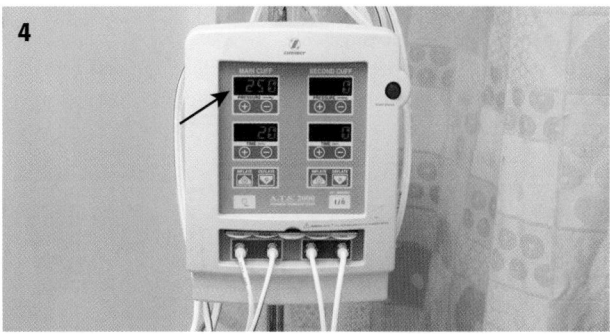

4

Inflate the tourniquet to 250 mm Hg or 100 mm Hg above systolic pressure. In the leg, inflate the cuff to 300 mm Hg or twice the systolic pressure measured in the arm.

5

Place the patient's arm by his side and remove the Esmarch bandage. The tourniquet remains inflated.

6

Slowly inject the 0.5% lidocaine solution into the infusion catheter at the calculated dose. See text for details and dosing information.

7

Remove the infusing needle/catheter, and tightly tape the puncture site to prevent extravasation of the anesthetic agent. Perform the procedure, including postreduction films and casting.

8

Once the procedure is complete, deflate the tourniquet in a cycling fashion (deflate for 5 seconds, reinflate for 1 to 2 minutes) 2 or 3 times. Then remove the tourniquet.

Figure 32-3 Intravenous regional anesthesia. A double cuff tourniquet is depicted in the figures. The procedure depicted demonstrates the use of a single tourniquet; refer to the text for details regarding the use of a double tourniquet.

Begin an intravenous (IV) line in the uninvolved extremity (optional).

Draw up and dilute 1% plain lidocaine (1.5- to 3-mg/kg total lidocaine dose) for a final concentration of 0.5% lidocaine.*

Place a padded tourniquet and inflate the upper cuff.

Insert a small plastic IV cannula near the pathologic lesion and secure it.

Deflate the tourniquet.

Elevate and exsanguinate the extremity.

Inflate the tourniquet (250 mm Hg), lower the extremity, and remove the exsanguination device. Inflate the proximal cuff only if a double-cuff system is used.

Infuse the anesthetic solution.

Remove the infusion needle and tape the site.

Perform the procedure.

If pain is produced by the tourniquet, *inflate the distal cuff first,* and then deflate the proximal cuff.

After the procedure has been carried out, deflate the cuff for 5 seconds and then reinflate it for 1 to 2 minutes. Repeat this step three times. Do not deflate the cuff if total tourniquet time is less than 20 to 30 minutes.

Observe 45 to 60 minutes for possible reactions.

From Roberts JR. Intravenous regional anesthesia. JACEP. 1977;6:263. Reproduced with permission.
Commercial preparations with or without preservatives are acceptable.

otherwise, the anesthetic will rapidly diffuse into the general circulation.

After 45 to 60 minutes of observation, the patient may be discharged (Box 32-1). Observation time depends on the use of other medications, procedural difficulties, and overall assessment of the patient. There are no standard or specific postprocedure instructions, but precautions similar to those given for conscious sedation are reasonable. Driving is best prohibited for 6 to 8 hours, and the patient should leave with a responsible adult. Delayed complications from lidocaine have not been reported.

MECHANISM OF ACTION

Some of the anesthesia is undoubtedly related to the ischemia produced by the tourniquet, but most of the anesthesia is secondary to the anesthetic agent itself. Although the exact mechanism by which anesthesia is produced is unknown, the site of action of the anesthetic may be at sensory nerve endings, neuromuscular junctions, or major nerve trunks.[13] Contrast-enhanced studies have demonstrated that the anesthetic agent does not diffuse throughout the entire arm, yet anesthesia of the entire limb is obtained. For example, when the anesthetic agent is injected into the elbow and kept in that region with both distal and proximal tourniquets, anesthesia of the entire arm develops.[14] Evidence indicates that the local anesthetic does not simply diffuse from the venous system into tissue but travels via vascular channels directly inside the nerve. Regardless of where the anesthetic is infused, the fingertips are the first area to experience anesthesia, thus suggesting that the core of the nerve is in contact with the anesthetic agent initially. After release of the tourniquet, a

considerable amount of the drug still remains in the injected limb for at least 1 hour.[15] This would suggest that at least a portion of the anesthetic leaves the vascular compartment and becomes fixed in tissue.

PROCEDURAL POINTS

Anesthetic Agent

Use of 0.5% plain lidocaine at a dose of 1.5 to 3 mg/kg is preferred for the upper extremity. A similar dose may be used in the leg if a *calf* tourniquet is used. For procedures in the leg, using a thigh cuff, 150 mL of 0.25% lidocaine (375 mg) has been used. The greater volume can augment drug distribution in the larger lower extremity. Other agents have been used without demonstrable advantage and are not recommended.[16] Bupivacaine (Marcaine, Sensorcaine) is *contraindicated* because of the potential for serious cardiovascular and neurologic complications.[17,18]

Some authors have suggested the use of IV ketorolac (60 mg) or clonidine (0.15 mg if the IV preparation is available) in addition to the lidocaine.[19,20] These additives are mixed with the lidocaine and injected into the operative arm. Both have been shown to be safe, and they decrease the need for postoperative analgesics and antiemetics. Tourniquet time is prolonged with these agents since pain under the tourniquet is the main reason for discontinuing the procedure. Opiates have not been found to be helpful when added to the lidocaine but may be given at a distant site (such as via the IV infusion in the opposite arm) for general pain control.

Dunbar and Mazze showed that patients with IVRA actually had significantly lower plasma lidocaine concentrations than did those with an axillary block or lumbar epidural anesthesia for similar procedures.[8] Peak plasma concentrations are reached 2 to 3 minutes after deflation of the tourniquet, and side effects are minimal if the deflation is cycled after the surgical procedure. The plasma half-life of lidocaine is approximately 60 seconds (see the excellent detailed discussion of pharmacokinetics by Covino[21]), but the drug demonstrates a theoretical three-compartment model similar to a direct IV infusion once the tourniquet is released.[22] Peak blood levels are related to the duration of vascular occlusion and to the concentration of the anesthetic.[21,22]

Peak plasma lidocaine levels after release of the tourniquet decrease as the time of vascular occlusion (tourniquet time) increases. If the tourniquet is inflated for at least 30 minutes and the deflation-reinflation technique is used when the procedure is finished, the plasma concentration of lidocaine should be approximately 2 to 4 μg/mL, below the 5- to 10-μg/mL level at which dose-related lidocaine reactions occur.[8] Tucker and Boas demonstrated a peak plasma lidocaine level of 10.3 μg/mL after a 10-minute period of vascular occlusion,[22] as opposed to 2.3 μg/mL if the tourniquet was inflated for 45 minutes.

More dilute solutions of lidocaine are associated with lower peak lidocaine levels. When equal doses of lidocaine are used, peak arterial plasma levels are 40% lower if the 0.5% solution is used than if the 1% solution is used.[22] For example, after 10 minutes of vascular occlusion, the peak plasma concentration of lidocaine has been demonstrated to reach 10.3 μg/mL with the 1% solution versus only 5.6 μg/mL when the drug was given under similar circumstances at a 0.5% concentration.[22]

Exsanguination

Many clinicians consider exsanguination of the extremity before injection of the anesthetic agent to be essential for success. Others do not believe that it is a critical factor. Exsanguination by simple elevation of the extremity should be done in all cases, but in certain instances one should consider avoiding the painful wrapping of the extremity with an elastic or Esmarch bandage. (Note that applying an Esmarch wrap over a fracture site is usually quite painful.) A pneumatic splint, such as the type used for prehospital immobilization, is also a reasonable alternative to painful wrapping. The process of exsanguination is believed to allow better vascular diffusion of the anesthetic.

Site of Injection

Anesthesia is usually achieved no matter where the local anesthetic is injected, but some evidence indicates that the procedure is more successful when the anesthetic is injected distally. Sorbie and Chacho noted the following failure rates associated with specific sites of anesthetic injection[23]: antecubital fossa, 23%; middle of the forearm or leg, 18%; and hand, wrist, or foot, 4%. In most cases a vein in the dorsum of the hand or foot is used. If local pathology precludes use of the hand, the midforearm or antecubital fossa of the elbow is an acceptable, albeit less desirable alternative as long as the infusion catheter is well below the tourniquet to avoid systemic injection.

Although most of the literature stresses use of this technique on the upper extremity, it may also be used successfully on the leg. It cannot, however, be used for procedures above the knee. Tourniquet pain appears to be a limiting factor when the procedure is used on the leg. One must be certain to avoid damage to the peroneal nerve by using the tourniquet in the midcalf area only.

COMPLICATIONS

Although IVRA is both safe and simple, one should not be lulled into complacency because complications do occur and are usually related to equipment failure or mistakes in technique.

Anesthetic Agent

Serious complications seldom occur if proper attention is paid to technique. True lidocaine allergy is very rare. Other reactions to lidocaine are rare and are usually systemic reactions from high blood levels.[8,18,24] High levels may result from miscalculation of dosages, from too rapid release of the tourniquet before the anesthetic has become fixed in tissue ("bolus effect"), or rarely, from advancement of the infusion catheter proximal to the tourniquet, thereby resulting in direct IV infusion.[25] To emphasize the safety of this procedure, note that the dose of lidocaine used in the minidose technique is similar to an IV bolus routinely given to patients with significant cardiovascular disease in the presence of ventricular dysrhythmias.

Generally, the central nervous system effects of lidocaine are minor and result in mild reactions such as dizziness, tinnitus, lethargy, headache, or blurred vision. This should not occur in more than 2% to 3% of patients and requires no treatment.[8] Transient hypotension and bradycardia may develop but are generally self-limited. Convulsions may occur but are extremely rare.

The most common complication related to the anesthetic agent is rapid systemic vascular infusion, which occurs when a blood pressure cuff explodes or slowly leaks, with consequent loss of anesthesia and high blood levels.[26] Similar complications may occur if the cuff is deflated earlier than 20 to 30 minutes after the induction of anesthesia. Both complications are the result of a bolus effect of the anesthetic, similar to an IV injection.

Van Neikerk and Tonkin reported three seizures in a series of 1400 patients.[24] Auroy and colleagues reported 23 seizures in 11,229 cases,[27] with no cardiac arrest or fatalities, and deemed IVRA safer than general anesthesia or peripheral nerve blocks. Seizures are generally not recurrent and are treated with oxygen and anticonvulsant drugs. Transient cardiovascular reactions, such as bradycardia and hypotension, are possible with large doses of lidocaine. Vasovagal reactions do occur. If resuscitation equipment is available and a precautionary IV line is started in the opposite arm, there should not be any serious sequelae.

One case of cardiac arrest 15 seconds after the use of 200 mg lidocaine has been reported, but the actual clinical scenario may have been a vasovagal reaction rather than a true cardiac arrest.[28]

Additional Complications

Thrombophlebitis can occur following the IV administration of anesthetics, and the formation of insignificant amounts of methemoglobin with the use of prilocaine hydrochloride (Citanest) has been reported.[29] Methemoglobinemia can also theoretically occur with lidocaine but has not been reported. Bupivacaine offers no benefit over lidocaine, has been associated with deaths, and should be avoided.[30]

A particularly bothersome problem is infiltration or dislodgement of the infusion catheter during exsanguination and tissue extravasation of the anesthetic agent. In addition, some leakage of anesthetic can occur after the infusion needle has been removed. Both problems may result in poor anesthesia but may be minimized if a small, well-secured plastic infusion needle is used instead of a metal scalp vein ("butterfly") needle and if the puncture site is tightly taped after withdrawal of the catheter.

This procedure cannot be used for manipulations or operations in which the pulse must be monitored as a guide to reduction (e.g., supracondylar fractures of the humerus) because the tourniquet occludes arterial flow. Use of the Bier block in patients with sickle cell disease is not well documented. It should be used with caution until the ischemic effect of the tourniquet on the red blood cells of such patients has been clarified. In all patients, tourniquet time should not exceed 90 minutes. Ischemia for less than this amount of time is not associated with serious sequelae.

An excellent summary of a very favorable experience with IVRA of both the arm and leg in 1900 outpatients is available.[31]

> References are available at www.expertconsult.com

CHAPTER 33

Systemic Analgesia and Sedation for Procedures

Baruch Krauss and Steven M. Green

Procedural sedation and analgesia (PSA) refers to the use of analgesic, dissociative, and sedative agents to relieve the pain and anxiety associated with diagnostic and therapeutic procedures performed in various settings. PSA is an integral element of emergency medicine residency and pediatric emergency medicine fellowship training and curricula, and graduates of these programs are skilled in the practice of PSA. Emergency clinicians are skilled in resuscitation, vascular access, and advanced airway management, which permits them to effectively recognize and manage the potential complications associated with PSA.[1]

In a recent study of all practitioners, the most common clinical errors associated with PSA were delayed recognition of respiratory depression and arrest, inadequate monitoring, and inadequate resuscitation,[2] mistakes that are unlikely to be made by emergency clinicians. The safety of PSA techniques by emergency clinicians has been well documented in numerous series in both children and adults.[3-7] Safe and successful application of PSA requires careful patient selection, customization of therapy to the specific needs of the patient, and careful monitoring of patients for adverse events. Emergency clinicians must ensure that all patients receive pain relief and sedation commensurate with their individual needs during any procedure.

TERMINOLOGY

The progression from minimal sedation to general anesthesia is a nonlinear continuum that does not lend itself to division into arbitrary stages. Low doses of opioids or benzodiazepines induce mild analgesia or sedation, respectively, with little danger of adverse events. If, however, clinicians continue administering additional medication beyond this initial level, progressively altered consciousness ensues with a proportionately increased risk for respiratory and airway complications. If further medications are administered, the patient will advance along this continuum until protective airway reflexes are lost and general anesthesia is ultimately reached. This continuum of sedation is not drug specific in that varying states from mild sedation to general anesthesia can be achieved with virtually all nondissociative PSA agents (e.g., opioids, benzodiazepines, barbiturates, etomidate, propofol).

In 1985, the American Academy of Pediatrics (AAP) and the National Institutes of Health issued guidelines for the management and monitoring of children receiving sedation for diagnostic and therapeutic procedures in response to the growing use of opioids and sedative-hypnotic agents in the outpatient setting and a number of sedation-related deaths.[8,9] In these documents, three levels of sedation were defined (conscious sedation, deep sedation, general anesthesia) to create a common language for describing drug-induced alterations in consciousness (Box 33-1).[10,11] A key development in the field of PSA has been revision of the original terminology and adoption of clearer descriptions of varying types and degrees of sedation (see Box 33-1). Though historically popular, the widely misinterpreted and misused term "conscious sedation" has fallen into disfavor[12]; it has been labeled as "confusing,"[13] "imprecise,"[12] and an "oxymoron"[12,13] and has been replaced with the term "moderate sedation."[10]

Despite improvements in PSA terminology, the system is imperfect and there is still no objective way to assess the depth of sedation. Levels of responsiveness remain at best crude surrogate markers of the respiratory drive and retention of protective airway reflexes. This is especially true for all levels of sedation in young children (infants and toddlers) who do not understand or are unreliable in following verbal commands. Although respiratory depression and respiratory arrest can be detected quickly with standard interactive and mechanical monitoring, there is no safe and practical way to assess the status of protective airway reflexes. Data are currently insufficient to determine whether deep sedation is associated with impairment of protective reflexes or whether such danger is encountered only when "pushing" deep sedation to the point at which it approaches or reaches general anesthesia.

PSA GUIDELINES

Before the promulgation of PSA guidelines by specialty societies and governmental agencies, clinicians simply administered sedatives in varied clinical settings and used individual judgment to determine the need for specific monitoring devices and supporting personnel. Since 1985, at least 27 sets of PSA guidelines have been published,[15] each crafted for the unique and differing settings in which PSA is practiced. Naturally, not all are in agreement.[5] The intent of each of these guidelines is to better standardize the manner in which PSA is performed to enhance patient safety. Those most pertinent to emergency clinicians are from the American College of Emergency Physicians,[3] the AAP,[16] and the American Society of Anesthesiologists (ASA).[14,17]

In the early 1990s, the Joint Commission on Accreditation of Healthcare Organizations, an independent, not-for-profit organization that evaluates and accredits hospitals in the United States, took a special interest in PSA, with the central theme being that the standard of sedation care provided should be comparable throughout a given hospital. Thus, patients sedated in the emergency department (ED) should not receive a significantly different level of attention or monitoring than those sedated for a similar-level procedure in the operating room or in the endoscopy suite. To ensure this, the Joint Commission requires specific PSA protocols to be applied consistently throughout each institution. These hospital-wide sedation policies will vary from site to site based on the specific needs and expertise available within each institution. In 2001, the Joint Commission released new standards for pain management, sedation, and anesthesia care.[10]

At each hospital accreditation survey the Joint Commission determines whether practitioners practice PSA consistently with their hospital-wide sedation policy and whether they provide sufficient documentation of such compliance. Clinicians must be familiar with their hospital's sedation policies and should work with their medical staff to ensure that

BOX 33-1 PSA: Terminology and Definitions

GENERAL

- **Analgesia**[10]: Relief of pain without intentional production of an altered mental state such as sedation. An altered mental state may be a secondary effect of medications administered for this purpose.
- **Anxiolysis**[10]: A state of decreased apprehension concerning a particular situation in which there is no change in a patient's level of awareness.
- **PSA**[3]: A technique of administering sedatives, analgesics, dissociative agents, or any combination of such agents to induce a state that allows the patient to tolerate unpleasant procedures while maintaining cardiorespiratory function. PSA is intended to result in a depressed level of consciousness but one that allows the patient to maintain airway control independently and continuously. Specifically, the drugs, doses, and techniques used are not likely to produce loss of protective airway reflexes.

CURRENT SEDATION STATE: TERMINOLOGY

- **Minimal sedation (anxiolysis)**[10]: A drug-induced state during which patients respond normally to verbal commands. Although cognitive function and coordination may be impaired, ventilatory and cardiovascular function is unaffected.
- **Moderate sedation (formerly conscious sedation)**[10]: A drug-induced depression of consciousness during which patients respond purposefully to verbal commands, either alone or accompanied by light tactile stimulation. Reflex withdrawal from a painful stimulus is not considered a purposeful response. No interventions are required to maintain a patent airway, and spontaneous ventilation is adequate. Cardiovascular function is usually maintained.
- **Dissociative sedation**[11]: A trancelike cataleptic state induced by the dissociative agent ketamine and characterized by profound analgesia and amnesia with retention of protective airway reflexes, spontaneous respirations, and cardiopulmonary stability.
- **Deep sedation**[10]: A drug-induced depression of consciousness during which patients cannot be easily aroused but respond purposefully after repeated or painful stimulation. The ability to independently maintain ventilatory function may be impaired. Patients may require assistance in maintaining a patent airway, and spontaneous ventilation may be inadequate. Cardiovascular function is usually maintained.
- **General anesthesia**[10]: A drug-induced loss of consciousness during which patients cannot be aroused, even by painful stimulation. The ability to independently maintain ventilatory function is often impaired. Patients frequently need assistance in maintaining a patent airway, and positive pressure ventilation may be required because of depressed spontaneous ventilation or drug-induced depression of neuromuscular function. Cardiovascular function may be impaired.

PSA, *procedural sedation and analgesia.*

---

such policies are suitably detailed, yet reasonable and realistic. Unduly restrictive policies do a disservice to patients by discouraging appropriate levels of analgesia and anxiolysis. Most hospitals pattern their sedation policies after the Joint Commission standards and definitions. It is important to note that the unique ketamine dissociative state does not fit into the existing Joint Commission definitions of sedation and anesthesia.[11] A ready solution is to assign a distinct definition for "dissociative sedation" (see Box 33-1).

The Joint Commission requires that PSA practitioners who are permitted to administer deep sedation be qualified to rescue patients from general anesthesia.[10] Emergency clinicians typically perform all levels of sedation except general anesthesia. Moderate sedation suffices for the majority of procedures in adults and cooperative children, although it will not be adequate for extremely painful procedures (e.g., hip reduction, cardioversion). Deep sedation can facilitate such procedures, but with greater risk for cardiorespiratory depression than is the case with moderate sedation. Moderate sedation is frequently insufficient for effective anxiolysis and immobilization in younger, frightened children, and deep or dissociative sedation is an appropriate alternative.

EVALUATION BEFORE PSA

The practice of PSA has three essential components performed in sequence: the initial presedation evaluation, sedation during the procedure, and postprocedure recovery and discharge from the ED. In all but the most emergency situations, perform a directed history and physical examination before PSA. If this evaluation suggests additional risk, reconsider the advisability of sedation. High-risk cases may be better managed in the more controlled environment of the operating room.

Presedation assessment is a Joint Commission requirement, and most hospitals have developed specific forms to facilitate consistent documentation of the involved items. In general, however, all the appropriate parameters are already documented in the general ED record or are obvious by simply evaluating the patient's complaint. Except in emergency situations, discuss the risks, benefits, and limitations of any PSA with the patient or parent or guardian in advance and obtain verbal agreement. Formal written informed consent is not required as a standard of care (unless a local institutional requirement), although documentation, as discussed earlier, is essential.

General

Assess the type and severity of any underlying medical problems. This is usually best documented by the standard ED medical record, history, physical examination, and nursing notes. Another tool used for this purpose is the ASA physical status classification for preoperative risk stratification (Table 33-1). Verify current medications and allergies. Inquire about previous adverse experiences with PSA or anesthesia.

Airway

Inspect the airway to determine whether any abnormalities (e.g., severe obesity, short neck, small mandible, large tongue,

TABLE 33-1   ASA Physical Status Classification

ASA CLASS	DESCRIPTION	EXAMPLES	SUITABILITY FOR SEDATION
1	Normal healthy patient	Unremarkable past medical history	Excellent
2	Patient with mild systemic disease—no functional limitation	Mild asthma, controlled seizure disorder, anemia, controlled diabetes mellitus	Generally good
3	Patient with severe systemic disease—definite functional limitation	Moderate to severe asthma, poorly controlled seizure disorder, pneumonia, poorly controlled diabetes mellitus, moderate obesity	Intermediate to poor; consider benefits relative to risks
4	Patient with severe systemic disease that is a constant threat to life	Severe bronchopulmonary dysplasia; sepsis; advanced degrees of pulmonary, cardiac, hepatic, renal, or endocrine insufficiency	Poor; benefits rarely outweigh risks
5	Moribund patient not expected to survive without the operation	Septic shock, severe trauma	Extremely poor

From Krauss B, Green SM. Sedation and analgesia for procedures in children. *N Engl J Med.* 2000;342:938.
ASA, American Society of Anesthesiologists.

trismus) are present that might impair airway management. Consider assessments such as Mallampati scoring or the distance between the chin and hyoid bone (see Chapter 4, Fig. 4-3).

Cardiovascular

Perform cardiac auscultation to assess for disturbances in rhythm or other abnormalities. In patients with known cardiovascular disease, evaluate their degree of reserve because most PSA agents can cause vasodilatation and hypotension.

Respiratory

Perform lung auscultation to assess for active pulmonary disease, especially obstructive lung disease and upper respiratory infections that may predispose the patient to airway reactivity.

Gastrointestinal

Assess the time and nature of the last oral intake because pulmonary aspiration of gastric contents is a dreaded complication of vomiting when protective airway reflexes are impaired. Figure 33-1 shows a four-step assessment tool to stratify the risk for aspiration before sedation and to identify prudent limits of targeted sedation,[18] although this tool has not yet been validated.

More conservative guidelines from the ASA for elective surgery or procedures in healthy patients specify an age-stratified fasting requirement of 2 to 3 hours for clear liquids and 4 to 8 hours for solids and nonclear liquids.[19] Nonetheless, they acknowledge that regarding PSA, "the *literature provides insufficient data to test the hypothesis that preprocedure fasting results in a decreased incidence of adverse outcomes.*"[14,17] The concept of preprocedure fasting is logistically difficult or impossible for emergency clinicians, who have no control over patients' oral intake before arrival at the ED. In actual practice, emergency clinicians routinely perform PSA safely on patients who are noncompliant with the ASA elective-procedure fasting guidelines.[18-20] Procedures can sometimes be delayed for a number of hours; however, this must be balanced against prolongation of pain and anxiety in the patient, inconvenience for the patient and family, and expenditure of room space and other finite ED resources. In addition, many ED procedures require urgent if not immediate attention (e.g., débridement and repair of animal bite wounds, acute burn management, arthrocentesis for suspected septic arthritis, reduction of joint dislocations, lumbar puncture in an uncooperative septic patient, hernia reduction, eye irrigation for ocular trauma or chemical burns, cardioversion in a hemodynamically unstable patient). Though uncommon, there may be occasions in which nonfasting patients require urgent procedures with a substantial depth of sedation that may be more safely managed in the operating room with endotracheal intubation to protect the airway.

Selecting agents that are less likely to produce vomiting, such as fentanyl instead of morphine or meperidine, may decrease the potential for aspiration. Concomitant antiemetic administration is an unproven adjunct but a common consideration. In summary, *common sense should apply and clinical judgment should prevail, but it is standard for PSA to be performed in the ED on patients in the nonfasting state.*

Hepatic and Renal

The implications of delayed metabolism or excretion of PSA agents in infants younger than 6 months, in the elderly, and in patients with hepatic or renal abnormality should be considered.

PERSONNEL AND INTERACTIVE MONITORING

The most important element of PSA monitoring is close and continuous observation of the patient by an individual capable of recognizing complications of sedation (Fig. 33-2). This person must be able to continuously observe the patient's face, mouth, and chest wall motion. Equipment or sterile drapes must not interfere with such visualization. Such careful observation allows prompt detection of adverse events such as respiratory depression, apnea, partial airway obstruction, emesis, and hypersalivation.

Standard-risk patient[a]

Oral intake in the prior 3 hours	Procedural urgency[b]			
	Emergeney procedure	Urgent procedure	Semiurgent	Nonurgent
Nothing	All levels of sedation	All levels of sedation	All levels of sedation	All levels of sedation
Clear liquids only	All levels of sedation	All levels of sedation	Up to and including brief deep sedation	Up to and including extended moderate sedation
Light snack	All levels of sedation	Up to and including brief deep sedation	Up to and including dissociative sedation, nonextended moderate sedation	Minimal sedation only
Heavier snack or meal	All levels of sedation	Up to and including extended moderate sedation	Minimal sedation only	Minimal sedation only

Higher-risk patient[a]

Oral intake in the prior 3 hours	Procedural urgency[b]			
	Emergeney procedure	Urgent procedure	Semiurgent	Nonurgent
Nothing	All levels of sedation	All levels of sedation	All levels of sedation	All levels of sedation
Clear liquids only	All levels of sedation	Up to and including brief deep sedation	Up to and including extended moderate sedation	Minimal sedation only
Light snack	All levels of sedation	Up to and including dissociative sedation, nonextended moderate sedation	Minimal sedation only	Minimal sedation only
Heavier snack or meal	All levels of sedation	Up to and including dissociative sedation, nonextended moderate sedation	Minimal sedation only	Minimal sedation only

Procedural sedation and analgesia targeted depth and duration

Increasing potential aspiration risk ↓

- Minimal sedation only
- Dissociative sedation; brief or intermediate-length moderate sedation
- Extended moderate sedation
- Brief deep sedation
- Intermediate or extended-length deep sedation

↓

Brief: <10 minutes
Intermediate: 10–20 minutes
Extended: >20 minutes

Figure 33-1 Prudent limits of targeted depth and length of emergency department procedural sedation and analgesia based on presedation assessment of aspiration risk.
[a]Higher-risk patients are those with one or more of the following present to a degree individually or cumulatively judged clinically important by the treating clinician:
- Potential for difficult or prolonged assisted ventilation should an airway complication develop (e.g., short neck, small mandible/micrognathia, large tongue, tracheomalacia, laryngomalacia, history of difficult intubation, congenital anomalies of the airway and neck, sleep apnea)
- Conditions predisposing to esophageal reflux (e.g., elevated intracranial pressure, esophageal disease, hiatal hernia, peptic ulcer disease, gastritis, bowel obstruction, ileus, tracheoesophageal fistula)
- Extremes of age (e.g., >70 years or <6 months)
- Severe systemic disease with definite limitation in function (i.e., American Society of Anesthesiologists physical status ≥3)
- Other clinical findings leading the emergency physician to judge the patient to be at higher than standard risk (e.g., altered level of consciousness, frail appearance)
[b]Procedural urgency:
- Emergency (e.g., cardioversion for life-threatening dysrhythmia, reduction of a markedly angulated fracture or dislocation with soft tissue or vascular compromise, intractable pain or suffering)
- Urgent (e.g., care of dirty wounds and lacerations, animal and human bites, incision and drainage of abscesses, fracture reduction, hip reduction, lumbar puncture for suspected meningitis, arthrocentesis, neuroimaging for trauma)
- Semiurgent (e.g., care of clean wounds and lacerations, shoulder reduction, neuroimaging for new-onset seizures, removal of foreign bodies, examination for sexual assault)
- Nonurgent or elective (e.g., nonvegetable foreign body in the external auditory canal, chronic embedded soft tissue foreign body, ingrown toenail)

(From Green SM, Roback MG, Miner JR, et al. Fasting and emergency department procedural sedation and analgesia: a consensus-based clinical practice advisory. Ann Emerg Med. 2007;49:454.)

PROCEDURAL SEDATION AND ANALGESIA

After a thorough presedation assessment, attach the patient to the monitoring system. Routine use of pulse oximetry, capnography, ECG monitoring, and blood pressure monitoring greatly enhances the safety of PSA.

Apply supplemental oxygen, especially for patients undergoing deep sedation with agents such as propofol. However, administration of oxygen precludes the use of pulse oximetry as an early warning device for apnea. Ideally, capnography should be used in all situations in which high-flow oxygen is administered.

Ensure that all necessary age-appropriate resuscitation equipment is available, including oxygen, a bag-valve-mask device, suction, reversal agents, and a defibrillator (for patients with significant cardiovascular disease).

Administer the agent selected. The choice of appropriate medications is discussed in detail in text. Here, propofol is being administered.

PSA requires a minimum of two experienced individuals: one to perform the procedure and one to continuously monitor the patient for potential complications. The person monitoring the patient must be focused on the patient's cardiopulmonary status.

Perform the procedure. Here, the patient is being cardioverted for new-onset atrial fibrillation. After the procedure, monitor the patient until there is no further risk for cardiorespiratory depression. Before discharge, be sure that the patient is alert and oriented with stable vital signs.

Figure 33-2 Procedural sedation and analgesia (PSA). *ECG,* electrocardiographic.

PSA personnel should understand the pharmacology of analgesic and sedative agents and their respective reversal agents. They must be proficient in maintaining airway patency and assisting ventilation if needed. PSA requires a minimum of two experienced individuals, most frequently one clinician and one nurse or respiratory therapist. The clinician typically oversees drug administration and performs the procedure, whereas the nurse or respiratory therapist continuously monitors the patient for potential complications. The nurse or respiratory therapist should also document the medications administered and the response to sedation and measure vital signs periodically. The nurse or respiratory therapist may assist in minor, interruptible tasks but must remain focused on the patient's cardiopulmonary status, and this responsibility must not be impaired. An individual with advanced life support skills should also be immediately available, which is a requisite easy to fulfill in the ED setting.

During deep sedation, the individual dedicated to patient monitoring should have experience with this depth of sedation and no other responsibilities that would interfere with the advanced level of monitoring and documentation appropriate for this degree of sedation.[16] Individual hospital-wide sedation policies may have additional requirements regarding how and when deep sedation is administered based on the patient's specific needs and the clinician's expertise.

It is not mandatory to have intravenous (IV) access in situations in which sedation is administered by the intramuscular (IM), oral, nasal, inhalational, or rectal routes, but it may be preferable based on the anticipated depth of sedation or comorbid condition or for additional drug titration. When sedation is performed without IV access, an individual skilled in initiating such access should be immediately available.

EQUIPMENT AND MECHANICAL MONITORING

The routine use of mechanical monitoring has greatly enhanced the safety of PSA. With current technology, oxygenation (via pulse oximetry), ventilation (via capnography), and hemodynamics (via blood pressure and electrocardiogram [ECG]) can all be monitored noninvasively in nonintubated, spontaneously breathing patients.

Pulse Oximetry

Mechanical monitoring for PSA should include continuous pulse oximetry with an audible signal. Pulse oximetry measures the percentage of hemoglobin that is bound to oxygen and is not a substitute for monitoring ventilation because of the variable lag time between the onset of hypoventilation or apnea and a change in the oxygen saturation of hemoglobin molecules.

Capnography

Capnography is a very useful tool that provides a continuous, breath-by-breath measure of the respiratory rate and CO_2 exchange. Importantly, capnography can detect the common adverse airway and respiratory events associated with PSA.[21-33] Capnography is the earliest indicator of airway or respiratory compromise and will show abnormally high or low end-tidal carbon dioxide pressure well before pulse oximetry detects falling oxyhemoglobin saturation, especially in patients receiving supplemental oxygen. Early detection of respiratory compromise is especially important in infants and toddlers, who have smaller functional residual capacity and greater oxygen consumption than older children and adults do.[34-36] Capnography provides a non–impedance-based respiratory rate directly from the airway (via an oral-nasal cannula). This is more accurate than impedance-based respiratory monitoring, especially in patients with obstructive apnea or laryngospasm, in whom impedance-based monitoring will interpret chest wall movement without ventilation as a valid breath.

Two recent randomized controlled trials have demonstrated that the use of capnography during procedural sedation decreases the incidence of hypoxic events.[37-39] Both studies randomized patients to standard monitoring alone (oximetry, ECG, and blood pressure) or standard monitoring with capnography, with hypoxia being the outcome measure. In both studies, the addition of capnography to standard monitoring alerted clinicians to ventilatory abnormalities before the development of hypoxia, and as a result, capnography significantly decreased the incidence of hypoxic events.[37,38]

At this time the American College of Emergency Physicians has no current standards for the use of capnography during PSA. Currently, the use of capnography in the ED for PSA varies widely.

ECG Monitoring

Although continuous ECG monitoring cannot be considered mandatory or standard of care in the absence of cardiovascular disease, such monitoring is simple, inexpensive, and readily available.

BIS Monitoring

The bispectral index (BIS) is a monitoring modality that uses a processed electroencephalogram signal to quantify the depth of anesthesia or sedation. A BIS value of 100 (unitless scale) is considered complete alertness, 0 represents no cortical activity at all, and the range of 40 to 60 is believed to be consistent with general anesthesia. Although this technology has been used widely to monitor the depth of sedation in the operating room, the ASA has judged that its clinical applicability for this purpose "has not been established."[40] Furthermore, a 2011 study found that patients in whom a modified minimum alveolar concentration protocol (i.e., the inhalational anesthetic concentration needed for 50% of patients to not move with the application of a noxious stimulus) was used had fewer awareness events than did those in whom a BIS protocol was used.[41] Even though PSA research has demonstrated statistical associations between BIS and standard sedation scores, these studies have also noted unacceptably wide ranges of BIS values at various depths of sedation.[21,42-46] Thus, although BIS is correlated with the depth of sedation in aggregate groups, it lacks sufficient capacity to reliably gauge such depth in individual patients and therefore cannot currently be recommended for ED PSA.

Resuscitation Equipment and Supplies

Gather all necessary age-appropriate equipment for airway management and resuscitation in the sedation area, including oxygen, a bag-valve-mask device, suction, and drug reversal agents. For subjects with significant cardiovascular disease, include a defibrillator as well.

Vital Signs

Measure vital signs periodically at individualized intervals, in most cases including measurements at baseline, after drug administration, on completion of the procedure, during early recovery, and at completion of recovery. During deep sedation it is reasonable to assess vital signs approximately every 5 minutes. Patients are at highest risk for complications 5 to 10 minutes after IV medications are administered and during the immediate postprocedure period when external stimuli are discontinued. Continuous monitoring of the ECG, blood pressure, pulse rate, and pulse oximetry via a standard monitor generally fulfills the monitoring requirements. Actual documentation in the medical record varies, and fewer entries on the record are necessary when continuous monitoring is used. There are no standards mandating the frequency of documentation of vital signs in the medical record, and guided by the specific patient scenario, medications used, and depth of sedation, common sense should prevail.

SUPPLEMENTAL OXYGEN

Substantial variation in practice exists with regard to the use of supplemental oxygen during PSA. The premise is a logical one—increasing systemic oxygen reserves should naturally delay or perhaps avert hypoxemia should an airway or respiratory adverse event occur. However, the price paid for this well-intentioned safeguard is the loss of pulse oximetry as an early warning device.[12,15,21] Hyperoxygenated patients will desaturate only after the apnea is prolonged—indeed, the time required for preoxygenated, apneic, healthy adults and adolescents to desaturate to 90% averages more than 6 minutes.[47,48]

Deitch and colleagues have shown in a series of randomized controlled trials that high-flow supplemental oxygen decreases the incidence of hypoxia during propofol sedation (number needed to benefit of 4)[49] whereas lesser amounts of oxygen (3 L/min) do so only marginally with propofol and not at all with lighter levels of sedation.[23,50] Thus, high-flow oxygen is strongly recommended with propofol or other deep sedation, assuming that interactive monitoring includes capnography to promptly identify respiratory depression.[51,52] For lighter levels of sedation, supplemental oxygen has no established benefit and may impair detection of respiratory depression when using pulse oximetry without capnography.[52]

DISCHARGE CRITERIA

Monitor all patients receiving PSA until they are no longer at risk for cardiorespiratory depression (Table 33-2). Before discharge be sure that patients are alert and oriented (or have returned to an age-appropriate baseline) with stable vital signs. Many hospitals have chosen to use standardized recovery scoring systems similar to those used in their surgical postanesthesia recovery areas (Table 33-3). Although no generally accepted minimum durations for safe discharge have been established, one large ED study found that in children with uneventful sedation, no serious adverse effects occurred more than 25 minutes after final medication administration.[53]

TABLE 33-2 Complications after Sedation

COMPLICATION	ETIOLOGY
Delayed awakening	Prolonged drug action Hypoxemia, hypercapnia, hypovolemia
Agitation	Pain, hypoxemia, hypercapnia, full bladder Paradoxical reactions Emergence reactions
Nausea and vomiting	Sedative agents Premature oral fluids

Cardiorespiratory events
  Tachycardia
 	
  Bradycardia
  Hypoxia
	
	Pain, hypovolemia, impaired ventilation
	Vagal stimulation, opioids, hypoxia
	Laryngospasm, airway obstruction, oversedation

From Krauss B, Brustowicz R, eds. *Pediatric Procedural Sedation and Analgesia.* Philadelphia: Lippincott, Williams & Wilkins; 1999:145.

This suggests that in most cases, prolonged observation beyond $\frac{1}{2}$ hour is unlikely to be necessary.

Make sure that all patients leave the hospital with a reliable adult who will observe them after discharge for postprocedural complications. Document the name of the individual in the hospital record. Give written instructions regarding appropriate diet, medications, and level of activity (Boxes 33-2 and 33-3). Even though patients may appear awake and able to comprehend instructions, they may not remember details once they leave the ED.

To be eligible for safe discharge, children are not required to walk unaided or demonstrate that they can tolerate an oral challenge because most PSA agents are emetogenic. Forcing fluids after sedation can lead to emesis before or after discharge. The AAP guidelines require only that "the patient can talk (if age-appropriate)" and "the patient can sit up unaided (if age-appropriate)."[16] When infants and young children are discharged after their evening bedtime, caution parents to position the child's head in the car seat carefully. Significant forward flexion might cause airway obstruction if the child falls asleep on the way home.

GENERAL PRINCIPLES

Therapeutic mistakes that result in inadequate analgesia and sedation include using the wrong agent, the wrong dose, the wrong route or frequency of administration, and poor use of adjunctive agents. With proper training and technique, adequate PSA can be provided in almost any circumstance. Understanding titration principles is critical to providing safe and effective PSA. Clinicians must have a thorough knowledge of the pharmacokinetics, dosing, administration, and potential complications of the PSA agents that they use. Time of onset from injection to the initial observed effect must be appreciated, especially when using drugs in combination, to avoid stacking of drug doses and oversedation.

The correct agent (or combination of agents) and the route and timing of administration depend on the following factors:

TABLE 33-3 Sample Recovery Scoring Systems

STEWARD RECOVERY SCORE	
Consciousness	
Awake	2
Responding to stimuli	1
Not responding	0
Airway	
Coughing on command or crying	2
Maintaining good airway	1
Airway requiring maintenance	0
Movement	
Moving limbs purposefully	2
Nonpurposeful movements	1
Not moving	0
MODIFIED ALDRETE SCORE	
Vital Signs	
Stable	1
Unstable	0
Respirations	
Normal	2
Shallow respirations or tachypnea	1
Apnea	0
Level of Consciousness	
Alert, oriented or returned to preprocedural level	2
Arousable, giddy, agitated	1
Unresponsive	0
Oxygen Saturation	
95-100% or preprocedural level	2
90-94%	1
<90%	0
Color	
Pink or preprocedural color	2
Pale or dusky	1
Cyanotic	0
Activity	
Moves on command or preprocedural level	2
Moves extremities or uncoordinated walking	1
No spontaneous movement	0

SEDATION SCORE	ACTION
>8	Consider discharge if no score = 0
7-8	Vital signs q20min
4-6	Vital signs q10min
0-3	Vital signs q5min— consider further evaluation if prolonged

From Krauss B, Brustowicz R, eds. *Pediatric Procedural Sedation and Analgesia.* Philadelphia: Lippincott, Williams & Wilkins; 1999:157.

BOX 33-2 Sample Adult Disposition Instructions after PSA

1. Do not drive or operate heavy machinery for 12 hours.
2. Eat a light diet for the next 12 hours.
3. Take only your prescribed medications as needed, including any pain medication you were discharged with. Avoid alcohol.
4. Do not make any important decisions or sign important documents for 12 hours. You may be forgetful because of the medications that were administered.
5. If you experience any difficulty breathing or persistent nausea and vomiting, return to the emergency department.
6. You should have a responsible person with you for the rest of the day and during the night.

PSA, *procedural sedation and analgesia.*

BOX 33-3 Sample Pediatric Disposition Instructions after PSA

Your child has been given medicine for sedation and/or pain control. These medicines may cause your child to be sleepy and less aware of the surroundings, thus making it easier for accidents to happen while walking or crawling. Because of these side effects, your child should be watched closely for the next few hours. We suggest the following:

1. No eating or drinking for the next 2 hours. Infants may resume half-normal feedings when they are hungry.
2. No playing for 12 hours that requires normal coordination, such as bike riding or jungle gym activities.
3. No playing without an adult to watch and supervise for the next 12 hours.
4. No baths, showers, cooking, or use of potentially dangerous electrical appliances unless supervised by an adult for the next 12 hours.

If you notice anything unusual about your child, call us for advice or return to the emergency department for reevaluation.

PSA, *procedural sedation and analgesia.*

How long will the procedure last? Will it be seconds (e.g., simple relocation of a dislocated joint, incision and drainage of a small abscess, cardioversion), minutes (e.g., complex manipulation of a fracture for reduction, breaking up loculations in a large abscess and then packing it), or prolonged (e.g., complex facial laceration repair)? How likely is it that the procedure will need to be repeated (e.g., fracture reduction)? Can topical, local, or regional anesthesia be used as an adjunct? Does the patient require sedation only for a noninvasive diagnostic imaging study?

Before drug administration, every effort should be made to minimize a patient's anxiety and distress, particularly in children. The emotional state of a patient on induction strongly correlates with the degree of distress on emergence and in the days immediately after the procedure.[54-57] Avoid being pressured by consultants to cut corners or rush PSA. Incorporating into the presedation preparation a discussion with the consultant about the sedation plan and the length of time required to safely prepare and sedate the patient can avoid the risks associated with hurried sedation.

For pediatric PSA, the clinician should appreciate the adult dose of the sedative being administered and consider this the maximum threshold. Understand that the initial dose of midazolam for PSA in a 100-kg patient on a milligram-per-kilogram basis is far less than the 0.1 mg/kg used in a child to avoid unexpected mishaps in drug dosing.

ROUTES OF ADMINISTRATION

For nondissociative agents, titrate the IV medications to the patient's response for the best method of achieving rapid and safe analgesia and sedation. Wait the appropriate time for the medications to produce the intended effect before adding more doses. When using opioids, administer doses in 2- to 3-minute increments and observe for side effects such as miosis, somnolence, decreased responsiveness to verbal stimuli, impaired speech, and diminished pain on questioning as appropriate initial end points. For sedative-hypnotics, use similar incremental dosing and end points such as ptosis (rather than miosis), somnolence, slurred speech, and alterations in gaze. Repeated doses may be given in a titrated fashion based on the patient's response during the procedure.

The oral, transmucosal (i.e., nasal, rectal), and IM routes are more convenient means of administration because IV access is not necessary, but they are much less reliable for timely dose titration to a desired response. New drug delivery systems, however, are expanding the effectiveness and ease of use of these routes of administration. The refinement of intranasal drug delivery has significantly increased the efficacy of this route of administration.[58,59] Before the development of metered-dose atomizers, the degree of absorption and effectiveness of intranasal drug administration were operator dependent. Furthermore, new drug formulations with concentrations appropriate for intranasal administration are becoming available for study.[60,61]

The main advantage of these other routes is for pediatric patients in whom IV access may be problematic or for procedures that may require only minimal sedation in conjunction with the use of local anesthetics. These routes are also advantageous for simple sedation during diagnostic imaging.

With the exception of ketamine, agents administered intramuscularly have erratic absorption and a variable onset of action. Accordingly, prolonged preprocedural and postprocedural observation may be necessary. When required, the IM route offers little advantage over oral or transmucosal administration.

Another PSA route is via inhalation of nitrous oxide. This gas can either be delivered by a demand-flow system using a handheld mask or be delivered to young children using a nose mask in a continuous-flow system under close clinician supervision.

Because individual needs may vary widely, the application of arbitrary ceiling doses of analgesic and sedative regimens is unwarranted. The true ceiling dose of an agent is the level that provides adequate pain relief or sedation without major cardiopulmonary side effects such as respiratory depression, apnea, bradycardia, hypotension, or allergic reactions.

There are two absolute contraindications to PSA: severe clinical instability requiring immediate attention and refusal by a competent patient. Relative contraindications include hemodynamic or respiratory compromise, altered sensorium, or an inability to monitor side effects (e.g., magnetic resonance imaging [MRI] without remote monitoring). However, even in many of these circumstances, appropriate agents can be given to provide analgesia and sedation while minimizing the chance for further deterioration. Although safely sedating patients at the extremes of age is challenging and requires additional care, as well as reductions in drug dosing (because of decreased drug metabolism and excretion), age is not a contraindication to PSA.

DRUG SELECTION STRATEGIES

The majority of nonpainful or minimally painful ED procedures in older children and adults can be performed without systemic sedation and analgesia. Skilled practitioners can frequently combine a calm, reassuring bedside manner with distraction techniques, careful local or regional anesthesia, or both.[62-64] Many procedures, however, cannot be technically or humanely performed without PSA. These situations can be divided into three categories.

Insufficient Analgesia. Despite a cooperative patient, for some procedures it is impossible to achieve effective pain control with local or regional anesthesia. Examples of procedures requiring systemic PSA include fracture reductions, dislocation reductions, incision and drainage of large loculated abscesses, wounds that require scrubbing such as "road rash," cardioversion, bone marrow aspiration/biopsy, and extensive burn débridement.

Insufficient Anxiolysis. Despite effective local or regional anesthesia, some patients will be so frightened that procedures cannot be technically or humanely performed without PSA. Young children requiring repair of lacerations are frequently terrified, and older children and adults may be highly anxious in anticipation of such repairs in sensitive or personal regions (e.g., face, genitalia, perineum).

Insufficient Immobilization. Despite effective local or regional anesthesia and anxiolysis, PSA may be indicated to prevent excessive motion during procedures that require substantial immobilization (e.g., repair of complex facial lacerations, diagnostic imaging studies). Immobilization is most commonly an issue with young children and the mentally challenged.

General Considerations. Clinicians must therefore base customization of their selection of drugs (e.g., anxiolysis, sedation, analgesia, immobilization) on the unique needs of the patient and their individual level of experience with specific agents (Table 33-4). A risk-benefit analysis should be performed before every sedation (Box 33-4). The benefits of reducing anxiety and controlling pain should be carefully weighed against the risk for respiratory depression and airway compromise. Factors influencing the extent of pharmacologic management are listed in Box 33-5. Some general drug selection strategies are discussed later and shown in Table 33-3.

MINOR PROCEDURES IN COOPERATIVE ADULTS AND OLDER CHILDREN.   Such procedures can usually be managed with topical, local, or regional anesthesia. Systemic PSA is typically unnecessary, although mild anxiolysis (e.g., nitrous oxide, oral midazolam) can make these patients more comfortable.

TABLE 33-4 Indications for PSA and Sedation Strategies*

CLINICAL SITUATION	INDICATION	PROCEDURAL REQUIREMENTS	SUGGESTED SEDATION STRATEGIES
Noninvasive procedures	CT Echocardiography Electroencephalography MRI Ultrasonography	Motion control Anxiolysis	Comforting alone Chloral hydrate PO (in patients <3 yr old) Methohexital PR Pentobarbital PO, IM, or IV Midazolam IV Propofol or etomidate IV
Procedure associated with low pain and high anxiety	Dental procedures Flexible fiberoptic laryngoscopy Foreign body removal, simple Intravenous cannulation Laceration repair, simple Lumbar puncture Ocular irrigation Phlebotomy Slit-lamp examination	Sedation Anxiolysis Motion control	Comforting and topical or local anesthesia Midazolam PO/IN/PR/IV Nitrous oxide
Procedures associated with a high level of pain, high anxiety, or both	Abscess incision and drainage Arthrocentesis Bone marrow aspiration and biopsy Burn débridement Cardiac catheterization Cardioversion Central line placement Endoscopy Foreign body removal, complicated Fracture or dislocation reduction Hernia reduction Interventional radiology procedures Laceration repair, complex Paracentesis Paraphimosis reduction Sexual assault examination Thoracentesis Thoracostomy tube placement	Sedation Anxiolysis Analgesia Amnesia Motion control	Propofol or etomidate IV Propofol and fentanyl IV Propofol and ketamine IV Ketamine IM/IV Midazolam and fentanyl IV

Modified from Krauss B, Green SM. Sedation and analgesia for procedures in children. *N Engl J Med.* 2000;342:938.

CT, computed tomography; *IM*, intramuscularly; *IN*, intranasally; *IV*, intravenously; *MRI*, magnetic resonance imaging; *PO*, orally; *PR*, per rectum; *PSA*, procedural sedation and analgesia.

*There is no universally accepted or clinically correct dose, medication, or combination. Many regimens are acceptable. This table is intended as a general overview. Sedation strategies should be individualized. Although the pharmacopoeia is large, clinicians should familiarize themselves with a few agents that are flexible enough to be used for the majority of procedures. In all cases it is assumed that practitioners are fully trained in the technique, appropriate personnel and monitoring are used as detailed in this chapter, and specific drug contraindications are absent.

BOX 33-4 Risk-Benefit Analysis for PSA

- Why is PSA needed in the first place? Is the procedure very painful, frightening, or requiring extreme cooperation?
- Are the risks of PSA appropriate for the procedure involved?
- If a child, do the parents or guardian consent to the use of PSA?
- How long will the procedure take? If it is a short procedure, is it worth the added risk and expense to the patient? If it is a longer procedure, is there an appropriate agent that can be titrated to allow adequate PSA throughout the entire length of the procedure?

- Are there significant side effects that limit a particular drug's usefulness?
- Are enough nurses and support personnel present to safely allow the use of PSA?
- What is the recovery period for a given agent? Are there enough treatment areas and staff in the ED to allow adequate observation during recovery?
- When did the patient last eat? Is a delay in waiting for a sufficient fasting time worth the time lost in performing the procedure?

From Krauss B, Brustowicz R, eds. Pediatric Procedural Sedation and Analgesia. *Philadelphia: Lippincott, Williams & Wilkins; 1999:294.*
ED, *emergency department*; PSA, *procedural sedation and analgesia.*

BOX 33-5 Factors Influencing the Extent of Pediatric Pharmacologic Management

AGE

Selected drugs and routes of administration have age limitations and are not recommended above or below a certain age (e.g., demand-flow nitrous oxide in children <5 years, nasal and rectal routes of administration in children >6 years).

TIME OF DAY

A toddler seen at naptime or at 9 PM who is tired and sleepy will usually require smaller dosing and possibly a lower level of PSA than required at 9 AM. Young children with facial lacerations at night, after their normal bedtime, may require only topical anesthesia and a quiet room for 20 to 30 minutes to achieve a painless laceration repair while the child sleeps.

FASTING STATUS

Young children can be extremely difficult and uncooperative when hungry, tired, or both. In anticipation of PSA, many children are kept without oral intake from the time that they are triaged in the ED. This can further increase hunger and irritability, especially if the child waits 1 to 2 hours to be seen by a clinician.

AVAILABILITY OF STAFFING AND EQUIPMENT

Staffing availability can affect the use and timing of sedation and is especially important in busy EDs with multiple sedations occurring concurrently and in smaller units that are set up for only one sedation at a time.

LOCATION OF THE INJURY

Injuries located in areas of cosmetic concern (especially on the face) or near sensory organs (e.g., ears, eyes, mouth, nose) will often require a high degree of agitation control and a concomitant level of PSA.

PREVIOUS MEDICATIONS

An accurate history of previous medication administration is important in situations in which a child is referred from another facility because this can affect the type and timing of PSA agents that can be given. In particular, a child may have received opioids or sedative-hypnotics before transfer and may still be sedated on arrival, thus necessitating an adjustment in the PSA regimen.

LEVEL OF ANXIETY

The level of anxiety of both the child and the accompanying adult or adults must be accurately assessed. Children manifest anxiety in many different ways, and emergency clinicians must be facile at recognizing the varying expressions of anxiety, especially in young children. A child with a facial laceration quietly sitting on the stretcher during the initial examination will not necessarily be a

calm and cooperative patient during repair of the laceration (infants and toddlers). The nursing assessment at triage of the state of the child and accompanying adult or adults can be very helpful in some cases in determining the need for PSA. A child who was frightened and uncooperative in triage may be calm and compliant during a procedure. Unfortunately, the reverse is also true. When confronted with an extremely anxious child, ED personnel should ascertain what the parents have told the child about the upcoming procedure. Many parents, in the hope of lessening their child's anxiety, will tell the child that she or he will get a "shot" or a "needle" and that the procedure will "only hurt for a minute." This type of parental preparation, especially in young children who do not have the cognitive ability to mediate their anxiety, often results in a significant increase in the child's anxiety and a decrease in the child's ability to cooperate, especially if the child has had a previous negative experience with a procedure in the ED. It is also important to assess the parents' level of anxiety because this will determine the degree to which they can assist during the procedure. An extremely anxious parent or a parent who must take care of other siblings during the procedure will find it difficult to assist in distracting the child or otherwise helping the child cope with the procedure.

PREVIOUS EXPERIENCE

Children's previous experience in hospitals can greatly affect their response to the current situation. Direct experience is not the only way to create anxious, frightened, and uncooperative patients, though. Images from television, stories from peers, or previous witness of a sibling being forcibly restrained for repair of a laceration can leave a powerful and lasting impression. This type of influence should be especially suspected in children whose anxiety seems out of proportion to the present situation. Eliciting from the parents a history of a previous difficult experience in the ED can be a decisive factor in determining the degree of sedation required. Children who have had a recent unpleasant laceration repair and who now have a new laceration may well require PSA as opposed to simple anxiolysis (either pharmacologic or nonpharmacologic) had there been no previous trauma.

CHILD'S BEHAVIOR AT ROUTINE PRIMARY CARE VISITS

Inquiring into how a child behaves during routine primary care visits can yield important information on how the child reacts to stressful situations, how cooperative the child will be with the anticipated procedure, and whether pharmacologic management is needed. Children who cry but hold still when vaccinated may be more compliant than children who are described by their parents as being "afraid of doctors" or "wild" during visits to the primary care physician.

ED, emergency department; PSA, procedural sedation and analgesia.

MORE COMPLEX PROCEDURES OF LONGER DURATION IN COOPERATIVE ADULTS AND OLDER CHILDREN. Supplementation of topical, local, or regional anesthesia with either nitrous oxide or IV midazolam and fentanyl permits customization of the depth of sedation and pain relief to the specific needs of each patient.

PROCEDURES IN UNCOOPERATIVE ADULTS OR THE MENTALLY CHALLENGED. Essentially all procedures in uncooperative

adult-sized patients are difficult without systemic PSA. Depending on operator experience, IV midazolam, IV propofol, IV etomidate, or IM/IV ketamine or midazolam may be used in these situations. Given that the sedatives midazolam, propofol, and etomidate lack specific analgesic properties, many emergency physicians attempt to control pain with an opioid such as fentanyl before the procedure. Midazolam can be titrated intravenously to a relatively deep level of sedation, although as discussed previously, the risk for adverse effects increases with the depth of sedation. Ketamine (typically with coadministered midazolam when used in adults) can also provide the profound analgesia and immobilization necessary to perform painful procedures. However, in adults there is a risk for unpleasant hallucinatory recovery reactions. Ketamine should be used with extreme caution in older adults because its sympathomimetic properties may aggravate any underlying coronary artery disease or hypertension. Occasionally, procedures in extremely uncooperative adults or the mentally challenged are best managed in the operating room with general anesthesia.

MINOR PROCEDURES IN UNCOOPERATIVE OLDER CHILDREN AND IN YOUNG CHILDREN. Minor procedures (e.g., small lacerations, IV cannulation, venipuncture, removal of superficial foreign bodies) in uncooperative children can frequently be managed by skilled practitioners with a combination of nonpharmacologic techniques (e.g., distraction, guided imagery, hypnosis, comforting, breathing techniques) in conjunction with topical anesthesia, careful local anesthesia, and when necessary, brief forcible immobilization (by personnel or a restraining device). In other cases, supplementing nonpharmacologic techniques with topical or local anesthesia and anxiolysis with oral midazolam may be sufficient to permit successful wound repair. Although oral administration is most popular and least invasive, the nasal or rectal routes can also be used depending on operator experience and preference.

MAJOR PROCEDURES IN UNCOOPERATIVE CHILDREN. Major painful procedures (e.g., fracture reduction, incision and drainage of large loculated abscesses, arthrocentesis of a major joint) require systemic PSA. Options include IM/IV ketamine, IV propofol, IV etomidate, or IV midazolam. Given that the sedatives midazolam, propofol, and etomidate lack specific analgesic properties, many emergency physicians attempt to control pain with an opioid such as fentanyl before the procedure. Ketamine may be the best option in such children because dissociative sedation can consistently provide immobilization and analgesia while maintaining protective airway reflexes and upper airway muscular tone.

PHARMACOPEIA

There is no universally correct or preferred medication or drug regimen. Many options are acceptable and successful. The best choice is an agent whose pharmacologic properties are familiar to the operator and that is used frequently by the operator, is easily titratable, and has a short duration of action or is readily reversible. All drugs should be given in adequate doses because underdosing of opioids or sedatives provides no useful purpose. Dosing recommendations for PSA drugs are provided in Table 33-5, and specialized protocols for midazolam or fentanyl, propofol, and ketamine are presented in Boxes 33-6, 33-7, and 33-8, respectively. Individual agents are discussed in the following sections.

Sedative-Hypnotic Agents

Chloral Hydrate
Pharmacology. Chloral hydrate is a pure sedative-hypnotic agent without analgesic properties. When administered orally, the average time to peak sedation is approximately 30 minutes,

with a recovery time of an additional 1 to 2 hours.[65,66] Residual motor imbalance and agitation may persist for several hours beyond this period.[67] Rectal administration is erratically absorbed and therefore not recommended.

Adult Use. Use of chloral hydrate is limited to diagnostic imaging studies in children. It has no current use in adults.

Pediatric Use. Chloral hydrate is widely used as a sedative to facilitate nonpainful outpatient diagnostic procedures such as electroencephalography and computed tomography (CT) or MRI.[66,68-72] IV pentobarbital appears to be more effective than chloral hydrate for the latter indication,[73] although many centers prefer chloral hydrate in younger children (e.g., <18 months) simply to avoid the need for IV access.[69,70,73]

Adverse Effects. Despite a wide margin of safety, chloral hydrate can cause airway obstruction and respiratory depression, especially at higher doses (75 to 100 mg/kg).[1,66,69,71,72] The incidence was 0.6% in one large series.[66] There is no known dosage threshold of chloral hydrate below which this potential complication can be consistently avoided,[1,71] and accordingly, standard interactive and mechanical monitoring precautions apply to chloral hydrate as they do to other PSA agents.

Because it is a halogenated hydrocarbon, overdoses of chloral hydrate can be arrhythmogenic and produce ventricular dysrhythmias. *β-Blockers may be most effective in terminating ventricular arrhythmias.* Despite reports of potential carcinogenicity, the AAP has judged that the evidence is currently insufficient to avoid single doses of chloral hydrate for this reason alone.[74]

Midazolam
Pharmacology. Benzodiazepines are a group of highly lipophilic agents that possess anxiolytic, amnestic, sedative, hypnotic, muscle relaxant, and anticonvulsant properties. They lack direct analgesic properties and thus are commonly coadministered with opioids. Caution must be exercised when using benzodiazepines and opioids together because the risk for hypoxia and apnea is significantly greater than when either is used alone.[75]

Midazolam is by far the most common benzodiazepine used for PSA and is preferred over the longer-acting lorazepam and diazepam. The time to peak effect for midazolam is approximately 2 to 3 minutes when given intravenously. Unlike diazepam, midazolam and lorazepam are water soluble, thus making parenteral administration less painful and mucosal absorption faster. *Midazolam is readily reversed with flumazenil,* and individuals undergoing PSA with midazolam are good candidates for this antidote should reversal be required.

Adult Use. Midazolam can be used effectively for moderate and deep sedation through careful IV titration to effect, typically together with fentanyl (see Box 33-6).

Pediatric Use. Advantages of midazolam over other benzodiazepines for pediatric PSA are its short duration of action, reversibility, and availability in multiple routes of administration. Midazolam may be used for the same indications and in the same manner as in adults. Some children require larger doses than would be typical for adults on a milligram-per-kilogram basis,[76] and paradoxical responses (e.g., hyperexcitability) are not uncommon.[67,77,78] Midazolam

TABLE 33-5 Drug Dosing Recommendations for PSA*

Sedative-Hypnotics

DRUG	CLINICAL EFFECTS	INDICATIONS	ADULT DOSE†	PEDIATRIC DOSE	ONSET (min)	DURATION (min)	COMMENTS
Choral Hydrate (Noctec)	Sedation, motion control, anxiolysis No analgesia Not reversible	Diagnostic imaging (age <3 yr)	Not recommended	PO: 25-100 mg/kg, after 30 min may repeat 25-50 mg/kg Maximum total dose: 2 g or 100 mg/kg (whichever is less) Single use only in neonates	PO: 15-30	PO: 60-120	Effects unreliable if age >3 yr Avoid in patients with significant cardiac, hepatic, or renal disease Rectal absorption is erratic May produce paradoxical excitement Because drugs cannot be titrated with the PO route, monitor closely for oversedation
Etomidate (Amidate)	Sedation, motion control, anxiolysis No analgesia Not reversible	Procedures requiring sedation and/or anxiolysis	Sedation: 0.1 mg/kg IV; repeat if inadequate response	Not FDA approved in children	IV: <1	IV: 5-15	Adverse effects include respiratory depression, myoclonus, nausea, and vomiting Adrenocortical suppression occurs but is of no clinical significance
Midazolam‡ (Versed)	Sedation, motion control, anxiolysis No analgesia Reversible with flumazenil	Procedures requiring sedation and/or anxiolysis	IV: Initial dose 1 mg, then titrated to max of 5 mg IM: 5 mg or 0.07 mg/kg	IV (0.5-5 yr): Initial dose of 0.05-0.1 mg/kg, then titrated to max of 0.6 mg/kg IV (6-12 yr): Initial dose of 0.025-0.05 mg/kg, then titrated to max of 0.4 mg/kg IM: 0.1-0.15 mg/kg PO: 0.5-0.75 mg/kg IN: 0.2-0.5 mg/kg PR: 0.25-0.5 mg/kg	IV: 2-3 IM: 10-20 PO: 15-30 IN: 10-15 PR: 10-30	IV: 45-60 IM: 60-120 PO: 60-90 IN: 60 PR: 60-90	Reduce the dose when used in combination with opioids May produce paradoxical excitement Because drugs cannot be titrated with the PO/PR/IN routes, monitor closely for oversedation
Methohexital (Brevital)	Sedation, motion control, anxiolysis No analgesia Not reversible	Diagnostic imaging	Anesthesia induction IV: 1 mg/kg (less for sedation) *Caution:* limited research	PR: 25 mg/kg IV (caution, limited research): 0.5-1 mg/kg	PR: 10-15	PR: 60	Avoid in patients with temporal lobe epilepsy or porphyria Because drugs cannot be titrated with the PR route, monitor closely for oversedation

Pentobarbital (Nembutal)	Sedation, motion control, anxiolysis No analgesia Not reversible	Diagnostic imaging	Not recommended	IV: 1-6 mg/kg, titrated in increments of 1-2 mg/kg to desired effect IM: 2-6 mg/kg, max of 100 mg PO/PR (<4 yr): 3-6 mg/kg, max of 100 mg PO/PR (>4 yr): 1.5-3 mg/kg, max of 100 mg	IV: 3-5 IM: 10-15 PO/PR: 15-60	IV: 15-45 IM: 60-120 PO/PR: 60-240	May produce paradoxical excitement Avoid in patients with porphyria Because drugs cannot be titrated with the PO/PR routes, monitor closely for oversedation
Propofol (Diprivan)	Sedation, motion control, anxiolysis No analgesia Not reversible	Procedures requiring sedation and/or anxiolysis	Load 1 mg/kg IV; may administer additional 0.5-mg/kg doses as needed to enhance or prolong sedation	Load 1-2 mg/kg IV; may administer additional 0.5-mg/kg doses as needed to enhance or prolong sedation	IV: <1	IV: 5-15	Frequent hypotension and respiratory depression Avoid with egg or soy allergies
Thiopental (Pentothal)	Sedation, motion control, anxiolysis No analgesia Not reversible	Diagnostic imaging	Not recommended	PR: 25 mg/kg	PR: 10-15	PR: 60-120	Avoid in patients with porphyria Because drugs cannot be titrated with the PR route, monitor closely for oversedation
Analgesic§							
Fentanyl (Sublimaze)	Analgesia Reversible with naloxone	Procedures with moderate to severe pain	IV: 50 µg, may repeat q3min, titrate to effect	IV: 1 µg/kg/dose, may repeat q3min, titrate to effect	IV: 3-5	IV: 30-60	
Dissociative Agent							
Ketamine (Ketalar)	Analgesia, dissociation, amnesia, motion control Not reversible	Procedures with moderate to severe pain or requiring immobilization	Limited experience in the ED setting IV: 1-1.5 mg/kg slowly over 30-60 sec, may repeat ½ dose q10min prn	IV: 1.5 mg/kg slowly over 30-60 sec, may repeat ½ dose q10 min prn IM: 4-5 mg/kg, may repeat after 10 min (½ dose)	IV: 1 IM: 3-5	IV: dissociation, 15; recovery, 60 IM: dissociation, 15-30; recovery, 90-150	Multiple contraindications[11]

Continued

TABLE 33-5   Drug Dosing Recommendations for PSA—cont'd

DRUG	CLINICAL EFFECTS	INDICATIONS	ADULT DOSE[†]	PEDIATRIC DOSE	ONSET (min)	DURATION (min)	COMMENTS
Inhalational Agent							
Nitrous oxide (Nitronox)	Anxiolysis, analgesia, sedation, amnesia (all mild)	Procedures requiring mild analgesia or sedation (age >4 yr)	Preset mixture with a minimum of 40% O₂ self-administered by a demand-valve mask (requires a cooperative patient)	Preset mixture for a cooperative child; continuous-flow nasal mask in an uncooperative child with close monitoring	<5	<5 following discontinuation	Requires specialized apparatus and gas scavenger capability Several contraindications[¶] Synergistic effect with recent opioids or sedative-hypnotics—use with caution in this setting
Reversal Agents (Antagonists)							
Naloxone (Narcan)	Opioid reversal	Opioid toxicity	IV/IM: 0.4-2 mg	IV/IM: 0.1 mg/kg/dose up to max of 2 mg/dose, may repeat q2min prn	IV: 2	IV: 20-40 IM: 60-90	If shorter acting than the reversed drug, serial doses may be required
Flumazenil (Romazicon)	Benzodiazepine reversal	Benzodiazepine toxicity	IV: 0.2 mg, may repeat q1min up to 1 mg	IV: 0.02 mg/kg/dose, may repeat q1min up to 1 mg	IV: 1-2	IV: 30-60	If shorter acting than the reversed drug, serial doses may be required Do not use in patients chronically taking benzodiazepines, cyclosporine, isoniazid, lithium, propoxyphene, theophylline, tricyclic antidepressants

Adapted from Krauss B, Green SM. Sedation and analgesia for procedures in children. *N Engl J Med.* 2000;342:938.

ED, emergency department; *FDA,* U.S. Food and Drug Administration; *IM,* intramuscularly; *IV,* intravenously; *PO,* orally; *PR,* per rectum; *prn,* as needed; *PSA,* procedural sedation and analgesia.

*Alterations in dosing may be indicated depending on the clinical situation and the practitioner's experience with these agents. Individual dosages may vary when used in combination with other agents, especially when benzodiazepines are combined with opioids.

[†]Use lower doses in geriatric patients and those with significant cardiopulmonary disease.

[‡]Midazolam is preferred over other benzodiazepines (e.g., diazepam, lorazepam) for procedural sedation and analgesia because of its shorter duration of action and multiple routes of administration.

[§]Fentanyl is preferred over other opioids (e.g., morphine, meperidine) for procedural sedation and analgesia because of its faster onset, shorter recovery, and lack of histamine release.

[‖]Generally accepted contraindications to ketamine include age younger than 3 months; history of airway instability, tracheal surgery, or tracheal stenosis; procedures involving stimulation of the posterior pharynx; active pulmonary infection or disease (including active upper respiratory infection); cardiovascular disease, including angina, heart failure, or hypertension; significant head injury; central nervous system masses, or hydrocephalus; glaucoma or acute globe injury; psychosis; porphyria; and thyroid disorder or thyroid medication.

[¶]Generally accepted contraindications to nitrous oxide include pregnancy (patient or personnel), preexisting nausea or vomiting, trapped gas pockets (e.g., middle ear infection, pneumothorax, bowel obstruction).

BOX 33-6 Procedure for Moderate to Deep Sedation with Intravenous Midazolam and Fentanyl

CAVEATS

- Do not consider this procedure if you lack experience with the drugs or do not have the time to perform procedural sedation and analgesia properly. Do not attempt this procedure if the pulse oximeter, suction, oxygen, or bag-mask device is not working, the intravenous line is not secured, or the room is too small or not set up for procedural sedation and analgesia.
- This is a two-person procedure, one to monitor the patient and one to perform the procedure.
- The individual response to the drugs is variable and dependent on the patient's underlying physiologic state and the presence of concomitant drugs and medications.
- The maximum drug effect occurs 2 to 3 minutes after administration. Proceed slowly and patiently and allow the medication to take full effect before giving the next dose.
- Have naloxone and flumazenil immediately available for oversedation or respiratory depression.
- If the patient seems overly sedated, begin the procedure. The pain of the procedure often stimulates respiration and lessens sedation.

CONTRAINDICATIONS—ABSOLUTE (RISKS ESSENTIALLY ALWAYS OUTWEIGH BENEFITS)

- Active hemodynamic instability
- Active respiratory distress or hypoxemia

CONTRAINDICATIONS—RELATIVE (RISKS MAY OUTWEIGH BENEFITS)

- Respiratory depression or altered level of consciousness
- Anticipated difficulty if ventilatory assistance should become necessary (e.g., facial deformity or trauma, small mandible, large tongue, trismus)

PROTOCOL

- Establish intravenous access.
- Preoxygenate the patient.

- Connect appropriate monitoring equipment to the patient. Administer supplemented oxygen if deep sedation is anticipated.
- The pulse, respiratory rate, blood pressure, and level of consciousness should all be recorded initially and periodically throughout the procedure, depending on the depth of sedation.
- Suction equipment, oxygen, a bag-valve-mask assembly, and reversal agents should be available immediately. An age-appropriate resuscitation cart with oral and nasal airways, endotracheal tubes, and a functioning laryngoscope must be nearby.
- The order of drugs is one of personal preference. The ratio of analgesia to sedation is determined by the nature of the procedure. Some procedures require primary analgesia and secondary anxiolysis or sedation (e.g., incision and drainage of an abscess, bone marrow aspiration, arthrocentesis, burn débridement, central catheter placement). In this case, administer fentanyl first. Others require primary anxiolysis or sedation with secondary analgesia (e.g., lumbar puncture, simple foreign body removal); administer midazolam first.
- Administer a local anesthetic if indicated after procedural sedation and analgesia are initiated (this often serves to help gauge the effectiveness of systemic analgesia).
- Perform the procedure. Additional doses of fentanyl or midazolam may be required if further pain or anxiety is noted based on the response and length of the procedure.
- If hypoxemia, oversedation, or slowed respirations are seen during or after the procedure, the patient should first be stimulated while oxygen is applied and the airway repositioned. If the patient's response is insufficient, assist ventilations with a bag-valve-mask device. Reversal agents should be considered if there is not a prompt response to assisted ventilation.
- Continue close observation until the patient is awake and alert, and release the patient with a friend, parent, or relative only after a sufficient discharge score has been attained.

does not reliably render a child motionless, and therefore methohexital or pentobarbital is generally preferred for neuroimaging.[73,79,80]

To avoid the need for IV access in frightened children, midazolam has been alternatively administered via the IM,[81] oral,[77,82-86] intranasal,[82,87-90] and rectal routes.[91] However, the inability to effectively titrate with these routes dictates that a reliable depth of sedation cannot be predictably or regularly achieved. Consequently, these non-IV routes are primarily reserved for pure anxiolysis or mild sedation (or both) for minimally painful procedures. Respiratory depression can also occur via these routes.[86]

Adverse Effects. When administered by skilled practitioners using standard precautions (see Box 33-6), the safety profile for midazolam is excellent.[5,6,92] However, when administering benzodiazepines, one must maintain continuous vigilance for respiratory depression.[1,67,75,92,93] Such respiratory depression is dose dependent and greatly enhanced in the presence of ethanol or other depressive drugs, especially opioids. These

effects are exaggerated in the elderly. Deaths from undetected apnea have occurred,[75] thus underscoring the critical role of continuous interactive and mechanical monitoring.

Benzodiazepines induce minimal cardiovascular depression. Although hypotension can occur, it is rare when the agents are carefully titrated. One reason that midazolam is ideal for painful procedures is its significant amnesic effect. Even though patients appear to feel pain during the procedure, it is often not remembered.

Pentobarbital

Pharmacology. Pentobarbital is a barbiturate capable of profound sedation, hypnosis, amnesia, and anticonvulsant activity in a dose-dependent fashion. It has no inherent analgesic properties. When carefully titrated intravenously, sedation is evident within 5 minutes with a duration of approximately 30 to 40 minutes.[79]

Adult Use. Pentobarbital has no advantage over midazolam for adult PSA and is rarely used for this purpose.

BOX 33-7 Procedure for Deep Sedation with Propofol

INDICATIONS

- Brief, painful procedures for which deep sedation is indicated, including fracture and dislocation reduction, incision and drainage of abscesses, cardioversion, tube thoracostomy, bone marrow aspiration or biopsy, and central line placement.

CONTRAINDICATIONS

Absolute (Risks Essentially Outweigh Benefits)

- Known or suspected allergy to soy or eggs.

Patients at Higher Relative Risk

- Patients older than 55 years, debilitated, or with significant underlying illness (i.e., ASA physical status score of 3 or 4) are at an increased risk for propofol-induced hypotension and other complications. When the benefits of using propofol outweigh the risks, administer lower doses more slowly. Patients should ideally have their volume status optimized before receiving propofol.
- Because there is no clear consensus on the optimal fasting time before sedation, decision making should balance the relatively low probability of aspiration with the patient's underlying risk factors, the timing and nature of recent oral intake, the urgency of the procedure, and the depth and length of sedation required.

PERSONNEL

- The minimum personnel present during deep sedation should be an emergency clinician and an ED nurse. When available, consider adding a separate emergency clinician who is solely dedicated to drug administration and patient monitoring.

PRESEDATION

- Physicians should perform a standard presedation assessment with special attention paid to the potential for airway management during deep sedation.
- Suction, airway, and resuscitation equipment should be available immediately.
- Preoxygenate the patient.
- Because propofol does not have analgesic properties, pretreatment with fentanyl (1 μg/kg) or coadministration with ketamine (0.5 mg/kg) should be considered for painful procedures.

ASA, *American Society of Anesthesiologists*; ED, *emergency department*.

- Assuming that capnography is in place to identify respiratory depression, high-flow oxygen is recommended because it has been shown to decrease the risk for hypoxia with propofol (number needed to benefit of 4).

PROPOFOL ADMINISTRATION: GENERAL

- Propofol induces sedation approximately 30 seconds after bolus injection, with typical resolution of clinical effects occurring within 6 minutes.
- The most common ED dosing is an initial bolus dose of 1 mg/kg followed by 0.5 mg/kg every 2 to 3 minutes as needed to achieve or maintain the desired level of sedation.
- Propofol is typically titrated to slurring of speech, lid ptosis, or both, depending on the depth of sedation and degree of relaxation needed for the procedure.

INTERACTIVE AND MECHANICAL MONITORING

- Patients should have their airway patency, oxygen saturation, electrocardiographic tracing, and level of consciousness monitored continuously.
- The addition of end-tidal carbon dioxide monitoring (capnography) can provide the earliest possible warning of impending airway and respiratory complications before clinical examination or pulse oximetry and is particularly important when supplemental oxygen negates pulse oximetry as a warning device.

POTENTIAL ADVERSE EFFECTS

- Respiratory depression or apnea leading to assisted ventilation (0% to 3.9%).
- Transient hypotension (2.2% to 6.5%).
- Emesis (0% to 0.5%).
- Pain with injection (2% to 20%).

RECOVERY AND DISCHARGE

- Patients receiving propofol should be monitored until they have returned to their baseline mental status.
- Qualified personnel should accompany patients who require transport before recovery.

Pediatric Use. Pentobarbital is the IV sedative of choice in many centers for diagnostic imaging in children.[70,73,79,94,95] It is regarded as superior to midazolam[73,79,80] or chloral hydrate for this indication.[73] Pentobarbital, like midazolam, is available in multiple routes of administration.

Adverse Effects. Like other barbiturates, pentobarbital can lead to respiratory depression and hypotension because it is a negative inotrope.[70,73,79,80]

Ultrashort-Acting Sedative-Hypnotic Agents

Ultrashort-acting sedatives (i.e., propofol, etomidate, thiopental, methohexital) can rapidly produce potent sedation when administered intravenously, and all exhibit rapid awakening (<5 minutes) after discontinuation of the drug. ED use

of these agents—propofol in particular—for a variety of common short, painful procedures has expanded dramatically in recent years because their brief yet profound obtundation creates superlative conditions.

Substantial controversy surrounded the early administration of these agents for ED PSA.[96] Proponents have cited their extremely rapid onset and recovery as enormous advantages over other sedatives. Critics have cited the level of continuous vigilance required to achieve a desired effect while simultaneously avoiding significant cardiopulmonary depression because these agents can result in rapid swings in levels of consciousness. Research that includes thousands of ED patients for propofol and hundreds for etomidate has subsequently demonstrated that the safety profiles of these agents are the same or better than those of other agents in the PSA

BOX 33-8 Procedure for Dissociative Sedation with Ketamine

DEFINITION OF DISSOCIATIVE SEDATION

- A trancelike cataleptic state induced by the dissociative agent ketamine and characterized by profound analgesia and amnesia with retention of protective airway reflexes, spontaneous respirations, and cardiopulmonary stability.

CHARACTERISTICS OF THE KETAMINE "DISSOCIATIVE STATE"

- Dissociation: After the administration of ketamine, the patient passes into a fugue state or trance. The eyes may remain open, but the patient does not respond.
- Catalepsy: Normal or slightly enhanced muscle tone is maintained. On occasion, the patient may move or be moved into a position that is self-maintaining. Occasional muscular clonus may be observed.
- Analgesia: Analgesia is typically substantial or complete.
- Amnesia: Total amnesia is typical.
- Maintenance of airway reflexes: Upper airway reflexes remain intact and may be slightly exaggerated. Intubation is unnecessary, but occasional repositioning of the head may be needed for optimal airway patency. Suctioning of hypersalivation may occasionally be necessary.
- Cardiovascular stability: Blood pressure and pulse rate are not decreased and are typically mildly increased.
- Nystagmus: Nystagmus is typical.

INDICATIONS

- Short, painful procedures, especially those requiring immobilization (e.g., facial laceration, burn débridement, fracture reduction, abscess incision and drainage, central line placement, tube thoracostomy).
- Examinations judged likely to produce excessive emotional disturbance (e.g., pediatric sexual assault examination).

CONTRAINDICATIONS: ABSOLUTE (RISKS ESSENTIALLY ALWAYS OUTWEIGH BENEFITS)

- Age younger than 3 months (higher risk for airway complications)
- Known or suspected schizophrenia, even if currently stable or controlled with medications (can exacerbate the condition).

CONTRAINDICATIONS: RELATIVE (RISKS MAY OUTWEIGH BENEFITS)

- Major procedures stimulating the posterior pharynx (e.g., endoscopy) increase the risk for laryngospasm, whereas typical minor ED oropharyngeal procedures do not.
- History of airway instability, tracheal surgery, or tracheal stenosis (presumed higher risk for airway complications).
- Active pulmonary infection or disease, including upper respiratory infection or asthma (higher risk for laryngospasm).
- Known or suspected cardiovascular disease, including angina, heart failure, or hypertension (exacerbation caused by the sympathomimetic properties of ketamine). Avoid ketamine in patients who are already hypertensive and in older adults with risk factors for coronary artery disease.
- Central nervous system masses, abnormalities, or hydrocephalus (increased intracranial pressure with ketamine).
- Glaucoma or acute globe injury (increased intraocular pressure with ketamine).
- Porphyria, thyroid disorder, or thyroid medication (enhanced sympathomimetic effect).

PERSONNEL

- Dissociative sedation requires two persons, one (a nurse) to monitor the patient and one (a physician) to perform the procedure. Both must know about ketamine's unique characteristics.

PRESEDATION

- Perform a standard presedation assessment.
- Educate accompanying family members about the unique characteristics of the dissociative state if they will be present during the procedure or recovery.
- Frame the dissociative encounter as a positive experience. Consider encouraging adults and older children to "plan" specific, pleasant dream topics in advance of sedation (believed to decrease unpleasant recovery reactions). Emphasize, especially to school-aged children and teenagers, that ketamine delivers sufficient analgesia, so there will be no pain.

KETAMINE ADMINISTRATION: GENERAL

- Ketamine is not administered until the physician is ready to begin the procedure because the onset of dissociation typically occurs rapidly.
- Ketamine is initially administered as a single IV loading dose or IM injection. There is no apparent benefit from attempts to titrate to effect.
- In settings in which IV access can be obtained with minimal upset, the IV route is preferable because recovery is faster and there is less emesis.
- The IM route is especially useful when IV access cannot be consistently obtained with minimal upset and in patients who are uncooperative or combative (e.g., the mentally disabled).
- IV access is unnecessary for children receiving IM ketamine. Because unpleasant recovery reactions are more common in adults, IV access is desirable in these patients to permit rapid treatment of these reactions should they occur.

KETAMINE ADMINISTRATION: IV ROUTE

- Administer an IV loading dose of 1.5 to 2.0 mg/kg in children or 1.0 mg/kg in adults, with this dose being administered during a 30- to 60-second period. More rapid administration produces high central nervous system levels and has been associated with respiratory depression or apnea.
- Additional incremental doses of ketamine may be administered (0.5 to 1.0 mg/kg) if initial sedation is inadequate or repeated doses are necessary to accomplish a longer procedure.

KETAMINE ADMINISTRATION: IM ROUTE

- Administer IM ketamine, 4 to 5 mg/kg in children; the IV route is preferred for adults.
- Repeat the IM ketamine dose (full or half dose) if sedation is inadequate after 5 to 10 minutes (unusual) or if additional doses are required.

COADMINISTERED MEDICATIONS

- Prophylactic anticholinergics are no longer recommended.
- Prophylactic benzodiazepines are no longer recommended for children; however, they should be available to treat rare, unpleasant recovery reactions should they occur. Prophylactic IV midazolam, 0.03 mg/kg, may be considered for adults (number needed to benefit, 6).

Continued

BOX 33-8 Procedure for Dissociative Sedation with Ketamine, cont'd

	ROUTE OF ADMINISTRATION	
	IV	IM
Advantages	Ease of repeated dosing, less vomiting, slightly faster recovery	No IV access necessary
Peak concentrations and clinical onset, minutes	1	5
Typical duration of effective dissociation (min)	5-10	20-30
Typical time from dose to discharge (min)	50-110	60-140

- Prophylactic ondansetron can slightly reduce the rate of vomiting (number needed to benefit, 9 or higher).

PROCEDURE
- Adjunctive physical immobilization may occasionally be needed to control random motion.
- An adjunctive local anesthetic is usually unnecessary when a dissociative dose is used.
- Suction equipment, oxygen, a bag-valve-mask device, and age-appropriate equipment for advanced airway management should be immediately available. Supplemental oxygen is not mandatory but may be used when capnography is used to monitor ventilation.

INTERACTIVE MONITORING
- Close observation of the airway and respirations by an experienced health care professional is mandatory until recovery is well established.
- Drapes should be positioned so that airway and chest motion can be visualized at all times.
- Occasional repositioning of the head or suctioning of the anterior pharynx may be indicated for optimal airway patency.

MECHANICAL MONITORING
- Maintain continuous monitoring (e.g., pulse oximetry, cardiac monitoring, capnography) until recovery is well established.

- The pulse and respiratory rate should both be recorded periodically throughout the procedure. Blood pressure measurements after the initial value are generally unnecessary because ketamine stimulates catecholamine release and does not depress the cardiovascular system in healthy patients.

POTENTIAL ADVERSE EFFECTS
Percent estimates are for children; corresponding adult estimates are not yet reliable enough to report.
- Airway misalignment requiring repositioning of the head (occasional)
- Transient laryngospasm (0.3%)
- Transient apnea or respiratory depression (0.8%)
- Hypersalivation (rare)
- Emesis, usually well into recovery (8.4%)
- Recovery agitation (mild in 6.3%, clinically important in 1.4%)
- Muscular hypertonicity and random, purposeless movements (common)
- Clonus, hiccupping, or short-lived nonallergic rash on the face and neck

RECOVERY
- Maintain minimal physical contact or other sensory disturbance.
- Maintain a quiet area with dim lighting, if possible.
- Advise parents or caretakers not to stimulate the patient prematurely.

DISCHARGE CRITERIA
- Return to the pretreatment level of verbalization and awareness
- Return to the pretreatment level of purposeful neuromuscular activity
- A predischarge requirement of tolerating oral fluids or being able to ambulate independently not required or recommended after dissociative sedation

DISCHARGE INSTRUCTIONS
- Nothing by mouth for approximately 2 hours
- Careful family observation and no independent ambulation for approximately 2 hours

Modified from Green SM, Roback MG, Kennedy RM, et al. Clinical practice guideline for emergency department ketamine dissociative sedation: 2011 update. Ann Emerg Med. 2011;57:449-461.
ASA, *American Society of Anesthesiologists*; ED, *emergency department*; IM, *intramuscular*; IV, *intravenous.*

pharmacopoeia.[21] Given the rapid onset and offset of propofol, consider (when available) an additional dedicated clinician (separate from the individual performing the procedure) to oversee administration of medication.[97]

Propofol

Pharmacology. Propofol is becoming an agent of choice for PSA in the ED because of its efficacy and safety profile (Fig. 33-3). When administered by IV bolus, its onset of action is typically within 30 seconds. The half-life for blood-brain equilibration is approximately 1 to 3 minutes, and its clinical effects typically resolve within 5 to 7 minutes. Longer procedures can be facilitated by repeated dosing. Patients are typically awake and alert within 15 minutes after discontinuation. Propofol exhibits inherent antiemetic and perhaps euphoric properties, and patient satisfaction is typically high. Propofol should be avoided in patients with known or suspected allergy to eggs or soy products.[22,97-104]

Figure 33-3 Propofol is emerging as an agent of choice for painful emergency department procedures. It is safe, effective, and very short acting. It can be cautiously combined with the short-acting narcotic fentanyl or with ketamine. All the safety caveats for procedural sedation and analgesia apply. The pain of a propofol injection can be minimized by choosing a large vein not on the dorsum of the hand and slowly injecting 2 to 3 mL of 2% lidocaine into the vein before injection of propofol.

Adult and Pediatric Use. Deep sedation can be achieved reliably in both adults and children with a single IV loading dose of propofol. Repeated bolus dosing is preferred, but an IV drip can be administered as needed to enhance or prolong sedation.[22,97-104]

Adverse Effects. Transient apnea and respiratory depression can occur with propofol but typically resolve spontaneously before intervention is necessary. Reported rates of assisted ventilation range from 0% to 4.6%.[97] Similarly, transient hypotension (via direct negative inotropy as well as arterial and venous dilation) is common but typically resolves spontaneously without treatment. Injection site pain is noted less frequently in the ED setting than in the operating room, where higher doses are generally administered.[22,97-104] Propofol usually causes pain on injection in awake individuals. Injecting slowly through a large vein, not a dorsal hand vein, and administering 2 to 3 mL of 2% lidocaine slowly into the vein before propofol infusion will lessen the pain of injection.

Etomidate
Pharmacology. When administered by IV bolus, the onset of action of etomidate is typically within 30 seconds, and patients are usually awake and alert within 30 minutes after discontinuation.

Adult Use. Deep sedation can be achieved reliably with single loading doses.[105-108] Dosing can be repeated as needed to enhance or prolong sedation. Etomidate may be somewhat less effective overall than propofol and, given its additional adverse effect of myoclonus, appears to be a less desirable choice than propofol for deep sedation.[21,38]

Pediatric Use. There is significantly less published experience with etomidate in children for ED PSA; however, its

safety and efficacy profile appears to be similar to that in adults.[109,110]

Adverse Effects. The primary adverse effects of etomidate are respiratory depression, myoclonus, nausea, and vomiting.[110,111] Respiratory depression has been reported to be less common with propofol PSA than with methohexital, fentanyl/midazolam, or etomidate.[112] Myoclonus is common yet generally benign, but it may be disconcerting and can interfere with the procedure. It consists of transient jerking or twitching movements that can be mistaken for seizure activity. Transient adrenal suppression occurs with etomidate in septic patients but appears to lack clinical significance for single doses when used for ED PSA.[21,111,113]

Thiopental and Methohexital
Pharmacology. Because of their lipid solubility, barbiturates are rapidly absorbed rectally. When given by the IV route, both thiopental and methohexital produce sedation within 1 minute. Clinical recovery is rapid ($\approx$15 minutes) as a result of rapid redistribution from the central nervous system to the periphery.

Adult Use. There is limited published experience using these IV barbiturates for ED PSA,[114] and propofol or etomidate would appear to be a better choice.

Pediatric Use. Rectal thiopental and methohexital can reliably produce sedation suitable for CT or MRI.[115-120] Respiratory depression is unusual when using typical doses (see Table 33-5) but can occur.[115,116,118-120] There is limited published experience using these IV barbiturates for ED PSA,[114] and propofol would appear to be a better choice.

Adverse Effects. Barbiturates cause potent respiratory depression; in one ED report, apnea occurred in 10% of patients.[121] Barbiturates also frequently cause hypotension at typical IV doses, so their use should be avoided whenever possible in patients with volume depletion or cardiovascular compromise.

Analgesic Agents
Fentanyl
Fentanyl is the most common opioid used for PSA because of its rapid onset, brief duration, rapid reversibility with naloxone, and lack of histamine release.[7] It is often combined with other agents such as propofol, etomidate, and midazolam to provide additional effect and pain relief. The effects of fentanyl can be reversed immediately with naloxone should excessive sedation or respiratory depression occur. The longer-duration opioids morphine and meperidine are preferred for nonprocedural or preprocedural pain control and are frequently given initially for acute analgesia followed by fentanyl to facilitate the needed procedure. Although longer-acting opioids can be readily used for analgesia during PSA, they will be associated with longer recovery times and a higher incidence of histamine-related effects (e.g., nausea and vomiting, hypotension, pruritus). Fentanyl lacks these effects and is therefore preferred.

Pharmacology. Fentanyl is 100 times more potent than morphine and has no intrinsic anxiolytic or amnestic properties. A single IV dose has a rapid onset (<30 seconds) with a peak at 2 to 3 minutes and brief clinical duration (20 to 40 minutes). This increase in potency and onset of action is in part related to its greater lipid solubility, which facilitates passage of the drug across the blood-brain barrier. The effects of fentanyl can be rapidly and completely reversed with opioid antagonists (e.g., naloxone, nalmefene).

Adult Use. Because of its pharmacokinetics, IV fentanyl is an ideal agent when analgesia is required for painful procedures; it can be easily and rapidly titrated.[7] Because anxiolysis and sedation do not occur at low doses (1 to 2 µg/kg), concurrent administration of a pure sedative, most commonly midazolam, is advisable, especially in children (see Box 33-6).

Pediatric Use. The combination of fentanyl and midazolam remains a popular PSA sedation regimen in children, with a strong safety and efficacy profile when both drugs are carefully titrated to effect.[6,92,122,123] Any necessary level of mild to deep sedation can be achieved with these agents.

Fentanyl is also available in an oral transmucosal preparation. Although this novel and noninvasive delivery route obviates the need for IV access, titration is difficult and its efficacy is variable.[124] Furthermore, the incidence of emesis is high (31% to 45%),[124,125] and consequently this formulation has never become popular for PSA.

Adverse Effects. Like all opioids, fentanyl can cause respiratory depression.[6,7,92,122,123] When used for PSA, standard interactive and mechanical monitoring is required. Because the opioid effect is most pronounced on the central nervous system respiratory centers, apnea precedes loss of consciousness. If apnea should occur, verbal or tactile stimulation should be attempted before the administration of opioid antagonists. As discussed earlier, caution must be exercised when using benzodiazepines and other PSA agents and opioids together because the risk for hypoxia and apnea is significantly greater than when either is used alone.[5,75]

In the absence of significant ethanol intoxication, hypovolemia, or concomitant drug ingestion, hypotension is rare, even with very large doses of fentanyl (doses of 50 µg/kg are common in adult and pediatric cardiac surgery). Because of its safe hemodynamic profile, fentanyl is an ideal analgesic agent for use in critically ill or injured patients. In addition, nausea and vomiting are rare in comparison to analgesia with morphine or meperidine. A commonly observed reaction to fentanyl is nasal pruritus, and patients frequently attempt to scratch their nose during the procedure.[7]

A rare side effect of fentanyl with potential for respiratory compromise is chest wall rigidity. This complication has not been problematic in the ED and is related to higher doses (>5 µg/kg as a bolus dose) than those used for PSA and has not been reported in any ED series.[6,7,122,123] If it should occur, chest wall rigidity can usually be reversed with opioid antagonists, positive pressure ventilation, or both. Equipment for urgent pharmacologic paralysis should be available if reversal and positive pressure ventilation are unsuccessful.

Diamorphine

Diamorphine is a nasal opioid that is currently available in the United Kingdom, Australia, New Zealand, and Canada, but not in the United States.[58,59,126] Diamorphine has an onset and duration of action similar to that of morphine; however, its higher water solubility permits potent doses to be delivered in the small (0.1 mL) volumes necessary for comfortable intranasal administration. In two studies of children and teenagers with fractures, intranasal diamorphine, 0.1 mg/kg, provided a similar level of analgesia with faster onset as IM morphine, 0.2 mg/kg. Intranasal spray administration was better tolerated than the injection, and there were no adverse events.[58,59,126] Diamorphine may prove to be a useful initial analgesic for children and teenagers with acute pain, although in practice, an IV line would most likely be established to permit titration to full pain relief and PSA for any procedures needed (e.g., fracture reduction). The role of diamorphine in adults remains to be determined.

Other Short-Acting Opioids

Sufentanil, alfentanil, and remifentanil are other short-acting opioids that have a potential role in PSA. Currently, however, there is insufficient published experience to warrant their routine use. Although intranasal sufentanil, 0.75 µg/kg, appeared promising in one small pediatric trial,[127] in another, doses of 1.5 µg/kg resulted in oxygen desaturation in 8 of the 10 children studied.[88] This low toxic-to-therapeutic ratio and inability to titrate would appear to limit the utility of intranasal sufentanil. In the one published report of IV remifentanil with midazolam for PSA, there was an unacceptably high incidence of hypoxemia.[128] Currently, there does not appear to be a clinically important advantage with these drugs versus fentanyl.

Ketamine

Pharmacology. Ketamine produces a unique state of cortical dissociation that permits painful procedures to be performed more consistently and effectively than with other PSA agents. This state of "dissociative sedation" is characterized by profound analgesia, sedation, amnesia, and immobilization (Fig. 33-4) and can be rapidly and reliably produced with IV or IM administration.[11] Ketamine is widely used worldwide and has demonstrated a remarkable safety profile in a variety of settings.[4,6,129-132] Clinicians administering ketamine must be especially knowledgeable about the unique actions of this drug and the numerous contraindications to its use (see Table 33-5).

Ketamine differs from other PSA agents in several important ways. First, it uniquely preserves cardiopulmonary stability. Upper airway muscular tone and protective airway reflexes are maintained. Spontaneous respiration is preserved, although when administered intravenously, ketamine must be given slowly (over a period of 30 to 60 seconds) to prevent respiratory depression. Second, it differs from other agents in that it lacks the characteristic dose-response continuum to progressive titration. At lower doses ketamine produces analgesia and disorientation. However, once a dosage threshold (≈1 to 1.5 mg/kg intravenously or 3 to 4 mg/kg intramuscularly) is achieved, the characteristic dissociative state appears. This dissociation has no observable levels of depth, and thus the only value of ketamine "titration" is to maintain the presence of the state over time. Finally, the dissociative state is not consistent with formal definitions of moderate sedation, deep sedation, or general anesthesia (see Table 33-1) and must therefore be considered from a different perspective than agents that exhibit the classic sedation continuum.[11,15]

Figure 33-4 A, Child undergoing insect removal from the ear under ketamine sedation. No child or adult can cooperate for this painful procedure, and general anesthesia is often the other option to ketamine. The blank stare is common. **B,** Insect successfully and atraumatically removed.

Ketamine is most effective and reliable when given intravenously or intramuscularly. Ketamine has a rapid circulation time when given intravenously, with onset of dissociation noted within 1 minute and effective procedural conditions lasting for about 10 to 15 minutes. When given intramuscularly, the same effect is achieved within 5 minutes, with effective procedural conditions for about 15 to 30 minutes. The typical duration from dosing to dischargeable recovery is 50 to 110 minutes when given intravenously and 60 to 140 minutes when given intramuscularly.[129,132]

Like the benzodiazepines, ketamine undergoes substantial first-pass hepatic metabolism. As a result, oral and rectal administration results in less predictable effectiveness and substantially higher doses are required. Clinical onset and recovery are considerably longer than when given parenterally, and thus these routes are rarely used in the ED.[91,133]

Ketamine can occasionally induce excessive salivation, and to combat this, some have historically coadministered atropine or glycopyrrolate. However, there is no evidence that either of these anticholinergic agents diminishes the risk for airway or respiratory adverse events,[134-136] and their routine prophylactic use is no longer recommended.[134] Instead, they can be reserved for treatment should excessive secretions occur.

Adult Use. The safety and efficacy of ketamine are well established in ED adults despite less published experience than in children.[134,137-143] Such experience is corroborated by the wide and successful use of ketamine in adults throughout the developing world for both minor and major surgery, particularly in areas lacking resources for inhalational anesthesia.[129,130,141,142]

Ketamine presents potential risk to patients with coronary artery disease because it is sympathomimetic and produces mild to moderate increases in blood pressure, heart rate, and myocardial oxygen consumption. Accordingly, other sedatives are preferred in the setting of known or possible ischemic heart disease, congestive heart failure, or hypertension.[134,142] There is no accepted maximum age for ketamine; instead, emergency physicians must weigh the risks and benefits of ketamine in older adults who may have unrecognized coronary artery disease.

Hallucinatory so-called emergence reactions have been reported in up to 30% of adults receiving ketamine (though rare in children) and can be fascinating and pleasurable or, alternatively, unpleasant and nightmarish.[129] In adults, coadministered IV midazolam (0.03 mg/kg) can modestly reduce their incidence (number needed to benefit of 6),[140] although not all such reactions are clinically important and this therapy should be considered optional.[144]

Pediatric Use. Ketamine is an ideal agent to facilitate short, painful procedures in children because of its superbly documented ED safety and efficacy.* The IM route is simple and effective, with venous access being unnecessary. IV administration is attractive because a lower cumulative dose can be used and recovery is faster than with the IM route. The primary caution with this route is that the initial bolus of ketamine must be administered slowly (over a 30- to 60-second period) or respiratory depression and transient apnea can occur.[132]

Unpleasant recovery reactions are uncommon in children and teenagers and are typically mild when they do occur.[146,147] Benzodiazepine coadministration does not measurably reduce the incidence of such reactions in children (unlike adults),[134,135,145-147] and these agents should be reserved for treating preprocedural anxiety or unpleasant reactions if they occur.[134]

Adverse Effects. In a metaanalysis of ketamine administration in 8282 pediatric patients, the overall incidence of airway and respiratory adverse events was 3.9%—primarily airway malalignment but also including transient laryngospasm (0.3%) and transient apnea (0.8%). None of these patients were intubated or had adverse sequelae.[134] The frequency of such events was slightly higher when unusually high doses of ketamine were administered; otherwise, there was no clinically important association with age, doses within the typically recommended range, or other clinical factors.

Vomiting was noted in 8.4% overall in this same metaanalysis, with early adolescence representing the greatest risk and a lower incidence of emesis occurring in younger and

---

*References 4, 6, 129, 132, 134, 135, 145.

older children.[145] It occurs more frequently with the IM route than with the IV route, and there is no evidence to support any dose relationship within the usual range of clinically administered doses.[145] When emesis occurs, it is typically late during the recovery phase when the patient is alert and can clear the airway without assistance.[134] Vomiting does occur in some patients after discharge, including some who do not vomit in the ED.[134] Although ondansetron prophylaxis (0.15 mg/kg up to a maximum of 4 mg intravenously) does reduce vomiting with ketamine, the magnitude of this effect is modest (number needed to benefit of 13), and thus it cannot be considered mandatory.[148]

In 40 years of regular use there have been no documented reports of clinically significant ketamine-associated aspiration in patients without established contraindications.[134] Because of its unique preservation of protective airway reflexes, ketamine may be preferred over other agents for urgent or emergency procedures when fasting is not ensured.[4,5,129]

Mild agitation (whimpering or crying) during recovery was noted in 7.6% of children in the large metaanalysis, with more pronounced agitation occurring in 1.4%. Such recovery reactions are not related to age, dose, or other factors to any clinically important degree, except for a higher incidence with subdissociative (<3 mg/kg intramuscularly) dosing.[145] In contrast to traditional thinking, adolescents are not at substantially higher risk.[145]

Despite the modest impact of prophylactic midazolam in reducing adult recovery agitation, in children, two controlled trials and a large metaanalysis failed to note even a trend toward a measurable benefit.[145-147] Children have far fewer recovery reactions than adults do, and their reactions are milder when they do occur. Midazolam is therefore not recommended for routine prophylaxis but is optimally reserved to treat unpleasant ketamine-associated recovery reactions when they do rarely occur.[134]

Ketamine is relatively contraindicated in patients with central nervous system masses, abnormalities, or hydrocephalus; however, there is no compelling evidence that it needs to be avoided in the setting of acute head trauma.[134,149,150] Repeated reports that ketamine can increase intracranial pressure have prompted traditional caution against use of this drug in the setting of real or potential neurologic compromise,[1,5,129,134,151-153] and there are case reports of deterioration in patients with hydrocephalus.[154,155] However, newer suggestive evidence indicates that in most patients the resulting increases in pressure are minimal, assuming normal ventilation,[149,150,154,156] and that the corresponding cerebral vasodilatory effect of ketamine may actually improve overall cerebral perfusion.[149,150]

Dissociative sedation may represent a risk in patients with acute globe injury or glaucoma given the inconclusive and conflicting evidence of increased intraocular pressure with ketamine.[157-161]

Ketamine-Propofol Combination (Ketofol) for Procedural Sedation and Analgesia in the ED

The PSA combination of ketamine and propofol, referred to by the portmanteau "ketofol," is both popular and controversial.[162] There is no doubt that ketofol is safe and effective in both adults and children[163-170]; instead, the dispute is whether the combination exhibits any clinically important advantage over use of either drug alone.[162]

An important allure to ketofol proponents is how these two completely different sedatives balance each other's deficits. Propofol is a superb sedative but lacks the analgesia that ketamine can amply provide. Ketamine mitigates propofol-induced hypotension, and propofol mitigates ketamine-induced vomiting and recovery agitation. The drugs exhibit synergistic and perhaps smoother sedation,[164] and the combination has the theoretical benefits of minimizing the propofol dose and obviating the need for coadministered opioids.[162]

Critics note that the existing ketofol literature fails to demonstrate superior procedural conditions or less respiratory depression than occurs with each drug alone[163] and question the added complexity of administering two drugs when one is sufficient. They argue that the purported advantages related to hemodynamics and the total propofol dose are not clinically important. Ketofol uses a subdissociative dose of ketamine, and thus ketamine may just be replacing fentanyl as an analgesic rather than as a sedative.[162]

Ketofol dosing is based on weight for both adults and children. One regimen uses an initial IV loading dose of ketamine of 0.5 mg/kg, followed by a 0.5- to 1.0-mg/kg IV propofol bolus, with subsequent titration of propofol alone.[164-166,168] A second strategy mixes propofol and ketamine together 1:1 in the same syringe (both at 10-mg/mL concentrations) and then titrates in increments of 0.25 mg/kg of each drug to a usual effective dose of about 0.75 mg/kg.[162,167,169,170]

Careful observation for respiratory depression is required, and the precautions listed for both agents should be stringently observed.

Nitrous Oxide

Pharmacology. Inhaled nitrous oxide provides anxiolysis and mild analgesia. It is commonly dispensed at concentrations between 30% and 50%, with oxygen composing the remainder of the mixture. Nitrous oxide quickly diffuses across biologic membranes and, accordingly, has a rapid onset of action (30 to 60 seconds). Its maximum effect occurs after about 5 minutes, and the clinical effect wears off quickly on discontinuation. At typical PSA concentrations, there is preservation of hemodynamic status, spontaneous respirations, and protective airway reflexes.[171-174] Nitrous oxide is widely used in dentistry at higher concentrations.[175]

Nitrous oxide has an excellent safety profile; however, as a sole agent, it cannot reliably produce adequate procedural conditions.[171-174] Given its relatively weak analgesic properties, in many cases nitrous oxide needs to be supplemented with an IV opioid or local or regional anesthesia (or both).

Adult and Cooperative Child Use. The safest method of administering nitrous oxide is via a self-administered demand-valve mask (Fig. 33-5).[172-174] Patients must generate a negative pressure of 3 to 5 cm H_2O within the handheld mask or mouthpiece to activate the flow of gas. They can thus self-titrate the dose by inhaling at will through the mask. Naturally, this will be effective only when the patient is cooperative. This technique provides a built-in fail-safe measure in that if patients become somnolent, the mask will fall from their face and gas delivery will cease.

Nitrous oxide can be used as an adjunctive anxiolytic during mildly painful procedures or during the administration

Figure 33-6 Nitrous oxide/oxygen continuous-flow system.

Figure 33-5 A, Demand-flow nitrous oxide/oxygen system. **B,** Example of a free mask for a nitrous oxide system. The patient must hold the mask in contact with the face. (*A, Courtesy of Nitronox delivery system by Matrx Medical, division of Henry Schein. matrx2@aol.com.*)

of local or regional anesthesia for other procedures. It may also be administered during difficult or high-anxiety procedures such as pelvic examination or during difficult IV attempts.

A double-tank system is commonly used to deliver the nitrous oxide and oxygen mixture. The system relies on a mixing valve preset to deliver a fixed ratio and will deliver gas only when oxygen is flowing. The double-tank system contains a fail-safe device that automatically stops the flow of nitrous oxide when the oxygen supply is depleted.

Uncooperative Child Use. The primary limitation of self-administration is that it is ineffective in uncooperative patients,

including most frightened young children. Continuous-flow nitrous oxide via a mask strapped over the nose or over the nose and mouth has been used in this population (Fig. 33-6).[176-179] Nitrous oxide can effectively produce moderate or deep sedation when administered in this manner; however, this technique necessitates an additional clinician dedicated to continuous gas titration to avoid oversedation. In addition, it appears that the continuous-flow technique is associated with a higher rate of emesis (10%) than self-administration is (0% to 4%),[171-174,176-179] which may be a potential hazard if a mask is strapped tightly over the child's mouth.[177]

Adverse Effects and Precautions. A number of generally minor adverse effects may be seen, including nausea, dizziness, changes in voice, euphoria, and laughter.[171-174] Nitrous oxide should be avoided in patients with closed-space disease such as bowel obstruction, middle ear disease, pneumothorax, or pneumocephalus. Because of its property of high diffusibility, it has the potential to increase the size of the closed space. This should be unlikely for short-term use in typical PSA concentrations.

Make sure that a scavenging system is in place to collect exhaled nitrous oxide, and take care to ensure compliance with occupational safety regulations. Avoid exposure of pregnant ED staff members to nitrous oxide because nitrous oxide is a known teratogen and mutagen.

Although the potential for abuse by ED staff exists, such abuse is rare if simple steps are taken. As with other agents, maintain a strict protocol of accountability. Add a simple locking device to the cylinders of gas. In addition, lock the delivery valve or mouthpiece in the same location as controlled substances.

Antagonists

Do not routinely administer reversal agents after the administration of opioids or benzodiazepines for PSA, but rather reserve them for the rare situations of oversedation or significant respiratory depression. The downside of reversal agents is that one must wait for the antagonist to dissipate before analyzing any residual effect of the PSA agent, with the caveat that long-acting PSA agents may last longer than the administered antagonist. Serious resedation after antagonism is not usually an issue with fentanyl or midazolam, but caution is advised, especially when large doses of PSA agents and large doses of antagonists have been used. Obviously, the length of observation varies with the amount of antagonist that has been administered.

Naloxone

Naloxone is an antagonist that competitively displaces opioids from opiate receptors. It rapidly reverses the analgesic and respiratory depressant effects of opioids. It may be administered intravenously, intramuscularly, subcutaneously, or even sublingually if needed,[163] and dosing has been standardized for infants and children.[180] Naloxone will not induce systemic opioid withdrawal symptoms in a patient without preexisting physiologic dependence. However, some patients will experience nausea with opioid reversal, and patients with persistent pain after their procedure will be quite uncomfortable. Rapid reversal may also lead to return of anxiety and stimulation of the sympathetic nervous system. If the situation permits, careful titration of small amounts of naloxone (0.1-mg aliquots intravenously) may permit partial rather than complete reversal. The only absolute contraindication to the use of naloxone is administration to a neonate born to an opioid-dependent mother because of the risk of precipitating life-threatening opioid withdrawal. The length of observation is dose related, but usually no more than 60 to 90 minutes after reversal will be sufficient if no more than 1 mg of naloxone has been administered intravenously.

Nalmefene

Nalmefene is a long-acting opioid antagonist with a duration of action significantly longer than that of naloxone.[181,182] Nalmefene may be given intravenously, intramuscularly, or subcutaneously, although intravenously is the preferred route.[182,183] Intravenously, it can be titrated in incremental doses of 0.25 µg/kg every 2 to 5 minutes until the desired effect is attained. Although either naloxone or nalmefene will reverse the analgesia of opioids, naloxone is the preferred agent. For ED PSA, short-acting opioids such as fentanyl are commonly used, and administration of a reversal agent with a duration of action as prolonged as that of nalmefene does not confer any additional benefit. Furthermore, nalmefene would interfere with postprocedure control of pain with opioids.

Flumazenil

Flumazenil is a benzodiazepine antagonist that can promptly reverse benzodiazepine-induced sedation and respiratory depression.[1,15,184,185] In the setting of PSA, flumazenil is a safe and effective method of reversing oversedation caused by benzodiazepines. It is not routinely used to reverse PSA because of the potential for resedation, and many clinicians prefer to allow patients to recover on their own. Flumazenil has not been shown to substantially decrease the time of observation in the ED required for a patient undergoing PSA. Flumazenil lowers the seizure threshold and may rarely lead to life-threatening seizures. It should be avoided in patients with known benzodiazepine dependence, seizure disorder, cyclic antidepressant overdose, and elevated intracranial pressure.[165] It should also be given cautiously to patients who are taking medications known to lower the seizure threshold (cyclosporine, tricyclic antidepressants, propoxyphene, theophylline, isoniazid, lithium).[186] These issues, however, are not usually involved in PSA in the ED. It has not been shown that simply taking therapeutic doses of these medications contraindicates the use of flumazenil, but flumazenil-induced seizures are generally associated only with drug overdose. Rapid reversal may also lead to return of anxiety and sympathetic stimulation. If the situation permits, careful titration of small amounts of flumazenil (0.1- to 0.2-mg aliquots intravenously) will reduce the risk for adverse effects and may permit partial rather than complete reversal. Observation times vary. For example, 1 hour after reversal will allow accurate assessment of residual sedation if less than 1 mg of flumazenil has been used to reverse conscious sedation with midazolam.

References are availabel at www.expertconsult.com

Soft Tissue Procedures

CHAPTER 34

Principles of Wound Management

Richard L. Lammers and Zachary E. Smith

Management of acute traumatic wounds is one of the most common procedures in emergency medicine. Although many aspects of traumatic wound management remain controversial, the clinician can follow some basic principles to maximize the chance for successful healing. The purpose of this chapter is to give the clinician a general approach to wound care and to describe appropriate indications and techniques for wound management.

Wound care involves much more than closure of divided skin. The primary goal of wound care is not technical repair of the wound but to provide optimal conditions so that the natural reparative processes of the wound may proceed. The cornerstones of wound care are cleaning, débridement, closure (when appropriate), and protection. The primary objectives in wound care are to

1. Preserve viable tissue and remove nonviable tissue
2. Restore tissue continuity and function
3. Optimize conditions for the development of wound strength
4. Prevent excessive or prolonged inflammation
5. Avoid infection and other impediments to healing
6. Minimize scar formation
7. Provide suitable anesthesia during wound management

Patients who seek care in the emergency department (ED) because of acute wounds report that their top priorities include prevention of infection, return to normal function, a good cosmetic outcome, and minimal pain during repair.[1,2] This chapter reviews the current strategies for attaining these goals.

BACKGROUND: WOUND HEALING

For centuries, victims of wounds commonly experienced inflammation, infection, and extreme scarring; in fact, these processes were considered part of normal wound repair. Only in the late 19th century did surgeons first realize that sepsis could be separated from healing.[3] Emergency clinicians should have a basic understanding of the process of wound healing. Highlights of this complex phenomenon as they relate to clinical decision making are presented here (Fig. 34-1).

Wounds extending beneath the epithelium heal by forming scar tissue. Inflammation, epithelialization, fibroplasia, contraction, and scar maturation constitute the five stages of this natural repair process.[3-5] Inflammation is a beneficial response that removes bacteria, foreign debris, and devitalized tissue, essentially a biologic débridement. Polymorphonuclear and mononuclear leukocytes concentrate at the site of injury and phagocytose dead and dying tissue, foreign material, and bacteria in the wound.[6]

As white blood cells die, their intracellular contents are released into the wound. When in excessive amount, the contents form the purulence characteristic of infected wounds. Some exudate is expected even in the absence of bacterial invasion, but infection with accumulation of pus interferes with epithelialization and fibroplasia and impairs wound healing. Wounds contaminated with significant numbers of bacteria or foreign material may undergo a prolonged or persistent inflammatory response and not heal. Granuloma formation surrounding retained sutures is an example of chronic inflammation.[7]

While white blood cells are removing debris within the wound, epithelial cells at the surface of the wound begin to migrate across the tissue defect. In most sutured wounds, the surface of the wound develops an epithelial covering impermeable to water within 24 to 48 hours. Surface debris, dead tissue, and eschar formation can impair this process. The epithelium thickens and grows downward into the wound along the course of skin sutures. Although there is some "adhesiveness" at the wound edges during the first few days, this is eventually lost because of fibrinolysis.

By the fourth or fifth day, newly transformed fibroblasts in the wound begin synthesizing collagen and protein polysaccharides, thereby initiating the stage of scar formation known as *fibroplasia*. Collagen is the predominant component of scar tissue. Wound strength is a balance between the lysis of old collagen and the synthesis of new collagen to "weld" the edges of the wound together. The amount of scar tissue that forms is influenced by physical forces (e.g., the stresses imposed by movement) acting across the wound. In contrast, a wound not physically closed by sutures or other means heals by secondary intention and closes by contraction. *Contraction* consists of movement of the skin edges toward the center of the defect, primarily in the direction of underlying muscle.

Significant gains in tensile strength do not begin until approximately the fifth day after the injury. Strength increases

HEALING BY FIRST INTENTION   HEALING BY SECOND INTENTION

Figure 34-1 Steps in wound healing by first intention (*left*) and second intention (*right*). Note the large amounts of granulation tissue and wound contraction in healing by secondary intention.

Figure 34-2 Graphic representation of the various phases of wound healing. Note that the tensile strength of scar tissue never reaches that of unwounded skin. The values of tensile strength displayed are approximate and demonstrate the general concept of wound healing.

rapidly for 6 to 17 days, more slowly for an additional 10 to 14 days, and almost imperceptibly for as long as 2 years (Fig. 34-2). The strength of scar tissue never quite reaches that of unwounded skin. Although the process of collagen formation is essentially completed within 21 to 28 days, the scar widens for another month, and collagen continues to remodel and strengthen the wound for up to 1 year.[3,7]

Decisions regarding the optimal time for suture removal and the need for continued support of the wound with tape are influenced by (1) the tensile strength of the wound, (2) the period of scar widening, and (3) the cosmetically unacceptable effect of epithelialization along the suture track. Scars are quite red and noticeable at 3 to 8 weeks after closure. The appearance of a scar should not be judged before the scar is well into its remodeling phase. The cosmetic appearance of wounds 6 to 9 months after injury cannot be predicted at the time of suture removal.[8] Therefore, scar revision, if necessary, should be postponed until 6 to 12 months after injury.

One of the most important factors in predicting the cosmetic result of a wound is its location.[9] In general, wounds on concave surfaces heal with better cosmetic results than do wounds on convex surfaces. Other factors that affect cosmesis include wound size, wound depth, and skin color.[10] Small, superficial wounds in lax, light-colored skin, especially areas where the skin is thin, result in less noticeable scars. Wounds on convex surfaces look better after primary closure than after secondary healing. Static and dynamic forces, along with the propensity toward keloid formation, may influence the long-term cosmetic appearance of wounds more than the surgical skills of the clinician who repaired the wound.[8] Repigmentation occurs over a period of 3 to 5 years, even in large wounds that heal by secondary intention.[10] In the patient care instructions it is important to emphasize the need for wearing sunscreen over the scar, especially during the early years, because unprotected exposure to the sun can alter the pigmentation as the wound heals and result in noticeably darker pigmentation than the surrounding skin.

INITIAL EVALUATION

The approach to management of a particular wound and the decision to close a wound immediately or after a period of observation are based primarily on factors that affect the risk for infection and secondarily on cosmesis and long-term functionality. The history and physical examination should be directed toward identifying these factors. Some wounds may appear benign but conceal extensive and devastating underlying tissue damage. The discovery that an extremity wound was produced by a roller or wringer device, a high-pressure injection gun, high-voltage electricity, heavy and prolonged compressive force, or the bite of a human or a potentially rabid animal radically alters the overall management of the patient. The American College of Emergency Physicians' "Clinical Policy for the Initial Approach to Patients Presenting with Penetrating Extremity Trauma" provides a useful approach to the evaluation of all wounds.[11]

History

In the initial evaluation of a wound, the clinician should identify all the extrinsic and intrinsic factors that jeopardize healing and promote infection, including (1) the mechanism of injury, (2) the time of injury, (3) the environment in which the wound occurred, and (4) the patient's immune status.

Wound Age

In general, the likelihood of a wound infection increases with time from the injury to definitive wound care.[12] Definitive wound care does not necessarily mean suturing. Some wounds should never be sutured, such as small contaminated lacerations on the bottom of the foot, whereas others can be sutured many hours after the injury without increasing infection rates. A delay in *wound cleaning* is the most important factor and may allow bacteria contaminating the wound to proliferate. A delay of only a few hours in the treatment of a heavily contaminated wound can increase the risk for infection. Although no scientific data exist to fully answer the question and there is no definitively accepted standard, it appears reasonable that most wounds that are not grossly contaminated can probably be closed safely 6 to 8 hours after injury if the wound can be adequately cleaned. In contrast, some evidence suggests that wounds in highly vascular regions such as the face and scalp can be closed without increased risk for as long as 24 hours after injury.[13] Contrary to popular belief, the "golden period"—the maximum time after injury that a wound may be closed safely without significant risk for infection—is not a fixed number of hours.[14]

Many factors affect risk for infection, and closure decisions should not be based solely on time considerations. Delayed primary closure is a reasonable alternative when there is clinical concern regarding closure at initial assessment. All data accumulated in the initial evaluation, both historical and physical, must be considered when making the decision to close a wound in a particular patient.[12] In addition, the techniques of wound care may extend the period; with skillful cleaning and débridement, a clinician may be able to convert a contaminated wound to a clean wound that can be safely closed in the ED.[5] *In summary, any time frames offered are suggestions, and clinical judgment and the potential for wound infection should be incorporated into the final decision making.*

Other Historical Factors

Other factors that affect wound healing or the risk for infection include the patient's age and state of health. Patient age appears to be an important factor in host resistance to infection, and individuals who are at the extremes of age, such as young children and the elderly, have the greatest risk for infection.[12,15] Infection rates are reported to be higher in patients with concurrent medical conditions, such as diabetes mellitus, immunologic deficiencies, malnutrition, anemia, uremia, congestive heart failure, cirrhosis, malignancy, alcoholism, arteriosclerosis, arteritis, collagen vascular disease, chronic granulomatous disease, smoking, chronic hypoxia, renal failure, liver failure, and morbid obesity, as well as in patients who are taking steroids or immunosuppressive drugs or undergoing radiation therapy. Shock, remote trauma, distant infection, bacteremia, retained foreign bodies, denervation, and peripheral vascular disease also increase wound infection rates and slow the healing process.[6,12,15-17]

In most instances the clinician cannot totally negate infection risks but can favorably affect the rate and extent of infection with adequate wound care. Unfortunately, simply prescribing antibiotics in the hope that infection will somehow be averted is an unrealistic expectation.

Additional information pertinent to decision making in wound management includes the following:

- *Current medications* (specifically, anticoagulants and immunosuppressive drugs)
- *Allergies* (especially to local anesthetics, antiseptics, analgesics, antibiotics, and tape)
- *Tetanus immunization status*
- *Potential exposure to rabies* (in bite wounds and mucosal exposures)
- *Potential foreign bodies* embedded in the wound, especially when the mechanism of injury is unknown or the injury was associated with breaking glass or vegetative matter[18]
- *Previous injuries and deformities* (especially with extremity and facial injuries)
- *Associated injuries* (underlying fracture, joint penetration)
- *Other factors* (availability for follow-up, patient understanding of wound care, compliance)

Physical Examination

All wounds should be examined for the amount of tissue destruction, degree of contamination, and damage to underlying structures. The examiner should wear clean or sterile gloves and avoid droplet contamination from the mouth. Examine the wound under good lighting and after the bleeding is controlled. Create a bloodless field, if necessary, with a tourniquet. Assess distal perfusion and motor and sensory function and document your findings during the evaluation of extremity wounds and before the use of anesthetics.

Mechanism of Injury and Classification of Wounds

The magnitude and direction of the injuring force and the volume of tissue on which the force is distributed determine the type of wound sustained. Three types of mechanical force—shear, tension, and compression—produce soft tissue injury. The resulting disruption or loss of tissue determines the configuration of the wound. Wounds may be classified into six categories:

1. *Abrasions.* Wounds caused by forces applied in opposite directions result in the loss of epidermis and possibly dermis (e.g., grinding of skin against a road surface).

2. *Lacerations.* Wounds caused by shear forces produce a tear in tissues. Little energy is required to produce a wound by shear forces (e.g., a knife cut). Consequently, little tissue damage occurs at the wound edge, the margins are sharp, and the wound appears "tidy." Tensile and compressive forces also cause separation of the tissues. The energy required to disrupt tissue by tensile or compressive forces (e.g., forehead hitting a dashboard) is considerably greater than that required for tissue disruption by shear forces because the energy is distributed over a larger volume. These lacerations often have jagged, contused, "untidy" edges, which have a higher risk for infection.[15]

3. *Crush wounds.* Wounds caused by the impact of an object against tissue, particularly over a bony surface, compress the tissue. These wounds may contain contused or partially devitalized tissue.

4. *Puncture wounds.* Wounds with a small opening whose depth cannot be entirely visualized are caused by a combination of forces. They are particularly prone to infection.

5. *Avulsions.* Avulsions are wounds in which a portion of tissue is completely separated from its base, which is lost, or left with a narrow base of attachment (a flap). Shear and tensile forces cause avulsions.[19] Skin tear avulsions often result from low-force friction or shearing forces that separate the layers of the skin (epidermis and dermis) from the underlying tissue. These wounds often occur in older adults as a result of minimal impact and vulnerable skin.

6. *Combination wounds.* Wounds can also have a combination of configurations. For example, a stellate laceration caused by compression of soft tissue against underlying bone can create wounds with elements of both crush injury and tissue separation. Missile wounds involve a combination of shear, tensile, and compressive forces that puncture, crush, and sometimes avulse tissue.[20]

Contaminants (Bacteria and Foreign Material)

Infection rates in studies of traumatic wounds range from 1% to 38%. Numerous factors affect the risk for wound infection, but the primary determinants of infection are the amount of bacteria and dead tissue remaining in the wound,[21] the patient's immune response, and local tissue perfusion.

Essentially all traumatic wounds are contaminated with bacteria to some extent. The number of bacteria remaining in the wound at the time of closure is directly related to the risk for infection. A critical number of bacteria must be present in a wound before a soft tissue infection develops. In experimental wounds, fewer bacteria are required to infect wounds caused by a compressive force ($\geq 10^4$ bacteria/g of tissue) than by a shear force ($\geq 10^6$).[22]

The nature and amount of foreign material contaminating the wound often determine the type and quantity of bacteria implanted. In general, visible contamination of a wound increases the risk for infection.[15] The presence of undetected, reactive foreign bodies in sutured wounds almost guarantees an infection. Although bullet or glass fragments by themselves rarely produce wound infection, these foreign bodies may carry particles of clothing, gun wadding, or soil into the wound. Minute amounts of organic or vegetative matter, feces, or saliva carry highly infective doses of bacteria. The bacterial inoculum from human bites often contains 100

million or more organisms per milliliter of saliva.[23] Inorganic particulate matter, such as sand or road surface grease, usually introduces few bacteria into a wound and has little chemical reactivity. These contaminants are relatively innocuous. Soil that contains a large proportion of clay particles or a high organic content (such as that found in swamps, bogs, and marshes), however, has a high risk for infection.[24]

In industrialized countries, most wounds encountered in the practice of emergency medicine have low initial bacterial counts. If wound cleaning and removal of devitalized tissue are instituted before bacteria within the wound enter their accelerated growth phase (3 to 12 hours after the injury), bacterial counts will generally remain below the threshold needed to initiate infection.[11,25]

Devitalized Tissue

Devitalized and necrotic tissue in a traumatic wound should be identified and removed. If left in place, it will allow bacteria to proliferate, inhibit leukocyte phagocytosis, and create an anaerobic environment suitable for certain bacterial species.[20,21]

Wound Location

The anatomic location of the wound has considerable importance in the risk for infection. Bacterial densities on the surface of the skin range from a few thousand to millions per square centimeter.[24] Distal extremity wounds are more at risk for the development of wound infections than are injuries on most other parts of the body.[12,26] The high vascularity in areas such as the scalp or perineum appears to offset the risk posed by the large numbers of endogenous microflora, whereas wounds in ischemic tissue are notoriously susceptible to infection.[27]

Underlying Structures

If injury to underlying structures such as nerves, vessels, tendons, joints, bones, or ducts is found, the clinician may choose to forego wound closure and consult a surgical specialist (Fig. 34-3). Procedures such as joint space irrigation, reduction and débridement of compound fractures, neurorrhaphy, vascular anastomosis, and flexor tendon repair are best accomplished in the controlled setting of the operating room, where optimal lighting, proper instruments, and assistance are available.[20]

CLEANING

Clean the wound as soon as possible after evaluation. Although most wounds are initially contaminated with less than an infective dose of bacteria, given time and the appropriate wound environment, bacterial counts may quickly rise to infective levels. The goals of wound cleaning and débridement are (1) to remove bacteria and reduce their numbers below the level associated with infection and (2) to remove particulate matter and tissue debris that would lengthen the inflammatory stage of healing or allow the growth of bacteria beyond the critical threshold.[17] There are two general wound-cleansing techniques—compression and irrigation. Compression involves gently pressing premoistened gauze to the wound to remove surface debris. If necessary, this can be followed by gentle and judicious scrubbing. Irrigation is recommended for most wounds and involves a steady flow of solution across the surface of the wound. This important step in wound management provides hydration to the wound, removes

Figure 34-3 This patient had weak, hesitant, but full flexion of the finger, thus suggesting at least a partial tendon laceration. The tendon was nearly 90% lacerated (*arrow*) and would have ruptured with any stress. Close examination of this wound, with careful blunt dissection down to the tendon itself *and the finger in the position of injury*, revealed significant trauma to the delicate flexor tendon that requires consultation with a specialist. Use of a proximal tourniquet for a bloodless field and instruments to explore finger wounds is mandatory to increase sensitivity for finding injury to deep structures. This wound can be repaired within a few days, but if discovered weeks later, problems are certain. When in doubt, always diagnose a potential tendon injury and seek consultation.

Figure 34-4 The ideal setup for evaluation and repair of a laceration is a supine patient, a seated clinician at the correct height for the procedure, and a bloodless field with good lighting.

deeper debris, and aids in visual examination while reducing the risk for infection. Normal saline or tap water is often used as the irrigation fluid.

Soaking a wound in a saline or antiseptic solution before the clinician arrives is of little value and may actually increase bacterial counts, so it is not recommended as a routine practice.[28]

Patient Preparation

Before examining, cleaning, exploring, or repairing a wound, explain the procedure to the patient to allay fears and encourage cooperation. In general, all wound care should be performed with the patient in a supine position because fainting is a common occurrence during wound preparation and repair (Fig. 34-4). Relatives and friends can be allowed to stay with the patient, but they should be cautioned to report any dizziness or nausea, and they should remain seated throughout the procedure.

Anyone cleaning, irrigating, or suturing wounds should wear protective eyewear, a mask, and gloves because virtually any patient may be seropositive for human immunodeficiency virus (HIV). Although mucosal exposure to blood or tissue products that are contaminated by HIV is considered a relatively low risk for subsequent infection, universal precautions are currently recommended.

Thorough cleansing of bacteria, soil, and other contaminants from a wound cannot be accomplished without the patient's cooperation. Scrubbing most open wounds is painful, and the patient's natural response is to withdraw the injured area away from the provider. Local or regional anesthesia should precede examination and cleansing of a wound. Despite adequate anesthesia, the patient may be too apprehensive to

cooperate. In this case, explain the wound-cleansing procedure and assure the patient that everything possible will be done to minimize pain. If reassurance does not alleviate the fears of young children, consider both sedation and physical restraining devices.

Mechanical Scrubbing

Initially, scrub a wide area of skin surface surrounding the wound with an antiseptic solution to remove contaminants that might be transferred into the wound by instruments, suture material, dressings, or the clinician's gloved hand during wound management. Minimal aseptic technique requires the use of gloves during the cleaning procedure. It is important to remove all nonabsorbable particulate matter; any such material left in the dermis may be retained in the healed tissue and result in a disfiguring "tattoo" effect.[7] Scrubbing the internal surface of a wound is controversial. Although scrubbing a wound with an antiseptic-soaked sponge does remove foreign particulates, bacteria, and tissue debris, an abrasive sponge may inflict more damage on the tissue and become a portal for inflammation and infection.[29,30]

Mechanical scrubbing should be reserved for wounds contaminated with significant amounts of bacteria or foreign material (Fig. 34-5A and B). If irrigation alone is ineffective in removing visible contaminants from a wound, scrub the wound. Because the amount of damage inflicted on tissues by scrubbing correlates with the porosity of the sponge, a fine-pore sponge (e.g., 90 pores/inch) should be used to minimize tissue abrasion.[29,31] Detergents have an advantage over saline in that they minimize friction between the sponge and tissue, thereby limiting damage to tissue during scrubbing. Detergents also dissolve particles and thus help dislodge them from the surface of the wound. Unfortunately, many of the detergents available are toxic to tissues.[29,32] Use caution when considering detergents.

Antiseptics during Cleaning

For many years, antiseptic solutions have been used for their antimicrobial properties in and around wounds (Table 34-1).

WOUND CLEANSING: MECHANICAL SCRUBBING AND IRRIGATION

Grossly contaminated wounds such as this need to be thoroughly cleansed prior to repair, by mechanical scrubbing and/or irrigation.

Reserve mechanical scrubbing for wounds contaminated with significant amounts of bacteria or foreign material. Use a fine-pore sponge (e.g., 90 pores/inch) to minimize tissue abrasion.

Top, ZeroWet splash shield attached to end of a syringe. The shield is held near or against the skin and protects the user from splashes from the high-pressure laminar flow nozzle. *Bottom*, a makeshift splash protector can be made from a medication cup.

Use of the ZeroWet device. Note that the clinician is holding the laceration open with forceps to allow irrigation of the deep structures.

Tap water and nonsterile gloves are commonly used to copiously irrigate wounds of the extremities by taking advantage of the volume and force parameters from the faucet. Anesthetize lacerations before cleaning. Be mindful of the potential for the patient to faint.

For foot wounds, the patient is placed on a stretcher and wheeled to the sink.

Figure 34-5 A-F, Wound cleansing: mechanical scrubbing and irrigation.

TABLE 34-1 Summary of Agents Used for Wound Care

AGENT	BIOLOGIC ACTIVITY	TISSUE TOXICITY*	SYSTEMIC TOXICITY*	POTENTIAL USES	COMMENTS
Povidone-iodine surgical scrub (Betadine 7.5%)	Virucidal; strongly bactericidal against gram-positive and gram-negative organisms	Detergent can be toxic to wound tissue	Painful to open wounds; other reactions extremely rare	Hand cleanser	Iodine allergy possible; systemic absorption of iodine from burns, open wounds; not routinely used in open wounds
Povidone-iodine solution (Betadine 10%)	Same as povidone-iodine scrub; virucidal, bactericidal	Minimally toxic to wound tissue at full strength; 1% solution has no significant tissue toxicity	Extremely rare	Wound periphery cleanser; dilute to 1% for wound irrigation	Probably the safest and most effective product currently available; iodine is the active agent, and povidone is the carrier molecule; iodine allergy possible; systemic absorption of iodine from burns, open wounds; dilute 10:1 (saline to Betadine) if used to irrigate wounds
Chlorhexidine gluconate (Hibiclens)	Strongly bactericidal against gram-positive organisms, less strong against gram-negative bacteria	Ionic detergent can be toxic to tissue and cellular components; eye and inner ear toxicity	Extremely rare	Hand cleanser	Generally avoid use in open wounds; not for use in the eye or ear
Poloxamer 188 (Shur-Clens; Pluronic F-68)	No antibacterial or antiviral activity	None known; does not inhibit wound healing	None known	Wound cleanser (particularly useful on the face)	Nonionic detergent used for its cleansing properties; nontoxic even with intravenous use; will not damage the eye or cornea; lack of antibacterial properties limits use
Hexachlorophene (pHisoHex)	Bacteriostatic against gram-positive bacteria, poor activity against gram-negative bacteria	Detergent can be toxic to wound tissue	Possibly teratogenic with repeated use	Alternative hand cleanser; not used on open wounds	Systemic absorption causes neurotoxicity
Hydrogen peroxide	Very weak antibacterial agent	Toxic to tissue and red cells	Extremely rare	Wound cleanser adjunct; very weak antiseptic properties	Breaks down to water and oxygen; foaming activity useful to remove debris and coagulated blood

*Based largely on in vitro studies and animal data. The true harm (or benefit) of these products for routine use in the emergency department is theoretical and probably of minimal clinical consequence for most wounds.

Studies of the use of antiseptics in wounds demonstrate that there is a delicate balance between killing bacteria and injuring tissue.[33] Intact skin can withstand strong microbicidal agents, whereas leukocytes and the exposed cells of skin and soft tissue can be damaged by these agents.[32] Many antiseptic solutions have been used for cleaning wounds, but the *true final benefit or harm from the multiple products introduced during ED wound preparation is difficult to assess or quantify.*

Povidone-iodine (Betadine) is widely available as a 10% stock solution. Although the undiluted solution may be used to prepare the skin surrounding a wound, it may be harmful to some tissue; therefore, it should not be placed within the interior of the wound. Diluted povidone-iodine solution in concentrations of less than 1% appears to be safe and effective for cleaning contaminated traumatic wounds, but the precise concentration that provides the most benefit is unclear. In contrast, povidone-iodine surgical scrub (Betadine scrub) and hexachlorophene (pHisoHex) both contain anionic detergents that are harmful to tissues. In vitro studies have demonstrated that chlorhexidine gluconate–alcohol (Hibiclens) is toxic to the cellular components of blood,[34] but its effect on wound infection rates is unknown. Many potentially harmful solutions (such as peroxide, alcohol, or commercial cleaning products) are commonly used by patients at home on their own wounds, usually without serious consequence. Hydrogen peroxide is hemolytic, and there is little reason to use it except to clean surrounding skin encrusted with blood and coagulum or to soak off adherent blood-saturated dressings. Peroxide should not be used on granulation tissue because oxygen bubbles lift newly formed epithelium off the wound surface.[35] Ethyl alcohol gel solutions are now used commonly as hand sanitizer agents, but their use as a wound antiseptic requires further study.

Nonantiseptic, nonionic surfactants are attractive alternatives to these toxic cleansing agents. In contrast to antiseptic solutions, these preparations cause no tissue or cellular damage, leukocyte inhibition, or impairment of wound healing. The solutions cause no corneal injury, conjunctival irritation, or pain on contact with the wound.[34,36] Poloxamer 188 (Pluronic F-68, Shur-Clens, and Pharma Clens) is non-toxic and nonallergenic.[29,32] This Pluronic polyol has no antibacterial activity, but scrubbing experimental wounds with poloxamer reduced infection rates, thus proving its ability to cleanse a wound effectively and atraumatically.[29] Pluronic polyols may be considered, especially if the wound is near mucous membranes. Even dilute povidone-iodine may be particularly irritating when used for scrubbing contaminated wounds. The use of antiseptic preparations in wounds remains controversial.

Irrigation

It is important to distinguish between skin antiseptics and irrigating solutions. As a general rule, commercially available antiseptics should be used only to clean intact skin and not exposed wound surfaces. Most open wounds can be irrigated effectively with copious amounts of saline or tap water.

Properly performed irrigation is effective in removing particulate matter, bacteria, and devitalized tissue that is loosely adherent to the edges of the wound and trapped within its depths. The effectiveness of irrigation is determined primarily by the hydraulic pressure at which the irrigation fluid is delivered.[37-39] Although some investigators have used port devices spiked into plastic intravenous bags and squeezed by hand to deliver a stream of fluid,[40,41] other studies have shown that such activities and bulb syringes or gravity flow irrigation devices deliver fluid at low pressure and are ineffective in ridding wounds of small particulate matter or lowering wound bacterial counts.[38] In an uncontrolled study, Hollander and coworkers[42] found comparable infection rates and cosmetic outcomes in facial and scalp wounds repaired with and without irrigation. Although irrigation may not be required for low-risk, highly vascular uncontaminated facial and scalp wounds, randomized, prospective trials are needed to answer this question.

The pressure that can be delivered with a syringe varies with the force exerted on the plunger and the internal diameter of the attached needle. A simple irrigation assembly consisting of a 19-gauge plastic catheter or needle attached to a 35-mL syringe produces 25 to 40 psi when the barrel of the syringe is pushed with both hands.[39] This high-pressure irrigation system removes significant numbers of bacteria and a substantial amount of particulate matter from the wound surface.

Wound irrigation is best achieved with a large-volume syringe and a 18- or 19-gauge catheter or needle to deliver irrigation volumes of at least 250 mL. Irrigation should continue until all visible, loose particulate matter has been removed. Warmed irrigant solutions are comfortable for patients, even after the wound is anesthetized.[43]

A potential complication of wound irrigation is that infectious material can be splashed into the face of the clinician, even when the tip of the irrigation device is held below the surface of the wound. Several commercial devices are available to contain the splatter, including devices that fit on the end of a syringe (see Fig. 34-5C and D) and devices that fit on the screw top of saline bottles (for this particular device the company reported variable pressure from 4 to 15 psi). An alternative strategy is to pierce the base of a small medicine cup with a large-bore needle. The cup can be placed upside down to cover the area to be irrigated and the syringe with the 19-gauge needle can be inserted through the base of the cup (see Fig. 34-5C). The wound should be positioned to allow continuous drainage of fluid during irrigation by any method.

Antibiotic Solutions for Irrigation

A variety of antibiotic solutions have been instilled directly into wounds or used as irrigation solutions, including ampicillin, a neomycin-bacitracin-polymyxin combination, tetracycline, penicillin, kanamycin, and cephalothin. Although there have been no reports of topical sensitization or toxic tissue levels of the antibiotic, studies have found inconsistent effectiveness in reducing infection rates.[44-47] The indications for using antibiotic solutions to clean wounds have not been defined, and this practice is not considered standard.

Recommendations for Cleaning the Wound

The prerequisites for any wound-cleaning technique are a calm or sedated patient, satisfactory anesthesia, and thorough cleaning of the skin surface adjacent to the wound. The primary goal of wound cleaning is to rid the wound of major contaminants and lower the infective dose of bacteria. Two strategies are recommended. A contaminated or "dirty" wound can be irrigated or both scrubbed and irrigated with a 0.9% saline solution. As an alternative, the wound can be scrubbed with Pluronic polyols and irrigated with normal saline solution. Only Pluronic polyols or saline should be used near the eyes. Perform scrubbing with a soft, fine-pore sponge, and use high-pressure techniques for irrigation. Avoid using hydrogen peroxide on open wounds. Either gentle scrubbing with poloxamer and normal saline high-pressure irrigation or irrigation alone appears to be a satisfactory method for cleaning minimally contaminated wounds.

A sterile bottle of saline solution can be used to irrigate the wounds of multiple patients until the bottle is empty, but once the bottle is opened, bacterial contamination occurs quite rapidly.[48] Use bottles opened only within the past 24 hours to irrigate wounds.[48,49] Patients frequently irrigate their wounds with tap water before going to the ED. Many clinicians routinely irrigate wounds, especially extremity wounds, with tap water instead of sterile saline, and infection rates have been found to be comparable to that of saline irrigation[50-53] (see Fig. 34-5*E* and *F*). The advantage of using tap water is that large volumes of irrigant can be quickly applied to an open wound. The disadvantages of this technique are that irrigation pressures are difficult to control and the patient may faint if allowed to stand at a sink. If tap water is used to irrigate wounds, deliver it through a syringe at the bedside.

Preparation for Wound Closure

Before débridement or wound closure, prepare and drape the wound. Avoid shaving body hair because preoperative wounds that were shaved demonstrated higher infection rates.[16,54-56] For wounds in hair-bearing areas, hair can be removed by clipping if it interferes with the procedure.[55] Stubborn hairs that repeatedly invade the wound during suturing can be coated with petrolatum jelly or a water-soluble ointment to keep them out of the field. Do not shave eyebrows because critical landmarks for exact approximation of the wound edges would be lost. Although shaved eyebrows will grow back eventually, shaving produces an undesirable cosmetic effect as well. Clip hair rather than shaving it. Use a petrolatum- or water-based ointment to keep the hair out of the wound field.

Disinfect the skin surface adjacent to the wound (not the wound itself) with a standard 10% povidone-iodine or chlorhexidine gluconate (Hibiclens) solution. Paint the solution widely on the skin surrounding the wound, but do not allow it to seep into the interior of the wound itself (Fig. 34-6*A*).

After hand washing, the clinician and any assistants involved in the procedure must wear sterile or nonsterile but clean gloves.[57] *Sterile gloves are not required, and their use does not decrease infection rates.* Wear face masks, especially if you have a upper respiratory bacterial infection. Because droplets of saliva may leak even from around the edges of a face mask, avoid talking in proximity to the wound.[58] Use a single fenestrated drape or multiple folded drapes around the wound site. Place a sterile glove on a patient who has a hand wound to provide a sterile field in lieu of a fenestrated drape (see Fig. 34-6*B*). The area to be sutured can then be exposed by cutting the glove, and the extremity can be placed on a sterile towel. This technique provides a clean field without the need to continually adjust the drape or to operate through a small opening.

Explore the entire depth and the full extent of every wound to locate hidden foreign bodies, particulate matter, bone fragments, or any injuries to underlying structures that may require repair (see Fig. 34-6*C*). Avoid the temptation to initially explore wounds and assess their characteristics with a finger in search of a foreign body because (see Fig. 34-6*E*) embedded glass, metal fragments, or sharp pieces of bone may cut the clinician and cause exposure to blood-borne infections. Visualize directly with good lighting in a bloodless field, explore the wound with a metal probe, and use radiographs as safer approaches to wound exploration. Despite these measures, lacerations through thick subcutaneous adipose tissue are treacherous because large amounts of particulate matter can be completely obscured in deep folds of tissue. Unless a careful search is undertaken, these contaminants may be left in the depths of a sutured wound, and infection usually follows. Some clinicians are reluctant to extend lacerations to properly clean or explore them; however, opening the wound

to permit adequate visualization may be necessary for successful wound exploration.

Débridement

Débridement of foreign material and devitalized tissue is of undisputed importance in the management of a contaminated wound. Use this technique to remove tissue embedded with foreign matter, bacteria, and devitalized tissue that otherwise impairs the ability of the wound to resist infection and also prolongs the period of inflammation. Débridement also creates a tidy, sharp wound edge that is easier to repair and results in a more cosmetically acceptable scar.

If the wound is already clean and the edges are viable, sharp débridement may not improve the outcome. Irregular wounds have greater surface areas than do linear lacerations. Because skin tension is distributed over a greater length, the width of the scar is usually less with jagged wounds than if the wound is converted to an elliptical defect with tidy edges. If the edges are devitalized or contaminated, though, the wound edges must be débrided (Fig. 34-7*A* and *B*). To avoid a wide scar in this situation, undermine the wound.

Excision

Excision is the most effective type of débridement because it converts a contaminated traumatic wound into a clean wound. If significant contamination occurs in areas in which there is laxity of tissues and if no important structures, such as tendons or nerves, lie within the wound, the entire wound may be excised[5] (see Fig. 34-7*C*). Complete excision of grossly contaminated wounds such as animal bites allows primary closure of such wounds with no greater risk for infection than occurs with relatively uncontaminated lacerations.[31]

When a puncture wound is excised, make the axis of the excision parallel to a wrinkle, a skin line, or a line of dependency or facial expression. Make the long axis of this lenticular excision three to four times as great as the short axis (see Fig. 34-7*D*). Premark the skin with a surgical marking pen or by making a superficial "scoring" mark (cutting only down to the epidermis) around the wound with a No. 15 scalpel blade. Place tension on the surrounding skin with a finger or a skin hook. While steadying your hand on the table or on the patient, use the No. 15 blade and cut through the skin at right angles or at slightly oblique angles to the surface of the skin. If complete excision of the entire depth of the wound is not necessary, use tissue scissors to cut the edge of the wound by following the path premarked in the epidermis with the scalpel blade. If complete excision is desired, incise each wound edge past the deepest part of the wound. Excise and remove the wedge of tissue carefully without contaminating the fresh wound surface.

Plan the excision carefully because excessive removal of tissue can create a defect that is too large to close. Wounds on the trunk, the gluteal region, or the thigh are amenable to excision. In contrast, simple excision of a wound on the palm or the dorsum of the nose will make approximation of the resulting surgical wound edges difficult. In hair-bearing areas of the face, particularly through the eyebrows, angle the incision parallel to the angle of the hair follicles to avoid linear alopecia (see Fig. 34-7*E*).

Selective Débridement

Complete excision is impossible for most wounds because of insufficient skin elasticity, so selective débridement must be

WOUND PREPARATION AND EXPLORATION

Disinfect the skin surface adjacent to the wound with 10% povidone-iodine or chlorhexidine gluconate, but do not allow it to seep into the wound.

A nonsterile clean glove on the hand with the finger cut out and a finger tourniquet to provide a bloodless field make examination and suturing of a wound easier.

Explore the depths of the wound and examine for injured structures, foreign bodies, and the extent of injury.

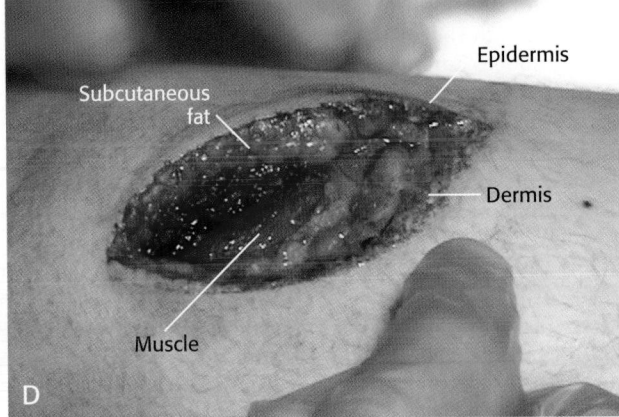

Anatomy of a deep laceration.

1, This patient punched out a window, a setup for retained glass. *2*, Do *not* explore this laceration with a finger. *3*, Instead, use radiographs and instruments to search for foreign bodies (the *arrow* defines a large piece of glass that could cut the examining finger). Many patients are unaware of the presence of large foreign bodies in a deep wound, although they should be questioned about the possibility or sensation of retained material.

Figure 34-6 A-D, Wound preparation and exploration.

used.[5,21] Stellate wounds and wounds with an irregular, meandering course have greater surface area and less skin tension per unit length than do linear lacerations. In some cases, excision of an entire wound would result in the loss of too much tissue (i.e., produce a gaping defect and excessive tension on the edges of the wound when closed). Avoid this problem by selective débridement and approximation of the irregular wound edges. This technique involves sharp débridement of devitalized or heavily contaminated tissue in the wound piece by piece and eventual matching of one edge of the wound to the other. Selective débridement is time-consuming but preserves more surrounding tissue.

Identifying devitalized tissue in a wound remains a challenging problem. Tissue with a narrow pedicle or base, especially distally based, narrow flaps on extremities, is unlikely to survive and should be excised. Sometimes, a sharp line of

WOUND DÉBRIDEMENT

Sharp débridement is the best way to remove devitalized tissue and create a more cosmetic result. Here, the wound edges are trimmed with iris scissors.

A scalpel can also be used. Alternatively, the skin is first sharply incised with a scalpel for a clean edge, and then the rest of the subcutaneous tissue is removed with scissors.

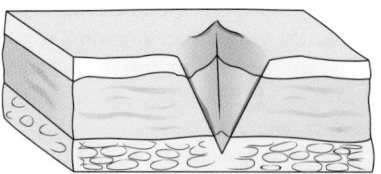

C

Excision is the most effective type of débridement because it converts a contaminated wound into a clean one. The entire wound may be excised if no important structures (such as tendons or nerves) are present. Grossly contaminated wounds may be excised and sutured primarily.

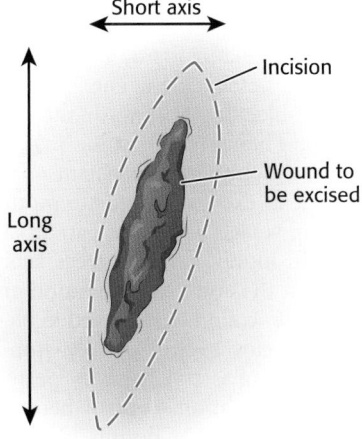

D

The long axis of an excision around a wound should be three to four times as great as the short axis.

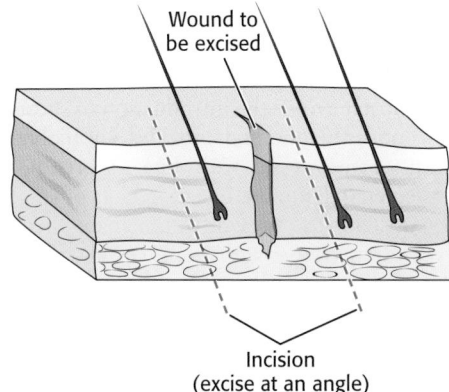

E

Excision through an eyebrow. Use an angled incision to remove tissue in the eyebrow, thus avoiding further injury to hair follicles.

Figure 34-7 A-E, Wound débridement.

demarcation distinguishes devitalized skin and viable skin, but in most wounds, usually only a subtle bluish discoloration is present. Try to predict tissue viability by comparing the capillary refill of injured tissue with that of the adjacent skin. If circulation is adequate, viable tissue also becomes hyperemic after the release of a proximal tourniquet.

In heavily contaminated wounds, especially those with abundant adipose tissue, remove all exposed fat and all fat impregnated with particulate matter. The subcutaneous adipose tissue attached to large flaps or to avulsed viable skin should be débrided before reapproximation of the wound; removal of this fatty layer allows better perfusion of the flap or the graft. Contaminated bone fragments, nerves, and tendons are almost never removed. Every effort should be made to clean these structures and return them to their place of origin because they may be functional later.[59] Fascia and tendons perform important functions despite potential loss of viability. If they can be cleaned adequately, these tissues should not be débrided. They may be left in wounds as free grafts and be covered by viable flaps of tissue.[60]

Instruments generally required for débridement include two fine single- or double-pronged skin hooks, a scalpel with a No. 15 blade, tissue scissors, hemostats, and a small tissue forceps. Using gentle tissue pressure, stabilize the jagged wound edges with skin hooks or forceps, and use the scalpel or scissors to cut away devitalized tissue from one end of the wound to the other. After débridement or excision, irrigate the wound again to remove any remaining tissue debris.

Control of Hemorrhage

Hemostasis is essential at any stage of wound care. Persistent bleeding obscures the wound and hampers exploration and closure of the wound. If bleeding is not a problem before wound débridement, it may become a complication during cleaning or after the edges of the wound are excised. If it is significant, hematoma formation in a sutured wound can separate the wound edges, impair healing, and cause dehiscence or infection.

Several practical methods of achieving hemostasis are available. Provide direct pressure with gloved fingers, gauze sponges, or packing material, and elevate the wound. This technique is usually effective in immediately controlling a single bleeding site or a small number of sites until the cut ends of vessels constrict and coagulation occurs. In a patient with multiple injuries and several urgent problems, control hemorrhage temporarily with a compression dressing. Apply several absorptive sponges directly over the bleeding site and secure them in place with an elastic bandage (e.g., Ace wrap) or elastic adhesive tape (Elastoplast). Apply pressure with the elasticity of the bandage. Elevate the bleeding part. Wound care can then be deferred while the clinician attends to more pressing matters.

Although simply crushing and twisting the end of a small vessel with a hemostat avoids the introduction of suture material into the wound, this method provides unreliable hemostasis. Ligation of the vessel with fine absorbable suture material is preferred. Clamp the bleeding ends of vessels with fine-point hemostats to provide immediate hemostasis. Because nerves often course with these vessels, clamp them only under direct visualization. The tip of the hemostat should project beyond the vessel to hold a loop of a ligature in place (Fig. 34-8*A*). With an assistant lifting the handle of the hemostat, pass a synthetic 5-0 or 6-0 *absorbable* suture around the hemostat from one hand to the other. Tie the first knot beyond the tip of the hemostat. Once the suture is securely anchored on the vessel, release the hemostat.[61,62] Three knots are sufficient to hold the ligature in place. Cut the ends of the suture close to the knot to minimize the amount of suture material left in the wound.

Ligate vessels with diameters greater than 2 mm. Vessels smaller than 2 mm that bleed despite direct pressure can be controlled by pinpoint, bipolar electrocautery. A dry field is required for an effective electrical current to pass through the tissues. If sponging does not dry the field, use a suction-tipped catheter. Minimize trauma by using fine-tipped electrodes to touch the vessel or touch the active electrode of the electrocautery unit to a small hemostat or fine-tipped forceps while gripping the vessel.[3] Keep the power of the unit to the minimum level required for thrombosis of the vessel.

Self-contained, sterilizable, battery-powered coagulation units are alternatives to electrocautery. These devices cauterize vessels by the direct application of a heated wire filament. Although these units may damage more surrounding tissue than electrocautery units do, they are compact, simple, and well suited for use in the ED (see Fig. 34-8*B*).

A cut vessel that retracts into the wall of the wound may frustrate attempts at clamping, ligation, or cauterization. First, control bleeding by downward compression on the tissue. Pass a suture through the tissue twice via a figure-of-eight or horizontal mattress stitch, and then tie it. This stitch will constrict the tissue containing the cut vessel (see Fig. 34-8*C*).

Large superficial varicosities may bleed spontaneously or from minor trauma. They may bleed profusely, especially when the patient stands up and increases venous pressure. Use a simple figure-of-eight suture to halt the bleeding (see Fig. 34-8*D*).

Epinephrine is an excellent vasoconstrictor. Place topical epinephrine (1 : 100,000) on a moistened sponge and apply it to a wound to reduce the bleeding from small vessels. When combined with local anesthetics, concentrations of 1 : 100,000 and 1 : 200,000 prolong the effect of the anesthetic and provide some hemostasis in highly vascular areas. Use vasoconstrictors only in situations in which widespread small-vessel and capillary hemorrhage in a wound cannot be controlled by direct pressure or cauterization. Hemostasis of a specific vessel may be achieved by directly injecting the soft tissues around the base of the bleeder with a small amount of lidocaine and epinephrine solution, even though the wound has previously been anesthetized. The combination of pressure and vasoconstriction may halt the bleeding long enough for the vessel to be ligated or cauterized or allow the wound to be closed and a compression dressing applied.

Fibrin foam, gelatin foam, and microcrystalline collagen may be used as hemostatic agents. Their utility is limited in that vigorous bleeding will wash the agent away from the bleeding site. Their greatest value may be in packing small cavities from which there is constant oozing of blood.[61]

Do not spend excessive time attempting to tie off several small bleeding vessels while the patient slowly exsanguinates (Fig. 34-9). In highly vascular areas such as the scalp, it is sometimes best to suture the laceration after exploration and irrigation of the wound despite active bleeding; the pressure exerted by the closure will usually stop the bleeding (Fig. 34-10). If bleeding is too brisk to permit adequate wound evaluation and irrigation, control hemorrhage by clamping and everting the galea or dermis of each wound edge with hemostats. Raney clamps or a large hemostat is an excellent way to stop scalp bleeding; they are used during neurosurgical procedures. If the edge of the entire scalp is compressed, the bleeding will generally stop (see Fig. 34-10*C*). In the majority of simple wounds with persistent but minor capillary bleeding, apposition of the wound edges with sutures, followed by a compression dressing, provides adequate hemostasis.

Tourniquets

If bleeding from an extremity wound is refractory to direct pressure, electrocauterization, or ligation or if the patient has exsanguinating hemorrhage from the wound, place a tourniquet proximal to the wound to control the bleeding temporarily. Tourniquets are also helpful in examining extremity lacerations by providing a bloodless field. However, they can also cause injury in three ways:

HEMORRHAGE CONTROL

1

2

A

When tying off a bleeding vessel, the tip of the hemostat should project beyond the clamped vessel. An assistant raises the handles of the hemostat as a ligature is passed under them.

Stretch the ligature thread between the index fingertips and carry it under the projecting tips of the hemostat.

B

Battery-powered cautery can be used to coagulate minor subcutaneous bleeders.

1   **2**

C

Ligation of a retracted, bleeding vessel. *1,* Horizontal mattress technique. *2,* Figure-of-eight technique.

D

This elderly patient experienced massive spontaneous bleeding from a ruptured varicose vein. Blood loss was substantial and recurrent when she walked.

After cautery, a figure-of-eight suture was placed. Simple cautery without suturing is not always effective. A pressure dressing is applied after hemostasis is verified by walking.

Figure 34-8 A-D, Hemorrhage control.

Figure 34-9 Scalp lacerations can bleed profusely. This patient's pressure dressing fell off while he was on a stretcher in the back hall, and he experienced significant blood loss from a large scalp laceration. His intoxication prevented him from supplying his history of hemophilia.

1. They can produce ischemia in an extremity.
2. They can compress and damage underlying blood vessels and nerves.
3. They can jeopardize the survival of marginally viable tissue.

Although problems rarely develop from the use of tourniquets in routine wound care, potential problems can be minimized if (1) a limit is placed on the total amount of time that a tourniquet is applied and (2) excessive tourniquet pressure is avoided. It is also imperative that all tourniquets be removed before releasing the patient. A small tourniquet may be overlooked if it is covered by a bulky dressing.

A single-cuff tourniquet (sphygmomanometer cuff) placed around an arm or a leg stops most distal venous or arterial bleeding without crushing any underlying structures. The length of time that a tourniquet may remain in place is limited by the development of pain underneath and distal to the tourniquet. This occurs within 30 to 45 minutes in a conscious patient, which is well within the limits of safety.[15]

Before application of the tourniquet, elevate the injured extremity and manually exsanguinate it to prevent persistent venous oozing (Fig. 34-11A). Wrap an elastic bandage (e.g., Ace wrap or Esmarch) circumferentially around the extremity, starting distally and moving in a proximal direction. Place a cuff that is 20% wider than the diameter of the limb around the arm proximal to the wound, inflate it to 250 to 300 mm Hg or 70 mm Hg higher than the patient's systolic blood pressure, and then clamp the tubing. Remove the bandage and lower the extremity. Because tourniquets impair the circulation and may produce neurapraxia, limit their use in the ED to a maximum of 1 hour.

Tourniquets on digits have a greater potential for complications. The maximum tourniquet time that is safe for a finger may easily be exceeded. Also, finger tourniquets can exert excessive pressure over a small surface area at the base of the finger and injure digital nerves or cause pressure necrosis of digital vessels. For this reason, standard rubber bands should not be used as tourniquets. Instead, place a 0.5-inch Penrose drain around the base of the finger and stretch it to no more than two thirds of its circumference (see Fig. 34-11B). This will provide safe and effective hemostasis. The pressure under a Penrose drain ranges between 100 and 650 mm Hg, but it can easily be controlled.[63] A few millimeters of difference in total stretch makes a large difference in the pressure applied by this type of tourniquet.[64] In digits, tourniquet pressures of only 150 mm Hg are needed for hemostasis.

A surgical glove placed over a patient's cleaned hand can also serve as a finger tourniquet (see Fig. 34-11C). Remove the tip of the glove covering the injured digit, and then roll it proximally along the patient's finger to form a constricting band at the base. Another advantage of this technique is that contamination of the wound during closure is less likely. Rolled surgical gloves produce pressures ranging from 113 to 363 mm Hg, depending on the thickness, the amount of glove finger removed, the number of rolls, and the size of the glove in relation to the size of the patient's hand.[64] Ring-shaped exsanguinating digit tourniquets are available commercially (Tourni-Cot, Mar-Med Company) (see Fig. 34-11D). There is a real danger of forgetting to remove such a small tourniquet and accidentally incorporating it into the dressing.

These techniques provide bloodless fields in which to examine, clean, and close extremity wounds. Maximum tourniquet time should not exceed 30 to 45 minutes on a finger.[63,64] Débridement of questionably devitalized tissue in a wound is best accomplished without a tourniquet or pharmacologic vasoconstriction because bleeding from tissues is often an indication of their viability.[59]

CLOSURE

The various techniques for wound closure are presented in Chapter 35. The remainder of this chapter addresses issues related to wound management (e.g., secondary closure, wound dressings, use of antibiotics, aftercare instructions, and suture removal).

Open versus Closed Wound Management

Wounds that heal spontaneously (i.e., by secondary intention) undergo much more inflammation, fibroplasia, and contraction than do those whose edges are reapproximated by wound closure techniques.[7,65] During wound healing, contraction covers the defect, but it may result in a deformity (contracture) or loss of function. Left to itself, the healing process may be unable to close a defect completely in areas in which the surrounding skin is immobile, such as on the scalp or in the pretibial area[7] (Fig. 34-12). Exposed tendons, bone, nerves, or vessels may desiccate in an open wound. If the patient is careless with an otherwise adequate dressing that covers an open wound, the wound may be further contaminated.[66] Surgical closure of wounds minimizes inflammation, fibroplasia, contracture, scar width, and contamination.

However, surgical closure of wounds can cause complications. Closure of contaminated wounds increases the probability of wound infection, with impaired healing, dehiscence, and sepsis being possible complications. For instance, raised

HEMORRHAGE CONTROL OF SCALP LACERATIONS

Scalp lacerations may bleed profusely, and arterial vessels may not retract if they are in tough fibrous tissue. This forceps was used to crush a small pumping artery. Placing large (3-0 nylon) sutures that incorporate all scalp layers, defined as all tissue between the thumb and index finger (*arrows*), is preferred to attempting to cauterize or ligate small bleeders.

A hemostat placed on the scalp edge can similarly be used on a single bleeder.

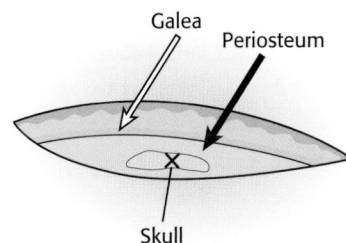

Note that the suture will incorporate all layers of the scalp. Both the galea and the periosteum are identified along with exposed skull (*x*). The periosteum is not sutured.

Load the Raney clip onto the applicator.

Lock the handles of the applicator to open the clip.

Slide the clip onto the wound edge.

Release the clip by unlocking the applicator.

Figure 34-10 A-C, Hemorrhage control of scalp lacerations. (*C, From Custalow CB.* Color Atlas of Emergency Department Procedures. *Philadelphia: Saunders; 2005:136-137.*)

HEMORRHAGE CONTROL: TOURNIQUETS

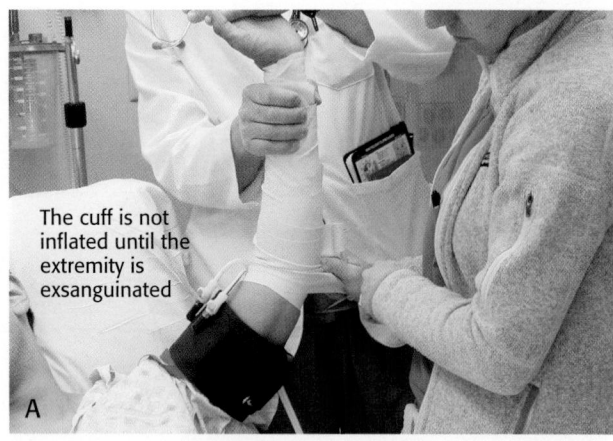

The cuff is not inflated until the extremity is exsanguinated

Before inflating a tourniquet such as a blood pressure cuff, wrap an elastic bandage (e.g., Ace wrap or Esmarch) around the extremity in a distal-to-proximal fashion. Inflate the cuff to 250 to 300 mm Hg or 70 mm Hg higher than systolic pressure. (The above photo is only a demonstration; gloves should obviously be worn in the case of a bleeding patient.)

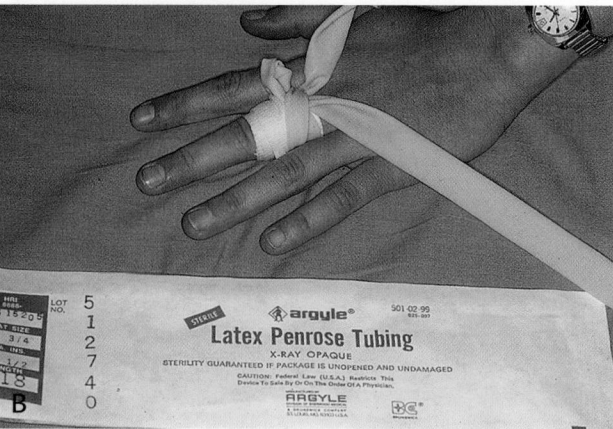

Use of a Penrose drain placed over padding for a finger tourniquet. Do not stretch the drain to more than two thirds of its circumference. This will provide safe and effective hemostasis.

Use of a sterile glove to provide a clean field and serve as a finger tourniquet. The distal end of the glove is clipped, and the glove finger is rolled proximally over the digit. A Penrose drain is also incorporated into this tourniquet.

Commercial tourniquet for finger lacerations (Tournicot Mar Med Company). Various sizes are available. The accompanying warning tag has been left exposed to remind the operator of the tourniquet device. Note how the tendon injury can be seen once a bloodless field is obtained.

Figure 34-11 A-D, Hemorrhage control: use of tourniquets.

pretibial flap lacerations in elderly patients often necrose when sutured but survive and heal well by secondary intention if taped back into position.

Sutures in themselves are potentially detrimental to healing and can increase the risk for infection.[67] Each suture inflicts a small intradermal incision that damages the surface epithelium, dermis, subcutaneous fat, blood vessels, small nerves, lymphatics, and epithelial appendages such as hair follicles, sweat glands, and ducts. Once divided and separated by a stitch, these appendages usually undergo inflammation and resorption.[68] Each suture is another piece of foreign material that can provoke inflammation.[7] When a suture is removed, bacteria that have settled on the exposed portion of the suture are pulled into the suture track and deposited there.[68]

The clinician must estimate the risk for infection. If the wound is judged to be clean or is rendered clean by scrubbing,

irrigation, and débridement, it may be closed. If the wound remains contaminated despite the best of efforts, it must be left open to heal by secondary intention. If the status of the wound is uncertain, delayed primary closure is another available option.

Delayed Primary or Secondary Closure

There is a common misconception that all wounds must be either sutured within a few hours or left open and relegated to slow healing and an unsightly scar. If there is a substantial risk that closure of a particular wound might result in infection, the decision to close or to leave the wound open can be postponed. After cleaning, wounds left unsutured appear to have higher resistance to infection than do closed wounds.

Figure 34-12 In areas in which the skin is immobile, as in the scalp, wounds left open may not heal.

Figure 34-13 Incidence of wound infection over time when delayed closure is performed. Delayed closure is best accomplished on the fourth or fifth day to minimize the risk for infection. *(From Edlich RF, Thacker JG, Rodeheaver GT, et al. A Manual for Wound Closure. St. Paul, MN: 3M Medical Surgical Products; 1979. Reproduced by permission. © 1979 by Minnesota Mining and Manufacturing Company.)*

The condition of the wound after 3 to 5 days will then determine the best strategy (Fig. 34-13).

Although cleaning and débridement should be accomplished as rapidly as possible, there is no urgency in closing a wound. Edlich and associates[20] pointed out that "the fundamental basis for delayed primary closure is that the healing open wound gradually gains sufficient resistance to infection to permit an uncomplicated closure." Despite its effectiveness, delayed primary closure is a technique that remains largely unappreciated and probably underused by many clinicians (Fig. 34-14). It is a highly effective means of managing wounds that have a sufficient risk for infection. After 4 to 5 days, a well-irrigated and cleaned wound may be closed primarily with very good results.

Open wound management is usually an outpatient procedure. The technique consists of careful cleaning and débridement, followed by packing of the wound with sterile, saline-moistened, fine-mesh gauze. The packed wound is covered with a thick, absorbent, sterile dressing. Depending on the specifics of the wound and the ability of the patient to perform his or her own wound care, the packing may be changed daily at home or in the ED or may be left

undisturbed for several days. Sterile saline-soaked packing is standard, and there is no need to impregnate wounds with antiseptics. Prophylactic antibiotics are occasionally prescribed, but their use is neither mandatory nor of proven benefit. On the fourth or fifth postoperative day, the wound is reevaluated for closure. If no evidence of infection is present, the wound margins can be approximated (delayed primary closure), or the wound can be excised and then sutured (secondary closure) with minimal risk for infection. Because the wound is closed before the proliferative phase of healing, there is no delay in final healing, and the results are indistinguishable from those of primary healing.

Certain wounds should almost always be managed open or by delayed closure (Fig. 34-15). Such wounds include those that are already infected and those heavily contaminated by soil, organic matter, or feces. Also included in this category are wounds associated with extensive tissue damage, such as high-velocity missile injuries, explosion injuries involving the hand, complex crush injuries, and most bite wounds. Deep or contaminated lacerations on the bottom of the foot, such as those occurring when the patient steps on an unknown object while wading in a stream or running through a field, or wounds that are deep punctures are ideal candidates for delayed closure. Some are never sutured but left open for primary healing. Human bite wounds (extending past the dermis) should probably never be closed and are *often opened or extended further for cleaning*. Clinicians disagree about which animal bite wounds may be closed initially. Most would suture cosmetically deforming injuries, including facial bites and bite wounds that can be excised completely.[69] Others would suture dog bites not involving an extremity.[70] In severe soft tissue injuries, delayed closure allows time for nonviable tissue to become demarcated from uninjured tissue. Débridement can then be accomplished with maximal preservation of tissue.[66]

PROTECTION

Dressings

At the conclusion of wound repair, wipe away dried blood on the surface of the skin with moistened gauze to minimize subsequent itching, and cover the wound with a nonadherent dressing. Depending on the specifics of the wound and the type of repair, a dressing can consist of a simple dry gauze pad or a complex multilayer dressing. Some wounds, such as sutured scalp lacerations, do not routinely require any dressing. Various specialized (and expensive) synthetic dressings are available, including vapor-permeable adhesive films, hydrogels, hydrocolloids, alginates, synthetic foam dressings, silicone meshes, tissue adhesives, barrier films, and collagen-containing dressings. However, little data exist to support their use over readily available, properly applied gauze dressings on acute, traumatic wounds managed in the ED.

Function of Dressings

Dressings serve various functions. They protect the wound from contamination and trauma, absorb excess exudate from the wound, immobilize the wound and surrounding area, exert downward pressure on the wound, and improve the patient's comfort.[14,71,72] Occlusive dressings on burns or abrasions maintain a moist environment and prevent painful exposure of the wound to air and dehydration of the wound's surface.[73] Sutured wounds are particularly susceptible to

DELAYED PRIMARY CLOSURE

This dirty and contused extremity wound, now 18 hours old, is an ideal candidate for delayed primary closure.

At arrival in the emeigency department, the wound is anesthetized, scrubbed, irrigated, and sharply débrided.

The wound is packed with sterile gauze and covered with a dry dressing. No antibiotics were prescribed and the wound was left undisturbed.

4 days later

Four days later the packing is removed and the wound is minimally débrided.

Interrupted sutures are placed as though this is a fresh, clean wound. At suture removal 10 days later, only a linear scar was evident.

Figure 34-14 Delayed primary closure.

infection from surface contamination during the first 2 days after wound repair. Dressings protect the wound from contamination during this vulnerable period.

One of the primary functions of a gauze dressing is to *absorb the serosanguineous drainage that exudes from all wounds*. Absorbent dressings also reduce the development of stitch abscesses to some extent. Surface sutures produce small indentations at their points of entrance; tiny blood clots and debris overlie these indentations and allow bacterial growth at the site. Small "stitch abscesses" can develop; they are initially undetectable but are nevertheless destructive to epithelium. Stitch abscesses rarely infect the entire wound but can slightly increase the width of the scar and produce noticeable, punctate suture marks.[14]

Figure 34-15 A, Human bites are never closed primarily and are often opened and extended to facilitate cleaning and a search for other injuries or foreign bodies such as fragments of teeth. **B,** Dog bites in a cosmetic area may be closed primarily. Large cosmetic defects are best closed in the operating room by a surgeon with adequate time to correctly prepare the wound. **C,** This wound on the bottom of the foot, sustained by stepping on an unknown object while running in a stream, should not be closed but rather left open to heal primarily. Always check for foreign bodies in such wounds. Note that an assistant holds the wound open while pressure irrigation is applied. This was initially a much smaller puncture wound that was extended for cleaning and initially packed open. Sutures were never required and the wound healed in 7 days.

The most common type of dressing is constructed in three layers: a nonadherent contact layer, an absorbent layer, and an outer wrap (Fig. 34-16*A*).[74] Ideally, this dressing provides nonadherence without maceration. The optimal appearance of an abrasion or an open wound under a dressing is a moist red surface with capillary and epithelial growth.

Contact Layer: Dry, Semiocclusive, and Occlusive Dressings

Wounds covered with permeable dressings such as plain gauze tend to dry out. Although this is acceptable for dressing sutured wounds, drying of the wound surface damages a shallow layer of exposed dermis, which impedes epidermal resurfacing of abrasions, burns, and incisions.[72] Wound desiccation results in further epidermal necrosis, crust formation, and increased inflammation.[75,76] Coarse weaves of gauze, usually available in the form of multilayered pads, absorb blood and exudate, but the dressing will adhere if the interstices of the fabric are relatively large. Capillaries, fibrin, and granulation tissue will penetrate and become enmeshed in the material. If the proteinaceous exudate from the wound dries by evaporation, the scab usually clings to the dressing.[74,75] Some clinicians use this effect to "débride" the wound when the gauze is removed. However, it may also destroy healing tissue, particularly the new epithelium. Even though débridement of the wound with wet-to-dry dressings is quick, careful débridement with surgical instruments is more controlled and less traumatic.

Adherence to the wound can be prevented if the dressing is nonabsorbent, occlusive, or finely woven. If the wound is kept moist by covering it with an occlusive film or nonadherent covering soon after wound management and if the film is left in place for at least 48 hours, the epidermis will migrate over the surface of the dermis faster than when a dry scab is allowed to form.[77-79] Protection of wounds that are healing by secondary intention with occlusive or semiocclusive dressings has several advantages,[10] including more rapid healing, less pain from exposure to air, better cosmetic result, few dressing changes, and protection from bacteria.

Petrolatum gauze (e.g., Adaptic, Xeroform, Betadine, Aquaflo) is commonly applied next to the surface of the wound to prevent the wound from sticking to the dry gauze in the absorbent layer and to protect the regenerating epithelium (Box 34-1). Always use nonadherent material to cover skin grafts. Some clinicians use fine-mesh gauze (41 to 47 warp threads/inch^2) rather than petrolatum gauze on abrasions, especially on wounds that are heavily contaminated, because removal of this type of dressing débrides only the small tufts of granulation tissue that become fixed in the mesh pores and leaves a clean, even surface. Once a healthy, granulating surface is present and reepithelialization is proceeding, nonporous dressings can be used.[75] Fine-mesh gauze is also used next to exposed tissue in wounds being considered for delayed primary closure; a protective and absorptive bulky dressing is placed on top of the wound.

Various polyurethane-derived membranes provide an occlusive effect, including Epi-Lock (Derma-Lock Medical Corporation), Op-Site (Smith and Nephew, Ltd.), Tegaderm (3M), Bioclusive (Johnson & Johnson), and Primaderm (ACCO, Inc.); those with soluble collagen or gelatin backing, such as DuoDERM (ConvaTec) and Biobrane (Woodroof Laboratories); products with hydrogels, such as Vigilon[75]; and other occlusive dressings such as Dermicel (Johnson & Johnson) and Telfa (Kendall). Silicon-based dressings (Mepitel Mölnlycke Health Care, Newton, PA) can be used for the treatment of skin tears.

One fear of using occlusive dressings is that microorganisms will proliferate in the moist environment beneath the occlusive film and increase wound infection rates.[72,80] However, occlusive dressings such as DuoDERM actually serve more as a barrier to external pathogenic bacteria.[81] Although skin bacteria under occlusive dressings can multiply,[82] even chronic wounds contaminated with large numbers of bacteria are routinely treated with occlusive dressings successfully.[83]

Adhesive-backed dressings (e.g., DuoDERM and Op-Site) may adhere to an open wound and remove new epidermis, macerate skin, or produce a thick eschar. The wound must

WOUND DRESSING

A common three-layer dressing consisting of antibiotic ointment, Adaptic, and gauze.

Snugness of the bandage is increased by 180° rotation of the bandage roll after each circular turn to create a reverse spiral.

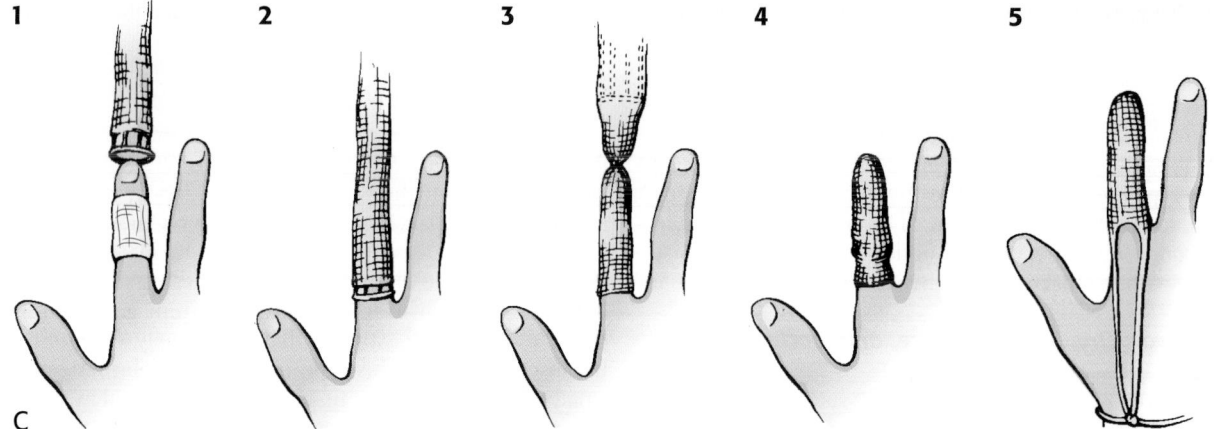

Tube gauze finger dressing applied loosely. Throbbing pain under this dressing mandates removal. *1,* The inner layer is nonadherent gauze. The middle layer is 2- × 2-inch gauze sponges wrapped circumferentially and held in place with tape. *2,* Begin with No. 2 tube gauze at the base of the finger. Hold this end with one finger while the tube gauze applicator is pulled toward the fingertip. A twisting motion firms the wrap about the digit; about 90° is necessary. Excessive stretch or twisting can compromise the circulation. *3,* When the fingertip is reached, make a 360° twist, but avoid placing a constricting twist around the finger itself. *4,* Pass the applicator toward the base of the finger with an additional 90° twist. Repeat once more; thus, three layers are in place. *5,* Cut enough gauze to reach the base of the finger, and tape it there. As an alternative, pull the final layer beyond the tip while leaving it long enough to reach to and around the wrist (about three times the finger length). Split this gauze into two strands; bring them dorsally to the wrist, knot, and loosely wrap around the wrist.

For a distal finger dressing, covering the gauze with a finger cut from a clean glove provides protection from dirt and wetness.

Figure 34-16 A-D, Wound dressings.

- More rapid healing
- Less pain from exposure to air
- Better cosmetic results
- Fewer dressing changes
- Better protection from bacteria

Data from Eaglstein WH. Effect of occlusive dressings on wound healing. Clin Dermatol. *1984;2:107.*

then epithelialize underneath the eschar.[84] These dressings do not allow exudate to drain out the edges of the dressing. Between dressing changes, coat the wound with petrolatum or an antibiotic ointment before applying these products.[10] Epi-Lock has the advantage of thermally insulating the wound by virtue of its thickness, but unlike Tegaderm and Op-Site, it is opaque and does not allow inspection of the underlying wound surface.[85] Because Epi-Lock allows drainage of exudate, it is better tolerated by patients if the overlying gauze bandage is changed daily. Wounds covered with certain occlusive dressings or with silver sulfadiazine (Silvadene, Marion Laboratories) appear to be blanketed with pus; this exudate actually represents the beneficial proliferation of macrophages and polymorphonuclear leukocytes.[79,85]

Absorbent Layer

When dressing wounds with considerable drainage, use sufficient gauze to cover the wound and absorb all the drainage. Change the dressing whenever it becomes soiled, wet, or saturated with drainage. Once a dressing becomes moist, pathogens can pass through it to the underlying wound.[72] Consequently, a dressing that is used to absorb exudate or débride the wound must be changed more frequently than one designed solely to occlude. Absorbent dressings on draining wounds can be changed daily to avoid bacterial overgrowth beneath the dressing.[7,75] Aspirate fluid accumulating under an occlusive dressing or change the dressing every 1 to 2 days during the first week or until the exudate no longer accumulates.[86]

Outer Layer

Bleeding may persist despite attempts to provide good hemostasis. Compressive dressings help prevent hematoma formation and eliminate dead space within a wound. They are particularly useful for wounds that have been undermined extensively and for facial wounds, in which subcutaneous capillary bleeding and swelling can exert tension on fine skin sutures and jeopardize skin closure. Pressure dressings should be used to immobilize skin grafts. Surgical tape can serve as a pressure dressing in areas on which bandages cannot be applied easily, such as fingertips.

Apply pressure dressings to all ear lacerations to prevent hematoma formation and subsequent deformation and destruction of cartilage. Envelop the ear in the dressing to distribute pressure from the outer bandage evenly across the irregular surface of the pinna. Pack moistened cotton into the concavities of the pinna until the cotton is level with the most lateral aspect of the helical rim. Cut square pieces of gauze to fit the curvature of the ear and place them behind (medial to) the pinna. Place several more gauze squares on the lateral

surface of the ear. Secure the packing in place with a circumferential head bandage, but do not encompass the opposite ear because it would just as easily cause pressure necrosis of that ear if left unprotected.

Bandage traumatic wounds to compress, immobilize, secure, and protect the wound and underlying dressing. Most bandaging is performed on extremities, where dressings are difficult to secure with tape alone. Rolls of cotton (Kerlix, Kling stretch gauze) are well suited for this purpose. Wind the bandage around the extremity and advance it proximally with circular, overlapping turns. Take care to avoid making wrinkles in the bandage, which may create pressure points, and also be careful to not make loose turns, which shorten the effective life of the dressing. When joint surfaces are crossed, anchor the cotton distally with several turns, then unroll it obliquely across the joint several times in a figure-of-eight pattern, and anchor it again proximally with two complete turns. Repeat this process until the bandage is securely in place. Fasten the ends of the bandage to the skin with strips of adhesive tape.

Bandages over the forearm and the lower extremities are particularly prone to slippage because of the constant motion of these parts and the marked changes in diameter of the extremity over a short distance. To help prevent this problem, rotate the roll of bandage 180 degrees after each circular turn to produce a reverse spiral and reduce the bandage's mobility (Fig. 34-16*B*). A simple dressing for a single digit is to use tube gauze or cover it with a finger cut from a surgical glove (see Fig. 34-16*C* and *D*).

Certain chemically treated wide-mesh weaves have the properties of cling and stretch, which holds it snugly in place but expands if edema develops.[74] An elastic cotton roll (Kerlix) allows the bandage to conform to body contours, provides some mobility to bandaged joints, and permits the wound to swell without the circumferential bandage constricting the extremity. An inelastic Kling bandage better immobilizes the part. Use rigid immobilization with plaster splints or braces to protect wounds in mobile areas, such as around large joints.

Most scalp wounds do well when left uncovered. Encourage the patient to shower daily to remove debris from a sutured scalp laceration. If a dressing is necessary, hold it in place with a bandage. Change the outer layer of the dressing when it becomes externally contaminated, it is saturated with exudate, or inspection and wound cleaning are required.

Dressings vary in their absorbency, adhesiveness, occlusiveness, opacity, and insulating properties. Further research may identify types of dressings that are best suited for different phases of the healing wound. Currently, a two- or three-layer dressing is used for most traumatic wounds. Base the choice of material for the contact layer on the characteristics of the individual wound.[87]

Splinting and Elevation

Wounds and sutured lacerations may be immobilized to enhance healing and to provide patient comfort (Fig. 34-17). *Immobilization of an injured extremity promotes healing* by protecting the closure and by limiting the spread of contamination and infection along lymphatic channels. Wounds overlying joints are subjected to repeated stretching and movement, which delays healing, widens the scar, and potentially disrupts

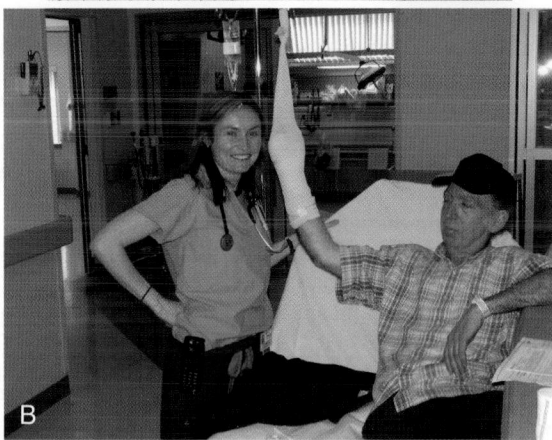

Figure 34-17 A, A pillow wrapped around a bandaged hand promotes elevation at home. Note that this sutured hand laceration also has a plaster splint for comfort. In general, immobilization promotes healing. **B,** Elevation of a severe hand injury in the emergency department with a stockinette, splint, and intravenous pole while awaiting the surgeon.

the sutures.[20] Short-term splints are almost always beneficial for lacerations that overlie joints and are frequently necessary for the protection of wounds involving the fingers, hands, wrists, volar aspect of the forearms, extensor surface of the elbows, posterior aspect of the legs, plantar surface of the feet, and the extremities when skin grafts have been applied. A plaster or aluminum splint may be incorporated into a bandage to reduce the mobility of the part.

Elevate injured extremities in all but the most trivial injuries. Elevation limits edema formation, allows more rapid healing,[20] and reduces throbbing pain. Patients given this information are often more motivated to elevate the extremity as instructed. Use slings to elevate wounds involving the forearm or the hand. The patient can also wrap a pillow around an injured hand to promote elevation at home (see Fig. 34-17A). With severe injuries, begin elevation in the ED (see Fig. 34-17B).

Figure 34-18 This patient used a neomycin-containing ointment on a minor wound, and redness, swelling, pruritus, and skin changes developed. The patient thought that it was an infection, but it was contact dermatitis from the neomycin. Plain bacitracin ointment will not cause this relatively common reaction. Bacitracin and Silvadene are alternative topicals, but any preparation is probably of minimal value.

Ointments

The safety and efficacy of topical antibiotic preparations used on wound surfaces are unproven, and no universal standard exists. Many clinicians routinely suggest the use of antibiotic ointments over sutured wounds, whereas others opt for a simple dry dressing. Use of a triple-antibiotic preparation containing neomycin, bacitracin, and polymyxin provides a broad spectrum of protection against infection in abrasions without systemic absorption, toxicity, or the emergence of resistant strains of bacteria. There is some evidence that Neosporin ointment, Silvadene cream, and mupirocin (Bactroban, GlaxoSmithKline, London), as well as their inert bases and vehicles, either improve wound healing or slightly reduce infection rates.[88] Although there is a risk for allergic sensitization or contact dermatitis with preparations containing neomycin, allergic reactions are uncommon unless the ointment is used repeatedly (Fig. 34-18).

One obvious benefit from the use of topical antibiotics is that ointments prevent adherence of the wound surface to the dressing. Use ointments to reduce the formation of a crust that covers and separates the edges of the wound. Lacerations surrounded by abraded skin are especially predisposed to coagulum formation. In such cases, instruct the patient to cleanse the wound frequently and to follow the cleansing with an application of ointment during the first few days.[20]

Strong topical corticosteroids have detrimental effects on healing. Application of 0.1% triamcinolone acetonide in an ointment retards healing in wounds by as much as 60%, whereas hydrocortisone probably does not interfere with epithelialization.[89] Some clinicians believe that single and low doses of oral corticosteroids probably have no effect on wound healing but that repeated, large doses of steroids (≤40 mg of prednisone per day) inhibit healing, particularly if used before the injury or during the first 3 days of the healing phase.[90] There is some evidence that topical vitamin A may reverse some of the antiinflammatory and immunosuppressive effects of corticosteroids.[91]

The exact value of ointments in the treatment of lacerations has yet to be determined. However, routine use of ointments after wound cleaning does encourage inspection of the wound by patients. Do not use ointments on wounds closed with tissue adhesive because the ointment will dissolve the adhesive.

Wound Cultures

Tissue taken for culture at the time of wound preparation and closure in the ED serves no useful purpose and is not recommended. The results of such cultures cannot logically guide future antibiotic selection. It is not necessary to routinely culture all minimally infected wounds after closure. Cultures should be considered if the infection is extensive, unusual, or otherwise concerning, if the patient is immunocompromised, or if there is suspicion of methicillin-resistant *Staphylococcus aureus*. All wounds that are grossly infected at the time of follow-up should be assessed for the presence of a foreign body.

It is not uncommon to encounter a minor suture track infection or inflammation of the suture tracks at the time of suture removal, as evidenced by a small drop of pus when the suture is removed. Such minor infections, so-called suture abscesses, usually do well with warm soaks or topical antibiotic ointments and do not require wound cultures or systemic antibiotics.

Systemic Antibiotics

Most traumatic soft tissue injuries sustain a low level of bacterial contamination.[56] Uncomplicated wound infection rates in ED patients range from 2% to 5%, *regardless of clinician intervention*. In a number of clinical studies of relatively uncontaminated and uncomplicated traumatic wounds (which represent the majority of wounds managed in the ED), prophylactic antibiotics administered in various routes and regimens did not reduce the incidence of infection.[92-98] Studies of antibiotic prophylaxis for animal bite wounds have produced variable results, and no large study providing stratification of the many prognostic factors has been conducted.[99]

Even after multiple studies on the use of prophylactic antibiotics for wounds treated in the ED, there is no clear practice standard.[100] Because no benefit has been established after multiple attempts with numerous antibiotic regimens, one would intuit that they have no benefit. In most soft tissue wounds in which the level of bacterial contamination after cleaning and débridement is low, antibiotics are not recommended. Heavily contaminated wounds (such as wounds in contact with pus or feces) often become infected despite antibiotic treatment. Nevertheless, antibiotics may have marginal benefit when the level of contamination is overwhelming or if the amount of questionably viable tissue left in the wound is considerable (e.g., with crush wounds). Antibiotics may be considered for extremity bite wounds, puncture-type bite wounds in any location, intraoral lacerations that are sutured, orocutaneous lip wounds, wounds that cannot be cleaned or débrided satisfactorily, and highly contaminated wounds (e.g., those contaminated with soil, organic matter, purulence, feces, saliva, or vaginal secretions). They may also be considered for wounds involving tendons, bones, or joints; for wounds requiring extensive débridement in the operating room; for wounds in lymphedematous tissue; for distal extremity wounds when treatment is delayed for 12 to 24 hours; for patients with orthopedic prostheses; and for patients at risk for the development of infective endocarditis.[20]

Although some consider prescribing prophylactic antibiotics for immunocompromised patients (diabetics and others), a true benefit has not consistently been demonstrated in any subset. The downside is selection of resistant organisms, and many resistant strains now encountered in clinical practice (patients and in the community) have been linked to the excessive use of needless antibiotics. It seems most prudent to eschew routine antibiotic prophylaxis and opt for meticulous wound care, close follow-up, and the selective use of antibiotics for proven infection. Other disadvantages of routine antibiotic use include needless expense and potential side effects (e.g., rash, anaphylaxis, diarrhea, vomiting). If antibiotics are considered useful in a specific case, give them as soon as possible after wounding and continue them for only 2 to 3 days in the absence of development of an infection. If the risk for infection is high enough to warrant antibiotics, delayed primary closure may also be considered.

Many patients have difficulty determining whether their wounds are infected and mistake the normal healing process for infection; therefore, in high-risk patients (a clinical judgment), mandatory follow-up would appear to be the best tactic.[101]

The choice of antibiotic, particularly for bite wound prophylaxis, is as controversial as the indications for use.[102] Many species of bacteria cause animal bite wound infections, thus making complete coverage impossible.[103] Antibiotic regimens vary with the species of the biter and with evolving bacterial resistance. The duration of antibiotic prophylaxis is also in question. It is common practice to provide antibiotics for 72 hours. (See additional comments on animal bites at the end of this chapter.)

Immunoprophylaxis

Although tetanus is rare, it still occurs in the United States and is a preventable disease. Therefore, any wound should be assessed for its potential to cause tetanus, and prophylaxis should be considered in the ED. About 70% of Americans older than 6 years have protective levels of tetanus antibodies, but levels decline as age increases, with elderly women having the lowest levels of protection. Hispanics (and probably other immigrants) were most likely to have inadequate immunity. Hence, efforts at preventing tetanus should especially be addressed in immigrants and the elderly. The recommendations of the Centers for Disease Control and Prevention for tetanus prophylaxis are listed in Figure 34-19.[104]

When questioning patients about their tetanus immunization status, ask whether they ever completed the primary immunization series and, if not, how many doses were given. Patients who have not completed a full primary series of injections may require both tetanus toxoid and passive immunization with tetanus immune globulin. Tetanus immune globulin will decrease, but not totally eliminate the subsequent development of clinical tetanus. Tetanus and diphtheria immunizations are often given together. The preferred preparation for active tetanus immunization in patients 7 years of age and older is 0.5 mL of tetanus toxoid (plus the lower, adult dose of diphtheria toxoid); the dose of tetanus immune globulin is 250 to 500 units given intramuscularly.[105]

Mild local reactions consisting of erythema and induration are common (≈20%) after tetanus toxoid injections; occasionally, they are accompanied by fever and mild systemic symptoms. Reactions are about twice as common if diphtheria

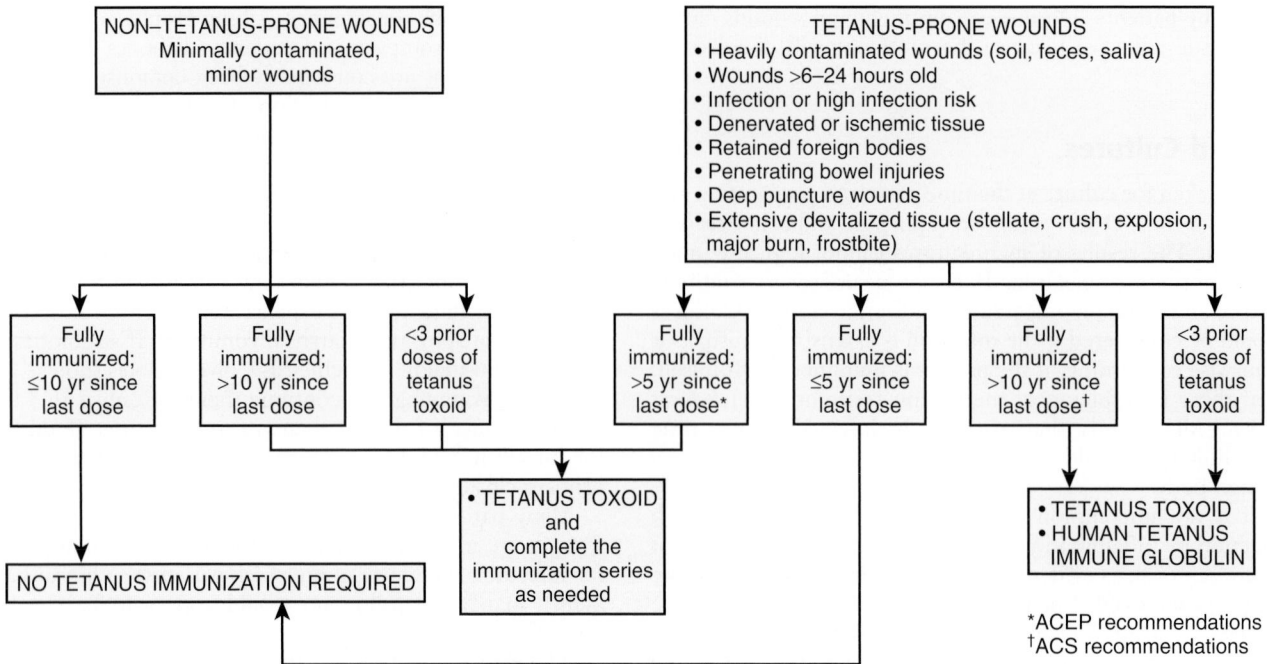

Figure 34-19 Tetanus immunization guidelines. *ACEP,* American College of Emergency Physicians; *ACS,* American College of Surgeons.

immunization is coupled with tetanus immunization. This is a hypersensitivity reaction, not an infection, and does not represent an absolute contraindication to further immunizations. A minor febrile illness, such as an upper respiratory infection, is not a reason to delay immunization. Although serious reactions are rare, a hypersensitivity reaction consisting of tenderness, erythema, and swelling or serum sickness develops in some patients with high antibody levels. Generalized urticarial reactions and peripheral neuropathy have also been reported.[106] The only absolute contraindication to tetanus toxoid is a history of anaphylaxis or a neurologic event. In such cases, tetanus immune globulin can be given safely. Pregnancy is not a contraindication to either toxoid or immune globulin, although some suggest that the toxoid be used with caution during the first trimester. Given the excellent amnestic response to the toxoid, it is likely that the primary immunization series, coupled with intermittent boosters, conveys immunity for most of one's life. However, a significant percentage of elderly patients fail to develop protective antitoxin antibody titers after 14 days when given tetanus toxoid boosters.

Base treatment decisions on the differentiation between clean and contaminated wounds. Even though any break in the skin can harbor *Clostridium tetani,* traditional definitions of tetanus-prone wounds include injuries more than 6 hours old; wounds contaminated by feces, saliva, purulent exudate, or soil; wounds with retained foreign bodies or containing devitalized or avascular tissue; established wound infections; penetrating abdominal wounds involving bowel; deep puncture wounds; and wounds caused by crush, burns, or frostbite.

Tetanus can develop despite prior immunization, and it can result from chronic skin lesions and apparently minor or clean wounds.[107] In 10% to 20% of cases, no previous wound can be identified. Patients' recall of past immunizations is imperfect, and immunity may be, on rare occasion, inadequate after a complete series of tetanus toxoid.[108] Tetanus boosters given more frequently than advised increase the incidence of adverse reactions to subsequent injections. However, the benefits of overtreatment seem to outweigh the risks.

PATIENT INSTRUCTIONS

Successful wound healing is partly dependent on the care given to the wound once the patient leaves the ED. Patient satisfaction depends not only on the cosmetic result but also on the expectation of that result.[10] Both are reasons why patients should receive thorough and clear instructions.

Inform the patient that no matter how skillful the repair, any wound of significance produces a scar. Most scars deepen in color and become more prominent before they mature and fade. The final appearance of the scar cannot be judged before 6 to 12 months after the repair.[8] Some wounds heal with wide, unattractive scars despite ideal management and closure. Wounds more likely to have significant scars are those that cross perpendicular to joints, wrinkle lines, or lines of minimum tension (Kraissel lines) and those that retract more than 5 mm. Wound that are likely to scar are those that are located over convexities or in certain anatomic locations (e.g., anterior upper part of the chest, back, shoulders) where hypertrophic scars are common. A wound crossing a concave surface may result in a bowstring deformity; one crossing a convexity may leave a scar depression. To avoid these complications, a Z-plasty procedure can be performed at the time of initial wound management, or the scar can be revised later. Tell the patient to expect suboptimal outcomes in these situations.[24]

Patients may experience dysesthesia in or around a scar, particularly about the midface. Gentle rubbing or pressing on the skin may relieve the symptoms. If wounds extending to subcutaneous levels lacerate cutaneous nerves, patients may be bothered by hypoesthesia distal to the wound. The dysesthesia and anesthesia usually resolve in 6 months to 1 year.[10]

After 48 hours the patient may remove the dressing on uncomplicated wounds and check for evidence of infection: redness, warmth, increasing pain, swelling, purulent drainage, or the "red streaks" of lymphangitis. Not all patients are able to identify these signs and often overlook an early infection or overcall an infection in the presence of normal healing. Patients with complicated or infection-prone wounds should be examined in 2 to 3 days by a clinician or nurse.[109] Inform patients that a painful wound is often a sign of infection or suture reaction, and pain should prompt inspection of the wound. If no sign of infection is present after 48 to 72 hours, the patient can care for the wound until it is time for removal of the sutures.

Because the edges of a wound are sealed by coagulum and bridged by epithelial cells within 48 hours, the wound is essentially impermeable to bacteria after 2 days.[14,110] Instruct the patient to protect the wound and keep the dressing clean and dry for 24 to 48 hours. In this initial period, change the dressing only if it becomes externally soiled or soaked by exudate from the wound. If possible, keep the injured part elevated.

Daily gentle washing with mild soap and water to remove dried blood and exudate is probably beneficial, especially in areas such as the face or the scalp,[109-111] but vigorous scrubbing of wounds should be discouraged. Patients may bathe with sutures in place but should not immerse the wound for a prolonged time. Although diluted hydrogen peroxide can be used to remove blood from the skin surface, it should not be repeatedly used as a cleaning agent on the healing wound itself.[35] Generally, a wound should be protected with a dressing during the first week and the dressing changed daily. If the wound is unlikely to be contaminated or traumatized, leave it uncovered. Sutured scalp lacerations are usually left open, and showering is encouraged.

If an injured extremity or finger is protected by a splint, it should be left undisturbed until the sutures are removed. Patients with intraoral lacerations can be instructed to use warm salt water mouth rinses at least three times a day.

Swimming is often prohibited while sutures are in place, but there are no data supporting this admonition. In general, showering and bathing are quite acceptable in the presence of sutured wounds. Common sense should prevail in making such decisions.

Patients may ask about the efficacy of various creams and lotions (e.g., vitamin E, aloe vera, cocoa butter) in limiting scar formation. At this time there are no data to evaluate the use of these substances. Their use is acceptable and may prompt some patients to participate in wound inspection and cleaning more regularly.

SECONDARY WOUND CARE

Reexamination

Patients with simple sutured wounds may be released with appropriate instructions for home care and be told to return for removal of the sutures at an appropriate time. Examine high-risk wounds, such as bite wounds and other infection-prone wounds, in 2 to 3 days for signs of infection. Inspect the wound if the patient experiences increasing discomfort, a fever develops, or the patient believes that the wound is infected.[71] Evaluate wounds being considered for delayed primary closure in 4 to 5 days.[65]

Figure 34-20 This patient was seen twice with a scalp wound infection and given two courses of antibiotics with initial improvement, all before the blade of a utility knife (*arrow*) was discovered in the wound. He was intoxicated during a bar fight and resisted wound closure in the emergency department, so it was done hastily and not thoroughly explored.

Wounds in which extensive dissection of subcutaneous tissue has been performed may develop an intense inflammation similar in appearance to low-grade, localized cellulitis. It is rarely necessary to open these wounds. Remove one or two stitches to relieve some of the tension caused by mild swelling, if necessary. Cleanse daily with water and a mild soap and apply warm compresses, and this type of wound reaction should subside within 24 to 48 hours.[71]

If a wound becomes infected, evaluate for the presence of a retained foreign body as the nidus of the infection (Fig. 34-20). Also, in most sutured wounds that become infected, remove the sutures to allow drainage. If a wound exhibits a minor infection, remove a few sutures or all of them. Pack grossly infected wounds open to allow further drainage. Infection around a suture can lead to the formation of a stitch mark.[112] Treat infected wounds with daily cleansing, warm compresses, and antibiotics. Leave wounds that have been opened to heal by secondary intention, which involves wound contraction, granulation tissue formation, and epithelialization.

Most wound infections can be treated in the outpatient setting with oral antibiotics and follow-up, but each case should be individualized. Lymphangitis does not mandate intravenous antibiotics or hospitalization.

Suture Removal

The optimal time for suture removal varies with the location of the wound, the rate of wound healing, and the amount of tension on the wound. Certain areas of the body, such as the back of the hand, heal slowly, whereas facial or scalp wounds heal rapidly. The speed of wound healing is affected by systemic factors such as malnutrition, neoplasia, and immunosuppression. Therefore, only general guidelines can be given for the timing of suture removal. At the time that suture removal is being considered, one or two sutures may be cut to determine whether the edges of the skin are sufficiently adherent to allow removal of all the sutures.[5] Removing

SUTURE REMOVAL

Skin surface   Skin surface   or   Skin surface   Skin surface

Skin pulled apart

Skin surface

CORRECT METHODS

A

INCORRECT METHOD

B

Figure 34-21 Technique for removal of sutures. Pull toward the wound line (**A**) rather than away from it (**B**), which causes the wound to tear apart. After suture removal, supporting the wound with surgical tape (Steri-Strips) may be advisable if tension or minor dehiscence is present.

sutures too early invites wound dehiscence and widening of the scar, whereas leaving sutures in longer than necessary may result in epithelial tracks, infection, and unsightly scarring.[113]

Percutaneous sutures stimulate an inflammatory reaction along the suture track. Factors that determine the severity of stitch marks include the length of time that stitches are left in place, skin tension, the relationship of the suture to the edge of the wound, the region of the body, infection, and the patient's tendency for keloid formation.[112,114] The skin of the eyelids, palms, and soles and the mucous membranes seldom show stitch marks. In contrast, oily skin and the skin of the back, the sternal area, the upper part of the arms, the lower extremities, the dorsum of the nose, and the forehead are likely to exhibit the permanent imprints of suture material on the skin surface.[112]

If sutures are removed within 7 days, generally no discernible needle puncture or stitch marks will persist.[114] However, at 6 days the wound is held together by a small amount of fibrin and cells and has minimal strength.[68] The tensile strength of most wounds at this time is adequate to hold the wound edges together, but only if there is no appreciable dynamic or static skin force pulling the wound apart.[5] Minimal trauma to an unsupported wound at this point could cause dehiscence. The clinician should decide on the proper time to remove the sutures after weighing these various factors. If early suture removal is necessary (such as on the face), wound repair can be maintained with strips of surgical skin tape. The key to wound tensile strength after suture removal is an adequate deep tissue layered closure.

Some general guidelines exist for suture removal. Remove sutures on the face on the fifth day after the injury or remove alternate sutures on the third day and the remainder on the fifth day. On the extremities and the anterior aspect of the trunk, leave sutures in place for approximately 7 days to prevent disruption of the wound. Leave sutures on the scalp, back, feet, hands, and joints in place for 10 to 14 days, even though permanent stitch marks may result.[112] Some clinicians recommend removal of the sutures used to repair eyelid lacerations as early as 72 hours to avoid epithelialization along the suture track along with subsequent cyst formation.[115]

Removing sutures is usually relatively simple. Cleanse the wound and any remaining crust overlying the surface of the wound or surrounding the sutures. Wipe the skin with an alcohol swab. Cut each stitch with scissors or the tip of a No. 11 scalpel blade at a point close to the surface of the skin on one side. Grasp the suture on the opposite side with forceps and pull it across the wound (Fig. 34-21). The amount of exposed suture dragged through the suture track is thereby minimized. It is difficult to remove sutures with very short ends. At the time of suture placement, cut the length of the suture ends so they generally equal the distance between sutures. This makes it easier to grasp the suture during subsequent removal while avoiding entanglement during the knotting of adjacent sutures.

Once the skin sutures are removed, the width of the scar increases gradually over the next 3 to 5 weeks unless it is supported. Support is provided by previously placed subcutaneous stitches that bring the edges of the skin into apposition or by the application of skin tape. A nonabsorbable subcuticular suture can be left in place for 2 to 3 weeks to provide continued support for the wound. Although complications such as closed epithelial sinuses, cysts, or internal tracts can occur from prolonged use of this stitch, they are unusual and can be avoided by placement of a buried subcuticular stitch with an absorbable suture.[14]

Small stitch abscesses may occur in wounds when sutures remain in place for more than 7 to 10 days. Localized stitch abscesses generally resolve after removal of the sutures and application of warm compresses and without antibiotics in simple cases.

If time and effort have been invested in cosmetic closure of the face, protect the repair with skin tape after the skin sutures have been removed. Wound contraction and scar widening continue for 42 days after the injury.[68] Because the desired result is a scar of minimal width, the tape can be used for as long as 5 weeks after removal of the sutures. With exposure to sunlight, scars in their first 4 months redden to a greater extent than the surrounding skin does. In exposed cosmetic areas and when prolonged exposure to the sun is anticipated, appropriate sun protection and avoidance strategies should be used (e.g., a hat and sunscreen). Sunscreen may have a role in protecting scars from the sun, but more studies are needed to better understand its impact.

COMPLICATIONS

There are several reasons why wounds fail to heal; some are related to decisions made at the time of wound closure, and others are consequences of later events. Some of the impediments to healing include ischemia or necrosis of tissue, hematoma formation, prolonged inflammation caused by foreign material, excessive tension on the edges of the skin, and immunocompromising systemic factors. A primary cause of delayed healing is wound infection. Wound cleaning and débridement, atraumatic and aseptic handling of tissue, and the use of protective dressings minimize this complication. Inversion of the edges of a wound during closure produces a more noticeable scar, whereas skillful technique can convert a jagged, contaminated wound into a fine, inapparent scar. The patient's actions also affect wound healing. Delay in seeking treatment of an injury may significantly affect the ultimate outcome of the wound. Furthermore, in the first few days after an injury, the patient must take responsibility for protecting the wound from contamination, further trauma, and swelling.

Infection is probably the most common cause of dehiscence. If the patient is careless or unlucky, reinjury can reopen a wound despite the protection of a thick dressing. If the size of the suture is too small, the stitch may break. A stitch that is too fine or tied too tightly may cut through friable tissue and pull out. Knots that have not been tied carefully may unravel. The suture material may be extruded or absorbed too rapidly. Finally, if a stitch is removed too early (i.e., before tissues regain adequate tensile strength), the wound loses support and falls open. If the wound edges show signs of separating at the time of suture removal, alternate stitches can be left in place and the entire length of the wound supported by strips of adhesive tape.

The final appearance of a scar is determined by several factors. Infection, tissue necrosis, and keloid formation widen a scar. Wounds located in sebaceous skin or oriented 90 degrees to dynamic or static skin tension lines result in wide scars.

Miscellaneous Aspects of Wound Care

Traumatic wounds are created by a wide variety of mechanisms, and clinicians must sometimes adjust wound management techniques to match special circumstances.

The ED Approach to Puncture Wounds

Puncture wounds are common, yet there are no universal treatment standards or prospective studies to identify the most effective and most appropriate way to manage puncture wounds in the ED. Aside from evaluating tetanus immunization status and considering the possibility of a foreign body, the clinician has few proven options to prevent infection in a puncture wound (Fig. 34-22). Clinical experience suggests that the course of a puncture wound is likely to be determined at the time of the injury. Scrubbing the surface of the puncture, evaluating the opening for retained foreign matter, and trimming jagged skin and tissue edges are suggested. The value or appropriateness of coring, probing, or irrigating the puncture track has not been established. Forcing an irrigation catheter into a small puncture wound is counterproductive and discouraged. Deep irrigation is impossible without extending the puncture site into a larger laceration, and there are theoretical risks of delayed healing and dissemination of contamination unless the full depth of the puncture is accessible and irrigated. In general, aggressive irrigation and routine enlargement of the puncture track are not recommended. For through-and-through punctures, the track can often be débrided by pulling gauze through the wound.

It is impossible to accurately predict the final outcome of a puncture wound, although most do well. No prospective randomized trials have evaluated the role of prophylactic antibiotic administration to prevent infection in puncture wounds. Hence there are no standards on the use, type, or duration of prophylactic antibiotic therapy, even in high-risk patients. Most clinicians take a conservative approach, forego routine antibiotics, and opt for simple cleaning and appropriate follow-up. Puncture wounds in immunocompromised patients are assessed individually and may receive alternative or more aggressive care. If a puncture is grossly contaminated or harbors foreign material, antibiotics will not prevent an infection; however, this scenario may not be appreciated for a number of days and does not mandate inappropriate aggressive interventions. Puncture wounds of the bottom of the foot may be an exception and are discussed in more detail in Chapter 51.

Gunshot Wounds

A subset of gunshot wounds may be definitively handled in the ED with outpatient follow-up. Studies by Ordog and colleagues[116,117] documented a very low infection rate in gunshot wounds treated with standard wound care on an outpatient basis, even when the missile was left in place and minor fractures were present. Because most gunshot wounds are puncture wounds, only minimal deep wound cleaning is possible. Superficial soft tissue wounds with entrance and exit wounds in proximity may be débrided by passing sterile gauze back and forth through the wound track (Fig. 34-23). Though prescribed frequently, no data support the routine use of antibiotics following gunshot wounds.

Animal Bites

Many aspects of the treatment of animal bites are controversial, and no universal standards exist. Most bites are caused by dogs or cats that are family pets. Numerous organisms can be cultured from an infected bite wound caused by a dog or cat, and cultures may guide antibiotic therapy in infected wounds.[103] Wound material taken for culture at the time of an animal bite is worthless. The predominant pathogens in animal bites are the oral flora of the biting animal and human skin flora. About 85% of bites harbor potential pathogens, and the average wound yields five types of bacterial isolates; 60% have mixed aerobic and anaerobic bacteria. Skin flora such as staphylococci and streptococci are isolated in about 40% of bites. The gram-negative rod *Pasteurella multocida*, *S. aureus*, and *Streptococcus viridans* are common culprits in bite wound infections. *Pasteurella* species are isolated from 50% of dog bite wounds and 75% of cat bite wounds. Cat bites are usually puncture wounds that cannot be completely cleaned. When compared with dog bites, cat bites may become infected rather quickly after the bite (within 24 hours), thus suggesting *Pasteurella* infection (Fig. 34-24). Cat bite wounds tend to penetrate deeply, with a higher risk for associated osteomyelitis, tenosynovitis, and septic arthritis than with dog bites, which are more likely to have associated crush injury and wound trauma. *Capnocytophaga canimorsus*, a fastidious gram-negative rod, can cause bacteremia and fatal sepsis after animal bites, especially in asplenic patients or those with underlying hepatic disease. Anaerobes isolated from dog and cat bite wounds include *Bacteroides*, fusobacteria, *Porphyromonas*, *Prevotella*, propionibacteria, and peptostreptococci. Puncture wounds from a dog can be problematic since they are difficult

Figure 34-22 Puncture wounds cannot be cleaned meticulously and the course is usually set at the time of the injury. This nail gun puncture of the distal finger joint (**A-C**) was able to be débrided by passing a small hemostat through the puncture wound and pulling gauze through the wound (**D**). A small piece of metal, used to attach the nails together (*arrows*), was removed with this maneuver (**E**). Note that nails from a nail gun clip are held together with a piece of metal that may hamper removal or be left in the wound (**F**). A splint and 3 days of cephalexin prophylaxis (because of the discovered foreign body) were provided, and this wound healed well.

to clean unless they are through-and-through wounds (Fig. 34-25) The incidence of infection after thoroughly cleaned dog bite lacerations may not be significantly greater than the incidence of infection in lacerations in general. Consequently, some clinicians have advocated primary closure of large dog bite lacerations that are centrally located on the body; however, markedly contused lacerations are good candidates for delayed primary closure (see Fig. 34-15*B*).

Treat infected animal bites with antibiotics, but the use of prophylactic antibiotics for animal bites is controversial (see earlier discussion). *Prophylactic* amoxicillin-clavulanate (875/125 mg twice daily) given for 3 to 5 days may reduce infection rates after cat or dog bites, especially for a puncture wound or if the patient is seen more than 8 hours after the bite and wound cleaning has been inadequate. Antibiotics given sooner seem to offer no benefit. Some clinicians

administer prophylactic antibiotics for all cat bites, for a dog bite that has been sutured, for hand wounds, for wounds close to a bone or joint, or for bites associated with deep tissue or crush injury. Although this is a reasonable and common approach, there are no data strongly supporting this practice. Alternative antibiotics include metronidazole (500 mg three times daily) *plus* moxifloxacin (400 mg daily), doxycycline (100 mg twice daily), or trimethoprim-sulfamethoxazole (1 double-strength tablet twice daily). Antibiotics lacking in vitro activity against *P. multocida* should be avoided; such antibiotics include first-generation cephalosporins (such as cephalexin), penicillinase-resistant penicillins (such as dicloxacillin), macrolides (such as erythromycin), and clindamycin. However, clindamycin may be used for anaerobic coverage if it is administered in conjunction with an additional agent that is active against *P. multocida*. The best way to approach bite wounds is

Figure 34-23 Patients with minor gunshot wounds may be treated as outpatients, even when bullet fragments remain and minor fractures are present. **A** and **B,** This through-and-through injury traversed the hypothenar eminence. No bullet remained and no bones were involved. **C,** Usually, it is impossible to irrigate a puncture wound, but in this case, note the saline at the exit site. **D,** After the entrance wound is débrided of the powder burn, pass an instrument through the wound. Grasp the gauze packing with the instrument and pull it into the wound. Pull the gauze *back and forth to débride the wound track.* Similarly, place clean packing. **E,** For a similarly cleansed gunshot wound of the leg, leave the gauze packing in the track for 48 hours. No antibiotics were given, the pack was removed at wound check in 48 hours, and the patient did well.

Human Bites

Human bite wounds are problematic because patients may not be truthful about the cause, wound care may be delayed, and these wounds may contain foreign material, human saliva contamination, and deep structural injury. Pathogens include aerobic bacteria (such as streptococci and *S. aureus*) and anaerobic bacteria (such as *Eikenella, Fusobacterium, Peptostreptococcus, Prevotella,* and *Porphyromonas* species). When cultured, most infected human bites harbor three to four pathogens, including both aerobes and anaerobes. Limited case reports suggest that viral pathogens, including hepatitis, HIV, and herpes simplex virus, may be transmissible by human bites; however, data are lacking to guide the clinician on the best approach in the ED for these potential infections. Generally, prophylaxis is not suggested if the wound does not penetrate the dermis.

Clenched fist injuries, caused by contact with another person's teeth during a fight, are the most serious human bite wounds. Lacerations typically occur over the third and fourth metacarpophalangeal or proximal interphalangeal joints of

Figure 34-24 Cat bite. Cat bites are puncture wounds that become infected rather quickly. See text for discussion of antibiotics.

simply to adhere to the basic principles of wound care. No specific intervention has been demonstrated to be superior for the preparation of bite wounds. Take care to search for underlying fractures or tooth fragments with deep animal bites. When a wound results from the bite or scratch of either a wild or a domestic animal, give rabies prophylaxis if indicated (Tables 34-2 and 34-3).

Figure 34-25 Dog bite. **A-D**, Dog bite puncture wounds are difficult to clean if not through and through. See text for discussion of the use antibiotics.

the dominant hand. Even small lacerations or punctures are highly prone to infection. Joint penetration is not uncommon. Relaxation of the fist may disseminate organisms into the deep compartments and the deep tendon spaces of the hand and predispose the patient to deep soft tissue infection, septic arthritis, and osteomyelitis. Many patients ignore these wounds until the onset of pain, swelling, or purulent discharge; as a result, these injuries are often complicated by established infection at the initial ED visit. In addition, some patients are not truthful about the origin of the wound, thereby leading to incorrect ED treatment of a seemingly minor injury (Fig. 34-26).

Irrigate bite wounds copiously with tap water or sterile saline, and remove grossly visible debris. Many clinicians will extend a small laceration to allow visualization of the underlying structures and better cleaning. Look for tooth chips, tendon injury, and joint penetration. Wounds involving tendons or joint spaces are more serious and require close follow-up.

In general, leave all human bite wounds open (unsutured), even when treated soon after the injury and with seemingly benign wound conditions. Pack them with gauze until follow-up, or loosely approximate the wound to facilitate closure by secondary intention. Do not use deep sutures. On reevaluation within a few days, perform delayed primary closure if desired. Facial bite wounds are a special exception, so consider primary closure for these wounds. Splinting of the hand in a position of function with a short-arm volar splint

for a few days is suggested, and elevation of the injured area is advised.

Most clinicians administer prophylactic antibiotics for 3 to 5 days for human bites that are not infected. There are no data demonstrating the need for this or trials to define the best antibiotic. Most infections are polymicrobial, but antibiotics with activity against *S. aureus*, *Eikenella corrodens*, *Haemophilus influenzae*, and β-lactamase–producing oral anaerobic bacteria are suggested. Amoxicillin-clavulanate (875/125 mg twice daily) is a common recommendation for monotherapy. Alternative empirical regimens include doxycycline (100 mg twice daily), trimethoprim-sulfamethoxazole (1 double-strength tablet twice daily), penicillin VK (500 mg four times daily), ciprofloxacin (500 to 750 mg twice daily), or moxifloxacin (400 mg once daily) plus metronidazole (500 mg three times daily) or clindamycin (450 mg three times daily).

Avoid agents that lack activity against *E. corrodens*, including first-generation cephalosporins (such as cephalexin), penicillinase-resistant penicillins (such as dicloxacillin), macrolides (such as erythromycin), clindamycin, and aminoglycosides. However, clindamycin may be used for anaerobic coverage if it is administered in conjunction with an additional agent that is active against *E. corrodens*.

Grossly infected wounds should be treated with intravenous antibiotics, but the need for hospitalization is based on the patient's profile and the clinician's assessment of the severity of the infection.

TABLE 34-2 Rabies Postexposure Prophylaxis Guide—July 1999

The following recommendations are only a guide. In applying them, take into account the animal species involved, the circumstances of the bite or other exposure, the vaccination status of the animal, and the presence of rabies in the region. Local or state public health officials should be consulted if questions arise about the need for rabies prophylaxis.

ANIMAL SPECIES	CONDITION OF ANIMAL AT TIME OF ATTACK	TREATMENT OF EXPOSED PERSON*
Domestic		
Dog and cat	Healthy and available for 10 days of observation Rabid or suspected rabid. Unknown (escaped)	None unless rabies develops in the animal[†] Local wound healing should be included in the treatment of exposed person for each category RIG[‡] and HDCV Consult public health officials. If treatment is indicated, give RIG[‡] and HDCV
Wild		
Skunk, bat, fox, coyote, raccoon, bobcat, and other carnivores	Regard as rabid unless proved negative by laboratory tests[§]	RIG[‡] and HDCV
Other		
Livestock, rodents, and lagomorphs (rabbits and hares)	Consider individually. Local and state public health officials should be consulted on questions about the need for rabies prophylaxis. Bites of squirrels, hamsters, guinea pigs, gerbils, chipmunks, rats, mice, other rodents, rabbits, and hares almost never call for antirabies prophylaxis	

From Human rabies prevention—United States, 1999. Recommendations of the Advisory Committee on Immunization Practices (ACIP). *MMWR Recomm Rep.* 1999;48(RR-1):1. Available at http://www.cdc.gov/mmwr/preview/mmwrhtml/00056176.htm.
*All bites and wounds should be immediately cleansed thoroughly with soap and water. If antirabies treatment is indicated, both rabies immune globulin (RIG) and human diploid cell rabies vaccine (HDCV) should be given as soon as possible, regardless of the interval after exposure. Local reactions to vaccines are common and do not contraindicate continuing treatment. Discontinue vaccine if fluorescent antibody tests of the animal are negative.
[†]During the usual holding period of 10 days, begin treatment with RIG and HDCV at the first sign of rabies in a dog or cat that has bitten someone. The symptomatic animal should be killed immediately and tested.
[‡]If RIG is not available, use antirabies serum, equine. Do not use more than the recommended dosage.
[§]The animal should be killed and tested as soon as possible. Holding for observation is not recommended. Vaccination may be discontinued if immunofluorescence tests of the animal are negative.

TABLE 34-3 Rabies Postexposure Prophylaxis Schedule, United States

VACCINATION STATUS	TREATMENT	REGIMEN*
Not previously vaccinated	Local wound cleansing RIG Vaccine	All postexposure treatment should begin with immediate thorough cleansing of all wounds with soap and water 20 IU/kg of body weight; if anatomically feasible, up to half the dose should be infiltrated around wounds and the rest administered IM in the gluteal area. Note: RIG should not be administered in the same syringe or into the same anatomic site as vaccine because RIG may partially suppress active production of antibody. No more than the recommended dose should be given HDCV or RVA, 1 mL IM (deltoid area[†]), one each on days 0, 3, 7, 14, and 28
Previously vaccinated[‡]	Local wound cleansing RIG Vaccine	All postexposure treatment should begin with immediate thorough cleansing of all wounds with soap and water RIG should not be administered. HDCV or RVA, 1 mL IM (deltoid area[†]), one each on days 0 and 3

From Human rabies prevention—United States, 1999 recommendations of the Immunization Practices Advisory Committee. *MMWR Recomm Rep.* 1991;40(RR-3):1.
HDCV, human diploid cell rabies vaccine; *IM,* intramuscularly; *RIG,* rabies immune globulin; *RVA,* rabies vaccine, adsorbed. Four formulations of three inactivated rabies vaccines are currently licensed for preexposure and postexposure prophylaxis in the United States.
*These regimens are applicable for all age groups, including children.
[†]The deltoid area is the only acceptable site of vaccination for adults and older children. For younger children, the outer aspect of the thigh may be used. The vaccine should never be administered in the gluteal area.
[‡]Any person with a history of preexposure vaccination with HDCV or RVA, previous postexposure prophylaxis with HDCV or RVA, or prior vaccination with any other type of rabies vaccine and a documented history of antibody response to the previous vaccination.

Figure 34-26 Human bite. This patient was seen on a Monday morning with a small puncture wound on the dorsal surface of his hand (*arrow*), and he claimed that it was an injury sustained at work. Hence, minimal wound care was given. In reality, it was a human bite from a bar fight the night before. In 3 days, a serious infection was obvious and hospitalization was required.

Serious Wound Infections

Most wound infections are easily recognized and can be treated in the outpatient setting with oral antibiotics, suture removal, consideration for a retained foreign body, and a commonsense follow-up schedule. Consider impatient treatment for a patient with systemic complaints (fever, malaise, nausea), worsening infection at follow-up, an unreliable patient, or an immunocompromised patient. Some infections, such as a subgaleal infection in a scalp laceration, can be quite serious and will require prompt aggressive treatment (Fig. 34-27).

Digital Nerves

Numbness in the area of digital innervation, concomitant injury to a digital artery (flash, pulsating bleeding), or an electric shock sensation when exploring a laceration should alert the clinician to a possible digital nerve injury. If there is uncertainty about nerve injury, the diagnosis can be established at the time of a follow-up visit. However, lacerations of digital arteries that impair the distal circulation must be identified early during the initial evaluation.

Débridement of hand and finger lacerations should be minimal, and wound cleaning should be gentle yet thorough. Digital nerves that are transected distal to the metacarpophalangeal joint may be candidates for surgical repair. It is unclear at which point along the course of a digital nerve a transection can be repaired successfully, so proper referral to a hand specialist is essential. Frequently, injuries proximal to the distal interphalangeal joint are not repaired, but many other factors will influence operative decisions. Repair of a digital nerve will often result in return of good sensory function, but it takes months, and repair can prevent painful neuromas from developing. Most hand surgeons will not repair digital nerves at the initial visit. Instead, they advise wound cleaning, skin closure, splinting, and outpatient follow-up in 24 to 36 hours, followed by delayed nerve repair.

Accidental Soft Tissue Injection with an EpiPen

An EpiPen provides self-injected subcutaneous epinephrine (0.3 or 0.15 mg) for emergency treatment of anaphylaxis (Fig. 34-28).

Figure 34-27 Scalp lacerations rarely become infected because of the excellent blood supply to the area. **A,** This patient had a painful swollen area under a sutured scalp laceration (*long arrow*) and impressive forehead and facial swelling (*short arrow*) from a laceration on top of the head. It was originally thought to be a hematoma. **B,** Removal of sutures revealed frank pus and an extensive subgaleal abscess that required drainage and intravenous antibiotics. This infection can drain into the brain, face, neck, or mediastinum.

Figure 34-28 The EpiPen and EpiPen, Jr. Each injector issues only one dose of epinephrine, and each delivers a total volume of 0.3 mL. The adult version injects 0.3 mg of epinephrine (it contains epinephrine in a 1:1000 concentration, so there is 1 mg of epinephrine in 1 mL of volume). The EpiPen, Jr., injects a similar 0.3-mL volume but uses a 1:2000 dilution of epinephrine, so only 0.15 mg of epinephrine is delivered with the injection.

Occasionally, the device is inadvertently discharged, usually into a finger, and intense distal vasospasm is produced (Fig. 34-29). The patient has a blanched finger and minor sensory disturbances. The natural history of untreated vasospasm is unknown, and although ischemia may last for an hour or two, it is probably self-limited given the pharmacology of epinephrine. Digit amputation from this event has not been reported. Nonetheless, clinicians may be faced with an obviously ischemic finger, and intervention is considered. Local heat and nitroglycerin ointment have been tried but are of no proven benefit. Placing a pulse oximeter on the

Figure 34-29 Accidental discharge of an EpiPen into a finger will usually cause intense distal vasoconstriction. **A,** This patient sustained such an injection into the volar tuft of the index finger (*arrow*) 2 hours before evaluation in the emergency department. **B,** Blanching of the distal end of the finger (*arrow*) caused by the vasoconstriction. **C,** A pulse oximetry probe was applied to the finger, and normal saturation (96%) (*arrow*) was found. She was simply observed for another hour, the blanching resolved, and she was discharged without intervention. **D,** This patient suffered from a similar injection on the volar surface of the middle finger. Blanching is obvious (*arrow*). **E,** Phentolamine and lidocaine were injected along the volar surface of the finger. **F,** Five minutes later the finger was hyperemic (*arrow*). No further intervention was required.

fingertip can indicate the degree of resultant hypoxia, an indirect quantification of ischemia, and can likewise be used to assess reversal therapy.

Injecting the digit with the α-adrenergic antagonist phentolamine (Regitine) will immediately and permanently reverse the ischemia and can be safely initiated in the ED (see Fig. 34-29D-F). A 5-mg vial of phentolamine is reconstituted and diluted at a 1% plain lidocaine– or saline-to-phentolamine ratio of 1:1. Inject a small aliquot of the mixture with a 25- to 27-gauge needle. Both a digital block and direct injection of the reversal agent into the site of epinephrine injection have been described. Injecting the actual site of penetration is intuitively the best option, but no studies have been performed. Within 5 to 10 minutes, the ischemia is reversed, and no further action is required.[118,119]

References are available at www.expertconsult.com

CHAPTER 35

Methods of Wound Closure

Richard L. Lammers and Zachary E. Smith

Not all wounds require definitive closure at the first emergency department (ED) encounter; however, once the decision to close a wound has been made, the clinician must select the closure technique best suited for the location and configuration of the wound. The most commonly used techniques include tape, tissue adhesive, metal staples, and sutures. All traumatic wounds should be cleaned, and wounds containing devitalized tissue should be débrided before closure (see Chapter 34).

WOUND TAPE

Surgical tape strips are now routinely used to close simple wounds. Tape strips can be applied by health care personnel in many settings, including EDs, operating rooms, clinics, and first aid stations. Advantages include ease of application, reduced need for local anesthesia, evenly distributed wound tension, no residual suture marks, minimal skin reaction, no need for suture removal, superiority for some grafts and flaps, and suitability for use under plaster casts. One main advantage of wound tape over standard sutures and wound staples is its greater resistance to wound infection.[1-4]

Background and Tape Comparisons

Currently, several brands of tape with different porosity, flexibility, strength, and configuration are available. Steri-Strips (3M Corporation, St. Paul, MN) are microporous tapes with ribbed backing (Fig. 35-1). They are porous to air and water, and the ribbed backing provides extra strength. Cover-Strips (Beiersdorf, South Norwalk, CT) are woven in texture and have a high degree of porosity. They allow not only air and water but also wound exudates to pass through the tape. Shur-Strip (Deknatel, Inc, Floral Park, NY) is a nonwoven microporous tape. Clearon (Ethicon, Inc, Somerville, NJ) is a synthetic plastic tape whose backing contains longitudinal parallel serrations to permit gas and fluid permeability. An iodoform-impregnated Steri-Strip (3M Corporation) is intended to further retard infection without sensitization to iodine.[3] Other tape products include Curi-Strip (Kendall, Boston), Nichi-Strip (Nichiban Co., Ltd, Tokyo), Cicagraf (Smith & Nephew, London), and Suture Strip (Genetic Laboratories, St. Paul, MN).

Scientific studies of wound closure tapes provide some comparisons of products. Koehn[5] showed that Steri-Strip tape maintains adhesiveness about 50% longer than Clearon tape does. Rodeheaver and coworkers[6] compared Shur-Strip, Steri-Strip, and Clearon tape in terms of breaking strength, elongation, shear adhesion, and air porosity. The tapes were tested in both dry and wet conditions. Steri-Strip tape had about twice the breaking strength of the other two tapes in both dry and wet conditions; there was minimal loss of strength in all tapes when wetted. Shur-Strip tape showed approximately two to three times the elongation of the other tapes at the breaking point, whether dry or wet. Shear adhesion (amount of force required to dislodge the tape when a load is applied at the place of contact) was slightly better for the Shur-Strip tape than for the Steri-Strip tape and approximately 50% better than for the Clearon tape. Of these three wound tapes, the investigators considered Shur-Strips to be superior for wound closure.

One comprehensive study of wound tapes compared Curi-Strip, Steri-Strip, Nichi-Strip, Cicagraf, Suture Strip, and Suture Strip Plus.[7] All tapes were 12 mm wide except for Nichi-Strip, which was 15 mm. Each tape was compared for breaking strength, elongation under stress, air porosity, and adhesiveness. Curi-Strip, Cicagraf, and Steri-Strip exhibited equivalent dry breaking strength. However, when wet (a condition that can occur in the clinical setting), Cicagraf outperformed all tapes. All the tapes tested had similar elongation-under-stress profiles with the exception of Suture Strip Plus. This tape did not resist elongation under low or high force. Excessive elongation may allow wound dehiscence. Nichi-Strip was the most porous to air, and Cicagraf was almost vapor impermeable. Nichi-Strip and Curi-Strip had the best adherence to untreated skin. When the skin was treated with tincture of benzoin, however, Steri-Strip dramatically outperformed all other products. When all study parameters were considered, Nichi-Strip, Curi-Strip, and Steri-Strip achieved the highest overall performance rankings.

Indications

The primary indication for tape closure is a superficial straight laceration under little tension. If necessary, tension can be reduced by placing deep closures. Areas particularly suited for tape closure are the forehead, chin, malar eminence, thorax, and non–joint-related areas of the extremities. Tape may also be preferred for wounds in anxious children when suture placement is not essential. In young children who are likely to remove the tape, tape closure must be protected with an overlying gauze bandage.

In experimental wounds inoculated with *Staphylococcus aureus*, tape-closed wounds resisted infection better than did wounds closed with nylon sutures.[2] Tape closure works well under plaster casts when superficial suture removal would be delayed. Tape closure effectively holds flaps and grafts in place, particularly over the fingers, the flat areas of the extremities, and the trunk (Fig. 35-2).[3,4] Wounds on the pretibial area are difficult to close, especially in the elderly because of tissue atrophy. Wound tape provides an alternative to suture closure in this situation. Tape closure can also be applied to wounds after early suture removal, particularly on the face, to maintain approximation of the wound edges while reducing the chance of permanent suture mark scarring. Finally, because of the minimal skin tension created by tape, it can be used on skin that has been compromised by vascular insufficiency or altered by prolonged use of steroids.

Contraindications

Tape closure has disadvantages as well. Tape does not work well on wounds under significant tension or on wounds that are irregular, on concave surfaces, or in areas of marked tissue laxity. In many cases, tape does not provide satisfactory apposition of the wound edges without concurrent underlying deep closure. Tape does not stick well to naturally moist areas, such as the axilla, the palms of the hands, the soles of the feet, and the perineum. Tape also has difficulty adhering to wounds that will have secretions, copious exudates, or persistent bleeding. It is of little value on lax and intertriginous skin, on the scalp, and on other areas with a high concentration of hair follicles. Tape strips are also at risk for premature removal by young children.

Do not place tape tightly and circumferentially around digits because it has insufficient ability to stretch or lengthen (Fig. 35-3). If placed circumferentially, the natural wound edema of an injured digit can make the tape act like a constricting band, which can lead to ischemia and possible necrosis of the digit. Use semicircular or spiral placement techniques if digits are to be taped.

Equipment

For simple tape closure, the equipment required includes forceps and tape of the proper size (see Fig. 35-1). Most taping can be done in the ED with $\frac{1}{4}$- × 3-inch strips. For wounds larger than 4 cm, however, $\frac{1}{2}$-inch-wide strips provide greater strength. Most companies manufacture strips up to 1 inch wide and 4 inches long.

Figure 35-1 Equipment required for the application of wound tape. Note that wound tape (3M Steri-Strip brand depicted here) comes in a variety of widths.

Figure 35-3 After suturing this proximally based flap, Steri-Strips are applied under a tourniquet to compress the flap, arrest motion of the flap, and lessen buildup of fluid. Tissue movement and fluid buildup are some reasons why flaps and avulsed skin fail to heal. Tape should be placed in a semicircular or spiral pattern on digits to avoid constriction.

Figure 35-2 Wound tape in the care of avulsion injuries. A skin avulsion in the elderly following minor trauma is an ideal wound to close with closure tape because such injuries cannot be closed with sutures. The goal is to provide approximation of the avulsed skin and *apply pressure to avoid movement of the skin flap or accumulation of fluid under the avulsion.* Tissue glue can augment this procedure. **A,** An elderly woman who was taking steroids had extremely thin skin and suffered a skin avulsion that could not be repaired with sutures. **B,** The skin edges are uncurled, stretched, and anatomically replaced. **C,** The wound should heal when closure tape keeps the skin in place. Tissue glue (Dermabond) was also dabbed on various parts of the edges to allow egress of fluid. **D,** Another elderly patient with a large avulsion injury on the forearm. **E,** Repair with Steri-Strips and skin glue. **F,** A compression dressing, such as an elastic bandage or a Dome paste (Unna) boot dressing, can be applied to minimize movement of the flap and decrease buildup of fluid under the flap.

Procedure

Proper wound preparation, irrigation, débridement, and hemostasis must precede tape closure. Fine hair may be cut short. Dry the area of tape application thoroughly to ensure proper adhesion. Do not attempt to apply tape to a wet area or over a wound that is slowly oozing blood because it will usually result in failure of the tape to stick to the skin. On fingers, tape can be applied to a wound that is kept dry by temporarily placing a tourniquet at the base of the finger (see Fig. 35-3).

The technique of applying tape is shown in Figure 35-4. After the wound has been dried, apply a liquid adhesive such as tincture of benzoin or Mastisol to the skin adjacent to the wound to increase adhesion of the tape.[2] All tape comes in presterilized packages. Open them directly onto the operating field. Handle tape with gloved hands. With the backing still attached, cut the tape to the desired length or long enough to allow approximately 2 to 3 cm of overlap on each side of the wound. After the end tab is removed, gently remove the tape from its backing with forceps by pulling straight back. Do not pull to the side because the tape will curl and be difficult to apply to the wound. Place half of the tape securely at the midportion of the wound. Gently but firmly appose the opposite wound edge to its counterpart. Apply the second half of the tape next. Hold the wound edges as close together as possible and at equal height to prevent the development of a linear, pitted scar. Apply additional tape by bisecting the remainder of the wound. Place a sufficient number of tape strips so that the wound is completely apposed without totally covering the entire length of the wound. Finally, place additional cross tapes to add support and prevent blistering caused by unsupported tape ends.[1]

Do not cover taped wounds with occlusive dressings. Adhesive bandages (e.g., Band-Aids) and other impermeable dressings promote excessive moisture, which can lead to premature separation of tape strips from the wound. An adhesive bandage may also adhere to the tapes and pull them off the skin during dressing changes. Keep the tape in place for approximately 2 weeks or longer, if necessary. Instruct the patient to clean the taped laceration gently with a slightly moist, soft cloth after 24 to 48 hours. However, emphasize that if excessive wetting or mechanical force is used, premature tape separation may result. Instruct patients to gently trim the curled edges of the closure tape with fine scissors to avoid premature loss of the tape.

Complications

Complications are uncommon with tape closure. The wound infection rate in clean wounds closed with tape compares favorably with rates for other standard closures.[1] However, some investigators believe that tape closure leads to inferior cosmetic results.[8] Premature tape separation occurs in approximately 3% of cases.[6] Other complications include (1) skin blistering, which occurs if the tape is not properly anchored with cross-strips or the tape is stretched too tightly across the wound, and (2) wound hematoma, which results if hemostasis is inadequate. Tape may loosen prematurely over shaved areas as hair grows back.

When tincture of benzoin is used, apply it carefully to the surrounding, uninjured skin. Be careful because if spillage into the wound occurs, there is a higher risk for infection.[9]

Benzoin vapor can cause pain when applied near an open wound that has not been anesthetized. Benzoin can also injure the conjunctival and corneal membranes of the eye.

Summary

Modern tape products and techniques serve a valuable role in the management of minor wounds in the ED. In selected wounds, tape closure is as successful as suture closure.[1,10] Closure tape should be considered for superficial wounds in cosmetically unimportant areas and for wounds on relatively flat surfaces that are too wide for simple dressings but do not require sutures.

TISSUE ADHESIVE (TISSUE GLUE)

Tissue adhesive (also called tissue "glue") provides a simple, rapid method of wound closure. Tissue adhesive has been approved for use in the United States since 1998. Two types of tissue adhesive are available: *N*-2-octylcyanoacrylate (Dermabond, Ethicon, Inc.) and *N*-butyl-2-cyanoacrylate (Indermil, Tyco Healthcare Group LP). Animal studies have shown octylcyanoacrylate-based adhesive to have significantly greater strength and flexibility than butylcyanoacrylate-based adhesive. Dermabond and Indermil are packaged in sterile, single-use ampules (Fig. 35-5). These bonding agents can be used on superficial wounds, even in hair-bearing areas. Tissue adhesives polymerize on contact with water. These substances are biodegradable but remain in the wound until well after healing.[11,12]

Procedure

Tissue adhesive can be used to approximate wounds that do not require deep-layer closure and do not have significant tension on the edges of the wound (Fig. 35-6). In preparation for closure, clean and anesthetize the wound. Débride the wound if necessary. *Control bleeding of the wound.*

Hold the wound edges together with forceps, gauze pads, or fingers. Squeeze the small, cylindrical plastic container to expel droplets of tissue adhesive through the cotton-tipped applicator at the end of the container. Apply the adhesive in at least three to four thin layers along the length of the wound's surface and extend it approximately 5 to 10 mm from each side of the wound. Alternatively, place the adhesive in strips perpendicular to the laceration (analogous to the placement of closure tape). The purple color of the solution facilitates placement of the droplets. Support and hold the edges of the wound together for at least 1 minute while the adhesive dries. Low-viscosity tissue adhesives may seep into the wound or trickle off rounded surfaces during application. This tendency toward migration or "runoff" can be minimized by using high-viscosity adhesives[13] (e.g., Dermabond HV Topical Skin Adhesive, Ethicon, Inc.), positioning the wound horizontally, or applying the adhesive slowly. Contain runoff with wet gauze or by creating a barrier of petrolatum.

Wound closures with tissue adhesive can be reinforced by pulling the edges of the wound into apposition with a few strips of porous surgical tape before application of the adhesive. Tissue adhesive can be placed on top of surgical tape, but tape should not be placed on top of dried tissue adhesive.

WOUND TAPE APPLICATION

1. After wound preparation (and placement of deep closures, if needed), dry the skin thoroughly at least 2 inches around the wound. Failure to dry the skin and failure to obtain perfect hemostasis are common causes of failure of tape to stick to the skin.

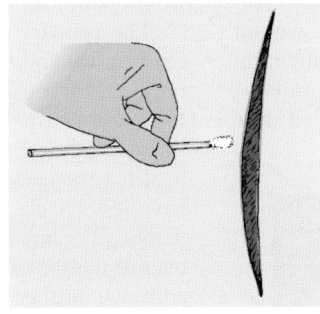

2. If desired, apply a thin coating of tincture of benzoin around the wound to enhance tape adhesiveness. Benzoin should not enter the eye because it causes pain if it seeps into an open wound.

3. Cut the tape to the desired length before removing the backing.

4. The tape is attached to a card with perforated tabs on both ends. Gently peel the end tab from the tape.

5. Use forceps to peel the tape off the card backing. Pull directly backward, not to the side.

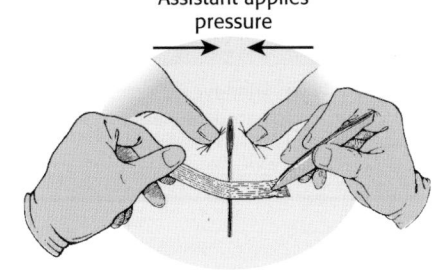

6. Place half of the first tape at the midportion of the wound; secure firmly in place.

7. Gently but firmly appose the opposite side of the wound with the free hand or forceps. If an assistant is not available, the operator can approximate the wound edges. The tape should be applied by bisecting the wound until the wound is closed satisfactorily.

8. Wound margins are completely apposed without totally occluding the wound.

9. Additional supporting strips of tape are placed approximately 2.5 cm from the wound and parallel to the direction of the wound. Taping in this manner prevents the skin blistering that may occur at the ends of the tap.

Figure 35-4 Proper technique for the application of wound tape.

Once the adhesive has dried completely, further protect the closure with a nonocclusive bandage.

Tissue adhesives can also be used to treat superficial skin tears that do not extend past the dermis. After the wound and skin flap are cleaned, lay the flap over the base of the wound and approximate the edges of the wound. Any remaining blood and serum are expressed from under the flap, and the entire area is dried. A thin layer of adhesive is applied over the wound margins and 1 to 2 cm beyond the margin. After the first layer dries, a second layer of adhesive is applied. A dressing is not required unless there is a reason to protect the wound from repeated injury."[14,15]

The primary advantage of tissue adhesive is the speed of closure. Wounds can be closed in as little as one sixth the time required for repair with sutures. Application is rapid and painless. Use of tissue adhesive avoids suture marks adjacent to the wound and reduces the risk for needlestick injuries to health care personnel. Wounds closed with tissue adhesive have less tensile strength in the first 4 days than do sutured wounds,[16,17] but 1 week after closure, the tensile strength and overall degree of inflammation in wounds closed with tissue adhesive are equivalent to those closed with sutures.[12,18] Cosmetic results are similar to those obtained with suture repair.[17,19-25] Tissue adhesive serves as its own wound dressing and has an antimicrobial effect against gram-positive organisms.[26,27] The material sloughs off in 5 to 10 days, thereby saving the patient from a clinician visit. Do not apply ointments or occlusive bandages on wounds closed with tissue adhesive.

Figure 35-5 Tissue adhesive, 2-octylcyanoacrylate, comes in a variety of commercially available dispensers.

Complications

Although tissue adhesive is classified as nontoxic and does not cause a significant foreign body reaction, some authors warn against placing it within the wound cavity.[17,18] However,

---

TISSUE ADHESIVE APPLICATION

1 To apply tissue adhesive (glue), the laceration must by dry. High-viscosity glue limits runoff. Squeeze the container to expel the adhesive through the cotton-tipped applicator at the end of the container. A precision tip applicator (see Fig. 35-5) is a useful adjunct.

2 Bring the edges together by using a gauze pad or fingers, and apply glue in a few layers, with drying between applications. Hold the wound edges together for at least 1 minute while the adhesive dries.

3 Near the eye, keep the patient supine, tilt the head to avoid eye contamination, and apply a layer of petroleum jelly as a barrier to the glue entering the eye. Do not apply the jelly to the area where the tissue adhesive must adhere.

4 Alternatively, use a gauze barrier. If the adhesive enters the eye or lids, wipe it off with the gauze and flush with saline. Lids glued shut may be loosened with antibiotic ointment or petroleum jelly. If unsuccessful, tell the patient to shower normally and the eye will open in a few days as the glue sloughs off the lid.

Figure 35-6 Application of tissue adhesive. Note: *Glue that touches a latex glove, gauze, or a plastic instrument (but not vinyl gloves or metal instruments) will glue them to the patient.*

various investigators have applied specially formulated octyl-2-cyanoacrylate ("liquid adhesive bandage") directly to open minor lacerations, abrasions, and partial-thickness wounds. When compared with adhesive bandages, wounds covered with this tissue adhesive had equivalent rates of healing and complications."[28,29]

If hemostasis is inadequate or an excessive amount of adhesive is applied too quickly, the patient can experience a burning sensation or sustain a local burn from the heat of polymerization. After polymerizing, tissue adhesive can fracture with excessive or repetitive movement. Although gentle rinsing is permitted, if the adhesive is washed or soaked, it will peel off in a few days, before the wound is healed.[17]

If the clinician's gloved fingers, gauze, or plastic instruments contact the tissue adhesive during application, the glove may adhere to the patient's skin. Tissue adhesive can be removed with antibiotic ointment or petrolatum jelly or more rapidly with acetone.[25] Indermil must be stored under refrigeration.

One risk involving the use of tissue adhesive is its ease of use—clinicians may fail to adequately clean wounds before closure with tissue adhesive.[30] Tissue adhesive should not be used to close infected wounds. *There is a slightly higher risk for wound dehiscence in closures with tissue glue than with sutures.*[31,32]

If the edges of the wound cannot be held together without considerable tension, tissue adhesive should not be used.[25] Percutaneous sutures provide a more secure immediate closure than tissue adhesive does.[12] Tissue adhesive should not be used near the eyes, over or near joints, on moist or mucosal surfaces, or on wounds under significant static or dynamic skin tension. See Figure 35-6 for information on managing eyelids that are accidentally glued shut.

WOUND STAPLES

Background

Automatic stapling devices have become commonplace for closure of surgical incisions and traumatic wounds (Fig. 35-7). Clinical studies of patients with stapled surgical incisions have found no significant difference between stapling and suturing when infection rates, healing outcome, and patient acceptance are compared.[33-37] Wound stapling and nylon suture closure of skin compared favorably in wound tensile strength, complication rates, patient tolerance, efficiency of closure, scar width, color, general appearance, suture or staple marks, infection rates, and cost. In animal models, staples caused less wound inflammation and offered more resistance to infection with contaminated wounds.[38-41]

The most significant advantage of wound stapling over suturing is speed of closure. The most significant downside is loss of the cosmetic effect that can be achieved with meticulous suture closure. On average, stapling is three to four times faster than suturing traumatic wounds.[42-44] When clinician time and cost of instruments are considered, the difference in cost between stapling and suturing is minimal[43] or favors stapling.[42,45]

Indications and Contraindications

The indications for stapling are limited to relatively linear lacerations with straight, sharp edges located on an extremity, the trunk, or the scalp. Staples may be especially useful for superficial scalp lacerations in an agitated or intoxicated patient. Because of their superficial placement in the adult scalp (usually above the galea), staples are not recommended for deep scalp lacerations. Staples may not provide the same hemostasis that is possible with deep sutures. They should not be placed in scalp wounds if computed tomography head scans are to be performed because staples produce scan artifacts. Similarly, staples should not be used if the patient is expected to undergo magnetic resonance imaging because the powerful magnetic fields may avulse the staples from the surface of the skin. Staples should not be used on the face, neck, hands, or feet.

Equipment

Standard wound care should precede wound closure. In many cases, when débridement and dermal (deep) closure are unnecessary, only tissue forceps are needed to assist in everting wounds.

Many stapling devices are commercially available. The most versatile and least expensive is the Precise stapler (3M Corporation). Different units that hold between 5 and 25 staples can be purchased. The 10-staple unit will suffice for most lacerations. Other devices include the Proximate 11 (Ethicon, Inc.), Cricket (US Surgical, Irvine, CA), and Appose (Davis & Geck, Columbus, OH).

Procedure

Before stapling, sometimes it is necessary to place deep, absorbable sutures to close deep fascia and reduce tension in the superficial fascia and dermal layers. To facilitate the stapling process, the edges of the wound should be everted, preferably by a second operator (Fig. 35-8, *step 1*). The assistant precedes the operator along the wound and *everts the edges of the wound with forceps or pinches the skin with the thumb and forefinger.* Stapling flattened wound edges may place the staple precisely but results in inversion of the wound. Once the edges are held in eversion, the staple points are gently placed across the wound. *It is imperative to place the center of the staple device over the center of the wound to ensure the best closure and to avoid overriding or misaligned edges* (difficult in an

Figure 35-7 Skin stapling device. Skin staples may be used for relatively linear lacerations with straight, sharp edges on the extremity, trunk, or scalp. Their main advantage is speed of closure. The main disadvantage is lack of the better cosmetic effect afforded by meticulous suture closure.

WOUND STAPLES

Approximate and evert the skin edges by hand or with forceps before they are secured with staples. If possible, have an assistant perform this duty. Failure to evert the wound edges is a common error that may cause an unacceptable result.

Align the stapler to the center of the wound

Align the center of the stapler over the center of the wound. Squeeze the stapler handle to advance one staple into the wound margins. Do not press too hard on the skin to prevent placing the staple too deeply.

As the handle is squeezed, an anvil automatically bends the staple to the proper configuration.

Allow a small space to remain between the skin and the crossbar of the staple. Excessive pressure created by placing the staple too deep causes wound edge ischemia, as well as pain on removal. Note that the staple bar is 2 to 3 mm above the skin line.

Supply the patient with a staple remover when being referred to an office for removal or for self-removal. To remove the staple, place the lower jaw of the remover under the crossbar of the staple.

Squeeze the handle gently, and the upper jaw will compress the staple and allow it to exit the skin.

Figure 35-8 Wound staples. Failure to align the center of the staple device directly over the center of the laceration is a common cause of a less than ideal staple closure. (*1-2, From Custalow C.* Color Atlas of Emergency Department Procedures. *Philadelphia: Elsevier; 2005;3-6, from Edlich RF.* A Manual for Wound Closure. *St. Paul, MN: 3M Medical-Surgical Products; 1979. Reproduced by permission.*)

Figure 35-9 A, A very poor result occurred when staples (some marked with *arrows*) were used to close this deep scalp laceration. The edges of the wound were not everted, staples were not in the midline, sections of the skin overlapped significantly, poor hemostasis was obtained, and the galea could not be closed by the superficial staples. The patient did not wash his hair as instructed. Three days later during inspection of the wound, the staples were removed (**B**) and the laceration was closed with 3-0 interrupted nylon sutures (**C**). The clinician should attempt to obtain a cosmetic closure on all scalp lacerations because as patients lose their hair, a previously hidden, unsightly scar emerges. In general, staples should not be used to close full-thickness scalp lacerations, especially wounds that are actively bleeding. **D,** Sloppy stapling on an extremity with *inversion* rather than *eversion of the edges of the wound. Some staples are totally misaligned and barely include the opposite skin edge.* **E,** The staples were left in too long, which caused a poor cosmetic result.

uncooperative patient). When the stapler handle or trigger is squeezed, the staple is advanced automatically into the wound and bent to the proper configuration (see Fig. 35-8, *steps 2 and 3*). The operator should not press too hard on the skin surface to prevent placing the staple too deeply and causing ischemia within the staple loop. When placed properly, the crossbar of the staple is elevated a few millimeters above the surface of the skin (see Fig. 35-8, *step 4*). A sufficient number of staples should be placed to provide proper apposition of the edges of the wound along its entire length. (One suggested method is to place a staple in the midpoint of the length of the wound and then bisect either side of the wound with additional staples. Continue the process until the edges of the wound are well opposed.) After the wound is stapled, an antibiotic ointment may be applied to minimize adherence of the dressing, and a sterile dressing is applied. If necessary, the patient can remove the dressing and gently clean the wound in 24 to 48 hours. *Scalp lacerations can be cleansed by showering within a few hours.*

Removal of staples requires a special instrument made available by each manufacturer of stapling devices. The lower jaw of the staple remover is placed under the crossbar, and the handle is squeezed (see Fig. 35-8, *steps 5 and 6*). This action compresses the crossbar and bends the staple outward, thereby releasing the points of the staple from the skin. Many primary care physicians do not routinely stock the instrument. If referred for office removal of staples, the patient can be given a disposable staple removal device. Motivated patients

can remove their own staples if given the removal device. The interval between staple application and removal is the same as that for standard suture placement and removal. Staples can cause significant scarring if left in place too long (Fig. 35-9).

Complications

Patient acceptance and comfort and wound infection and dehiscence are similar with staple-closed wounds and sutured wounds. However, removal of staples can be somewhat more uncomfortable than removal of sutures.

A common error during insertion of staples is failure to evert the edges of the skin before stapling (see Fig. 35-9). Eversion avoids the natural tendency of the device to invert the closure. Eversion may be accomplished with forceps or by pinching the skin with the thumb and index finger, a procedure that requires some practice. Another common error is to fail to align the middle of the staple exactly in the midline of the wound. Staples do cause marks in the skin similar to sutures. In patients who tend to scar more easily, the scar resulting from staples may be more pronounced than that produced by sutures, especially if the staples are left in place for prolonged periods.

Wound stapling achieves results that are generally comparable to those of sutures for the closure of traumatic, linear lacerations in noncosmetic areas, such as the scalp, trunk, and extremities. Stapling is much faster than suturing. Wound stapling does not differ significantly from suturing in terms

Figure 35-10 Basic suturing equipment includes a needle driver, forceps, and suture scissors.

Figure 35-11 A wide variety of both absorbable and nonabsorbable suture material is available. Other variables include suture size (e.g., 4-0, 5-0, 6-0), needle size, and type (e.g., PS-2, reverse cutting, conventional cutting). These variables are discussed in detail in text.

of cost, infection rates, wound healing, and patient acceptance. Cosmesis does, however, suffer, especially if the staples are left in too long (see Fig. 35-9*D* and *E*).

SUTURES

In the United States, most traumatic wounds are closed by suturing.

Equipment

Instruments

In addition to the instruments used for débridement, a needle holder and suture scissors are required for suturing (Fig. 35-10). The mechanical performance of disposable needle holders distributed by different surgical instrument companies varies considerably.[46] The size of the needle holder should match the size of the needle selected for suturing—that is, the needle holder should be large enough to hold the needle securely as it is passed through tissue, yet not so large that the needle is crushed or bent by the instrument.

Instruments used to débride a grossly contaminated wound should be discarded and replaced with fresh instruments for closure. Instruments covered with coagulated blood can be cleansed with hydrogen peroxide, rinsed with sterile saline or water, and then used for suturing.

In addition, 2.5 loupe magnification may improve inspection of wounds and facilitate the repair of facial and hand wounds.[47]

Suture Material

A wide variety of suture material is available (Fig. 35-11). Clinician preference varies widely, and there are no definitive standards on which to base the use of suture material for a particular wound or particular site. For most wounds that require closure of more than one layer of tissue, the clinician must choose sutures from two general categories: an absorbable suture for the deeper, subcutaneous (SQ) layer and a nonabsorbable suture for surface (percutaneous) closure.

Sutures can be described in terms of four characteristics:

1. Composition (i.e., chemical and physical properties)
2. Handling characteristics and mechanical performance
3. Absorption and reactivity
4. Size and retention of tensile strength

TABLE 35-1   Examples of Suture Material

ABSORBABLE SUTURE	NONABSORBABLE SUTURE
Monofilament	
Plain gut	Dermalon (nylon)
Chromic gut	Ethilon (nylon)
PDS (polydioxanone)	Prolene (polypropylene)
Maxon (polyglyconate)	Silk
	Steel
	Surgilene (polypropylene)
	Tevdek (Teflon coated)
Multifilament	
Dexon (polyglycolic acid)	Ethibond (polyethylene)
Coated Vicryl (polyglactin)	Mersilene (braided polyester)
	Nurolon (nylon)
	Surgilon (nylon)
	Ti-Cron (polyester)

Composition

Sutures are made from natural fibers (cotton, silk), from sheep submucosa or beef serosa (plain gut, chromic gut), or from synthetic material such as nylon (Dermalon, Ethilon, Nurolon, Surgilon), Dacron (Ethiflex, Mersilene), polyester (Ti-Cron), polyethylene (Ethibond), polypropylene (Prolene, Surgilene), polyglycolic acid (Dexon), and polyglactin (Vicryl, coated Vicryl). Stainless steel sutures are rarely, if ever useful in wound closure in the ED setting because of handling difficulty and fragmentation. Some sutures are made of a single filament (monofilament); others consist of multiple fibers braided together (Table 35-1).[48]

Handling and Performance

Desirable handling characteristics in a suture include smooth passage through tissue, ease in knot tying, and stability of the knot once tied (Table 35-2). Smooth sutures pull through tissue easily, but knots slip more readily. Conversely, sutures with a high coefficient of friction have better knot-holding capacity but are difficult to slide through tissue. Smooth sutures will loosen after the first throw of a knot is made, and thus a second throw is needed to secure the first in place. However, the

TABLE 35-2 Characteristics of Suture Material

SUTURE MATERIAL	KNOT SECURITY	TENSILE STRENGTH	TISSUE REACTIVITY	DURATION OF SUTURE INTEGRITY (DAYS)	TIE ABILITY (HANDLING)
Absorbable					
Surgical gut	Poor	Fair	Greatest	5-7	Poor
Chromic gut	Fair	Fair	Greatest	10-14	Poor
Coated Vicryl	Good	Good	Minimal	30	Best
Dexon	Best	Good	Minimal	30	Best
PDS	Fair	Best	Least	45-60	Good
Maxon	Fair	Best	Least	45-60	Good
Nonabsorbable					
Ethilon	Good	Good	Minimal		Good
Prolene	Least	Best	Least		Fair
Silk	Best	Least	Greatest		Best

Modified with permission from Hollander J, Singer A. Laceration management. *Ann Emerg Med.* 1999;34:351.
PDS, dioxanone.

clinician may want to tighten a knot further after the first throw is made. This is difficult with rougher types of suture.

Multifilament sutures have the best handling characteristics of all sutures, whereas steel sutures have the worst. In terms of performance and handling, significant improvements have been made in the newer absorbable sutures. Gut sutures have many shortcomings, including relatively low and variable strength, a tendency to fray when handled, and stiffness despite being packaged in a softening fluid.[49,50] Multifilament synthetic absorbable sutures are soft and easy to tie and have few problems with knot slippage. Polyglactin 910 (coated Vicryl) sutures have an absorbable lubricant coating. The "frictional drag" of these coated sutures as they are pulled through tissue is less than that of uncoated multifilament materials, and resetting of knots after the initial throw is much easier. This characteristic allows retightening of a ligature without knotting or breakage and with smooth, even adjustment of suture line tension in running subcuticular stitches.[51] Synthetic monofilament sutures have the troublesome property of "memory"—a tendency of the filament to spring back to its original shape, which causes the knot to slip and unravel. Some nonabsorbable monofilament sutures are coated with polytetrafluoroethylene (Teflon) or silicone to reduce their friction. This coating improves the handling characteristics of these monofilaments but results in poorer knot security.[42]

Three square knots will secure a stitch made with silk or other braided, nonabsorbable material, and four knots are sufficient for synthetic, absorbable, and nonabsorbable monofilament sutures.[52] Five knots are needed for the Teflon-coated synthetic Tevdek.[53] When coated synthetic suture material is used, attention to basic principles of knot tying is even more important. An excessive number of throws in a knot weakens the suture at the knot. If the clinician uses square knots (or a surgeon's knot on the initial throw, followed by square knots) that lie down flat and are tied securely, knots will rarely unravel.[54]

Absorption and Reactivity

Sutures that are rapidly degraded in tissue are termed *absorbable*; those that maintain their tensile strength for longer than 60 days are considered *nonabsorbable* (see Table 35-1). Plain gut may be digested by white blood cell lysozymes in 10 to 40 days; chromic gut will last 15 to 60 days. Remnants of both types of suture, however, have been seen in wounds more than 2 years after placement.[49,52,55] Ethicon catgut is rapidly absorbed within 10 to 14 days and is associated with less inflammation than chromic catgut is.[56] Vicryl is absorbed from the wound site within 60 to 90 days[49,52] and Dexon, within 120 to 210 days.[57,58] When placed in the oral cavity, plain gut disappears after 3 to 5 days, chromic gut after 7 to 10 days, and polyglycolic acid after 16 to 20 days.[59] In contrast, SQ silk may not be completely absorbed for as long as 2 years.[52] The rate of absorption of synthetic absorbable sutures is independent of suture size.[57]

Sutures may lose strength and function before they are completely absorbed in tissues. Braided synthetic absorbable sutures lose nearly all their strength after about 21 days. In contrast, monofilament absorbable sutures (modified polyglycolic acid [Maxon, Davis & Geck] and polydioxanone [PDS, Ethicon]) retain 60% of their strength after 28 days.[60,61] Gut sutures treated with chromium salts (chromic gut) have prolonged tensile strength; however, all gut sutures retain tensile strength erratically.[49,52] Of the absorbable types of suture, a wet and knotted polyglycolic acid suture is stronger than a plain or chromic gut suture subjected to the same conditions.[50,62]

Polypropylene remains unchanged in tissue for longer than 2 years after implantation.[63] In comparison testing, sutures made of natural fibers such as silk, cotton, and gut were the weakest; sutures made of Dacron, nylon, polyethylene, and polypropylene were intermediate in tensile strength; and metallic sutures were the strongest.[50] Comparison of suture strength versus wound strength is a measure of the usefulness of a suture. Catgut is stronger than the soft tissue of a wound for no more than 7 days; chromic catgut, Dexon, and Vicryl are stronger for 10 to 21 days; and nylon, wire, and silk are stronger for 20 to 30 days.[64]

All sutures placed within tissue will damage host defenses and provoke inflammation. Even the least reactive suture impairs the ability of the wound to resist infection.[63] The magnitude of the reaction provoked by a suture is related to the quantity of suture material (diameter × total length) placed in the tissue and to the chemical composition of the suture. Among absorbable sutures, polyglycolic acid and polyglactin sutures are the least reactive, followed by chromic gut. Nonabsorbable polypropylene is less reactive than nylon or Dacron.[50,65,66] Significant tissue reaction is associated with catgut, silk, and cotton sutures. Absorbable polyglycolic acid sutures are less reactive than those made of nonabsorbable silk.[67] Highly reactive material should be avoided in contaminated wounds.

The chemical composition of sutures is a factor in early infection. The infection rate in experimentally contaminated wounds closed with polyglycolic acid sutures is lower than the rate when gut sutures are used.[63] However, other authors have compared plain gut and nonabsorbable nylon sutures for skin closure in children and found comparable cosmetic results and infection rates.[68] Lubricant coatings on sutures do not alter suture reactivity, absorption characteristics, breaking strength, or the risk for infection.[51,63] Multifilament sutures provoke more inflammation and are more likely than monofilament sutures to produce infection if left in place for prolonged periods.[69,70] Monofilament sutures elicit less tissue reaction than do multifilament sutures, and multifilament materials tend to wick up fluid by capillary action. Bacteria that adhere to and colonize sutures can envelop themselves in a glycocalix that protects them from host defenses,[71] or they can "hide" in the interstices of a multifilament suture and, as a result, be inaccessible to leukocytes.[69] PDS provides the advantages of a monofilament suture in an absorbable form, thus making it a good choice as a subcuticular stitch. Polypropylene sutures have a low coefficient of friction, and subcuticular stitches with this material are easy to pull out.[72]

Size and Strength

The size of suture material (thread diameter) is related to the tensile strength of the suture; threads with greater diameter are stronger. The strength of the suture is proportional to the square of the diameter of the thread. Therefore, a 4-0 suture of any type is larger and stronger than a 6-0 suture. The correct suture size for approximation of a layer of tissue depends on the tensile strength of that tissue. The tensile strength of the suture material should be only slightly greater than that of the tissue because the magnitude of damage to local tissue defenses is proportional to the amount of suture material placed in the wound.[52,73]

Synthetic absorbable sutures have made the older, natural suture material unnecessary for most wound closures. Polyglycolic acid (Dexon) and polyglactin 910 (coated Vicryl) have improved handling characteristics, knot security, and tensile strength. Their absorption rates are predictable, and tissue reactivity is minimal.[74,75] The distinct advantages of synthetic nonabsorbable sutures over silk sutures are their greater tensile strength, low coefficient of friction, and minimal tissue reactivity.[63,74] They are extensible and elongate without breaking as the edges of the wound swell in the early postoperative period.[73,74] In contrast to silk sutures, synthetics can easily and painlessly be removed once the wound has healed. The monofilament synthetic suture Novafil has elasticity that allows a stitch to enlarge with wound edema and to return to its original length once the edema subsides. Stiffer materials lacerate the encircled tissue as the wound swells.[76]

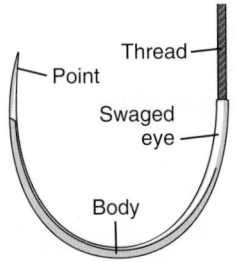

Figure 35-12 The eyeless, or "swaged," needle. (*From* Suture Use Manual. Use and Handling of Sutures and Needles. *Somerville, NJ: Ethicon, Inc.; 1977:29. Reproduced by permission.*)

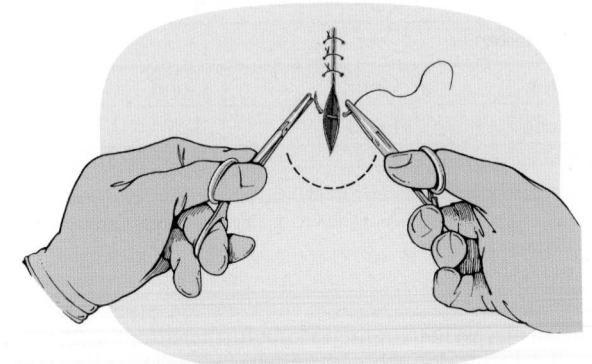

Figure 35-13 The needle should be large enough to pass through tissue and should exit far enough to enable the needle holder to be repositioned on the end of the needle at a safe distance from the point.

The suture material most useful to emergency clinicians for wound closure is Dexon or coated Vicryl for SQ layers and synthetic nonabsorbable suture (e.g., nylon or polypropylene) for skin closure. Fascia can be sutured with either absorbable or nonabsorbable material. In most situations, 3-0 or 4-0 suture is used for the repair of fascia, 4-0 or 5-0 absorbable suture for SQ closure, and 4-0 or 5-0 nonabsorbable suture for skin closure. The lips, eyelids, and skin layer of facial wounds are repaired with 6-0 suture, whereas 3-0 or 4-0 suture is used when the edges of the skin are subjected to considerable dynamic stress (e.g., wounds overlying joint surfaces) or static stress (e.g., scalp).

Needles

The eyeless, or "swaged," needle is used for wound closure in most emergency centers (Fig. 35-12). Selection of the appropriate needle size and curvature is based on the dimensions of the wound and the characteristics of the tissue to be sutured. The needle should be large enough to pass through tissue to the desired depth and then to exit the tissue or skin surface far enough that the needle holder can be repositioned on the distal end of the needle at a safe distance from the tip of the needle (Fig. 35-13). Although it is tempting to use the fingers to grasp the tip of the needle to pull it through the skin, this practice risks a needlestick. The clinician should either reposition the needle holder or use forceps to disengage the needle from the laceration.

In wound repair, needles must penetrate tough, fibrous tissue—skin, SQ tissue, and fascia—yet should slice through this tissue with minimal resistance or trauma and without bending. The type of needle best suited for closure of SQ tissue is a conventional cutting needle in a three-eighths or

Figure 35-14 One-half and three-eighths circle needles, used for most traumatic wound closures.

Figure 35-15 Types of needles. **A,** The conventional cutting needle has two opposing cutting edges and a third edge on the inside curvature of the needle. The conventional cutting needle changes in cross-section from a triangular cutting tip to a flattened body. **B,** The reverse cutting needle is used to cut through tough, difficult-to-penetrate tissue such as fascia and skin. It has two opposing cutting edges and a third cutting edge on the outer curvature of the needle. The reverse cutting needle is made with a triangular shape extending from the point to the swage area, with only the edges near the tip being sharpened. (*From* Suture Use Manual. Use and Handling of Sutures and Needles. *Somerville, NJ: Ethicon, Inc.; 1977:31. Reproduced by permission.*)

one-half circle (Fig. 35-14). Double-curvature needles (coated Vicryl with PS-4-C cutting needles, Ethicon) may be easier to maneuver in narrow, deep wounds. For surface closure, a conventional cutting-edge needle permits more precise needle placement and requires less penetration force (Fig. 35-15).[77,78]

Suturing Techniques (Figs. 35-16 and 35-17)

Skin Preparation

Before suturing, the clinician should ensure adequate exposure and illumination of the wound and placement of the patient at the appropriate height. The clinician should assume a comfortable standing or sitting position at one end of the long axis of the wound.

The skin surrounding the wound is prepared with a povidone-iodine solution and covered with sterile drapes. A clear plastic drape (Steri-Drape, 3M Corporation) can be used to provide a sterile field and a limited view of the area surrounding the wound. Some surgeons do not drape the face but prefer to leave the facial structures and landmarks adjacent to the wound uncovered and within view. If no drapes are used on the face, the skin surrounding the wound should be widely cleansed and prepared. Wrapping the hair in a sheet or placing the patient's hair in an oversized scrub hat prevents stray hair from falling into the operating field. For a finger laceration, a sterile glove can be placed on the patient's hand to avoid using a drape.

Closure Principles

Clinician preference varies widely, and there are no definitive standards on the exact method of wound preparation, manipulation of tissue, or closure technique that is preferred for any given wound. There is a tendency to overuse sutures for minor lacerations that will heal nicely with no intervention.

Therefore, before suturing, one must assess the need for the procedure (Fig. 35-18).

Three principles apply to suturing lacerations in any location: (1) minimize trauma to tissues, (2) relieve tension exerted on the edges of the wound by undermining and layered wound closure, and (3) accurately realign landmarks and skin edges by layered closure and precise suture placement.

Minimizing Tissue Trauma

The importance of careful handling of tissue has been emphasized since the early days of surgery. Skin and SQ tissue that has been stretched, twisted, or crushed by an instrument or strangled by a suture that is tied too tightly may undergo necrosis, and increased scarring and infection may result. When the edges of a wound must be manipulated, the SQ tissues should be lifted gently with toothed forceps or a skin hook while avoiding the surface of the skin.

When choosing suture size, the clinician should select the smallest size that will hold the tissues in place. Skin stitches should incorporate no more tissue than is needed to coapt the wound edges with little or no tension. Knots should be tied securely enough to approximate the edges of the wound but without blanching or indenting the skin surface.[79]

Relieving Tension

Many forces can produce tension on the suture line of a reapproximated wound. Static skin forces that stretch the skin over bones cause the edges of a new wound to gape, and they also continuously pull on the edges of the wound once it has been closed. Traumatic loss of tissue or wide excision of a wound may have the same effect. The best cosmetic result occurs when the long axis of a wound happens to be parallel to the direction of maximal skin tension; such alignment brings the edges of the wound together.[76]

Muscles pulling at right angles to the axis of the wound impose dynamic stress. Swelling after an injury creates additional tension within the circle of each suture.[79] Skin suture marks result not only from tying sutures too tightly but also from failing to eliminate any underlying forces distorting the wound. Tension can be reduced during wound closure in two ways: undermining of the wound edges and layered closure.

Undermining. The force required to reapproximate the edges of a wound correlates with the subsequent width of the scar.[80] Wounds subject to significant static tension require the undermining of at least one tissue plane on both sides of the wound to achieve a tension-free closure. To undermine a wound, the clinician frees a flap of tissue from its base at a distance from the edge of the wound approximately equal to the width of the gap that the laceration presents at its widest point (Fig. 35-19).

The depth of the incision can be modified, depending on the orientation of the laceration to skin tension lines and the laxity of skin in the area. A No. 15 scalpel blade held parallel to the surface of the skin is used to incise the adipose layer or the dermal layer of the wound. The clinician can also accomplish this technique by spreading scissors in the appropriate tissue plane. Undermining allows the edges of the skin to be lifted and brought together with gentle traction.[81] Potential complications of this procedure include injury to cutaneous nerves and creation of a hematoma under the flap. Because undermining may harm the underlying blood supply, this technique should be reserved for relatively uncontaminated

GENERAL SUTURING TECHNIQUE

Cleanse the skin surrounding the wound with an antiseptic such as chlorhexidine or providone-iodine. Avoid introducing antiseptic into the wound because it may be toxic to tissue.

Anesthetize the wound prior to exploration and irrigation. Introduce the needle through the wound (as opposed to through the epidermis).

Explore the wound to exclude the presence of foreign bodies, gross contamination, or injuries to deep structures. Débride grossly contaminated or devitalized tissue.

Irrigate the wound thoroughly until it is visibly clean. Use of a large syringe with a splash guard is ideal. Retract the wound edges with an instrument to facilitate thorough irrigation.

Apply a sterile drape, gather the instruments, and ensure that the field is appropriately lit.

Place the first suture at the center of the wound so that it bisects the laceration into two equal segments.

Tie the knot. The first throw should be a double throw (i.e., surgeon's knot) to prevent it from loosening. Place an additional three (single) throws and then cut the sutures while leaving 1- to 2-cm tails.

Continue to place additional sutures by further bisecting each segment of the laceration. After the last stitch has been placed, cleanse the area and apply an appropriate dressing.

Figure 35-16 General suturing technique.

INSTRUMENT TIE

Place the needle driver parallel to the wound, and wrap the suture end twice over the needle driver. This forms the surgeon's knot, which prevents the first throw from loosening.

Rotate the needle driver 90°, and grasp the short suture end on the opposite side of the laceration.

Gently pull the suture ends to the side of the laceration opposite their origin. Tighten only enough to approximate the skin edges; avoid overtightening, which may lead to tissue strangulation.

To begin the second throw, again place the needle driver parallel to the laceration. Wrap the long suture end over and around the needle driver once. (Only one wrap is used on throws 2 to 4).

Rotate the needle driver 90°, and grasp the short suture end on the opposite side of the laceration.

Pull the suture ends to the side of the laceration opposite their origin. On the second and subsequent throws, you can tighten the knot down snugly.

Place an additional 2 throws (for a total of 4), as depicted in *steps 4 through 6*. Remember to place the needle driver parallel to the wound and pull the long suture end *over* the driver; this will ensure that all knots tied are square knots.

After the last throw, cut the ends of the suture while leaving 1- to 2-cm tails. Avoid cutting the ends too short, which may lead to knot unraveling or difficulty during suture removal.

Figure 35-17 Instrument tie. *(From Custalow C. Color Atlas of Emergency Department Procedures. Philadelphia: Elsevier; 2005.)*

Figure 35-18 There is a tendency to overuse sutures. **A,** This child sustained a superficial forehead laceration just through the epidermis. The swelling accentuated the defect. Treatment was simply keeping the laceration clean. **B,** Four months after the injury, an excellent result was achieved. As the laceration was healing, it became red and more noticeable, *as do all scars,* but eventually faded.

wounds when no other methods adequately relieve wound tension.[77]

Layered Closure. The structure of skin and soft tissue varies with the location on the body (Fig. 35-20). Most wounds handled in an ED require approximation of no more than three layers: fascia (and associated muscle), SQ tissue, and skin surface (papillary layer of the dermis and epidermis).[82] Any "dead space" (or unapposed edges) within a wound may fill with blood or exudate and enhance the development of infection. Closure of individual layers obliterates this dead space (Fig. 35-21).

Separate approximation of muscle and layers hastens healing and return of function to the muscle. However, the fascia, not muscle, should be sutured. Muscle tissue itself is too friable to hold a suture. Layered closure is particularly important in the management of facial wounds; this technique prevents scarring of muscle to the SQ tissue and consequent

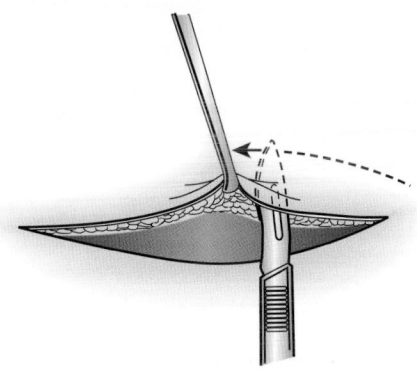

Figure 35-19 The technique of undermining is underused and can markedly improve cosmetic results by relieving wound tension. The scalpel is used to find an appropriate site; a natural plane often exists at the junction of the epidermis and dermis.

Figure 35-20 Variation in the structure of skin. **A,** Section of the skin of the scalp, ×15. **B,** Section of human sole perpendicular to the free surface, ×100. **C,** Section through human thigh perpendicular to the surface of the skin. Blood vessels are injected and appear black (low magnification). (*A, Courtesy of H Mizoguchi; **B** and **C,** after Maximow AA. From Bloom W, Fawcett DW. A Textbook of Histology. 10th ed. Philadelphia: Saunders; 1975. Reproduced by permission.*)

deformation of the surface of the wound with contraction of the muscle. If a deep, gaping wound is closed without approximation of underlying SQ tissue, a disfiguring depression may develop at the site of the wound. Finally, layered closure provides support to the wound and considerably reduces tension at the skin surface.

Several exceptions exist to the general rule of multilayered closure. The adipose layer of soft tissue should not be closed separately. A "fat stitch" is not necessary because little support is provided by closure of the adipose layer and additional suture material may increase the possibility of infection.[2,83] Scalp wounds are generally closed in a single layer. For lacerations penetrating the dermis in the fingers, hands, toes, and feet and the sebaceous skin of the nasal tip, the amount of SQ tissue is too small to warrant layered closure; in fact, SQ stitches may leave tender nodules in these sensitive locations. Layered closure is not recommended for wounds without tension, those with poor vascularity, and those with a moderate or high risk for infection. With single-layer closure, the surface stitch should be placed more deeply.[64]

Figure 35-21 Note how a subcutaneous suture almost closes the wound with minimal tension on the edges of the skin while obliterating any subcutaneous space. Tie and bury the knot by pulling the *sutures in the long axis of the wound.*

Suture Placement
SQ Layer Closure

Once the fascial structures have been reapproximated, the SQ layer is sutured. Although histologically the fatty and fibrous SQ tissue (hypodermis) is an extension of (and continuous with) the reticular layer of the dermis,[84] suturing of these layers is traditionally referred to as a *SQ closure.* One approach is to close the length of this layer in segments by placing the first stitch in the middle of the wound and bisecting each subsequent segment until closure of the layer has been completed.[48] This technique is useful for the closure of wounds that are long or sinuous, and it is particularly effective for wounds with one elliptical and one linear side. The needle is grasped with the needle holder close to the end of the suture. The clinician can suture more rapidly if the fingers are placed on the midshaft of the needle holder rather than in the rings of the instrument (Fig. 35-22).

The suture enters the SQ layer at the bottom of the wound (Fig. 35-23A) or, if the wound has been undermined, at the base of the flap (see Fig. 35-23B) and exits in the dermis. Once the suture has been placed on one side of the wound, it can be pulled across the wound to the opposite side (or the edges of the wound pushed together) to determine the matching point on the opposite side. The needle is then advanced into this point. The needle should enter the dermis at the same depth as it exited from the opposite side, pass through the tissue, and exit at the bottom of the wound (or the base of the flap). The edges of the wound can be closely apposed by pulling the two tails of the suture in the same direction along the axis of the wound (see Fig. 35-23C). Some clinicians place their SQ suture obliquely rather than vertically to facilitate knot tying. When the knot in this SQ stitch is tied, it will remain inverted, or "buried," at the bottom of the wound. Burying the knot of the SQ stitch avoids a painful, palpable nodule beneath the epidermis and keeps the bulk of this foreign material away from the surface of the skin. Most emergency clinicians construct knots with the instrument tie technique (see Fig. 35-17). Hand and instrument knot-tying techniques are described and illustrated in wound care texts.[85,86]

Once the knot has been secured, the tails of the suture should be pulled taut for cutting. The scissors are held with the index finger on the junction of the two blades. The blade of the scissors is slid down the tail of the suture until the knot

Figure 35-22 A, Thenar grip technique of handling the needle holder. The index finger is placed on the side of the needle holder, where it guides placement of the needle. Neither the index nor the middle finger is placed in the ringlet hole. This method allows more rapid suturing. **B,** An alternative method is the thumb-ring finger grip. **C,** Hold the forceps in your nondominant hand as you would hold a pencil or a dart.

SUBCUTANEOUS SUTURES

Dermis

Subcutaneous layer

A Place the suture in the subcutaneous layer at the bottom of the wound, and pass it upward so that it exits in the dermis. Pull the suture across the wound to determine the correct level of dermal entry on the opposite side. Pass the needle downward through the dermis on the opposite side so that it exits at the bottom of the wound.

Start here

B If the wound has been undermined, the needle enters at the base of the flap and is passed upward through the dermis.

C Pull the two tails of the suture in the same direction along the axis of the wound to appose the wound edges, and then tie the knot. Subcutaneous knots are "buried" at the bottom of the wound to prevent painful nodules beneath the epidermis and to keep the bulk of the foreign material away from the skin surface.

Figure 35-23 Subcutaneous sutures.

is reached. With the cutting edge of the blade tilted away from the knot, the tails are cut. This technique prevents the scissors from cutting the knot itself and leaves a 3-mm tail, which protects the knot from unraveling.[87] The entire SQ layer is sutured in this manner.

After the SQ layer has been closed, the distance between the skin edges determines the approximate width of the scar in its final form. If this width is acceptable, surface sutures can be inserted.[88] Despite undermining and placement of a sufficient number of SQ sutures, on occasion a large gap between the edges of the wound may persist. In such cases, a horizontal dermal stitch may be used to bridge this gap (see Fig. 35-29).

Surface Closure

The epidermis and the superficial layer of dermis are sutured in a single layer with nonabsorbable synthetic suture. The choice of suture size, the number of sutures used, and the depth of suture placement depend on the amount of skin tension remaining after SQ closure.

If the edges of the wound are apposed after closure of the deeper layers, small 5-0 or 6-0 sutures can be used simply to match the epithelium on each side. Wounds with greater tension and separation should have skin stitches placed closer to each other and closer to the edge of the wound; layered closure is important in such wounds. If the edges of the wound remain retracted or if SQ stitches were not used, a larger-size suture placed deeply may be required.

The number of sutures used in closing any wound will vary with the wound's location, the amount of tension on the wound, and the degree of accuracy required by the clinician and patient. For example, sutures on the face would probably be placed between 1 and 3 mm apart.[69] Unless the edges of the wound are uneven, sutures should be placed in a mirror-image fashion such that the depth and width are the same on both sides of the wound.[52] In general, the distance between each suture should be approximately equal to the distance from the exit of the stitch to the edge of the wound.[48,85]

Skin closure may be accomplished by placing the appropriate number of sutures in segments (Fig. 35-24). When suturing the skin, right-handed operators should pass the needle from the right side of the wound to the left. The needle should be driven through tissue by flexing the wrist and supinating the forearm; *the course taken by the needle should result in a curve identical to the curvature of the needle itself* (see Fig. 35-24, *steps 1 and 2,* and Fig 35-25). *The angle of exit for the needle should be the same as its angle of entrance so that an identical volume of tissue is contained within the stitch on each side of the wound* (see Fig. 35-24, *steps 3 and 4*).

Once the needle exits the skin on the opposite side of the wound, it is regrasped with the needle holder and advanced through the tissue; care should be taken to avoid crushing the point of the needle with the instrument. Forceps are designed for handling tissue and thus should not be used to grasp the needle. Forceps can stabilize the needle by holding it within the tissue through which the needle has just passed. An assistant can keep excess thread clear of the area being sutured, or the excess can be looped around the clinician's fingers. If the point of the needle becomes dull before all the attached thread has been used, the suture should be discarded.

SIMPLE INTERRUPTED SUTURES

1

Hold the needle pointing down-ward by excessively pronating the wrist so that the needle tip initially moves farther from the laceration as the needle penetrates deeper into the skin. Drive the needle tip downward and away from the cut edge into the subcutaneous layer.

2

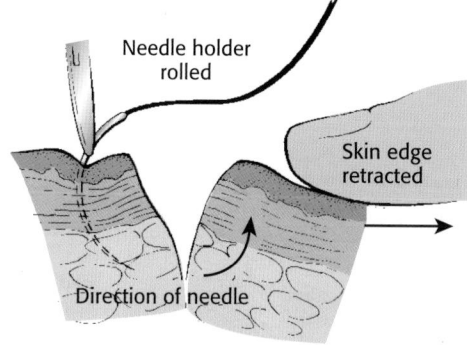

Advance the needle into the laceration. The needle tip is directed toward the opposite side at the same level by rolling the needle holder. The arc of the needle pathway is controlled by retracting the skin edge. This method incorporates more tissue within the stitch in the deeper layers of the wound than at the surface. As an alternative, if a small needle is used in thick skin or the distance across the wound is great, the needle can be removed from the first side, remounted on the needle holder, and advanced to the opposite side.

3

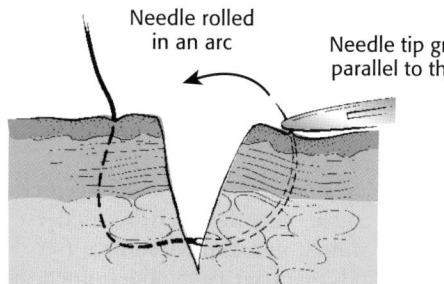

Advance the needle upward toward the surface so that it exits at the same distance from the wound edge as on the contralateral side of the wound. Grasp the needle behind the tip and roll it out in the arc of the needle.

4

The final position, with more tissue in the depth than in the surface. The distance from each exit of the suture to the laceration is half the depth of the dermis.

5

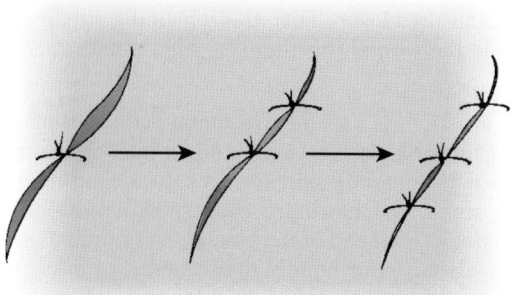

Close the surface of the wound in segments rather than from one end. Place the first suture in the center of the wound for a straight suture line.

6

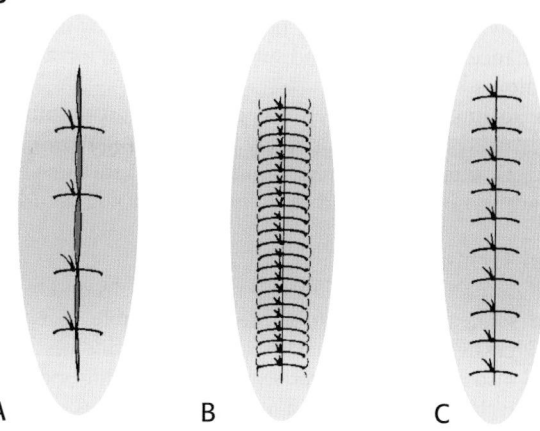

A, Too few stitches used. Note the gaping between the sutures. **B,** Too many stitches used. **C,** Correct number of stitches used for a wound under an average amount of tension.

Figure 35-24 Simple interrupted sutures. See also Figures 35-16 and 35-17. *(1-4, Redrawn from Kaplan EN, Hentz VR.* Emergency Management of Skin and Soft Tissue Wounds: An Illustrated Guide. *Boston: Little, Brown; 1984:86. Reproduced by permission.)*

Sutures placed   Sutures removed

Figure 35-25 Motion of the needle holder mimics the curve of the needle. Rotate the wrist (pronate) so that the needle enters the skin perpendicularly, not at an angle, as the wrist supinates. This helps evert the edge of the wound. *(From Anderson CB. Basic surgical techniques. In: Klippel AP, Anderson CB, eds.* Manual of Outpatient and Emergency Surgical Techniques. *Boston: Little, Brown; 1979. Reproduced by permission.)*

Figure 35-26 Skin edges that are slightly *everted* will gradually flatten to produce a level wound surface when the sutures are removed. An inverted wound catches the light in a shadow and is more visible. In addition, eversion allows subcutaneous tissue to heal. *(From Grabb WC. Basic technique of plastic surgery. In: Grabb WC, Smith JW, eds.* Plastic Surgery: A Concise Guide to Clinical Practice. *Boston: Little, Brown; 1979. Reproduced by permission.)*

Complications

Sutures act as foreign bodies in a wound, and any stitch may damage a blood vessel or strangulate tissue. Therefore, the clinician should use the smallest size and the least number of sutures that will adequately close the wound.[63] However, if spaced too widely, surface stitches will leave a "crosshatch" pattern of marks.

Encompassing too much tissue with a small needle is a common error. Forcefully pushing or twisting the needle in an effort to bring the point out of the tissue may bend or break the body of the needle. Using a needle of improper size will defeat the best suturing technique.

If sutures are tied too tightly around the edges of the wound or if individual stitches are under excessive tension, blood supply to the wound may be impeded, thereby increasing the chance of infection, and suture marks may form even after 24 hours.[52,89]

If the techniques described are applied to most wounds, the edges will be matched precisely in all three dimensions, and the least number of sutures required to appose the edges and relieve tension but avoid excessive scarring will be used.

Eversion Techniques

If the edges of a wound invert or if one edge rolls under the opposite side, a poorly formed, deep, noticeable scar will result. Excessive eversion that exposes the dermis on both sides will also result in a larger scar than if the edges of the skin are perfectly apposed, but inversion produces a more visible scar than eversion does. Because most scars undergo some flattening with contraction, optimal results are achieved when the epidermis is slightly everted without excessive suture tension (Fig. 35-26). Wounds over mobile surfaces, such as the extensor surfaces of joints, should be everted. In time, the scar will be flattened by the dynamic forces acting in the area.

Numerous techniques can be used to avoid inversion of the edges of the wound. If the clinician angles the needle obliquely away from the laceration, a surface stitch can be placed so that

it is *deeper than it is* wide[81] and the stitch encircles more tissue in the SQ layer than at the surface. If this "bottle-shaped stitch" is intended to produce some eversion of the wound edges, the stitch must include a sufficient amount of SQ tissue (see Fig. 35-24, *step 4*).

Eversion can be accomplished by lifting and turning the edge of the wound outward with a skin hook or fine-toothed forceps before insertion of the needle on each side (Fig. 35-27, *plate 1*). Eversion can also be achieved simply by pressing on the skin adjacent to the wound with closed forceps (or a thumb and finger as long as a needlestick is avoided) (see Fig. 35-27, *plate 2*).

Vertical mattress sutures are particularly effective in everting the edges of the wound, and they can be used exclusively or alternated with simple interrupted sutures (see Fig. 35-27, *plate 3*).[90] In wounds that have been undermined, an SQ stitch placed at the base of the flap on each side can in itself evert the wound (Fig. 35-27, *plate 4*).

Interrupted Stitch

The simple interrupted stitch is the most frequently used technique for closure of skin. It consists of separate loops of suture tied individually. Although tying plus cutting each stitch is time-consuming, the advantage of this method is that if one stitch in the closure fails, the remaining stitches continue to hold the wound together (see Fig. 35-24).

Continuous Stitch

A continuous stitch is an effective method for closing relatively clean, low-risk wounds that are under little or no tension and are on flat, immobile skin surfaces. In a continuous, or "running," stitch, the loops are the exposed portions of a helical coil tied at each end of the wound. A continuous suture line can be placed more rapidly than a series of interrupted stitches. A continuous stitch has the additional advantages of strength (with tension being evenly distributed along its entire length), fewer knots (which are the weak points of stitches), and more effective hemostasis. This stitch will accommodate mild wound swelling. The continuous technique is useful as an epithelial or "surface" stitch in cosmetic closures; however, if the underlying SQ layer is not stabilized in a separate closure, a continuous surface stitch tends to invert the edges of the wound.

The continuous suture technique has some disadvantages. This technique should not be used to close wounds overlying joints. If a loop breaks at one point, the entire stitch may

EVERSION TECHNIQUES

1

Use of forceps or a skin hook to evert the wound edge. This technique allows the operator to see the needle path, thereby ensuring that the proper depth has been reached, and promotes eversion of the skin edges.

2

Eversion of the wound edge by thumb and finger pressure. Great care must be taken to avoid a needlestick.

3

Only a small bite of the skin edge taken here

Begin here with a deep bite of tissue

A vertical mattress suture is the best technique for producing skin edge eversion. **A,** The usual type of mattress suture for approximating and everting wound edges. **B,** "Tacking" type of vertical mattress suture extending into the deep fascia to obliterate dead space under the wound. Note that only a small bite of skin is included on the inner suture.

4

Deep dermis suturing technique. The suture enters the base of the flap, is brought up into the dermis, and exits just proximal to the wound edge along the base of the flap to be tied and cut.

Figure 35-27 Eversion techniques. *(2 and 3, From Converse JM. Introduction to plastic surgery. In: Converse JM, ed.* Reconstructive Plastic Surgery: Principles and Procedures in Correction, Reconstruction, and Transplantation. *Vol 1. 2nd ed. Philadelphia: Saunders; 1977. Reproduced by permission; 4, from Stuzin J, Engrav LH, Buehler PK. Emergency treatment of facial lacerations.* Postgrad Med. *1982;71:81. Reproduced by permission.)*

unravel. Likewise, if infection develops and the incision must be opened at one point, cutting a single loop may allow the entire wound to fall open. A simple continuous stitch has a tendency to produce suture marks if used for the closure of large wounds and if left in place for more than 5 days.[79] However, if all tension on the wound can be removed with SQ sutures, stitch marks are seldom a problem.

Among the variations of the continuous technique, the simple continuous stitch is the most useful to emergency clinicians (Fig. 35-28*A*). An interrupted stitch is placed at one end of the wound, and only the free tail of the suture is cut. As suturing proceeds, the stitch encircles the tissue in a spiral pattern. After each passage of the needle, the loop is tightened slightly, and the thread is held taut in the clinician's nondominant hand. The needle should travel perpendicularly across the wound on each pass. The last loop is placed just beyond the end of the wound and the suture is tied, with the last loop being used as a "tail" in the process of tying the knot. A

locking loop may be used with continuous suturing to prevent slippage of loops as the suturing proceeds (Fig. 35-28*B*). The interlocking technique allows use of the continuous stitch along an irregular laceration.[81]

Continuous Subcuticular Stitch

Nonabsorbable sutures used for surface closure outlast their usefulness and must be removed. On occasion, wounds require an extended period of support, longer than that provided by surface stitches. Some patients with wounds that require skin closure are unlikely or unwilling to return for removal of the sutures. Some sutured wounds are covered by plaster casts. On occasion, the patient (child or adult) is likely to be as frightened by and uncooperative with suture removal as for suture placement. Surface sutures are more likely to produce stitch marks in children because the wounds are under greater tension than those in adults. The continuous subcuticular (or "dermal") suture technique is ideal for these situations; the

CONTINUOUS SUTURES

Place a suture at one end of the laceration in an analogous fashion to a simple interrupted stitch. However, *cut only the distal end of the suture* while leaving the needle end attached.

Cross over the wound at a 45° angle, and reenter the wound parallel to the first pass. Do not tie the suture or cut the ends.

Advance the needle back to the original side and exit the skin at an equal distance from the previous suture pass.

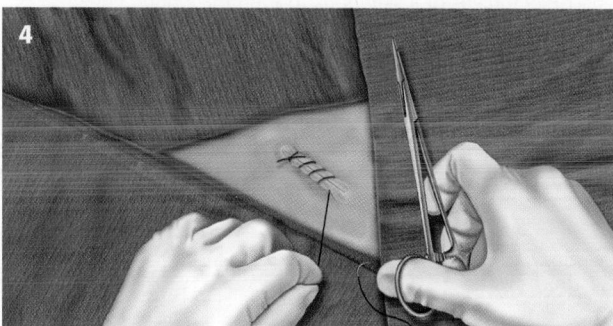

Continue in this fashion until the wound edges are closed and the end of the wound is approached.

On the last pass, leave a loop of suture. Use this loop as a free end to tie.

Tie the loop to the needle end of the suture with an instrument tie, and then cut the knot.

A

Figure 35-28 A, Continuous sutures.

wound can be closed with an absorbable subcuticular stitch, thereby obviating the need for later suture removal. In patients prone to keloid formation, the subcuticular technique can be used in lieu of surface stitches to avoid disfiguring stitch marks. Buried, absorbable subcuticular stitches do not appear to provoke more inflammation than percutaneous running stitches with monofilament nylon.[78] Because stitch marks are not a problem, a nonabsorbable subcuticular suture can be left in place for a longer period than a surface suture can.[90]

Although this technique is commonly used for cosmetic closures, closure of the subcuticular layer alone may not alter the width of the scar.[91] This technique does not allow perfect approximation of the vertical height of the two edges of a

wound,[92] and in cosmetic closures it is often followed by a surface stitch. The subcuticular stitch requires a 4-0 or 5-0 suture made of either absorbable material or nonabsorbable synthetic monofilament. An absorbable suture can be "buried" within the wound, whereas a nonabsorbable suture is used for a "pullout" stitch. The absorbable synthetic monofilament suture PDS (Ethicon) is designed for subcuticular closure. It passes through tissues as easily as nonabsorbable monofilament sutures do and is absorbed if left in the wound.

Before the subcuticular stitch is begun, the SQ layer should be approximated with interrupted sutures to minimize tension on the wound. The pullout subcuticular stitch is started at the skin surface approximately 1 to 2 cm away from one end of

CONTINUOUS LOCKED SUTURES

Begin the repair as you would a regular continuous stitch (Fig. 35-28A, *steps 1 and 2*). As the needle exits the near side, "lock" the suture by passing through the circle of the previous suture loop.

As the suture is pulled through the circle (*arrow*), it will become locked.

Keep tension evenly distributed across the suture as it is pulled down to the skin. The lock should be parallel to the wound edge (*arrow*).

Continue in this fashion by locking each throw along the way. On the last pass, leave a loop of suture and use it to tie to the needle end of the suture.

B

Figure 35-28, cont'd B, Continuous locked sutures.

Continued

the wound. The needle enters and exits the dermis at the apices of the wound (Fig. 35-28C, *plate 1*). Bites through tissue are taken in a horizontal direction, with the needle penetrating the dermis 1 to 2 mm from the skin surface. These intradermal bites should be small, of equal size, and at the same level on each side of the wound.[75,90] Each successive bite should be placed 1 to 2 mm behind the exit point on the opposite side of the wound so that when the wound is closed, the entrance and exit points on either side are not directly apposed. Small bites should be taken to avoid puckering of the skin surface, and the stitch should not be accidentally interlocked. Some clinicians prefer to place a fine (6-0) running skin suture on the surface, in addition to the subcuticular suture, for meticulous skin approximation. The skin suture is removed in 3 to 4 days to avoid suture marks.

If a subcuticular stitch is used on lengthy lacerations, it is difficult to remove. Placement of "reliefs" consisting of periodic loops through the skin every 4 to 5 cm along the length of the stitch facilitates later removal (see Fig. 35-28C, *plate 2*). The suture is crossed to the opposite side, and the needle is passed from SQ tissue to the surface of the skin. The suture is carried over the surface for approximately 2 cm before reentering the skin and SQ tissue. The subcuticular stitch is then continued at approximately the point at which the next bite would have been placed had the relief not been used.

At the completion of the stitch, the needle is placed through the apex and exits the skin 1 to 2 cm away from the end of the wound. The stitch should be tightened by pulling each end taut. If reliefs have been used, pulling on the reliefs will take up any slack in the stitch. The clinician can secure the two ends of the stitch by taping them to the skin surface with wound closure tape, by placing a cluster of knots on each tail close to the skin surface, or by tying the two ends of the suture to each other over a dressing. The subcuticular stitch will become lax as tissue swelling subsides 48 hours after wound closure. The stitch can be tightened at this time.

Subcuticular closure can be accomplished with absorbable sutures that do not penetrate the skin. Closure is begun with a dermal or SQ suture placed at one end of the wound and secured with a knot. After placement of the continuous subcuticular stitch from apex to apex, the suture is pulled taut, and a knot is tied with a tail and a loop of suture (see Fig. 35-28C, *plate 3*). The final knot can be buried by inserting the needle into deeper tissue; the needle exits several millimeters from the edge of the wound. By pulling on the end of the needle, the knot disappears into the wound.[74] The advantage of this technique is that there are no suture marks on the skin.

Nonabsorbable subcuticular sutures can be left in place for 2 to 3 weeks, thus providing a longer period of support than

CONTINUOUS SUBCUTICULAR SUTURES

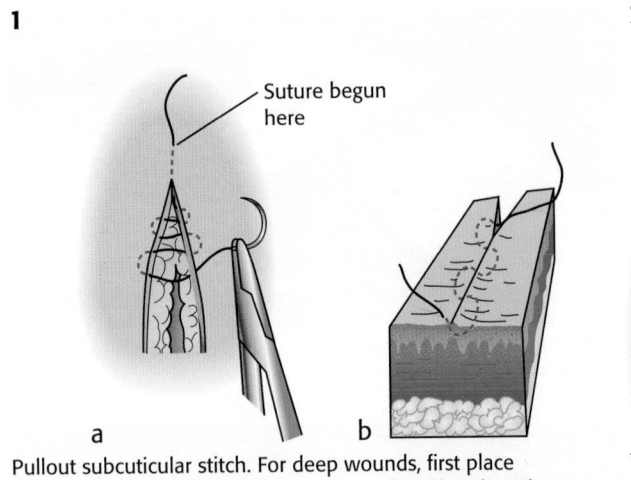

1

Suture begun here

a   b

Pullout subcuticular stitch. For deep wounds, first place interrupted sutures to relieve tension on the skin edge. The suture is introduced into the skin in line with the incision, approximately 1 to 2 cm away.

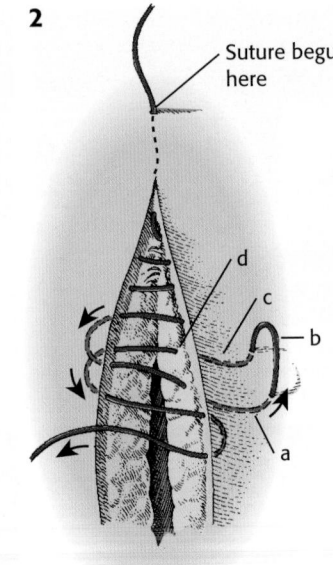

2

Suture begun here

d

c

b

a

In constructing the relief to facilitate suture removal, the suture is crossed to the opposite side by going into the subcuticular area beneath the skin for approximately 2 cm before exiting (*a*). The suture is then carried over the epidermis for approximately 2 cm (*b*) and then back under the dermis again (*c*). Reentry is made into the wound area (*d*) at approximately the same location where the next "bite" would have been placed had the relief not been used.

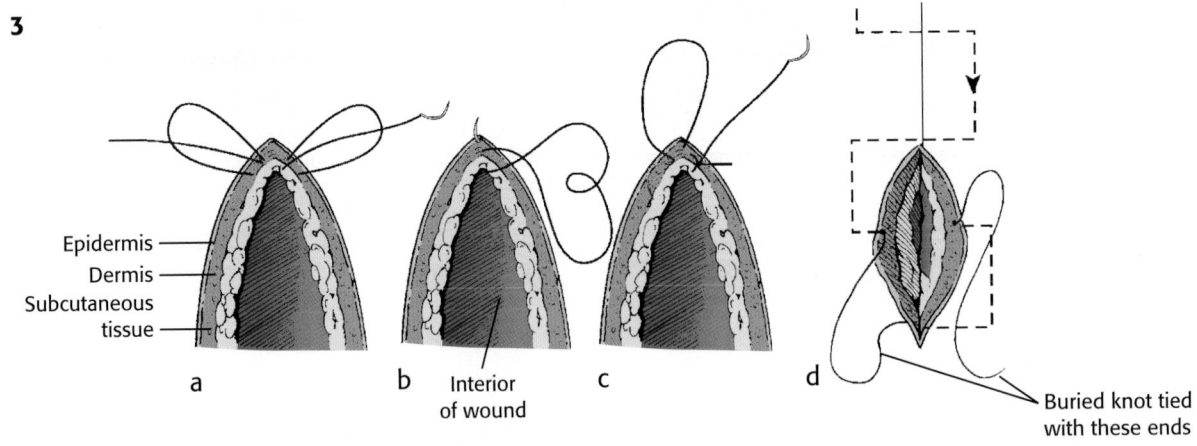

3

Epidermis

Dermis

Subcutaneous tissue

a   b   Interior of wound   c   d

Buried knot tied with these ends

Subcuticular closure without epidermal penetration. **a,** The initial knot is secured in dermal or subcutaneous tissue. **b,** The short strand is cut, and the needle is inserted into the dermis at the apex of the wound. **c,** The needle in the dermis close to the corner of the wound and exiting the wound at the same horizontal level. **d,** After the subcuticular stitch has been completed, a knot is tied with the tail and the loop of the suture.

C

Figure 35-28, cont'd C, Continuous subcuticular sutures. (*A and B, From Custalow C.* Color Atlas of Emergency Department Procedures. *Philadelphia: Elsevier; 2005; C, 1-2, from Grimes DW, Garner RW. "Reliefs" in intracuticular sutures.* Surg Rounds. *1978;1:47. Reproduced by permission; 3, modified from Stillman RM. Wound closure: choosing optimal materials and methods.* ER Rep. *1981;2:43.)*

with surface sutures and without the problem of stitch marks.[79] If skin sutures are used in conjunction with a subcuticular stitch, they are removed in 3 to 4 days. A subcuticular closure in itself is stronger than a tape closure. If the subcuticular technique is used exclusively to approximate the skin surface, skin tape can be applied to correct surface unevenness and to provide more accurate apposition of the epidermis.

The primary disadvantage of the subcuticular stitch is that it is time-consuming, especially when supporting surface stitches are used. Another, faster method that avoids penetrating the skin is the interrupted subcuticular stitch (Fig. 35-29). Wounds with strong static skin tension may benefit from a few interrupted dermal stitches placed horizontal to the skin surface instead of a continuous subcuticular stitch.

Mattress Stitch

The various types of mattress stitches are all interrupted stitches. The *vertical mattress stitch* is an effective method of everting skin edges (Fig. 35-30*A*; see also Fig. 35-27, *plate 3*). A vertical mattress stitch may be used to take a deep bite of skin, thereby eliminating the need for layered closure in areas where excessive tension does not result. If the superficial loop is placed first, the tails can be pulled upward while the deep loop is placed; this technique ensures eversion of the wound in less time than needed with the traditional technique.[93]

The *horizontal mattress stitch* is an SQ stitch that is oriented 90 degrees to the interrupted SQ stitch described previously (Fig. 35-30*B*). The horizontal mattress stitch apposes the skin

Horizontal
dermal stitch

Figure 35-29 Interrupted subcuticular stitch (also called a horizontal dermal stitch). Absorbable sutures are used. (A vertical suture also closes the deep tissue.)

edges closely while providing some degree of eversion.[79] A horizontal mattress suture may be ideal for areas where eversion is desirable but there is little SQ tissue.

The *half-buried horizontal mattress stitch* is particularly useful in suturing the easily damaged apex of a V-shaped flap (see Fig. 35-30*B*). In performing the "corner stitch," the suture needle penetrates the skin at a point beyond the apex of the wound and exits through the dermis. The corner of the flap is elevated, and the suture is passed through the dermis of the flap. The needle is then placed in the dermis at the base of the wound and returned to the surface of the skin. All dermal bites should be placed at the same level. The suture is tied with sufficient tension to pull the flap snugly into the corner without blanching the flap.[79,94] If the tip of a large flap with questionable viability may be further jeopardized by postoperative swelling, a cotton stent can be placed underneath the knot of the corner stitch. The cotton absorbs the tension produced by swelling.

VERTICAL MATTRESS SUTURES

1 Pass the needle through both sides of the wound in the same manner as the first pass in a simple interrupted suture. This "inner" pass should be very close to the wound edge.

2 Reinsert the needle vertical to the previous exit site at a greater distance from the wound edge.

3 Pass the needle deeper than the previous pass, and exit about 0.5 cm vertical to the previous entrance site. Pull the suture through so that 2 cm of the short end remains outside the skin.

4 Tie the ends of the suture with an instrument tie, while everting the edges of the wound. Place subsequent sutures until the wound edges are apposed.

a b c d e

Steps in the vertical mattress stitch. The key to close apposition and exact alignment of edges is to place the inner sutures very close to the suture line (wound edge). *Note:* in steps 1–4 at the top of this figure the inner pass was placed first, whereas in steps a–e at the bottom the outer pass was placed first. Either method is acceptable.

A

Figure 35-30 A, Vertical mattress sutures.   *Continued*

HORIZONTAL MATTRESS SUTURES

Standard Horizontal Mattress

Pass the needle through both sides of the wound in the same manner as the first pass in a simple interrupted suture.

Reinsert the needle about 5 mm from and horizontal to the previous exit site. Exit the wound on the opposite side, parallel to the first pass and at the same distance from the wound edge.

Pull the suture through so that approximately 2 cm of the short end of the suture remains outside the skin.

Tie the ends of the suture with an instrument tie, while everting the edges of the wound. Place subsequent sutures until the wound edges are apposed.

Half-Buried Horizontal Mattress

a

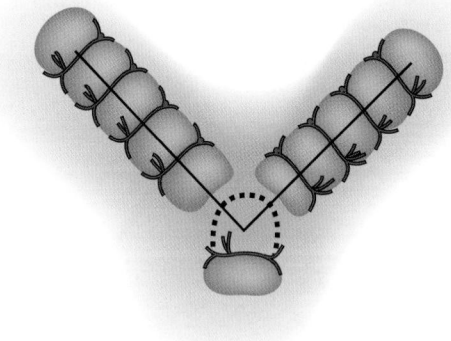

b

a and *b*, Corner stitch: Approximation of a flap with a half-buried horizontal mattress stitch, followed by interrupted sutures for the rest of the wound.

B

Figure 35-30, cont'd B, Horizontal mattress sutures. (*A and B, From Custalow C.* Color Atlas of Emergency Department Procedures. *Philadelphia: Elsevier; 2005.*)

The only disadvantage of the horizontal and vertical mattress stitches is that they cause more ischemia and necrosis inside their loops than do either simple or continuous stitches.[95]

Figure-of-Eight Stitch

A figure-of-eight stitch is useful for wounds with friable tissue, on the eyelids where the skin is too thin for buried sutures, or in areas in which buried sutures are undesirable (Fig. 35-31, *plate 1*).[96] This stitch reduces the amount of tension placed on the tissue by the suture, which allows the stitch to hold in place when a simple stitch would tear through the tissue. The disadvantage of this technique is that more suture material is left in the wound. A vertical variation of the figure-of-eight stitch is sometimes used to approximate close, parallel lacerations (see Fig. 35-31, *plate 2*).[97] Another technique involves a vertical mattress stitch (Fig. 35-32).

FIGURE-OF-EIGHT SUTURES

1

2

Start here

Figure-of-eight stitch, two methods. These stitches are useful in wounds with friable tissue or in areas where buried sutures are undesirable. This stitch reduces the amount of tension placed on the tissue by the suture.

Vertical figure-of-eight suture technique. It can be used to close parallel lacerations.

Figure 35-31 Figure-of-eight sutures. *(1, Modified from Dushoff IM. About face.* Emerg Med. *1974;6:11. Reproduced by permission; 2, from Mitchell GC. Repair of parallel lacerations [letter].* Ann Emerg Med. *1987;16:924.)*

Start here

Figure 35-32 Technique for closure of parallel lacerations in which the central tissue island has an intact base. *(Redrawn from Samo DG. A technique for parallel lacerations.* Ann Emerg Med. *1988;17:297.)*

Correction of Dog-Ears

When the edges of a wound are not precisely aligned horizontally, there will be excess tissue on one or both ends. This small flap of excess skin that bunches up at the end of a sutured wound is commonly called a *dog-ear*. This effect also occurs when one side of the wound is more elliptical than the opposite side or when excision of a wound is not sufficiently elliptical because it is either too straight or too nearly circular.[48,90]

If a dog-ear is present, it can be eliminated on one side of the wound in the following manner. The flap of excess skin is elevated with forceps or a skin hook, and an incision is made at an oblique angle from the apex of the wound toward the side with the excess skin. The flap is then undermined and laid flat. The resulting triangle of skin is trimmed, and the closure is completed (Fig. 35-33, *plate 1*).[88,94] An alternative

method consists of carrying the incision directly from the apex in line with the wound. The flap of excess tissue is pulled over the incision while skin hooks are used to retract the extended apex of the wound. Excess tissue is excised, and the remainder of the wound is sutured.[90] If dog-ears are present on both sides of one end of the wound, the bulge of excess tissue can be excised in an elliptical fashion and the wound closed (see Fig. 35-33, *plate 2*).[94]

Stellate Lacerations

Repair of a stellate laceration is a challenging problem. Usually a result of compression and shear forces, these injuries contain large amounts of partially devitalized tissue. The surrounding soft tissue is often swollen and contused. Much of this contused tissue cannot be débrided without creating a large tissue defect. Sometimes tissue is lost, yet the amount is not apparent until key sutures are placed. In repairing what often resembles a jigsaw puzzle, the clinician can remove small flaps of necrotic tissue with iris scissors; large, viable flaps can be repositioned in their beds and carefully secured with half-buried mattress stitches. If interrupted stitches are used to approximate a thin flap, small bites should be taken in the flap and larger, deeper bites in the base of the wound. A modification of the corner stitch can be used to approximate multiple flaps to a base (Fig. 35-34). Thin flaps of tissue in a stellate laceration with beveled edges may be more easily repositioned and stabilized with a firm dressing.[79]

Closure of stellate lacerations cannot always be accomplished immediately, especially if considerable soft tissue

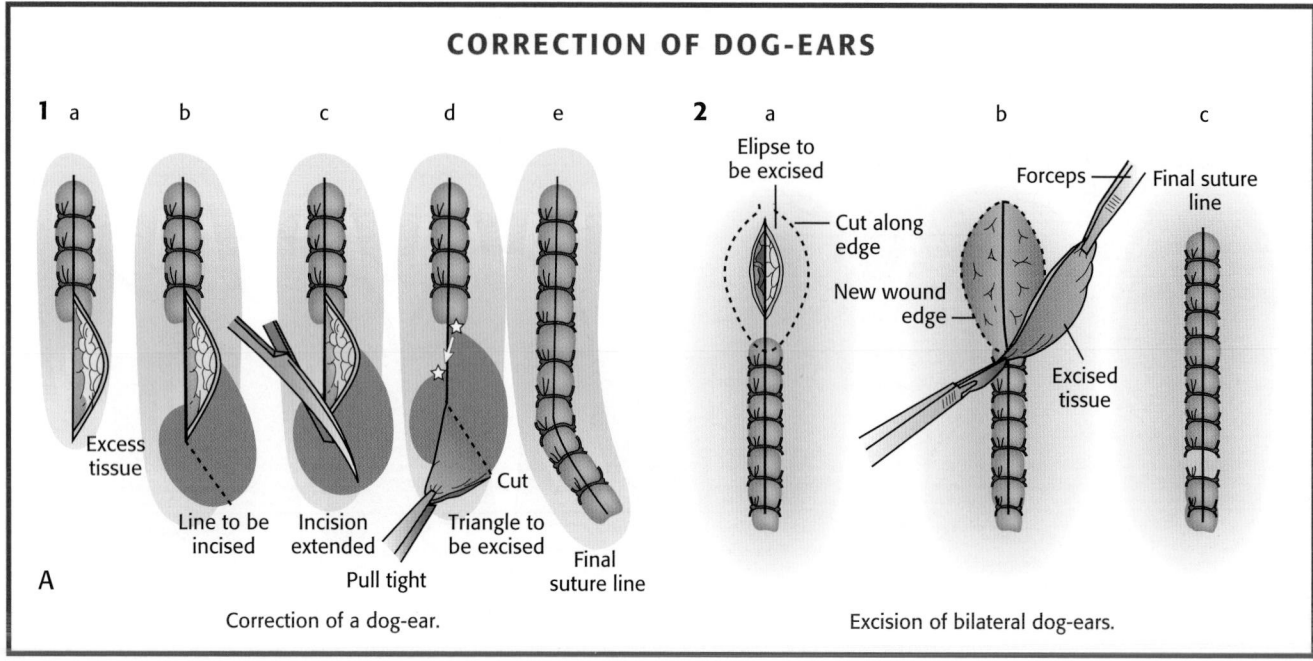

CORRECTION OF DOG-EARS

Figure 35-33 Correction of a dog-ears. The critical maneuver is *1d,* where the skin is pulled tight to align the starred areas and identify the triangular piece of excess tissue to be excised. Note that a straight laceration becomes somewhat curved with this technique. (*A, From Dushoff IM. A stitch in time. Emerg Med. 1973;5:1. Reproduced by permission.*)

MANAGEMENT OF STELLATE LACERATIONS

View from above a stellate laceration showing closure with half-buried mattress stitches. For some stellate lacerations it is best to cover with Steri-Strips and revise the scar later or, if small, excise the laceration and convert it to a linear repair.

Left, significant soft tissue contusion with stellate lacerations. *Right,* the result at 1 year. No tissue was débrided; instead, meticulous attention was paid to accurate soft tissue realignment with fine suture (7-0).

Figure 35-34 Management of stellate lacerations.

swelling is present. It may be best in some instances to consider delayed closure or revision of the scar at a later date. In complicated lacerations, inexact tissue approximation may be all that is possible initially. For small stellate lacerations, it may be possible to excise the lesion totally and turn it into a linear repair.

Repair of Special Structures

Facial Wounds (General Features)

The ideal result in the repair of a facial laceration is an extremely narrow, flat, and inapparent scar. Facial and forehead lacerations that follow natural skin creases or lines will heal with a less noticeable scar than those that are oblique or perpendicular to the natural wrinkles of the skin (Fig. 35-35). In addition to basic wound management, a few additional techniques can be used to achieve satisfactory cosmetic results.

Although necrosis of partially devitalized wound edges contributes to wide scars, facial skin with apparently marginal circulation may survive because of excellent vascularity. SQ fat, which in other locations may be débrided thoroughly, *should be preserved if possible in facial wounds* to prevent eventual sinking of the scar and to preserve normal facial contours. Therefore, débridement of most facial wounds should be conservative[82] (Fig. 35-36).

A *layered closure* has long been considered essential in the cosmetic repair of many facial wounds. However, the importance of layered closure in facial wounds was called into question by Singer and associates.[98] These investigators found similar cosmetic outcomes and scar widths in facial wounds less than 3 cm in length and 10 mm in width that were repaired with and without deep dermal sutures. Further confirmation of these results is needed.

If a layered closure is undertaken, approximation of the dermis with an SQ stitch or with a combination of SQ and subcuticular stitches should bring the edges of the wound together or to within 1 to 2 mm of apposition—close enough that the use of additional sutures seems almost unnecessary.[88] If an SQ stitch is the only stitch used to close the deeper layers, it should pass through the dermal-epidermal junction, or within 1 to 2 mm of the surface of the skin, without causing a dimpling effect. The stitch should be tied snugly by pulling the two ends of the suture in the same direction (see Fig. 35-23*C*).

In cosmetic areas, a surface stitch should not be used to relieve a wound of significant tension. A surface stitch on the

Figure 35-35 Lacerations following natural skin lines (shown here) heal with a less noticeable scar than do those that are oblique or perpendicular to natural lines (or wrinkles).

Figure 35-36 A, This woman was punched in the face, suffered a laceration of her cheek, and went to the emergency department 35 hours later. The wound was not infected, but it had contracted and was beginning to heal by granulation. Under local anesthesia, the wound was opened, irrigated, and minimally débrided, and the skin edges were trimmed. **B,** Using a No. 15 blade, a 1-mm-deep incision was made in the skin along the edges of the wound border. **C,** The incised edges were then cut away with tissue scissors. **D,** The wound was undermined to relieve tension on the skin. **E,** The wound is clean, undermined, and ready to close. **F,** The wound was closed with 6-0 interrupted sutures, which were removed in 5 days. No antibiotics were used, and only a small linear scar resulted.

face is most appropriately used to match the epidermal surfaces precisely along the length of the wound. If the edges of the wound are separated more than about 2 to 4 mm after closure of the SQ layer, a 5-0 or 6-0 subcuticular suture can be used to eliminate the tension produced by this separation and to provide prolonged stability. An alternative approach is the use of a few *guide stitches* to hold sections of the wound together before definitive closure with surface stitches. Guide stitches allow the surface sutures to be placed with little tension on each individual stitch, they match irregular edges, and they protect the SQ stitches from disruption. The first guide stitch is placed at the midpoint of the wound, and subsequent guide stitches bisect the intervening spaces. Once the definitive surface stitches have been placed, the guide stitches, if slack, can be removed. Because a needle damages tissue with each passage through the skin, guide stitches should be used only when necessary.

In a straight laceration, better apposition during surface closure is achieved if the wound is stretched lengthwise by finger traction or with skin hooks. When the needle is placed on one side of the wound, if that side is higher than the opposite side, a shallow bite is taken. The needle is used to depress the edges of the wound to the proper height, after which the needle "follows through" to the other side to pin the two sides together. If the first side entered is lower, the needle is elevated when entering the second side to match the epithelial edges.

If the skin edges are apposed closely by the SQ stitch or a subcuticular stitch, a small, shallow "*epithelial*" stitch can be used in lieu of the standard, deeper, surface stitch to correct discrepancies in vertical alignment (Fig. 35-37).[81] Precise alignment of wound edges is achieved by inserting the needle as close to the edge as possible without tearing through the

tissue. A 6-0 synthetic nonabsorbable suture is an excellent material for this stitch. A continuous stitch is preferable because it can be placed quickly, but interrupted stitches are acceptable. Epithelial stitches should be spaced no more than 2 to 3 mm apart and should encompass no more than 2 to 4 mm of tissue.[81] Once skin closure is complete, final adjustments in the tension on a continuous suture line are made before the end of the stitch is tied. If any discrepancies in level persist, interrupted sutures or tape can be used to flatten these few irregularities. The disadvantages of epithelial stitches are that they are time-consuming and add more suture material to the wound. Discrepancies in level can often be corrected with surgical tape.

Surgical tape is useful as a secondary support to protect the surface stitch from the stress produced by normal skin movement (Fig. 35-38). Facial wounds have a tendency to swell and place excessive stretch on a surface stitch. This can be minimized by applying a pressure dressing and cold compresses to the wound after closure. Surgical tape can serve to a limited extent as a small pressure dressing. In simple, low-tension facial wounds, wound closure with surgical tape provides results that are equivalent to closure with tissue adhesive.[99]

Forehead

Although the forehead is actually a part of the scalp, lacerations in this region are treated as facial wounds. Vertical lacerations across the forehead are oriented 90 degrees to skin tension lines, and the resulting scars are more noticeable than those from horizontal lacerations. Midline vertical forehead lacerations may result in cosmetically acceptable scars with standard closure techniques; uncentered lacerations may benefit from S-plasty or Z-plasty techniques during the initial repair or during later revision of the scar.

Superficial lacerations may be closed with skin stitches alone, but deep forehead lacerations must be closed in layers. Significant periosteal defects should be approximated before the closure of more superficial layers (Fig. 35-39). If skin is directly exposed to bone, adhesions might develop that in time may limit the movement of skin during facial expressions. The frontalis muscle fascia and adjacent fibrous tissue should be closed as a distinct layer; if left unsutured, the retracted ends of this muscle may bulge beneath the skin. If the gap in a muscle belly is later filled with scar tissue, movement of the muscle may pull on the entire scar and make it more apparent.[82]

Figure 35-37 Epithelial stitches. If the skin edges are well apposed by a subcutaneous or subcuticular stitch, epithelial stitches can be used to correct discrepancies in vertical alignment. Achieve precise alignment by inserting the needle as close to the edge as possible without tearing the tissue, no more than 2 to 3 mm apart and encompassing no more than 2 to 4 mm of tissue. This wound should be carefully evaluated for an occult globe injury.

Figure 35-38 Wound closure tape can be used to provide additional support while sutures are in place and after they are removed. This may be especially useful in cosmetic areas such as the face.

A U-shaped flap laceration with a superiorly oriented base poses a difficult problem. Immediate vascular congestion and later scar contraction within the flap produce the "trapdoor" effect, with the flap becoming prominently elevated (Fig. 35-40, *plates 1 and 2*). This effect can be minimized by approximation of the bulk of the SQ tissue of the flap to a deeper level on the base side of the wound; the skin surfaces of the two sides are apposed at the same level (see Fig. 35-40, *plate 3*). A firm compression dressing helps eliminate dead space and hematoma formation within the wound. Despite these efforts, secondary revision is sometimes necessary.[79] Frequently, swelling of the flap resolves over a 6- to 12-month period. Because flap elevation can be quite disconcerting, the clinician should forewarn the patient and family about a possible trapdoor effect.

When a forehead laceration borders the scalp and the thick scalp tissue must be sutured to thinner forehead skin, a horizontal or vertical mattress stitch with an intradermal component can be used (see Fig. 35-40, *plates 3E and 3F*).[90]

Note that even a minor forehead contusion or laceration may bleed subcutaneously and, in a few days, *produce blackness around the eyes* (Fig. 35-41). Patients should be forewarned about this. So-called raccoon eyes were once thought to represent a fracture, and although associated with fractures, this is usually a common benign finding, albeit occasionally a striking one.

Windshield injuries involving the forehead can be problematic (see Fig. 35-41*C*) to the extent that multiple superficial cuts harbor small glass particles and the injuries do readily not lend themselves to closure with suture. Supraorbital blocks can be used to anesthetize the forehead while the clinician meticulously looks for glass in each skin defect, often feeling pieces only with forceps or a small hemostat. Some pieces of glass are best felt; others are appreciated as shining objects under a good light source.

Eyebrow and Eyelid Lacerations

Jagged lacerations through eyebrows should be managed with little, if any, débridement of untidy but viable edges. The hair shafts of the eyebrow grow at an oblique angle, and vertical excision may produce a linear alopecia in the eyebrow, whereas with simple closure, the scar remains hidden within the hair.

If partial excision is unavoidable, the scalpel blade should be angled in a direction parallel to the axis of the hair shaft to minimize damage to the hair follicles.

Points on each side of the lacerated eyebrow should be aligned precisely; a single percutaneous stitch on each margin of the eyebrow should precede SQ closure. The edges of the eyebrow serve as landmarks for reapproximation; therefore, the eyebrow must not be shaved because these landmarks will be lost. Shaved eyebrows grow back slowly and sometimes incompletely, and shaving them often results in more deformity than caused by the injury itself. Care must be taken to not invert hair-bearing skin into the wound.[92]

The thin, flexible skin of the upper eyelid is relatively easy to suture. A soft 6-0 suture (or smaller) is recommended for closure of simple lacerations. Traumatized eyelids are susceptible to massive swelling; compression dressings and cool compresses can be used to minimize this problem.

The emergency clinician must recognize complicated eyelid lacerations that require the expertise of an ophthalmologist with experience in ocular plastic surgery. Lacerations that traverse the lid margin require exact realignment to avoid entropion or ectropion. Injuries penetrating the tarsal plate frequently cause damage to the globe (Fig. 35-42*A*).

Figure 35-39 A, This patient suffered a full-thickness flap avulsion type of forehead laceration. **B,** The surface of the skull is visible in the upper portion of the wound. Injuries such as these must be closed in layers. **C,** The galea aponeurosis is repaired with absorbable suture. **D,** Additional subcuticular and subcutaneous stitches were placed meticulously, which resulted in excellent apposition of the wound edges. **E,** The surface is repaired with a combination of simple interrupted and continuous epithelial sutures.

REPAIR OF "TRAPDOOR" INJURIES

1

Flap
Base

Sutured wound

Bulge or "trapdoor" swelling in a healed laceration

Final result

Elevation of a forehead flap. The "trapdoor effect" is a natural healing process of elliptical or round lacerations. Patients should be advised of this phenomenon.

2

This flap-type laceration of the forehead will heal with a puffed-up center (trapdoor), even under the best of circumstances.

3

Flap   A   Base

Flap   D   Base
A B   C

E

F

Repair of a U-shaped flap laceration with a superiorly oriented base to minimize the trapdoor effect. **A**, Excision of edges. **B**, Undermining. **C**, Approximation of subcutaneous tissue on the flap to subcutaneous tissue at a deeper level on the base. **B** and **C**, When a laceration in the thin skin of the forehead borders the thicker skin of the scalp, a horizontal mattress suture with an intradermal component can enhance healing by bringing tissues to the same plane. These figures show eversion of thinner skin to obtain adequate approximation with thicker scalp tissue. **D-F**, Skin closure.

Figure 35-40 Repair of "trapdoor" injuries. *(1, From Grabb WC, Kleinert HE.* Technics in Surgery: Facial and Hand Injuries. *Somerville, NJ: Ethicon, Inc; 1980. Reproduced by permission; 3, from Converse JM.* Introduction to plastic surgery. *In: Converse JM, ed.* Reconstructive Plastic Surgery: Principles and Procedures in Correction, Reconstruction, and Transplantation. *Vol 1. 2nd ed. Philadelphia: Saunders; 1977. Reproduced by permission.)*

Figure 35-41 A, Patients should be informed that minor forehead or nasal bridge trauma can produce benign blackness around the eyes in a few days. **B,** "Raccoon eyes" are most often benign; however, this phenomenon can be impressive. **C,** Under bilateral supraorbital nerve blocks, multiple small lacerations from this windshield injury are explored with a metal instrument and good lighting to remove tiny pieces of glass. Most superficial cuts can be left alone and others sutured with 6-0 nylon suture (a clinical call on which require closure).

DIRECT CLOSURE OF A MARGINAL EYELID LACERATION

| Placement of intial margin suture | Partial-thickness lamellar sutures in the tarsus | Margin sutures tied through skin sutures |

Orbicularis muscle — Tarsus — Skin

A

Eyelid retractors — Tarsus sutures

Skin sutures

Severed canaliculus

1

Silicone tube

Sutured canaliculus

2

B

C

Figure 35-42 A, A laceration of the eyelid margin is a complicated repair usually done by an ophthalmologist or plastic surgeon. The principles of repair are demonstrated here. 1, The suture is placed precisely in the plane of the meibomian glands at the eyelid margin, approximately 2 mm from the edges of the wound and 2 mm deep. This placement should provide adequate eversion of the margins. 2, Partial-thickness lamellar sutures are placed across the tarsus and tied anteriorly. 3, The anterior skin and muscle lamella are closed with fine sutures, and these are tied over the long marginal sutures to prevent them from touching the cornea. **B,** A method of identifying and repairing the canaliculus. This repair is best left to the ophthalmologist, but the emergency clinician must recognize the potential for a canaliculus injury. **C,** Deep laceration of the left upper lid with herniation of orbital fat. For fat to prolapse, the orbital septum (and potentially the globe itself) must have been perforated. This is a wound requiring operating room exploration and repair.

A deep horizontal laceration through the upper lid that divides the thin levator palpebrae muscle or its tendinous attachment to the tarsal plate can result in ptosis. In most cases an ophthalmologist should repair the injury primarily. A laceration through the portion of the upper or lower lid medial to the punctum frequently damages the lacrimal duct or the medial canthal ligament and requires specialized techniques for repair (see Fig. 35-42B). Adipose tissue seen within any periorbital laceration may be retrobulbar fat herniating through the wound, and further evaluation is required (see Fig. 35-42C). Repair of lid avulsions, extensive lid lacerations with loss of tissue, and complex types of lid lacerations should be left to ophthalmologists.

Ear Lacerations

The primary goals in the management of lacerations of the pinna are expedient coverage of exposed cartilage and prevention of wound hematoma (see Fig. 35-43). Cartilage is an avascular tissue, and when ear cartilage is denuded of its protective, nutrient-providing skin, progressive erosive chondritis ensues. The initial step in the repair of an ear injury involves trimming away jagged or devitalized cartilage and

Figure 35-43 A, Lacerations of the ear require a special repair aimed at covering cartilage and preventing hematoma formation. With this through-and-through laceration of the margin of the pinna, the cartilage is trimmed just enough to allow the skin to be approximated to cover all exposed cartilage. Sutures are not used in the cartilage itself for this laceration, but the edges are approximated by skin sutures that incorporate the perichondrium. **B,** The repair is easiest if the posterior pinna is sutured first. **C** and **D,** Lacerations of the helical rim that traverse the two skin surfaces and the cartilage require a three-layer repair with accurate reapproximation of the auricular cartilage, as is done for the nose, to avoid notching. The cartilage is repaired by placing 5-0 or 6-0 clear monofilament through the perichondrium and cartilage. The skin is repaired with 6-0 or 7-0 monofilament. **E,** An ear compression dressing should be used to prevent hematoma (see Chapter 63 for discussion of anesthesia and dressing for this injury).

skin. If the skin cannot be stretched to cover the defect, additional cartilage along the wound margin can be removed. Depending on the location, as much as 5 mm of cartilage can be removed without significant deformity. Cartilage should be approximated with 4-0 or 5-0 absorbable sutures initially placed at folds or ridges in the pinna representing major landmarks. Sutures tear through cartilage; therefore, the anterior and posterior perichondrium should be included in the stitch. No more tension should be applied than is needed to touch the edges together.

In through-and-through ear lacerations, the posterior skin surface should be approximated next with 5-0 nonabsorbable synthetic suture. Once closure of the posterior surface is completed, the convoluted anterior surface of the ear can be approximated with 5-0 or 6-0 nonabsorbable synthetic suture, with landmarks joined point by point (see Fig. 35-43C and D). On the free rim, the skin should be everted to avoid later notching. Care should be taken to cover all exposed cartilage. In heavily contaminated wounds of the ear (e.g., bite wounds)

that already show evidence of inflammation, the necrotic tissue should be débrided, the cartilage covered by a loose approximation of skin, and the patient given antibiotics.[79,100] After a lacerated ear has been sutured, it should be enclosed in a compression dressing (see Chapter 63).

Nose Lacerations

Lacerations involving the margin of the nostril are complicated and should be repaired accurately to ensure that unsightly notching does not occur (Fig. 35-44). In the medial portion of the nostril and superior columella, the lower lateral cartilages are quite close to the margin and relatively superficial. If the extent of the laceration is not recognized and not repaired, wound healing may cause superior retraction of the margin of the nostril. Secondary repair of complications is difficult.

In repairing superficial lacerations of the nose, reapproximation of the edges of the wound is difficult because the skin is inflexible. Even deeply placed stitches will slice through the

Figure 35-44 **A,** Initially benign-appearing laceration of the left nostril of a 2-year-old patient. **B,** However, further investigation shows a full-thickness injury with a laceration of the lower lateral cartilage. A three-layer closure with reapproximation of the cartilage was performed.

Figure 35-45 *Check all lip lacerations for tooth fragments embedded in the wound.* **A,** This superficial mucosal laceration produced by the teeth can be cleaned, minimally trimmed, and left open to heal. Note the broken upper teeth (*arrow*); fragments may be embedded in the laceration. Healing produces a whitish tissue that can be mistaken for infection. **B,** This extensive laceration of the mucosa requires a layered suture closure. **C,** Small through-and-through lacerations made by the teeth can be irrigated and closed with skin and mucosal sutures in two layers. Small defects in the mucosa may be left open. Large through-and-through injuries and lacerations of the tongue margins require sutures to achieve anatomic healing. The muscle layer should be closed separately (with absorbable sutures) to prevent hematoma formation. In general, buried sutures are better tolerated by the patient.

epidermis and pull out. When the edges of the wound cannot be coapted easily, 6-0 absorbable sutures can be placed in the fibrofatty junction in an SQ stitch before skin closure. Because it is difficult to approximate gaping wounds in this location, débridement must be kept to a minimum. Nasal cartilage is frequently involved in wounds of the nose, but it is seldom necessary to suture the cartilage itself.

The free rim of the nostril must be aligned precisely to avoid unsightly notching. Many clinicians recommend early removal of stitches to avoid stitch marks, yet the oily nature of skin in this area makes it difficult to keep the wound closed with tape. If the wound is gaping before closure, a subcuticular stitch is recommended to provide support for a prolonged period.[101] If there is significant tissue injury, consultation with a facial plastic surgeon may be warranted.

Lip and Intraoral Lacerations

Lip lacerations are cosmetically deforming injuries, but if the clinician follows a few guidelines, these lacerations usually heal satisfactorily.

The contamination of all intraoral and lip wounds is considerable, and they must be thoroughly irrigated. Regional nerve blocks are preferred over local anesthetic injection because the latter method distends tissue, distorts the anatomy of the lip, and obscures the vermilion border. Loss of less than 25% of the lip permits primary closure with little deformity. The following types of wounds require initial surgical consultation or later reconstructive surgery: loss of more than 25% of the lip, extensive lacerations directly through the

commissure of the mouth,[100] and deep scars in the vermilion of the upper lip (which can later result in a redundancy of tissue).[100]

Small puncture-type lacerations heal well only if the skin is closed and the small intraoral laceration is left open (Fig. 35-45*A*). Such injuries commonly occur as a result of a punch in the face when the victim's tooth lacerates the lip. *Check all lip lacerations for retained tooth fragments.* In general, small lacerations of the oral mucosa heal well without sutures. If a mucosal laceration creates a flap of tissue that falls between the occlusal surfaces of the teeth or if a laceration is extensive enough to trap food particles (e.g., ≥2 to 3 cm in length), it should be closed. Small flaps may be excised. Closure is easily accomplished with 4-0 Dexon or Vicryl in a simple interrupted suturing technique. These materials are soft and less abrasive than gut sutures, which become hard and traumatize adjacent mucosa. Nylon sutures have sharp ends that are annoying and painful; thus, this suture material should be avoided inside the mouth. Muscle and mucosal layers should be closed separately. Sutures in the oral cavity easily become untied by the constant motion of the tongue. Each suture should be tied with at least four square knots. These sutures need not be removed; they either loosen and fall out within 1 week or are rapidly absorbed.[82,102,103]

Small through-and-through lacerations can be thoroughly cleaned and closed in two layers (skin and mucosa). It is acceptable to leave the mucosal side open if the defect is small (see Fig. 35-45*C*). Large through-and-through lacerations of the lip should be closed in three layers. With a multilayer

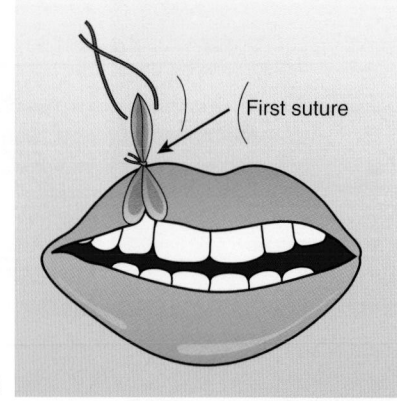

Figure 35-46 A, A poorly aligned vermilion border (*arrow*) distorts the lip contour. **B,** To prevent this complication, place the first stitch at the vermillion-cutaneous border to obtain proper alignment.

Figure 35-47 A, This patient sustained a large through-and-through lip laceration that will require a layered closure. A submental nerve block may be used, or a local anesthetic (lidocaine with epinephrine) can be injected if it does not distort the tissue landmarks. The muscle layer should be repaired with 4-0 or 5-0 absorbable suture. **B,** The vermillion border (*arrow*) must be repositioned precisely to prevent permanent disfigurement. A 5-0 or 6-0 guide stitch should be placed at the border before any other closure. Nonabsorbable monofilament sutures are then used to close the skin. **C,** Absorbable sutures are used to close the buccal mucosa.

closure, the muscle layer is approximated with a 4-0 or 5-0 absorbable suture securely anchored in the fibrous tissue located anterior and posterior to the muscle. The vermilion-cutaneous junction of the lip is a critical landmark that if divided, must be repositioned with precision; a 1-mm step-off is apparent and cosmetically unacceptable. The vermilion border should be approximated with a 5-0 or 6-0 nonabsorbable guide suture before any further closure to ensure proper alignment throughout the remainder of the repair (Fig. 35-46*A*). The vermilion surface of the lip and the buccal mucosa are then closed with interrupted stitches of 4-0 or 5-0 absorbable suture. Finally, the skin is closed with 6-0 nonabsorbable suture (Fig. 35-47).[102]

All lacerations that penetrate the oral mucosa should be evaluated for the presence of a tooth fragment, especially if a tooth is missing or chipped. The search should be intensified if the patient returns with an infection of a sutured wound. Probing the wound with forceps may identify fragments not seen directly in the wound. In the setting of marked facial swelling, a radiograph of the soft tissue may help identify an embedded tooth fragment.

Tongue Lacerations

Some controversy exists regarding when to suture tongue lacerations. Simple, linear lacerations, especially those in the central portion of the tongue, heal quickly with minimal risk

for infection. Many small tongue lacerations that occur in children or from falls or seizures do not require sutures. In general, lacerations that involve the edge or pass completely through the tongue, flap lacerations, and all lacerations bisecting the tongue need to be sutured[102] (Fig. 35-48). Small flaps on the edge of the tongue may be excised, but large flaps should be sutured. When dilute peroxide mouth rinses and a soft diet are used for a few days, healing can be rapid. Persistent bleeding from minor lacerations brings most patients to the ED, and closure with deep sutures may be necessary to prevent further bleeding.

Repair of a tongue laceration in any patient is somewhat difficult, but in an uncooperative child, the procedure may prove impossible without general anesthesia. A Denhardt-Dingman side mouth gag aids in keeping the patient's mouth open. A localized area of the tongue may be anesthetized topically by covering the area with 4% lidocaine-soaked gauze for 5 minutes; the maximum safe dose of local anesthetic should be determined and exposure to greater doses avoided. Large lacerations require infiltration anesthesia (1% lidocaine with buffered epinephrine) or a lingual nerve block. If the tip of the tongue has been anesthetized, a towel clip or suture can be used to maintain protrusion of the tongue in an uncooperative patient. Further anesthesia and subsequent wound cleansing and closure are possible while an assistant applies gentle traction on the tongue.

Figure 35-48 A, A lacerated tongue usually heals well without sutures, but they were placed in this patient because of a large rent in the middle of the tongue. Dexon, Vicryl, or silk sutures (avoid nylon) are ideal for suturing the surface of the tongue. Bleeding is usually controlled with direct pressure and local infiltration of lidocaine with epinephrine; others require deep sutures for hemostasis. Many seemingly large central tongue lacerations (such as occur during a seizure) heal well with no suturing if the margins of the tongue are intact. **B,** When a forked tongue is possible or flaps are pronounced, the tongue requires anatomic repair. **C,** This laceration will heal well without sutures.

Figure 35-49 Anatomy of the scalp. The skin, superficial fascia, and galea constitute the outer layer. *Blood vessels in the fascia are the major source of the bleeding noted with scalp lacerations.*

Size 4-0 absorbable sutures should be used to close all three layers—inferior mucosa, muscle, and superior mucosa—in a single stitch, or the stitch should include half the thickness of the tongue, with sutures placed on the superior and inferior surfaces, as well as on the edge of the tongue. Sutures on the tongue frequently become untied. This problem can be prevented if the stitches are buried. Nylon sutures should be avoided because the sharp edges are uncomfortable.[82] Closure of the lingual muscle layer with a deep absorbable suture alone may be sufficient to control bleeding and return motor function to the lacerated tongue; mucosal healing is rapid.

Scalp Lacerations

The scalp extends from the supraorbital ridges anteriorly to the external occipital protuberances posteriorly and blends with temporalis fascia laterally. The scalp has five anatomic layers: skin, superficial fascia, galea aponeurotica, subaponeurotic areolar connective tissue, and periosteum (Fig. 35-49); however, clinically, the scalp may be divided into three distinct layers. The outer layer consists of the skin, superficial fascia, and galea (the aponeurosis of the frontalis and occipitalis muscles), which are firmly adherent and surgically considered as one layer. The subaponeurotic layer and the periosteum form the second and third layers. The integrity of the outer layer is maintained by inelastic, tough, fibrous septa, which keep wounds from gaping open unless all three portions have been traversed. Wounds that gape open signify a laceration extending beneath the galea layer (Fig. 35-50). The galea itself is loosely adherent to the periosteum by means of the slack areolar tissue of the subaponeurotic layer. The galea is firmly attached to the underside of the SQ fascia and is rarely identified as a distinct layer in the depths of a wound. The periosteum covers the skull. The tissue-thin periosteum is often mistakenly identified as the galea, but the periosteum is flimsy and adherent to the skull and cannot be sutured.

Several unique problems are associated with wounds of the scalp. Multiple scalp wounds that are hidden by a mat of hair are easily overlooked. Stellate lacerations are common in this region, not only because the scalp is vulnerable to blunt trauma but also because its superficial fascial layer is inelastic and firmly adherent to the skin. Stellate lacerations pose additional technical problems in closure and have a greater propensity for infection. Shear-type injuries can cause extensive separation of the superficial layers from the galeal layer. Debris and other contaminants can be deposited several centimeters from the visible laceration; therefore, careful exploration plus cleaning of scalp wounds is important. When scalp

Figure 35-50 A, The galea has been transected in wounds that gape open like this one, and to achieve hemostasis and obtain the best closure, the galea should be sutured. **B,** This nongaping wound does not include the galea and can be closed with superficial sutures.

Figure 35-51 To temporarily control bleeding from vessels in the fascia, the galea can be everted to compress the fascia.

wounds are débrided, obviously devitalized tissue should be removed, *but débridement should be conservative* because closure of large defects on the scalp is difficult.

The presence of a rich vascular network in the superficial fascia results in profuse bleeding from scalp wounds. Severed scalp vessels tend to remain patent because the fibrous SQ fascia hinders the normal retraction of blood vessels that have been cut and allows persistent or massive hemorrhage with simple lacerations. The subgaleal layer of loose connective tissue contains "emissary veins" that drain through diploic vessels of the skull into the venous sinuses of the cranial hemispheres. In scalp wounds that penetrate this layer, bacteria may be carried by these vessels to the meninges and the intracranial sinuses. Thus, a scalp wound infection can result in osteomyelitis, meningitis, or a brain abscess.[101] Closure of galeal lacerations not only ensures control of bleeding but also protects against the spread of infection.

Profuse bleeding, especially from extensive scalp lacerations, is best controlled by suturing[94] (see also Chapter 34). Unless the vessels are large or few, ligation of multiple scalp vessels seldom provides effective hemostasis, and considerable blood loss can occur during the attempt. Ask an assistant to maintain compression around the wound while you complete closure of the wound. A simple procedure that often provides

hemostasis of scalp wounds is to place a wide, tight rubber band or Penrose drain around the scalp from the forehead to the occiput. You can also control bleeding temporarily in some cases by grasping the galea and the dermis with a hemostat and everting the instrument over the edge of the skin (see Fig. 35-51). The disadvantage of this technique is that tissue grasped by the hemostat may be crushed and devitalized.[94] If the SQ tissue is also everted for a prolonged period, necrosis can occur.

If an assistant is not available to apply direct pressure, use local anesthetics containing epinephrine because this is sometimes effective in controlling persistent bleeding from small vessels in a scalp wound. If bleeding from the edge of the scalp wound is vigorous and definitive repair must be postponed while the patient is resuscitated, Raney scalp clips or a hemostat can be applied quickly to the edge of the scalp wound to control the hemorrhage.

Before wound closure, visually examine the underlying skull and palpate it for skull fractures (Fig. 35-52). In wounds that can be *visualized* or *explored*, more small skull fractures are detected with the clinician's eyes and gloved finger than with radiographs. However, a common error is to mistake a tear in the galea or the periosteum for a fracture during palpation inside the wound. Direct visualization of the area should resolve the issue. Of particular importance are stab or puncture wounds in the scalp and forehead, such as from a nail, spike, screwdriver, knife, or ice pick. Without a laceration to explore, such wounds may seem benign, and the patient can initially appear relatively asymptomatic, yet the skull or brain has been penetrated. When evaluating a puncture or stab wound to the head, a computed tomography scan may provide unexpected findings of a skull fracture, linear or depressed, or an underlying brain injury or early hemorrhage. In wounds that expose bone but do not penetrate the skull, prolonged exposure may leave a nidus of dead bone in which osteomyelitis could develop. If exposed bone is visibly necrosed, remove the bone with rongeurs until active bleeding appears.[94] Clip hair surrounding the scalp wound far enough from the edge of the wound so that suturing can proceed without entangling the hair or burying it in the wound. If hairs along the wound edges become embedded in the wound, they will stimulate excessive granulation tissue and delay healing.[104] Place Vaseline or tape on stubborn hairs that persistently fall into the wound to help hold them back. Although clipping scalp hair is not popular with some patients, failure to

Figure 35-52 A, A finger and direct vision can be used to identify skull factures. Do not mistake a rent in the soft tissues as a fracture. **B,** Puncture wounds in the forehead and scalp from such objects as a knife, nail, screwdriver, or ice pick can penetrate the skull and brain, and initially the patient appears well and the wound looks benign. This patient was in a bar fight and was "stabbed" in the forehead. He had no complaints. The wound could not be fully explored but appeared to be benign. **C,** Computed tomography scan demonstrating a depressed skull fracture (*arrows*).

CLOSURE OF SCALP LACERATIONS

1

Needle

3-0 nylon suture

Galea — Skin

All layers included with one suture

Fascia

Skull

Periosteum

Potential space (obliterated by the illustrated suture)

To close a scalp laceration that extends through the galea, use a long needle, forceps, and 3-0 sutures (blue polypropelene sutures make removal easier). Incorporate the skin, subcutaneous tissue, and galea in a single stitch. If this technique is used, individual buried sutures in the galea are not required, and hemostasis is ensured. At the base of this wound is the periosteum, a thin, tissue-like covering of the skull that is often mistaken for the galea. Periosteum is not sutured. The galea is actually adherent to the avulsed flap.

2

A good way to include all layers of the scalp in the closure is to use forceps to manipulate the tissue so that the needle can penetrate the galea as it transverses to the skin.

Figure 35-53 Closure of scalp lacerations.

---

adequately expose an area is a common cause of improper cleaning and closure of scalp wounds. Because of the extensive collateral blood supply of the scalp, most lacerations in this area heal without problem, even after delayed treatment. Nonetheless, wound cleaning must be sufficient to avoid the devastating complication of scalp infection.

Unlike most wounds involving multiple layers of tissue, scalp wounds can usually be closed with a single layer of sutures that incorporate skin, SQ fascia, and the galea (see

Fig. 35-53). The periosteum does not need to be sutured; in fact, sutures will not hold in this tissue. Separate closure of the galea introduces additional suture material into the wound and may increase the risk for infection. However, in extremely large wounds, separate closure may be necessary to provide a more secure approximation of the galea than can be obtained with a large-needle, single-layer closure. In this situation, an inverted stitch (with an absorbable 3-0 or 4-0 suture) will "bury" the knot beneath the galea.

In superficial wounds, approximate the skin and SQ tissue with simple interrupted or vertical mattress stitches using nonabsorbable 3-0 nylon or polypropylene suture on a large needle. Avoid smaller suture material because it tends to break when firm knots are being tied. Leave the ends of the tied scalp sutures at least 2 cm long to facilitate subsequent removal. The use of blue nylon rather than black may make suture removal easier.

With microvascular techniques, large sections of skin avulsed from the scalp can be reimplanted. Use the same techniques in salvaging avulsed scalp as those used for amputated extremities.[105]

Sutured scalp lacerations need not be bandaged. Instruct patients that they can wash their hair in 2 hours (Fig. 35-54). If bleeding persists, use an elastic bandage as a compression dressing. Place gauze sponges over the laceration to provide direct local pressure beneath the elastic bandage.

Nail Bed Lacerations

Injuries to the nail and nail bed (also called the nail matrix) are common problems in emergency medicine, yet controversy exists over proper management (Fig. 35-55). As a general rule, repair nail bed lacerations unless they are well

Figure 35-54 Once the scalp is sutured, the patient is encouraged to wash the hair at home that day to remove blood and debris. Prohibiting bathing with sutures in place in any part of the body has no scientific merit.

approximated. An exception is a nail bed laceration that causes a simple subungual hematoma.

Subungual Hematomas

Subungual hematomas develop from a nail bed laceration. Some nail bed lacerations are minor and of no consequence, whereas others portend a poor outcome unless the bed is repaired.[106,107] *A simple subungual hematoma (even in the presence of a tuft fracture) in which the nail is firmly adherent and disruption of the surrounding tissue is minimal is not an indication to remove the nail to search for nail bed lacerations* (Fig. 35-56).[108] Despite the presence of a nail bed laceration, a good result can be expected as long as the tissue is held in anatomic approximation by the intact fingernail. Nail trephination is discussed in Chapter 37.

Suture the nail bed if a large subungual hematoma is associated with an unstable or avulsed nail. Remove the nail completely and repair the nail bed under a bloodless field (Fig. 35-57). Always use *absorbable sutures* in the nail bed so they do not have to be removed. A good outcome depends on maintaining the space under the eponychium (cuticle) as the laceration heals and the new nail grows out, which is a slow process.

Partial Nail Avulsions

If the nail is partly avulsed (especially at the base) or loose, lift the nail to assess and potentially repair the nail bed. If the nail is intact, it is best to leave it in place if the nail bed laceration can be repaired (Fig. 35-58). The method for atraumatically removing a nail is demonstrated in Figure 35-60.

Nail Bed Repair

When the integrity of the nail bed is significantly disrupted, a rippled nail may develop (see Fig. 35-58*F*). Anatomic repair of the nail bed may minimize subsequent nail deformity. Approximate a simple nail bed laceration with 6-0 or 7-0 absorbable suture (to obviate the need for suture removal). If available, use loupe magnification and a finger tourniquet to maintain a bloodless field (Fig. 35-59). Repair the proximal and lateral nail (onychial) folds first. Attach a sturdy needle to a 4-0 thread for suturing lacerated nails. Insert the needle tangentially to the nail because the needle penetrates most easily in this position. The point of the needle carves a rigid path through the nail. Unless the entire length of the needle

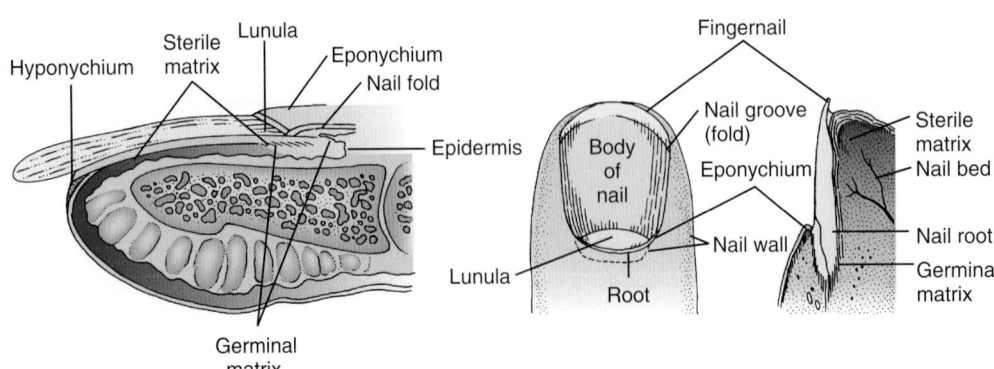

Figure 35-55 Anatomy of the fingernail. The fingernail rests on the nail bed, also termed the matrix. The distal end of the nail covers the sterile matrix; the proximal end arises from and covers the germinal matrix. The tissue adherent to the proximal dorsal surface of the nail is the eponychium (also termed the cuticle), and the potential space between the nail and the eponychium is the nail fold.

is allowed to follow this path as it passes through the nail, the needle is likely to bend or break. Alternatively, use an electrical cautery instrument or a heated paper clip to perforate the nail and permit easy passage of the needle.

Protect the exposed nail bed by reapplying the avulsed nail (best choice) or by applying a nonadherent dressing, Silastic sheet, or gauze packing for approximately 2 to 3 weeks. Reinsertion of the nail occasionally results in infection, so clean the nail carefully. After cleaning, suture the avulsed nail in place or secure it with wound closure tape. If only the distal portion of the nail has been avulsed, it can still be used as a temporary splint or "dressing" to protect and maintain the integrity of the underlying nail bed (see Fig. 35-59).

Complete Nail Avulsions

If the entire nail is avulsed but intact, replace it after repairing the nail bed laceration for three reasons: (1) it acts as a splint or mold to maintain the normal anatomy of the nail bed, (2) it covers a sensitive area and facilitates dressing changes, and (3) it maintains the fold for new nail growth. If the proximal portion of the nail is not replaced, either of two complications may result: (1) longitudinal scar bands may form between the proximal nail fold and the germinal matrix and cause a permanent split or deformity of the nail, or (2) the space between the proximal nail fold and the germinal matrix of the nail bed may be obliterated within a few days.[109] Consequently, splint for 2 to 3 weeks. The proximal portion of the traumatized nail often needs to be trimmed so that it

will fit more easily into the nail fold. It is usually necessary to suture the nail in place. A replaced nail may grow normally and act as a free graft, but it is often dislodged by a new nail. If the nail was lost or irreparably destroyed, insert a piece of nonadherent, petrolatum-impregnated gauze (such as Adaptic or Xeroform) between the proximal nail fold and the germinal matrix. Nails grow at a rate of 0.1 mm/day, and approximately 6 months is required for a new nail to reach to the fingertip.

Complicated Nail Bed Injuries

If the germinal matrix of the nail bed is avulsed but intact, reimplant the nail with a 5-0 or 6-0 absorbable suture via a mattress stitch.[82,110] If an open fracture exists, allow the matrix to remain trapped in the fracture line.[111]

If the nail bed is found to be extensively lacerated, it may be prudent to refer the patient to a hand surgeon, who can raise a flap of tissue extending from the proximal nail fold, explore the wound for foreign bodies, and clean under the nail bed. A fingertip avulsion that involves the nail bed or an isolated nail bed avulsion should not be allowed to heal on its own (i.e., by secondary intention). If the exposed nail bed is left open to granulate, it will form scar tissue that could produce a distorted and sensitive digit. Therefore, if part of the nail bed has been lost, refer the patient to a surgical consultant for a matrix graft.[82,112,113]

Recheck wounds 3 to 5 days after repair. At that time, remove and replace any nonadherent material that was

Figure 35-56 A, This subungual hematoma occupies most of the nail and should be drained by simple nail trephination. The injury does not require nail removal or repair of the nail bed because the nail is still firmly attached to the matrix. Even though a nail matrix laceration (the source of the bleeding) is present, the cosmetic result will be excellent. The presence of an underlying digital tuft fracture does not change management. This hole is too small and did not evacuate all the blood. **B,** There are two issues with this injury. First, an inadequately sized hole was placed (too small) and did not drain the subungual hematoma. All blood should be drained in the emergency department before discharge to ensure proper treatment. N ote the subtle ecchymosis under the eponychium (*arrows*). This can occur only if the nail base was avulsed. The base of the nail is lying just under the skin. Compare it with **A,** where no blood is seen in the paronychial area since the nail base remains intact. **C,** After the hole is enlarged and the blood is totally drained and without removing the nail, a hemostat is used to pull the nail forward and manipulate the base back into its proper position under the eponychium.

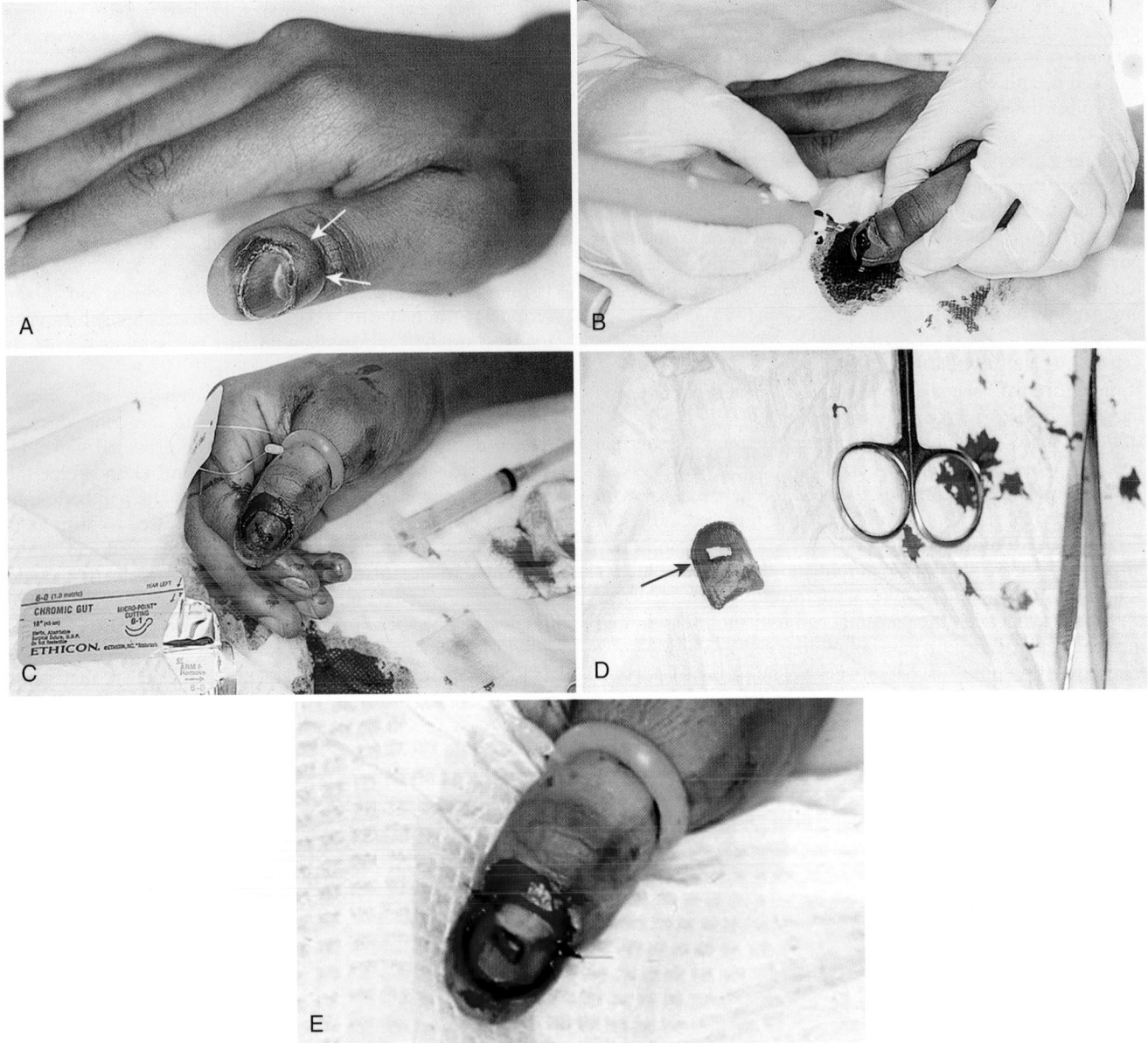

Figure 35-57 **A,** Classic "finger slammed in a door" with forced flexion and avulsion of the base of the nail. This large subungual hematoma can be misleading, but it is associated with blood under the cuticle (*arrows*) proximal to the nail, a clue that this is not a simple injury. **B,** When the blood is drained, the extent of the injury is more obvious. **C,** Careful removal of the nail exposes a laceration of the nail bed, which is sutured with absorbable suture. **D,** A drainage hole is placed in the nail (*arrow*) because it will be used as a temporary splint for the nail bed and to keep the cuticle space open to prevent scarring. **E,** The avulsed nail is placed under the eponychium to its base and sutured in place for 3 to 4 weeks while a new nail grows. This replaced nail may be removed or is pushed out by the new nail.

inserted under the proximal nail fold, and assess the wound for infection. The use of absorbable suture for nail bed repair makes suture removal unnecessary. Sutures that were used to reattach the nail are removed in 2 weeks, and the old nail is allowed to fall off as the new nail grows. The value of antibiotics is unproved. Advise all patients with nail injuries of a possible cosmetic defect in the new nail that may occur regardless of the repair technique.

Removal of a Nail

If a partially avulsed or intact nail requires removal, take care to not injure the nail bed. The nail is usually firmly attached to the bed but can be separated by advancing and opening small scissors in the plane between the nail and the bed.

Once loosened, pull the nail from its base with a hemostat (Fig. 35-60).

Tuft Fractures

Once the nail bed has been lacerated, a tuft fracture is considered an open fracture. The use of antibiotics for nail bed laceration is open for discussion, and no rigid standards exist. Most do well with good wound care and reasonable follow-up. Antibiotics are usually eschewed after nail trephination, even in the presence of a tuft fracture. Infection is rare, but antibiotics may be considered for significant crush or highly contaminated injuries. A tuft fracture, technically an open fracture, generally heals well. The approach to an open tuft fracture varies from formal operating room débridement and

Figure 35-58 A, This fingernail was avulsed at the base, a common result of having a door slam on the digit. The nail is tightly adherent to the nail bed, so it is not removed but simply replaced under the eponychium to its former position. **B,** Sutures are placed in the nail to keep it stable. This nail may simply start to grow on its own. **C,** A saw-induced laceration of the fingertip with an open fracture, nail bed laceration, and skin laceration. **D,** Only part of the nail was removed and the nail bed repaired through the window. The skin is closely approximated. Such injuries usually heal well with attention to detail, and infection is unusual despite the open fracture. Oral antibiotic therapy for 5 to 7 days is reasonable. **E,** Because this avulsed nail is unstable and subungual bleeding is present, the nail can be removed and the nail bed inspected. Any large nail bed laceration should be repaired meticulously with absorbable suture (6-0). After repair of the nail bed, a drainage hole is placed in the nail, and the nail is replaced under the eponychium (cuticle) and fixed in place with sutures that incorporate the nail edge and the skin bilaterally. In 2 to 3 weeds, the new nail will begin to push out the old nail (usually growing under it while maintaining the eponychium), and the old nail is removed. The exposed nail bed will be sensitive for a while. See Figure 35-60 for a simple technique to remove the fingernail. **F,** This nail is permanently deformed with ridges. Although crush injury to the nail bed is probably responsible for this deformity, repair of the nail bed might have minimized the resultant deformity.

intravenous antibiotics to thorough ED cleaning and oral antibiotics with close follow-up. Splinting is protective. Search for a traumatic mallet finger with flexion (door slam) injuries.

Drains in Sutured Wounds

Drains are used primarily to keep wounds open for drainage of existing purulence or blood that may otherwise collect in the wound. Drains do not prevent infection. When no infection exists, the use of drains in soft tissue wounds "prophylactically" is controversial in the ED setting. Drains in uninfected wounds may wick surface bacteria into the wound

and impair resistance of the wound to infection.[73] Drains placed in experimental wounds contaminated with subinfective doses of bacteria behave as foreign bodies by enhancing the rate of infection, regardless of whether the drain is placed entirely within the wound or brought out through the wound.[114]

If the wound is considered to be at high risk for infection, instead of suturing the wound with a drain in place (in anticipation of infection), it may be more prudent to leave the wound open and consider delayed primary closure later when the risk for infection subsides. Furthermore, drains should not serve as substitutes for other methods of achieving hemostasis in traumatic wounds.

NAIL BED REPAIR

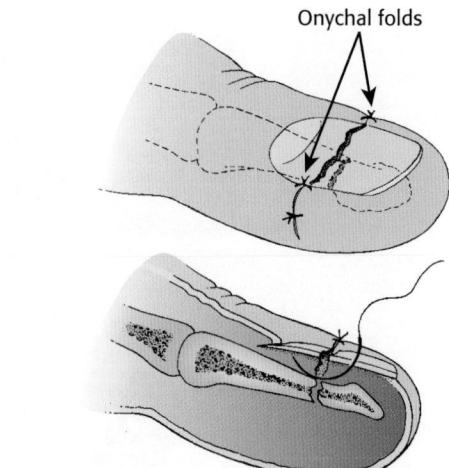

A laceration involving the nail bed, germinal matrix, and skin fold must be carefully approximated. First, the nail is completely removed. **A**, Fine, absorbable sutures are used to repair the nail bed under a bloodless field provided by a finger tourniquet. The avulsed nail (trimmed at the base) or a gauze pack is gently placed between the matrix and the eponychium for 2 to 3 weeks to prevent scar formation. **B**, If the original nail is replaced (the best option), it may be sutured or taped in place. A large hole in the nail will allow drainage. The old nail is gradually pushed out by a new one. If the nail matrix is replaced quickly and atraumatically, the nail may act as a free graft and grow normally. Note: Only absorbable sutures are used to repair the nail bed.

Repair of a distal finger laceration involving the nail and the onychial fold. In this case, the nail is still adherent to the nail matrix and acts as a natural splint. If the nail is loose or completely transected, it is prudent to remove the entire nail and then carefully suture the nail bed under direct vision.

This nail was removed and the nail bed repaired with absorbable suture.

Because the nail was macerated and unable to be replaced, gauze is used to maintain the eponychial space for 2 to 3 weeks. A small piece of gauze is placed with forceps to gently pack open the space to prevent scar formation.

Figure 35-59 Nail bed repair. *(2, from Dushoff IM. Handling the hand. Emerg Med. 1976;8:111. Reproduced by permission.)*

Lacerations over Joints

Lacerations over joints may enter the joint itself or injure tendons or muscle groups. It may be difficult to determine whether the joint has been violated. If so, greater attention to cleaning is required, occasionally with open débridement, but the approach varies with the joint involved. In the knee, for example, a plain radiograph may demonstrate air in the knee joint, which is evidence of joint penetration (Fig. 35-61).

Fingertip Amputations

Treatment of fingertip amputations has undergone evolution from complicated grafts and flaps to nonsurgical conservative follow-up and primary healing (Figs. 35-62 and 35-63). If bone is not involved, a good result can be expected with attentive wound care, occasional minimal débridement, and protective dressing changes. It may take 6 to 12 weeks for healing to occur, but acceptable length, function, and sensation can be expected. A motivated patient and good follow-up are

required. There is no standard that mandates long-term antibiotics for such injuries, and recommendations vary or are nonexistent. It is reasonable to provide gram-positive antibiotic coverage for 7 to 10 days, but no helpful data exist.

DISTALLY AND PROXIMALLY BASED FLAP LACERATIONS

There are few data in the literature concerning the care of minor flap lacerations in the ED. Large flaps, such as scalping lacerations, are best handled by a consultant, but many proximally and distally based flaps are treated primarily in the ED. It is important to note that these are not always simple lacerations and general wound healing principles may not apply. The major issue is vascularity, both perfusion pressure and venous drainage at the end of the flap and the potential for ischemic necrosis. The body has the ability to augment the

NAIL REMOVAL

To remove a fingernail or toenail atraumatically, the blades of iris scissors are held parallel to the nail bed to avoid lacerating the matrix. A digital block is necessary. The closed blades are slowly advanced in the plane between the nail and the nail bed and then gently spread to loosen the nail. The scissors are advanced and spread in stages until the base of the nail is reached and the entire nail is loose. The nail is grasped with a hemostat and pulled from the base.

Once the nail is removed, repair any nail bed lacerations with absorbable suture.

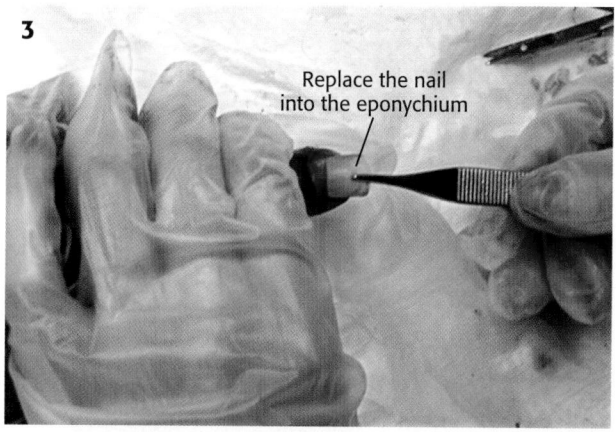

Replace the nail into the eponychium

Replace the nail into the eponychial fold.

Suture the nail in place with nonabsorbable stitches.

Figure 35-60 Nail removal.

circulation in some flaps (Fig. 35-64*A*). Contrary to common belief, the length-to-width ratio of the flap is not the main variable in survival of the flap (see Fig. 35-64*B*). Perfusion pressure is the most critical factor. Intravascular perfusion pressure decreases along the length of the flap. At the distal end of the flap, intravascular perfusion pressure will become less than interstitial pressure, thereby causing the capillaries to collapse (the critical closing pressure). As edema is generated by ischemia and inflammation, interstitial pressure increases, which results in a decrease in tissue survival.

Many proximally and distally based flaps (see Fig. 35-64*C*) may be closed in the ED and monitored on an outpatient basis. Healing of a distally based flap is hampered by loss of venous and lymphatic drainage and subsequent edema of the flap causing decreased capillary flow. Warn the patient about the possibility of flap necrosis and the need for revision or even skin grafting at a later date. *Partial take is better than total loss of the flap, and seemingly nonviable flaps should not be removed.*

Figure 35-61 A, This laceration looks benign but may involve the knee joint or quadriceps tendon. A radiograph to look for air in the joint or a saline arthrogram (see Chapter 53) should be performed. **B,** Air in the joint space (*arrows*) on a plain radiograph proved joint space violation.

Figure 35-62 A and **B,** Guillotine amputation of the fingertip through the distal end of the nail (*arrow*). The distal phalanx is not involved. Approaches vary widely, and referral can be made in a few days if not immediately available. Although it is tempting to replace the amputated tip (**C**), many would allow this wound to heal spontaneously, albeit slowly (8 to 12 weeks), and not perform skin grafts or flaps. **D,** The amputated nail is placed under the eponychium and sutured into place. A rounded but shortened tip with sensation can be expected. Periodic débridement and use of the nail as a splint resulted in a good final appearance. **E** and **F,** In only 4 weeks this amputation has nearly healed to the original length and contour with only dressing changes and minimal débridement. Note that a new nail is growing (*arrow*) and the replaced nail has been removed.

Figure 35-63 A and **B,** This macerated tip has islands of skin left and good tissue volume and will do quite well with sutures to restore the basic anatomy. Healing will take 4 to 5 weeks.

Flaps are similar to free skin grafts, and the keys to a more successful outcome include undermining the flap to relieve tension, limiting buildup of fluid under the flap with a compression dressing, and decreasing movement of the flap as it heals. Minor defatting may be performed on the underside of the flap. Tissue adhesive instead of multiple sutures can be helpful.

Self-inflicted wounds with a vague or inaccurate history may be encountered in the ED. Characteristic self-mutilation patterns are depicted in Figure 35-65. No specific treatment is required other than recognizing these patterns of injury.

References are available at @ www.expertconsult.com

Figure 35-64 A, Vascular territories in skin flaps. Multiple perforating vessels exist and are interconnected at the periphery of their vascular territory. When some of these vessels are cut, the blood supply can be replaced with nearby perforating vessels, and then tissue necrosis does not occur. **B,** Fallacy of the length-to-width ratio. The slope of decreasing perfusion pressure versus length does not change with the incorporation of additional vessels (flap a versus flap b) at the same perfusion pressure. Flap necrosis occurs when perfusion pressure decreases below the critical closing pressure of the capillary bed. **C,** This distally based flap is at risk for necrosis because of impaired venous and lymphatic drainage rather than from loss of the arterial supply. As with all flap repairs, it should be replaced by undermining the base to relieve tension (if possible), a compression dressing to limit movement and fluid buildup under the flap, and elevation of the extremity. Even if it undergoes only partial take, closure can be performed in the emergency department. Impaired venous drainage from a proximally based flap is less problematic.

Figure 35-65 A-C, These patients had minor lacerations and were brought to the emergency department simply for tetanus prophylaxis or for other vague or unrelated reasons. Obviously, these are classic self-inflicted wounds that are representative of serious underlying psychiatric issues, and further evaluation is required. **D,** These cigarette burns are also self-inflicted, but the patient initially stated that she got burned with grease while cooking.

CHAPTER 36

Foreign Body Removal

Daniel B. Stone and David J. Scordino

EVALUATION AND DIAGNOSIS

A foreign body (FB) is any substance that is not naturally part of the body. These cases are common in the clinical setting. An FB should be suspected whenever the skin is broken. A thorough history and physical examination are essential to assess the risk for an FB. During assessment, remember that FBs may not be obvious and that the wound may appear closed, but they should be considered whenever the history is particularly concerning. For example, a patient who is walking without shoes and experiences a sharp, sudden pain in the foot may have a needle, toothpick, or any other similar type of FB, even when a "sprained foot" seems obvious (Fig. 36-1). Certain mechanisms of injury, such as punching or kicking out a window or stepping on an unknown object while walking in a field or stream, are associated with a retained FB. Mechanisms that make FBs less likely include lacerations from metal objects; however, if considerable force was applied during the injury and the object is not available for inspection, radiographic imaging may be warranted since bone may have been encountered and a small section might have splintered off the offending object. The history should also include asking whether the patient perceives or suspects an FB. Steele and associates found that the negative predictive value of patient perception was 89% but that the positive predictive value was just 31%.[1] Importantly, the patient's past medical history should be explored for allergies to local anesthetics, bleeding diatheses, diabetes mellitus, vascular disease, uremia, immunocompromised state, or other diseases that would affect wound healing or management.

Before the physical examination be sure to have *enough examination time, as well as proper space and equipment. It is important to confirm that the patient is willing to undergo the procedure because cooperation is essential to optimize success.* Attempts at removing an FB in an overtly uncooperative patient, such as one who is intoxicated, drugged, cognitively limited, or confused, is potentially injurious to both the examiner and the patient. In most noncritical situations, if a patient is uncooperative, perform the examination again when the patient is able to cooperate. In benign cases, follow-up can occur a few days later.

During the physical examination, carefully palpate the periphery of all wounds to elicit tenderness because retained FBs often produce pain. Also, some FBs can migrate away from the wound or perceived entry point. Some superficial FBs may be palpated through the skin, but surprisingly large FBs may be found in seemingly minor wounds without much external evidence. In some cases, the external characteristics of the wound do not yield firm evidence regarding the presence or absence of an FB. Deeper FBs may not be palpable and must be localized by other techniques.

Exploration is an important part of the bedside evaluation, whether done initially or after further imaging studies (Fig. 36-2). This requires adequate pain control, good lighting, proper equipment, a bloodless field, a cooperative patient, and appropriate positioning to visualize as much of the wound as possible (Figs. 36-3 and 36-4). A metal probe may help identify the FB by feel or sound. Glass, as an example, is difficult to identify by sight in soft tissue, but touching it with metal causes a characteristic grating sound. *Probing a wound with a gloved finger to locate or identify an FB is strongly discouraged* because of the risk of the FB penetrating the glove and exposing the clinician to human immunodeficiency virus (HIV) and hepatitis (Fig. 36-5). Alternatively, some authors have suggested injecting the entrance wound with methylene blue to outline the track of the FB.[2] The blue line of injected dye is followed into the deeper tissues. This technique is of limited value because the track of the FB often closes tightly and does not allow passage of the methylene blue.

Augmenting the Physical Examination: Imaging Techniques

Many emergency clinicians mistakenly believe that in the absence of adipose tissue, if the base of the wound can be clearly visualized and explored, an FB can always be ruled out. Orlinsky and Bright found the reliability of exploration to be related to the depth of the wound.[3] In their study, only 2 of 133 superficial wounds, deemed adequately explored, had an FB on plain films, but 10 of 130 wounds had FBs beyond the subcutaneous fat despite negative explorations. Anderson and coworkers reported that 37.5% of the foreign bodies were initially missed by the treating physicians.[4] In many of these cases, a radiograph of the injured area was not taken. Avner and Baker detected glass with routine radiographs in 11 of 160 wounds (6.9%) that were inspected and believed by the clinician to be free of glass.[5] Clinicians evaluating for FBs should maintain a low threshold for ordering or performing imaging studies. Options for imaging include plain radiographs, ultrasound (US), computed tomography (CT), magnetic resonance imaging (MRI), and fluoroscopy. See Table 36-1 for a summary.

Plain Radiography

Plain radiographs are readily available, are easily interpreted, and cost significantly less than CT, formal US, and MRI do.[7] The ability of plain films to detect FBs in soft tissue depends on the object's composition (relative density), configuration, size, and orientation (Fig. 36-6). Detection of FBs on plain films can be enhanced by requesting an underpenetrated soft tissue technique and by *obtaining multiple views to prevent FBs from being obscured by superimposed bone or soft tissue folds.*[8] Plain films are often sufficient; however, digitized radiographs may be manipulated to enhance identification of a suspected FB. Indirect evidence of an FB may include trapped or surrounding air, a radiolucent filling defect, or secondary bony changes such as periosteal elevation, osteolytic or osteoblastic alterations, or pseudotumors of bone.[8]

Metallic objects are readily visualized on radiographs. Despite a common misconception that glass must contain lead to be visualized on a plain radiograph, *almost all glass objects in soft tissue (bottles, windshield glass, lightbulbs, microscope cover slips, laboratory capillary tubes) are at least somewhat radiopaque and can be detected by plain radiographs unless they are obscured by bone or are very small (<1 mm)* (Fig. 36-7).[7,9,10] The absence of a glass FB on multiple projections is strong, though not

Figure 36-1 **A,** A common foreign body (FB) in the foot is a splinter, toothpick, pin, or needle that is impaled while walking barefoot on a carpet. This sewing needle (*arrow*) was obvious, but in the absence of a history of an FB, some FBs may be mistaken for a simple puncture wound, heel spur, stress fracture, contusion, or tendinitis. **B,** A commonly missed FB is the second one. Postoperative radiographs demonstrate complete removal. **C,** This patient fell, landed on a metal pipe, and suffered a deep laceration in the thigh. A radiograph was taken to rule out a fracture, and the key was seen but thought to be an artifact (i.e., an item left on the backboard). During the examination the key was found embedded in the wound. It had been in the patient's pants pocket and was forced into the wound by the pipe during the injury.

absolute evidence that glass is not contained in a wound. Other nonmetallic objects readily visualized include teeth, bone, pencil graphite, asphalt, and gravel.[7,11] Aluminum, which has traditionally been deemed radiolucent, can occasionally be visualized on plain films if the object is projected away from the underlying bone. Ellis demonstrated that pure aluminum fragments as small as $0.5 \times 0.5 \times 1$ mm could be identified in a chicken wing model simulating a human hand or foot.[12] Ellis cautioned that other aluminum FBs, such as pull tabs from cans, may not be visualized in other parts of the body such as the esophagus or stomach.[12]

Certain FBs such as vegetative material (thorns, wood, splinters, and cactus spines) are radiolucent and not readily visualized on plain radiographs. These materials absorb body fluids as they sit in situ and become isodense with the surrounding tissue. Because of their varying chemical composition and density, plastics may or may not be visible on plain films.[13]

Besides simply diagnosing FBs, radiographs can also be used to estimate the general location, depth, and structure of radiopaque FBs. If one strategically attaches a marker (needle or paper clip) to the skin surface at the wound entrance before taking a radiograph, the FB will be seen in relation to the entrance wound (Fig. 36-8). This also helps identify the path

that leads to the FB and the relative distance from the surface to the FB.[14] Needles at two angles may also be used to aid in localization (Fig. 36-9).

Liberal use of plain film radiography makes sound medicolegal practice. A review of 54 wound FB claims against 32 physicians from 22 institutions found glass, a radiopaque substance, to be the most common material. However, in only 35% of the cases involving glass were plain films taken. Cases with a glass FB without a radiograph ordered were associated with unsuccessful defense (60%) and higher indemnity payments.[15]

US

US has become the modality of choice for imaging radiolucent FBs such as wood and thorns because most soft tissue FBs are hyperechoic on US. In addition, if in place for more than 24 hours, most FBs will be surrounded by a hypoechoic area corresponding to granulation tissue, edema, or hemorrhage, which may aid in making the diagnosis.[16] Metal will leave a linear trail of echoes deep to the FB, referred to as the "comet tail artifact." A wooden object leaves an acoustic shadow without artifact.[17,18]

US may be performed at the bedside. To do so, use a high-frequency transducer (at least 7.5 MHz, such as a

Figure 36-2 Some wound mechanisms are classic for the presence of a foreign body (FB). **A,** This intoxicated patient kicked out a window and sustained seemingly minor puncture wounds. He did not believe that glass was in the wound, there was little pain, and no FB could be palpated externally. **B,** A radiograph revealed a large shard of glass (*arrows*) deeply embedded in the wound. **C,** The shard of glass was removed, but only after 20 minutes of exploration. **D,** Another classic scenario for a retained glass FB is putting the arm through a window. An FB was not suspected or sensed by the patient or clinician. **E,** When a radiograph was taken, a large shard of glass (*arrow*) was readily detected. Despite its size, removal was difficult and time-consuming.

Figure 36-3 A, This patient has an obvious wooden foreign body on the dorsal aspect of the proximal part of the forearm. **B,** Manual removal of the object was not difficult. **C,** However, thorough exploration of the wound cavity via an incision over the entire length of the FB tract revealed multiple small wooden fragments. Proper exploration requires adequate analgesia, good lighting, hemostasis, and a cooperative patient. Use of a metal probe may help identify the foreign object by feel or sound (see Fig. 36-17).

Figure 36-4 A windshield forehead injury usually harbors multiple retained pieces of glass that are difficult to find. Probing with a needle or forceps to feel or hear contact with the fragments may help find them. A supraorbital nerve block is ideal to facilitate probing.

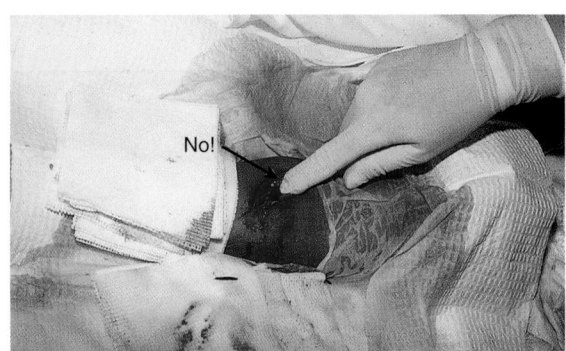

Figure 36-5 What's wrong here? Though historically suggested as a useful technique to find foreign bodies, probing the depths of a wound with a gloved finger may result in a puncture wound in the operator. The practice is strongly discouraged because of the prevalence of hepatitis and human immunodeficiency virus infection.

TABLE 36-1 Imaging Summary

	RADIOGRAPHY	US	CT	MRI	FLUOROSCOPY
Materials visualized	Metal Glass Graphite Plastic (variable)	Wood Thorns Organic matter Metal Glass	Metal Glass Wood (late) Plastic (variable) Organic material (variable)	Glass Plastic Organic matter	Metal Glass Plastic (variable)
What type of material cannot be visualized	Wood Thorns Organic matter Plastic (variable)	Deep FBs	Wood (early) Plastic (variable) Organic material (variable)	Wood (variable) METAL!	Wood Thorns Organic matter Plastic (variable)
Pros	Cheap Available Easy to interpret	Bedside use for real-time extraction Relatively inexpensive	3D images with some improved visualization of FBs vs. plain film	Improved detection of radiolucent objects vs. CT	Useful for real-time bedside extraction
Cons	Unable to visualize all material May miss small FBs in areas adjacent to bone	Results vary based on operator experience Difficult visualization in the hands and potential for false positives	Expensive Increased exposure to ionizing radiation	Expensive Not readily available in all EDs Dangerous for metallic FBs	Unfamiliar technique to most ED clinicians Not widely available
Conclusions	Reasonable initial approach, particularly for metal and glass Obtain multiple views via a soft tissue technique	Recommended for radiolucent structures such as vegetative material (wood, thorns, etc.) Allows direct visualization Can assist with operative removal Potentially a bedside procedure depending on the clinician's skill level	Recommended approach for intracranial, intraorbital FBs Has a role for repeated visits and concerns for retained FBs Limited role during initial evaluation	Role limited on initial evaluation Has a role with repeated visits and concern for retained FBs	Use limited to individual clinicians with experience and availability

3D, three dimensional; *CT*, computed tomography; *ED*, emergency department; *FB*, foreign body; *MRI*, magnetic resonance imaging; *US*, ultrasonography.
A reasonable initial approach for localizing nonvisualized FBs in the ED is to obtain multiple-projection plain radiographs with a soft tissue technique. This technique will visualize the majority of FBs, especially metal and glass. US should be considered for objects known to be radiolucent, such as wood or thorns. The role of CT and MRI for evaluation of FBs in the ED is limited, but they are the definitive imaging tests in confusing cases. For suspected intraorbital or intracranial FBs, CT is recommended. CT or MRI is also warranted *when a previously negative explored wound exhibits recurrent infection, poor healing, or persistent pain*. CT or MRI may be the appropriate initial test for patients with nonspecific swelling to define FBs and possible alternative diagnoses such as abscesses, masses, or other inflammatory processes.[6] Bedside US and fluoroscopy (for radiopaque FBs) may be used to guide difficult FB extractions if initial attempts at removal are unsuccessful and the proper equipment and experienced personnel are available.

Figure 36-6 Radiographic appearance of various foreign bodies. *Arrows* point to glass (**A**), pencil lead (**B**) (graphite, but not wood, is radiopaque), and a metallic pin (**C**). Plain radiographs should be taken in multiple projections. Do not ignore subtle soft tissue irregularities. Generally absent on radiographs are aluminum, plastic, wood, thorns and other organic objects such as fish spines, and small pieces of gravel.

high-frequency linear vascular probe) since most FBs are small and superficial. A lower frequency may also be necessary if a deeper FB is suspected, but it may miss small FBs.[19] A spacer may be needed to adjust the "focal zone"—where the beam is the narrowest and signal intensity is the highest. US may be particularly difficult in the hand or foot, which have many echogenic structures and web spaces that may limit visualization when the FB is adjacent to bone.[16,18,20] Keep in mind that the presence of air, scars, calcification, sutures, and sesamoid bones in surrounding tissue may lead to false-positive results.[20,21]

Figure 36-7 *Almost all glass is visible on a plain radiograph, regardless of its lead content.* Do not ignore small white specs on a radiograph. If glass is superimposed on bone, it may be missed, so multiple projections are recommended. Plain film radiography shows sharp corners characteristic of glass. Proximity of the foreign body to the bone may be deceiving.

Figure 36-8 A, This patient had an obvious diabetic foot abscess. **B**, A radiograph was taken to rule out osteomyelitis or soft tissue gas. To everyone's surprise, including the patient's, a sewing needle (*arrow*), origin and timing unknown, was the source of the infection. **C** and **D**, A paper clip was taped to the skin to localize the depth and position of the foreign body (FB; *arrow*) on the radiograph. An anteroposterior radiograph (not shown) also localized the FB.

Advantages of US include low cost, no ionizing radiation, the ability to define the object in three dimensions, and real-time imaging, which may be used during removal.[8] Many studies report that US is highly sensitive for the detection of FBs by adequately trained personnel, either radiologists, technicians, or emergency physicians.[3] It is difficult to cite a precise sensitivity or specificity because of the wide variation in these studies with regard to FB size, material, and location; operator experience; and the models used in these studies.[21-23]

CT

CT depends on x-ray absorption; thus, it generally visualizes the same material detected on plain films, but subtle differences in soft tissue densities may help identify FBs not seen on radiographs.[7,11] Also, CT produces a better three-dimensional image than plain films do and may visualize objects embedded in or behind bone. However, CT is more costly and exposes the patient to more ionizing radiation than radiography or US does, and its use should therefore be judicious.

As an example, wood is unlikely to be visible initially on CT, but after 1 week, the wood absorbs surrounding blood products and may become higher in attenuation than muscle and fat. It may then appear on CT as a linear area of increased attenuation on a wide window setting such as a bone window.[6]

MRI

Although MRI is expensive and not as readily available to emergency clinicians as plain films and CT are, it may be superior to CT in detecting small, nonmetallic, radiolucent FBs such as plastic, particularly in the orbit.[24] MRI may not visualize wood, which may appear as a linear signal with associated inflammation and looks hypointense with respect to muscle on T1- and T2-weighted sequences, on which it appears as a signal void.[6] Plastic is more easily visualized with MRI than with CT. *MRI cannot be used for metallic objects and gravel*, which contain various ferromagnetic particles that produce signal artifacts and a theoretical risk of shifting within the magnetic field and causing structural damage.[7] This is particularly important when evaluating FBs in the eye, brain, or deep structures of the neck, face, or extremities. FBs may be difficult to differentiate from other low-signal structures on MRI, such as tendon, scar tissue, and calcium.[25]

Fluoroscopy

More recently, portable, low-power, C-arm fluoroscopy has become available in some emergency departments (EDs), particularly for orthopedic reductions. Its use has also been

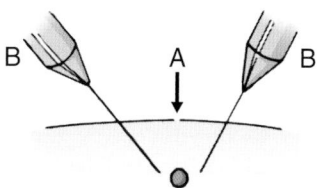

Figure 36-9 When a small entrance wound (*A*) is noted but the foreign body (FB) is not seen, noninvasive localization is preferable to blind probing. Metal markers taped to the skin or needles inserted close to the FB under local anesthesia (*B*) and radiographed at different angles provide a guide to localization and extraction of the FB. (*Reproduced from* Hospital Medicine, *January 1981, with permission of Cahner's Publishing Co.*)

Figure 36-8, cont'd E, For orientation, the outline of the paperclip was traced on the foot. A dot marks a possible entrance site. **F,** A generous incision was made over the projected site of the FB. **G,** The needle (*arrow*) was felt and extracted with a hemostat. **H,** The wound was left open and packed with a cotton wick.

ULTRASOUND: Foreign Body Removal

by Christine Butts, MD

Many foreign bodies are radiopaque and can easily be seen with traditional radiography. Such foreign bodies include glass, metal, and some plastics. Other foreign materials, such as splinters, spines, and thinner plastics, are radiopaque and easily missed on radiographs. Ultrasound is an optimal modality for both identifying retained foreign bodies and aiding in their removal. A number of studies have evaluated the sensitivity and specificity of ultrasound in identifying foreign bodies in soft tissue. The findings have been variable, depending on the type and size of foreign body.[1-3]

General Considerations

A preliminary radiograph may be helpful in narrowing down the area to be evaluated with ultrasound, particularly when there is a large area where the foreign body may be found. Asking the patient to identify the point of maximal tenderness may also be helpful in narrowing down the overall area to be examined. Once the area has been clarified, a high-frequency (10 to 12.5 MHz) transducer should be selected. Higher frequencies will convey sufficient resolution to distinguish foreign material from normal soft tissue structures.

Each type of foreign body has specific identifiable characteristics; however, certain general findings suggest the presence of foreign material. The finding of soft tissue edema, represented by anechoic (black) or hypoechoic (dark gray) areas within the normal soft tissue, is highly suggestive of recent tissue disruption (Fig. 36-US1).

The area in question should be evaluated from a number of different angles to find the object in its long axis. A small foreign body may easily be overlooked if only a small portion of it is seen.

Additionally, the use of a "stand-off" pad may be helpful, especially when dealing with superficial structures such as the hand or foot. A slim, fluid-filled structure, such as a 100-mL bag of saline or a glove filled with water, is placed over the area of interest. The transducer is then placed on top of this pad. This extra layer creates an acoustic window to allow greater resolution and eliminate some superficial artifacts that may impede the examination.

Metallic foreign bodies are strongly echogenic and are very straightforward to locate. They will appear bright white and often give off strong reverberation artifacts (Fig. 36-US2).

Glass foreign bodies appear very similar to metallic objects in that they are highly echogenic (white). Glass may cause a reverberation artifact but more typically will cause acoustic shadowing to extend deep to the object (Fig. 36-US3).

Wooden objects (such as splinters) are more challenging to locate, particularly with very small foreign bodies. Wooden foreign bodies do not create as strong an echogenic focus as other types of material do and may appear only slightly brighter than normal tissue (Fig. 36-US4). Very subtle shadowing may be seen extending deep to the object. The presence of surrounding edema is often key to locating the foreign body.

Figure 36-US2 Metallic foreign body identified as a brightly echogenic (*white*) object (*arrow*) with a comet tail artifact seen extending deep into the soft tissue (*arrowhead*).

Figure 36-US3 Glass foreign body (*arrow*) identified as a hyperechoic (*white*) object causing a strong shadow (*arrowhead*) within the otherwise normal-appearing soft tissue.

Figure 36-US1 Wooden foreign body in the foot. The foreign body is hyperechoic (*arrow*), whereas the surrounding hypoechoic region (*arrowhead*) is indicative of edema or pus. (*From Rumack CM. Diagnostic Ultrasound. 4th ed. St. Louis: Mosby; 2010.*)

ULTRASOUND: Foreign Body Removal, cont'd

Figure 36-US4 Sonographic appearance of a retained wooden foreign body.

Removal

Once the object has been localized, it can be removed either blindly or under direct sonographic guidance.

Another technique that may be helpful, particularly with smaller objects, is to insert two 25-gauge needles under sonographic guidance. These needles should be inserted at right angles to each other so that the tips of each of them rest at the foreign body. The clinician can then cut the skin and overlying soft tissue and dissect down to the intersection of these two needles.

REFERENCES

1. Orlinsky M, Knittel P, Feit T, et al. The comparative accuracy of radiolucent foreign body detection using ultrasonography. *Am J Emerg Med.* 2000;18:401-403.
2. Schlager D, Sanders A, Wiggins D, et al. Ultrasound for the detection of foreign bodies. *Ann Emerg Med.* 1991;20:189-191.
3. Dean AJ, Gronczewski CA, Costantino TG. Technique for emergency medicine bedside ultrasound identification of a radiolucent foreign body. *J Emerg Med.* 2003;24:303.

reported for the removal of BB pellets, metal, glass, and coins from patients.[26] Like radiography, fluoroscopy can visualize objects that are radiopaque but not radiolucent such as wood and plastic.[26,27] By using correct technique and shielding, radiation scatter to imaging personnel is minute, less than 0.0001 R/hr.[28] Fluoroscopy also offers the advantage of real-time bedside imaging.[26,28] Fluoroscopic image-intensifying equipment may be used to follow a wound's entrance, localize the material, grasp the FB, and remove it without making a larger incision. Ariyan described a technique in which two needles are placed in the soft tissue from opposite directions and pointing toward the FB.[29] The extremity is rotated while the clinician watches the image under the image intensifier to obtain a three-dimensional effect. An incision is made perpendicular to the plane of the needles, and the object is removed. Although the technique to use fluoroscopy is relatively easy to learn, the lack of instruction and availability is the major limitation to its use in the ED.[28-30]

FB REMOVAL

Removal Decisions

One should judiciously evaluate and manage each FB scenario individually. The composition and location of an FB, as well as the patient's medical status and vocational and avocational activities, greatly affect decision making related to FB removal, including the best time and place for removal. Reactive material, such as wood, should be removed immediately when accessible because retained wood will invariably lead to inflammation and infection. Other inert material, such as glass or plastic, may often be removed on an elective basis. Some innocuously located glass and metallic FBs may frequently be left permanently embedded in soft tissue. With deeply embedded, small, inert material (BB, bullets, etc.) that is not located near any vital structures, the time, effort, and trauma involved in removal may be excessive when compared with the possible adverse effects of the foreign material

remaining in place. An ill-conceived extended search for an elusive but otherwise harmless FB often results in frustration for the clinician and discomfort, dissatisfaction, and possible injury for the patient.

If localization is certain and removal can be accomplished within a manageable period without worsening of the injury, an attempt at removal is generally indicated on the initial visit (given the availability of clinicians and support staff).

When reviewing the decision regarding when and how to remove the FB, the possibility of the FB migrating to involve vital structures, though quite remote, should be discussed with the patient. Cases of reported missile embolization in the vascular system are influenced by missile caliber, impact velocity, physical wound characteristics, point of vessel entrance, body position and movement, and velocity of blood flow.[31] Retained bullets usually remain in soft tissue but can rarely make their way into the vascular system. Schurr and colleagues reported a paradoxical bullet embolization from the left external iliac vein to the left iliac artery via a patent foramen ovale.[32] When clinicians first examined the patient, a bullet was noted on the chest radiograph, and an isolated chest wound was suspected. However, the bullet had apparently entered the chest, traversed the abdomen to the iliac vein, and then embolized back to the chest and arterial system.

After the initial history, examination, and preoperative and preanesthetic documentation of the neurovascular status of the patient, a decision must be made regarding the time and place of removal. Thirty minutes is a reasonable self-imposed limit for the provider when attempting removal of an FB in the ED. More difficult procedures should be referred. Many FBs appear superficial on radiographs, thus suggesting that removal will be quite easy. However, surprisingly large or presumed superficial FBs still often prove quite elusive.

If an FB is left in place, inform the patient why it was not removed. If the patient is referred for delayed removal, this should also be carefully explained and documented. Regardless of whether the FB is removed, clean all wounds appropriately and update tetanus prophylaxis if indicated.

Equipment and Preparation

Good space and lighting, a comfortable patient and operator position, a standard suture tray, and a scalpel are usually adequate equipment for the removal of most simple FBs (Fig. 36-10). Tissue retractors, special pickups, and loupes may be added if needed.

Local soft tissue injection or selected nerve blocks with buffered bupivacaine or lidocaine (or both) are the recommended anesthesia for the removal of most soft tissue FBs. Judicious use of sedation (parenteral, rectal, or oral) is advised if the clinician senses undue apprehension or anxiety in the patient. Sedation may be especially helpful in children, with ketamine often being an excellent choice. If the patient is totally uncooperative, postpone exploration to a more appropriate time and setting (e.g., under regional or general anesthesia in the operating room).

To successfully remove an FB in the soft tissue of an extremity, a time-limited arterial tourniquet can help provide a bloodless field. Inflate a blood pressure cuff or portable self-contained pneumatic cuff above arterial pressure on the upper part of the arm, forearm, leg, or thigh. To limit bothersome backbleeding, elevate the extremity and wrap it with an elastic bandage to exsanguinate the extremity before inflating the tourniquet. A Penrose drain or specialized tourniquet may be used as a tourniquet at the base of a finger or toe. Alternatively, use a sterile glove as a finger tourniquet. Cut the fingertip of the glove on the involved finger and roll the glove down to the base of the finger. Most patients can tolerate an ischemic tourniquet for 15 to 30 minutes, and it is safe to stop the circulation to an extremity for this length of time.

Operative Technique

The specific technique for removal of an FB is tailored to each clinical situation. In general, FBs should be removed only under direct vision. Grasping blindly into a wound with a hemostat to remove an FB should be avoided. This technique is especially dangerous in the hand, foot, neck, or face, where sensitive or vital structures may easily be damaged.

After obtaining appropriate informed consent and following sterile preparation, *consider enlarging the entrance wound with an adequate skin incision, which can be advantageous.* Numerous techniques are used, depending on the clinical scenario (Fig. 36-11). Attempting to remove an FB through a puncture wound or an inadequate skin incision is a common error that is both frustrating and self-defeating. After a proper skin incision, explore the wound carefully by spreading the soft tissue with a hemostat. Frequently, the FB can be felt with an instrument before it can be seen (see Fig. 36-11, *plate 1*). After placing a tourniquet on an extremity, follow the track of the FB, although it often cannot be identified when surrounded by muscle or fat. If the FB, such as one that is made of fiberglass or plastic, is difficult to visualize, is located in the superficial soft tissue, or has contaminated the surrounding soft tissue, excising a small block of tissue rather than removing the FB alone may be necessary. Excise the block of tissue only under direct vision and after nerves, tendons, and vessels have been identified and excluded from the excision area.

If an FB such as a thorn or needle enters the skin perpendicularly, a linear incision may pass to one side or the other of the FB, and it may be difficult to determine where the FB lies in relation to this incision (see Fig. 36-11, *plate 2*). For

Figure 36-10 The contents of a standard suture tray, with the addition of a scalpel, are usually adequate for the removal of most foreign bodies.

this reason the search must then be extended into the walls of the incision rather than simply through the skin.[33] In such cases, excise a small ellipse of skin and undermine the skin for 0.5 to 1.0 cm in all directions. Next, compress the tissue from the sides in the hope that the FB will extrude and can then be grasped with a hemostat.

After removal of the FB, it is important to irrigate and cleanse the wounds. If a small incision has been made in a noncosmetic area (such as the bottom of the foot), leave the incision open and bandaged. The area may be periodically soaked in hot water for a few days. A return visit is necessary only if signs of infection develop. If a large incision has been made, the skin may be sutured primarily as long as no other contraindications are present. In cases in which gross contamination has occurred or there is significant tissue injury, do not close the wound on the initial visit. Leave the wound open but packed. Suture the skin after 3 to 5 days if the wound is free of inflammation or infection (known as delayed primary closure; see Chapters 34 and 35 for details).

Special Scenarios and Techniques

Puncture Wounds in the Sole of the Foot

Puncture wounds in the feet from unknown objects and under unknown circumstances present problems to the clinician. In general, puncture wounds in the feet are at risk for retained FBs and infection. It is impossible to adequately explore a puncture wound. In noncosmetic areas, therefore, a puncture wound can be converted to a laceration to adequately explore and clean it (Fig. 36-12). Under most circumstances, delayed primary closure is recommended (see Chapter 34). This topic, including stepping on a nail and puncture wounds in the sole of the foot, are discussed extensively in Chapter 51.

Subungual FBs

Once a subungual FB has been identified, perform a digital block before manipulation of the nail or nail bed. Pay special attention to deeply embedded subungual FBs.[34] Some cases may require removing a small portion of the nail with double-pointed heavy scissors to expose the FB and grasp the foreign material with splinter forceps (Fig. 36-13).

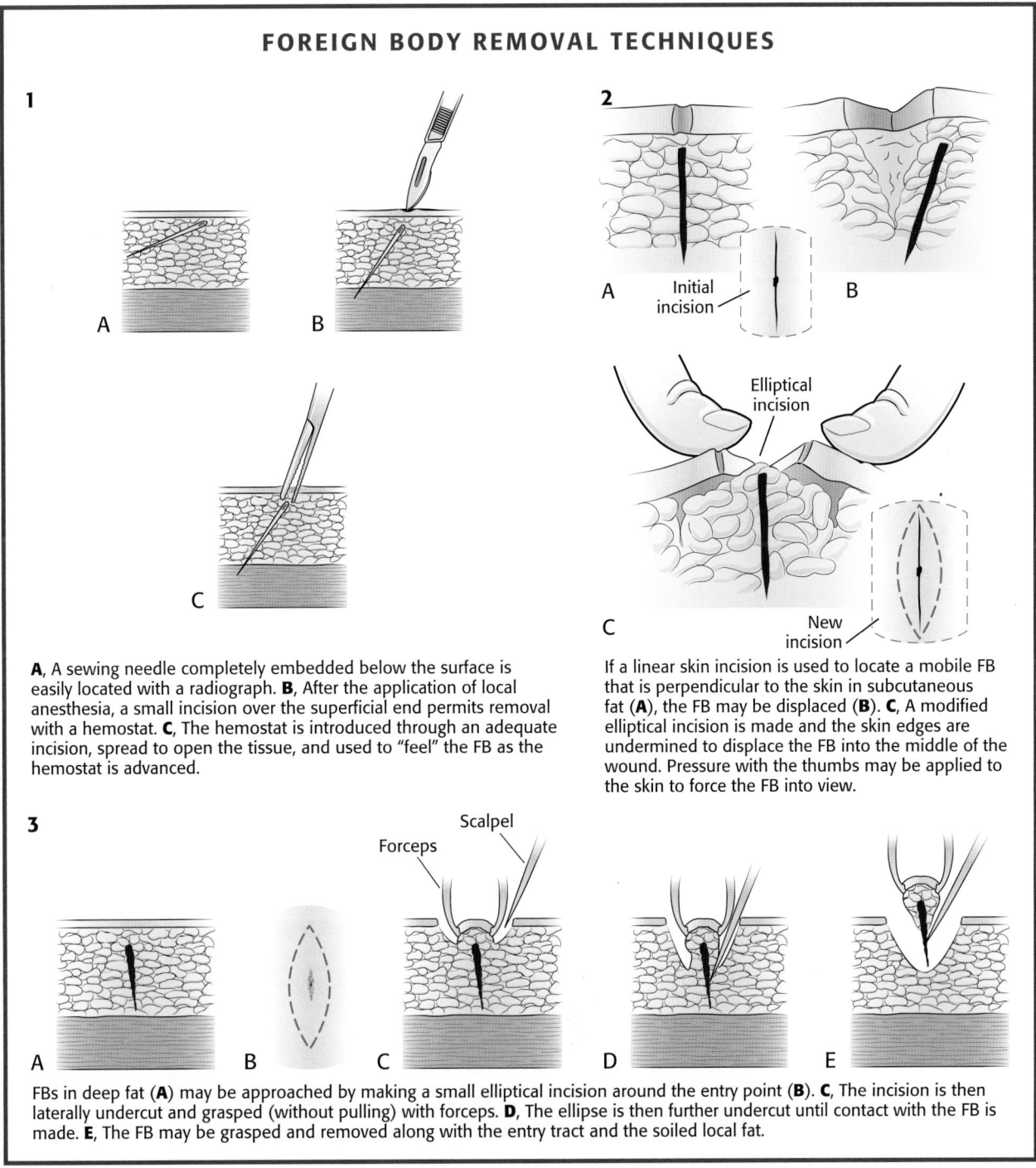

FOREIGN BODY REMOVAL TECHNIQUES

1

A, A sewing needle completely embedded below the surface is easily located with a radiograph. **B**, After the application of local anesthesia, a small incision over the superficial end permits removal with a hemostat. **C**, The hemostat is introduced through an adequate incision, spread to open the tissue, and used to "feel" the FB as the hemostat is advanced.

2

If a linear skin incision is used to locate a mobile FB that is perpendicular to the skin in subcutaneous fat (**A**), the FB may be displaced (**B**). **C**, A modified elliptical incision is made and the skin edges are undermined to displace the FB into the middle of the wound. Pressure with the thumbs may be applied to the skin to force the FB into view.

3

FBs in deep fat (**A**) may be approached by making a small elliptical incision around the entry point (**B**). **C**, The incision is then laterally undercut and grasped (without pulling) with forceps. **D**, The ellipse is then further undercut until contact with the FB is made. **E**, The FB may be grasped and removed along with the entry tract and the soiled local fat.

Figure 36-11 Foreign body (FB) removal techniques. (*1 and 3, Reproduced from* Hospital Medicine, *January 1981, with permission of Cahner's Publishing Co; 2, From Rees CE. The removal of FBs: a modified incision.* JAMA. *1939;113:35. Copyright 1939, American Medical Association. Reproduced with permission.*)

One technique is to bend the tip of a sterile hypodermic needle and slide it under the nail. Hook the FB and then remove it. Alternatively, slide a 19-gauge hypodermic needle under the nail to surround a small splinter. Bring the needle tip against the underside of the nail and secure the splinter. Remove the needle and splinter as a unit.[35] Another possible technique is to shave the overlying nail plate with a No. 15 scalpel blade via light strokes in a proximal-to-distal direction.

This creates a U-shaped defect in the nail and exposes the entire length of the sliver.[36]

Wooden splinters are commonly embedded under the fingernail. Such FBs must be removed completely because subsequent infection is almost certain. If complete removal cannot be achieved with the techniques described earlier, remove the entire nail (see Chapter 35). This allows all the fragments to be visualized and removed. The proximity of the distal phalanx to the subungual area is a constant concern for the development of osteomyelitis and requires follow-up.

Metallic Fragments and Bullets

High-velocity fragments (e.g., bullets, BBs) are easy to visualize radiographically and relatively simple to remove if embedded in areas that are anatomically accessible (Fig. 36-14). Before removal, assess the area in which the fragments are embedded to determine which structures are involved and which structures might be encountered during removal. Defer removal of deeply embedded metallic FBs unless symptoms of infection develop. Infection is rare because such FBs usually become encysted over time.

Surgery is rarely performed solely for the purpose of removing bullets. Retained bullets rarely cause complications or infection, and aggressive attempts to find and remove bullets generally cause more harm than good. Retrieval is often quite difficult unless the fragments are very superficial. Gunshot wounds themselves need no intervention beyond simple cleaning and perhaps minor débridement of the entrance or exit wound. Gunshot wound tracks do not need débridement unless there is gross contamination or significant tissue devitalization. Entrance or exit wounds should not be closed. Antibiotics are unnecessary for minor uncomplicated gunshot wounds but may be beneficial in patients with multiple injuries, gross wound contamination, significant tissue devitalization, large wounds, or delay in treatment.

A caveat is lead toxicity from bullet fragments. If a bullet is bathed in synovial, pleural, peritoneal, or cerebrospinal fluid, the lead may leach out over time and produce a significant elevation in blood lead levels. Though rare, lead fragments in contact with synovium are a reason for concern and potentially a reason for removal (see the previous discussion). In one study, Farrell and associates found that patients with

Figure 36-12 This patient stepped on "something" while walking through a polluted urban creek, a setup for a foreign body and infection. Mandatory radiographs were negative. **A,** Under proper lighting (and a calf blood pressure cuff for a tourniquet), the patient is placed prone. Local lidocaine with epinephrine is infiltrated *through the cut skin edges*, not via the intact sensitive skin. (Alternatively, a posterior tibial nerve block could be used.) **B,** Inspection reveals a dirty skin flap that is cut off. **C,** Because a puncture wound cannot be explored or irrigated, this wound should be lengthened with a scalpel to allow further care. **D,** The depths of the wound are explored. **E,** An assistant holds the wound open with a hemostat so that copious irrigation can be accomplished. This wound should be *packed open* and checked in 24 to 48 hours, *not closed primarily with sutures.* Delayed closure can be performed in 4 to 5 days if necessary, but this injury healed well without sutures. Prophylactic antibiotics are of no proven value but may be given.

retained lead FBs had statistically significant elevated blood lead levels.[37] The study did not differentiate the location of the FB and whether patients were, in fact, symptomatic from plumbism. Nevertheless, it may be prudent for the patient's primary care provider to monitor blood lead levels in patients with known lead FBs to prevent the future development of lead toxicity. The value of routine prophylactic antibiotics for metallic FBs left in soft tissue has not been proved.

For superficial metallic FBs, a sterile magnet can be used to facilitate the removal of small metallic fragments.[38] Introduce the magnet into the entry site, with a small scalpel and hemostat used to extend and open the wound as needed. When the magnet comes in contact with the metal, a click is heard and the FB is removed while attached to the magnet. If resistance to extraction occurs, exploration can be done with the FB attached to the magnet. Sometimes, instead of introducing the magnet directly into the wound it can be placed on the overlying skin to guide superficial small FBs out of the wound.[39] Make an effort to not grasp or touch the bullet because it can interfere with ballistics evidence during any subsequent legal investigation.

FBs in Fatty Tissue

Remove FBs in fatty tissue by making an elliptical incision around the entrance wound. Grasp the incised skin loosely

Remove
wedge of nail

Figure 36-13 For a foreign body (FB) deep in the nail bed, take as small a wedge of nail as will allow access to the proximal end of the splinter, and then extract the FB with splinter forceps. All wood particles should be removed. A digital nerve block is usually necessary.

with Allis forceps. Undercut the incision until the FB is contacted. Remove the FB, skin, and entrance track in one block. Remove a small portion of subcutaneous fat along with the FB to minimize infection. FBs in fat are very mobile, and probing may displace them even further. FBs that are embedded in fat and are perpendicular to the skin can also be removed, as shown in Figure 36-11.

Pencil Lead/Graphite

Use careful judgment in removing pencil graphite when it is lodged in the skin. Graphite invariably leaves a pigmented tattoo in the soft tissue, and it is preferable to excise the material en bloc (see Fig. 36-11) when pencil lead is found in a cosmetic area. The graphite specks cannot be irrigated or scrubbed off, and tattooing results if they are not removed. Furthermore, a pencil lead FB may resemble a malignant melanoma over time. US has been shown to be useful in differentiating between pencil lead FBs and melanoma.[40]

Fishhooks

Traditionally, four fishhook removal techniques have been described: advance and cut, string-yank, needle cover, and retrograde.[41] The preferred method depends on the location, depth of penetration, and conditions under which the removal is to take place (Fig. 36-15).[42-44] Initially, note whether the fishhook is single or multiple. In addition, note the number and location of barbs. Remove or cover any remaining exposed hooks to prevent subsequent injury. As with most injuries, document the patient's vascular and neurologic status before and after removal. As with all wounds, administer tetanus prophylaxis if indicated. Prophylactic antibiotics are not generally necessary.

Advance and Cut Technique

To perform the advance and cut technique for removal, advance the fishhook and cut proximal to the barb (Fig. 36-16, *plate 1*). This method is particularly well suited for superficially embedded fishhooks. Generally, infiltrate local anesthetic (1% lidocaine) into the tissue overlying the barb. Force the barb through the anesthetized skin and clip it off. Move the rest of the hook retrogradely, along the direction of entry. Because this technique is almost always successful, it can be considered a first-line option.

Figure 36-14 A and **B,** High-velocity fragments such as bullets or BBs are often easy to locate and visualize radiographically. Here, a BB is found embedded in the volar tuft of a finger. **C,** After a digital block, a small linear incision is made with a scalpel. **D,** The BB is removed without difficulty.

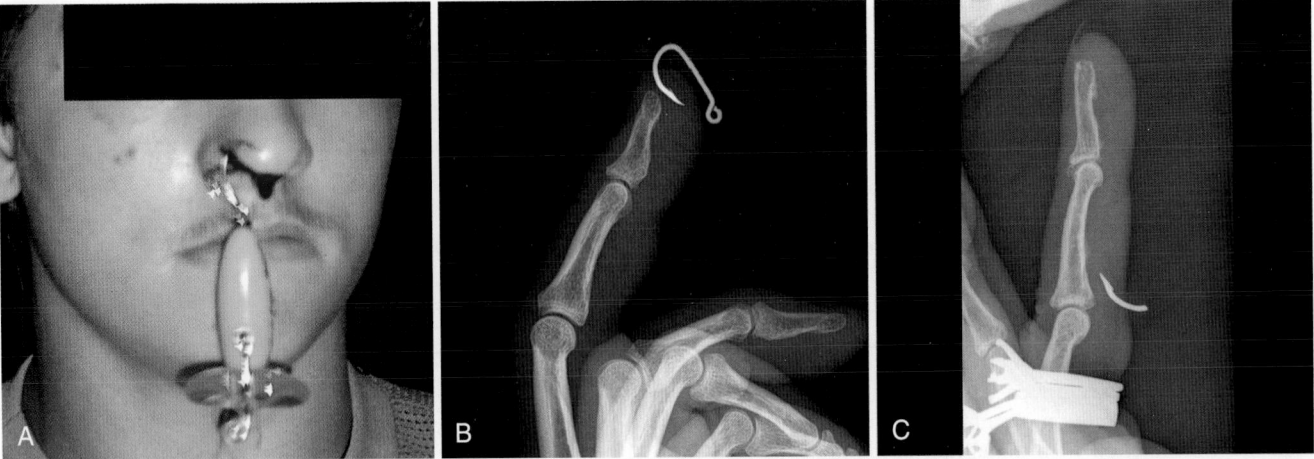

Figure 36-15 Fishhooks. **A,** Fishing lure embedded in the nasal ala. This type of injury may occur while casting the line. **B,** Fish hook embedded in the distal tuft of the finger. Note that the barb is completely embedded in subcutaneous tissue, thus making removal by simply pulling the hook out impossible. **C,** This patient cut off the portion of the embedded hook external to the skin before coming to the emergency department. Patients will commonly do this; however, it makes removal more difficult because there is very little hook exposed that can be manipulated during attempts at removal.

String-Yank Technique

In the field or stream, removal of a fishhook may be accomplished without local anesthesia by using the string-yank technique. This technique may be used in the ED as well. Some clinicians prefer to use local 1% lidocaine to facilitate removal. For the "stream" technique (see Fig. 36-16, *plate 2*), pass a looped string or fishing line around the belly of the hook at the point where it enters the skin. Wrap approximately 1 ft of string around the dominant hand to provide strong traction. Hold the shank of the hook parallel to and in approximation to the skin with the index finger of the opposite hand. Use the thumb and middle finger of the opposite hand to stabilize and depress the barb, which helps the index finger disengage the barb from the subcutaneous tissue. When the barb has been disengaged, give a sharp pull (i.e., a quick tug with a snapping motion) with the dominant hand to remove the hook. Take care to keep bystanders out of the expected path of the hook because it often flies out of the patient. A commercial fishhook extractor device is available that is based on this method. It is used to grasp the hook during removal (Minto Research and Development, Inc., Redding, CA).

Needle Cover Technique

For this technique use an 18-gauge needle to cover the barb (see Fig. 36-16, *plate 3*). After adequate local anesthesia has been achieved, pass the needle through the entrance wound of the hook parallel to the shank of the hook to sheath the barb and allow the hook to be backed out while the barb is covered. An alternative to this procedure is to insert a No. 11 blade parallel to the shank of the hook down to the barb and use the point of the blade to free the subcutaneous tissue that is engaged on the barb. Cover the barb with the point of the No. 11 blade and back the hook out, with the blade protecting the barb.

Retrograde Technique

This is the simplest, but least effective method. By applying downward pressure on the shank of the hook, disengage the barb to allow successful removal (see Fig. 36-16, *plate 4*). If resistance is encountered, abandon the procedure and attempt removal with another technique. If the barb is not already protruding from the skin, the retrograde technique may cause less tissue trauma.

Wooden Splinters

Removal of wooden splinters is a common FB removal procedure. By simply grasping the end of a superficial, protruding splinter, it may be adequately removed, but care should be taken to not leave small pieces of material in the wound. Some splinters cannot be visualized at the point of entry but can easily and readily be palpated beneath the skin. When a wood FB is in subcutaneous tissue, it is advisable to cut down on the long axis of the FB to remove it via a skin incision rather than pulling it out through the entrance wound (Figs. 36-17 and 36-18). Although an incision may seem extensive and creates a laceration where only a puncture wound existed, opening the track allows thorough cleaning and removal of all the small pieces of the splinter that might otherwise remain. If the incision is linear, it may be sutured. Occasionally, the fastest method of removing small wooden splinters is to completely excise the entrance track and the FB en bloc, followed by linear closure. Particular mention should be made of certain wood splinters that are pliable and reactive, such as California redwood and northwest cedar. Any wood that is easily fragmented requires meticulous care to ensure removal of all material.

Traumatic Tattooing

Ground-in foreign material or tattooing of the skin is a difficult problem because permanent disfigurement may occur (Fig. 36-19). These injuries occur most often from falls on blacktop surfaces or asphalt or falls from bicycles or motorcycles on a variety of surfaces. Many cases may be managed with adequate local anesthesia and meticulous débridement with a sponge, scrub brush, or toothbrush. If all foreign material cannot be removed with these methods, give careful consideration to secondary excision of the tattooed area and primary closure with subsequent plastic surgery to repair the defect. However, it is usually impossible to completely remove traumatic tattooing in the ED. Referral for more extensive surgical treatment after local wound care is quite acceptable. Dermabrasion may be an acceptable delayed treatment when the tattooing is superficial.[45] An alternative is to refer patients to a dermatologist for laser removal of traumatic tattoos. Certain lasers, such as a yttrium-aluminum-garnet (YAG) laser, have proved to be an excellent alternative.[46] The process is more specific in removing embedded material without harming the surrounding tissue. The type of material will determine the number of treatments required. Not all tattoos can be removed completely.[47]

Marine FBs

Although most marine FBs, such as shell fragments, may be treated like other FBs, a number of marine animals carry toxins and may leave FBs that require special consideration. Saltwater marine FBs may be contaminated with *Vibrio* species, which are usually sensitive to tetracyclines, aminoglycosides, or third-generation cephalosporins. Even if all foreign material has been removed, stings from marine animals may initiate a prolonged local irritation that simulates cellulitis. However, the presence of a wound infection on a subsequent visit strongly raises concern for an occult retained FB rather

---

FISHHOOK REMOVAL

1   Advance and Cut Technique

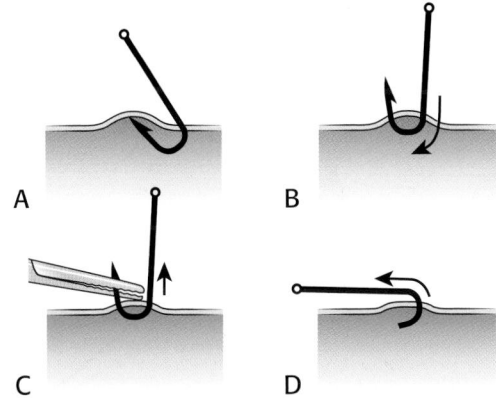

Method of removing an embedded fishhook when anesthesia is available and the point of the fishhook (**A**) is close to the skin. **B**, Force the point through the anesthetized skin. **C**, Clip off the barb. **D**, Remove the rest of the hook by reversing the direction of entry.

2   String-Yank Technique

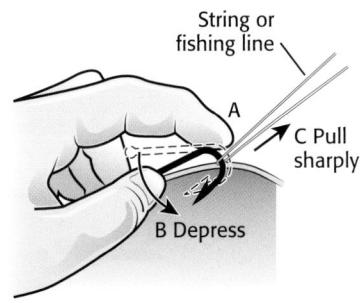

Method of removing an embedded fishhook when anesthesia is unavailable or when the barb of the fishhook lies too deep to force it out through a second wound without causing significant additional damage. *A*, Loop a piece of string (or thick suture material) around the belly of the hook and hold it down against the skin with the index finger of the left hand. Depress the shaft of the hook against the skin with the middle finger and thumb while applying light downward pressure with the index finger of the left hand to disengage the barb from subcutaneous tissue (*B*), and pull sharply on the ends of the string with the right hand (*C*) to remove the hook through its entry wound. Be careful of the flying hook.

3   Needle Cover Technique

Method of removing an embedded fishhook using anesthesia when the hook is large and not too deep in the skin. **A**, After anesthetizing the area with 1% lidocaine, insert a short-bevel 18-gauge needle through the entry wound of the hook and attempt to sheathe the barb of the hook within the needle. **B**, If this is done correctly, the hook and needle may then be backed out together.

4   Retrograde Technique

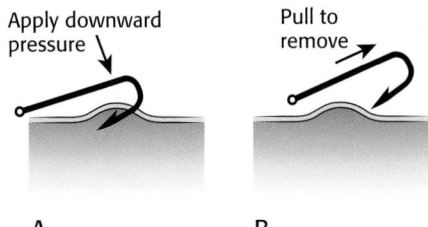

This is the simplest but least effective method. **A**, First apply downward pressure on the shank of the hook to disengage the barb. **B**, Pull the hook out. If resistance is encountered, abandon the attempt and try another technique.

Figure 36-16 Fishhook removal. *(Reproduced from* Hospital Medicine, *July 1980, with permission of Cahner's Publishing Co.)*

Figure 36-17 A, The course and depth of penetration of this large wooden splinter in the leg are uncertain, but it is axiomatic that all pieces of wood must be removed to prevent infection. **B-D,** To ensure complete removal of foreign bodies, an incision is made over the entire course of the splinter. **E-G,** All pieces of wood are carefully removed under direct vision. **H,** The laceration is sutured primarily. Although it may be tempting to simply pull the splinter out and irrigate the puncture track, such actions often lead to retained particles and complications.

than the simple conclusion that the wound is merely infected by bacteria introduced during the initial insult.

Coelenterates

Coelenterates, including the Portuguese man-of-war, true jellyfish, fire coral, box jellyfish, and sea anemones, inject several different toxins that are responsible for many marine envenomations by embedding venom-containing organelles, called *nematocysts*, into the victim's skin (Fig. 36-20). The tentacles of coelenterates may contain thousands of nematocysts, which allows many to be deposited by even minor skin contact. After deposition, nematocysts discharge their venom. Reactions

may be local or systemic, and the pain may be severe and is often described as "shocklike," "itching," "burning," or "throbbing." Substances such as tetramine, histamine, and 5-hydroxytryptamine are thought to be responsible for this localized reaction, whereas proteinaceous substances are implicated in the systemic response. Systemic reactions usually consist of fever, chills, and muscle spasm, but severe reactions may result in neurologic sequelae ranging from malaise and headache to paralysis and coma. Potential cardiopulmonary manifestations include dysrhythmias, hypotension, syncope, bronchospasm, laryngeal edema, and cardiorespiratory failure.[48,49]

Figure 36-18 A, A splinter was removed from the foot of this 3-year-old 7 days earlier, and a few days after removal it began to swell. A retained foreign body (FB) was suspected. Plain radiographs were negative. A small pyogenic granuloma is seen. After ketamine sedation a 5-mm core of tissue was removed, but no FB was found on extensive exploration. This was an abscess from the puncture. The wound was packed open and cephalexin was given. **B,** It healed well (1 week later), but if it recurs, computed tomography or magnetic resonance imaging would be indicated to search for an occult FB.

Figure 36-19 Traumatic tattoos. **A,** This patient was seen approximately 1 week after a blast injury. Traumatic tattoos are evident. The patient subsequently underwent successful laser removal of most of the pigment. **B,** Traumatic tattoo of the chin. Bluish discoloration and slight erythema, predominantly caused by silica, are apparent. (*A, From Flint PW, Haughey BH, Lund VJ, et al, eds.* Cummings Otolaryngology: Head & Neck Surgery. *5th ed. St. Louis: Mosby; 2010; B, from Bolognia JL, Jorizzo JL, Shaffer JV, eds.* Dermatology. *3rd ed. St. Louis: Saunders; 2012.*)

Initial wound care should focus on decontamination and removal of unfired nematocysts, which will decrease the pain and systemic reactions. Vinegar (5% acetic acid) is the initial decontaminating agent of choice because it will inactivate the unfired nematocysts of most (but not all) species of jellyfish, Portuguese man-of-war, and sea anemones.[48,50,51] Apply it continuously for 30 minutes or until the pain is gone.[49] *Do not apply fresh water* to the area because the osmotic shock will activate any remaining unfired nematocysts and cause them to discharge toxin and increase pain and toxicity. Other suggested, but unproven remedies include meat tenderizer, ammonia, baking soda, urine, olive oil, sugar, and papaya latex.

After the wound has been decontaminated, remove any remaining tentacle fragments. Extract large fragments with forceps; however, individual nematocysts are very small (<1 mm in length) and are not easily visible. To remove the remaining nematocysts, scrape the skin with a hard edge, such

as a credit card held perpendicular to the skin. An alternative is to apply shaving cream and shave the area gently to eliminate the remaining fragments.[49] Do not used sand to remove nematocysts because sand can increase the discharge of venom. If the pain persists, it should be assumed that organelles still remain and further cleansing is required.

After decontamination, use topical anesthetics or steroids, but prophylactic antibiotics are not necessary. Follow routine wound care. Treat allergic and systemic reactions appropriately. The application of warm or cold packs to the area has not been shown to reduce pain.[50] Antivenin is available only for box jellyfish envenomation, but its use remains incompletely understood and controversial.

Coral

Coral is composed of a calcium carbonate core and thousands of small marine animals. Fire coral, a specific type of coral, is another type of coelenterate that produces toxicity with

NEMATOCYST IN RESTING STATE

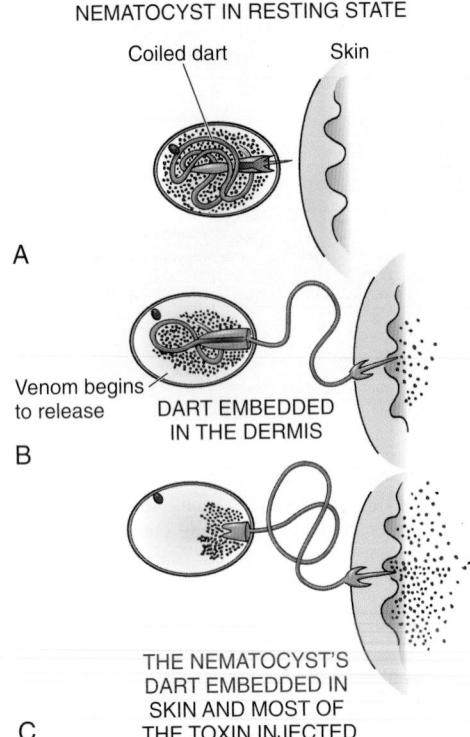

Figure 36-20 A, Magnified view of a venom-containing nematocyst in its resting or "cocked" state. After contact with the skin, a dartlike tail is extended and penetrates the dermis (**B**), and venom is injected (**C**). Further stimulation of the attached nematocyst can expel more venom (see text for the decontamination and removal technique).

Figure 36-21 Fire coral stings. (*From James WD, Berger TG, Elston DM, eds.* Andrews' Diseases of the Skin: Clinical Dermatology. *11th ed. St. Louis: Saunders; 2011.*)

stinging nematocysts. After contact, a burning and intense pruritus may occur along with a series of skin eruptions. Within minutes of contact, pruritus, erythema, and urticaria-like lesions may appear, and blister formation may result within hours (Fig. 36-21). Eventually, the lesions will become lichenoid, but complete resolution may not take place for 15 weeks after contact. Ultimately, hyperpigmented areas will form at the point of initial contact. Immediate care with oral antihistamines and topical steroids tends to reduce, but not prevent the symptoms.

"Coral cuts," which can be deep lacerations, occur in divers and snorkelers exploring coral reefs. With these wounds, delayed healing may take place with the secondary development of cellulitis or ulceration, perhaps as a result of contamination of the wound with bacteria or microparticles of coral.[48] Treatment consists of saline irrigation. Hydrogen peroxide may be used to help remove small coral particles from the wound.[48] Do not close the wound; wet-to-dry dressings are advised instead.

Sponges
Sponges produce both an irritant and a contact dermatitis. The irritant dermatitis occurs as a result of sponge spicules embedded in the victim's skin. Remove the spicules with adhesive tape (applied to the skin and then peeled back), and then bathe the area with vinegar.[48] Contact dermatitis, which is believed to be caused by a toxin, produces erythema, pruritus, and vesicles similar to those with poison oak.[48] Treatment is initial immersion in vinegar followed by local steroid creams.

Sea Urchins and Starfish
Sea urchins and starfish are free-living echinoderms covered with venomous, sharp, brittle spines and with venom-secreting pincers located near the mouth. If sea urchins or starfish are handled or inadvertently stepped on, these spines may become embedded in the patient and a severe local reaction may result from venom in the spines. Systemic symptoms occur and include muscle weakness; paralysis of the lips, tongue, and face; hypotension; abdominal pain; and respiratory distress. Local pain responds quite well to immersion in hot water (43.3°C to 46.1°C [110°F to 115°F]) for 30 to 90 minutes. Retained spines may become infected or cause delayed (≤1 to 2 months) FB granulomas. This reaction is not adequately understood, but it may be due to an intense and persistent inflammatory reaction. Spines that penetrate joints may induce synovitis. Echinoderm spines may discharge a purple dye that may be mistaken for a retained spine (Fig. 36-22).[49] Spines are usually visible on radiographs and should be removed if possible, although they are brittle and can break off in the skin. A YAG laser may be an effective alternative to remove sea urchin spines. If spines are located in a joint or near a nerve, surgical extraction using an operative microscope may be necessary.[48] Otherwise, if removal is difficult, leave the spine in place until it is resorbed or a local reaction takes place. Open the wound and drain it to allow it to close by secondary intention.

Catfish
Several species of catfish in North America contain toxic venom, and a sting from the dorsal or pectoral spines can embed an FB. The spine secretes venom from an epidermal gland at the base of the spine.[52] The pain is usually ephemeral, and because no specific antitoxin exists, treatment consists of local care and analgesics. Immerse the affected part in hot water (≈43.3°C [110°F]) for at least 30 minutes if the pain is

Figure 36-22 A, Multiple sea urchin punctures in the hand soon after injury and following a soak in hot water. **B,** The same hand after 6 days without intervening therapy other than soaking. Lack of discoloration indicates absorption of dye from the sea urchin spines and probable absence of retained fragments. *(From Auerbach PS, ed.* Wilderness Medicine. *6th ed. St. Louis: Mosby; 2011.)*

severe. This is believed to provide relief of symptoms by decreasing vascular and muscle spasm.[53] Local injection of the wound with alkalized bupivacaine provides local analgesia and may also neutralize the toxin.[52] Inspect the wound and remove any remaining spines (Fig. 36-23). A radiograph may be taken to confirm the absence of FBs, but catfish spines and cartilage may be radiolucent. Bedside US may be helpful, depending on the clinician's level of experience. Thoroughly clean and irrigate the wound. Update the patient's tetanus prophylaxis if necessary. Some authors recommend empirical antibiotic therapy to cover gram-negative bacilli (e.g., *Aeromonas hydrophila*), but infection is quite rare and routine antibiotic prophylaxis is not standard.[52]

Stingrays

Stingray envenomation usually occurs in a person who accidentally steps on a creature that is resting on the bottom in shallow water and covered by sand (Fig. 36-24). This causes the stingray to lash out its whiplike caudal appendage, or tail, which contains one to four venom-containing serrated spines. Portions of the spine may become buried in the victim's skin. Each spine is covered with a sheath containing venom glands, and in addition to immediate toxin-induced pain, pieces of the spine or sheath may remain embedded in the wound. These fragments, though often difficult to locate, do not dissolve and must therefore be removed. Persistent pain and inflammation, even weeks to months after the attack, mandate consideration of a retained FB, but a *persistent and difficult-to-treat irritative process can occur in the absence of a retained spine or sheath.* Immediate local and systemic reactions develop as a result of injection of a complex toxin. Systemic reactions may be severe and can include muscle cramps, vomiting, seizures, hypotension, arrhythmias, and (rarely) death.[54]

Treatment consists of irrigation with saline followed by immersion in hot water at 42°C to 45°C for 30 to 90 minutes to inactivate the heat-labile toxin. Local digital blocks without vasoconstrictors provide effective analgesia for hand wounds.

Figure 36-23 To ensure total removal, remove the spine of a catfish by incising the puncture site as opposed to simply pulling it out.

Explore and débride all wounds, and remove all remnants of the spine and integumentary sheath.[48] Wounds should heal by secondary intention. The venom can cause significant local tissue necrosis, and surgical débridement may be required.

Tetanus and Antibiotic Therapy

Prophylactic antibiotic therapy for marine injuries is common, although there are no convincing data to support or refute this practice. Unlike other soft tissue infections, marine injuries become infected with unusual gram-negative organisms, particularly *Vibrio* species. Although few studies have evaluated the effects of specific antibiotics, it is recommended that quinolones, trimethoprim-sulfamethoxazole, tetracyclines, third-generation cephalosporins, or aminoglycosides be used in lieu of penicillin, ampicillin, erythromycin, or first-generation cephalosporins.[49] It is always difficult to differentiate chronic inflammation caused by toxins and foreign material from true infection, and surgical exploration is often required in persistent cases. Administer tetanus prophylaxis as per routine recommendations.

Figure 36-24 A, Stingray resting on the bottom of the ocean, usually covered by a layer of sand. **B,** An unsuspecting victim steps on the stingray, and the whiplike tail impales the foot (even through a heavy boot) with one or more spines. The spine has backward-facing barbs covered by a sheath with venom-containing cells (**C**), which causes a toxic envenomation and the potential for multiple foreign bodies.

Cactus Spines

The size of cactus spines fluctuates considerably. The difficulty of removal is generally inversely proportional to the size of the FB.[55] Larger embedded cactus spines are managed like wood splinters and sea urchin spine FBs. More advanced imaging techniques (US, CT, or MRI) may be required for localization of deeply embedded spines.

Figure 36-25 A thousand or more glochids may become affixed to the skin by contact with a single pad of polka dot cactus. **A,** To remove them, professional facial gel is spread with a fan brush, thin at the edges. **B,** The gel rollup is started by picking at the edge with the fingernails. When the gel is peeled off, all the very small spines come with it. *(From Lindsey D, Lindsey WE. Cactus spine injuries. Am J Emerg Med. 1988;6:362. Reproduced by permission.)*

Deeply embedded cactus spines generally produce granulomatous reactions, but infections are rare.[56] Dermatitis from embedded cactus spines is a well-described phenomenon. Hence, make an effort to remove deeply embedded spines after carefully weighing the benefit and potential harm related to deep exploration, especially in a sensitive location.[55] Using forceps, remove superficially embedded, medium to large cactus spines by direct axial traction on each spine. Smaller spines (glochids) may be difficult and tedious to remove individually. Apply an adherent facial mask gel to remove the spines en masse with the gel (Fig. 36-25). Depilatory wax melted in a microwave oven and applied warm, commercial facial gels, and household glue (Elmer's Glue-All, Borden, Inc., Columbus, OH) have all been recommended for this purpose.[55,57-59] Over-the-counter "home use" facial mask gels are not adherent enough to be effective without multiple (eight or more) applications.

Ring Removal

Frequently, a ring must be removed to prevent laceration of tissue or vascular compromise. Thoroughly lubricate (with a water-soluble lubricant, e.g., K-Y jelly) the finger and use a circular motion with traction on the ring. However, the string-wrap method or physically cutting the ring off may be necessary. Preferably, remove all rings before the edema is extensive enough to cause pain or vascular compromise.

String-Wrap Method

An occasional patient can remain calm during this procedure, but if the swelling is significant or the digit has been traumatized, anesthesia is necessary. Perform a proximal digital or metacarpal block to provide sufficient anesthesia and to minimize tissue distention at the ring site. Before removal of the ring, wrap a wide Penrose drain circumferentially in a distal-to-proximal direction to reduce the soft tissue swelling (Fig. 36-26). Leave the wrap in place for a few minutes to reach the maximum effect. Some nonanesthetized patients panic during the procedure because of increasing pain from compression and unwinding.[60]

First, pass a 20- to 25-inch piece of string, umbilical tape, or thick silk suture between the ring and the finger. Shorter lengths are discouraged because one may need to repeat the wrapping procedure midway. If marked soft tissue swelling is present, pass the tip of a hemostat under the ring to grasp the string and pull it through. Wrap the distal string clockwise around the swollen finger (proximal to distal) to include the proximal interphalangeal (PIP) joint and the entire swollen finger. Start the wrapping next to the ring. Wrap it snugly enough to compress the swollen tissue. Place successive loops of wrap next to each other to keep any swollen tissue from bulging between the strands. When the wrapping is complete, carefully unwind the proximal end of the string in the same clockwise direction to force the ring over that portion of the finger that has been compressed by the wrap. The PIP joint is the area that is most difficult to maneuver over and causes the most pain.

Occasionally, the finger must be rewrapped if it was not done carefully the first time. It is not uncommon to produce abrasions or other kinds of trauma in the skin during this procedure. If the finger with the ring is lacerated or there are underlying fractures, it is prudent to cut the ring off instead of attempting this technique.

Certain rings are made of extremely hard material such as tungsten carbide or ceramic. In these cases, cracking the material with standard locking pliers can break the ring. Place the pliers on the ring and adjust the jaws to fit tightly, and then remove and readjust them while increasing tension with each subsequent adjustment. Continue until the material cracks and falls apart. Some rings may be lined with a metal band. Use a standard ring cutter to remove the band.

Ring Cutter

A ring cutter should be used when the swelling is excessive or other methods fail (Fig. 36-27). A ring cutter has a small hook that fits under the ring and serves as a guide for the saw-toothed wheel that cuts the metal. The cut ends of the ring are spread with large hemostats (e.g., Kelly clamps), and the ring is removed. If the tension is too great to spread the ring, another cut 180 degrees apart from the original ring cut can be performed. This will allow the ring to fall off in two pieces. A jeweler can subsequently repair cut rings.

Certain hardened metal rings, such as tungsten carbide, may not be amenable to the use of a ring cutter. Case studies have demonstrated that a dental-tipped drill or dental volvere can be used successfully. However, because of the nature of these instruments and the possibility of injury from them, such as lacerations from the blade, thermal burns, or ocular FBs, take precautions to limit further damage to the finger, as well as the use of eye protection to shield the patient's and operator's eyes.

Body Piercing and Removal

The art of body piercing predates most history books. Over the last decade an enormous increase in the practice of body piercing has occurred. Accordingly, so have the complications associated with the practice.[61] For centuries the ears were the most common place. Today, the lips, tongue, eyebrow, nose, navel, nipples, and genital areas have become sites of body piercing. To date, there are only a limited number of studies on infection after piercings in areas other than the ears. Three major types of jewelry are used: (1) barbell studs, which are straight bars with a ball threaded onto both ends; (2) labret studs, which are straight bars with a ball threaded on one end and a disk permanently fixed on the other end (more commonly used on the lips); and (3) a captive bead ring, which consists of a bead with small dimples on opposite sides and an incomplete ring with rounded ends to fit into the dimples (Fig. 36-28). The bead is held "captive" by tension from both sides of this incomplete ring. The bead ring is a variation of this: one bead is permanently fixed to one end, and an opening is made by removing the free end of the ring.[62]

The most common reason for removal is infection (Fig. 36-29). Other symptoms such as bleeding, edema, allergic reaction, and keloid formation may also prompt removal. Occasionally, tongue piercings must be removed to permit intubation. To remove barbell- and labret-type studs, hold the bar with forceps and unscrew the bead on the other end. To remove a captive bead ring, hold the ring on both sides of the captive bead to release tension on the bead. This will dislodge the bead from the ring, which is holding it in place. If the jewelry is near the mouth or nose, take care to prevent aspiration of the bead. The complete microbiology of infections related to body piercing has not yet been determined. However, organisms such as *Staphylococcus epidermidis* and *Staphylococcus aureus*, along with *Pseudomonas aeruginosa*, have been commonly implicated pathogens. Other infectious complications from body piercing such as septic arthritis, endocarditis, hepatitis B and C, and HIV have been reported.[63,64]

Most commonly, however, local wound infections predominate and can be managed with warm compresses, antibacterial soap, and topical antibacterial ointment once the FB is removed. The possibility of leaving the piecing in place while treating the infection has yet to be studied.

Postoperative Suture Removal

FBs in the form of nonabsorbed suture material are frequently encountered in the postoperative period. Drainage, localized pain, tenderness, and an inflammatory reaction along the suture line are characteristic of a retained FB (suture abscess). In this instance, probing the wound with a sterilized needle bent into the shape of a crochet hook is frequently successful. Hooking the suture material through the sinus tract and removing it allows the wound to heal over the tract.

Tick Removal

It is important to remove ticks early because the hard tick of the Ixodid family is likely to transmit disease. Rocky Mountain spotted fever, Lyme disease, tularemia, and ascending paralysis are among the many infections identified as tick-borne diseases. It is important to note that the rate of disease transmission before 48 hours of attachment is exceedingly low.[65] Removal of Ixodid ticks is difficult because the mouthparts become cemented within 5 to 30 minutes of contact with the host's skin. Removal will become more difficult the longer the tick is attached. Inadequate or partial removal of the tick may cause infection or chronic granuloma formation. Removal

RING REMOVAL: STRING-WRAP METHOD

Lessen the edema by compressing the finger with a Penrose drain left tightly wrapped for 3 to 5 minutes.

Slide a small hemostat under the ring, grab a long piece of umbilical tape, and pull it under the ring.

Begin to carefully wrap the tape around the finger in a proximal-to-distal fashion.

Even rows, no skin bulging

Wrap clockwise

Continue winding the distal strand to compress the skin distal to the ring. Take time to place successive loops next to each other, and keep tissue from bulging between the strands.

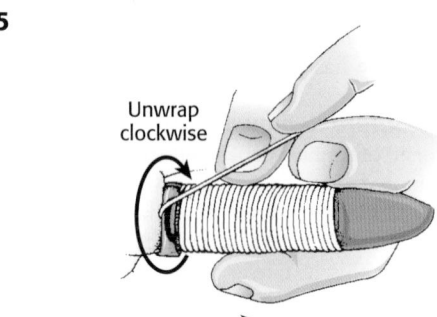

Unwrap clockwise

Remove the ring by unwrapping the proximal strand in the same direction that it was wrapped. The most difficult area to negotiate is the proximal interphalangeal joint. You may have to repeat the wrapping procedure to totally remove the ring.

Successful removal of the rings.

Figure 36-26 Ring removal: string-wrap method.

by mechanical means is recommended.[66] Nonmechanical, traditional, and folk methods of forcing the tick to disengage (e.g., the use of petroleum jelly, fingernail polish, a hot match, or alcohol) are not advised and can cause the tick to regurgitate, thereby increasing the possibility of transmission of infection.

The use of straight or curved forceps or tweezers is the recommended method of removal. If these instruments are not available, use a gloved hand. Grasp the tick as close to the patient's skin surface as possible and gently apply steady axial traction (Fig. 36-30). Take care to not squeeze, crush, twist, or jerk the tick's body because this may expel infective agents or

RING REMOVAL: RING CUTTER METHOD

1

This ring is too tight to be removed by the string-wrap technique. Note that the skin is deeply indented.

2

An electric ring cutter is the best option.

3

When the ring is cut through, grab the cut ends with hemostats and separate the sides. This ring can be repaired by a jeweler to a nearly new condition.

4

Note the macerated tissue under the ring.

Figure 36-27 Ring removal: ring cutter method.

leave mouthparts in the skin. If mouthparts are left behind after removal of the body, they may be removed with tweezers. If one is still unable to remove the mouthparts, consider excision under local anesthesia to prevent local infection.

Many patients have great anxiety about the development of tick-borne diseases after tick removal. Some studies have demonstrated that single-dose doxycycline (200 mg) may prevent the development of Lyme disease.[65] Children younger than 8 years may be given a single dose of doxycycline (4 mg/kg). However, prophylactic antibiotic treatment of all tick bites is not recommended. Amoxicillin prophylaxis is not effective. When a patient is in an area where the incidence of Lyme disease is high or when a partially engorged deer tick in the nymphal stage is discovered on the body, the patient is more likely to benefit from prophylaxis. Regardless of whether prophylaxis is given, instruct patients about the symptoms and signs of Lyme disease and encourage them to return or seek medical evaluation if these symptoms develop.

Barbell studs

Labret studs

Captive bead ring

Bead ring

Figure 36-28 Various types of piercing jewelry. To remove a barbell stud or labret stud, unscrew the ball that is threaded onto the bar. To remove a captive bead ring, snap the ball out of the incomplete ring (it is held in place simply by tension and is not screwed in.) You may need to insert needle-nose pliers into the center of the ring and spread it to pry the ring open. To remove a bead ring, unscrew the ball from one end of the ring.

BODY PIERCING REMOVAL

This patient has a labret stud piercing. Note that the ball is visible externally (*short arrow*); however, the disk portion has migrated internally and the buccal mucosa has closed over it (*long arrow*).

Infiltrate the region with local anesthetic. Alternatively, an infraorbital nerve block could be used (see Chapter 30).

Next, unscrew the ball on the end of the bar.

Make an incision in the buccal mucosa over the embedded disk.

Use a hemostat to find and remove the bar from the lip.

The labret stud, successfully removed and reassembled.

Figure 36-29 Body piercing removal. This piercing became infected when the mucosal portion of the metal bar migrated into tissue. An incision was required to find and grasp the metal bar.

Zipper Entrapment

The skin of the penis may become painfully entangled in a zipper mechanism (Fig. 36-31). Unzipping the zipper frequently lacerates the skin and increases the amount of tissue caught in the mechanism. Although the clinician may anesthetize the skin and excise the entrapped tissue, a less invasive method can be considered.

Cutting the median bar between the faceplates of the zipper mechanism remains the most common method. The interlocking teeth of the zipper then fall apart when the median bar (diamond or bridge) of the zipper is cut in half (Fig. 36-32), and the skin is subsequently freed. A bone cutter or wire clippers and a moderate amount of force may be required to break the bar. The addition of mineral oil followed by traction has been demonstrated to achieve some success. Patients with penile lacerations warrant urologic follow-up to assess for urethral injury.

Infiltration of Radiographic Contrast Material

The infiltration of high-osmolality intravenous contrast material has the potential to cause skin necrosis, but the use of low-osmolality dye, which is well tolerated in soft tissues, has essentially eliminated this problem (Fig. 36-33). The use of high-pressure power injectors, with the technologist out of the room, calls for careful inspection of the intravenous site before injection. However, because of the high-pressure rapid auto-injection of contrast material and the absence of a technician in the room, extravasation of contrast material is not a rare event and occurs even with meticulous technique. Infiltration occurs in about 0.5% to 1% of auto-injections. Once contrast material has infiltrated, no intervention has been demonstrated to ameliorate the local reactions, which are usually mild. Swelling, erythema, and mild discomfort at the infiltration site may occur. It is best to resist the temptation to use excessive heat or cold. Elevation of an extremity is

TICK REMOVAL

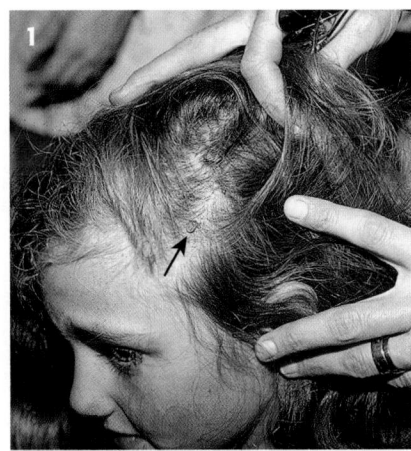

Ticks should be removed as soon as possible to minimize the transmission of tick-borne pathogens and to limit their fixation to the skin by a secreted cement compound. This engorged tick has been attached for about a day and has burrowed under the skin. Most home remedies are worthless.

Grasp the head, not the body

A recommended approach is to grasp the tick with forceps near its head where it enters the skin (avoid the soft body) and gently pull it out. Some advise twisting the head counterclockwise, but this has not objectively been found to be more effective.

If pieces of the tick remain (*arrow*), they should be dug out. Anesthetize the area and use a scalpel with a No. 11 blade to excise the embedded mouthparts. The erythema surrounding this tick bite is not erythema chronicum migrans (which is characteristically an oval-shaped rash, with or without central clearing), but rather local irritation from the initial removal attempt.

Figure 36-30 Tick removal.

Figure 36-31 Penile skin caught in a zipper creates a rather painful and embarrassing situation for the patient. Instead of anesthetizing and excising the skin, consider cutting the zipper as demonstrated in Figure 36-32.

appropriate but of unproven value. Injection of steroids and other agents has no known benefit. Low-osmolality dye is usually totally resorbed in a few days, with no serious consequences in the vast majority of cases. Progress of the dye's egress may be followed with radiographs. The majority of contrast material extravasations resolve with no long-term consequences with conservative management. If large volumes of contrast material are injected (>75 to 100 mL), especially

in confined areas such as the dorsum of the hand, it is possible that skin necrosis from the pressure or a compartment syndrome may develop, but this is rare. The clinician should resist attempts to routinely remove even large volumes of extravasated contrast material by incision or aspiration. Although some contrast material may be removed with surgical techniques during fasciotomy, the actual benefit is unknown. Surgical intervention is rarely required and is based on measurement of compartment pressure and clinical evaluation. Patients with small-volume and minimally symptomatic extravasations may be discharged. Large-volume extravasations warrant consultation or further observation.

TASER Darts
The Thomas A. Swift Electric Rifle, or "TASER," is a conducted electrical weapon used in many areas by police to subdue violent patients (see Chapter 70). The TASER fires two barbed electrodes on long copper wires (Fig. 36-34). The barbs attach to skin or clothing and create an arc that delivers an electrical jolt that causes overwhelming pain and involuntary muscle contraction and incapacitates the subject. The electricity is of such high frequency that it is believed to stay near the surface and not penetrate to the depth of internal organs. The barbs are designed to not penetrate deeper than 4 mm, and police are taught to remove them by stretching the surrounding skin and tugging sharply. If this fails, cutting down on the dart after local anesthesia should facilitate removal.[67,68] Patients may need medical evaluation after ED removal of the darts for the underlying state of agitation that required the use of a TASER, complications of electrical injury, injury from the fall after incapacitation, and injury

Figure 36-32 Zipper removal. (*From* Emergency Medicine, *October 15, 1982, p. 215. Used by permission.*)

from the barb, especially if struck in the mouth, eye, neck, or groin. Most patients do well with minimal intervention and proper wound management if the patient is not unduly agitated and the TASER did not involve the critical areas of the body just mentioned.

Human and Animal Bite FBs
The most common FB after a human bite is a piece of tooth. These FBs can be difficult to find and may not be appreciated if the patient does not admit or disclose the bite wound. Usually, the bite puncture is small and not easily cleaned or visualized. The puncture can be widened with a formal incision to aid in cleaning and evaluation for tendon integrity, injury to the joint capsule, fracture, or an FB (Fig. 36-35). Occasionally, small pieces of teeth can become embedded in a wound, such as with dog, cat, or snake bites (Fig. 36-36). Radiographic detection is variable, and exploration is often the only alternative.

Pyogenic Granuloma (Lobar Capillary Hemangioma)
A pyogenic granuloma is a benign acquired polypoid, friable vascular lesion of the skin (hand, neck, foot, fingers, and trunk) and mucous membranes (Fig. 36-37). They are common in children; in pregnancy the lesion is termed *epulis gravidarum* (pregnancy tumor). The cause is unknown, but there is some association with topical retinoids and the protease inhibitor indinavir; they are not due to infection, and they are not granulomas. They grow rather rapidly over a period of a few weeks, are occasionally associated with minor trauma, have a glistening dark red appearance, and may bleed.

Histologically, a pyogenic granuloma is a hemangioma. A variety of topical therapies (silver nitrate, cryotherapy), laser, or cautery is available, but removal by sharp dissection with primary suturing is usually curative (Fig. 36-38). The recurrence rate may be as high as 40% with nonsurgical intervention.[69]

Hair-Thread Tourniquet
Hair or thread fibers adherent to infants' clothing occasionally become tightly wrapped around a child's digits or genitals (Fig. 36-39).[70] If they are left in place, amputation may eventually occur. The offending fibers may be difficult to visualize, and the child is often brought for evaluation only after signs of distal ischemia appear. Occasionally, the fiber can be grasped with toothless forceps or a small hemostat and then be unwrapped. More commonly, fibers cannot be identified because they are deeply embedded in swollen tissue. Removal not requiring minor surgery includes use of a chemical depilatory, such as the over-the-counter product Nair (calcium thioglycolate), to dissolve or weaken the hair. A generous amount of depilatory cream is worked into the involved area and allowed to dissolve or weaken the hair, which is then removed mechanically. If a depilatory is not successful in 30 to 60 minutes, surgical removal is indicated.

A No. 11 blade can be used to cut the constricting bands under a regional nerve block.[71] It may be difficult to identify individual hairs that are deeply embedded in a swollen digit and even more difficult to assess the success of the intervention. Frequently, multiple hairs are involved. Because the bands may be quite deep, the incision should avoid known

Figure 36-33 The entire volume (100 mL) of nonionic low-osmolality contrast material (Isovue) for a computed tomography scan was pressure-injected into the antecubital soft tissue when the intravenous line infiltrated. High-volume injections are automatically administered by a programmed autoinjector; the technician is not in the room to stop it. **A,** There was only mild pain but considerable soft tissue swelling, and most of the redness and blistering occurred when the technician taped an unprotected ice pack directly to the skin and nearly caused frostbite. **B,** X-ray evidence of the infiltration. **C,** Within 36 hours, the dye was absorbed, without further treatment. No skin necrosis occurred, as has been seen when older ionic high-osmolality agents infiltrate. There is no known proven way to ameliorate the potential soft tissue injury. The antecubital fossa is the preferred site for an intravenous live for injection of contrast material, and such an extravasation on the dorsum of the hand may be more serious. Do not attempt to remove the contrast material by aspiration or surgical incisions.

Figure 36-34 A and **B,** Barbed TASER darts can be removed by a quick pull or through a small incision made over the barb.

Figure 36-35 This human bite puncture wound was enlarged with an incision to aid in cleaning and search for a foreign body, usually a piece of tooth.

neurovascular tracts. Barton and coworkers recommend a dorsal, rather than a lateral incision on the digits.[70] If the soft tissue on the distal end of the digit has been rotated after a circumferential dermal laceration from the tourniquet, the distal tissue can be realigned with the proximal tissue and two dorsolateral sutures placed or tissue adhesive glue applied to maintain the digit in alignment.

Generally, conservative wound care is sufficient once the band has been removed. Application of an antibiotic ointment may enhance healing and allow easier removal of serous drainage from the circumferential laceration. Clinical reassessment in 24 hours will indicate whether any constricting bands remain.

DISPOSITION MANAGEMENT

Tetanus

Wounds with FBs should be considered contaminated wounds, and tetanus status should be updated according to the recommendations for patients with contaminated wounds.

Antibiotics

There is no consensus or standard for the use of antibiotics after removal of wound FBs. Antibiotics may be indicated for immunocompromised patients, but there are no data to support the routine use of antibiotics in patients with

Figure 36-36 A, The bite of a boa constrictor, though not poisonous, may contain small tooth fragments (**B**). As with cat and dog bites, radiographic evaluation is variable and exploration may be required.

Figure 36-37 Pyogenic granuloma. Despite their name, these lesions are neither pyogenic (i.e., infectious) nor granulomas. Rather, they are a type of hemangioma. Pyogenic granulomas can develop rapidly over a period of weeks and are common in pregnant women.

wounds that have been thoroughly cleaned and from which all foreign material has been extracted. Prophylaxis may be considered if there was excessive time between injury and removal or obvious contamination or when it is difficult to adequately clean the wound. Under these circumstances it is more prudent to opt for an open wound and delayed closure.

If prophylactic antibiotics are prescribed, a first-generation cephalosporin or penicillinase-resistant penicillin has traditionally been the first-line choice. In patients with contraindications to penicillins and cephalosporins and with the increasing incidence of community-acquired methicillin-resistant *S. aureus* in many areas, clindamycin, trimethoprim-sulfamethoxazole, or tetracycline may provide alternative coverage.[72] However, infections associated with FBs are not likely to be from methicillin-resistant *S. aureus*. Under certain circumstances, alternative antibiotics may be indicated. For infected plantar punctures through a shoe, a fluoroquinolone to cover *P. aeruginosa* is appropriate coverage, although most *Pseudomonas* infections are complex and may need extensive débridement and intravenous antibiotics. Saltwater marine FBs may be contaminated with *Vibrio* species, which are usually sensitive to tetracyclines, aminoglycosides, or third-generation cephalosporins. Freshwater FBs, on the other hand, are more likely to harbor *A. hydrophila*, which can be treted with tetracyclines.

FB Reactions

If the FB is not removed or cannot be removed, an FB reaction may occur. Some FBs produce an inflammatory reaction or infection a few days after introduction into the body. Other objects may not cause problems for weeks, months, or even years until they flare up for no apparent reason. The primary factors that affect the extent of tissue reactions are contamination and whether the material is inert or reactive with human tissue. Reactive FBs, such as wood, will always produce inflammation eventually, whereas inert FBs, such as bullets, rarely do. Some inert FBs carry dirt particles, pieces of clothing, or other sources of bacterial contamination. Expeditious removal may be necessary, even if the FB itself is relatively small and unlikely to cause a reaction.

A purulent bacterial infection may develop in the presence of any FB; therefore, any abscess or cellulitis that recurs or wounds that do not heal as expected should always be investigated for retained FBs.[73,74] Karpman and coworkers found a 15% rate of infection (*S. aureus* and Enterobacteriaceae) in a series of 25 patients treated for cactus thorn injuries on the extremities.[56] Certain thorns (black thorns, rose thorns), redwood and northwest cedar splinters, toothpicks, hair, and stingray or sea urchin spines are noted for their ability to initiate chronic FB reactions. Sea urchin spines and other marine FBs are covered with slime, calcareous material, and other debris that commonly initiate an FB granuloma. The inflammatory reaction seen with cactus thorns may be an allergic reaction to fungus found on the cactus plant.

Many FB reactions are thought to result from an inflammatory response to organic material, or they may represent infection from bacteria introduced at the time of the wound. Clinically evident reactions may be delayed for weeks or even years after injury (Fig. 36-40). The chronic infection or inflammatory reaction may not be accompanied by the production of pus, but it may be quite painful or result in loss of

Figure 36-38 A-D, Pyogenic granuloma removed by sharp dissection under ketamine anesthesia and primary suturing.

Figure 36-39 This child has multiple hair tourniquets compromising the circulation to two toes. The hairs are deeply embedded in the skin creases and cannot be visualized. An over-the-counter depilatory (such as Nair) smeared into the fold may dissolve the hair in 30 to 45 minutes, but if unsuccessful, an incision must be performed. The best way to ensure removal of the constriction is to cut the depth of the folds with a scalpel blade (using a dorsal incision to avoid the neurovascular bundle) and attempt to extricate individual fibers. A digital nerve block may be performed for anesthesia. Return of circulation should be obvious by the change in temperature and color in the affected digit or digits before it is assumed that all the fibers have been cut.

function. FBs may also be associated with the formation or development of a chronic pseudotumor, a sinus tract, or an osteomyelitis-like lesion of bone and soft tissue.[73] In addition, organic material has been noted to induce chronic tenosynovitis, chronic monarticular synovitis, and chronic bursitis.

Rapidly traveling projectiles with considerable inherent heat (e.g., bullets) are less likely to cause infection but are more apt to cause other difficulties. Damage to surrounding areas can occur during passage through tissue. Rarely do retained lead FBs, such as bullets or shotgun pellets, leach out lead into the general circulation and produce systemic lead poisoning unless they are in contact with synovium (Fig. 36-41). If this process does occur, it may take years to develop and can result in vague or nondescript symptoms (e.g., fatigue, arthralgia, headache, or abdominal pain) many years after the initial injury. Elevated blood lead levels are more likely to occur if body fluids such as joint, pleural, peritoneal, or cerebrospinal fluid bathe the lead. Bullets retained in muscle or other soft tissue are not likely to produce any sequelae related to their lead content. However, Farrell and colleagues reported unsuspected elevated lead levels in patients with retained lead fragments who were seen in the ED with a variety of complaints.[75] Lead levels of up to 50 μg/dL were reported. Levels greater than 45 μg/dL are generally considered an indication for chelation therapy. The relationship between the retained lead and the symptoms was unclear, but this report verifies the observations of others that retained lead FBs in selected areas can significantly elevate blood lead levels and may produce symptomatic plumbism.

Discharge Instructions

The patient should be informed that despite every effort there can be no absolute guarantee that all foreign material has been identified or extracted, regardless of whether some or any FB was removed during the initial exploration. Prudent clinicians should always suggest close follow-up and should leave open the option that an occult FB may still remain in the wound. Discharge instructions should also include the signs and

Figure 36-40 This foreign body (FB) granuloma developed after the FB was stable for 6 months. There was no gross infection and it was dissected en masse.

symptoms of problems related to retained material. Some centers routinely add this caveat on all discharge instructions to patients treated for lacerations or soft tissue defects. Assure patients that additional steps may be undertaken if foreign material is subsequently suspected.

Acknowledgment

The authors and editors wish to thank Ted Koutouzis and Matthew Levine for contributions to this chapter in previous editions

References are available at www.expertconsult.com

Figure 36-41 There is no need to routinely remove retained bullets. Most lead foreign bodies are well tolerated, but if a bullet is bathed in synovial, pleural, peritoneal, or cerebrospinal fluid (CSF), the lead may leach out over time and produce a significant elevation in blood lead levels. The symptoms are often vague, and the relationship between the retained lead and the patient's clinical scenario may be difficult to sort out. **A,** This patient had chronic neurologic findings, including wristdrop, and was wheelchair bound. **B,** The symptoms were due to chronic lead poisoning from a 20-year-old retained bullet (*arrows*) in or near the spinal canal, possibly being bathed by CSF. **C,** Note the lead lines in the gingiva, indicative of lead poisoning.

CHAPTER 37

Incision and Drainage

Liam C. Holtzman, Eveline Hitti, and Jeffrey Harrow

Incision and drainage (I&D) procedures in the emergency department (ED) are most commonly performed for soft tissue abscesses (Fig. 37-1).[1,2] The total number of ED visits increased from 90 million to 115 million over a 10-year period, with visits for abscess-related complaints increasing faster than overall ED visits.[3]

The emergence and predominance of methicillin-resistant *Staphylococcus aureus* (MRSA) as the cause of cutaneous abscesses during the past several decades have necessitated major revisions in long-standing guidelines for antibiotic administration. In light of this significant etiologic change, MRSA should be considered as a probable cause in most skin and soft tissue infections.

ABSCESS ETIOLOGY AND PATHOGENESIS

Localized pyogenic infections may develop in any region of the body. Abscesses generally begin as a localized superficial cellulitis. Some organisms cause necrosis and liquefaction, as well as the accumulation of leukocytes and cellular debris. This is followed by loculation and subsequent walling off of these products, all of which results in the formation of one or more abscesses. Any process or event that causes a breach in the skin's defensive epithelial barrier increases risk for the development of an abscess. The lymph tissues may be involved in this form of lymphangitis. Systemic signs of toxicity or fever suggest deeper tissue involvement, bacteremia, or both. As the process progresses, the area of liquefaction increases until it "points" and eventually ruptures into the area of least resistance. This may be toward the skin or the mucous membrane, into the surrounding tissues, or into a body cavity. If the abscess is particularly deep seated, spontaneous drainage may occur. In some cases a fistulous tract can arise and lead to the formation of a chronic draining sinus. This development—or the recurrence of an abscess that was previously drained—should broaden the etiologic differential. For example, recurrent abscesses in the perineal or lower abdominal area should raise suspicion for inflammatory bowel disease as the trigger, and recurring abscesses in the axilla or groin should raise the possibility of hidradenitis suppurativa. Chronic abscesses may also be associated with an immunocompromised state. Recurrent abscesses may suggest the possibility of a retained foreign body, underlying osteomyelitis, or the presence of an atypical or drug-resistant organism.

An abscess typically starts as a local superficial cellulitis. Various organisms that colonize normal skin can cause necrosis and liquefaction with subsequent accumulation of leukocytes and cellular debris. Loculation and subsequent walling off of these products lead to abscess formation. The cause of localized abscesses depends on the anatomic location, and they are usually caused by the flora indigenous to that area. Different organisms cause disease based on environmental exposure. For example, direct inoculation of extraneous organisms may occur during a mammalian bite (e.g., *Eikenella*, *Pasteurella*), exposure to saltwater (e.g., various *Vibrio* strains) or freshwater (e.g., *Aeromonas*), or meat or fish exposure (e.g., *Erysipelothrix rhusiopathiae*). *Pseudomonas* folliculitis has been associated with the use of whirlpools.[4]

Staphylococcal strains, which are normally found on the skin, produce rapid necrosis, early suppuration, and localized infections with large amounts of creamy yellow pus—the typical manifestation of an abscess. Conversely, group A β-hemolytic streptococcal infections tend to spread through tissues and cause a more generalized infection characterized by erythema, edema, a serous exudate, and little or no necrosis—typical manifestations of cellulitis. Anaerobic bacteria, which proliferate in the oral and perineal regions, produce necrosis with profuse brownish, malodorous pus[5] and may cause both abscesses and cellulitis.

Normal skin is extremely resistant to bacterial invasion, and few organisms are capable of penetrating intact epidermis. In a normal healthy host with intact skin, the topical application of even very high concentrations of pathogenic bacteria does not result in infection. The requirements for infection usually include a high concentration of pathogenic organisms, such as in hair follicles in the adnexa; occlusion of glands or other structures that prevent desquamation and normal drainage; a moist environment; adequate nutrients; and trauma to the corneal layer, which allows organisms to penetrate into deeper tissues.[6] Tissue perfusion may also play a role in the ability to prevent infection. Trauma may be the result of abrasions, shaving, insect bites, hematoma, injection of chemical irritants, incision, or occlusive dressings that macerate the skin. The presence of a foreign body can potentiate skin infections by enabling a lower number of bacteria to establish an infection. For example, abscesses occasionally develop at suture sites in otherwise clean wounds. In addition, abscesses can develop at any site used for body piercing. "High" ear piercings (through the cartilage of the pinna) seem to be at particular risk for infection because of the avascularity of auricular cartilage.[7]

When favorable factors are present, the normal flora that colonize cutaneous areas flourish and infect the skin and deeper structures. In persons performing manual labor, the arms and the hands are infected most frequently. In women, the axilla and submammary regions are frequently infected because of minor trauma from shaving, contact with garments, a moist environment, and an abundance of bacteria in these areas. Infections may develop anywhere on the body in intravenous (IV) drug users, although the upper extremities are most commonly affected.[8,9] Deep soft tissue abscesses can be caused by an addict's attempts to access deep venous structures when peripheral venous access sites are exhausted.[10] In addition, areas with compromised blood supply are more prone to infection because normal host defenses, including cell-mediated immunity, are less available.[7]

Bacteriology of Cutaneous Abscesses

Although most abscesses contain bacteria, 5% of abscesses are sterile, especially those associated with IV drug use. Clinically, sterile abscesses cannot be differentiated from those caused

Figure 37-1 Cutaneous soft tissue abscesses such as this are commonly encountered in the emergency department. Incision and drainage are required for definitive treatment; antibiotics alone are not sufficient. Readily drained abscesses do not benefit from antibiotics after incision, and the surrounding cellulitis of the abscess will be cured with incision and drainage alone. Multiple recurrent abscesses in the same area raise suspicion for a foreign body or underlying osteomyelitis.

by bacteria. Somewhat atypical abscesses develop in parenteral drug users. Injection of a cocaine-heroin mixture ("speedball") may predispose users to abscesses by inducing soft tissue ischemia.[11] Bergstein and coworkers[9] found anaerobes in 143 of 243 isolates from 57 drug-abusing patients. Abscesses at the site of injection tend to contain predominantly staphylococcal and streptococcal species. However, some drug users lubricate their hypodermic needles with saliva, which potentially explains the isolation of oral pathogens such as *Eikenella corrodens* from injection site abscesses.

The microbiology and the underlying cause of skin and soft tissue abscesses are related to their location. Abscesses involving the extremities are generally the result of a breach in the skin's integrity from trauma such as cuts, abrasions, or needle punctures. Abscesses involving the head, neck, and perineal region are usually associated with obstruction of the apocrine sweat glands. These types of abscesses increase in frequency after puberty because of the increased apocrine and sebaceous gland activity. Perirectal abscesses are typically the result of bacterial spread from adjacent anal glands. Vulvovaginal abscesses usually result from obstruction of a Bartholin gland, which then causes duct and gland edema and subsequent infection. Pilonidal abscesses are hypothesized to be caused by sacrococcygeal infections from ingrown hairs in the intergluteal cleft.

In 2002, Brook[12] compiled the findings from more than 15 bacteriologic studies of 676 polymicrobial abscesses. *S. aureus* and group A β-hemolytic streptococci were the most prevalent aerobes in skin and soft tissue abscesses and were isolated in specimens from all body sites. Gastrointestinal and cervical flora (enteric gram-negative bacilli and *Bacteroides fragilis*) were found most often in intraabdominal, buttock, and leg lesions. Group A β-hemolytic streptococci, pigmented *Prevotella*, *Porphyromonas* species, and *Fusobacterium* species—all normal residents of the oral cavity—were most commonly found in lesions of the mouth, head, neck, and fingers.

In a study of the bacteriology of cutaneous abscesses in children, Brook and Finegold[13] found aerobes (staphylococci

and group A β-hemolytic streptococci) to be the most common isolates from abscesses of the head, neck, extremities, and trunk, with anaerobes predominating in abscesses of the buttocks and perirectal sites. Mixed aerobic and anaerobic flora was found in the perirectal area, head, fingers, and nail bed. This study noted an unexpectedly high incidence of anaerobes in nonperineal abscesses. Anaerobes were found primarily in areas adjacent to mucosal membranes (e.g., the mouth), where these organisms tend to thrive, and in areas that are easily contaminated (e.g., by sucking fingers, which causes nail bed and finger infections or bite injuries).

If an unexpected or atypical organism is found in an abscess culture, the clinician should consider an underlying process not readily apparent from the history or physical examination. For example, tuberculosis or fungal isolates are sometimes found in immunocompromised patients (e.g., those with diabetes or acquired immunodeficiency syndrome). Finding *Escherichia coli* suggests an enteric fistula or even self-inoculation of feces in some patients with a psychiatric illness such as Munchausen's syndrome. Recurrent abscesses without an obvious underlying cause could indicate clandestine drug use. What appears to be a typical recurrent abscess may be a manifestation of an underlying septic joint, osteomyelitis, or rarely, metastatic or primary cancer (Fig. 37-2).

Special Considerations

Parenteral drug users, insulin-dependent diabetics, hemodialysis patients, cancer patients, transplant recipients, and individuals with acute leukemia have an increased frequency of abscess formation when compared with the general population. At initial evaluation the patient may emphasize an exacerbation of the underlying disease process or an unexplained fever, with symptoms of an abscess being a secondary complaint. In this situation, abscesses tend to have exotic or uncommon bacteriologic or fungal causes and typically respond poorly to therapy.[14-17] Patients with diabetes-induced ketoacidosis (DKA) should be evaluated extensively for an infectious process; a rectal examination should be included with the physical examination to rule out a perirectal abscess as the infectious trigger of DKA. This is also true for patients who are immunocompromised. There are several reasons why patients with diabetes and parenteral drug users are at increased risk for abscess formation: intrinsic immune deficiency, an increased incidence of staphylococcal carriage, potentially compromised tissue perfusion, and frequent needle punctures, which allow a mode of entry for pathogenic bacteria.[18]

Drug users frequently use veins in the neck and in the femoral areas, which can produce abscesses and other infectious complications at these sites.[19] Any abscess near a vein of the antecubital fossa or dorsum of the hand should alert the clinician to possible IV drug use; however, substance users may also inject directly into the skin ("skin popping"), which can cause cutaneous abscesses distant from veins (Fig. 37-3).

A foreign body may serve as a nidus for abscess formation. IV drug users frequently break needles off in skin that has been toughened by multiple injections, so the clinician should maintain a high index of suspicion for retained needle fragments. If an abscess is recurrent or if the patient is a known or suspected IV drug user, consider radiographs or other techniques to search for foreign bodies, an underlying septic joint, or osteomyelitis.[20] Ultrasound is also a useful adjunct to evaluate for foreign bodies that are not radiopaque.

Figure 37-2 *An abscess that appears in an atypical place or recurs after successful initial treatment should raise the possibility of rare or underlying conditions.* **A,** This patient had a large "abscess" on the lateral chest wall that initially drained unusual gelatinous material, not frank pus. **B,** At follow-up 3 days later, the abscess was much improved. The contents of the abscess had been sent for pathologic analysis because it had an unusual consistency, and a highly undifferentiated soft tissue malignancy was demonstrated. The fluid was sterile. Normally, analyzing or culturing the contents of an abscess will not yield helpful information, but in this case, the unusual consistency of the collection prompted further analysis. **C,** This intravenous drug user had an "abscess" of the chest wall drained in various emergency departments several times over a 2-month period, and it seemed to initially respond to drainage and antibiotics. He still had an area of cellulitis, minor fluctuance, and continued drainage near the center of the chest. This is an atypical place for a simple cutaneous abscess. Magnetic resonance imaging demonstrated osteomyelitis and an abscess of the sternoclavicular joint that was draining to the skin and simulating a recurrent cutaneous abscess. He required extensive surgical débridement and prolonged antibiotics. The etiologic organism was never ascertained, but *Pseudomonas* is often present. **D,** This patient underwent a sternotomy for bypass surgery a few months ago. She had been treated sporadically for a minor wound infection, but then a draining fluctuant mass developed at the inferior border of the sternum. This is the external manifestation of extensive sternal osteomyelitis.

MRSA

First acknowledged in the 1960s as a cause of infection in patients in health care settings, MRSA has now become the most common identifiable cause of community-acquired skin and soft tissue infections in many metropolitan areas in the United States. The spread of this organism is considered an epidemic, and it is a very virulent and aggressive.[21,22]

Virulent community-acquired MRSA (CA-MRSA) causes rapid and destructive soft tissue infection because of the presence of two bacterial toxins elaborated by the omnipresent VSA-300 and VSA-400 strains. Panton-Valentine leukocidin enhances tissue necrosis, and phenol-soluble modulin is toxic to neutrophils. A small pustule can become a large abscess in 24 to 48 hours (Fig. 37-4). Such lesions are often mistaken for a spider bite or drug use because of their rapid progression and seemingly spontaneous onset in an otherwise healthy person. Methicillin resistance is mediated by PBP-2a, a penicillin-binding protein encoded by the *mecA* gene that permits the organism to grow and divide in the presence of methicillin and other β-lactam antibiotics. *S. aureus* acquires methicillin resistance through a mobile staphylococcal cassette chromosome (SCC) that contains the *mecA* gene complex (SCCmec). MRSA probably arose as a result of antibiotic selective pressure.[23,24]

A single clone probably accounted for most MRSA isolates discovered during the 1960s; by 2004, six major MRSA clones had emerged.[25] The spread of resistance is thought to be mediated by horizontal transfer of the *mecA* gene and related regulatory sequences thereon.[26]

In 1980, the spread of MRSA from hospitals into communities became evident. More recently, community-acquired infections have occurred more frequently, even in people without known risk factors. These observations have led to the identification of some risk factors for CA-MRSA (Box 37-1), including skin trauma (e.g., lacerations, tattoos, IV and intradermal drug use, shaving), incarceration, shared razors or towels, and close contact with others colonized or infected with MRSA.[27-35] Animals can also carry MRSA and can function as a source of transmission.[36] Importantly, many patients with CA-MRSA have no identifiable risk factors for acquisition of the disease.[37]

Figure 37-3 This patient had a large abscess in the deltoid area (*arrow*) and could offer no explanation for it. This is a typical scenario for a drug user who injects directly into the skin. **B,** The characteristic circular skin lesion from "skin popping" found on the arms (*arrows*) confirmed the clinical suspicion. Even though a drug screen was positive for opioids, the patient denied drug use and attributed the leg lesions to frequent trauma on the job. Drug users with abscesses are at risk for numerous infections, including brain abscess, endocarditis, and occult osteomyelitis.

Figure 37-4 A-C, Examples of community-acquired methicillin-resistant *Staphylococcus aureus* (CA-MRSA) infections. These aggressive infections can spread rapidly. The patient frequently describes a small pustule that becomes an abscess in 24 to 48 hours. Patients often believe that it is a spider bite because of its rapid onset in an otherwise healthy person with no other reason for the lesion. A CA-MRSA abscess, though clinically aggressive, is usually treated like any other cutaneous abscess.

BOX 37-1   Risk Factors for Infection with MRSA

Contact sports	Invasive indwelling devices	Chronic illness
Previous antibiotic use	Mechanical ventilation	Previous isolation of MRSA
Day care attendance	Endotracheal tube	Sexual contact
Health care worker	Intravenous drug abuse	MRSA, methicillin-resistant *Staphylococcus*
Diabetes mellitus	Hemodialysis	*aureus.*
Hospitalization	Immunosuppression	

Based on Cohen PR, Grossman ME. Management of cutaneous lesions associated with an emergency epidemic: community-acquired methicillin-resistant Staphylococcus aureus *skin infections. J Am Acad Dermatol. 2004;51:132.*

CA-MRSA tends to be more virulent than health care–associated MRSA (HA-MRSA) and is associated with more frequent serious complications such as osteomyelitis, joint infections, sepsis, and death. However, these organisms fortunately tend to be susceptible to a broader array of antibiotics.[38]

The prevalence of MRSA has increased in both health care and community settings. For example, the prevalence of methicillin resistance among *S. aureus* isolates in intensive care units in the United States was 60%,[21] and more than 90,000 invasive infections by MRSA occurred in the United States in 2005.[39]

HA-MRSA and CA-MRSA differ with respect to their clinical epidemiology and molecular structures.

HA-MRSA is defined as MRSA infection that occurs following hospitalization (hospital onset, formerly "nosocomial") or MRSA infection that occurs outside the hospital within 12 months of exposure to a health care setting (e.g., history of surgery, hospitalization, dialysis, or residence in a long-term care facility—community onset instead of community acquired).[21]

HA-MRSA is usually associated with severe, invasive disease, including skin and soft tissue infection, bloodstream infection, and pneumonia.[6,40] In fact, *S. aureus* continues to be a significant cause of surgical site infections.[39] HA-MRSA strains tend to be resistant to multiple drugs. MRSA is one of the few pathogens routinely implicated in nearly every type of hospital-acquired infection. This is probably related in part to the organism's capacity for biofilm formation on indwelling lines and tubes in hospital settings.[24]

Biofilm facilitates survival and multiplication of MRSA on these surfaces, thereby prolonging the duration of exposure of the organism to antibiotics, as well as promoting the potential for the development of genetic resistance.[27]

CA-MRSA is defined as MRSA infection that occurs in the absence of health care exposure. It is often associated with skin and soft tissue infections in young, otherwise healthy individuals.[27]

Most CA-MRSA strains are sensitive to non–β-lactam antibiotics, although a multidrug-resistant isolate has been described in men who have sex with men.[41,42] This strain contains the pUSA03 plasmid and carries resistance genes for β-lactams, fluoroquinolones, tetracycline, macrolides, clindamycin, and mupirocin.

The CA-MRSA and HA-MRSA classifications are no longer distinct since MRSA colonization can develop in one realm and manifestations of infection in another. In the mid-2000s in San Francisco, the annual incidence of CA-MRSA surpassed that of HA-MRSA.[43]

Furthermore, community-onset HA-MRSA infections have been observed with increasing frequency. This was illustrated in a study of 209 patients discharged from hospitalized care; within 18 months following hospital discharge, 49% of new MRSA infections began outside the hospital.[44]

In another series of 102 patients with CA-MRSA infections, 29% had molecular typing consistent with HA-MRSA.[45]

CA-MRSA was initially reported in injection drug users in the early 1980s and has since become the most frequent cause of skin and soft tissue infections seen in U.S. EDs and ambulatory clinics. In an assessment of the prevalence of MRSA across the United States, Moran and colleagues[46] compiled data from adults who sought treatment of acute skin and soft tissue infections in EDs in 11 American cities in August 2004. *S. aureus* was isolated from three fourths of the 422 patients who met the study criteria. Seventy-eight percent of the *S. aureus* isolates were resistant to methicillin. MRSA was isolated from 59% of patients in the study. The prevalence of MRSA ranged from 15% to 74% in the participating EDs (Table 37-1). MRSA was the most common

TABLE 37-1 Bacterial Isolates from Purulent Skin and Soft Tissue Infections in U.S. EDs*

SITE	PATIENTS (N)	MRSA[†]	MSSA	OTHER BACTERIA[‡]	NO BACTERIAL GROWTH
Albuquerque	42	25 (60)	10 (24)	3 (7)	4 (10)
Atlanta	32	23 (72)	4 (12)	3 (9)	2 (6)
Charlotte	25	17 (68)	0	4 (16)	4 (16)
Kansas City, MO	58	43 (74)	6 (10)	4 (7)	5 (9)
Los Angeles	47	24 (51)	6 (13)	8 (17)	9 (19)
Minneapolis	28	11 (39)	4 (14)	9 (32)	4 (14)
New Orleans	69	46 (67)	11 (16)	9 (13)	3 (4)
New York	20	3 (15)	8 (40)	5 (25)	4 (20)
Philadelphia	58	32 (55)	12 (21)	12 (21)	2 (3)
Phoenix	30	18 (60)	8 (27)	4 (13)	0
Portland, OR	13	7 (54)	2 (15)	3 (23)	1 (8)

From Moran GJ, Krishnadasan A, Gorwitz RJ, et al, for the EMERGEncy ID Net Study Group. Methicillin-resistant *S. aureus* infections among patients in the emergency department. *N Engl J Med.* 2006;355:666-674.

ED, emergency department; *MRSA*, methicillin-resistant *Staphylococcus aureus*; *MSSA*, methicillin-susceptible *Staphylococcus aureus*.

*Thirty-one cultures, including 10 from which MRSA was isolated, were polymicrobial. Because of rounding, percentages may not total 100.

[†]*P* < 0.001 for the test for homogeneity of MRSA prevalence across sites.

[‡]Other bacterial isolates were as follows: MSSA (17%), *Streptococcus* species (7%), coagulase-negative staphylococci (3%), and *Proteus mirabilis* (1%).

identifiable cause of skin and soft tissue infections in all but one of the EDs.

Frazee and associates,[38] reporting from an ED in northern California, found that half of the 137 patients in their study were either infected with or colonized by MRSA. Three fourths of all *S. aureus* isolates were MRSA. In addition, 76% of cases met a strict clinical definition of CA-MRSA.

The incidence of CA-MRSA, genetically unrelated to nosocomial isolates, increased steadily from 1990 to 2001 and then dramatically in 2002 and each year thereafter.[47,48]

MRSA has also emerged as a potential sexually transmitted disease. Roberts and colleagues described their treatment of two patients who came to their urban ED with abscesses probably transmitted by heterosexual oral-genital contact. Both tested positive for MRSA.[22] A 2010 case report drew a similar conclusion. It reported orogenital transmission of MRSA to an immunocompetent 22-year-old man who tested orally positive for MRSA and group B (genital) *Streptococcus* after oral contact with a female partner in whom MRSA-positive gluteal lesions had previously been diagnosed.[48]

In a retrospective chart review, Roberts and colleagues found that 18% of the 524 subcutaneous abscesses treated in their urban ED in 2006 were confined to the genital area. Almost three fourths of the 272 outpatient wound cultures performed on that year's patient population were positive for MRSA.[22]

MANIFESTATIONS OF CUTANEOUS ABSCESSES

The diagnosis of cutaneous abscess formation is usually straightforward. The presence of a fluctuant mass in an area of induration, erythema, and tenderness is clinical evidence that an abscess exists (see Fig. 37-1). An abscess may appear initially as a definite tender soft tissue mass, but in some cases, a distinct abscess may not be readily evident. If the abscess is deep, as is true of many perirectal, pilonidal, and breast abscesses, the clinician may be misled by the presence of a firm, tender, indurated area without a definite mass. If the findings on physical examination are equivocal, needle aspiration or ultrasound examination may be performed to assist in the diagnosis.[49] This approach may also identify a mycotic aneurysm or an inflamed lymph node simulating an abscess. A specific entity commonly mistaken for a discrete abscess is the sublingual cellulitis of Ludwig's angina (see Chapter 64).

Parenteral injection of illicit drugs can produce simple cutaneous abscesses that unpredictably advance to extensive necrotizing soft tissue infections. The emergency clinician must maintain a high index of suspicion to avoid missing this potentially life-threatening condition.[8] Cellulitis and abscess formation can lead to bacteremia and sepsis, especially in immunocompromised patients.

The pain of an abscess often brings the patient to the hospital before it spontaneously ruptures, or the patient can have a draining abscess that appears to have undergone spontaneous rupture and is self-resolving. The patient may have punctured the abscess in an attempt to drain it. In most cases, a formal I&D and packing procedure will be necessary to eliminate the process, even though copious drainage may not be encountered. Although no formal drainage may be required after the spontaneous rupture of a simple cutaneous abscess, conditions such as a perirectal abscess, Bartholin gland abscess,

and breast abscess are usually best managed with further drainage and packing.

IMAGING

Ultrasound-Guided Needle Aspiration

Radiologists have performed needle aspiration of abscesses for some time, and emergency clinicians are now becoming more comfortable with the procedure. High-resolution ultrasound technology is being used to obviate "blind" procedures done in the ED (e.g., joint aspiration and central line placement).

For ultrasound-guided drainage of a cutaneous abscess, use a high-resolution probe (5 or 7.5 MHz), and maintain sterility throughout the procedure. Place the sterile transducer over the main body of the abscess, and insert the needle through the skin adjacent to the transducer. Adjust their relative relationships in keeping with the depth and location of the abscess cavity. Guide the needle—seen as a bright artifact—directly into the abscess. Watch the abscess cavity collapse as pus drains out. Scan the entire area of the suspected abscess to capture unexpected extensions. Be sure to drain all pockets.

LABORATORY FINDINGS

A complete blood count (CBC), blood cultures, and Gram stain are not standard or required for the treatment of straightforward cutaneous abscesses in the ED. Recommendations for culturing abscesses encountered in the ED are confusing, and clinical practice varies. Firm recommendations for the emergency clinician are difficult to standardize, partly because of insufficient data but also because the recommendations promulgated are not confined to ED abscess treatment. In addition, "complicated" and "uncomplicated" criteria are somewhat arbitrary. Traditionally, culturing the contents of a readily drainable cutaneous abscess was not indicated, nor standard. It simply provided no useful information to the clinician under most circumstances. Many clinicians still forgo *routine culturing*, even in the CA-MRSA milieu. Currently, there is no agreed on standard concerning routine culturing, and reasonable arguments can be made for a culture or no-culture approach to most abscesses treated in the ED. The authors support selective, not routine culturing but acknowledge that some now consider cultures to be indicated for all abscesses drained in the ED. A culture will potentially identify an unusual or resistant organism, especially if I&D is not curative. Culture will also permit identification of antibiotic susceptibility and assist in customization of antibiotic therapy. Cohort results also provide a framework for local epidemiology and resistance patterns. Culturing the abscess contents will distinguish between MRSA and nonresistant abscesses and will provide useful sensitivity information when managing complicated cases. Culturing should be performed for recurrent, unusual, or atypical abscesses. This information could be useful if the patient responds poorly to initial surgical drainage, if secondary spread of the infection occurs, or if bacteremia develops.[50,51] It also appears prudent to obtain cultures from abscesses and other purulent skin and soft tissue infections in patients already taking antibiotics, in immunosuppressed patients, in those with signs of systemic illness, in patients who have not responded adequately to initial

ULTRASOUND: Cellulitis and Abscesses

by Christine Butts, MD

Ultrasound offers a distinct advantage when evaluating a patient with suspected soft tissue infection and may change management. A recent study from *Academic Emergency Medicine* by Tayal and colleagues evaluated the effect of soft tissue ultrasound on the management of cellulitis in the emergency department.[1] The authors found that in patients with a low suspicion for abscess, ultrasound changed management in 56% of cases. Peritonsillar abscesses are difficult to diagnose from the physical examination alone, and some clinicians may feel hesitant to attempt blind drainage. Ultrasound of suspected peritonsillar abscesses has been found to be reliable in making the diagnosis. The overall size of the abscess, as well as its proximity to the carotid artery, can be evaluated with ultrasound, which will perhaps improve the confidence of the clinician in attempting drainage.[2,3]

General Considerations

Typically, a high-frequency (7.5 to 10 MHz) transducer should be used to evaluate the superficial soft tissues. The higher frequency will allow the clinician sufficient resolution to identify changes consistent with soft tissue infection. The entire area should be scanned in detail, in multiple planes, to identify fluid pockets. Surrounding structures in the area should also be evaluated , especially when incision and drainage are planned. When evaluating the posterior pharynx for a potential paratonsillar abscess, an intracavitary transducer should be used.

Normal Soft Tissue

Normal soft tissue is characterized by well-defined layers, with clear demarcation between these layers (Fig. 37-US1). The top of the screen corresponds to the most superficial soft tissue, including the epidermis and dermis. It should appear hyperechoic (light gray to white), thin, and clearly separate from the underlying layers. Subcutaneous tissue is found beneath the dermis and is of varying thickness. However, as with the most superficial layers, this layer should appear thin and well demarcated from the surrounding layers. Underneath the subcutaneous tissue, muscle will typically be seen as layers of striated tissue separated by bright layers of fascia.

Cellulitis

Cellulitis is recognized on ultrasound by thickening of the skin and subcutaneous layers (Fig. 37-US2). The tissue may also appear more hyperechoic than normal soft tissue. When a significant amount of edema is present within the tissue, bands of hypoechoic (dark gray) or anechoic (black) fluid may be seen within the area of thickened tissue. This is known as "cobblestoning" (Fig. 37-US3). Cobblestoning appears as thin bands of fluid throughout the tissue and can be distinguished from an abscess by the lack of a discrete fluid collection.

Abscess

An abscess is seen as a focal, discrete fluid collection within an area of cellulitis (Fig. 37-US4). The presence of surrounding cellulitis is the key to distinguishing an abscess from other fluid collections such as cysts.

Figure 37-US2 Ultrasound image of cellulitis. Thickening of subcutaneous tissue can be seen with loss of organized tissue planes. A small artifact is seen at the center of the image.

Figure 37-US1 Ultrasound image of normal soft tissue. In this image the tissue planes are clearly defined, with well-demarcated boundaries between the layers. This clean, organized appearance is lost with soft tissue edema and cellulitis.

Figure 37-US3 Ultrasound appearance of cobblestoning. Thickened subcutaneous tissue can be seen in this image with strands of hypoechoic (*dark gray*) fluid interwoven between the tissue (*arrow*). This interweaving gives the appearance of a "cobblestoned" street and is consistent with soft tissue edema.

Continued

ULTRASOUND: Cellulitis and Abscesses, cont'd

Figure 37-US4 Ultrasound appearance of an abscess. A large, well-contained hypoechoic (*dark gray*) fluid collection (*arrow*) can be seen surrounded by thickened subcutaneous tissue.

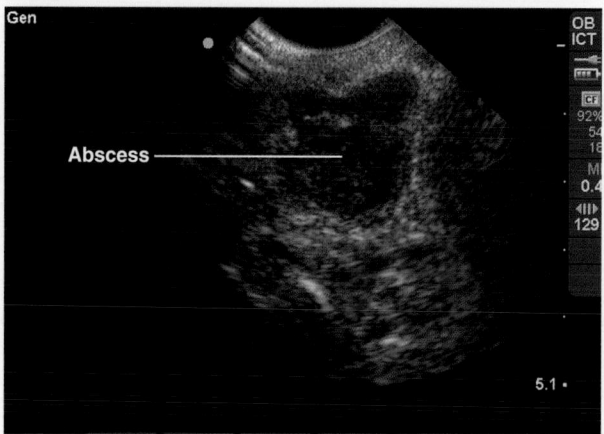

Figure 37-US5 Ultrasound image of a peritonsillar abscess. A rounded area of mixed density (both anechoic and hypoechoic areas) is seen in the center of the image.

The character of the fluid may be variable, depending on the content of the abscess. Collections that are completely fluid will appear as anechoic (black) areas, whereas areas with more solid components will appear to have "internal echoes" within the collections (Fig. 37-US5). Once a focal fluid collection has been located, it can be evaluated in detail to determine the overall size and depth from the surface. Peritonsillar abscesses appear as rounded hypoechoic (dark gray) to anechoic (black) collections of variable size. In addition to confirming the presence of an abscess, the location and depth of the carotid artery can also be judged before an attempt at aspiration.

REFERENCES:

1. Tayal VS, Hasan N, Norton HJ, et al. The effect of soft-tissue ultrasound on the management of cellulitis in the emergency department. *Acad Emerg Med.* 2006;13:384-388.
2. Blaivas M, Theodoro D, Duggal S. Ultrasound-guided drainage of peritonsillar abscess by the emergency physician. *Am J Emerg Med.* 2003;21:155-158.
3. Lyon M, Blaivas M. Intraoral ultrasound in the diagnosis and treatment of suspected peritonsillar abscess in the emergency department. *Acad Emerg Med.* 2005;12:85-88.

treatment, if there is concern for a cluster or outbreak of infection, or in patients with severe local infection.[51] Severe local infection can be defined as an abscess larger than 5 cm in diameter, multiple lesions, or extensive surrounding cellulitis. However, the degree of surrounding cellulitis qualifying as "extensive" is ill defined.

When obtaining a specimen for culture, the most accurate and complete culture results will be obtained if one aspirates pus with a needle and syringe before I&D. The material should be cultured for aerobic and anaerobic bacteria. Most clinicians, however, still culture free-flowing purulent material obtained with a cotton swab during I&D. For uncomplicated ED abscesses, this culture technique is standard and adequate to isolate aerobic organisms, including MRSA. A "sterile" culture from a specimen collected with a standard cotton swab after incision is frequently the result of improper anaerobic culture technique. In selected patients, such as immunocompromised hosts or IV drug users, isolation of possible anaerobic organisms by needle aspiration with a syringe through appropriately cleaned (e.g., with chlorhexidine) skin before I&D will enhance the results of culture and can add information that may be clinically relevant to subsequent therapy. There is a general misconception that foul-smelling pus is a result of *E. coli*. This foul odor is actually caused by the presence of anaerobes; the pus associated with *E. coli* is odorless.

The discovery of solid or suspicious material in an abscess should prompt histologic evaluation since a malignancy may mimic cutaneous abscesses (see Fig. 37-2*A* and *B*).

The majority of patients with an uncomplicated cutaneous abscess will have a normal CBC and will not experience fever, chills, or malaise. Therefore, in the absence of extenuating circumstances, it is not standard to analyze blood from patients with typical cutaneous abscesses because laboratory test results do not lead to a specific therapeutic path. An abscess may produce leukocytosis, depending on the severity and duration of the purulent process; however, *the presence or absence of leukocytosis has virtually no diagnostic or therapeutic implications.* Bacteremia may occasionally be manifested as a peripheral abscess resulting from septic emboli, and it usually produces clinical characteristics dissimilar to those associated with cutaneous abscesses. A cutaneous abscess itself rarely produces bacteremia.

Gram stain is neither indicated nor standard in the care of uncomplicated simple abscesses. However, patients who appear "toxic" or immunocompromised and those who require prophylactic antibiotics (see the section "Prophylactic Antibiotics" later in this chapter) may benefit from Gram stain in addition to cultures. Gram stain results have been shown to correlate well with subsequent culture results, so in compromised hosts the test can be used to direct the choice of antibiotic therapy. Anaerobic infections should be suspected when multiple organisms are noted on Gram stain, when a foul odor is associated with the purulence, when free air is noted on radiographs of the soft tissue, and when no growth is reported on cultures.[12]

INDICATIONS FOR AND CONTRAINDICATIONS TO I&D

Surgical I&D is the definitive treatment of a soft tissue abscess[52]; antibiotics alone are often inadequate. Drainage of a suppurative focus generally results in marked resolution of the symptoms in most uncomplicated cases. In the initial stages, only induration and inflammation may be found in an area destined to produce an abscess. Premature incision, before localization of pus, will not be curative and may theoretically be deleterious because extension of the infectious process and, rarely, bacteremia can result from manipulation. In some cases, the application of heat to an area of inflammation may ease the pain, speed resolution of the cellulitis, and facilitate the localization and accumulation of pus. Nonsurgical methods are not a substitute for surgical drainage and should not be continued for more than 24 to 36 hours before the patient is reevaluated.

PROPHYLACTIC AND THERAPEUTIC ANTIBIOTIC THERAPY

The utility of antibiotics remains unproven for prophylaxis against and for treatment of uncomplicated and adequately drained cutaneous abscesses in immunocompetent hosts. For simple abscesses, I&D alone is likely to be quite adequate and curative, even if the causative organism is MRSA. Routine administration of antibiotics after I&D is not currently standard, although the topic is subject to ongoing investigations. Simply stated, drainage alone for uncomplicated abscesses is usually curative.

Furthermore, the use of antibiotics may in fact be harmful. Antibiotic misuse has also been shown to complicate resistance patterns, both in general and in specific patients.

Even though no randomized controlled trial data definitively demonstrate the need for antibiotic therapy in conjunction with I&D of uncomplicated cutaneous abscesses in healthy, immunocompetent patients (without the specific types of valvular heart disease discussed below), there is strong consensus for antibiotic treatment of abscesses associated with the following conditions: severe or extensive disease (e.g., involving multiple sites of infection) or rapid progression in the presence of associated cellulitis, signs and symptoms of systemic illness, associated comorbid conditions, immunosuppression, extremes of age, abscess in an area difficult to drain (e.g., face, hand, and genitalia), associated septic phlebitis, and lesions that are unresponsive to I&D alone.

Antibiotic use is indicated for abscesses with associated severe cellulitis (not well defined and generally a clinical judgement) and those with *purulent cellulitis*. Purulent cellulitis is defined as cellulitis associated with purulent drainage or exudate in the absence of a drainable abscess. Purulent cellulitis is usually caused by MRSA. Nonpurulent cellulitis, defined as cellulitis with no purulent drainage or exudate and no associated abscess, is usually due to β-hemolytic streptococci. Empirical therapy for MRSA pending culture results is recommended for patients who have failed non-MRSA treatment, for those with a previous history of or risk factors for MRSA, and for those with severe infection or systemic signs and symptoms. Empirical therapy for infection with β-hemolytic streptococci is likely to be unnecessary under these circumstances.

The duration of therapy for skin and soft tissue infections has not been well defined, although no differences in outcome were observed in adult patients with uncomplicated cellulitis receiving 5 versus 10 days of therapy in a randomized, controlled trial.[53] In the Food and Drug Administration licensing trials for complicated skin and soft tissue infections, patients were typically treated for 7 to 14 days. However, in the outpatient setting of uncomplicated infections, 3 to 5 days of antibiotic therapy is reasonable but should be individualized on the basis of the patient's clinical condition and response to treatment. Accordingly, a return wound inspection or primary care follow-up is an important component of the care plan.

IV drug users with an abscess and fever require parenteral antibiotic therapy after blood has been drawn for culture until bacterial endocarditis can be ruled out.[50] Additionally, patients who have extensive cellulitis or are clinically septic require immediate IV antibiotics, as well as aggressive surgical drainage of pus. By administering IV ampicillin/sulbactam (2 g/1 g) every 6 hours, Talan and colleagues[51] achieved 100% eradication of pathogens from major abscesses in hospitalized IV drug users and non–drug users.

Therapeutic Antibiotics

In contrast to prophylaxis before surgery, the routine use of therapeutic oral antibiotics after I&D of simple cutaneous abscesses in otherwise healthy patients who are not immunocompromised appears to have no value, and their empirical use cannot be scientifically supported. Llera and Levy[52] performed a randomized, double-blind study to compare the outcomes of patients treated with a first-generation cephalosporin after the drainage of cutaneous abscesses in the ED with those who received placebo. They found no significant difference in clinical outcome between the two groups and concluded that antibiotics are unnecessary for abscesses in individuals with normal host defenses. This is in agreement with several previous studies.[54-56] It should be noted that high-risk patients were often excluded from these studies. Immunocompromised patients have not been adequately studied in this situation and are therefore often given antibiotics empirically, but this practice, though common, has not been supported by rigorous prospective studies.

For empirical coverage of CA-MRSA in outpatients with skin and soft tissue infection, oral antibiotic options include the following: clindamycin, trimethoprim-sulfamethoxazole (TMP-SMX), a tetracycline (doxycycline or minocycline), and linezolid. If coverage of both β-hemolytic streptococci and CA-MRSA is desired, options include the following: clindamyacin alone or the use of TMP-SMX or a tetracycline in combination with a β-lactam (e.g., amoxicillin or cephalexin), or linezolid alone. The use of rifampin as a single agent or as adjunctive therapy for the treatment of skin and soft tissue infections is not recommended.

Facial abscesses should be handled cautiously and checked frequently. Any abscess above the upper lip and below the brow may drain into the cavernous sinus, so manipulation may predispose to septic thrombophlebitis of this system.

Treatment with antistaphylococcal antibiotics and warm soaks after I&D has been recommended pending resolution of the process. Areas not in this zone of the face can be treated in a manner similar to that used for other cutaneous abscesses.

A relatively unstudied but a common and currently accepted strategy for patients with soft tissue infections (especially CA-MRSA infections) that are borderline, by clinical judgment, for hospital admission and therapeutic IV antibiotics is to administer a single dose of an IV antibiotic in the ED, followed by oral antibiotics and close outpatient follow-up. When a CA-MRSA infection is likely, IV vancomycin or linezolid is a reasonable option. Oral linezolid may be as effective as the IV form.

Prophylactic Antibiotics

Prophylaxis for Endocarditis

The precise risk for endocarditis after I&D of a cutaneous abscess remains unknown, and it is difficult to predict in which patients an infection will develop and which particular therapeutic procedures subject the patient to the highest risk for infection. However, bacteremia clearly occurs with manipulation of infected tissue, and mortality rates are substantial for MRSA-associated endocarditis (30% to 37%).[57,58]

Given this risk, it is reasonable that patients at highest risk for cardiac complications related to transient bacteremia be pretreated with appropriate antibiotics within 1 hour preceding the procedure.[59-61]

Guidelines issued by the American Heart Association (AHA) in 2007 recommend antibiotic prophylaxis for procedures involving the respiratory tract or involving infected skin or musculoskeletal tissue only in patients with cardiac conditions that carry the highest risk for an adverse outcome from infective endocarditis.[60] These conditions are listed in Box 37-2. Most skin infections are polymicrobial, but only staphylococci and β-hemolytic streptococci are likely to cause

---

BOX 37-2 Cardiac Conditions with the Highest Risk for Adverse Outcome from Endocarditis

Prosthetic cardiac valve
Previous infective endocarditis
Congenital heart disease (CHD)*
  Unrepaired cyanotic CHD, including palliative shunts and conduits
  Completely repaired congenital heart defect with prosthetic material or a device, whether placed via surgery or catheter intervention, during the first 6 months after the procedure†
  Repaired CHD with residual defects at the site of or adjacent to the site of a prosthetic patch or prosthetic device (which inhibits endothelialization)
Cardiac transplantation with the development of cardiac valvulopathy

From Wilson W, Taubert KA, Gewitz M, et al. Prevention of infective endocarditis. Circulation. 2007;116:1736.
*Except for the conditions listed previously, antibiotic prophylaxis is no longer recommended for any other form of CHD.
†Prophylaxis is recommended because endothelialization of prosthetic material occurs within 6 months after the procedure.

---

infective endocarditis. Therefore, the therapeutic regimen should include an agent active against these organisms, such as an antistaphylococcal penicillin or a cephalosporin. For patients who cannot tolerate a β-lactam or if MRSA is suspected, vancomycin or clindamycin can be substituted.

Two clinical situations deserve special mention. First, because of the frequent incidence of valvular damage in IV drug users, prophylactic antibiotics may be indicated before I&D of abscesses in these patients; however, no standards exists. It is prudent to inquire about previous endocarditis or auscultate for a heart murmur if IV drug abuse is suspected or known and administer antibiotics under these circumstances. Second, any patient with a documented history of endocarditis must receive prophylactic antibiotics before the I&D procedure.

Cutaneous abscesses may result from active endocarditis and prophylactic antibiotics may obscure subsequent attempts to identify the causative organism. With this in mind, two or three blood cultures (aerobic and anaerobic) should be considered before antibiotic therapy for those at risk for endocarditis. Patients with a diagnosis of mitral valve prolapse have traditionally been included for treatment with prophylactic antibiotics, but the indication for this is unclear, and antibiotic prophylaxis for uncomplicated mitral valve prolapse is no longer part of the AHA guidelines.[62]

Kaye[63] suggested prophylaxis only for patients who have a holosystolic murmur secondary to mitral valve prolapse.

Prophylaxis for Bacteremia in Other Conditions

Conflicting results have been reported from the few studies investigating the relationship between I&D of cutaneous abscesses and bacteremia. For example, in 1985 Fine and associates[64] concluded that I&D of cutaneous abscesses is often accompanied by transient bacteremia. They compared blood culture results from specimens obtained before and at 1, 5, and 20 minutes after I&D procedures in 10 patients with soft tissue infections. None of the cultures of blood obtained before I&D were positive; however, six patients had at least one positive culture after the procedure. Eleven of the 30 postprocedure cultures yielded growth. In contrast, in 1997 Bobrow and coworkers[65] concluded that I&D of a localized cutaneous abscess is unlikely to result in transient bacteremia in afebrile adults. Their study included 50 patients with localized cutaneous abscesses. Blood samples were collected before and at 2 and 10 minutes after I&D. In addition, specimens from the wound were collected after drainage. None of the blood cultures were positive, even though 64% of the wound cultures were positive, primarily for *S. aureus*. Bobrow and coworkers[65] noted that prophylactic antibiotics should be given to patients at high risk for bacterial endocarditis. In a discussion of the differences between these findings and those reported by Fine and associates,[64] Bobrow and coworkers[65] noted that Fine and associates' cultures were obtained from indwelling, heparinized IV catheters, a practice that allows ample opportunity for contamination. Furthermore, half the patients in Fine's group had perirectal abscesses, and if these abscesses involved mucosal surfaces, the risk for bacteremia was potentially increased.[64]

Immunocompromised patients may benefit from the prophylactic administration of antibiotics in preparation for I&D of cutaneous lesions. In contrast to patients with risks for endocarditis, immunocompromised patients are at risk for septicemia secondary to brief bacteremia. IV drug users have a high incidence of diseases associated with human immunodeficiency virus (HIV),[61,66,67] and the treating clinician must anticipate various degrees of immunodeficiency among them. Because no specific standard of care exists, clinical judgment must guide the use of antibiotics in these situations.

No specific guidelines have been offered for the antibiotic regimen to be used before I&D of infected cutaneous tissue in patients at risk for conditions other than endocarditis. The choice of antimicrobial agent is based on the organism anticipated to cause the bacteremia. Although the location of the abscess will give some clue to the organism involved, most abscesses contain multiple strains of bacteria. Not all bacteria are potent pathogens, so their mere presence does not predict their role in subsequent morbidity. Because *Staphylococcus* continues to be the most common cause of cutaneous abscesses, a broad-spectrum antistaphylococcal drug is indicated. Prophylaxis can consist of a single IV dose given half an hour before I&D. A first-generation cephalosporin or penicillinase-resistant penicillin is a good initial choice. Vancomycin may also be considered. Others may prefer cefazolin (Ancef, Kefzol), 1 g intravenously, for adults. This regimen covers staphylococcal and streptococcal species, many gram-negative organisms, and many anaerobes.

Although it has not been studied, it is reasonable to also give antibiotics before I&D to all patients who will subsequently be administered therapeutic antibiotics. The ideal duration of therapeutic antibiotics is unknown. As a general guideline, immunocompromised patients should receive antibiotics for 5 to 7 days and immunocompetent patients for 3 to 5 days after the procedure, depending on the severity of the condition and their clinical response at follow-up.

RECURRENT INFECTIONS

The first-line approach to the prevention of recurrent soft tissue infections is education regarding personal hygiene and appropriate wound care. Patients should be directed to keep wounds covered with clean, dry bandages. Maintain good personal hygiene with regular bathing and frequent hand washing with soap and water or an alcohol-based hand gel, especially after touching the wound or items that came in contact with the wound. Avoid reusing or sharing personal items that have contacted the infected area.

Environmental hygiene measures should be considered in patients with recurrent skin and soft tissue infections in the household or community setting. Focus cleaning efforts on high-traffic surfaces (i.e., surfaces that come in frequent contact with skin each day, such as counters, door knobs, and toilet seats) that may contact bare skin or uncovered infections.

An approach to individual treatment of recurrent CA-MRSA soft tissue infections is outlined in Box 37-3.

Oral antimicrobial therapy is recommended for the treatment of active infection only and is not routinely recommended for decolonization. In the case of multiple recurrent infections, consider infectious disease expert consultation.

I&D PROCEDURE

Procedure Setting

Definitive I&D of soft tissue abscesses is performed in either the ED or the operating room (OR). When abscesses are drained in the ED, some centers prefer to use a special area to avoid contamination of general treatment rooms, but protocols vary greatly.

The choice of the locale for the procedure depends on a number of important factors. The location of the abscess may dictate management in the OR. Large abscesses or abscesses located deep in soft tissues require a procedure involving a great degree of patient cooperation, which might be achieved only under general or regional anesthesia. Proximity to major neurovascular structures, such as in the axillae or antecubital fossa, may necessitate specific management. Infections of the hand (with the exception of distal finger infections) have traditionally been managed in the OR because of the many important structures involved and the propensity for limb-threatening complications.

Lack of adequate anesthesia is the most common factor limiting I&D in the ED. The current increased use of ED procedural sedation (see Chapter 33) has changed previous OR cases to ones that can be managed well in the ED. If the clinician believes that the abscess cannot be fully incised and drained because of inadequate anesthesia, the patient should

---

BOX 37-3 **Strategies to Eradicate CA-MRSA Carrier States in Patients with Recurrent CA-MRSA Soft Tissue Infections**

Recurrent community-acquired methicillin-resistant *Staphylococcus aureus* (CA-MRSA) soft tissue infections have been linked to a carrier state in affected individuals, with the nose and skin being areas colonized. It may be difficult to totally or permanently eradicate colonization, and there are no proven methods to accomplish this. The following strategies have been used in an attempt to eradicate the carrier state in individuals with recurrent CA-MRSA soft tissue infections. The appropriate time to implement these procedures is not known, but it would be reasonable to institute first-line techniques if more than two to three episodes of proven CA-MRSA infection are documented.

FIRST LINE

Apply 1 cm of mupirocin (Bactroban) ointment (an intranasal form is available) to the anterior nares three times a day for 7 days,* plus

Daily total body wash with (4%) chlorhexidine (Hibiclens) for 5 to 7 days.†

SECOND LINE

Obtain specimens for culture to ascertain sensitivity to various antibiotics.

Repeat mupirocin and chlorhexidine as above.

Rifampin, 300 mg twice a day, *plus*, if sensitivities dictate, trimethoprim-sulfamethoxazole DS or doxycycline (100 mg) twice a day for 1 to 2 weeks.‡

Note: For multiple recurrent infections, consider consultation with an infectious disease expert.

*May cause burning, pruritus, dry membranes, and erythema. Avoid long-term use. Do not substitute bacitracin.
†May cause skin and eye irritation. Apply for 5 minutes and then rinse thoroughly.
‡Do not use rifampin alone since resistance may develop. It can cause an orange color of urine and tears and stain contact lenses. Adjust the dose for patients with renal impairment. Do not use in those with impaired hepatic function.

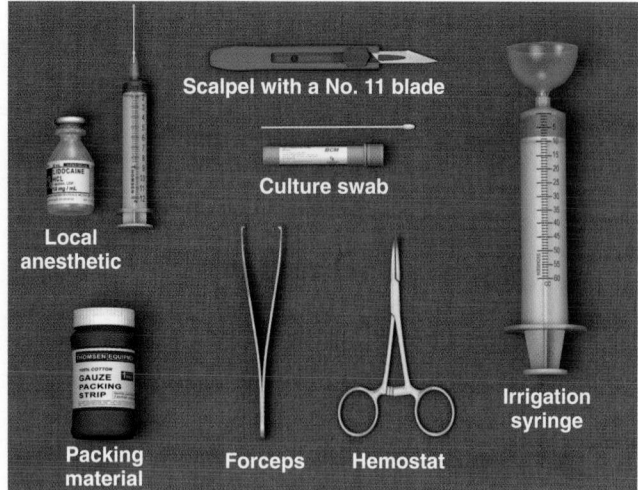

Figure 37-5 Equipment required for incision and drainage. Most items can be found in a routine suture kit. The scalpel, culture swab, and packing material need to be gathered separately.

be taken to the OR for management under general anesthesia. In addition to limiting proper drainage, it is inhumane and unethical to subject a patient to extreme pain when alternatives are available.

Equipment and Anesthesia

A standard suture tray provides adequate instruments if a scalpel and packing material are added (Fig. 37-5). Although sterility is impossible during the procedure, one should avoid contamination of surrounding tissue. Some clinicians prefer to use an obligatory skin scrub with an antiseptic solution, but the value of this step is dubious. Most clinician use nonsterile gloves while draining pus, but practice varies.

It is often quite difficult to achieve local anesthesia by direct infiltration because of the poor function of local anesthetic agents in the low pH of infected tissue. Furthermore, distention of sensitive structures by a local injection is quite painful and hence poorly tolerated by most patients. Skin anesthesia is usually possible, but total anesthesia of the abscess cavity itself cannot generally be achieved. If a regional block can be performed (see Chapters 30, 31, and 32), this type of anesthesia is preferred. Alternatively, a field block may be used. It should be noted that infected tissue is very vascular and local anesthetics are therefore absorbed quickly. Strict adherence to maximum safe doses of local anesthetics is required.

The skin over the dome of an abscess is often quite thin, thus making skin anesthesia difficult. If a 25-gauge needle is used carefully, one can frequently inject the dome of the abscess subcutaneously. Without moving the tip of the needle, the anesthetic solution spreads over the dome through the subcutaneous layers into the surrounding skin and provides excellent skin anesthesia. If the needle is in the proper plane (best accomplished by holding the syringe parallel rather than perpendicular to the skin), the surrounding skin blanches symmetrically during infiltration without having to reposition the needle (Fig. 37-6, *step 2*). In an extremely anxious or uncomfortable patient, judicious use of preoperative sedation (see Chapter 33) with IV opioids and sedatives or with nitrous oxide makes the procedure easier for both the patient and

clinician. Ketamine, propofol, or a combination of these drugs is a popular option in the ED setting.

Some clinicians recommend the use of topical ethyl chloride or Fluori-Methane spray for the initial skin incision, but although this is an attractive concept to patients, the pain relief offered by these agents is variable and fleeting. Ethyl chloride is also highly flammable. These vapocoolant sprays may be useful to provide momentary anesthesia for injection of a local anesthetic or for the initial skin incision if the injection or incision is made immediately after blanching of the skin. In general, however, these agents are of minimal benefit as a stand-alone anesthetic agent for all but the smallest of superficial abscesses (e.g., purulent folliculitis).

Incision

One should make all incisions conform with skin creases or natural folds to minimize visible scar formation (Fig. 37-7). Care should be taken in areas such as the groin, the posterior aspect of the knee, the antecubital fossa, and the neck so that vascular and neural structures are not damaged.

A No. 11 or 15 scalpel blade, held perpendicular to the skin, is used to nick the skin over the fluctuant area, and then a simple linear incision is carried the total length of the abscess cavity (see Fig. 37-6, *step 3*). This will afford more complete drainage and facilitate subsequent breakup of loculations. *Attempting to drain an abscess with an inadequate incision is counterproductive and makes packing changes more difficult.* A cruciate or X-shaped incision and an elliptical skin excision are to be avoided in the routine treatment of cutaneous abscesses. The tips of the flaps of a cruciate incision may necrose and result in an unsightly scar (Fig. 37-8). A timid "stab" incision may produce pus but is not generally adequate for proper drainage. The scalpel is used only to make the skin incision and is not used deep in the abscess cavity.

Exceptions to the rule regarding aggressive incision are abscesses in cosmetic areas, in areas under significant skin tension (e.g., extensor surfaces), and in areas with extensive scar tissue (e.g., sites of multiple previous drainage procedures). In these special circumstances, a stab incision or simple aspiration alone may be attempted initially, with the goal of limiting tissue injury and resultant scar formation. Use of this less aggressive approach requires that the patient be counseled that multiple decompressions (e.g., via needle aspiration) or delayed aggressive I&D may be required. The abscess will need to be reassessed in 24 to 48 hours to determine whether additional intervention is needed.

Wound Dissection

Following a standard incision, the operator should probe the depth of an abscess to assess its extent and ensure proper drainage by breaking open loculations (see Fig. 37-6, *step 5*). An ideal instrument for this procedure is a hemostat, optionally wrapped in gauze (or a cotton swab for small abscesses), which is placed into the abscess cavity and spread and manipulated throughout the cavity (Fig. 37-9). Traditionally, the operator's gloved finger has been suggested as an ideal way to assess the depth of the abscess cavity and to break up loculations, but this is a potentially dangerous practice that should be avoided unless it is certain that the abscess contains no sharp foreign body. Of particular concern is an abscess caused by skin-popping of IV drugs. These abscesses occasionally

INCISION AND DRAINAGE

Identify and confirm the location of the abscess. This patient has a pilonidal abscess, which is found at the superior portion of the gluteal cleft.

Anesthetize the region. Use a 25-gauge needle to inject the dome of the abscess. Hold the needle parallel to the skin during injection. Blanching will occur as the anesthetic spreads.

Use an 11-blade scalpel to make a linear incision over the total length of the abscess cavity. If possible, the incision should conform to skin creases or natural folds.

Culture the purulent drainage.

Probe the depth of the abscess and use a hemostat to break open loculations. This can be painful; inject additional anesthetic if needed through the cut skin edges and into the deeper tissues.

Irrigate the abscess cavity to assist with removal of residual debris.

Loosely pack the abscess cavity with gauze wick. The purpose of the packing is to keep the incision open, which allows continued drainage of the cavity. Avoid overpacking the abscess.

Place an absorbent gauze dressing over the packed abscess. Arrange for follow-up care, which usually entails a repeat exam in 1 to 3 days.

Figure 37-6 Incision and drainage. Routine culturing and irrigation are optional and left to the discretion of the clinician.

Figure 37-7 Relationship of the elective lines of tension in the face to the underlying mimetic musculature. Only in the lower eyelid are these lines not perpendicular to the muscles. The *left side* of the drawing shows the use of this principle when common facial lesions are excised or a facial abscess is drained. *(From Schwartz SI, Lillehei RC, eds.* Principles of Surgery. *2nd ed. New York: McGraw-Hill; 1974. Reproduced with permission.)*

harbor broken needle fragments (see Fig. 37-9D and E). In addition, patients who engage in this practice have a high incidence of hepatitis and HIV infection. Clinicians are often surprised at the depth or extent of abscesses discovered during probing. Sharp curettage of the abscess cavity is not usually required and may produce bacteremia. Although tissue probing is generally the most painful aspect of the technique and total local anesthesia is difficult to attain, this portion of the procedure should not be abbreviated. If pain persists,

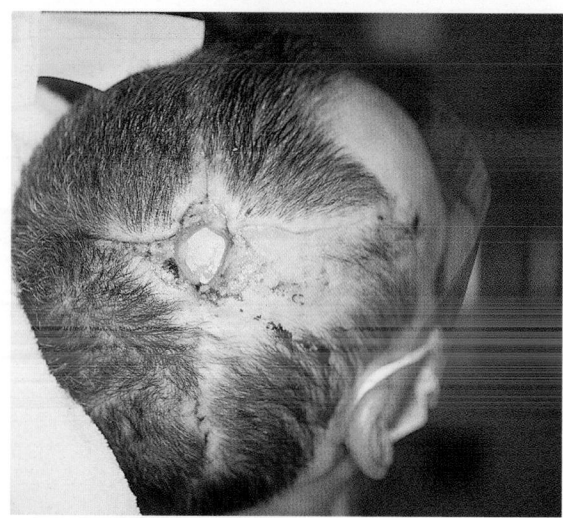

Figure 37-8 A simple linear incision is preferred over an X-shaped or crosshatched incision. In this case a cutaneous postsurgical scalp abscess was drained by an X incision and the tips of the flap necrosed, which left a slowly healing, full-thickness wound.

Figure 37-9 Options for wound dissection. **A,** A hemostat wrapped with gauze is an ideal instrument to break up loculations. **B,** Alternatively, cotton-tipped swabs can be used. **C,** Traditionally, fingers have been used to identify and open the cavity. However, this practice must be avoided if there is any chance of a foreign body. **D** and **E,** This intravenous drug user had an abscess (*arrow*) in the antecubital fossa. After the incision, the clinician attempted to break up the loculations with his finger. When a radiograph was obtained, three needle fragments (*arrows*) were found embedded in the wound. The patient was positive for human immunodeficiency virus and claimed no knowledge of the presence of the needles. Instead of using a finger, break up loculations with an instrument.

additional local anesthetic can be *administered through the cut skin edges* and into deeper tissues to provide additional anesthesia (Fig. 37-10*A*). If the procedure is limited because of pain, use of appropriate analgesia or anesthesia is mandated. Failure to adequately pack the abscess on the first visit makes follow-up packing changes more problematic.

A blunt-ended suction device can be used to extract copious pus from large or deep abscesses while also assisting in breakup of loculations (see Fig. 37-10*B*).

Wound Irrigation

Following the breakup of loculations, some clinicians advocate copious irrigation of the abscess cavity with normal saline to ensure adequate removal of debris from the wound cavity (see Fig. 37-6, *step 6*). Though intuitively beneficial, irrigation of the abscess cavity is not universal and has not been experimentally demonstrated to significantly augment healing or affect outcome. Hyperemic tissue may bleed profusely, but the bleeding usually stops in a few minutes if packing is used.

Figure 37-10 A, If pain persists while an abscess is being drained, pull the skin open and inject additional anesthetic into the subcutaneous tissue under direct vision. **B,** This large abscess is draining copious pus. A tonsil suction device is used to both break up loculations and extract pus. Note the copious pus in the tubing (*arrows*).

Abscesses of the extremities can be drained with the use of a tourniquet to provide a bloodless field.

Packing and Dressing

Multiple studies, most from countries outside the United States, suggest that *primary suture closure* of incised and drained abscesses results in faster healing than after packing and secondary closure and in similar low abscess recurrence rates. Many of the reported cases involved abscesses in the anogenital region, a site teeming with bacteria. Acute superficial abscesses can be cured with incision, curettage, and *primary suture closure* without antibiotics or packing, which is safe and cost-effective. This clinical approach is not currently in wide practice in the United States.

Although the specific technique and the clinical value of routine packing of abscesses have not been well studied, packing is a traditional intervention and is often performed in the ED. Some, however, advocate that packing is not needed nor beneficial for easily drained abscesses, and the intervention adds to cost and patient discomfort. As noted above, some advocate curettage and irrigation of the abscess cavity and then primary suture closure, without packing. Overall, it appears reasonable to avoid packing of small, easily drained abscesses. The loop drainage technique described below is evidence that formal packing is not a prerequisite for abscess healing. Hence, clinical judgment, common sense, and individualized treatment based on the particular scenario should prevail. Simple stated, no packing standard is universally accepted.

When used, a loose packing of gauze or other material is placed gently into the abscess cavity to prevent the wound margins from closing and to afford continued drainage of any exudative material (see Fig. 37-6, *step 7*). The packing material should make contact with the cavity wall so that on removal, gentle débridement of necrotic tissue will occur spontaneously. A common error is to attempt to pack an abscess too tightly with excessive packing material. In essence, the pack merely keeps the incision open, and its main purpose is not to absorb all drainage—a dressing accomplishes this goal. Care must be exercised to ensure that the packing does not exert significant pressure against the exposed tissue and lead to further tissue necrosis. Some prefer to use plain gauze, some use gauze soaked in saline or povidone-iodine, and some use gauze impregnated with iodine (iodoform). For large abscess cavities, gauze pads (without cotton backing) are ideal packing material (Fig. 37-11). If gauze pads are used, the number of pads placed in the wound should be counted and charted—ideally, the corner of each pad should exit from the wound. The clinician must ensure that all gauze pads will be removed when the packing is changed or discontinued. More commonly, thin (0.6 to 1.2 cm) packing strip gauze, either plain or iodoform, is used. The iodoform gauze may sting the patient for a few minutes after it is inserted. Packing, especially packing strips containing iodine, will be radiopaque on a plain radiograph. If a foreign body is considered, a radiograph should be obtained before packing. The value of antibiotic-impregnated gauze is uncertain.

An absorbent gauze dressing should be placed over the packed abscess, or if an extremity is involved, a lightly wrapped circumferential dressing should be used (see Fig. 37-6, *step 8*). Generous amounts of dry gauze are used over the packing to soak up any drainage or blood. The affected part should be splinted if possible, and elevation should be routine. The dressing and splint should not be disturbed until the first follow-up visit. Drainage relieves most of the pain of an abscess, but postoperative analgesics may be required.

After treatment, packing is often changed periodically (Fig. 37-12*A*). Most patients require a repeated visit to the clinician for packing change, but if the original packing is to be removed and not replaced (as with a paronychia or hair follicle abscess), selected patients may remove the packing and perform their own wound care totally at home. Motivated patients can provide total follow-up, and a cotton-tipped applicator swirled in the base of the wound for a few days can replace formal packing (see Fig. 37-12*B*).

FOLLOW-UP EXAMINATION

A drained abscess should be reevaluated in 1 to 3 days, depending on a number of factors. Most lesions are reevaluated 48 hours after the procedure, with the first but possibly the only packing change occurring at this time. Some wounds

warrant closer monitoring. Diabetic patients or other patients with impaired healing capacity, mental impairment, or physical disabilities may require a home care nurse or hospital admission for more frequent wound care and packing changes. Wounds that are at high risk for complications, such as those about the face or hands or those with significant cellulitis, require close follow-up depending on the specific scenario. The patient should be encouraged to play an active role in wound care. During the first follow-up visit, compliant and able patients should be taught to change the packing and dressing. If this is anatomically impossible, a friend or family member can be instructed in the technique. If long-term packing or complicated wound care is required, referral to wound care centers rather than multiple repeated ED visits may be more practical.

The technique for changing packing material is usually one of personal preference. It should be emphasized that patients often fear a repeated visit and expect significant pain with subsequent wound care, especially if the initial I&D was difficult. Therefore, the specifics of packing change should be addressed before release home after the initial drainage procedure. Ideally, the initial procedure will have been accomplished without undue pain to allay subsequent fears. Some clinicians suggest that an oral opioid be taken 30 to 40 minutes before the next visit or the use of local anesthesia

Figure 37-11 Wound packing. **A,** The traditional packing material is ¼- to ½-inch gauze, plain or with iodoform. **B,** A 4- × 4-cm gauze pad soaked in povidone-iodine (Betadine) can be used to pack a large abscess, but be careful to avoid losing or forgetting about packing material in the base of a large abscess. Use an instrument to introduce the packing into the *bottom of the abscess.* Use only enough gauze to keep the incision open, and avoid tight packing. Some clinicians do not use packing at all for easily drained abscesses, and packing is not an absolute standard. See discussion about the vessel loop abscess drainage technique (see Fig. 37-13).

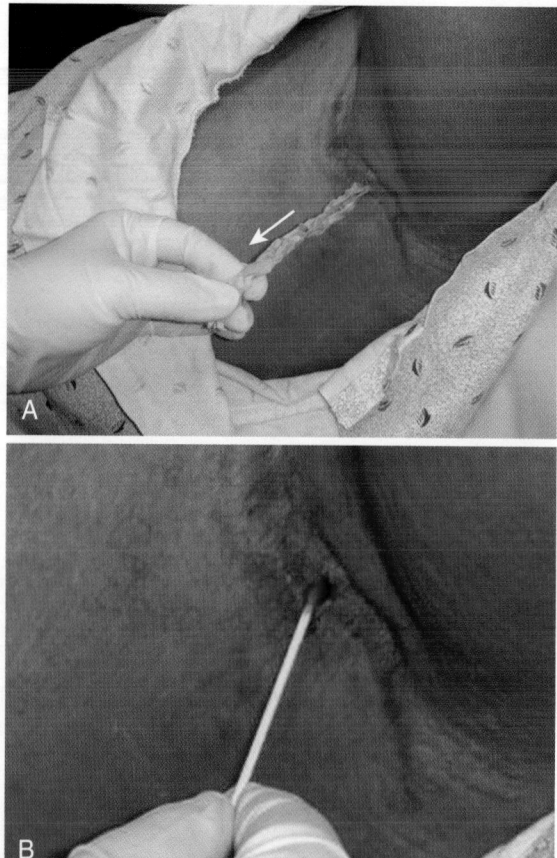

Figure 37-12 Wound check. **A,** Packing gauze is removed from the abscess on the first wound inspection. If drainage is present, the abscess is repacked. **B,** Small abscesses can be cleaned with a cotton swab swirled in the cavity, which is left open. This care can be continued at home.

or parenteral analgesia if significant pain is anticipated. Removal of packing material is frequently painful, but if the packing is moistened with saline before removal, it may be less traumatic. If the original incision was of the proper length, loculations were adequately removed, and packing was adequate, subsequent packing changes will be considerably easier. Once the packing is removed, the wound is inspected for residual necrotic tissue. The cavity may be irrigated with saline before replacing the pack if significant exudate is present, but this is not often required because the packing absorbs most debris.

The frequency of packing or dressing changes is also clinically guided. Some wounds require multiple packing changes, whereas other wounds require only the initial packing. For most facial abscesses, the packing should be removed after only 24 hours, at which time warm soaks should be started. Wounds large enough to require repeated packing should be repacked at least every 48 to 72 hours (occasionally daily for the first few visits) until the drainage stops or healing continues in a deep-to-superficial direction.

In general, once healthy granulation tissue has developed throughout the wound and a well-established drainage tract is present, packing may be discontinued. The patient should then be instructed to begin warm soaks of the wound. Gentle hydrostatic débridement may be performed by the patient in the shower at home: the patient holds the skin incision open and directs the shower or faucet spray into the abscess cavity. Appropriate dressing changes should then follow until healing is completed. When all signs of infection (e.g., erythema, drainage, pain, and induration) have resolved and healthy granulation tissue is present, the patient may be discharged from medical care.

SPECIFIC ABSCESS THERAPY
Folliculitis, Furuncles, and Carbuncles

Folliculitis, furuncles, and carbuncles can develop in healthy individuals with no predisposing risk factors other than skin, nasal, perineal, or gut colonization with a *Staphylococcus*

Abscess Drainage by the Loop Drainage Technique[68]

Historically, drainage of an abscess has involved the creation of a large skin incision to ensure adequate initial drainage of purulent material, followed by filling the abscess cavity with packing to promote continued drainage. The loop drain technique, an old technique now undergoing renewed interest, confers several advantages over the classic I&D. There are no packing changes, smaller incisions result in better cosmesis, and incisions drain as long as the loop is in place. This technique, though perhaps counterintuitive to classic teaching, provides excellent results for abscesses that previously would have been subjected to traditional incision, drainage, and packing and repacking protocols.

WHAT TYPE OF DRAIN TO USE
The original article describing this technique used a silicone vessel loop, a small Penrose drain, or a sterile rubber band. A readily available product is a vessel loop used by surgeons (Fig. 37-13, *step 1*).

TECHNIQUE
Step 1: Make a small (5 to 10 mm) incision with a No. 11 scalpel blade at the periphery of the abscess but still within its borders (see Fig. 37-13, *step 2*). Make the first incision where the abscess is pointing or already draining. Then probe the cavity with a hemostat and break up loculations (see Fig. 37-13, *step 4*). Pus should flow out of this puncture incision.

Step 2: With the hemostat inside the abscess cavity, find the opposite edge of the abscess cavity and position the tip of a hemostat underneath the area where you will make the second incision (see Fig. 37-13, *step 5*). Tent the skin from underneath. Make another stab with a No. 11 scalpel blade over the hemostat tip. Slide the tip of the hemostat through the new incision.

At this stage you should have two small incisions with a hemostat going into one, tunneling through the abscess cavity, and coming out of the other incision. There should be a maximum separation between the two incisions of up to 4 cm. If the abscess is

larger than this, you can place more loops, depending on the shape of the abscess cavity.

Step 3: Using the hemostat that has traversed the cavity, grab the end of the loop drain and pull it back through the wound (see Fig. 37-13, *steps 7 and 8*). There should be a long end of the loop drain exiting each incision.

Step 4: Tie the two ends of the drain together without tension. Too much tension is painful and can necrose the skin between the incisions. One way to avoid excessive skin tension is to place a syringe between the skin and the drain while you are tying it (see Fig. 37-13, *step 9*). Tie the knots flush with the syringe, and when the syringe is pulled away, there will be a loosely placed loop that will exert no tension on the incision sites. A finger should be able to be passed between the skin and loop. The drain is going to be slippery, so make about five knots. Tie the last two very tightly by stretching the loop almost to the breaking point. Trim the ends of the drain (see Fig. 37-13, *step 10*). An option at this point is to irrigate the abscess cavity through the stab incision. Cover the operative site with gauze since drainage will continue.

DISCHARGE INSTRUCTIONS
With the dressing removed and the loop still in place, the patient should bathe or shower twice a day for the first 3 days to promote continued drainage. Change the dressing at least twice daily or whenever saturated. Gently pull the loop back and forth once or twice a day to help keep the wound open.

WHEN TO REMOVE THE DRAIN
Remove the drain when the discharge stops and cellulitis improves. Simply cut the loop and pull it out. The loop is generally removed in about 5 to 10 days but may be removed sooner with a small abscesses or rapid healing. The patient now has only two small puncture sites that will heal over rather than a large scar that must heal by secondary intention.

From Tsoraides SS, Pearl RH, Stanfill AB, et al. Incision and loop drainage: a minimally invasive technique for subcutaneous abscess management in children. J Pediatr Surg. 2010;45:606-609.

VESSEL LOOP METHOD OF INCISION AND DRAINAGE

Instead of traditional gauze packing, a sterile silicone loop is used. This is commonly referred to simply as a "vessel loop", and is readily available from the OR (this device is used by vascular surgeons).

After sterile preparation and anesthetic infiltration, make a small (5–10 mm) incision at the periphery of the abscess. If possible, make the incision where the abscess is already pointing.

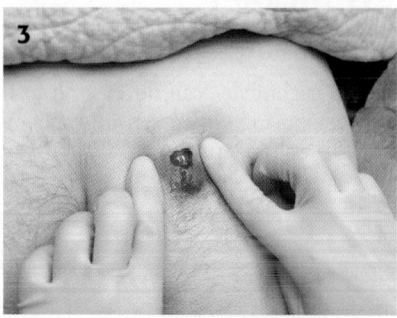

Express as much pus as possible from the incision. Obtain cultures if clinically indicated.

Use a hemostat to probe the abscess cavity and break up loculations.

Probe with the hemostat to find the opposite edge of the abscess cavity. Position the tip of the hemostat underneath the area of the second incision, tent the skin, and make another stab incision over the hemostat tip.

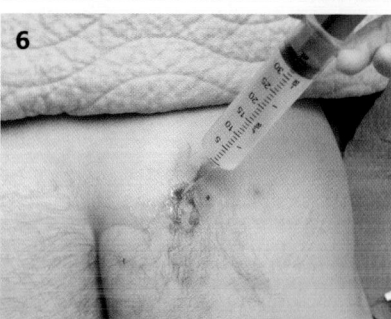

Optionally irrigate the cavity with a syringe and plastic IV catheter.

Place the hemostat through the cavity so that it exits the second incision. Grab the end of the vessel loop (*arrow*).

Pull the vessel loop through the abscess cavity so that it exits through the first incision.

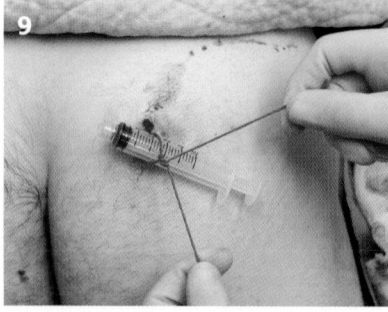

Tie the two ends of the vessel loop together. To avoid excessive skin tension, tie the loops over a syringe. Tie at least five knots, as the loop material is slippery. Tie the last two knots tightly, by stretching the loop almost to the breaking point.

Remove the syringe, and then trim the ends of the vessel loop. Note that it is not tied tightly against the skin. Refer to the text for information on discharge instructions and loop removal.

Figure 37-13 Vessel loop method of incision and drainage. For more details, refer to McNamara WF. An alternative to open incision and drainage for community-acquired soft tissue abscesses in children. *J Pediatr Surg*. 2011;46:502-506; Ladd AP. Minimally invasive technique in treatment of complex, subcutaneous abscesses in childfren. *J Pediatr Surg*. 2010;45:1562-1566; and Tsoraides SS, Pearl RH, Stanfill AB, et al. Incision and loop drainage: a minimally invasive technique for subcutaneous abscess management in children. *J Pediatr Surg*. 2010;45:606-609.

Figure 37-14 A, *Staphylococcus aureus* is a common cause of folliculitis, although other bacteria such as *Pseudomonas* may be responsible. Treatment consists primarily of local measures such as warm compresses and antibacterial soaps and ointments. **B,** Furuncles are circumscribed abscesses of the skin and subcutaneous tissue that usually involve a hair follicle. **C,** A carbuncle is a complicated abscess on the nape of the neck. It is very common in diabetics. Carbuncles are usually caused by *S. aureus*, including community-acquired methicillin-resistant *S. aureus*. Because of its many crypts, loculations, and intercommunicating small abscesses, treatment by simple incision and drainage is often not readily curative. When fluctuance is appreciated, incision is indicated. One should avoid multiple small incisions because tissue circulation may be compromised. Antibiotics may augment healing of this abscess, but wide surgical excision may be required. (*A, from Weston WL, Lane AT, Morelli JG, eds.* Color Textbook of Pediatric Dermatology. *4th ed. St. Louis: Mosby; 2007; B, from Long SS, Pickering LK, Prober CG, et al.* Principles and Practice of Pediatric Infectious Diseases Revised Reprint. *3rd ed. Philadelphia: Churchill Livingstone; 2009.*)

bacterium. The umbilicus of neonates is also commonly colonized. Individuals in close contact with others who have active disease in the form of abscesses, furuncles, or carbuncles are at increased risk for similar infections. The pathogenesis of staphylococcal disease is a complex host-bacterium interaction. *S. aureus* invades the skin by way of the hair follicles or an open wound (abrasions, shaving, or insect bites) and produces local tissue destruction followed by hyperemia of vessels. Subsequently, an exudative reaction occurs, during which polymorphonuclear cells invade. The process then extends along the path of least resistance. The abscess may "point" or form sinus tracts. The process can disseminate by invasion of vessels and thus can infect other distant organs. Most cases of staphylococcal osteomyelitis, meningitis, and endocarditis occur by this mechanism.[2,69]

Folliculitis represents inflammation of hair follicles in response to infection, chemical irritation, or skin injury (Fig. 37-14A). An area of purulence often forms after superficial bacterial invasion of the hair follicle and is generally isolated to the epidermis. *S. aureus* is commonly found, although other bacteria are also responsible for specific follicular infections. *Pseudomonas* is an important pathogen in cases caused by exposure to hot tubs, pools, or whirlpools that are not adequately chlorinated.[4] In persons with broad-spectrum antibiotic use or immunosuppression, consider *Candida* as well.[70] Individuals exposed to whirlpool foot baths at nail salons are at risk for mycobacterial infection. Treatment generally involves local measures, including warm compresses, antibacterial soaps and ointments, and avoidance of the source of contaminated water in the case of hot tub or whirlpool footbath folliculitis. These measures usually suffice, but systemic antibiotics may be required if multiple sites are involved or if the patient is a chronic staphylococcal carrier. Shaving of involved areas should be temporarily avoided.

Furuncles, or boils, are acute circumscribed abscesses of the skin and subcutaneous tissue that usually involve the hair follicle (see Fig. 37-14B). They most commonly occur on the face, neck, buttocks, thigh, perineum, breast, and axilla. Carbuncles are aggregates of interconnected furuncles that frequently occur on the back of the neck (see Fig. 37-14C). In this area the skin is thick, so extension occurs laterally rather than toward the skin surface. *S. aureus* species, both methicillin susceptible and methicillin resistant, are the usual culprits.[40] Carbuncles may become large and can cause systemic symptoms and complications. All patients with a carbuncle should be evaluated for diabetes because this is a common risk factor. Treatment should consist of surgical drainage and administration of systemic antibiotics. Large carbuncles may be difficult to drain adequately in the ED and could require operative management. Carbuncles usually consist of many loculated pockets of pus, so simple I&D is often not curative. Occasionally, wide excision and skin grafting are required.

Most recurrent staphylococcal skin infections are caused by autoinfection from skin lesions or nasal reservoirs. Prevention is directed at eliminating the organism. This is accomplished by the application of bacitracin to the nares, chlorhexidine baths, and good hygiene, including frequent cleansing with antibacterial soap. If these measures are unsuccessful, systemic oral antistaphylococcal treatment is instituted for 2 to 3 weeks. Detection and treatment of infection in family members may be necessary.[2,71,72]

S. aureus can cause suture abscesses. A suture abscess is often misdiagnosed as a wound infection, but in fact it is a local nidus of inflammation, infection, or both caused and potentiated by suture material. Such an abscess usually appears after sutures have been in place for 3 to 5 days, with single or multiple discrete areas of erythema and tenderness being noted at the site where the suture penetrates the skin. Simply removing the suture (a drop of pus may be expressed) and providing warm compresses and topical antibiotic ointment is generally all that is required. Wide opening of the wound and systemic antibiotics are seldom required. When the suture is buried, a small incision should be followed by probing the wound with a small hook or bent needle (see Chapter 35) to snare the suture for removal.

Hidradenitis Suppurativa

Hidradenitis suppurativa (Greek *hidros*, or "sweat," and *aden*, or "gland") is a chronic, relapsing, inflammatory disease process that affects the apocrine sweat glands in the axilla, the inguinal region,[73] and the perineum (Fig. 37-15). Its prevalence is 0.3% to 4% in industrialized countries; most affected individuals are young women.[74] The condition results from follicular inflammation and subsequent occlusion of the apocrine ducts by keratinous debris, which leads to ductal dilation, inflammation, and rupture into the subcutaneous area. Most commonly, the disease is manifested as an episodic appearance of localized pain, edema, pruritus, burning, swelling, and purulence. Dysregulation of the immune response is thought to play a role, with some studies showing a response to immunosuppressive agents.[75] Occlusion of the hair follicle predisposes to secondary bacterial infection and subsequent abscess formation. In its early stages it is indistinguishable from a simple furuncle. Progression and recurrence, however, lead to the distinctive appearance of multiple foci coupled with areas of induration and inflammation that are in various stages of healing. This chronic process can create draining fistulous tracts, often involving large areas that are not amenable to simple I&D procedures (see Fig. 37-15C).[72]

Genetic factors may play some role in hidradenitis suppurativa.[76] Fitzsimmons and Guilbert[77] proposed a single dominant gene transmission. Some authors have suggested an increased incidence in patients of African descent, although this does not seem to be substantiated by studies.[78] A hormonal association has also been postulated. More women than men are affected, and onset after menopause and before puberty is rare.[79] Other factors thought to be related include obesity and smoking. A matched-pair case-control study found an odds ratio of 9.4 in smokers versus controls (95% confidence interval, 3.7 to 23.7).[80] Environmental factors, including antiperspirants and shaving,[81] were implicated in the past, but more recent studies have not found any association.[82]

Bacterial cultures of specimens from suppurative hidradenitis lesions are frequently sterile or reflect organisms seen in other soft tissue abscesses. *Staphylococcus* is the most commonly isolated organism,[82] with *E. coli* and β-hemolytic streptococci being other important pathogens. In the perineal region, enteric flora are often found. Many of these abscesses have multiple isolates, and anaerobic bacteria are frequently cultured. CA-MRSA is an increasing cause of such abscesses.

Initial outpatient management of an acute suppurative lesion usually involves ED intervention. Any fluctuant area requires drainage, as described in the section "I&D Procedure." In patients with extensive cellulitis, a broad-spectrum, antistaphylococcal antibiotic should be used. Unfortunately, hidradenitis suppurativa cannot be cured with localized I&D. If I&D is required for relief of a secondary abscess, it should

Figure 37-15 **A,** Axillary abscesses are common and recurrent. Community-acquired methicillin-resistant *Staphylococcus aureus* is an increasing cause. **B,** Vessel loop drainage of an axillary abscess. **C,** Hidradenitis suppurativa of the groin or axilla is a complicated series of abscesses that may not be amenable to simple incision and drainage. In this patient with involvement of the groin, extensive surgery was required to excise recurrent infection.

be made clear to the patient that this procedure does not cure the underlying disease.[83] The chronic nature of the disease produces multiple areas of inflammation and subcutaneous fistulous tracts that induce routine recurrences. The patient must be informed of this unfavorable prognosis and should be referred to a dermatologist or surgeon for long-term care.

Milder forms of the disease are initially treated with conservative measures. Many different approaches have been tried, with only limited degrees of success. Few controlled studies of treatment strategies have been performed. Patients are often counseled to lose weight, stop smoking, refrain from shaving, stop using deodorants, and improve personal hygiene. The benefits of these efforts are unknown. Oral antistaphylococcal antibiotics are most commonly used, with varying results.[84] Retrospective reviews looking at the efficacy of combination therapy (clindamycin and rifampin) have been promising, with some patients experiencing long-term remission, although diarrhea is a common side effect.[85,86] There have been reports of success with topical clindamycin,[87,88] hormone therapy in females,[89] and laser therapy.[90] Finally, immunosuppressive therapy with tumor necrosis factor-α inhibitors (infliximab, adalimumab[91,92]) has been successful in treating a few intractable cases.

Advanced stages of the disease are managed by wide or local excision. Smaller excisions are more likely to recur than wider excisions.[93] Delayed closure[94,95] may offer better results, but this has not been directly compared with primary closure. Wide excision may warrant skin grafting.[96]

Breast Abscess

Breast abscesses can occur in lactating (14%) and nonlactating breasts (86%).[97] They are caused by normal skin bacteria that enter through a break or crack in the skin, usually the nipple (Fig. 37-16). The infection becomes established in parenchymal tissue and causes pain, swelling, and localized hyperthermia. In its early stages, when cellulitis predominates, a breast abscess can be difficult to diagnose. In equivocal cases, antibiotics may be curative. Cellulitis may progress to frank abscess formation. Women with this condition can be quite ill and appear toxic.

The estimated incidence of inflammatory processes of the breast (mastitis) in lactating women ranges from 2% to 33%.[98] In lactating women the infection is usually precipitated by milk stasis after weaning or missed feedings and usually occurs in the first 6 weeks of breastfeeding or during the weaning phase. The cause is usually bacterial invasion through a cracked or abraded nipple by *S. aureus*, including MRSA, or streptococci originating from the mouth of the nursing child.[99-101] Manifestations include redness, heat, pain, fever, and chills. Treatment consists of antistaphylococcal antibiotics, continued breast emptying with a breast pump, and application of heat. It is important to encourage continued breast emptying to promote drainage. Nursing can be continued with the noninfected breast.[102]

Breast abscesses in nonlactating women are more common. People at risk are smokers and diabetics. These are also risk factors for recurrence. In addition, abscesses may be a complication of nipple piercing or breast implants inserted under appropriate medical care,[103] as well as via illicit cosmetic procedures.[104,105] In nonpuerperal infections, *S. aureus* and streptococci are common causative organisms, as are *Bacteroides* species and anaerobic streptococci.[105] Mixed flora are more commonly found in recurrent abscesses (20.5% in those with recurrence versus 8.9% in those with a single episode).[106] Recommended antibiotics include amoxicillin and clavulanic acid or, in patients with penicillin allergies, combination therapy with erythromycin and metronidazole. If the community prevalence of MRSA is high, treatment with clindamycin, tetracycline, or TMP-SMX should be considered.[107]

Ultrasound-guided needle aspiration is becoming the standard of care for most breast abscesses. When compared with I&D, aspiration causes less scarring, does not interfere with breastfeeding, and does not require procedural sedation.[107] Christensen and associates[108] recommended that ultrasound-guided needle drainage replace surgery as first-line treatment

Figure 37-16 Breast abscess. These abscesses are more common in nonlactating than in lactating women. Initial treatment recommendations call for ultrasound-guided needle aspiration. *(From Bland KI, Copeland EM III, eds. The Breast. 4th ed. Philadelphia: Saunders; 2009.)*

of uncomplicated puerperal and nonpuerperal breast abscesses. Emerging treatment parameters are ultrasound-guided needle aspiration for abscesses less than 3 cm in diameter and ultrasound-guided catheter drainage for abscesses 3 cm in diameter or larger.[109] Ultrasound images of breast abscesses appear as inhomogeneous, hyperechoic masses (Fig. 37-17). Repeat aspiration every other day to achieve complete resolution, with a mean of 3.5 aspirations being required.[109]

Recurrent abscesses are a common, troublesome complication after traditional treatment with I&D and antibiotics.[110,111] Fortunately, the reported recurrence rate associated with ultrasound-guided aspiration or drainage procedures is quite low.[112,113] Patients with persistent recurrences should be managed by a surgeon for total excision of the involved area.

Although a breast abscess is rarely a harbinger of malignancy, it could be the initial manifestation of a metastatic process.[112,114] After needle aspiration or catheter drainage, send the aspirate for culture and cytologic examination, and perform a postdrainage mammogram and ultrasound to evaluate for underlying or coexistent malignancy.[113]

A breast abscess in a male is an unusual occurrence, so consider malignancy and underlying bone or joint infection in these cases (see Fig. 37-2A and B).

Bartholin Gland Abscess

The Bartholin glands (or greater vestibular glands) are located at the 4- and 8-o'clock positions on each side of the vestibule of the vagina (Fig. 37-18A). These mucus-secreting glands maintain the moisture of the vaginal mucosa. When the ostium becomes blocked by inflammation or trauma, a cyst or abscess may form, which occurs in 2% of women.[115]

Asymptomatic cysts (no pain, no discharge) frequently occur as a result of duct blockage and retention of secretions. Symptomatic cysts (vulvar pain, dyspareunia, and discomfort while walking or sitting) can be managed with warm sitz baths and compresses. Abscesses involve an acute inflammatory reaction within the stroma of the duct and are usually accompanied by pain, rubor, and occasionally discharge. The majority of cases (80%) are caused by mixed vaginal flora (*Bacteroides*, *E. coli*, *S. aureus*).[116] *Neisseria gonorrhea* and, less commonly, *Chlamydia* can also be involved. Examination reveals a tender,

Figure 37-17 Longitudinal images of ultrasound-guided drainage of an abscess in the lower inner quadrant of a 27-year-old woman's right breast 8 weeks after delivery. **A,** Well-defined, slightly loculated, inhomogeneous hypoechoic abscess measuring 6 × 4 cm. *Dots extend across the abscess, with the cursor at one margin of the abscess.* **B,** Pigtail catheter (7 Fr) containing a trocar *(arrows)* in the abscess cavity. **C,** After removal of the trocar and aspiration of 70 mL of pus. The parallel lines represent the walls of the catheter *(arrows). (From Ulitzsch D, Nyman MKG, Carlson RA. Breast abscess in lactating women: US-guided treatment.* Radiology. *2004;232:904.)*

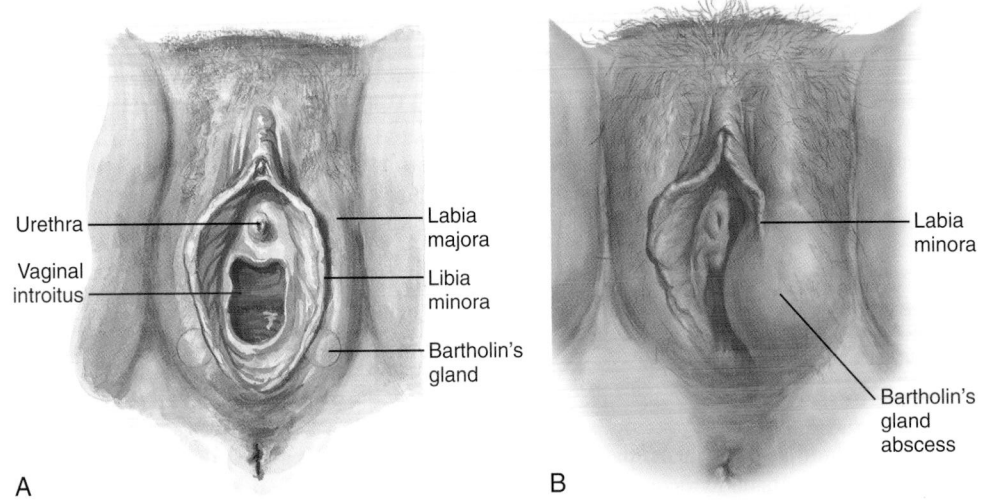

Figure 37-18 Bartholin's gland and abscess. **A,** Anatomy of the female external genitalia. Note the location of Bartholin's glands at 5 and 7 o'clock. **B,** Bartholin gland duct cysts and abscesses are recognized by the presence of a fluctuant mass of variable size within the posterior vestibule, with the labia minora transecting the cyst. *(Netter illustration from* www.netterimages.com. © *Elsevier Inc. All rights reserved.)*

fluctuant mass in the posterior of the labia that can be palpated between the thumb and index finger (see Fig. 37-18*B*).

The most common procedure for treating a Bartholin abscess is insertion of a drainage catheter, as described by Word in 1968.[117] This single-barreled, sealed-stopper, balloon-tipped catheter serves as initial and long-term therapy (Fig. 37-19*A*). In his original description, Word reported only 2 recurrences in 72 lesions, both of which were treated successfully with a second catheter. None of the patients required marsupialization. The Word catheter procedure involves fistulization of the duct cavity by a 1-inch catheter with an inflatable balloon tip.[118] Though not a traditional I&D procedure, the technique permits continued drainage of the gland.

In preparation for insertion of the catheter, place the patient in the standard dorsal lithotomy position and drape the perineum (Fig. 37-20, *step 1*). Cleanse the area with povidone-iodine solution. If an anesthetic is deemed necessary for patient comfort and cooperation, infiltrate with lidocaine just external to the hymenal ring, where the distal duct opening should be located (at the 5- or 7-o'clock position) (see Fig.

37-20, *step 2*).[119] Test the balloon of the Word catheter by filling it with 3 mL of water via a 25-gauge needle. Aspirate the water back and keep the needle on the catheter to serve as a handle for insertion. Make a small incision in the mucosa, not the cutaneous surface (see Fig. 37-20, *step 3*). Use a scalpel or a hemostat to puncture the abscess cavity (see Fig. 37-20, *step 4*). It can be difficult to enter this deep abscess cavity. Failure to obtain frank pus or to appreciate a "pop" when entering the abscess usually prognosticates failure of the procedure. Stabilize the abscess with the thumb and forefinger, hold the hemostat in place, and skewer the abscess onto the hemostat (Fig. 37-21). Pushing the hemostat into the immobilized abscess is technically more difficult. Make a stab incision large enough to accommodate the catheter but small enough to prohibit the inflated balloon from being extruded. Once the abscess has been entered (signaled by a palpable pop or the free flow of pus), place the deflated balloon in the abscess cavity (see Fig. 37-20, *step 5*). Inflate the balloon with 2 to 4 mL of water (not air). Persistent pain indicates that too much fluid has been used. Most abscesses drain for a few days,

Figure 37-19 Word catheter. **A,** Inflatable bulb-tipped catheter. Left, uninflated; right, inflated with 4 mL water. **B,** Use of the Word catheter for outpatient drainage of a Bartholin gland abscess. This is a fistulization procedure rather than standard incision and drainage. **B,** *1,* A stab incision is made on the mucosal surface. *2,* The catheter is inserted into the cyst cavity. *3,* The catheter is filled with 3 to 4 mL of water. Vessel loop drainage is an alternative to use of a Word catheter. (*B, From Word B. Office treatment of cyst and abscess of Bartholin gland.* JAMA. *1964;190:777*).

and the Word catheter often falls out within a week. Ideally, the device is left in place for 2 to 4 weeks to allow fistula formation, so follow-up is required. If the catheter falls out prematurely, it should be replaced quickly to allow fistulization. Some clinicians do not reinsert the catheter if healing has progressed significantly after the first drainage procedure.

Alternative treatment strategies have also been explored. Gennis and coworkers[120] designed a rubber ring catheter called the Jacobi ring from an 8-Fr T-tube threaded with 2-0 silk suture material (Fig. 37-22). The catheter enters and exits the abscess through separate incisions, and a closed ring is formed when the ends of the suture are tied (Fig. 37-23). The device was tested in a randomized study involving 38 women,

25 of whom received a ring catheter and 13 received a Word catheter. The catheters were rated similarly in terms of successful placement, abscess resolution (all resolved within 3 weeks), and recurrence rates (no recurrences at 6 months and two [one in each treatment group] at 1 year). However, the ring catheter outperformed the Word catheter in patient satisfaction.

A loop device similar to the Jacobi ring can be created from butterfly Vacutainer tubing and 2-0 suture. The availability of such equipment in most institutions makes this an attractive option. Jacobi rings or similar loop devices have the advantage of a lower risk for dislodgment than with the Word catheter. Disadvantages include the creation of two drainage tracts in comparison to one. Additionally, loop devices require pelvic rest, whereas the patient may resume intercourse with the Word cathether.[121]

Standard I&D can give the patient immediate relief, but this procedure is not recommended because the abscess recurrence rate is so high.[122] However, if neither a Word catheter nor equipment for a loop device are available, I&D can be performed, with the caveat that the clinician and the patient must appreciate the likelihood of an unfavorable long-term outcome. Make the incision over the medial surface of the introitus (on the mucosa, not on the skin) in a line parallel to the posterior margin of the hymenal ring. The abscess cavity is slightly deeper than most cutaneous abscesses, so the clinician must be certain to enter the actual abscess cavity to achieve complete drainage. This is most easily accomplished by inserting a hemostat through the mucosal incision and spreading the tips of the instrument in the deeper soft tissue. After the contents have drained, pack the abscess for 24 to 48 hours, and start sitz baths thereafter.

CO_2 laser vaporization is another technique described whereby laser technology is used to create an opening in the area of the duct's orifice. The abscess is then evacuated and either excised, vaporized, or left intact.[123] Lack of available equipment, however, precludes using this method in the ED. Silver nitrate sticks have also been used to ablate the cyst after I&D. Complications of this method include postoperative vulvar burning, labial edema, and cauterization of the surrounding mucosa.[124]

Empirical antibiotics are indicated only for patients with a frank abscess and local cellulitis. More than 80% of cultures from Bartholin's cysts show no growth, and the same is true for a third of cultures from abscesses.[125] Cultures that are positive typically show polymicrobial growth, usually anaerobes and especially *Bacteroides* species and other colonic bacteria. Much less often, *N. gonorrhoeae* or *Chlamydia trachomatis* is cultured from the abscess cavity. Chronic low-grade inflammation from a gonococcal infection has been implicated as a causative factor in cyst formation and occasionally in the development of an abscess; therefore, choose an antibiotic that will provide coverage for *N. gonorrhoeae*. It is reasonable to culture cervical and anal specimens for gonorrhea and chlamydia from women with a Bartholin gland abscess because of the association of these infections with sexually transmitted disease.[126] However, empirical treatment of gonorrhea or chlamydia is not necessary unless the clinician has a high suspicion that a sexually transmitted organism is the infectious cause. At the current time, CA-MRSA infections of the Bartholin glands are uncommon.

Particular care must be taken when treating a pregnant woman with a Bartholin gland abscess because she is at high

BARTHOLIN ABSCESS DRAINAGE (WORD CATHETER)

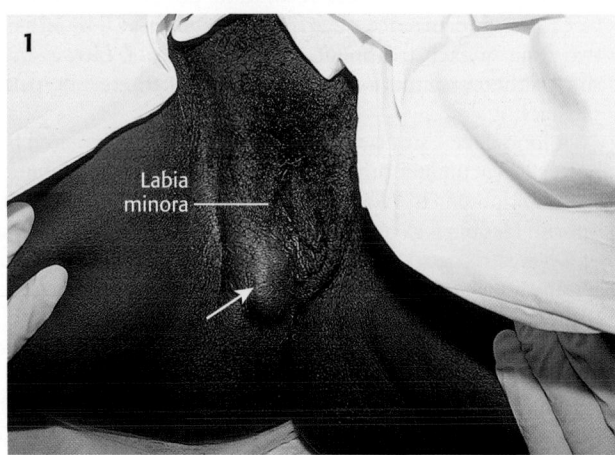

Place the patient in the dorsal lithotomy position and identify the abscess, which will be located at either the 5- or 7-o'clock position, with the labia minora transecting the abscess.

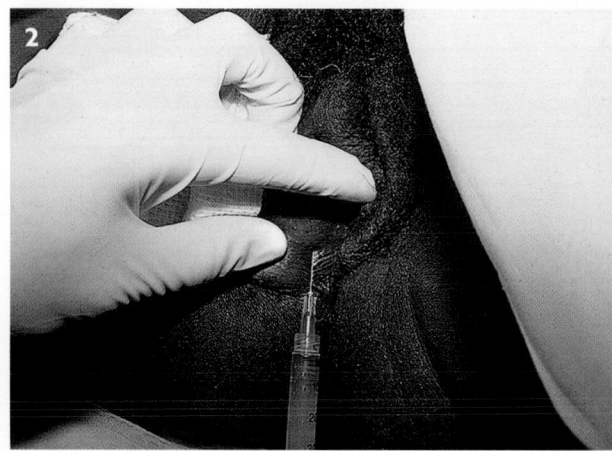

Cleanse the area with antiseptic solution. While stabilizing the abscess with your thumb and index finger, inject local anesthetic through the mucosal surface (not through the skin).

Use a No. 11 scalpel blade to make an incision in the mucosal surface of the abscess. Make the incision large enough to accomodate the catheter, but small enough to prevent extrusion of the inflated balloon.

Alternatively, a hemostat can be used to puncture the abscess cavity. Stabilize the abscess with your thumb and index finger and skewer the abscess onto the hemostat (see Fig. 37-21).

Once the abscess has been entered (heralded by a palpable pop or the free flow of pus), insert the Word catheter to the hilt and inflate with 3 to 4 mL of saline. Use a 25-gauge needle to fill the balloon.

The catheter is left in place for 2 to 4 weeks to form a fistula. Antibiotics are of no proven value once drainage is performed, but practice varies.

Figure 37-20 Drainage of a Bartholin abscess (Word catheter insertion.) Loop drainage (Fig. 37-13) or the Jacoby ring (Fig. 37-23) are alternative techniques.

Figure 37-21 It is technically easier to enter the Bartholin gland abscess cavity if the hemostat is held steady and the abscess, held with the thumb and index finger, is skewered onto the hemostat. Attempting to puncture a deep immobilized abscess by stabbing with the hemostat may be more difficult. Expect a palpable pop or drainage of frank pus when entering the abscess.

Figure 37-22 Equipment needed for the Jacobi ring method of drainage of a Bartholin gland abscess.

BARTHOLIN ABSCESS DRAINAGE (JACOBI RING)

1 Make an incision into the mucosal surface of the Bartholin gland abscess. Lyse any adhesions and allow the abscess to drain.

2 Pass a hemostat into the abscess cavity.

3 Tunnel the hemostat through the abscess cavity, and a make a second incision.

4 Grasp the silk suture at one end of the Jacobi ring with the hemostat.

5 Pull the Jacobi ring through the abscess cavity while taking care to not pull the suture out of the tube.

6 Tie the two ends of the suture to form a closed ring.

Figure 37-23 Drainage of a Bartholin gland abscess (Jacobi ring insertion). This is essentially a loop drainage method. *(Redrawn from Gennis P, Li SF, Provataris J, et al. Jacobi ring catheter treatment of Bartholin's abscesses. Am J Emerg Med. 2005;23:414-415.)*

risk for complications. Sepsis in a pregnant woman following marsupialization of an abscess has been reported.[127] Post-menopausal women with what appears to be a Bartholin gland abscess should be referred to a gynecologist to rule out malignancy. A vulvar abscess in an HIV-positive woman should raise suspicion for Kaposi's sarcoma.[128]

Recurrence is a complication with all the aforementioned techniques. If the abscess recurs, more definitive therapy in the form of marsupialization or complete excision of the gland may be required; however, these procedures are not performed initially and, when chosen, should be done in an OR.

Pilonidal Abscess

Pilonidal sinuses are common malformations that occur in the sacrococcygeal area (Fig. 37-24). The cause of the sinus formation is unclear, and the malformation may occur during embryogenesis. Pilonidal cyst formation is thought to be secondary to blockage of a pilonidal sinus. The result of this obstruction is repeated soft tissue infection, followed by drainage and partial resolution, with eventual reaccumulation. The blockage is most commonly the result of hair in the region, and the lesion may in part be a foreign body (hair) granuloma. Although pilonidal sinuses are present from birth, they are not usually manifested clinically until adolescence or the early adult years. Pilonidal abscess formation most frequently affects young (often white) adult males. The sinuses and cysts are lined with stratified squamous epithelium and, after excision, may be found to contain wads of hair and debris. When cultured, pilonidal abscesses generally yield mixed fecal flora with a preponderance of anaerobes.[129] Poor hygiene and repeated trauma (called "jeep bottom" in World War II) may precipitate acute infection. It is postulated that as a patient sits, microtrauma in the intergluteal cleft acts as a suction that draws hair into the superior gluteal folds. Subsequently, hairs become ingrown, bacteria invade, and an abscess developsin the sacrococcygeal region. At the current time, CA-MRSA infections are not common.

Patients with a pilonidal abscess will seek care for back pain and local tenderness. On physical examination the area is found to be indurated. Frank abscess formation may not be appreciated in this deep abscess. One will usually see barely perceptible dimples or tiny openings at the rostral end of the gluteal crease (Fig. 37-25). A hair or slight discharge may be noticed at the opening. One may find a more caudal cyst or abscess, possibly with a palpable sinus tract connecting the two. The sinus and cyst may be draining chronically, or they may become infected as the size increases and blockage occurs.[130]

Treatment of an acutely infected cyst is the same as previously discussed for any fluctuant abscess: all hair and pus should be removed, and the lesion should be packed (see Figs. 37-6 and 37-13). The abscess cavity may be quite large and thus necessitate a lengthy incision to ensure complete drainage. There is some evidence to support lateral, off-midline incisions. A retrospective study looked at 48 patients who had undergone lateral incisions and matched them with 48 patients who had undergone midline incisions. Those who had undergone midline incisions took approximately 3 weeks longer to heal than did those drained with a lateral incision.[131] In general, reported median healing times after I&D vary between 12 and 63 days.[132,133] The area may be repacked at 2- to 4-day intervals as an outpatient procedure, although

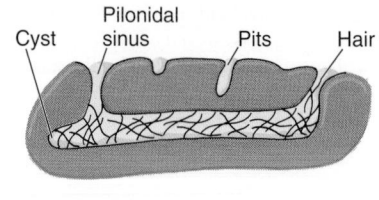

Figure 37-24 Pilonidal sinus. **A,** Sinuses occur in the midline some 5 cm above the anus in the natal cleft. **B,** Longitudinal section showing sinuses and pits. *(From Hill GJ II, ed. Outpatient Surgery. 3rd ed. Philadelphia: Saunders; 1988. Reproduced with permission.)*

Figure 37-25 Pilonidal abscess. An erythematous, indurated, fluctuant, and tender mass is found at the superior gluteal cleft. Small dimples or openings (*arrow*) can be seen on the surface of the abscess.

some prefer to discontinue packing after the first week. Antibiotic therapy is not generally required.

Simple I&D is not usually curative, with recurrence rates of 5% to 13% reported[134,135]; therefore, the patient should be referred to a surgeon for removal of the cyst and sinus after the inflammatory process has resolved. Small abscesses may be incised and drained as an outpatient procedure performed under local anesthesia, but the disease process is often extensive, and general anesthesia may be required to achieve complete drainage. The extent of the cyst cavity and the volume of pus encountered on initial incision can be surprising.

Closure strategies for these potentially large wounds vary. Gencosmanoglu and Inceoglu[133] concluded that a modified lay-open technique is superior to excision with primary

Figure 37-26 Perirectal abscess. **A,** If a perirectal abscess spontaneously ruptures and drains, formal incision, drainage, and packing should still be performed. **B,** A deep, poorly localized perirectal abscess of this size simply cannot be adequately drained in the emergency department (ED). *Arrows* outline the area of induration. This patient requires extensive drainage under general anesthesia. A computed tomography scan may further evaluate the location of the abscess. Broad-spectrum intravenous antibiotics may be started in the ED before definitive surgical intervention. A stab incision in the ED to initiate drainage is also optional, especially if definitive operating room treatment is delayed.

closure for chronic pilonidal sinuses with regard to morbidity and recurrence rates. Other closure options after extensive resection of complex or recurrent sinus tracts are Z-plasty, an advancement flap, or a rotational flap. When primary closure is chosen, administration of a broad-spectrum regimen of antibiotics (e.g., preoperative infusion of cefuroxime and metronidazole followed by 5 days of oral co-amoxiclav[136]) offers protection against wound infections.

Perirectal Abscesses

Most anorectal infections originate in the cryptoglandular area located in the anal canal at the level of the dentate line. Abscesses within these glands can penetrate the surrounding sphincter and track in a variety of directions, with larger abscesses occurring within the perianal, intersphincteric, ischiorectal, and supralevator spaces. A small number of anorectal abscesses have a noncryptoglandular cause such as Crohn's disease, atypical infection (e.g., tuberculosis, lymphogranuloma venereum), malignancy, or trauma.[137]

Perirectal infections can range from minor irritation to fatal illness. Surprisingly, clandestine infections often occur in diabetics. Successful management depends on early recognition of the disease process and adequate surgical therapy. Small abscesses can initially be managed on an outpatient basis with simple I&D, described previously. Because of the morbidity and mortality associated with inadequate treatment of these conditions, patients with large and deep abscesses should be promptly admitted to the hospital for evaluation and treatment under general or spinal anesthesia (Fig. 37-26).

It is important to understand the anatomy of the anal canal and the rectum to appreciate the pathophysiology of these abscesses and their treatment (Fig. 37-27). The mucosa of the anal canal is loosely attached to the muscle wall. At the dentate line, where columnar epithelium gives way to squamous epithelium, there are vertical folds of tissue called the rectal columns of Morgagni that are connected at their lower ends by small semilunar folds called anal valves. Under these valves are invaginations termed anal crypts. Within these crypts are collections of ducts from the anal glands. These glands are believed to be responsible for the genesis of most, if not all perirectal abscesses. These glands often pass through the internal sphincter but do not penetrate the external sphincter.

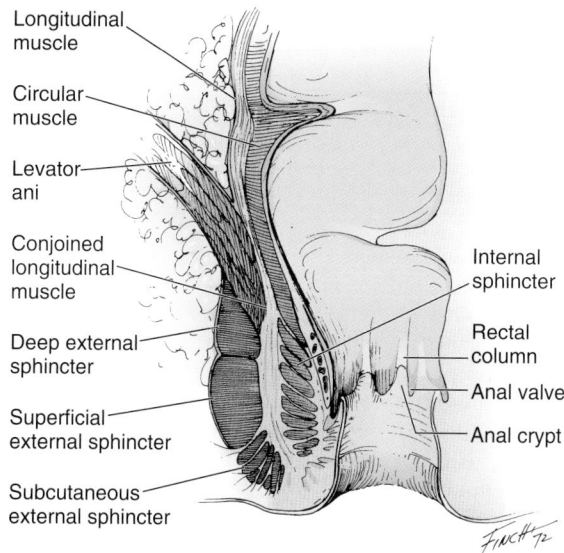

Figure 37-27 Schematic coronal section of the anal canal and rectum. (*From Schwartz SI, Lillehei RC, eds.* Principles of Surgery. *2nd ed. New York, McGraw-Hill, 1974. Reproduced with permission.*)

The muscular anatomy divides the perirectal area into compartments that may house an abscess, depending on the direction of spread of the foci of the infection (Fig. 37-28).[136,138]

The circular fibers of the intestinal coat thicken at the rectum-anus junction to become the internal anal sphincter. The muscle fibers of the levator ani fuse with those of the outer longitudinal fibers of the intestinal coat as it passes through the pelvic floor. These conjoined fibers are connected by fibrous tissue to the external sphincter system, which consists of three circular muscle groups.

Pathophysiology

As described previously, the anal glands are mucus-secreting structures that terminate in the area between the internal and external sphincters. It is believed that most perirectal infections begin in the intersphincteric space secondary to blockage and subsequent infection of the anal glands. Normal host defense mechanisms are overwhelmed, and this results in invasion and overgrowth by bowel flora.[139]

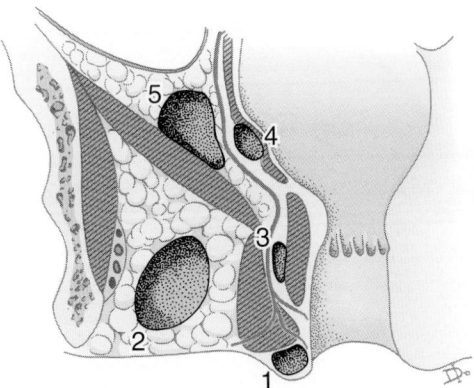

Figure 37-28 Classification of perirectal abscesses. *1,* Perianal. *2,* Ischiorectal. *3,* Intersphincteric. *4,* High intramuscular. *5,* Pelvirectal. *(From Hill GJ II, ed.* Outpatient Surgery. *3rd ed. Philadelphia: Saunders; 1988. Reproduced with permission.)*

If the infection spreads across the external sphincter laterally, an ischiorectal abscess is formed. If the infection dissects rostrally, it may continue between the internal and external sphincters and give rise to a high intramuscular abscess. The infection may also dissect through the external sphincter over the levator ani to form a pelvirectal abscess.[140]

When infection of an anal crypt extends by way of the perianal lymphatics and continues between the mucous membrane and the anal muscles, a perianal abscess forms at the anal orifice. A perianal abscess is the most common variety of perirectal infection. A perianal abscess lies immediately beneath the skin in the perianal region at the lowermost part of the anal canal. It is separated from the ischiorectal space by a fascial septum that extends from the external sphincter and is continuous with the subcutaneous tissues of the buttocks. The infection may be small and localized or it may be very large, with a wall of necrotic tissue and a surrounding zone of cellulitis.[2] Perianal abscesses may be associated with a fistula in ano. A fistula in ano is an inflammatory tract with an external opening in the skin of the perianal area and an internal opening in the mucosa of the anal canal. A fistula in ano is usually formed after partial resolution of a perianal abscess, and its presence is suggested by recurrence of these abscesses with intermittent drainage. The external opening of the fissure is usually a red elevated piece of granulation tissue that may exhibit purulent or serosanguineous drainage on compression. In many cases the tract can be palpated as a cord. Patients with anal fistulas should be referred for definitive surgical excision.[140]

Ischiorectal abscesses are fairly common. They are bounded superiorly by the levator ani, inferiorly by the fascia over the perianal space, medially by the anal sphincter muscles, and laterally by the obturator internus muscle. These abscesses may commonly be bilateral, and if so, the two cavities communicate by way of a deep postanal space to form a "horseshoe" abscess.[2]

Intersphincteric abscesses are less common. They are bounded by the internal and external sphincters and may extend rostrally into the rectum, thereby separating the circular and longitudinal muscle layers.

Causes of perirectal abscesses other than the cryptoglandular process have been documented but are fairly rare. It is believed that hemorrhoids, anorectal surgery, episiotomy, or local trauma may cause abscess formation by altering the local anatomy and thus destroying natural tissue barriers to infection.[141,142] Perirectal abscesses may serve as a portal of entry for organisms responsible for necrotic soft tissue infections such as Fournier's gangrene.[143]

Physical and Laboratory Findings

A perianal abscess is not generally difficult to diagnose. The throbbing pain in the perianal region is acute and aggravated by sitting, coughing, sneezing, and straining. There is swelling, induration, tenderness, and a small area of cellulitis in proximity to the anus. Rectal examination of a patient with a perianal abscess reveals that most of the tenderness and induration are located below the level of the anal ring. Deeper abscesses may be difficult to localize and identify. Computed tomography is often the first imaging study given its ready availability. The sensitivity of computed tomography for anorectal abscesses, however, is only 77%.[144] Therefore, when clinical suspicion is high, magnetic resonance imaging should be considered.

Patients with ischiorectal abscesses have fever, chills, and malaise, but at first there is less pain than with a perianal abscess. Initially on physical examination, one will see an asymmetry of the perianal tissue; later, erythema and induration are apparent. Digital examination reveals a large, tense, tender swelling along the anal canal that extends above the anorectal ring. If both ischiorectal spaces are involved, the findings are bilateral.

Patients with intersphincteric abscesses usually have dull, aching pain in the rectum rather than in the perianal region. No external aberrations of the perianal tissues are noted, but tenderness may be present. On digital examination one frequently palpates a soft, tender, sausage-shaped mass above the anorectal ring; if the mass has already ruptured, the patient may give a history of passage of purulent material during defecation.[142,145]

Diagnosis of pelvirectal abscesses may be very difficult. Usually, fever, chills, and malaise are present, but because the abscess is so deeply seated, few or no signs or symptoms are present in the perianal region. Rectal or vaginal examination may reveal a tender swelling that is adherent to the rectal mucosa above the anorectal ring.

Laboratory findings do not always aid in the diagnosis. Kovalcik and colleagues[139] found that less than 50% of their patients had a white blood cell count greater than 10.0×10^9/L. Cultures of perirectal abscesses usually show mixed infections involving anaerobic bacteria, most commonly *B. fragilis* and gram-negative enteric bacilli. MRSA, though less common, should also be considered in endemic areas.[140]

Treatment

Successful management of perirectal abscesses depends on adequate surgical drainage. Complications from these infections may necessitate multiple surgical procedures, prolong hospital stays, and result in sepsis and death. Bevans and associates[141] retrospectively studied the charts of 184 patients who were treated surgically over a 10-year period. These patients were evaluated primarily to identify factors that contributed to morbidity and mortality. Initial drainage was performed under local anesthesia in 38% of the patients and under spinal or general anesthesia in 62%. The authors identified three key factors in those with excessive morbidity and mortality: (1) delay in diagnosis and treatment, (2) inadequate initial examination or treatment, and (3) associated systemic disease. They believed that the only way to effectively examine and adequately drain all but superficial well-localized perirectal abscesses was under spinal or general anesthesia. This assessment was supported by evidence of an increased incidence of recurrence, sepsis, and death in patients treated under local anesthesia. Drainage of deep abscesses under local anesthesia generally does not allow drainage of all hidden loculations. In addition, local anesthesia is not adequate for the treatment of associated pathologic conditions.

Small, well-defined perianal abscesses without deeper perirectal involvement are the only perirectal infections that lend themselves to outpatient therapy. All other perirectal abscesses should be drained in the OR. The result of I&D is almost immediate relief of pain and rapid resolution of infection. Indications for inpatient drainage are failure to obtain adequate anesthesia, systemic toxicity, extension of the abscess beyond a localized area, or recurrence of a perianal abscess. Recurrence may be caused by the presence of a fistula in ano.

Drain a perianal abscess through a cruciate incision because if a simple linear incision is used, the abscess cavity has a propensity to close prematurely without adequate drainage. With either technique, make an incision over the area that is most fluctuant. If a simple linear incision is used, lightly pack the abscess cavity for at least 24 hours to ensure adequate drainage. It is extremely painful to probe a perianal abscess and to break up loculations, so liberal analgesia is advised and conscious sedation should be considered. Advise the patient to begin sitz baths at home 24 hours after surgery. Replace the packing at 48-hour intervals until the infection has cleared and granulation tissue has appeared. This usually occurs within 4 to 6 days. Antibiotics are not generally required.

Use of de Pezzer catheters in anorectal abscesses has been described as an alternative to traditional incision and packing. In a series of 91 patients treated in this manner, Kyle and Isbister[142] found equivalent rates of subsequent fistula surgery, less need for general anesthesia, and a shorter postoperative hospital stay than in patients treated with traditional incision and packing. Beck and coworkers[146] reported successful use of catheter drainage in 55 patients with an ischiorectal abscess. Because of the complexity of ischiorectal abscesses, this technique is probably best left to the surgeon who is providing ongoing care.

Perirectal abscesses are currently recognized as a fairly common cause of fever in granulocytopenic patients. These abscesses have a different bacteriologic profile: *Pseudomonas aeruginosa* organisms are isolated most frequently. These patients are initially seen later because pain develops later in the course, and fever may be the first manifestation. Therefore, any patients who are granulocytopenic with vague anorectal complaints, especially those with fever, should be examined carefully for perirectal abscesses. Any abscess that is found should be drained immediately under appropriate anesthesia, and extensive IV antibiotic coverage should be initiated.

Patients with a spontaneously ruptured perirectal abscess may appear to have experienced a self-cure, but under most circumstances they should still undergo formal I&D and packing. Treatment should be individualized.

Infected Sebaceous Cyst

A common entity that appears as a cutaneous abscess is an infected sebaceous cyst. Such infections are increasingly being caused by CA-MRSA. Sebaceous cysts, caused by obstruction of sebaceous gland ducts, can occur anywhere on the body. The cyst becomes filled with a thick, cheesy, sebaceous material, and the contents frequently become infected. Sebaceous cysts can be quite large and may persist for many years before they become infected. When infected, they appear clinically as tender, fluctuant subcutaneous masses, often with overlying erythema.

The initial treatment of an infected sebaceous cyst is simple I&D (Fig. 37-29). The loop drainage technique may not be suited for this abscess. The thick sebaceous material must be expressed because it is too thick to drain spontaneously. An important difference exists between infected sebaceous cysts and other abscesses. A sebaceous cyst has a definite pearly white capsule that must be excised to prevent recurrence. Traditionally, in the presence of significant inflammation it is preferable to drain the infection initially and remove the shiny capsule on the first follow-up visit or at a later visit, when it can be more easily identified. Alternatively, the entire cyst can be removed during the initial incision. At the time of capsule removal, the edges are grasped with clamps or hemostats, and the entire capsule is removed by sharp dissection with a scalpel or scissors. After excision of the capsule, the area is treated in the same manner as a healing abscess cavity. Simple drainage without excision of the capsule often leads to recurrence.

Kitamura and colleagues[147] reported a randomized study of 71 patients treated by either traditional I&D or primary resection of the cyst, followed by irrigation and wound closure. In this study the patients treated by primary resection had faster healing, fewer days of pain, and less scarring.

Paronychia

Paronychia is an infection localized to the area around the nail root (Fig. 37-30). It is a common infection probably caused by frequent trauma to the delicate skin around the fingernail and the cuticle. These type of infections have also been linked to "insults" induced by nail cosmetics (mechanical trauma, irritant reactions, and allergic reactions)[148] and to a number of occupations (e.g., hair cutting and meat handling).[149] When a minor infection begins, the nail itself may act like a foreign body. Usually, the infectious process is limited to the area above the nail base and underneath the eponychium (cuticle), but occasionally, it may spread to include tissue under the nail as well and form a subungual abscess. Lymphadenitis and lymphadenopathy are not usually seen. Generally, a paronychia is a mixed bacterial infection. *Staphylococcus* is commonly cultured from these lesions; however, anaerobes and numerous gram-negative organisms may be isolated.[150] Paronychia in children is often caused by anaerobes, and it is believed that this is the result of finger sucking and nail biting. Occasionally, a group A β-hemolytic streptococcal infection will develop in a paronychia in a child with streptococcal pharyngitis who engages in thumb sucking.[151,152] Paronychias involving CA-MRSA have been reported.[153,154]

A paronychia appears as a swelling and tenderness of the soft tissue along the base or the side of a fingernail (Fig. 37-31). Pain, often around a hangnail, usually prompts a visit to the ED. The infection begins as a cellulitis and may form a frank abscess. If the nail bed is mobile, the infectious process has extended under the nail, and a more extensive drainage procedure should be performed. Although no comparative trials of surgical management versus oral antibiotics have been performed,[155] some general guidelines for the management of

SEBACEOUS CYST EXCISION

This patient has an infected sebaceous cyst on the posterior of the earlobe (*arrow*). These lesions are typically tender, fluctuant, subcutaneous masses, often with overlying erythema.

Drain the cyst as you would a typical abscess. The thick sebaceous material must be expressed manually, because it is too thick to drain spontaneously.

Sebaceous cysts differ from simple abscesses in that they have a distinct capsule with a pearly white appearance (*arrow*). This capsule must be removed to prevent recurrence. This may be done initially or on a return visit once the inflammation has subsided.

Appearance of the cavity after excision of the capsule. Treat the lesion as you would any other abscess, with wound packing and timely follow-up care.

Figure 37-29 Excision of an infected sebaceous cyst. Loop drainage is not applicable to this abscess due to the need for capsule removal.

Figure 37-30 Paronychia. *1,* Abscess at the side of the nail. *2,* The infection has extended around the base of the nail. It has raised the eponychium but has not penetrated under the nail. *3,* End stage of paronychia, with a subeponychial and subungual abscess. (*From Wolcott MW, ed.* Ferguson's Surgery of the Ambulatory Patient. *5th ed. Philadelphia: Lippincott; 1974. Reproduced with permission.*)

paronychias have become established in clinical practice. If soft tissue swelling is present without fluctuance, remission may be achieved with frequent hot soaks (six to eight times a day) and a short course of oral antibiotics (3 to 4 days).[156] Incision will be of little value at this early cellulitic phase. Antibiotic treatment of localized infection is summarized in Table 37-2. If significant cellulitis is present, a broad-spectrum antistaphylococcal antibiotic (cephalosporin or semisynthetic penicillin) may be tried. Splint and elevate the digit.[156,157]

When a definite abscess has formed, drainage is usually curative quickly. A number of invasive operative approaches have been suggested. Actual skin incision or removal of the nail is rarely required, and neither procedure should be the initial form of treatment. One can invariably obtain adequate drainage by simply lifting the eponychial fold away from the nail matrix to allow the pus to drain. This is usually curative because a paronychia is not a cutaneous abscess per se, but rather a collection of pus in the potential space between the cuticle and the proximal end of the fingernail. Drainage may

Figure 37-31 Paronychia in various degrees of severity. **A,** Paronychia of the index finger. In this early stage of abscess formation, the collection is limited to the lateral nail fold (*arrow*). **B,** More advanced paronychia of the great toe. The abscess has spread around the base of the nail and lifted the eponychium (*arrows*) but has not yet spread under the nail. There is associated cellulitis on the distal portion of the toe. **C,** Even more advanced paronychia, with subungual extension (*black arrow*) and cellulitis extending up the finger and onto the dorsum of the hand (*white arrow*). This patient required removal of the nail and intravenous antibiotics.

TABLE 37-2 Common Hand Infections, Usual Offending Organisms, and Appropriate Therapeutic Regimens

CONDITION	MOST COMMON OFFENDING ORGANISMS	RECOMMENDED ANTIMICROBIAL AGENTS	COMMENTS
Paronychia	Usually *Staphylococcus aureus* or streptococci; *Pseudomonas*, gram-negative bacilli, and anaerobes may be present, especially in patients with exposure to oral flora	First-generation cephalosporin or antistaphylococcal penicillin; if anaerobes or *Escherichia coli* is suspected, oral clindamycin (Cleocin) or a β-lactamase inhibitor such as amoxicillin-clavulanate potassium (Augmentin)	I&D should be performed if infection is well established If infection is chronic, suspect *Candida albicans* Early infections without cellulitis may respond to conservative therapy
Felon	*S. aureus*, streptococci	First-generation cephalosporin or antistaphylococcal penicillin	I&D should be performed if infection is well established Oral antibiotic therapy is usually adequate
Herpetic whitlow	Herpes simplex virus	Supportive therapy	Antivirals may be prescribed if infection has been present for <48 hr For recurrent herpetic whitlow, suppressive therapy with an antiviral agent may be helpful Consider antibiotics if secondarily infected I&D contraindicated

Adapted from Clark DC. Common acute hand infections. *Am Fam Physician*. 2003;68:167.
I&D, infection and drainage.

be accomplished without anesthesia in selected patients,[158] but a digital nerve block is frequently required. After softening the eponychium by soaking, advance a No. 11 scalpel blade, scissors, or a 21- to 23-gauge needle parallel to the nail and under the eponychium at the site of maximal swelling (Fig. 37-32).[157,159,160] Pus escapes rapidly, with immediate relief of pain. A tourniquet placed at the base of the finger may limit bleeding and aid the clinician in determining the exact extent of the infection during the drainage procedure.

If more than a tiny pocket of pus is present, fan the knife tip or needle or spread the scissors under the eponychium while keeping the instrument parallel to the plane of the fingernail (see Fig. 37-32, *steps 5 and 6*). When a large amount of pus is drained, slip a small piece of packing gauze under the eponychium for 24 hours to provide continual drainage. Cultures are generally not indicated. Antibiotics are frequently prescribed, although they are not essential if drainage is complete or the surrounding area of cellulitis is minimal.

PARONYCHIA DRAINAGE

In selected patients the procedure can be completed without anesthesia. After softening the eponychium by soaking, advance a No. 11 scalpel blade under the eponychium parallel to the nail.

Pus escapes rapidly, with immediate relief of pain. Antibiotics are not required for minor cases. Instruct the patient to frequently soak the digit in warm water at home.

Many patients, especially those with a large paronychia, will require a digital block before the procedure. (See Chapter 31 for details on digital blocks.)

Lift the eponychial fold away from the nail. Here, the blunt side of a No. 15 blade is being used. No sharp incision is required; simply lifting the eponychium away from the nail is sufficient.

Pus will readily escape as the fold is lifted.

Keep the scalpel parallel to the nail and continue to lift the eponychium to release all the pus. Place a small piece of packing gauze under the eponychium for 24 hours, encourage warm soaks, and prescribe antibiotics if cellulitis is present.

Figure 37-32 Paronychia drainage.

An alternative to systemic antibiotics is to keep the operative site bathed in antibiotic ointment. After the anesthesia has worn off, start the patient on frequent soaks in warm tap water at home. In most cases the patient may easily remove the packing. At 24 to 36 hours, soak the finger in hot water and pull the gauze out; a repeated visit to a clinician is not required if healing is progressing, but follow-up examinations should always be encouraged. Once the packing is removed, cover the area with a dry, absorbent dressing. Apply an antibiotic ointment to the site for a few days. The benefit of antibiotic ointments in reducing infection is unproven, but instruct the patient on detailed use of the ointment. The ointment helps keep the bandage from sticking.

An alternative technique called the Swiss roll technique was described by Pabari and colleagues for severe acute paronychia with a run-around or contiguous infection of both nail folds. With a No. 15 scalpel blade pointing away from the nail bed, make an incision on both sides of the nail fold. The nail fold, after thorough irrigation with saline, is then rolled proximally over nonadherent dressing, like a swiss roll, and sutured to the skin with a nonabsorbable dressing. Apply a finger dressing. Remove the sutures in 48 hours and unfold the nail fold back to its original position to allow it to heal by secondary intention.[161] The authors argue that this technique spares the nail plate and allows rapid healing, although no controlled studies have compared this technique with simple incision followed by packing gauze described above.

If the infection has produced purulence beneath the nail (subungual abscess), remove a portion of the nail or trephinate the nail to ensure complete drainage. As an alternative to nail removal, place a hole in the proximal part of the nail with a hot paper clip or a portable electrocautery device. Make a large opening or multiple holes to ensure continued drainage. The proximal portion of the nail is involved in most cases. Treat this by bluntly elevating the eponychium to expose the proximal edge of the nail. Elevate the proximal third of the nail from the nail bed and resect it with scissors. Leave the distal two thirds of the nail in place to act as a physiologic dressing and to decrease postoperative pain (Fig. 37-33). If purulence is found below the lateral edge of the nail, gently elevate the affected part and excise it longitudinally.[162] Exercise care during this procedure to avoid damage to the nail matrix. Place a wick of gauze beneath the eponychium for 48 hours to ensure continued drainage.

Most paronychias resolve in a few days, and one to two postoperative visits should be scheduled to evaluate healing and reinforce home care. For compliant patients with a small paronychia, home care alone may suffice after the initial drainage. Clinical infection lasting longer than a few weeks should prompt evaluation for osteomyelitis of the distal phalanx, a well-known but rare complication of even a properly drained paronychia.

Patients occasionally come to the ED complaining of a chronic, indolent paronychial infection. These seldom respond to ED intervention. Frank purulence is rarely present, and conservative treatments are often unsatisfactory. Many causes of this frustrating condition have been described, including fungal, bacterial, viral, and psoriatic conditions. Screen patients for malignancy if they have chronic paronychia that is unresponsive to therapy.[159] Treatment modalities are varied, and controlled studies evaluating the various techniques are lacking. Meticulous hand care, oral and topical antimicrobial medications, and occasionally aggressive

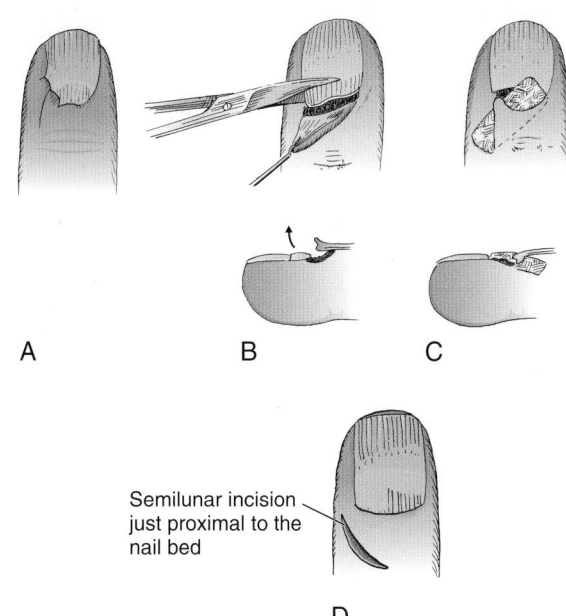

Figure 37-33 **A-C,** Aggressive treatment of recurrent paronychia or subungual abscess includes removal of a portion of the proximal part of the nail and incision of the eponychium. **D,** Some physicians prefer to use a semilunar incision proximal to the eponychium rather than directly incising and potentially injuring the cuticle permanently. These aggressive therapies are seldom required and are not first-line interventions.

Semilunar incision just proximal to the nail bed

surgical intervention have been suggested.[160] Refer these patients to a dermatologist or hand surgeon because of the prolonged treatment required.

Herpetic Whitlow

Herpetic whitlow is an extremely contagious infection of the distal phalanx caused by herpes simplex virus (type 1 or 2) (Fig. 37-34). In children, herpetic whitlow tends to be associated with gingivostomatosis caused by herpes simplex 1, whereas adults most commonly harbor herpes simplex 2. Inoculation occurs through a discontinuity in the skin.[163] Health care providers exposed to oral secretions (e.g., dental hygienists and respiratory therapists) and patients with other herpes infections are most commonly infected.[164,165] After a 2-day to 2-week incubation period, an infected individual may experience prodromal signs and symptoms such as fever, malaise, lymphadenitis, and axillary lymphadenopathy. In the affected finger the infection is characterized by tenderness followed by throbbing pain (out of proportion to the findings on physical examination), edema, and erythema. Vesicles containing clear, bloody, or cloudy fluid form and mark the most infectious stage of the process. Viral vesicles typically involve the digits but can also involve other areas of the hand.[166] The lesions are usually quite painful but are self-limited and resolve in 2 to 3 weeks. I&D of herpetic whitlow is contraindicated because it may induce a secondary bacterial infection and delay healing.[164,167] Treatment is symptomatic and consists of splinting, elevation, and analgesia as needed. Oral antiviral agents effective against herpes infections (acyclovir, famciclovir, or valacyclovir) can shorten the course of the disease if given early (see Box 37-3). After an accidental needlestick in health care

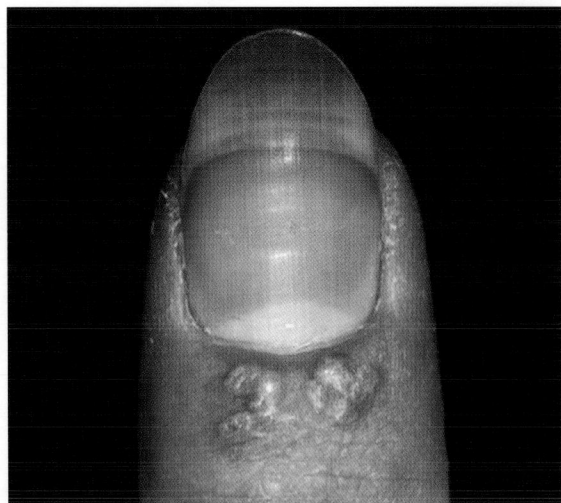

Figure 37-34 Herpetic whitlow. Clinical findings include pain out of proportion to the results of examination, erythema, and vesicular lesions. Herpetic whitlow may be confused with paronychia. However, incision plus drainage is contraindicated because it may lead to bacterial superinfection. *(From Habif TP. Clinical Dermatology. 5th ed. St. Louis: Mosby; 2009.)*

Figure 37-35 A well-developed felon. In this advanced case the patient had little pain at initial evaluation. The distal phalanx was almost completely resorbed because of pressure, inflammation, and chronic osteomyelitis. This infection is extensive and warrants consultation with a hand specialist.

workers, oral famciclovir may be used as a preventive.[168] Infection recurs in 30% to 50% of cases, but the initial infection is usually the most severe. Acyclovir, 200 mg taken orally three to four times a day, can decrease recurrence rates.[165]

Consideration must be given to preventing spread of the infection. An occlusive dressing decreases the chance of viral transmission, but health care providers with herpetic whitlow should limit and perhaps even refrain from patient contact, especially until all lesions have crusted over and viral shedding has stopped.[169,170] Compliance with universal precautions will decrease the likelihood of patient-to-provider transmission.

Felon

A felon is an infection of the pulp of the distal end of the finger (Fig. 37-35). The usual cause is trauma with secondary invasion by bacteria. A felon may develop in the presence of a foreign body, such as a thorn or a splinter, but often a precipitating trauma cannot be identified. An important anatomic characteristic of this area is that many fibrous septa extend from the volar skin of the fat pad to the periosteum of the phalanx; these septa subdivide and compartmentalize the pulp area. When an infection occurs in the pulp, these structures make it a closed-space infection. The septa limit swelling, delay pointing of the abscess, and inhibit drainage after incomplete surgical decompression. Pressure may increase in the closed space and initiate an ischemic process that compounds the infection. The infection can progress to osteomyelitis of the distal phalanx, septic arthritis, and flexor tenosynovitis. Although the septa may facilitate an infection in the pulp, they also provide a barrier that protects the joint space and tendon sheath by limiting proximal spread of the infection.

In most cases the offending organism is *S. aureus*, but mixed infections and gram-negative infection may also occur. A study looking at the bacteriology of hand infections over an 11-year period found that of 159 hand infections, 48 (30%) harbored CA-MRSA, the incidence of CA-MRSA increased by 41% per year, and IV drug use and felon infections in particular were risk factors for CA-MRSA.[162] These changing patterns, along with the often protracted course of felons and concern for osteomyelitis, make this one of the few soft tissue infections in which culture may be helpful.

A patient in whom a felon is developing will describe a gradual onset of pain and tenderness of the fingertip. In a few days the pain becomes constant and throbbing and gradually becomes severe. In the initial stages, physical examination may be quite unimpressive because the fibrous septa limit swelling in the closed pulp space. As the infection progresses, swelling and redness become obvious. Occasionally, one may elicit point tenderness, but frequently, the entire pulp space is extremely tender. The patient characteristically arrives with the hand elevated over the head because the pain is so intense in the dependent position. Cessation of pain indicates necrosis and nerve degeneration.

During the early stages of cellulitis, a felon may be controlled by treatment consisting of elevation, oral antibiotics (see Box 37-3), and warm water or saline soaks. For more developed felons, proper treatment consists of early and complete I&D.[164] Antibiotics alone are not curative once suppuration has occurred. Delaying surgery may result in permanent disability and deformity.

A minor felon can usually be drained on an outpatient basis with a digital nerve block (Fig. 37-36). A long-acting anesthetic (bupivacaine) will prolong the anesthesia. A tourniquet (1.25-cm Penrose drain) can be used to allow an incision into a bloodless field. Surgical drainage must be performed carefully to avoid injury to nerves, vessels, and flexor tendons. Most felons can be managed with a limited procedure, but many surgical options have been advocated, none of which has been proved to be superior for all circumstances.[164] Traditional incisions ("hockey stick" or "fish mouth") have a propensity for complications such as sloughing of tissue and postoperative fat pad anesthesia or instability and are rarely used. The preferred initial treatment is a simple longitudinal incision over the area of greatest fluctuance,[171,172] 3 to 5 mm distal to the distal interphalangeal joint. The incision may be made laterally or along the volar surface (see Fig. 37-36A), although injury to the sensory nerve or digital artery is more of a

FELON DRAINAGE

1

Preferred approach

Lateral incision may be through and through

2 Avoid digital nerves

Alternative approach

3 Avoid the flexor tendon

A, The preferred initial incision for draining a felon is made directly into the area of most fluctuance (*1*). More aggressive incisions should be reserved for complicated cases because they have greater morbidity and require more complicated wound care. The unilateral longitudinal approach is a good first choice. Some prefer a similarly located through-and-through incision (see below).

A fat pad incision is generally avoided but can be acceptable for localized infections. They may be associated with a painful scar in an area that is often traumatized. The transverse fat pad incision should avoid the digital nerves (*2*), and the longitudinal fat pad incision should avoid the flexor tendon (*3*).

A

1

This patient has an extensive paronychia (*arrow*) but did not seek medical attention.

2

The infection has spread volarly and progressed to a felon. Drainage of both areas is required.

3

The eponychium is lifted, which resulted in immediate drainage of large quantities of pus.

4

A hemostat is placed under the eponychium to facilitate complete evacuation of the pus.

5

To drain the felon, a through-and-through incision is made on the volar side. A hemostat is used to break up loculations in the fat pad and then to grab gauze for a pull-through pack.

6

The gauze pack is pulled through the incision and left in place for 24 to 48 hours to ensure continued drainage.

B

Figure 37-36 Felon drainage. For a felon the authors prefer the through-and-through drainage procedure shown in **B.** Antibiotics should be used postoperatively. Culture can aid in the selection of long-term antibiotics, but most initially cover for community-acquired methicillin-resistant *Staphylococcus aureus*.

concern with the lateral incision given its proximity to these structures. Frank pus may be encountered during incision, but usually only a few drops are expressed. One more often drains a combination of necrotic tissue and interstitial fluid. A foreign body should be sought even if the history is not known. A potential drawback to an incision in the middle of the fat pad is the production of a scar in a very sensitive and commonly traumatized area. The incision must not extend to the distal interphalangeal crease because of the danger of injuring the flexor tendon. The subcutaneous tissue is bluntly dissected with a hemostat to provide adequate drainage. A gauze pack may be placed in the wound for 24 to 48 hours to ensure continued drainage. Recurrent or more severe infections may require a more aggressive approach by a hand specialist. Follow-up recommendations for patients with a diagnosis of felon should include referral to a hand surgeon.

No matter which incision is made, it must not be carried proximal to the closed pulp space because of the danger of entrance into the tendon sheath or the joint capsule. A snug dressing, splinting, elevation, and adequate opioid analgesics are prerequisites for a successful outcome. Most felons are treated empirically with antibiotics for at least 5 days. A broad-spectrum cephalosporin is a reasonable choice pending cultures (if done). Antibiotics effective against CA-MRSA should also be considered given its increasing incidence. MRSA infections can be treated with vancomycin, 1 g twice a day, or linezolid and may require weeks until resolution.[173] Oral linezolid may allow outpatient treatment.

The patient should be rechecked in 2 to 3 days. On the first postoperative visit, perform a digital block and remove the packing if present. Irrigate the incision copiously with saline, and remove any additional necrotic tissue. If there is continued drainage at this time, replace the drain for 24 to 48 hours, but it can usually be removed and a dressing reapplied. Soaking may be advised. At the first revisit, check the sensitivities of the bacterial cultures, and make a decision to continue or change antibiotics.

Some clinicians advocate radiographic evaluation for retained foreign bodies at the initial visit, as well as a baseline evaluation of the bone for subsequent evaluation of osteomyelitis. Other clinicians reserve radiographs for wounds not showing significant improvement in 5 to 7 days. Evidence of osteomyelitis, however, may not be found radiographically for several weeks after the appearance of the lesion. Persistent infections necessitate more radical I&D and may require IV antibiotics. After adequate drainage, osteomyelitis may respond surprisingly well to outpatient antibiotic therapy, with almost complete regeneration of bone being achieved if the I&D procedure has been adequate.

Fingertip infections can be stubborn. Difficult or persistent cases require evaluation and care by a hand surgeon. In these cases, early consultation is advisable to avert catastrophic complications such as loss of function or amputation.

SEROMA AND HEMATOMA DRAINAGE

Although most I&D procedures are performed for decompression of purulent collections, drainage of sterile hematomas or seromas may be required in the ED. In general, the same principles used for formal drainage of pus in the soft tissues apply to drainage of a sterile fluid collection, and hence one can directly apply the principles of this chapter to the drainage of sterile fluids. In addition, when a sterile fluid collection is drained, the operator has the option of primarily closing the incision site after wound irrigation (see Chapters 34 and 35 for wound management techniques). Drainage of a soft tissue hematoma is generally best postponed for several days after the initial injury to permit hemostasis and to minimize the risk for reaccumulation of the hematoma after drainage. The procedure is generally reserved for soft tissue hematomas that are large and painful (secondary to tissue distention), and they are expected to either resolve slowly or result in soft tissue deformity if not drained. Seromas and hematomas rarely become infected if the overlying skin remains intact. It is best to avoid needle aspiration because this procedure rarely drains the collection completely and it has the potential to introduce infection into a good culture medium in a closed space. If a hematoma becomes infected, treat it as a cutaneous abscess.

Although it is tempting to drain a small, seemingly fluctuant noninfected hematoma that has persisted for many days, a conservative nonoperative approach is usually best. A persistent mass after trauma usually causes concern in patients, so a thorough explanation should be provided. Most hematomas will resolve, albeit slowly (weeks), and incision is often disappointing in its yield (unless the hematoma is large and superficial) and leaves a scar. Drainage of a subungual hematoma represents a special case of hematoma drainage.

Subungual Hematoma

Subungual hematomas are typically caused by hitting a fingertip with a hammer, slamming a finger in a door (Fig. 37-37), or dropping a weight on a foot. The patient's main concern is obtaining relief from the terrible throbbing pain that increases with the pressure under the nail.

When describing the injury, the clinician should estimate the percentage of nail bed that is affected by the hematoma and discuss associated trauma to the nail margins or surrounding tissue. The examination should include tests of the extensor and flexor tendons, of circulation by capillary refill, and of the sensitivity of the area.[174]

If fracture of the distal phalanx is suspected (e.g., if the fingertip is unstable or the mechanism of injury suggests a fracture), obtain anteroposterior and lateral x-ray films. Radiographs differentiate tendinous from bony mallet-type injuries. Crush injuries are associated with three types of distal phalanx fractures: longitudinal, transverse, and comminuted. If the fracture is angulated, displaced, unstable, or intraarticular or involves a third or more of the articular surface, refer the patient to a hand surgeon.[175] Because trephination in patients with a distal phalanx fracture converts a closed fracture into an open one, there is concern about infectious and cosmetic complications. In the two studies that examined this possible association,[176,177] with fracture subsets totaling 26, no infections occurred. The presence of an underlying fracture does not contraindicate nail trephination for fear of converting a closed fracture into an open one.

Nail removal is unnecessary, even if there is an underlying distal phalanx fracture, as long as the nail margins and nail are intact.[178,179] If the nail is split, avulsed or disrupted or a nail bed laceration extends to the skin, the nail should be removed and the underlying nail bed repaired (see further discussion in Chapter 35). Simple trephination of an uncomplicated subungual hematoma, even if it involves the entire subungual

Figure 37-37 Subungual hematoma. **A,** Subungual hematoma with a totally blackened nail bed. Do not remove this intact nail even though the nail bed is lacerated or there is a total hematoma and underlying minor tuft fracture. In this example, blood accumulated only under the nail, not in any paronychial areas. **B,** Subungual hematoma of the great toe after dropping a heavy object on the foot (a common injury).

area, results in a good outcome functionally and cosmetically.[180] Trephination should also be considered if the hematoma covers more than half the intact nail or if it is smaller but painful.

Prophylactic antibiotics are not necessary for patients with uncomplicated subungual hematomas that have been trephinated. For more serious injuries, a slight risk for infection exists, but in most cases, rigorous wound cleaning and careful soft tissue repair constitute adequate treatment.[181,182]

Methods of Trephination

All methods of trephination require aseptic technique. Clean the nail thoroughly and place the digit in a sterile field. Follow universal precautions because the fluid under the nail is under pressure and can spurt.[183] Ensure that adequate analgesia has been achieved. Anesthesia is not always required, but a digital block can be used to calm an anxious patient and is commonly performed.

Hot cautery is the most common form of trephination and is usually done with a paper clip that has been straightened and heated in a flame (Figs. 37-38 and 37-39). Place the hot end on the nail above the center of the hematoma and apply gentle pressure until the nail is breached and the hematoma expressed. A "give" is felt as the instrument passes through the nail. Stop the pressure at this point to avoid damage to the nail bed. Blood exits rapidly, and the blackened nail regains its normal color (see Fig. 37-39, *step 3*). The blood usually remains fluid for 24 to 36 hours and can easily be expressed with slight pressure. Multiple holes may be needed for continued drainage. Do not use hot cautery trephination on artificial nails because they are flammable.[178] Hot cautery with a paper clip is easy to perform, but hematomas treated in this way tend to reform. A cold lancet has the benefits of reducing the pain immediately, as well as reducing the likelihood of infection.[179] A portable hot-wire electrocautery unit can be used, but it is difficult to obtain an adequate drainage hole without adapting the instrument (see Fig. 37-39). It can be modified to burn a larger hole by "fattening" the end of the wire loop and rotating the device slowly as the nail is penetrated or by removing a small rectangle of nail. In addition to being convenient, the cautery device is desirable because the wire stays hotter longer, thereby enhancing nail penetration.

Figure 37-38 A straightened paper clip, held with a hemostat and heated with a flame, can be used for hot cautery trephination.

The PathFormer (Path Scientific, Carlisle, MA) is a new device that allows controlled nail trephination ("mesoscission") and therefore minimizes patient discomfort during the procedure.[183] It uses electrical resistance in the nail bed as feedback to stop and retract the drill when it penetrates the nail plate. The nail bed, with its blood supply and nerve endings, is not disturbed.

An 18- or 21-gauge needle can be rotated between the thumb and the index finger while gentle pressure is applied so that the sharp end of the needle corkscrews through the nail.[183] When using a needle, the give is harder to feel, so the clinician should proceed slowly until blood is drawn. Because the hole made with a needle is small, a second hole may be required.

An alternative needle-based approach is being used by a group of Turkish dermatologists. Kaya and associates[184] use extra fine, 29-gauge insulin syringes for evacuation of hematomas. After the nail is trimmed, the needle is inserted parallel to the nail plate and advanced to the distal edge of the hematoma. This technique is especially effective for small hematomas of the second, third, and fourth toenails, which are hard to trephine.

A No. 11 scalpel blade can be used to score and then cut through the affected nail. This approach is painful for the patient because the hole is usually larger than what is required.

NAIL TREPHINATION

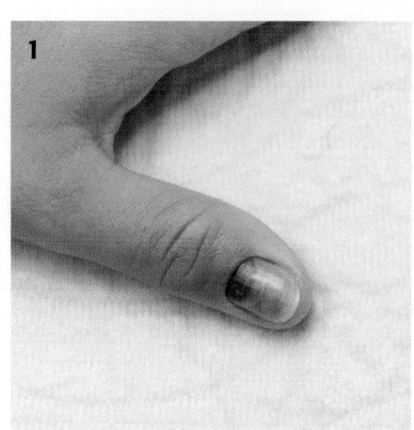

This patient has a painful subungal hematoma and requires trephination. Cleanse the area with antiseptic prior to trephination. Anesthesia with a digital block can optionally be used.

Place the hot cautery device (here, a disposable cautery pen) over the center of the hematoma and apply gentle pressure. A "give" is felt and blood is rapidly expressed as the hematoma is released. Multiple holes may be required.

Successful trephination is demonstrated by relief of pain and return of the normal color of the nail bed.

Figure 37-39 Nail trephination.

Outcome

It is difficult to predict the fate of the fingernail after drainage of a subungual hematoma. Obviously, there must be a nail bed laceration if bleeding occurs, but with a stable nail bed, repair is unnecessary. Even if a small tuft fracture is present, most do well with simple drainage. Some patients will lose the nail, but if the nail root or nail bed is not significantly disrupted and the nail remains implanted, a normal-appearing nail is the usual final result.

After a hematoma has been drained, the nail should be cleaned thoroughly and a dry dressing applied. Patients should be advised to keep the digit dry for 2 days. Any fracture should be splinted and given appropriate follow-up at a surgical clinic.

Conditions with a Similar Appearance

One condition that may be mistaken for a simple subungual hematoma is closed avulsion of the base of a fingernail occurring in conjunction with a subungual hematoma from a nail bed laceration. A common mechanism is slamming a finger in a car door, which causes sudden flexion of the distal phalanx in conjunction with a crush injury of the nail bed. The nail itself is usually stable, so generally no repair of the nail bed appears to be required. However, if the subungual hematoma extends past the confines of the nail bed, such as in the paronychial space (under the skin of the cuticle), there must be a communication between the nail bed and this space. This produces a paronychial hematoma, with blood occupying the space where pus would be located in an infectious paronychia (Fig. 37-40). When this condition is present, the avulsed proximal portion of the fingernail overlies the nail fold of the cuticle but is appreciated only after the overlying skin is opened. Open reduction (replacement) of the nail must be performed. The replaced nail often grows normally, but a lost or deformed nail is possible. Repair of the

nail bed laceration is optional at this juncture but may not be required if the nail is stable. Once the injury is anatomically aligned, splinting and soaking follow as for a simple subungual hematoma. These injuries rarely become infected, and there is no evidence that the prophylactic use of antibiotics is necessary.

Subungual hematomas can be manifestation of diseases such as Kaposi's sarcoma and melanoma. These conditions should be considered when no trauma has occurred and the findings on physical examination are not consistent with a simple subungual hematoma.

MUCOCELE

Sometimes mistaken for infection, a mucocele of the mucous membranes of the mouth is a nontender pearl-colored small lump that is felt by the patient's tongue. It is a plugged saliva gland, and it becomes evident when it fills up with a gel-like substance. Occasionally, the patient will squeeze it to express the gel, but the mucocele may return unless excised. Under local anesthesia, the entire mass is removed by sharp dissection with a scalpel. The ulcer is left open and will heal quickly (Fig. 37-41).

Acknowledgments

The authors acknowledge the significant contributions of Todd M. Warden, Mark W. Fourre, Howard Blumstein, and Ken Butler to this chapter in previous editions and Jeff Harrow for his help with this edition.

References are available at www.expertconsult.com

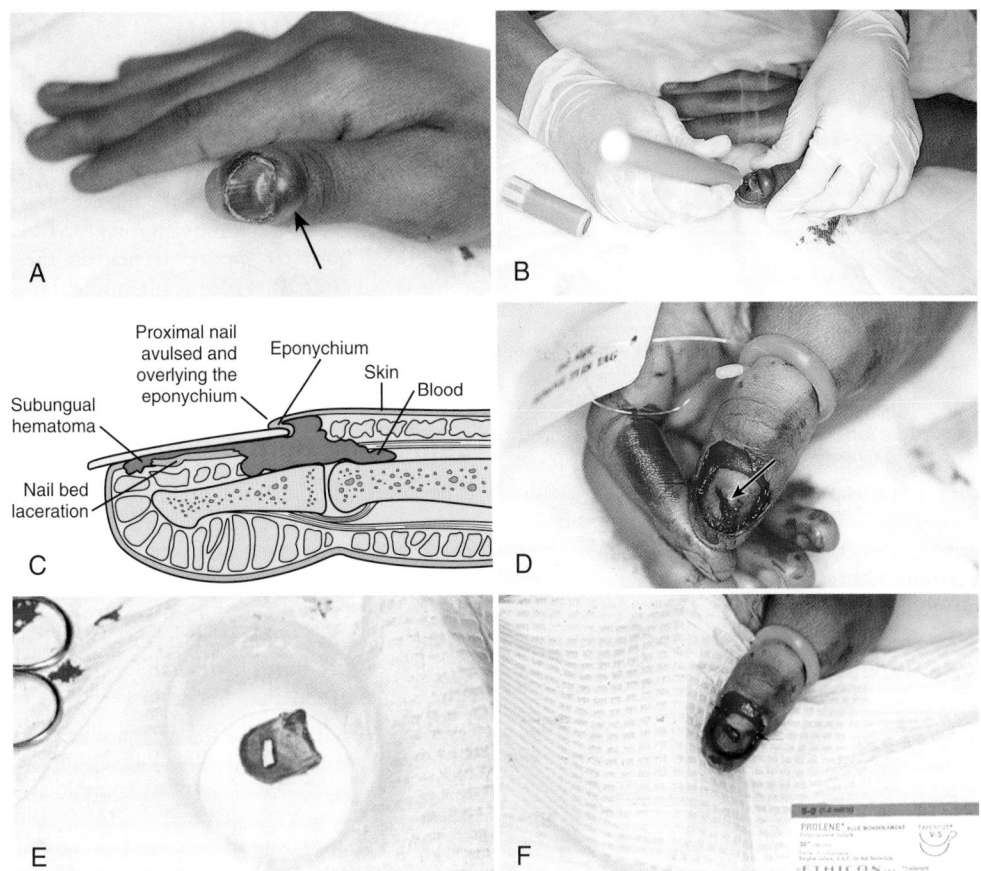

Figure 37-40 Complicated subungual hematoma. **A,** This patient slammed his finger in a car door and sustained acute flexion of the distal phalanx and a crush injury. It appears to be a simple subungual hematoma, but note the blood in the paronychial space (*arrow*). There is communication between the nail bed laceration and the eponychium. **B,** All the blood did not drain when the nail was trephinated. **C,** Blood accumulated in this area because the base of the fingernail has been avulsed from its origin and now lies between the eponychium (cuticle) and skin. This is appreciated when the skin is débrided. Note the white avulsed base of the fingernail just under the skin. The closed nature of the injury causes the confusion. **D,** With the nail removed, the nail bed laceration (*arrow*) can be seen and repaired. The old trephined nail (**E**) can now be replaced and sutured in its original position (**F**) to keep the eponychial space open, or the space can be packed with gauze for a few weeks to discourage scar formation and subsequent nail deformity. Note the drainage hole in the original nail.

Figure 37-41 A mucocele is a nontender lump filled with a gel-like substance that often appears on the mucosa of the lip. Lidocaine with epinephrine is injected locally. **A,** The entire structure is excised. **B,** The operative site is left open and heals rapidly. Simple aspiration of a mucocele is not usually curative.

CHAPTER 38

Burn Care Procedures

Anthony S. Mazzeo, Leigh Ann Price, and Kevin B. Gerold

Two million people suffer a burn-related injury every year in the United States. The American Burn Association (ABA) estimates that approximately 450,000 of these patients received medical evaluation and treatment in 2011 and approximately 10% (45,000) required hospitalization.[1] Patients who suffer burn injuries are predominately male (70%), and their mean age is 32 years old. Children younger than 5 years account for 18% of burns, and patients older than 60 years account for an additional 12%. Seventy percent of all burns involve less than 10% of the total body surface area (TBSA). Nearly 80% of all burns are caused by flame or fire or by scalds, with scald injury occurring most in children younger than 5 years.

Advances in resuscitation, surgical and anesthetic techniques, intensive care, infection control, nutrition, and metabolic support have all contributed to dramatic improvements in the preservation of body function, physical appearance, and emotional outcomes of patients with this injury. The initial care provided to burn patients by emergency medical providers can improve outcomes by preventing the conversion of superficial burns to deep burns requiring surgery and by improving the long-term functional and cosmetic outcomes of the affected tissues.

The classification of burns is based on three criteria[2]: depth of skin injury, percentage of TBSA involved, and source of injury (thermal, chemical, electrical, or radiation). The seriousness of a burn injury is determined by the characteristics and temperature of the burning agent, the duration of exposure, the location of the injury, the presence of associated injuries, and the age and general health of the victim (Table 38-1).

The ABA defines minor burns as uncomplicated partial-thickness burns involving less than 5% TBSA in children (<10 years old) or the elderly (>50 years old), less than 10% TBSA in adults, or full-thickness burns less than 2% TBSA.[3] Moderate or major burns include injuries that involve a greater TBSA, as well as burns in areas of specialized function, such as the face, hands, feet, and perineum. More serious burns also include those caused by a high-voltage electrical injury or those with associated inhalation injuries or other major trauma.

Throughout the course of history, clinicians have experimented with burn therapies to relieve pain and promote healing. Many treatment regimens and home remedies have been successful, largely because of the fact that minor burns generally do well with a modicum of intervention and commonsense wound care. Although little has changed in the care of minor ambulatory burns over the past 3 decades, treatment of major burns has significantly improved, including the development of sophisticated burn centers, increased knowledge of burn wound physiology, and prevention of infection.

WOUND EVALUATION

Emergency clinicians should be aware that the depth of a burn wound cannot always be determined accurately on clinical grounds alone at initial evaluation and that burn injury is a dynamic process that may change over time, particularly during the 24 to 48 hours after the burning process has been arrested. It is common, for example, for a seemingly minor or superficial burn to appear deeper on the second or third return visit (Fig. 38-1). This phenomenon is not a continuation of the burning process that can be altered by clinician intervention but is considered to be a pathophysiologic event related to tissue edema, dermal ischemia, or desiccation.[4]

Estimating Burn Depth

The depth of a burn is commonly classified by degree.[5] First degree involves the epidermis only, second-degree (or partial-thickness) burns extend into the dermis, and third-degree (or full-thickness) burns destroy the entire skin. An additional fourth degree is sometimes used to describe injuries to the underlying muscle, tendon, or bone (Fig. 38-2).

First-degree burns involve the epidermis only (Fig. 38-3A). The skin is reddened but is intact and not blistered. This injury ranges from mildly irritating or even pruritic to exquisitely painful. Minor edema may be noted. Causes include ultraviolet light (as in sunburn) and brief thermal "flash" burns. First-degree burns may blister within 24 to 36 hours, and the patient should be warned about this possibility. Frequently, the epidermis flakes or peels within 5 to 10 days. Healing occurs spontaneously, usually without scarring.

Second-degree burns involve the epidermis and extend into the dermis to include the sweat glands and hair follicles. Superficial second-degree burns involve only the papillary dermis (see Fig. 38-3B). These burns are pink, moist, and extremely painful. Blisters are common and the skin may slough. The burn blanches with pressure, and mild to moderate edema is common. Hair follicles are often intact. Superficial second-degree burns are the most common burns seen in the emergency department (ED). The usual causes are scalds, contact with hot objects, or exposure to chemicals. Barring infection or repeated trauma, these burns heal spontaneously and without scarring in about 2 weeks. These areas may be sensitive to sunburn, windburn, and skin irritation for months after the original injury has healed.

Deep second-degree burns involve the reticular dermis and appear mottled white or pink (see Fig. 38-3C). There is obvious edema and sloughing of the skin, and any blisters are usually ruptured. Blanching is absent. These burns are not generally painful initially and may have decreased sensation, but pressure may be perceived. Within a few days, however, these burns can become exquisitely painful. This type of burn may be converted to a full-thickness injury by further trauma or infection.

Third-degree burns result from complete loss of the dermis and may extend into subcutaneous (SQ) tissue (see Fig. 38-3D). These burns usually appear dry, pearly white, or charred. They are initially painless, with a leathery texture. Circumferential third-degree burns on an extremity or the torso cause a loss of elasticity that may impair the circulation or ventilation and necessitate an escharotomy.

Fourth-degree burns extend deeply into SQ tissue, muscle, fascia, or bone (see Fig. 38-3E). These burns are

TABLE 38-1   Characteristics of Burns, by Depth

CLASSIFICATION OF BURN	ETIOLOGY	APPEARANCE	SENSATION	TIME TO COMPLETE HEALING	SCARRING
First Degree					
Superficial epidermal layers	Sunburn, other UV exposure Short flash flame burns	Dry, red Blanches with pressure	Present May be quite painful	3-7 days	No
Second Degree					
Varying depth, blisters, or bullae formation Dermal appendages spared (e.g., sweat glands, hair follicles) Includes entire epidermis and some portion of the dermis					
Superficial partial thickness	Water scald Longer flash burn	Blisters, peeling skin Blanches with pressure Skin red and moist under blisters	Painful Exposure to air and temperature painful	7-21 days	Unusual if no infection and proper follow-up Pigment change may be seen Burned area may be sensitive to frostbite, windburn, and sunburn for many months Itching may be problematic for weeks after healing
Deep partial thickness	Flame Water immersion Oil, grease, hot foods (e.g., soup)	Variable color Wet or waxy dry, does not blanch Blisters easily removed, skin peeling off	Pressure only	>21 days	Severe; risk for contracture
Third Degree					
Loss of all skin elements, thrombosis and coagulation of vessels	Flame, steam, oil grease Immersion, scald Caustic chemical, high voltage	Leathery appearance, white or charred, dry, inelastic; blanching with pressure May be present under blisters	Deep pressure only	Never heals Requires grafting	Very severe, high risk for contracture

Modified after Clayton MC, Solem LD. No ice, no butter: advice on management of burns for primary care physicians. *Postgrad Med.* 1995;97:151; and Morgan ED, Bledsoe SC, Barker J. Ambulatory management of burns. *Am Fam Physician.* 2000;62:2015.
UV, ultraviolet.

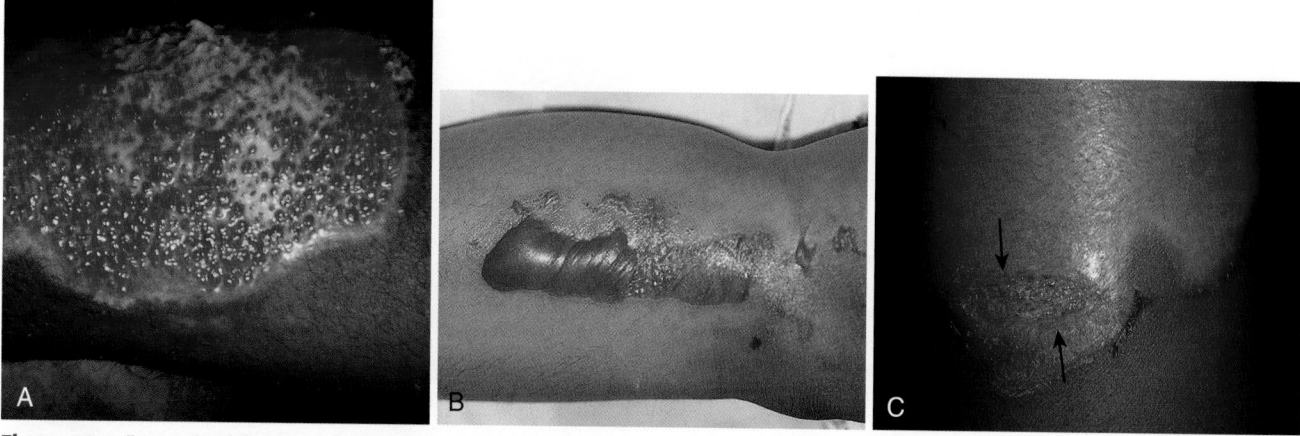

Figure 38-1 It may be difficult to accurately assess the depth or severity of a burn on the first visit. **A,** This full-thickness burn will not heal without a skin graft. **B,** This blistered hot water burn is probably second degree, but full-thickness burns can develop under blisters. **C,** At 2 weeks, a second-degree burn and small area of third-degree burn (*arrows*).

Figure 38-2 Depths of a burn. First-degree burns are confined to the epidermis. Second-degree burns extend into the dermis (dermal burns). Third-degree burns are full thickness through the epidermis and dermis. Fourth-degree burns involve injury to underlying tissue structures such as muscle, tendons, and bone. (*From Townsend CM, Beauchamp RD, Evers BM, et al, eds.* Sabiston Textbook of Surgery. *19th ed. St. Louis: Saunders; 2012.*)

Figure 38-3 Depth of thermal injury. **A,** Patient with sunburn on the lower extremity (a superficial or first-degree burn with associated blisters on the anterior tibial surface). **B,** Partial-thickness injury of the hand (superficial second-degree burn). **C,** Partial-thickness injury extending beyond the subcutaneous layers (deep second-degree burn). **D,** Full-thickness (third-degree) burn. **E,** Full-thickness injury with extensive tissue loss (fourth-degree burn). (*From Davis PJ, Cladis FP, Motoyama EK, eds.* Smith's Anesthesia for Infants and Children. *8th ed. St. Louis: Mosby; 2011.*)

TABLE 38-2 American Burn Association's Grading System for Burn Severity and Disposition of Patients*

	TYPE OF BURN		
	Minor	Moderate	Major

Criteria	<10% TBSA burn in adult
	<5% TBSA burn in young or old
	<2% full-thickness burn
		10-20% TBSA burn in adult
		5-10% TBSA burn in young or old
		2-5% full-thickness burn
		High-voltage injury
		Suspected inhalation injury
		Circumferential burn
		Concomitant medical problem
		   predisposing the patient to infection
		   (e.g., diabetes, sickle cell disease)
			>20% TBSA burn in adult
			>10% TBSA burn in young or old
			>5% full-thickness burn
			High-voltage burn
			Known inhalation injury
			Any significant burn involving the face,
			   eyes, ears, hands, feet, genitalia, or
			   joints
			Significant associated injuries (e.g.,
			   fracture, other major trauma)

Disposition	Outpatient management	Hospital admission	Referral to a burn center

Adapted with permission from hospital and prehospital resources for optimal care of patients with burn injury: Guidelines for development and operation of burn centers. American Burn Association. *J Burn Care Rehabil.* 1990;11:98; with additional information from Hartford CE. Care of outpatient burns. In: Herndon DN, ed. *Total Burn Care.* Philadelphia: Saunders; 1996:71.

TBSA, total body surface area (percentage) affected by the injury.

*Burn, partial-thickness or full-thickness burn, unless specified; young, patient younger than 10 years; adult, patient 10 to 50 years of age; old, patient older than 50 years.

characteristically caused by contact with molten metal, flame, or high-voltage electricity.

A more practical method of classifying burns is to describe them as either superficial or deep because this approach defines both treatment and prognosis. Superficial burns involve the papillary dermis, with its rich vascular plexus, and the epidermis, which permits spontaneous healing by reepithelialization from the dermal appendages, including hair follicles, sebaceous glands, and sweat glands. This usually occurs within 2 weeks with minimal scarring. Superficial burns appear wet, pink, and blistered and blanch with pressure. They are painful. Deep burns involve the reticular dermis and SQ fat and generally lack sufficient epithelial appendages for spontaneous healing. If healing does occur, it will occur slowly and produce unstable skin, hypertrophic scarring, and contracture. Deep burns are best treated by excision and skin grafting. The initial appearance of deep burns ranges from cherry red, mottled, white, and nonblanching to leathery, charred, brown, and insensate (Table 38-2).

Although bedside evaluation of very superficial or deep wounds presents little diagnostic difficulty, clinical assessment of a mid-dermal or "indeterminate" burn is accurate only about two thirds of the time.[6] Even though it is useful to initially characterize the extent of the burn, it must be noted that the early appearance of a burn wound may not accurately reflect the true extent of the soft tissue injury. Reexamination and follow-up are critical because burn wounds may change during the 24 to 72 hours following injury. Indeterminate burns may eventually heal spontaneously, or they may convert to deeper wounds requiring excision and skin grafting (see Fig. 38-1).

Estimating Burn Size

Estimating burn size assists practitioners in determining the initial fluid requirements and prognosis. Several formulas are available to estimate TBSA in burn patients. In 1944, Lund and Browder published the now famous Lund-Browder chart (Fig. 38-4).[7,8] In their landmark paper, they used direct measurements and body surface area formulas to produce a chart

that clinicians can use to estimate %TBSA. The initial Lund-Browder chart was developed from human anatomic studies derived from 11 adults (3 women and 8 men) and produced a unisex chart. A more recent study involving 60 volunteers determined that the Lund-Browder chart significantly underestimates the size of chest burns in large-breasted women. The investigators developed a table that incorporates a correction using brassiere cup size.[9]

The simplest method for estimating TBSA in adults is the "rule of nines." This formula was developed in the late 1940s by Pulaski and Tennison, who observed that the percentage of each body segment was approximately a multiple of nine (Fig. 38-5).[10] Similar formulas for children adjust estimates for their disproportionately large head surface area.

In a study of obese patients it was determined that this formula underestimates %TBSA of the legs and torso and overestimates %TBSA of the arms and head. The authors suggested replacing the "rule of nines" with a "rule of fives" for obese patients heavier than 80 kg.

The size of a burn can also be estimated by using the patient's hand as representing approximately 1% TBSA. With this method, the hand is a rectangle. However, two studies using planimetry have determined that the hand actually represents from 0.5% to 0.78% of a patient's TBSA.[11]

HISTOPATHOLOGY OF BURNS

One thermal wound theory describes three zones of injury in burns (Fig. 38-6)[12]:

1. Zone of coagulation: dead, avascular tissue that must be débrided.
2. Zone of stasis: injured tissue in which blood flow is impaired. Desiccation, infection, or mechanical trauma may lead to cell death.
3. Zone of hyperemia: minimally injured, inflamed tissue that forms the border of the wound. The hyperemia usually resolves within 7 to 10 days but may be mistaken for cellulitis.

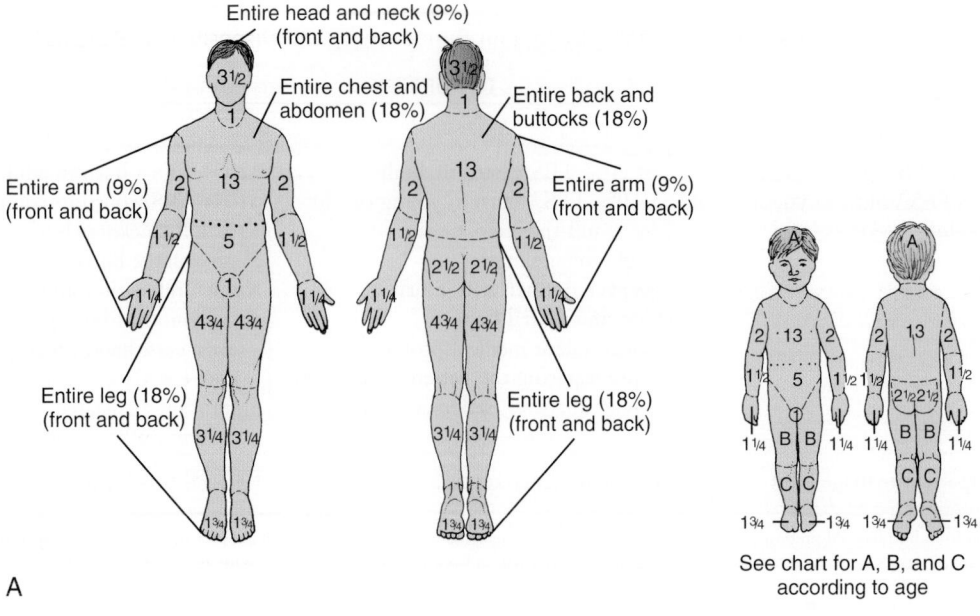

A

AGE	Birth–1 yr	1–4 yr	5–9 yr	10–14 yr	15 yr	Adult
Head	19	17	13	11	9	7
Neck	2					
Ant trunk	13					
Post trunk	13					
R buttock	2½					
L buttock	2½					
Genitalia	1					
R U arm	4					
L U arm	4					
R L arm	3					
L L arm	3					
R hand	2½	6½	8	8½	9	9½
L hand	2½	6½	8	8½	9	9½
R thigh	5½	5	5½	6	6½	7
L thigh	5½	5	5½	6	6½	7
R leg	5					
L leg	5					
R foot	3½					
L foot	3½					

B BODY AREA

Figure 38-4 Lund-Browder charts. **A,** The Lund-Browder charts are somewhat more accurate than the rule of nines in estimating the total body surface area (TBSA) burned. **B,** Proportion of TBSA of individual areas according to age. When compared with adults, children have larger heads and smaller legs. Other areas are relatively equivalent throughout life. The rule of nines is not accurate in determining the percentage of TBSA burned in children.

Histologically, full-thickness burns are characterized by confluent vascular thrombosis involving arterioles, venules, and capillaries. Edema secondary to loss of microvascular integrity results not only from the effects of direct thermal injury but also from the release of vasoactive mediators. The increase in vascular permeability is linked to activation of complement and release of histamine. Histamine increases catalytic activity of the enzyme xanthine oxidase, with resultant production of hydrogen peroxide and hydroxyl radicals. These by-products increase the damage to dermal vascular endothelial cells and result in progressive vascular permeability.[13]

The cellular debris and denatured proteins of the eschar provide a substrate for the proliferation of microorganisms. The devitalized tissue (eschar) sloughs spontaneously, usually as a result of the proteolytic effect of bacterial enzymes. The greater the degree of wound bacteriostasis, the greater the delay in sloughing.

Partial-thickness burns result in incomplete vascular thrombosis, usually limited to the upper dermis. The dermal circulation is restored gradually, generally over a period of several days, thus resulting in a significant interval of relative ischemia. The eschar in deep partial-thickness burns is thinner than in a full-thickness burn and sloughs as a result of reepithelialization rather than bacterial proteolysis.

OUTPATIENT VERSUS INPATIENT CARE

One of the first steps in minor burn care is to select patients for whom outpatient care is appropriate. For patients determined to require inpatient care, the admit or transfer decision

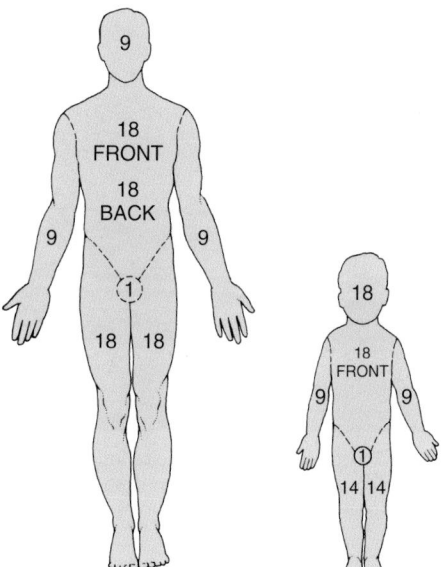

Figure 38-5 The "rule of nines." The rule of nines is a rough estimate of the total body surface area (TBSA) burned. Note that adults
and children are different. This formula frequently overestimates the
extent of a burn in clinical practice. As a rough guide, the area
covered by the individual's palm is approximately 1.25% TBSA. See
Figure 38-4 for a more accurate method of determining TBSA
burned in children.

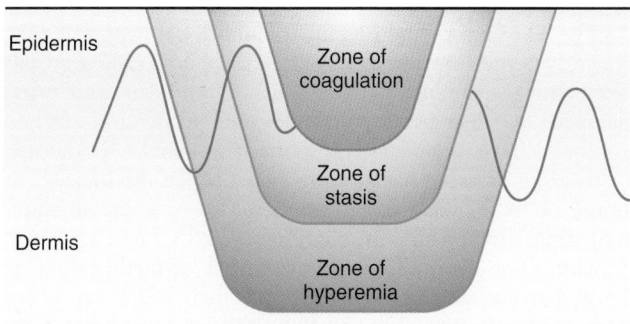

Figure 38-6 Zones of injury after a burn. The zone of coagulation
is the portion irreversibly injured. The zones of stasis and hyperemia
are defined in response to the injury. (*From Townsend CM, Beauchamp
RD, Evers BM, et al, eds.* Sabiston Textbook of Surgery. *19th ed. St.
Louis: Saunders; 2012.*)

depends on the burn care capabilities of the initial treating
facility. Guidelines set forth by the ABA[14] regarding criteria
for referral to a burn center are listed below. Burn injuries
that should be referred to a burn center include the
following:

1. Partial thickness burns greater than 10% TBSA
2. Burns involving the face, hands, feet, genitalia, perineum,
   or major joints
3. Third-degree burns in any age group
4. Electrical burns, including lightning injury
5. Chemical burns
6. Inhalation injury
7. Burn injury in patients with preexisting medical disorders
   that could complicate management, prolong recovery, or
   affect mortality

8. Any patient with burns and concomitant trauma in which
   the burn injury poses the greatest risk for morbidity or
   mortality after emergency or surgical stabilization of the
   traumatic injuries
9. Burned children in hospitals without qualified personnel
   or equipment for the care of children
10. Burn injury in patients who will require special social,
    emotional, or rehabilitative intervention

The decision to admit a patient with an acute burn injury
is rarely inappropriate. Candidates who can be considered for
outpatient treatment are generally adults and children meeting
the ABA criteria for minor burn criteria. Burns usually better
managed initially on an inpatient basis are large or deep burns
involving the hands, face, feet, neck, or perineum; burns
resulting from abuse or attempted suicide; burns occurring in
association with other trauma or inhalation injuries; and
chemical or electrical burns.

Poor candidates for outpatient care of even minor burns
include patients with concomitant medical problems such as
diabetes mellitus, peripheral vascular disease, congestive heart
failure, and end-stage renal disease; patients taking steroids or
other immunosuppressive agents; patients who are very young
or very old; those who are mentally impaired or have drug and
alcohol dependency; homeless persons; those who are malnourished; and patients without a sufficient home support
system. Inpatient treatment should be considered in these
circumstances even though the burn might be considered
"minor" by ABA criteria. Other admission considerations
include pain control, the ability to return for follow-up care,
the degree of incapacity, the ability to receive wound care at
home, and the overall social situation—all should influence the
final decision of whether admission is warranted.[15]

Additional guidelines that can guide emergency physicians
in determining the need for admission following an acute
burn injury include the following:

1. *Patients requiring intravenous (IV) access.* Following a burn
   there is an immediate capillary leak of plasma-like fluid
   that can last for 18 to 24 hours. In burns involving greater
   than 20% TBSA, the leak occurs in both burned and non-
   burned tissues. If not replaced, this fluid loss can lead to
   hypovolemic shock and renal failure. IV fluid resuscitation
   is indicated for all patients with second- and third-degree
   burns greater than 10% TBSA, in patients younger than
   10 or older than 50 years, and for burns greater than 20%
   TBSA in all other age groups.
2. *Anticipated surgery.* Deep burns are best treated by early
   surgical excision and skin grafting. This permits faster
   wound healing, provides more stable skin, and reduces
   contractures. Hospital admission facilitates wound care
   and preparation for surgery.
3. *Respiratory problems.* Patients with respiratory distress
   requiring oxygen therapy and those suspected of inhaling
   toxic fumes or vapors should be admitted for observation
   or intubation and mechanical ventilation (Box 38-1).
   Direct bronchoscopic evaluation of the airway may assist
   in the evaluation and diagnosis of tracheobronchitis or
   pneumonitis from a smoke inhalation injury.
4. *Need for special nursing care.* Specialized wound care, dressings, and nursing care are often required for burns involving the face, hands, feet, perineum, and genitalia and are
   best treated on an inpatient basis. Patients unable to care

---

BOX 38-1   General Approach to Blisters with Minor Burns*

IF TREATED LESS THAN 48 HOURS AFTER THE BURN

1. Leave all intact blisters alone.
2. If blisters have ruptured, treat them as dead skin and débride them completely.
3. Needle aspiration is not generally advised but may be used to decompress large burn blisters that appear ready to burst.

ON FOLLOW-UP OR MORE THAN 48 TO 72 HOURS AFTER THE BURN

1. Débride large (>6 cm in diameter) intact blisters and all blisters that have ruptured. Large, firm blisters on the palms and soles may be left intact longer. Do not aspirate blisters.
2. Do not débride small or spotty blisters until they break or until 5 to 7 days after the burn.

FIVE TO 7 DAYS AFTER THE BURN

1. Débride all blisters completely.

Note: *Intact blisters provide significant pain relief. Be prepared for an exacerbation of pain immediately after débridement. Prophylactic analgesia is recommended.*
All blisters and burned skin are débrided in the presence of infection. Note: Multiple approaches to blisters are acceptable, and practice varies considerably.

Figure 38-7 This patient suffered from circumferential third-degree burns on the arm, and compartment syndrome developed. Escharotomy was required.

for themselves or those lacking family and friends able to assist them may also require admission.

5. *Special burn injuries.* Chemical injuries are often more severe than the initial examination would suggest. Unlike thermal burns, tissue destruction may continue many hours after injury. Patients with chemical injuries should be admitted whenever the injuries are of indeterminate depth, affect a large area, or are deep and require surgical excision or if there are systemic manifestations of chemical toxicity or when the chemical responsible for injury requires a specific antidote. Swelling from deep circumferential burns may constrict the chest or limbs and result in compartment syndrome. Such burns should monitored frequently to determine the need for escharotomy or fasciotomy (Fig. 38-7). Whenever the patient's condition prevents a reliable clinical examination, direct measurement of compartment pressures can provide an objective measurement of intracompartmental pressure and assist in the decision to perform these surgical procedures (see Chapter 54). Patients with extensive burn injuries that require fluid resuscitation with large volumes of crystalloid should be monitored closely for the development abdominal compartment syndrome. Patients with mechanical burns involving large areas of skin loss and with significant frostbite injuries are generally admitted for specialized wound care and parenteral pain management. Patients with electrical injuries are often admitted for cardiac monitoring, specialized wound care, or both.

PROCEDURE

Emergency Treatment

Home or field treatment and ED care overlap. Initial treatment of a thermal injury begins immediately following the burn. If safe to do so, patients should be rapidly removed from the source of injury. Flames are extinguished by smothering the fire with a blanket, jacket, or equivalent item; by dousing the fire with water; or by using a chemical fire extinguisher. Most chemical injuries are best treated by irrigating the affected area with copious quantities of clean water. Patients with electrical injuries are removed from contact with the electrical source as soon as it is safe to do so.

Cooling is most beneficial for small burns if started within 3 minutes of injury and possibly of additional benefit if continued for the first few hours after the burn. Doing so has been shown to reduce pain significantly and can limit tissue damage by decreasing thromboxane production. When cooling a burn wound, it is important to avoid hypothermia or freezing of tissue because this may deepen the injury.[16] At home or in the field, room-temperature or cold tap water irrigation, immersion, or compresses (20°C to 25°C) will provide some pain relief without the risk of further injuring burned tissues and inducing hypothermia, which can occur with iced solutions (Fig. 38-8).[17,18] Placing ice on a burn should not be done. Sterile dressings are not required for field treatment; a moist towel or nonadherent sheet may be used. Nonmentholated shaving cream makes an excellent temporary covering for out-of-hospital use if a dressing is not available.[19] Home remedies, such as butter or Vaseline, are best avoided but are probably benign.[20] Remove jewelry and gross debris in the field if possible.

Initial Care of Major Burns

Major burns require the specialized resources of a burn center. Emergency physicians should initiate the resuscitation, consult the burn center for referral, and transfer the patient as soon as practically possible. Initial resuscitation should follow standardized trauma protocols, including a primary and secondary survey, and provide immediate interventions directed at airway management, breathing, and cardiovascular support, as needed. IV catheters can be inserted initially through burned skin when unburned sites are unavailable. Early IV access permits the administration of resuscitative fluids, medications, and parenteral narcotics to relieve the pain. Patients with burns exceeding 20% TBSA should receive IV fluid resuscitation with lactated Ringer's solution based on

Figure 38-8 To cool a burn that cannot easily be immersed in water, cover the area with unfolded gauze pads that have been soaked in room-temperature saline. Continue to frequently soak the gauze with cool saline or tap water drawn up in a syringe. Adding a few ice chips to the liquid is helpful, but do not cover the burn with ice. Towels are generally too bulky for this procedure. Narcotics are the best way to control pain in any burn.

BOX 38-3 Simplified ED Burn Fluid Resuscitation: The Rule of 10

1. Estimate burn size (%TBSA) to the nearest 10.
2. %TBSA × 10 = initial fluid rate in mL/hr (for adult patients weighing 40 to 80 kg).
3. For every 10 kg above 80 kg, increase the rate by 100 mL/hr.

From Chung KK, Salinas J, Renz EM, et al. Simple derivation of the initial fluid rate for the resuscitation of severely burned adult combat casualties: in silico validation of the rule of 10. J Trauma. 2010;69:S49-S54.
ED, *emergency department;* TBSA, *total body surface areal*

BOX 38-2 ED Burn Fluid Resuscitation

FIRST 24 HOURS

Fluid of choice: lactated Ringer's solution

Adults

2 to 4 mL/kg/%BSA burned (excluding first-degree burns)
Half of the fluid to be infused in the first 8 hours after the injury
Half of the fluid to be infused over the next 16 hours

Pediatrics

4 mL/kg/%BSA burned (excluding first-degree burns)
Half of the fluid to be infused in the first 8 hours after the injury
Half of the fluid to be infused over the next 16 hours
Add normal maintenance fluids to the burn resuscitation fluid

BSA, *body surface area;* ED, *emergency department.*
The above calculations are only a guide. Adjust fluids to maintain urine output at 0.5 mL/kg/hr in adults and 1 mL/kg/hr in children.

---

the Parkland or Brooke formulas (Box 38-2). More recently, the U.S. Army Institute of Surgical Research has advocated a simpler formula for estimating hourly fluid requirements in burn patients. This simpler formula may be more useful for prehospital providers or ED resuscitation (Box 38-3). The formulas estimate hourly fluid requirements and must be adjusted up or down to achieve a urine output of 0.5 to 1.0 mL/hr. Insertion of a Foley catheter is usually necessary to accurately measure hourly urine output.

Patients exposed to carbon monoxide should have carboxyhemoglobin levels measured and empirically receive 100% oxygen for 6 hours. Once considered a traditional empirical treatment, there is no evidence-based proven benefit from hyperbaric oxygen therapy for carbon monoxide poisoning. A recent Cochrane review (http://summaries.cochrane.org/CD002042) concluded that there is insufficient evidence to support the use of hyperbaric oxygen for the treatment of patients with carbon monoxide poisoning. The Cochrane review of published trials found conflicting, potentially biased,

and generally weak evidence regarding the usefulness of hyperbaric oxygen for the prevention of neurologic injury. Per an evidence-based analysis, existing randomized trials do not establish whether the administration of hyperbaric oxygen to patients with carbon monoxide poisoning reduces the incidence of adverse neurologic outcomes. Because there may still be advocates of hyperbaric oxygen therapy, consultation with a local hyperbaric center is reasonable, but it is not standard that this intervention be routinely implemented. Critically ill and pregnant patients are still often offered hyperbaric treatment, but controversy over the efficacy and safety persists even for these subgroups.

Patients suspected of having been exposed to significant levels of cyanide and manifesting symptoms should receive hydroxocobalamin (Cyanokit). If not available, the Cyanide Antidote Package may be used despite lack of proven benefit of this traditional cyanide therapy. It is reasonable to empirically administer hydroxocobalamin or the sodium thiosulfate portion of the cyanide kit to burn victims in coma or to those exhibiting metabolic (lactic) acidosis after smoke exposure.

Burn patients have an impaired ability to regulate their core body temperature and will quickly become hypothermic if untreated. Core temperature should be measured frequently, and active and passive warming strategies should be implemented to prevent hypothermia from developing. This can include minimizing exposure by covering patients with sheets and blankets, warming IV fluids, warming the room, or applying radiant or convective warming systems. In anticipation of transfer to a burn center or before surgical consultation, remove any wet cooling dressings that may have been applied initially and cover the wounds with dry gauze dressings.

Initial Care of Minor Burns

Prompt cooling of the burned part is an almost instinctive response and is one of the oldest recorded burn treatments, having been recommended by Galen (AD 129-199) and Rhazes (AD 852-923).[4] In the ED, room-temperature or cold tap water irrigation, immersion, or compresses (20°C to 25°C) are optimal in obtaining pain relief and providing some measure of protection for burned tissues without the problems of hypothermia that iced solutions can cause.[8,9] If not done before ED treatment, immediate cold water immersion may still have some ability to limit the extent of a burn and will provide significant pain relief. It is acceptable to add a few ice chips to the water, but packing the wound in ice must be avoided.

BOX 38-4 **Advantage of Prompt Burn Cooling**

Reduction or cessation of pain
Elimination of local hyperthermia
Inhibition of postburn tissue destruction
Decreased edema
Reduced metabolism and toxin production

All involved clothing and jewelry (such as rings), along with any gross debris, should be removed from the burned area. Chemical burns involving the skin or eyes require prolonged tap water irrigation. The burn should otherwise be covered with a moist, sterile dressing. In the ED and prehospital phase, appropriate analgesics, usually narcotics, are the best way to control pain and should not be forgotten in the initial phase of burn care. The burned area may be immersed immediately in room-temperature water or covered with gauze pads soaked in room-temperature water or saline (see Fig. 38-8). The gauze may be kept cool and moist to provide continued pain relief; the patient will let the clinician know when additional cooling is desired. Many clinicians use sterile saline for cooling, but it has no proven benefit over tap water, even when the skin is broken. It is acceptable to add ice chips to water or saline to lower the temperature. As stated previously, immersion of burned tissue in ice or ice water should be avoided because ice immersion increases pain and risks frostbite injury or systemic hypothermia.

The potential benefits of burn cooling are listed in Box 38-4. Because most patients with minor burns seek medical attention after initial self-instituted prehospital cooling, it is unlikely that the clinician can favorably affect the burned tissue with any intervention in the ED. With the exception of pain relief and removal of debris, the primary benefits of burn cooling are probably experienced only if the burn is cooled promptly, within the first 3 minutes after injury, thus making home care important.[21,22] Minor burns are considered tetanus prone, and tetanus toxoid should be administered if patients are unsure of their tetanus immunization status or when it has been more than 10 years since the last immunization. Nonimmunized patients should receive human tetanus immune globulin, 250 units intramuscularly, along with tetanus toxoid and a booster injection of toxoid in about 3 weeks.

Outpatient Care of Minor Burns

Minor burns are generally those that will heal spontaneously and do not require surgery or specialized wound care. These wounds are not associated with immunosuppression or hypermetabolism, nor are they highly susceptible to infection, a quality associated with larger burns.[23,24] Treated conservatively, most minor burns will heal without significant scarring. Many complications seen with minor burns are thought to result from overtreatment rather than undertreatment. Examples include the use of dry dressings that can adhere to newly forming skin and secondary infections from the overzealous use of topical or systemic antibiotics.

The most important characteristic of a dressing is that it controls fluids within the wound. Burn dressings that keep the surface of the wound moist and avoid pooling of fluids will speed healing.[25] The best material for this purpose is a generous amount of simple dry gauze applied over a nonadherent dressing or topical preparation. The outer layer of dressing should be porous to permit evaporation of water from the absorbent dressing material. Some clinicians prefer to eschew a nonadherent portion of the dressing so that subsequent dressing removal aids in minor débrident. Wound preparation and basic bandaging should include the following steps (Fig. 38-9):

1. Cleanse the burned area gently with a clean cloth or gauze and a mild antibacterial wound cleaner such as chlorhexidine, and irrigate the wound with saline or water. It is not necessary to shave the hair in or around the wound. There is no benefit to vigorously washing a minor wound with strong antiseptic preparations (such as povidone-iodine [Betadine] and others).[24]

2. Débride blisters and sloughed skin initially by peeling the devitalized skin from the wound (Fig. 38-10*A-C*). Blisters can be opened with scissors and forceps. If necessary, analgesia should be provided for any painful débrident. The initial débrident should attempt to remove only grossly devitalized tissue. Additional débrident of the wound can take place, if needed, during subsequent follow-up visits when the wound has matured.

3. Consider applying a layer of antibiotic cream or ointment such as 1% silver sulfadiazine (Silvadene) or bacitracin directly to the wound (see Fig. 38-10*D*).

4. Apply fine-mesh gauze or commercial nonadherent gauze such as Adaptic or petrolatum gauze impregnated with 3% bismuth tribromophenate (Xeroform) to the burn wound.

5. Cover and pad the wound with loose gauze fluffs. If fingers and toes are involved, pad the web spaces and the digits individually and separate them with strips of gauze (see Fig. 38-9*D* and 38-10*E* and *F*). The entire dressing is wrapped snugly (but not tightly) with an absorbent, slightly elastic material such as Kerlix.

6. The patient should be instructed to elevated the affected limb to prevent swelling, which may cause delayed burn conversion or wound infection.

Open Burn Care

Following cleansing of the wound with chlorhexidine soap and débrident of blisters and any loose skin, wounds that are not amenable to a dressing, such as those on the face, can be managed initially by the application of a bland topical antibiotic such as bacitracin. The wound can be washed two or three times per day, followed by reapplication of the topical agent. This is the preferred method for managing burns on the face and neck.

Burn Dressings
Biologic Dressings

Biologic dressings are natural tissues, including skin, that consist of collagen sheets containing elastin and lipid. They are not routinely used in the emergency care of minor wounds. The benefits of biologic dressings include a reduction in surface bacterial colonization, diminished fluid and heat loss, avoidance of further wound contamination, and prevention of damage to newly developed granulation tissue. Examples of biologic dressings include cadaveric

Figure 38-9 Outpatient burn dressing of the hand. Patients with serious hand burns should be admitted to the hospital, but minor burns can be treated in the outpatient setting. After the application of an antibiotic ointment or a dry, nonadherent dressing, the fingers are separated with fluffs in the web spaces (**A**), and the entire hand is enclosed in a position of function (**B**) (here with the help of a roll of Kerlix). **C,** If the wrist is involved, a removable plaster splint may be applied over the dressing. **D,** The result of a minor burn involving the hand when the fingers were not wrapped individually. Initially, there were only a few blisters, but this patient now has second-degree skin loss because of an improper burn dressing that caused maceration of normal skin between the fingers. Not only were the fingers incorrectly wrapped together in one gauze wrap, but the first wound check was also incorrectly scheduled in 6 days, too long for the first wound inspection of a hand burn.

human skin and commercially available porcine xenograft or collagen sheets.

Synthetic Dressings

Synthetic dressings are manufactured in various forms. Film-type dressings have a homogeneous structure and are usually polymers. Because these dressings are nonpermeable, problems with retention of wound exudates have occurred. Some second-generation dressings have been developed to address these problems. These products include Tegaderm, Vigilon, DuoDERM, Biobrane, Op-Site, Omniderm, and Sildimac.[25,26] These preparations have theoretical benefits under certain circumstances, but none has proved to have superior performance over simple gauze dressings for minor outpatient burns. These products are most often used by burn centers and have little applicability for minor burns in patients discharged from the ED. For patients admitted or transferred to a burn center, simple gauze dressings are appropriate. Some burn centers prefer that topical agents not be applied before transfer so that the full extent of the burn can be assessed immediately.

Specific Clinical Issues in Minor Burn Care
Analgesia

Pain is a critical feature of any burn injury. Relief of pain by the appropriate and judicious use of narcotic analgesics is of the utmost importance in the initial care of all burn patients. Prehospital narcotics are very appropriate when standard contraindications do not exist. Analgesia should be provided before extensive examination or débridement is performed. Inadequate analgesia is probably the most common ED error in the treatment of burn injuries, especially when burns occur in children. Parenteral narcotic analgesics have been erroneously relegated to pain control only for major burns, but it is suggested that narcotics be generously administered in the initial treatment of even minor painful burns.

Parenteral opioids (fentanyl, 1 to 2 µg/kg, or morphine, 0.1 to 0.2 mg/kg) are usually required, especially if painful procedures such as débridement and dressing changes are planned. We prefer to use IV opioids (occasionally supplemented with a short-acting benzodiazepine such as midazolam) for all painful procedures. For complicated

Figure 38-10 Débridement and dressing of a blistering burn. **A,** Exactly when to débride burn blisters is controversial and probably of no consequence to the final outcome (see text). Eventually, however, all dead tissue must be removed. **B** and **C,** The easiest and quickest way to débride blisters is to grasp the dead loose skin with dry 4- × 4-inch gauze and pull it off quickly rather than use slow meticulous instrument techniques. Analgesia is used as per the clinical condition. **D,** An appropriate ointment is applied to the denuded tissue. (Silvadene is shown here, although bacitracin can also be used.) **E** and **F,** The débridement itself is not especially painful, but when the underlying tissue is exposed, pain increases. Hence, dress the burn quickly after débridement.

débridement or dressing changes, adequate analgesia and sedation (see Chapter 33) is strongly advocated.

Regional or nerve block anesthesia is an excellent alternative when practical, and if feasible, nitrous oxide analgesia may be used. Ketamine may also be a reasonable alternative. Oral opioids may be inappropriate for the initial treatment of significant pain but can be used for continued outpatient analgesia. Local anesthetics may be injected in small quantities when appropriate, such as for the débridement of a deep ulcer or other small burn. Topical analgesics have no role in burn care. A properly designed dressing will do much toward preventing further discomfort after release home; however, home burn care and dressing changes may be quite painful. For this reason, an adequate supply of an oral opioid analgesic should be provided, and responsibility in analgesic use should be encouraged.

Pruritus

Postburn pruritus is one of the most common and distressing complications of burn injury and is estimated to affect 87% of burns.[27] It typically develops in the subacute phase and is therefore not a common issue for the emergency clinician in the acute treatment phase. Despite the limited literature on the treatment of postburn pruritus, available therapies include oral antihistamines, topical antihistamines, and topical moisturizers. The use of topical therapies should be withheld until sufficient wound healing has occurred.

Edema

Minor burns lead to immediate inflammation mediated by the release of histamine and bradykinins, which cause localized derangements in vascular permeability with resultant burn wound edema. This edema may be harmful in several ways. First, the increase in interstitial fluid increases the diffusion distance of oxygen from capillaries to cells and thereby increases hypoxia in an already ischemic wound. Second, the edema may produce untoward hemodynamic effects by a purely mechanical mechanism: compression of vessels in muscular compartments. Third, edema has been associated with the inactivation of streptococcidal skin fatty acids, thus predisposing the patient to burn cellulitis.[28,29]

Successful management of burn edema hinges on immobilization and elevation. Most patients are unfamiliar with the medical definition of elevation and are not aware or convinced of its value. Patient education in this regard is critical; however, certain burns (e.g., burns in dependent body areas) are prone to edema despite everyone's best intentions. It is for this reason that lower extremity burns in general and foot burns in particular are prone to problems. Major burns of the hand should be elevated while the patient is still in the ED. This is most readily accomplished by hanging the injured hand from an IV pole with a stockinette to support the bandaged hand (Fig. 38-11).

Use of Topical Preparations and Antimicrobials

Minor burns result in insignificant impairment of normal host immunologic defenses, and burn wound infection is not usually a significant problem. Topical antimicrobials are often used; however, some believe that these agents may actually impair wound healing.[29] Although the procedure is of unproven value, many clinicians routinely use antibiotic creams or ointments on even the most minor burns. Most patients expect some type of topical concoction, so a discussion of their use—or nonuse—is prudent.

Topical antimicrobials were designed for the prevention and care of burn wound sepsis or wound infection, primarily in hospitalized patients with major burns, and there is no convincing evidence that their use alters the course of first-degree burns and superficial partial-thickness injuries. As noted, the burn dressing is the key factor in minimizing complications in all burns. Nonetheless, topical antimicrobials are often soothing to minor burns, and their daily use prompts the patient to look at the wound, assess healing, perform prescribed dressing changes, or otherwise become personally involved in the care. Keep in mind that if a topical antimicrobial is used, its effectiveness is decreased in the presence of proteinaceous exudate, thus necessitating regular dressing changes if the antimicrobial benefit of topical therapy is to be realized. In reality, once-daily dressing changes are most practical and are commonly prescribed, and no data indicate that this regimen is inferior to more frequent dressing changes.

Figure 38-11 Elevation of a burned hand should begin in the emergency department. After a hand dressing is applied, the arm is suspended from an intravenous pole with a stockinette. A plaster or fiberglass splint may also be incorporated into the dressing.

All full-thickness burns should receive topical antimicrobial therapy because the eschar and burn exudate are potentially good bacterial culture media and deep escharotic or subescharotic infections may not be easily detected until further damage is done. All deep partial-thickness injuries likewise benefit from the application of a topical antimicrobial. As stated, this intervention can await definitive therapy in a burn unit.

Criteria for choosing a specific topical agent include its in vitro and clinical efficacy, toxicity (absorption), superinfection rate, ease and flexibility of use, cost, patient acceptance, and side effects. It is important to note that no firm scientific data convincingly support the use of any specific topical antimicrobial for minor outpatient burns.

Specific Topical Agents

Silver Sulfadiazine (Silvadene). This poorly soluble compound is synthesized by reacting silver nitrate with sodium sulfadiazine. It is the most commonly used topical agent for outpatients, and it is well tolerated by most patients (Fig. 38-12A; also see Fig. 38-10D). It has virtually no systemic effects and moderate eschar penetration, and it is painless on application. Although silver sulfadiazine is commonly used, many burn specialists prefer plain bacitracin ointment as the topical of choice because of its cost, equal efficacy, and good patient acceptance.

Silver sulfadiazine is available as a "micronized" mixture with a water-soluble white cream base in a 1% concentration that provides 30 mEq/L of elemental silver. It does not stain clothes, is not irritating to mucous membranes, and washes

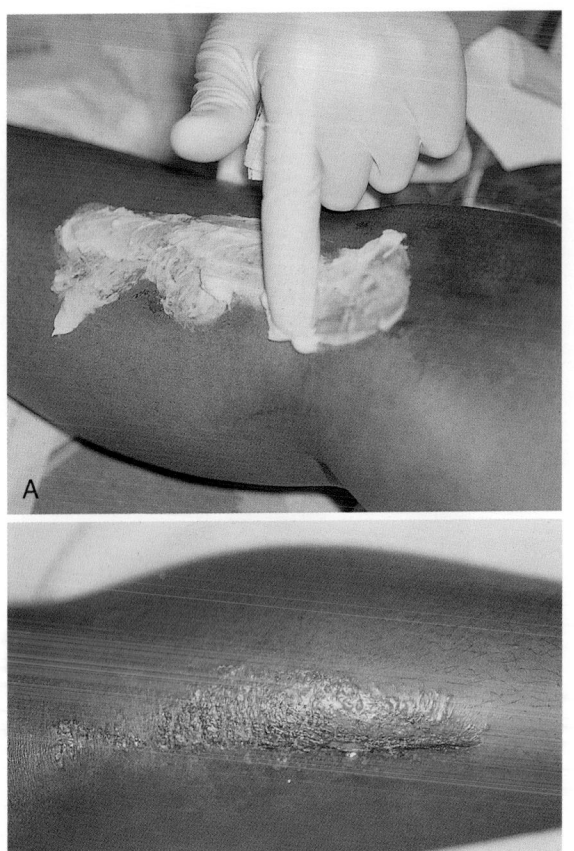

Figure 38-12 A, The most popular topical burn preparation is Silvadene cream. Though commonly used on minor burns, it probably has little beneficial effect on healing, and minor burns rarely become infected. Nonetheless, Silvadene is a standard intervention that at least causes the patient to look at the burn and become involved in dressing changes. **B,** Some clinicians suggest inexpensive topical antibiotic ointments (such as bacitracin and polymyxin B sulfate, neomycin sulfate [Neosporin]) for all outpatient burns. They are commonly used on face and neck burns. Bacitracin is preferred because contact dermatitis can occur from the neomycin portion of some topical agents, as depicted in the photograph.

off easily with water. It may be used on the face, but such use may be cosmetically undesirable for open treatment. Its broad gram-positive and gram-negative antimicrobial spectrum includes β-hemolytic streptococci, *Staphylococcus aureus* and *Staphylococcus epidermidis*, *Pseudomonas* spp., *Proteus* spp., *Klebsiella* spp., Enterobacteriaceae, *Escherichia coli*, *Candida albicans*, and possibly herpesvirus hominis.

Silver sulfadiazine often interacts with wound exudate to form a pseudomembrane over partial-thickness injuries. This pseudomembrane is often difficult and painful to remove.

Except for term pregnancy and in newborns (i.e., because of possible induction of kernicterus), there are no absolute contraindications to the use of silver sulfadiazine. Allergy and irritation are unusual, although there is potential cross-sensitivity between silver sulfadiazine and other sulfonamides.

Other Topical Preparations. Mafenide acetate (Sulfamylon), gentamicin, chlorhexidine, povidone-iodine, and silver nitrate are products that have been replaced with newer topicals, but they are mentioned for historical interest. These products are not used in modern burn therapy, although they are generally acceptable alternatives.

BROAD-SPECTRUM ANTIBIOTIC OINTMENTS. Many nonprescription topical antimicrobials are used for minor burn therapy despite a paucity of data attesting to specific benefits. Included are bacitracin zinc ointment, polymyxin B–bacitracin (Polysporin), and nitrofurazone (Furacin). These are all soothing, cosmetically acceptable for open treatment (such as on the face), and effective antiseptics under burn dressings. Some researchers caution against agents containing neomycin because of a potential for sensitization (see Fig. 38-12B). Though commonly applied by patients without adverse effects, we advise against the use of topicals that contain neomycin (Neosporin) because of the potential for contact dermatitis. The authors suggest plain bacitracin ointment as the routine topical agent, although Silvadene is a very acceptable, albeit more expensive alternative.

ALOE VERA CREAM. Aloe vera cream is commercially available in a 50% or higher concentration with a preservative. It exhibits antibacterial activity against at least four common burn wound pathogens: *Pseudomonas aeruginosa*, *Enterobacter aerogenes*, *S. aureus*, and *Klebsiella pneumoniae*. Heck and coworkers and others[30,31] compared a commercial aloe vera cream with silver sulfadiazine in 18 patients with minor burns. Healing times were found to be similar, and there was no increase in wound colonization in the aloe vera group in comparison to patients treated with silver sulfadiazine. Other authors have promulgated the use of aloe gel preparations for minor burns.[31] Aloe vera cream is an acceptable, inexpensive option for open or dressed outpatient care of minor burns.

HONEY. Honey has long been advocated as an inexpensive and effective topical for minor outpatient burns. The physicochemical properties of honey (osmotic effect, pH) give this substance the antibacterial and antiinflammatory properties that support its use. It may be superior to silver sulfadiazine with regard to minor burn wound healing. Honey is not widely used, but it has been promulgated as a safe, effective, and inexpensive dressing for the outpatient management of burn wounds.[32-34]

CORTICOSTEROIDS. High-potency topical steroid preparations have no beneficial effects on the rate of healing or limitation of scarring of thermal burns. Though probably not harmful, their use is not supported.[35]

FOLLOW-UP CARE OF MINOR BURNS

The specifics of outpatient follow-up of minor burns are controversial and often based on clinician preference and personal bias rather than on firm scientific data. Follow-up should be individualized for each patient and should be based on the reliability of the patient, the extent of the injury, the frequency and complexity of dressing changes, and the amount of discomfort anticipated during a dressing change. Some EDs have a "fast track" for inspecting burns that requires only a few visits. Physical therapy departments or wound care centers often have excellent facilities to monitor outpatient burns with periodic clinician oversight.

Figure 38-13 Providing patients with burn dressing material on discharge encourages proper home care. Dispensing only limited supplies of the items may enhance compliance with follow-up visits.

BOX 38-5 How to Change a Burn Dressing at Home: Patient Instructions

1. Take pain medicine ½ hour before dressing change if you find dressing changes to be painful.
2. If the burn is on the hand, foot, or other area that is difficult to reach, have someone help you.
3. Have all materials available. Gloves may be worn.
4. Remove the dressing and rinse off all burn cream or ointment with tap water, under a shower, or in the bathtub. The area can be gently washed with mild soap and a clean cloth or gauze pads.
5. Look at the burn and assess the healing, blistering, and amount of swelling. Note any signs of infection.
6. Gently exercise the area through range of motion.
7. Apply the burn ointment with a sterile tongue blade.
8. Cover the cream with fluffed-up gauze.
9. Wrap the area in bulky gauze.
10. Repeat this dressing change daily.

If a topical antibiotic agent is used, the dressing should be changed daily with removal and reapplication of the topical preparation. The wound should be rechecked by a clinician after 2 to 3 days and periodically thereafter, depending on wound size, compliance, healing, and other social issues. If a dry dressing is chosen, follow-up every 3 to 5 days is usually adequate. The purpose of any burn dressing changes or home care regimen is defeated if the patient cannot afford the material or is not instructed in the specifics of burn care. Many EDs supply burn dressing material on patient release. A complete pack includes antibiotic ointment or cream, gauze pads (fluffs), an absorbent gauze roll, a sterile tongue blade to apply the cream, and tape (Fig. 38-13). Providing limited supplies of the items necessary for dressing changes may enhance compliance with follow-up if the patient has to return for additional supplies. Writing a prescription and merely stating that the dressing should be changed daily may not be sufficient.

Daily home care can be performed by the patient with help from a family member or visiting nurse (Box 38-5). The dressing may be removed each day and gently washed with a clean cloth or a gauze pad, tap water, and a bland soap. Sterile saline and expensive prescription soaps are not required. A tub or shower is an ideal place to gently wash off burn cream. The affected area may be put through a gentle range of motion during dressing changes. After the burn is cleaned, the patient inspects it in the hope that complications can be recognized and prompt further follow-up. After complete removal of the old cream, a new layer is applied with a sterile tongue blade and covered with absorbent gauze.

If the undermost fine-mesh gauze of a dry dressing is dry and the coagulum is sealed to the gauze, the patient should allow the dressing to remain and simply reapply the overlying gauze dressing. If the wound is moist and macerated, the fine-mesh gauze should be removed and the wound cleaned and redressed. The patient should be instructed to not remove dry adherent fine-mesh gauze from the underlying crust. When epithelialization is complete, the crust will separate, and the gauze can be removed at that time.

In the postacute phase, dryness in healing skin may be treated with mild emollients such as Nivea (Beiersdorf, Inc., Norwalk, CT), Vaseline Intensive Care Lotion (Chesebrough

Ponds, Inc., Greenwich, CT), or other readily available over-the-counter skin care moisturizing lotions. Natural skin lubrication mechanisms usually return by 6 to 8 weeks.[23] Excessive sun exposure should be avoided during wound maturation because this may lead to hyperpigmentation. When the patient is outdoors, sun avoidance strategies should be used, or at the very least, a commercially available sunblock should be applied. Exposure of the recently healed burned area to otherwise minor trauma (chemicals, heat, sun) may result in an exaggerated skin response. Pruritus is common and may be treated with oral antihistamines or a topical moisturizing cream.

Outpatient Physical Therapy for Burn Care

When the hospital's outpatient physical therapy department or wound care center is equipped to treat minor burns, it is prudent to consider this option as a means of longitudinal follow-up. Many centers make available daily or periodic burn treatment consisting of dressing changes, whirlpool débridement, and range-of-motion exercises. An additional advantage is that medically trained personnel evaluate the burn daily, thereby decreasing clinician visits and enabling identification of problems before serious complications develop. Generally, all that is required from the clinician is to write a prescription for "burn care and dressing changes" and set up the appointment.

Burn Wound Healing

Burn wound healing differs from healing of other soft tissue wounds.[2] The duration is variable but is often proportional to burn depth. Within 1 to 3 weeks and following the initial inflammatory response, neovascularization of the burn occurs and is accompanied by fibroblast migration. Collagen production begins but it is often deposited randomly, thereby leading to scar formation. Reepithelialization follows collagen deposition. The persistence of necrotic tissue and eschar in the wound will impede all aspects of healing. The extent of scar formation is related directly to healing time. Wound healing that occurs in fewer than 16 days often results in decreased scar formation.[2] Proper wound débridement is also associated with faster wound healing and minimizes scar formation.

Healing of superficial burns occurs by reepithelialization from the wound edge and from residual dermal elements containing epithelial cells. This process generally requires 10 to 14 days. After healing, the initial epithelial layer is often fragile and is easily reinjured. The application of bland, lanolin-containing creams for 4 to 8 weeks after initial healing may reduce dryness and cracking of the healing wound.

Deep burns lack residual dermal elements within the wound and heal by reepithelialization from the wound edge. Healing is slow and often unsatisfactory; it frequently takes longer than 3 weeks, and an unstable epithelium is produced that is prone to hypertrophic scarring and contractures. This is a particular problem in burns that extend across joints and limit motion. Burns that take longer than 2 to 3 weeks to heal are also prone to infection, which may be reduced by using topical antimicrobial agents. Deep wounds should be referred for surgical consultation and generally require early excision, grafting, and physical therapy.

SPECIAL MINOR BURN CARE CIRCUMSTANCES

Blisters

Management of blisters in minor burns is controversial. In reality, there is little one can do wrong when it comes to a clinical approach to blisters in minor burns (Fig. 38-14). Management arguments are generally theoretical or based on local tradition; the ultimate outcome of a minor burn is rarely determined by how one treats blisters. Intact blisters do offer a physiologic dressing that rarely becomes infected; however, most large blisters spontaneously rupture after 3 to 5 days and eventually require débridement. When the integrity of the blister is breached, the fluid becomes a potential culture medium. Clinical choices for blister management include débridement, aspiration, or simply leaving the blister intact.

Some studies suggest that intact burn blisters may allow reversal of capillary stasis and less tissue necrosis.[2] Madden and colleagues[36] showed that burn exudate (as contained within intact blisters) is beneficial in stimulating epidermal cell proliferation.

Swain and associates[37] demonstrated that the density of wound colonization with microorganisms was much lower in minor burns with blisters left intact. They also found that 37% of patients with aspirated blisters experienced a reduction in pain versus none of those whose blisters were unroofed. Other investigators believe that undressed wounds with débrided blisters are subject to additional necrosis secondary to desiccation, which can convert a partial-thickness burn to a full-thickness injury.[3] Finally, intact blisters clearly provide some pain relief, as evidenced by the sudden increase in pain immediately after débridement. Increased pain should be anticipated and analgesia offered as appropriate when débridement is necessary. We suggest the guidelines in Box 38-3 as a general approach to burn blisters.[2,3,36-38]

Minor Burn Infections

Prophylactic systemic antibiotics are not warranted in the routine treatment of outpatient burns. It may be difficult to separate the erythema of the injury or healing process from

Figure 38-14 It is difficult to do anything wrong with minor burn blisters, and many regimens are acceptable. Eventually, however, the blisters will have to be débrided. An expeditious and relatively painless way to débride a burn is to use a dry gauze pad to grasp the dead skin (**A**) and peel it off (**B**). Meticulous instrument débridement is often time-consuming and stressful to the patient. Be aware that pain occurs when air comes in contact with the débrided skin, and prophylactic analgesia should therefore be provided. Large burns can be débrided under procedural sedation.

cellulitis, but minor burns rarely become infected, with infection rates being well under 5%.[39] There are bacteria on the skin at all times—normal skin usually harbors nonvirulent pathogens such as *S. epidermidis* and diphtheroids. Therefore, all burns are contaminated but not necessarily infected. Because thermal trauma results in coagulative necrosis, burn wounds contain a variable amount of necrotic tissue, which if infected, acts much as an undrained abscess and prevents access of antibiotics and host defense factors.

The microbial flora of outpatient burns varies with time after the burn. Shortly after injury, the burn becomes colonized with gram-positive bacteria such as *S. aureus* and *S. epidermidis*. After this period there is a gradual shift toward inclusion of gram-negative organisms, 80% of which originate from the patient's own gastrointestinal tract.[4] Common organisms seen on days 1 to 3 include *S. epidermidis*, β-hemolytic streptococci, *Bacillus subtilis*, *S. aureus*, enterococci, *Mima polymorpha*, *Enterobacter* spp., *Acinetobacter* spp., and *C. albicans*. One week after the burn these organisms may be seen along with *E. coli*, *P. aeruginosa*, *Serratia marcescens*, *K. pneumoniae*, and *Proteus vulgaris*.

Anaerobic colonization of burn wounds is rare unless there is excessive devitalized tissue, as occurs with a high-voltage electrical injury.[40] For this reason, routine anaerobic cultures are generally unnecessary in an assessment of infective organisms that produce minor infections.

A healing burn may produce leukocytosis and a mild fever in the absence of infection, especially in children. Early (days 1 to 5) burn infections are generally caused by gram-positive cocci, especially β-hemolytic streptococci. Streptococcal cellulitis is characterized by marked spreading erythema extending outward from the wound margins. Despite the plethora of organisms and the presence of some gram-negative pathogens in superficial burn cultures, first-line treatment in a normal host is oral penicillin, 1 to 2 g/day. Alternatives include erythromycin, cephalosporins, and dicloxacillin.

Effective topical treatment at the time of initial burn care and subsequent dressing changes is meant to delay bacterial colonization, maintain the bacterial density of wounds at low levels, and produce a less diverse wound flora. Because outpatient management of burns should be attempted only when the risk for infection is minimal, the use of systemic antibiotics is unnecessary for minor burns, even in the setting of delayed treatment, diabetes, and steroid use.[41] Unnecessary antibiotic use may select for resistant organisms. Antibiotics in the management of minor burns have been recommended for patients undergoing an autograft procedure.[42] There are no data on the use of antibiotics as prophylaxis for patients with burns in the setting of valvular heart disease.

In minor burn care, wound cultures are not required or recommended. It is useless, for example, to culture blister fluid in a patient who arrives for emergency care immediately after a thermal injury. Cultures are necessary only when overt infection develops, especially when it occurs while a topical or systemic antibiotic is being used. Cultures may also be of benefit when the infected wound is old, when hygiene is poor, or when there are preexisting abrasions nearby.[43] Although they may adequately reflect wound flora, falsely sterile cultures are relatively frequent. In general, superficial cultures do not reflect deep burn flora and provide no quantitative information.

Sterile wound biopsy for culture is most satisfactory for the assessment of intraescharotic, subescharotic, or invasive infections and allows quantification of bacterial flora.

Foot Burns

Despite their relatively small surface area, foot burns tend to heal poorly, usually because of excessive edema; therefore, they are generally considered major burns. Foot burns are the most common burn category to fail outpatient therapy and subsequently require admission and inpatient care (Fig. 38-15). Zachary and coworkers[44] reported on a series of 104 patients with foot burns. In no patient admitted on the day of injury did burn cellulitis develop; in contrast, 27% of delayed-admission patients had cellulitis. Their study also noted a higher incidence of hypertrophic scarring and need for skin grafting in the delayed-admission group. Overall, fewer days of hospitalization were required for the initially admitted group.

Specific problems in the care of foot burns include pain, wound drainage, difficulty changing dressings without help, inability of even motivated patients to comply with the requirements for elevation, and prolonged convalescence. The benefits of hospital admission include splinting, intensive local burn care, physical therapy, and bed rest with elevation, which minimizes edema. For these reasons, initial admission is advised for all but the most minor of foot burns. Close

Figure 38-15 Burns of the feet are specialized burns that require careful evaluation and an individualized treatment plan, even if the burn surface area is relatively small. It is difficult for most patients to provide ideal burn care at home when the feet are involved. **A,** It is tempting to initially treat this seemingly minor superficial second-degree foot burn in an outpatient setting, but the patient's compliance and social situation must be ideal for a successful outcome. Hospitalization until home health care can be established is prudent. **B,** Example of a foot burn that is a potential disaster, in this case because of late treatment of a diabetic patient.

outpatient follow-up wound checks are required for foot burns appropriate for outpatient care.

Hand Burns

Because of its functional significance, burns involving the hand can result in significant functional loss even when the TBSA burned is small. Losing the use of one or both hands can become seriously disabling and affect the patient's activities of daily living regardless of whether the cause of the loss is a burn dressing, the late onset of scar contractures, or loss as a result of amputation.[45]

As with other burns, the depth and extent of the burn determine the severity of the injury. The entire surface of one hand represents only 2.5% TBSA, yet even small burns can cause a disproportionate loss of function. Deep partial- or

Figure 38-16 This badly burned hand requires referral to a surgeon or burn center and should not be definitively handled in the emergency department. Note the very tight ring (*arrow*).

full-thickness hand burns, even if quite small, often warrant referral for early excision and grafting to limit scarring and maintain function. The skin on the dorsum of the hand is thinner than that on the palm and is more susceptible to burn injury but must remain flexible to allow finger motion. Any exposed tendon or bone, such as may be seen with an electrical burn, constitutes a true fourth-degree injury, and either flap closure or amputation is required to heal the wound.

Many of the issues complicating outpatient management of foot burns are relevant to the care of hand burns. After initial burn cooling, the wound should be gently cleansed with mild soap. Any loose skin or ruptured blisters should be gently débrided, rinsed, patted dry, and covered with a topical antimicrobial agent and a nonadherent, bulky gauze dressing. The fingers should be carefully separated and bandaged individually. Small, intact blisters that do not interfere with hand function should be left intact to serve as a biologic dressing. Elevation of the hand is very important in the first few days after a burn injury to minimize edema. Deep partial- or full-thickness burns on the dorsum of the hand should be splinted[46,47] after bandaging to avoid the development of contractures or a boutonnière deformity.

Hospital admission or burn center referral should be considered for all significant hand burns, particularly full-thickness injuries and circumferential burns involving the digits (Fig. 38-16). If outpatient treatment is attempted, the patient must be given comprehensive instructions and should have the resources available to perform daily dressing changes and range-of-motion exercises of the fingers and wrist during these dressing changes. An initial follow-up visit should be arranged in 48 to 72 hours, but the patient should be encouraged to return if burn cellulitis, worsening pain, fever, or lymphangitis develops. Ideally, the patient should be seen twice in the first week after injury and then once a week until the burn is healed.

Facial Burns

Facial burns commonly result from unexpected ignition flash burns (e.g., from a stove, oven, or charcoal grill) or from car radiator accidents (Fig. 38-17*A* and *B*).[48,49] Facial burns from these sources usually do well, but singeing of facial hair, significant edema, and pain often result. However, facial burns from these causes may produce airway problems and might require skin grafting. Singed nasal hairs or any sign of significant heat exposure to the face should prompt an evaluation of airway injury, which may result in airway compromise at a time later than the initial incident (see Fig. 38-17*C*).

Concurrent globe or corneal injury is quite rare because of protective blinking reflexes. If the eye is burned, it is usually in the setting of a life-threatening concomitant burn injury.[50] Burns involving the eyelids can cause significant scarring. Fluorescein staining and slit-lamp examination should be performed to confirm or exclude the diagnosis of corneal injury (Fig. 38-18). Treatment of a corneal injury can involve irrigation, topical ophthalmic antibiotics, and consideration of eye patching versus protective soft contact lens (see Chapter 62). Referral to an ophthalmologist is usually prudent. Facial burns are otherwise treated in the usual fashion and with an open (no dressing) technique. Patients are instructed to wash their face two or three times a day with a mild soap and then apply a thin layer of antibiotic ointment, such as bacitracin zinc. Car radiator burns result from the combination of a hot liquid and steam burn (see Fig. 38-17*B*). Antifreeze does not produce a caustic injury, nor is it systemically absorbed. Neck burns are treated similarly.

A flash burn in a patient smoking cigarettes while using nasal oxygen causes a facial burn that is not uncommonly seen in the ED (see Fig. 38-17*D*). These burns may involve the nose and lips, may have melted plastic particles onto the skin, and can be quite painful. Although such patients generally do well, facial burns can make the continued use of nasal cannula oxygen problematic until healing takes place. Though not generally an inhalation burn issue, careful evaluation of the upper airways and assessment of lung function are prudent. Many patients using oxygen are immunocompromised. They cannot tolerate even minor physical insults and have fragile conditions that require careful evaluation, short-term observation in some cases, and close follow-up for delayed healing and infection. Hospitalization for burn care and general supportive measures are suggested for all but minor burns. Minor burns can be treated on an outpatient basis in an open fashion with topical ointments, such as bacitracin.

All patients with head or neck burns should be evaluated carefully for a concomitant inhalation injury. Such patients may have direct evidence of injury, such as oral burns, blisters, soot, or hyperemia and a history of being in an enclosed space, or have indirect evidence, such as dyspnea, wheezing, arterial hypoxemia, or an elevated carboxyhemoglobin level. The definitive diagnostic test for inhalation injury is fiberoptic bronchoscopy.[51] Flash ignition burns involving the face do not pose a problem with carbon monoxide poisoning, and although inhalation injuries generally do not occur with minor flash ignition burns, airway management should remain a consideration.

Inpatient care should be considered for all patients with significant facial burns. Outpatient pain control may be difficult in those with facial burns, the degree of edema may be difficult to predict, and home care can be problematic. There are no universally agreed standards for admission versus outpatient treatment of facial burns.

Corneal contact burns, as from accidental contact with a curling iron, are often manifested rather dramatically as

Figure 38-17 A, Flash burns on the face from lighting a gas stove. These burns are painful and may cause edema, but they usually do well. Note the singed facial hair. The eyes are usually protected by rapid reflex blinking, and carbon monoxide poisoning and pulmonary burns are not an issue. Most can be handled in the outpatient setting with bacitracin ointment and no dressing. Pain control may be problematic unless opioids are prescribed. **B,** Facial and neck burns when a radiator cap was removed and the victim was sprayed with steam and hot antifreeze. **C,** This patient has a severe facial burn with smoke inhalation, as evidenced by soot in the pharynx and singed nasal hairs. Tracheal intubation is in the near future for this patient. **D,** Flash burn in a patient who was smoking a cigarette while using nasal oxygen.

opacified, "heaped-up" corneal epithelium (see Fig. 38-18). Despite their appearance, the end result is usually excellent. Treatment is the same as for a corneal abrasion.[52]

Abuse of Children and Elderly Individuals

Recognition of the possibility of deliberate abuse by burning in the pediatric and geriatric populations is essential. In addition, children younger than 2 years have a thinner dermis and a less well-developed immune system than adults do. Elderly patients (>65 years) likewise tolerate burns poorly. These two populations are the most prone to abuse, often by family members (Fig. 38-19). For these reasons, both these groups of patients often require inpatient care.[18]

The majority of abused children are 18 to 36 months old, and for unknown reasons, the majority are male.[29] Immersion burns are a common type of abuse and are characterized by circumferential, sharply demarcated burns on the hands, feet, buttocks, and perineum. Cigarette burns and burns from hot objects such as irons should be obvious. Contact burns on

Figure 38-18 Thermal burn of the cornea. Note the opacified, "heaped-up" appearance of the epithelium. *(From Kanski JJ, ed. Clinical Diagnosis in Ophthalmology. St. Louis: Mosby; 2006.)*

Figure 38-19 Burns can be a manifestation of child abuse, spouse abuse, or abuse of the elderly. **A,** Abuse burns from contact with a hot metal grate as a result of a child allegedly falling. **B,** This burn was the result of spouse abuse caused by throwing hot soup during an argument. Domestic abuse is often denied initially, but the delayed arrival at the hospital was a clue. **C,** Burns of the face and neck are common when a toddler pulls hot liquid from a stove. This case was never proved to be child abuse, but burns in young children are often due to abuse, especially if they are in atypical places. Although the body surface area of this burn is relatively small, the patient's age and the burn's location, coupled with the possibility of child abuse, require that this child be hospitalized. **D,** This infant received a severe blistering sunburn at the beach despite being in the shade most of the day. Reflection of sunlight from the sand and water can injure the delicate skin of an infant, who should have sunscreen applied. **E,** Self-inflicted cigarette burns in a psychiatric patient.

"nonexploring" parts of the child also warrant suspicion. A delay in seeking treatment may be a tip-off that a burn resulted from abuse. In older populations, the presence of confirmed self-inflicted burns such as cigarette burns suggests psychiatric disease (see Fig. 38-19*E*).

Burns in Pregnancy

There is little information in the literature concerning the special problems of pregnant burn victims. Ying-bei and Ying-jie[53] reported on 24 pregnant burn patients representing a wide range of burn severity. Complications of the burn injuries included abortion and premature labor, although all patients in this series with burns covering less than 20% TBSA did well and delivered living full-term babies.

Because the resistance of pregnant women to infection is lower than that of nonpregnant women, control of burn wound infection is paramount. Gestational age appears to have no direct bearing on prognosis. Silver sulfadiazine cream should be avoided near term because of the potential for kernicterus.

SPECIFIC BURNING AGENTS

Hot Tar Burns

Asphalt is a product of the residues of coal tar and is commonly used in roofing and road repair. It is kept heated to approximately 450°F. When spilled onto the skin, the tar cools rapidly, but the retained heat is sufficient to produce a partial-thickness burn. Fortunately, full-thickness burns are unusual. Cooled tar is nonirritating and does not promote infection. When cooled tar is physically removed, the adherent skin is usually avulsed (Fig. 38-20). Careless removal of the tar may inflict further damage on burned tissues. Agents such as alcohol, acetone, kerosene, or gasoline have been used to remove the tar, but these are flammable and may cause additional skin damage or a toxic response secondary to absorption.

There is no great need to meticulously remove all tar at the first visit. Obviously devitalized skin can be débrided, but adherent tar should be emulsified or dissolved rather than manually removed (Fig. 38-21). Polyoxyethylene sorbitan (Tween 80 or polysorbate 80) is the water-soluble, nontoxic, emulsifying agent found in Neosporin and several other topical antibiotic creams. Note that the cream formulations, not the ointments, contain the most useful tar dissolvers. The creams contain a complex mixture of ethers, esters, and sorbitol anhydrides that possess excellent hydrophilic and lyophilic characteristics when used as nonionic, surface-active emulsifying agents. With persistence, most tar can be removed (emulsified) on the initial visit.

Another household product (De-Solv-It multiuse solvent) also appears logical for topical ED use.[43,54] De-Solv-It has a surface-active moiety that wets the chemical's surface and emulsifies tar and asphalt. Because De-Solv-It is itself a petroleum-based solvent, it should be applied only briefly, and the operator should wear gloves and protective eyewear during application. It should be used only for external exposure to tar or asphalt.

Many clinicians instead prefer to emulsify the majority of tar on an outpatient basis. A generous layer of polysorbate-based ointment can be applied under a bulky absorbent gauze dressing. The patient is then released home, and the residual tar is easily washed off after 24 to 36 hours (see Fig. 38-20*B*). A number of dressing changes may be required. Once the residual tar is removed, the wound is treated as any other burn.

Shur-Clens, a nontoxic, nonionic detergent, also works well for tar burn wound cleansing, as do mineral oil, petrolatum, and Medi-Sol (Orange-Sol, Inc, Chandler, AZ), a petroleum-citrus product. Butter-soaked gauze has been suggested as an emulsifier of tar.

Figure 38-20 A, There is no compelling reason to remove all tar on the first visit. Physical removal of cooled tar usually results in avulsion of the underlying skin. Skin that is obviously loose should be débrided, but adherent tar is best liquefied with an emulsifying agent. Neomycin cream, not ointment, is a suggested emulsifier, but others are acceptable (see text). Final removal may be delayed for several days to permit loosening of the tar. Frequent dressing changes and application of an emulsifying agent can be performed by the patient to remove the tar over a period of a few days. **B,** This extremity was covered with an emulsifying agent and with gauze, and the residual tar was washed off easily 36 hours later.

Chemical Burns

Chemical burns generally occur in the workplace, and the offending substance is usually well known. More than 25,000 chemicals currently in use are capable of burning the skin or mucous membranes. Commonly used chemical agents capable of producing skin burns are shown in Box 38-6.

Injury is caused by a chemical reaction rather than a thermal burn.[55] Reactions are classified as oxidizing, reducing, corrosive, desiccant, or vesicant or as protoplasmic poisoning. The injury to skin continues until the chemical agent is physically removed or exhausts its inherent destructive capacity. The degree of injury is based on the strength, concentration, and quantity of the chemical; duration of contact; location of contact; extent of tissue penetration; and mechanism of action.

Immediate flushing with water is recommended for all chemical burns, with the exception of those caused by alkali

Figure 38-21 Tar stuck to the face (**A**) can be emulsified with various agents and a lot of patience and persistence (**B**). Fortunately, tar burns are not usually full-thickness burns.

BOX 38-6	Commonly Used Acids and Alkalis

ACIDS	ALKALIS
Picric	Sodium hydroxide
Tungstic	Ammonium hydroxide
Sulfosalicylic	Lithium hydroxide
Tannic	Barium hydroxide
Trichloroacetic	Calcium hydroxide
Cresylic	Sodium hypochlorite
Acetic	
Formic	
Sulfuric	
Hydrochloric	
Hydrofluoric	
Chromic	

metals. Flushing serves to cleanse the wound of unreacted surface chemical, dilute the chemical already in contact with tissue, and restore lost tissue water. Leonard and colleagues[56] clearly demonstrated that patients receiving immediate copious water irrigation for chemical burns had less full-thickness burn injury and a 50% or greater reduction in hospital stay.

Acid and Alkali Burns

Chemical burns cause progressive tissue damage until the chemical is inactivated or removed. Acids damage tissue by coagulation necrosis, a process that limits the depth of penetration into tissue. Alkalis react with lipids in skin and result in liquefaction necrosis. This process permits penetration of the chemical into tissues until neutralized. Thus, exposure to alkali is more likely to produce deep tissue wounds. Skin exposed to caustic substances should be decontaminated aggressively until neutralized and the resulting wounds considered deep until demonstrated otherwise.

Desiccant acids, such as sulfuric acid, create an exothermic reaction with tissue water and can cause both chemical and

thermal injury. With extensive immersion injuries, acids may be absorbed systemically, thereby leading to systemic acidosis and coagulation abnormalities.

Chemical burns may be excruciatingly painful for long periods. Discomfort can be out of proportion to what one might expect from the depth or extent of the burn. When caring for a chemical burn, the emergency care team should remove all potentially contaminated clothing. Any dry (anhydrous) chemical should be brushed off the patient's skin. The involved skin should then be irrigated with large amounts of water under low pressure. Any remaining particulate matter should be carefully débrided during irrigation.

Strong alkali burns may require irrigation for 1 to 2 hours before tissue pH returns to normal. Some recommend that if the burn continues to feel "slippery" or tissue pH has not returned to normal after extensive irrigation, chemical neutralization may be helpful.[57,58] Given that any heat of neutralization will be carried away with the irrigation solution,[59] prompt irrigation with a dilute acid (e.g., vinegar, or 2% acetic acid) may hasten neutralization and patient comfort.

Contact Burns from Wet Cement

The major constituent of Portland cement, an alkaline substance, is calcium oxide (64%), combined with oxides of silicon, aluminum, magnesium, sulfur, iron, and potassium. There is considerable variability in the calcium oxide content of different grades of cement, with concrete having less and fine-textured masonry cement having more.[56] The addition of water exothermically converts the calcium oxide to calcium hydroxide (Ca[OH]$_2$), a strongly corrosive alkali with a pH of 11 to 13. As the cement hardens, the calcium hydroxide reacts with ambient carbon dioxide and becomes inactive.

Both the heat and the Ca(OH)$_2$ produced in this exothermic reaction can result in significant burns. Because of its low solubility and consequent low ionic strength, long exposure to Ca(OH)$_2$ is required to produce injury. This usually occurs when workers spill concrete into their boots or kneel in it for a prolonged period. The burn wound and the resultant protein denaturation of tissues produce a thick, tenacious, ulcerated

Figure 38-22 Alkali burns from wet cement develop insidiously, are extremely painful, and are frequently full-thickness injuries. They are most common on the feet when cement leaks over the top of the boots (**A**) or from kneeling in wet cement while working (**B**). The alkali can penetrate clothing.

Figure 38-23 A burn on the forearm from a first-generation air bag can be a combination of friction and chemicals. They are usually minor.

eschar. Concrete burns are insidious and progressive. What may appear initially as a patchy, superficial burn might in several days become a full-thickness injury requiring excision and skin grafting.[60] The pain associated with these burns is often severe and more intense than the appearance of the wound might suggest (Fig. 38-22). Interestingly, many workers are not warned of the dangers of prolonged contact with cement, and because the initial contact with cement is usually painless, exposure may not be realized until the damage is done.

Treatment is as follows. Any loose particulate cement or lime should be removed, usually by brushing off, contaminated clothing is removed, and the wound is copiously irrigated with tap water (the pH of the effluent is tested and irrigation continued if the effluent is still alkaline). Compresses of dilute acetic acid (vinegar) may be applied to neutralize the remaining alkali and provide relief of pain after irrigation, and antibiotic ointment is applied to the eschar during the early postburn period.

Sutilains ointment (Travase, Flint Pharmaceuticals, Deerfield, IL) is often recommended because it contains proteolytic enzymes that help speed eschar separation, but any common

topical burn preparation is acceptable. The depth of burns from wet cement can be difficult to assess in the first several days. If it becomes apparent that the burns are full-thickness burns, early excision and skin grafting are recommended.

Cement burns should be differentiated from cement dermatitis, which is far more common. The latter is a contact sensitivity reaction, probably from the chromates present in cement. The contact dermatitis can initially be treated as a superficial partial-thickness burn.

Air Bag Keratitis and Thermal Burns

Safety legislation has mandated increased use of air bags to protect automobile occupants in the event of collision (Fig. 38-23). Burns from air bags can be thermal, friction, or chemical. The automobile air bag is a rubberized nylon bag that inflates on spark ignition of sodium azide to yield nitrogen gas, ash, and a small amount of sodium hydroxide. Within seconds, the superheated air is vented, and this can produce a thermal burn if it contacts an extremity, the face, or the upper part of the torso.[5,61,62] If the air bag ruptures, the alkaline contents of the bag are dispersed as a fine, black powder that usually causes no problems unless the eyes are exposed. Patients with eye exposure exhibit clinical evidence of a chemical keratoconjunctivitis, including photophobia, tearing, redness, and decreased visual acuity. Tear pH is usually elevated, and there may be a small amount of particulate material in the fornices.[63]

The severity of an ocular alkaline burn is related to the duration of exposure and the concentration and pH of the chemical. For this reason, prompt, copious irrigation of the eyes with frequent assessment of tear pH is essential to prevent or minimize the injury (see Chapter 62). A rising pH suggests that trapped particulate matter is releasing additional chemical. Corneal edema and conjunctival blanching are signs of serious injury and can necessitate immediate ophthalmologic consultation.

Hydrocarbon Burns

Hydrocarbons are capable of causing severe contact injury by virtue of their irritant, fat-dissolving, and dehydrating properties. Cutaneous absorption may cause even more dangerous systemic effects. Gasoline, the usual agent involved, is a complex mixture of C_4 to C_{11} alkane hydrocarbons and benzene; the hydrocarbons appear to be the major toxic agent. Lead poisoning caused by either absorption through intact skin or burns from exposure to leaded gasoline have been reported previously but are currently quite rare because unleaded gasoline has virtually replaced the leaded version for most purposes.[64]

The depth of injury is related to the duration of exposure and the concentration of the chemical agent. Gasoline immersion injuries resemble scald burns and are usually partial thickness.[65] Occasionally, gasoline-injured skin exhibits a pinkish brown discoloration, possibly related to dye additives. A common source of gasoline exposure is motor vehicle collisions in which a comatose patient has been lying in a pool of gasoline.

The lungs are the usual site of systemic absorption and are often the only major route of excretion. The resultant high pulmonary concentrations may lead to pulmonary hemorrhage, atelectasis, and acute respiratory distress syndrome. Treatment of hydrocarbon burns includes removal of contaminated clothing, prolonged irrigation or soaking of the contaminated skin, early débridement of significant burns caused by lead-containing gasoline (to reduce systemic lead absorption), and the use of topical antibiotic ointments.

Phenol Injury

Phenol is a highly reactive aromatic acid alcohol that acts as a corrosive. Carbolic acid, an earlier term for phenol, was noted to have antiseptic properties and was used as such by Joseph Lister in performing the first antiseptic surgery. Hexylresorcinol, a phenol derivative, is in current use as a bactericidal agent. Phenols, in strong concentrations, cause considerable eschar formation, but skin absorption also occurs and can result in systemic effects such as central nervous system depression, hypotension, hemolysis, pulmonary edema, and death. Interestingly, phenol acts differently from other acids in that it penetrates deeper when in a dilute solution than when in a more concentrated form.[55] Therefore, irrigation with water is suboptimal for phenol burns, but because water is commonly readily available, it is frequently used for irrigation.

Full-strength polyethylene glycol (PG 300 or 400) is more effective than water alone in removing phenolic compounds and should be obtained and used after water irrigation has begun. Polyethylene glycol is nontoxic and nonirritating and may be used anywhere on the body. When immediately available, polyethylene glycol can be used to remove the surface chemical before water irrigation (and chemical dilution) is begun.

Hydrofluoric Acid Injury

Hydrofluoric acid (HFA) is one of the strongest inorganic acids known; it has been widely used since its ability to dissolve silica was discovered in the late 17th century.[66] Currently, HFA is used in masonry restoration, glass etching, and semiconductor manufacturing; for control of fermentation in breweries; and in the production of plastics and fluorocarbons. It is also used as a catalyst in petroleum alkylating units. It is available in industry as a liquid in varying concentrations up to 70%. It is also readily sold in home improvement and hardware stores. Significant concentrations of HFA are present in many home rust removal products, aluminum brighteners, automobile wheel cleaners, and heavy-duty cleaners in concentrations of less than 10%. Despite its ability

Figure 38-24 A, Initially, this very painful hydrofluoric acid burn of the thenar and hypothenar eminence appeared minimal. **B,** Despite infiltration with calcium gluconate, a deep burn developed 3 days later.

to cause serious burns, unregulated and poorly labeled HFA products are recklessly used on a regular basis in the home and in small businesses. The public and many clinicians are generally unaware of the potential problems with this acid (Fig. 38-24).

Although HFA is quite corrosive, the hydrogen ion plays a relatively insignificant role in the pathophysiology of the burn injury. The accompanying fluoride ion is a protoplasmic poison that causes liquefaction necrosis and is notorious for its ability to penetrate tissues and cause delayed pain and deep tissue injury. This acid can penetrate through fingernails and cause nail bed injury. With home products, the unwary user does not realize that the substance is caustic until the skin (usually the hands and fingers) is exposed for a few minutes to hours, at which time the burning begins and becomes progressively worse. At this point the damage is done and the absorbed HFA cannot be washed off. With higher-strength industrial products, symptoms are almost immediate.

The initial corrosive burn is due to free hydrogen ions; secondary chemical burning is due to tissue penetration of fluoride ions. Fluoride is capable of binding cellular calcium, which results in cell death and liquefaction necrosis. The ionic shifts that result, particularly shifts of potassium, are believed to be responsible for the severe pain associated with HFA burns.

In high concentrations, the fluoride ions may penetrate to bone and produce demineralization. Exposure of skin to concentrated HFA involving as little as 2.5% TBSA can lead to systemic hypocalcemia and death from intractable cardiac arrhythmias; it has been calculated that exposure to 7 mL of anhydrous HFA (HFA gas) is capable of binding all the free calcium in a 70-kg adult.[67,68] Hyperkalemia and hypomagnesemia can also develop. If the hands are exposed, the acid characteristically penetrates the fingernails and injures the nail bed and cuticle area. As with most caustics, the pain is generally out of proportion to the apparent external physical injury. HFA burns produce variable areas of blanching and erythema, but rarely are blisters or skin sloughing seen initially. Skin necrosis and cutaneous hemorrhage may be noted in a few days.

Immediate treatment should begin with copious irrigation with water. Another approach is to wash the area with a solution of iced magnesium sulfate (Epsom salts) or a 1:500 solution of a quaternary ammonium compound such as benzalkonium chloride (Zephiran) or benzethonium chloride (Hyamine 1622). Magnesium and calcium salts form an insoluble complex with fluoride ions, thus preventing further tissue diffusion. Though frequently recommended, topical preparations are often ineffective in limiting injury or controlling pain.

If there is no or only minimal visible evidence of skin injury and minimal pain, the burn may be dressed with topical calcium gluconate paste. This is not commercially available in the United States but is easily compounded in the pharmacy by mixing 3.5 to 7 g of pulverized calcium gluconate with 5 oz of a water-soluble lubricant such as K-Y jelly. This will form a thick paste with a calcium gluconate concentration of 2.5% to 5.0%. Some have suggested dimethyl sulfoxide as a vehicle to aid in skin penetration of the calcium. Plastic wrap (e.g., Saran Wrap) is used over a standard dry burn dressing to cover the calcium paste on the limbs; a vinyl or rubber glove is used to cover the paste when used on the hands. The wound should be completely redressed and the paste reapplied every 6 hours for the first 24 hours. As with most topical treatments of HFA burns, calcium gluconate is only minimally effective in relieving pain, and its value is probably overestimated in the literature.

A digital or regional nerve block with long-acting bupivacaine is an excellent way to provide prolonged pain relief if the hands are involved, but this does nothing to ameliorate the injury. In most cases, oral opioids are required. If bullae or vesicles have formed, they should be débrided to decrease the amount of fluoride present, and the wound should then be treated as any partial-thickness burn. Burns with HFA of less than 10% strength will heal spontaneously, usually without significant tissue loss, but pain and sensitivity of the fingertips may persist for 7 to 10 days. In addition, the fingernails may become loose.

The presence of significant skin injury or intense pain implies penetration of the skin by fluoride ions. This scenario is particularly common with exposure to HFA solutions in concentrations of 20% or greater, but tissue injury can occur with prolonged exposure to less concentrated products.

Initial treatment of a more concentrated exposure begins as described earlier and includes immediate débridement of necrotic tissue to remove as much fluoride ion as possible.[69] After débridement, a 10% solution of calcium gluconate (note: avoid calcium chloride for tissue injections) is injected intradermally and subcuticularly with a 30-gauge needle about the exposed area, with about 0.5 mL per square centimeter of burn being used. Pain relief should be almost immediate if this therapy is adequate. Because the degree of pain is a measure of the effectiveness of treatment, the use of anesthetics, especially by local infiltration, may be deleted if the burn is on the arm or leg. HFA can penetrate fingernails without damaging them. Soft tissue can be injected without prior anesthesia, but if the fingertips or nail beds are involved, they may be injected after a digital nerve block has been performed (Fig. 38-25). Before anesthesia and injection of calcium, the patient can outline the affected areas with a pen to ensure accurate injection of the antidote (see Fig. 38-25C). Although some investigators recommend that the fingernails be removed routinely, we strongly advise against this unless the nails are very loose or there is obvious necrosis of the nail bed. Fingers are best injected with a 25- or 27-gauge needle (a tuberculin syringe works well).[58] Nails frequently become loose in a few days, but they often return to normal and do not require removal, particularly when lower-concentration nonindustrial products are involved.

Although infiltration of calcium gluconate is somewhat effective, the technique has certain limitations. Injections are painful, and the calcium gluconate solution itself causes a burning sensation. Because of the volume restrictions, not enough calcium may be delivered to bind all the free fluoride ions present. For example, 0.5 mL of 10% calcium gluconate contains 4.2 mg (0.235 mEq) of elemental calcium, which will neutralize only 0.025 mL of 20% HFA.

Several authorities have advocated intraarterial calcium infusions in the treatment of serious HFA burns of the extremities.[70,71] Though very effective, this technique is not recommended for burns secondary to dilute HFA (i.e., concentrations <10%) because the morbidity is usually quite mild. When using this technique, 10 mL of 10% calcium gluconate is diluted in 50 mL of a 5% dextrose and water solution. The dilute solution is administered by slow infusion into an arterial catheter. It is unclear which artery best delivers the calcium to injured tissues. If only the radial three digits are involved, probably only the radial artery need be cannulated. Otherwise, a percutaneous catheter is inserted into the brachial artery. However, some investigators have advocated use of the radial artery in all cases, and because the arterial supply of the hand is interconnected, this may be a reasonable recommendation.[72] The radial artery is usually more easily cannulated than the brachial artery. When arterial access has been accomplished, the solution is infused slowly over a 4-hour period. At this point the catheter is left in place and the patient is observed. If pain returns at any time over the next 4 hours, the infusion is repeated. If the patient is pain free over the 4-hour observation period, the burn is dressed and the patient is released home. This technique may be initiated in the ED, but many clinicians are reluctant to cannulate an artery and infuse calcium in the ED. Such patients require hospitalization or burn center referral for further evaluation and observation.

Advantages of the intraarterial method are elimination of the need for painful SQ injections and avoidance of the

Figure 38-25 A, Hydrofluoric acid (HFA) burns of the fingertips are extremely painful despite minimal clinical findings; initially only hyperemia and minor ecchymosis are apparent. HFL can penetrate the intact fingernail and produce a significant injury to the nail bed. **B,** The area of burn can be injected with calcium gluconate minimally diluted with plain lidocaine. Using a small-gauge needle, generously infiltrate the entire area of the burn. **C,** Before performing digital block anesthesia to painlessly infiltrate the fingertips with calcium gluconate, the patient outlines the painful areas with a felt-tipped marker to ensure accurate placement of the antidote. In the treatment of HFA burns, topical therapy is often ineffective. Calcium gluconate may be injected subcutaneously with a 25- to 27-gauge needle into the nail bed via the fat pad under a digital nerve block. Fingernails should not be removed routinely if burns are mild, such as those seen with household products containing less than a 10% concentration of the acid. Intraarterial calcium infusions are often quite successful in relieving pain and limiting necrosis. **D,** Calcium gluconate is combined with a small amount of lidocaine for injection.

volume limitations of the SQ route while providing substantially more calcium to neutralize the fluoride. Disadvantages of intraarterial calcium therapy include the possibility of local arterial spasm (which can be treated with vasodilators such as phentolamine or removal of the catheter), local arterial injury or thrombus, and the long duration of treatment required.

Infusing calcium into the general venous circulation is of no benefit for HFA burns. Some authors have advocated the use of regional IV calcium gluconate, similar to the method used with the Bier block for regional anesthesia (see Chapter 32).[73] Case reports have noted variable success, but this technique has neither been well studied nor rigorously compared with other options. This method would be useful only for upper extremity burns. To perform regional calcium therapy, an IV catheter is placed in the dorsum of the hand on the involved extremity. The arm is partially exsanguinated by elevation, wrapping with an elastic bandage, or both. A Bier block tourniquet or a heavy-duty blood pressure cuff is applied

proximal to the burn and inflated 20 to 30 mm Hg above systolic pressure to stop blood flow to and from the arm. Because slow deflation of a regular blood pressure cuff may thwart success of the procedure, use of a specialized tourniquet is recommended. Then, 10 mL of 10% calcium gluconate, diluted with 30 to 40 mL of saline, is infused into the venous catheter, and the solution is kept in the arm by the tourniquet for 20 to 30 minutes. Some patients cannot tolerate arm ischemia for this period, thus limiting the effectiveness of this procedure. Theoretically, the calcium diffuses out of the venous system and into the injured tissues. After 20 to 30 minutes, the cuff is deflated and normal circulation to the extremity is restored. It may require 10 to 20 minutes after deflation of the tourniquet before the patient experiences relief of pain. This procedure is safe, but its efficacy is variable.

HFA burns involving the eye are potentially devastating injuries that deserve special mention. Ophthalmologist referral is mandatory. Ocular exposure to liquid or gaseous HFA will result in severe pain, tearing, conjunctival inflammation, and corneal opacification or erosion. Complications include decreased visual acuity, globe perforation, uveitis, glaucoma, conjunctival scarring, lid deformities, and keratitis sicca. Optimal therapy for ocular HFA burns, other than initial irrigation, is unknown. Irrigation may be performed with water, isotonic saline, or magnesium chloride.[74] We advise copious saline irrigation. Topical antibiotics and cycloplegics, along with light pressure patching, are also recommended. The use of topical steroids has been advocated by some to lessen corneal fibroblast formation, but other attempted therapies such as subconjunctival injections of calcium gluconate and ocular irrigation with quaternary ammonium compounds have been associated with additional injury.[75]

Chromic Acid Injury

Chromium compounds are used extensively in industry, mainly in metallic electroplating. Chromic acid is commonly used in concentrated solutions containing up to 25% sulfuric acid. It causes sufficient skin damage to allow absorption of the toxic chromium ion if intensive irrigation is not undertaken immediately. Heated (60°C to 80°C) chromic acid makes the problem of chromium absorption much worse.

Dichromate salts containing hexavalent chromium are the most readily absorbed and the most toxic because they can cross cell membranes. The mortality rate from these burns is very high if the burn exceeds 10% TBSA. Chromium absorption leads to diarrhea, gastrointestinal bleeding, hemolysis, hepatic and renal damage, coma, encephalopathy, seizures, and disseminated intravascular coagulation.

Treatment includes immediate excision of the burned tissues to lessen the total body dichromate burden. Wounds should be washed with a 1% sodium phosphate or sulfate solution and dressed with bandages soaked in 5% sodium thiosulfate solution. These actions reduce the hexavalent chromium ion to the less well absorbed trivalent form.[76]

Chelation therapy with ethylenediaminetetraacetic acid should be instituted and IV sodium thiosulfate and ascorbic acid given. Hemodialysis, peritoneal dialysis, or exchange transfusion may be indicated.

Phosphorus Burns

White phosphorus is a translucent, waxy substance that ignites spontaneously on contact with air. For this reason, it is usually stored under water. It is used primarily in fireworks, insecticides and rodenticides, and military weapons.

Phosphorus causes both thermal burns from the flaming pieces and acid burns from the oxidation of phosphorus to phosphoric acid. The burns classically emit a white vapor with a characteristic garlic odor.[77]

These burns are treated first by immersion in water, followed by débridement of any gross debris. The wound is then washed with a 1% copper sulfate solution, which reacts with the residual phosphorus to form copper phosphate; the latter appears as black granules and allows easy débridement. After débridement, the residual copper is removed by a thorough water rinse, and the wound is dressed and treated as any other burn.

Elemental Alkali Metal Burns

The commonly encountered alkali metals (sodium, lithium, and potassium) are highly reactive with water and with water

TABLE 38-3 Chemical Burn Treatment

Water lavage	Chromic acid	Tannic acid
	Potassium permanganate	Tannic acid
	Cantharides	Sulfosalicylic acid
	Lyes (hydroxide salts)	Trichloroacetic acid
	Clorox	Cresylic acid
	Dichromate salts	Acetic acid
	Picric acid	Formic acid
Calcium salt infection	Oxalic acid Hydrofluoric acid	
Oil immersion	Sodium metal White phosphorus Mustard gas	
Avoid water lavage	Sodium metal Potassium metal Lithium metal	
Specific approaches	Sodium metal Lyes (hydroxide salts)	Excision Weak acid lavage (vinegar)
	Hydrofluoric acid	Calcium gluconate injection
	White phosphorus	Copper sulfate solution

vapor in air and produce their respective hydroxides with liberation of hydrogen gas. Therefore, water should never be used for extinguishing or débridement of the metal. A class D fire extinguisher or plain sand may be used for smothering the fire, followed by the application of mineral oil or cooking oil to isolate the metal from water and allow safe débridement. The burn is then treated as an alkali burn.

Magnesium burns in a less intense fashion but otherwise acts as other alkali metals do. These burns may be particularly injurious, however, because if all the metallic debris is not removed, the small ulcers that form will slowly enlarge until they become quite extensive.

The initial topical treatment of unusual chemical burns is outlined in Table 38-3.

Electrical Burns

Electrical burn wounds occur when energy traveling through the body across a potential difference is converted to heat. This energy has the ability to destroy deep tissues, including muscles, tendons, and nerves (Fig. 38-26). In addition, electrical injuries can arise from the arc produced when electricity passes through the air and from flames caused by the ignition of clothing. Electrical injuries from high-voltage or high-current sources (>1000 V and >5000 mA) are more likely to result in deep soft tissue damage, whereas low voltage or low current (<1000 V and 5 to 60 mA) causes less soft tissue damage but is more likely to result in cardiac arrhythmias.[78]

TEN and SJS

Toxic epidermal necrolysis (TEN) and Stevens-Johnson syndrome (SJS) are severe blistering diseases. They are usually associated with the intake of drugs that cause apoptosis of keratinocytes, which results in the separation of large areas of skin at the dermal-epidermal junction and produces the appearance of a scald. A major factor in improving outcomes has been high-quality intensive support and trained nursing care with expertise in wounds. Thus these disorders are ideally suited to treatment at burn centers.

The distinction between TEN and SJS is one of extent, with lesions occupying less than 10% TBSA qualifying as SJS (Fig. 38-27) and lesions involving greater than 30% TBSA being called TEN (Fig. 38-28); when the extent of involvement lies between 10% and 30%, an intermediary term is coined, SJS-TEN overlap. These disorders are rare with an annual incidence of 0.4 to 1.2 and 1.2 to 6.0 per million persons, respectively, and are more common in females and the elderly.[79] Patients at risk are those who are severely immunocompromised (e.g., human immunodeficiency virus

infection, lymphoma). Death occurs on average in every third patient with TEN. More than 100 drugs, including antibiotics (particularly sulfonamides), nonsteroidal antiinflammatory drugs, and anticonvulsants, have been implicated.

Various theories exist to explain the precise sequence of molecular and cellular events responsible for the development of TEN. The 1- to 3-week interval between the onset of TEN and the commencement of drug therapy favors an immune etiology. Cytotoxic T cells are seen in cutaneous lesions, and it is hypothesized that necrolysis is due to their recognition of complexes between drug metabolites and major histocompatibility complex class I molecules on the surface of keratinocytes. Exfoliation is due to the death of keratinocytes via apoptosis, and recent data suggest that the latter is mediated by interaction of the death receptors, transmembrane proteins, Fas, and its ligand FasL. This activates the proteolytic cascade (caspases), which leads to cellular disintegration.[80] Evidence has shown upregulation of FasL in patients with TEN.

Figure 38-26 Electrical burn. The patient experienced a contact burn across the dorsa of the toes from an exposed electrical wire. (*From Davis PJ, Cladis FP, Motoyama EK, eds.* Smith's Anesthesia for Infants and Children. *8th ed. St Louis: Mosby; 2011.*)

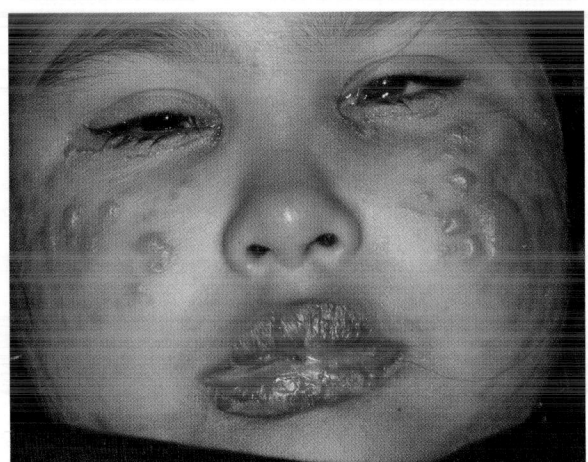

Figure 38-27 Stevens-Johnson syndrome (SJS). Purpuric macules became bullous. Note the inflammation of the conjunctivae and lips. By definition, in SJS the lesions occupy less than 10% of total body surface area. (*From Paller AS, Mancini AJ, eds.* Hurwitz Clinical Pediatric Dermatology. *4th ed. St. Louis: Saunders; 2011.*)

Figure 38-28 Toxic epidermal necrolysis. **A,** Detachment of large sheets of necrolytic epidermis (>30% body surface area) led to extensive areas of denuded skin. A few intact bullae are still present. **B,** Hemorrhagic crusts with mucosal involvement. **C,** Epidermal detachment of the palmar skin. (*From Bolognia JL, Jorizzo JL, Rapini RP, eds.* Dermatology. *3rd ed. St. Louis: Saunders; 2012.*)

Clinical Features

TEN and SJS are usually characterized by fever, corneal irritation, and painful swallowing (representing oral mucocutaneous involvement). These symptoms can precede the rash by 1 to 3 days. In more than 99% of patients, erythema and erosions of the buccal, ocular, and genital mucosa develop and are painful. The epithelium of the respiratory tract is involved in 25% of cases of TEN, and gastrointestinal lesions can occur. The skin lesions first appear as erythematous, dusky red, or purpuric macules, irregular in size and shape, that tend to coalesce. Nikolsky's sign (blistering following pressure with the finger) may be evident. A gray appearance of the macule heralds necrosis of the epidermis, which soon separates from the dermis and leaves a raw painful area. Wound infections (*S. aureus* and *P. aeruginosa*) and fluid and electrolyte loss often follow. Death is mainly due to sepsis, acute respiratory distress syndrome, and multiorgan failure. Reepithelialization and healing of wounds can occur within 3 weeks but may be prolonged. There are, however, late sequelae such as scarring and pigmentary abnormalities, as well as serious ophthalmic complications (e.g., symblepharon, conjunctival synechiae, entropion), which can range from sicca syndrome to blindness.

Management

Initial management of TEN requires immediate discontinuation of all medications, including antibiotics, if there are no signs of infection. Supportive care is similar to that required in the treatment of thermal burns. Attention is therefore paid to correction of fluid and electrolyte abnormalities, renal insufficiency, nutrition, and sepsis. Involvement of respiratory mucosa may warrant intubation and ventilation. The wounds are carefully débrided and a biopsy specimen is taken to confirm the diagnosis. Regular hydrotherapy and topical antimicrobials are used to decrease infection. Silvadene and mafenide are best avoided because they may be implicated in causing the disorder, but alternative dressings include the various silver products (e.g., Acticoat), as well as bacitracin and Xeroform. Synthetic dressings such as Biobrane and biologic materials, including allograft, have all been used with various success.[81]

Regular examination by an ophthalmologist is also recommended. The eyelids should be cleansed daily and followed with a daily application of antibiotic ointment. Attention to oral hygiene is also mandatory because oral lesions are common. Several case reports and uncontrolled series suggest the utility of specific therapies for the treatment of TEN/SJS; however, thus far there are no strong evidence-based standards to promote any particular therapy. Promising studies have included cyclosporine, cyclophosphamide, plasmapheresis, and *N*-acetylcysteine, but these therapies are not established standard of care.[82] The use of systemic corticosteroids remains controversial, and they may even increase mortality. Promising results were shown with the use of IV immunoglobulins that contain antibodies against Fas that can block the binding of Fas with FasL.[83]

Frostbite

Frostbite is the result of exposure to low environmental temperatures (Fig. 38-29). The formation of ice crystals within extracellular fluid causes direct cellular injury and cellular dehydration through transmembrane osmotic shifts. In addition, a secondary vascular effect of cooling leads to endothelial damage and progressive dermal ischemia.[84]

Initial management of acute frostbite should entail determination of the core temperature and a full physical examination. The frostbitten part should be rapidly rewarmed in a water bath (temperature of 40°C to 42°C) with adequate analgesia for 15 to 30 minutes. Treatment of deep injury consists of elevation of the injured part to control edema, adequate analgesia, splinting, and the application of topical antibiotics. Traditionally, white blisters are débrided. They generally represent superficial injury, and débridement is thought to be beneficial because it helps in the removal of thromboxane A_2 and prostaglandin $F_{2\alpha}$. Hemorrhagic blisters, however, are said to represent deeper injury and are best left intact to protect tissues against desiccation. The use of antithromboxane drugs such as aspirin or ibuprofen has been shown to be useful, as has the application of aloe vera. Premature amputation should be avoided but may be necessary for definitive closure. Long-term consequences include a predilection for future frostbite, vasospastic syndromes, and cold hypersensitivity.

Radiation Burns

Accidents involving ionizing radiation are not common, but when they occur, the clinical findings may range from

Figure 38-29 Frostbite. Initial management includes rapid rewarming in a water bath (temperature of 40°C to 42°C) for 15 to 30 minutes. Hemorrhagic blisters should be left intact; white or clear blisters may be débrided.

erythema to charring of the superficial layers of skin. Whole-body exposure of more than 100 rad causes acute radiation syndrome within hours of exposure. This is characterized acutely by nausea, vomiting, diarrhea, fever, fatigue, and headache. The symptoms may resolve transiently during a latent period only to recur as hematopoietic, gastrointestinal, or vascular complications.[85,86]

EMERGENCY ESCHAROTOMY

Full-thickness burns result in an eschar that is inelastic and may become restrictive and result in compartment syndrome. Intracellular and interstitial edema can develop and progress, both because of fluid resuscitation and as a direct result of transcapillary extravasation of fluid from the thermal injury. As the soft tissues become edematous and pressure rises under the unyielding eschar, first venous and then lymphatic, capillary, and ultimately arterial flow to the underlying and distal unburned tissue may be compromised. Full-thickness and extensive partial-thickness circumferential extremity burns are most likely to impede peripheral blood flow. Circumferential chest burns may restrict chest wall movement and impair ventilation, and circumferential neck burns may result in tracheal obstruction. In such cases, immediate escharotomy may be indicated.

On occasion, because of high-volume fluid resuscitation, noncircumferential and deep partial-thickness burns require surgical decompression to prevent the complications of nerve or muscle damage. Once signs and symptoms of vascular impairment are present, the clinician must act quickly to prevent tissue hypoxia and cellular death. This pathophysiology may be manifested within a time frame that requires an emergency clinician to intervene. Clinical assessment of tight compartments may be aided by measurements such as capillary refill, Doppler signals, pulse oximetry, and direct measurement of compartment pressures. Escharotomy, when required, is usually performed within the first 2 to 6 hours of a burn injury. The need for non–burn specialists to identify the need for and perform an adequate escharotomy is illustrated by the report of Brown and associates,[87] who found that 44% of pediatric burn cases were inadequately decompressed before arrival at a referral burn unit.

It is not standard of care that emergency clinicians be skilled in emergency escharotomy, nor can it be expected that this procedure will be done in the ED. The technique is described here for circumstances when escharotomy must be performed by a non–burn specialist.

Indications

The indications for escharotomy are based on clinical examination, compartment pressure, or both. A high index of suspicion and a low threshold for intervention are essential for a successful outcome. Skin temperature and palpation of pulses are unreliable and imprecise indicators of the adequacy of circulation because of peripheral vasoconstriction and local edema. A patient with circulatory embarrassment significant enough to warrant escharotomy may complain of deep aching pain, progressive loss of sensation, or paresthesias, but these parameters are difficult to quantitate in a severely burned, sedated, or mechanically ventilated patient. However, motor

activity and peripheral pulses may remain intact despite severe underlying muscle ischemia. In the series by Brown and associates,[87] peripheral pulses were present in 74% of the limbs that required decompression. Muscle compartments with pressures in excess of 30 mm Hg should be decompressed. Measurements should be taken before and after escharotomy to ensure adequate decompression.

In a patient with absent distal arterial flow (as determined with a Doppler ultrasonic flow meter) but otherwise adequate blood pressure, immediate escharotomy is indicated. Bardakjian and coworkers[88] suggested that an oxygen saturation below 95% in the distal end of the extremity as demonstrated by pulse oximetry (in the absence of systemic hypoxia) is also a reliable indicator of the need for emergency escharotomy.

Technique of Escharotomy

Because full-thickness burns are insensible to pain and involve coagulation of superficial vessels, no anesthesia is needed. Patients with deep partial-thickness burns may still possess pain sensation, and escharotomy may be performed with local anesthesia or systemic analgesia. A properly executed escharotomy releases the eschar to the depth of SQ fat only. This results in minimal bleeding, which can be controlled with local pressure or electrocautery. These incisions, even though life or limb saving, represent potential sources of infection for the burn patient and should be treated as part of the burn wound. The wounds should be loosely packed with sterile gauze impregnated with an appropriate topical antimicrobial such as silver sulfadiazine cream. Fasciotomy, which involves a deeper incision, may be needed for thermal or electrical burns.

Limbs

Under sterile conditions, the lateral and medial aspects of the involved extremity are incised with a scalpel or electrocautery 1 cm proximal to the burned area and 1 cm distal to the involved area of constricting burn (Fig. 38-30). The incision is carried through the full thickness of skin only and should result in immediate separation of the constricting eschar to expose SQ fat. Because joints are areas of tight skin adherence and potential vascular impingement, incisions should cross these structures (Fig. 38-31). Care must be taken to avoid vital structures, such as the ulnar nerve at the elbow, the radial nerve at the wrist, the superficial peroneal nerve near the fibular head, and the posterior tibial artery at the ankle. In circumferential burns of the feet, if escharotomy is indicated, the incision should extend to the great toe medially and the little toe laterally. In circumferential burns of the hands in which escharotomy is indicated, the incisions should extend to the thenar and hypothenar aspects of the hands (see Figs. 38-30 and 38-31). Softening of the compartment, improved distal tissue perfusion, return of sensation, Doppler flow signal strength, and oximetry values indicate adequate release.[88]

Chest

Full-thickness circumferential chest or upper abdominal burns may impair respiration. Nearly all these patients would expected to be intubated and mechanically ventilated. Evidence of the need to release the eschar is increasing airway pressure or an inability to ventilate. Escharotomy of the chest wall should extend from the clavicle to the costal margin in the anterior axillary line bilaterally while avoiding breast

Figure 38-30 Escharotomy. **A,** Patients with deep, nearly circumferential or circumferential chest wall burns may require escharotomy to facilitate ventilation. If performed properly, escharotomy of the torso will markedly enhance compliance. **B,** Properly performed escharotomy will result in immediate improvement in extremity blood flow. *(From Vincent J-L, Abraham E, Moore FA, et al, eds.* Textbook of Critical Care. *6th ed. St. Louis: Saunders; 2011.)*

Figure 38-31 Preferred sites for escharotomy incisions. *Dotted lines* indicate the escharotomy sites. *Bold lines* indicate areas where caution is required because vascular structures and nerves may be damaged by escharotomy incisions. *(From Davis JH, Drucker WR, Foster RS, et al.* Clinical Surgery. *St. Louis: Mosby; 1987.)*

tissue in females, and it may be joined by transverse incisions to result in a chevron-shaped subcostal incision (see Fig. 38-30).

Neck
Neck escharotomy should be performed laterally and posteriorly to avoid the carotid and jugular vessels.

Penis
Penile escharotomy is performed midlaterally to avoid the dorsal vein.

Complications
Complications of escharotomy include bleeding, infection, and damage to underlying structures. Complications of inadequate decompression include muscle necrosis, nerve injury (such as footdrop), and even amputation of the limb. Systemic complications of inadequate decompression include myoglobinuria and renal failure, hyperkalemia, and metabolic acidosis.

CONCLUSION
Patients with circumferential or nearly circumferential burns should be evaluated for the risk of compartment syndrome and deep tissue ischemia developing. Emergency clinicians should not hesitate to perform an escharotomy before transfer of the patient to a burn center if there is evidence of reduced limb perfusion or impaired ventilation.

Acknowledgment
The significant contributions of Courtney A. Bethel, MD, to earlier editions are appreciated.

References are available at www.expertconsult.com

Gastrointestinal Procedures

CHAPTER 39

Esophageal Foreign Bodies

David W. Munter

Patients with foreign bodies (FBs) lodged in the esophagus commonly go to the emergency department (ED) for evaluation and treatment. Though most commonly accidental, FBs may sometimes be swallowed purposefully. Patients may have a sensation of a recently passed FB, minor irritation, life-threatening airway obstruction, or other significant complications. Because of the anatomic and physiologic features of the esophagus, FBs in this area of the gastrointestinal (GI) tract present unique clinical issues to the clinician.

GENERAL FEATURES

Anatomy

The esophagus is a muscular tube 20 to 25 cm in length. There are three anatomic areas of narrowing in which FBs are most commonly entrapped: in the upper esophageal sphincter, which consists of the cricopharyngeus muscle; in the midesophagus at the crossover of the aortic arch; and in the lower esophageal sphincter (LES) (Fig. 39-1). *The LES is the narrowest point of the esophagus and the entire GI tract.*

Epidemiology

Patients with retained esophageal FBs generally fall into one of the following categories: pediatric patients, psychiatric patients, prisoners, and adults who either are edentulous or have underlying esophageal pathology.

Children account for 75% to 85% of esophageal FBs seen in the ED, with the peak incidence occurring at the age of 18 to 48 months.[1-9] The incidence is equal in boys and girls. Inquisitive children frequently place objects in their mouth and unintentionally swallow them. As a result, children most commonly ingest coins, but they also swallow buttons, marbles, beads, screws, and pins.[1,2,4,9-13] Unlike adults, chil-

dren who have entrapped, accidentally swallowed FBs do not normally have underlying esophageal disorders.[14] However, this is not the case in children with esophageal meat impaction, and these patients will need further evaluation for underlying esophageal disease.[15]

Patients with an anatomic abnormality of the esophagus or a motor disturbance are more prone to FB entrapment.[12,15,16] Anatomic abnormalities include strictures, webs, rings, diverticula, and malignancies. Motor disturbances include achalasia, scleroderma, and esophageal spasm. Adults who have dentures or underlying esophageal anatomic or motor abnormalities may accidentally ingest food boluses, chicken bones, fish bones, glass, toothpicks, fruit pits, or pills while in the act of eating.[13]

Prisoners and psychiatric patients ingest a wide variety of objects, some of which may be quite unusual: spoons, razor blades, pins, nails, or practically any other object.[12]

Complications

Impacted FBs of the esophagus must be removed or dislodged. The time frame under which this mandate must be carried out varies widely and depends on many circumstances. In general, however, the esophagus does not tolerate FBs well or for prolonged periods because it is prone to pressure, edema, necrosis, infection, and eventually perforation. FBs can transit the esophagus in a matter of seconds or minutes or may adhere to the mucosa. Retained objects may become less symptomatic after time, and the clinician must resist the urge to allow esophageal FBs to "pass by themselves" or "dissolve." Once FBs become stuck in the mucosa, *they may become less symptomatic, but they rarely pass on their own.* The one exception may be children with coins, especially those lodged at the LES. Approximately one third of these coins may pass spontaneously within 24 hours, and some authors have advocated an observational approach, although this is more poorly accepted by parents.[17-21]

A wide array of complications can arise from retained esophageal FBs (Box 39-1), including benign mucosal abrasions, lacerations, esophageal stricture, and necrosis from corrosive agents such as button batteries. Esophageal perforation[21-27] can lead to life-threatening conditions such as retropharyngeal abscess,[28] mediastinitis, pericarditis, pericardial tamponade,[29] pneumothorax, pneumomediastinum, tracheoesophageal fistula, and vascular injuries, including injuries to the subclavian vein and aorta.[20,30,31] Complications are more

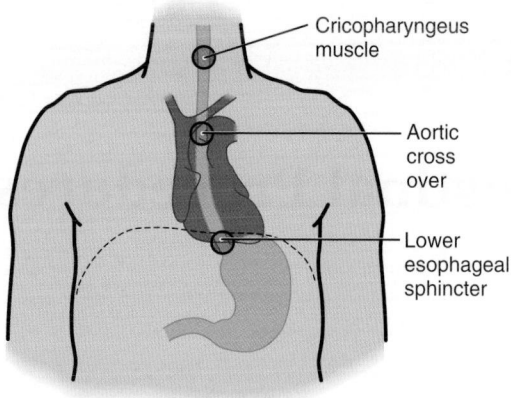

Figure 39-1 Blunt esophageal foreign bodies are most commonly lodged at one of three anatomic areas of narrowing: the cricopharyngeus muscle, the level of the aortic crossover, and the lower esophageal sphincter.

TABLE 39-1   Level of Entrapment of Esophageal FBs

LEVEL	PEDIATRIC (%)	ADULT (%)
Cricopharyngeus muscle	74	24
Aortic crossover	14	8
Lower esophageal sphincter	12	68

FB, foreign body.

all be caused by an underlying esophageal FB in a child, especially a young infant.[15,37-39]

Dysphagia is a common initial complaint with esophageal FBs. Drooling is suggestive of high-grade obstruction, and complete inability to handle oral secretions is a sign of total obstruction. Infants with a clandestine esophageal FB can exhibit wheezing or a chronic cough. They may appear to have bronchospasm and may be treated for asthma. Stridor from an FB can mimic epiglottitis.

The esophagus is well innervated proximally, and patients can typically accurately localize FBs in the oropharynx or upper third of the esophagus. However, scratches or abrasions of the esophagus can create a persistent FB sensation. Upper esophageal FBs often cause gagging or vomiting. In rare cases, an upper esophageal FB can impinge on the trachea, especially in children, and mimic infection by inducing wheezing, stridor, or frank respiratory distress. The lower two thirds of the esophagus is not as well innervated, and FBs in this location typically cause vague symptoms of discomfort, fullness, or nonlocalizing pain. Swallowed coins that lodge in the lower part of the esophagus in children may cause no overt symptoms until feeding is attempted.

The location of retained esophageal FBs is related to age (Table 39-1). Children more typically have objects entrapped in the upper part of the esophagus at the level of the cricopharyngeus muscle, whereas adults more commonly have entrapment at the LES.[18,38,40-42]

Evaluation

The most useful aspect of the evaluation is the history. The time of the ingestion, size and shape of the ingested object, and any current symptoms should be ascertained. Findings on physical examination are frequently normal in patients with esophageal FBs, unless complete obstruction is present. In this case they will be drooling, spitting, and unable to handle oral secretions. Even though a patient may be asymptomatic at initial encounter, transient coughing or gagging should raise the index of suspicion for an esophageal FB. Examination of the oropharynx, neck, respiratory system, cardiac system, and abdomen is essential in the evaluation of potential complications.

After attending to life-threatening conditions such as airway compromise, the goal of ED evaluation is to localize the FB to determine what, if any, interventions need to be undertaken to remove it or assist its transit into the stomach. Once an FB passes into the stomach, it has a greater than 90% likelihood of passing through the entire GI tract without any further problems.[34] Even large, irregular, and seemingly dangerous FBs will often transit the entire GI tract with relative ease.

BOX 39-1   Complications of Esophageal FBs

Airway compromise secondary to tracheal compression
Aspiration pneumonia
Esophageal necrosis
Esophageal perforation
Esophageal stricture
Failure to thrive
Mediastinitis
Mucosal abrasion
Paraesophageal abscess
Pericardial tamponade
Pericarditis
Pneumothorax
Pneumomediastinum
Retropharyngeal abscess
Tracheoesophageal fistula
Vascular injury, including aortic perforation
Vocal cord paralysis

FB, foreign body.

common when FBs are entrapped for longer than 24 hours[2,32,33] and when they are sharp.[34] An estimated 1500 deaths occur annually as a result of esophageal FBs, primarily from complications of esophageal perforation.[9]

Clinical Findings

Esophageal FB impaction is usually an acute condition, particularly in adults who have a clear history of ingestion. Children also commonly remember an ingestion, but some will have a vague history or symptoms. As many as one third of children with proven esophageal FBs are asymptomatic on initial evaluation[20,34-36]; therefore, a high index of suspicion is indicated, especially in children who were seen with an object in their mouth that subsequently disappeared. This is particularly true if transient coughing or gagging occurred, even though the actual ingestion was not witnessed. Poor feeding, irritability, fever, stridor, cough, wheezing, and aspiration can

RADIOLOGY OF ESOPHAGEAL FBS

Background

Radiographic imaging of a patient with a suspected esophageal FB is a common practice and is particularly useful for detecting radiopaque FBs. Traditionally, an inability to quickly identify the object by physical examination encouraged the use of plain radiography in an attempt to verify and localize the retained FB. However, the limitations of plain radiography require that other diagnostic approaches be considered as well.

Indications

Interactive, verbal patients can provide valuable information about the ingested object and can typically localize the retained FB with reliable accuracy.[43] In such cases the diagnostic workup should be tailored to localization of the symptoms and ingested material. However, nonverbal patients, including preschool children and those who are demented or debilitated, warrant a low threshold for screening radiography in cases with a suspicious history. Examples include a child seen with an object in the mouth that "disappeared" or a patient with symptomatology suggestive of an esophageal FB, such as drooling, gagging, or unexplained respiratory symptoms.

Plain Radiographs

Plain radiographs reliably verify and localize radiopaque FBs such as glass and metal of sufficient size and are indicated as the main method of radiologic evaluation for these objects.

Unfortunately, many ingested FBs are nonopaque, including nonbony food, plastic, wood, and aluminum. Some pull tabs from beer cans may be seen if oriented in the coronal plane. A metal detector has been reported to help localize radiolucent aluminum pull tabs.[44,45] Calcification of fish and chicken bones is often incomplete, but cooking alters the structure of bones and makes them radiolucent on plain films. The degree of bony calcification varies with the fish species and between different samples of the same species, thus preventing useful guidelines.[46-49] For these reasons, *plain films provide little substantive evidence in the majority of cases of fish or chicken bone dysphagia.* They detect only 25% to 55% of endoscopically proven bones and carry a high rate of false-negative and false-positive interpretations.[43,48-53] Because of the lack of diagnostic value for detecting bones, *many clinicians do not routinely order plain radiographs and instead initially opt for computed tomography (CT) in cases in which radiographic evaluation is required.*[54,55]

When used, a complete oropharyngeal radiographic series includes the nasopharynx to the lower cervical vertebra in both lateral and anteroposterior views. Optimum-quality radiographs are mandatory. Patients should be positioned upright with the neck extended and the shoulders held low. Use of a soft tissue technique enhances the discrimination of weak radiopaque FBs. Phonation of "eeeee" during radiography prevents motion artifact from swallowing, distends the hypopharynx, and enhances soft tissue landmarks. As previously mentioned, FBs are most frequently entrapped at one of three locations in the esophagus: the cricopharyngeus muscle (Fig. 39-2), the aortic crossover (Fig. 39-3), and the LES (Fig. 39-4).

Figure 39-2 Posteroanterior radiograph of an esophageal foreign body (coin) lodged at the level of the cricopharyngeus muscle. This is the most common area of the esophagus to harbor a coin in children. Coins remaining in the upper tract are usually removed unless there is steady progression with observation. This coin would probably be symptomatic in an infant and cause respiratory distress, drooling, wheezing, and perhaps stridor. *Note:* The chance of spontaneous passage is about 20% to 25%.

Figure 39-3 Posteroanterior radiograph of an esophageal foreign body (coin) lodged at the level of the aortic crossover. *Note:* The chance of spontaneous passage is about 20% to 25%.

Figure 39-4 Posteroanterior radiograph of an esophageal foreign body (coin) lodged at the level of the lower esophageal sphincter. Coins in this area are most likely to pass and be favorably manipulated by medication (see Table 39-2). *Note:* The chance of spontaneous passage is about 25% to 60%; chances increase with prolonged observation. *(From Waltzman ML, Baskin M, Wypij D, et al. A randomized clinical trial of the management of esophageal coins in children.* Pediatrics. *2005;116:614; and Soprano JV, Fleisher GR, Mandl KD. The spontaneous passage of esophageal coins in children.* Arch Pediatr Adolesc Med. *1999;153:1073.)*

Figure 39-5 A, Lateral neck radiograph showing a chicken bone (*arrow*) lodged in the pharynx with associated soft tissue swelling. Plain radiographs have poor diagnostic accuracy for detecting bones in the esophagus, and they are often eschewed in favor of a computed tomography scan if radiographic evaluation is deemed necessary. **B,** A chicken bone in the proximal end of the esophagus (*arrow*), where it is more readily seen on a radiograph. **C,** Another example of a chicken bone in the proximal end of the esophagus (*arrow*).

Plain radiography of the neck is limited by the radiographic properties of ingested materials and the complicated anatomy of the upper aerodigestive tract. The base of the tongue, palatine and lingual tonsils, vallecula, and piriform recesses are common regions for entrapment of small, sharp objects and deserve careful interpretive attention (Fig. 39-5). Superimposition of the mandible contributes to suboptimal resolution of this region on lateral neck films. Calcified airway cartilage often masquerades as FBs and contributes to false-positive rates as high as 25%.[43,48,50,52,56-58] Normal ossification of airway cartilage begins in the third decade and progresses with age.[59] The typical curvilinear contour and well-defined margins of bony FB fragments may help distinguish them from normal laryngeal calcifications. The orientation of bony FBs is variable. The C6 vertebra approximates the level of the cricopharyngeus, a common site of FB impaction. Increased prevertebral soft tissue width, air within the cervical esophagus, and soft tissue emphysema are rare indirect findings that may help identify radiolucent objects.[49,60]

Posteroanterior (PA) and lateral views of the chest are used to evaluate the remainder of the esophagus. Both projections are indicated to identify multiple objects and FBs visible in only one plane. Esophageal FBs typically lie in the vertical plane and are differentiated from airway bodies or calcifications by their location posterior to the tracheal air column on lateral radiographs. As a rule, flat objects such as coins perch in the coronal plane in the esophagus and in the sagittal orientation in the trachea. Intraesophageal air and air-fluid levels represent indirect evidence of esophageal obstruction and may aid in the verification of radiopaque FBs. Soft tissue swelling, extraluminal air, and aspiration pneumonitis can occasionally help identify complicated impactions radiographically.

Figure 39-6 A, Barium swallow demonstrating complete esophageal obstruction in the proximal to midportion of the esophagus (*arrow*). **B,** Barium esophagogram demonstrating a large piece of meat (*long arrow*) lodged above an esophageal stricture (*short arrow*). Many patients with lodged meat have underlying esophageal pathology. **C,** Bolus of meat seen in the distal end of the esophagus with an endoscope. The scope provides a means for removal and esophageal evaluation simultaneously. This young person had a ringed esophagus as his pathology.

In children, a film from the nasopharynx to the anus is frequently obtained to allow visualization of the entire nasopharynx, throat, and esophagus, as well as the abdomen in case the FB has passed into the stomach or beyond. Radiation exposure can be minimized if adult-sized radiograph cassettes are used. Swallowed coins or other FBs may become lodged in the nasopharynx, usually after gagging or vomiting, and could be missed if this area is not included on the radiograph. In adults, if neck or chest films are negative, abdominal films are sometimes obtained for reassurance of the presence of the FB in the stomach.

Contrast-Enhanced Esophagograms

Background

A contrast-enhanced esophagogram is a test with limited utility in the ED as a routine intervention to evaluate for an esophageal FB. It may be considered when plain radiographs are negative, but esophagography has largely been replaced by CT and endoscopy for evaluation of FBs. This technique uses swallowed contrast material to help identify the presence and location of an impacted radiolucent FB, the degree of obstruction, any underlying anatomic abnormalities, and the presence of perforation. A variation of this technique is to have the patient swallow contrast-soaked cotton pledgets. This technique uses smaller contrast loads and may identify impacted FBs by the impeded progression of the cotton or by tagging sharp irregular objects with radiopaque cotton threads as the bolus passes. Theoretically, this variation might interfere less with follow-up endoscopy because of the attenuated contrast loads. Unfortunately, ingestion of liquid contrast agents yields overall results no better than those of plain film radiography. More importantly, contrast material may interfere with the detection and extraction of FBs at endoscopy (barium) and may increase the risk for aspiration pneumonitis (diatrizoate meglumine and diatrizoate sodium [Gastrografin]).[40,61,62] Therefore, routine, serial contrast-enhanced esophagograms after negative plain radiography in patients with known or suspected FBs are unnecessary for diagnostic purposes in most cases. Selective use is reasonable, but CT or endoscopy is the intervention with the best and most cost-effective yield.[63]

Procedure

Esophagograms couple voluntary ingestion of an enteric contrast agent (Gastrografin or barium) and plain radiography. Immediately after ingestion, erect and horizontal radiographs are performed at right-angle projections (PA and lateral or right and left anterior oblique). In addition to anatomic abnormalities, radiolucent FBs may be identified by contrast delineation or filling defects within the contrast column (Fig. 39-6).

The initial choice of contrast agent is debated and should be individualized according to the threat of aspiration and perforation. Other logistic concerns, listed later, have relegated this test to minimal use in the ED. Water-soluble Gastrografin is indicated first in most cases of suspected perforation because it causes less mediastinal inflammation when extravasated; however, it can give rise to severe chemical pneumonitis if aspirated and is relatively contraindicated in patients with complete esophageal obstruction.[12] Patients without evidence of complete esophageal obstruction are instructed to swallow progressively larger aliquots of contrast agent up to approximately 50 mL. If these films are normal, the procedure is repeated with half-strength and then full-strength barium to delineate small esophageal injuries. Note that water-soluble contrast material (Gastrografin) causes more pulmonary reaction than barium does when inadvertently aspirated and should be used in small aliquots if aspiration or complete esophageal obstruction is a concern. Contrast-enhanced esophagograms coupled with fluoroscopy are seldom used for acute esophageal FB impactions, although slowed progression or abnormal peristalsis may suggest a retained FB or an anatomic abnormality. Barium interferes with endoscopy and should not be used when endoscopy is anticipated.

Figure 39-7 Computed tomography scan demonstrating an esophageal foreign body.

Figure 39-8 Esophageal foreign body (*arrow*) seen on nasopharyngoscopy.

CT

Non–contrast-enhanced CT of the neck and mediastinum is an easy, rapid, cost-effective, and noninvasive means of detecting or ruling out upper GI FBs (Fig. 39-7)[48,49,51,54,55] and has garnered support in the clinical setting of suspected FB entrapment.[64-66] CT further excels at localization and characterization of the impacted FB and identification of associated complications such as perforation.[49,64,67-69]

CT clearly provides improved diagnostic utility for fish bone FBs over plain radiography with or without barium enhancement.[48,49,51,54] Use of CT in patients in whom clinical suspicion for a retained FB is high has the potential to reduce the number of unnecessary endoscopies.[51]

Conclusions

Diagnostic radiography for esophageal FBs requires individualization of cases. Plain radiographs clearly assist the clinician in several situations: (1) screening of children, adults with dementia, and nonverbal patients with a history or symptoms suspicious for purposeful or inadvertent FB ingestion that *can be assumed to be radiopaque* and (2) localization of known radiopaque ingestants to clarify the necessity for and means of FB extraction. Conversely, attempts to verify radiolucent FBs, including bones, by plain radiography are often misleading. Contrast-enhanced esophagograms may be used in special situations but have largely been replaced by CT and direct endoscopy. The use of CT to exclude fish bones and other FBs is effective when initial routine plain films are avoided.[63]

VISUALIZATION OF ESOPHAGEAL AND PHARYNGEAL FBS

Patients with an FB sensation in their oropharynx typified by a "fish bone" or "chicken bone" sensation need to have some form of visualization of their oropharynx performed as part of the physical examination. The three procedures are direct pharyngoscopy, which is simply direct visualization or examination using a tongue blade with a light source that may be a pen light, wall light, or head light; indirect laryngoscopy, which involves using a handheld mirror reflecting a light to allow visualization of the epiglottis, vallecula, arytenoids, arytenoids folds, and vocal cords—a procedure that requires experience and a cooperative patient; or nasopharyngoscopy, a procedure using a flexible nasopharyngoscope. If an FB is visualized (Fig. 39-8), it should be removed with forceps and the oropharynx carefully reexamined for any injury or additional FB. All three of these procedures are discussed in detail in Chapter 63.

ESOPHAGOSCOPY

Esophagoscopy is the definitive diagnostic and therapeutic procedure for impacted esophageal FBs.[9,41] Although esophagoscopy is not a procedure performed by the emergency clinician, its proper role in the ED evaluation of FBs must be understood. With esophagoscopy, the clinician can document the presence and location of the FB along with any underlying lesion. The clinician can then remove the object and reevaluate the esophagus after removal of the FB to rule out perforation or underlying pathology. Esophagoscopy may be necessary even if a radiologic contrast-enhanced study does not reveal complete obstruction because x-ray studies are not always conclusive.[8,70] Esophagoscopy may be necessary to exclude predisposing pathology or resultant perforation, even when symptoms presumed to be due to an esophageal FB have resolved.

Esophagoscopy is the preferred method for removal of sharp or pointed objects such as bones, open safety pins, and razors. In the case of sharp objects prone to causing esophageal perforation, intravenous antibiotics should be administered before the procedure. Endoscopy is the preferred way to remove an impacted meat bolus and to evaluate for possible esophageal pathology at the same time. Esophagoscopy is also indicated for an FB retained for more than 24 to 48 hours, both to remove it and to examine for esophageal wall erosion or perforation. Esophagoscopy is the only appropriate removal

TABLE 39-2 Recommended Pharmacologic Therapies for Esophageal FBs

CLASS AND AGENTS	SITE OF ACTION	DOSE AND ROUTE	ADVERSE EFFECTS
Spasmolytics			
Glucagon	LES	1-2 mg IV*	Nausea, vomiting, hyperglycemia, hypersensitivity
Nitroglycerin	Body and LES	0.4-0.8 mg SL[†]	Hypotension, tachycardia, bradycardia
Nifedipine	LES	5-10 mg SL[‡]	Hypotension, tachycardia *Use with caution*
Gas-Forming Agents			
Tartaric acid	Distal and proximal	15 mL tartaric acid (18-20 g/100 mL)[§]	Vomiting, increased intraesophageal pressure
Sodium bicarbonate	Distal and proximal	15 mL sodium bicarbonate (10 g/100 mL)[§]	Vomiting
Carbonated beverage	Distal and proximal	100 mL PO	Increased intraesophageal pressure

FB, foreign body; *IV*, intravenously; *LES*, lower esophageal sphincter; *PO*, per os (orally); *SL*, sublingually.
*May be repeated once or used in conjunction with nitroglycerin.
[†]One to 2 inches of nitroglycerin paste applied under an occlusive dressing may be an alternative.
[‡]A capsule is punctured, chewed, held in the mouth for 3 minutes, and then swallowed. Because of *hypotension*, a 5-mg dose may be used in the elderly. *Do not use if the patient has cardiovascular disease, is hypotensive, or has also recently been given nitroglycerin.*
[§]Alternatively, dissolve 2 to 3 g tartaric acid and 2 to 3 g sodium bicarbonate in 30 mL water.

technique for multiple or large esophageal FBs. This technique is also indicated for patients with an FB proved to have passed into the stomach and for those who have persistent symptoms possibly caused by esophageal wall injury. Flexible endoscopic procedures can usually be performed without general anesthesia, even in most children.[71] The success rate of flexible endoscopy in patients with retained esophageal FBs exceeds 96%.[41,72]

Traditionally, esophagoscopy is more expensive than other maneuvers such as Foley catheter removal or esophageal bougienage (described later),[3,7,73,74] largely because of charges for the surgical suite, but it has a higher success rate than the other two techniques do. ED removal of esophageal FBs in children by experienced endoscopists, while the child is under ketamine sedation administered by the emergency clinician, has been reviewed.[75] In selected cases this approach can shorten the interval to completion of the procedure and reduce expense.

ESOPHAGEAL PHARMACOLOGIC MANEUVERS
Background

Since the LES is the narrowest portion of the entire GI tract, most FBs that reach the stomach eventually move through the GI tract without further problems. Because a large number of entrapped esophageal FBs are lodged at the LES, especially in adults, several therapeutic maneuvers have been developed to assist transit into the stomach, including pharmacologic relaxation of the LES. In theory, agents that promote smooth muscle relaxation should improve mobility through the LES. Although many clinicians use pharmacologic adjuncts for all esophageal FBs, objects lodged at the LES will probably benefit most from such interventions. *Nonspecific pain relief, anxiolysis, vomiting, and spontaneous passage over time may account for the success attributed to many pharmacologic manipulations of esophageal FBs.*

Several pharmacologic agents, including diazepam, meperidine, and atropine, have been shown to be *unsuccessful* in removing or resolving esophageal impaction by FBs.[13] These agents, alone or in combination, have success rates below 10%, which is no better than observation alone.[2] Glucagon, nitroglycerin, nifedipine, and gas-forming agents (Table 39-2) are described later and are the most effective pharmacologic agents for treatment of distal esophageal food impaction.

Indications and Contraindications

The indication for pharmacologic relaxation of the LES is the presence of a smooth or blunt FB such as a coin or food bolus. Angulated, abrasive, or sharp FBs should not be treated with pharmacologic modalities but instead should be removed by esophagoscopy. Analgesics and sedatives are routinely indicated if pain is present or the patient is excessively anxious.

Glucagon
Pharmacology

Glucagon has been a prototype for the spasmolytic agents.[76-78] Glucagon theoretically relaxes esophageal smooth muscle and decreases LES resting pressure. One study of normal subjects found that glucagon significantly lowers mean LES resting pressure but causes no significant difference in the mean amplitude of contraction in the distal end of the esophagus.[79] Glucagon has no effect on the upper third of the esophagus, a common site of coin impaction in children, where striated muscle is present and some voluntary control is operative. It only minimally affects the middle third of the esophagus. Peristalsis is not affected by glucagon. Results with glucagon have been mixed, and the only randomized study, done in children, showed no better results than those achieved with placebo.[80] A nonrandomized study in adults showed that glucagon is about equivalent to placebo, with a 33% success rate, and that the addition of a benzodiazepine increases the success rate slightly.[81] Its use, however, is still advocated by some authorities and has little downside. Glucagon may cause vomiting, and this action may be responsible for some of the drug's success.[82]

Indications and Contraindications

Glucagon is most useful for smooth FBs or food impactions at the LES that are suspected because of a patient's complaint of pain or "something stuck" in the lower part of the chest or epigastrium. The clinical diagnosis is usually straightforward, especially if complete esophageal obstruction is present and the patient is unable to tolerate oral secretions. Nevertheless, some clinicians recommend that the FB be localized first with radiographs (with or without contrast enhancement) to establish that the impaction is indeed there. The radiographs can then serve as the baseline study for comparison after administration of glucagon. However, with classic findings on the history and physical examination, most investigators agree that an initial contrast-enhanced study can be omitted. Glucagon is not effective in relieving upper and middle esophageal obstruction, and it is not widely recommended for use in children. In addition, glucagon is not usually effective in patients with fixed fibrotic strictures or rings at the gastroesophageal junction.[77] Glucagon is contraindicated if the patient has an insulinoma, pheochromocytoma, Zollinger-Ellison syndrome, hypersensitivity to glucagon, or a sharp esophageal FB.

Administration of Glucagon

Some reports recommend a small test dose to check for hypersensitivity to glucagon. In practice, this is rarely done. The therapeutic dose is 0.25 to 2 mg administered intravenously over a period of 1 to 2 minutes in a seated patient, although one study found that in normal subjects, 1 mg of glucagon provides no significant additive benefit over 0.5 mg.[79] The patient is given water orally within 1 minute after the injection of glucagon to stimulate normal esophageal peristalsis; this helps push the food through the relaxed LES into the stomach. Glucagon has a rapid onset and short duration of action: GI smooth muscle relaxes within 45 seconds, and its duration of action is about 25 minutes. If no results are seen within 10 to 20 minutes, a second administration of 0.25 to 2 mg may be tried. Success rates are higher when glucagon is combined with gas-forming agents or even carbonated beverages.[83,84] It is recommended that a small volume of some oral fluid be routinely given to enhance the activity of glucagon.

Complications

Glucagon is associated with a few minor side effects. If administered too rapidly, it causes nausea and vomiting. Therefore, adult patients must be alert and mobile enough to avoid aspiration. Occasionally, vomiting dislodges the impacted food bolus. Theoretically, there is a risk for rupture of the obstructed esophagus during induced emesis, so slow injection is preferred to minimize this side effect.

Administration of glucagon is also associated with dizziness. Mild elevation of blood glucose levels is also common but not of clinical concern, and blood glucose levels do not need to be monitored. No fatalities have been reported. Although theoretically glucagon can stimulate release of catecholamine in patients with pheochromocytoma and can induce hypoglycemia from reflex release of insulin with an

insulinoma, these endocrine tumors are rare. Nonetheless, precipitation of either profound catecholamine or insulin reactions with the use of glucagon should direct a workup for these underlying tumors.

Further Evaluation and Therapy

If the patient experiences relief of symptoms after the administration of glucagon, a postprocedure radiograph or contrast-enhanced study may be obtained to confirm passage of a radiopaque object, but this is not mandatory (Fig. 39-9). Adult patients with successful FB passage into the stomach may also be discharged home, but careful follow-up should be obtained to rule out coexistent esophageal pathology because a significant number of patients (65% to 80%) will have underlying esophageal disorders.[9,16] Pediatric patients with food boluses lodged in the esophagus also have a high rate of underlying esophageal disease and need referral for further evaluation; this is not the case for accidentally swallowed FBs in children.[15] If glucagon fails to produce relief of the symptoms or resolve the radiograph findings, its use does not preclude other methods from being used.

Nitroglycerin and Nifedipine Pharmacology

Both sublingual nitroglycerin and nifedipine have been used in a manner similar to glucagon to relieve LES tone and

Before   After

Figure 39-9 This patient had meat impacted in the distal end of the esophagus, clearly visible on the "before" contrast-enhanced esophagogram (*arrow*). He was treated successfully with simultaneous administration of glucagon and an effervescent sodium bicarbonate drink. On the "after" esophagogram, the contrast material can be seen flowing down the distal end of the esophagus and into the stomach (*arrows*). (*Note:* Gastrografin contrast medium was used in this study.)

allow the passage of a distal esophageal FB.[85-87] Although these two agents have been used less than glucagon for the treatment of esophageal FBs, both are useful for the relief of chest pain associated with esophageal smooth muscle spasm[64] and may be administered concurrently with glucagon. Manometric and radiographic studies after the administration of nitroglycerin have revealed abolition of the repetitive high-pressure wave contractions characteristic of esophageal spasm. Nifedipine, conversely, significantly reduces LES pressure without changing contraction amplitudes in the body of the esophagus. Thus, nitroglycerin may relieve partial or complete obstruction of the middle or lower part of the esophagus secondary either to intrinsic esophageal disease or to simple FB impaction, and nifedipine, like glucagon, is most likely to succeed when the bolus is lodged at the gastroesophageal junction.

Indications and Contraindications

Similar to clinical indications for the use of glucagon, any patient with an impacted smooth esophageal FB, especially a food bolus, may be a candidate for nitroglycerin or nifedipine (or both). Also, similar to the mode of action of glucagon, neither of these agents is expected to relax a fixed fibrotic stricture or ring at the gastroesophageal junction.[77] Nevertheless, because both agents have a relatively benign side effect profile, if the patient has no contraindication to their use, they may be tried with or without previous documentation of the distal esophageal obstruction with a contrast-enhanced study. Contraindications to their use include a history of allergic reactions, a sharp esophageal FB, hypovolemia, and hypotension.

Use and Complications

Doses of 1 or 2 (0.4 mg) sublingual nitroglycerin tablets, 1 to 2 inches of nitroglycerin paste, or 5 to 10 mg of nifedipine have been reported.[85-87] Remember that some patients with esophageal FBs may have some degree of dehydration because of the inability to swallow liquids or their own saliva. These patients may be prone to hypotension from the vasodilation associated with the use of either agent. Ideally, rehydration should precede therapy with these agents. Sublingual nifedipine (5- to 10-mg capsule punctured, chewed, and swallowed) has been implicated in cerebral or coronary insufficiency in patients with cardiovascular disease, so caution is warranted. *Do not use both agents simultaneously.* The smaller dose of nifedipine is suggested in the elderly or those with cardiovascular disease.

Further Evaluation and Therapy

As with the use of glucagon, if nitrate therapy fails to produce relief of the symptoms or resolve the radiographic findings, its use does not preclude trying another method. If a patient experiences symptomatic relief, a postprocedure radiograph may be obtained to confirm passage of a radiopaque object, but this is not mandatory. Adult patients may be discharged home, but careful follow-up should be obtained to rule out coexistent esophageal pathology because a significant number of patients will have underlying esophageal disorders.

Gas-Forming Agents

Pharmacology

The use of gas-forming agents for the treatment of distal esophageal food impaction, especially meat boluses, was first described in 1983.[88] The combination of tartaric acid solution followed immediately by a solution of sodium bicarbonate or even carbonated beverages has been reported. In theory, use of this acid-base mixture or a carbonated beverage may produce sufficient carbon dioxide to distend the esophagus, relax the LES, and push impacted food through the gastroesophageal junction into the stomach.[89,90]

Indications and Contraindications

Gas-forming agents are indicated for the relief of smooth distal esophageal FB impaction, with or without prior FB confirmation by a radiographic study (see Fig. 39-9). They are often given to patients with food impaction or retained coins. Although gas-forming agents are more likely to succeed with distal esophageal impactions, they have also been successful in relieving obstructions in the proximal part of the esophagus. Concurrent administration of spasmolytic agents may improve the effectiveness of gas-forming agents.[84]

Use and Complications

A solution of 15 mL of tartaric acid (18.7 g/100 mL), followed by 15 mL of a sodium bicarbonate solution (10 g/100 mL), or 1.5 to 3 g of tartaric acid and 2 to 3 g of sodium bicarbonate dissolved in 15 mL of water can be used.[88,89] Carbonated beverages (100 mL) have also been successful in the transit of FBs into the stomach[89,90] and are more readily available in the ED. Many patients with esophageal FB impaction have been noted to retch after receiving gas-forming agents, which theoretically puts patients at risk for esophageal trauma, including rupture. Gas-forming agents should not be given to patients with impactions of greater than 6 hours' duration or to patients with chest pain that might be indicative of an esophageal injury.

Further Evaluation and Therapy

As with the use of glucagon, nitroglycerin, or nifedipine, even if administration of the gas-forming agent is successful, as judged by relief of symptoms, follow-up evaluation is necessary to determine the underlying esophageal abnormality that potentially led to the FB impaction.

Papain

Papain is not recommended for treatment of an esophageal FB. It is a proteolytic enzyme that has been touted for its ability to dissolve meat impactions.[91] Papain is available commercially in a variety of meat tenderizers. This therapy has never been tested in a clinical trial. Although it is harmless when in brief contact with a normal esophagus, if it is left in an obstructed esophagus too long, papain may begin to dissolve the esophageal mucosa underlying an FB. This is likely to occur when the esophageal wall is ischemic secondary to FB impaction and the resultant wall pressure, when esophageal injury results from small bony spicules in the FB, or when an underlying lesion is responsible for the obstruction. The subsequent rupture and leakage of proteolytic enzymes result in a self-perpetuating mediastinitis. Patients with esophageal FBs are at increased risk for aspiration, and pulmonary aspiration of papain results in acute hemorrhagic pulmonary edema. Papain is not currently recommended because of the unacceptable risk for complications and the availability of safer, more effective interventions.

REMOVAL OF ESOPHAGEAL FBS IN THE ED

In the United States the most prevalent method for removing FBs lodged in the esophagus is referral for removal under direct visualization via endoscopy, normally done in either an endoscopy suite or operating room under sedation. Endoscopy is costly[7,74,92,93] and time-consuming, and if the patient is being seen after hours, the procedure requires additional personnel to come into the hospital to care for the patient. With procedural sedation becoming more common in EDs, procedures to remove lodged esophageal FBs, when appropriate, are becoming more common. Currently, three procedures are used in the ED to remove FBs lodged in the esophagus, and these are somewhat dependent on the type and location of the FB. These procedures include Magill forceps removal, Foley catheter removal, and esophageal bougienage. Each will be described separately. Another strategy, "watchful waiting," is reserved for single, smooth, asymptomatic FBs typically at the LES in children and will also be discussed.

Magill Forceps Removal of Esophageal FBs

Background

In children, the most common accidentally ingested FB is a coin, and the most common location for the FB to be lodged is at the cricopharyngeus muscle (Fig. 39-10). Given these facts, when children have a single coin at the level of the cricopharyngeus muscle confirmed by radiographs, they are candidates for Magill forceps removal. The procedure requires sedation (see Chapter 33), and thus all airway equipment must be available, as well as monitoring equipment and expertise in its use. In centers that are using this procedure, success rates have ranged from 95% to 100%.[94-97] All centers reporting this procedure used sedation and visualization with a laryngoscope or video-assisted system. The procedure was rapidly

Figure 39-10 Coin lodged at the level of the cricopharyngeus muscle in a 2 year-old toddler.

performed, usually in less than a minute.[94,97] Complications were rare and typically consisted of minor bleeding or vomiting. In the one center that intubated patients before the procedure, complications were higher and associated with the intubation.[96] Magill forceps removal seems to be ideally indicated for stable children with a coin at the cricopharyngeus muscle in a facility that is well equipped and staffed and experienced in managing procedural sedation and airways in children.

Procedure (Fig. 39-11)

1. Ensure that adequate procedural sedation and appropriate monitoring are both implemented (refer to Chapter 33). Place the patient supine on the stretcher with the head slightly extended in the "sniffing position."
2. Insert the laryngoscope or video-assisted laryngoscope. Suction as necessary.
3. Visualize the upper part of the esophagus, where the FB is normally lodged.
4. Grasp the FB with the Magill forceps and then slowly remove it.
5. Visualize the esophagus after removal for any injuries such as erosion or bleeding.
6. Recover the patient from procedural sedation.

Aftercare

No specific aftercare is necessary if no complications have occurred from the procedure. If there is any evidence of esophageal injury, the patient needs to be referred to gastroenterology immediately. Children who ingest FBs are at risk for future ingestions, with the "repeat offender" rate being as high as 18% to 20%.[34]

Foley Catheter Removal of Esophageal FBs

Background

Foley catheter removal of esophageal FBs was first described in the thoracic surgery literature in 1966[98] and in the emergency medicine literature in 1981.[99] The technique has essentially been unchanged since the first reports and is now used by emergency clinicians, radiologists, otolaryngologists, and general surgeons.[100-103] The classic patient for this technique is a small child who is brought to the hospital shortly after swallowing a coin that is documented by radiography, but the procedure may be used for a wide variety of smooth FBs in patients of all ages. Success rates for Foley catheter removal of FBs have been cited from 85% to 100%, with complication rates of 0% to 2%.[7,72,104-108] Many of the reported complications were due to nasal insertion of the catheter, and complication rates are lower when the catheter is inserted orally and at centers that perform the procedure frequently. Foley catheter extraction of FBs costs significantly less than endoscopy.[7,92,109] Fluoroscopic assistance may be preferable, but it is not essential. Whether the procedure is performed in the ED or the radiology department, equipment and personnel capable of emergency pediatric airway management must be present.

Indications

Recently ingested smooth, blunt objects that are radiographically opaque are most suitable for balloon catheter extraction. Recently ingested FBs carry little likelihood of causing pressure necrosis, perforation, or other significant injury; however,

24 to 48 hours' duration of impaction should be the upper limit for consideration of this technique.[7,33,92]

Coins are particularly amenable to Foley manipulation, but food boluses and button batteries have also been extracted successfully.[99] Radiographically opaque objects are most easily located with plain radiographs. Radiolucent objects can be manipulated, but uncertainty about location mandates contrast-enhanced esophagography.

Contraindications

Contraindications to catheter removal of esophageal FBs include total esophageal obstruction, as manifested by an air-fluid level on a plain radiograph or contrast-enhanced esophagogram or when patients are unable to handle oral secretions. The presence of a total obstruction prevents passage of the tip of the catheter distal to the FB. Esophageal perforation, as recognized by the typical symptoms and signs, requires immediate surgical consultation and precludes blind esophageal manipulation, as does airway distress. The presence of multiple esophageal FBs also precludes use of the Foley catheter. Sharp, irregularly shaped FBs should not be removed with this technique because esophageal perforation or laceration can result and the balloon may burst during the procedure. Finally, lack of expertise or equipment to handle an airway problem arising during the procedure is a contraindication.

Procedure (Fig. 39-12)

1. Coach the patient on the procedure. Topical oropharyngeal anesthesia may be used (although this increases the risk for aspiration). Light sedation may be used.
2. Place the patient in the Trendelenburg, lateral decubitus, or prone position.
3. Insert an uninflated catheter (10 to 16 Fr in children) so that the tip is past the FB (as visualized on fluoroscopy or as estimated on radiographs).
4. Fill the catheter balloon slowly with 3 to 5 mL of saline or contrast material (if fluoroscopy is used). Stop inflating the balloon if the patient complains of increased pain.
5. Use steady, gentle traction to withdraw the catheter.
6. Once the FB and the tip of the catheter reach the hypopharynx, grasp the object with forceps, or instruct the patient to spit it out.
7. Obtain another radiograph to ensure that multiple FBs were not present.

MAGILL FORCEPS REMOVAL OF ESOPHAGEAL FOREIGN BODY

1

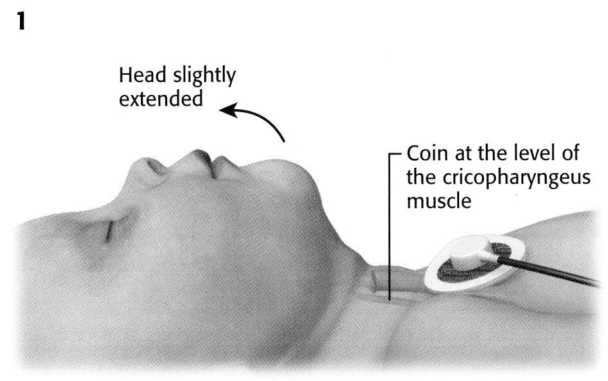

Ensure that adequate procedural sedation and appropriate monitoring are implemented. Place the patient in the supine position with the head slightly extended in the "sniffing position."

2

Insert the laryngoscope or video-assisted laryngoscope. Suction as necessary. Visualize the upper part of the esophagus, where the foreign body is normally lodged.

3

Grasp the foreign body with the Magill forceps, and then slowly remove the foreign body.

4

After removal, visualize the esophagus for any injury such as erosion or bleeding. Recover the patient from procedural sedation.

Figure 39-11 Removal of an esophageal foreign body with Magill forceps.

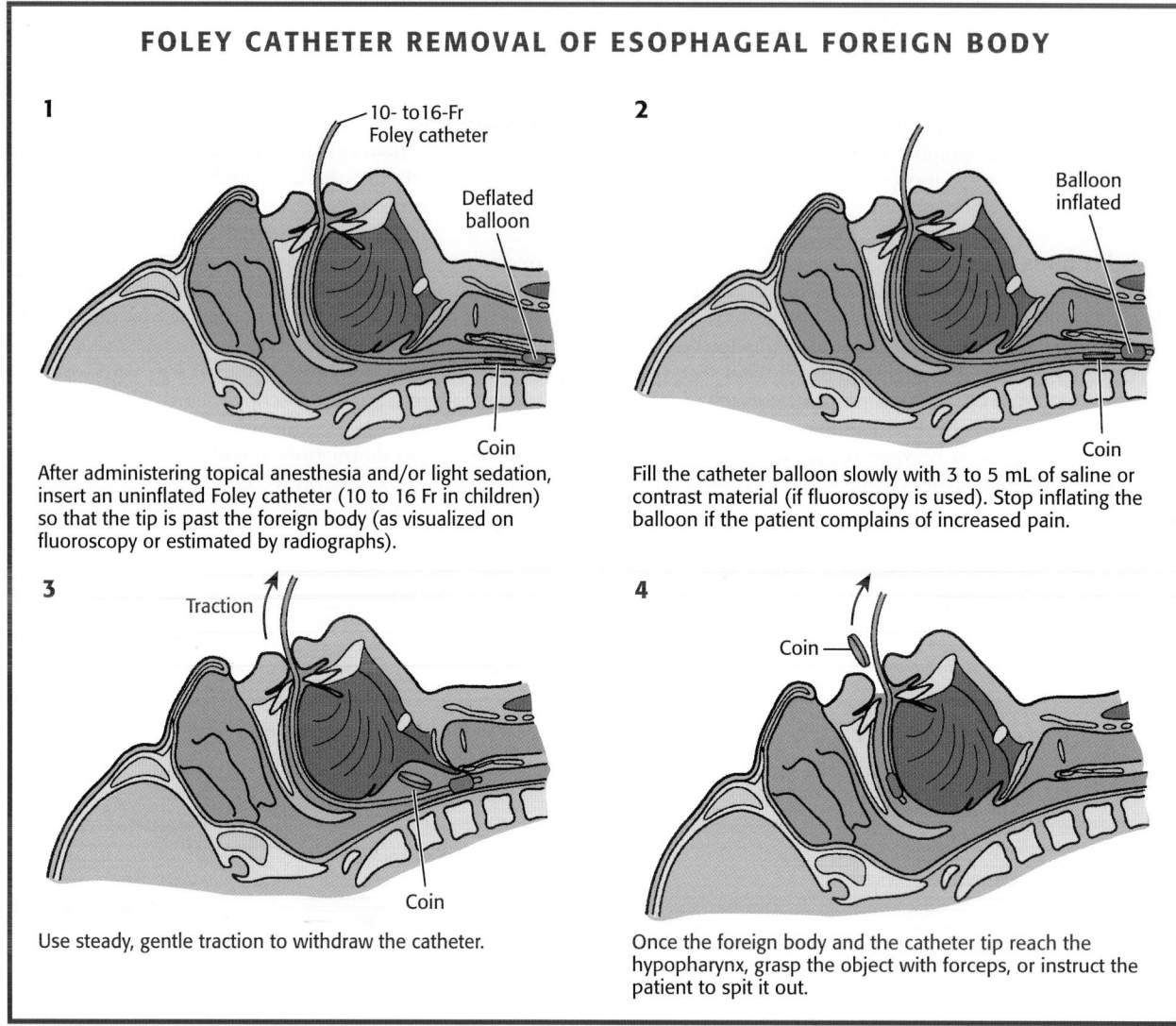

FOLEY CATHETER REMOVAL OF ESOPHAGEAL FOREIGN BODY

1

10- to16-Fr
Foley catheter

Deflated
balloon

Coin

After administering topical anesthesia and/or light sedation, insert an uninflated Foley catheter (10 to 16 Fr in children) so that the tip is past the foreign body (as visualized on fluoroscopy or estimated by radiographs).

2

Balloon
inflated

Coin

Fill the catheter balloon slowly with 3 to 5 mL of saline or contrast material (if fluoroscopy is used). Stop inflating the balloon if the patient complains of increased pain.

3

Traction

Coin

Use steady, gentle traction to withdraw the catheter.

4

Coin

Once the foreign body and the catheter tip reach the hypopharynx, grasp the object with forceps, or instruct the patient to spit it out.

Figure 39-12 Removal of an esophageal foreign body with a Foley catheter.

8. If the catheter slips by the FB, reinsert the catheter, inflate it with an additional 2 to 3 mL of fluid, and make one additional attempt at withdrawal.
9. If fluoroscopy is not used and no FB is retrieved, another radiograph should be obtained because 10% to 20% of the time the FB will pass distally into the stomach.

Complications

Complication rates of 0% to 2% have been reported.[7,72,104-108] Many complications (nosebleeds or displacement of the FB into the nose) have been related to nasal insertion of the catheter. Complication rates are lower when the catheter is inserted orally and generally lower at centers that perform the procedure frequently. No deaths have been reported. Laryngospasm and aspiration are rare complications. Failure to either remove the object or displace it into the stomach occurs in approximately 2% to 10% of carefully selected patients,[104,106-109] but success rates are lower in adults or patients with underlying esophageal disorders.[108]

Aftercare

Children who have an FB removed successfully with a Foley catheter need no further follow-up if they remain asymptomatic. If the FB was moved into the stomach, clinical follow-up should be adequate to verify movement of gastric FBs through the alimentary tract. Discharge instructions should include warnings about the potential symptoms of GI obstruction, perforation, and hemorrhage. Parents of children who swallow coins can be instructed to watch for coins in their stool. Adults with esophageal FBs that have been removed successfully must be referred for evaluation of possible esophageal pathology, as should children with food impactions. Should an FB remain lodged in the esophagus, immediate referral for endoscopy is necessary.

Esophageal Bougienage

Background

Displacement of esophageal FBs into the stomach can be done with nasogastric or orogastric tubes or via esophageal bougienage. Esophageal bougienage is a technique for dislodging impacted esophageal coins by blind mechanical advancement of the coin into the stomach, a procedure first described in 1965.[110] The technique has greater than a 95% success rate with essentially no reported complications when used for the proper indications.[7,73,74,111,112] Rates as high as

ESOPHAGEAL BOUGIENAGE

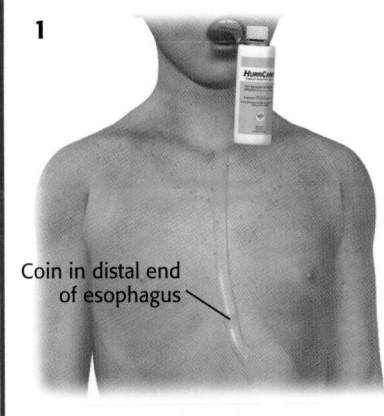

1 Place the patient in the upright position. Achieve topical anesthesia with gargled 2% to 4% viscous lidocaine, atomized 2% lidocaine, or topical benzocaine spray.

Coach the patient (and parents!) on the procedure.

Coin in distal end of esophagus

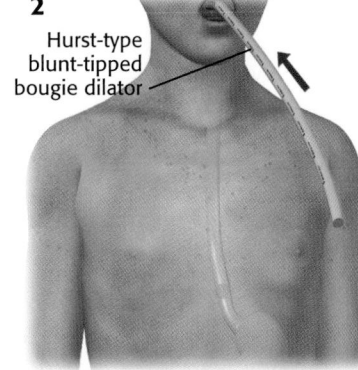

2 Pass the lubricated bougie posteriorly along the roof the mouth and caudally to the hypopharynx.

Hurst-type blunt-tipped bougie dilator

The patient may gag momentarily; ask him to swallow, and then gently pass the dilator past the cricopharyngeus muscle.

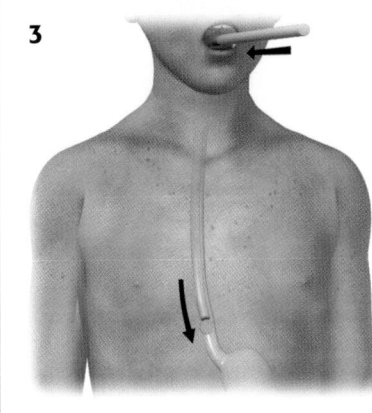

3 Once past the cricopharyngeus, extend the head to enable the bougie to pass distally to the stomach with little resistance.

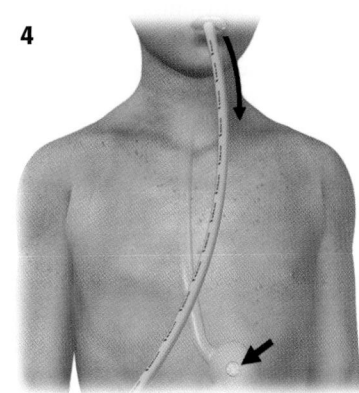

4 Withdraw the bougie after a single pass.

Terminate the procedure immediately for pain or resistance to advancement.

Figure 39-13 Esophageal bougienage.

those with endoscopy have been reported.[92] Furthermore, bougienage is unrivaled in overall cost-effectiveness since it is approximately 10% of the cost of endoscopic removal.[7,74,92,113]

This technique does not allow visualization of the esophagus or retrieval of the object. There have traditionally been warnings against forceful advancement of esophageal FBs, but growing evidence verifies the efficacy and safety of blind esophageal bougienage as first-line therapy for coin ingestions in properly selected patients. Although early articles suggested that esophageal bougienage should be performed exclusively by pediatric surgeons, the technique is easily mastered and used by emergency clinicians.[74,112]

Indications and Contraindications

Strict patient selection is paramount for successful and uncomplicated bougienage. The criteria have changed little since initially proposed and define a group in whom a round, smooth object can be forcibly passed into the stomach with little risk.[93,111] Although many swallowed objects meet this description, only coins hold clear supportive evidence in the literature. *Since many patients with impacted food or meat have underlying esophageal pathology, we do not suggest that it be used in the ED for this condition.* Selection criteria are the following: a single, smooth FB lodged less than 24 hours in a patient with no respiratory distress or history of esophageal disease, including previous FBs or surgery. The FB should be likely to pass beyond the stomach without complications. The procedure is contraindicated in patients who do not satisfy all the

criteria. It is important to ascertain the duration of esophageal impaction to avoid performing the procedure when there may be underlying esophageal injury. For this reason, some advocate the requirement that the ingestion be clearly witnessed less than 24 hours before arrival at the ED.[113] Plain radiographs are indicated to verify coin location and the absence of multiple esophageal bodies. Preprocedure esophagograms are not required.

Procedure (Fig. 39-13)

1. Coach the patient (and parents) on the procedure. Place the patient in an upright position.
2. Achieve topical anesthesia with gargled 2% to 4% viscous lidocaine, atomized 2% lidocaine, or topical benzocaine spray.
3. Flex the patient's head, open the mouth, and ask the patient to protrude the tongue. Use a tongue blade if necessary.
4. Pass a well-lubricated, appropriately sized bougie posteriorly along the roof of the mouth and caudally to the hypopharynx.
5. The patient may gag momentarily—ask the patient to swallow and gently pass the dilator past the cricopharyngeus muscle.
6. Ask the patient to phonate while passing the bougie at this point.
7. Once past the cricopharyngeus, extend the head to enable the bougie to pass distally to the stomach with little resistance.

8. Withdraw the bougie after a single pass.
9. Terminate the procedure immediately if pain or resistance to advancement is encountered.

Complications

Gagging and self-limited nonbloody vomiting are not uncommon after the procedure and may reveal the dislodged coin. Patients may experience a residual FB sensation for several hours. Pulmonary aspiration and inadvertent passage into the airway are potential complications. Likewise, traumatic pharyngeal and esophageal injury, ranging from mild self-limited bleeding to frank esophageal perforation with concomitant infection, are possible but rare.

Aftercare

Plain radiographs of the chest and abdomen are indicated to verify passage of the FB into the stomach and to check for any potential complications. Discharge asymptomatic patients with appropriate precautions, including the need to return if signs of respiratory compromise, chest or abdominal pain, dysphagia, hematemesis, persistent vomiting, or other concerns are present. Follow-up abdominal radiographs may be performed to document passage of the coin if it is not identified in feces within 1 week. For adult patients, follow-up is mandated because of the 65% to 80% chance of underlying esophageal disorders.[9]

SPECIAL SITUATIONS

Childhood Coin Ingestion

Coins are among the most commonly ingested objects by preschool-age children. In most cases, the ingestion is quickly realized by a caretaker, and in the majority of cases the coins pass uneventfully.[114] Rarely, an esophageal coin can be clandestine for many weeks or months and produce a variety of vague respiratory or GI symptoms.[115] In addition, many coin ingestions are not witnessed,[39] so maintain a high index of suspicion for children with dysphagia, drooling, or crying, who may have esophageal FBs, most likely coins.

Most coins pass from the esophagus to the stomach with only transient symptoms. The child may be in pain for a few minutes as the coin migrates, but on arrival at the ED, the child is often asymptomatic. Coins that remain in the esophagus are likely to but do not always produce continued symptoms (e.g., drooling, pain, dysphagia, refusal to eat or drink). Rarely, esophageal coins can cause airway distress by external compression of the trachea and simulate an asthmatic attack. Coins below the diaphragm are asymptomatic, and the presence of pain or symptoms requires further evaluation. Coins in the trachea produce immediate and obvious respiratory distress.

The first clinical decision is whether to obtain a radiograph. Although some authors recommend that asymptomatic children not be radiographed, it is important to remember that up to 44% of children with esophageal coins may be asymptomatic. Therefore, it is prudent to obtain plain radiographs in all children with a suggestive history.[35] In most cases a single film that includes the pharynx, esophagus, and stomach will suffice to prove or exclude an ingested coin (Fig. 39-14). Another advantage of obtaining radiographs is to rule out multiple FB ingestions, which are not uncommon in children.[116] Only a single PA chest film is needed to prove the

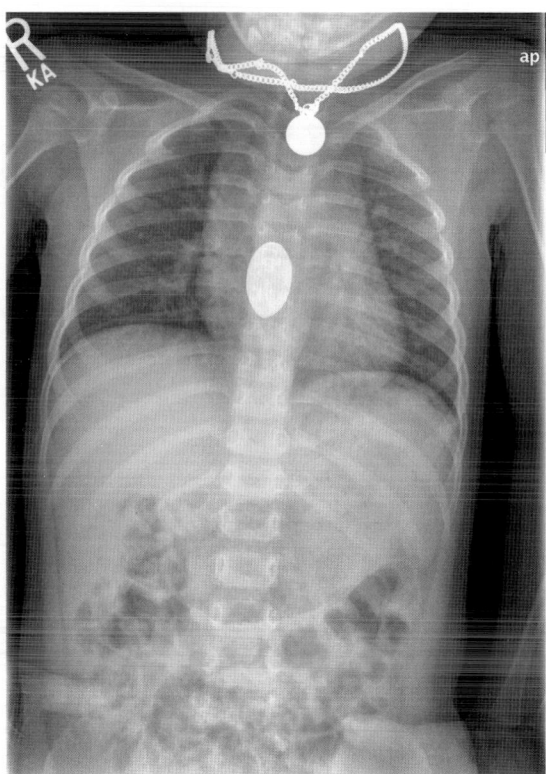

Figure 39-14 For children who are suspected of having ingested a coin, a single radiograph that includes the pharynx, esophagus, and stomach will usually suffice to prove or exclude an ingestion. Here, the child swallowed a souvenir penny, which is seen in the region of the aortic crossover.

presence of a coin, but a lateral projection is also suggested. If the flat surface of the coin is seen (see Figs. 39-2 to 39-4), this orientation ensures an esophageal position. If the edge of the coin is seen, this orientation suggests that it has traversed the vocal cords, but a coin in the airway *is not subtle and produces obvious distress.* It is advisable to also routinely obtain a lateral radiograph to determine whether multiple coins are stacked on top of each other (Fig. 39-15).

Once a coin's presence has been documented, a decision concerning removal must be made. The approach varies, and there is no agreed standard. *Overall, about 25% of coins will pass spontaneously, even if the coin is located proximally.* Observation for 8 to 16 hours is a reasonable approach for asymptomatic children if the ingestion has taken place within 24 hours. Coins in the upper and middle third of the esophagus are less likely to pass spontaneously, and some prefer to remove them as soon as the diagnosis is made.[18] Coins in the distal end of the esophagus will pass spontaneously in one third to one half of patients within 24 hours.[18,35,117]

The decision regarding management of these patients depends on various factors: clinician comfort and experience with removal techniques, local protocols and procedures developed by the medical staff of each institution, and comfort level of the caretakers with various therapeutic options. Regardless of the approach, a radiograph should be taken just before removal to ensure that spontaneous passage has not occurred.

One suggested protocol (Fig. 39-16) involves radiologically localizing the coin and, if the child is symptomatic, immediately removing the coin. If the patient is asymptomatic, the

Figure 39-15 A, Lateral radiograph of a child showing *four stacked coins* at the same location. A posteroanterior (PA) view suggested a single coin. Multiple swallowed coins are common in children. It is important to obtain both PA and lateral films to ascertain the exact number and location of swallowed coins. **B,** A single coin was seen on the PA chest film, but this lateral film suggests *three coins*. However, they do not seem to be stacked directly on top of each other. This digital radiograph was accidentally exposed three times; actually, only one coin was swallowed and x-rayed three times during minimal movement.

coin may be removed immediately or the patient may be observed either as an inpatient or at home. If the child is asymptomatic, one common practice is to allow the child to drink a carbonated beverage and eat a small amount of soft food in the ED, wait about 1 to 2 hours, and obtain another radiograph. If sent home with an asymptomatic retained FB, the patient is allowed to eat or drink but should be rechecked in 12 to 24 hours with the knowledge that up to 50% of asymptomatic coin FBs will pass into the stomach spontaneously.[18,35,118]

The techniques of Magill forceps removal, esophageal bougienage, and Foley catheter removal have been described earlier. All are options for single coins present in the esophagus for less than 24 to 48 hours. Another option for coins impacted at the LES is pharmacologic relaxation of the sphincter to aid passage into the stomach. The most common method to remove esophageal coins in use today is esophagoscopy.

About half of ingested coins are in the stomach at the time of first investigation, and such patients can be released home safely to allow almost certain spontaneous passage with a normal diet. Spontaneous passage of a coin from the stomach to the anus usually requires 3 to 7 days. There is no need for routine cathartic use. Parents should be advised to check the stool for the coin and return for repeated radiographs if the coin is not found in 1 to 2 weeks. Most coins are passed unknowingly by the patient. Any abdominal discomfort or

distention warrants reevaluation in the ED. If a follow-up radiograph demonstrates a persistent coin in the intestines for more than 3 to 4 weeks, an obstructive lesion may be present, and further evaluation is warranted.

Finally, there are theoretical concerns about U.S. pennies, which contain 97.5% zinc. Theoretically, zinc can lead to mucosal ulceration from the caustic nature of zinc[119]; however, the evidence to date suggests no increased risk from ingested pennies.[120]

Fish or Chicken Bones in the Throat

Patients who complain of a "bone" in their throat usually arrive at the ED within several hours of the onset of symptoms and have generally tried a home remedy, such as swallowing a piece of bread. These patients are typically able to pinpoint the location of their discomfort and have an FB sensation that is exacerbated by swallowing. Patients who are markedly symptomatic, vomiting, or unable to swallow require definitive therapy. Those with minor complaints may be evaluated safely over a period of a few days, often as outpatients.

In cooperative patients, careful examination of the oropharynx by either direct or indirect laryngoscopy, or both, should be done. If the bone is seen, it should be removed with forceps.

If the patient feels pain in the upper part of the throat, special attention is directed to the tonsils because bones often

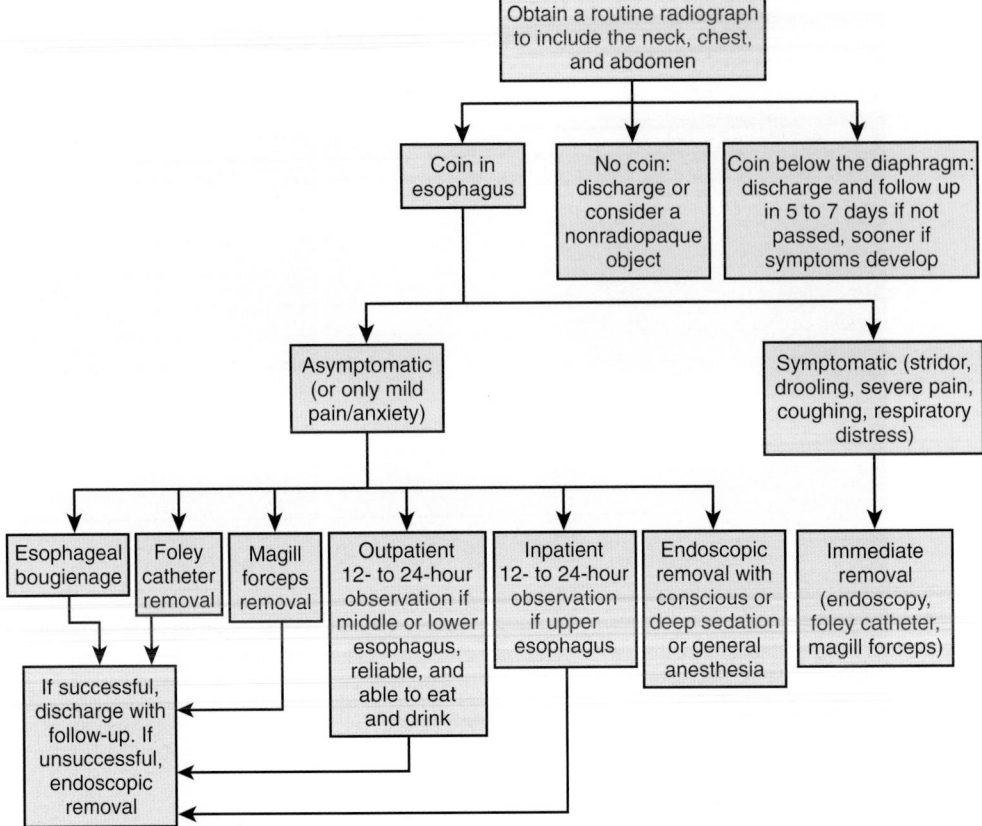

Figure 39-16 Flow diagram outlining an approach to the management of swallowed coins.

lodge in this area (Fig. 39-17). Strands of saliva may mimic a bone, and small bones may be difficult to see. More commonly, the area of complaint is below the oropharynx. In these patients, indirect laryngoscopy or nasopharyngoscopy should be the first step, once again removing the bone if one is seen. This can also be accomplished with local oropharyngeal anesthesia by topical spray and direct visualization with a laryngoscope blade or commercial videoscope blade and then removal of any bone with forceps.

Most patients with an oropharyngeal FB will not have an easily identified or visualized object on examination. These patients present a diagnostic dilemma for several reasons. *Only 17% to 25% of patients complaining of an FB sensation after eating chicken or fish have an endoscopically proven bone present,* and only 29% to 50% of endoscopically proven bones are seen on plain films.[64,121,122] The symptoms in patients with an FB sensation but no FB on endoscopy are believed to be due to esophageal abrasions.

For these reasons, a two-tiered, but individualized approach to managing these patients is proposed.[6,9,34] The patient receives a physical examination and the bone is removed if seen. Carefully examine the tonsils, posterior pharynx, and base of the tongue, *which are common places for bones to lodge.* If the bone is removed and the symptoms disappear, no further intervention is required and follow-up is instituted as needed. *Removal of a bone usually provides immediate and complete relief of symptoms.* Persistent symptoms are cause for further evaluation based on individual circumstances.

If no bone is seen on physical examination, the bone may have passed after causing local irritation that persists, or the bone is present and not visualized because of location or consistency. Minor symptoms in the upper part of the throat probably represent persistent local irritation. Minimally symptomatic patients can be discharged and reevaluated in 24 hours. Those with complaints of an FB below the visualized pharynx or with very bothersome persistent symptoms should be evaluated with a CT scan of the neck or possibly the chest if the symptoms are distal. Positive scans are an indication for endoscopic removal of the bone. If the CT scan reveals no FB or postbone complication and the patient is stable, the patient is discharged home with follow-up within 24 hours. Patients with oropharyngeal abrasions will usually be asymptomatic at that time. If still symptomatic on follow-up, endoscopy is advocated.

A small bone lodged in the esophagus for a few days is annoying and painful, but it is not generally an emergency. However, impacted bones can cause serious sequelae, often weeks later, and continued complaints cannot be ignored. Importantly, a *lodged bone will not dissolve and rarely passes spontaneously once lodged in the mucosa.* Referral and possible endoscopy are necessary if complaints persist for more than 2 to 3 days, even if the examination and CT scan are negative.

Sharp Objects in the Esophagus

Sharp objects cause the majority of complications seen in patients with esophageal FBs. Such objects include tacks, pins, open paper clips, bobby pins, toothpicks, and razor blades (Fig. 39-18). They will not usually pass spontaneously and should be removed. The only appropriate removal technique is under direct visualization with endoscopy. Swallowed dentures or partial plates are a particular hazard in elderly,

Figure 39-17 Many fish bones become impaled in the soft tissues of the upper digestive tract. **A,** This woman felt a bone catch in her throat while eating fish. As is often the case, she was able to consistently localize the foreign body to the right submandibular area, thus suggesting that it could be seen by direct visualization. **B,** With only a tongue blade, local anesthetic spray, and good lighting, a fish bone was found embedded in the tonsil and was easily removed with forceps. Removal provided immediate and total relief, as is usually the case. Strands of saliva can mimic a fish bone, so be careful when probing and grasping. **C,** Fishbone visualized (*arrow*) embedded in a patient's right tonsil. **D** and **E,** This patient felt a fish bone in her left pharynx, and a small bone (*arrow*) was removed from her left tonsil, a common place to find a bone with such symptoms. (*C, Courtesy of Geoff deLaurier, MD, and Jerahme Posner, MD.*)

demented, or mentally challenged patients. Frequently, there is no history of such, and patients have a variety of complaints, such as a sore throat or persistent vomiting (Fig. 39-19). Prisoners and psychotic patients are well known to clandestinely swallow multiple bizarre and sharp objects.

Attempts at radiographic localization are appropriate for metallic or radiopaque FBs. Most objects in the stomach, even those considered problematic, will transit the remainder of the GI tract if less than 6 cm in length or 2 cm in diameter. If larger than this, consult a gastroenterologist. If radiographs show the FB in the esophagus, endoscopic removal is indicated, and attempts to remove such objects in the ED by other methods are not indicated. Complication rates for endoscopic removal of sharp FBs range from 0% to 3%.[8,40]

Nonradiopaque Objects in the Esophagus

Objects such as toothpicks, aluminum pull tabs from beverage cans, plastic, and food boluses cannot be visualized on plain radiographs and will normally not pass spontaneously. *Toothpicks cause a higher percentage of complications than any other type of esophageal FB.* As with fish bones, toothpicks often lodge in the tonsils or posterior pharynx and can be seen on direct

vision. The imaging modality of choice is CT. Removal is mandatory and time-sensitive for sharp objects, especially toothpicks.

Impacted Food Bolus

A large bolus of food may become impacted in the esophagus, usually at the LES. This occurs most frequently in the elderly, those intoxicated while eating, or those with dentures. Frequently, underlying esophageal pathology is present, such as a stricture or web, even in the young (see Fig. 39-6). The diagnosis is usually straightforward, and patients may be in significant distress, gagging, and unable to swallow. A barium swallow may be used to confirm the diagnosis, but this is rarely necessary. Proceeding directly to endoscopy appears most reasonable. Food boluses may be amenable to pharmacologic relaxation of the LES, but the definitive intervention is endoscopy to both *remove the bolus and evaluate the esophagus for pathology.* The specific approach, however, is varied and not standard.

The most logical ED approach is initial aggressive relief of symptoms (judicious narcotics, sedatives, antiemetics), followed by attempts at pharmacologic manipulation of the LES.

Figure 39-18 A, Posteroanterior radiograph of an open safety pin lodged in the upper part of the esophagus. Sharp foreign bodies (FBs) in the esophagus are best removed by endoscopic visualization. **B,** This 10-year-old child was brought to the emergency department (ED) with severe chest pain. No history of an FB was given. Even when the radiograph demonstrated this metallic object in the esophagus, how it got there remained a mystery. Objects such as this are removed under anesthesia with an endoscope, and no ED intervention, except for relief of pain, is indicated.

Figure 39-19 This elderly nursing home patient was seen in the emergency department twice for a sore throat and inability to eat. He had swallowed his partial denture (*arrow*), but this history could not be obtained and the foreign body was discovered when a chest x-ray was taken. Endoscopic removal was indicated.

If the bolus passes, esophageal evaluation can be performed at follow-up. *Papain is contraindicated.* An esophagogram can be performed but seems unnecessary if the diagnosis is obvious (it usually is) and endoscopy is available or planned. A barium swallow should not be used because it can delay definitive treatment. Removal of impacted food is an urgent issue but need not be done immediately on arrival at the ED or in the middle of the night with inadequate resources. Frequently, pain relief and a few hours of relaxation will allow the bolus to slowly break up. Vomiting occasionally dislodges the impaction.

Button Battery Ingestion

Button batteries lodged in the esophagus should be considered an emergency because of the potential for serious morbidity and mortality.[22,24,123,124] These batteries range in size from 7 to 25 mm and are radiopaque (Fig. 39-20). Batteries appear as round densities, similar to an impacted coin, but some demonstrate a "double-contour" configuration. It is important to distinguish between a coin and a button battery because button batteries require immediate removal. Batteries consist of two metal plates joined by a plastic seal. Internally, they contain an electrolyte solution (usually concentrated sodium or potassium hydroxide) and a heavy metal such as mercuric oxide, silver oxide, zinc, or lithium.

If ingested, these batteries often lodge in the esophagus. Mechanisms of injury include electrolyte leakage, injury from electrical current, heavy metal toxicity, and pressure necrosis. Of particular concern is the development of corrosive esophagitis or perforation as a result of caustic injury and prolonged mucosal pressure. Though essentially harmless in the stomach and intestines, batteries lodged in the esophagus should be considered an emergency situation because even new batteries are subject to corrosion and leakage, which can result in mucosal necrosis within a few hours of contact with the esophagus.[23,24,123,124]

Esophageal impaction mandates immediate removal. Options include Magill forceps removal, Foley catheter removal, esophageal bougienage, or esophagoscopy. Esophagoscopy allows direct esophageal evaluation and a more controlled extraction. In addition, the "invasive" nature of batteries may lead to rapid edema, thus making the catheter technique more difficult.

Once in the stomach, button batteries do not require removal. They may be monitored radiographically to demonstrate passage, with little risk for GI injury or heavy metal poisoning, even if the battery opens.[125-128]

Magnets

Swallowed small magnets from toys and household items have become a serious health hazard in children. Some children with complications from multiple magnet ingestion have

Figure 39-21 Buckyballs are strong round toy magnets that when swallowed, aggregate strongly in the bowel and may cause intestinal perforation or necrosis if the bowel wall is compressed. They should be removed if in the esophagus or stomach. Careful observation is acceptable for asymptomatic patients with multiple magnets that are not readily removed, but symptomatic patients require surgical removal if bowel pathology is suspected.

Figure 39-20 Button batteries have a wide range of sizes and can mimic coins on radiographs. Note that the battery (**A**) has a double-density circular appearance at the border whereas the coin (**B**) has a homogeneous density with smooth borders. **C,** Button batteries range from 7 to 25 mm and are similar in size to coins. **D,** An example of the potentially rapid, destructive, and caustic power of button batteries in the esophagus. In this model, intact batteries of different sizes were inserted into a hot dog. Larger batteries with greater areas of surface contact caused damage within 30 minutes, and after 3 hours (image shown) caustic changes were seen with each of batteries tested. Immediate removal of all batteries from the esophagus seems prudent. (*A and B, From Kost KM, Shapior RS. Button battery ingestion. A case report and review of the literature.* J Otolaryngol. *1987;16:4.* **D,** *Pictures courtesy of Adnan Ameer, Rais Vohra, Christian Tomaszewski, and Steve Marcus.*)

underlying conditions such as developmental delay or autism, but older children can inadvertently swallow magnets when using them to imitate a pierced tongue. In 2011 the U.S. Consumer Safety Product Commission issued an alert describing the safety risks from swallowed magnets (http://www.cpsc.gov/cpscpub/prerel/prhtml12/12037.html). Bucky-ball magnets are small round strong magnets used to make toys of various shapes, and if multiple balls are swallowed, they will become adherent inside the bowel (Fig. 39-21). Multiple magnets, especially if ingested at different times, may attract each other across layers of bowel and lead to pressure necrosis, fistula, volvulus, perforation, infection, or obstruction. A piece of bowel may be pinched by two magnets that are swallowed simultaneously. Hence, suspected magnet ingestion requires urgent evaluation. Radiographs of the neck

and abdomen should be obtained to prove magnet ingestion, but radiographs cannot determine whether bowel wall is compressed between the magnets. Identification of magnets that appear to be stacked but slightly separated raises concern for bowel entrapment.

Management of swallowed magnets depends on the timing, location, type, and number of magnets. Because even single magnets have some risk, endoscopic removal should be considered if the magnet is accessible. Magnets in the esophagus or stomach should be promptly removed via endoscopy. Single magnets passed beyond the stomach can generally be managed conservatively initially, but serial outpatient radiographs should be obtained to confirm that the magnet is progressing through the gastrointestinal tract. Theoretically, the child should be kept away from any magnetic or metallic material (such as metallic buttons or buckles in clothing) until the magnet has passed. Ingestion of multiple magnets is associated with a high risk for complications and warrants preemptive removal. Management of patients with multiple magnets beyond the stomach depends on the symptoms and progression. Asymptomatic patients who have swallowed multiple magnets should be admitted and monitored closely with serial radiographs and physical examination every 4 to 6 hours. Alternatively, magnets can be removed by enteroscopy or colonoscopy if accessible. Symptomatic patients or any patient with multiple magnets that do not progress on serial radiographs should undergo surgery for operative removal of the magnets.

The Patient in Distress

Pharyngeal or upper esophageal FBs can cause respiratory distress or respiratory arrest, usually in infants and the elderly.

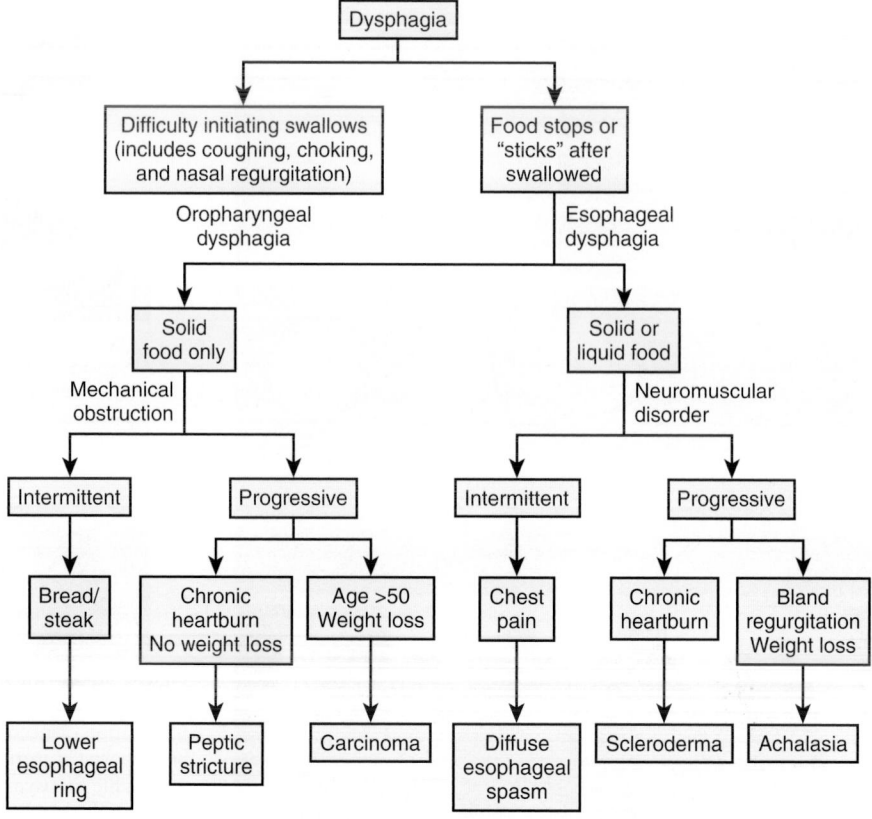

Figure 39-22 Diagnostic algorithm for assessment of a symptomatic patient with dysphagia. *(Adapted from Saud BM, Szyjkowski RD. A diagnostic approach to dysphagia. Clin Fam Pract. 2004;6:525.)*

The Heimlich maneuver can be attempted in the prehospital setting or the ED when the situation is appropriate. The first intervention is to ensure an adequate airway, which can be obvious by the situation or may require laryngoscopy or other means of direct visualization. Forceps may be required to remove obstructions under direct vision. Because FBs may mimic multiple other pathologies, the approach to an acutely choking patient is challenging and every situation individual. Upper esophageal FBs can compress the trachea and cause stridor and respiratory compromise; these are indications for immediate removal.

ED Evaluation of FB Sensation in the Throat

FB impactions in the esophagus are usually straightforward, but patients may seek treatment in the ED because of a lump in the throat or difficulty swallowing with no apparent reason or history of FB ingestion. Such complaints require an examination and an investigation based on the clinical encounter and individual circumstances. Complete evaluation of these complaints is beyond the scope of this chapter, but initial modalities available to the clinician to evaluate these complaints are barium swallow, CT, and pharyngoscopy or laryngoscopy. The need for consultation is based on the clinical scenario. Figure 39-22 is a suggested approach to patients with dysphagia without an FB found on evaluation.

If no cause is suspected by the history or examination, globus pharyngeus may be the etiology. This may be associated with anxiety or a panic attack. The sensation of a painless lump in the throat is called globus pharyngeus or globus hystericus. It has many causes other than FBs. Palpate, visualize, or review the anatomic structures in the area: the chin, laryngeal cartilage, cricothyroid cartilage, tracheal rings, sternum, and cricopharyngeal muscle.

FB sensation may be caused by infection, acid reflux, esophageal spasm, esophageal strictures, pill esophagitis, benign and malignant tumors, hiatal hernia, scleroderma, and many other causes. Globus sensations may also persist after an FB has been completely removed because of mucosal injury. Neurologic causes include botulism, myasthenia gravis, cerebrovascular accident, and amyotrophic lateral sclerosis. If the patient otherwise appears well and is able to drink liquids and keep hydrated, referral to a gastroenterologist as an outpatient is standard.

References are available at www.expertconsult.com

CHAPTER 40

Nasogastric and Feeding Tube Placement

Leonard E. Samuels

Nasogastric (NG) intubation is commonly used to evaluate or treat bowel obstruction, ileus, or gastric hemorrhage, preoperatively or postoperatively, or to administer food or medication into the gastrointestinal (GI) tract. Patients with long-term feeding tube complications and those requiring replacement or other manipulation of tubes are frequently seen and treated in the emergency department (ED).

PROPERTIES OF NG AND FEEDING TUBES

Polypropylene is the material most commonly used for Levin and Salem sump NG tubes (Fig. 40-1), but it is too rigid for long-term use as a feeding tube. Polypropylene tubes are less likely to kink than others but are more capable of creating a false passage during placement. Latex (rubber) tubes are moderately firm, require greater lubrication for passage, are relatively thick walled, and induce a greater foreign body reaction than do tubes made of other common materials. Latex, especially in latex balloons, deteriorates more rapidly than other material does.[1] Foley catheters are primarily latex, although silicone Foley catheters are available for patients with latex allergies. Silicone tubes are thin walled, pliable, and nonreactive; however, the walls of silicone tubes are weaker and may rupture if fluid is introduced into a kinked tube.[2] Polyurethane tubes are nonreactive and relatively durable. Rigidity varies from manufacturer to manufacturer, depending on the thickness of the tube. A stylet may aid in the passage of polyurethane and silicone tubes, but it increases rigidity and the potential for tissue dissection, especially with tubes that have a small distal end-bulb.[3] Some feeding tubes have weights, which are usually made of tungsten and are nontoxic if released into the GI tract.

NG TUBE PLACEMENT

Indications and Contraindications

The simplest NG tube is the Levin tube, which has a single lumen and multiple distal "eyes." The advantage of the Levin tube is its relatively large internal diameter (ID) in proportion to its external diameter. The theoretical disadvantage is that a Levin tube should not be left hooked up to suction after the initial contents of the stomach have been drained because the suction will cause the stomach to invaginate into the eyes of the tube and thereby blocking future tube function and potentially cause injury to the stomach lining. Levin tubes are therefore rarely used in the ED. The Salem sump tube is preferred over the Levin tube for chronic use as a drainage device because it has a separate (blue-colored) channel that vents the distal main lumen to the atmosphere (Fig. 40-2). This vent helps prevent excessive vacuum from forming at the tip of the tube. Note that both intermittent suction and wall unit vacuum can exceed the venting capacity of the second lumen, so the vacuum setting should be less than 120 mm Hg.

The major indication for NG tube placement and suction is to aspirate the stomach contents in patients with gastric outlet or intestinal obstruction, gastric or bowel distention,

Nasogastric Tube Placement

Indications
Decompression of stomach (e.g. obstruction or perforation)
Reduce incidence and risk of vomiting
Monitor and evaluate upper gastrointestinal bleeding
Prolonged ileus
Administration of medication or oral contrast in a patient
   unable to swallow
Detection of transdiaphragmatic stomach herniation

Contraindications
Midface injury, basilar skull fracture, or coagulopathy
   (Orogastric placement may be a better option)
History of gastric bypass or lap banding
Esophageal strictures or alkali injury

Complications
Bleeding	Vomiting/retching
Intracranial placement	Perforation
Pulmonary placement	Sinusitis
Pneumothorax	Aspiration

Equipment

Review Box 40-1 Nasogastric tube placement: indications, contraindications, complications, and equipment.

Figure 40-1 Salem sump tube. This tube contains a second lumen that allows venting during continuous suction. *1*, Pigtail extension (blue) of the air vent lumen; *2*, connector for attachment of the suction lumen to the vacuum line; *3*, gastric end with suction eyes; *4*, insertion depth markers.

Figure 40-2 Diagram of the Salem sump tube. **A,** General design. **B,** Diagram of the double-lumen principle for suction. (*A and B, Courtesy of the Argyle Division of Sherwood Medical, St. Louis.*)

prolonged ileus, or gastric, esophageal, or bowel perforation. Draining the dilated stomach of excessive contents lessens the chance of vomiting and possibly aspiration and provides marked relief of symptoms in patients with intestinal obstruction. The presence or anticipation of depressed mentation potentially justifies NG tube placement to protect the airway, especially if the stomach is full or vomiting is uncontrolled. Bag-valve-mask ventilation often distends the stomach with air, and a postintubation NG tube can improve ventilation, prevent vomiting, and increase patient comfort.

Trauma patients may need an NG tube as part of the evaluation for GI injury or to decompress the stomach before surgery or peritoneal lavage. A radiopaque NG tube may help delineate transdiaphragmatic hernia of the stomach after trauma. A deviated NG tube is a nonspecific sign of traumatic aortic rupture. An NG tube may be used to instill air into the stomach for documentation of a suspected gastric perforation by enhancing visualization of free air under the diaphragm on an upright chest film. In patients unable to swallow, an NG tube may be passed to administer medications or oral contrast material for a computed tomography (CT) scan.

For the evaluation and treatment of upper GI bleeding, indications for NG tubes differ among clinicians, and practices vary widely. Clinical judgement prevails as the best arbitrator, but the true clinical value of an NG tube in patients with GI bleeding is probably less than traditionally promulgated. Although insertion of an NG tube may prompt earlier endoscopy, the procedure has not been demonstrated to improve clinical outcomes.[4] NG aspiration can help localize bleeding in only a minority of patients with GI hemorrhage. Patients who vomit a significant amount of proven bloody material have had upper GI bleeding; they do not need an NG tube for diagnosis. Such patients are best evaluated by endoscopy, although when a history of bleeding is suspected, stomach aspiration may have a role in diagnosis to confirm the presence of blood. In patients without hematemesis, NG aspiration uncovers less than half the patients with upper GI hemorrhage and thus cannot be used to unequivocally rule out upper GI bleeding. Even a rapidly bleeding duodenal ulcer may not produce blood in the stomach. Some contend that emptying a markedly dilated stomach of blood and stomach contents may reduce the rate of bleeding, but data are lacking. Patients with presumptive upper GI bleeding, which includes those with melena, those younger than 50 years old, and those with a hematocrit lower than 30, need upper endoscopy.[5,6] Patients passing clots or blood per rectum or those with known previous lower GI bleeding are usually experiencing lower GI bleeding.[6] Except when frankly bloody fluid is obtained, a nasogastric aspirate is diagnostically unhelpful. Small bits of darkish material, bloody mucus, or positive Gastroccult or guaiac tests probably represent sequelae of the procedure, whereas a clear appearance and negative tests still miss most bleeding distal to the stomach. Patients with a bleeding pattern indicative of a Mallory-Weiss tear may need neither an NG tube nor endoscopy.

NG tubes can provide the earliest indication of high-volume esophageal or gastric bleeding. Although variceal rupture may potentially be caused by insertion of instruments into the esophagus, several studies suggest that passage of an NG tube is generally safe, even in patients with esophageal varices. Use of NG tubes for the evaluation and monitoring of upper GI bleeding should be judicious rather than universal.

Increasingly, the literature suggests that most other causes of vomiting are best controlled with medication. Postoperative ileus ends sooner and patients recover faster without an NG tube after various studied abdominal surgeries.[5] NG tubes prolong the hospital stay, pain, and hyperamylasemia in those with mild to moderate pancreatitis.[7,8] Many patients are better off without an NG tube from the point of view of safety, comfort, and speed of recovery.

In an awake and alert patient with a preserved gag reflex, passage of a NG tube has not been demonstrated to result in

Figure 40-3 A nasogastric (NG) tube may enter the cranium or facial soft tissues in patients with severe head or facial trauma. Those with a coagulopathy may experience significant bleeding from nasal or pharyngeal trauma during passage of an NG tube. In such cases, a standard NG tube inserted *through the mouth* (as shown above) may be a better alternative.

significant pulmonary aspiration, even when vomiting occurs during passage. NG tubes are, however, contraindicated in patients with a special predisposition to injury from placement of the tube. Patients with facial fractures who have sustained an injury to the cribriform plate may suffer intracranial penetration with a blindly placed nasal tube.[9] Severe coagulopathy is a relative contraindication to passage of an NG tube. In patients with a coagulopathy or significant facial or head trauma, an NG tube passed through *the mouth* may be a better alternative (Fig. 40-3). Patients who have esophageal strictures or a history of alkali ingestion may suffer esophageal perforation. Gagging will decrease venous return and increase cervical and intracranial venous pressure. Comatose patients may vomit during or after NG tube placement. Indwelling NG tubes predispose patients to pulmonary aspiration because of tube-induced hypersalivation, depressed cough reflex, or mechanical or physiologic impairment of the glottis.[7] Aspiration is also quite common with nasoenteral feedings in debilitated patients, hence the use of a gastrostomy feeding tubes for this condition. An NG tube should be avoided when possible in patients who have undergone gastric bypass surgery or lap banding procedures.

Extended irrigation of the stomach with water in a patient with upper GI hemorrhage can lower serum potassium levels,[10] and animal studies suggest that cold water lavage can cause rather than control bleeding.[11,12] No study has shown irrigation to be effective in the control of bleeding,[13,14] and vigorous lavage with cold water may lower the body temperature. Erythromycin has been demonstrated to be effective in clearing the stomach for endoscopy,[15,16] and its success is better substantiated than irrigation.

Equipment

Passage of standard NG or feeding tubes can be messy and may be accompanied by coughing, retching, sneezing, bleeding, and spilled water or stomach fluid. For this reason, both the patient and clinician should be gowned; cleanup may be reduced if the bib area is covered with a towel and a supply of tissues or washcloths is available. For standard NG tube placement, a piston or bulb syringe (with a catheter slip-tip)

should be available. NG feeding tubes should have a compatible 50- or 60-mL syringe (some are Luer compatible and others are slip-tip compatible).

Tape torn into 4-inch strips or a commercial NG tube holder (e.g., Suction Tube Attachment Device, Hollister, Libertyville, IL) should be handy for securing the tube after placement. Cotton-tipped applicators and tincture of benzoin may be helpful in securing the tube to the nose if the skin is greasy. Make sure that the feeding tube is designed for duodenal passage if this is desired—such tubes are usually longer than regular feeding tubes.

Procedure

Explain the procedure to the patient. Written informed consent is not standard. If the patient is alert, raise the head of the bed so that the patient is upright. Place a towel over the patient's chest to protect the gown, and place an emesis basin on the patient's lap.[17] Position the tube (typically a 16- or 18-Fr sump) so that the insertion distance can be estimated, and mark the distance with tape or by noting the markers printed on the proximal end of the tube. A simple method is to measure the tube from the xiphoid to the earlobe and then to the tip of the nose. Then add 15 cm (6 inches) to this number (Fig. 40-4, *step 5*).[18] *It is a common error to fail to estimate the proper length of tube before passage*, which can result in the tip of the tube positioned in the esophagus or coiled excessively in the stomach. Check the nares for obstruction. Assess patency by direct visualization, by gentle digital nasal examination, and by having the patient sniff while first one and then the other nostril is occluded. Pass the tube down the more patent naris.

Relief of Discomfort

Ameliorate the pain and gagging associated with tube placement by using vasoconstrictors, topical anesthetics, and antiemetics. Because patients rate NG tube placement as very painful, one of the most painful procedures performed in the ED, *use these adjuncts whenever time and the clinical situation permit* (Fig. 40-5). Spray topical vasoconstrictors, such as phenylephrine (0.5% Neo-Synephrine) or oxymetazoline (0.05% Afrin), into both nares at first in case one side proves to be problematic (see Fig. 40-4, *step 2*). The nares, nasopharynx, and oropharynx should all be anesthetized *at least 5 minutes before the procedure*. Gagging is reduced if the pharynx is anesthetized as well as the nose. Combinations of tetracaine, butyl aminobenzoate, and benzocaine (Cetacaine), nebulized or atomized (spray cans or bottles) lidocaine (4% or 10%), and lidocaine gels (2%) are most commonly used. Lidocaine preparations of 10% are most useful. Lidocaine may be nebulized and delivered by face mask with the equipment used to administer bronchodilators to asthmatics (see Fig. 40-4, *step 3*). This method has been found to be superior to lidocaine spray for reducing gagging and vomiting and increasing the chance of successful passage.[19,20] Cullen and coworkers concluded that nebulized nasal and pharyngeal lidocaine (4 mL of a 10% solution) reduces the discomfort associated with passage of an NG tube better than placebo does and without any lidocaine-related toxicity.[21]

After a topical vasoconstrictor and anesthetic are administered, lubricate the tube with viscous lidocaine or lidocaine jelly.[22] Lubrication and anesthesia of the nares can be facilitated by using a syringe (without needle) filled with 5 mL of

NASOGASTRIC TUBE PLACEMENT

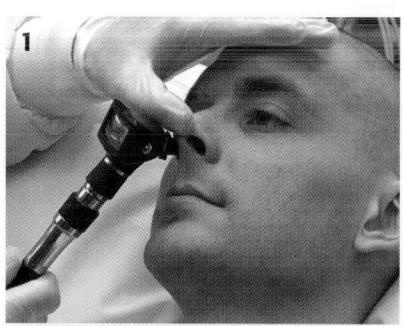
Choose the most patent naris by visual inspection and the sniff test. Alternatively, insert a gloved finger into each nostril to assess patency.

Apply a topical vasoconstrictor, such as phenylephrine or oxymetazoline.

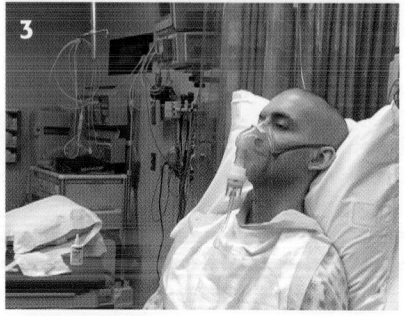
Anesthetize the naris, nasopharynx, and oropharynx *at least 5 minutes before the procedure.*

Nebulized lidocaine is ideal because it reduces both nasal and pharyngeal discomfort.

Apply 2% viscous lidocaine along the floor of the nasal cavity, and allow it to drip into the nasopharynx and be swallowed.

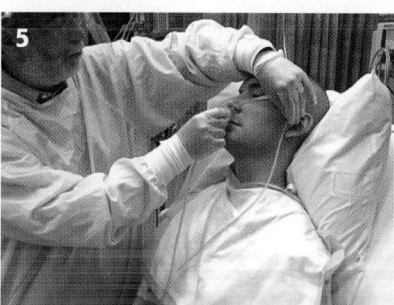
Measure the distance from the tip of the nose to the earlobe to the xiphoid process.

Add another 15 cm to this distance.

Note the total distance on the nasogastric tube markers.

Slowly insert the nasogastric tube along floor of the nostril under direct vision until it passes into the oropharynx.

While the patient sips water from a straw, rapidly pass the tube to the predetermined depth. Coordinate tube advancement with the swallowing mechanism to promote easy passage.

Assess tube placement with air insufflation and aspiration.

Attach the tube to intermittent wall suction.

Secure the tube to the nose with tape.

Figure 40-4 Nasogastric tube placement.

Figure 40-5 Insertion of a nasogastric (NG) tube has been termed one of the most painful and unpleasant procedures performed in the emergency department, and it should not be used unless specifically indicated. Whenever possible, some form of topical anesthesia for *both the nose and the pharynx* should be used *at least 5 minutes before passing an NG tube.*

A = Inferior turbinate
B = Nasal septum
C = Pathway of the NGT

Figure 40-6 Endoscopic view of the nasal cavity before and after the application of oxymetazoline nasal spray. The nasogastric tube (NGT) is passed under the inferior turbinate, which is made more patent after the application of topical vasoconstrictors. The operator should actually *look into the nose during insertion to properly guide the tube*, not force it blindly. (*From Thomsen T, Setnik G, eds.* Procedures Consult—Emergency Medicine Module. *Copyright 2008, Philadelphia, Elsevier Inc. All rights reserved.*)

an anesthetic lubricant, such as 2% lidocaine gel (Fig. 40-4, *step 4*). Simply putting anesthetic jelly *on the tube* just before insertion will not provide any anesthesia. Topical anesthetics are generally quite safe, but pay attention to the total dose of anesthetic administered to avoid toxicity.[23] Note that each milliliter of a 10% lidocaine solution contains 100 mg of lidocaine and can be absorbed systemically. In rare cases, topical benzocaine has caused methemoglobinemia even with the relatively small amounts used for endoscopy.[24]

Although no standard exists and supportive data are sparse, some clinicians administer ondansetron (Zofran, 4 mg) or metoclopramide (Reglan, 10 mg) intravenously 5 minutes before passage of an NG tube to potentially reduce nausea and gagging and, secondarily, to improve the pain and prolongation of the procedure that gagging engenders. Metoclopramide may have additional benefits on the discomfort associated with NG tube insertion, unrelated to its antinausea effects. Ondansetron is preferred for nausea because metoclopramide can cause agitation or facial and tongue spasm, but these effects can be reversed rapidly with the administration of 25 mg diphenhydramine intravenously.

Under direct vision, not blind forcing, insert the tube gently into the naris along the floor of the nose *under the inferior turbinate* and not upward toward the nasal bridge (Fig. 40-6; also see Fig. 40-4, *step 6*). If mild resistance is felt in the posterior nasopharynx, apply gentle pressure to overcome this resistance. If significant resistance is encountered, it is better to try the other nostril because bleeding or dissection into retropharyngeal tissue may occur if force is used. Once the tube passes into the oropharynx, pause to help the patient

regain composure and enhance the chance for cooperation with the rest of the procedure.

If the patient is alert and cooperative, a common option is to ask the patient to sip water from a straw and swallow while you advance the tube into and down the esophagus (see Fig. 40-4, *step 7*). This may facilitate passage of the tube. Once the tube is in the nasopharynx, flex the patient's neck to direct the tube into the esophagus rather than the trachea. In an intubated, anesthetized, or paralyzed patient, two stacked positive pressure breaths lasting 1 to 2 seconds each via a face mask provide similar relaxation of the upper esophageal sphincter for a brief 4- to 5-second window, and this markedly increases successful tube placement.[25]

Some gagging during the procedure is common and is not an indication to halt attempts at passage. Withdraw the tube promptly into the oropharynx if the patient has excessive choking, gagging, coughing, or a change in voice or condensation appears on the inner surface of the tube because this indicates the possibility of passage of the tube into the trachea. Inspect the tube by way of the mouth to detect coiling or respiratory passage. If the tube is lateral to the midline, this suggests correct position in the esophagus.[26] Once the tube is in the esophagus, *advance it rapidly* to the previously determined depth. Passing the tube slowly prolongs discomfort and may precipitate more gagging.[17]

Confirmation of Tube Placement

Before the NG tube is secured, confirm successful placement by nonradiographic means or by auscultation. Use more than one method when in doubt because all methods of confirmation have some possibility of error. Radiographic evaluation is the most definitive way to confirm the position of an NG tube, but it is not standard to routinely obtain radiographic confirmation.

A quick and simple method of confirmation is to insufflate air into the NG tube and auscultate for a rush of air over the stomach (see Fig. 40-4, *step 8*). If increased pressure is required to instill the air or if no sounds are heard, the tube may be malpositioned or kinked. Suspect an esophageal location if the patient immediately burps on insufflation.

If alert and cooperating, the patient will feel whether the tube is entering the trachea or lungs and can notify the inserter. Unfortunately, if the patient is comatose, struggling, or demented, the tube may pass into the lungs unrecognized. Insufflation is often insufficient to detect this type of malpositioning.[3] The insufflation test is also unreliable in detecting a tube that has advanced past the stomach and into the small bowel.[27] In such patients, radiographic verification may be prudent.

Aspiration of stomach contents, especially if pH-tested, is more reliable and can be performed if positioning is in question. If the pH is less than 4, there is an approximately 95% chance that the tube is in the stomach and nonrespiratory placement is almost guaranteed.[28] Although aspirated fluid can occasionally be obtained from the lung or pleural space, the pH should be 5.5 or higher.[29] Approximately 4% of correctly placed tubes have aspirates with a pH higher than 5.5. Causes include duodenal reflux, antacids, H_2 blockers, or recent instillation of formula or medications.[29]

If awake and cooperative, ask the patient to talk. If the patient cannot speak, suspect respiratory placement. Note that with small-bore tubes, patients may still be able to speak despite tracheal placement.[30]

Once correct tube position is tentatively confirmed, secure the tube. If the patient requires abdominal or chest radiographs for other diagnostic purposes, place the NG tube before obtaining the films. An NG tube deviated to the right may occasionally be seen in patients with traumatic rupture of the aorta, but this is not a reliable indicator.

Securing the Tube

The NG tube is generally secured to the patient with tape attached to both the tube and nose (Fig. 40-4, *step 10*). A butterfly bandage (or tape on each side of the nose) that coils around the NG tube is a typical approach. The nose and tube should both be clean and prepared with tincture of benzoin if possible. If the tape should let go or require repositioning, both the tape and the tincture of benzoin must be replaced. It is wise to also secure the tube to the patient's gown so that a tug on the tube will encounter this resistance before pulling on the tape securing the tube to the patient's nose. A rubber band tied around the tube with a slipknot (Fig. 40-7) and pinned to the gown near the patient's shoulder is effective. It is critical to ensure that the tube is secured in such a way that it *does not press on the medial or lateral aspect of the nostril*. Necrosis or bleeding can result if a tube is not secured correctly.

When a Salem sump is used, the blue pigtail must be kept above the level of the fluid in the patient's stomach or the stomach contents may leak back through the vent lumen. If a patient needs to ambulate with a sump tube in place, fit the blue pigtail into the plastic connector at the end of the suction lumen. This creates a closed loop that should not leak.

Placement Issues

If the patient is intubated, deflate the balloon of the endotracheal (ET) tube briefly to allow passage of the NG tube. In a nonintubated unconscious patient, the NG tube is easily

Figure 40-7 Attach the nasogastric tube to the patient's gown with a rubber band and a safety pin so that a tug on the tube pulls the gown and not the tape holding the tube in the patient's nose.

misplaced into the pulmonary tree. This complication may be missed during the procedure in cases in which the gag and cough reflexes are suppressed and the patient cannot talk. In addition, the absence of swallowing may prevent successful passage of the tube. In comatose or ventilated patients, several techniques have been studied to aid in passage of the NG tube. Using Magill forceps to grip the tube or stenting the end of the tube with a gum bougie passed into the most distal tube eye can help stiffen and control the tube. The combination and sequence of techniques used will depend on the clinician's expertise, the equipment available, and the level of sedation.

If less traumatic strategies fail, an ET tube can be prepared with an ID that is slightly larger than the external diameter of the NG tube. Slit it along its lesser curvature from the proximal end to a point 3 cm from its distal end. Pass the NG tube through a naris into the oropharynx. Visualize the tip of the tube with a laryngoscope, grasp it with Magill forceps, and pull it out of the mouth. Pass the slit ET tube (generally 8 mm in ID) through the mouth into the esophagus.[31] Alternatively, pass a 7-mm-ID slit ET tube directly through the nose into the esophagus.[32] Passage into the esophagus is facilitated by the stiffness of the larger ET tube and does not require active swallowing. Thread the tip of the NG tube into the ET tube and advance it into the stomach (Fig. 40-8). Remove the slit ET tube from the esophagus. When the distal part of the ET tube is visible, slit the unslit 3-cm distal part with scissors. Remove the ET tube, and the NG tube will remain in place.[33] Advance any slack tubing with forceps or pull it back nasally, depending on the final depth required for the NG tube. The technique can also be performed by passing the slit ET tube nasally, which saves the trouble of orally advancing or nasally retracting any slack in the tubing.[33,33] Make sure that the NG tube can pass into the 7-mm-ID tube and that the ET tube is well lubricated inside and out.

In a particularly passive, intubated, sedated, unconscious, or toothless patient, guiding the NG tube with fingers into the pharynx is occasionally successful (Fig. 40-9*A*).[34] Displacing the larynx forward by manually gripping and lifting the thyroid cartilage can aid in inserting the tube,[35] as can simple jaw elevation. A soft nasopharyngeal airway, well lubricated, is at times easier to pass nasally than an NG tube, and then the lubricated NG tube can be passed through it. In addition, it affords some protection to the nasal mucosa if multiple

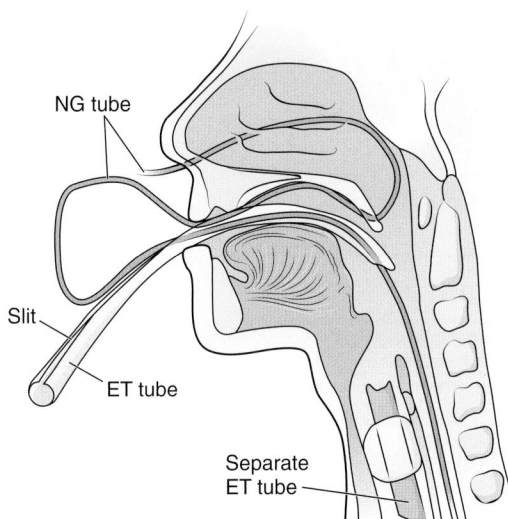

Figure 40-8 Diagrammatic representation of separation of the naso-gastric (NG) tube from the guiding endotracheal (ET) tube through the slit in the guiding ET tube. The NG tube has first been passed through the nose and is pulled out through the mouth. The tip of the tube is then threaded into the guiding ET tube to ensure passage down the esophagus. The guiding ET tube is removed from the esophagus before being separated from the NG tube. Note the previous placement of another ET tube in the trachea (partially shown) to avert passage of the guiding ET tube into the trachea. *(Modified from Sprague DH, Carter SR. An alternate method for nasogastric tube insertion.* Anesthesiology. *1980;53:436.)*

Figure 40-9 A, Passage of a nasogastric (NG) tube through the nose of an intubated patient can be difficult. An endotracheal tube is in the trachea via the mouth. Place the second and third fingers in the posterior pharynx. Depress the tongue with the fingers. Guide the NG tube down the esophagus by passing it through the second and third fingers, which are in the posterior pharynx. *Importantly, place the thumb under the jaw and pull the jaw forward.* **B,** In this intubated patient, a video laryngoscope (GlideScope, Verathon, Bothell, WA) can be used to manipulate the larynx and visualize the passage of the nasogastric tube.

attempts at passing the NG tube are necessary or if it is particularly important to minimize bleeding or trauma. Cooling an NG tube increases its rigidity, and coiling it can increase the curvature of the tube, both of which may help pass the tube. Alternatively, the NG tube and larynx can be visualized with a laryngoscope, endoscope, or the GlideScope (Fig. 40-9*B*).[35] Under laryngeal visualization, manipulation and lifting of the jaw and neck flexion can help align the tube for passage under direct vision into the esophagus.

Ultimately, if all other methods fail, place a flexible fiberoptic bronchoscope or esophagoscope into and through the esophagus under direct visualization.[36] Thread a guidewire into the stomach. Place the NG tube over the guidewire into the stomach and then remove the guidewire.[37]

Complications

Complications of standard NG tube placement are similar to the problems noted with placement of an NG feeding tube. The complications related to tube misplacement are discussed in that section. In addition, clinicians placing an NG tube in a patient with neck injuries should be cautious of potentiating cervical spine injuries with excessive motion during passage (especially in association with coughing and gagging in an awake patient). Furthermore, passage of an NG tube in an awake patient with a penetrating neck wound may exacerbate hemorrhage should coughing or gagging result. Particularly serious forms of tube misplacement are pulmonary placement (Fig. 40-10) and intracranial placement (Fig. 40-11). In confusing cases, a CT scan will clarify most misplacement issues (Figs. 40-12 and 40-13). NG tubes, when in place for

prolonged periods, are a common cause of innocuous gastric bleeding and gastric erosions.

Tension gastrothorax can develop in patients with an intrathoracic stomach. It can occupy much of the left hemithorax and thus displace the heart and lungs and cause a clinical syndrome identical to tension pneumothorax. Even though successful passage of an NG tube will relieve tension gastrothorax, the high pressures of a tension gastrothorax often develop because torsion of the stomach in the chest prevents egress of air; such torsion may also prevent ingress of the therapeutic NG tube. The condition is rare enough that

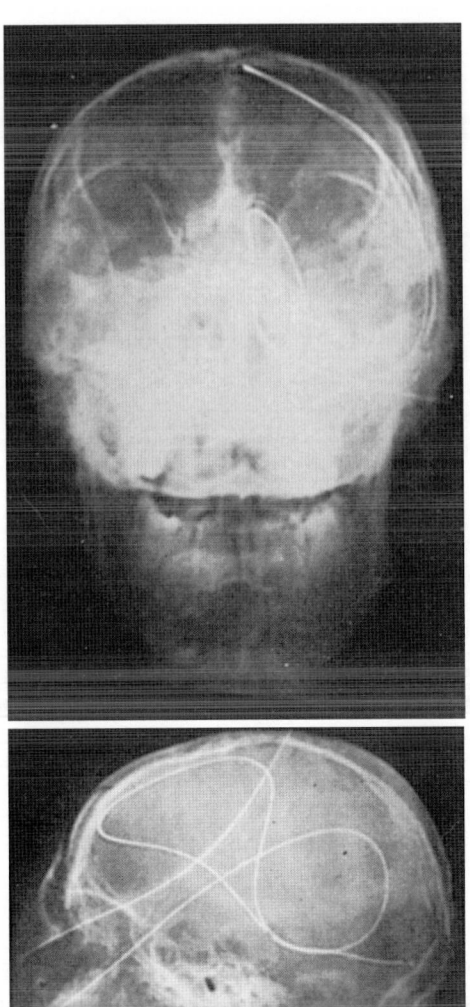

Figure 40-10 A, Levin tube inadvertently placed in the right main stem bronchus; an alveolar infiltrate consistent with early pneumonia is also shown. **B,** Proper position of the nasogastric (NG) tube (*arrow*) is best verified with a radiograph. (*A, From Johnson JC. Letter to the editor: back to basics for morbidity-free nasogastric intubation.* JACEP. *1979;8:289;* **B,** *from Thomsen T, Setnik G, eds.* Procedures Consult—Emergency Medicine Module. *Copyright 2008, Philadelphia, Elsevier Inc. All rights reserved.*)

Figure 40-11 Anteroposterior and lateral skull radiographs demonstrate intracranial insertion of a nasogastric tube in a patient with multiple skull fractures. (*From Johnson JC. Letter to the editor: back to basics for morbidity-free nasogastric intubation.* JACEP. *1979;8:289.*)

further emergency therapy is based on case reports rather than substantial series. Relief of tension gastrothorax has been accomplished by transthoracic puncture of the stomach with a 16-gauge catheter-over-the-needle device inserted into the second intercostal space in the midclavicular line and then removing the needle. The catheter was left in place attached to intravenous tubing with the distal end under a water seal.[38] A single 16-gauge puncture of the stomach is unlikely to leak and cause pleuritis; such punctures have long been used for placement of percutaneous endoscopic gastrostomy (PEG) tubes. Inserting a chest tube into the stomach is not advisable because gastric fluid may leak into the pleural space. Once the tension on the stomach is relieved, it may be possible to pass the NG tube to prevent reoccurrence of the problem. The stomach, no longer tense and wedged in the chest, can twist to allow the tube to pass. Surgical correction of the condition permitting intrathoracic herniation of the stomach is the

definitive treatment to prevent recurrence of tension gastrothorax.

REPLACEMENT OF NASOENTERIC FEEDING TUBES

Indications and Contraindications

The most common indication for replacement of a feeding tube in the ED is unintentional removal of a preexisting feeding tube. In one prospective study, 38% of tubes were removed unintentionally. Although some of these tubes had fallen out or had been coughed out, more than half were pulled out by the patient.[39] Tube rupture, deterioration, or clogging may also necessitate replacement. Management of a clogged or nonirrigating feeding tube is discussed in the later section on clogged feeding tubes.

Figure 40-12 A, In this scout view of a thoracic computed tomography scan, the tip of the nasogastric tube descends only to the level of the T7 vertebrae (*arrow*). The stomach is overinflated with air (*asterisk*). **B,** An axial image from the neck reveals that the nasogastric tube is coiled multiple times in the pharynx (*arrows*) and thus never reached the stomach. Also seen is an endotracheal tube (ETT) and oropharyngeal airway (OPA).

Figure 40-13 This axial computed tomography (CT) scan at the superior thoracic level demonstrates tracheal placement of a naso-gastric tube (NGT). The NGT is seen twice in the esophagus (*small red arrows*), which suggests that it first descended and then coiled and ascended in the esophagus. It then coiled again, turned downward, and ultimately came to rest in the trachea (*large red arrow*) anterior to the endotracheal tube (*yellow arrow*). Luckily, no oral contrast media was injected through the NGT before the CT scan.

Feeding Tube Site

Three major classes of enteral feeding tubes are in common use and are classified according to the site of insertion. Tubes can enter through the nares (a cervical ostomy) or the abdomen (an abdominal ostomy). Enteral tubes are often categorized by the location of the tip of the tube. Tubes may terminate primarily in the stomach, such as a gastrostomy (G) or PEG tube (Fig. 40-14). They may terminate in the jejunum (J tube) (Fig 40-15) or in both the stomach and the small intestine (a PEG-J tube). To confuse the issue, *some tubes enter the stomach and terminate in the stomach (G tube) or in the proximal part of the small bowel (J tube), whereas others enter the GI tract directly through the wall of the small bowel (J tube)*. Practically speaking, almost all gastric tubes are PEG tubes. They are placed endo-scopically with local anesthesia and without a surgical

incision. J tubes that enter the small bowel directly are inserted surgically under general anesthesia, require a surgical inci-sion, and result in a surgical scar at the insertion site. Gastric feeding results in better digestion than intestinal feeding does. Jejunal feeding reduces reflux and aspiration.[40] Normally, about 20% of the gastric antral contents pass into the duode-num, with 80% refluxing back into the body of the stomach for further mixing, so proximal duodenal feeding is of limited benefit in preventing aspiration.[41,42] If the feeding tube is placed in the antrum of the stomach or in the small bowel, enteral feeding solution passing into the small bowel may not be tolerated and can result in diarrhea and paradoxical decreased nutrition.[41,42]

Procedure

The clinician should explain the procedure to the patient before passage of the tube. Replacement of a nasoenteric feeding tube requires greater time and effort if the patient is uncooperative or has a physically obstructing lesion. It is generally advisable to restrain the hands of demented, impaired, or otherwise uncooperative patients. Prepare the nares before passage of the tube similar to the procedure for primary NG tube placement. If a feeding tube stylet is used, lubricate and insert it into the feeding tube before introducing it into the naris. Tube stylets can be lubricated with water-soluble jelly. If using the Dobhoff, Entri-Flex (Biosearch), or another tube with preapplied lubricant, you may need to acti-vate the lubricant with a 5-mL flush of water. Never allow the stylet to protrude beyond the end of the feeding tube because these stiff, small-diameter wires have the capacity to scratch the esophagus and allow the creation of a false passage. The stylet may lock into position on the tube at the proximal end and should be properly secured.

When the patient is uncooperative or cannot drink, intro-duce 5 to 15 mL of water into the mouth or into the proximal end of the feeding tube with a syringe; this may induce

Figure 40-14 Placement of a percutaneous endoscopic gastrostomy tube. **A,** Under conscious sedation, pass a lighted endoscope into the stomach. Indent the skin with a finger to determine the optimal puncture site where the stomach and abdominal wall are closest, with no bowel between. **B,** Fill a syringe with saline and advance it percutaneously to the selected entry point until the tip of the needle is seen entering from the gastric lumen through the endoscope. If air is aspirated and no needle tip is seen, the needle is in the bowel, not the stomach. **C,** Push and pull the scope/snare/feeding tube combination into position. **D,** Pull the head of the feeding tube into contact with the gastric mucosa. **E,** Use an external bolster or crossbar to keep the tube snug against the skin and gastric wall, but not so tight that it causes ischemia of the intervening tissue.

Figure 40-15 Formation of a Witzel tunnel and final permanent placement of a jejunal catheter. *(From Wiedeman JE, Smith VC. Use of the Hickman catheter for jejunal feedings in children.* Surg Gynecol Obstet. *1986;162:69.)*

swallowing and facilitate passage of the tube. Although the patient may not swallow for several minutes, wait for swallowing because this may mean the difference between a coiled or pulmonary tube placement and successful passage.

Confirmation of Placement

Auscultatory confirmation of tube placement can be misleading, so confirm proper placement of the tube with a radiograph before feeding.[3] However, radiographic confirmation of tube placement may also be misleading. In viewing the radiograph, it is particularly important to study the area around the carina. An esophageal tube shows at most a mild change in course, whereas a tracheally placed tube usually deviates significantly as it travels into the right or left main stem bronchus. The end of an NG tube may appear to be in the stomach yet may actually be in the left lung behind and below the top of the diaphragm.[43] When a stylet has been used for passage, leave it in the feeding tube for the radiograph because the tube's course is not always visible without it. The stylets of most tubes are designed to allow insufflation and

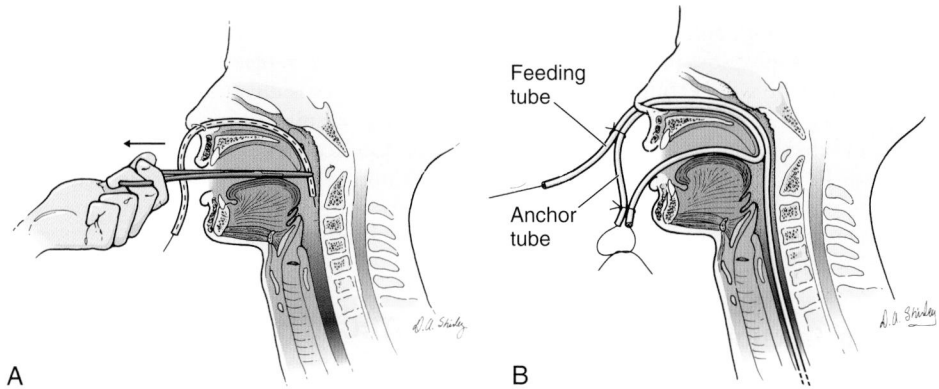

Figure 40-16 Placement of a nasogastric (NG) tube anchor to secure a companion NG or feeding tube in an uncooperative patient who repeatedly pulls out the feeding tube. **A,** Using forceps, grasp the tube in the pharynx and pull it out through the mouth. This will serve as an anchor tube. **B,** Tie the ends of the short anchor tube together to form a loop, and tie the companion NG or feeding tube to the anchor loop.

aspiration while in place. Even when stomach entry is certain, the intestinal location may be misleading on a radiograph. A nasoenteric tube may lie completely to the left of midline and yet have its tip in the duodenum, or it may occupy a position overlying the right side of the abdomen yet not have entered the duodenum. A contrast-enhanced study is necessary to ascertain duodenal position when pulmonary placement has been ruled out.[44,45]

Examine the radiograph also for the presence of mediastinal air or pneumothorax, which may suggest pulmonary or esophageal puncture. An esophageal puncture should be evaluated with endoscopy and may require surgery, depending on the size of the rent.

The end-bulb of many nasoduodenal tubes will pass into the duodenum after positioning the patient in the right decubitus position for an hour. Some researchers recommend pretreatment with metoclopramide to enhance gastric emptying.[46-48] One investigator found that metoclopramide enhances duodenal passage of nasogastrically placed feeding tubes in diabetic but not in nondiabetic patients.[44] Gastric antral motility in diabetics is often impaired; metoclopramide helps restore normal synchronized activity in these patients but has little effect on emptying in subjects with normal antral function. The usual dose of metoclopramide is 10 mg administered intravenously. Also, 3 mg/kg of erythromycin lactobionate given intravenously over a 1-hour period works similarly and may be effective even if metoclopramide fails.[49] Endoscopy or fluoroscopy may be necessary if positioning and metoclopramide are not successful.

Complications

Pulmonary intubation is an uncommon but well-known and potentially fatal complication of insertion of nasal feeding tubes (see Fig. 40-10*A*). Coughing and respiratory distress are the most common symptoms of respiratory passage of an NG tube, but there may be relatively few apparent symptoms in a demented or comatose patient.[50] Decreased mentation and an absent cough reflex are predisposing factors for unrecognized nasopulmonary intubation with NG tubes.[3] Misplacement is far more likely in patients with ET or tracheostomy tubes, conscious or not, perhaps because tracheal stimulation by a misplaced tube is less likely to be appreciated or

communicated. A small end-bulb (e.g., 2.7 mm in diameter) can slip past a tracheal high-volume, low-pressure cuff and easily pass to the periphery of the lung.[3,50-54] Pneumothorax may result when an NG tube dissects into or is withdrawn from the pulmonary parenchyma.[55] Bloody aspirate from a tube should heighten awareness of possible tissue damage.

A clogged or nonfunctional NG tube may be difficult to remove. Fluoroscopy may allow careful insertion of a guidewire or stylet into an in situ tube to facilitate removal. Fluoroscopy may also identify the mechanical problem interfering with removal of the tube. Segments bent double are probably the most common cause. Knots, though uncommon, do occur. Do not use excessive force to remove an NG tube because serious injury to the patient may result.

Premature removal of an NG tube is the most frequent complication of the use of feeding tubes. For long-term use or frequent removal of an NG tube by a patient, a gastric feeding tube will probably be inserted. To help prevent removal by an uncooperative patient, secure the NG tube to a loop anchor passed in the same naris. The anchor works by aversive stimulation of the soft palate and nose with distraction of the NG tube rather than by mechanical stabilization of the tube.

Sax and Bower recommend a technique for creating a separate NG tube anchor.[56] Cut a soft weighted nasoenteric tube approximately 12 inches from the top. Pass a heavy (2-0) silk suture through the tube to exit the side hole. Insert the guidewire with care because it must not protrude from the inserted end. Sedate the patient if uncooperative. Insert the tube through the anesthetized naris into the nasopharynx, grasp it with Magill forceps, and pull to remove it through the mouth (Fig. 40-16*A*). Trim excess tubing without cutting the silk suture. Make a closed loop by tying the silk suture in front of the nose. Leave the loop long enough that it does not apply continuous pressure to the nose or palate while at rest. Pass the nasal feeding tube through the same nostril and secure it to the loop (Fig. 40-16*B*). This anchor is simpler to construct and more comfortable than anchors that pass through the opposite nostril.[56]

Complications of properly placed nasoenteric tubes include nasopharyngeal erosion, esophageal reflux, tracheoesophageal fistula, gagging, rupture of esophageal varices, and otitis media.[57] One survey of nasogastrically fed patients found that the most distressing features of having an NG tube for feeding were deprivation of tasting, drinking, and chewing of food; soreness of the nose; rhinitis; esophagitis; mouth breathing; and the sight of other patients who were eating.[58]

Checking feeding tolerance is difficult with small-gauge feeding tubes. Aspiration of tubes to check for residuals is not recommended with tubes 9 Fr in size or smaller. Aspiration is likely to clog the tubes because they collapse under pressure and relatively small particles can occlude the tube. For the same reasons, the residual is likely to be inaccurate.[59]

Patient or Nursing Instructions

To maintain patency of the catheter, small tubes should be flushed with 20 to 30 mL of tap water at least two to three times daily and after the administration of medication.[45,59] Water is a more effective irrigant than cranberry juice.[60] Medications should be in liquid form or be completely dissolved or they may clog the tube. Methods of dealing with a clogged tube are discussed subsequently. The tube should be anchored to the nose and face in such a way that it is not in contact with the skin at the nasal opening. This reduces tube discomfort and prevents necrosis of the alae, nares, and distal septum. Patients who exhibit a tendency to pull on their tubes need adequate restraints. Patients receiving tube feedings should have their head elevated to at least 30 degrees above the horizontal.[59]

PHARYNGOSTOMY AND ESOPHAGOSTOMY FEEDING TUBES

Cervical pharyngostomy and cervical esophagostomy have both been developed relatively recently. Cervical esophagostomies are generally performed at the time of cervical or maxillofacial operations. Malignant growths in the proximal part of the esophagus, head, or neck are the primary indications for esophagostomy. Cervical esophagostomies may

eventually evolve into a permanent sinus, thereby allowing the feeding tube to be removed between meals. Such tubes are unlikely to be replaced in the ED, but the concept of these feeding tubes is illustrated in Figure 40-17. Complications of pharyngostomy and esophagostomy include local soft tissue irritation, accidental extubation because of excessive length of the external tube, pulmonary aspiration from vomiting, arterial erosion with exsanguination, and esophagitis or stricture of the esophagus from reflux.

GASTROENTEROSTOMY AND JEJUNOSTOMY TUBES

A nursing home patient with a nonfunctioning or displaced feeding tube represents a common ED scenario. The clinician cannot always determine the location of the original feeding tube by simply looking at a patient who arrives in the ED for replacement of the tube. Nevertheless, the emergency clinician should attempt to ensure that the terminal end of a replaced tube is in the same viscus as the original was. External inspection may or may not reveal where a feeding tube should terminate. Contrast-enhanced studies and fluoroscopy usually provide such information (Fig. 40-18). Gastrotomy tubes are available in various types (Fig. 40-19). Tubes are kept in place by either a modified end (such as a mushroom tip) or an inflatable balloon. A de Pezzer (mushroom) tube, a Corflo tube, or a Foley G tube is designed only for intragastric termination. Some tubes have two lumens, one terminating in the stomach for decompression and the other in the small bowel for feeding. These can be confused with tubes that have two entrances to one lumen (one for continuous feeding and the other for medications) and tubes that have a second lumen leading to an inflatable balloon. An original tube is not usually a Foley or balloon-tipped tube. An original PEG tube is pictured in Figure 40-20. Note that on cross section this original long tube has no balloon or port to inflate a balloon but has a mushroom end that is removed by traction.

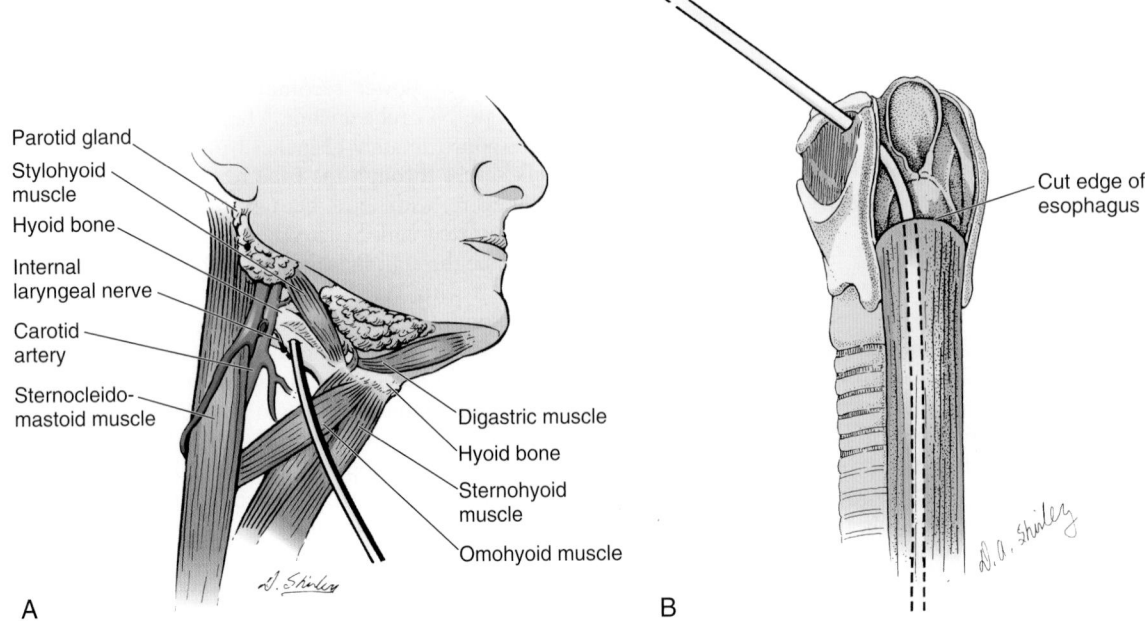

Parotid gland
Stylohyoid muscle
Hyoid bone
Internal laryngeal nerve
Carotid artery
Sternocleido-mastoid muscle

Digastric muscle
Hyoid bone
Sternohyoid muscle
Omohyoid muscle

Cut edge of esophagus

A   B

Figure 40-17 A, Pharyngostomy feeding tube. **B,** Pathway for an esophagostomy or pharyngostomy feeding tube.

Foley catheters are not ideal as long-term feeding tubes. They clog easily, and the balloon disintegrates in stomach acid. They may be used temporarily but should be replaced with specialized feeding tubes when feasible (Fig. 40-21). A call from a nursing home indicating that a tube has been pulled out should be answered by the advice that a Foley catheter be used immediately to keep the stoma open. Always inflate the balloon with saline and use a bolster to prevent migration of the tube. The clinician has a few options when faced with the task of replacing a feeding tube. Unfortunately, old records or nursing home personnel rarely give specific information that is helpful to the emergency clinician. If only a stoma exists, one may request that the nursing home *describe or send the prior tube to the ED.* If no surgical scar is seen at the stoma site, the tube is almost certainly a G tube or a G tube that terminated in the jejunum. When in doubt, pass a Foley catheter without balloon inflation, tape it to the skin, and refer the patient to a consultant or the original referring clinician. *Some type of tube must be placed to stent the stoma, or the stoma will quickly close (in a matter of hours) and the patient might require a more complicated procedure to regain access.* The only real concern of placing a gastric tube into the jejunum is that

Figure 40-18 A, Without old records, the exact type and positioning of this nonfunctioning feeding tube are unknown. The operative scar on the abdominal wall suggests an implanted tube, not a simple gastric tube. **B,** Injection of contrast material before removal of the tube demonstrates the tip of the tube ending in the small bowel, not the stomach. **C,** If the tube has been removed and questions remain about the type of tube and circumstances of placement, a new tube is best placed under fluoroscopy with guidewire assistance.

Figure 40-19 A, Various types of gastrostomy tubes. *1,* Silicone catheter (American Endoscopy, Bard Interventional Products, Billerica, MA). *2,* Polyurethane catheter with a collapsible foam flange (to collapse, the tube should be cut) (VIASYS MedSystems, Wheeling, IL). *3,* Latex catheter with a movable external bolster and an internal mushroom or de Pezzer–type flange on the end (American Endoscopy, Bard Interventional Products, Billerica, MA). *4,* Balloon (Foley) catheter (Wilson-Cook Co., Winston-Salem, NC). **B,** A user-friendly gastrostomy tube is supplied by VIASYS MedSystems (Wheeling, IL). The CORFLO-DUAL GT gastrostomy tube is packaged with lubricant, a prefilled syringe for inflating the balloon, and an extension set. The color-coded inflation valve indicates tube size (12 to 24 Fr). The silicone tube uses a retention balloon and a movable bolster. Note that the retention bolster is designed to prevent inward migration of the tube and not to be an anchoring device sutured to the skin. **C,** A gastric balloon jejunal feeding tube enters the stomach and delivers feedings into the jejunum.

the balloon will produce intestinal obstruction if it is fully inflated.

If the tube is nonfunctioning yet still in place, the clinician must make a judgment regarding the risk versus benefit of removal and replacement versus an attempt at unclogging the tube (see the subsequent discussion on unclogging). The major concern is that a new tube may be misplaced (i.e., into the peritoneal cavity). If it appears that a skin incision was used to place the tube, it is unlikely that the patient has an easily removable tube. If the patient has signs of a complication (e.g., infection, ileus, intestinal obstruction), surgical consultation is warranted. Note that a migrated tube, with the balloon or tube obstructing the gastric outlet, *is a common cause of gastric distention, persistent vomiting, or signs of intestinal obstruction.* This is easily remedied (see procedural description in "Complications" and Fig. 40-22).

Most PEG tubes do not have sutures joining the stomach with the abdominal wall, so there is potential for a replaced tube to end up in the peritoneal cavity. Adhesions, however, usually keep the stomach appropriately positioned, but only after the tract has matured. Nonoperative tube replacement techniques are safe only through an established tract between the skin and the bowel. *Catheter replacement should not be attempted in the immediate postoperative period.* A simple gastrostomy takes about a week to form a tract.[61] A stable

tract may take 2 or 3 weeks longer to form if healing is compromised.

Poor nutrition is the most common element compromising wound healing in patients requiring a feeding tube. A Witzel tunnel may take up to 3 weeks after the operation to mature sufficiently for safe nonoperative tube replacement (see Fig. 40-15).

Equipment for Replacing a Dislodged Tube

Equipment for replacing a feeding tube *through a matured site* includes gloves, a stethoscope, a feeding tube, an external bolster, lubricant, a basin, and a syringe that fits the tube. Tincture of benzoin, tape, and absorbent dressing material may be used to dress the wound, although many are better left undressed.[62] Some feeding tubes require special plugs or connectors. Others need to be pinched with a clamp when not in use to prevent leakage. Some tubes are placed with the aid of accompanying guidewires or stents.

The easiest tube to replace is one that has been removed in the ED or dislodged for only a few hours (Fig. 40-23). The stoma closes quite quickly, so replacement is best done as soon as possible. Gently probe the stoma site with a cotton-tipped applicator to determine patency and direction of the tract. In selected cases, a hemostat can gently dilate the opening to

Figure 40-20 A, This type of tube serves as the original percutaneous endoscopic gastrostomy (PEG) device. It has a mushroom head, not a balloon. **B,** When replaced, a balloon-type tube (*upper tube*) is used in place of the original mushroom tip tube (*lower tube*). **C,** This original tube is leaking because the mushroom tip has been pulled out of the stomach lumen and is lodged in the soft tissue of the abdominal wall. **D,** If the tube tract has matured (at least 2 weeks after placement), it may be removed by traction/countertraction. Significant force may be required, and be prepared for a pop and splattering of gastric contents. **E,** It is easy to determine whether there is a balloon at the end of a PEG tube that cannot be removed. Simply cut the tube, and if there is no additional port or channel to inflate the balloon (**F**), it must be the type of tube that can be removed by traction.

accept a replacement tube. *Do all such attempts carefully to avoid creating a false tract.* Use local anesthetic around the stoma if exploration causes pain. Bleeding is common. After the tube is passed, restrain the hands to avoid removal of the tube by uncooperative patients.

Removal of a Transabdominal Feeding Tube

A feeding tube may need to be removed because it is irreversibly clogged, leaking, or broken; persistently develops kinks; is too large or too small; causes a hypersensitivity reaction; is associated with an abscess; or is not the appropriate length for

feeding into the desired viscus. Before a new transabdominal feeding tube is inserted, remove the old tube. Most, but not all tubes can be removed without endoscopy. It is imperative to know whether the tube in place is safe to remove before attempting to remove it. Standard de Pezzer or mushroom catheters that have been modified with bolsters or rings at the time of endoscopic or surgical insertion may no longer be safe to remove with traction. Tubes are occasionally secured with sutures or rigid internal bumpers or stays. It is rare, however, to encounter a tube that cannot be removed with traction/countertraction. Modest force may be required. Use a hand for countertraction, and be prepared for a pop and splattering

G-TUBE REPLACEMENT (WITH FOLEY CATHETER)

 To make a bolster, cut a 3-cm segment of tubing from the proximal end of another Foley catheter. (A red rubber catheter is used in this case). A bolster will prevent migration of the tube, which can cause gastric obstruction.

 Cut a small hole (on each side) in the middle of the 3-cm segment.

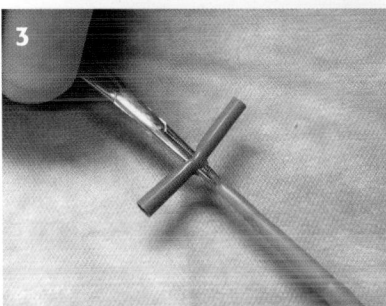 Insert a hemostat through the holes in the new bolster and grasp the feeding tube.

 Pull the feeding tube through the bolster

It should be placed 1 cm above the external abdominal skin.

 Identify and inspect the stoma

Surrounding scars may suggest that the tube is in fact an implanted jejunal tube, not a simple G tube.

 Lubricate the tube and gently pass it into the stoma.

 Inflate the balloon with saline once it is in proper position.

 Advance the bolster so that it is 1 cm above the skin.

 Confirm proper tube placement with auscultation and aspiration

A contrast-enhanced radiograph may be also be obtained.

 Remember that Foley catheters are not ideal feeding tubes but are useful in temporarily maintaining stoma patency.

Disintegration of the catheter latex may occur in a few months.

Figure 40-21 G-tube replacement (with a Foley catheter).

Figure 40-22 A, Whenever possible, use a formal feeding tube instead of a Foley catheter. **B,** A common dilemma. This patient had persistent vomiting after tube feedings and gastric distention. The tube had simply migrated distally (note the comparison of the new tube and positioning of the indwelling one) because the bolster was too far proximal. Withdrawing the tube and repositioning the bolster alleviated the problem.

of gastric contents (Fig. 40-24). This causes the tube and end mushroom to narrow, and the tube should come out easily. The inner crossbar, if present, may remain in the stomach when the rest of the feeding tube complex is removed by traction. The crossbar will pass in stool, and obstruction from it has yet to be reported in adults. In small children, obstruction is a possibility, and the crossbar should be removed by endoscopy.[63,64]

Recently placed feeding tubes may need to be left in until a tract has formed (1 to 3 weeks, depending on the procedure), even if the tube is nonfunctional.

A simple Foley catheter G tube is the easiest to remove. Deflate the Foley balloon and the tube should slide right out. If the Foley balloon cannot be deflated, cut the tube to allow the balloon to deflate. Do not cut the catheter so close to the abdomen that it will be impossible to maintain a grip on it for removal by traction if the balloon still does not deflate. The balloon may also be punctured to cause it to deflate. To puncture a Foley balloon, apply traction on the catheter to draw the balloon up against the ostomy (Fig. 40-25). Using the taut feeding tube as a guide, pass a small-gauge needle along the tube to puncture the balloon. It may be necessary to try again on the other side of the catheter because the balloon may be inflated asymmetrically and contact with the needle may be established on one side and not the other. Be careful to not track away from the ostomy into the patient's abdominal wall or to cause separate punctures of the stomach. Allow a minute for the balloon to deflate before making another attempt at removal by traction. Large, nondeflating balloons should

probably be punctured, whereas small balloons may be removed with traction.

If it is not possible to pull the inner bolster or mushroom out through the ostomy, cut the tube at the skin, push the remaining short stump into the stomach, and rely on later rectal passage. Although obstruction or impaction is infrequent, it can occur, and this alternative has the potential to be problematic in children or patients who have had previous impaction, potential for bowel obstruction, or stool-passing problems. Rigid or large internal mushrooms and bolsters, the very kind that cause the most difficulty with percutaneous removal, are also more likely to cause difficulty with rectal passage. In no case should a device be released into the gut with a long length of tubing attached. Remember that double-part tubes may have an additional length of tubing for duodenal or jejunal feeding that extends far past the inner bolster. Korula and Harma reported successful intestinal elimination of 63 of 64 gastrostomy tubes that were cut at the skin entrance and advanced into the stomach through the stoma.[65] These cases included tubes with internal bumpers, and success occurred regardless of the nature of the patient's underlying medical disorder, age, or method of original tube placement. However, no patient had suspected obstruction or potential for obstruction (e.g., no previous radiotherapy, inflammatory bowel disease). The one lodged tube required endoscopic removal from the pylorus. In most cases, passage of the tube was documented by sequential radiographs, with a mean interval of 24 days until passage (range, 4 to 181 days).

Some clinicians and surgeons strongly condemn cutting off the tube at the skin, even when the risks posed by the procedure are very low. It is always advisable to contact the patient's private clinician before cutting the tube. In some cases, endoscopic retrieval of the tube remnant is preferred over allowing rectal passage, and the tube should not be cut until just before or during endoscopy to ensure that migration does not occur before endoscopy.

Securing a Transabdominal Feeding Tube

If a bolster is used, no additional means of securing the tube is necessary if the patient is not prone to pulling it out. Some clinicians tape tubes to the skin rather than using a bolster or use special adhesive devices designed to control the tube and prevent ingress, such as the Drain/Tube Attachment Device (Hollister, Inc., Libertyville, IL) or Flexi-Trak (ConvaTec, Skillman, NJ). Tape is particularly vulnerable to problems because the stress that the tape places on the skin as the tube pulls on the tape can lead to skin damage. Strong adhesive tape can also damage the skin on removal. Tape that is not sufficiently adhesive can let go, particularly if it gets wet. Because tape is less durable, home or nursing home caregivers who are less skilled may retape the tube (Fig. 40-26). If the tape is replaced at home, it may be placed under too much tension and cause thinning of the abdominal wall at the stoma. If too much slack is allowed, the tube may get pulled in. Strong tape can also damage the tube during tape changes if it comes to adhere too strongly to the tube. Special adhesive devices or bolsters are preferred.

Verification of Placement

There is no universally agreed-on standard with regard to performing a confirmatory contrast-enhanced study for all

Figure 40-23 A, The feeding tube was dislodged at 11 PM, and by 9 AM the stoma was too tight for easy replacement of the tube. It was accomplished under fluoroscopic guidance, always the best option in questionable cases. **B,** The stoma opening and direction of the tract can be investigated by gently probing the site and tract with a Q-tip; in this case it easily entered the stomach. **C,** This tight stoma was carefully dilated with a hemostat under local anesthesia. A false passage can easily be created, and this area usually bleeds readily. **D,** To give a Foley catheter sufficient rigidity to aid in passage, the end of a Q-tip was inserted in the side port of the distal end of the catheter, and traction was applied to the catheter. **E,** If a de Pezzer catheter is used, an endotracheal tube stylet distends the flange for passage, and the tip re-forms once in the stomach. **F,** This patient removed her recently replaced feeding tube, with the balloon inflated, while still in the emergency department awaiting transfer. This could have been avoided if her hands were restrained.

easily replaced feeding tubes. Some clinicians verify position routinely with a contrast-enhanced radiograph, whereas others use the clinical criteria outlined earlier. The authors advocate radiographic verification in the majority of cases, a procedure easily performed and interpreted in the ED. Routine use of postplacement contrast-enhanced radiography to confirm proper placement should be mandatory when the tube tract is immature (i.e., <1-month duration),[66] when passage of the replacement catheter has been difficult, when the clinician is unable to aspirate intestinal contents, or when the patient is unable to communicate any symptoms that might occur with tube misplacement. Peritoneal infusion of feeding solution can be fatal.

The position of the G tube may be checked by air insufflation and aspiration of gastric fluid, as is done with nasoenteric tubes. Air should enter the stomach without resistance and should produce immediate borborygmi. Gastric fluid should return with aspiration. It may be necessary to insert a small volume of water to obtain good return. Water pooling in soft tissue may be aspirated back through a misplaced catheter. Good tube placement is indicated when more fluid returns with aspiration than was originally placed into the catheter.

Correct tube placement is easy and readily verified radiographically with a small amount of contrast material passed into the tube (Fig. 40-27). Use a catheter-tipped syringe to introduce *water-soluble contrast solution* (e.g., diatrizoate meglumine–diatrizoate sodium [Gastrografin]) into the tube. Barium is contraindicated because of the potential for peritoneal contamination. Inject 20 to 30 mL of water-soluble solution to document the intraluminal tube position. Take a supine abdominal film 1 to 2 minutes after instillation of dye to optimize visualization of the gut. Because the film must be

Figure 40-24 Gentle, firm traction using the flat part of the opposite hand for countertraction will remove most percutaneous endoscopic gastrostomy tubes, even those with internal mushroom bumpers. Modest force may be required, and be prepared for a sudden pop and splattering of gastric contents.

Figure 40-26 Tape is best avoided to minimize skin maceration. If needed, this is a simple but less secure technique for securing a gastrostomy tube to the skin.

Figure 40-25 A, If a Foley balloon will not deflate, use traction to bring the balloon against the abdominal wall. Gently pass a small needle along the course of the catheter while puncturing the balloon as many times as necessary. Wait a few minutes for the fluid to egress. **B,** Once the balloon is deflated, it can be withdrawn. Note the encrusted condition of this long-standing Foley catheter used as a percutaneous endoscopic gastrostomy tube. **C,** Occasionally, the wire from a central line kit can clear the inflation lumen and allow deflation. **D,** If the valve mechanism malfunctions, cut the catheter and attempt to drain the balloon by placing a needle in the inflation channel and flushing and withdrawing fluid.

Figure 40-27 A, Although this feeding tube seemed to be replaced easily in an uncommunicative nursing home patient, gastric contents could not be aspirated; therefore, a contrast-enhanced study was performed. **B,** Note the free flow of contrast material throughout the abdomen, especially outlining the liver (*arrows*). This film indicates placement of the feeding tube into the peritoneum. Placing food through this tube could be disastrous. It is prudent to routinely obtain a contrast-enhanced study after replacement of a percutaneous endoscopic gastrostomy tube in the emergency department. Instill 20 mL Gastrografin/10 mL saline into the tube and take a radiograph in 3 to 5 minutes. **C,** Contrast-enhanced study demonstrating correct placement of a feeding tube. Note the outline of the gastric rugae and the characteristic mucosal folds of the small intestine.

obtained quickly, *it is easiest to perform the injection in the radiology suite, followed by a radiograph in only a few minutes.* If the contrast material does not flow freely into the tube, the procedure should be terminated immediately and the position of the tube questioned. With proper positioning, contrast material will outline the part of the gut containing the tube (e.g., stomach with a G tube). An irregular or rounded blotch with wispy edges or streamers suggests peritoneal leakage. In questionable cases, injection of dye can be performed under fluoroscopy.

Complications

Viscus puncture, viscus–abdominal wall separation, and creation of a false tract with subsequent misplacement of the tube are risks associated with dilation procedures. Complications of gastrostomy include wound infection around the catheter, performance of an unnecessary laparotomy for suspected

leakage, gastrocolic fistula, pneumatosis cystoides intestinalis, bowel obstruction, peritonitis, and hemorrhage.[64] Jejunostomies can cause most of these complications, as well as other types of fistulas and small bowel obstruction from adhesions or volvulus around the jejunostomy site.[48,67] The most common complications of gastrostomy and gastroenterostomy are local skin erosion from leakage, wound infection, hemorrhage, and dislodgment of the tube.[59] Peritonitis and aspiration are the most critical complications of gastrostomy feedings.[59,67] Jejunostomies are less prone to stomal leakage and cause less nausea, vomiting, bloating, and aspiration than do gastrostomies.[68,69]

Dislodgment of G and J tubes is most common in the 2 weeks after creation of the ostomy.[70] Extrusion of the G tube is usually caused by excessive tension applied to the tube. Only gentle contact of the gastric and abdominal walls is desirable. Uncooperative patients should be restrained, and mittens are often particularly helpful. Sutures and large mushrooms or balloons do not prevent purposeful removal of the G tube by an uncooperative patient.

A small amount of drainage is to be expected at the tube entry site. Local leakage of gastric juices may macerate and irritate the skin, which can predispose the site to local infections and abscesses and encourage the development of small granulomas.[68,71] Granulomas are particularly common in children. They can be treated with silver nitrate at the time of dressing changes. Any dressing used around the entry site of an enteral nutrition tube should absorb fluid and not encourage persistent moisture.[62] An unusually large stoma may promote a leak. Although insertion of a larger tube or firmer traction on the tube might be transiently effective, these measures often result in further enlargement of the stoma. Rigid gastrostomies promote leakage by widening the stoma as they pivot. Insertion of a soft, pliant feeding tube through the widened stoma is often easy and allows later contraction of the stoma.[1] If these techniques are ineffective, temporary removal of the feeding tube may allow the stoma to shrink. Large amounts of drainage around the stoma site may occur with high residual volumes.[72] The residual should be checked and feedings withheld until residuals are less than 100 mL. Feeding residuals should be checked every 4 hours when a patient is receiving continuous-drip feeding.[73]

Pneumoperitoneum after percutaneous gastrostomy is neither unusual nor dangerous. Benign pneumoperitoneum may be present as long as 5 weeks after PEG.[64,72] Pneumatosis cystoides intestinalis can occur through the defect in the bowel wall created for the enterostomy tube. Though often clinically insignificant, its occurrence suggests air under pressure in the small bowel. NG suction and diet change generally permit resolution of the problem. Catheter or feeding tube removal is not usually required.[74]

Clinically significant pulmonary aspiration can occur with G-tube feeding. Methods of checking for silent pulmonary aspiration include assessing tracheal aspirates with a glucose oxidant reagent strip or placing methylene blue in the formula and monitoring tracheal aspirates for pigmentation.[57,75,76]

A Foley balloon accidentally inflated in the small bowel or esophagus can lead to perforation or obstruction.[77] Carefully inflate the balloon soon after it has entered the stomach to prevent perforation of the viscus. A G tube may migrate in the stomach and obstruct the gastric outlet. This complication is manifested clinically by vomiting and high residuals of feeding solution. Volvulus and jaundice may also occur as a result of balloon migration. To correct inward migration, first deflate the balloon. Pull the tube back just deep to its final position. Reinflate the balloon and pull it the rest of the way back into position.[29] The external bolster should be repositioned or one made and positioned, or inward migration will probably reoccur.[63,72] If the balloon is not deflated before repositioning, the bowel in which it is wedged may be drawn back with it, thereby preventing relief of the obstruction and possibly precipitating intussusception.

A gastrocolic fistula is usually manifested as copious diarrhea. Once it is confirmed, treatment consists of removal of the G tube. Later creation of a gastrostomy in a different location may be possible. The patient may require hospital admission for nutritional support and monitoring of fluid and electrolyte status.

An external bolster that is snugged down too tightly might result in a short stoma and embedding of the internal bolster in the abdominal wall. An abscess may result. Overly tight external bolsters should be loosened. The correct position is 1 cm from the external surface of the abdomen.

CLOGGED FEEDING TUBES

Clogging, leaking, fracture, and kinking are problems common to all feeding tubes. Whenever feasible, replace nonfunctioning or leaking tubes with new ones. Although it may be only a temporary solution, it is prudent to attempt to unclog a tube before it is replaced, especially if the tube has a complex placement or the clinician is unsure how the tube is secured internally. Large G tubes are the least likely to clog. G tubes at least 28 Fr in size can tolerate home blenderized foods and viscous feeding solutions. Isosmotic feeding solutions are tolerated by fairly narrow tubes and cost one sixth of what elemental feedings cost. Isosmotic feedings will clog needle catheters.[46] When tube lumens are 14 Fr or smaller, all pills and the contents of all capsules should be dissolved in water to prevent obstruction of the tube.[62]

Kinking is a frequent cause of tube blockage during the immediate period after reinsertion. Withdrawing the tube a few centimeters usually relieves the kink and obstruction. A persistently recurring kink requires removal of the tube and insertion of a fresh tube.

Accumulated feeding solution or medication precipitates are very difficult to clean or remove. Milking a pliant tube backward may remove some of the cheesy precipitates. Guidewires or stylets may clear the proximal portion of a clogged tube lumen but are unsafe to use in subcutaneous areas of the lumen because they can puncture the tube and injure the patient or create a leak in the tube. Bionix Medical Technologies supplies tube decloggers in two lengths and several diameters for clearing clogs in G and J tube (Fig. 40-28). After selecting a declogger shorter than the feeding tube, insert it gently into the tube until the end of the screw hits the clog and then rotate it clockwise to bury the end in the clog. Next, slide the declogger up and down to break up and dislodge the clog. Insertion, rotation, and sliding might have to be repeated several times until the dislodged material can be flushed into the patient with saline or water. Gravity alone should be sufficient to allow fluid to pass through the feeding tube into the patient and is a better test of successful declogging than is passage of fluid with a syringe. Theoretically, the pointed screw end of the declogger can puncture the tube, or if a declogger is put in that is too long, it may puncture the bowel or stomach directly. According to the company, no cases have been reported.

Fogarty arterial embolectomy catheters can be used to unclog J and G tubes.[78] Insert the soft tip of the Fogarty catheter into the feeding tube and advance it while monitoring the insertion distance to avoid penetrating farther than the length of the feeding tube. Premeasure the allowable length of insertion. A No. 4 embolectomy catheter is suitable for a 10- or 12-Fr feeding tube, and a No. 5 embolectomy catheter is suitable for a 14-Fr feeding tube. When the catheter meets an obstruction, inflate the balloon. This usually opens the obstruction sufficiently for passage of the catheter. Once the Fogarty has been manipulated to a point just proximal to the internal feeding opening, withdraw it while gently inflating and deflating the balloon intermittently. Do not withdraw the catheter while the balloon is inflated because the catheter and feeding tube tend to move as a unit. Repeat

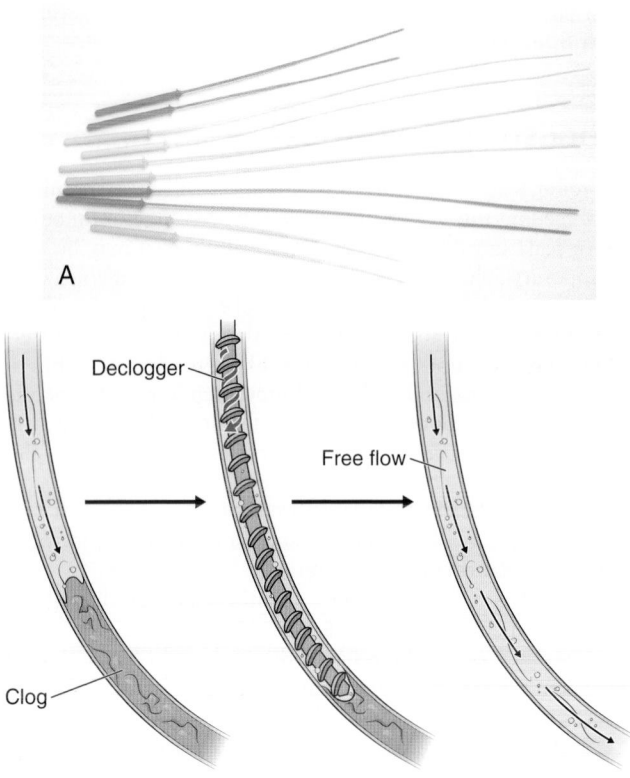

A

Declogger

Free flow

Clog

B

Figure 40-28 A and **B,** The Bionix tube declogger. *Note:* Two lengths and several diameters are available. Caution must be observed any time that the screw end of the declogger passes from view because the potential exists to extend or puncture out of the tube and into the patient. (*A and B, Redrawn courtesy of Bionix Medical Technologies. Bionix Enteral Feeding DeCloggers are a registered trademark of Bionix Medical Technologies. www.BionixMed.com. Accessed June 21, 2012.*)

this procedure several times if necessary. Once declogging is successful, inject contrast material to confirm the position and integrity of the tube.[78]

Irrigation with carbonated beverages and high-pressure irrigation with small-volume syringes have also been recommended as techniques for unclogging feeding tubes. Although irrigation seems like a straightforward and simple solution, these techniques are generally ineffective; furthermore, the possibility exists for dangerous tube rupture with internal leakage. Broviac catheters are especially prone to tube aneurysms, which can rupture under pressure.[71] Tubes unclogged by forceful irrigation or by deep luminal probing should be radiographed after injection of contrast material to check the integrity of the tube.

References are available at www.expertconsult.com

CHAPTER 41

Balloon Tamponade of Gastroesophageal Varices

Michael E. Winters and Edward A. Panacek

INTRODUCTION

Managing patients with acute gastrointestinal bleeding from gastroesophageal varices can be one of the most challenging scenarios in emergency medicine. These patients often have advanced liver disease and can arrive at the emergency department (ED) with massive hematemesis, airway compromise, hemodynamic instability, critical anemia, thrombocytopenia, and coagulopathy. Gastroesophageal varices are the fourth most common cause of upper gastrointestinal bleeding (UGIB) and account for almost 12% of cases (Fig. 41-1).[1] In patients with cirrhosis, varices account for up to 80% of cases of UGIB.[2,3] In patients with established gastric or esophageal varices, the annual incidence of acute hemorrhage ranges from 4% to 15%.[2,4]

Over the past 3 decades, advances in resuscitation, critical care, pharmacology, and endoscopy have significantly reduced the mortality rate associated with acute variceal bleeding. In fact, mortality rates in patients with acute variceal bleeding currently range from 15% to 20%.[1,5-7] Despite advances in management, a small number of patients with acute variceal bleeding fail standard therapy. Rescue therapies for this group of patients are limited and include balloon tamponade,

surgery, and placement of a transjugular intrahepatic portosystemic shunt. This chapter details the indications and contraindications for balloon tamponade in patients with acute variceal bleeding, the techniques for placement of the various devices, and the potential complications of this intervention. Although this procedure is rarely needed and placement in the ED is not considered a standard intervention, emergency physicians with knowledge of the technique can attempt to place these critical and potentially lifesaving devices.

BACKGROUND

In 1950, Sengstaken and Blakemore developed and described the use of a double-balloon device to control variceal hemorrhage.[8,9] Since that time, the Sengstaken-Blakemore tube has become the most widely known balloon tamponade device. The Sengstaken-Blakemore tube has an esophageal and a gastric balloon, along with a gastric aspiration port that allows continuous suction of stomach contents (Fig. 41-2). In 1968, Edlich and colleagues, from the University of Minnesota, modified the Sengstaken-Blakemore tube by adding an esophageal aspiration port and increasing the capacity of the gastric balloon.[10]

Currently, three balloon tamponade devices are commercially available: the Linton-Nachlas, the Sengstaken-Blakemore, and the Minnesota tubes. In contrast to the Sengstaken-Blakemore and Minnesota tubes, the Linton-Nachlas tube is a single-balloon device that consists of a gastric balloon and two ports (esophageal and gastric) for aspiration and lavage. Because placement of these tubes remains a relatively rare procedure, most hospitals stock only one type of device. Regardless of the type of device, success rates for the control of hemorrhage with balloon tamponade tubes range from 60% to 90%.[11]

Balloon Tamponade of GE Varices

Indications

Unstable patients with massive variceal bleeding in the following scenarios:
  Endoscopy is not available
  Endoscopy is unsuccessful at controlling bleeding
  Consultant physicians are unavailable and vasoactive agents have failed to stop bleeding

Contraindications

History of esophageal stricture
Recent esophageal or gastric surgery

Complications

Airway obstruction
Esophageal rupture
Aspiration pneumonitis
Pain
Ulceration of lips, mouth, tongue, or nares
Esophageal and gastric mucosal erosions

Equipment

Viscous lidocaine
Nasal spray
60 mL syringe (catheter-tip)
Manometer
Bulb inflator
Sengstaken Blakemore tube
Tube clamps
"Y" tube
Scissors

Review Box 41-1 Balloon tamponade of gastroesophageal varices: indications, contraindications, complications, and equipment.

Figure 41-1 Endoscopic appearance of esophageal varices. **A,** Upper gastrointestinal endoscopy demonstrating dilated and straight veins (small esophageal varices) in the distal end of the esophagus (*arrows*). **B,** Upper gastrointestinal endoscopy demonstrating large esophageal varices, greater than 5 mm in diameter, with a fibrin plug (*arrow*) representing the site of recent bleeding. (*From Feldman M, Friedman LS, Brandt LJ, ed.* Sleisinger and Fordtran's Gastrointestinal and Liver Disease. *9th ed. Philadelphia: Saunders; 2010*).

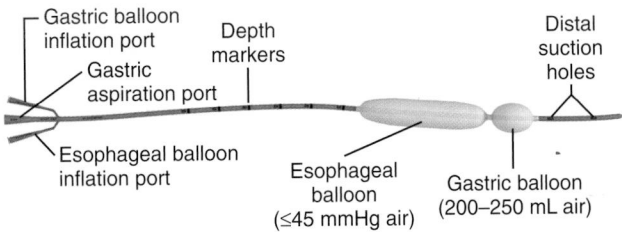

Figure 41-2 The Sengstaken-Blakemore (SB) tube. Note that this tube does not have esophageal aspiration ports; a nasogastric tube must be attached to the SB tube to allow esophageal suctioning (see text for details.)

INDICATIONS

The general management of unstable patients with acute variceal bleeding is described in detail elsewhere. In brief, initial resuscitation should focus on early endotracheal intubation; circulatory resuscitation, including blood transfusion and administration of vasoactive agents and antibiotics; and early endoscopy. Vasoactive agents should be given as soon as possible in cases of confirmed or suspected variceal hemorrhage. Vasoactive medications reduce portal pressure and have been shown to decrease or stop variceal bleeding.[12-17] Somatostatin and its synthetic analogue octreotide decrease release of the vasodilator hormone glucagon, thereby indirectly resulting in splanchnic vasoconstriction and reduced portal blood flow. Vasopressin and its synthetic analogue terlipressin are direct vasoconstrictors and can be given systemically or locally during angiography. These two medications, however, can cause significant coronary, cerebral, and splanchnic ischemia and are typically used in patients who fail somatostatin or octreotide therapy.

Endoscopy by a gastroenterologist remains the "gold standard" for the diagnosis and treatment of acute variceal hemorrhage.[2] Sclerotherapy and band ligation are the two endoscopic techniques used to control bleeding esophageal or gastric varices. Endoscopic band ligation has been shown to be superior to sclerotherapy in initially controlling hemorrhage and improving survival.[18] In fact, endoscopic band ligation is considered the treatment of choice for esophageal varices.[2,18,19]

Balloon tamponade is indicated in unstable patients with massive hemorrhage in whom endoscopy either cannot be performed or is unsuccessful in controlling the bleeding. Balloon tamponade is also indicated when consultant physicians are unavailable and pharmacologic therapy with vasoactive agents has failed to stop the bleeding. In cases in which consultants are unavailable, balloon tamponade can be used to stabilize a patient for transfer to another institution with the resources to continue care.

It is important to recognize that balloon tamponade is only a temporizing measure. Even though success rates in controlling the initial hemorrhage are high, up to 50% of patients rebleed when the device is deflated.[20] Although rebleeding rates can be reduced with the concomitant use of vasoactive agents, arrangements must be made for more definitive control of varices in patients with a balloon tamponade device in place.

CONTRAINDICATIONS

Because gastroesophageal balloon tamponade devices are typically placed as a final attempt to control hemorrhage and prevent imminent death, contraindications to the device are few. They are limited primarily to conditions that predispose patients to esophageal rupture with balloon inflation and include a history of esophageal stricture and recent esophageal or gastric surgery.

PROCEDURE

Patients with an acute variceal hemorrhage that requires a balloon tamponade device are critically ill. Because these patients are at high risk for vomiting, aspiration, and airway compromise, endotracheal intubation should be strongly considered in all patients before placement of a balloon tamponade tube.[21] For the rare patient who is not intubated, use of soft restraints and administration of appropriate analgesia and sedation are critical for a successful procedure.

For placement of a balloon tamponade tube, begin by testing the esophageal and gastric balloons for air leaks (Fig. 41-3, *step 1*). If there is any concern about a leak, submerge the balloons in water during inflation. If time permits, inflate the gastric balloon in 100-mL increments to the maximal recommended volume while measuring the pressure. Importantly, do not exceed a pressure of 15 mm Hg within the gastric balloon with each successive instillation of 100 mL. Note the pressure at full inflation of the gastric balloon. If no air leaks are detected, fully deflate the esophageal and gastric balloons and clamp the inflation ports. If the kit comes with plastic plugs, they may be used in lieu of clamps to occlude the ports and maintain deflation of the balloon during insertion (see Fig. 41-3, *step 2*). Once fully deflated, coat the balloons with a thin layer of water-soluble lubricating jelly.

When using the Sengstaken-Blakemore tube, it is important to recall that the device does not have an esophageal aspiration port. To construct a makeshift aspiration port, secure a nasogastric tube (NGT) to the tamponade tube with silk sutures such that the distal tip of the NGT is placed approximately 3 cm proximal to the esophageal balloon (see Fig. 41-3, *step 3*).

Position the patient properly for insertion of the tube, with the head of the bed elevated to at least 45 degrees. For patients who are unable to tolerate this position, use the left lateral decubitus position. For nonintubated patients, anesthetize the nasopharynx and oropharynx adequately. Accomplish this by using a topical anesthetic spray or jelly combined with a nebulized lidocaine solution.

Orogastric passage of the tamponade tube is the preferred route of insertion, especially in intubated patients. Nasogastric insertion can be attempted in nonintubated patients. Pass the tube at least to the 50-cm mark and preferably to the maximum depth allowed by the length of the tube (see Fig. 41-3, *step 4*). After the tube is inserted, apply continuous suction to its gastric and esophageal aspiration ports (see Fig. 41-3, *step 5*). Inflate the gastric balloon with approximately 50 mL of air and obtain a chest radiograph to confirm that the gastric balloon is below the diaphragm (Fig. 41-4; also see Fig. 41-3, *step 6*). Confirm the location of the gastric balloon, which is essential to reduce the risk for esophageal rupture from inflation of a misplaced gastric balloon.

Once the location of the gastric balloon is confirmed, connect a manometer to the pressure-monitoring outlet of the gastric balloon (see Fig. 41-3, *step 7*). Inflate the gastric balloon to the recommended total volume of air in 100-mL increments. Compare the pressure at each 100-mL increment with the values obtained during testing of the gastric balloon. If the pressure during inflation is more than 15 mm Hg higher than the testing pressure at an equivalent volume, it is likely that the gastric balloon has migrated to the esophagus. At this point deflate the gastric balloon and advance it further into the stomach. Obtain another chest radiograph before reinflation.

When the gastric balloon is fully inflated, clamp the inflation and pressure-monitoring ports (see Fig. 41-3, *step 8*). Slowly pull the device back until resistance is encountered (see Fig. 41-3, *step 9*). Resistance indicates that the gastric balloon

has engaged the cardia and fundus of the stomach (Fig. 41-5). To maintain proper position of the gastric balloon, apply continuous traction. Accomplish this by using an overhead frame and pulley system, a football helmet or catcher's mask, or the sponge rubber cuff (provided in most kits) for patients who underwent nasogastric insertion. Of these methods, the pulley system is preferred to deliver the recommended 0.5 to 1.0 kg of traction. If the emergency physician does not have the weights required for a pulley system, a 1-L bag of crystalloid solution conveniently provides 1 kg of traction (Fig. 41-6).

After traction is applied, connect the esophageal and gastric aspiration ports to continuous suction (see Fig. 41-3, *step 10*). If blood is obtained from either port, inflate the esophageal balloon to approximately 35 to 40 mm Hg. Similar to the gastric balloon, monitor inflation of the esophageal balloon with a manometer connected to the esophageal pressure–monitoring outlet (see Fig. 41-3, *step 11*). In general, do not inflate the esophageal balloon to more than 45 mm Hg. Keep esophageal balloon pressure at the lowest inflation pressure that achieves hemostasis. Occasionally, esophageal pressure may *transiently* spike to values approaching 70 mm Hg. This can occur with respiratory variation or esophageal contraction and is not indicative of overinflation. Once hemostasis is achieved, clamp the esophageal inflation port to prevent air leaks (Fig. 41-3, *step 12*).

If blood continues to be obtained from the gastric aspiration port despite maximal inflation of the esophageal balloon, it is usually indicative of an uncontrolled gastric varix. In this case, increase the traction gradually to a maximum of 1.2 kg.

AFTERCARE

Although the primary objective is to control variceal bleeding, the emergency physician must continue care of the patient with a balloon tamponade device until transfer to an intensive care unit, an operating room, a radiology suite, or another facility. Patients should be maintained in a position with the head of the bed elevated to approximately 45 degrees. In addition, continued administration of sedative and analgesic medication is critical. Connect the esophageal and gastric aspiration ports to continuous suction for approximately the first 12 hours.

Mucosal ulceration from direct pressure of the balloons can occur within just a few hours after tube placement. Accordingly, examine the tube, nares, mouth, tongue, and lips frequently, along with periodic monitoring of esophageal balloon pressure. Once the bleeding has been controlled for several hours, decrease the pressure in the esophageal balloon by approximately 5 mm Hg every 3 hours until a pressure of 25 mm Hg is reached. Regardless of the pressure, periodic deflation of the esophageal balloon for several minutes every 5 to 6 hours can decrease the incidence of mucosal ischemia and necrosis. Once hemorrhage is controlled and the patient is stabilized, balloon tamponade devices are generally left in place for approximately 24 hours.

COMPLICATIONS

Complications from balloon tamponade can be severe and occur in up to 14% of patients.[20] Major complications include

BALLOON TAMPONADE OF ESOPHAGEAL VARICES

Test the esophageal and gastric balloons for air leaks, by submerging under water during inflation. If time permits, record pressures during gastric balloon inflation (see text for details).

Fully deflate the esophageal and gastric balloons. Clamp the inflation ports with a tube clamp, or insert the plastic plugs supplied with the tube into the tube lumen. Lubricate the tube and balloons with water-soluble jelly.

Construct a makeshift esophageal aspiration port by securing a standard nasogastric tube to the SB tube with silk sutures. The distal tip of the NG tube should be 3 cm proximal to the esophageal balloon.

Pass the tube orally (preferred) or nasally, to at least the 50-cm mark, or to the maximum depth allowed by the tube.

After the tube is fully inserted, apply continuous suction to the gastric and esophageal aspiration ports.

Inflate the gastric balloon with 50 mL of air and obtain a chest radiograph to confirm the position of the gastric balloon below the diaphragm.

Figure 41-3 Balloon tamponade of gastroesophageal varices with the Sengstaken-Blakemore (SB) tube. *NG,* nasogastric.

airway obstruction, esophageal rupture, and aspiration pneumonitis. Airway obstruction can be catastrophic and usually results from migration of a dislodged esophageal balloon into the oropharynx.[10,22] Prevent proximal migration of the tube by maintaining adequate inflation of the gastric balloon,

radiographic confirmation, and periodic monitoring of inflation pressure. Treat respiratory distress in nonintubated patients with a balloon tamponade device as airway obstruction until proved otherwise. In these patients use surgical scissors to cut across the lumen of the tube just distal to the

7
Connect a manometer to the gastric inflation port via the Y-tube. Inflate the gastric balloon to the recommended total volume in 100 mL increments. Compare pressure at each 100 mL increment to values obtained during testing. High pressures suggest the gastric balloon has migrated into the esophagus. (See text for details).

8
When the gastric balloon is fully inflated, clamp the gastric inflation port. Note that bare metal hemostats should not be used, as they may damage the tube. Cover the clamping surfaces with cut pieces of red rubber tubing or tape (*arrow*).

9
Slowly pull back the device until resistance is encountered. Apply continuous traction to the tube. (See text and Fig. 41-6).

10
After traction is applied, continuously suction the gastric aspiration port and the attached NG tube which is in the esophagus. If blood is obtained from either source, then esophageal balloon inflation is required.

11
Inflate the esophageal balloon using the same configuration as in *Step 7*. In general, do not inflate the balloon >45 mmHg (see text). The use of a bulb inflator is helpful for this step.

12
Once hemostasis is achieved, clamp the esophageal inflation port to prevent air leaks.

Figure 41-3, cont'd

inflation and aspiration ports. This will result in deflation of both balloons and allow immediate extraction of the device. Given the risk for airway obstruction, always keep surgical scissors at the bedside of patients who have a balloon tamponade device in place.

Esophageal perforation is another catastrophic complication of balloon tamponade that is almost universally fatal. This dreaded complication can occur from a misplaced gastric balloon, an overinflated esophageal balloon, or prolonged inflation of the esophageal balloon and result in decreased

Figure 41-4 Chest radiograph showing a fully inflated gastric balloon (*arrow*) of a Sengstaken-Blakemore tube properly positioned under the diaphragm and in the stomach. Before inflation, obtain a radiograph to confirm that the gastric balloon is indeed in the stomach. Inflation of the gastric balloon in the esophagus can lead to esophageal rupture. (*Courtesy of Dr. Frank Gaillard, www.radiopaedia.org.*)

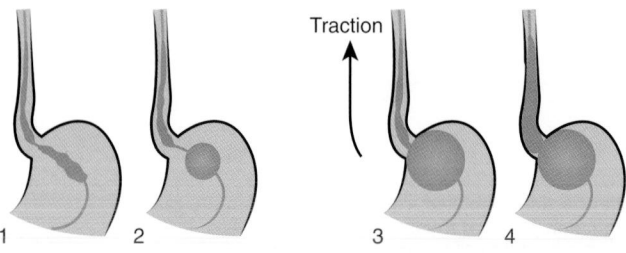

Figure 41-5 The Sengstaken-Blakemore tube in position: (*1*) with both balloons deflated, (*2*) after partial inflation of the gastric tube to confirm proper position, (*3*) after full inflation of the gastric balloon with appropriate traction applied to engage the cardia and fundus of the stomach, and (*4*) after full inflation of the gastric and esophageal balloons.

mucosal blood flow, ischemia, and necrosis. To minimize the risk for esophageal perforation, obtain radiographic confirmation of gastric balloon placement before full inflation. In addition, keep the esophageal balloon at the minimum pressure necessary to control hemorrhage. If the device is required for longer than 24 hours, periodically deflate the esophageal balloon to limit mucosal damage and decrease the risk for necrosis.

Aspiration pneumonitis can result from the aspiration of blood, oral secretions, and gastric contents and is a frequent complication of balloon tamponade.[23] The incidence of pneumonitis can be decreased by evacuating the stomach and intubating the patient before placement of the tamponade device.[21]

Additional complications of balloon tamponade include pain; ulceration of the lips, mouth, tongue, and nares; and esophageal and gastric mucosal erosions.[23] As discussed, patients with a tamponade device should receive adequate analgesia and sedation. Frequent monitoring of tube placement and pressure can decrease the incidence of esophageal or gastric mucosal erosions.

Figure 41-6 To maintain proper position of the gastric balloon and tamponade on the gastric fundus, apply continuous traction to the tube. Traditional methods of applying traction include the use of an overhead frame and pulley system, a football helmet, or a catcher's mask. A more simple solution uses a roll of Kerlix and a bag of intravenous (IV) fluid. **A,** Make a lark's head knot around the proximal portion of the tube with the Kerlix. **B,** Tie the end of the Kerlix to a 1-L bag of IV fluid, and suspend it from an overhead IV pole. The liter bag of fluid will provide the appropriate 1 kg of traction.

CONCLUSION

Balloon tamponade is a critical, lifesaving procedure that may be required in the ED management of unstable patients with bleeding gastroesophageal varices. Indications for placement of a balloon tamponade tube include unsuccessful control of hemorrhage with endoscopy and vasoactive medications, unavailability of consultant physicians when bleeding cannot be controlled with vasoactive therapy, and massive hemorrhage preventing endoscopy. Although complications of balloon tamponade can be fatal, their incidence can be markedly reduced through a stepwise approach to tube placement. Once bleeding is controlled, the emergency physician must continue to monitor tube position and measure balloon pressure until the patient is transferred from the ED.

References are available at www.expertconsult.com.

Decontamination of the Poisoned Patient

Christopher P. Holstege and Heather A. Borek

In 2009, the National Poison Data System of the American Association of Poison Control Centers reported 2,479,355 human toxic exposures and 1452 resultant fatalities.[1] Of these total exposures, 24.1% were managed in a health care facility. Massive exposure to some toxic agents (e.g., calcium channel blockers, tricyclic and other antidepressants, antipsychotics, β-blockers, colchicine, chloroquine, cyanide, *Amanita phalloides* mushrooms, paraquat) *will probably result in severe morbidity or fatality regardless of even the most sophisticated and timely medical interventions*. With general supportive care and the use of a few specific antidotes, however, the mortality rate in unselected overdose patients is less than 1% if the patient arrives at the hospital in time for the clinician to intervene.

Key management of poisoned patients seen in health care facilities initially focuses on confirming the diagnosis of possible exposure to a toxin, providing standard cardiovascular and respiratory supportive care, and using a small cadre of specific antidotes. In rare and yet undefined selected instances, prevention of further absorption of toxin by various decontamination procedures may theoretically ameliorate the morbidity or reduce mortality. Although a better final outcome after gastric decontamination may seem intuitively reasonable, *there is no definitive evidence from prospective clinical trials that the use of various decontamination techniques positively alters the morbidity or mortality of a poisoned patient.*[2]

Before the availability of objective or experimental evidence addressing gastric-emptying procedures, most clinicians instituted previously performed unproven decontamination procedures in the emergency department (ED) as a reflex response for the majority of patients suspected of drug overdose, often without much forethought and certainly without confirming data. Mounting evidence relegates any benefit from any form of gastric decontamination to selected cases and specific individual scenarios. In fact, because of the lack of demonstrable benefit and the mounting evidence for potential harm, syrup of ipecac, once a mainstay in the management of poisonings, is no longer recommended; the American Heart Association and American Red Cross International Consensus on First Aid Science state that syrup of ipecac should not be used in first aid treatment of acute poisonings,[3] and parents have been instructed by the American Academy of Pediatrics to remove it from the home.[4] Parents and health care providers appear to be heeding this recommendation since less than 0.01% of poisoned patients received ipecac in 2009.[1]

Nonetheless, a selective role for other methods of gastric decontamination exists, and there will always be a role for real-time clinical judgment. Because compelling circumstances may prospectively clinically support gastric decontamination, this chapter discusses specific clinical procedures. These techniques include gastric lavage, oral administration of activated charcoal, and whole-bowel irrigation (WBI). In addition, dermal decontamination as a result of a toxic exposure is also addressed. Before performing these techniques, the clinician responsible for the care of a poisoned patient

Gastric Lavage

Indications

Potentially life-threatening poisonous ingestions, but only if the procedure can be performed within 60 minutes

Contraindications

Compromised airway protective reflexes (unless patient is intubated)
Ingestion of corrosive substances (acids or alkalis)
Hydrocarbons (unless containing highly toxic substances such as pesticides)
Known esophageal strictures
History of gastric bypass surgery

Complications

Trauma due to tube insertion
Instillation of lavage fluid into lungs/aspiration
Cardiac dysrhythmias
Hypoxia
Laryngospasm
Fluid and electrolyte disturbances
Hypothermia

Equipment

Review Box 42-1 Gastric lavage: indications, contraindications, complications, and equipment.

must clearly understand that these procedures are not without hazard and that any decision on their use must consider whether the benefit of decontamination outweighs any procedure-related harm.

GASTRIC DECONTAMINATION

Gastric Lavage

Background

The use of gastric lavage in poisoned patients has decreased significantly since the 1990s, and in the United States it is currently reported to be used in less than 1% of overdose case.[1,5,6] Numerous animal and human volunteer studies have been conducted to examine the effectiveness of gastric lavage in removing toxins from the stomach, especially with respect to other gastrointestinal decontamination methods.[7-18] The reported efficacy of gastric lavage in removing markers from the stomach varies significantly in these studies. The difference in these study results is due in part to the variability of the methods used (different fluid-instilled markers, animal models, positioning, amount of lavage, and lavage tube size) and the time that elapsed from instillation of the marker in the stomach until gastric lavage was performed. Even within individual studies, the range of effectiveness of gastric lavage in removing the marker varied considerably. For example, Tandberg and coworkers performed gastric lavage 10 minutes after ingestion of the marker and reported that its effectiveness in removing the marker varied from 18.9% to 67.7%.[13]

Many of these studies do not replicate the typical clinical scenario encountered in emergency medicine.[2,19] The efficiency of gastric lavage in removing a marker significantly decreases with increasing time after ingestion. This is due to the fact that as time increases after ingestion, there is more time for the marker to be absorbed and pass out of the stomach. For example, Shrestha and colleagues reported that more than 70% of the marker used in their study passed out of the stomach by 60 minutes.[20] It is rare that gastric lavage can be performed within the first hour after toxic ingestion. Not only does it take time for these patients to arrive at the ED, but it also takes time for evaluation, stabilization, and performance of gastric lavage. Watson and associates reported that the mean time required by experienced emergency medicine nurses to perform lavage was 1.3 hours.[16] Gastric lavage may also propel the marker from the stomach into the small intestine, thereby decreasing the effectiveness of removing the toxin from the stomach and actually enhancing the rate of absorption.[21]

Three major studies have examined whether gastric lavage positively influences the outcome of poisoned patients.[22-24] In a study performed by Kulig and coworkers, there was no difference in outcome in patients who received gastric lavage followed by charcoal versus charcoal alone when these interventions were performed more than 1 hour after ingestion.[22] In patients who were treated within 1 hour of ingestion, gastric lavage followed by charcoal provided a small but statistically significant advantage over activated charcoal alone. Merigian and colleagues demonstrated that in symptomatic patients, the rate of intensive care admission and need for intubation was significantly higher in patients who received gastric lavage followed by charcoal than in those who received charcoal alone.[23] This increased admission and intubation rate was directly attributed to the aspiration of gastric contents as

Figure 42-1 Position statement: gastric lavage. *(From Vale JA. Position statement: gastric lavage. American Academy of Clinical Toxicology; European Association of Poisons Centres and Clinical Toxicologists. J Toxicol Clin Toxicol. 1997;35:711-719.)*

a result of gastric lavage. Pond and associates replicated the Kulig and colleagues' study.[24] They found no difference in outcome between patients who received gastric lavage followed by charcoal and those receiving charcoal alone, regardless of the time of performance of gastric lavage. They concluded that "gastric emptying procedures can be omitted from the treatment regimen for adults after acute overdose, including those who present within 1 hour of overdose and those that manifest severe toxicity."

Indications

Based on the literature available, gastric lavage should not be routinely used in the management of poisoned patients (Fig. 42-1).[25] There is no universally accepted standard of care that can be applied to the use of gastric lavage in unselected poisoned patients in the ED. Under certain circumstances, however, there may be a theoretical benefit from gastric emptying, and the local poison center should be contacted to assist in making a decision whether gastric lavage may be of benefit. Whether specific subsets of overdose patients may benefit from gastric lavage has not been clearly defined.

Only patients who have ingested a potentially life-threatening amount of poison and in whom the procedure can be performed within 60 minutes are the primary candidates for gastric lavage. Oral charcoal alone is considered superior to gastric lavage if a drug is adsorbed by charcoal.

Contraindications

Though generally safe, gastric lavage is not an innocuous procedure. Performance of gastric lavage is contraindicated in any person who demonstrates compromised airway protective reflexes, unless that person is intubated.[26] Many clinicians opt for lavage in a seriously ill patient who is intubated because airway protection is already accomplished. Tracheal intubation, however, does not ensure a totally protected airway. Paralyzing plus intubating a patient merely to initiate gastric lavage is generally eschewed.

Gastric lavage is contraindicated in persons who have ingested corrosive substances (acids or alkalis) or hydrocarbons (unless they contain highly toxic substances such as pesticides) or have known esophageal strictures or a history of gastric bypass surgery.[27] Caution should be exercised in performing gastric lavage in combative patients and in those who have medical conditions such as bleeding diatheses that could be compromised by performing this procedure.

Equipment and Preparation

If the decision is made to perform gastric lavage, careful attention to the details of the procedure results in increased safety for the patient and more effective removal of the ingested poison. Before lavage, the patient should have intravenous access secured and continuous cardiac monitoring and pulse oximetry initiated (Fig. 42-2, *step 1*). A large, rigid suction catheter should be available immediately.

If the patient is highly anxious or agitated, give a small dose of a benzodiazepine (e.g., 1 to 2 mg midazolam intravenously). If the patient's level of consciousness is significantly depressed, airway status is questionable, or the airway is likely to be compromised during the procedure, consider rapid-sequence induction and intubation with a cuffed endotracheal tube before initiating gastric lavage. If the patient is fully awake and alert, proceed to lavage without tracheal intubation. The procedure should proceed deliberately without significant patient resistance. It is intended to be therapeutic, not punitive. Antiquated arguments promulgating that a noxious lavage procedure will keep patients from overdosing again should be abandoned.

The position of the patient during gastric lavage is important. Place all patients in the left lateral decubitus, Trendelenburg position (≈20-degree tilt on the table) (Fig. 42-3). This position diminishes the passage of gastric contents into the duodenum during lavage and decreases the risk for pulmonary aspiration of gastric contents should vomiting or retching occur. Restrain the hands of an uncooperative patient to prevent removal of the gastric or endotracheal tube. Intubated patients on a ventilator may be lavaged in the supine position because of logistic reasons (Fig. 42-4). Under no circumstances should a nonintubated patient undergo lavage in the restrained supine position. Such positioning invites aspiration and diminishes the patient's natural protective maneuvers, such as coughing and sitting up.

Most clinicians prefer the oral route for gastric lavage, but in selected circumstances a standard large-bore nasogastric (NG) tube (Salem sump pump) may be used. Large-diameter gastric hoses with extra holes cut near the tip have traditionally been recommended for gastric lavage. There are no convincing data on humans to refute or support this recommendation, and one study of a small number of dogs failed to show any difference in efficacy with lavage through a 32-Fr tube versus a 16-Fr lavage tube.[28] It is generally held that large-diameter NG or orogastric tubes (>1 cm) are more likely to retrieve particulate matter successfully, but the tube size is such that whole pills are unlikely to pass (Fig. 42-5). Smaller, more flexible tubes may kink and are significantly more difficult to pass. An NG tube may be passed through the mouth or nose, but orogastric hoses should not be passed through the nose. Because most pills disintegrate in the stomach in a few minutes, significant amounts of particulate matter may be retrieved with a large-bore NG tube such as an 18-Fr Salem sump tube. NG tubes are considerably easier to pass and less traumatic for the patient. NG tubes are preferred for liquid ingestions and in children (Fig. 42-6).

In most cases, a 36- to 40-Fr or a 30-English gauge tube (external diameter, 12 to 13.3 mm) should be used in adults and a 24- to 28-Fr gauge (diameter, 7.8 to 9.3 mm) tube in children.[25] Before passage, estimate the length of tube required to enter the stomach by approximating the distance from the corner of the mouth to the midepigastrium. Premeasurement avoids the curling and kinking of excess hose in the stomach (see Fig. 42-2, *step 2*). Passage of an excessive length of hose may cause gastric distention, bruising, and perforation, whereas passage of an insufficient length of hose may result in lavage of the esophagus and increased risk for emesis and aspiration. Commercial lavage systems are available and often use either a gravity fill-and-empty system with a Y connector or a closed irrigation syringe system. Alternatively, an irrigation syringe can be used for intermittent input and withdrawal of lavage fluid.

Technique

Lubricate the gastric tube and pass it gently to avoid damage to the posterior pharynx (see Fig. 42-2, *step 3*). Use of a bite block or an oral airway may prevent the patient from chewing on the orogastric tube and biting the fingers of the inserter. If the patient is obtunded or paralyzed, extend the jaw to facilitate passage. Never use force to pass the tube. Once the pharynx has been entered, put the patient's chin on the chest to facilitate passage of the tube into the esophagus (see Fig. 42-2, *step 4*). Cough, stridor, or cyanosis indicates that the tube has entered the trachea; withdraw the tube immediately and reattempt passage. Once the tube is passed, confirm that it is in the stomach. Intragastric placement is usually evident on clinical grounds by the spontaneous egress of gastric contents but may be confirmed by auscultation of the stomach during injection of air with a 50-mL syringe followed by successful aspiration of gastric contents (see Fig. 42-2, *step 5*). In an intubated or obtunded patient or a young child, confirm tube position radiographically before lavaging, although this is not routinely performed (Fig. 42-7*A*). A misplaced tube may irrigate the esophagus with a tube that has doubled back on itself during passage (see Fig. 42-7*B*). The most serious complication, other than esophageal perforation, is inadvertent passage of the tube into the lungs. Tracheal passage of a lavage tube should be readily obvious in an awake patient before lavage, and obtunded patients are intubated, thereby obviating this problem. If an awake patient begins to vomit during lavage, immediately remove the tube to allow the patient to protect the airway.

Before gastric irrigation, remove the gastric contents by careful gastric aspiration with repeated repositioning of the tip of the tube (see Fig. 42-2, *step 6*). With the Y-connector closed system, perform lavage by clamping the drainage arm of the Y adapter and infusing aliquots of fluid into the stomach from a reservoir. Clamp the reservoir arm of the Y, and then open the drainage arm to permit drainage of the stomach contents by gravity. Repeat this procedure. Some resistance is produced by the Y connector and tubing. Apply suction intermittently to the drainage tubing to enhance emptying of the stomach.

Lavage can be performed adequately with tap water in adults. Because electrolyte disturbances have occurred in children who underwent lavage with tap water, prewarmed (45°C) normal saline is generally recommended for children.[29-31] Warmed lavage fluid increases the solubility of most substances, delays gastric emptying, and should theoretically increase the effectiveness of the procedure.[32,33] Repeatedly introduce small aliquots of lavage solution (200 to 300 mL in

GASTRIC LAVAGE

Before lavage, obtain intravenous access and place the patient on a continuous cardiac monitor and pulse oximeter. Restrain the hands of uncooperative patients.

Measure and mark the appropriate depth of the gastric lavage tube before passage. This ensures that the tip is in the stomach and that there is no excess tubing that may kink or knot the tube.

Lubricate the gastric tube and pass it gently to avoid damage to the posterior pharynx. Use a bite block or an oral airway to prevent the patient from biting the tube or inserter.

Once the tube enters the pharynx, put the patient's chin on the chest to facilitate passage of the tube into the esophagus. Pass the tube into the stomach.

Once the tube is passed, confirm that it is in the stomach via auscultation and aspiration of gastric contents. A radiograph may be obtained if deemed clinically necessary.

Before gastric irrigation, remove the gastric contents by careful gastric aspiration with repeated repositioning of the tip of the tube.

Repeatedly introduce small aliquots (200–300 mL in adults) into the stomach and then remove them. Perform this step with the patient in the left lateral decubitus position.

After gastric aspiration and lavage are completed, administer a slurry of activated charcoal through the gastric tube. When no longer needed, clamp off the gastric tube before removal.

Figure 42-2 Gastric lavage.

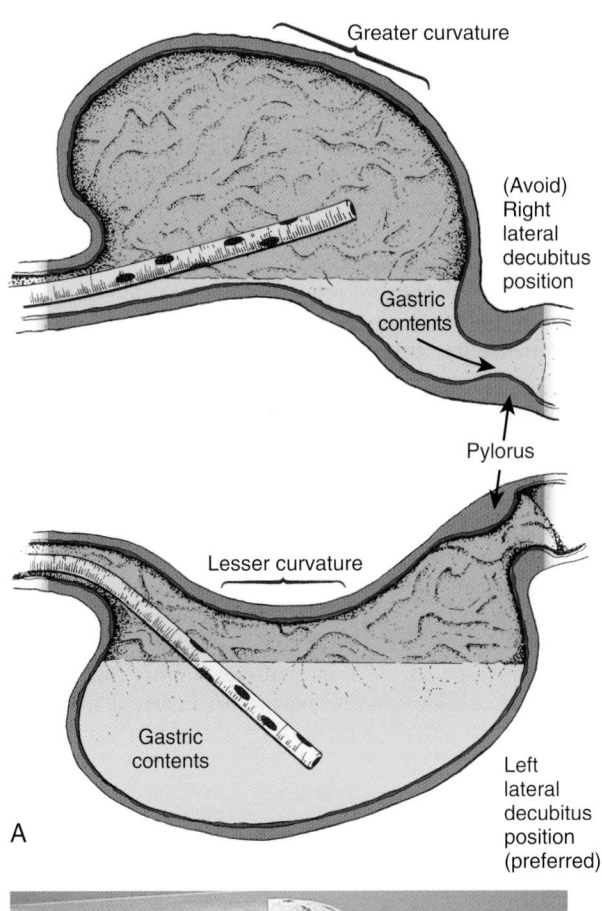

Greater curvature

(Avoid)
Right
lateral
decubitus
position

Gastric
contents

Pylorus

Lesser curvature

Gastric
contents

Left
lateral
decubitus
position
(preferred)

A

Figure 42-4 Patients on a ventilator or intubated with airway protection may undergo lavage while supine for logistic reasons, but an awake nonintubated patient should never undergo lavage in the supine position.

B

Figure 42-3 A, Effect of patient positioning on lavage. **B,** The left lateral decubitus position is preferred.

Figure 42-5 This large-diameter gastric lavage tube demonstrates the size of the holes and the size of some typical pills. Extra holes can be cut in the side of the tube to facilitate the removal of large fragments.

adults and 10 mL/kg body weight in children up to a maximum of 300 mL) into the stomach and then remove them (see Fig. 42-2, *step 7*). Larger amounts of fluid create the potential for an increased risk of washing the gastric contents into the duodenum or lungs. Much smaller amounts are not clinically practical because of the dead space in the tubing (≈50 mL in a 36-Fr hose) and the increased time required. The amount of fluid that is returned should approximate the amount introduced. Manual agitation of the patient's stomach by gently "kneading" it with a hand placed on the abdomen may increase recovery.[32] Continue lavage until the fluid becomes clear.

After gastric aspiration and lavage have been completed, administer a slurry of activated charcoal through the gastric tube (see Fig. 42-2, *step 8*). When no longer needed, clamp off the gastric tube during removal to avoid "dribbling" fluid into the airway. With the increasing use of repetitive doses of activated charcoal, an NG tube may be left in place, or passed, after the lavage procedure is completed. A patient who remains obtunded may receive additional doses via a standard NG tube. Because the large gastric tube is irritating and may predispose the patient to gagging, drooling, or aspiration, it

Figure 42-6 Gastric lavage in a child is always problematic. Obviously, an adult-sized large-bore oral gastric tube cannot be used, but a nasogastric (NG) tube may suffice. Some pediatric textbooks recommend a 24-Fr oral gastric tube for toddlers and a 36-Fr tube for adolescents. In this case, a child was found with an open bottle of digoxin, and it could not be determined whether ingestion had occurred. She would not drink charcoal. An 18-Fr NG tube was used in an attempt to aspirate digoxin from the stomach (none was recovered) and to instill charcoal. Some would suggest an oral route for this tube, but it was passed rather easily through the nose. An NG tube is not ideal for some ingestants (iron, sustained-release products), but most pills quickly dissolve in the stomach and the small particles can easily be removed with an NG tube. Although lavage may have been reasonable in this scenario, a potent and safe antidote for digoxin does exist. The common routine practice of passing an NG tube in a child who is unwilling to drink charcoal is controversial, and though intuitively reasonable, it is of unproven value and probably done far too often for benign ingestions.

should be removed. Alert patients should take subsequent doses of charcoal orally as necessary.

Complications

A correctly performed procedure in the appropriate environment is generally safe, but numerous complications have been associated with gastric lavage.[26] The complications can be divided into those caused by mechanical trauma and those resulting from the lavage fluid.

Depending on the route selected for insertion of the tube, damage to the nasal mucosa, turbinates, pharynx, esophagus, and stomach has been reported.[34-37] After insertion of the tube, it is imperative to confirm correct placement. Scalzo and associates found radiographically that 7 of 14 children had improper tube placement (too high or too low) despite positive gastric auscultation in all cases, although the clinical effects of such misplacement was not evaluated. Radiographic confirmation of tube placement should be considered in young children and intubated patients (see Fig. 42-7).[38] Instillation of lavage fluid and charcoal into the lungs through tubes inadvertently misplaced within the airways has been reported.[39]

During lavage, changes in cardiorespiratory function have been noted. Thompson and coworkers reported that during lavage 36% of patients had atrial or ventricular ectopy, 4.8% had transient ST elevation, and 29% had a fall in oxygen tension to 60 mm Hg or lower.[40] Laryngospasm may also occur during gastric lavage.[25]

The lavage fluid itself is a potential source of complications. The large amount of fluid administered during lavage has been reported to cause fluid and electrolyte disturbances. These disturbances have been seen with the use of both hypertonic and hypotonic lavage fluid in the pediatric population.[29-31] Hypothermia is a possible complication if the lavage fluid is not prewarmed.

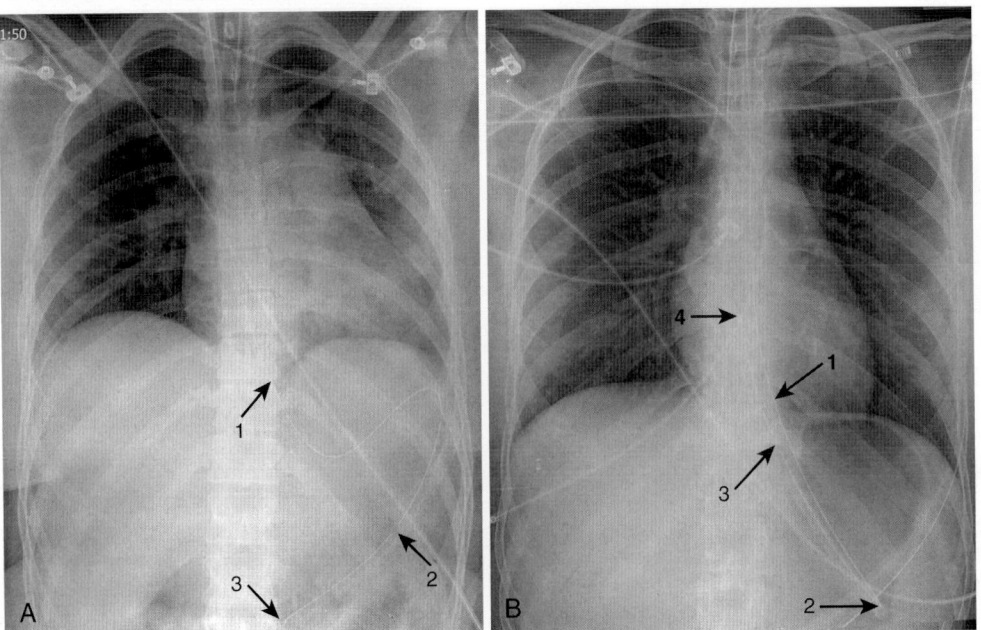

Figure 42-7 Radiographic confirmation of gastric lavage tube placement. **A,** This radiograph confirms proper placement of the lavage tube. It can be seen descending below the diaphragm (*1*), and the interruption in the radiopaque line (which signifies the most proximal hole) is in the stomach (*2*). The tip of the tube (*3*) is also visible. **B,** The lavage tube in this patient is misplaced! The tube can be seen descending beneath the diaphragm (*1*) but is kinked in the stomach (*2*) and has doubled back on itself. The gap in the radiopaque line (*3*) is at the level of the gastroesophageal junction, and the distal tip of the tube is in the midesophagus (*4*). Proper measurement of the tube before insertion would probably have prevented this misplacement. *If there is any doubt about proper positioning of the tube, a radiograph should be obtained before lavage!*

Pulmonary aspiration of gastric contents or lavage fluid is the primary potential risk during gastric lavage, especially in patients with compromised airway protective reflexes.[41-43] Merigian and colleagues reported a 10% incidence of aspiration pneumonia in patients who underwent gastric lavage.[23] This risk is reduced by using small aliquots of lavage fluid, adequately positioning the patient, and intubating patients with compromised airway protective reflexes.

If the lavage tube cannot be removed easily, do not force it. Kinking or knotting of the tube can occur, but occasionally a tube may become stuck because of lower esophageal spasm. If fluoroscopy or radiography demonstrates no deformation of the lavage tube, 1 to 2 mg of intravenous glucagon can be infused in an attempt to relieve lower esophageal spasm.[44] Surgical removal may be necessary if the gastric tube is deformed by kinking or knotting.

Activated Charcoal

Background

Activated charcoal is a carbon product that is subjected to heat and oxidized to increase its surface area (Fig. 42-8). It has the capacity to adsorb substances onto the porous surface of the charcoal. The use of activated charcoal for poisoning has been recognized for almost 2 centuries. To demonstrate charcoal's effectiveness, in 1930 French pharmacist Touery ingested several times the lethal dose of strychnine mixed with 15 g of activated charcoal. He performed this act in front of a class of colleagues and exhibited no ill effects.

Activated charcoal acts both by adsorbing a wide range of toxins present in the gastrointestinal tract and by enhancing elimination of toxin if systemic absorption has already occurred. It enhances elimination by creating a concentration gradient between the contents of the bowel and the circulation, but it also has the potential of interrupting enterohepatic circulation if the particular toxin is secreted in bile and enters the gastrointestinal tract before reabsorption.[45] Oral activated charcoal is given as a single dose or in multiple doses. The adsorptive capacity of charcoal depends on the inherent properties of the toxin and the local milieu, such as pH. Adsorption begins within minutes of contact with a toxin but may not reach equilibrium for 20 to 30 minutes. Desorption of toxins from charcoal occurs over time, although this has little clinical significance for most patients and can be overcome by administering additional charcoal.

Indications

For years, administration of a single oral dose of activated charcoal for essentially all overdoses has been routine. However, with the emergence of new guidelines in overdose management,[6] use of charcoal has declined to less than 5% of all potential toxin exposures (Fig. 42-9).[1] Clearly, charcoal binds many toxins in the gut, thereby decreasing some systemic absorption. Despite a lack of scientific data demonstrating a decrease in morbidity and mortality and firm evidence to support its widespread use, charcoal is a reasonable intervention for most poisoned patients encountered in the ED if it can be administered easily and safely. The exact indications are not established, and no universally accepted standard of care has been promulgated.[46] A single dose of activated charcoal is indicated if the clinician estimates that a clinically significant fraction of the ingested substance remains in the gastrointestinal tract, the toxin is adsorbed by charcoal, further absorption may result in clinical deterioration, and it can be administered safely. This will usually be a clinical decision because adequate historical data may often be lacking. It may also be administered by multiple dosing if the clinician anticipates that the charcoal will result in increased clearance of an already absorbed drug. It is most effective within the first 60 minutes after an oral overdose and decreases in effectiveness over time. Charcoal is generally considered to provide superior gut decontamination over gastric lavage. There is no definitive evidence, however, that administration of activated charcoal improves outcome.

Contraindications

Administration of charcoal is contraindicated in any person who demonstrates compromised airway protective reflexes unless already intubated.[46] It is absolutely contraindicated in persons who have ingested corrosive substances (acids

Figure 42-8 Activated charcoal. Because the contents may settle with time, shake the bottle vigorously before administration. Rinse the container with a small amount of tap water as well to ensure that the patient receives the full dose. Plain charcoal, without sorbitol, is preferred.

POSITION STATEMENT: SINGLE-DOSE
ACTIVATED CHARCOAL

American Academy of Clinical Toxicology; European Association of Poisons Centres and Clinical Toxicologists

Single-dose activated charcoal should not be administered routinely in the management of poisoned patients. Based on volunteer studies, the effectiveness of activated charcoal decreases with time; the greatest benefit is within 1 hour of ingestion. The administration of activated charcoal may be considered if a patient has ingested a potentially toxic amount of a poison (which is known to be adsorbed to charcoal) up to 1 hour previously; there are insufficient data to support or exclude its use after 1 hour of ingestion. There is no evidence that the administration of activated charcoal improves clinical outcome. Unless a patient has an intact or protected airway, the administration of charcoal is contraindicated.

Figure 42-9 Position statement: single-dose activated charcoal. *(From Chyka PA, Seger D. Position statement: single-dose activated charcoal. American Academy of Clinical Toxicology; European Association of Poisons Centres and Clinical Toxicologists. J Toxicol Clin Toxicol. 1997;35:721-741.)*

or alkalis). Not only does charcoal provide no benefit in a corrosive ingestion, but its administration could also precipitate vomiting, obscure endoscopic visualization, and lead to complications if a perforation developed and charcoal entered the mediastinum, peritoneum, or pleural space. Charcoal should be avoided with ingestion of a pure aliphatic petroleum distillate. Hydrocarbons are not well adsorbed by activated charcoal, and its administration could lead to further risk for aspiration. Many hydrocarbons are potential systemic toxins (e.g., carbon tetrachloride and benzene) or are mixed with other potentially significant toxins such as pesticides. In these cases data are lacking, but charcoal administration can be considered. Caution should be exercised in using charcoal in patients with medical conditions that could be further compromised by charcoal ingestion, such as gastrointestinal perforation or bleeding. Charcoal is not indicated for isolated ingestion of ethanol or metals (e.g., iron, lithium) because these substances are not adsorbed. If the airway is not secure, charcoal should be given with caution to minimally symptomatic patients who have ingested a toxin that may suddenly induce seizures. Because it is often impossible to determine the exact nature of an ingestion, a liberal use policy is advocated for potentially mixed overdoses.

Charcoal administration by paramedics and other emergency response personnel should be performed with caution.[47] There is insufficient evidence to recommend for or against administration of activated charcoal in the prehospital setting.[3] The same indications and contraindications apply as for patients who are in the hospital. The motion of the ambulance during transport may make the patient more prone to emesis. Either spilling of charcoal or vomiting of charcoal may result in significant contamination of the transport vehicle and subsequently place that vehicle out of commission until it can be cleaned.

Technique

There is no universally accurate dose for charcoal. A 10:1 ratio (charcoal to toxin) is recommended if the amount of ingestion is known. Dosing of charcoal should be considered in light of the specific ingestion, but the following empirical doses of single-dose activated charcoal (standard aqueous products such as Liqui-Char) are recommended[46]:

- Up to 1 year: 1 g/kg of body weight
- 1 to 12 years: 25 to 50 g
- Older than 12 years: 25 to 100 g

If the ingestion were, for example, clonidine (0.1-mg tablets) or digoxin (0.25-mg tablets), this regimen would be more than adequate for even a massive overdose to achieve the desired 10:1 ratio. If the ingestion consisted of a large number of 325-mg aspirin tablets or 240-mg verapamil tablets, the dosing regimen could be insufficient. If toxic medications with a high-milligram dosage are ingested, it would be prudent to administer more charcoal than indicated by these guidelines. There is no known benefit of mixing charcoal with a cathartic (i.e., sorbitol), and the combination is not suggested. Sorbitol increases the incidence of vomiting.

Because in many charcoal formulations the contents settle with time, shake the preparation vigorously before administering it to the patient. Follow this by rinsing the container with a small amount of tap water before administering it to the patient to allow ingestion of the full dose.[48] Aqueous

activated charcoal has a gritty texture that most patients find unpleasant, but attempts have been made to improve its taste and texture. Mixing activated charcoal with chocolate milk, chocolate- or cherry-flavored syrup, or ice cream may increase palatability, but mixing with these additives has been suggested, though not proved, to cause a decrease in the adsorptive capacity of activated charcoal.[49] Rangan and colleagues reported no decrease in adsorption after mixing superactivated charcoal with a noncaffeinated cola.[50] Scharman and associates demonstrated that a regular, sugared cola was favored by children over a diet cola, but only 20% of the time were they able to cajole even nonpoisoned children younger than 3 years to drink a therapeutic amount of flavored charcoal.[51]

Give activated charcoal orally if the patient is awake and cooperative and by NG tube if the patient is unconscious. If an NG tube is inserted, it is imperative that correct placement be verified. Confirm correct tube placement radiographically before administering charcoal, especially in obtunded or intubated patients (see Fig. 42-7). Instillation of charcoal into the lungs has been reported after inadvertent misplacement within the airways, and massive aspiration can be fatal (Fig. 42-10).[39,52] Intubation is protective, but it is not uncommon to see some charcoal in the airway even if the patient has been intubated.

A clinical conundrum exists when a patient refuses to drink charcoal and an NG tube must be passed without consent if charcoal is deemed advisable. The common tactic of passing an NG tube in an awake but uncooperative patient merely to administer charcoal is controversial, and no standards exist. Such a scenario is more likely to result in trauma from placement of the tube, a misplaced tube, or subsequent emesis from the rapid administration of charcoal. Given the unproven efficacy of charcoal, the authors advise against routine insertion of an NG tube simply to administer charcoal in an awake and minimally symptomatic patient. Such a decision is, however, a clinical one that must be made by the health care provider and be based on the entire clinical milieu (Fig. 42-11).

Complications

Administration of activated charcoal is not without risks and complications. Published reports have demonstrated adverse effects associated with activated charcoal therapy, including childhood deaths.[53] The most common complications of charcoal administration include constipation, diarrhea, and vomiting.[54,55] Bowel perforation has been described in a patient with diverticular disease.[56] Pulmonary aspiration of activated charcoal is a dreaded complication that can result in pneumonitis, obstruction of the respiratory tree, bronchiolitis obliterans,[36,57-59] acute lung injury, and barotrauma.[53] Risk factors for serious aspiration are large amounts of charcoal instilled over a short period, multiple-dose charcoal in the setting of ileus, charcoal administration in a patient who becomes obtunded, charcoal that is inappropriately diluted, or forced administration of charcoal via an NG tube, especially in a restrained supine patient. These complications can be prevented by prudent dosing of charcoal and associated cathartic therapy, as well as by monitoring the patient's fluid and electrolyte status and clinical condition and performing abdominal examinations. Trivial aspiration of charcoal is common and usually innocuous even if the patient is intubated. Studies show a 4% to 39% incidence of aspiration pneumonia in intubated

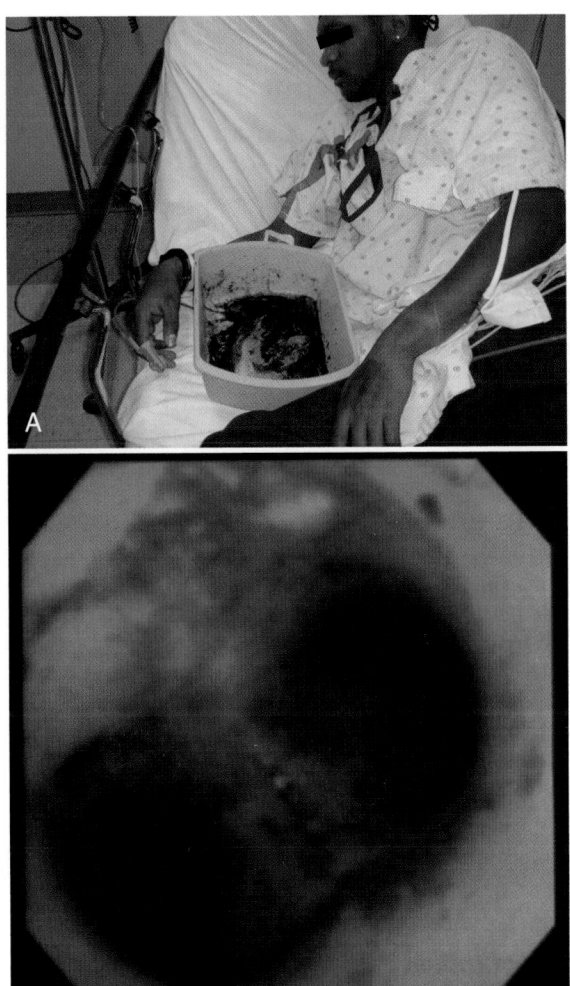

Figure 42-10 A, Vomiting can be expected following charcoal administration, especially if sorbitol is added (not recommended). This patient rapidly became drowsy after administration of charcoal, vomited, but fortunately did not aspirate. **B,** In another patient who aspirated, the charcoal can be seen at the carina with a fiberoptic scope. Massive aspiration can be fatal. Intubation does not totally protect against minimal charcoal aspiration.

patients who received activated charcoal while intubated.[60] It has been shown that even in patients with a protected airway and a cuffed endotracheal tube, vomiting can lead to pulmonary aspiration of the charcoal.[53] This can result in a significant increase in lung microvascular permeability and lead to lung edema and pulmonary compromise.[61]

Multiple Doses of Activated Charcoal

Indications

The use of multiple-dose activated charcoal (MDAC) may be indicated in selected cases (Fig. 42-12).[62] Its use has been advocated for two purposes: first, to prevent continued absorption of a drug that may still be present in the gastrointestinal tract and, second, to increase serum clearance of a drug that has already been absorbed (Box 42-1).

MDAC prevents continued absorption by either binding a drug that may be present throughout the gastrointestinal tract or binding a drug that exists as extended-release or enteric-coated preparations. MDAC enhances elimination of a drug

Figure 42-11 A, If an overdose patient will voluntarily drink charcoal, there are few reasons to withhold it, even though a definite clinical benefit in routine cases cannot be proved. If a patient will not drink charcoal, patient management becomes controversial. Passing a nasogastric (NG) tube in a struggling patient or in a recalcitrant child merely to instill the unproven, but theoretically useful antidote is not supported by scientific data. Nonetheless, it remains a common procedure. Though not always easy or pleasant, such an intervention is usually safe. Pulmonary aspiration, even in an awake patient, is the major downside. *Restrained supine patients are at greatest risk for aspiration,* and that position should be avoided, even in an initially awake patient. **B,** Charcoal that is voluntarily swallowed or instilled via an oral-gastric lavage tube or an NG tube can induce emesis. This occurs in both obtunded and awake patients. In this instance the patient was unconscious from the overdose and the airway was protected with prior tracheal intubation. Although the intubation procedure does not totally exclude pulmonary aspiration and it carries some morbidity in its own right, it is recommended before use of charcoal in patients who are not able to fully protect their airway. Patients who are initially asymptomatic or minimally affected but have ingested drugs that have the potential to produce rapid deterioration, seizures, or loss of airway protection make decisions on the use of charcoal difficult for the clinician. In borderline cases, some experienced clinicians avoid the use of charcoal altogether.

POSITION STATEMENT: POSITION STATEMENT AND PRACTICE GUIDELINES ON THE USE OF MULTI-DOSE ACTIVATED CHARCOAL IN THE TREATMENT OF ACUTE POISONING

American Academy of Clinical Toxicology; European Association of Poisons Centres and Clinical Toxicologists

Although many studies in animals and volunteers have demonstrated that multiple-dose activated charcoal increases drug elimination significantly, this therapy has not yet been shown in a controlled study in poisoned patients to reduce morbidity and mortality. Further studies are required to establish its role and the optimal dosage regimen of charcoal to be administered.

Based on experimental and clinical studies, multiple-dose activated charcoal should be considered only if a patient has ingested a life-threatening amount of carbamazepine, dapsone, Phenobarbital, quinine, or theophylline. With all of these drugs there are data to confirm enhanced elimination, though no controlled studies have demonstrated clinical benefit.

Although volunteer studies have demonstrated that multiple-dose activated charcoal increases the elimination of amitriptyline, dextropropoxyphene, digitoxin, digoxin, disopyramide, nadolol, phenylbutazone, phenytoin, piroxicam, and sotalol, there are insufficient clinical data to support or exclude the use of this therapy.

The use of multiple-dose charcoal in salicylate poisoning is controversial. One animal study and 2 of 4 volunteer studies did not demonstrate increased salicylate clearance with multiple-dose charcoal therapy. Data in poisoned patients are insufficient presently to recommend the use of multiple-dose charcoal therapy for salicylate poisoning. Multiple-dose activated charcoal did not increase the elimination of astemizole, chlorpropamide, doxepin, imipramine, meprobamate, methotrexate, phenytoin, sodium valproate, tobramycin, and vancomycin in experimental and/or clinical studies.

Unless a patient has an intact or protected airway, the administration of multiple-dose activated charcoal is contraindicated. It should not be used in the presence of an intestinal obstruction. The need for concurrent administration of cathartics remains unproven and is not recommended. In particular, cathartics should not be administered to young children because of the propensity of laxatives to cause fluid and electrolyte imbalance. In conclusion, based on experimental and clinical studies, multiple-dose activated charcoal should be considered only if a patient has ingested a life-threatening amount of carbamazepine, dapsone, Phenobarbital, quinine, or theophylline.

Figure 42-12 Position statement and practice guidelines on the use of multidose activated charcoal in the treatment of acute poisoning. *(From Position statement and practice guidelines on the use of multi-dose activated charcoal in the treatment of acute poisoning. American Academy of Clinical Toxicology; European Association of Poisons Centres and Clinical Toxicologists.* J Toxicol Clin Toxicol. *1999;37:731-751.)*

BOX 42-1 Drugs Whose Serum Clearance May Be Enhanced by Multiple Doses of Activated Charcoal

Aspirin	Phenobarbital
Caffeine	Phenytoin
Carbamazepine	Quinine
Cyclosporine	Sotalol
Dapsone	Sustained-release thallium
Digoxin	Theophylline
Disopyramide	Valproate
Nadolol	Vancomycin

MDAC has been shown to increase total-body clearance of multiple drugs, including carbamazepine,[65] dapsone,[66] phenobarbital,[67] quinine,[68] and theophylline.[62] Despite the reported increase in drug clearance associated with the use of MDAC, improved clinical outcomes have not been definitively demonstrated. For example, Pond and coworkers described 10 comatose patients following phenobarbital overdose who were randomized to receive either single-dose activated charcoal or MDAC.[69] Despite the fact that the MDAC group had a significantly shorter phenobarbital serum half-life, no difference was found between the groups with regard to the duration of intubation or hospitalization. In a rural, developing world setting, routine use of MDAC was not found to alter mortality rates.[70]

Contraindications

MDAC is contraindicated in patients with evidence of bowel obstruction. Ileus is a relative contraindication.[71] Many ill patients in whom ileus develops may be candidates for MDAC if the airway is protected. Administration of MDAC is contraindicated in any patient who does not have an intact or protected airway. MDAC should be avoided in patients with repetitive emesis, especially when associated with decreased mental status or a decreased gag reflex. Concurrent use of cathartics with MDAC remains unproved and is not recommended.[72] MDAC with cathartics should not be administered to young children because of the propensity for laxatives to cause fluid and electrolyte imbalance. For example, MDAC with sorbitol has been associated with hypernatremia and dehydration,[73,74] and MDAC with magnesium cathartics has been associated with hypermagnesemia, neuromuscular weakness, and coma.[75,76]

Technique

Give 1 g/kg (≤100 g) for the first dose of charcoal. If a cathartic is used, administer it only with the first dose of charcoal to decrease the potential risk for cathartic-induced electrolyte abnormalities, especially in children.[73-76] Follow the initial dose of charcoal with 0.5 g/kg (≤50 g) every 4 hours. Stop giving MDAC if repeated examination reveals an absence of bowel sounds or a distended abdomen. In this case, consider placing an NG tube and put it on low intermittent suction. Patients receiving MDAC may be at increased risk for emesis because of the larger total dose of activated charcoal received. The use of antiemetics may help decrease the incidence of vomiting associated with MDAC.[77,78] Charcoal therapy should

by interrupting enterobiliary recirculation or augmenting enterocapillary exsorption.[54] By interrupting enterobiliary recirculation, charcoal binds to an active drug that is secreted by the biliary system, thus subsequently preventing reabsorption. By augmentation of enterocapillary exsorption, charcoal produces sink conditions that drive diffusion of the drug from capillaries into the entraluminal space, where it is subsequently eliminated. This process is called *intestinal dialysis*.[63] Drug characteristics associated with enhanced systemic clearance via MDAC include a low intrinsic clearance, a prolonged distributive phase, low protein binding, and a small volume of distribution.[64]

be continued until clinical improvement is evident and plasma drug levels have fallen to acceptable levels.

Complications

The complications encountered with single-dose activated charcoal are also encountered with MDAC. In addition, there have been reports of gastrointestinal obstruction and perforation with MDAC therapy, especially in conjunction with the ingestion of drugs that have anticholinergic properties.[79-83]

Cathartics

Background

The use of cathartics is intended to decrease the absorption of substances by accelerating expulsion of the poison from the gastrointestinal tract. Cathartics are often used in conjunction with activated charcoal because of charcoal's side effect of constipation. The mechanism of action of cathartics is such that theoretically, it would minimize the possibility of desorption of drug bound to activated charcoal. There is little evidence that a single dose of aqueous activated charcoal is significantly constipating; however, cathartics are often given for this potential problem. The majority of data suggest negligible clinical benefit from the use of cathartics.[84,85]

Indications

Routine administration of a cathartic in combination with activated charcoal is not endorsed by the American Academy of Clinical Toxicology or the European Association of Poison Centres and Clinical Toxicologists.[86] Administration of a cathartic alone has no role in the management of a poisoned patient.

Contraindications

Cathartics are contraindicated in patients with volume depletion, hypotension, significant electrolyte imbalance, ingestion of a corrosive, ileus, recent bowel surgery, and intestinal obstruction or perforation. Administration of cathartics is also contraindicated in patients who do not have an intact or protected airway. They should be avoided in those with repetitive emesis, especially when associated with decreased mental status or a decreased gag reflex. Cathartics should be used cautiously in young children and the elderly because of the propensity for laxatives to cause fluid and electrolyte imbalance.

Technique

There are two types of osmotic cathartics: saccharide cathartics (sorbitol) and saline cathartics (magnesium citrate, magnesium sulfate, and sodium sulfate). The optimal dose of sorbitol or magnesium citrate remains to be determined. The recommended dose of sorbitol is approximately 1 to 2 g/kg of body weight or 1 to 2 mL/kg of 70% sorbitol in adults and 4.3 mL/kg of 35% sorbitol in children (single administration only).[86] Many charcoal formulations come premixed with sorbitol, but the sorbitol content varies considerably. The recommended dose of magnesium citrate is 250 mL of a 10% solution in an adult and 4 mL/kg body weight of a 10% solution in a child. Multiple doses of cathartics should be avoided.

Complications

Administration of sorbitol has been associated with vomiting, abdominal cramps, nausea, diaphoresis, and transient hypotension.[87-89] Because the sorbitol content varies between different charcoal-sorbitol combination products, pay attention to the sorbitol content in each brand to avoid excessive sorbitol administration. Be aware that multiple doses of sorbitol have been associated with volume depletion.[73] Multiple doses of magnesium-containing cathartics have been linked to severe hypermagnesemia.[75,76] Children are particularly susceptible to the adverse effects of cathartics, and therefore use caution or totally avoid using cathartics in children.

Whole Bowel Irrigation

Background

WBI involves the enteral administration of an osmotically balanced polyethylene glycol electrolyte solution (PEG-ES) in a sufficient amount and rate to physically flush ingested substances through the gastrointestinal tract, thereby purging the toxin before absorption can occur.[14] PEG-ES (CoLyte, GoLYTELY) is isosmotic, is not systemically absorbed, and will not cause electrolyte or fluid shifts. The data available suggest that the large volumes of this solution needed to mechanically propel pills, drug packets (such as in body packers or stuffers), or other substances through the gastrointestinal tract are safe, including use in pregnant women and young children.[90-92]

Clinical data on the efficacy of WBI remain limited. Ly and colleagues found that the effect of WBI on reduction of acetaminophen concentration versus time was not statistically significant.[93] However, WBI did have a mechanical effect on radiopaque markers in the gastrointestinal tract, with 8 of 10 subjects' markers congregating in the right hemicolon after WBI. WBI was shown to mobilize lead BB pellets in a child to the large bowel, where less absorption occurs and the foreign bodies could be removed by colonoscopic intervention.[94] In addition, PEG-ES may play a role in the pharmacologic conversion of some toxins. For example, it has been shown that the relatively high pH of PEG-ES increases the rate of spontaneous conversion of cocaine to its inactive metabolite benzoylecgonine.[95]

Indications

WBI may be considered for the ingestion of exceedingly large quantities of potentially toxic substances, toxins that are poorly adsorbed to activated charcoal (e.g., iron, lithium), and delayed-release formulations; late arrival at the ED after ingestion of a toxin; the presence of pharmacobezoars; and body stuffers or packers (Fig. 42-13).[95-97] WBI remains a theoretical option for these ingestions and is often performed on body packers who have ingested many times the lethal amount of heroin or cocaine (Fig. 42-14). No definitive evidence exists that WBI improves the outcome of poisoned patients.[98] Though not a proven procedure, WBI is often suggested by toxicologists, and its use in selected cases is intuitively reasonable and supported by the authors. The most common indication for WBI in the ED is for the treatment of toxic sustained-release medications (such as iron, calcium channel blockers, β-blockers, theophylline, and lithium) and iron tablets (Fig. 42-15).[98]

Contraindications

WBI is contraindicated in patients with gastrointestinal obstruction, perforation, ileus, and ingestion of a corrosive

POSITION STATEMENT: WHOLE BOWEL IRRIGATION

American Academy of Clinical Toxicology; European Association of Poisons Centres and Clinical Toxicologists

Whole bowel irrigation (WBI) should not be used routinely in the management of the poisoned patient. Although some volunteer studies have shown substantial decreases in the bioavailability of ingested drugs, no controlled clinical trials have been performed and there is no conclusive evidence that WBI improves the outcome of the poisoned patient. Based on volunteer studies, WBI may be considered for potentially toxic ingestions of sustained-release or enteric-coated drugs. There are insufficient data to support or exclude the use of WBI for potentially toxic ingestions of iron, lead, zinc, or packets of illicit drugs; WBI remains a theoretical option for these ingestions. WBI is contraindicated in patients with bowel obstruction, perforation, ileus, and in patients with hemodynamic instability or compromised unprotected airways. WBI should be used cautiously in debilitated patients, or in patients with medical conditions that may be further compromised by its use. A single dose of activated charcoal administered prior to WBI does not appear to decrease the binding capacity of charcoal or to alter the osmotic properties of WBI solution. Administration of charcoal during WBI appears to decrease the binding capacity of charcoal.

Figure 42-13 Position statement: whole-bowel irrigation. (*From Tenenbeim M. Position statement: whole bowel irrigation. American Academy of Clinical Toxicology; European Association of Poisons Centres and Clinical Toxicologists. Clin Toxicol. 1997;35:753-762.*)

agent. It should also be avoided in patients with hemodynamic instability or an unprotected airway.[98] WBI should likewise be avoided with patients who have repetitive emesis, especially when associated with decreased mental status or a decreased gag reflex. WBI should be used cautiously in debilitated patients.

Technique

PEG-ES is marketed in a powder form. Add tap water to make a total volume of 4 L. The recommended rate of administration is as follows[98]:

- 9 months to 6 years: 500 mL/hr
- 6 to 12 years: 1000 mL/hr
- Older than 12 years: 1500 to 2000 mL/hr

Cooperative patients with intact airway protective reflexes may drink the solution. The large volume and taste often limit even the most motivated patient's ability to comply. If the patient is unable or unwilling to drink this solution, administer it through a small-bore NG tube after placement is confirmed. Even cooperative patients have difficulty drinking adequate fluid for effective WBI. Because it is common for WBI to be delayed while the patient and medical personnel attempt to administer the large volumes of oral WBI solution required to be effective, it is suggested that NG instillation be instituted early in the ED course (Fig. 42-16). Unconscious patients with protected airways may receive WBI via an NG tube. In one study, patients vomited shortly after beginning WBI infusion at a rate of 1.5 to 2 L/hr. Antiemetics such as ondansetron, as well as gradually advancing the infusion rate over a 60-minute period, can help ease this

Figure 42-14 A, This body packer attempted to smuggle more than 50 packets of heroin. All packets were passed intact after 12 hours of whole-bowel irrigation. **B,** Note the integrity of the carefully wrapped packets that were passed.

side effect. Prewarming the irrigant to a temperature of approximately 37°C avoids the potential complication of hypothermia. To collect the waste products, ask an awake patient to sit on a commode. In an obtunded patient, insert a rectal tube to collect the waste. Many toxicologists recommend adding two to three bottles of activated charcoal to each liter of WBI solution. The benefit is unproved, but there is little theoretical downside to this technique, and it is supported by the authors. The binding capacity of charcoal is decreased when combined with PEG-ES, but the clinical consequences of this observation are unknown and probably minimal. Empirically, metoclopramide (10 to 20 mg intravenously) may be coadministered to decrease nausea and facilitate gastrointestinal passage.

Figure 42-15 Whole-bowel irrigation (WBI) is commonly recommended for the treatment of iron ingestion. These radiographs depict the effect of 5 hours of WBI. Note the marked decrease in radiopaque pills (*arrows*) in the gastrointestinal tract. Intact pills were recovered in the rectal effluent.

The end point of WBI is the arrival of clear rectal effluent or resolution of the toxic effect (or both).[98] There are rare case reports of late purging of drug packets, plant parts, and tablets after the arrival of clear effluent.[96,99] Radiographic studies may also be beneficial to determine the end point in body packers or in patients who have ingested radiopaque medications.

Complications

Few complications from WBI therapy, especially pertaining to acute poisonings, have been reported. Nausea, vomiting, abdominal cramps, bloating, and aspiration have been described.[71,100] Nausea and vomiting may make administration of WBI difficult. Antiemetics and a 15- to 30-minute break followed by a slower rate may allow readministration. As discussed with the other methods of decontamination, attention should be directed to the airway and the potential for aspiration. Administration of a large amount of chilled or room-temperature WBI fluid to pediatric patients could potentially cause hypothermia. Consider warmed fluids in these patients. If activated charcoal is administered concurrently with WBI, desorption of toxin from charcoal might occur.[101-103]

DERMAL DECONTAMINATION

Background

Numerous hazardous material (HAZMAT) incidents occur each year in the United States. In the first 6 months of 2009, 3458 HAZMAT events occurred in 13 states as reported to the Hazardous Substances Emergency Events Surveillance System.[104] HAZMAT events frequently result in injuries, and ED treatment of contaminated HAZMAT patients is not a rare event. Many of these patients, including those involved in past terrorist events, transport themselves to the ED. For example, in the Tokyo sarin gas attack, 93% of 498 patients reporting to St. Luke's Hospital arrived by means other than ambulance.[105] The risk for injury to medical personnel incurred while treating contaminated patients is significant. After the Tokyo attack, 13 of 15 clinicians (87%) reported symptoms while treating patients in the ED, and 23% of involved hospital staff complained of acute poisoning

Figure 42-16 It is very difficult for even the most motivated patient to drink an effective volume of whole-bowel irrigation (WBI) solution. To enhance compliance and to decrease vomiting, polyethylene glycol electrolyte solution (PEG-ES) may be slowly and continuously administered via a nasogastric (NG) tube. An empty bag of saline is hung on an intravenous pole, the corner of the bag is removed, and the PEG-ES is poured into the bag. Standard intravenous tubing is connected to the proximal end of an NG tube (*arrow*) and the solution is infused continuously via a pump (1 L/hr). In this picture (**A**), charcoal has been added to the WBI solution. Metoclopramide (IV) was coadministered to reduce nausea, a common side effect of WBI.

symptoms.[106] Burgess and associates reported that 13% of Washington state emergency care facilities had evacuated their ED or another part of the hospital because of contamination during a 5-year period.[107] Ghilarducci and coworkers surveyed level 1 trauma centers in the United States and reported that only 6% had the necessary equipment required for safe decontamination.[108] Less than 36% of emergency medicine staff had received appropriate training in handling contaminated patients, and 5.6% had experienced injuries to their staff from contact with contaminated patients during a 1-year period. It is imperative that EDs have plans in place to handle patients who have been exposed to potential toxins, provide adequate decontamination facilities, and ensure the safety of the treating medical staff.[109]

Technique

There are a number of key components in the management of HAZMAT incidents and the care of contaminated patients seen in the ED.[110] These components should include early recognition of a HAZMAT event, rapid activation of a plan to manage contaminated patients, initiation of primary triage, appropriate patient registration, patient decontamination, secondary triage, and final treatment.

First, the ED must be able to recognize that an event has occurred before contaminated patients gain entrance into the health care facility (Fig. 42-17, *step 1*). Communication with the local fire, police, and paramedic systems provides early detection of such events and allows preparation before patients arrive. Security should be arranged to prevent contaminated patients from entering the hospital, and "lockdown" of the facility should be considered.

Second, the ED should have the authority to activate a plan expeditiously to prepare the decontamination facility and allow appropriate preselected personnel to don personal protective equipment (PPE) (see Fig. 42-17, *step 2*). If necessary, the hospital disaster plan should be activated quickly at the discretion of the ED clinician who is in contact with scene operations and incoming patients. Specific data to determine

---

MANAGEMENT OF HAZARDOUS MATERIALS (HAZMAT) INCIDENTS

The ED recognizes that an incident has occurred before patients gain entry into the facility, via communication with police and EMS officials. Security prevents contaminated patients from entering the hospital.

The ED activates its disaster plan. The decontamination facility is prepared and trained individuals don personal protective equipment. Shown here are providers in Level C splash-proof, chemical-resistant suits.

The ED staff, with the assistance of EMS providers, performs primary triage. A brief initial assessment of each patient is performed, and the patient's name and date of birth are recorded. Contaminated clothing is placed in an impervious bag.

Decontamination is performed. A portable decontamination facility as shown here is ideal, although may not be available at many institutions. Simpler solutions, such as a warm shower nozzle and a wading pool outside the ED, may be used.

Figure 42-17 During a hazardous materials (HAZMAT) incident, a decontamination tent with personnel in protective gear is assembled outside the emergency department (ED) entrance. *EMS,* emergency medical service.

the appropriate level of PPE to maintain protection of hospital workers remain limited. The minimum PPE for hospital-based decontamination (level C) consists of a splash-proof, chemical-resistant suit with tape, double-layer protective gloves, and a powered air-purifying respirator per the National Institute of Occupational Safety and Health. Higher levels of protection, such as a level A self-contained breathing apparatus (SCBA), fully encapsulated chemical-resistant suit, or level B SCBA chemical-resistant suit, are recommended with unknown chemical and biologic exposures and for entering hot zones, but these levels of protection are not readily available in EDs.[111,112] Fortunately, most chemical exposures are known. For those that occur in the workplace, Material Safety Data Sheets can be obtained and either the local poison center or the Agency for Toxic Substances and Disease Registry (ATSDR) can be contacted for advice on what level of protection is appropriate.

Third, appropriate primary triage should take place (see Fig. 42-17, *step 3*). Contaminated patients should not enter the ED until proper decontamination has occurred to ensure that the hospital staff will not be subjected to secondary contamination. Appropriate triage should then take place, with experienced personnel performing an initial brief assessment of each patient. The triage and decontamination areas should be organized into several "zones" to prevent further contamination. The "hot" zone is the location with the highest level of contaminant or where the incident occurred. In most cases of hospital-based decontamination, there is no hot zone because patients have been removed from the initial chemical insult. On average, patients arrive at the ED 20 minutes after the event and have had significant off-gassing by this time; however, the majority of patients will have transported themselves and will not have received any prehospital decontamination by emergency medical services/HAZMAT personnel. Basic lifesaving treatments, airway and hemorrhage control, antidote administration (e.g., for cyanide or nerve agents), and decontamination occur in the "warm" zone. The "cold" zone is safe from contaminant.[112]

Fourth, a brief sign-in process in the warm zone should capture the patient's name and date of birth, with full registration to occur after decontamination. Contaminated clothing and valuables should be placed in an impervious bag to avoid potential off-gassing.[113,114]

Fifth, decontamination should be performed (see Fig. 42-17, *step 4*). The hospital ED should have preexisting HAZMAT incident protocols that designate the decontamination area and the triage and decontamination team. Ideally, a hospital should have a permanent decontamination facility capable of handling a small number of chemically exposed patients and, in addition, a large portable unit for mass casualties. The decontamination area should meet several qualifications: (1) it should be secured to prevent spread to other areas of the hospital, (2) the ventilation system should be separate from the rest of the hospital or it should be shut off to prevent airborne spread of contaminants, and (3) provisions must be made to collect the rinse water from contaminated patients to prevent contamination of the facility and water supply. At most facilities the best place to begin initial treatment and

evaluation is outdoors. Portable decontamination facilities are available, but their cost may be prohibitive for many institutions. A practical alternative is to have a warm shower nozzle, soap, and a wading pool available outside the entrance to the ED. A tent or screen can provide privacy.

The first priority in decontaminating patients is to remove their clothing while both maintaining privacy and preventing hypothermia. This step is the most important in the decontamination process and can reduce the level of contaminant by 75% to 90%. Cut the clothes off rather than pulling them off if possible. Place all clothing and valuables in labeled bags, as mentioned earlier. Brush off solids with a soft brush or towel. Irrigate the skin with copious amounts of warm water and cleanse the skin with soap. Although some agents (e.g., metallic sodium, potassium, cesium, and rubidium) may react with water, it is still more beneficial to immediately irrigate and decontaminate the skin than to delay treatment. Starting from head to toe, irrigate the exposed skin and hair for 10 to 15 minutes. Scrub with a soft surgical sponge while being careful to not abrade the skin. Irrigate wounds for an additional 5 to 10 minutes with water or saline. Remove contact lenses and irrigate the eyes for 10 to 15 minutes with saline. Direct irrigation away from the medial canthus to avoid forcing contaminants into the lacrimal duct. With strongly alkaline substances, irrigate for longer times. Irrigate the nares and ear canals with frequent suctioning if contamination is suspected. Clean underneath the fingernails with a brush. Avoid using stiff brushes and abrasives because they may enhance dermal absorption of the toxin and can produce skin lesions that may be mistaken for chemical injuries. Sponges and disposable towels are effective alternatives.

Secondary triage should occur after decontamination. Transfer patients with major or moderate injuries to areas designated for such cases. Send patients with minor or no injuries to appropriate holding areas for further evaluation. Medical care at this stage depends on the toxin to which the patient has been exposed and the potential toxicity of that agent. Wounds, after copious irrigation, may need thorough exploration and possibly surgical removal of the contaminant.

For the ED to care for contaminated patients, protocols should be in place and be regularly rehearsed by the facility. Train staff in the procedures and protocols, establish communication between community agencies and hospitals, regularly inspect equipment, and rehearse setups. Obtain template protocols from both the peer-reviewed medical literature and the government literature if needed.[115,116] For example, guidelines for managing HAZMAT incidents are available from ATSDR. In addition, prompted by the 2001 terrorist attacks, the U.S. Department of Veterans Affairs and several policy experts have developed a "comprehensive hospital-wide emergency mass casualty decontamination program." This program has been applied at most Veterans Affairs medical centers and has been demonstrated to be a cost-effective protocol suitable for implementation at other U.S. hospitals.[117]

References are available at www.expertconsult.com

CHAPTER 43

Peritoneal Procedures

Michael S. Runyon and †John A. Marx

Paracentesis and diagnostic peritoneal lavage (DPL) constitute the two primary intraperitoneal procedures. They are fundamentally similar in purpose and design; however, the former is generally reserved for medical concerns and the latter for evaluation of traumatic pathology.

DPL

Root and colleagues introduced DPL in 1964.[1] It has withstood the passage of several decades and remains a useful diagnostic adjunct for the management of penetrating torso trauma. Following a blunt mechanism of injury, its greatest utility is as a triage tool in the assessment of hemodynamically unstable, multiply injured patients. The intent is to rapidly discover or exclude the presence of intraperitoneal hemorrhage (IPH). The advent and availability of ultrasound (US) in the emergency department (ED) have rendered this purpose complementary to that of US in the diagnostic armamentarium of emergency clinicians evaluating blunt trauma patients.[2]

Though commonly referred to as diagnostic peritoneal *lavage*, this procedure has two distinct components: peritoneal aspiration and peritoneal lavage. Peritoneal aspiration, in which an attempt is made to retrieve free intraperitoneal blood, precedes lavage. A finding of intraperitoneal blood is a marker for intraperitoneal organ injury and obviates the need for subsequent lavage. In the lavage portion, normal saline is introduced by catheter into the peritoneal cavity, recovered by gravity, and analyzed for evidence of significant intraperitoneal injury.

Peritoneal lavage can be used as a therapeutic tool in patients with hypothermia and as a means of removing toxins.[3] It has also been used as a diagnostic instrument for suspected intraabdominal infection and nontraumatic sources of hemorrhage.[4,5] Although the steps of the procedure are the same regardless of the indication, the primary use of DPL is to determine the need for laparotomy after trauma, and this chapter focuses on that indication.

Indications

Blunt Trauma

Before the advent of computed tomography (CT) and US, DPL was the sole diagnostic option to supplement physical examination for predicting the need for operative intervention (Table 43-1). It was integral to both reduction of unnecessary laparotomies and discovery of unsuspected and life-threatening intraabdominal hemorrhage in patients with significant closed-head injury.[6,7]

This procedure may be undertaken by the emergency physician, but its use is not mandated and often relegated to the trauma service or consulting surgeon. In a number of respected

---

†Deceased.

Diagnostic Peritoneal Lavage

Indications
Rapidly determine presence of intraperitoneal hemorrhage
Determine the presence of hollow viscus injury
Determine diaphragmatic violation

Contraindications
When clinical mandates for urgent laparotomy already exist

Complications
Infection, hematoma, and dehiscence
Solid organ or hollow viscus injury
Vascular injury

Equipment

Semi-open technique

Antiseptic | Sterile drape | Local anesthetic
11- and 15-blade scalpels | Peritoneal catheter and trocar
Army Navy retractors | Towel clips

Closed technique

Antiseptic | Sterile drape | Local anesthetic
11-blade scalpel
Syringe and needle | Flexible guidewire | Peritoneal catheter

Review Box 43-1 Diagnostic peritoneal lavage (semi-open and closed techniques): indications, contraindications, complications, and equipment.

centers in the United States, DPL continues to be a focal diagnostic instrument.[2,8] It serves two primary functions.[9] First, it can be used to rapidly determine or exclude the presence of IPH (Table 43-2). Thus, a patient with a critical closed-head injury, an unstable motor vehicle crash victim with multiple potential sources of blood loss, or a patient with

TABLE 43-1 Clinical Indications for Laparotomy after Blunt Trauma

MANIFESTATION	PITFALL
Unstable vital signs with strongly suspected abdominal injury	Alternative sources of shock
Unequivocal peritoneal irritation	Unreliable
Pneumoperitoneum	Insensitive; may be due to a cardiopulmonary source or invasive procedures (diagnostic peritoneal lavage, laparoscopy)
Evidence of diaphragmatic injury	Nonspecific
Significant gastrointestinal bleeding	Uncommon, unknown accuracy

From Marx J, Isenhour J. Abdominal trauma. In: Marx JA, Hockberger RS, Walls RM, et al, eds. *Rosen's Emergency Medicine: Concepts and Clinical Practice.* 6th ed. St. Louis: Mosby; 2006:509.

TABLE 43-2 Likelihood of Injury by Entry Site

	INTRAPERITONEAL	RETROPERITONEAL	DIAPHRAGM
Anterior abdomen	++	+	+
Flank	+	++	+
Back	+	++	+
Low chest	+	+	++

From Marx JA. Diagnostic peritoneal lavage. In: Ivatury RR, Cayten CG, eds. *The Textbook of Penetrating Trauma.* Baltimore: Williams & Wilkins; 1996:336.

pelvic fractures and retroperitoneal hemorrhage can be appropriately routed to lifesaving laparotomy.[10,11] Furthermore, given its exquisite sensitivity, a negative peritoneal aspiration allows the clinician to proceed to alternative management steps and the patient to forego unnecessary laparotomy. Second, DPL has been used in less exigent circumstances as a means of predicting solid or hollow visceral injury requiring laparotomy.[12,13] However, in this venue its sensitivity to the presence of hemorrhage may prompt unnecessary laparotomy in patients with self-limited lacerations of the liver, spleen,[14-17] or mesentery.[17] CT specifically evaluates all intraperitoneal structures, as well as the retroperitoneum, a region inaccessible to DPL. Because the resolution and the speed with which it can be undertaken have vastly improved, CT has become an invaluable adjunct in the management of blunt trauma and has largely replaced DPL in stable patients. It is most useful in identifying injury to solid organs with accompanying IPH and greatly assists nonoperative management of these injuries. The ability of CT to discern hollow viscus and pancreatic pathology has continued to improve as the modality has evolved.[11] With regard to hollow viscus injury, it is when serial clinical evaluations cannot be performed that gut

perforation leads to preventable mortality. This is especially true in patients with severe closed-head injury or high spinal cord injury, in whom physical assessment of the abdomen is quite compromised. It is for these express scenarios that some authorities recommend the performance of DPL. The clinician's concern for hollow viscus injury should be heightened if US or CT demonstrates minimal amounts of free intraperitoneal fluid without evidence of solid organ damage.[18]

Two paradigms have brought US to the forefront. First, this modality has been adopted as the primary triage instrument, in lieu of DPL, for the detection of IPH on the basis of identifying which pouches and gutters are filled with fluid.[19-21] Clinical success in this role has been mixed, with reported sensitivity for IPH of 65% to 95%.[22-28] In addition, to be useful in this role, a competent technician and interpreter and the appropriate equipment must be present in real time. It has been demonstrated that emergency clinicians and surgeons can be trained in this technique to a level of competence sufficient for this need.[29] In centers that rely on US, DPL should serve as a reliable study when US equipment is unavailable, performance of US is technically difficult, or the results of US are indeterminate, especially when the patient demonstrates hemodynamic compromise.

DPL is a readily available procedure that can be conducted rapidly in the safe confines of the ED. The ability to undertake CT in particular or, to a lesser extent, US in a similar manner requires careful consideration of the clinical circumstances, location of equipment, and capabilities of the personnel available (Fig. 43-1 and Table 43-3).[2,11]

Penetrating Trauma

The advent of DPL was seminal in the promotion of selective management for penetrating abdominal injury. Here its role is more dominant than for blunt trauma because of the far greater likelihood of occult injury to hollow viscera and the diaphragm after a penetrating mechanism.[30,31]

Instruments and missiles may penetrate the abdominal cavity via the anterior abdominal wall, flank, back, or low chest region.[32] The intraperitoneal space is vulnerable if penetration occurs as high as the fourth intercostal space anteriorly and the sixth or seventh space laterally and posteriorly because the diaphragm may rise to these levels in the expiratory phase of respiration.[33] Coincident thoracic penetration occurs in up to 46% of patients with abdominal injuries.[34-36] The likelihood of retroperitoneal injury increases when the entry site is over the flank or back, but the prospect of intraperitoneal pathology remains considerable, with cited incidences of up to 43% for the flank and 14% for the back (Table 43-4).[37-39]

Stab Wounds

Because only one fourth to one third of patients who sustain stab wounds to the anterior aspect of the abdomen require laparotomy, diagnostic algorithms are used to decrease the rate of unnecessary surgery.[30,35,40] An optimal approach would not sacrifice sensitivity for morbid intraperitoneal injury. A pathway using a combination of clinical mandates, local wound exploration, and DPL is well established (Fig. 43-2).[41] These clinical mandates are reasonably accurate predictors of significant intraperitoneal injury (Table 43-5). Thus, the presence of one or more mandates suggests the need for urgent laparotomy and precludes the undertaking of other diagnostic studies.

BLUNT ABDOMINAL TRAUMA ALGORITHM

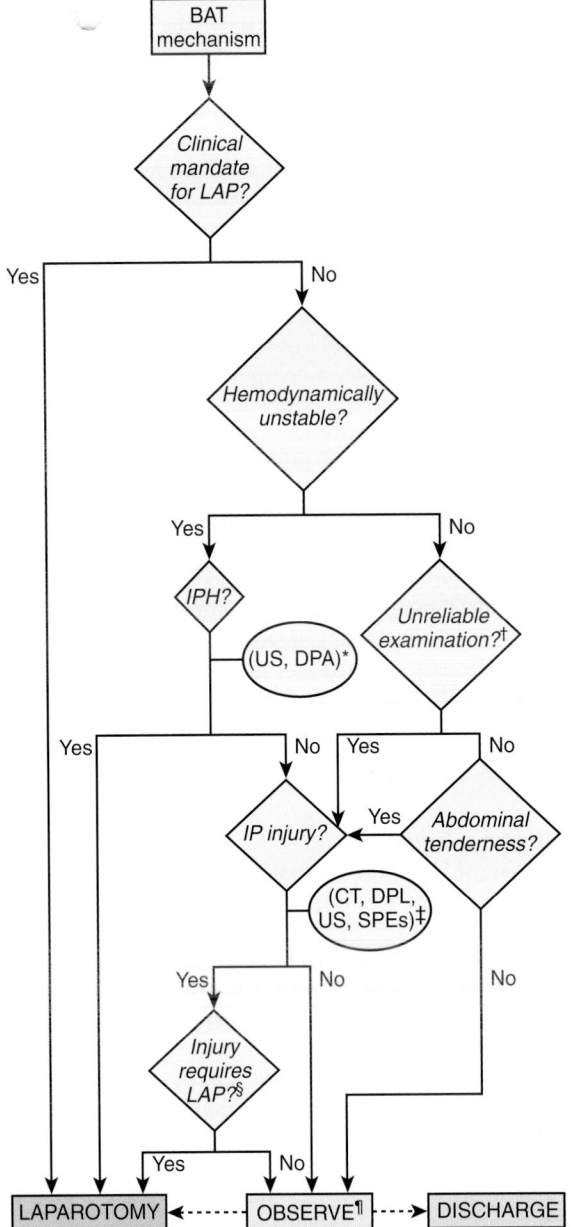

Figure 43-1 Algorithm for blunt abdominal trauma (BAT). *Determined by unequivocal free IP fluid on US or positive peritoneal aspiration on DPA. †May be unreliable because of closed-head injury, intoxicants, distracting injury, or spinal cord injury. ‡One or more studies may be indicated. §The need for LAP is based on the clinical scenario, diagnostic studies, and institutional resources. The duration of observation should be 6 to 24 hours, depending on whether diagnostic tests have been performed, the results of the tests, and clinical circumstances, including the absence of factors rendering the examination unreliable. *CT,* computed tomography; *D/C,* discharge; *DPA,* diagnostic peritoneal aspiration; *DPL,* diagnostic peritoneal lavage; *IP,* intraperitoneal; *IPH,* intraperitoneal hemorrhage; *LAP,* laparotomy; *SPE,* serial physical examination; *US,* ultrasound. *(From Marx J, Isenhour J. Abdominal trauma. In: Marx JA, Hockberger RS, Walls RM, et al, eds.* Rosen's Emergency Medicine: Concepts and Clinical Practice. *6th ed. St. Louis: Mosby; 2006:508.)*

DPL fills three roles in the evaluation of patients with abdominal stab wounds (see Table 43-2): (1) rapid determination of the presence of hemoperitoneum, (2) discovery of intraperitoneal injury requiring surgery in stable patients, and (3) establishment of diaphragmatic violation. As is the case in blunt trauma patients, DPL can be invaluable as a rapid triage tool when the source of hemodynamic instability is not known. Pericardial tamponade, intrathoracic hemorrhage, and IPH may be contributory to hemodynamic instability or wholly causal. Again, as for blunt trauma evaluation, US is the only bedside diagnostic modality for IPH that is competitive

TABLE 43-3   Diagnostic Studies in Patients with Blunt Abdominal Trauma

SCENARIO	STUDY PURPOSE	PRIMARY STUDY	ALTERNATIVE OR COMPENSATORY
Hemodynamically Unstable			
General	IPH	US	DPA
Pelvic fracture	IPH	US	DPA*
Hemodynamically Stable			
General	OI†‡	CT	SPEs, DPL
Nonoperative management§	OI	CT‖	SPEs, DPL¶
CHI	OI, HVI	CT,‖ DPL¶	SPEs**
BAI	IPH	US, DPL	CT††

Adapted from Marx J, Isenhour J. Abdominal trauma. In: Marx JA, Hockberger RS, Walls RM, et al, eds. *Rosen's Emergency Medicine: Concepts and Clinical Practice.* 6th ed. St. Louis: Mosby; 2006:507.
BAI, blunt aortic injury; *CHI,* closed-head injury; *CT,* computed tomography; *DPA,* diagnostic peritoneal aspiration; *DPL,* diagnostic peritoneal lavage; *HVI,* hollow viscus injury; *IPH,* intraperitoneal hemorrhage; *OI,* organ injury; *SPEs,* serial physical examinations; *US,* ultrasonography.
*A positive peritoneal aspirate mandates laparotomy; a positive red blood cell count warrants attention only to the pelvic fracture.
†To discover fluid or blood suggesting injury.
‡US for OI is much less reliable than for IPH.
§Institutional capability should be carefully considered.
‖CT is less reliable for HVI than for solid visceral injury.
¶Complementary to CT if HVI is suspected.
**SPEs are unreliable in patients with CHI.
††May be more appropriate if helical CT is the primary study for BAI or can be acquired rapidly.

TABLE 43-4   Likelihood of Injury by Entry Site

	INTRAPERITONEAL	RETROPERITONEAL	DIAPHRAGM
Anterior abdomen	++	+	+
Flank	+	++	+
Back	+	++	+
Low chest	+	+	++

From Marx JA. Diagnostic peritoneal lavage. In: Ivatury RR, Cayten CG, eds. *The Textbook of Penetrating Trauma.* Baltimore: Williams & Wilkins; 1996:336.

in this role, and it carries the added advantage of scanning for intrapericardial and intrathoracic hemorrhage.[35] In determining injury after stab wounds, DPL has 90% accuracy.[42-44] Serial examinations,[45-47] CT, and laparoscopy[48-51] are alternative modalities in specific circumstances and centers.[52] The diaphragmatic rents created by stab wounds are generally small; thus, at the outset they do not create apparent clinical or radiologic abnormalities.[53,54] However, morbidity from delayed herniation of bowel is common and substantive.[55] Physical examination is notoriously insensitive and DPL is currently the most sensitive means of discerning this injury in the immediate posttrauma phase.[42] There is some evidence that coronal reconstruction of CT images provides greater sensitivity for detecting small diaphragmatic tears, and as CT technology continues to evolve, it may surpass DPL for evaluation of these subtle injuries.[56] For these small wounds, magnetic resonance imaging may be diagnostic, but because of safety and accessibility concerns, it should be reserved for the nonacute phase of management. Laparoscopy has demonstrated promise in experienced hands.[48,49]

Gunshot Wounds

Injury to multiple organs is the rule after gunshot wounds, and mortality is significantly greater than after stab wounds.[52] The diagnostic approach is more conservative for gunshot wounds because in some studies the likelihood of intraperitoneal injury requiring operative intervention has exceeded 90% when the projectile has entered the intraperitoneal cavity (Fig. 43-3).[57] If clinical mandates are met (see Table 43-5) or if peritoneal violation has occurred, most centers proceed to laparotomy.[41] One series, however, cited intraabdominal injury in 70% to 80% of cases, thus supporting the contention that nonoperative management could be applied to a substantial percentage of patients.[58] In a separate cohort of 152 patients sustaining solid organ injury from penetrating abdominal trauma (70% gunshot wounds and 30% stab wounds), 27% were successfully managed without laparotomy after selection by a protocol combining clinical examination and CT scanning.[59] DPL is reserved for two circumstances: (1) the wound tract is neither obviously superficial nor intraperitoneal, and (2) penetration occurred in the low chest region, where diaphragmatic injury is more likely yet the possibility of intraperitoneal injury also exists.

ANTERIOR ABDOMEN STAB WOUND ALGORITHM

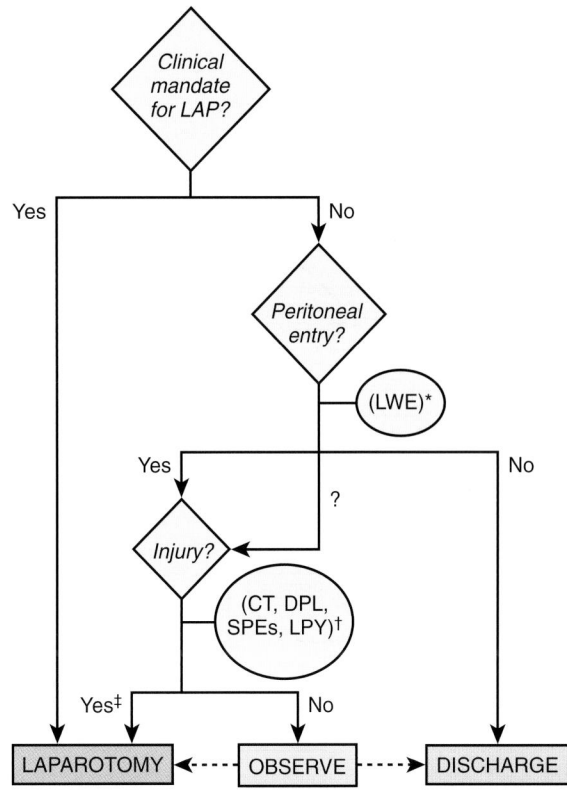

Figure 43-2 Algorithm for anterior abdominal stab wounds. *Plain films, ultrasonography, LPY, and CT can also assess peritoneal entry. †CT, DPL, SPEs, or LPY can be used in singular or complementary fashion depending on the clinical scenario. ‡Expectant management of injuries is infrequently attempted. *CT,* computed tomography; *D/C,* discharge; *DPL,* diagnostic peritoneal lavage; *LAP,* laparotomy; *LPY,* laparoscopy; *LWE,* local wound exploration; *SPE,* serial physical examination. *(From Marx J, Isenhour J. Abdominal trauma. In: Marx JA, Hockberger RS, Walls RM, et al, eds.* Rosen's Emergency Medicine: Concepts and Clinical Practice. *6th ed. St. Louis: Mosby; 2006:503.)*

TABLE 43-5 Clinical Indications for Laparotomy after Penetrating Trauma		
MANIFESTATION	**PREMISE**	**PITFALL**
Hemodynamic instability	Major solid visceral or vascular injury	Thorax, mediastinum
Peritoneal signs	Intraperitoneal injury	Unreliable, especially immediately after injury
Evisceration	Additional bowel, other injury	No injury in one fourth to one third of stab wound cases
Diaphragmatic injury	Diaphragmatic herniation	Rare clinical, radiographic findings
Gastrointestinal and vaginal hemorrhage	Proximal gut or uterine injury	Uncommon, unknown accuracy
Impalement in situ	Vascular impalement	High operative risk, pregnancy
Intraperitoneal air	Perforation of a hollow viscus	Insensitive; may be caused by intraperitoneal entry only or be due to a cardiopulmonary source

Modified from Marx JA. Diagnostic peritoneal lavage. In: Ivatury RR, Cayten CG, eds. *The Textbook of Penetrating Trauma.* Baltimore: Williams & Wilkins; 1996.

ABDOMINAL GUNSHOT WOUND ALGORITHM

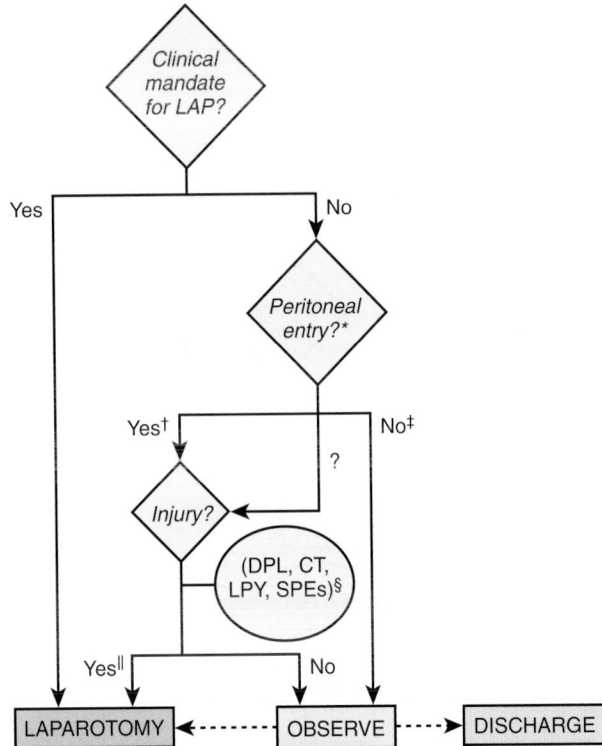

Figure 43-3 Algorithm for abdominal gunshot wounds. *Can be assessed by the path of the missile, plain films, local wound exploration, ultrasonography, and LAP. †Most centers proceed to LAP if peritoneal entry is suspected. ‡Patients with documented superficial and low-velocity injuries can be discharged; high-velocity injuries or those of unknown depth require further tests or observation. § DPL, CT, LPY, or SPEs can be used in singular or complementary fashion depending on the clinical scenario. Expectant management of injuries caused by gunshot wounds is rarely attempted. *CT*, computed tomography; *D/C*, discharge; *DPL*, diagnostic peritoneal lavage; *LAP*, laparotomy; *LPY*, laparoscopy; *SPE*, serial physical examination. *(From Marx J, Isenhour J. Abdominal trauma. In: Marx JA, Hockberger RS, Walls RM, et al, eds. Rosen's Emergency Medicine: Concepts and Clinical Practice. 6th ed. St. Louis: Mosby; 2006:506.)*

Contraindications

DPL can be undertaken in virtually any patient irrespective of age or comorbid illness. Adjustment of the technique and site of performance allows relative contraindications to be overcome. Relative contraindications include previous abdominal surgery or infections, obesity, coagulopathy, and second- or third-trimester pregnancy. The sole absolute contraindication is when clinical mandates for urgent laparotomy already exist.

Procedure

Decompress the stomach and bladder to prevent inadvertent injury. Place the patient in the supine position and administer sedatives and analgesics as appropriate. Perform DPL according to compliance with standards for body fluid precautions. Observe sterile technique throughout the procedure. Before making the skin incisions described later, prepare the site with standard skin antiseptics and drape appropriately.

Prophylactic antibiotics are not indicated for routine DPL because local and systemic infections are rare.[60]

Infiltrate the area for incision and dissection with a local anesthetic such as 1% lidocaine *with* epinephrine (Fig. 43-4, *step 1*). Delay the incision for more than 30 seconds after infiltration of local anesthetic to permit local vasospasm, which minimizes bleeding of the wound during the procedure.

Placement of the Catheter

There are two basic methods for DPL: open and closed. The two open techniques are *semi-open* and *fully open*, and both typically require an assistant. DPL is clearly within the diagnostic armamentarium of the emergency clinician and surgeon. Either may undertake it in keeping with clinical policies established at the particular trauma center.

Semi-open Technique

Make a skin incision 4 to 6 cm in length with a No. 11 scalpel blade. Using Army-Navy retractors, proceed with blunt dissection to expose the *rectus fascia* (Fig. 43-4, *steps 2 and 3*). With the infraumbilical incision in the midline, continue blunt dissection until the *linea alba* is seen. Its crossing bands of crural fibers may be apparent.[61] Make a small 2- to 3-mm opening in the linea alba with a No. 15 scalpel blade (Fig. 43-4, *step 4*). You may notice a tough, gritty sensation when cutting the linea alba with the scalpel. Place towel clips through this opening to grasp each side of the rectus fascia (Fig. 43-4, *step 5*). Ask an assistant to lift the two towel clips and carefully advance the catheter and trocar in a 45- to 60-degree caudad orientation. Proceed through the peritoneum into the peritoneal cavity (see Fig. 43-4, *steps 6 and 7*).[62]

One method to decrease the likelihood of penetrating any underlying viscera is to hold the fingers low on the catheter/trocar instrument such that on entering the abdominal peritoneum, the fingers prevent deep penetration. Excessive pressure during penetration with the trocar is a common error. Apply steady one-finger pressure to the handle sufficient to "pop" through the peritoneum. After controlled peritoneal penetration of 0.5 to 1.0 cm in the midline, retract the trocar 1.0 to 2.0 cm within the catheter, and advance the catheter carefully toward the pelvis. Some operators advance the catheter toward the right or left side of the pelvis. Use a slight twisting motion during advancement to minimize visceral or omental injury.

The fully open technique extends the semi-open technique by one step. Lengthen the opening in the linea alba to open the peritoneum, and use direct visualization to advance the catheter into the peritoneal cavity. The trocar is unnecessary with the open technique.

The two open techniques can be accomplished by a single technician, but it is useful to have an assistant help with retraction and handling of the instruments. The fully open method is the more technically demanding and time-consuming. Reserve this method for clinical circumstances in which neither the closed nor the semi-open technique is deemed safe or they have been attempted and failed. Examples of such circumstances include pelvic fracture, pregnancy, previous abdominal surgery, adhesions, infections, and obesity.

Closed Technique

For the closed technique, introduce the catheter into the peritoneal space in a blind percutaneous fashion.[63] Use the simple Seldinger (guidewire) method, in which a small-gauge

DIAGNOSTIC PERITONEAL LAVAGE: SEMI-OPEN TECHNIQUE

1 Anesthetize the skin with lidocaine with epinephrine.

2 Make a 4- to 6-cm infra-umbilical midline skin incision with a No. 11 scalpel.

3 Using Army-Navy retractors, bluntly dissect to the linea alba.

Subcutaneous fat
Rectus fascia
Army-Navy retractor

4 Make a small 2- to 3-mm opening in the linea alba with a No. 15 scalpel blade.

5 Place towel clips through this opening to grasp and lift each side of the rectus.

Towel clamps lift peritoneum
Traction
Incision

6 Advance the catheter and trocar 45° to 60° caudally into the peritoneum.

Traction

7 Retract the trocar within the catheter, and advance the catheter toward the pelvis.

8 Withdraw the trochar and aspirate for blood using a 10-cc syringe.

9 If lavage is necessary, infuse 1 L of warm normal saline and recover under gravity.

Figure 43-4 Semi-open technique of diagnostic peritoneal lavage. Note that the stomach and bladder have been decompressed under most circumstances.

guide needle is inserted into the peritoneal cavity in the midline just inferior to the umbilicus (Fig. 43-5, *step 2*). Pass a flexible wire through the needle (Fig. 43-5, *step 3*), and remove the needle but not the wire. Advance a soft catheter over the wire and into the peritoneal cavity. Make a small stab with a No. 11 scalpel blade at the entry site of the wire to allow easier passage of the catheter through the abdominal wall (Fig. 43-5, *step 4*). Rotate the catheter while pushing it over the guidewire to facilitate entry into the peritoneal cavity. Place the catheter into the right or left pelvic gutter.

Always control the guidewire to avert intraabdominal migration of the wire. Withdraw the wire and aspirate for blood with a 10-mL syringe. Follow this with peritoneal lavage when necessary. Proponents of the guidewire technique promote its ease and rapidity.[64-68] Those who prefer the semi-open method argue that the time until peritoneal aspiration, the more critical interval, is minimally different and that this method may have fewer complications and thus be more accurate than the guidewire technique.[69-73] Note that for both the semi-open and closed approaches, the time until aspiration is performed should be no more than 2 to 5 minutes.

Site

The optimum location for DPL is at the infraumbilical ring at the inferior border of the umbilicus (Table 43-6). Here, between the rectus abdominis muscles there is adherence of the peritoneum and relative lack of vascularity and preperitoneal fat.[61] Closed DPL should always be conducted here. In the event of second- or third-trimester pregnancy, a suprauterine approach is used. If midline scarring is present, a fully open technique at the lateral border of the rectus abdominis in the left lower quadrant may be necessary. The left side is preferred to avoid later confusion about whether an appendectomy has been performed. It is interesting to note that Moore and associates found no increase in complications or misclassified lavage when the closed technique was used in a small series of patients with previous abdominal surgery.[74] In the presence of a pelvic fracture, use a fully open supraumbilical approach. This greatly decreases the likelihood of passing the catheter through a retroperitoneal hematoma that has dissected from the fracture anteriorly and across the abdominal wall.[75] In patients with penetrating trauma, do not perform DPL through the stab or missile entry site. This approach can contaminate the intraperitoneal cavity, potentially exacerbate

the abdominal wall bleeding, and lead to a false-positive result.

Aspiration and Lavage

Once the catheter has been placed successfully into the peritoneal cavity, attach the right-angle adapter, extension tubing, and a non–Luer-Lok syringe and attempt aspiration (see Fig. 43-4, *step 8*). If 10 mm of blood is aspirated, the test is positive and the procedure is terminated. With penetrating trauma, acquisition of lesser amounts may be meaningful because of the tendency for the diaphragm and bowel to hemorrhage minimally when injured. However, no rules have been established in this regard.

If little to no blood is aspirated, lavage the peritoneal cavity with either normal saline or lactated Ringer's solution (see Fig. 43-4, *step 9*). Apply a blood pressure cuff or blood infusion pump around the plastic intravenous (IV) bag to speed the influx (i.e., decrease lavage time) if necessary. Large-bore infusion tubing (e.g., urologic irrigation tubing sets, such as the Abbott No. 6543 cystoscopy/irrigation set) also shortens fluid influx time. Infuse 1 L of fluid in adults or 15 mL/kg in children. When possible, roll or shift the patient from side to side after the infusion to increase mixing. Place the IV bag or bottle on the floor (or below abdominal level), and allow the fluid to return by gravity.

If the fluid does not return, there may be several reasons. Some IV tubing contains a one-way valve. If tubing with a valve was used in error, replace it with valveless tubing and reattach it to the IV bag. Another reason for poor return is inadequate suction. To correct this problem, insert a needle into the second opening at the bottom of the IV bag or into the head of the IV bottle for aspiration of 10 mL of air. Alternatively, the catheter may be adherent to the peritoneum. If so, try to relieve some of the pressure in the IV bottle by gently wiggling and twisting the catheter or applying abdominal pressure to aid in the return of flow.

Return of 700 mL or more in an adult is generally accepted as adequate for interpretation of the findings. However, as little as 10% to 20% of the infusate may give a representative sample for both gross and microscopic determination. Send 10 mL of fluid from the return to the laboratory for cell count analysis, and send another 10 mL for enzyme analysis (see the section "Interpretation" later in this chapter). Some operators prefer to leave the catheter in place until the returned fluid is analyzed so that lavage may be repeated if the initial results are borderline or an occult bowel perforation is suspected.

Complications

Local and Systemic

Local wound complications, including infection, hematoma, and dehiscence, occurred in only 0.3% of patients in two large series.[42,76] Dehiscence with evisceration is an even rarer condition.[77] Systemic infection has been described rarely (Table 43-7).

Intraperitoneal

Iatrogenic intraperitoneal injury can be inflicted by the trocar, wire, and rarely, the catheter. Virtually any structure in the peritoneal cavity can be breached, including the small and large bowel, the bladder, and major vessels. Typically, if the needle is the culprit and even if the trocar is responsible,

TABLE 43-6 Preferred Site for DPL		
CLINICAL CIRCUMSTANCE	**SITE**	**METHOD**
Standard adult	Infraumbilical midline	C or SO
Standard pediatric	Infraumbilical midline	C or SO
Second- and third-trimester pregnancy	Suprauterine	FO
Midline scarring	Left lower quadrant	FO
Pelvic fracture	Supraumbilical	FO
Penetrating trauma	Infraumbilical midline*	C or SO

C, closed; *DPL*, diagnostic peritoneal lavage; *FO*, fully open; *SO*, semi-open.
*The stab wound or gunshot wound site should be avoided.

injury to these structures is minimal and self-limited, and observation of the patient is sufficient.

Technical Failure

Inability to recover peritoneal aspirate or lavage fluid can result in a false-negative interpretation. This can occur in several circumstances. It follows unwitting placement of the catheter into the preperitoneal space, which is less likely to occur with either open technique. Compartmentalization of fluid by adhesions or obstructing omentum can impede the egress of fluid. When a fully open supraumbilical or suprauterine technique is used, the catheter may be too short to access the depths of the intraperitoneal cavity. Finally, the large diaphragmatic tears typical of blunt pathophysiology allow flow of lavage fluid from the intraperitoneal to the thoracic cavity. Saunders and coworkers compared percutaneous DPL and the open technique in a prospective, randomized trial.[78] Fluid obtained by the two techniques had similar test performance for intraabdominal pathology. The open technique took, on average, more than 4 minutes longer, but the percutaneous approach had an 11.2% technical failure rate (versus 3.8% with the open approach).

DIAGNOSTIC PERITONEAL LAVAGE: CLOSED TECHNIQUE

1 Anesthetize the skin with lidocaine with epinephrine.

2 Access the peritoneal cavity with a needle and syringe in the infra-umbilical midline.

3 Guidewire — Pass the guidewire through the needle into the peritoneum and remove the needle.

4 Guidewire — Make a small stab with a No. 11 scalpel blade at the site of entry of the wire. Small puncture

5 Pass the catheter over the guidewire and into the peritoneal cavity. Direct the catheter into the left or right pelvic gutter.

6 Withdraw the wire and aspirate for blood with a 10-mL syringe.

7 If lavage is necessary, infuse 1 L of warm normal saline and recover under gravity.

Figure 43-5 Closed technique of diagnostic peritoneal lavage. Note that the stomach and bladder are decompressed under most circumstances.

TABLE 43-7   Complications of DPL

CATEGORY	COMMENTS
Local and Systemic	
Hematoma incision site	Local wound care
Dehiscence incision site	Local wound care
Local wound infection	As indicated
Systemic infection	As indicated
Intraperitoneal Injury	
Bowel	Observe, usually self-limited
Bladder	Observe, usually self-limited
Vascular	Observe, usually self-limited
Technical Failure	
*Inability to Recover Fluid**	
Preperitoneal catheter placement	Repeat DPL
Compartmentalization of fluid	US, CT
Obstructed catheter	Gentle catheter manipulation
Diaphragm injury	Reverse Trendelenburg; consider US, CT
"Short" catheter (supraumbilical or suprauterine approach)	Trendelenburg
Intraperitoneal Hemorrhage†	
Iatrogenic injury	As indicated by clinical markers
Stab wound, abdominal wall bleeding	As indicated by clinical markers
Pelvic fracture (RBC count)	Complementary CT

CT, computed tomography; *DPL*, diagnostic peritoneal lavage; *RBC*, red blood cell; *US*, ultrasound.
*May lead to false-negative DPL results.
†May lead to false-positive DPL results.

TABLE 43-8   Diagnostic Peritoneal Lavage RBC Criteria (per mm³)

	POSITIVE	INDETERMINATE
Blunt trauma	100,000*	20,000-100,000
Stab wound		
Anterior abdomen	100,000	20,000-100,000
Flank	100,000	20,000-100,000
Back	100,000	20,000-100,000
Low chest	5000-10,000	1000-5000
Gunshot wound	5000-10,000	1000-5000

From Marx J, Isenhour J. Abdominal trauma. In: Marx JA, Hockberger RS, Walls RM, et al, eds. *Rosen's Emergency Medicine: Concepts and Clinical Practice*. 6th ed. St. Louis: Mosby; 2006:500.
RBC, red blood cell.
*In a hemodynamically stable patient with a pelvic fracture and a positive or equivocal red blood cell count, computed tomography should be obtained to corroborate or refute intraperitoneal injury.

False-positive findings can occur in two ways. First, iatrogenic misadventure may be responsible. Second, in penetrating trauma, particularly stab wounds, bleeding from the abdominal wall injury site into the peritoneal cavity can lead to positive findings when no injury to intraperitoneal structures has occurred.[44]

Interpretation

Gross Blood

Recovery of 10 mL or more of blood via aspiration is considered a positive finding. Aspirates with lesser volume are generally discarded and are not factored into analysis of the lavage fluid. Grossly bloody aspirates are typically indicative of solid visceral or vascular injury, with a positive predictive value of greater than 90%.[79,80] Aspiration of blood is responsible for approximately 80% of true-positive DPL findings with blunt trauma and for 50% with stab wounds.[43]

A positive aspiration in a blunt trauma patient who is hemodynamically stable or has been resuscitated to apparent stability need not mandate urgent surgery. Unnecessary laparotomy will occur if there has been minimal and self-limited damage to the liver, spleen, bowel serosa, or mesentery.[81] In this situation, CT and clinical indicators should be used in concert with the findings on DPL.

RBC Count

The recommended red blood cell (RBC) threshold varies according to the mechanism and, in the case of stab wounds, the external site of injury (Table 43-8). The optimum criterion will deliver excellent sensitivity, a high positive predictive value, and a minimal incidence of unnecessary laparotomy. Negative laparotomy incurs a prolongation of hospitalization and increases the cost of care, in addition to creating the potential for procedural complications.[82,83] RBC counts greater than $10^5/mm^3$ ($10^5/\mu L$) are generally considered positive with a blunt mechanism or after stab wounds in the anterior part of the abdomen, flank, or back. Counts of 20,000 to 100,000/mm³ should be considered indeterminate.[43,45,84,85] For stab wounds in the low chest region, where the diaphragm is at increased risk for injury, the RBC criterion should be lowered to 5000/mm³ to maximize sensitivity for isolated injury to this structure.[36,43,86,87] With gunshot wounds involving the abdomen or low chest region, the same RBC criterion of 5000/mm³ is applied. This is intended to increase the sensitivity of the test because intraperitoneal entry by a missile carries a 90% or greater likelihood of intraperitoneal injury.[36,60,88] An uncomplicated DPL should not result in more than several hundred to several thousand RBCs in the peritoneal lavage fluid.

The incidence of false-positive RBC interpretation in the setting of pelvic fracture is considerable. However, aspiration of free blood in patients with critical pelvic fractures predicts active IPH in more than 80% of cases. A positive RBC count should generally prompt corroboration or refutation of intraperitoneal injury by CT. In this fashion, needed pelvic angiography and embolization will not be delayed unnecessarily

PELVIC FRACTURE AND BLUNT ABDOMINAL TRAUMA ALGORITHM

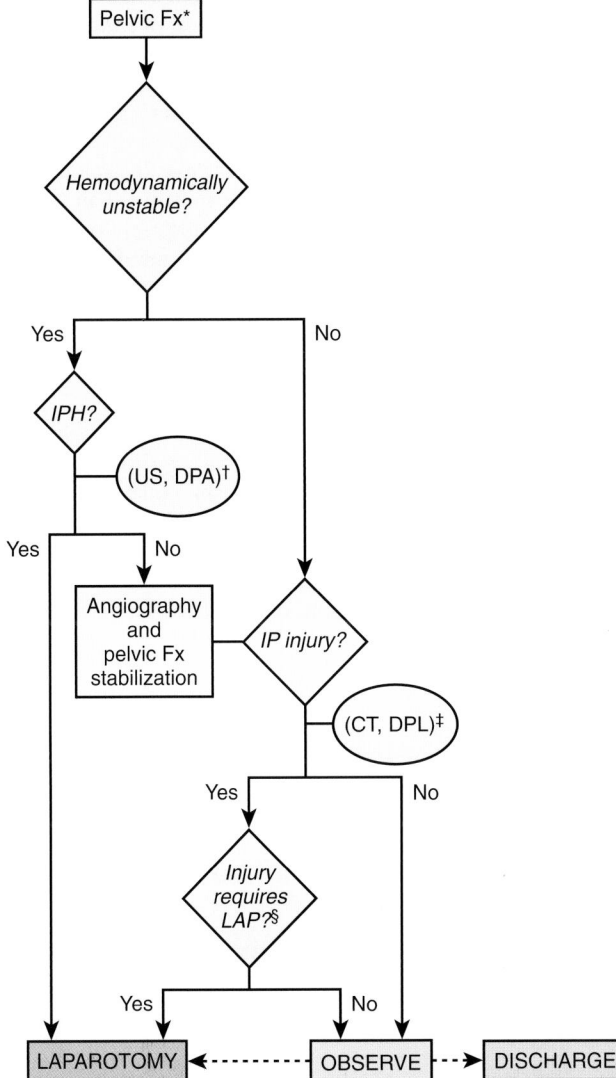

Figure 43-6 Algorithm for the management of pelvic fractures and blunt abdominal trauma. *Certain pelvic fractures are more likely to cause pelvic vascular disruption and subsequent retroperitoneal hemorrhage. †Determined by unequivocal free intraperitoneal fluid on US or positive peritoneal aspiration on DPA. ‡One or more studies may be indicated. SPEs are generally considered unreliable because of the presence of a pelvic fracture. §The need for LAP is based on the clinical scenario, diagnostic studies, and institutional resources. ¶D/C from the perspective of need for further consideration for LAP. *CT*, computed tomography; *D/C*, discharge; *DPA*, diagnostic peritoneal aspiration; *DPL*, diagnostic peritoneal lavage; *Fx*, fracture; *IP*, intraperitoneal; *IPH*, intraperitoneal hemorrhage; *LAP*, laparotomy; *SPE*, serial physical examination; *US*, ultrasonogram. (*From Marx J, Isenhour J. Abdominal trauma. In: Marx JA, Hockberger RS, Walls RM, et al, eds.* Rosen's Emergency Medicine: Concepts and Clinical Practice. *6th ed. St. Louis: Mosby; 2006:510.*)

should active intraperitoneal bleeding not be found (Fig. 43-6).

WBC Count

An inflammatory peritoneal response to a multitude of stimuli can occur, including stool, blood, and enzymes.[89] The white blood cell (WBC) count in lavage effluent was formerly touted

TABLE 43-9 DPL Non–RBC Criteria		
	POSITIVE	**INDETERMINATE**
LAM (IU/L)	>20	10-19
LAP (IU/L)	≥3	NA
WBCs (per mm³)	>500	250-500

From Marx JA. Diagnostic peritoneal lavage. In: Ivatury RR, Cayten CG, eds. *The Textbook of Penetrating Trauma.* Baltimore: Williams & Wilkins; 1996:337. *DPL*, diagnostic peritoneal lavage; *LAM*, lavage amylase; *LAP*, lavage alkaline phosphatase; *NA*, not applicable; *RBC*, red blood cell; *WBCs*, white blood cells.

to predict small bowel injury but has since been proved unreliable.[90] It is insensitive in the immediate postinjury period because 3 to 5 hours is necessary before the test becomes positive (Table 43-9).[91,92] Moreover, a positive finding is likely to be falsely so.[91,93] Therefore, the WBC level in and of itself should not determine the need for laparotomy.

Enzymes

Alkaline phosphatase is contained intramurally in the small bowel, as well as in hepatobiliary secretions released into the proximal part of the intestine. Amylase is contained in the latter only. Perforation of the small bowel allows access of these two markers to the peritoneal cavity, where they can be recovered by peritoneal lavage.[94-96] Although levels of the two markers usually rise in tandem, lavage amylase has been shown to be a more accurate marker than lavage alkaline phosphatase (see Table 43-9). In contradistinction to the WBC count, these tests will be positive in the immediate postinjury period. However, they may not be economical if used on a mandatory rather than a selective basis. Neither is helpful in discerning the presence of pancreatic pathology.

Miscellaneous

Routine bile staining, Gram staining, and microscopy to identify vegetable fibers are rarely productive and are of untested accuracy. Deck and Porter reported that finding urine in the lavage fluid, as evidenced by a straw color, and creatinine in the peritoneal fluid should suggest an intraperitoneal bladder or collecting system injury.[97]

Conclusion

In the current era of readily available advanced imaging techniques such as CT and US, DPL maintains a diminished, but important role in the evaluation of injured patients. It can identify life-threatening IPH in unstable patients when US is unavailable, indeterminate, or negative for free fluid. In addition, DPL can identify hollow viscus injury when CT is nondiagnostic in patients in whom serial clinical evaluations are impractical or unreliable, as in those with severe traumatic brain and spinal cord injuries. Finally, DPL remains more accurate than CT in identifying occult diaphragmatic injuries and is useful in high-risk patients without other indications for surgical abdominal exploration. It should be used in commonsense fashion. The noted laboratory parameters are guidelines and should not be embraced to the exclusion of pertinent clinical features. Optimal strategies depend largely on the capability of an institution's resources and personnel in each clinical scenario.

PARACENTESIS

Therapeutic abdominal paracentesis is one of the oldest medical procedures and dates to approximately 20 BC. Paracentesis was first described in the modern medical literature by Saloman at the beginning of the 20th century, and it became a valued decompressive therapy.[98] With the advent of diuretics in the early 1950s, paracentesis fell out of favor as a treatment option. Controlled clinical trials in the late 1980s up to the present have restored its reputation by demonstrating the safety and efficacy of large-volume paracentesis (LVP) in adults and children.[99-105] Because this mode is invasive and consumes clinician hours, it is generally reserved for the treatment of patients with chronic ascites who have tense ascites or whose condition is refractory to diuretic therapy.[102] However, paracentesis remains an important diagnostic agent for patients with new-onset ascites or to determine the presence of worrisome conditions, notably infection, in those with preexistent ascites.[106]

Clinical Features

Determination of Ascites

Small amounts of ascites may be asymptomatic. Larger collections typically cause a sense of abdominal fullness, anorexia, early satiety, and perhaps nausea and abdominal pain. Substantial accumulations create symptoms of respiratory distress by virtue of restricting lung capacity.[107]

The most predictive history and physical examination findings for excluding the diagnosis of ascites are the absence of ankle swelling and increased abdominal girth and an inability to demonstrate bulging flanks, flank dullness, or shifting dullness.[108] Positive predictors for the diagnosis are a positive fluid wave, shifting dullness, or peripheral edema.[108,109]

Patients who lack obvious clinical markers may benefit from the performance of US, which can discern the presence of as little as 100 mL of fluid.[110] Endoscopically guided US may detect as little as 10 mL. It is more sensitive than CT in this respect and can assist in the identification of malignancy.[111] In addition, it is a useful adjunct for determining the location of fluid that may be compartmentalized by preexistent infection or surgical adhesions.

Differential Diagnosis

Causes of ascites can be categorized in several ways. On a structural basis the causes are divided into diseases of the peritoneum and diseases not involving the peritoneum. The former group includes infection, neoplasm, collagen vascular disease, and idiopathic causes. The latter includes cirrhosis, congestive heart failure, nephrotic syndrome, protein-losing enteropathy, malnutrition, myxedema, pancreatic disease, ovarian disease, chylous effusion, Budd-Chiari syndrome, and hepatic venous occlusive disease. Pathophysiologic categories are listed in Box 43-1. In the United States, parenchymal liver pathology is overwhelmingly the most likely cause. Within this group, alcoholic liver disease is responsible for

---

Abdominal Paracentesis

Indications

New onset ascites
Suspected spontaneous bacterial peritonitis
To relieve the cardiorespiratory and gastrointestinal
   manifestations of tense ascites

Contraindications

Uncorrected coagulopathy AND clinically evident fibrinolysis
   or disseminated intravascular coagulation
Bowel dilation or obstruction
Pregnancy (technique should be altered as noted below)
Abdominal hematoma, engorged veins, or superficial infection
   at puncture site

Complications

Systemic
Hyponatremia
Renal dysfunction
Hepatic encephalopathy
Hemodynamic compromise
Significant bleeding
Death

Local
Persistent ascitic fluid leak
   at the wound site
Abdominal wall hematoma
Localized infection

Intraperitoneal
Perforation of vessels and viscera
Generalized peritonitis
Abdominal wall abscess

Equipment

Antiseptic

Sterile drape

Local anesthetic

Over-the-needle catheter system

18g 1.5" needle

3.5" spinal needle

Large syringe

High pressure tubing

Evacuated container

Review Box 43-2 Abdominal paracentesis: indications, contraindications, complications, and equipment.

approximately 80% of cases (Table 43-10).[112] Finally, ascites can be classified on the basis of a serum-ascites albumin gradient, that is, the difference between albumin values obtained simultaneously from serum and ascites samples (Box 43-2).[113]

Indications and Contraindications

Therapeutic paracentesis is often undertaken in the ED setting to relieve the cardiorespiratory and gastrointestinal manifestations of tense ascites.[114-116] LVP, or removal of more than 5 L, ameliorates the shortness of breath and early satiety that these patients experience. It may also be associated with collateral advantages, such as a reduction in hepatic venous pressure gradients, intravariceal pressure, and variceal wall tension. These parameters are considered important predictors of variceal bleeding, and the improvement after LVP may decrease the risk for bleeding. Diagnostic paracentesis, often relegated to inpatient services, is indicated in any patient whose ascites is of new onset or to disclose the presence of infection in patients with known or suspected ascites, particularly in the context of alcohol-related cirrhotic liver disease.[117,118] Diagnostic paracentesis is also useful in the management of patients with acquired immunodeficiency syndrome (AIDS), in whom the etiology of ascites will be non–AIDS related in three quarters of cases.[119] There are few relative contraindications to abdominal paracentesis. Certain systemic and anatomic risks should be considered, however.

Systemic

Given the predominance of alcohol-related cirrhotic liver disease as the cause of ascites, as many as two thirds to three quarters of patients who undergo paracentesis will have a coagulopathy. However, the only prospective study that evaluated the complications of paracentesis determined that transfusion-requiring abdominal hematomas occurred in less than 1% of cases despite the fact that 71% of the patients had

an abnormal prothrombin time (PT).[120] Because transfusion-requiring hematoma is so unlikely, even in this population, prophylactic administration of fresh frozen plasma or platelets is not standard, nor mandated, and imposes considerable cost, in addition to the risk for posttransfusion hepatitis, with little net gain.[121] Therefore, for patients undergoing repeated therapeutic paracentesis, in the absence of previous problems or obvious clotting issues, obtaining a platelet count and international normalized ratio (INR) before the procedure is not routine. In an investigation of 628 patients undergoing outpatient LVP, the procedure was safely performed when the PT INR was as high as 8.7 (mean value, 1.7) and the platelet count as low as 19,000/mm^3 (mean value, 50/mm^3).[122] These data countermand older and more conservative recommendations to administer platelets to patients with levels of less than

---

BOX 43-2 Classification of Ascites by the Serum-Ascites Albumin Concentration Gradient

HIGH GRADIENT (≥1.1 G/DL)	LOW GRADIENT (<1.1 G/DL)
Cirrhosis	Peritoneal carcinomatosis
Alcoholic hepatitis	Tuberculous peritonitis
Cardiac ascites	Pancreatic ascites
Massive liver metastases	Biliary ascites
Fulminant hepatic failure	Nephrotic syndrome
Budd-Chiari syndrome	Serositis in connective tissue
Portal vein thrombosis	diseases
Venous occlusive disease	
Fatty liver of pregnancy	
Myxedema	
Mixed ascites	

From Runyon BA. Ascites. In: Schiff L, Schiff ER, eds. Diseases of the Liver. *7th ed. Philadelphia: Lippincott-Raven; 1993:997.*

BOX 43-1 Pathophysiologic Classification of Ascites

I. Elevated hydrostatic pressure
  A. Cirrhosis
  B. Congestive heart failure
  C. Constrictive pericarditis
  D. Inferior vena cava obstruction
  E. Hepatic vein obstruction (Budd-Chiari syndrome)
II. Decreased osmotic pressure
  A. Nephrotic syndrome
  B. Protein-losing enteropathy
  C. Malnutrition
  D. Cirrhosis or hepatic insufficiency
III. Fluid production exceeding resorptive capacity
  A. Infections
    1. Bacterial
    2. Tuberculosis
    3. Parasitic
  B. Neoplasms

From Runyon BA. Diseases of the peritoneum. In: Wyngaarden JB, Smith LH, eds. Cecil Textbook of Medicine. 18th ed. Philadelphia: Saunders; 1988:790-793.

TABLE 43-10 Causes of Ascites*

CAUSE	PATIENTS (%)
Parenchymal liver disease	80
"Mixed"	5
Malignancy	10
Heart failure	5
Tuberculosis	2
Pancreatic	1
Nephrogenous ("dialysis ascites")	<1
Chlamydia	<1
Nephrotic	<1
Surgical peritonitis in the absence of liver disease	<1

From Runyon BA. Ascites and spontaneous bacterial peritonitis. In: Sleisenger MH, Fordtran JS, eds. *Gastrointestinal Disease: Pathophysiology/Diagnosis/Management.* 5th ed. Philadelphia: Saunders; 1993:1977.
*Based on a series of 1500 paracenteses performed in a predominantly inpatient hepatology/general internal medicine setting (B. A. Runyon, unpublished observations).

50,000/mm³ or to give fresh frozen plasma to those with a PT exceeding 20 seconds (1.5 times the therapeutic level).[123] These blood products should be reserved for clinically evident fibrinolysis and disseminated intravascular coagulation.

Anatomic

Structural impediments to the safe introduction of a paracentesis needle can include the bladder, bowel, and pregnant uterus. The bladder is normally tucked into the recess of the pelvis. However, bladders that are neuropathologically distended as a result of pharmacologic agents or medical conditions should preferably be emptied by voiding or by catheterization to avoid puncture. The intestines typically float in ascitic fluid and will move safely away from a slowly advancing paracentesis needle.[123] Therefore, US guidance may be indicated in cases of suspected adhesions or bowel obstruction. Even if penetrated by an 18- to 22-gauge needle, leakage of intestinal contents will not occur unless intraluminal pressure is 5- to 10-fold greater than normal conditions.[124] In second- and third-term pregnancy, an open supraumbilical or US-assisted approach is preferred. The abdomen should be inspected carefully for evidence of abdominal hematoma, engorged veins, or superficial infection, and these sites should be strictly avoided.

Technique

Preliminary Actions

Paracentesis should be performed after the patient has voided. It is not standard to decompress the stomach with a nasogastric tube or the bladder with a catheter before paracentesis. Place the patient in the supine position. The supine lateral decubitus position is preferred by some clinicians. Perform paracentesis according to compliance with standards for body fluid precautions. Observe sterile technique throughout the procedure to prevent the iatrogenic introduction of bacteria into the abdominal wall tract or peritoneal cavity. Before making the skin incisions described later, prepare the site with standard skin antiseptics and drape appropriately.

Site of Entry

The best site of entrance for repeated paracentesis is determined by the patient's previous experience, so this question should be asked of the patient. Theoretically, most sites on the abdominal wall can be used, but in absence of previous experience with the individual patient, two sites are preferred. One site is approximately 2 cm below the umbilicus in the midline (Fig. 43-7), where the fasciae of the rectus abdominis muscle join to form the fibrous, thin, avascular linea alba. Large collateral veins may occasionally be present and should be avoided (Fig. 43-8), as should suspected areas of skin infection. If the patient has midline scarring or if previous experience has been positive, the preferred alternative site is in either the right or left lower quadrant, approximately 4 to 5 cm cephalad and medial to the anterior superior iliac spine (see Fig. 43-7). The importance of remaining lateral to the rectus sheath is to avoid the inferior epigastric artery. Patients with a large quantity of ascites can readily undergo the procedure in the supine position with the head of the bed slightly elevated. Those with lesser amounts of fluid may benefit from a lateral decubitus position with introduction of the needle into the midline or dependent lower quadrant (Fig. 43-9). Some clinicians prefer to use the lateral decubitus position

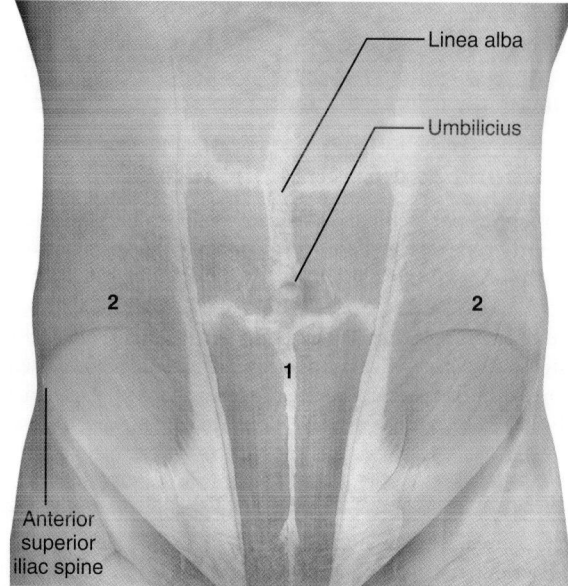

Figure 43-7 The best site for drainage of recurrent ascites is based on success in previous similar procedures on the patient or ultrasound evaluation. The following are the preferred sites for paracentesis. *1,* The primary site is infraumbilical in the midline through the linea alba. *2,* The preferred alternative (lateral rectus) site is in either lower quadrant, approximately 4 to 5 cm cephalad and medial to the anterior superior iliac spine.

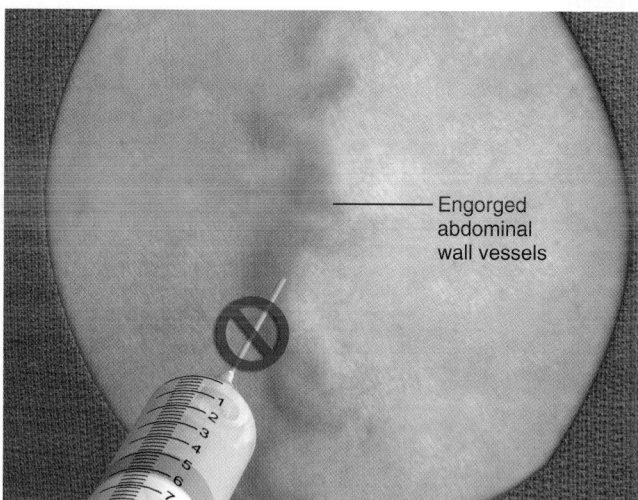

Figure 43-8 Avoid sites on the abdominal wall with engorged veins.

routinely because the bowel tends to float upward and away from the path of the needle. Hence, the site of needle entrance is in the midline or on the side closest to the bed. Rarely, patients may need to be placed in a facedown, hands-on-knees position.[120] In patients with multiple abdominal scars or suspicion of compartmentalized abdominal fluid for any reason, US guidance is prudent.[125]

Procedure

A prepackaged kit, such as the Saf-T-Centesis system, is a convenient way to perform the procedure (Fig 43-10). Following sterile preparation of the skin, inject local anesthetic at the paracentesis site (Fig. 43-11, *step 4*). Use a standard

Figure 43-9 An alternative to the sitting or supine position for diagnostic or therapeutic needle paracentesis is to place the patient in the lateral decubitus position. In this example the midline is aspirated, although lateral rectus sites may also be used. Some prefer the lateral decubitus position routinely because the bowel tends to float upward and out of the path of the needle. Note the cloudy fluid seen with spontaneous bacterial peritonitis. The patient had vague abdominal pain only, a subtle manifestation of a serious problem.

Red safety indicator

Pig-tail catheter

Blunt-tipped obturator needle

Figure 43-10 Paracentesis can be performed with a prepackaged kit. The Saf-T-Centesis system depicted here includes safety features such as a blunt-tipped obturator needle, a color-changing indicator, and a pigtail catheter. The blunt-tipped obturator needle retracts with pressure to expose the sharp needle tip. This causes the color in the device to change from white to red. Once the abdominal cavity is entered and there is no longer pressure on the tip, the spring-loaded obturator covers the sharp tip of the needle to prevent damage to the underlying organs. This will cause the color to revert back to white.

3.8-cm (1.5-inch) metal needle in most cases. If necessary, use a longer 8.9-cm (3.5-inch) spinal needle in obese patients. Plastic sheath cannulas tend to kink and run the risk of being sheared off into the peritoneal cavity, but a steel needle can be left in the abdomen during a therapeutic tap for intervals of an hour or longer without injury. The 15-gauge, 3.25-inch Caldwell needle/cannula is an alternative for LVP that has been shown to perform similar to a steel needle in terms of

procedural complications and the volume of fluid removed.[126] Use a smaller-gauge (20- to 22-gauge) needle for diagnostic taps because such needles lessen the likelihood of leakage of ascitic fluid through the wound site after the procedure. However, for therapeutic LVP, use an 18-gauge needle because it permits expeditious outflow.[104,127]

Insert the needle directly perpendicular to the skin at the preferred site (Fig. 43-11, *step 5*). Alternatively, use the "Z-tract" method. For this method, pull the skin approximately 2 cm caudad to the deep abdominal wall with the non–needle-bearing hand while slowly inserting the paracentesis needle (Fig. 43-12). Release the skin when the needle has penetrated the peritoneum and fluid flows. This technique also holds the draining needle in place without suture or tape. Remove the needle after the procedure, and the skin will slide to its original position and help seal the tract. In any case, insert the needle slowly in 5-mm increments to detect undesired entry of a vessel and to help prevent unnecessary puncture of the small bowel. Avoid continuous suction because it may attract bowel or omentum to the end of the paracentesis needle with resultant occlusion. Once fluid is flowing, stabilize the needle to ensure a steady flow. If flow ceases, gently rotate the needle and advance it inward in 1- to 2-mm increments. When fluid removal is complete, remove the needle and place an adhesive bandage over the puncture site. If there is persistent leakage of fluid, a pressure bandage may be required.

Ultrasound Guidance

US-guided paracentesis may be performed by a radiologist or an experienced emergency clinician ultrasonographer (see the specific US box in this chapter). This technique clearly delineates the pocket of ascitic fluid and allows visualization of loculated collections and avoidance of bowel adherent to the anterior abdominal peritoneum. The ultrasonographer scans the abdomen and marks the skin at the point overlying the optimal puncture site (see Fig. 43-11, *step 2*). Once the entry site is marked, keep the patient immobile and perform the procedure (as detailed previously) as soon as practical to avoid shifting of the fluid, which may decrease the utility of US guidance.

Volume of Fluid Removed

Many patients with chronic ascites are well versed on the procedure and have experienced it many times. Some undergo paracentesis on a regular basis in the outpatient setting. Therefore, the best guide to the volume of fluid to be removed for recurrent ascites is based on the patient's previous experience, and this question should be asked. Up to 5 or 6 L is routine and well tolerated, and for therapeutic purposes, at least this volume should be removed. Patients seen in the ED are probably less compliant with outpatient regimens and seek care only when in extremis. Hence, their ascites is likely to be much more voluminous than in those treated regularly. In general, the paracentesis volume consists of as much fluid as can be removed without excessive manipulation of the patient. Volumes greater than 5 L are termed LVP. Up to 10 to 12 L may be removed safely in most patients with chronic ascites (Fig. 43-13). For first-time paracentesis and for diagnostic purposes (ruling out bacterial peritonitis, screening for cancer), 200 to 500 mL is usually sufficient, but more can be drained if it flows easily.

ABDOMINAL PARACENTESIS

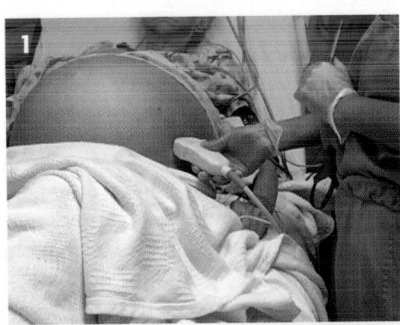

Localize the fluid collection by percussion or by ultrasound. Mark the entry site.

With ultrasound, identify free pockets of ascitic fluid, as well organs such as the liver, spleen, kidney, or bowel.

See details of ultrasound techniques at the end of this chapter.

Cleanse the overlying skin with antiseptic and apply a sterile drape.

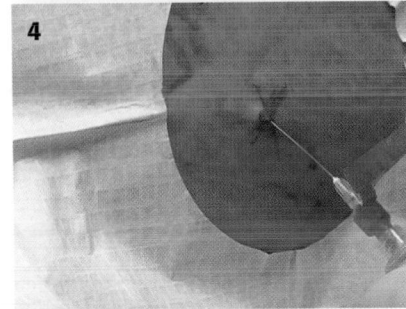

Anesthetize the skin and the proposed tract of the paracentesis needle with local anesthetic.

Insert the needle perpendicular to the skin and slowly advance.

See text and Figure 43-12 for details on the Z-tract method of paracentesis.

Advance the needle in 5-mm increments until fluid is returned in the syringe. Advance the catheter over the needle and into the peritoneal cavity (if a catheter-over-the-needle system is being used).

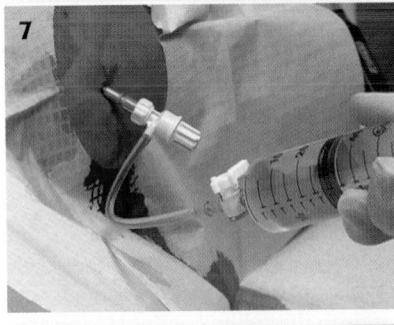

Aspirate peritoneal fluid into a 20- to 60-mL syringe for a diagnostic sample.

If large-volume (therapeutic) paracentesis is desired, attach the high-pressure tubing to the catheter hub.

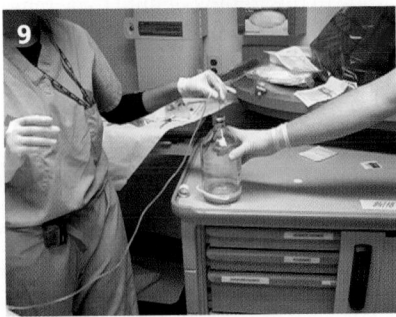

Insert the high-pressure tubing needle into the evacuated container to withdraw the fluid.

After fluid collection is completed, remove the catheter and apply an adhesive bandage (or a pressure dressing if there is persistent fluid leakage).

Figure 43-11 Abdominal paracentesis.

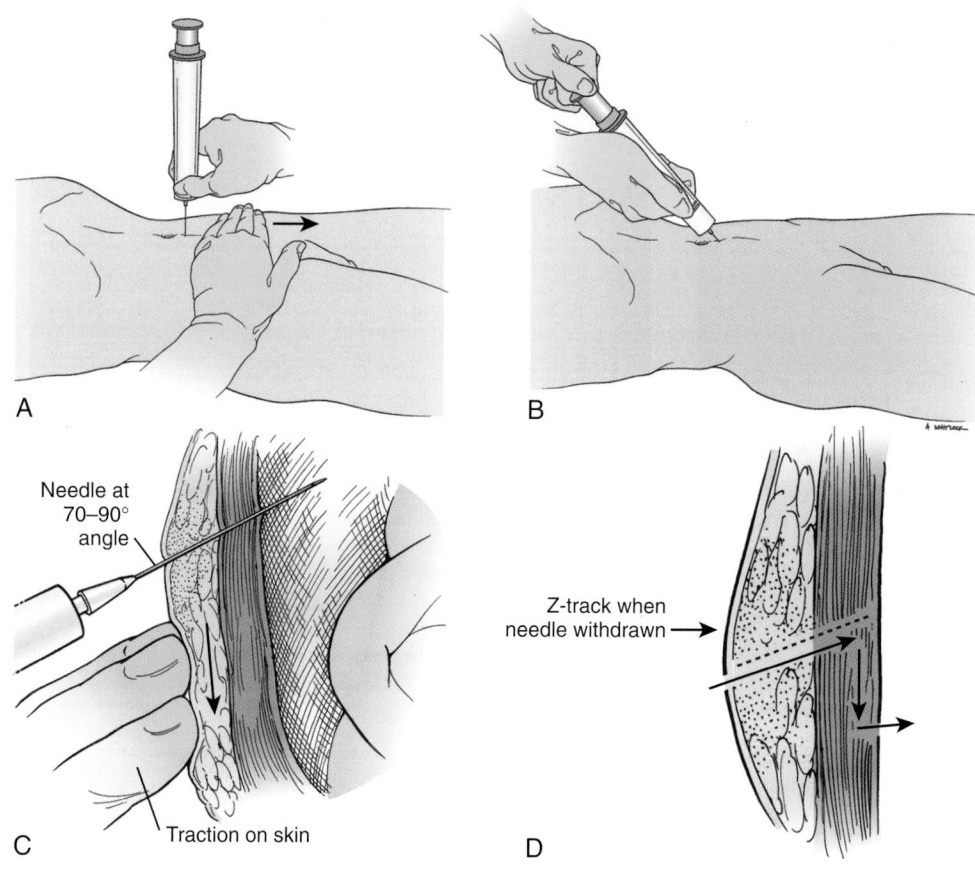

Figure 43-12 A, Z-tract method of needle paracentesis. Pull the skin approximately 2 cm caudad in relation to the deep abdominal wall with the non–needle-bearing hand while slowly inserting the paracentesis needle perpendicular to the skin. **B,** After penetrating the peritoneum and obtaining return of fluid, release the skin. Note that the needle is now angled caudally. **C** and **D,** Use of the Z-tract method helps seal the tract and prevent persistent fluid leaks.

 # ULTRASOUND: Abdominal Paracentesis   *by Christine Butts, MD*

Although paracentesis has traditionally been performed "blindly," use of ultrasound allows the physician to confirm the presence of ascites. Also, it allows the clinician to evaluate the most optimal location to attempt the procedure, which can be less straightforward in patients with smaller fluid collections or in whom physical examination alone is insufficient to make the diagnosis.

Equipment

Use a low-frequency transducer (2 to 5 mHz) to obtain a sufficient depth of penetration to visualize the area of interest. It is frequently helpful to set the initial depth to 20 to 25 cm to ensure that the entire abdomen is visualized.

Image Interpretation

The location of ascites is variable and depends on the amount of fluid present, as well as the position of the patient. The dependent areas of the abdomen, those evaluated with the focused abdominal sonography for trauma (FAST) examination, are ideal initial areas of evaluation. Evaluate the right upper quadrant by placing the transducer in either the transverse or the longitudinal orientation in the 8th to 11th intercostal space at the anterior axillary line (Fig. 43-US1). The transducer will probably need to be adjusted slightly to allow an optimal view of this area, either by moving up or down a rib space or by adjusting the angle of the transducer. Ascitic fluid will appear anechoic (black) and may be seen in Morison's pouch (in the hepatorenal space), near the inferior

aspect of the liver, or at the superior aspect of the liver (Fig. 43-US2). Once this area has been evaluated in detail, evaluate the left upper quadrant in much the same fashion. Because the spleen is typically slightly more superior and posterior than the liver, place the transducer in the 8th to 11th intercostal space in the posterior axillary line

Figure 43-US1 Placement of the ultrasound transducer in the right upper quadrant to evaluate for the presence of free fluid.

Continued

Figure 43-US2 Free fluid in the right upper quadrant. The liver can be seen as the hypoechoic (*dark gray*) object *on the left* of the image, with anechoic (*black*) fluid seen between the liver and kidney (*on the right* of the image).

Figure 43-US4 Free fluid in the left upper quadrant. Anechoic (*black*) free fluid can be seen surrounding the spleen at the right of the image. The diaphragm is seen as the bright white arcing structure on the far right of the image.

Figure 43-US3 Placement of the ultrasound transducer in the left upper quadrant to evaluate for the presence of free fluid.

Figure 43-US5 Placement of the ultrasound transducer to evaluate the pelvis for free fluid.

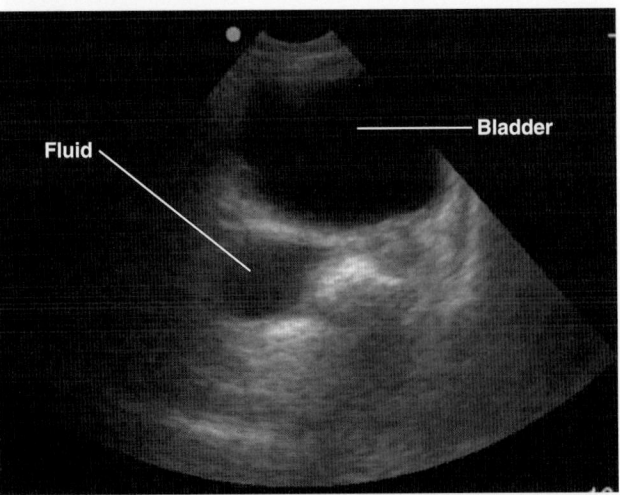

Figure 43-US6 In this ultrasound image of the pelvis, the bladder can be seen as the rectangular object filled with anechoic (*black*) urine. An area of free fluid can be seen posterior to the bladder.

(Fig. 43-US3). Again, make slight adjustments as needed to fully evaluate the area in question. Ascitic fluid will appear as anechoic (black) areas in the splenorenal space, as well as the potential space between the diaphragm and the spleen (Fig. 43-US4). Once these areas have been evaluated, look at the pelvis and lower part of the abdomen by placing the transducer just superior to the pubic symphysis (Fig. 43-US5). First identify the bladder to avoid any confusion. The bladder is typically seen as a well-demarcated area that is rectangular in shape in the transverse orientation and slightly triangular in shape in the longitudinal orientation (Fig. 43-US6). In contrast, free fluid will appear to have irregular borders and may seem to "seep" into the crevices of the lower part of the abdomen and pelvis. Additionally, bowel may be seen to float freely within free fluid (Fig. 43-US7). If free fluid is not appreciated in this area, evaluate the right and left aspects of the lower part of the abdomen as well. To do this, place the transducer in either the transverse or longitudinal orientation over the right and left lower quadrants, or near the areas

ULTRASOUND: Abdominal Paracentesis, cont'd

Figure 43-US7 Large area of free fluid seen with ultrasound. Bowel loops are seen to "float" within the fluid.

Figure 43-US8 Place the paracentesis needle at the site that ultrasound had previously identified as being free of bowel loops and containing a large amount of fluid.

where the traditional "blind" approach to paracentesis would be performed.

Procedure and Technique

Once free fluid has been seen, identify the area with the largest collection of fluid. Use ultrasound to identify the areas that contain the least number of loops of bowel. If the fluid collection appears to be large, use ultrasound to "mark the spot" and then put it aside. Proceed with the procedure in the typical sterile fashion in the area that has been identified and marked (Fig. 43-US8).

In cases in which the fluid collection is smaller, cover the transducer with a sterile cover to guide direct placement of the catheter.

Before

11.5 liters of fluid removed

After

Figure 43-13 Large-volume paracentesis in a patient with a history of recurrent ascites. See text for guidelines on the volume to remove and potential complications of removing large volumes. Note the use of blood pressure monitoring.

Complications

Complications of paracentesis can be divided into systemic, local, and intraperitoneal categories.

Systemic

Retrospective studies have suggested a risk for deterioration in hospitalized patients following LVP. However, the risk attributable to paracentesis is unclear given the difficulty in adjusting for the underlying severity of illness and comorbid conditions in these patients. The risk in ambulatory ED patients has not been investigated but is clearly less since paracentesis is often an outpatient procedure. Most systemic complications of paracentesis are merely temporally related or seen in seriously ill patients with end-stage liver failure who have a plethora of comorbidities.

Oft-cited but poorly documented concerns include hemodynamic compromise and other physiologic conditions caused by the overzealous removal of large volumes of ascitic fluid (greater than 5 L). This has been termed postparacentesis circulatory dysfunction (PCD), and it may occur in 15% to 20% of patients undergoing LVP. It may not occur for a number of hours or days after paracentesis and is characterized primarily by hypovolemia (often asymptomatic), hyponatremia, and impaired renal function. The actual clinical significance of the associated disorders is unclear. Hypotension, for example, is common after paracentesis and is often asymptomatic.

Because upward of 6 L has been reportedly removed in less than 15 minutes without complication, certain authorities decry this issue as folklore.[128] Others believe that rapid total paracentesis is accompanied by marked cardiovascular and humoral changes, some of which are explained by mechanical factors directly or indirectly related to relief of abdominal pressure.[129,130] Other changes, including systemic vasodilation and humoral deactivation, are of a nonmechanical nature. Hepatic encephalopathy, hyponatremia, hepatorenal syndrome, and rapid reaccumulation of ascitic fluid have also been ascribed to LVP. In the editor's clinical experience, PCD of varying degrees is a real syndrome, and it may occur more often than suspected because many patients are discharged after the procedure. The consequences of LVP in ED patients have not been well studied, and the implications are somewhat obscure in this subset of patients. Because many patients require therapeutic paracentesis on a regular basis, ask the patient about previous experience and the usual volume of fluid removed to help guide treatment.

Because fluid and electrolyte shifts tend to be minimal after the removal of large amounts of fluid,[131] colloid infusion is considered strictly optional by some for patients with paracentesis of more than 5 L and is universally *not recommended* for paracentesis of lesser volume.[106,132,133] Others support the routine administration of albumin if more than 5 L is removed. When colloid is indicated, albumin has been the de facto choice. Being a blood product, albumin has been associated with rare complications, including anaphylaxis. The recommended infusion is 6 to 8 g of IV albumin per liter of ascitic fluid removed, or 50 g.[132,134] However, colloid dextran 70 is favored by some authorities because of cost and concern for infection.[135-137]

The necessity of routine plasma expansion after LVP remains controversial. No study has shown a direct survival advantage of one expander over another or in comparison

to no expander. Postparacentesis plasma volume expansion does not prevent asymptomatic laboratory abnormalities. The mere fact that controversy still exists suggests that no clear indications can be promulgated to the emergency physician. The authors suggest *not* using IV albumin after taps of less than 5 L. We suggest that it may be used (6 to 8 g of albumin per liter of fluid removed, or 50 g) when more than 6 to 8 L is removed. Twenty-five percent albumin can be given if the patient is hypervolemic, whereas 5% albumin can be given if dehydration is suspected. If used, albumin is generally given immediately after the procedure, although administering it immediately before the procedure also seems reasonable.

Local

Local complications include persistent leakage of ascitic fluid at the wound site, abdominal wall hematoma, and localized infection. Persistent fluid leaks can be corrected with a single suture at the site of puncture.[127] An abdominal wall hematoma requiring transfusion is very uncommon, but careful observation in such cases is necessary.

Intraperitoneal

Intraperitoneal complications include perforation of vessels and viscera.[138] In experienced hands these complications are uncommon, and in most circumstances they are self-sealing and clinically inconsequential. However, generalized peritonitis and abdominal wall abscess have been reported after paracentesis in rare cases. The most common cause of postparacentesis IPH is bleeding as a result of a coagulopathy rather than large-vessel injury per se.[139]

Interpretation

Ascitic fluid should undergo gross inspection. Routine laboratory testing includes a differential cell count, albumin assay, and cultures (Box 43-3). The prevalence of occult infection of ascitic fluid in asymptomatic outpatients undergoing therapeutic LVP for resistant ascites is low. As a result, in the absence of concerning symptoms or cloudy fluid, routine laboratory tests and culture of fluid during outpatient or ED paracentesis are not warranted.

BOX 43-3   Ascitic Fluid Laboratory Data to Be Obtained on Patients with Ascites

ROUTINE	UNUSUAL
Cell count	Tuberculosis smear and culture
Albumin	Cytology
Culture in blood culture bottles	Triglyceride
	Bilirubin

OPTIONAL	UNHELPFUL
Total protein	pH
Glucose	Lactate
Lactate dehydrogenase	Cholesterol
Amylase	Fibronectin
Gram stain	

From Runyon BA. Ascites. In: Schiff L, Schiff ER, eds. Diseases of the Liver. 7th ed. Philadelphia: Lippincott-Raven; 1993:997.

TABLE 43-11 Ascitic Fluid Characteristics in Various Disease States

CONDITION	GROSS APPEARANCE	SPECIFIC GRAVITY	PROTEIN (g/dL)	CELL COUNT		OTHER TESTS
				RBCs (>10,000/μL)	WBCs/μL (WBCs/mm³)	
Cirrhosis	Straw colored or bile stained	<1.016 (95%)*	<25 (95%)	1%	<250 (90%),* predominantly mesothelial	
Neoplasm	Straw colored, hemorrhagic, mucinous, or chylous	Variable, >1.016 (45%)	>25 (75%)	20%	>1000 (50%); variable cell types	Cytology, cell block, peritoneal biopsy
Tuberculous peritonitis	Clear, turbid, hemorrhagic, or chylous	Variable, >1.016 (50%)	>25 (50%)	7%	>1000 (70%); usually >70% lymphocytes	Peritoneal biopsy, stain and culture for acid-fast bacilli
Pyogenic peritonitis	Turbid or purulent	If purulent, >1.016	If purulent, >2.5	Unusual	>250; mainly polymorphonuclear leukocytes	Positive Gram stain, culture
Congestive heart failure	Straw colored	Variable, <1.016 (60%)	Variable, 15-53	10%	<1000 (90%); usually mesothelial, mononuclear	
Nephrosis	Straw colored or chylous	<1.016	<25 (100%)	Unusual	<250; mesothelial, mononuclear	If chylous, ether extraction, Sudan staining
Pancreatic ascites (pancreatitis, pseudocyst)	Turbid, hemorrhagic, or chylous	Variable, often >1.016	Variable, often >25	Variable, may be blood stained	Variable	Increased amylase in ascitic fluid and serum

From Glickman RM, Isselbacher KJ. Abdominal swelling and ascites. In: Isselbacher KJ, Braunwald E, Wilson JD, et al. eds. *Harrison's Principles of Internal Medicine*. 13th ed. New York: McGraw-Hill; 1994:234.
RBC, red blood cell; *WBC*, white blood cell.
*Because the conditions of examining fluid and selecting patients were not identical in each series, the percentages (in parentheses) should be taken as an indication of the order of magnitude rather than as the precise incidence of any abnormal finding.

Inspection

Ascitic fluid is typically translucent and yellow. A dark greenish brown hue may reflect biliary perforation. Cloudy fluid generally indicates particulate matter, including neutrophils; fluid with WBC counts greater than 5000/μL (i.e., >5000/mm³) are cloudy, and those greater than 50,000/μL are purulent. An opaque, milky appearance may indicate elevated triglyceride levels.[140] A blood-tinged appearance requires at least 10,000 RBCs/μL. This may reflect an iatrogenic complication, malignancy, hemorrhagic pancreatitis, or tuberculous peritonitis, although the last diagnosis creates hemorrhagic-appearing fluid in less than 5% of cases.[120]

Cell Count

Several milliliters of ascitic fluid is sufficient to obtain a differential cell count. Cirrhotic ascites should generally contain less than 250 WBCs/μL (Table 43-11). However, because cells may exit through the peritoneal cavity more slowly than fluid does, the WBC count can rise in the ascitic fluid during the procedure.[141] Thus, an upper limit for uncomplicated cirrhotic ascites is reported as 500 cells/μL.[142-144] Lymphocytes should predominate, and clinical signs or symptoms of peritoneal infection should be absent.[145] In cases in which

spontaneous bacterial peritonitis is a clinical consideration, the WBC criterion is 250/μL with greater than 50% polymorphonuclear leukocytes.[115,117,145,146]

Albumin

A serum-ascites albumin gradient can be obtained by simultaneously measuring albumin in ascites and serum and calculating the gradient. A serum-ascites albumin gradient greater than 1.1 g/dL indicates portal hypertension with greater than 95% accuracy (see Box 43-2).[147-149]

Culture and Gram Stain

The most valuable method for determining the presence of infection is culture. The sensitivity of this test is markedly increased by direct inoculation of blood culture bottles at the bedside as opposed to simply delivering the ascitic fluid to the laboratory.[150,151] Gram staining of peritoneal fluid is rarely helpful in the evaluation of ascites.[118] Approximately 10 bacteria/μL of fluid is required for a positive Gram stain. Thus, the Gram stain is notoriously insensitive in patients with spontaneous bacterial peritonitis, in whom the medium concentration of bacteria is 10^{-3} organisms/μL of fluid.[152] Gram stain can be expected to be helpful only in cases of free gut perforation.

Miscellaneous

Optional tests include measurement of total protein, glucose, lactate dehydrogenase, and amylase. These tests will be beneficial in selected circumstances and need not be obtained on a routine basis. Immunosuppressed patients, including those with AIDS, should undergo microbiologic testing for opportunistic infections, including tuberculosis.[119] Cytologic analysis is recommended in patients with suspicious constitutional symptoms and signs.[152,153] Triglyceride and bilirubin studies are indicated if the gross appearance of the fluid is suggestive of increased levels.[154]

Medical Therapy and Disposition

Total paracentesis may be performed safely in the ED, even in cirrhotic patients with large volumes of ascitic fluid (>5 L). However, the immediate relief provided by the procedure is temporary, and medical therapy is indicated to prevent or slow the reaccumulation of fluid. Measures include reduction of dietary sodium intake (<2000 mg/day) and the use of diuretics (spironolactone and furosemide) to promote natriuresis. It is prudent to observe patients undergoing LVP in the ED for 2 to 4 hours for hemodynamic compromise. In the absence of other indications for hospital admission, these patients may then be managed in the outpatient setting with close follow-up to ensure adequacy of their medical regimen. Overall, the clinician should base the decision to admit or discharge on the initial scenario, individual patient characteristics, and response to paracentesis.

Chronic Ambulatory Peritoneal Dialysis

Patients undergoing chronic ambulatory peritoneal dialysis are at an increased risk for peritonitis because of the presence of a chronic indwelling peritoneal catheter. Culture yield is maximized by obtaining a sample of greater than 10 mL of the peritoneal effluent under sterile conditions after a dwell time of at least 2 to 4 hours.[155,156] Peritonitis is defined by cloudy fluid with more than 100 WBCs/mm^3 and greater than 50% polymorphonuclear cells.[156] Although Gram stain is often negative in patients with bacterial peritonitis, it may reveal the presence of yeast and prompt timely initiation of antifungal therapy. Intraperitoneal antibiotics are superior to IV dosing, and removal of the catheter may be required for refractory or recurrent infections. Initial, empirical intraperitoneal therapy usually includes a first-generation cephalosporin along with an aminoglycoside, ceftazidime, cefepime, or carbapenem.[156] Vancomycin should be considered in patients with a previous history of methicillin-resistant *Staphylococcus aureus* colonization or infection, in those who are seriously ill, or in areas with an increased local rate of methicillin resistance. The optimal treatment strategy should be discussed with the consulting nephrologist.

Acknowledgment

This chapter is dedicated to the memory of John A. Marx, MD, editor, author, educator, researcher, leader, humanitarian, and friend.

References are available at www.expertconsult.com

Abdominal Hernia Reduction

Michael T. Fitch and David E. Manthey

When a patient is seen in the emergency department (ED) with a suspected abdominal hernia, the emergency clinician must consider three issues: (1) Is a palpable mass truly a hernia? (2) Is the hernia easily reducible or incarcerated? (3) Is the vascular supply to the bowel strangulated? A patient with an easily reducible hernia can be discharged safely for outpatient follow-up and elective repair, whereas incarcerated and strangulated hernias are a surgical emergency. Some seemingly incarcerated hernias can be reduced by careful manipulation in the ED. Any patient with symptoms of bowel obstruction should also be evaluated for the possible presence of an abdominal hernia (Fig. 44-1).[1]

Hernias in the groin area have been the subject of medical diagnosis and treatment as long ago as 1550 BC. Throughout history, treatment of this condition has been the focus of ongoing discussion and debate.[2-7] This chapter addresses abdominal and groin hernias, which are amenable to diagnosis and potential manual reduction in the ED. These types include ventral hernias of the abdominal wall, direct and indirect groin hernias, femoral hernias, and pantaloon hernias.

BACKGROUND

A *hernia* is defined as protrusion of any viscus from its normal cavity through an abnormal opening. Abdominal hernias are characterized by protrusion of intraabdominal contents (usually bowel, with or without mesentery) through an abnormal defect in the abdominal wall musculature. Hernias can develop along a congenital tract that fails to close (e.g., indirect inguinal hernia) or along an area of weakness in the muscular and fascial wall layers (e.g., direct inguinal hernia or incisional hernia). This weakness may be due to aging and the accompanying loss of tissue elasticity, increased intraabdominal pressure, or trauma involving the abdominal wall itself. It is estimated that hernias develop in 5% of the male population and 2% of the female population[8,9] and that 75% of them occur in the groin.[10] In children and young adults, the majority of hernias are indirect inguinal hernias of congenital origin,[11] whereas direct hernias are acquired and become more common as the patient ages.[12]

CLASSIFICATION

One of the first priorities for the emergency clinician is to determine whether a suspected hernia is reducible, incarcerated, or strangulated. A *reducible hernia* is one whose contents can be returned through the fascial defect back into the abdominal cavity without surgical intervention. Patients often have rather large reducible hernias for years and are able to reduce them themselves, but such hernias can also become strangulated or incarcerated. An *incarcerated hernia* is one whose contents are not reducible without surgical intervention and is often associated with swelling of the hernia sac contents. A *strangulated hernia* is an incarcerated hernia whose blood supply to the herniated structures is compromised. Hernias with a small neck are more likely to strangulate. A strangulated hernia is a surgical emergency because gangrene will result if blood flow is not returned.

The anatomic location of the hernia will help one determine which type is most likely to be found. A *ventral hernia* of the abdominal wall may be umbilical, epigastric, or spigelian, depending on its location. An *incisional hernia* is found along a previous surgical scar. An *inguinal hernia* is found within the inguinal triangle, which is formed by the inguinal ligament on the inferior side, the inferior epigastric artery on the superolateral side, and the lateral edge of the rectus abdominis muscle on the medial side. Direct and indirect inguinal hernias occur superior to the inguinal ligament, whereas a femoral hernia is located inferior to the inguinal ligament.

Indirect Inguinal Hernia

An indirect inguinal hernia passes through the internal (deep) inguinal ring and into the inguinal canal (Fig. 44-2). It is located lateral to the inferior epigastric vessels. During fetal development, the processus vaginalis allows descent of the testes into the scrotum. Failure of it to close before birth leads to a hernia or hydrocele.

An indirect inguinal hernia is the most common type overall. This type of hernia occurs more frequently in males than in females and is commonly found in children and young adults. Approximately 5% of full-term infants and 30% of preterm infants will have an inguinal hernia.[13,14] Incarceration occurs more commonly in patients younger than 1 year, and 30% of hernias in children younger than 3 months become incarcerated.[15,16] For incarcerated inguinal hernias in children that are successfully reduced, surgical repair within 24 to 48 hours should be considered because of the risk for recurrent incarceration.[17] When an inguinal hernia is diagnosed, even without incarceration or strangulation, it is important to make a referral for elective repair. Studies have shown that even asymptomatic and painless inguinal hernias can cause symptoms over time if they are not surgically repaired,[4] although watchful waiting may also be appropriate in some patients.[18] Clinical studies demonstrate increased morbidity with emergency versus elective repair of inguinal hernias.[19]

Direct Inguinal Hernia

A direct inguinal hernia comes directly through the muscular and fascial wall of the abdomen. It is located within the inguinal triangle and is thus medial to the inferior epigastric vessels (Fig. 44-3). It can be differentiated from an indirect inguinal hernia in that it does not travel along the inguinal canal.

A direct inguinal hernia is the second most common groin hernia. It is an acquired hernia and occurs later in life secondary to weakening of the fascial and muscular wall as a result of aging and the repetitive stress of increased abdominal pressure. This hernia carries minimal risk for incarceration because the neck of the hernial orifice is typically wide.

Pantaloon Hernia

A pantaloon hernia is a combination of a direct and an indirect hernia and resembles the two legs of a pair of pants. This

Figure 44-1 A, This patient was admitted with the diagnosis of bowel obstruction. **B,** It was not until the physician carefully examined the groin area that an incarcerated inguinal hernia was found. Symptoms of the obstruction, the impressive radiographic findings, and an incomplete physical examination led to initial failure to diagnose the obvious hernia.

Figure 44-2 Indirect inguinal hernia.

Figure 44-3 Direct inguinal hernia.

variation of an inguinal hernia is difficult to diagnose in the ED and is often discovered during surgical exploration. Successful treatment depends on correctly identifying the hernia and subsequent reduction of each "leg" of the hernia separately.

Femoral Hernia

A femoral hernia occurs inferior to the inguinal ligament through a defect in the transversalis fascia. The contents protrude into the potential space in the femoral canal located medial to the femoral vein and lateral to the lacunar ligament (Fig. 44-4). Because of the small fascial defect and constriction by the inguinal ligament, this hernia becomes incarcerated in up to 45% of cases.[20] A femoral hernia is relatively uncommon, occurs more frequently in women than in men, and is an uncommon condition in children.[21]

Incisional Hernia

An incisional hernia commonly follows abdominal surgery in an area of postincisional weakness in the abdominal wall (Fig. 44-5A). Poor wound healing (e.g., because of infection)

Figure 44-4 Femoral hernia.

Figure 44-5 Ventral hernias. *A,* Incisional hernia. *B,* Umbilical hernia. *C,* Epigastric hernia. *D,* Spigelian hernia.

increases the likelihood of forming this type of hernia.[22,23] An incisional hernia occurs after 3% to 13% of all abdominal surgeries and carries a recurrence rate of 20% to 50%.[24] Because the lines of tension pull this hernia open, the size of the defect is usually sufficient to prevent incarceration.

Umbilical Hernia

An umbilical hernia traverses the fibromuscular ring of the umbilicus (Fig. 44-5*B*). This hernia is most commonly found in infants and children, is congenital in origin, and often resolves without treatment by the age of 5.[25] If the hernia persists beyond this age, is larger than 2 cm, or becomes incarcerated or strangulated, it may be repaired surgically.[19,26] An acquired umbilical hernia may also be seen in an adult, particularly with increased abdominal pressure (such as with obesity, ascites, or pregnancy). An umbilical hernia is more prone to incarceration and strangulation in an adult than in a child.

Epigastric Hernia

This hernia occurs in the midline through the linea alba of the rectus sheath (see Fig. 44-5*C*). It is usually located in the epigastric region between the xiphoid and the umbilicus. Though previously considered rare in infants, one study found epigastric hernias in 4% of all pediatric patients evaluated for hernias.[27]

Spigelian Hernia

A spigelian hernia is rare and courses through a defect in the lateral edge of the rectus muscle at the level of the semilunar line (Fig. 44-5*D*). It is caused by a partial abdominal wall defect in the transverse abdominal aponeurosis or the spigelian fascia. Patients are typically 40 to 70 years of age, but the hernia has also been reported in younger patients.[1] Incarceration rates (often with omentum) have been reported to be as high as 20% with these uncommon hernias.[25,28] Some reports suggest that ultrasound may be a valuable adjunct for the diagnosis of these hernias and may be helpful during attempted reduction procedures.[29,30]

DIAGNOSIS

History and Physical Examination

A patient with a symptomatic hernia may seek treatment in the ED because of swelling or pain in the region of the hernia or abdomen. Ask whether the patient has a history of heavy lifting. Inquire about signs of infection and systemic illness, such as fever, chills, and malaise. Determine whether the patient has signs of bowel obstruction, including nausea and vomiting. Occasionally, the signs and symptoms of intestinal obstruction can be so prominent that the clinician does not suspect the hernia to be the culprit. Document a record of previous surgeries and hernia repairs, including the presence of synthetic mesh.

On physical examination, palpate the inguinal canal in males by inverting the scrotal skin and passing a finger into the external ring. Ask the patient to cough or perform a Valsalva maneuver, which increases intraabdominal pressure and facilitates detection of a hernia. Palpation of the external ring is more difficult in females because it is narrower. An indirect inguinal hernia is manifested as a swelling in the area of the inguinal ligament or as scrotal swelling in male patients. It is often painless and may be noted as an incidental finding. On examination this hernia can be differentiated from a direct hernia in two distinct ways. First, it begins lateral to the inferior epigastric arteries. Second, on palpation of the inguinal canal, the contents of the hernia will strike the tip of the finger instead of the pad. This occurs as the hernia protrudes down the canal to meet the finger instead of across a fascial and muscular defect. This effect can be accentuated by applying pressure over the internal ring after hernia reduction. Bulging will recur with straining if the hernia is direct, but the pressure over the internal ring should block distention of the hernia into the inguinal canal. A hernia that fills the scrotum is most likely an indirect hernia. The peritoneal contents may become incarcerated if there is swelling of the internal or external ring.

An asymptomatic hernia may be manifested as a mass that is found incidentally on physical examination of the abdomen or groin. If a hernia is easily reducible, no specific intervention is required in the ED, but give patients instructions for appropriate outpatient surgical follow-up for potential elective repair. This is particularly important for inguinal hernias because elective repair is associated with much less morbidity than emergency repair for strangulation.[4,19,20]

A child with an inguinal hernia may have a reducible inguinal or scrotal mass that occurs with straining or crying. Such a child may be brought to the ED because of vomiting, poor eating, lethargy, or irritability. Always consider incarcerated or strangulated hernias in the differential diagnosis of vague complaints such as these.

Figure 44-6 Incarcerated spigelian hernia identified on abdominal computed tomography. **A,** Dilated loops of small bowel with air-fluid levels (AFL) are noted in the abdomen. Loops of both small bowel (SB) and large bowel (LB) are seen outside the peritoneal cavity in a lateral position, which is diagnostic of a spigelian hernia. **B,** A cut lower in the abdomen shows the site of the hernia. The efferent loop of small bowel is of normal caliber; however, the afferent loop is decompressed, thus suggesting a transition point within the hernia. Operative repair was required.

Figure 44-7 Strangulated hernia in a 56-year-old man. An axial contrast-enhanced, reformatted computed tomography image of the abdomen shows a strangulated left inguinal hernia with a C-shaped configuration (*arrows*). Note the bowel wall thickening, severe fat stranding, mesenteric engorgement, and extraluminal fluid confined to the hernia sac, findings that suggest strangulation. (*Reprinted with permission from Aguirre DA, Santosa AC, Casola G, et al. Abdominal wall hernias: imaging features, complications, and diagnostic pitfalls at multidetector row CT. Radiographics. 2005;25:1501-1520.*)

Radiologic Imaging

When findings on physical examination are equivocal and the emergency clinician suspects an occult hernia, several options are available for diagnostic imaging.[31] Magnetic resonance imaging has a high positive predictive value for patients with clinically uncertain herniations,[32] and computed tomography can also be helpful for the diagnosis of hernias and any associated complications (e.g., bowel obstruction or perforation)[33] (Figs. 44-6 and 44-7). Ultrasound examination has been shown to have good sensitivity and specificity for the diagnosis of groin hernias[34] and may decrease the rate of emergency surgery by improving the ability to reduce hernias.[35] Ultrasound may also have good specificity and a high positive predictive value for diagnosing postoperative incisional hernias.[31]

Diagnosis of Incarcerated Versus Strangulated Hernias

When the patient or emergency care provider cannot manually reduce the contents of the hernia back into the abdominal cavity, the hernia is described as *incarcerated*. Although hernias are a leading cause of bowel obstruction, patients with incarcerated hernias do not necessarily have associated bowel obstruction. Incarceration is more common with femoral hernias, small indirect inguinal hernias, and abdominal wall hernias. Incarceration can be caused by the presence of a small fascial defect, by constriction of the defect by outside musculature, or by swelling of the hernia contents.

In contrast, a strangulated hernia is a hernia in which the vascular supply to the herniated bowel is compromised, thus leading to ischemia. Strangulated hernias will most commonly also be incarcerated, but this is not a universal finding. Ischemic injury of the bowel is suggested by a red, purple, or bluish discoloration of the skin over the hernia, significant abdominal tenderness with peritoneal signs, and radiographic findings of extraluminal air.[25] Patients with strangulated hernias may exhibit bowel obstruction, peritonitis, viscus perforation, intraabdominal abscess, or septic shock. Associated symptoms may include nausea, vomiting, fever, or abdominal distention.

In rare instances a strangulated or incarcerated hernia may inadvertently be reduced en masse to a preperitoneal location (Fig. 44-8), thus making the hernia sac and contents no longer palpable.[36-38] In this case the hernia has not been reduced into the peritoneal cavity and the incarceration and ischemia have not been relieved. Because the clinician believes that the hernia has been appropriately reduced, this can result in delay in the diagnosis of incarcerated or ischemic bowel. Fortunately, this occurs in less than 1% of hernias.[39] One case report described a 3-month-old patient whose gangrenous intestines were completely reduced into the peritoneal cavity (not the preperitoneal fat), thereby leading to delayed diagnosis and significant morbidity.[40] Persistent pain after reduction of a hernia, especially more than at the orifice of the fascial defect, should alert the physician to the possibility of either properitoneal reduction or reduction of ischemic bowel.

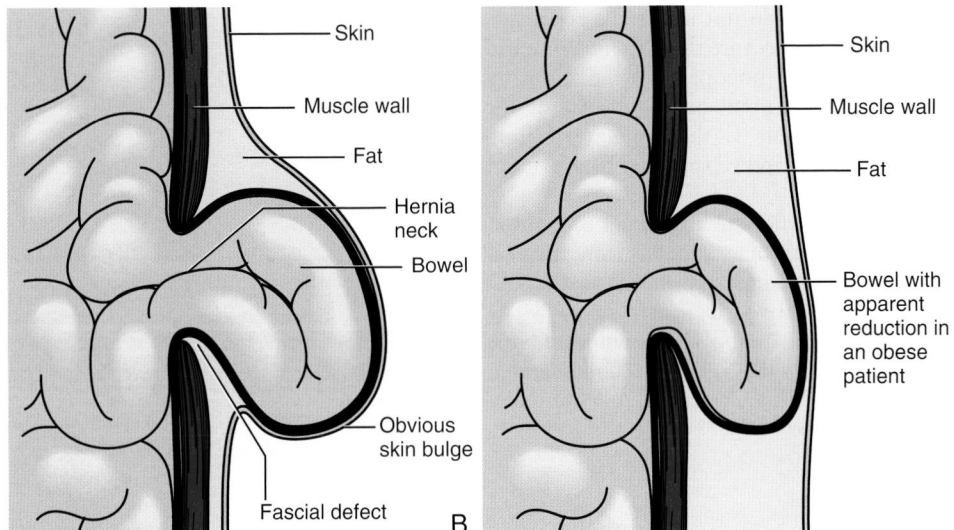

Figure 44-8 En masse reduction. **A,** When a hernia forms, it projects from the fascia into subcutaneous fat. The object of reduction is to replace the hernia into the peritoneal cavity. **B,** If the hernia sac is partially reduced into the subcutaneous fat of an obese patient, it may appear reduced and not be palpable because of the patient's body habitus. However, the hernia is still susceptible to incarceration or ischemia because it has not been returned to the peritoneal sac.

BOX 44-1 **Differential Diagnosis of Groin Masses**	
Hernia	Epididymitis
Testicular torsion	Hidradenitis suppurativa
Retracted or undescended	Groin abscess
testicle	Hematoma
Hydrocele	Lipoma
Spermatocele	Epidermal inclusion cyst
Venous varix	Tumor
Pseudoaneurysm	Tracking of intraperitoneal
Lymphadenopathy	blood
Lymphogranuloma venereum	

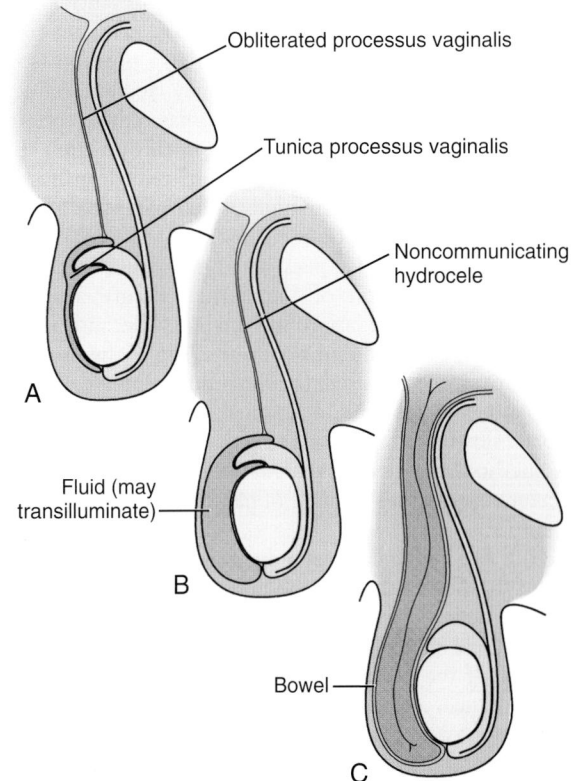

Figure 44-9 Hydrocele versus hernia. **A,** Normal anatomy. **B,** Noncommunicating hydrocele (which may transilluminate) that may be confused with a hernia. **C,** Indirect hernia that can be palpated from the inguinal ring to the testicle.

Differential Diagnosis

The differential diagnosis for a groin mass is large. Box 44-1 lists a number of disease processes that may masquerade as hernias. For example, testicular torsion can be mistaken for a hernia, especially if there is an associated reactive hydrocele. The clinician must examine the testicle for tenderness, swelling, lie, and cremasteric reflex. If there is concern for testicular torsion, urology should be notified immediately while diagnostic studies are undertaken simultaneously. A hydrocele can also be confused with a hernia because both can occupy the same anatomic space (Fig. 44-9). A hydrocele may transilluminate, whereas a hernia generally does not. Differentiation can be difficult and may require ultrasound to define the contents of the scrotum.

REDUCTION

Indications and Contraindications

The indications for reducing a hernia are the presence of a hernia and the absence of strangulation. Because many patients require sedation for successful reduction, it may be helpful to have a surgeon available while reduction is attempted and the patient is under sedation in the ED. This may be facilitated by discussing the treatment plan with the consultant before sedating the patient and attempting reduction. If reduction proves to be difficult, do not undertake repetitive attempts at reducing the hernia because this may increase the swelling and limit the chance of nonoperative reduction by the surgical consultant. An important prognostic factor for patients requiring surgical repair is the amount of time between the onset of symptoms and repair of an incarcerated hernia.[7]

In addition to incarceration despite attempted reduction, several other clinical situations may benefit from surgical consultation. Reduction of a strangulated hernia in the ED is contraindicated and operative management will be required. Surgical consultation in the ED is indicated for bowel obstruction associated with a hernia, undescended testicles, ovaries within the hernia contents, or traumatic hernias.

Procedure

The first step in successful hernia reduction is to position the patient properly because increases in intraabdominal pressure will work against efforts to reduce a hernia. Place the patient in a position so that gravity can work to pull the contents of the hernia sac back into the peritoneal cavity. Ensure patient comfort to decrease voluntary or involuntary muscle contraction and guarding, which subsequently increases intraabdominal pressure. For ventral abdominal hernias, place the patient in the supine position. The Trendelenburg position (supine with the head 20 degrees downward) may facilitate reduction of inguinal hernias. Many of these hernias reduce spontaneously if the patient is left comfortably in this position for 10 to 20 minutes. In children, spontaneous reduction has been reported in up to 80% of inguinal hernias over a 2-hour period without manipulation.

A cool compress or ice pack may help reduce the swelling and facilitate reduction of the hernia. Before attempting reduction, consider sedation and analgesia because this will help the patient relax and minimize the pain of the procedure. Options for procedural sedation include etomidate, propofol, midazolam, and fentanyl. If manual reduction is necessary, approach slowly with soft, ongoing dialogue and warm hands. This method encourages patient relaxation and minimizes muscular contractions because of pain, cold, or other physical discomfort.

Before beginning hernia reduction, identify the components of the hernia that will be manipulated during the procedure. A hernia consists of a defect in the existing wall of tissue (muscle and fascia) that makes up the neck of the hernia sac. If the neck is small, the hernia will be more difficult to reduce, and a higher incidence of incarceration and strangulation will result. When attempting to reduce the hernia, take care to not allow the contents of the hernia sac to override the edge of the hernia orifice because this will cause "ballooning" of the contents of the hernia sack around the hernia neck. Attempt to find the edge of the hernia defect and *position your hand or fingers opposite the reducing hand*. This will help reduce ballooning and stabilize the edge of the fascial defect.

Begin the reduction procedure by gently guiding *the proximal contents of the hernia sac back through the neck of the hernia first*. In other words, reduce the hernia in the opposite order from which the contents protruded. Guiding the distal end of the contents or the hernia sac itself through the fascial defect

Figure 44-10 A, This very large hernia is challenging to reduce. **B,** Merely pushing on the distal end of the mass, as shown here, will not be successful. **C,** Instead, try to first reduce the contents that are more proximal by stabilizing the neck and first replacing the portion of bowel closest to the fascial defect.

first may cause the proximal contents to be displaced around the opening (ballooning) and prevent reduction. Apply gentle, steady pressure *on the tissue at the neck of the hernia* to overcome this problem and then gradually reduce the hernia (Figs. 44-10 and 44-11). *Failure to perform this important procedure is a common error that precludes reduction.*

When attempting to reduce inguinal hernias in children, place the patient supine in about a 20-degree Trendelenburg position, which may allow spontaneous reduction. Another option is to place the patient in the "unilateral frog-leg" position[41] (Fig. 44-12). Stabilize the patient by grasping the anterior superior iliac spines to prevent lateral movement of the pelvis. Abduct the ipsilateral leg, externally rotate and flex the hip, and flex the knee to obtain the classic frog-leg position. The purpose of this position is to allow the greatest reapproximation of both the internal and external rings. After achieving this position, use the fingers of one hand to prevent the hernia contents from overriding the external ring while using the other hand to provide steady but gentle pressure on the contents of the hernia sac. Repeated forceful attempts are not recommended.

HERNIA REDUCTION

A The hernia can be divided into several sections. The proximal portion is closest to the neck or fascial defect, through which the hernia protrudes. The distal portion is farthest from the neck.

B When attempting to reduce the hernia, be careful to not invaginate the distal portion first or the proximal portion may obstruct the opening as it is pushed over the sides.

— Ballooning of the proximal part of the hernia prevents reduction

Incorrect

Correct

Stabilize the neck to avoid ballooning

C By placing fingers along the edge of the hernia neck, one can direct the contents into instead of over the fascial defect.

Figure 44-11 Hernia reduction (see Fig. 44-10).

HERNIA REDUCTION: FROG-LEG TECHNIQUE

1

Hernia —

Stabilize the patient by grasping the anterior superior iliac spines.

2

Abduct the ipsilateral leg, and externally rotate and flex the hip to obtain the classic frog-leg position.

3

Use the fingers of one hand to prevent the hernia contents from overriding the external ring while using the other hand to provide steady but gentle pressure on the contents of the hernia sac.

Figure 44-12 Frog-leg technique of hernia reduction.

POTENTIAL COMPLICATIONS

Major complications may occur during the reduction of hernias. Underlying bowel may be injured from overzealous attempts at reduction. Repetitive and overaggressive attempts may aggravate the swelling and make the hernia irreducible. This complication can be avoided with appropriate patient preparation, positioning, sedation, and reduction techniques. Reduction of ischemic bowel in the setting of an undiagnosed strangulated hernia is a potential complication. It may occur when the clinician inadvertently reduces ischemic bowel back into the peritoneal cavity or en masse into the preperitoneal space and then ignores or does not search for signs of ischemic tissue.

INTERPRETATION

In general, successful reduction can be identified by the absence of a mass, palpation of the hernia ring, and relief of pain. Continued significant pain suggests the possibility that strangulated bowel has been reduced back into the peritoneal cavity. Inability to palpate the hernia ring after reduction suggests that the hernia is in the preperitoneal position, is not completely reduced, or is not palpable because of body habitus.

References are available at www.expertconsult.com

CHAPTER 45

Anorectal Procedures

Wendy C. Coates

Patients with anorectal disorders are frequently encountered in the emergency department (ED). In some cases the condition is isolated, whereas in others, the anorectal complaint may be an outward manifestation of a serious underlying illness. A thorough history and physical examination must precede any procedure. Because of the nature of these conditions, extreme sensitivity and professionalism must be applied.

Patients may be anxious about anorectal examination or associated procedures, including the simple digital rectal examination (DRE). The results of DRE may lead to performing diagnostic or therapeutic procedures, such as anoscopy, excision of thrombosed external hemorrhoids, drainage of anorectal abscesses or pilonidal cysts, reduction of rectal prolapse, or removal of rectal foreign bodies (FBs). For these procedures, analgesia, sedation, or both may be useful adjuncts.

ANATOMY

The rectum and anus compose the most distal portion of the gastrointestinal tract. The rectum begins at the level of the third sacral vertebra and extends distally 12 to 15 cm. Blood supply to the anorectum is derived from the superior, middle, and inferior hemorrhoidal arteries. Venous drainage from the rectum and anus returns to both the portal and systemic systems (Fig. 45-1). The dentate or pectinate line marks the transition from the rectum to the anus and contains submucosal glands in anal crypts. Occlusion with subsequent infection of these glands is the etiology of anorectal abscesses. Sensory innervation to the rectum is primarily visceral, whereas the anus is innervated by cutaneous fibers. Therefore, patients are often unaware of rectal pathology because the pain associated with it may be vague or absent. By contrast, anal lesions are usually very painful and well localized.[1]

DRE

Indications and Contraindications

The physical examination should be performed in a private location and the patient should be completely draped and relaxed. Generally, a calm atmosphere and caring examiner preclude the need for analgesic or anxiolytic agents, although they may be needed to facilitate a thorough examination. In some extremely painful conditions, such as thrombosed or gangrenous hemorrhoids, DRE may be postponed until the patient is anesthetized. If a sharp-edged foreign body (e.g., metal blade or broken glass) is suspected, performing a DRE may cause injury to the clinician, as well as the patient. In these cases, radiologic evaluation with subsequent operative management may be indicated.

Procedure

The examiner should place the patient in the lateral decubitus position and wear protective gloves. The examination begins with a preliminary visual inspection of the perianal area for important information regarding patient hygiene, trauma, or sexually transmitted diseases. Next, ask the patient to perform a Valsalva maneuver and note any prolapsing rectal mucosa or hemorrhoids. When the patient relaxes, prolapsed structures may retreat or remain external to the anus. By placing a finger firmly against the anal sphincter, it will relax and allow entry of the examiner's gloved, lubricated finger (Fig. 45-2A). Once inserted into the anus, make a 360-degree sweep to identify any irregularities in the anorectum and prostate. On withdrawal of the examining finger, examine stool remaining on the glove for the presence of visible or occult blood (see Fig. 45-2B and C).[2] Testing for blood in stool is discussed in detail in Chapter 67.

Complications

Although DRE causes some vasovagal depression, it is safe to perform in patients with acute myocardial infarction.[3] Although not a firm contraindication in patients whose absolute neutrophil count is dangerously low, some would defer routine DRE, especially avoiding vigorous prostate manipulation, to minimize the likelihood of bacteremia.

ANOSCOPY

Indications and Contraindications

When evaluating a patient for anal pathology, some practitioners use anoscopy as an adjunct to DRE. Internal hemorrhoids, tears in the distal rectal mucosa, FBs, and distal anorectal masses may be visualized. An imperforate anus is the only absolute contraindication to anoscopy; however, severe rectal pain, a common complaint in the ED, may preclude awake anoscopic examination in anxious patients or those suffering from thrombosed hemorrhoids or other painful conditions. Internal visual inspection in these patients is better performed with sedation. In many cases a more definitive study such as sigmoidoscopy or colonoscopy is being planned by the treating physician, and thus anoscopy can be deferred in the acute care setting.

Equipment and Setup

The anoscope is a plastic or stainless steel tube with a removable obturator (Fig. 45-3). It may have an integrated light source or require an external light or head lamp. An appropriate examination table, topical anesthetics, lubricant, gauze, and forceps may also be required.

Positioning

Ideally, place the patient in a prone position on a proctoscopic examination table. The prone or lateral decubitus position with the knees and hips flexed may also be adequate and is sometimes tolerated better. In the lateral decubitus position, place the patient on the left side if the examiner is right-handed (Fig. 45-4, step 1).

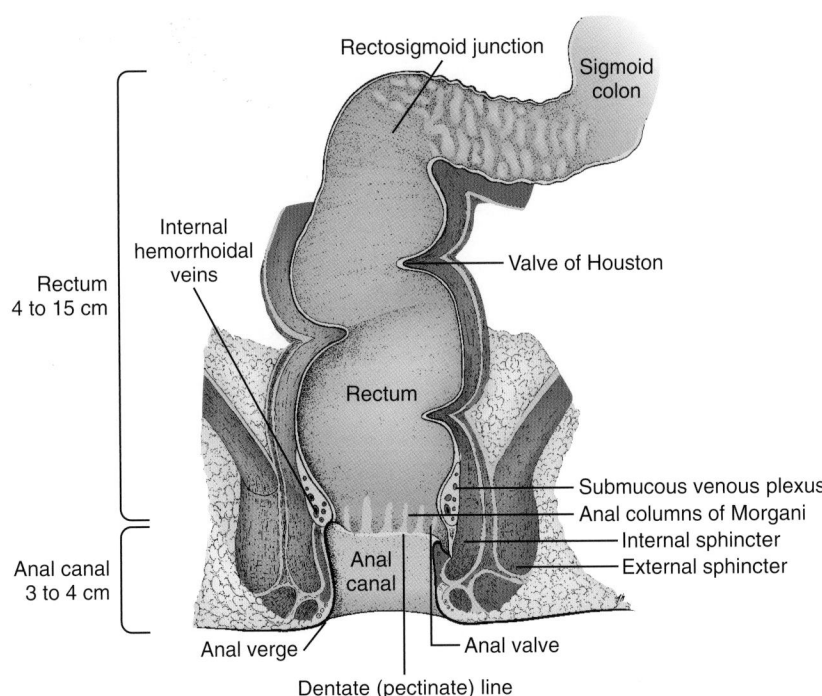

Figure 45-1 Anatomy of the terminal gastrointestinal tract. *(Redrawn from Abrahams PH, Webb PJ. Clinical Anatomy of Practical Procedures. London: Pitman; 1975.)*

Figure 45-2 Digital rectal examination. **A,** Insert a gloved, lubricated finger into the anus and perform a 360-degree sweep to check for any irregularities in the anorectum and prostate. **B,** Examine the stool for visible and occult blood. This patient had melena, which is very dark and tarry in consistency and indicative of upper gastrointestinal hemorrhage. **C,** This sample is positive for blood. The *large arrow* points to the blue coloration on the test area of the card, whereas the *small arrow* points to the control.

Procedure

Although most patients do not require intravenous sedation and analgesia, administer these agents as needed to keep the patient relaxed and comfortable. Before anoscopy, perform a routine DRE to identify sources of bleeding or pain and to locate any palpable masses. After DRE and with the obturator inserted completely into the anoscope, carefully introduce the scope into the anus. Use gentle, constant pressure to overcome resistance from involuntary contraction of the external anal sphincter. Gently advance the anoscope while asking the patient to bear down slightly. Pass the anoscope gently into the anorectum (see Fig. 45-4, *step 2*). If the obturator falls back during insertion, remove the anoscope completely and replace the obturator to avoid pinching the anal mucosa. Advance the anoscope until the outer flange impinges on the anal verge. Unless the anoscope has an internal light, use an external light source such as a penlight, otoscope, or pelvic examination light.

When the anoscope is fully inserted, remove the obturator (see Fig. 45-4, *step 3*). While gradually *withdrawing the anoscope*, visualize the anal canal (see Fig. 45-4, *step 4*). Swab away blood or debris to aid in visualization, and culture any abnormal discharge that is found. Note whether there is rectal bleeding or an FB beyond the reach of the anoscope. Withdraw the anoscope slowly as the entire circumference of

Figure 45-3 Reusable stainless steel (**A**) and disposable plastic (**B**) anoscopes are available. Regardless of the type of anoscope used, the obturator must be fully inserted and held in place with the thumb during advancement of the device into the anorectum.

ANOSCOPY

1 Left lateral or Sims' position

Place the patient in the left lateral position (**A**), prone position (**B**), or ideally prone on a proctoscopic examination table (**C**).

2

Thumb pressure

With the obturator fully inserted into the anoscope, carefully introduce the scope into the anus. Hold the obturator in place with your thumb. Use gentle, constant pressure to pass the anoscope into the anorectum. Advance until the outer flange impinges on the anal verge.

3

Remove the obturator

Remove the obturator when the anoscope is fully inserted.

4

Evaluate as the scope is withdrawn

Gradually withdraw the anoscope and visualize the anal canal. Swab away blood or debris to aid in visualization, culture any discharge, and inspect for hemorrhoids, anal fissures, ulcerations, abscesses, or tears.

Figure 45-4 Anoscopy. Remember to keep your thumb on the obturator during passage of the instrument until it is fully inserted. (*Step 1, From Hill GJ II.* Outpatient Surgery. *3rd ed. Philadelphia: Saunders; 1988.*)

mucosa is inspected for hemorrhoids, anal fissures, ulcerations, abscesses, or tears. Near the last stage of withdrawal, be aware of reflex spasm of the anal sphincter, which may cause the anoscope to be expelled quickly. Use firm counterpressure to prevent such rapid expulsion.

Complications

Although complications are rare, patients often complain of increased pain after the examination. Local mucosal irritation with subsequent bleeding is the most common complication. To prevent transmission of infectious diseases, dispose of or sterilize instruments after each use.

MANAGEMENT OF HEMORRHOIDS

Hemorrhoids are a common affliction and have been described and treated for more than 4000 years. The refined, low-fiber diet of Western nations makes hemorrhoids extremely common in the United States, where 1 in 25 to 30 individuals is afflicted. One million patients annually seek medical attention for this condition.[4]

Hemorrhoidal tissue is composed of vascular, mucosal, and muscular tissue. Though frequently attributed to varicosities, all three elements are included in hemorrhoids (Fig. 45-5). There are two types of hemorrhoids: internal and external. *Internal hemorrhoids* originate above the dentate line, are covered with mucosa, and lack sensory innervation. They can

be identified by noting that their covering differs in appearance from the surrounding perianal skin. Internal hemorrhoids may prolapse and bleed, which usually produces bright red blood on toilet paper or in the toilet bowl. This bleeding is arterial from presinusoidal arterioles and is mostly associated with brown stool and bleeding only with a bowel movement. Atypical bleeding requires further investigation. Internal hemorrhoids are rarely felt by digital palpation unless they are very large or thrombosed. Internal hemorrhoids are usually painless unless gangrenous, strangulated, extruded, or thrombosed, and then they may be extremely painful. Anal pain in the absence of such pathology suggests a problem other than simple internal hemorrhoids.[5]

Internal hemorrhoids can be further classified as first through fourth degree. First-degree hemorrhoids do not prolapse but may be identified on anoscopic examination. Second-degree hemorrhoids prolapse on straining but reduce spontaneously. Third-degree hemorrhoids prolapse on straining and can be reduced manually, whereas fourth-degree hemorrhoids prolapse and are irreducible. Fourth-degree hemorrhoids are prone to thrombosis, strangulation, and eventually gangrene (see Fig. 45-5*C*).

External hemorrhoids originate below the dentate line and are covered with squamous epithelium. This makes them easily recognizable because their covering matches the surrounding skin. A thrombosed external hemorrhoid appears as a bluish mass covered by epidermis. Acute thrombosis occurs suddenly and is generally very painful because external hemorrhoids are innervated by the inferior rectal nerve. Many

Figure 45-5 A, Anatomic location of internal and external hemorrhoids. **B,** Thrombosed external hemorrhoid. **C,** Thrombosed prolapsed internal hemorrhoids. These hemorrhoids cannot be permanently reduced and are quite painful; occasionally, partial relief can be obtained by manual reduction if they are not gangrenous. They should not be incised in the emergency department; formal hemorrhoidectomy is required if conservative measures are not successful. They are often mistaken for a partial "rectal prolapse." Sitz baths and stool softeners are frequently futile in such severe cases. **D,** This small external hemorrhoid ruptured and produced minor but persistent bleeding and pain. Conservative treatment consisting of topical corticosteroids or Preparation H and frequent sitz baths will be curative in 5 to 7 days. (*A, From Hill GJ II. Outpatient Surgery. 2nd ed. Philadelphia: Saunders; 1980.*)

patients feel a tender mass and are unable to sit comfortably. Significant bleeding is uncommon but may occur with spontaneous rupture. Increased pressure from straining or trauma from constipation or diarrhea may exacerbate external hemorrhoids. Distention and trauma predispose the hemorrhoidal venous plexus to stasis with ensuing clot formation and edema.[2,4,6-9]

Conservative Treatment

ED management of minor *internal hemorrhoids* is conservative. Prolapsing internal hemorrhoids will not benefit long-term from conservative intervention and should receive surgical consultation. A useful mnemonic for managing hemorrhoids is WASH: water (increase fluid intake, warm water contacting the hemorrhoid via bath or directed shower), analgesics, stool softeners, and a high-fiber diet.[2] Psyllium (e.g., Metamucil) is often prescribed as a dietary supplement to increase fiber. Hemorrhoids that fail to respond to medical management may be treated on an outpatient basis with rubber band ligation, sclerosis, and thermotherapy consisting of an infrared beam, electric current, CO_2 laser, or ultrasonic energy. Patients who must push hemorrhoids back in after a bowel movement have symptomatic third-degree internal hemorrhoids and would benefit from elective surgical referral. This condition can easily be demonstrated by having the patient strain before DRE. *Nonreducible prolapsed internal hemorrhoids* should receive prompt surgical consultation and, frequently, admission to the hospital.[6]

Without treatment, thrombosed *external hemorrhoids* and those that have spontaneously ruptured will generally resolve over a period of 1 to 3 weeks. Residual skin tags may persist. During the interim, however, they are quite painful and may bleed. Small ruptured or nonruptured hemorrhoids that are seen acutely with minimal discomfort may be managed conservatively with warm water baths or a directed stream of water, topical corticosteroids (Anusol HC), or Preparation H. These topical agents may promote skin breakdown from the corticosteroid or local anesthetic if used for more than a couple of days. Since the pain is most severe within the first 48 hours, patients evaluated within this time window benefit from excision (not incision and drainage) of the contents of the thrombosed external hemorrhoid and its overlying skin. Patients seen after this time are usually best managed with conservative treatment because the thrombosis begins the reabsorption process and may be liquefied (see Fig. 45-5D).[2,4,8,9]

Surgical Excision of Thrombosed External Hemorrhoids

Indications and Contraindications

Indications for surgical excision of acutely (<48 hours) thrombosed external hemorrhoids in the ED include relief of symptoms and prevention of the formation of permanent perianal skin tags. These appendages remain as loose skin after the body reabsorbs the thrombosis and serve as a nidus for poor perianal hygiene and local irritation. Surgical consultation should be obtained in the ED for multiple painful external hemorrhoids and for profuse bleeding that is hemodynamically significant. Bleeding disorders, serious systemic illness, and hemodynamic instability are all relative contraindications to excision in the ED.

Procedure

Place the patient in the prone or lateral decubitus position. Tape the buttocks apart to aid in visualization (Fig. 45-6, *step 1*). An assistant is often needed. Administer parenteral analgesics and sedatives as an adjunct to local anesthesia if necessary. Infiltrate with a local anesthetic (such as 0.5% bupivacaine or buffered 1% lidocaine with epinephrine at 1:100,000) just under the skin and over the dome of the hemorrhoid (Fig. 45-7; also see Fig. 45-6, *step 2*). The overlying skin should blanch, which indicates that anesthesia has been introduced at the appropriate depth. Inject additional anesthetic through the incised tissue into the base of the hemorrhoid rather than through the intact skin if needed (see Fig. 45-7C).

Grasp the skin overlying the thrombosis with forceps. Make an elliptical incision around the clot and direct it radially from the anal orifice (Fig. 45-8; also see Fig. 45-6, *step 3*). Elevate the edges of the skin with forceps and excise from the edges to expose the underlying thrombosis. Remove the clot with forceps or by applying digital pressure (see Fig. 45-6, *steps 4 and 5*). Frequently, multiple individual clots will be present. If any skin ulceration is noted over the hemorrhoid, include it in the excised portion. Pack the wound loosely with standard cotton gauze to prevent the skin edges from reapproximating prematurely.

For the trip home, place a gauze pad between the buttocks and tape the buttocks together to hold the gauze in place (see Fig. 45-6, *step 6*). Advise the patient to avoid prolonged standing or straining for the next few days. Minor bleeding may occur. Hygiene with a directed stream of warm water or sitz baths can be started a few hours after the procedure. The gauze may fall out or can be removed at the first sitz bath. After the packing has been removed, the patient may apply a soothing cream to the area for a couple of days (such as Preparation H, Anusol HC, or witch hazel pads). Instruct the patient to avoid using toilet paper after a bowel movement for a few days but to wash the area with mild soap and water in the shower. Most patients are relatively asymptomatic in 48 hours and do not need a routine wound check unless the pain or bleeding persists. Once the clot has been removed, recurrent thrombosis is unlikely, but these patients are predisposed to future episodes. Long-term therapy should be directed toward avoiding constipation by increasing dietary fiber and fluid intake. Antibiotics are not routinely indicated.[2,10]

If an invasive procedure would not be well tolerated by the patient, alternative nonoperative treatments include topical nitrates or topical nifedipine. Applied to the thrombosed hemorrhoid, these creams relax the anal sphincter, relieve pain, and promote healing. Systemic absorption is minimal, and the application is usually well tolerated.[7]

Complications

Although complications are rare, bleeding and infection do occur. The bleeding usually stops with direct pressure. When simple incision plus drainage is performed instead of an elliptical excision or when the ellipse of skin is not removed completely, the edges of the skin can close prematurely and result in infection and a permanent perianal skin tag. Premature closure can also result in incomplete evacuation of the clot.

MANAGEMENT OF ANORECTAL ABSCESS AND PILONIDAL CYST AND ABSCESS

These topics are covered in detail in Chapter 37.

EXCISION OF THROMBOSED EXTERNAL HEMORRHOIDS

Place the patient in the prone or lateral decubitus position. Tape the buttocks apart to aid in visualization.

Infiltrate with a local anesthetic just under the skin and over the dome of the hemorrhoid (see Fig. 45-7).

Make an elliptical incision around the clot and direct it radially from the anal orifice (see Fig. 45-8).

Remove the clot with digital pressure. Often, multiple individual clots will be present.

Use forceps to remove residual clots.

Pack the wound loosely with standard cotton gauze. Place a gauze pad between the buttocks and tape the buttocks together to hold the gauze in place.

Figure 45-6 Excision of thrombosed external hemorrhoids.

MANAGEMENT OF RECTAL FBS

Causes of rectal FBs include autoeroticism (most common), iatrogenic or self-administered placement (thermometer, enema tip), assault, accidental ingestion, and concealment (body packing). The myriad of objects that have been removed include vibrators, sex toy phalluses, aerosol cans, light bulbs, glass bottles, billiard balls, fruits, vegetables, and small animals (Fig. 45-9). Many of these objects can be removed successfully in the ED. By following some simple guidelines, outpatient treatment can be practical and cost-effective.

Diagnosis of a rectal FB is usually made from the history. The physical examination should therefore concentrate on excluding anorectal or intestinal perforation and determining

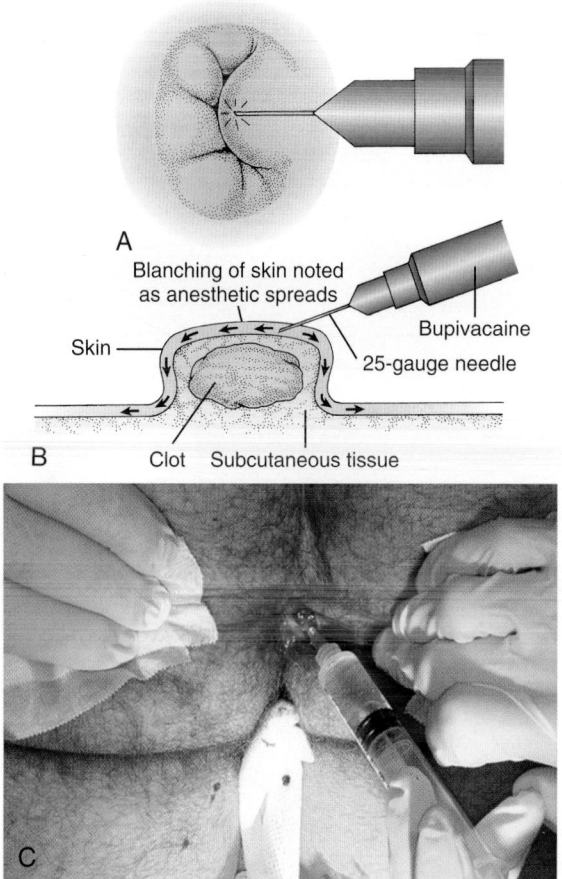

Figure 45-7 A, For surgical treatment of a thrombosed external hemorrhoid in the emergency department, anesthesia usually can be obtained with a *single injection* of buffered long-acting bupivacaine with epinephrine. In elective cases, apply a eutectic mixture of local anesthetics (EMLA) cream for 1 hour before the procedure. Parenteral sedation is optional. Using a 25-gauge needle, inject an anesthetic solution into the middle of the swollen hemorrhoid just below the surface of the skin. **B,** Do not move the tip of the needle. With slow injection, the anesthetic will spread over the surface of the dome and into the surrounding tissue. Avoid deep field blocks at the base of the hemorrhoid because they are unnecessary and very painful. **C,** If pain persists, inject additional anesthetic into deeper tissues *through the cut edges, not through the intact skin.*

Figure 45-8 Schematic technique as described in Figure 45-6. **A,** For the unroofing technique, make an elliptical incision to remove a piece of the overlying skin. To prevent skin tags, do not use a simple linear incision. **B,** Blood clots may extrude spontaneously, but remove the remaining ones with forceps or express them with the fingers (**C**). **D,** Frequently, multiple clots are present, and they should all be removed. Ask an assistant to provide exposure with forceps if necessary.

Removal of FBs in the ED is contraindicated in patients who have severe abdominal pain or signs of perforation, a nonpalpable FB, or broken glass in the rectum. Other situations precluding ED removal include a rectal FB that is unusually difficult to remove (a set time limit has elapsed or the patient cannot tolerate removal) or when there is insufficient experience or equipment to perform the procedure. Patients who arrive at the ED under these conditions require surgical consultation.[11-13]

Equipment

The specific equipment required will often depend on the nature of the FB (Fig. 45-11). In general, the clinician will need a speculum with a light source and an instrument to grasp the FB. The speculum can be an anoscope, a rigid sigmoidoscope, a vaginal speculum, or a retractor. Instruments useful for grasping the FB include ring forceps, tenaculum forceps, and obstetric forceps. In some instances, a Foley catheter or endotracheal tube will be helpful. A suction dart, vacuum extractor, and plaster of paris have also been used to aid in FB retrieval. Individual situations may lead to creative use of standard medical equipment, but one must ensure safety before using a device to remove a rectal FB.

which objects will be accessible in the ED. DRE will identify objects that are low lying or palpable. Such objects are most likely to be removed successfully in the outpatient setting. Plain radiographs can supplement the examination by delineating the shape, position, and number of objects. If an FB with a sharp edge is suspected from the history or radiograph, omit the DRE to prevent injury to the provider.[11-13]

Indications and Contraindications

Although some objects may pass spontaneously, delayed removal may lead to obstipation, pain, infection, and perforation. For these reasons, FB removal is indicated according to the algorithm included in this chapter (Fig. 45-10). *Rectal FB removal can lead to rectal perforation. Although many FBs can be removed safely in the ED, complicated or prolonged attempts may be better performed under general anesthesia.*

Procedure

The technique for removal depends on the size, location, orientation, and composition of the FB. Place the patient either prone in the knee-chest position or in a lateral decubitus position. Alternatively, if the patient is in the lithotomy position, pressure can be placed on the abdomen to help maneuver the FB toward the distal end of the rectum. Parenteral analgesia is often required to relieve the pain from anal

Figure 45-9 Rectal foreign bodies. **A,** Two large tungsten spheres, one on top of the other, gave a snowman-like appearance on the radiograph. They were removed manually in the emergency department (ED) with the aid of a Foley catheter and large-volume balloon. **B,** A vibrator that migrated into the sigmoid colon. It required removal in the operating room under general anesthesia. **C,** A small glass jar that the patient had tried to remove multiple times over a period of hours at home. On arrival at the ED, he had signs of peritonitis and was taken to the operating room, where perforation of the distal colon was discovered. Diverting colostomy was required. **D,** A toothbrush that was removed manually in the ED.

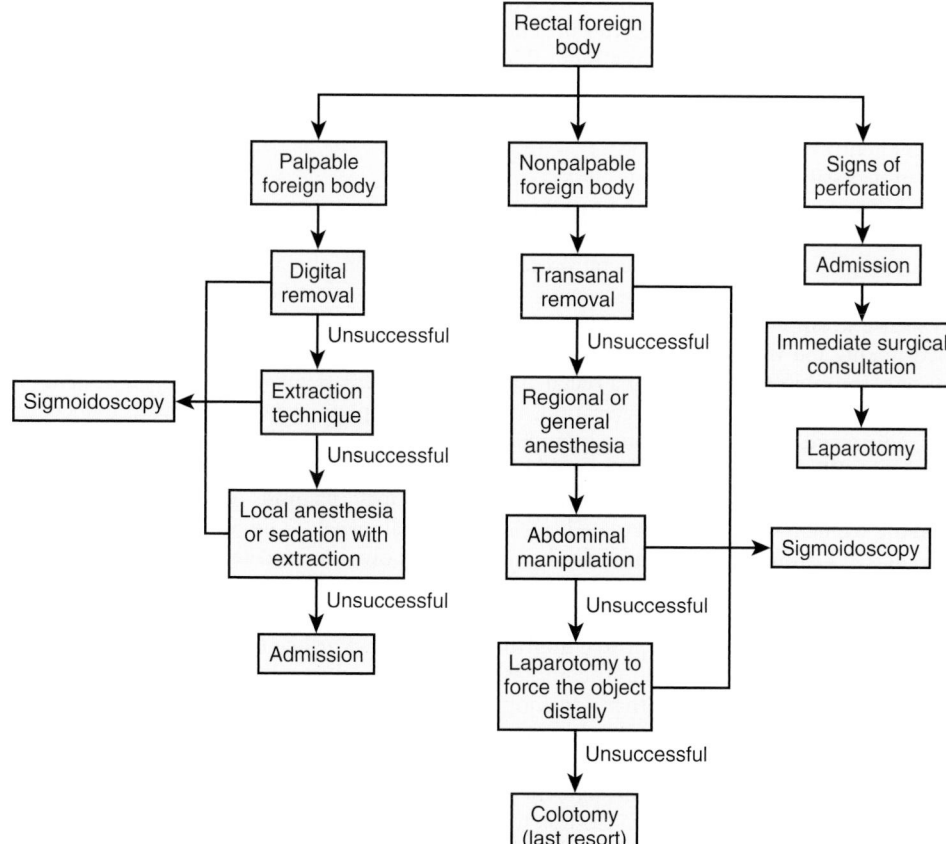

Figure 45-10 Emergency approach to the removal of rectal foreign bodies. Foreign bodies that are fragile or associated with rectal spasm are generally managed with regional or general anesthesia. The use of supplemental analgesic, anxiolytic, and local anesthetic medications is recommended.

Figure 45-11 A variety of equipment may be required to remove a rectal foreign body, and the choice of specific equipment will depend on the clinical scenario. Individual situations may lead to creative use of standard medical equipment, but one must ensure safety before using a device to remove a rectal foreign body.

stretching and manipulation. Intravenous sedation is almost always required to calm the patient and facilitate relaxation of the anal sphincter. Perform a perianal block to allow greater dilation of the sphincter. As described earlier, local infiltration with 0.5% bupivacaine or 1% lidocaine with epinephrine at 1:100,000 may be administered circumferentially around the anus in the submucosal tissue.

After analgesia and sedation of the patient, perform a DRE to gauge the position and orientation of the FB. Suprapubic pressure from above, the examiner's finger from below, and the patient performing a Valsalva maneuver may successfully deliver the object without instrumentation. If the FB is lodged against the sacrum posteriorly, redirect it by cradling its posterior aspect between two fingers and directing it slightly proximally and anteriorly while the patient gently bears down.

If DRE reveals that the object has an accessible edge or lip, use an instrument to extract it under direct visualization (Fig. 45-12). First, insert an anoscope, rigid sigmoidoscope, vaginal speculum, or retractor into the anus as described previously in the section "Anoscopy." If an intact object is visualized clearly, use a blunt instrument to secure it. Apply gentle traction to remove the object, the instrument, and the anoscope or speculum as a single unit. Grasp the object under direct visualization to avoid pinching or tearing the mucosa.

Rigid sigmoidoscopes offer a unique advantage in that air can be insufflated into the rectum around the FB. This technique can be particularly helpful when retrieving glass objects. Glass rectal FBs often create a vacuum in the segment of bowel just proximal to where they lie. This makes removal with simple traction almost impossible. The vacuum can be released by distending the rectal wall around the object with air. If a sigmoidoscope cannot be used to retrieve a glass object, pass one or two Foley catheters or an endotracheal tube beyond the FB and inflate the balloon or cuff. Then remove the object with the inflated balloons and gentle traction. Often, specific equipment is not available to remove all FBs, and the clinician must improvise depending on the circumstances. Something as simple as two large spoons or an endotracheal tube may be used in lieu of complicated forceps and clamps.

Besides creating a vacuum, glass objects are especially difficult to remove because they can break and cause a tear or perforation in the rectal wall. If forceps are used for retrieval of a glass object, coat the grasping edge with rubber or plastic or pad it with gauze. Plaster of Paris has been used to remove a hollow glass object if the object has an open end facing distally. Insert a hollow tube (e.g., an endotracheal tube or small chest tube) into the open end. Fill the FB with plaster by injecting it through the hollow tube with a large irrigation syringe. Once the plaster cools around the tube, it can be used as a handle to remove the object with gentle traction. Be careful to not leak plaster onto the mucosa. In addition, heat is released as the plaster hardens and may cause the glass to crack or shatter. After removal, perform sigmoidoscopy to evaluate for edema and possible perforation of the mucosa. Patients with normal findings on postextraction examination and no evidence of perforation may be released home safely after a period of observation.[11-13]

FBs that are positioned proximal to the rectum warrant surgical consultation. Management options include observation to enable passage to the rectum or surgical removal. Enemas or cathartics should not be used because they may increase the impaction of a rectal FB or cause it to move higher into the colon.

Complications

The most common complication is an inability to remove the rectal FB, which should prompt surgical consultation. The most serious complication of rectal FB retrieval is perforation or a deep mucosal tear, which may necessitate surgery. Cracking or shattering of glass may also require surgical exploration and retrieval. Mild mucosal edema and rectal bleeding are common sequelae of prolonged rectal FB presence and retrieval. These complications may not require any specific treatment. However, the presence of postprocedural abdominal pain, fever, sustained or profuse rectal bleeding, or discharge warrants surgical consultation.

MANAGEMENT OF RECTAL PROLAPSE

Rectal prolapse is protrusion of some or all of the layers of the rectal wall through the anal orifice. Prolapse is not usually an emergency, and manual reduction is often easily accomplished in the ED. The most common complaint is protrusion of a rectal "mass" or tissue. Patients may complain of pain on defecation, itching, incomplete evacuation, incontinence, or bloody mucosal discharge and mistake the condition for "hemorrhoids." Rectal prolapse is diagnosed by visual inspection of the anus. DRE may diagnose occult prolapse that is situated inside the anal canal. The differential diagnosis includes hemorrhoids, polyps, cystocele, and carcinoma.

There are three types of prolapse. (1) Complete prolapse, or procidentia, involves all layers of the rectum protruding through the anal orifice (Figs. 45-13 and 45-14). (2) Incomplete, or occult, prolapse describes internal prolapse that does not reach the orifice. This type is difficult to diagnose in the ED and requires no emergency intervention. (3) Mucosal prolapse is limited to protrusion of mucosa through the anal opening.

Complete and partial prolapse can be distinguished from each other by digital palpation. A thick muscular layer of

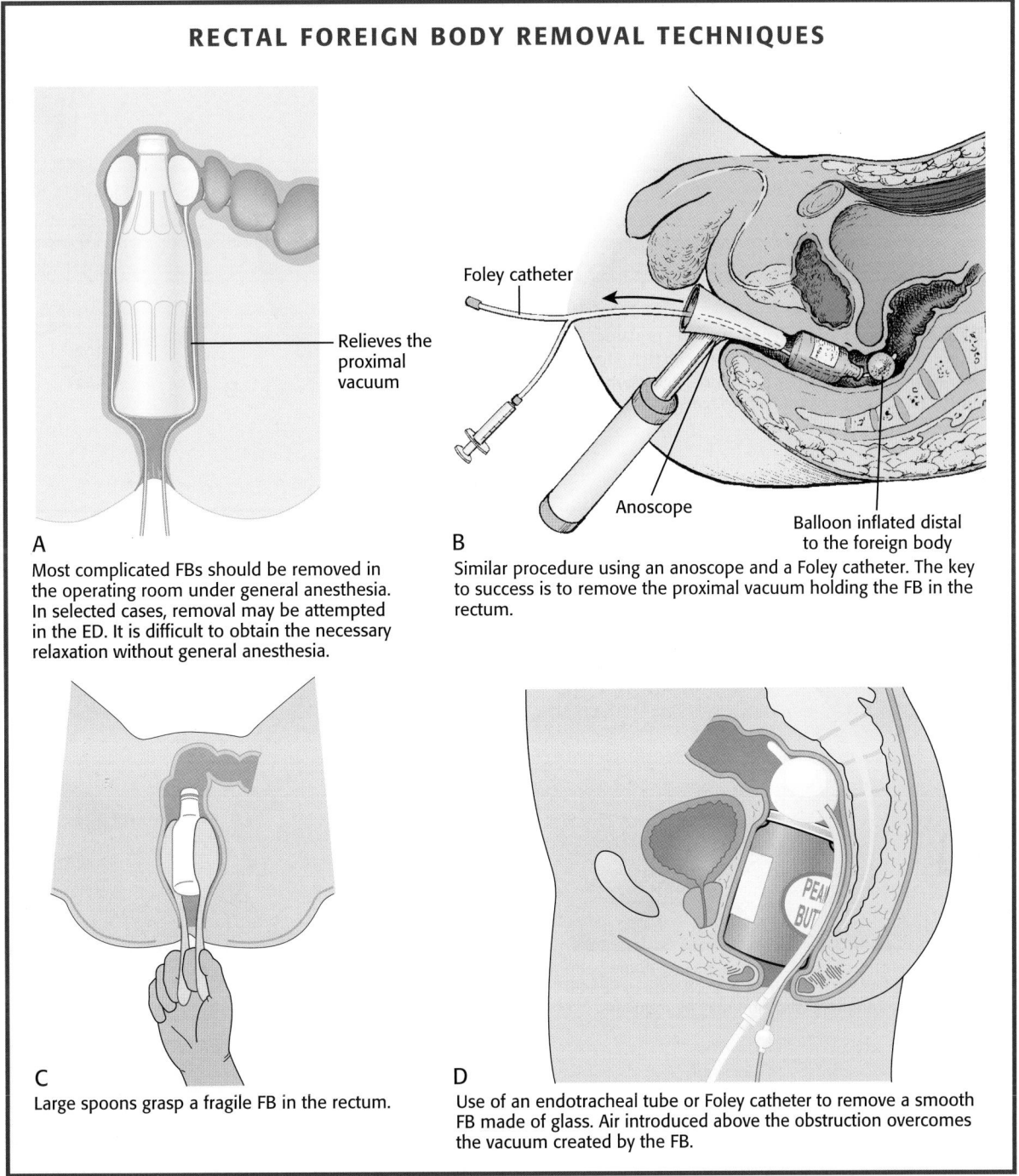

RECTAL FOREIGN BODY REMOVAL TECHNIQUES

A
Most complicated FBs should be removed in the operating room under general anesthesia. In selected cases, removal may be attempted in the ED. It is difficult to obtain the necessary relaxation without general anesthesia.

Relieves the proximal vacuum

B
Similar procedure using an anoscope and a Foley catheter. The key to success is to remove the proximal vacuum holding the FB in the rectum.

Foley catheter

Anoscope

Balloon inflated distal to the foreign body

C
Large spoons grasp a fragile FB in the rectum.

D
Use of an endotracheal tube or Foley catheter to remove a smooth FB made of glass. Air introduced above the obstruction overcomes the vacuum created by the FB.

Figure 45-12 Rectal foreign body (FB) removal techniques. *ED*, emergency department.

tissue between the examiner's thumb and forefinger suggests complete prolapse. With partial or mucosal prolapse, radial rectal folds may be seen protruding through the rectum. This type of prolapse rarely extends more than 3 to 4 cm from the anus. Complete prolapse can extend 10 to 15 cm outside the anal verge.

Rectal prolapse is most common in children and older adults. Prolapse in children is typically incomplete, or mucosal. It usually affects children younger than 3 years and is often associated with cystic fibrosis, parasitic infection, chronic diarrhea, or malnutrition or occurs as a sequela of chronic neurologic disease. Prolapse is usually self-limited; outpatient

management (after manual reduction) includes correcting constipation, avoiding straining, and referring for testing to exclude cystic fibrosis. Rectal prolapse in adults occurs most often in older women and may be recurrent. The etiology is poorly understood, but it is associated with chronic constipation, chronic neurologic conditions, or pudendal neuropathies that weaken the anal sphincter.[14-16]

Indications for Reduction

Rectal prolapse may be reduced in the ED. If unsuccessful, outpatient surgical referral is appropriate. Definitive surgery

Figure 45-13 A, Type I procidentia (rectal prolapse). **B,** Intussusception of the sigmoid colon beyond the anus. *(A and B, From Kratzer GL, Demarest RJ.* Office Management of Colon and Rectal Disease. *Philadelphia: Saunders; 1985.)*

A

B

RECTAL PROLAPSE REDUCTION

Complete (recurrent) rectal prolapse in a nursing home patient. To reduce the prolapse, place the patient in the prone or lateral decubitus position. Parenteral sedation may be required.

Tape the buttocks apart (or enlist the help of an assistant to spread the buttocks) to aid in reduction.

Apply constant, gentle circumferential pressure to the prolapsed area, beginning with the portion closest to the lumen (the most distal segment). Apply pressure with the thumbs while rolling the walls inward to force the prolapse back through the anus.

Successful reduction of the rectal prolapse.

Figure 45-14 Reduction of rectal prolapse.

may be attempted, but occasional prolapses in debilitated patients are usually treated conservatively. Patients should be referred for outpatient proctoscopy to search for a polyp or malignancy that may have acted as a lead point. If the prolapse is incarcerated, surgical consultation should be obtained.

Procedure

Reduce a mucosal prolapse by applying gentle, constant pressure on the mass for a few minutes. In children, intravenous sedation may be necessary to allow reduction. Children are often more relaxed if they are allowed to remain in the parent's lap during the procedure. After reduction, send the child home with a pressure dressing and stool softeners. Counsel the parents on the use of dietary fiber and increased fluid intake to prevent constipation and straining. Refer the child for outpatient follow-up.[17]

For reduction of a complete prolapse, place the patient in the prone or lateral decubitus position (see Fig. 45-14, *step 1*). Parenteral sedation may be required if the patient is anxious or has difficulty relaxing the sphincteric muscles. Tape the buttocks apart or have an assistant aid in reduction (see Fig. 45-14, *step 2*). Apply constant, gentle circumferential pressure to the prolapsed area, beginning with the portion closest to the lumen (the most distal segment). Place the thumbs on either side of the lumen while grasping the exterior walls with the fingers. Apply pressure with the thumbs while rolling the walls inward to force the prolapse back through the anus (see Fig. 45-14, *step 3*). Care should be taken to avoid poking at the tissue with the fingertips. If substantial tissue edema has developed, application of gauze soaked in sugar water may promote shrinkage and subsequent manual reduction.[16]

Complications

Complications after successful reduction are uncommon but may include bleeding and ulceration. Failure to reduce a prolapse requires surgical consultation. Apply saline-moistened gauze over the rectal tissue while awaiting consultation. A persistently prolapsed rectum can result in ulceration, strangulation, and perforation of the bowel wall. Moreover, the possibility of loss of anal sphincter tone and incontinence increases with delays in reduction of rectal prolapse.

ANAL FISSURE

An anal fissure is a small laceration or ulcer at the anal verge.[5] Anal fissures are the most common cause of anorectal pain. Though appearing trivial on examination, fissures can be extremely painful, even hours after a bowel movement, because of persistent spasm (Fig. 45-15). The condition is quite difficult to eradicate, is debilitating, and can last for months. It is occasionally associated with bright red rectal bleeding. An anal fissure is most commonly found in young adults, men and women equally. In children it can be a sign of child abuse. Anal fissures are usually associated with constipation, a hard or strained stool, or chronic diarrhea, but the exact etiology is unknown. The diagnosis is relatively easy to make, and the fissure is readily seen by spreading the buttocks. The vast majority of anal fissures occur in the posterior midline, 10% to 15% occur in the anterior midline, and less

Figure 45-15 A posterior midline anal fissure is the most common type. Although some topical preparations may be helpful (see text), these lesions are painful and difficult to heal. In a child, an anal fissure may arouse suspicion of child abuse. (*By permission of Mayo Foundation.*)

than 1% occur in lateral positions. Fissures occurring in atypical locations should prompt consideration of other diseases. Multiple or recurrent fissures are associated with Crohn's disease, tuberculosis, syphilis, human immunodeficiency virus infection, and malignancy. Conservative therapy with the WASH regimen (see the section on hemorrhoids) may promote gradual healing in 4 to 6 weeks.

Most patients with acute anal fissures and almost half of patients with chronic fissures will experience healing with medical therapy. Therapy is aimed at breaking the cycle of pain, spasm, and ischemia, factors thought to be responsible for the development of the fissure. Therapies include relaxation of the internal sphincter, institution and maintenance of atraumatic passage of stool, and relief of pain. Simple measure include bulk agents, stool softeners, and probably most helpful, warm sitz baths following bowel movements to relax the sphincter. Based on the theory that anal fissures are caused by ischemia through a spasmodic internal sphincter, pharmacological agents, including glyceryl trinitrate (GTN), diltiazem, and botulinum toxin, may be useful as alternatives to surgical sphincterotomy for chronic fissures. GTN ointment applied two to four times per day to the anus results in various healing rates, but a major side effect is dose-related headaches. Nitroglycerin 0.2% ointment applied twice daily may heal chronic ulcers via a reduction in resting anal pressure and an increase in anoderm blood flow. Diltiazem ointment (2%) appears to have efficacy similar to that of GTN but may cause fewer side effects. Diltiazem may be associated with the development of pruritus. Both diltiazem and GTN are first-line therapies. Botulinum toxin causes temporary muscle paralysis by preventing the release of acetylcholine from presynaptic nerve terminals, thereby decreasing pressure in the internal sphincter. Surgical treatment is generally reserved for fissures that have failed medical therapy and is usually curative.

References are available at www.expertconsult.com

Musculoskeletal Procedures

CHAPTER 46

Prehospital Immobilization

Anne Klimke and Molly Furin

Modern emergency medical service (EMS) was created in 1966 as a result of the National Highway Safety Act. Since then, provision of medical care in the prehospital setting has undergone considerable change. Today's EMS providers can start intravenous lines, administer intravenous medications and fluids, and perform lifesaving procedures. Nonetheless, the task of immobilizing the spine, pelvis, and extremities has remained a primary EMS function. This chapter reviews basic prehospital immobilization techniques and equipment, including spinal immobilization, pelvic stabilization, extremity splinting, and removal of protective equipment.

SPINE IMMOBILIZATION

Background

The first recommendations for spinal immobilization following blunt trauma came from the American Academy of Orthopaedic Surgeons in 1971.[1] These guidelines called for spinal immobilization of patients with symptoms or physical findings suggestive of spinal injuries.[1,2] Since then, recommendations for spinal immobilization have evolved considerably. During the 1980s and 1990s, indications for spinal immobilization were based primarily on the mechanism of injury, regardless of the presence or absence of symptoms or physical findings suggestive of a spine injury.[2,3] This resulted in routine prehospital spinal immobilization for all but the most trivial injuries and an abundance of unnecessary radiographs. Such wide-scale prehospital immobilization was initiated despite scant scientific evidence of improved patient outcomes. As a result, efforts were initiated to determine whether historical or clinical data could reasonably identify who had and who did not have serious injuries that would theoretically benefit from prehospital immobilization.

Growing concern over the cost of cervical spine radiographs and excessive radiation exposure led to the development of easily applied low-risk criteria that could identify the vast majority of significant injuries in an attempt to safely reduce the overuse of cervical spine radiography.[4] In early 2000, two large prospective studies validated the use of clinical criteria to rule out injury to the cervical spine in victims of blunt trauma.[5,6] These studies dramatically reduced the number of unnecessary cervical spine radiographs following blunt trauma and led some investigators to question the prehospital practice of spinal immobilization based solely on mechanism of injury.[2,7-9]

In 1998, Hauswald and colleagues[7] published the results of a 5-year retrospective review comparing patients from Malaysia, where cervical spine immobilization was nonexistent, to patients from New Mexico, where cervical spine immobilization based on the mechanism of injury was standard practice. Based on their results, the authors concluded that out-of-hospital immobilization has little or no effect on neurologic outcome in patients with blunt spinal injuries.[7] More recently, researchers sought to determine whether prehospital providers could apply a set of clinical decision rules (Box 46-1) to selectively immobilize patients after blunt trauma.[10,11] A 4-year prospective study in two Michigan counties found that the use of a selective immobilization protocol resulted in spine immobilization for most patients with spinal injury without causing harm to patients in which spine immobilization was withheld.[10] A larger study in New York demonstrated that selective immobilization based on a statewide protocol resulted in only one nonimmobilized unstable cervical spine fracture in more than 32,000 patient encounters.[11] Several other trials supported the use of clinical criteria for cervical spine clearance by prehospital care providers and hence supported the safety of avoiding routine immobilization for injuries that are extremely unlikely to be clinically significant.[12,13]

Although spinal fracture and spinal cord injury (SCI) can have devastating results, the incidence of such injuries in trauma patients is relatively low, about 2% to 5% in most reviews. Unfortunately, most final neurologic outcomes after spinal cord trauma can be prognosticated by the initial evaluation, and lifelong disability has been set by the primary insult, not by prehospital or emergency department (ED) interventions. Sundheim and Cruz[14] calculated that only 0.03% to 0.16% of all out-of-hospital trauma patients may be expected to have *secondary SCI* that may be helped by immobilization. The number needed to immobilize to prevent one secondary injury is between 625 and 3333 trauma patients, but wholesale dismissal of any benefit from immobilization is not justified. It is important to note, however, *that despite*

> BOX 46-1 **Clinical Criteria for Prehospital Spine Immobilization**

Concerning mechanism of injury (such as axial loading, car roll-over, fall from a significant height)
Spine pain or tenderness
Focal neurologic deficit
Unreliable patient examination (not awake, alert, oriented, calm, and cooperative)
Head injury (including severe head and facial trauma)
Altered mental status:
    No history available
    Found in the setting of possible trauma (e.g., lying at the bottom of a staircase)
    Near-drowning with a history or high probability of a diving injury
Distracting injury
Communication barriers
Extremes of age

> BOX 46-2 **Spinal Immobilization for Trauma Patients***

Spinal cord damage from injury causes long-term disability and can dramatically affect quality of life. The current practice of immobilizing trauma patients before hospitalization to prevent more damage may not always be necessary because the likelihood of further damage is low. From studies of healthy volunteers it has been suggested that patients who are conscious might reposition themselves to relieve the discomfort caused by immobilization, which could theoretically worsen any existing spinal injuries.

AUTHORS' CONCLUSIONS

We did not find any randomized controlled trials that met the inclusion criteria. The effect of spinal immobilization on mortality, neurologic injury, spinal stability, and adverse effects in trauma patients remains uncertain. Because airway obstruction is a major cause of preventable death in trauma patients and because spinal immobilization, particularly of the cervical spine, can contribute to airway compromise, the possibility that immobilization may increase mortality and morbidity cannot be excluded. Large prospective studies are needed to validate the decision criteria for spinal immobilization in trauma patients at high risk for spinal injury. Randomized controlled trials in trauma patients are required to establish the relative effectiveness of alternative strategies for spinal immobilization.

From Kwan I, Bunn F, Roberts IG. Spinal immobilization for trauma patients. Cochrane Database Syst Rev. *2001;2CD002803.*
Published online January 21, 2009.

zealous use of prehospital cervical spine immobilization and countless medical and legal attempts to prove worsening of injury from its absence, there is little scientific evidence quantifying the effect of spinal immobilization in trauma patients or the possible adverse effects of its application (Box 46-2). Simply stated, the effect of spinal immobilization on mortality, neurologic injury, spinal stability, and adverse effects in trauma patients remains uncertain by evidence-based medicine, and no randomized prospective trials have been conducted.

Clinical judgment remains an acceptable and prudent approach, and it is most logical to consider the mechanism of injury and initial complaints or findings of neurologic dysfunction as reasonable indications for spine immobilization in the prehospital setting. However, despite growing questions regarding the efficacy and safety of routine prehospital spinal immobilization and despite a lack of scientific evidence demonstrating improved patient outcomes, it remains common practice for prehospital providers to immobilize most patients with traumatic mechanisms. Consequently, emergency medicine providers should be familiar with the devices and potential complications associated with spinal immobilization.

Epidemiology

According to the National Spinal Cord Injury Statistical Center (NSCISC), an estimated 12,000 new, survivable SCIs occur in the Unites States annually.[15] The NSCISC estimates that 265,000 people were living with SCI in the United States in 2010.[15] Since 2005, the most common cause of SCI is motor vehicle collision, which accounts for just more than 40% of cases, followed by falls and acts of violence, primarily gunshot wounds.[15] Sports such as American football, rugby, swimming and diving, gymnastics, ice hockey, track and field (specifically pole vaulting), cheerleading, and baseball all place participants at increased risk for spinal injuries.[15] The cost of care in both the immediate and extended care setting can be exorbitant, especially among the young. The average lifetime cost of medical care for patients with SCI varies depending on the level of injury but ranges from 500,000 to more than 3 million dollars.[15]

Pathophysiology

The direction and strength of the injurious force may help predict the type of injury sustained. Generally speaking, the basic forces that can be exerted on the spine are flexion, extension, rotation, lateral bending, distraction (stretching), and compression (axial loading).[16,17] Of course, complex mechanisms may exert multiple forces. For example, high-speed rollover motor vehicle collisions could easily exert all the aforementioned forces.

Injuries to the upper cervical spine (C1 and C2) (Fig. 46-1) occur more often in older, osteoporotic patients than in younger patients. The spectrum of injuries in the cervicocranium includes occipital condyle fractures, occipitoatlantal dislocations, dislocations and subluxations of the atlantoaxial joint, fractures of the ring of the atlas, odontoid fractures, fractures of the arch of the axis, and fractures of the lateral mass of the axis (Fig. 46-2). Involvement of the spinal cord at this high level can cause devastating neurologic injury, and it is reasonable to believe that many of these injuries are not reported because they result in death.[18] Subaxial cervical spinal injuries involving C3-7 have a broad spectrum of clinical implications. Approximately two thirds of cervical injuries causing quadriplegia occur within the lower cervical spine, with fractures occurring most often in C6 and C7 and dislocations most commonly occurring between C5-6 and C6-7.[19]

The orientation of the facets in the thoracic spine allows significantly less flexion and extension than in the cervical or lumbar spine. In addition, the free space between the thoracic spinal cord and the borders of the spinal canal is relatively

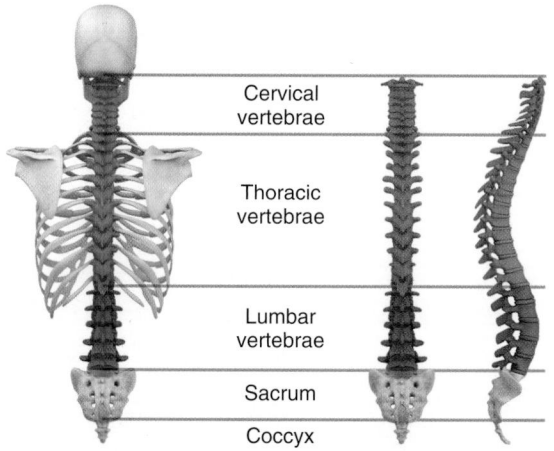

Figure 46-1 The human spinal column.

Cervical vertebrae

Thoracic vertebrae

Lumbar vertebrae

Sacrum

Coccyx

Figure 46-2 Type III odontoid (C2) fracture (*arrow*). A common scenario for this type of injury is an elderly woman who falls from a standing height.

small, and the blood supply is less robust. These factors increase the susceptibility of the spinal cord to injuries at this level. At the thoracolumbar junction there is an acute transition in stability because of the loss of rib restraint, which increases the risk for flexion-extension and rotational injuries. Disk size and shape also change, thus making this section of the spine particularly susceptible to injury. Approximately half of all vertebral body fractures and 40% of all SCIs occur between T11 and L2.[20]

The lumbar spine is protected only by the abdominal and paraspinous musculature, which makes it subject to distraction and shear forces, such as seen with lap belt injuries. There is also a higher prevalence of compression and burst fractures in the lumbar spine. These fractures commonly occur when axial loading forces straighten the natural lordosis at the moment of impact.[21]

The sacrum forms both the terminal portion of the spine and the central portion of the pelvis, which gives it added stability and makes isolated sacral fractures uncommon. Such fractures are usually caused by direct trauma or falls from a height or occur as a result of sacral insufficiency secondary to osteopenia, chronic steroid use, or previous pelvic irradiation.

BOX 46-3 Contraindications to Prehospital Spine Immobilization*

May be potentially harmful (e.g., prevents identification of airway compromise)
Need for a surgical airway
Presence of a preexisting airway (e.g., tracheostomy tube)
Obesity
Impaled objects
Chronic respiratory diseases (e.g., congestive heart failure) or acute respiratory distress from any cause (e.g., ascites)
Altered mental status (e.g., intoxicated patients)
Cervical dislocation or anatomic limitation because of preexisting conditions (e.g., ankylosing spondylitis)
Logistically impractical (e.g., mass casualty incident)
Unsafe scene:

- Exposure to hazardous material, fire, or smoke
- Building explosion or collapse
- Deep or fast moving water that poses a risk for drowning
- Risk for injury from assault (e.g., gunshot, stabbing, blunt trauma)
- Any other circumstance that the emergency medical service provider deems an immediate danger to the life or health of the patient, provider, or both

Situations listed in this table can often be managed with an improvised cervical immobilizer (e.g., towel roll or manual in-line stabilization [see text for details].

More often, sacral fractures occur as a result of high-energy mechanisms and are associated with major pelvic disruption.[22]

Indications

The National Association of EMS Physicians recommends spinal immobilization of prehospital trauma patients who sustain an injury with a mechanism that has the potential for causing spinal injury and who have at least one of the following clinical criteria: altered mental status, intoxication, a distracting painful injury (e.g., long-bone fracture), a neurologic deficit, and spinal pain or tenderness.[2]

Extremes of age and the presence of communication barriers (e.g., language, hearing impairment) may affect the ability to accurately assess the patient's perception and communication of pain and should lower one's threshold for spinal immobilization.[2,3] It is also important to remember that serious cervical cord injuries can occur in the absence of demonstrable fractures. SCI is common in elderly patients with cervical spondylosis, in whom an arthritic osteophyte may sever a portion of the cord as permanently as a fracture or dislocation. In such cases there may be little subjective pain, and the mechanism of injury may appear seemingly minor.[23]

Contraindications

Spinal immobilization is contraindicated (or may require modification) when its use could harm the patient, when it is logistically impossible, or when the scene is unsafe (Box 46-3). Good clinical judgment, not blind application of protocols, is essential. For example, if application of a cervical collar will cause or mask airway compromise secondary to swelling, an expanding hematoma, or other process, it should not be used. Obviously, if a patient requires a surgical airway, the EMS provider will need immediate, unencumbered access to the anterior aspect of the neck. Sometimes preexisting airways (e.g., tracheotomy tube) and associated equipment prohibit proper application of a cervical collar. These situations can often be managed with an improvised cervical immobilizer, such as a collar fashioned from a towel roll or prolonged manual stabilization without traction.

Other conditions that may prevent spinal immobilization or require modification of standard techniques and equipment (e.g., towel roll and manual in-line stabilization) include obesity, impaled objects, underlying respiratory problems or acute respiratory distress (e.g., from congestive heart failure or ascites), altered mental status (e.g., combative patients because of intoxication or psychiatric illness), and cervical dislocation with fixed angulation or anatomic limitations from preexisting conditions such as ankylosing spondylitis and kyphosis.[24]

There are also scenarios when spinal immobilization is logistically difficult or impossible. In a mass casualty incident, for instance, spinal immobilization of multiple victims with a low probability of spinal injury is impractical (Fig. 46-3).

Finally, spinal immobilization may need to be delayed or modified when the scene poses a significant threat to the patient or providers (see Box 46-3).[16] In these situations, the prehospital provider may opt for rapid extrication of the patient from the scene without immobilization of the spine (Fig. 46-4).

Equipment

Cervical Collars

Traditionally, cervical collars have used a four-point support structure at the bottom of the collar—at the two trapezius muscles posteriorly and at the two clavicles anteriorly. Most modern collars are modified rigid head-cervical-thoracic devices that use the sternum as a fifth support structure. Current collar designs support the head with winglike flaps on the collar's upper posterior edges. Anteriorly, the collar supports the mandible. The collar's flaring design generally prevents compression of the thyroid cartilage and cervical vessels, even when applied firmly. Some collars come as single units that conform to the neck once a chin support has been assembled, whereas others come in two parts, with a front and a back that are secured with Velcro (Fig. 46-5). Some manufacturers have developed collars that have adjustable heights to account for different neck lengths. Soft collars, though comfortable, have no role in spinal immobilization because they provide minimal support and do not reduce cervical motion to any significant degree.[25,26]

Investigators have attempted to evaluate cervical collars in an objective fashion. The accepted "gold standard" for comparison is the halo brace, which restricts motion to 4% flexion-extension, 1% rotation, and 4% lateral bending.[27] Unfortunately, even the best cervical collars (when used independently) restrict flexion and extension by only 70% to 75% and overall neck movement by 50% or less.[28] A number of studies have evaluated neck motion in volunteers immobilized supine on a backboard with various collars in place.[25,26,29-32] Although these studies demonstrated small differences among some of the collars, overall they merely confirm the fact that

Figure 46-3 Though often performed as a reflex for even minor trauma that has little or no chance of associated spinal injury, the true value of formal spinal immobilization in preventing initial, further, or secondary neurologic damage remains uncertain by evidence-based medicine, and no randomized prospective trials have been conducted. It is always prudent to be overly cautious, but during a mass casualty incident such as a train accident, spinal immobilization of multiple victims with a low probability of spinal injury may not be practical and may delay other more pressing interventions if resources are limited.

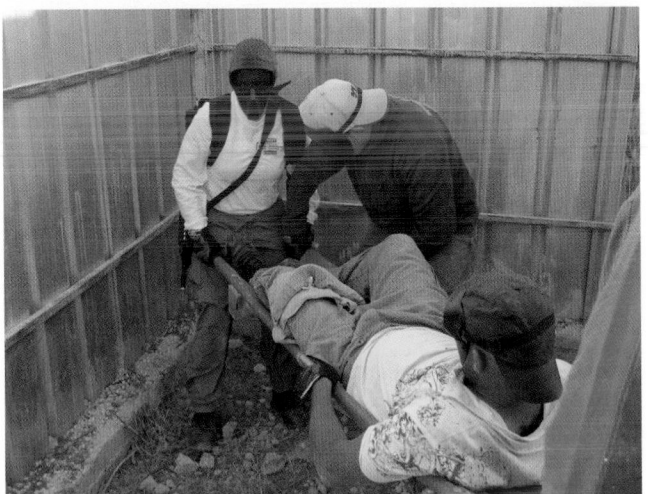

Figure 46-4 Spinal immobilization may need to be delayed or modified when the scene poses a significant threat to the patient or providers, such as evacuating a wounded soldier during a sniper attack. Rescue from a toxic or poisonous environment, such as hydrogen sulfide or carbon monoxide, is a similar situation.

cervical collars alone are inadequate to immobilize the cervical spine completely. Thus, it is important to keep in mind that for effective cervical spine immobilization, differences among the various types of cervical collars are less important than proper application, a snug but comfortable fit, and most importantly, use of adjunctive equipment.

Cervical Extrication Splints

A large variety of short spine boards (Fig. 46-6) and intermediate-stage extrication devices are available for

Figure 46-5 Cervical collars. **A,** Philadelphia collar. This two-piece, high-type collar comes in four sizes. The collar supports the head in a dish-shaped contour that is formed when the front and rear halves are joined by Velcro fasteners. When properly sized for a patient, this collar provides excellent support. When applied too tightly, it tends to force the mandible backward and can cause compression of the thyroid in some patients. **B,** Stifneck collar. This collar is made of high-density polyethylene (a hard material) and padded with semi-flexible foam margins. Note the low-reaching anterior panel, which contacts the sternum for additional support.

Fig. 46-6 Cervical extrication splints. **A,** Rigid short boards. **B,** Kendrick Extrication Device. *(Courtesy of Ferno-Washington, Inc., Wilmington, OH.)*

Figure 46-7 The LSP half-back. This cervical extrication splint resembles a Kendrick Extrication Device but is more rugged and durable. In addition to providing spinal immobilization, it also acts as a harness that can be used for hauling patients over flat surfaces and vertical lifts.

prehospital use. Generally, these devices are manufactured from rigid lightweight material. They have a narrow board design that permits easy application in automobiles or confined spaces and are constructed with multiple openings along the edges to allow a variety of strapping options. Ideally, these devices should also be translucent so that radiographs can be readily obtained in the ED, and they should allow repeated use and easy clean up. When not in use, store extrication splints with their straps secured in their individual retainers to reduce the likelihood of becoming entangled during application.

Application of a cervical extrication splint should not produce unnecessary movement or change the position of the head, neck, shoulders, or torso. In conjunction with a good cervical collar, a properly applied cervical extrication splint should effectively limit flexion, extension, and lateral and rotational motion of the head, neck, and torso.

One commonly used device that meets all these criteria is the Kendrick Extrication Device (KED) (see Fig. 46-6B). This device consists of two layers of nylon mesh impregnated with plastic and sewn over plywood slats to provide rigidity. It has a nylon loop behind the patient's head that is continuous with the pelvic support straps for additional strength. Part of its anterior thoracic panels can be folded backward to fit obese, pregnant, or pediatric patients.[33] When properly applied, the KED is a snug-fitting, highly adaptable immobilizer that can be used in even the most adverse circumstances.

When patients require immobilization or extrication (or both) in more difficult or treacherous environments, many EMS providers prefer the LSP half-back, which resembles a KED but is more rugged and durable. In addition to providing spinal immobilization, it also acts as a harness and can be used for hauling patients over flat surfaces, as well as vertical lifts (Fig. 46-7).[34]

Mosesso and coworkers[35] compared six prehospital cervical immobilization devices and concluded that the devices were similar in their ability to immobilize the cervical spine.

Full-Body Spine Immobilizers
Full-Body Spine Boards (Backboards)

Backboards are made of wood or plastic composites and can be either rectangular or tapered in shape (Fig. 46-8A). Most rescuers prefer the tapered type because it takes up less horizontal room when angled into a narrow opening or doorway. In addition, the slight narrowing of these boards on either end enhances the effectiveness of strapping.

Most backboards have strategically placed openings along the edges that can be used to secure head-stabilizing devices, strap the patient to the board, or lift the patient. Many also feature runners, usually about 2.5 cm thick, on their undersides that serve both as stiffeners and as spacers. They raise the board slightly off the ground so that rescuers can get

Iron Duck long spine board. *(Courtesy of Iron Duck — A Division of Fleming Industries, Chicopee, MA.)*

Ferno-Washington model 65 orthopaedic (scoop) stretcher. *(Courtesy of Ferno-Washington, Inc. Wilmington, OH.)*

CombiCarrier. *(Courtesy of Hartwell Medical, Carlsbad, CA.)*

Scoop EXL. *(Courtesy of Ferno-Washington, Inc. Wilmington, OH.)*

Miller body splint. *(Courtesy of Life Support Products, Inc., Irvine, CA.)*

Evac-U-Splint mattress. *(Courtesy of Hartwell Medical, Carlsbad, CA.)*

Figure 46-8 Full-body spine boards (backboards.)

their fingers under the board during lifting. The runners, however, may make it more difficult to slide a patient onto the board.

Advantages of boards over full-body splints include their ease of storage, low cost, and extreme versatility. The backboard can be used to slide a victim out of an automobile or to protect a victim during removal of a windshield.

The biggest drawback of using backboards as immobilizers is lack of patient comfort. Board splints, as a class, are the least comfortable of all immobilizers. Studies have demonstrated that spinal immobilization on a hard backboard causes head, back, and jaw pain.[36,37] Pain in these areas may become severe if patients are left immobilized on these boards for extended periods.[38-40] In addition, the pain caused by application of a backboard may be difficult to separate from other sources of pain in a trauma patient and might lead to unnecessary and costly radiographs.[2] Discomfort may be minimized by using padding at points of contact between a bony prominence and the board. This concept was reaffirmed by Hauswald and colleagues,[41] who found that increasing the amount of padding on a backboard decreases the amount of ischemic pain caused by immobilization.

Scoop Stretchers

If an injured person has to be extricated from a tight location, a smooth backboard is probably the best device to immobilize and move the victim. If the victim is not in a tight location, the scoop stretcher is an ideal field immobilizer (see Fig. 46-8B). In fact, one recent study found that using the Sterno scoop stretcher caused less spinal motion than did a traditional long backboard and logroll technique.[42]

The scoop stretcher is designed to split into two or four pieces. It is comfortable, rigid, and adaptable to patients of various lengths and provides unobstructed radiographic transparency of the entire spine. If necessary, it can be applied almost instantly or removed without disturbing the position of the victim. The scoop stretcher also provides good lateral stability because of the troughlike shape of its top surface, and it is stable enough to be used for carrying. For optimal protection of a potential spinal injury, the spine should be completely immobilized (e.g., cervical collar, lateral supports, and secure strapping) and the scoop stretcher should be placed on a backboard before moving the patient. In addition, the scoop stretcher should be carefully reassembled to avoid trapping clothes, skin, or other objects between interlocking parts.

The scoop interferes slightly with the ischial section of a half-ring traction splint but works well with Sager-type devices. The Ferno-Washington model 65 scoop (Ferno-Washington, Inc., Wilmington, OH) is the most widely used stretcher of this type. Other devices such as the Combi-Carrier (Hartwell Medical, Carlsbad, CA) and the Scoop EXL (Ferno-Washington, Inc., Wilmington, OH) offer lightweight polymer construction and additional spine support (see Fig. 46-8C and D).

Full-Body Splints

Various devices take the concept of full-body immobilization one step further than the spine board. One popular device is the Miller body splint, which consists of a polyethylene shell injected with closed-cell foam that is radiographically translucent and provides buoyancy in water (see Fig. 46-8E). This full-body splint features a removable head harness and a thoracic harness, as well as pelvic and lower extremity belts. The space between the lower extremities facilitates wrapping with bandage material in the event of fractures. In addition, it is shaped so that it can easily fit into a basket-type rescue stretcher. Similar spine immobilization systems are available for pediatric patients (e.g., Pedi-Pac, Ferno-Washington, Inc., Wilmington, OH).

An important innovation in the area of spine immobilization in the United States has been the vacuum mattress splint (e.g., EVAC-U-SPLINT, Hartwell Medical, Carlsbad, CA, and Immobile-Vac, MDI, Gurnee, IL) (see Fig. 46-8F). It consists of a vinyl-coated polyester envelope filled with thousands of 1.1-mm-diameter polyester foam spheres. A manual or electric vacuum pump is used to evacuate the interior to a pressure of about 0.25 atm. This reduction in internal pressure causes the mattress to conform to the contours of the patient's body. Vacuum splints have been shown to produce lower sacral interface pressure and lower mean pain scores than traditional hard backboards[37,43] and may provide better immobilization in patients with known SCI.[44,45] It should also be pointed out, however, that vacuum splints are larger and more cumbersome than backboards, thus making ambulance storage more difficult.

Lateral Neck Stabilizers

Lightweight objects such as blocks (10 × 10 × 15 cm) made of medium-density foam rubber are commonly used to provide additional lateral stabilization of the head and neck. Foam blocks are inexpensive and disposable and do not slip on the backboard. Disposable cardboard devices that have the same advantages as foam blocks are also available (Fig. 46-9A).

Another commercial device is the Universal Head Immobilizer. It is a lateral neck stabilizer designed to quickly and easily fasten the patient's head to a scoop stretcher or spine board (see Fig. 46-9B). The Universal Head Immobilizer is made of a Herculite nylon and polyethylene foam platform fastened to the stretcher with Velcro straps. The lateral pillows are then attached to the nylon platform by means of large Velcro interfaces.

It should be noted that although sandbags are effective devices for lateral immobilization, they may cause significant movement of the neck if the board is suddenly tilted (e.g., to decrease the risk for aspiration in a vomiting patient). Therefore, their use is no longer recommended.

A

B

Figure 46-9 Lateral neck stabilizers. **A,** The HeadBed, a cervical immobilization device made of a water-resistant corrugated board. **B,** Universal Head Immobilizer. (*A, Courtesy of Laerdal Medical Corporation, Wappingers Falls, NY; B, courtesy of Ferno-Washington, Inc., Wilmington, OH.*)

Figure 46-10 Padding. Padding increases comfort and theoretically may prevent further injury. It can also help support an injured extremity or impaled object or allow an obese or kyphotic patient to lie supine on a long backboard.

Foam Padding

Padding increases comfort and can help prevent further injury. It can also help support an injured extremity or impaled object or allow an obese or kyphotic patient to lie supine on a long backboard (Fig. 46-10).[29] Pregnant women may benefit from padding under the right hip to help shift the gravid uterus off the inferior vena cava and increase venous return.[46]

Padding applied under the neck and shoulders prevents hyperflexion in children with large occiputs (Fig. 46-11) or in individuals wearing certain types of helmets (e.g., bicycle, motorcycle, rock climbing) that cannot be removed in the field.

Procedure

Cervical Spine Immobilization

It is important to remember that the continuous nature of the spinal column means that movement of one part of the column is transmitted to the other areas, so to protect the injured area the entire spine must be immobilized. This requires the head, neck, and torso to be fastened into a single common plane. Hence, in addition to a rigid cervical collar, the patient must also be secured to an intermediate spine-immobilizing device (e.g., short spine board, KED), a full-length spine board (e.g., backboard, scoop stretcher, full-body splint), or both (see later) to ensure complete cervical spine immobilization.

The first priority in cervical spine immobilization is providing manual in-line stabilization in the neutral position. This can be done with the patient standing, seated, supine, or prone and consists simply of placing both hands on the sides of the patient's head to prevent flexion, rotation, or bending. Do not apply cervical traction because it can increase the risk for SCI, and be sure to maintain manual in-line stabilization during application of the cervical collar and until the patient can be fully immobilized in an intermediate-stage corset-type device or on a long backboard (see later in this section). Once the cervical spine has been manually stabilized in the neutral position, examine the neck for swelling, ecchymosis, deformity, bony tenderness, or penetrating wounds. Application of a cervical collar follows and is generally a straightforward procedure (Fig. 46-12). The rescuer's intentions should be thoroughly explained to the patient throughout the procedure.

Figure 46-11 A, Young child immobilized on a standard backboard. Note how the large head forces the neck into flexion. Backboards can be modified by an occiput cutout (**B**) or a double mattress pad (**C**) to raise the chest, the actual clinical consequences of which are unknown. (*A-C, Adapted from Herzenberg JE, Hensinger RN, Dedrick DK, et al. Emergency transport and positioning of young children who have an injury of the cervical spine. J Bone Joint Surg Am. 1989;71:15.*)

Once the collar is in place, conscious patients should be cautioned repeatedly against movement of the head. Investigate any persistent complaints of pain or dyspnea by removal and possible replacement of the device while manual stabilization is maintained. The size of collar should be determined from the manufacturer's suggested guidelines. For example, the Stifneck collar (Laerdal Medical Corp., Wappingers Falls, NY) is available in various sizes and uses the distance from the top of the shoulder to the chin to determine the appropriate size. Use the tallest collar that does not cause hyperextension. For extremely short necks, a special cervical collar such as the No-Neck (Laerdal Medical Corp., Wappingers Falls, NY) is recommended. In cases in which a cervical collar of the proper size is not available, an improvised device should be made from available material (Fig. 46-13).

It should also be remembered that application of a cervical collar should not be attempted until the patient's head has been brought into a neutral position and manual in-line stabilization has been applied.[28] If the patient experiences cervical muscle spasm, increased pain, neurologic complaints (e.g., paresthesias, weakness), or airway compromise, immediately halt any further movement of the head and neck. In these situations, immobilize in the position that the patient was found by using an alternative technique (e.g., blanket, towel roll, manual in-line stabilization).

Thoracolumbar Spine Immobilization

Despite the presence of a field cervical collar, manual in-line cervical stabilization should be continued until the patient is fully immobilized with either a cervical extrication splint or a full-body splint (e.g., a backboard or vacuum stretcher). The immobilization technique used will depend on the patient's position of origin.

Sitting Position

To immobilize patients who are in a sitting position, use a short backboard or commercially available cervical extrication device (e.g., KED). At least two rescuers should be present to apply an extrication splint to a sitting patient. Interestingly, a recent study by Shafer and Naunheim found that healthy volunteers who were allowed to extricate themselves from the front seat of a car and lie down on a long spine board while wearing a cervical collar had less spinal movement than did those who were placed in cervical collars and moved onto the board directly or after application of a KED.[47] Nevertheless, use of KEDs or short boards remains the most common method for vehicle extrication.

Open the device butterfly style and gently slide it behind the victim via a rocking motion (Fig. 46-14, *step 1*). If necessary, carefully rock the patient forward a few degrees to facilitate placement of the splint. Once behind the victim, free the splint's pelvic support straps from their retainers and allow them to dangle at the patient's sides. Next, bring the lateral thoracic panels around the chest just beneath the patient's shoulders. Grasp these panels and slide the splint upward until the top edges of the panels firmly engage the patient's axillae. Now use the thoracic straps to secure the splint, beginning with the middle strap, then the bottom strap, and finally the top strap (see Fig. 46-14, *step 2*).

This procedure may need to be modified depending on injuries and preexisting conditions. For example, patients with pelvic fractures may not tolerate placement of the pelvic support and bottom straps, and the gravid abdomen of a pregnant patient may prevent placement of the middle strap. The straps should be snug, but not so tight that they interfere with respiration.

Fasten the pelvic support straps next. They can be slipped one at a time beneath the patient's lower extremities and brought directly beneath the pelvis with a back-and-forth motion. If the pelvic straps are not applied properly, considerable slippage may occur when the patient is lifted. Connect the free end of each pelvic strap to buckles located at the patient's hip on the outside of the splint. Once a strap is ready to be buckled, it can be either attached to the buckle on its own side or moved across the patient's lap and engaged with the opposite buckle. Most prehospital care providers prefer the latter method because it allows the patient's knees to remain together without discomfort. It is also a good idea to pad the groin area when placing the pelvic support straps because these straps may cause the patient considerable discomfort.

Next, secure the head to the device (see Fig. 46-14, *step 3*). When using the KED, wrap the head panels snugly around the head and neck while another rescuer applies the diagonal head straps. It may be necessary to place padding behind the

Figure 46-13 Horse collar. Most extrication collars are available in three to five factory sizes. If a collar is not sized properly to fit a particular patient, it performs no function. Patients with extremely long necks or especially short ones can be immobilized by means of a horse collar fashioned from a blanket or towel. The blanket (or towel) is rolled to the thickness desired and slid under the patient's neck while a bystander applies manual stabilization; the ends of the blanket (or towel) are then brought across the anterior aspect of the patient's chest. (*Courtesy of AtlantiCare Regional Medical Center, Emergency Medical Services, Atlantic City, NJ.*)

CERVICAL COLLAR APPLICATION

A Posterior-First Method

While one provider applies in-line stabilization (*not* traction!), slide the posterior portion of the collar behind the patient's neck. Maintain in-line stabilization in the neutral position until the patient is fully immobilized.

Bring the front portion of the collar around, under the patient's chin. Ensure that the chin is well supported by the chin piece. Difficulty positioning the chin piece may indicate the need for a shorter collar.

Attach the loop Velcro from the posterior portion of the collar to the hook Velcro on the anterior portion. Recheck the position of the patient's head for proper alignment. Tighten the collar as needed until proper support is obtained.

B Anterior-First Method

While in-line stabilization is provided, position the chin piece under the patient's chin.

Slide the posterior portion of the collar behind the patient's neck.

Secure the collar and assess proper placement as described above.

Figure 46-12 Cervical collar application.

head to maintain a neutral position. Use the forehead as a point of engagement for one strap and the cervical collar for the other.

As a final step, tighten all buckles until the entire splint is firmly in place. The patient can now be moved. If the patient is to be lifted from a vehicle, bring the ambulance cot with a spine board on it as close to the patient as possible (see Fig. 46-14, *step 4*). While one rescuer supports the patient's knees, the other rescuer uses the handholds on the splint to lift the patient. The patient should be rotated and laid in a supine position onto a backboard. Loosen the pelvic straps to allow the legs to be lowered onto the backboard. The legs can then be extended and secured to the backboard or left in the flexed position with a pillow placed under the knees for support.

Apply a lateral immobilizer to help prevent movement of the head and neck, and strap the body into place on the backboard. Once the patient is on the board, the thoracic straps of the cervical extrication splint may need to be readjusted.

Recumbent Position

A patient who is found in a recumbent position should be placed in a supine position, if not already in one. If repositioning is necessary, examine the back during the process. Physical examination, spinal immobilization, airway management, and transport are easier to accomplish with the patient in the supine position.

Patients who are found supine do not require the use of a cervical extrication splint. They should, however, receive initial manual in-line cervical stabilization and a cervical collar. The patient should then be fastened to a full-body spinal immobilizer, such as a scoop stretcher, backboard, or full-body splint.

Scoop Stretcher. A patient who is in a supine position can be moved by means of a scoop stretcher. In a conscious patient, rescuers should explain that they are about to apply a scoop-type stretcher, which may be cold to the touch, beneath the patient's body. Apply a cervical collar and

KENDRICK EXTRICATION DEVICE (KED)

Apply a cervical collar and maintain in-line stabilization throughout the procedure. Gently slide the KED behind the patient; it may be necessary to rock the patient forward a few degrees to facilitate placement of the device.

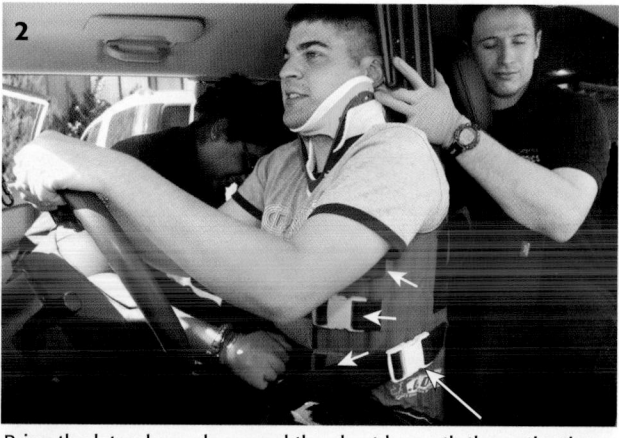

Bring the lateral panels around the chest beneath the patient's shoulders. First secure the thoracic straps (*short arrows*), and then fasten the pelvic support straps (*long arrow*). See text for details.

Next, secure the patient's head to the device. Wrap the head panels snugly around the head and neck while another rescuer applies the diagonal head straps (*arrows*).

Bring the ambulance stretcher (with a backboard on it) as close to the patient as possible. Rotate the patient out of the vehicle and onto the backboard. Loosen the pelvic straps, and secure the patient to the board.

Figure 46-14 Kendrick Extrication Device. Use of other short boards follows the same principles as depicted here.

maintain manual in-line cervical stabilization until the patient is completely secured to the stretcher.

Place the scoop on the ground next to the patient and open the latches that regulate its length. Adjust the length to fit the full length of the patient's body and reengage (lock) the latches. Next, release the latches at each end and separate the stretcher into two halves. Place each half next to the patient. One rescuer then gently pushes half the stretcher under one side of the patient. In some cases it may be necessary to have another rescuer rock the patient to allow proper positioning. Repeat the procedure with the opposite half of the scoop until both halves are aligned beneath the patient. Engage the latch at the head of the device first. Then bring the lower ends together and engage the foot latch to complete the integrity of the stretcher. Strap the patient's torso into place and immobilize the head with a suitable lateral neck stabilizer. The patient can then be lifted onto another device for transport (e.g., Stokes stretcher or backboard). After placement on another device, the scoop stretcher can be removed without disturbing the patient's position, if necessary.

Full-Body Spine Boards (Backboards). There are several ways of placing a patient onto a spine board. The precise technique used will depend on the space available and the position of the patient within that space. For lengthwise extrication, as from an automobile seat, the patient can be slid, either feet first or head first, onto the backboard. It is important that the patient be moved as a unit during this process. Place one end of the backboard on the seat or doorsill of the automobile. One rescuer stabilizes the opposite end of the board while at least two other rescuers lift and slide the patient's body onto the board. Once the patient is secured to the board, slide the board out of the vehicle and onto a waiting stretcher. Maintain manual cervical in-line stabilization throughout the procedure and avoid spinal compression or traction.

When space permits, lateral extraction is preferred. If the patient is in the recumbent position, logroll or slide the patient onto the board. The *logroll maneuver* requires the presence of at least three rescuers. Position one rescuer at the patient's head to apply manual in-line cervical stabilization (Fig. 46-15, *step 1*). It is this person's responsibility to oversee and direct body movement throughout the procedure. Next, position the backboard next to the patient's body (see Fig. 46-15, *step 2*). To minimize thoracolumbar movement, extend the patient's arms at the sides with the palms resting on the lateral aspect of the thighs.[48] To keep the patient from reaching for a rescuer or object during transfer, some rescuers prefer to have patients cross their arms across the thorax. However, this maneuver has not been shown to prevent or minimize thoracolumbar movement. If one arm is injured, place the backboard against this side so that the patient can be rolled onto the uninjured extremity. Position the other rescuers on the side that the patient will be rolled toward, with one rescuer at the midchest level and the other at the legs. The rescuer at the chest should reach across the victim and take hold of the shoulder and hips while the other rescuer grasps the hips and lower part of the legs. When everyone is ready, the rescuer at the head gives the command to roll the patient onto the side (see Fig. 46-15, *step 3*). If possible, examine the patient's back at this point. Slide the backboard under the patient, and when everyone is ready, the rescuer at the head gives the command to roll the patient back onto the

board (see Fig. 46-15, *step 4*). Before applying straps, it is often necessary to center the patient on the board.

To safely center the patient on the long spine board, support the cervical spine, shoulders, and hips and slide the patient first caudally, then cephalad, in a zigzag pattern to avoid applying uneven lateral or rotational force onto the spine. Alternatively, during lateral extraction, a recumbent patient can be slid sideways onto the spine board. This improvised technique also requires the presence of three or four rescuers, one of whom can maintain control of the patient's head and neck.

Various techniques can be used to secure a patient to the backboard. In addition to the standard thoracic, pelvic, and lower extremity straps, use of an abdominal strap significantly reduces lateral motion without compromising respiration.[49] Proper strap placement and firm contact between the straps and the patient are also important in limiting lateral motion (see Fig. 46-15, *step 5*).[50]

After the body has been strapped to the board, the head can be secured. If necessary, padding can be placed under the occiput to maintain the head in the neutral position. Apply a lateral neck stabilizer (e.g., foam blocks, HeadBed device) and secure the head in place with tape or straps (see Fig. 46-15, *step 6*). Most taping techniques involve the use of one piece across the forehead and one piece across the cervical collar. Note that this method of securing a patient to a backboard is designed for horizontal lifting only.

Standing Position

A standing patient with a potential spine injury must be immobilized and placed in the supine position. One technique for placing these patients on a backboard that is quick, safe, and effective is presented here.[51] Position the tallest rescuer behind the patient to manually stabilize the head while a second rescuer applies a cervical collar (Fig. 46-16, *step 1*). The first rescuer must maintain manual in-line cervical stabilization until the patient is completely secured to the board. Center the backboard behind the patient between the arms of the rescuer who is stabilizing the head and neck (see Fig. 46-16, *step 2*). Facing the patient, a rescuer on each side reaches under the patient's arms and grabs the backboard by a handhold at or above the patient's axillae (see Fig. 46-16, *step 3*). The patient's elbows are then brought closer to the body. If additional personnel are available, position a rescuer at the feet to prevent the board from sliding out. Slowly tilt the patient back by lowering the head of the backboard (see Fig. 46-16, *step 4*). The rescuer at the head should step back during this process while maintaining the patient's head and neck in neutral alignment. When the backboard is completely horizontal, secure the patient to the backboard in the usual fashion.

Pediatric Patients

Little information is available on the proper selection and application of spinal immobilization devices for children. Most of the data available were derived from studies of adults and might not be applicable to children. Half of the total growth in head circumference is achieved by the age of 18 months, thus giving children a disproportionately large head in comparison to the rest of the body. Before 8 years of age, these anatomic and developmental differences result in a higher incidence of upper cervical spine injuries (C1-2).

FULL-BODY SPINE BOARD (BACKBOARD): LOGROLL MANEUVER

Position one rescuer at the patient's head to apply manual in-line stabilization. This rescuer oversees and directs all body movement throughout the procedure.

Position the backboard next to the patient's body. Note that a lateral neck stabilizer has been pre-applied to the board.

When the rescuer at the patient's head gives the command, roll the patient onto his side, examine the patient's back, and slide the backboard under the patient.

Roll the patient back onto the board when the head rescuer gives the command. Center the patient on the board before applying the straps.

Strap the patient to the board. Proper strap placement (chest, pelvis, and legs) and firm contact between the straps and the patient are important in limiting lateral motion.

Apply a lateral neck stabilizer, like the Ferno Universal Head Immobilizer shown above. Secure it in place using the supplied straps or tape.

Figure 46-15 Full-body spine board (backboard): the logroll maneuver.

Because injuries in this area are frequently unstable, proper cervical immobilization in the neutral position is critically important.

In the neutral position, the pediatric cervical spine is normally lordotic or extended.[52] However, because the occiput is large, positioning the child's body on a standard backboard may force the neck into flexion or a relative kyphosis. The clinical significance of this is currently unclear, but theoretically it may be hazardous for young children. Therefore, the standard backboard should be modified to adapt to the child's larger head size. As a rough guide, the external auditory meatus should be on the same level as the midpoint of the

FULL-BODY SPINE BOARD (BACKBOARD): STANDING POSITION

Position the tallest rescuer behind the patient to provide manual in-line stabilization while a second rescuer applies a cervical collar.

Center the backboard behind the patient, in between the arms of the first rescuer.

A rescuer on each side of the patient reaches under the patient's arms and grabs the backboard by a handhold at or above the patient's axillae.

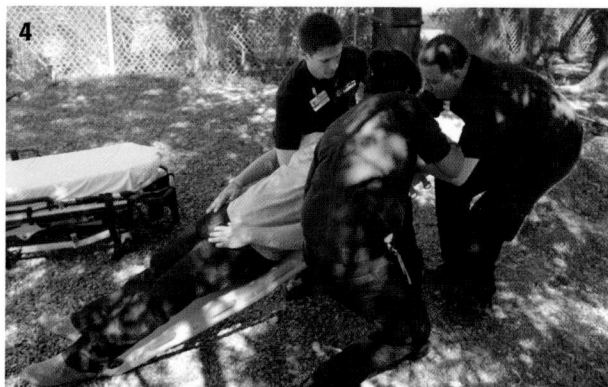

Slowly tilt the patient back by lowering the head of the backboard. The rescuer at the patient's head steps back during this process. Secure the patient to the board as depicted in Figure 46-15.

Figure 46-16 Full-body spine board: securing the patient from a standing position.

shoulder. Suggested modifications include a cutout in the backboard that accommodates the occiput or a pad under the back at the level of the chest (see Fig. 46-11). If not modified, the standard backboard in conjunction with the disproportionately large head of a child may force the neck into hyperflexion and potentially aggravate an underlying cervical spine injury. Nypaver and Treloar[53] showed that all children required elevation of the back (mean height, 25.4 ± 6.7 mm) for correct neutral position on a spine board. Children younger than 4 years required more elevation than did those 4 years or older. It must be pointed out, however, that there have been no published reports of a cord lesion resulting from the use of standard immobilization techniques and equipment in children.[52]

Complications

Cervical Immobilization

Improper application of a cervical collar can occur if the wrong size is used or too little care is exercised during placement. The best means of preventing either error is strong clinician involvement in training and continuing education of EMS crews together with vigorous feedback regarding correct

and incorrect application. In addition, adherence to the manufacturer's collar-specific recommendations for size and application should be emphasized.

A collar that is too small for a patient may be either too tight for the girth of the neck (with obvious complications) or too short to provide adequate immobilization. Too large a collar commonly results in hyperextension, which can exacerbate a preexisting spinal injury. Underlying spinal abnormalities from conditions such as ankylosing spondylitis, rheumatoid arthritis, or kyphosis can also contribute to exacerbation of injuries with cervical collar application.[24]

Improper or prolonged application of an extrication collar may impede venous return and raise intracranial pressure (ICP).[54] Although the clinical significance of increased ICP produced by cervical immobilization is still unknown, two studies have confirmed that application of a rigid cervical collar causes a statistically significant and sustained rise in ICP.[55,56] Kolb and colleagues[55] reported a 24.8–cm H_2O increase in cerebrospinal fluid pressure in 20 adult patients undergoing lumbar puncture. Hunt and associates[56] reported a 4.6–mm Hg mean rise in ICP in 30 patients with severe traumatic brain injury. The largest rise in ICP was noted in patients with a baseline ICP higher than 15 mm Hg. The

Figure 46-17 This seizure patient was initially postictal and combative and did not allow prehospital cervical spine immobilization. Although this is a dilemma for all involved, it is best to avoid forcing such immobilization (see Box 46-1). Sedation may be an alternative if injury is suspected and immobilization is deemed clinically necessary. Despite a now clear mental status and no neck pain (and National Emergency X-radiology Utilization Study rules negative), an unneeded collar was subsequently applied in the emergency department, to the annoyance of the patient, who then became very agitated and tried to leave. Note that the patient is now physically restrained and is *incorrectly still upright.*

authors of these studies concluded that the elevation in ICP produced by cervical immobilization might have deleterious effects in patients with acute or sustained intracranial hypertension.[55,56]

Long-term use of the Philadelphia extrication collar (Philadelphia Cervical Collar Co., Westville, NJ) as part of the treatment plan for an underlying cervical spine injury has been associated with pressure ulcers of the scalp.[57] Because some collars (e.g., Philadelphia and Stifneck) have been shown to exert higher capillary closing pressure at contact points, it is suggested that collars with favorable skin pressure patterns and superior patient comfort (e.g., Nec-Loc, Jerome Medical, Moorestown, NJ) be used for long-term application.

One final complication should be mentioned. A patient who, for whatever reason, actively resists placement of a cervical collar or other splint *should not be forced to wear it* (Fig. 46-17). Postictal and intoxicated patients may present such a dilemma. Immobilization of a combative patient cannot be accomplished without considerable muscular exertion, not only by rescuers but also by the patient. If fractures do exist, it is possible that struggling can cause further damage. If the patient permits manual stabilization, this should be used as an alternative. Sedation may be used judiciously to enhance compliance.

Thoracolumbar Immobilization

In general, complications are more likely to occur from failure to immobilize spinal injuries before movement than from the technique of immobilization. When complications do arise, they may be related to improper choice or use of equipment or prolonged immobilization.

Victims are generally strapped in place on a spine board to prevent sliding during transport. If too few straps are used or if the straps are loosely applied, motion during transport can

occur. Moreover, even when applied correctly, spinal immobilization on a hard board may be extremely uncomfortable for patients and may induce pressure-related tissue damage. In one study, 100% of healthy volunteers reported significant pain after only 30 minutes on a long spine board.[36] Occipital headaches, as well as mandibular, lumbar, and sacral pain, developed in these subjects. Other studies have demonstrated elevated tissue interface pressure in patients on spine boards without air mattress padding.[38,58,59] These studies underscore the need to use adequate padding and remove patients from the board as soon as possible.

Excessive strapping can interfere with respiratory function in both children[60] and adults.[61-63] In healthy children 6 to 15 years old, forced vital capacity (FVC) has been shown to decrease from 4% to 59% during spinal immobilization.[60] Totten and Sugarman[63] evaluated the effect of two spinal immobilization methods (wooden backboard and vacuum mattress) on eight respiratory function measurements in healthy volunteers. In comparing baselines for each method, six of the eight measures (FVC, FVC%, forced expiratory volume in 1 second [FEV_1], FEV_1%, peak expiratory flow [PEF], and forced expiratory flow [FEF_{25-75}%]) were reduced an average of 15%. Although this may not be a problem in healthy volunteers, the effects on patients with chest trauma or preexisting respiratory disease may be significant.[63]

Patients immobilized on a backboard are also at risk for aspiration if they vomit. If this does occur, the patient and board should be logrolled as a unit to the side. Although this procedure may be associated with some spinal movement, airway protection takes precedent.

Conclusion

Even though spinal immobilization has not been shown to decrease the likelihood of spinal injury and may actually increase morbidity because of complications, it remains a mainstay of prehospital trauma treatment. Prehospital providers will continue its practice until further evidence leads to a widespread paradigm shift and modification of trauma protocols. In the meantime, emergency medicine practitioners should know when its continued use is indicated, recognize properly and improperly applied devices, and minimize unnecessary immobilization time.

EXTREMITY IMMOBILIZATION

Upper Extremity

Background

The earliest evidence of upper extremity splinting comes from the Egyptians circa 300 BCE. In 1903 archaeologists from the Hearst expedition discovered two specimens whose open fractures had been treated with wooden splints and bandages. Their bones showed no signs of healing, so the subjects probably died soon after their injuries; however, numerous other ancient Egyptian specimens that have been discovered show evidence of well-healed forearm fractures.[64]

The purpose of splinting is to prevent motion of broken or dislocated bone ends. Carefully applied splints decrease pain while minimizing further damage to muscles, nerves, and blood vessels. Splinting also reduces the risk of converting a closed injury to an open one.[65] Nevertheless, injuries to adjacent structures may still occur, so circulation, motor function, and sensation distal to the injury must be assessed early and monitored closely during transport.

Over the last 3 decades, prehospital splinting materials, equipment, and techniques have evolved considerably. Today's prehospital providers can choose from a wide assortment of ready-to-use splints made from a variety of sturdy lightweight material.

Indications and Contraindications

Indications for splinting an extremity are usually clear. Pain after trauma, with or without deformity, should arouse suspicion of underlying bone or joint injury. Other signs include swelling, discoloration, deformity, crepitus, and loss of neurovascular function. However, absence of these findings does not rule out an underlying fracture or dislocation. Thus, whenever a musculoskeletal injury is suspected, a splint should be applied and maintained.

There are no absolute contraindications to splinting suspected upper extremity fractures or dislocations. However, in the setting of multisystem trauma with life-threatening injuries, rapid transport may be more important than extremity splinting. Averting loss of life takes precedence over loss of limb.

Equipment

Various types of splints are currently available for immobilizing upper extremity injuries. Emergency care providers should be well trained and familiar with their equipment. The type of splint used is less important than the expertise of the provider applying the splint. Upper extremity splints can be divided into two basic types: rigid and soft.[66]

Rigid Splints

Rigid and semirigid splints are the mainstays of EMS fracture care (Fig. 46-18*A-C*). These splints are made of many different material, including cardboard, plastic, aluminum, wire, and wood. They are fastened to the injured extremity with tape, gauze, cravats, or Velcro straps. Rigid splints are generally nonflexible (some commercially available splints may have some flexibility in their design) and, when applied properly, immobilize the limb in a rigid fashion to maintain stability. Although most commercial rigid splints are prepadded, many will still benefit from additional soft padding to cushion the splint and increase comfort. This is particularly true over bony prominences. When applying rigid splints, leave the fingertips exposed so that the distal circulation can be continuously monitored.

Cardboard splints are excellent for long-bone fractures in the upper part of the arm. They can be formed into many shapes and are easy to apply, inexpensive, lightweight, radiolucent, and compatible with magnetic resonance imaging. Splints made from wax-impregnated cardboard are also water resistant. Plastic, aluminum, wire, and wood splints, though less malleable, are also good choices. An inexpensive aluminum splint that is popular with emergency care providers and can be found in many wilderness medical kits is the SAM Splint (Sam Medical Products, Portland, OR) (see Fig. 46-18*D*). The SAM Splint is built from a thin core of soft aluminum alloy sandwiched between two layers of closed-cell foam. The SAM Splint is extremely pliable. Bent into any of three simple curves, it is extremely strong and provides support for any fractured or injured extremity. In addition, it is water resistant, lightweight, radiolucent, reusable, and not affected by extreme temperatures or altitudes. These characteristics make it an ideal tool for emergency care providers and outdoor enthusiasts.

Vacuum splints (see Fig. 46-18*E*) are a special type of rigid splint in which the air is evacuated from a closed bag containing tiny foam beads. This compresses the contents into a solid mass and results in a rigid splint. Injuries can be encased and immobilized in the position in which they are found, thereby reducing patient discomfort. Flexibility of the splint before removal of the air allows molding of the splint to conform to the patient's position. Vacuum splints are radiolucent and do not apply external pressure, thus ensuring maximum circulation to the injured extremity.

Soft Splints

Soft splints include air splints, pillows, slings, and swaths. Depending on the type of injury being treated, immobilization with pillows, slings, or swaths alone may be inadequate because they allow significant flexibility and motion. Therefore, when treating fractures and dislocations, these splints are most effective when used with some form of a rigid device. However, even when used alone, pillows, slings, or swaths provide cushioning and some limitation of motion that may be adequate for less severe injuries such as sprains and contusions.

Air splints are soft splints that become rigid when inflated. Besides providing immobilization, they help compress the underlying soft tissue to reduce local hemorrhage. These devices are sensitive to differences in atmospheric pressure and temperature. Therefore, constantly monitor their inflation to ensure that the underlying tissue is not being subjected to pressure-induced ischemia and the development of a compartment syndrome. One study suggested a maximum splint pressure of 15 mm Hg to reduce the risk for ischemia.[67] With long ambulance transport times, deflate the splint for 5 minutes every 1.5 hours.[68]

Disadvantages include an inability (with most air splints) to continuously monitor pulses once the air splint is in place and susceptibility of the air splint chambers to puncture. Air splints are designed to conform to a specific shape when inflated and should not be used on angulated fractures. In addition to being radiolucent, some types can be inflated with a refrigerant to provide concurrent cooling.

Pillow splints (see Fig. 46-18*F*) can be fashioned from any soft bulky material and are excellent choices for hand or wrist injuries. These splints are extremely comfortable and can be applied easily.

Slings and swaths are generally used in combination with a rigid or a soft splint. When used alone, they can effectively immobilize injuries to the shoulder, clavicle, or humerus (see Fig. 46-18*G*).

Procedures

To properly apply a splint to an injured extremity, several guidelines should be followed. Communication is important to ensure that the patient understands what is being done at all times. When possible, administer an appropriate analgesic to make splint application less painful. Remove any unnecessary clothing to adequately visualize the injured extremity. Stabilize the fracture site manually to help limit unnecessary movement and prevent further injury. Check the patient's neurovascular status (i.e., pulse, motor, and sensation) before and after the application of a splint. For a severely angulated

GENERAL SPLINTING GUIDELINES:
• Remove unnecessary clothing and visualize the extremity.
• Check neurovascular status before and after splinting.
• Cover open wounds with a dry sterile dressing.
• Immobilize the joint above and below the fracture site.
• Cool and elevate the injured area if possible.
• Frequently reassess neurovascular status and pain.

Figure 46-18 Upper extremity splints. **A-C,** Padded rigid splints. **D,** SAM Splint. **E,** Evac-U-Splint vacuum splint. **F,** Soft towel splint. (A pillow can be used in a similar manner.) **G,** Sling and swath. (*D, Courtesy of SAM Medical Products, Portland, OR; E, courtesy of Hartwell Medical, Carlsbad, CA.*)

TABLE 46-1 Management of Specific Upper Extremity Orthopedic Injuries

SITE	SUGGESTED IMMOBILIZATION TECHNIQUES
Clavicle	Sling and swath
Shoulder	Sling and swath as it lies
Humerus	Cardboard or vacuum splint with a sling and swath
Elbow	Cardboard or vacuum splint as it lies
Forearm	Cardboard, malleable metal, air, or vacuum splint with a sling and swath
Wrist	Pillow, cardboard, malleable metal, or vacuum splint applied in the position found
Hand	Pillow, cardboard, or malleable metal splint in the position of function
Finger	Tongue depressor or small malleable metal splint

AIR SPLINT APPLICATION

A
If the splint does not have a zipper, place the splint over your arm. Use this hand to grasp the hand of the patient's injured extremity and your other hand to stabilize the arm.

B
Instruct an assistant to slide the splint onto the patient's arm, and smooth out any wrinkles.

C
Inflate the splint until finger pressure makes a slight dent. Continuously assess the distal circulation while the splint is inflated.

Figure 46-19 Air splint application.

extremity with neurovascular compromise, reduce the deformity with gentle longitudinal traction (but not exceeding 10 lb of pressure) before splinting. Make only one attempt at fracture reduction. If resistance or pain is encountered, splint the extremity in the position found. Cover open wounds with a dry sterile dressing before applying the splint. Apply the splint (Table 46-1) by using the orthopedic principle of immobilizing the joint above and below a suspected fracture site. Cool and elevate the injured area to help reduce local swelling and pain. Once the splint has been applied, assess distal neurovascular status frequently. Any deterioration requires immediate evaluation of the splint to determine whether excessive pressure is being applied. In addition, frequently assess and treat pain.

Rigid Splints
To apply a rigid splint, have an assistant provide support and gentle traction above and below the injury. Apply the splint on the side of the extremity away from any open wounds. The splint should be large enough to immobilize the joint above and below a suspected fracture or the bone above and below a dislocation and be well padded to reduce the risk for pressure necrosis. Secure the splint to the extremity with gauze, tape, cravats, or Velcro straps (see Fig. 46-18A-C).

Apply vacuum splints in much the same manner as other rigid splints. While an assistant stabilizes the injured site and applies traction, wrap the splint around the extremity and secure it in place with the attached straps. Evacuate the air from the splint with a hand pump until the splint becomes rigid.

Soft Splints
The application procedure for an air splint depends on whether the splint is equipped with a zipper. If the splint does not have a zipper, first place the splint over the rescuer's arm until the bottom edge lies above the wrist. Use this hand to grasp the hand of the patient's injured extremity and use the free hand to provide support and gentle traction above the injury (Fig. 46-19A). An assistant then slides the splint onto

the patient's arm (see Fig. 46-19B). Smooth out any wrinkles and inflate the splint until finger pressure makes a slight dent (see Fig. 46-19C). Open a zippered air splint and place it around the injured area. Close the zipper and inflate the splint as described previously. With air splints that completely enclose the hand, continuously assess the distal circulation by checking fingertip color, temperature, and capillary refill.

Apply pillow splints by encasing the injury in the pillow and securing it with tape, cravats, or gauze (see Fig. 46-18F). If possible, keep the nail beds exposed to allow frequent neurovascular checks.

To apply a sling, have an assistant support the injured arm in a flexed position across the patient's chest (Fig. 46-20). Place the long edge of the triangular bandage lengthwise along the patient's side opposite the injury with its tip over the uninjured shoulder. Bring the other tip over the injured shoulder to enclose the arm in the sling. Adjust the sling so that the arm rests comfortably with the hand higher than the elbow. Tie the ends of the sling together at the side of the neck and pad the knot for comfort. Finally, wrap the point of the sling at the elbow around the front of the forearm and pin. With the sling properly applied, rest the patient's arm comfortably against the chest with the fingertips exposed.

To apply a swath, place a cravat of sufficient length under the uninjured arm and over the injured arm at the level of the midhumerus. Tie the ends circumferentially around the

SLING APPLICATION

First, place tip *A* over the uninjured shoulder. Next, bring tip *B* over the injured shoulder to enclose the arm. Then, draw tip *C* around the front and secure with a pin.

The completed sling. A swath may be added to provide further immobilization (see Fig. 46-18*G*).

Figure 46-20 Sling application. Note that the wrist is supported by the sling (*arrow*) since the tendency is to flex the wrist with any upper extremity injury.

thorax so that the injured extremity is secured snugly to the chest (see Fig. 46-18*G*). In adults, two cravats may have to be tied together in an end-to-end fashion to produce a swath of sufficient length.

Complications
Potential complications of upper extremity splinting include pressure necrosis, conversion of a closed injury to an open one, and loss of neurovascular function. With the use of air splints, there is the additional risk of pressure-induced tissue ischemia and compartment syndrome.[67]

Conclusion
Injuries to the upper extremities, though not life-threatening, may be limb-threatening and can have significant immediate or long-term effects. Maintain a high index of suspicion for underlying neurovascular injury; check neurovascular status before and after applying a splint and frequently during transport. When possible, administration of appropriate analgesia will be greatly appreciated by the patient.

Lower Extremity

Background
Injuries to the lower extremities, including sprains, fractures, and dislocations, are also commonly encountered by prehospital care providers. As with upper extremity injuries, application of a splint is an essential part of the prehospital management of lower extremity injuries. Many of the principles, techniques, and complications discussed for upper extremity splinting also apply to injuries to the lower extremity; the SAM Splint (see Fig. 46-18*D*) and pillow splint (Fig. 46-18*F*) are just two examples (Fig. 46-21; also see Fig. 46-18). Table 46-2 provides recommendations for immobilizing a variety of lower extremity injuries. One fundamental difference between splinting upper and lower extremity injuries is use of a traction splint in the management of femoral fractures. The remainder of this section focuses on the use of traction splints.

The use of traction and countertraction for alignment and reduction of fractures dates from the time of Hippocrates.[69] In the late 1800s, Sir Hugh Owen Thomas developed the first full-ring traction splint for the definitive management of fractured femurs.[64,69] However, because the Thomas full-ring splint was difficult to apply on the battlefield, it was later modified by his nephew, Sir Robert Jones, and other surgeons to a half-ring design that made it easier to apply during battle. During World War I, the modified splint was credited with reducing the mortality rate associated with fractured femurs from 80% to 15%.[69] Since then, several additional modifications that carry the name of their inventors (e.g., Glenn Hare, Joseph Sager, Allen Klippel) have furthered the development

Figure 46-21 Prefabricated padded leg splint. Similar to the arm splints described earlier, many prefabricated leg splints are commercially available. Their application and use mirror the general principles of splinting described in Figure 46-18.

TABLE 46-2 Management of Specific Lower Extremity Orthopedic Injuries

SITE	SUGGESTED IMMOBILIZATION TECHNIQUES
Hip	Traction splint and long backboard or secure the injured leg to the uninjured leg Long backboard with the limb supported by pillows
Femur	Traction splint or pneumatic antishock garment
Knee	Cardboard or vacuum splint in the position found
Tibia/fibula	Cardboard, air, or vacuum splint
Ankle	Pillow or air splint
Foot	Pillow or air splint
Toe	Tape to the adjacent toe

Figure 46-22 Femur fracture. Anteroposterior and lateral views of the right femur demonstrate a displaced, angulated, and foreshortened femoral fracture. Such injuries may result in substantial hemorrhage into the thigh, even to the point of hemorrhagic shock.

Indications

Application of a lower extremity traction splint is indicated whenever a fractured femur is suspected.[66,72,73] Clinical signs of a fractured femur include thigh pain associated with limb shortening, angulation, crepitus, swelling, or ecchymosis.

Contraindications

Do not use traction splints on patients with pelvic fractures, hip injuries with gross displacement, significant injuries involving the knee, or avulsion or amputation of the ankle or foot.[73] Use of traction splints is not recommended in the presence of an associated distal tibia-fibula or ankle fracture in the same extremity. In these circumstances, the amount of traction required to realign the fractured femur can distract the distal fracture site. A variety of rigid splints may be considered in these settings.

There has been some controversy over whether a traction splint should be applied to an open femoral fracture. Concern has been expressed that the use of traction may allow contaminated bone fragments to retract into the wound. Should this occur, it must be relayed to the receiving clinician. As an alternative, a variety of rigid splints can be used to immobilize the bony fragments in the position that they were found initially. In any case, stabilization of the fracture site to prevent

of lower extremity traction splints. Today, traction splints are a nearly universal piece of equipment found on most ambulances, and their application is an integral part of the prehospital care provider's skill set. The main purpose of the traction splint is to immobilize a fractured femur.[70,71]

In the setting of a fractured femur, muscle spasm and overlap of fragments may cause the thigh to lose its cylindrical shape and adopt a more spherical appearance (Fig. 46-22).[69] The resultant decreased tissue pressure and increased volume may allow 1 to 2 L of blood to accumulate at the fracture site. Traction splints are designed to align fracture segments and restore the cylindrical shape of the thigh (Fig. 46-23). This in turn increases tissue pressure, decreases the potential space for blood loss, and inhibits further hemorrhage. In addition, traction splints help reduce pain, prevent further damage to neurovascular structures, and lower the incidence of fat embolism.[70,71]

further hemorrhage, neurovascular damage, or soft tissue injury should take precedence over the theoretical risk for increased contamination.

Equipment

Regardless of the type or manufacturer, the basic traction splint consists of a metal frame that extends from the proximal end of the thigh to an area distal to the heel. The padded proximal end fits against the ischial tuberosity and serves as the anatomic fixation point. The proximal portion of the splint may be a ring that encircles the proximal end of the thigh, a partial ring, or a padded bar. At the distal end of the splint is typically a ratchet-type device that when engaged, creates traction on the distal end of the femur. All traction splints also have several soft elastic straps that support the thigh and leg.[73]

Commonly used traction splints include the Hare Traction Splint, Kendrick Traction Device, Sager Emergency Traction Splint, and the Ferno-Trac (Fig. 46-24). Each of these splints

Figure 46-23 Use of a traction splint helps restore femoral fractures to a more natural anatomic alignment, which may reduce hemorrhage, pain, and damage to surrounding neurovascular structures.

has its own advantages, disadvantages, and unique method of application. For example, traction splints that use a half-ring design apply countertraction to the ischial tuberosity from below the shaft of the femur. This produces flexion at the hip joint of up to 30 degrees and will not allow complete fracture alignment unless the patient is in a reclining position about 30 degrees from horizontal or the injured extremity is elevated to create the same angle. Traction splints that do not use a half ring do not cause hip flexion.

Procedure

Application of the Ferno-Trac Traction Splint (Ferno-Washington, Wilmington, OH) and the Sager Emergency Traction Splint (Minto Research and Development, Redding, CA) is illustrated in Figures 46-25 and 46-26, respectively.

When possible, explain the splinting procedure to the patient. Pain is always associated with the application of a traction splint, so make every effort to provide appropriate analgesia (e.g., parenteral opiates) before application of the splint. In addition, reassure the patient that although the initial application of traction is often quite painful, stabilization of the fracture site will help reduce subsequent discomfort. Expose the area of injury and remove the patient's shoe and sock to assess distal neurovascular status before and after splint application. Manage open fractures as discussed previously. If the injured leg is markedly deformed, an assistant should first attempt to straighten it with manual traction and maintain that position until a splint has been applied. The amount of traction necessary to straighten a badly deformed extremity will vary but rarely exceeds 15 lb. If the patient strongly resists while traction is being applied, stop the procedure and splint the injured extremity in the position in which it was found.

If the splint has an adjustable bar, determine the appropriate length by measuring the uninjured leg. The splint should extend beyond the ankle by approximately 6 inches (15 cm). With the extremity slightly elevated, place the traction splint

Hare Traction Splint
(Dyna-Med, Lexington, KY)

Kendrick Traction Device
(Ferno-Washington, Inc., Wilmington, OH)

Sager Emergency Traction Splint
(Minto Research & Development, Redding, CA)

Ferno-Trac Traction Splint
(Ferno-Washington, Inc., Wilmington, OH)

Figure 46-24 Traction splints. A wide variety of devices are commercially available, each with their own advantages, disadvantages, and unique method of application.

(e.g., Ferno-Trac Traction Splint) under the injured leg and rest it firmly against the ischial tuberosity. To ensure that the injured extremity will remain elevated once manual traction has been released, unfold the heel stand and lock it into place. Place the Sager Emergency Traction Splint against the symphysis pubis or laterally against the greater trochanter of the femur. When the padded end of a Sager Emergency Traction Splint is placed in the groin, ensure that the genitalia are carefully protected.

Next, place the ankle harness immediately above the medial and lateral malleoli and attach it to the distal end of the traction splint. Ferno-Trac and other similar traction splints use a ratchet mechanism to apply constant (static) traction on the ankle strap. For Sager-type devices, gently extend the inner shaft of the splint until the desired amount of traction is achieved. The newest Sager model, the SX405, uses a handle to lengthen the inner shaft until the fractured leg is the same length as the uninjured leg. This traction handle also enables providers to set and document the traction force applied. The Sager Emergency Traction Splint is unique in that it provides gentle, quantifiable traction that is dynamic in nature. This dynamic function permits the traction to decrease automatically as muscle spasm decreases and leg length increases.[69] Regardless of which splint is being used, apply traction gradually to approximately 10% of body weight or a maximum of 15 lb. Only rarely will more traction be required.[72,73] The goal is to stabilize the fracture and maintain proper limb alignment. Use the least amount of force necessary to accomplish this task.[74]

Before moving the patient, place supportive straps around the thigh, knee, and distal end of the leg to vertically stabilize the extremity. After application of the splint, be sure to recheck distal neurovascular status and then secure the patient and splint firmly on a backboard. Take extra care while moving the patient and when closing any transport vehicle door to avoid unnecessary movement or further injury. If the splint extends beyond the dimensions of the backboard or stretcher, additional support for the splint may be needed (e.g., short spine board or cardiopulmonary resuscitation [CPR] board) to ensure that the injured extremity remains elevated throughout transport. Loss of pulses with application of a traction splint requires that the position of straps and the amount of traction applied be reassessed immediately. Also, recheck the position of the splint and the patient's neurovascular status after moving the patient. Remove the traction splint in reverse order of application.

FERNO TRACTION SPLINT APPLICATION

1
Place the ankle hitch around the posterior of the heel so that the traction strap hangs inferiorly, under the foot.

Traction strap

2
Secure the velcro on the ankle hitch (*arrow*). Ensure that the D-ring is present. This will be used to receive the hook from the traction device.

D-ring

3
While one rescuer gently applies traction and lifts the leg, slide the splint under the patient. The ischial pad should be firmly seated against the ischial tuberosity. Secure the ischial strap around the proximal and of the femur.

4
Maintain manual traction on the leg, and attach the traction device hook to the D-ring on the ankle hitch. Turn the traction dial counterclockwise to apply traction. Manual traction should be continued until mechanical traction takes over.

5
Stop applying traction once the leg has resumed its normal length (compare with the uninjured side). Secure the 4 remaining Velcro straps (2 above and 2 below the knee). Repeat a neurovascular examination.

Figure 46-25 Application of the Ferno Traction Splint. Note that the splint should be adjusted so that it is 12 inches longer than the uninjured leg before application. (*Reproduced and modified with permission. Ferno-Washington, Inc., Wilmington, OH.*)

SAGER TRACTION SPLINT APPLICATION

1

Prior to application of the splint, get a rough measure of the length of splint needed. Extend the splint so that the wheel is at the heel.

2

Grasp the Kydex buckle and slide the thigh strap up under the leg so that the perineal cushion is snug against the perineum and ischial tuberosity.

3

Tighten the Kydex buckle thigh strap to draw the perineal-ischial pad to the lateral portion of the crotch.

4

Apply the ankle harness tightly around the ankle above the medial and lateral malleoli of the ankle. Check the posterior tibial and dorsalis pedis pulses before hitch application and after traction is established.

5

Shorten the loop of the harness connected to the cable ring by pulling on the strap threaded through the square "D" buckle.

6

Extend the inner shaft of the splint by opening the shaft lock and pulling the inner shaft out until the desired amount of traction is noted on the calibrated wheel. As a rough guide to determine the amount of traction needed, apply 10% of body weight to a maximum of 22- to 25-1b (10- to 25-kg) traction.

7

Apply the longest 6-inch wide thigh strap as high up the thigh as possible.

8

Apply the second longest thigh strap around the knee. Use padding as needed. Next, apply the shortest 6-inch wide strap over the ankle harness and lower the leg.

9

Apply figure-eight strap around both ankles. The patient's leg is now secured, traction is controlled, medial and lateral shift of the distal fragment and internal and external rotation is prevented.

Figure 46-26 Application of the Sager traction splint. Note that the splint can alternatively be strapped to the outer portion of the leg. Also, it is possible to splint both legs with a single splint.

Special Considerations

The Sager Models S304 (Form III Bilateral) and SX404 (Extreme Bilateral) offer a unique advantage in that they can be used to immobilize both legs simultaneously with only one splint. In addition, neither splint extends beyond the patient's heels, thus making them ideal for use in helicopters, fixed-wing aircraft, and smaller van-type ambulances.

Complications

Complications are generally the result of incorrect application and include pain, ongoing hemorrhage, peroneal nerve injury, perineal injury, movement at the fracture site, or further neurovascular compromise.

Conclusion

When properly applied, traction splints reduce the pain, hemorrhage, and injury to adjacent structures that is associated with femoral fractures. Close attention to the manufacture's application instructions and frequent patient reassessment will help reduce complications. Once the fracture site is stabilized, additional traction is unnecessary and potentially dangerous.

PELVIC IMMOBILIZATION

Background

Pelvic fractures cause significant morbidity and mortality, especially in the elderly. The decreased bone density in older individuals contributes to the likelihood of sustaining pelvic fractures from low- to moderate-energy mechanisms, such as falls from a standing height. The findings on physical examination may be subtle, such as slight asymmetry of the lower extremities, so a high index of suspicion is important. In younger individuals, pelvic injuries are usually associated with high-energy mechanisms, with the most common being motor vehicle collisions.[75] Major pelvic trauma can lead to severe, uncontrollable hemorrhage, hypovolemic shock, and multisystem organ failure (Fig. 46-27).[76]

In the prehospital setting, early stabilization of fracture segments to control hemorrhage, along with gentle handling and immediate transport to a trauma center, is the

cornerstone of treatment.[77] However, even the most experienced prehospital provider may find it difficult to identify pelvic injuries in the field (the exception being an open-book fracture).

Indications and Contraindications

For any patient with significant pelvic pain or tenderness or evidence of pelvic instability after trauma, apply a pelvic circumferential compression device, especially if the patient is hypotensive.[78,79] There are no contraindications to pelvic stabilization in patients with presumed pelvic fractures.

Procedure

Several methods exist for stabilizing pelvic fractures in the prehospital setting, including pelvic sheeting, commercially available pelvic circumferential compression devices (also known as *pelvic binders*) such as the SAM Sling (Fig. 46-28), vacuum "beanbag" mattress splints, and pneumatic antishock garments (PASGs). However, with the advent of commercial pelvic binders and their well-documented list of complications and disadvantages, application of a PASG for pelvic fracture stabilization is no longer recommended.[80,81] When using any pelvic stabilizing device it must be remembered that aggressively moving patients or palpating the injured pelvis (e.g., pelvic rock) can precipitate further vascular injury or clot disruption and lead to life-threatening hemorrhage.

Stabilization of the pelvis consists primarily of compressing the bony ring. This can be accomplished by using a sheet or commercially available pelvic binder. To apply a sheet, place it over a long spine board and then gently logroll the patient (but no more than 15 degrees) into position on the board.[78] Alternatively, lift the patient with a scoop stretcher and then slide the sheet beneath the patient. Regardless of which method is used, wrap the sheet around the greater trochanters and tie the ends into a knot to compress the bony pelvis (Fig. 46-29). Pelvic binders are designed for quick and easy application in the field or ED. They are easy to maintain, reusable, and sized to fit 95% of the adult population. The pelvic binder acts similar to a bed sheet and, when placed properly (over the area of the greater trochanters), provides a safe and effective force to stabilize pelvic fractures.[82,83] Application of one such device, the SAM Sling, is illustrated in Figure 46-30.

Complications

Application of any pelvic compression device can damage the underlying soft tissue, as well as organs enclosed within the bony pelvis, including the bladder, urethra, and vagina.[84]

Figure 46-27 Traumatic internal hemipelvectomy. Major pelvic trauma such as this can lead to uncontrollable hemorrhage and hypovolemic shock. Early stabilization and immediate transport are mandatory. (*From Asensio JA, Trunkey DD, eds.* Current Therapy of Trauma and Surgical Critical Care. *St. Louis: Mosby; 2008.*)

Figure 46-28 The SAM Sling may be used to stabilize a fractured pelvis. (*Courtesy of SAM Medical Products, Portland, OR.*)

Figure 46-29 Pelvic stabilization using a sheet. Note that the sheet is wrapped firmly around the greater trochanters and tied to compress the bony pelvis.

However, the potential benefits of pelvic stabilization far outweigh these rare potential complications and should not discourage one from applying a pelvic stabilization device.[84]

Conclusion

Pelvic fractures can be quickly and easily stabilized with a sheet or commercially available pelvic circumferential compression device. Early recognition and stabilization of pelvic injuries, along with gentle manipulation of the patient and rapid transport, will help reduce morbidity and mortality.

REMOVAL OF HELMETS AND PROTECTIVE EQUIPMENT

Background

Though originally developed for protection of the head during combat, helmets are commonly worn by motorcyclists, athletes (e.g., football, hockey, lacrosse, motor sports), and individuals participating in a host of recreational activities (e.g., cycling, skiing, snowboarding, in-line skating, skateboarding). Emergency care providers must therefore be equipped and trained to remove a helmet safely.

The majority of modern sports helmets consist of a hard polycarbonate shell lined with foam padding, adjustable air cells, or both. Density, strength, and rigidity vary depending on the type of impact that the helmet is designed to protect against (Fig. 46-31). Many helmets are considered multisport

and meet the requirements for several potential mechanisms of injury and varying degrees of impact.[85]

Most helmets may be modified with additional padding so that they conform tightly to the individual's head. In addition, helmets used in contact sports (e.g., football, hockey, lacrosse) typically have some type of face mask secured to the front of the helmet to provide additional protection for the athlete's eyes and face. These athletes also use a variety of additional pads that may complicate or hinder helmet removal, such as shoulder pads and neck orthoses. Shoulder pad configuration varies from sport to sport and even from player to player. Cervical orthoses limit neck motion when paired with helmets and shoulder pads and protect against spinal and brachial plexus injuries. Commonly used cervical orthoses include neck rolls, cowboy collars, and butterfly restrictors.

Motorcycle helmets may or may not have a full face guard, but in either case they have been shown to reduce the incidence of severe head injury and death and are associated with shorter hospital stays and reduced hospital cost.[86-88] Although early studies suggested that the use of motorcycle helmets might be associated with an increased incidence of cervical spine injuries,[89,90] this concern has not been substantiated.[91-93]

Most of the early research in the area of helmet removal focused on the removal of motorcycle helmets. More recently, the spotlight has turned to football helmet removal because football players commonly sustain head and neck trauma, and their care is frequently complicated by the presence of additional protective equipment.[94]

Helmet removal requires a careful, methodical approach to avoid compounding a possible injury to the spinal cord.[95,96] Fluoroscopic studies have detected spinal motion even in the best of circumstances when removing hockey and football helmets.[95-97] As with all trauma victims, the initial management of an injured athlete is to address the ABCs (airway, breathing, circulation). However, it is important to note that a properly fitting sports helmet holds the head securely in a neutral position of alignment and minimizes any motion, provided that the athlete is also wearing shoulder pads. In this case, removing the face mask but leaving the helmet and shoulder pads in place will allow adequate airway control while maintaining proper alignment of the cervical spine and reducing the risk for further injury.[94,98]

Motorcycle and motor sport helmets do not usually have a removable face mask, do not always fit properly, and are worn without shoulder pads. Thus, in contrast to helmets worn by athletes, motorcycle and motor sport helmets should be removed routinely to properly immobilize the spine.[94]

Indications

For years, the proper management of a spine-injured athlete prompted much debate and disagreement among various health care professionals. In 1998, the National Athletic Trainers' Association formed the Inter-Association Task Force (IATF) for the Appropriate Care of the Spine-Injured Athlete, which in 2001 released a comprehensive set of guidelines and recommendations titled *Prehospital Care of the Spine-Injured Athlete*.[99] This consensus document outlines the current recommendations for removal of helmet and shoulder pads, which include the following[99]:

- If the helmet and chin strap fail to hold the head securely so that immobilizing the helmet does not also adequately immobilize the head

SAM SLING APPLICATION

1

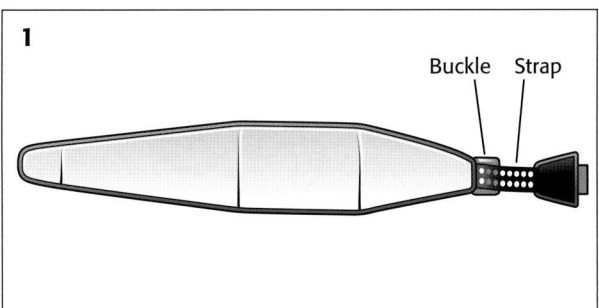

Buckle   Strap

Remove objects from the patient's pockets or pelvic area. Unfold the SAM Pelvic Sling with the nonprinted side facing up. *Keep the strap attached to the buckle.*

2

Place the nonprinted side of the SAM Pelvic Sling beneath the patient at the level of the buttocks (greater trochanters).

3

Wrap the nonbuckle side of the SAM Pelvic Sling around the patient.

4

FIRMLY WRAP the buckle side of the sling around the patient and position the buckle in the midline. Secure by pressing the flap to the sling.

5

Lift the black strap away from the sling by pulling upward.

6

"click"

With or without assistance, firmly pull the orange and black straps in opposite directions until you hear and feel the buckle click. MAINTAIN TENSION!

7

IMMEDIATELY press the black strap onto the surface of the SAM Pelvic Sling to secure it.
Note: Do not be concerned if you hear a second "click" after the sling is secured.

8

To remove it, lift the black strap by pulling upward. Maintain tension and slowly allow the SAM Pelvic Sling to loosen.

Figure 46-30 Application of the SAM Sling. *(Courtesy of SAM Medical Products, Portland, OR.)*

Full face coverage – motorcycle, auto racer   Full face coverage – motorcross   Partial face coverage – motorcycle, auto racer   Light head protection – bicycle, kayak   Football

Figure 46-31 Types of helmets.

- If the helmet and chin strap design prevent adequate airway control or ventilation, even after removal of the face mask
- If the face mask cannot be removed after a reasonable period
- If the helmet prevents proper immobilization for transportation in an appropriate position

If the athlete's helmet is not removed, maintain cervical spine immobilization with a properly fitting helmet by using tape, commercially available foam blocks, and a backboard. If it does become necessary to remove the helmet, the principle of "all or nothing" should apply. That is, remove the helmet and shoulder pads (if present) at the same time to avoid hyperextension of the cervical spine.[94,95,100] If in doubt regarding the need for removal of a sport helmet, the National Athletic Trainers' Association suggests remembering two overarching principles: (1) exposure and access to vital life functions (e.g., airway, chest for cardiopulmonary resuscitation or use of an automated external defibrillator) must be established or easily achieved in a reasonable and acceptable manner, and (2) neutral alignment of the cervical spine should be maintained while allowing as little motion of the head and neck as possible.[100]

In contrast to athletic helmets, motorcycle and motor sport helmets should be removed in the prehospital setting.[66] Motorcycle helmets with a full face guard make it very difficult to assess and manage the airway and to evaluate injuries to the head and neck. The helmet's large size and design may cause significant neck flexion if left in place when the patient is placed on a backboard. Though thought to reduce the risk for head and cervical spine injury, the increasing use of head and neck restraint devices (e.g., the HANS device; Fig. 46-32) in professional motor sports has further complicated cervical spine management and helmet removal.

In the ED, stable patients typically undergo imaging studies of the cervical spine before removal of the helmet and shoulder pads. The National Collegiate Athletic Association and the IATF recommend that the helmet (with the face mask removed) and shoulder pads remain in place until the initial radiographic evaluation is completed.[99] However, two small studies involving healthy volunteers found that the helmet and shoulder pads worn by athletes may interfere with standard cervical spine radiographic evaluation.[101,102] The authors of these studies recommend incorporating procedures for controlled and cautious removal of equipment before initial radiographic evaluation.[101,102] A study by Wanninger and associates[103] evaluated the use of computed tomography (CT) as a viable alternative to cervical spine clearance in an injured helmeted athlete. Although the findings in this small study require further validation, the use of CT for initial triage and diagnosis seems promising.

Figure 46-32 The HANS device. (*Courtesy of HANS Performance Products, Atlanta, GA.*)

Contraindications

The only absolute contraindication to helmet removal is neck pain or paresthesias associated with the procedure or an inability to remove the helmet because of an impaled object (e.g., deer antler through a motorcycle helmet).[104,105] Relative contraindications to helmet removal include unfamiliarity with the technique and lack of sufficient assistance.[106,107]

Procedure

Sport Helmet Removal

Whenever possible, treat injured athletes with a suspected cervical spine injury with their equipment (e.g., helmet, chin strap, shoulder pads) left in place to minimize any risk for further cervical spine motion.[96] However, when present, remove face masks at the earliest opportunity, before transportation and despite the absence of any respiratory complaints.[99,100,106,108]

A variety of tools (e.g., FM Extractor, Trainer's Angel, anvil pruner, polyvinyl chloride pipe cutter, or power screwdriver) and techniques are used for face mask removal.[96] All emergency care providers should have tools for face mask removal

FOOTBALL HELMET AND SHOULDER PAD REMOVAL

One rescuer manually stabilizes the patient's head and neck in the neutral position by placing his or her hands on each side of the helmet, with the thumbs pointing up.

A second rescuer then removes the chin strap by cutting or unsnapping it.

The second rescuer then takes over in-line immobilization of the head by using one hand to grasp the patient's mandible between the thumb and the first two fingers while placing the other hand under the occiput.

The first rescuer then places a thumb inside each ear hole of the helmet and curls his or her fingers along the bottom edge of the helmet. Without pulling laterally, the helmet is removed by gently rotating it off the head.

The shoulder pads are removed by cutting the straps underneath the arms and the anterior straps holding the pads together.

The hands of the second rescuer stabilize the head as the shoulder pads are removed. When possible, the helmet (with the face mask removed) and shoulder pads should remain in place until the initial clinical and radiographic evaluation is completed in the ED.

Figure 46-33 Football helmet and shoulder pad removal. Proper removal of a helmet and shoulder pads requires at least two rescuers. (Note: *This figure does not demonstrate removal of the face mask and cheek/jaw pads, which is recommended before helmet removal. See text for details.*) ED, emergency department. (*Courtesy of AtlantiCare Regional Medical Center, Emergency Medical Services, Atlantic City, NJ.*)

readily available and be familiar with their use. The choice of equipment is less important than the skill and experience of the personnel using it.[109] To remove the face mask of a football helmet, cut the four plastic loop straps that secure the face mask to the helmet. Similarly, remove hockey and lacrosse face masks by unscrewing the external screws holding them in place. Maintain in-line stabilization to keep the head and neck in the neutral position during the entire procedure. With practice, the face mask of any helmet can be quickly and safely removed with minimal risk of extraneous movement of the cervical spine.[98]

The National Athletic Trainers' Association protocol for helmet and shoulder pad removal discussed in this chapter has been shown to effectively limit motion of the cervical spine during removal of equipment.[110] Proper removal of a helmet and shoulder pads requires at least two (and preferably three or four) individuals along with in-line stabilization of the cervical spine throughout the procedure.[86,106,111]

One rescuer manually stabilizes the head and neck in the neutral position by placing her or his hands on each side of the helmet with the thumbs pointing up (Fig. 46-33, *step 1*). A second rescuer then removes the chin strap by cutting or

Figure 46-34 Riddell Revolution football helmet. These helmets are padded with a number of air-filled bladders that must be deflated (rather than removed) before removal of the helmet. **A,** Frontal view. **B,** Inside view. See text for details. (*A and B, Courtesy of Riddell, Elyria, OH.*)

unsnapping it (see Fig. 46-33, *step 2*). Next, this rescuer removes the left or right cheek and jaw pads from the helmet by first slipping the flat blade of a screwdriver or bandage scissors between the pad snaps and the helmet's inner surface and twisting slightly. Once separated from the helmet, remove the pads by sliding them out firmly and slowly. Remove the opposite side in the same manner. Note that some helmet models (e.g., Riddell Revolution) are padded with a number of air-filled bladders that must be deflated (rather than removed) before removal of the helmet (Fig. 46-34).[112] In this case, the second rescuer deflates the air inflation system by releasing the air at the external ports with the inflation needle that comes with the helmet. Alternatively, an 18-gauge needle or air pump needle may be tried. If an inflation needle is not available (or an 18-gauge needle or air pump needle does not work), directly puncture the bladders with an 18-gauge needle.

The second rescuer then takes over in-line immobilization of the head by using one hand to grasp the patient's mandible between the thumb and the first two fingers while placing the other hand under the occiput (see Fig. 46-33, *step 3*). The first rescuer then places a thumb inside each ear hole of the helmet and curls his or her fingers along the bottom edge of the helmet (see Fig. 46-33, *step 4*). At this point some experts recommend easing the helmet off by pulling laterally and longitudinally in line with the head and neck.[111] However, this maneuver may actually tighten the helmet at the occiput and the forehead.[113] The IATF recommends rotating the helmet off the head in a gentle fashion without pulling laterally.[99] Remove shoulder pads by cutting the straps underneath the arms and the anterior straps holding the pads together (see Fig. 46-33, *step 5*). If a cervical orthosis (e.g., neck roll, cowboy collar, or butterfly restrictor) is present, disconnect it from the helmet and shoulder pads before removal.

When possible, remove the shoulder pads and helmet simultaneously to prevent the head from falling into extension. If the shoulder pads cannot be removed simultaneously, manually stabilize the head in the neutral position during the procedure. The hands of the second rescuer can be moved superiorly as the helmet is being removed so that the thumb and first fingers grasp the maxilla at each side of the nose in the maxillary notch (see Fig. 46-33, *step 6*).

After removal of the helmet, place a cervical collar while maintaining in-line stabilization. Remember that if the helmet cannot be removed and access to the chest area is required, remove the anterior half of the shoulder pads and leave the posterior portion to maintain cervical position with the helmet in place.

Motorcycle Helmet Removal

For the reasons described earlier, motorcycle helmets should be removed in the prehospital setting. The removal method endorsed by the American College of Surgeons in 1997 is the method most often used today (Fig. 46-35).[114] Providers should be aware that unacceptable cervical motion can occur during removal of a motorcycle helmet if the shoulders are not properly elevated; a folded sheet or jacket placed behind the patient's shoulders may help limit any cervical motion associated with the procedure.[115]

If attempts to remove the helmet result in pain or paresthesias, the advanced trauma life support guidelines recommend removing the helmet via a technique described by Aprhamian and coworkers.[116] This technique uses a cast saw to bivalve the helmet in the coronal plane. Following division of the outer rigid shell, incise the inner foam material and remove it with the head and neck in neutral alignment. Although this approach does provide an alternative method of removing the helmet, the intense vibrations produced during use of the cast cutter may exacerbate an underlying spinal injury. In addition, even with the proper equipment available to the prehospital care provider, the technique may be slow and difficult with modern, well-fitting, high-quality helmets.[106,117,118]

The preferred method of helmet removal in organized motor sports is the Eject Helmet Removal System (formerly the Hats Off System), which consists of an inflatable air bladder that can be placed into the helmet before use or introduced into the crown of the helmet with a specially designed insertion tool. When inflated with a hand pump or CO_2 cartridge, it purportedly loosens the helmet to allow easy removal (Fig. 46-36).[117] Despite little scientific data supporting its use, the Indycar Racing League, American Speed Association, and American Motorcycle Association have made the Eject Helmet Removal System mandatory at all of their events. In addition, the Championship Auto Racing Teams and National Association for Stock Car Auto Racing have strongly recommended its use.

Complications

Underlying cervical spine injuries may be exacerbated by failure to adhere to proper helmet removal techniques. Although this is not supported by conclusive evidence, the few related studies seem to suggest that there may be a risk with helmet removal.[96] In a cadaveric model, Donaldson and colleagues[118] demonstrated that even in the best clinical setting, there is a significant amount of motion during removal of helmets and shoulder pads. Larger studies are needed to determine whether there is a real and significant risk in the clinical setting.

Conclusion

Prehospital care providers must take extreme caution when evaluating and treating an athlete with a suspected head and

MOTORCYCLE HELMET REMOVAL

One rescuer maintains in-line immobilization by placing his or her hands on each side, of the helmet with the fingers on the victim's mandible. This position prevents slippage if the strap is loose.

A second rescuer cuts or loosens the strap at the D-ring.

The second rescuer places one hand on the mandible at the angle, the thumb on one side and the long and index fingers on the other. With the other hand the rescuer applies pressure from the occipital region. This maneuver transfers the in-line immobilization responsibility to the second rescuer.

The rescuer at the top moves the helmet. Three factors should be kept in mind:
• The helmet is egg shaped and therefore must be expanded laterally to clear the ears.
• If the helmet provides full facial coverage, glasses must be removed first.
• If the helmet provides full facial coverage, the nose may impede removal. To clear the nose, the helmet must be tilted backward and raised over it.

Throughout the removal process the second rescuer maintains in-line immobilization from below to prevent unnecessary neck motion.

After the helmet has been removed, the rescuer at the top replaces his or her hands on either side of the victim's head with the palms over the ears.

Figure 46-35 Motorcycle helmet removal. *(Reproduced with permission from Norman E. McSwain, Jr., MD, FACS, and Richard L. Garrnelli, MD, FACS—American College of Surgeons Committee on Trauma, April 1997.)*

Figure 46-36 The Eject Helmet Removal System. This device uses a small air bladder that is neatly folded in an accordion fashion and placed underneath the helmet liner. A small tube runs under the padding and fastens to the bottom of the rim of the helmet to provide easy access. The device may be prefitted into the rider's helmet or inserted at the time of removal by using an insertion tool that allows the airbag to be slid up inside the top of a helmet. *(Courtesy of Shock Doctor, Minneapolis, MN. Available at* http://www.ejectsafety.com. *Accessed September 2012.)*

neck injury. Unless absolutely necessary, helmets and shoulder pads should not be removed in the prehospital setting. However, face masks should be removed early in the management of these patients. In contrast, motorcycle and motor sport helmets should be removed routinely to provide access to the patient's airway and allow proper spinal immobilization. When indicated, prehospital helmet removal can be accomplished in a safe and effective manner by well-trained prehospital care providers.

The primary complication of removing helmets and protective padding is causing additional injury to the patient. It may also prolong on-scene time and delay transport to the hospital.

SPECIAL CIRCUMSTANCES

Clinical Clearance of Immobilized Patients in the ED

Patients with low-risk injuries who have been immobilized by EMS personnel in the field often remain in uncomfortable positions while unattended or unevaluated in a busy ED. Many of these patients do not have a spinal injury yet often undergo prolonged immobilization before their complaints can be addressed or spinal injury can be clinically excluded and they can be removed from a backboard or other immobilization. Backboard immobilization by itself, for 30 to 60 minutes, will often result in iatrogenic backboard-initiated pain, even in healthy pain-free noninjured volunteers.[119] Such new or additional pain can prompt unnecessary imaging studies, result in patient inconvenience, and initiate the use of unneeded analgesics. It is therefore desirable to attend to immobilized patients in a prompt manner to avoid such problems. However, the average backboard time reported in one university hospital ED study was 54 minutes (range, 10 to 201) in patients eventually cleared clinically. Immobilization times averaged 181 minutes (range, 133 to 239) in patients not removed from a backboard until after radiographic clearance.[119] Since the average time spent in backboard immobilization in an ED may exceed times associated with iatrogenic injury, the clinical criteria used by nurses and house staff to clear the patient of a spinal injury can be implemented.

Numerous studies have concluded that nurse clearance of spine injuries agrees closely with physician decisions to clinically clear an immobilized patient.[120,121] Criteria used to clinically clear an immobilized patient can be based on absence of the following: altered level of consciousness, drug or alcohol impairment, pain or posterior cervical spine tenderness, distracting injuries, or new focal subjective or objective neurologic deficits. These are similar to various validated clinical criteria such as the Canadian C-Spine Rule or the National Emergency X-radiography Utilization Study criteria.

Gunshot Wounds to the Head

An isolated gunshot wound to the head is not an indication for routine cervical spine immobilization. Such intervention may lead to missed injuries under the collar and airway compromise and delay resuscitation or impede intubation because

Figure 46-37 A gunshot wound (GSW) to the head is not an indication for routine cervical spine immobilization, and such intervention may lead to missed injury under the collar, airway compromise, and delay in resuscitation for fear of manipulating the spine. There is no meaningful recovery from GSW injuries to the spinal cord.

of unwarranted concern for manipulating the spine (Fig. 46-37). In one study of 215 patients with gunshot wounds to the head, no bony or ligamentous injuries unrelated to direct bullet injury were identified in any patient, and none sustained indirect blast- or fall-related injuries to the spinal cord.[122] In this study, cervical spine immobilization was deemed to compromise securing of the airway. There is no meaningful recovery from gunshot injuries to the spinal cord.

Seizure Patients

Patients who have had a seizure in the field are at some risk for a spine injury, albeit it quite low and poorly characterized. They may be immobilized by EMS personnel or in the ED because of a presumed risk for spinal injury (see Fig. 46-17). Frequently, the patient's postictal mental status does not allow meaningful clinical evaluation, and attempts at immobilization can prompt further patient confusion and agitation, or struggling may exacerbate injuries that do exist. There are sparse data on this subject, but McArthur and Rooke, in a retrospective study of 1656 seizure patients, found no spinal fractures but did note a mandibular, tibial, and nasal fracture.[123] This study questioned the need for full spinal precautions in patients sustaining uncomplicated seizures. It would be prudent to consider sedation of agitated seizure patients who will not tolerate immobilization of the neck or spine when there is clinical concern for a spinal injury based on the mechanism of injury, physical findings, an obvious motor deficit, significant facial trauma, or patient complaints.

References are available at www.expertconsult.com

CHAPTER 47

Management of Amputations

Dean Moore II

"The first person caring for an injured hand will probably determine the ultimate stage of its usefulness."[1] Consequently, rapid and appropriate emergency care of a patient with an amputated part is crucial to the salvage and preservation of function. This chapter discusses the acute care of amputated parts before they are replanted and specifically addresses the management of distal digit amputations and dermal "slice" wounds.

Amputation may be partial or complete. Injuries with any interconnecting tissue between the distal and proximal portions, even if it is only a small piece of bridging skin, are considered incomplete (or partial) amputations. Complete amputations are replanted, whereas partial amputations are revascularized. This distinction is arbitrary; for emergency clinicians, treatment of both injuries is very similar. The prognosis and outcome of both types of amputations are similar, although partial amputations often have better venous and lymphatic drainage and functional recovery may be more complete if there is less anatomic damage.

The peak incidence of traumatic amputations occurs between the ages of 20 and 40 years.[2,3] Men predominate over women at a ratio of 4:1. Local crush injuries are the most common mechanism of injury, and sharp guillotine amputations are the least common.[4,5] Partial amputations occur as often as total amputations.[6] Proximal amputations are less common than distal amputations.

The media has somewhat exaggerated the success of replantation and has often generated unrealistic expectations from the public. The technical limitations of successful repair of vessels that are less than 0.3 mm in diameter usually preclude replantation of digits distal to the distal interphalangeal (DIP) joint.[7] Successful revascularization of amputated parts often ensures viability, but neurologic, osseous, and tendinous healing is critical for ultimate function. If there is incomplete neurologic recovery, limited range of motion, and intolerance to cold, the replanted part may have little functional value for the patient. Rehabilitation from replantation surgery may be prolonged, with more than 1 year often required, as well as repeated surgical procedures. The emergency clinician should be aware of the limitations of replantation surgery and *should not encourage unrealistic expectations in injured patients or their families*.[8]

BACKGROUND

The possibility of restoring viability and function to traumatically severed parts has fascinated clinicians for centuries. Clinicians have attempted to replant parts with little more than a few sutures and secure bandaging and have occasionally had spectacular results. One of the earliest medical reports was by Fioravanti,[9] who in 1570 reported successful replantation of a soldier's nose that had been severed by a saber. He first

Management of Amputations

Indications
Young stable patient
Thumb
Multiple digits injured
Sharp wounds with little associated damage
Upper extremity (children)

Contraindications
Absolute
  Associated life threats
  Severe crush injuries
  Inability to withstand prolonged surgery
*Relative**
  Single digit, unless thumb
  Avulsion injury
  Prolonged warm ischemia (>12 hr)
  Gross contamination
  Prior injury or surgery to part
  Emotionally unstable patient
  Lower extremity

Complications
Infection
Poor function

Equipment

Saline · Gauze · Kerlix

Styrofoam cooler with ice · Plastic bag

Review Box 47-1 Management of amputations: indications for reimplantation, contraindications, complications, and equipment.
*If the victim is a child or if there are multiple losses, salvage reimplantations are attempted and the relative contraindications are ignored.

cleansed it with urine and then carefully bandaged it. In 1814, Balfour[10] reported successful replantation of a finger that was severed with a hatchet by using only meticulous alignment and secure bandaging.

The ability to consistently replant amputated parts awaited the development of modern microvascular surgical techniques. The first reported successful upper limb replantation was by Malt and McKhann in 1962.[11] Later that year, Chen and Pao[12] reported successful replantation of a hand and arm. Developments in microsurgical techniques, advanced optics, and microsurgical instruments have created the ability to consistently replant amputated parts with a high degree of success. Since 1965, when Kleinert and Kasdan[13] reported the first successful microvascular anastomosis of a digital vessel, several large series of replantations have reported success rates ranging from 70% to 90%.[5,6,14-20] To the original pioneers in replant surgery, survival of the replanted tissue was the criterion for success, but with further technological and surgical refinements, today's surgeons emphasize functional recovery as well as viability. Replantation of a part that is painful or useless or that interferes with function is a disservice to the patient and is less desirable than early restoration of function without replantation.[21,22]

INDICATIONS

Preservation of the amputated part is generally indicated whenever there is a potential for replantation or revascularization. Revascularization and reanastomosis of partially and completely amputated parts should be provided when there is hope of preservation or restoration of function. Aesthetic considerations, patient avocations, and occasionally the patient's religious or social customs may also influence the decision to proceed with surgery.[21,23,24] In the end, the microsurgical team and patient must reach the decision together after a rational explanation of the potential results and successes.

Indications for replantation of fingers and hands have been proposed and are generally accepted, although they should not be applied rigidly in all circumstances. Successful functional recovery is more likely with distal than with proximal extremity amputations and more likely with multidigit amputations, single-digit thumb amputations, or transmetacarpal amputations.[25] Generally, these are the indications for replantation (Review Box 47-1). Single-digit amputations that are both proximal to the DIP joint and distal to the flexor digitorum superficialis may be replanted successfully with good functional recovery (Fig. 47-1).

Successful replantations have been reported in patients from the ages of 7 months to 84 years.[26,27] There are no fixed age limits for replantation, although particularly good functional results have been reported in children because of their regenerative capacity and adaptability to rehabilitation.[2,28,29] The decision to replant is made on a case-by-case basis by the microsurgical team, who must weigh all the factors involved.

CONTRAINDICATIONS

There is no contraindication to managing the amputated part and stump as though replantation were going to occur, even when replantation is considered unlikely. In addition, ancillary personnel can often handle care of the amputated

Figure 47-1 **A** and **B,** Single-digit amputations are not usually replanted unless the thumb is involved. This sharp amputation with little associated damage in a 20-year-old may qualify, but it is best to discuss this with the hand surgery team before giving unrealistic expectations to the patient, who may anticipate a normal result by simply "sewing it back on." Avulsion of the tendons proximal to the amputation greatly complicates this case.

part and stump during resuscitation and transportation of the patient. However, it must be remembered that evaluation and treatment of life-threatening injuries always take precedence over care of the amputated part. Contraindications to replantation are listed in Review Box 47-1 and are discussed in the following sections. Note that even when replantation is contraindicated, tissue (skin, bone, tendon) from the amputated part may be useful in restoring function to other damaged parts. *Never discard amputated tissue until all possible uses of the severed parts are considered.* For example, even an amputated fingertip not suitable for replantation may be an ideal donor source for a skin graft on the stump.

GENERAL CONSIDERATIONS
Mechanism of Injury

Severe extremity trauma is a significant cause of morbidity, and the potential for successful replantation in terms of survival, as well as useful function, is directly related to the mechanism of injury. Guillotine-type injuries are the least common but have the best prognosis because of the limited area of destruction. Crush injuries are the most common but produce more tissue injury and therefore have a poorer prognosis. Avulsion injuries have the worst prognosis because a significant amount of vascular, nerve, tendon, and soft tissue injury invariably occurs.[2,4-6,30]

Ischemia Time

The time that an amputated part can survive before replantation has not been determined. After 6 hours, additional delay may decrease the success rate of revascularization and lead to diminished function. Skin, bone, tendons, and ligaments tolerate ischemia much better than do muscle and connective tissue. As a general rule, the more proximal the amputation, the less ischemia time that the amputated part can tolerate. Attempts to extend viability during ischemia have shown that the most important controllable factor is the *temperature* of the amputated part. Warm ischemia may be tolerated for 6 to 8 hours.[31] When the part is cooled properly to 4°C, 12 to 24 hours of ischemia may be tolerated with distal amputations.[2,4,6,14,15,32] There is a report of successful digital replantation after 33 hours of cold ischemia.[33] Hypothermia limits the metabolic demand of tissues, thereby preserving intracellular energy and reducing the production of toxic metabolites caused by ischemia.[33-36] It also retards the development of acidosis[37] and may prevent the no-reflow phenomenon that can follow ischemic and low-flow states.[21,33,34,38]

Delay in replantation of proximal arm and leg amputations containing significant amounts of muscle tissue can lead to the buildup of toxic products. In such cases, when the blood supply is restored, the absorbed toxins have been reported to cause respiratory failure, renal failure, cardiovascular collapse, and even death.[21,24,33,34,39-42]

Intraoperative perfusion techniques such as those used for organ transplants to extend anoxic time are being used to help cool amputated parts before replantation. However, emergency clinicians should not attempt perfusion because the risk of damaging vessels, as well as the potential delay in care and rapid transport, overrides the theoretical benefits of cold perfusion in the emergency department (ED).[21,43]

ASSESSMENT OF THE PATIENT

The initial care and treatment of a patient who has had a body part amputated are the same as those for any trauma patient. The amputated extremity or the excitement of others must not distract the clinician from assessing and stabilizing the patient's airway, breathing, and circulation. Amputations are not generally life-threatening injuries, and other potentially more serious injuries must first be assessed and treated. Hemorrhage from completely amputated limbs is often limited by the retraction and spasm of severed vessels. Partial amputations may result in more serious hemorrhage than if the vessels were totally severed. Control hemorrhage with direct pressure and elevation. *Avoid using vascular clamps and hemostats in the ED when possible.* A proximally placed blood pressure cuff inflated 30 mm Hg above systolic pressure can be used for short periods (<30 minutes) to control severe bleeding, if necessary.

After the initial primary assessment and treatment and subsequent stabilization of the patient, care of the stump and amputated part can be initiated safely. In addition to the general history obtained from all trauma patients, focus attention on the exact mechanism of injury, the time and duration of the injury, handedness, allergies, medications, illness, previous injury to the affected part, care of the stump and amputated part before arrival in the ED, occupation, avocations, and tetanus history.

Initiate tetanus prophylaxis and broad-spectrum systemic antibiotic therapy (e.g., cephalosporins). Intravenous opioids are usually required for pain; titrate the dose to the clinical condition. With fingertip amputations, digital or regional nerve blocks are ideal for pain relief but may make functional and neurologic evaluation by a consultant impossible (see Chapters 31 and 32). Aspirin, low-molecular-weight dextran, or both have been administered in an attempt to maintain small-vessel perfusion[44] but have not proved beneficial in the ED management of these injuries.

Patients who have suffered an amputation often experience denial, shock, disbelief, and feelings of hopelessness about their injury; some have even become suicidal. Treat patients with supportive and realistic reassurance, and avoid unrealistic medical promises. It is important that the emergency clinician (or other non-replantation specialist) not speculate on the specifics of the ultimate prognosis.

Examination of the stump may be brief and should primarily be an assessment of the degree of damage to surrounding tissue (Fig. 47-2). Remove gross contamination by irrigating

Figure 47-2 A, Blast injury resulting in amputation. Remove gross contamination by irrigating with normal saline. Avoid using antiseptics because they may damage viable tissue. Assess the degree of contamination, the level of the injury, and any concomitant injury. **B,** Obtain radiographs of the amputated part (if available) and the proximal stump to include at least one joint proximal to the injury site. *(Courtesy of Stephen Pap, MD.)*

with normal saline. Do not use local antiseptics, especially hydrogen peroxide or alcohol, because they may damage viable tissue. Similarly, tissue should not be manipulated, clamped, tagged, or further traumatized in any way. Assess the degree of contamination, the level of the injury, and any concomitant injury. Examine the amputated part for the degree of tissue injury, level of contamination, and the presence of distal injuries. Obtain radiographs of the amputated part and proximal stump that include at least one joint proximal to the injury site (see Fig. 47-2*B*). If not already done, obtain preoperative laboratory studies and intravenous access in an uninjured extremity.

Assess the neurologic status of the stump or distal end of the extremity in partial amputations via pinprick and two-point discrimination tests. The presence of sweat may indicate autonomic neurologic functioning. Record vascular competence, motor and tendon function, and neurovascular status in the medical record. Contact the regional replantation resource center as soon as possible to arrange transportation and provide adequate time for mobilization of the replantation team.

CARE OF THE STUMP AND AMPUTATED PART

The stump should be dealt with during the secondary assessment of the trauma victim (Box 47-1). If replantation is proposed, the goals of initial care include control of hemorrhage and prevention of further injury or contamination. Remove all jewelry and irrigate the stump with normal saline to remove gross contamination; only the replantation team should perform manual débridement and dissection. Do not clamp arterial bleeders. Cover the stump wound with a *saline-moistened* sterile dressing to prevent further contamination and to limit damage from desiccation. Splint the stump for protection and to prevent further injury from concomitant fractures or compromised blood flow from a change in position. Splinting and elevation may also reduce swelling and help control bleeding.

Care of the amputated part follows the same general guidelines as for the stump. Remove all jewelry and irrigate the

---

BOX 47-1 Axioms for Care of Amputations

DO'S

Splint and elevate
Apply a pressure dressing
Protect from further trauma or injury
Protect from further contamination
Provide analgesia
Supply tetanus prophylaxis and antibiotic therapy
Obtain radiographs

DON'TS

Apply dry ice or freeze tissue
Place tags on tissue
Place sutures in tissue
Sever skin bridges
Initiate perfusion of the amputated part
Place tissue in formalin or water

---

amputated part with normal saline to remove gross contamination. Wrap the amputated part in a saline-moistened sterile dressing; do not handle the part any more than necessary to prevent further damage. *Avoid direct prolonged immersion in saline or hypotonic fluids* because it may cause severe maceration of the tissue and make replantation technically more difficult. Cool the amputated part as soon as possible. The ideal temperature is 4°C, but care must be taken to prevent freezing of tissues. To best accomplish this, wrap the amputated part in saline-moistened gauze, place the gauze-wrapped part in a watertight plastic bag, and then immerse the bag in a container of ice water (Fig. 47-3). Do not place amputated parts directly on ice because tissue in contact with ice may freeze. A guideline is to use half water and half ice. Avoid excessive ice. Cooling coils and refrigeration devices have occasionally been used but are not generally available and offer no significant advantage. Label the tissue containers with the patient's name, the amputated part contained within, the time of the original injury, and the time that cooling began.

Treatment of *partial amputations* with vascular compromise is the same as that just described. Irrigate the wound with normal saline. Place a saline-moistened sponge on the open tissue, and wrap the injury in a sterile dressing in which a splint has been incorporated to protect it from further injury. Place ice packs or commercial cold packs over the dressing to cool the devascularized area (see Fig. 47-3, *step 6*).

SPECIAL CONSIDERATIONS

Hand Function

Determine hand function in part by testing pinch and grasp functions. If the index finger is amputated, the middle finger can often adequately perform the pinching function formerly provided by the index finger. Power in grasping and gripping is primarily an ulnar function of the fourth and fifth digits. An effective grip that provides the ability to hold a variety of objects is a central function of the ring and middle fingers. In addition to its function in pinching, the thumb is the major opposing force for successful grip and grasp. The thumb is the most important digit for adequate hand function, and its loss results in 40% to 50% disability. For this reason, such disability requires aggressive attempts to replant amputated thumbs. If this is impossible or unsuccessful, secondary alternatives are pollicization of other digits or toe transfers.[45,46] Pollicization is a plastic surgery technique in which a thumb is created by using another finger.

Lower Extremity Amputations

There are few reports of successful replantation of amputated parts of the lower extremity.[47-49] Indications for replantation of lower extremity parts are different from those of amputated upper extremity parts. Isolated toe amputations are not replanted. It is generally held that if replantation does not restore function, a patient may be substantially better off with a prosthesis because lower limb prostheses, especially those used below the knee, are well tolerated and functional.[50] Prostheses provide a secure stance and permit locomotion. Lower extremity replantation generally requires skeletal shortening, and distal nerve regeneration is often imperfect, with both deficits producing dysfunction. Extracellular matrix scaffolds and muscle regeneration with stem cells are promising

CARE OF THE STUMP AND AMPUTATED PART

 Irrigate the wound with saline solution.

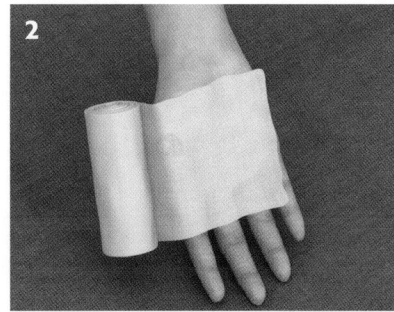 Wrap the wound with Kerlix or Kling for pressure, then elevate.

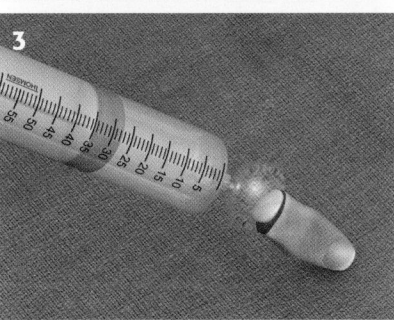 Rinse the amputated part with saline solution.

 Wrap the amputated part in a moist sterile gauze or towel, and place it in a plastic bag or container. Do not immerse the amputated part in saline.

 Place the amputated part in a container (preferably Styrofoam) and cool with separate plastic bags containing ice or in a container of ice water.

 For partial amputations, begin by irrigating the wound with saline solution.

 Place parts in a functional position, then apply a saline-moistened sterile dressing over the wound.

 Apply a coolant bag outside of the dressing.

— Cold pack

 Splint and elevate the extremity.

NOTE: Do not scrub or apply antiseptic solution to the wound.

Control any bleeding with pressure.

If a tourniquet is required, place it close to the amputation site.

Figure 47-3 Care of the stump and amputated part.

			TREATMENT
TYPE I Soft-tissue loss: Minimal Bone loss: None Nail/nail bed injury: None			Conservative management
TYPE II Soft-tissue loss: Moderate Bone loss: None Nail/nail bed injury: None			Conservative management or split-thickness skin graft
TYPE III Soft-tissue loss: Major Bone loss: Minimal Nail/nail bed injury: None			Split-thickness skin graft, operative procedure*
TYPE IV Soft-tissue loss: Major Bone loss: Moderate Nail/nail bed injury: Minor to major			Operative procedure
TYPE V Soft-tissue loss: None Bone loss: Minimal Nail/nail bed injury: Minor to major			Conservative management, split-thickness skin graft

Figure 47-4 Clinical classification of fingertip injuries and treatment of each type. *Note*: Though traditionally treated with various flaps and advancement techniques, type III guillotine amputations often do well with conservative management, even if some bone is exposed (see Fig 47-5). *(From Newmeyer WL. Managing fingertip injuries on an outpatient basis. J Musculoskel Med. 1985;2:17. CMP Medica.

technologies. However, the functional limitations that result from loss of the muscle needed to cover bone and provide limb function are a major factor in the decision to amputate a salvaged limb.[51,52] A patient with a replanted lower extremity with significant shortening and without sensation would function better with a prosthesis. This is not necessarily true of someone with an upper extremity replant. For these reasons, lower limbs are not generally replanted except under particularly ideal circumstances, usually in children. The final decision regarding replantation should be left to the replantation team.

Fingertip Amputations and Dermal "Slice" Wounds

Proper treatment of distal fingertip injuries is controversial, but good results are often achieved with conservative management. Fingertip amputations frequently heal by normal wound contracture, but occasionally this results in loss of the functional ability to palpate. The basic goals of treatment are to provide tissue coverage, an acceptable cosmetic result, and early functional recovery. Distal amputations with a wound area smaller than 10 mm² are not a problem (Figs. 47-4 and 47-5). Larger dorsal wounds also heal well by secondary intention. However, when loss of skin and soft tissue from the finger pad is significant, the clinician is faced with a more challenging situation. Volar skin is unique because of its combination of toughness and sensitivity. Wounds with significant loss of volar tissue frequently require additional treatment. Children, with their regenerative capacity, often progress very well when significant volar wounds are allowed to heal primarily. For older people and for amputations that involve a more significant amount of the distal digit, a wide variety of techniques for managing the injured fingertip have

Figure 47-5 This very minimal amputation of a fat pad with a mandolin slicer that does not involve bone or the nail bed is a common injury and will heal well with conservative therapy (see Fig. 47-5). *Note*: The ring should be removed as soon as possible.

been advocated, including partial-thickness skin grafts; full-thickness skin grafts; V-Y, Kutler, Kleinert, and island advancement flaps; and various local and distal flap coverage techniques. These procedures are designed to preserve length, soft tissue coverage of exposed bone, and sensation of the finger pad. Each of these procedures has its own indications, complications, and limitations.[53,54] Although traditionally some type of grafting or advancement techniques have been used for distal guillotine amputations, conservative management is now more common, even if some portion of bone is exposed (Fig. 47-6). Further discussion of these procedures is beyond the scope of this chapter. Most of these techniques are best performed by a specialist in the operating room at the time of the injury or as delayed procedures when necessary.

In most complete fingertip amputations distal to the DIP joint, the emergency clinician can provide adequate care initially with conservative wound management. Despite a considerable change in thinking over the years, many hand surgeons still advise skin grafting to shorten the time for wound healing. Although complete transverse amputations could be handled conservatively, wound healing may take several weeks, and these patients may benefit from operative treatment and skin grafting. Refer patients with complete transverse amputations distal to the DIP joint for consultation to coordinate their initial care and subsequent follow-up. Regardless of the type of injury, definitive care is usually provided on a delayed basis, and ED intervention is conservative with subsequent consultation considered to be standard treatment.

Incomplete transections and small distal amputations without significant soft tissue loss may heal well with conservative therapy started by the emergency clinician. Nonoperative treatment in selected patients provides excellent functional and cosmetic results, minimizes recovery time, and has few complications.[54-60] Children have excellent regenerative capacity and also respond extremely well to conservative treatment. Débride necrotic and grossly contaminated tissue. Irrigate the wound thoroughly with normal saline. If bone is left exposed without soft tissue coverage, the patient will probably need an operative procedure. Alternatively, the bone may be rongeured (shortened) to allow soft tissue coverage and primary healing with better functional recovery. The nail bed tissues should be preserved, if possible, because the presence of a nail affects the cosmetic appearance. After cleansing and careful débridement, apply an occlusive dressing directly over the wound and then bandage and splint the finger for protection. Provide tetanus prophylaxis if needed. Amputations that involve the distal phalanx are frequently treated as contaminated open fractures. In these cases, a recent Cochrane review supports the early use of antibiotics to reduce the incidence of infection.[61] Wounds managed conservatively must undergo serial dressing changes and cleansing. This helps provide superficial débridement, which may aid healing and minimize the chance of secondary infection. Wound contraction and healing usually result in acceptable cosmetic and functional recovery in 2 to 3 weeks. Arrange appropriate follow-up to ensure adequate healing and recovery.

The emergency clinician can also manage partial fingertip amputations distal to the DIP joint. These wounds are treated in a manner similar to complete amputations. However, when the amputation has a substantial amount of undamaged tissue connecting the fingertip, use sutures or bandaging and protective splinting to carefully align and stabilize the injured fingertip. Partially amputated fingertips, especially in children, may occasionally survive and regain vascularization and

Figure 47-6 A, This young man with no medical problems had his fingertip cut off by a metal press, a guillotine-type amputation that has traditionally been treated with various surgical techniques. A conservative approach is now advocated, especially in children. Note that the nail bed is exposed because of avulsion of the nail. The distal phalanx was not injured but was felt in the stump. **B,** The avulsed tip has skin and the avulsed nail attached. **C,** After the tip was cleaned by gentle scrubbing and minor débridement of macerated tissue, the nail was dissected from the tip and sutured back under the eponychium. The amputated tip was discarded. **D,** A protective splint and a pressure dressing were applied. Cephalexin was given for 7 days. The patient was seen weekly for dressing changes and minor débridement. **E,** At 4 weeks the finger has healed well with good sensation and an almost normal appearance. **F,** The old nail was removed to reveal the growth of a new nail. At 8 weeks there was no deformity or problem except minor shortening of the tip.

sensation. If the distal tissue becomes ischemic and necrotic, the amputation becomes complete.

Injury to the nail bed requires special attention to ensure proper alignment. If the nail bed tissues are not aligned properly, permanently disfigured nails may result. Complete or partial nail removal may be required for the placement of sutures.

Manage dermal "slice" wounds (see Figs. 47-4 type I and 47-5) by gently cleansing the wound and applying antibiotic ointment and a nonadherent dressing, followed by a pressure dressing. The patient should return in 48 to 72 hours for the wound to be inspected and the dressing changed. At that time, instruct the patient on the use of nonadherent dressings and to change them daily for 10 to 14 days until functional epithelialization of the wound takes place. A protective finger splint or guard also minimizes the risk for further injury and pain from trauma to the sensitive wound area. Protection allows earlier return to functional use and employment. Wounds larger than 10 mm^2 and those with deep loss of digit pulp tissue may be candidates for skin grafting.

Conservative Management of Fingertip Amputations

An amputation of the fingertip that does not involve significant injury to bone or massive tissue maceration generally does well with conservative treatment. In the past, skin grafts, flaps, and advancement techniques were used for the type II and type III injuries depicted in Figure 47-4, but currently, such interventions are uncommon for simple fingertip amputations. The common transverse guillotine amputation from machinery heals with good cosmesis and adequate sensation, but 6 to 8 weeks may be required for complete healing. Such injuries may simply be cleaned and bandaged in the ED and appropriately referred. However, if ED follow-up is available, patients may be reevaluated and the wound selectively débrided at 1-week intervals. Figure 47-6 outlines such a conservative course.

Penis, Ear, and Nose Amputations

Replantation of the penis, ear, and nose generally results in better function and cosmesis than a prosthesis or reconstructive surgery does. The amputated parts and wounds should be handled in the same manner as digital replantations.

Penile amputations are an uncommon problem. Most cases result from self-inflicted trauma in patients who are severely psychologically disturbed. Successful replantation with microsurgical techniques has been reported. Preservation or reconstruction of the urethra to maintain a competent urinary stream is critical for success.[62,63] Ears and noses are frequently partially amputated and occasionally totally amputated. Whenever possible, these body parts should be replanted unless they are severely traumatized and gross contamination is present. These wounds frequently heal well, and patients with such wounds have a high tissue survival rate and a low incidence of total necrosis. Replantation of these parts requires good suture technique and careful placement but does not necessarily require skill in microsurgical techniques.[63-66]

COMPLICATIONS

The care of amputated parts should not lead to avoidable complications if the aforementioned principles are followed. Avoid improper management of the parts or stump and subsequent additional injury to the tissue from overzealous hemostasis or cleansing. Furthermore, avoid desiccation, maceration, or freezing of tissue from improper storage. *Expedite the preoperative workup of the patient and immediately notify the replantation team because these are crucial factors in the patient's care.*

Despite optimal initial care, replantation itself may be associated with acute or long-term complications. There is the usual risk associated with anesthesia and protracted surgery. Moreover, it is not unusual for patients to need second and third emergency operations to reestablish adequate blood flow. Postoperative complications include vascular thrombosis, hemorrhage, infection, and reaction to accumulated toxins.[67] Toxins accumulate in the ischemic amputated parts despite cooling. The amount of toxin is directly proportional to the amount of muscle mass and the duration of ischemia. Significant pulmonary failure, electrolyte disturbance, and even death have been reported in replantation efforts. Finally, anticoagulants are often prescribed, which creates additional risk.

Later complications include a significant percentage (60%) of patients with cold intolerance, limited function, anesthesia, pain, paresthesias, malunions, and nonunions. Also, repeated operative procedures may be required to achieve a functionally useful result.

FIELD AMPUTATIONS

Emergency physicians may be called upon to perform field amputation of an extremity as a life-saving intervention. Such circumstances are usually related to disaster situations or other trauma where a victim is trapped or unable to be extricated from the scene because an extremity is covered or held immobile due to debris or other heavy objects or is lodged in narrow spaces. The procedure is not detailed in this text but is contained in the video library.

Acknowledgment

The contributions by William C. Dalsey, MD, Jeffrey Luk, MD, and Maria Halluska-Handy, MD, to earlier editions are appreciated.

References are available at www.expertconsult.com

Extensor and Flexor Tendon Injuries in the Hand, Wrist, and Foot

Peter E. Sokolove and David K. Barnes

EXTENSOR TENDONS

Extensor tendons are quite superficial, covered only by skin and a thin layer of fascia, and are thus highly susceptible to injury by commonly experienced trauma. Such injuries may result from lacerations, bites, or burns, but they may also be caused by closed injury with even seemingly superficial lacerations. Whereas some extensor tendon injuries must be managed by a hand surgeon, others may be treated in the emergency department (ED). The emergency clinician must understand the anatomy, principles of treatment, repair technique, and postrepair care of these injuries to ensure the best possible patient outcome.

Functional Anatomy

There are 12 extrinsic extensors of the wrist and digits, all of which are innervated by the radial nerve. The muscles that give rise to these tendons originate in the forearm and elbow (Fig. 48-1). The extrinsic extensor tendons reach the hand and digits by passing through a fibroosseous tendon sheath (retinaculum) located at the dorsal surface of the wrist. This synovium-lined sheath provides smooth gliding of the tendons and prevents bowstringing when the wrist is extended.[1] The dorsal retinaculum contains six compartments or subdivisions (Fig. 48-2). These compartments are numbered from the radial to the ulnar side of the wrist.

The first compartment contains two tendons, the abductor pollicis longus (APL) and the extensor pollicis brevis (EPB). The APL tendon is the most radial of the extensor tendons and inserts on the base of the first metacarpal. It can be palpated just distal to the radial tubercle. The APL tendon causes thumb abduction and extension and some radial wrist deviation. The EPB travels with the APL through the first compartment but inserts at the base of the proximal phalanx of the thumb. The EPB tendon can be palpated over the dorsum of the first metacarpal when the thumb is extended against resistance. Both tendons can be tested by having the patient spread the fingers apart against resistance.

The second compartment also contains two tendons: the extensor carpi radialis brevis (ECRB) and the extensor carpi radialis longus (ECRL). These two tendons arise from the lateral epicondyle of the elbow. The ECRL inserts on the base of the second metacarpal, and the ECRB inserts on the base of the third metacarpal. Both tendons are powerful wrist extensors, and the ECRL also allows some radial wrist deviation. Wrist extension plays an especially important role in the mechanics of the hand because hand grip strength is maximal only when the wrist is extended.

The third compartment contains only one extensor tendon, the extensor pollicis longus (EPL). This tendon crosses over the ECRB and ECRL and travels along the dorsum of the thumb to insert on the distal phalanx. The EPL forms the top of the anatomic "snuffbox," and the bottom is formed by the EPB. The EPL can be visualized when the thumb is extended, and its strength can be tested by having the patient hyperextend at the interphalangeal (IP) joint against resistance. The intrinsic extensor of the thumb can provide some degree of extension at the IP joint. Therefore, if an EPL injury is suspected, it is important to compare extension at the IP joint with that of the unaffected thumb.

The fourth and fifth compartments contain the six tendons that extend the index through the little fingers. Each finger has its own extensor digitorum communis (EDC) tendon. The index and little fingers have an additional independent extensor tendon—the extensor indicis proprius (EIP) for the index finger and the extensor digiti minimi (EDM) for the little finger. The fourth compartment contains the EIP and EDC tendons, and the fifth compartment contains only the EDM tendon. These six tendons can be seen over the dorsum of the hand, where they are poorly protected and prone to injury. In this region the tendinous, ligamentous, and fascial connections between these tendons are known as the *juncturae tendinum*. Because of these interconnections, a patient may be able to extend a digit, albeit weakly, even when there is a complete laceration of its EDC tendon. To avoid missing a tendon injury on the dorsum of the hand, it is important that the examiner test for tendon strength and not just for active extension.

The course of the extensor tendons along the fingers is more complex, but a basic understanding of this anatomy is essential for the emergency clinician to evaluate and treat extensor tendon injuries (Fig. 48-3). The EIP tendon joins the EDC tendon at the level of the metacarpophalangeal (MCP) joint in the index finger. The EDM tendon parallels the course of the EDC tendon; the four EDC tendons eventually insert at the base of the proximal, middle, and distal phalanges. The most proximal insertion of the EDC tendon is at the level of the base of the proximal phalanx. The tendon actually inserts in two ways. First, there is a loose dorsal insertion just distal to the MCP joint. In addition, the EDC tendon inserts into the volar plate via the sagittal bands. The sagittal bands are circumferential structures at the level of the metacarpal head that serve to keep the EDC tendon centered over the metacarpal head, as well as to provide a stable connection with the volar plate located on the palmar side of the hand. After its primary insertion at the level of the MCP joint, the EDC tendon then extends dorsally along the digit. The EDC trifurcates over the proximal phalanx (Fig. 48-4). Its major central slip inserts on the base of the middle phalanx (Fig. 48-5). The lateral branches of the EDC tendon join with the lateral bands from the interossei and lumbricals to form the conjoined lateral bands. The two conjoined lateral bands then fuse together over the middle phalanx to form the terminal extensor mechanism (TEM), which inserts into the base of the distal phalanx (Fig. 48-6). The triangular ligament is a connection between the two conjoined lateral bands that assists in keeping these structures on the dorsal aspect of the digit.

The sixth dorsal compartment of the wrist contains only one tendon, the extensor carpi ulnaris (ECU). This tendon originates at the lateral epicondyle of the elbow and inserts at

Posterior (dorsal) view

Extensor carpi ulnaris – Compartment 6

Extensor digiti minimi – Compartment 5

Extensor digitorum
Extensor indicis } Compartment 4

Extensor pollicis longus – Compartment 3

Extensor carpi radialis brevis
Extensor carpi radialis longus } Compartment 2

Abductor pollicis longus
Extensor pollicis brevis } Compartment 1

Radial artery in anatomical snuffbox

Dorsal interosseous muscles

Plane of cross section shown below

Extensor retinaculum

Abductor digiti minimi muscle

Intertendinous connections

Transverse fibers of extensor expansions (hoods)

A

Cross section of most distal portion of forearm

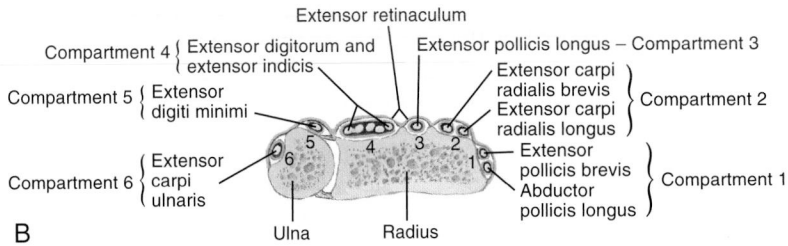

Extensor retinaculum

Compartment 4 { Extensor digitorum and extensor indicis

Extensor pollicis longus – Compartment 3

Compartment 5 { Extensor digiti minimi

Extensor carpi radialis brevis
Extensor carpi radialis longus } Compartment 2

Compartment 6 { Extensor carpi ulnaris

Extensor pollicis brevis
Abductor pollicis longus } Compartment 1

Ulna   Radius

B

Posterior view

Radial nerve (C5, 6, 7, 8, T1) Inconstant contribution

Superficial (terminal) branch

Deep (terminal) branch

Lateral epicondyle

Anconeus muscle

Brachioradialis muscle

Extensor carpi radialis longus muscle

Supinator muscle

Extensor carpi radialis brevis muscle

Extensor carpi ulnaris muscle

Extensor digitorum muscle and extensor digiti minimi muscle

Extensor indicis muscle

Extensor pollicis longus muscle

Abductor pollicis longus muscle

Extensor pollicis brevis muscle

Extensor-supinator group of muscles

Posterior interosseous nerve (continuation of deep branch of radial nerve distal to supinator muscle)

Superficial branch of radial nerve

Dorsal digital nerves

C

Figure 48-1 Extensor muscles and tendons of the right wrist and hand. **A,** Posterior (dorsal) view. **B,** Cross section of the most distal portion of the forearm. **C,** Radial nerve in the forearm: posterior view. (*A-C, Netter illustrations used with permission of Elsevier Inc. All rights reserved.*)

Figure 48-2 A, The extensor mechanism at the wrist and dorsum of the right hand. The six extensor compartments at the wrist contain (*1*) the abductor pollicis longus (APL) and extensor pollicis brevis (EPB), (*2*) the extensor carpi radialis longus (ECRL) and brevis (ECRB), (*3*) the extensor pollicis longus (EPL), (*4*) the extensor digitorum communis (EDC) II to V and the extensor indicis proprius (EIP), (*5*) the extensor digiti quinti (EDQ), and (*6*) the extensor carpi ulnaris (ECU). An important anatomic detail is the presence of a synovial sheath around each tendon unit within each fibroosseous canal. Note that the EDQ is also called the extensor digiti minimi (EDM) by some authors. **B,** Note that the juncturae tendinum allow some weak extension of the finger when the proximal extensor is completely lacerated. (*A, Adapted from Thomas JS, Peimer CA. Extensor tendon injuries: acute repair and late reconstruction. In: Chapman MW, ed.* Operative Orthopaedics. *3rd ed. Philadelphia: JB Lippincott; 2001:1487.*)

the base of the fifth metacarpal. The ECU functions as a wrist extensor and ulnar deviator. It can be palpated just distal to the tip of the ulna, and its strength can be tested by forced ulnar deviation of the wrist.

General Approach to Extensor Tendon Injuries

The key to detecting extensor tendon injuries in the ED is to perform a careful and thorough history and physical examination. Closed injuries may appear innocuous at first but can result in tendon injuries that may lead to severe deformities or dysfunction if undetected (Figs. 48-7 to 48-9). Closed injuries are also commonly associated with fractures. A hand radiograph is recommended for closed-hand injuries when a fracture is suspected or for open-hand injuries in which a fracture or foreign body is suspected. It is generally accepted that all open injuries that result from glass should be radiographed. Plain radiographs have a sensitivity of approximately 98% for detecting radiopaque foreign bodies (e.g., gravel, glass, metal).[2]

Injuries to extensor tendons from lacerations are quite common, especially on the dorsum of the hand, where they are located superficially. All dorsal wrist, hand, and digit lacerations should be assumed to have an underlying tendon laceration until proved otherwise. Digital extension, albeit weak, can still occur with partial tendon lacerations of up to 90%, so visualization of the tendon and careful strength testing are required to definitively rule out a partial injury. In some cases the specific diagnosis simply cannot be made on the first examination (see later). Complete laceration of an EDC tendon on the dorsum of a hand can also still allow digital extension through the juncturae tendinum.

After assessing the strength and neurovascular status of the injured hand it is imperative that the emergency clinician visually inspect the wound thoroughly. Inspection should include an assessment of the degree of wound contamination, as well as a search for foreign bodies and occult tendon lacerations. It is often necessary to extend the skin laceration to aid in the visualization of a possible tendon injury. Some investigators have advocated for the use of ultrasound in the diagnosis of suspected extensor (and flexor) tendon lacerations in the hand.[3] This is a potentially attractive tool since it is easy to use and noninvasive and provides point-of-care analysis, but the use of sonography for detection of hand and digit tendon injuries cannot yet be advocated for routine use by emergency physicians. Because an extensor tendon is a mobile structure, it is imperative that if it is exposed, it be visualized in its entirety through a full range of motion. It is especially important to examine the tendon in the position that it occupied at the time of injury because the tendon injury frequently does not lie directly under the external skin wound (see Fig. 48-8).

Posterior (dorsal) view

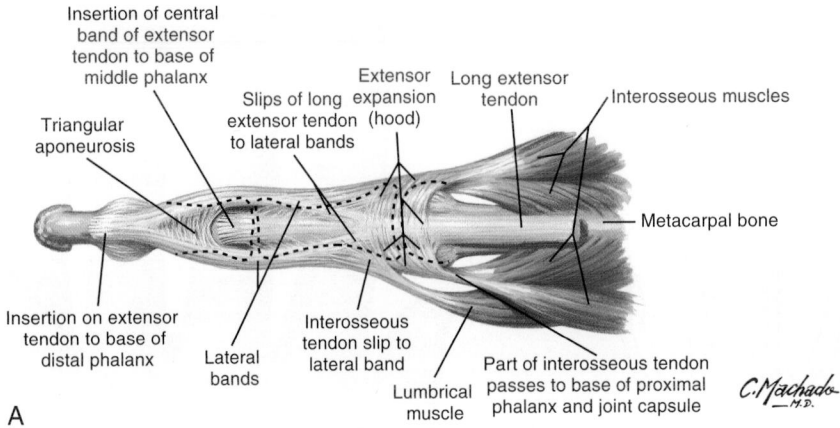

A

Finger in extension: lateral view

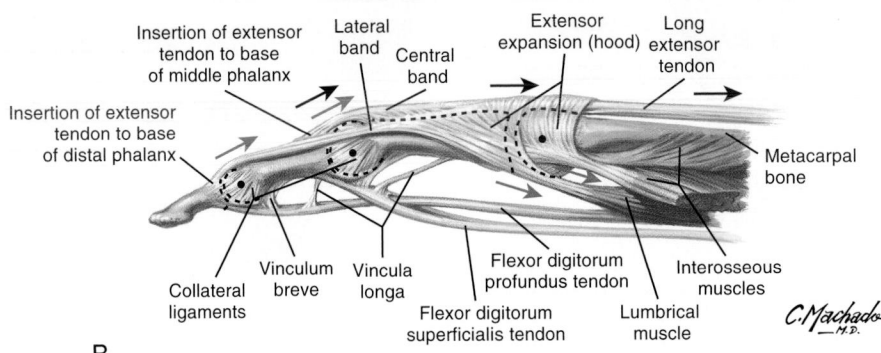

B

Finger in flexion: lateral view

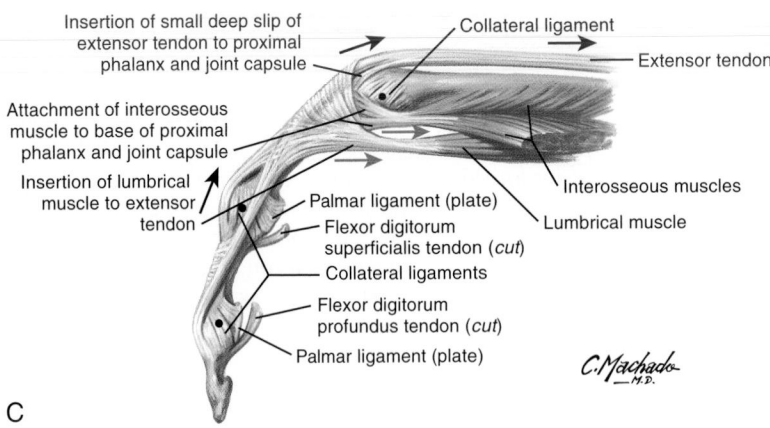

C

Figure 48-3 Flexor and extensor tendons in the fingers. **A,** Posterior (dorsal) view. **B,** Finger in extension: lateral view. **C,** Finger in flexion: lateral view. (*A-C, Netter illustrations used with permission of Elsevier Inc. All rights reserved.*)

Definitive examination of any wound must occur under the best possible conditions—with a good light source, a bloodless field, adequate local anesthesia, and a cooperative patient. *It may be impossible to adequately assess some patients completely during the first ED visit. In this case, final diagnosis must be delayed until the proper circumstances permit the required conditions.* Occasionally, patient noncompliance thwarts even the most carefully planned follow-up. Frequently, the patient's pain, swelling, anxiety, or degree of intoxication or altered sensorium limits the clinician's diagnostic ability; therefore, *it would not be considered standard to diagnose the presence or the*

full extent of all extensor tendon injuries immediately. Whenever logistically possible, consult a specialist when an extensor tendon injury is suspected by mechanism, location of the wound, or tendon dysfunction. Under most circumstances, however, there is no value in obtaining an immediate on-site consultation with a hand or orthopedic surgeon because the intrinsic scenario would similarly limit any clinician's diagnostic acumen.

If the examining clinician suspects but is unable to locate a tendon laceration or if a patient is uncooperative with the examination and the circumstances prohibit ideal initial care,

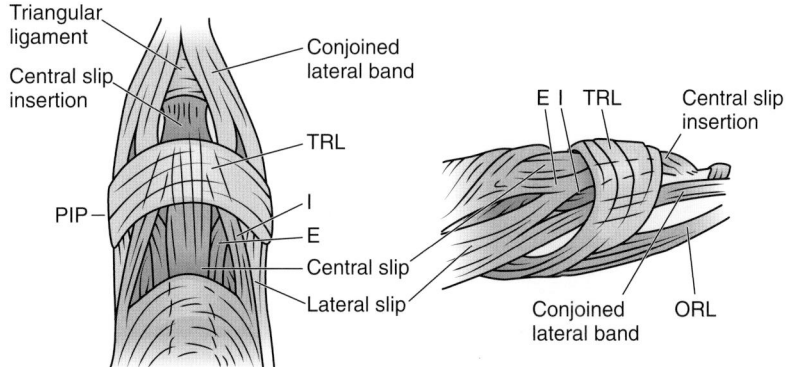

Figure 48-4 Zone of convergence of the digital extensor mechanism, which begins at about the midportion of the proximal phalanx and ends at the level of the insertion of the central slip into the dorsal base of the middle phalanx. Proximal to the zone of convergence, the extrinsic and intrinsic components of the extensor mechanism are separate: the central slip is extrinsic, whereas the lateral slips are intrinsic. Within the zone of convergence there is complete reciprocal crossover of fibers from the central slip and lateral slips. The products of the completed convergence are the central slip insertion and the conjoined lateral bands, both of which have dual muscular activity. *E,* extrinsic contribution to the conjoined lateral bands; *I,* intrinsic contribution to the insertion of the central slip; *ORL,* oblique retinacular ligament; *PIP,* proximal interphalangeal joint; *TRL,* transverse retinacular ligament. *(From Thomas JS, Peimer CA. Extensor tendon injuries: acute repair and late reconstruction. In: Chapman MW, ed.* Operative Orthopaedics. *3rd ed. Philadelphia: JB Lippincott; 2001:1500.)*

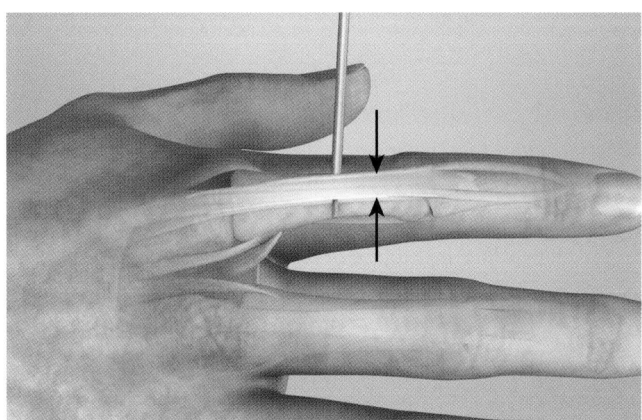

Figure 48-5 The extensor mechanism on the dorsum of a finger. Arrows point to the radial and ulnar lateral band portions of the extensor mechanism, and the probe is lifting the entire structure up off the phalanx.

Figure 48-7 Because of their superficial location, it is difficult to avoid at least partial injury to the extensor tendons with even superficial lacerations of the dorsum of the wrist, hand, or fingers. **A,** This complete extensor tendon laceration is obvious since the index finger cannot be extended. **B,** This partial tendon laceration was not appreciated on initial examination, which seemingly demonstrated full tendon function. The entire tendon could not be visualized because of an uncooperative patient. The unappreciated partial laceration progressed to a complete rupture by the time of suture removal. Expeditious delayed primary repair resulted in a good outcome.

Figure 48-6 The terminal extensor mechanism.

Figure 48-8 To examine for tendon injury, use a bloodless field. Note the sterile glove on the patient to maintain a clean field. *It is almost impossible to cut the dorsum on the hand or fingers and avoid at least a partial tendon injury.* **A,** The location and depth of this laceration suggest an extensor tendon injury. On examination, the patient had full extension. **B,** Note that no tendon injury is visualized when the laceration was examined with the fingers in extension. When the laceration was *extended and probed with the finger flexed,* a 60% laceration of the extensor tendon could be viewed in the depths of the wound. **C** and **D,** Note the typical shiny white appearance of fully exposed tendons (*arrows*).

Figure 48-9 Given the superficial location of extensor tendons, suspect a tendon injury even with seemingly superficial lacerations of the dorsum of the hand and fingers. Full function is possible with a significant tendon laceration, and delayed total rupture can occur days to weeks later if the injury is not repaired or splinted. Most partial extensor tendon lacerations do well with 3 to 4 weeks of splinting and no surgical repair. When in doubt, clean the laceration, suture the skin, splint, and refer for subsequent examination in a few days.

refer the patient for follow-up in 1 to 3 days for a repeated examination. Close the skin and apply a splint for interim wound care. A delay of a few days for definitive diagnosis, surgical repair, or both does not result in any significant alteration in the final outcome. Delayed primary repair, without the need for tendon grafting or tendon transfer, is a well-accepted technique. In fact, many hand surgeons are reluctant to immediately repair even a complete extensor tendon laceration in a contused, potentially contaminated wound. The exact time frame under which such delayed repair results in an outcome similar to that of immediate repair is not well defined and depends on the clinical scenario. Usually, repair delayed for up to 7 to 10 days will still ensure an outcome similar to that of an immediate repair, but this varies depending on the injury. Clearly document the inability to rule out a tendon injury in the ED and the mandate for follow-up within a specified time frame on the medical record and discharge instructions.

Use of Antibiotics

There are no data to support or refute the use of prophylactic antibiotics as a routine adjunct after tendon injury. In general, prophylactic antibiotics have not been demonstrated to reduce infection rates after soft tissue injury in the setting of proper wound cleaning. Nor have they been proved to reduce infection rates in the absence of gross contamination, retained foreign material, extensive contusion, or a delay in cleaning. Many clinicians opt for antibiotics with gram-positive (including antistaphylococcal) coverage if the tendon has been injured or sutured, but no universally accepted standard of care exists. An individualized approach is advocated. Prophylaxis is generally used for only 3 to 5 days after injury unless there are extenuating circumstances (such as lack of immunocompetency, a human bite, an unusual source of contamination, or peripheral vascular disease). If the sterility of a wound is in doubt, do not attempt tendon repair.

Preparation for Repair

Before attempting repair of an open extensor tendon injury in the ED, be prepared and have the proper equipment available. Place the patient supine on a gurney that ideally has an arm board attached. Bright overhead lighting is important for wound exploration so that the presence of tendon injuries and foreign bodies can be adequately assessed. Instruments should include, at a minimum, a needle holder, two skin hooks and retractors, sharp (i.e., iris) and blunt-nosed scissors, several small hemostats, and one pair of small single-toothed (i.e., Adson) forceps.

The choice of suture material depends on the location of the tendon injury. For repair of complete tendon injuries on the dorsum of the hand, nonabsorbable, synthetic braided sutures are preferred.[4] Polyester sutures, such as Ethibond or Mersilene, are recommended. Nylon sutures are acceptable but are less ideal because colored nylon may be visible under the skin. Chromic and plain gut should be avoided because they will dissolve before adequate tendon healing has occurred. Silk is not desirable because of its reactivity. Most extensor tendons on the dorsum of the hand will accommodate 4-0 sutures, but 5-0 suture material may be needed for smaller tendons. Small, "plastic repair" tapered needles should be used to avoid tearing the tendon. Partial tendon injuries in the digits are best repaired with fine, synthetic absorbable sutures such as polyglactin (Vicryl). Complex lacerations that involve tissue loss and fraying of the tendon margins (e.g., table saw injuries) represent a particularly challenging clinical scenario that may make an otherwise straightforward tendon repair very difficult. In these cases, Lalonde and Kozin recommend closing the lacerated skin and tendon together (i.e., dermatotenodesis). Take large, composite bites of skin and tendon together, 5 to 10 mm on either side of the wound, with 3-0 or 4-0 nylon sutures tied outside the skin. Tighten the sutures until the digit is in full extension.[5]

Before repairing a tendon injury, it is imperative that the clinician use adequate anesthesia so that thorough wound exploration can occur. A field block or regional nerve block can be used on the dorsum of the hand, whereas local anesthesia or a digital nerve block can be used on the fingers. The choice of anesthetic composition has been the subject of long-standing controversy. Traditional teaching admonishes the use of epinephrine in anesthetics for fear of digital ischemia; however, many clinicians readily use lidocaine with epinephrine in the hand and fingers without complications. There is ample anecdotal and clinical evidence supporting the safety profile of epinephrine in digital anesthesia. Epinephrine has the benefit of prolonging the anesthetic effect and promoting a bloodless field during wound exploration and repair.[6] It is important that the digits be fully anesthetized or, in the case of more proximal wounds on the hand, that the area around the wound be liberally anesthetized because many lacerations must be extended to afford access to the surgical field. It is a common error to avoid extending a laceration and to attempt

examination, cleaning, or repair through a small initial skin laceration.

Following the administration of an anesthetic, place a tourniquet on the involved limb if hemostasis is problematic. It is absolutely essential that adequate control of blood flow be obtained before attempting to repair a tendon laceration. It is very difficult to find the proximal end of a retracted tendon in a bloody field. Before applying a tourniquet, wrap the patient's arm in several layers of cast padding as a comfort measure, and elevate the arm for at least 1 minute to allow blood to drain by gravity. Place a blood pressure cuff on the middle to upper part of the arm, wrap several more layers of cast padding around the cuff, and then inflate it to 260 to 280 mm Hg. Once inflated, clamp the tubes tightly with a hemostat. The use of cast padding during inflation helps avoid inadvertent unraveling of the cuff. Use of a hemostat to clamp the blood pressure cuff tubes helps avoid a slow leak in the cuff with resultant deflation. A blood pressure cuff tourniquet is generally well tolerated by patients for approximately 15 to 20 minutes. If tendon repair cannot be accomplished in this time, it is likely that the injury is too complex for repair in the ED. When necessary, use parenteral sedation to help the patient tolerate a longer tourniquet time.

Atraumatic technique is essential for minimizing adhesions and scar tissue formation. Tendons should be handled delicately, with crushing force or excessive punctures with forceps and needles avoided. Forceps should be used only on the exposed, cut end of the tendon whenever possible.[7]

Patterns of Injury and Management

Treatment of extensor tendon injury depends primarily on whether the injury is open or closed, as well as the anatomic location of the injury. The most widely accepted classification system is that developed by Verdan,[8] which divides the hand and wrist into eight anatomically based zones (Fig. 48-10). It is quite useful for emergency clinicians to become familiar with this classification because in many instances the zone of injury can help determine whether tendon repair should be

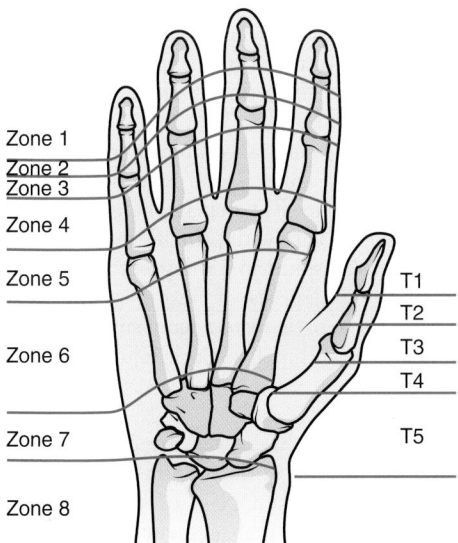

Figure 48-10 Dorsum of the left hand. The injury classification system recommended by Verdan[8] includes eight anatomically based zones. *(Adapted from Blair WF, Steyers CM. Extensor tendon injuries.* Orthop Clin North Am. *1992;23:142.)*

Figure 48-11 An effective way to fully immobilize a finger with a tendon laceration is to incorporate an aluminum foam splint into the middle layers (*arrow*) of a standard dorsal plaster/fiberglass short-arm dorsal splint.

attempted in the ED. One must keep in mind that repair of lacerated extensor tendons within 72 hours of injury is still considered primary closure. Therefore, although emergency clinicians may repair many extensor tendon injuries immediately, some injuries are best managed with delayed repair. In these cases, initial care in the ED should consist of sterile skin preparation, copious wound irrigation and inspection for foreign bodies, skin closure, splint application, and referral to a hand specialist for further care in 1 to 5 days. A dorsal plaster or fiberglass splint in which a metal foam finger splint is incorporated is an ideal way to totally immobilize a finger (Fig. 48-11) (see Chapter 50).

Zone 7 and 8 Injuries[1]

Zones 7 and 8 consist of the area over the wrist and the dorsal aspect of the forearm, respectively. Extensor tendon lacerations in these regions can be quite complex and are therefore not repaired in the ED. Because of the close proximity of extensor tendons in the distal part of the forearm, lacerations such as stab wounds may appear innocuous but often result in multiple tendon lacerations. At the wrist level, the extensor tendons are covered by a retinaculum that is lined with synovium. Although this tissue allows smooth gliding of tendons during normal activity, the presence of synovium increases the risk for adhesions after tendon repair. In addition, lacerated tendons in the wrist and distal part of the forearm may retract away from the site of initial injury. This may make tendon retrieval and repair quite difficult and necessitate incision of the retinaculum and exploration of one or more compartments.

As a result of the potential complexity of these injuries, all tendon lacerations in zones 7 and 8 require formal surgical exploration and repair. ED management of these patients includes local wound care with primary repair of the skin and placement of a volar splint in 35 degrees of extension at the wrist and 10 to 15 degrees of flexion at the MCP joints. Promptly refer these patients to a hand surgeon so that repair may be undertaken within 1 week of injury.

Zone 6 Injuries[1,4,9]

Zone 6 consists of the area over the dorsum of the hand. Extensor tendon injuries in this region are frequently caused by lacerations from broken glass or another sharp object. Common pitfalls in ED management of these injuries are usually related to failure to recognize that the tendon has been injured. It is important to remember that these tendons are superficially located, partial tendon lacerations may occur, and weak extension of a digit is possible with a complete tendon

laceration because of transfer of extensor function through the juncturae tendinum. Lacerations of the EIP or EDM tendons are evidenced by an inability to independently extend the index or little finger, respectively. In most cases, missing zone 6 injuries can be avoided if a careful physical examination is performed, including thorough wound exploration under sterile conditions using a tourniquet, adequate local anesthesia, and good lighting.

Extensor tendon injuries in zone 6 are generally appropriate for repair in the ED. Because of the juncturae tendinum, extensor tendons in zone 6 are less likely to retract than those in zone 7 or 8; however, the severed tendon may retract when the injury is more proximal. The distal end of a severed tendon is usually easy to find by passively extending the patient's affected digit to bring the end into view. Retrieval of the proximal portion of a severed tendon is sometimes required and can usually be accomplished in the ED. Before searching for the proximal end of the tendon, the clinician should have a 4-0 nylon suture loaded onto a needle holder. When the proximal end is located, place this suture as a holding suture as far proximal as possible so that the tendon is not lost again. It is often necessary to use a scalpel to extend the wound proximally in a direction parallel to the course of the injured tendon to obtain adequate exposure. One should then begin to search for the tendon by lifting up this overlying skin with forceps and inspecting the proximal portion of the wound. Sometimes, the blood-stained end of a tunnel can be seen; this may contain the proximal end of the tendon. By gently placing a small hemostat or toothed forceps up this tunnel, the tendon stump can often be pulled into view.

Once both ends of the injured tendon have been located, the technique used for repair depends on the size and shape of the tendon. Whereas larger, round tendons can accommodate sutures that pass through the core of the tendon, smaller or flat tendons are difficult to repair with this technique. Most of the tendons in zone 6 can be repaired with either a modified Kessler or a modified Bunnell core suture technique using 3-0 or 4-0 nonabsorbable suture (Fig. 48-12). Both these techniques involve first placing a single suture in half of the cut tendon. Place the suture in the tendon core by inserting the suture needle into the exposed, cut end and then weaving the suture through the lateral tendon margins. Next, place the same suture through the core of the opposite half of the cut tendon. Tie the suture ends in a square knot in between the cut ends of the tendon to bring the two halves together.

Smaller tendons may be repaired with a figure-of-eight or horizontal mattress suture (see Fig. 48-12). Small, tapered needles should be used to avoid tearing the tendon. In a cadaver study comparing these multiple suture techniques, it was found that the modified Bunnell technique provided the strongest extensor tendon repair.[10] In addition, this technique produced no gapping between the repaired tendon ends and minimized the postrepair restriction of flexion at the MCP and proximal interphalangeal (PIP) joints. It is important to passively test the degree of flexion at the MCP joint after a zone 6 tendon repair to be certain that the tendon has not been excessively shortened.

To improve the tensile strength of the repair, a number of other suture techniques may be used.[4] One option is to increase the number of suture strands that cross the repair site (e.g., four strands rather than two). A cadaver study that compared various four-strand tendon repair techniques concluded

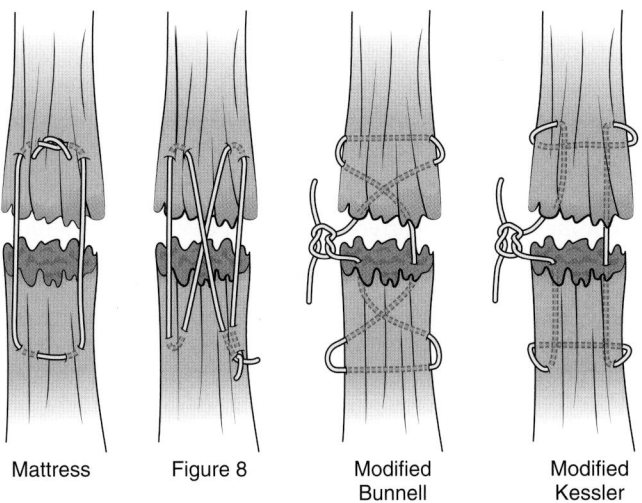

| Mattress | Figure 8 | Modified Bunnell | Modified Kessler |

Figure 48-12 Suture techniques used for extensor tendon repair.

Figure 48-13 Regardless of this patient's history, this wound is infected and highly suggestive of a human bite injury, which was vehemently denied by this patient. Human bites cause *extensor tendon injuries, fractures, and joint capsule injuries and can harbor foreign bodies.*

that the Massachusetts General Hospital technique was more resistant to gap formation than either the Krackow-Thomas or the four-strand modified Bunnell technique.[11] However, this cadaver model could not assess tendon shortening or subsequent range of motion.[12] Another way to improve tensile strength is to place a peripheral suture in addition to the core suture. Place a running cross-stitch suture of synthetic, absorbable material (e.g., 5-0 polyglycolic acid, polyglactin, polydioxanone) circumferentially around the repair site or just on the dorsal surface of the tendon across the laceration site. Alternatively, place sutures laterally along both sides of the tendon, starting at about 1 cm on either side of the repair site. The ultimate choice of repair technique will depend largely on the treating clinician's familiarity with extensor tendon repair, as well as the size of the tendon.

The approach to partial extensor tendon lacerations is not well defined, and no definitive standard of care exists. One evidence-based analysis identified 141 papers in its literature search, but none were relevant to the question of repair of partial extensor tendon injuries.[13] The authors concluded that there is no direct evidence to assist in answering this question. Given the lack of literature on the subject, a reasonable approach may be to extrapolate from data on flexor tendon injuries. It has been demonstrated that many partial flexor tendon lacerations do well without repair,[14] but hand surgeons still disagree on the need for repair of these injuries. In a survey of hand surgeons, 30% of respondents repaired all partial flexor tendon lacerations and 45% repaired only lacerations with greater than 50% involvement of the cross-sectional area.[15] Except at the wrist level, extensor tendons are not covered with synovium and are less likely than flexor tendons to form adhesions after repair. This encourages some authors to recommend repair of most partial extensor tendon lacerations. Although the ideal approach to these injuries is not known, it is reasonable to consider repair of partial extensor tendon lacerations to be optional if less than 50% of the cross-sectional area is involved. However, if not repaired, such injuries must be splinted for 3 to 4 weeks to ensure that a partial laceration is not converted into a complete injury. Skin closure, splinting, and referral for follow-up is a standard approach to unsutured partial extensor tendon lacerations.

After repair of a lacerated EDC tendon in zone 6, apply a plaster or fiberglass volar splint so that the wrist is in 30 to 45 degrees of extension, the affected MCP joint is in neutral (0 degrees of flexion), and the unaffected MCP joints are in 15 degrees of flexion. The PIP and distal interphalangeal (DIP) joints should be allowed full range of motion. After 10 days, the MCP joints are allowed 20 to 30 degrees of flexion. If there is an isolated EIP or EDM tendon injury, only the index or little finger must be included in this splint. Dynamic extension splinting may be used as early as 2 days after tendon repair, so close follow-up is recommended.[16]

Zone 5 Injuries[17,18]
Zone 5 consists of the area over the MCP joint. Open injuries in this region should be considered secondary to a human tooth bite until proved otherwise (Fig. 48-13), especially if the injury occurs over the first or second MCP joint because this is frequently the location of a clenched-fist ("fight-bite") injury. ED evaluation must begin with a careful and persistent history and physical examination, although patients' reluctance to admit to punching someone in the mouth is notorious. The wound should be inspected through its full range of motion because the position of the EDC tendon changes with hand position. It is generally recommended that radiographs be obtained for all these injuries to evaluate for metacarpal head fractures, air in the joint space, or the presence of a foreign body such as a tooth fragment (Fig. 48-14).[16]

If after a thorough evaluation it is determined that a human bite in this region has resulted in a superficial skin laceration only, without injury to the underlying tendon or joint, outpatient management is appropriate. The wound should be copiously irrigated and left open. A volar splint is applied with the wrist in 45 degrees of extension, the MCP joints in the neutral position (0 degrees of flexion), and the hand dressed with a bulky dressing. The use of prophylactic antibiotics for these "low-risk" human bites on the hand is controversial, and clinical trials have yielded mixed results.[19,20] Despite the lack of compelling clinical evidence for either approach, many authors recommend that 3 to 5 days of prophylactic antibiotics be given to these patients. Regardless of whether antibiotics are prescribed, patients should be seen in 24 to 36 hours for a repeated examination to evaluate for wound infection.

If a human bite results in tendon damage, including partial or complete laceration, some clinicians opt for admission and intravenous antibiotics. However, no specific standard of care exists. Outpatient therapy is acceptable in a reliable patient who has access to follow-up. Delayed closure with evaluation and repair of the tendon should be undertaken by a hand surgeon after 7 to 10 days of antibiotic therapy.[4,16] Primary closure of even seemingly clean and well-irrigated human bites in this region is not advisable because of the increased risk for wound infection, as well as the potential for septic destruction of the MCP joint if it is violated. If an open joint is noted on physical examination, a more aggressive approach is warranted. Such patients are generally admitted for intravenous antibiotics after copious irrigation.[4,16]

If a patient suffers a zone 5 tendon injury and it can be determined with complete certainty that it was caused by a relatively clean, sharp object rather than by a human bite, primary closure is appropriate. Referral of these injuries to a hand surgeon is common practice given the complexities of the injury and possible sequelae. Careful repair of lacerations

Figure 48-14 This patient stated that he sliced his hand on a piece of metal at work (expecting a workers' compensation claim) but was unable to explain the chipped bone and *piece of tooth* that was found in the wound on exploration. Note that this puncture-type wound had to be significantly extended to adequately visualize the extent of the injury.

involving both the EDC tendon and the sagittal bands is necessary to prevent subluxation of the EDC tendon away from the center of the metacarpal head. Initial ED management of non–human bite injuries is often limited to skin closure, splinting as described earlier, and referral to a hand surgeon within 1 to 5 days.

Closed extensor tendon injuries in zone 5 usually result from the acute or recurrent application of compressive force to the MCP joint capsule. Closed injuries in this region are sometimes referred to as a *boxer's knuckle*. Repetitive closed injury to the MCP joint region can produce small tears in the EDC tendon, the sagittal bands, or the joint capsule. These patients tend to have chronic and recurrent pain and swelling in the MCP joint region but usually have normal radiographic findings. Acute trauma may result in the same injuries or cause more severe damage to the extensor hood. Such patients may have complete disruption of the extensor mechanism, including damage to the central tendon and the sagittal bands. The MCP joint is swollen, has decreased mobility, and may exhibit an extensor lag. Traumatic subluxation of an EDC tendon may be present and usually involves the middle finger with subluxation to the ulnar side (Fig. 48-15). Dislocation to the radial side is less common, probably because of the juncturae tendinum on the ulnar side, which can compensate for injuries to the ulnar sagittal band.[21] The subluxation becomes more prominent with flexion at the MCP joint. Controversy exists regarding the initial management of closed injuries in this region. Whereas some authors prefer initial surgical repair,[18] others use an initial trial of extension splinting in some or all cases.[4,16,17,21] Splinting the MCP joint in neutral or slight flexion for 6 weeks has been recommended for dislocations initially seen within 3 weeks of injury, with operative repair being reserved for more delayed manifestations or patients who fail splint therapy.[16]

Zone 4 Injuries[17]

Zone 4 consists of the area over the dorsal aspect of the proximal phalanx between the MCP and PIP joints. The extensor tendon is a broad, flat structure in this region and is relatively easy to repair. Because the extensor tendon is flat and conforms to the roundness of the proximal phalanx,

Figure 48-15 Traumatic ulnar dislocation of the extensor digitorum tendon at the metacarpophalangeal (MCP) joint of the long finger. **A,** No swelling or tenderness. The tendon is centralized. Tendon instability is not evident with MCP joint extended. **B,** Ulnar displacement of the extensor tendon increases with MCP joint flexion. *(From Skirven TM. Rehabilitation of the Hand and Upper Extremity. 6th ed. St. Louis: Mosby; 2011.)*

tendon injuries in this area generally result from a laceration and are almost always incomplete. As a result, extension at the PIP joint is not usually impaired. It is therefore imperative that all these wounds be explored carefully while remembering that the extensor tendon lies immediately beneath the thin overlying skin. Tendons tend to not retract in this area, so close inspection will usually result in location of the injured tendon.

A hand surgeon generally repairs central slip lacerations or any laceration that results in an extension lag at the PIP joint. The decision whether to repair a partial tendon laceration in zone 4 and whether it should be repaired by the emergency clinician is best discussed with the consulting hand surgeon. In general, because of the duality of the extensor system in this region, lacerations of a single lateral slip can either be repaired with 5-0 nonabsorbable suture or be left unrepaired and splinted. Placement of a running suture or simple interrupted sutures with buried knots is appropriate for this area. Postrepair splinting depends on the presence of tension at the repair site. Minor lacerations in zone 4 that do not result in tension on the repair site can be treated with a finger guard for 7 to 10 days and early range of motion. Treat larger lacerations or those that result in tension at the repair site with a splint that extends from the forearm to the digit for 3 to 6 weeks. The splint should be applied so that the wrist is in 30 degrees of extension, the MCP joint is at 30 degrees of flexion, and the PIP joint is in neutral position. Group the fingers so that either digits 2 and 3 or digits 3 through 5 are immobilized.

It is important to recognize that complex partial tendon lacerations (e.g., laceration of a lateral slip with a saw) in zone 4 may result in damage to the gliding layer located between the tendon and the bone. If the patient is still able to actively extend the digit at the PIP joint, these complex partial tendon lacerations are best managed by débriding the frayed tendon ends and splinting the digit in extension rather than attempting to suture the damaged tendon. The splint should be worn for 10 days, followed by active range of motion.

Zone 3 Injuries[1,16,18]

Zone 3, the area over the PIP joint, is a common site of both closed and open injuries. An open injury usually results from laceration with a sharp object. It is imperative that these wounds be carefully explored in the ED to rule out penetration of the joint capsule. Patients with wounds that are suspected of penetrating the joint are generally taken to the operating room for surgical exploration, irrigation, and treatment with intravenous antibiotics, but protocols vary.

Zone 3 tendon lacerations can result in long-term deformity if not carefully repaired, and patients with such injuries are commonly referred to a hand surgeon. Partial lacerations of the central slip or lateral bands are managed variably, and it is advisable to discuss these injuries with the consulting hand surgeon. Lacerations in this area may sometimes result in a complete central slip injury. This may manifested as an acute boutonnière ("buttonhole") deformity in which the PIP joint rests in 60 degrees of flexion. The signs may be subtler, however, and may be noticeable only by weakened extension at the PIP joint or incomplete extension by only a few degrees.

A boutonnière deformity develops when the central slip is ruptured by an open or closed mechanism that leads to unopposed action of the flexor digitorum superficialis tendon (Fig. 48-16). This results in flexion at the PIP joint, protrusion of

the head of the proximal phalanx between the two lateral bands, and disruption of the triangular ligament. When this occurs, the lateral bands are displaced volar to the axis of motion of the PIP joint. The lateral bands then paradoxically become flexors of the PIP joint. In addition, the extensor hood mechanism is pulled more proximally, which results in increased tension on the TEM and hyperextension at the DIP joint. Thus, a boutonnière deformity consists of flexion of the PIP joint with hyperextension at the DIP joint.

Open central slip injuries are usually managed operatively, and complex injuries may require direct attachment of the tendon to bone or tendon reconstruction. If the consulting hand surgeon chooses not to repair the tendon injury immediately, close the skin and apply a splint in the same fashion as described for zone 4 injuries. Thermoplastic splints allow splinting of the hand without involvement of the wrist but are generally not available in the ED setting. Promptly refer these patients to a hand surgeon so that repair may be undertaken within 1 week of injury.

Patients with closed injuries in zone 3 are commonly encountered in the ED. They may complain of a direct blow to the dorsal PIP joint or a "jammed" finger. This injury occurs when an object such as a ball delivers a sudden axial loading force with forced flexion of the PIP joint while it is extended. These patients commonly complain of a painful, swollen PIP joint, which often makes the examination difficult. Some of these injuries may represent PIP joint dislocations that were spontaneously or manually reduced before arrival of the patient at the ED. The tendon injury that is important to recognize in this setting is an occult isolated central slip rupture. Patients may have decreased extension at the PIP joint, but extension is generally normal because the lateral bands are the primary extenders of this joint. With forced extension against resistance, patients usually have pain and may have decreased strength. To eliminate pain as the cause of the decreased mobility, it may be helpful to test PIP extension against resistance after performing a digital block. With acute central slip rupture, PIP joint extension may be particularly weak when the MCP and wrist joints are held in maximal flexion. In this position, a 15-degree or greater loss

Figure 48-16 Boutonnière deformity. This can be an open or a closed injury. Note the flexion of the proximal interphalangeal joint and extension of the distal interphalangeal joint from a laceration of the central slip mechanism (see Fig. 48-17).

Figure 48-18 A, Boutonnière splint. **B,** This splint allows active flexion at the metacarpophalangeal and distal interphalangeal joints.

Figure 48-17 A, Diagram of a boutonnière deformity. **B-E,** The Elson test for early diagnosis of an acute rupture of the central slip of the extensor digitorum communis tendon. Such rupture results in a boutonnière deformity in which the distal interphalangeal joint is hyperextended, as shown. **B,** With the patient's finger flexed (over a straight edge) at the proximal interphalangeal (PIP) joint, the examiner palpates the dorsal surface of the middle phalanx. **C,** If the central slip is intact, PIP joint flexion causes the slip to tighten distally, thereby relaxing the lateral bands and leaving the distal phalanx flail (*arrows*). Thus, when the patient is asked to extend the digit, the examiner feels pressure that is being exerted by an intact central slip. **D** and **E,** If the central slip is disrupted, however, the examiner feels no pressure on the dorsum of the middle phalanx as the patient tries to extend the digit. It is possible for the patient to extend the injured finger successfully only by hyperextending (by action of the lateral bands) (*arrows*).

of active extension is highly suggestive of a central slip injury.[18] The Elson test may also help identify this injury (Fig. 48-17).[22]

A boutonnière deformity does not usually develop in patients with closed zone 3 injuries until 10 to 21 days after injury. The only way to prevent this deformity is to have a high index of suspicion for its presence and treat these patients conservatively. It is advisable that all patients with a swollen, tender PIP joint and pain with flexion or extension be splinted and referred for close follow-up. Apply a dorsal splint overlying the PIP joint while keeping it in full extension. This can

be accomplished with an aluminum foam-backed splint or a Bunnell ("safety pin") splint, although the latter may not be available in the ED.[16] The MCP and DIP joints should be left free to have full, active range of motion (Fig. 48-18). If a central slip attachment fracture is present, orthopedic consultation is recommended because these patients may require surgical internal fixation.[23]

Zone 1 and 2 Injuries[1,4,16,18]

Zones 1 and 2 consist of the area over the DIP joint and the middle phalanx, respectively. In zone 2 the conjoined lateral bands come together to form the TEM and are held together, in part, by the triangular ligament. The TEM inserts on the base of the distal phalanx and allows extension at the DIP joint. Complete disruption of the TEM results in an inability to extend at the DIP joint. Because of the unopposed action of the flexor digitorum profundus (FDP) tendon, the DIP joint rests in the flexed position. This is known as a *mallet deformity* of the finger (Fig. 48-19*A*). When evaluating DIP motion, it is important to isolate the function of the extensor tendon by holding the PIP joint in full extension (Fig. 48-19*B* and *C*). Normally, full active extension is possible.

Tendon lacerations in zones 1 or 2 that result in a partial or complete mallet deformity generally warrant discussion with a hand surgeon (Fig. 48-20). Management consists of repair of the lacerated tendon and postrepair immobilization. Some surgeons will use only an external splint; others prefer placement of a Kirschner wire (K-wire) through the distal phalanx into the middle phalanx to help stabilize the joint. One technique for tendon repair involves placement of a roll-type suture (dermatotenodesis) that incorporates the tendon and overlying skin into a single suture (Fig. 48-21).[1,16] The DIP joint is then splinted in full extension for at least 6 weeks.

Figure 48-19 A, Mallet finger deformity. **B** and **C,** When evaluating distal interphalangeal (DIP) motion for a mallet finger, isolate the function of the extensor tendon by holding the proximal interphalangeal (PIP) joint in full extension. This minimizes the contribution of the central slip to DIP extension. With the PIP joint stabilized, test active extension at the DIP joint. A patient with a mallet finger will be unable to extend the distal phalanx actively, but the joint can usually be extended passively. (*A, From Leddy JP, Dennis TR. Tendon injuries. In: Strickland JW, Rettic AC, eds.* Hand Injuries in Athletes. *Philadelphia: Saunders; 1992:180.*)

Occult partial tendon lacerations are important to recognize to prevent the development of a mallet deformity. If there is a partial tendon laceration in zone 1 or 2 that does not result in any extension lag, the approach to repair is variable, and it is advisable to discuss the repair with the consulting hand surgeon. In general, partial tendon lacerations involving less than 50% of the tendon area that do not result in an extension lag may be splinted in extension for 7 to 10 days with or without repair of the tendon itself.[16] Partial tendon lacerations involving more than 50% that do not result in an extension lag may be repaired by a hand surgeon or an emergency

Figure 48-20 An open mallet finger can be repaired surgically.

Figure 48-21 Dermatotenodesis technique for zone 1 extensor tendon repair. **A,** Fresh lacerations of the extensor mechanism over the distal joint with a mallet finger deformity are repaired with a running-type suture, which simultaneously approximates the skin and tendon (**B** and **C**). A small dressing is applied along with a splint to maintain the joint in full extension. The sutures are removed at 10 to 12 days, but the splint is continued for a total of 6 weeks. (*A-C, Adapted from Baratz ME, Schmidt CC, Sugar AM, et al. Extensor tendon injuries. In: Green DP, ed.* Operative Hand Surgery. *5th ed. Philadelphia: Churchill Livingstone; 2005:190. Ccopyright 2005 by Churchill Livingstone, an imprint of Elsevier Inc.*)

clinician who is experienced in the repair of these injuries. In either case it is advisable to discuss with the consultant hand surgeon whether the tendon will be repaired in the ED or the operating room.

If a zone 1 or 2 partial tendon laceration is repaired in the ED, it can be approximated by using a combination of running and cross-stitch sutures[16] with 5-0 nonabsorbable (e.g., Prolene) suture material. In general, given the diminutive size of the extensor tendon in this region, placement of core sutures is not possible. It is important that the tendon ends be approximated but not pulled too tightly; otherwise, joint stiffness and limitation of flexion will occur. After repair of a partial tendon laceration, splint the DIP joint in extension for 6 to 8 weeks, followed by 2 to 4 weeks of night splinting and active range-of-motion exercises. Patients should be warned after tendon repair that there is likely to be some residual loss of flexion at the DIP joint, even in the best case.

Closed injuries in zones 1 and 2 may result in a partial or complete mallet deformity, depending on the injury pattern. These injuries are usually caused by an axial loading force with forced flexion of the DIP joint while it is being held in extension. A common ED scenario involving this injury is a patient who complains of pain and swelling at the DIP joint after a ball strikes the fingertip.

Closed tendon injuries in this region can generally be classified into three types. The first type of injury consists of closed rupture of the TEM. The second type of injury is an avulsion fracture of the dorsal lip of the distal phalanx. This fracture is intraarticular, but there is no volar displacement of the remaining portion of the distal phalanx. Avoid attempting to reduce displaced fractures before splinting because any reduction is unlikely to be maintained without surgery; mallet fingers with associated fractures are best splinted and referred.

Treat both type 1 and type 2 injuries with splinting in full extension for 6 to 8 weeks. Either a dorsal or palmar splint should hold the DIP joint in extension or slight hyperextension (5 to 10 degrees) *while allowing free range of motion of the PIP joint* (Fig. 48-22). With a properly fitted splint, no flexion of the DIP joint should occur. The splint can be constructed from an aluminum, foam-backed splint or from a prefabricated Stack splint. A Cochrane review of treatment of mallet finger injuries found inadequate data to establish the most effective type of splint, but the Stack splint is the editor's preference for ease of application and patient comfort.[24] Be careful to avoid excessive sustained pressure from the splint on the DIP joint area because skin necrosis may occur. Strictly maintain the DIP joint in full extension for 6 to 8 weeks, including during sleep and splint changes. Adherence to this instruction is essential since patients have a tendency to test its function on their own, thus tearing the healing tendon fibers. The most common reason for failure of treatment is patient noncompliance with prolonged splinting. Whenever the splint is removed, support the distal fingertip in full extension at all times. Should DIP joint extension be lost at any point during the initial treatment period, reset the treatment clock for an additional 6 weeks.

The third type of closed injury is an intraarticular avulsion fracture of the dorsal lip of the distal phalanx with volar displacement of the remaining portion of the distal phalanx (Fig. 48-23). Such injuries are best referred for definitive treatment consisting of either surgery or more complex splinting. Normally, the DIP collateral ligaments hold the distal phalanx in place; however, if there is a large enough fracture fragment (usually >50% of the articular surface), the remaining distal phalanx fragment displaces in the volar direction secondary to unopposed action of the FDP tendon. When volar displacement of the distal phalanx occurs, this injury may require more aggressive treatment to achieve an optimal outcome.[18] Unfortunately, there are no adequate published randomized, controlled trials comparing operative versus conservative treatment of these injuries.[24] Operative repair usually involves open reduction and internal fixation of the fracture with placement of a K-wire for additional stabilization. It is important to remember that it is the presence of volar subluxation, not the size of the avulsion fracture, that is most often considered when determining the need for operative management.

Any injuries, whether open or closed, that result in complete disruption of the TEM may result in a swan neck deformity (Figs. 48-24 and 48-25). This deformity consists of flexion at the DIP joint (a mallet finger) and hyperextension at the PIP joint. It results from increased extension force on the middle phalanx caused by dorsal and proximal displacement of the lateral bands. This complication can often be

Figure 48-22 Mallet finger splints. Care should be taken to avoid direct sustained pressure from the splint on the skin in the area of the distal interphalangeal (DIP) joint. Excessive pressure or hyperextension can cause skin necrosis. The splint should allow easy motion of the proximal interphalangeal joint *with no flexion of the DIP joint*. Immobilize the DIP joint in full extension or slight hyperextension (5 to 10 degrees). Splints are maintained continually for 6 to 8 weeks, including during sleep, with strict avoidance of any flexion during hand washing or splint changes. **A,** Commercially available and an *ideal and preferred* volar plastic splint (Stack mallet finger splint); **B,** dorsal aluminum foam splint; **C,** volar aluminum foam splint; **D** and **E,** Kleinert mallet finger splint. The Kleinert splint provides modest hyperextension and avoids pressure on the skin by removing the middle third of the foam padding, thereby eliminating all direct pressure on the injury site. All give good results.

avoided if disruption of the TEM is diagnosed and treated correctly in the ED.

Complications

All extensor tendon repairs are subject to the usual complications of wound infection and skin breakdown secondary to prolonged splinting. Tendon rupture is a rare complication after tendon repair and may result from inadequate suture technique or premature motion against resistance. It is important when extensor tendons are repaired that at least five throws be used and a square knot be tied. All extensor tendon repairs require some period of complete immobilization

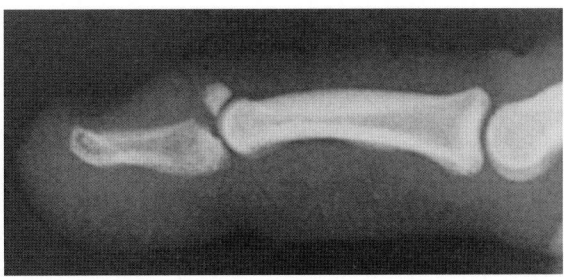

Figure 48-23 A mallet fracture with volar subluxation of the distal phalanx. Avoid attempts to reduce any displaced fractures before splinting because any reduction is unlikely to be maintained without surgery; mallet fingers with associated fractures are best referred.

Figure 48-24 Swan neck deformity. *(From Skirven TM. Rehabilitation of the Hand and Upper Extremity. 6th ed. St. Louis: Mosby; 2011.)*

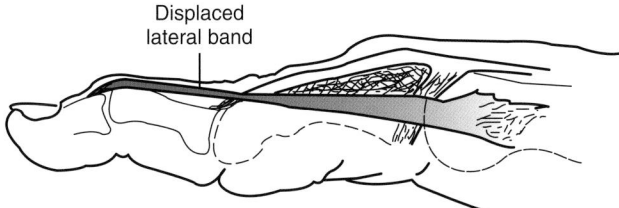

Figure 48-25 Diagram of the swan neck deformity. Lateral bands have displaced dorsal to the axis of the proximal interphalangeal joint, where they extend the joint and allow the distal interphalangeal joint to flex. *(From Rizio L, Belsky MR. Finger deformities in rheumatoid arthritis. Hand Clin. 1996;12:531.)*

during tendon healing, and the emergency clinician must stress the necessity for patient compliance.

Extensor tendon injuries in zone 7 tend to have the worst prognosis. Because of the presence of a synovial lining, postrepair adhesions may develop. Adhesions may lead to decreased excursion of the extensor tendons with resultant decreased mobility at the wrist. There may also be limitation of finger flexion when the wrist is flexed, as well as limitation of finger extension when the wrist is extended. Because of the lack of synovium, the low risk for adhesions, greater tendon excursion, the relatively simple anatomy, and the usual lack of associated injuries, zone 6 tendon injuries tend to have fewer complications than other areas of the hand. The tendons in zone 6, however, do have a tendency to shorten if the ends are approximated too tightly. This may result in restriction of PIP and MCP joint flexion. In addition, worse outcomes may

occur with complex zone 6 tendon injuries when additional soft tissue or bony injuries are present.[16,25]

Zone 5 injuries are particularly prone to infection because injuries in this region commonly occur from a human bite. In addition, if the extensor hood covering the MCP joint is not repaired carefully, subluxation of the EDC tendon may occur.[9] If complex partial tendon lacerations in zone 4 are managed too aggressively, tendon shortening and stiffness may result. As discussed previously, these injuries are often best managed by splinting alone. A common complication of zone 3 extensor tendon injury is the development of a boutonnière deformity, which usually results from failure to diagnose or adequately immobilize a central slip injury. Similarly, undiagnosed or improperly treated extensor tendon injuries in zones 1 and 2 may lead to either a swan neck or a chronic mallet deformity of the digit. DIP joint splinting itself may result in skin ulceration or tape allergy, often occurring in the second week of treatment.[16] Skin breakdown may ensue if the DIP joint is splinted in hyperextension because of decreased skin perfusion.

Postrepair Care and Rehabilitation

Proper care after diagnosis and repair of an extensor tendon injury is extremely important for optimal patient outcome. Even the best initial tendon repair can have a poor result if subsequently treated improperly. Rehabilitation of tendon injuries has evolved since 1980 to include dynamic splinting and active range-of-motion exercises to achieve maximal motion of the affected digit.

Zone 1 and 2 injuries are usually treated with static splinting, as described previously. After 6 weeks, active range-of-motion exercises should begin. Night splinting is recommended for an additional 2 to 6 weeks.[1,16,18] Some authors also recommend wearing the splint during the day when performing heavy tasks.[16] It is advisable to give the patient a number of extra splints so that the patient (or family) can change the splint frequently to avoid pressure injury. During splint changes it is important that the DIP joint be held in full extension either by using the other hand or by placing the finger against a table. If an extension lag develops at any time, continuous splinting must be repeated. Closed injuries of the central slip (zone 3) are often treated with a boutonnière splint for 4 to 6 weeks, followed by 2 to 6 weeks of gradual flexion exercises and night splinting. During the initial period of immobilization, the patient should be instructed to passively flex the DIP joint every hour to maintain gliding and proper position of the lateral bands.

Lacerations in zones 3 and 4 have traditionally been treated with static splinting from the forearm to the digits. An alternative approach is to splint only the DIP and PIP joints in extension and begin a "short-arc-motion" protocol within 1 to 2 days of repair.[26] This consists of active motion at the PIP joint progressing from 0 to 30 degrees the first 2 weeks to 0 to 50 degrees in the fourth week. When compared with static splinting, this protocol may lead to better PIP and DIP joint flexion without resulting in tendon rupture or a boutonnière deformity. Dynamic extension splints are also proving to be useful for rehabilitation of zone 3 and 4 tendon injuries.[16,26,27]

Early motion after extensor tendon repair has been found to be most useful in zones 5 through 7. A dynamic extension splint in which the wrist is extended 45 degrees and all finger joints rest in the neutral position is commonly used. A volar block allows 30 to 40 degrees of MCP joint flexion, whereas a dynamic traction mechanism passively extends the digits. Dynamic splinting is started 1 to 3 days after repair. Active motion is added at 3 to 4 weeks, and resistance is added at 7 weeks. A randomized, controlled trial of zone 5 and 6 extensor tendon repairs found total active motion with dynamic splinting to be superior to static splinting at 4 to 8 weeks, but not at 6 months. However, grip strength in the affected hand was improved at 6 months with dynamic splinting.[28] A short-arc-motion protocol with controlled active motion at the MCP joint has also been shown to be safe and effective when started 24 to 48 hours after repair.[9] One comparative trial reported that dynamic extension splinting and controlled active mobilization worked equally well for zone 5 and 6 tendon injuries.[29] All early range-of-motion protocols are most beneficial when managed closely by a skilled hand therapist. Patient age, associated injuries, suture type, and repair technique all affect the choice of rehabilitation protocol.[9] Most importantly, patients must be reliable and motivated to take advantage of early range-of-motion techniques. It is best to refer patients to a hand surgeon or hand therapist as soon as possible after repair so that rehabilitation can begin in a timely manner.

EXTENSOR TENDON INJURIES OF THE FOOT

The extensor tendons of the foot are less commonly injured than the extensor tendons of the hand and wrist. The most important extensors of the foot and ankle that may be injured and encountered in the ED are the tibialis anterior, extensor hallucis longus (EHL), and extensor digitorum longus (EDL) tendons.

The tibialis anterior muscle originates on the shaft of the tibia and interosseous membrane and inserts on the medial cuneiform and the base of the first metatarsal. The tibialis anterior extends the foot at the ankle joint and inverts the foot at the subtalar and transverse tarsal joints. Spontaneous rupture of the tibialis anterior tendon may be seen in both elderly and young patients who have been injured during athletic activity. Injury to this tendon commonly results from forceful attempted dorsiflexion of the ankle while it is held fixed in the plantar-flexed position.[28] Patients generally have decreased strength of foot dorsiflexion because the toe extensors are used to accomplish this motion. Rupture or laceration of the tibialis anterior tendon should be promptly referred to an orthopedic surgeon for consideration of formal operative repair. In some cases, closed injuries of the tibialis anterior tendon may be managed nonoperatively, depending on the extent of the patient's symptoms and functional impairment.[30]

The EDL and EHL tendons both originate from the shaft of the fibula and interosseous membrane. The EHL tendon inserts into the base of the distal phalanx of the great toe, and the EDL tendon divides into four branches that insert on toes 2 through 5 (Fig. 48-26). Both the EHL and the EDL tendons primarily result in extension of the toes and dorsiflexion at the ankle. The extensor digitorum brevis (EDB) and extensor

Figure 48-26 Muscles of the dorsum of the foot: superficial dissection. (*Netter illustrations used with permission of Elsevier Inc. All rights reserved.*)

hallucis brevis (EHB) muscles originate from the upper part of the calcaneus. The EHB tendon joins the lateral aspect of the EHL tendon before inserting on the great toe. The EDB muscle gives rise to three tendons that join the lateral side of the EDL tendons going to toes 2 through 4 (see Fig. 48-26).

Injury to the EHL and EDL tendons may result from a sharp object lacerating the dorsum of the foot. Patients may have weakness of or an inability to extend the involved toe. The examiner may be unable to palpate the injured tendon. Whether one should repair EHL or EDL tendon lacerations is controversial. However, many authors favor repair because failure to repair EDL tendons may result in a claw deformity of the adjacent toes.[31] Lacerations of the EHL and EDL tendons at the level of the ankle are usually repaired, whereas lacerations on the dorsum of the foot and the toe are managed variably. If the patient has significant pain or any flexion deformity of the involved toe, one should probably repair the lacerated tendon. Repair is also favored when both ends of the tendon are easily visualized in the wound and the patient is willing to undergo prolonged immobilization after repair.[32] Because management of these injuries is controversial, it is advisable to discuss the care of these patients with the consulting orthopedic surgeon. Extensor tendon repair of the foot is not usually performed in the ED setting. Superficial cutaneous nerves are easily injured on the dorsum of the foot during wound exploration, which can lead to the formation of a chronic, painful neuroma. If the injury is repaired in the ED, the technique for repair is similar to that used for the dorsum of the hand (zone 6). A posterior splint that includes the toes should be applied after tendon repair. Splint the ankle in 90 degrees with the toes in the neutral position.

FLEXOR TENDON INJURIES

Flexor tendon injuries are more difficult to diagnose and more challenging to treat than extensor tendon injuries. In general, repair of flexor tendons is not performed by emergency clinicians. Anatomic and biomechanic issues, the physiology of flexor tendons and tendon healing, and follow-up rehabilitation and physical therapy are complex and formidable. A satisfactory outcome is more difficult to achieve with an injured flexor tendon than with a similar degree of injury to an extensor tendon. Unlike extensor tendons, flexor tendons are influenced by a number of pulley mechanisms. The tendon must glide through delicate tendon sheaths, so even a minor defect in tendon integrity is physiologically magnified (Fig. 48-27). In addition, flexor tendon injuries are often associated with nerve and vascular injuries.

The main clinical mandates for emergency clinicians are to diagnose or consider flexor tendon injuries, provide initial proper wound care, and expedite appropriate consultation and follow-up. Unlike the more superficial extensor tendons, flexor tendons are often buried deep within the hand and forearm, and it is frequently not readily possible to visualize the tendon in the recesses of a wound. Puncture wounds of the palm often injure flexor tendons, but deep puncture wounds prohibit visualization of the injured structures (Fig. 48-28). Therefore, a partial flexor tendon injury may be clinically silent until rupture occurs days or weeks later. Delayed repair of undiagnosed flexor tendons may be complicated by tendon retraction or scar formation, and tendon transfer and grafting may be necessary.

It may not be possible on the initial visit for the emergency clinician to diagnose the presence of all flexor tendon injuries, nor the full extent of such injuries. Help may be obtained from a specialist if logistically possible, but generally, there is no mandate for such immediate on-site examination when questions about tendon integrity exist. Even though consultation is advised before definitive disposition, the same limitations in the examination would similarly confront a specialist. Individual scenarios and local protocols will guide the timing and degree of consultation in the ED.

Notwithstanding the previous discussion, complete flexor tendon injuries are often apparent on physical examination, either by testing individual tendons or by the resting posture of the injured hand. In contrast, partial tendon lacerations are commonly clinically unappreciated because no functional deficit is evident. Clinical clues to a potential flexor tendon injury are weakness of flexor tendon function (difficult to evaluate in an acutely injured extremity), pain at the site of injury when performing active range of motion against resistance, and an abnormal resting posture of the hand (Fig. 48-29A and B), which can be determined by careful examination but is always difficult in a child or uncooperative patient (see Fig. 48-29C and D). However, the emergency clinician may not be able to arrive at a complete or accurate diagnosis without surgical exploration. Moreover, it is counterproductive and potentially harmful to attempt extensive exploration of the deep recesses of the hand or forearm in the ED merely to visualize a suspected flexor tendon injury.

Completely transected flexor tendons are surgically repaired by a consultant, usually on an elective basis. Most hand surgeons are reluctant to perform primary repair of a flexor tendon injury on ED patients and prefer to have the wound cleaned, the skin closed, and the patient scheduled for subsequent definitive repair. The final outcome of flexor tendon surgery depends on multiple factors; however, surgical repair of most flexor tendons accomplished within 10 to 21 days of injury (delayed primary repair) generally produces final outcomes similar to those with immediate repair.[33-35] Therefore, if a partial tendon laceration is not diagnosed at the initial visit and rupture is noted at the time of removal of the skin sutures or inspection of the wound, immediate referral to a hand surgeon would be expected to provide a similar result as that expected had the injury been diagnosed at the time of the initial ED visit.

Partial flexor tendon lacerations, if appreciated, are usually treated by careful wound cleaning, skin closure, splinting, and referral for reevaluation in 1 to 5 days. Definitive treatment of partial lacerations remains quite controversial. Some surgeons will repair all partial tendon lacerations, whereas others take a more conservative approach. The conservative approach is supported by experimental evidence suggesting that surgical repair of partially lacerated tendons results in weaker tendons than if the tendons were not surgically repaired.[36] Wray and colleagues suggest forgoing suturing in favor of splinting, followed by early mobilization of tendons with lacerations involving 25% to 95% of the cross-sectional area.[37] Without conclusive evidence either way, a reasonable approach would be to suture tendon lacerations involving greater than 50% of the cross-sectional area with special surgical techniques, suture tendon lacerations involving 25% to 50% of the cross-sectional area with simple or special suture techniques, and simply trim injuries that affect less than 25% of the cross-sectional area to promote normal gliding function.[35] All

Figure 48-27 A, Muscles of the forearm (deep layer): anterior view. **B,** Muscles of the forearm (intermediate layer): anterior view.

Palmar view

Transverse cross section of wrist demonstrating carpal tunnel

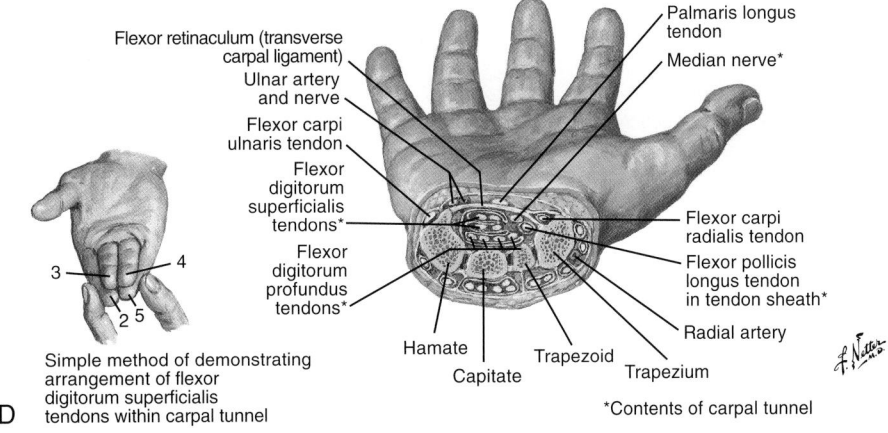

Figure 48-27, cont'd C, Flexor tendons, arteries, and nerves at the wrist: palmar view. **D,** Transverse cross section of the wrist demonstrating the carpal tunnel. (**A-D,** *Netter illustrations used with permission of Elsevier Inc. All rights reserved.*)

decisions concerning the type and timing of repair should be made in concert with a consultant while keeping in mind that some decisions regarding surgical repair of partial injuries cannot be made for weeks or months.

Following evaluation of a known or suspected flexor tendon injury, suture the skin and splint the hand to protect the tendon and minimize retraction. Techniques vary, and the initial splinting positions are probably inconsequential to the final outcome if the duration of splinting does not exceed 7 to 14 days. As a guideline, splinting with the wrist in 30 degrees of flexion, the MCP joints in 70 degrees of flexion, and the IP joints in 10% to 15% of flexion has been recommended.[38] There are no data to support or refute the value of prophylactic antibiotics for any soft tissue injury that has been properly cleaned. Although no definitive standard of care has been promulgated, many clinicians prescribe 3 to 5 days of antibiotics effective against gram-positive organisms (including *Staphylococcus aureus*) if the tendon is injured. Antibiotics are recommended if the degree of contamination

is significant, cleaning has been delayed, there are unusual sources of injury, or the patient is immunocompromised. Specific written instructions with a definite follow-up time frame outlined and assistance in patient referral will probably improve the final outcome, but *flexor tendon injuries often produce lifelong disability despite even ideal care in the ED.*

ACHILLES TENDON RUPTURE

An Achilles tendon rupture can lead to serious morbidity. Although definitive care of such injuries is not performed in the ED, it is important to make the correct diagnosis and institute proper and prompt referral. This injury is easy to miss, and it is not always diagnosed on the first visit. In a recent case series the diagnosis was missed in more than 20% of cases.[39] It is usually initially considered a minor ankle sprain by both the patient and clinician. Rupture often occurs with steroid use, with degenerative conditions, and in the elderly,

Figure 48-28 Deep puncture wounds of the palm may injure the flexor tendons. **A,** The depth of this wound precludes extensive exploration to visualize the tendon. Partial tendon lacerations may still initially allow full function. Clues to a partial flexor tendon laceration include weakness of flexion or pain with attempts at flexion against resistance, but many partial lacerations are clinically silent. Despite full function, this wound's location and depth suggest the possibility of at least a partial tendon injury. The prudent course would include meticulous wound care, splinting, skin closure, and contact with a hand specialist to arrange reexamination in a *few days* while cautioning the patient that a flexor tendon injury may be present and delayed repair for up to 1 to 3 weeks yields results comparable to immediate repair. Immediate repair is often eschewed because of swelling and wound contamination. Further care may be required. **B,** This palm laceration from the sharp top of a metal can seemed superficial. Function was normal. **C,** When examined with the fingers in extension, the tendon was readily visualized, a surprise to the clinician given the benign and superficial appearance of the laceration. The visualized tendon was intact. **D,** When the fingers were flexed (*arrow*), *the position of the hand when the injury occurred*, a 20% to 30% laceration of the tendon was demonstrated. **E,** This injury will do well with 3 weeks of splinting and no tendon repair. Follow-up with a hand surgeon in a few days is prudent. Note the outrigger aluminum splint incorporated into a short-arm plaster splint (*arrow*; see Fig. 48-11).

but Achilles tendon rupture can also occur in healthy athletic patients with no history of heel pain and often with seemingly *minor trauma*. Fluoroquinolone antibiotics have been implicated in Achilles tendon rupture, especially in the elderly. This led the Food and Drug Administration to issue a "black box" warning on the use of all fluoroquinolones for this condition in 2008. Mechanisms for rupture include sudden overload of the tendon by forceful plantar flexion of the foot, as in recreational sports involving jumping (basketball), pushing a heavy object, or stepping up. The injury is usually a *complete as opposed to a partial tear*, and rupture occurs in a region 2 to 6 cm proximal to the tendon's insertion on the calcaneus. Occasionally, a snap or pop may be appreciated by the patient. Pain may not be perceived in the tendon itself; instead, heel or diffuse ankle pain may be experienced. Because multiple structures plantar-flex the foot, the initial result is weakness

of the ankle, and importantly, *complete loss of motion of the foot does not occur*. Characteristic ecchymosis may be evident in 48 to 72 hours after injury.

The diagnosis may be suggested by a palpable defect in the tendon, *but this can be subtle or absent* (Fig. 48-30). The calf squeeze test (Thompson's test) is a physical finding that is 96% to 100% sensitive. To perform this test, have the lie patient prone on a stretcher with the feet overhanging the edge. Squeeze the calf and observe for strong passive plantar flexion of the foot. If the foot does not move, a complete tear is diagnosed (Fig. 48-31). When the diagnosis is not clinically certain or when the possibility of other injuries exists, emergency imaging should be performed. With isolated Achilles tendon rupture, standard radiographs will be normal. Magnetic resonance imaging (MRI) is diagnostic but not usually indicated in the ED. Some practitioners have recently

Figure 48-29 A, Note the obvious abnormal resting posture of the hand. This boy's palm laceration involved the flexor tendons to his index finger. With his hand at rest, his index finger lies in extension, in contrast to his other fingers, which are partially flexed. **B,** Loss of the digital cascade in the middle finger illustrated here should be indicative of a flexor tendon laceration without further examination. The small glass laceration in the palm accounts for the profundus laceration, apparent only at follow-up. Children are difficult to fully examine in the emergency department. Splinting and follow-up in a few days are prudent based on the injury mechanism and location. **C,** The flexor digitorum profundus tendon is examined by immobilizing the digit in question and asking the patient to flex the distal interphalangeal joint against resistance. **D,** The flexor digitorum superficialis tendon is examined by immobilizing the digits not being tested and asking the patient to flex the proximal interphalangeal joint against resistance. Pain and weakness associated with flexion against resistance may suggest a partial tendon laceration, but this is often a very subtle or inaccurate evaluation that must be repeated when the pain and swelling have subsided. (*A, Courtesy of Robert Hickey, MD, Children's Hospital of Pittsburgh.*)

advocated using ultrasound to diagnose both complete and partial tendon ruptures.[40] Sonography is an appealing diagnostic tool given its relatively low cost, portability, safety profile, and the ability to perform static and dynamic evaluations and compare the contralateral side. A *sonographic Thompson test* can also be performed by directly visualizing the tendon with a high-frequency, linear ultrasound probe while the calf muscle of the prone patient is gently squeezed. The Achilles tendon is assessed, proximally to distally, for synchronous movement. Complete tears are recognized by retraction of the proximal tendon end; echogenic adipose tissue (Kager's fat) may be seen to herniate between the torn ends of the

tendon (Fig. 48-32). No studies have evaluated the diagnostic accuracy of ultrasound performed by emergency physicians for Achilles tendon rupture.[39] Treatment varies from conservative splinting to surgery and is controversial. Splinting the foot in mild plantar flexion (gravity equinus) can protect the tendon for follow-up in 1 to 5 days.

KNEE EXTENSOR TENDON RUPTURE[41]

The extensor mechanism of the knee is composed of the four strong quadriceps muscles, the femoral quadriceps tendon,

Figure 48-30 This patient complained of a sprained ankle of 3 day's duration after jumping in a basketball game. There was moderate weakness of plantar flexion, but not complete loss. A defect in the Achilles tendon may be appreciated in some cases of Achilles tendon rupture, but not in this case. Note the characteristic bruising.

Figure 48-31 A, To perform the calf squeeze test (Thompson's test) place the patient prone on the stretcher with the feet overhanging the edge. **B,** Squeeze the calf and look for forceful passive plantar flexion of the foot. In this case the left foot (note the swelling and ecchymosis) did not move, thus confirming a complete Achilles tendon rupture.

Figure 48-32 Longitudinal ultrasound of a complete Achilles tendon rupture. There is a 2.6-cm separation between the proximal (left) and distal (right) torn tendon ends (indicated by the dotted line between plus marks). The calcaneus is located far to the right. Herniated echogenic fat can be seen between the injured tendon edges. *(From Fessell DP, Jacobson JA. Ultrasound of the hindfoot and midfoot.* Radiol Clin North Am. *2008;46:1027.)*

the patella, the patellofemoral and patellotibial ligaments, the medial and lateral retinacula, the patellar tendon, and the tibial tubercle. Both the quadriceps and patellar tendons are subject to rupture. Quadriceps tendon rupture is more common in the elderly and in those with systemic degenerative disease, arthritis, and steroid use and is associated with significant morbidity regardless of treatment. It may also be seen in younger patients, such as occurs after taking a basketball jump shot. Performance-enhancing steroid use is likewise a risk factor in these patients. Patella tendon rupture is also a serious injury but occurs more commonly in healthy patients younger than 40 years participating in sporting events.

As with Achilles tendon rupture, rupture of the knee extensor mechanism is *not always initially suspected or diagnosed*; it is missed by primary care providers in 20% to 30% of cases. The mechanism of quadriceps tendon rupture is usually a deceleration injury with the knee partially flexed, coupled with a strong quadriceps muscle contraction when the foot is fixed. The trauma may be seemingly minor, such as missing a step or jumping from a low height. A common history is an elderly patient who is descending steps or walking off a curb, misses a step, and attempts to keep from falling. A popping or tearing sensation may be elicited. The pain may be deceptively minor. The rupture may be partial but is more often complete. Quadriceps tendon rupture usually occurs transversely just proximal to the patellar insertion, with or without an avulsion fracture of the superior pole of the patella. A suprapatellar gap may be palpated. The mechanism of patella tendon rupture is usually an excessive load on the flexed knee during athletic activities. The patient complains of pain and inability to extend the knee or ambulate. Patella tendon ruptures generally occur at the inferior patella pole. Athletic patients may continue to play with a partial tear, but a

complete rupture does not allow ambulation. Bilateral complete rupture has been described, but the condition is generally unilateral.

With either type of rupture, a large hemarthrosis is usually produced and often prompts the incorrect diagnosis of a ligamentous injury (such as an anterior cruciate ligament rupture). A palpable defect superior or inferior to the patella may be appreciated, but diffuse swelling can hide this finding (Fig. 48-33). Lack of the expected defect can be misleading in the presence of a large hemarthrosis. In cases in which the history consists of only minor trauma and the findings on physical examination are subtle, malingering or noncooperation with

Figure 48-33 A, This elderly man lost his footing going down the stairs and missed only a single step. He felt a pop and was unable to walk. Arthrocentesis yielded a grossly bloody effluent. An obvious suprapatellar soft tissue defect and an inability to perform a straight-leg raise while supine made the diagnosis of a complete quadriceps tendon rupture obvious. **B,** This man landed on both feet while jumping off a low curb and then collapsed. Pain was minimal and malingering was suspected. Diffuse soft tissue swelling, bilateral knee effusions, normal radiographic findings, and the ability to walk *with bilateral knee immobilizers* delayed the diagnosis of bilateral quadriceps tendon rupture until follow-up. **C,** A step-off above the knee readily identified a complete quadriceps tendon rupture. The patient was unable to lift the leg off the stretcher, an activity that made the soft tissue defect obvious.

the examination may be incorrectly contemplated by the clinician. With complete rupture, a *supine* patient is *unable to actively extend the knee* or lift a straightened leg off the stretcher, and the knee flexes when posterior thigh support is removed from the raised leg. Weak extension, especially in the sitting position, may be possible if portions of the medial and lateral retinacula are intact, even with a complete rupture of the central rectus femoris. With complete rupture the patient cannot walk, and the knee gives way immediately. As one would intuit, however, a knee immobilizer allows the patient to apparently walk normally. Partial tears may allow the patient to walk with a peculiar forward-leaning gait that helps support the knee in extension.

Plain radiographs have normal findings except for the occasional patellar avulsion fracture. With quadriceps tendon ruptures, a low-riding patella (*patella baja*) may be present as the patella falls inferiorly. Conversely, a high-riding patella (*patella alta*) is often seen with patella tendon ruptures as the

quadriceps tendon and patella retract superiorly. MRI is definitive in identifying nuances of the process. As with Achilles tendon rupture, sonography is an emerging diagnostic imaging tool used by some ED providers to assess for ruptures of the quadriceps and patella tendons.[40] Partial tears of either tendon may be treated conservatively; complete tears require surgical repair, usually as soon as the diagnosis is made. Although definitive treatment is not undertaken in the ED, early diagnosis may improve the long-term outcome. A 2- to 3-week delay in diagnosis makes recovery less complete and repair more problematic. The postoperative period of recovery for the elderly is prolonged and difficult. Acute injuries diagnosed in the ED may be treated with a knee immobilizer and crutches with 1- to 2-day follow-up, but admission is often warranted to expedite definitive intervention.[36]

References are available at www.expertconsult.com

CHAPTER 49

Management of Common Dislocations

Amanda E. Horn and Jacob W. Ufberg

Joint dislocations are frequently encountered in patients seen in the emergency department (ED). They can range from a simple finger joint dislocation to limb- or life-threatening consequences of high-energy trauma. Keys to clinical assessment and radiographic evaluation of these injuries are discussed along with methods of reduction. The emphasis of the chapter is on simple dislocations that should be diagnosed and initially managed in the ED. Fracture-dislocations that commonly require operative intervention and emergency orthopedic consultation are not discussed.

PREPARATION OF THE PATIENT

Although many authors claim that their reduction method is well tolerated without premedication, they have not usually measured the discomfort of their patients quantitatively.[1-5] There are no rigid, generally accepted guidelines for the use of pharmacologic adjuncts in the management of dislocations. Each patient and each dislocation is unique, and the treating clinician must use judgment regarding whether premedication is required, which agent or agents to use, and what dose to give. In general, the authors suggest the judicious use of analgesia with or without sedation for the majority of reductions performed in the ED. A calm, cooperative patient may tolerate attempts at gentle reduction of a major joint such as the shoulder, but even the most stoic of patients may be quite uncomfortable with the manipulations necessary for reduction of a dislocated finger. A radial head dislocation in a child is usually easily treated without analgesia; however, reduction of a hip dislocation is unlikely to be successful without a significant amount of sedation and analgesia. Attempting any reduction technique in an extremely anxious patient without premedication will generally frustrate the operator and further upset the patient and may hinder a successful outcome. When multiple attempts are required and significant force must be exerted because of muscle spasm or an uncooperative patient, there is an additional chance of producing complications during the reduction.

Verbal techniques for alleviating anxiety and discomfort are not to be discounted because they can be of great assistance during joint reduction. In field settings, simple hypnosis techniques have been used successfully for major joint dislocations.[6] In the ED, verbal reassurance and distracting conversation are useful adjuncts.

In most circumstances, analgesia or sedation of some sort, or both, will be required; the intravenous (IV) route of drug administration is usually the method of choice because it allows rapid relief of patient discomfort and facilitates repetitive dosing for titration to the desired effect (see Chapter 33). Alternatives to procedural sedation and analgesia include intraarticular injection of local anesthetics, hematoma blocks, peripheral nerve blocks, and regional anesthesia (see Chapters 29, 31, and 32).

GENERAL PRINCIPLES

Clinical assessment of a patient with a dislocation must include a search for fractures or other serious injuries, especially if the mechanism involved high energy. This is generally most important for hip, knee, and posterior sternoclavicular dislocations. For all dislocations, perform a detailed neurovascular examination of the extremity before focusing attention on the injured joint.

Although many dislocations are clinically obvious, some may escape detection for some time while other injuries or issues dominate the clinical picture. A knee dislocation may be quite obvious in a 170-lb man who displays a deformity of the knee, but in a 400-lb patient, the knee may look deceivingly normal on first glance. The history and mechanism of injury can be quite helpful in certain circumstances. For example, a painful shoulder joint in a seizure patient should prompt assessment for a posterior shoulder dislocation, whereas a history of the knee striking the dashboard is a clue to the potential for a hip dislocation.

Carpal dislocations in the hand are often radiographically clandestine to an inexperienced clinician but are clinically suggested by severe pain and swelling. Some dislocations will have been reduced before clinician assessment. A careful history will uncover these injuries and prompt the necessary assessment of the ligamentous integrity of the joint and the possibility of an associated vascular injury and guide proper immobilization and follow-up care. *A dislocated and then spontaneously reduced knee is a severe injury that often escapes detection by even a seasoned clinician's initial evaluation.* Other dislocations that are commonly first seen in a reduced state include finger dislocations, patellar dislocations, and radial head subluxations.

Although the chance that a gentle attempt at reduction will cause a fracture or neurovascular injury is extremely low, careful evaluation before and after reduction, as well as documentation of the patient's neurovascular status, is important. Frequently, the initial pain of the dislocation is distracting, and paresthesias or a weak pulse may not be readily apparent until the joint has been reduced. When the integrity of the pulse is in question, *blood pressure* at the wrist or foot may be compared with that in the uninjured extremity, or a *pulse oximeter* may be applied to the distal end of the fingers (Fig. 49-1).

Prereduction radiographs are generally recommended. Reasons include difficulty distinguishing a fracture-dislocation by clinical examination and the potential for medicolegal problems if the fracture is not identified before attempts at reduction. More importantly, certain associated fractures predict a poor outcome with closed reduction and make orthopedic consultation a consideration before such attempts. Obvious exceptions to this rule include suspected radial head subluxation in young children and clinical circumstances in which radiographs are not readily available (e.g., in the wilderness). Obvious clinical conditions (i.e., vascular compromise or threatened skin penetration) may dictate the need for immediate reduction without radiographs; however, the few minutes required for initial radiographic evaluation rarely

Figure 49-1 Significant vascular injuries from dislocations, such as knee, elbow, or ankle dislocations, are usually obvious, but impaired distal circulation may be subtle or delayed because of a slowly increasing intimal flap arterial lesion. Standard techniques to assess vascular injury are the strength of the pulse and capillary refill; this should detect most arterial injuries. Taking a blood pressure reading distal to the injury with a cuff and Doppler ultrasound (**A**) or applying a pulse oximeter distal to the injury and comparing the results with those of the uninjured extremity (**B**) may give some helpful clues to underlying vascular injuries.

increases vascular or neurologic complications and provides very useful information to the consultant.

Some authors question the need for prereduction films in certain patients with obvious or recurrent anterior shoulder dislocation.[7,8] Although postreduction radiographs are traditionally obtained, the need for this in a clinically obvious successful shoulder joint relocation has been questioned.[8,9] The authors suggest that postreduction films be taken in virtually all patients who have had a dislocation reduced in the ED. Patients who have received sedatives and opioids may not remember the actual successful reduction or the immediate postreduction period. Reinjury after release from the ED without radiographic corroboration of a successful reduction can raise questions about the adequacy of the initial procedure. Occasionally, a fracture is detected on postreduction radiographs that was not obvious on the initial films, or a previously noted minor fracture may be found to reside in an intraarticular location.[8]

In general, dislocations of all types are less common in children than in adults because of the relative weakness of the epiphyseal growth plate with respect to the ligamentous support of the joint. Therefore, in children the epiphysis will tend to fracture before dislocation occurs, except in the case of radial head dislocation (nursemaid's elbow). Reduction techniques for pediatric dislocations are generally similar to those used for adults.

The proper terminology for dislocations describes the relationship of the distal (or displaced) segment relative to the proximal bone or the normal anatomic structure. The terms *anterior* and *posterior* are used for most dislocations. Therefore, if the head of the humerus lies anterior to the glenoid fossa, the injury is an anterior shoulder dislocation. Similarly, if the olecranon lies behind the distal end of the humerus, the injury is a posterior elbow dislocation. In the hand, wrist, and foot, one uses the terms *dorsal* and *volar*. *Palmar* and *plantar* are sometimes used in place of volar to describe the position of the dislocated part. Dislocations can be *open* or *closed* and may have associated fractures, which requires a separate description.

It is generally accepted that the sooner a dislocation is reduced, the better. This alleviates the patient's discomfort and corrects distortion of the surrounding soft tissues. In some studies the success rate of reduction is higher when attempted closer to the time of injury.[2] However, there is no reason to forego an attempt at closed reduction of an "old injury" in the vast majority of dislocations. Chronic dislocations persisting several days, weeks, or longer are often difficult to reduce in a closed manner, but such cases are infrequent.

A certain percentage of all types of dislocations are not amenable to closed reduction. Inability to complete a closed reduction is generally the result of interposition of soft tissue structures or fracture fragments and not necessarily due to improper technique. If sedation and analgesia are adequate to permit relaxation of the patient's muscle tone, reduction should be relatively straightforward. When reduction under adequate sedation and analgesia is unsuccessful after several attempts, further attempts at closed reduction are inappropriate. Generally, orthopedic consultation should be obtained after two or three failed attempts.

Once an attempt at reduction is completed, recheck the neurovascular status that was documented before the reduction was performed. For the elbow, hand, and forefoot joints, perform passive range of motion to assess the stability of the reduction and to ensure a smoothly gliding joint that is free of intraarticular obstruction. In addition to close monitoring of the medicated patient, proper aftercare involves adequate immobilization of the injured joint for comfort and to prevent repeated dislocation. Recommendations for follow-up care depend on the injury and its severity.

Timing of Reduction

Questions often arise concerning the necessity of immediate reduction versus delayed reduction, with the clinician fearing disastrous neurovascular consequences if a dislocation is not manipulated immediately on arrival at the ED. In reality, there is rarely an instance in which prereduction radiographs, even portable films, cannot be obtained before treatment. Even if the pulse is weak or the fingers are numb, a few minutes' delay is usually acceptable to gain important radiographic information on the type of dislocation and the presence of an associated fracture and to provide documentation for follow-up clinicians. Important clinical information may be difficult to obtain, or the specific initial injury may be

Figure 49-2 A and **B,** Because the distal pulse is weak and the toes are numb, it may be tempting—and is commonly advocated and acceptable—to immediately reduce these obvious dislocations while the patient is still on the ambulance stretcher. Because proper analgesia or sedation (or both) is required, it is often prudent, although not mandatory, to take a few minutes to also obtain at least a portable radiograph. **C,** Note the very significant fracture-dislocation on the prereduction radiograph. **D,** Once the reduction is accomplished, there is a remarkable difference that suggests a less impressive injury. *The specific initial injury will be impossible to reconstruct from the postreduction physical examination alone.* The few minutes required to properly prepare the patient for reduction and to document the initial injury will not result in a more serious adverse outcome than has been prognosticated by the initial injury. However, when the patient has sustained multiple trauma and extremity films are a low priority, early reduction without radiographs may be warranted.

impossible to reconstruct once the joint has been reduced (Fig. 49-2). Of equal importance, a dislocation with concomitant neurovascular injury should be reduced with the least amount of trauma possible, which often requires a few minutes for induction of analgesia and sedation, a time during which radiographs can be obtained. If a vascular or neurologic abnormality is documented before reduction, the joint should be reduced by the most timely and least traumatic procedure available. Each case should be handled individually by taking the specific injury, available resources, and the clinician's experience into account. Although multiple unsuccessful or forceful attempts at reduction in the ED should be avoided with all dislocations, this is especially important in patients with vascular or neurologic compromise. Occasionally, the more prudent course is reduction under general anesthesia, but this decision must take into consideration the availability of consultation and other resources.

This chapter covers dislocations of the various joints with the exception of wrist dislocations, which are complex and

require orthopedic consultation, and temporomandibular joint dislocations, which are discussed in Chapter 63.

SHOULDER DISLOCATIONS

The human shoulder joint is remarkable for its degrees of motion, but the anatomic features that allow this mobility, contribute to its instability. The glenohumeral joint has the greatest range of motion of any joint in the body, largely because of the loose joint capsule and the shallow nature of the glenoid fossa.[10] Posterior dislocation is uncommon, mainly because of the anatomic support of the scapula and the thick muscular support in this area. Anterior support is less pronounced, with the inferior glenohumeral ligament serving as the primary restraint to anterior dislocation.[11] The depth of the glenoid fossa is somewhat increased by the fibrocartilaginous glenoid labrum, which forms the rim of this structure.

Most shoulder dislocations are anterior (i.e., the humeral head becomes situated in front of the glenoid fossa). Posterior dislocations are the next most common, but they generally account for less than 4% of shoulder dislocations.[12] Uncommon variations include inferior (luxatio erecta), superior, and intrathoracic dislocations.

Anterior Shoulder Dislocations

Anterior dislocations of the shoulder are the most common major joint dislocation encountered and reduced in the ED. The usual mechanism of injury is indirect and consists of a combination of abduction, extension, and external rotation.[10,11] Only rarely is the mechanism a direct blow to the posterior aspect of the shoulder. Occasionally, *especially with recurrent dislocations*, the mechanism is surprisingly minor and can be puzzling to the clinician. An anterior dislocation can be induced by mere external rotation of the shoulder while rolling over in bed or raising the arm overhead. When the first dislocation occurs at a younger age, the recurrence rate is higher. If the first dislocation occurs before 20 years of age, there is an 80% to 92% rate of recurrence. If the first dislocation takes place after 40 years of age, the rate of recurrence is 10% to 15%.[10] Rotator cuff injuries, however, occur more frequently in older patients with anterior shoulder dislocations.[13]

The four types of anterior dislocations are classified according to where the humeral head comes to rest. Subcoracoid dislocations account for more than 75% of anterior dislocations. Other shoulder dislocations include subglenoid dislocation and the uncommon subclavicular and intrathoracic dislocations (Fig. 49-3).[10]

Clinical Assessment

The presence of an anterior shoulder dislocation is usually obvious (Fig. 49-4). A posterior dislocation is more subtle in terms of both clinical and radiographic findings. It can be misdiagnosed as a severe contusion (Table 49-1). A patient with an anterior shoulder dislocation supports the injured extremity and leans toward the injured side while holding the arm in abduction and slight external rotation. The patient cannot adduct or internally rotate the shoulder. Visual inspection reveals loss of the rounded appearance of the shoulder because of absence of the humeral head beneath the deltoid region. The acromion is prominent and an abrupt drop-off below the acromion can be seen or palpated. An anterior fullness in the subclavicular region is visible in thinner individuals and is easily palpable in most others. Comparison with the uninjured side is a useful aid for both visual examination and palpation. Any attempt at internal rotation is quite painful and resisted by the patient. An inability to place the palm from the injured extremity on the uninjured shoulder is consistent with an anterior shoulder dislocation; after reduction, this maneuver should be possible.

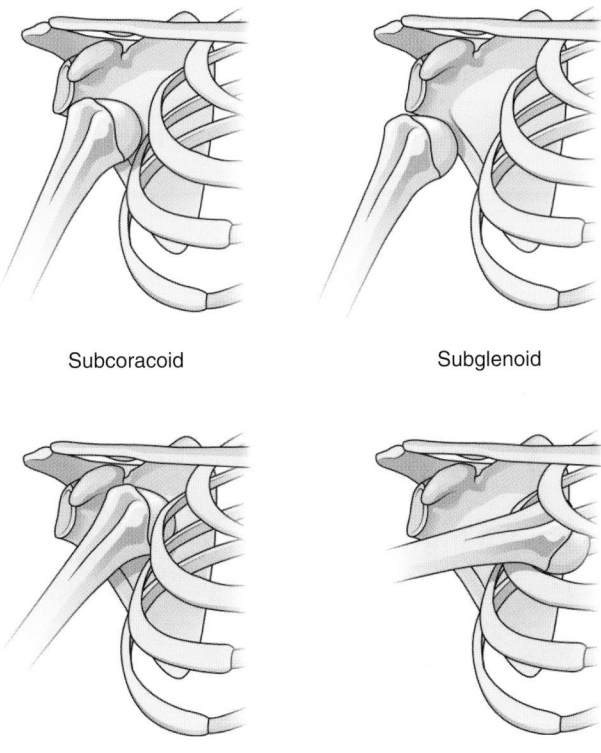

Subcoracoid   Subglenoid

Subclavicular   Intrathoracic

Figure 49-3 Types of anterior shoulder dislocations.

Figure 49-4 A, Typical manifestation of an anterior right shoulder dislocation. The shoulder is very painful, and thus the patient resists movement. The outer round contour of the shoulder is obviously flattened, and the displaced humeral head may be appreciated in the subcoracoid area. Frequently, the patient abducts the arm slightly, bends the torso toward the injured side, and supports the flexed elbow on the injured side with the other hand. **B,** Obvious left shoulder dislocation. This chronic dislocation occurred frequently with minimal trauma, and the patient was able to dislocate it at will, feign a new injury, and obtain narcotics from multiple emergency departments.

Careful assessment of the neurovascular status of the affected extremity is essential (Figs. 49-5 and 49-6). Injury to the axillary artery is rare. It usually occurs in the elderly[13] and can be quickly assessed by a decreased or absent radial pulse or by the appearance of an expanding hematoma. It is important to evaluate the status of the axillary nerve because this is the most common nerve injury resulting from anterior dislocations.[14] Assess the sensory component of the axillary nerve by testing for sensation over the lateral aspect of the upper part of the arm in the "regimental badge" area over the deltoid muscle. Test the motor component of the axillary nerve by assessing the strength of the deltoid muscle; however, this is a difficult undertaking in a patient with a dislocated shoulder. Less commonly, the brachial plexus may be injured by a stretch injury and produce variable nerve deficits. Perform a complete assessment of all the major nerves to the arm because other nerve injuries may occur, such as injuries to the ulnar and radial nerves.[14] A neurologic deficit does not preclude closed reduction, but in patients with a nerve injury, avoid multiple forceful attempts at reduction.

Brachial plexus injuries require an especially atraumatic reduction. If generous sedation and analgesia do not permit easy reduction in the ED, reduction of a dislocation with a nerve injury may be more prudently performed in the operating room with the patient under general anesthesia. Nerve injuries in this setting generally have a good prognosis, but the patient should be informed of the findings and the need for follow-up. The symptoms may require many months to resolve.

Vascular injuries, such as axillary artery disruption, are rare but usually quite obvious because of dysesthesias and coolness of the involved arm. An expanding axillary hematoma, pulse deficit, peripheral cyanosis, and pallor can be seen. Collateral circulation may produce a faint pulse in the extremity, so comparison with blood pressure on the uninjured side may be helpful. Specific lesions include complete disruption, linear tears, and thrombosis. Axillary artery injuries can occur at all ages, but they are more prominent in the elderly. The artery is particularly at risk with anterior dislocations, and dislocation with spontaneous reduction can produce the injury. Arteriography with surgical repair of the artery is required, occasionally with fasciotomy of the forearm if the ischemia is long-standing.[15]

Some portion of the rotator cuff will be injured in many shoulder dislocations. Rotator cuff tears are easier to evaluate

TABLE 49-1 Comparison of Anterior and Posterior Shoulder Dislocations: Classified According to Displacement of the Humeral Head

TYPE OF DISLOCATION	FEATURES	OTHER CLINICAL CLUES	RADIOGRAPHS
Anterior 99% subcoracoid and subglenoid Humeral head anterior to the glenoid	Arm held in *abduction* and *slight external rotation* (abduction more prominent with subglenoid dislocation) The patient cannot adduct or *internally* rotate the shoulder	Seen from the front, the shoulder appears "squared off" Distal acromion prominent on a side view	*On AP view*: obvious dislocation *On lateral or "Y" view*: humeral head appears anterior to the glenoid fossa
Posterior 95% subacromial 5% subglenoid and subspinous Humeral head posterior to the glenoid	Arm held in the sling position with adduction and internal rotation Attempts at *abduction* and *external rotation* cause extreme pain	Coracoid process prominent, glenoid fossa empty anteriorly, and humeral head bulging posteriorly	*On AP view*: vacant glenoid sign, 6-mm sign, light bulb sign *On lateral or "Y" view*: humeral head appears posterior to the glenoid fossa

AP, anteroposterior.

Figure 49-5 Neurovascular evaluation of the upper extremity with a shoulder dislocation. **A,** Axillary (circumflex) nerve palsy is the most common neurologic complication. The axillary nerve has sensory and motor function. Test the integrity of the nerve by assessing sensation to pinprick in its distribution over the "regimental badge" area. (The shoulder is usually too painful to allow assessment of deltoid activity with certainty.) **B,** Look for (rare) involvement of the radial nerve by testing wrist extension and, **C,** involvement of the axillary artery by palpating the radial pulse.

after reduction, often days later when the pain and swelling have subsided.

Radiologic Examination

Associated fractures are detected in 15% to 35% of anterior shoulder dislocations, with fractures of the greater tuberosity being the most common.[10] The presence of a fracture of the greater tuberosity does not change the initial management of anterior shoulder dislocations, and these fractures usually heal well after closed reduction in routine fashion.[10] The Hill-Sachs deformity, a sign of repeated dislocations, produces a groove in the posterolateral aspect of the humeral head and may be seen on prereduction or postreduction films (Fig.

49-7). The Hill-Sachs deformity is caused by impaction of the humeral head against the glenoid rim after dislocation. It rarely has any clinical significance but may result in a loose body within the joint.[13] Impaction of the humeral head against the glenoid during dislocation may also cause disruption of the anteroinferior portion of the cartilaginous labrum of the glenoid or the inferior aspect of the bony glenoid, an injury known as a *Bankart lesion*. It has been implicated as one source of recurrent dislocations but does not affect immediate ED management.[13]

Fractures of the humeral neck are frequently displaced with attempts at closed reduction, which can lead to avascular necrosis of the humeral head.[16] The fact that humeral neck fractures are a known complication of shoulder relocation[10] suggests the value of prereduction radiographs of anterior shoulder dislocations. However, some argue that clinically obvious recurrent dislocations and first-time anterior dislocations without a blunt traumatic mechanism (information usually offered by the patient) can be reduced without prior radiographs because fracture is quite unlikely in these situations.[7,8] Hendey and coworkers[17] performed a prospective validation study of an algorithm for selective radiography that incorporated the mechanism of injury, previous dislocations, and the clinician's certainty of joint position. In this study, 24 patients with recurrent atraumatic anterior shoulder dislocations who received neither prereduction nor postreduction radiographs had no clinically significant fractures found on follow-up. These patients had much shorter ED lengths of stay than did patients who received only prereduction or postreduction films, or both.[17]

One retrospective case-control study found that the presence of any of three risk factors (age >40 years, first episode of dislocation, traumatic mechanism of injury defined as a fall greater than one flight of stairs, a fight or assault, or a motor

Figure 49-6 Anatomy about the shoulder demonstrating the possibility of neurovascular damage after dislocation. *(Reproduced by permission from Thomsen T, Setnik G, eds. Procedures Consult—Emergency Medicine Module. Copyright 2008 Elsevier Inc. All rights reserved.)*

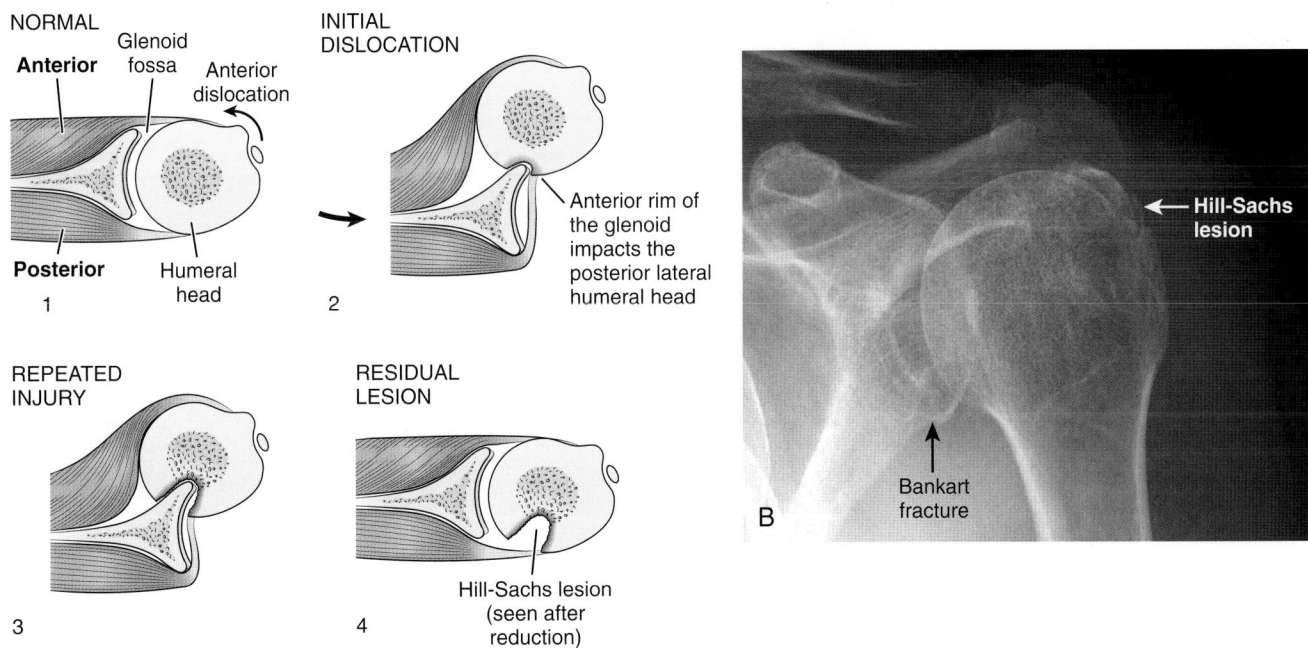

Figure 49-7 A, *1,* Normal. With repeated anterior shoulder dislocations, a Hill-Sachs lesion may form. *2,* During dislocation, the humeral head is damaged by the sharp anterior rim of the glenoid. *3,* With repeated dislocation, a lesion called the "hatchet sign" develops. *4,* On the reduction film the lesion is apparent. **B,** Radiograph demonstrating a Hill-Sachs lesion and a Bankart fracture: a fracture of the inferior glenoid rim from impaction of the dislocated humeral head.

vehicle collision) predicted clinically important fractures with a sensitivity of 97.7%.[18] This study has not yet been prospectively validated.

Anterior dislocations are not subtle on routine anteroposterior (AP) radiographs, and this view detects the most important fracture to identify, that of the humeral neck (Fig. 49-8). An adequate AP view, when combined with the typical clinical examination, allows successful management of most anterior shoulder dislocations. A true AP view of the shoulder is taken at a right angle to the scapula and requires rotation of the patient to 30 to 45 degrees.

The typical lateral views obtained include a scapular Y view (see Fig. 49-8), a transthoracic view, and an axillary view. These views rarely add to the AP film in patients with an obvious anterior dislocation, but they are of value in posterior dislocations (Fig. 49-9). The usefulness of additional views for anterior shoulder dislocations is primarily to detect fractures, and the previously mentioned lateral views (especially the transthoracic view) are quite limited in this respect.[19] The apical oblique view has been found to be more valuable than the oblique scapular projection for acute shoulder trauma.[19] This view is obtained by angling the beam 45 degrees caudad with the patient in a 45-degree oblique position (Fig. 49-10).

Postreduction radiographs are obtained to document the success of the reduction. Occasionally, they will reveal a fracture not detected on prereduction radiographs. In one series, 8% of patients with anterior shoulder dislocations had Hill-Sachs deformities noted only on postreduction films.[8] More recent reports have highlighted the role of ultrasound in

G = glenoid, C = coracoid, HH = humeral head, S = scapular body, Sp = scapular spine

Figure 49-8 Anteroposterior (AP) and scapular "Y" views of an anterior subcoracoid dislocation. The AP views (*top row*) are fairly easy to interpret. On the prereduction film, the humeral head is clearly dislocated from the glenoid fossa and is seen underneath the coracoid process. The correct anatomic relationship of the humeral head and glenoid is demonstrated on the postreduction film. Note the presence of a Hill-Sachs lesion (*arrow*) on the superior aspect of the humeral head. The scapular "Y" view (*bottom row*) is more difficult to understand. The limbs of the "Y" are composed of the scapular spine, the coracoid process, and the scapular body (*gray lines*). The glenoid fossa is found at the convergence of these limbs in the center of the scapula. On the prereduction view, the humeral head is found *anterior*, or *medial*, to the glenoid and under the coracoid, thus confirming the presence of an anterior dislocation. In a posterior dislocation, the humeral head is *posterior*, or *lateral*, to the glenoid (see Fig. 49-9). On the postreduction view, the humeral head is correctly positioned in the middle of the "Y," over the glenoid. (*Diagrams from Heppenstall RB. Fracture Treatment and Healing. Philadelphia: Saunders; 1980:374.*)

Figure 49-9 Posterior shoulder dislocation. **A,** Anteroposterior (AP) view of a patient with a posterior dislocation. A *posterior dislocation* may be difficult to appreciate on an AP view because it is *not inferiorly displaced and may appear to be in the glenoid fossa*. Note the space between the glenoid fossa and the humeral head (*arrow*). It does not look normal. **B,** The scapular Y view reveals that a posterior dislocation is present. Note that the humeral head lies *posterior, or lateral, to the glenoid fossa* rather than being centered over it. *G,* glenoid; *HH,* humeral head.

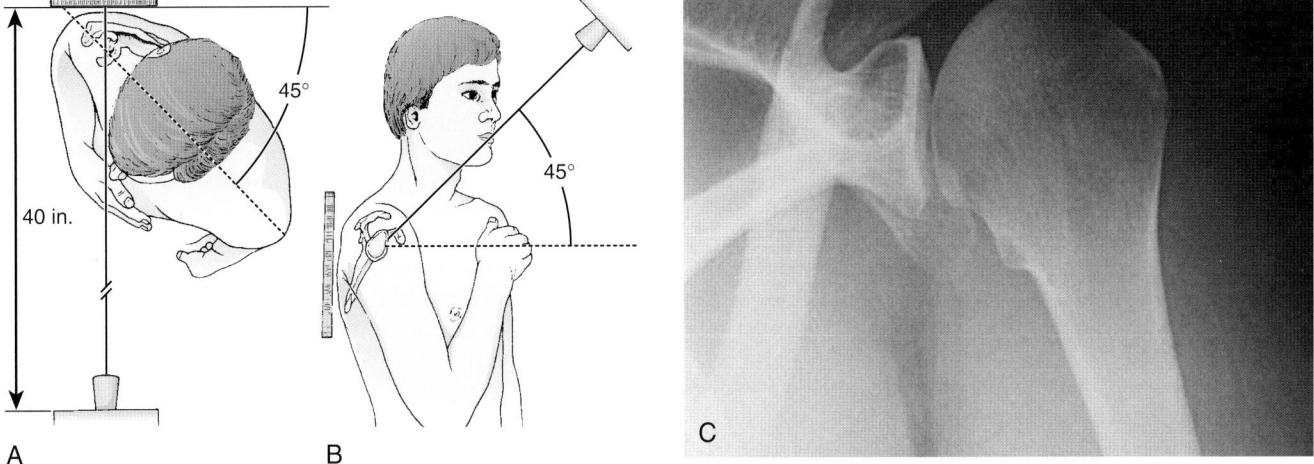

Figure 49-10 A and **B,** Positioning for an apical oblique view. The affected shoulder is placed at a 45-degree oblique position and the central ray is angled 45 degrees caudad. The affected arm is adducted. **C,** Normal apical oblique view. *(From Heppenstall RB.* Fracture Treatment and Healing. *Philadelphia: Saunders; 1980:392. Reproduced with permission.)*

shoulder dislocation, both for diagnosis[19,20] and for confirmation of reduction.[21]

Reduction Techniques

Hippocrates (450 BC) is generally credited with the first detailed description of reduction techniques, and it is believed that a drawing in the tomb of Upuy (1200 BC) is the earliest depiction of such a method.[10] The Hippocratic technique involves placement of the operator's foot in the axilla to allow countertraction. This technique is problematic and not recommended by some authors.[3,11] Likewise, the Kocher method, which involves forceful leverage of the humerus, is associated with an increased rate of complications and is generally discouraged in favor of other techniques.[10,11]

This section discusses several methods of reduction that are well studied, proven to be safe, and easy to master. Regardless of the reduction technique used, gradual, gentle application of the technique is essential. Although all the techniques

discussed are generally acceptable and many authors state that their techniques are quite painless,[1-5] few studies have quantified the actual pain reported by patients.[22] As noted previously, intraarticular lidocaine may also be used to reduce the pain accompanying reduction (Fig. 49-11). In studies by Matthews and Roberts[23] and Kosnick and colleagues,[24] intraarticular injection of lidocaine was found to offer significant relief of pain during reduction of anterior shoulder dislocations. In addition, a recent metaanalysis showed that intraarticular lidocaine had similar success rates as procedural sedation and led to decreased ED length of stay, decreased personnel times, and reduced overall health care cost, thus making it a useful alternative to procedural sedation and analgesia.[25] A Cochrane review reported similar results.[26] When using intraarticular lidocaine, any blood present should be aspirated from the glenohumeral joint before injecting the anesthetic. Note that 10 to 20 mL of 1% lidocaine has been used with the intraarticular technique and that it may take as

Figure 49-11 A, Intraarticular injection for the reduction of an acute anterior shoulder dislocation can be very effective. After aspirating blood from the joint, 10 to 20 mL of 1% plain lidocaine is injected slowly through the lateral sulcus. Allow 15 to 20 minutes for the lidocaine to take effect. **B,** The empty glenoid fossa is easily identified when considering an injection of lidocaine into the joint to facilitate reduction of a dislocated shoulder.

long as 15 to 20 minutes for adequate analgesia. Recently, Blaivas and Lyon[27] reported the ED use of ultrasound-guided interscalene blocks for analgesia before reduction of shoulder dislocations (see Chapter 31). It is important to note that neither local nor regional anesthesia produces muscle relaxation, but they may obviate the need for IV access and prolonged observation. Operator judgment is an important part of the decision whether reduction should be attempted without premedication. Advantages of such an approach include avoidance of potential complications from drug therapy, reduced staff requirements, and theoretically, more rapid patient disposition. Certainly, a patient who is markedly intoxicated may require little, if any supplemental sedative therapy. However, all patients who are reluctant or too anxious to cooperate with an attempt at reduction without medication and those with a high degree of muscle spasm should receive premedication. Generally, only one attempt is made; if unsuccessful, further attempts at reduction are made after the IV administration of sedatives. When in doubt, it is best to use pharmacologic adjuncts (see Chapter 33).

Several factors will help in deciding which reduction technique is best in each clinical situation. Do not use forceful techniques such as traction-countertraction in patients who are not being sedated. The clinician's comfort level with a given technique is always a factor since the greatest success rates will probably result from techniques with which the clinician is most familiar. The time and resources available to the clinician must also be considered because methods such as the Stimson maneuver require more time and the availability of weights and straps. In addition, certain reduction techniques can be performed without assistance, whereas others require an additional person to apply countertraction or to help with manipulation of the scapula or humeral head. Ideally, the emergency clinician should become familiar with a number of different techniques for reducing anterior shoulder dislocations because no single method has a 100% success rate nor is any technique ideal in every situation.

Stimson Maneuver (Fig. 49-12*A*)

The Stimson maneuver is a classic technique that offers the advantage of not requiring an assistant. Place the patient prone on an elevated stretcher and suspend about 2.5 to

5.0 kg (5 to 10 lb) of weight from the wrist.[10,11] The weights can be strapped to the wrist, or a commercially available Velcro wrist splint can be placed and the weights hung from the strap with a hook.[28] The slow, steady traction produced with this method often permits reduction, but 20 to 30 minutes may be required. If needed, facilitate reduction by externally rotating the extended arm.

Variations of this method include the recommendation for flexion of the elbow to further relax the biceps tendon and the application of manual traction instead of weights.[29,30] Rollinson[31] allowed the arm to hang under its own weight after a supraclavicular block and reported a 91% success rate with usually no more than a gentle pull on the arm after 20 minutes in this position. Each variation of the Stimson method can be used in combination with the scapular manipulation technique described later. Indeed, a success rate of 96% has been reported with the combined prone position, hanging weights, IV analgesia and sedation, and scapular manipulation.[28]

Disadvantages of the Stimson method include the time required to achieve reduction and possible dangers to the patient associated with the positioning required for this technique. There is a potential danger of patients slipping off the elevated bed. A "seat belt" strap or bedsheet may be placed around the patient and stretcher to avoid movement of the patient off the stretcher. Airway access to a patient in the prone position may be more difficult in the setting of an overly intoxicated patient or one who becomes overly sedated iatrogenically. In addition, it can be difficult to find a bed that elevates to a suitable height for length of the patient's arm, a convenient method to hang the weights, or the weights themselves in a busy ED.

Scapular Manipulation Technique (see Fig 49-12*B*)

This method is popular because of its ease of performance, reported safety, and acceptability to patients. To date, no complications from the scapular manipulation technique have been reported in the literature.[22,28,32] Shoulder reduction via this method focuses on repositioning the glenoid fossa rather than the humeral head, and less force is required than with many other methods.[23] Its success rate is high, generally greater than 90% in experienced hands.[28,32,33] Some studies report higher success rates in patients who have had repeated dislocations and lower rates in patients with an associated greater tuberosity fracture.[33] The initial maneuver for scapular manipulation is traction on the arm as it is held in 90 degrees of forward flexion. This may be performed with the patient prone and the arm hanging down, as described for the Stimson method, with or without flexion of the elbow to 90 degrees. Alternatively, this traction may be applied by placing an outstretched arm over the seated patient's midclavicular region while pulling the injured extremity with the other arm. Regardless of the means of arm traction, slight external rotation of the humerus may facilitate reduction by releasing the superior glenohumeral ligament and presenting a favorable profile of the humeral head to the glenoid fossa.[34]

The prone patient position is recommended for those not familiar with the technique because it facilitates identification of the scapula for manipulation (medial rotation of the tip). Nonetheless, the technique can be performed with the patient supine given that the patient's shoulder is flexed to 90 degrees and the scapula is exposed during gentle upward traction on the humerus.[35] Although seated scapular manipulation offers the advantage of not requiring the patient to go through the awkward and potentially uncomfortable assumption of the prone position, it is a technically more difficult variation of scapular manipulation, especially if sedation is going to be necessary. When using the prone position, place the injured shoulder over the edge of the bed to allow the arm to hang perpendicular for the application of traction (see Fig. 49-12A).[32]

After the application of traction, manipulate the scapula to complete the reduction. Anderson and associates[32] recommended manipulation of the scapula after the patient's arm is relaxed; however, success is possible with no delay in performing this second step.[22] Manipulate the scapula by stabilizing the superior aspect of the scapula with one hand and pushing the inferior tip of the scapula medially toward the spine. Place the thumb of the hand stabilizing the superior aspect of the scapula along the lateral border of the scapula to assist the pressure applied by the thumb of the other hand. A small degree of dorsal displacement of the scapular tip is recommended as it is being pushed as far as possible in the medial direction.[32]

When the patient is properly positioned with the affected arm hanging perpendicularly, the lateral border of the scapula may be difficult to find in larger patients. This border is generally located quite laterally with the patient in this position, and it must be properly located before any attempt at reduction. The reduction itself is occasionally so subtle that it may be missed by both the patient and operator. A minor shift of the arm may be the only clue that reduction has been successful. Careful palpation of the subclavicular area to locate the position of the humeral head before repositioning the patient may be used to determine the success of the reduction.

BOB Technique (see Fig. 49-12C)
A recently described variation of the seated scapular manipulation technique is the "best of both" (BOB) maneuver.[36] To perform the BOB maneuver, position the patient seated sideways on the stretcher with the unaffected shoulder and hip against the fully elevated head of the stretcher. Stand on the foot end of the gurney at the patient's affected side and use one hand to apply downward force on the proximal end of the patient's bent forearm. Use the other hand to grasp the patient's hand and gently rotate the arm internally or

externally as needed. Once downward force is being applied, ask an assistant to perform the scapular manipulation maneuver described earlier.[36]

External Rotation Method (see Fig. 49-12D)
This method offers the advantage of requiring only one person and no special equipment. The technique needs no strength or endurance on the part of the operator and is well tolerated by patients.[3] The actual pain experienced by patients with this technique has not been quantified, but Plummer and Clinton[3] stated that it can be performed with "little, if any sedation." In this technique, the basic maneuver is slow, gentle external rotation of the fully adducted arm. In 1957, Parvin[37] described a self-reduction external rotation technique in which the patient sits on a swivel-type chair and grasps a fixed post positioned waist high and slowly turns the body to enact external rotation. Parvin[37] reported that the reduction usually takes place at 70 to 110 degrees of external rotation.

Since Parvin's initial study, this method has been described with the patient supine and the affected arm adducted tightly to the side of the patient.[1,38] Flex the elbow to 90 degrees and hold it in the adducted position with the operator's hand closest to the patient. Use the other hand to hold the patient's wrist and guide the arm into slow and gentle external rotation. The procedure may require several minutes because each time that the patient experiences pain, the procedure is halted momentarily. Although the report of Mirick and coworkers[1] mentioned using the forearm as "a lever," a later description clearly recommends allowing the forearm to "fall" under its own weight.[3] No additional force should be applied to the forearm, and no traction is exerted on the arm.

The end point of the reduction may be difficult to identify because reduction is frequently very subtle. It is therefore recommended that external rotation be continued until the forearm is near the coronal plane (lying on the bed, perpendicular to the body), a process that usually takes 5 to 10 minutes.[3] If the patient's dislocation persists after full external rotation, apply steady gentle traction at the elbow. Reduction may occasionally be noted when the arm is rotated back internally.[38] The success rate of this technique in three series performed by emergency clinicians was around 80%.[1,38,39]

Milch Technique (see Fig. 49-12E)
Proponents of this method praise its gentle nature, high success rate, lack of complications, and tolerance by patients.[2,5] It can be described as "reaching up to pull an apple from a tree." The basic steps of this technique are abduction, external rotation, and gentle traction of the affected arm. Finally, if needed, the humeral head can be pushed into the glenoid fossa with the thumb or fingers.

In describing this technique, Milch[40] wrote that the fully abducted arm was in a natural position in which there was little tension on the muscles of the shoulder girdle. He postulated that this was related to our ancestral "arboreal brachiation" (swinging from trees). The primary step in this technique is to abduct the affected arm to an overhead position. Russell and colleagues[34] had their patients raise their arm and put their hand behind their head as a first step. Although this seems odd, patients can usually do this quite readily with little assistance and be quite comfortable in this position. Alternatively, abduct the arm by grasping the patient's arm at the elbow or the wrist. Lacey and Crawford[41] found that the prone position, with the patient's shoulder close to the end of the bed, facilitated this step.

ANTERIOR SHOULDER DISLOCATION REDUCTION

A. Stimson Maneuver

Place the patient prone on the edge of the stretcher. Be careful that a sedated or intoxicated patient does not fall off the table. Belts or sheets can be used to secure the patient to the stretcher, 5-kg weights are attached to the arm, and the patient maintains this position for 20 to 30 minutes, if necessary.

The addition of scapular manipulation and/or gentle external and internal rotation of the shoulder with manual traction may aid in reduction.

B. Scapular Manipulation

Rotate the inferior tip of the scapula medially and dorsally toward the spine with the tips of your thumbs.

The procedure can take place with the patient prone (as in the Stimson technique) or with the patient seated. For the latter, have an assistant apply traction on the arm while applying countertraction on the ipsilateral clavicle.

C. Best-of-Both Technique

Position the patient seated sideways with the unaffected shoulder and hip against the upright head of the stretcher. Apply downward force on the patient's flexed forearm, and gently rotate the arm internally or externally as needed.

Once downward force is applied, instruct an assistant to perform scapular manipulation as described above.

Figure 49-12 Anterior shoulder dislocation reduction methods. *ED*, emergency department.

ANTERIOR SHOULDER DISLOCATION REDUCTION

D. External Rotation

Fully adduct the arm and flex the elbow to 90°. Hold the patient's wrist and guide the arm into slow and gently external rotation. Halt momentarily if the patient experiences pain. Continue the rotation until the forearm is laying on the bed. No traction is applied.

E. Milch Technique

First abduct the arm to an overhead position by grasping the patient's arm at the elbow or wrist. Once fully abducted, apply gentle longitudinal traction with slight external rotation. If reduction does not occur quickly, push the humeral head upward into the glenoid fossa.

F. Traction-Countertraction Method

Wrap one sheet around the affected axilla and the assistant's waist. The assistant leans back to apply countertraction. Wrap another sheet around the patient's flexed arm and your waist. Lean back to apply traction.

Reduction can be facilitated by gently adducting the arm (after traction is applied) while a second assistant provides gentle lateral traction on the humerus.

G. Spaso Technique

With the patient supine, gently lift the arm toward the ceiling while applying gentle vertical traction. Instruct an assistant to apply countertraction. Apply gentle external rotation during the procedure.

H. Eskimo Method

While the patient lies on the unaffected side, lift him a short distance off the ground by grasping the abducted arm of the injured side. This is a field technique and should not be used in the ED.

Figure 49-12, cont'd

Once the arm is fully abducted, apply gentle longitudinal traction with slight external rotation. If reduction does not occur quickly, push the humeral head upward into the glenoid fossa with the thumb or fingers of the other hand. Beattie and associates[2] reported a success rate of 70% with the Milch technique, but others have achieved success rates of 90% or greater.[5,34]

Traction-Countertraction (see Fig. 49-12*F*)

This method is commonly used in the ED, largely because of tradition, clinician comfort, and a high success rate. Clinician familiarity is an advantage of this technique, but it requires more than one operator, some degree of force, and occasionally, endurance. This technique is usually quite uncomfortable for the patient, and premedication is recommended before any attempt.

With the patient supine, wrap a sheet or strap around the upper part of the patient's chest and under the axilla of the affected shoulder. Ask an assistant to hold the sheet, preferably by wrapping it around the assistant's waist to take advantage of body weight rather than arm strength to apply the countertraction. Do not place a foot in the axilla to provide countertraction. Traction may then be applied onto the extended arm by the clinician, but this generally results in operator fatigue, especially if the operator relies on biceps strength to provide continuous traction. Instead, flex the elbow of the affected side to 90 degrees and wrap a sheet or strap around the proximal part of the forearm and then around the operator's back. Elevate the bed to the point at which the sheet can sit at the level of the operator's ischial tuberosities. This allows the operator to comfortably lean back and use body weight to supply the force of traction, thereby eliminating the possibility of operator fatigue. The portion of the sheet that is positioned on the patient's forearm has a tendency to ride up; flexion of the elbow beyond 90 degrees will minimize this problem. Alternatively, the operator merely leans backward with the arms fully extended, again using the continuous weight of the body rather than the strength of the biceps to provide constant traction.

Once traction has been applied, the operator must be patient because the procedure may take a number of minutes to be successful. The premedication is probably inadequate if the patient resists the procedure or is notably uncomfortable during attempts at reduction. Do not hesitate to order supplementary medications. Gentle, limited external rotation is sometimes useful to speed reduction.[10] Applying traction to an arm that is slightly abducted from the patient's body is often successful, but some operators prefer to slowly bring the arm medial to the patient's midline while maintaining traction or to have an assistant apply a gentle lateral force to the midhumerus to direct the humeral head laterally. Successful reduction is usually presaged by slight lengthening of the arm as relaxation occurs, and a noticeable "clunk" may occur at the point of reduction. A brief wave of fasciculations in the deltoid may also be seen at the time of reduction.

Spaso Technique (see Fig. 49-12*G*)

This technique was first reported by Spaso Miljesic as a simple, single-operator technique requiring minimal force.[42] One published series reported an 87.5% success rate in premedicated patients when performed by junior house officers.[43] Place the patient in the supine position and grasp the affected arm around the wrist or distal end of the forearm. Gently lift the affected arm vertically toward the ceiling and apply gentle vertical traction. While maintaining traction continuously, externally rotate the arm. Reduction may be subtle but is generally signaled by hearing or feeling a "clunk." Completion of this technique may require several minutes of gentle traction to allow the muscles of the patient's shoulder to relax.[43]

Other Methods

Poulsen[44] reported a method termed the *Eskimo technique* that may be performed in field settings (see Fig. 49-12*H*). In this technique the patient lies on the unaffected side and is lifted a short distance off the ground by grasping the abducted arm on the injured side. The patient's body weight acts to effect the reduction. Poulsen's success rate was 74% in a series of 23 patients, all of whom were premedicated. However, the author[44] also postulated that this technique could place undue stress on the brachial plexus or axillary vessels. Use of this technique, when other options are available, should probably be reserved until more data are obtained.

Noordeen and coworkers[45] reported a simple method in which the patient sits sideways in a chair with the affected arm draped over the backrest. The operator holds the arm with the wrist supinated, and the patient is instructed to stand up. The success rate was 72% in 32 patients treated in this manner. A variation of the chair technique, which was successful in 97% of 188 anterior shoulder dislocations, involves operator-applied traction on the patient's flexed elbow by means of a cloth loop or stockinette.[46] Standing beside the patient, the operator holds the involved elbow in 90 degrees of flexion while stepping down on the cloth loop. The patient sits in the chair, and an assistant may help support the patient by applying countertraction under the involved arm.

Postreduction Care

After an attempt at reduction, the neurovascular status of the affected extremity should be rechecked and the results documented on the patient's record. Indirect evidence that the reduction has been successful includes an immediate decrease in pain, restoration of the round shoulder contour, and increased passive mobility of the shoulder. No harm is done by putting the joint through a limited range of motion. If the patient can tolerate placement of the palm from the injured arm on the opposite shoulder, it is quite likely that the shoulder reduction was successful (see Fig. 49-13*A*). For patients with possible axillary nerve injury, close to 90% will recover with expectant management. Nevertheless, it is prudent to refer these patients for early orthopedic follow-up.[47]

Postreduction radiographs are often recommended to make a careful search for new fractures. Although most greater tuberosity fractures do not alter patient management, patients with greater tuberosity fractures displaced more than 1 cm after closed reduction almost always have an associated rotator cuff tear[48] and should receive prompt orthopedic consultation because they may require operative repair.

Traditional postreduction treatment focuses on the importance of preventing the shoulder from dislocating again after the patient is discharged. This is best accomplished by immobilizing the joint with a commercially available shoulder immobilizer or a sling and swath to limit external rotation and abduction (see Chapter 50). Orthopedic follow-up is recommended for all anterior shoulder dislocations because the incidence of rotator cuff injury is as high as 38% and it might complicate restoration of normal function.[49] Younger patients are usually immobilized for approximately 3 weeks and can

Figure 49-13 A, If a patient with a shoulder injury can place the palm of the injured arm on top of the contralateral shoulder, it is unlikely that a shoulder dislocation is present. Alternatively, completion of this maneuver after an attempt at reduction provides strong evidence that the reduction was successful, even if the patient is still sedated. **B,** The best way to immobilize any reduced shoulder dislocation is uncertain and unlikely to be of consequence for a few days (see text). A typical shoulder immobilizer or a simple sling is appropriate pending orthopedic referral and follow-up.

be instructed to follow up within 1 or 2 weeks of the event. As a general rule, the older the patient, the shorter the recommended time of immobilization[10] because it is important to maintain mobility in joints of the elderly. Those older than 60 years should have early follow-up (e.g., 5 to 7 days) to allow early mobilization and avoid persistent shoulder joint stiffness or adhesive capsulitis.

Since the early 2000s, the wisdom of immobilization in internal rotation has been questioned. Several studies have shown that placing the arm in internal rotation actually increases labral detachment from the glenoid rim whereas some degree of external rotation maximizes contact between the detached labrum and the glenoid rim.[50-52] In one study, cadavers were used to measure the force of contact between the labrum and the glenoid rim in different arm positions. The authors of this study found that maximum contact force was actually generated in 45 degrees of external rotation whereas no contact force was generated with the arm in internal rotation.[52] One prospective study showed that of 20 patients immobilized in external rotation, none had recurrent dislocation after more than 1 year, whereas of 20 patients immobilized in internal rotation, 6 had recurrent dislocation.[51]

Despite this growing body of evidence, very few scientific data are available to guide the clinician on the most appropriate position for postreduction immobilization of anterior shoulder dislocations. A recent literature review was designed to assess (1) whether traumatic anterior shoulder dislocations should be immobilized, (2) how long they should be immobilized, and (3) whether the position of immobilization affects outcome. Unfortunately, the study was unable to provide any definitive answers.[53] According to the author of this study, "much of this uncertainty is due to the limited size of the evidence base [and] numerous methodologic weaknesses (e.g., small sample sizes, no control groups, and not evaluating findings against statistical tests)."[53] More recent studies and reviews have shown conflicting results on whether immobilization in external rotation is preferable to immobilization in internal rotation.[54-57] As a result, it is not unreasonable to immobilize the extremity in a manner consistent with the recommendations of the orthopedic surgeons at one's institution until further evidence is presented. When in doubt, a simple sling or the traditional shoulder immobilizer will certainly suffice pending 5- to 7-day follow-up (see Fig. 49-13B).

It is appropriate to prescribe oral analgesics (either nonsteroidal antiinflammatory drugs or narcotics) to minimize patient discomfort. Instruct the patient to return if the clinical condition worsens. Periodically, one may encounter a return visit from a successfully treated patient who is in severe pain from hemarthrosis. In a series of patients older than 60 years, Trimmings[58] reported that excellent pain relief was achieved by aspirating the hemarthrosis 24 to 48 hours after shoulder reduction. This can be accomplished by using the technique of arthrocentesis described in Chapter 53. In addition, intraarticular instillation of 10 to 20 mL of 1% lidocaine (or a longer-acting local anesthetic) may be helpful for further pain relief.

Posterior Shoulder Dislocations

Posterior shoulder dislocations account for less than 4% of all shoulder dislocations.[12] Because they are so uncommon, posterior dislocations have the potential to be missed. The emergency clinician must be knowledgeable about these injuries to avoid a misdiagnosis. Delays in diagnosis for weeks to months have been reported with posterior dislocations.[59,60] This may lead to increased rates of dislocation arthropathy and chronic pain.[13] The mechanism of injury is almost always indirect and consists of a combination of internal rotation, adduction, and flexion.[10] Classic precipitating events include seizure, electrical shock, and falls. The patient may also be initially seen at a point long past the original event.[60] In addition, patients with seizures may not experience obvious problems in the immediate postictal period because of their altered mental status.

Clinical Assessment

Though clinically less obvious than anterior dislocations, posterior shoulder dislocations do occur in a typical, recognizable manner. Mistakes may be made if the clinician is overly reliant on AP radiographs, which are potentially misleading[60] and may result in misdiagnosing the injury as a soft tissue contusion or acromioclavicular (AC) strain. The principal sign of a posterior dislocation is an arm that is somewhat fixed in adduction and internal rotation (Fig. 49-14). Abduction and external rotation are limited, and attempts to perform these movements generally elicit pain.[10,12] Inspection and palpation reveal loss of the normal anterior contour of the shoulder, as well as a prominent coracoid and acromion. The shoulder is flattened anteriorly and rounded posteriorly, and the humeral head may be palpable.[10,12]

Comparison with the opposite shoulder should be undertaken with caution because this injury may occasionally occur bilaterally. Perform neurovascular assessment in the standard manner, but such complications are unusual with posterior dislocations.

Radiologic Examination

The key point regarding radiographs for posterior shoulder dislocations is the subtle nature of this dislocation on a single

Figure 49-14 A posterior dislocation may be difficult to appreciate on radiographs. A clue to a posterior shoulder dislocation is the arm locked in adduction and internal rotation and the patient's inability to rotate the shoulder externally with the elbow flexed at 90 degrees.

AP film (Figs. 49-15A and 49-16A) and the diagnostic importance of the scapular Y view (see Fig. 49-15B) or the axillary view (see Fig. 49-16B). Diagnosis of posterior shoulder dislocation is quite easy with the axillary view, whereas the routine AP and lateral views are difficult to interpret in around half the cases.[60] The axillary view is generally available in the radiology department and can be obtained with as little as 20 to 30 degrees of abduction and the plate placed on the shoulder.[60] In addition to easy visualization of the posteriorly situated humeral head, the axillary view often reveals an impression fracture of the humeral head (see Fig. 49-16B). The scapular Y view is produced by superimposing the head of the humerus over the coracoid, acromion, and body of the scapula, which form a Y shape. In the event of a posterior shoulder dislocation, the head of the humerus will lie posterior to the glenoid (away from the chest wall) (see Figs. 49-9B and 49-15B).

Even though axillary and scapular Y views are diagnostic, clues to posterior dislocation do exist on AP films. The internally rotated humeral head appears symmetric on an AP film and is in the shape of a light bulb, as opposed to the normal club-shaped appearance created by the greater tuberosity (Fig. 49-17).[61] With posterior dislocation, the space between the articular surface of the humeral head and the anterior glenoid rim is widened, and there is a decrease in the half-moon–shaped overlap of the head and the fossa.[59,61] There may also be a compression fracture on the medial aspect of the humeral head, as indicated by a dense line. This is known as the trough sign.[61] A fracture of the lesser tuberosity should always prompt a search for the presence of a posterior shoulder dislocation.

Reduction Technique (Fig. 49-18A)

Reduce an acute posterior dislocation by applying traction on the internally rotated and adducted arm combined with anteriorly directed pressure on the posterior aspect of the humeral

Figure 49-15 Posterior shoulder dislocation seen on a scapular Y view (see also Figs. 49-8 and 49-9). **A,** The anteroposterior view does not definitively show the dislocation. Because the dislocation is directly posterior, there is no superior or inferior displacement of the humeral head. On superficial observation, the head of the humerus appears to maintain a normal relationship with the glenoid fossa and the acromion process. However, definite abnormalities exist on this film. The space between the humeral head and the glenoid fossa is abnormal, and because of the extreme internal rotation of the humerus, the head and neck are seen end on and resemble a light bulb. **B,** On the scapular Y view it becomes obvious that the humeral head is posteriorly dislocated. It projects posteriorly under the scapular spine rather than in its normal location, centered over the glenoid fossa. *G,* glenoid fossa; *HH,* humeral head; *Sp,* scapular spine.

head.[10,60] Generous premedication is usually indicated, and countertraction may be applied with a sheet looped in the affected axilla, very much similar to the procedure described for anterior dislocations. Kwon and Zuckerman[10] recommended applying lateral traction on the upper part of the humerus if the humeral head is locked on the posterior glenoid. Hawkins and colleagues[60] suggested that posterior dislocations with an impression defect of the humeral head greater than 20% of the articular surface require open reduction. Posterior dislocations that have been diagnosed late are difficult to reduce in a closed manner, but an attempt with adequate premedication is generally indicated.[60]

Postreduction Care

As with anterior dislocations, neurovascular examination and radiographs should be repeated after attempts at reduction. Successful reduction is suggested by a patient's ability to place the palm of the injured arm on the opposite shoulder. Given the rarity of these injuries, orthopedic consultation is often sought early in the care of these patients. Certainly in

Figure 49-16 Posterior shoulder dislocation, seen on axillary view. **A,** The dislocation is not immediately evident on the anteroposterior view. The humeral head appears as a light bulb, which indicates internal rotation and is a subtle sign that a posterior dislocation might be present (*arrow*). **B,** On the axillary view the humeral head is seen to lie posteriorly and is impacted on the rim of the glenoid (*arrow*). When viewing axillary films, use the coracoid process to orient yourself to anterior and posterior (the coracoid is an anterior structure). *(From Andrews JR, Wilk PE, Reinold MM. The Athlete's Shoulder. 2nd ed. Philadelphia: Churchill Livingstone; 2008.)*

Figure 49-17 Anteroposterior views comparing posterior dislocation and a normal shoulder joint. Posterior shoulder dislocation causes internal rotation of the humeral head, which makes the head appear as a light bulb rather than its normal club-shaped appearance. Also, note that the space between the articular surface of the humeral head and the anterior glenoid rim is widened (*arrows*), and there is a decrease in the overlap between the head and the fossa.

POSTERIOR AND INFERIOR SHOULDER DISLOCATION REDUCTION

A.   Posterior Dislocation

Apply traction, internal rotation, and adduction to the affected arm. Instruct one assistant to apply countertraction (with a sheet wrapped around the waist) and another assistant to apply anteriorly directed pressure on the posterior aspect of the humeral head.

B.   Inferior Dislocation (Luxatio Erecta)

Apply overhead traction with the arm in abduction. With your free hand, exert cephalad pressure over the humeral head. Instruct an assistant to apply countertraction toward the patient's feet with a sheet placed over the injured shoulder.

Figure 49-18 Posterior and inferior shoulder dislocation reduction methods.

Figure 49-19 Luxatio erecta. **A,** This is a rare inferior shoulder dislocation, and patients may hold their arm in marked abduction with the elbow flexed and the forearm resting on their head. **B,** Radiographic appearance of luxatio erecta.

a training environment, involvement of orthopedic residents is of benefit to their education and should be considered early.

Unusual Shoulder Dislocations

Luxatio Erecta

Inferior dislocations of the shoulder, known as *luxatio erecta*, are quite rare but also quite obvious. The patient has the arm locked in marked abduction with the flexed forearm lying on or behind the head[62] (Fig. 49-19). Occasionally, the humerus may have less abduction, thus potentially obscuring the diagnosis.[63] The humeral head can be palpated along the lateral chest wall. With this injury, the inferior capsule is almost always torn. Associated injuries include fractures of the greater tuberosity, acromion, clavicle, coracoid process, and glenoid rim. Neurovascular compression may be present, but this is usually reversed once reduction is accomplished.[10] Long-term

complications include adhesive capsulitis and recurrent dislocations.

Apply overhead traction (generally with the arm in full abduction) in the longitudinal direction of the arm, and exert cephalad pressure over the humeral head much as with the Milch technique (see Fig. 49-18*B*).[10,63] If needed, apply countertraction toward the patient's feet by using a sheet placed over the injured shoulder. After reduction, bring the abducted arm into adduction against the body and supinate the forearm.[64]

Alternatively, use the "two-step" maneuver described by Nho and associates[65] to reduce inferior dislocations. In this technique, convert the luxatio erecta to an anterior dislocation. To perform this maneuver, place one hand on the medial condyle of the elbow and the other hand around the shaft of the humerus. Push anteriorly on the shaft of the humerus while stabilizing the medial condyle of the elbow, and rotate

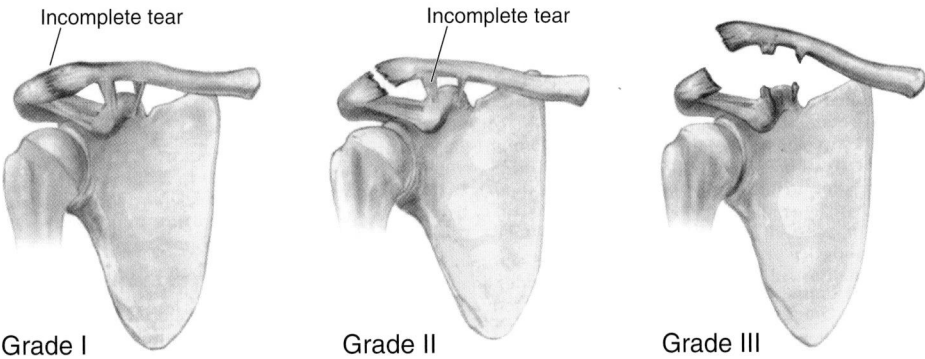

Incomplete tear   Incomplete tear

Grade I   Grade II   Grade III

Figure 49-20 Grade I to III acromioclavicular separation. (See text for description.) *(From Heppenstall RB. Fractures and dislocations of the distal clavicle. Orthop Clin North Am. 1975;6:480.)*

the humeral head from an inferior to an anterior position. The authors then describe using the external rotation method to reduce what is now a typical anterior dislocation.[65]

Scapular dislocation or "locked scapula" is a rare condition characterized by obvious protrusion of the lateral border of the scapula and significant swelling of the medial border because of tearing of the musculature.[66] To reduce the scapula, apply traction on the abducted arm and apply medial pressure on the scapula.[66]

AC JOINT SUBLUXATION AND DISLOCATION

The AC joint is a true diarthrodial joint that consists of a synovial cavity surrounded by a relatively lax capsule and the weak AC ligament. This structure allows the gliding motion necessary for shoulder movement. The major stability of the AC joint comes from two ligaments. The AC ligament is primarily responsible for joint stability in the AP direction. The coracoclavicular ligament, which has posterior (conoid) and anterior (trapezoid) components, anchors the distal end of the clavicle to the coracoid process of the scapula and therefore supports the joint in a superior-inferior direction. In general, AC injuries arise from a direct force such as a fall on the point of the shoulder with the arm adducted.[67] AC joint injuries are categorized according to the Rockwood classification (types I to VI) (Fig. 49-20).

First Degree (Type I)

This injury consists of a minor tear in the AC ligament. The coracoclavicular ligament is intact. The clinical findings are limited to tenderness in the area of the AC joint. Radiographs show little, if any change in position of the clavicle in relation to the acromion.[48] Management of this condition consists of a sling for comfort, ice, and mild analgesics. Generally, the symptoms subside with 7 to 10 days of rest.[10] Orthopedic referral is not usually necessary unless return to normal function is delayed beyond 2 weeks.

Second Degree (Type II)

In addition to a complete tear of the AC ligament, the coracoclavicular ligament is stretched or incompletely torn.[48] The patient generally supports the injured arm and has slight swelling and definite tenderness over the AC joint. Radiographs demonstrate a definite change in the relationship of

Figure 49-21 Third-degree acromioclavicular (AC) separation. In a third-degree AC separation, the clavicle is seen riding high above the acromion. This is due to disruption of both the AC and coracoclavicular ligaments.

the distal end of the clavicle to the acromion. However, in type II injuries the inferior edge of the clavicle should not be separated from the acromion by more than half its diameter,[48] and on radiographic examination the coracoclavicular distance is the same as that on the uninjured side.[10] This injury can be treated in closed fashion with a sling.[10] Orthopedic referral is recommended, and some will use a sling-strap device that elevates the arm and depresses the clavicle for these injuries.[48]

Third Degree (Type III)

In this injury, the distal end of the clavicle is essentially free floating because both the AC and coracoclavicular ligaments are completely disrupted.[48] The arm is supported by an uncomfortable-appearing patient, and the distal end of the clavicle is usually seen to be riding high above the acromion. The diagnosis is generally obvious, and radiographs are used mainly to rule out an associated fracture. Radiographic criteria for this degree of injury include the inferior border of the clavicle raised above the acromion or a discrepancy in the coracoclavicular distance between the normal and affected sides (Fig. 49-21).[10] These injuries require orthopedic referral, and a fair bit of controversy exists regarding their subsequent management.[10,68] Larsen and coworkers[69] conducted a prospective, randomized trial of conservative versus operative management of significant AC separations and concluded that conservative management was generally better, with possible exceptions made for patients with significant cosmetic deformity and for those who frequently keep their arm at 90 degrees of abduction. Even though optimal therapy is still unclear, a logical approach would include ED treatment with a sling and early orthopedic referral.

Fourth, Fifth, and Sixth Degrees (Types IV to VI)

In type IV injury, the distal end of the clavicle is free floating and posteriorly displaced into or through the trapezius muscle. Type V injury is characterized by inferior displacement of the scapula with a marked increase (two to three times normal) in the coracoclavicular interspace.[10] Type IV and V dislocations generally require surgery, and orthopedic referral is necessary. Type VI injury involves dislocation of the distal end of the clavicle inferiorly. Because this is usually the result of major trauma, multiple other fractures are often present and should be pursued.[10]

Radiographic Examination

The diagnosis is usually made clinically by noting pain and local tenderness at the AC joint in the absence of other findings. Radiographs are generally indicated to rule out associated fractures and to aid in assessing the degree of injury. A single radiograph of the injured shoulder often suffices, but some clinicians prefer to obtain comparison views of the opposite shoulder. Although their efficacy has never been proved, it has traditionally been recommended that "weighted" films be obtained for suspected type I or II injuries. Weighted films are generally performed after routine "unweighted" radiographs and are obtained by strapping about 4.5 to 7.0 kg (10 to 15 lb) of weight to the patient's wrists and repeating the radiographs. Weighted films are of questionable value in mild injuries and superfluous in obvious type III to VI injuries. Their use has essentially been abandoned in emergency medicine practice.[70] In a prospective study of 70 type I or II

injuries, the use of weights was associated with less evident separation in 7 cases, essentially producing a false-negative study in comparison to plain unweighted films. Only three injuries were recategorized as type III after the performance of weighted films.[70]

STERNOCLAVICULAR DISLOCATIONS

Despite the fact that the sternoclavicular joint is the least stable joint in the body, sternoclavicular dislocations are rare.[71] The primary supports of this joint are the sternoclavicular and costoclavicular ligaments. Anterior dislocations are much more common and usually the result of an indirect mechanism involving a blow thrusting the shoulder forward,[48] or they may be atraumatic and be caused by ligamentous laxity in teens and young adults.[71] Posterior dislocations also usually result from a blow to the shoulder but can be the result of a direct superior sternal or medial clavicular blow.[71] Indeed, athletic injuries and those resulting from motor vehicle accidents account for the vast majority of sternoclavicular dislocations.[47,72] Posterior sternoclavicular dislocation (also known as retrosternal dislocation because the medial end of the clavicle dislocates both posteriorly and medially) is potentially life-threatening because injury to the great vessels or compression of the airway might occur.[71] Patients may complain of dyspnea, choking, or hoarseness with tracheal compression; dysphagia with esophageal compression; ipsilateral upper extremity pain and swelling with subclavian vessel occlusion; or paresthesias if the brachial plexus is compromised.[72] Any suggestion of these complications should prompt immediate surgical consultation.

The clinical manifestation of these injuries is usually straightforward and consists of pain, swelling, tenderness, and deformity of the joint. Patients may complain of pain that is worse with arm movement and when they are supine. Plain radiographs of this joint are difficult to interpret and generally include an apical lordotic-type view with the radiographic tube angled 45 degrees cephalad. Confirmation of the diagnosis is best made with a thoracic computed tomography (CT) scan, which may also identify high rib fractures, pulmonary contusion, or pneumothorax (Fig. 49-22).[71,73] CT angiography will

Figure 49-22 Sternoclavicular joint: posterior dislocation. **A,** Frontal chest radiograph showing asymmetry in the position of the medial margins of the clavicle, with the right clavicle (on the injured side) being located inferior to the left clavicle. **B,** An axial computed tomography scan confirms posterior dislocation of the right sternoclavicular joint. *(From Resnick D Kransdorf MJ, eds.* Bone and Joint Imaging. *3rd ed. Philadelphia: Saunders; 2005.)*

also show vascular injury associated with posterior dislocations. Children may have epiphyseal disruption with retrosternal displacement of the medial aspect of the clavicle.[74]

To reduce both types of sternoclavicular dislocation, place a rolled blanket or a sandbag between the scapula and spine in to separate the medial aspect of the clavicle from the manubrium. Apply traction on the 90-degree abducted, 10-degree extended arm in line with the clavicle and then push (anterior dislocation) or lift (posterior dislocation) the clavicle back into position.[71] Posterior dislocations may be difficult to reduce and to maintain via closed reduction. Therefore, some authors recommend reduction in an operating suite unless complications necessitate immediate reduction.[71] Given the rarity of this injury and the potential for major underlying complications, early consultation is recommended for suspected posterior sternoclavicular dislocations. Once reduced, a clavicle strap may be used to immobilize both anterior and posterior dislocations for up to 6 weeks.[72]

ELBOW DISLOCATIONS

The elbow is second only to the shoulder as a site of major joint dislocations in adults; it is the most commonly dislocated joint in children. Anatomically, the principal articulation of the humerus and ulna is a stable hinge joint with the intercondylar groove of the distal end of the humerus nestled in the olecranon fossa. Because of the stability of the elbow, any dislocation is expected to be accompanied by considerable soft tissue damage, and associated fractures of the radial head and coronoid process of the ulna are common. Elbow dislocations are often simply divided into posterior and anterior dislocations (Fig. 49-23). However, there are actually several different types of elbow dislocations in addition to posterior and anterior, including lateral, divergent, and isolated dislocations of the radius.[75] In the rare divergent dislocations, the radius and ulna are dislocated in opposite directions, either anterior and posterior or medial and lateral.[75]

Recent studies have shown that many patients report long-term problems with residual pain and joint stiffness after elbow dislocation.[76,77] However, the most serious complication of elbow dislocation is injury to the brachial artery. This injury is possible with any type of elbow dislocation and is a frequent occurrence with open dislocations.[75] Vascular compromise can be delayed in onset and result from either unsuspected arterial injury or progressive soft tissue swelling. The circulatory status of the arm must be carefully monitored even after successful reduction.[75] Though not absolute, patients with these injuries who have significant or immediate soft tissue swelling or hematoma formation or those who have questionable vascular integrity or neurologic findings are often admitted to the hospital or ED observation unit. In most cases, orthopedic consultation should be sought before disposition.

Injury to the median and ulnar nerves may be the result of stretch, severance, or entrapment. It is difficult to clinically distinguish these causes; therefore, management of nerve injuries is frequently expectant.[75] It is imperative to conduct a careful neurologic examination before and after reduction because any increase in findings may indicate entrapment and the need for surgical intervention.[75] Myositis ossificans is also a potential complication of elbow dislocations secondary to hemarthrosis, which underscores the advisability of orthopedic consultation early in the course of care.

Posterior Dislocations

Posterior dislocations make up the vast majority of elbow dislocations.[48] The usual mechanism is a fall on an outstretched hand with the elbow in extension. Findings on clinical examination are usually diagnostic unless severe soft tissue swelling is present. The patient has a shortened forearm that is held in flexion, and the olecranon is prominent posteriorly. The normally tight triangular relationship of the olecranon and the epicondyles of the distal end of the humerus is disturbed in a posterior dislocation. A defect may also be palpated above the prominence of the olecranon.

Radiologic Examination
Two radiographic views, an AP and a true lateral, should be obtained (Fig. 49-24). The diagnosis is obvious with proper

Figure 49-23 Classification of elbow dislocations.

Posterior dislocation   Anterior dislocation

Figure 49-24 Posterior elbow dislocation. *Top row,* prereduction films; *bottom row,* postreduction films.

POSTERIOR ELBOW DISLOCATION REDUCTION

A. Initial Recommended Approach

1, Position the patient prone and hang the flexed elbow over the bed. Instruct an assistant to grasp the humerus with both hands and apply pressure on the olecranon with the thumbs (*black arrow*). Apply longitudinal traction on the humerus (*white arrow*).

2, If reduction is not accomplished, try to further flex the elbow while applying traction (*white arrows*), or instruct the assistant to lift the humerus while pushing down on the olecranon (*black arrows*). Reduction is generally noted by a definitive "clunk."

B. Traction-Countertraction

C. Chair/Back of Bed Method

With the patient supine, instruct an assistant to stabilize the humerus. Grasp the wrist and apply in-line traction. Slightly flex the elbow, and hold the wrist supinated as traction is applied.

Hang the patient's arm over the padded back of a chair or over the edge of the bed. Apply pressure to the posterior aspect of the olecranon to achieve reduction. Traction may be applied to the forearm.

Figure 49-25 Posterior elbow dislocation reduction methods.

radiographs. A careful search for fractures of the distal end of the humerus, radial head, and coronoid process must be undertaken since they commonly occur in this injury.[75] In children younger than 14 years, the fracture is usually a medial epicondyle separation because the epiphyseal plate gives way before the medial collateral ligament of the elbow. Postreduction radiographs are also necessary to confirm reduction and disclose any associated fractures.[78]

Reduction Techniques and Postreduction Care

As with shoulder reductions, some authors claim that their method of elbow reduction is virtually painless,[37,79] but this has not been objectively documented. In general, patients with posterior elbow dislocations are quite uncomfortable, and it is beneficial to administer IV analgesics early in the course of care, preferably before positioning for radiographs. In addition to or in lieu of parenteral sedation and analgesia, some clinicians inject the elbow joint with a local anesthetic

(e.g., 3 to 5 mL of 2% plain lidocaine) before attempting reduction. Before injection, the joint should be aspirated to remove blood.

Traditional Traction Method

Place the patient in the supine position and have an assistant stabilize the humerus with both hands[80] (Fig. 49-25B). Grasp the wrist and apply slow and steady in-line traction. Slightly flex the elbow to keep the triceps mechanism loose, and hold the wrist supinated while applying traction. Reduction is usually signified by a "clunk" that is heard or felt. If this method is not successful after a reasonable period of traction (10 minutes), gently flex the forearm to effect reduction. Alternatively, apply downward pressure on the proximal volar surface of the forearm to free up the coronoid process.

Alternatives

Several authors have described variations of a prone method of reduction that are reportedly well tolerated by patients.[37,79,80]

ANTERIOR ELBOW DISLOCATION REDUCTION

Apply in-line traction and backward pressure on the proximal end of the forearm while an assistant provides countertraction on the humerus. A clunk usually indicates that reduction is achieved.

Flex the arm beyond 90° to ensure that the joint has been reduced. Splint the elbow in at least 90° of flexion with a posterior long-arm splint.

Figure 49-26 Anterior elbow dislocation reduction method.

In the method described by Minford and Beattie,[79] position the patient with the arm hanging over the padded back of a chair or over the edge of the bed (see Fig. 49-25C). Apply pressure to the prominent posterior aspect of the olecranon to achieve reduction. Alternatively, apply traction with the elbow flexed over the edge of a chair. Pull down on the hand while using the thumb to guide the olecranon into place.[80] Parvin[37] positioned the patient as for the Stimson method of shoulder relocation, prone on a stretcher with the arm hanging down, and applied gentle downward traction on the wrist.

Recommended Initial Approach

A prone technique is advantageous because patients tolerate this position quite well. Hang the flexed elbow over the edge of the bed and position an assistant with his or her back toward the patient such that the patient's humerus can be encircled with both hands and pressure applied with the thumbs on the posterior aspect of the olecranon (see Fig. 49-25A). This pressure on the olecranon is intended to lift it up and away from the humerus. Apply longitudinal traction on the arm with the elbow in slight flexion. If reduction is not accomplished, an attempt may be made to further flex the elbow, or the assistant can be instructed to lift the humerus. Reduction is generally noted by a definite "clunk."

Postreduction Care

Once reduction is achieved, put the elbow through a gentle range of motion to ensure that the reduction is stable and there is no mechanical block to movement.[75] An inability to move the elbow through a smooth range of motion after reduction is often caused by an entrapped medial epicondyle fracture fragment, which requires operative intervention.[75] Immobilize the elbow in at least 90 degrees of flexion with the forearm in slight pronation by using a long arm posterior splint (see Chapter 50). A randomized trial is currently under way to assess the long-term outcome of immobilization versus early range of motion.[81] After immobilizing the joint, recheck the neurovascular status of the extremity and obtain postreduction radiographs.

After reduction, *any signs of delayed vascular compromise are first addressed by loosening the splint and decreasing the degree of flexion.* This may restore adequate blood flow.[75] If not, immediate surgical consultation is necessary for emergency arteriography, exploration of the brachial artery, or both.[78] Delayed brachial arterial injury may not be immediately apparent because of the presence of collateral circulation. The risk for vascular compromise is a reason to consider in-hospital observation. Alternatively, observe the patient in the ED or ED observation unit for 2 to 3 hours after reduction to evaluate for delayed neurovascular compromise before discharge.

Anterior Dislocations

Anterior dislocations of the elbow are quite rare; they usually result from a direct posterior blow onto the olecranon with the elbow flexed.[75] On physical examination, the arm is elongated and extended with anterior tenting of the proximal end of the forearm and prominence of the distal end of the humerus posteriorly.[75] These injuries are the result of a great deal of force; they are frequently open and accompanied by significant neurovascular injury. An avulsion of the triceps mechanism may also occur.[75]

To reduce anterior dislocations of the elbow, apply in-line traction and backward pressure on the proximal end of the forearm (Fig. 49-26). An assistant provides countertraction by grasping the humerus with both hands. Given the infrequent nature of anterior dislocations and the high probability of a severe associated injury, the emergency clinician should consider early orthopedic consultation for such dislocations.

RADIAL HEAD SUBLUXATION (NURSEMAID'S ELBOW)

Radial head subluxation is a common pediatric orthopedic issue that generally occurs between the ages of 1 and 3 years. The mean age is just older than 2 years, but this entity has

Figure 49-27 Radial head subluxation (nursemaid's elbow). **A,** The classic mechanism for this injury is longitudinal traction on the arm with the wrist in pronation. **B,** The pathologic lesion is usually a torn piece of the annular ligament becoming trapped between the radial head and the capitellum of the humerus. (*From Fleisher GR, Ludwig S, eds.* Textbook of Pediatric Emergency Medicine. *Baltimore: Williams & Wilkins; 1988:1322. Reproduced by permission.*)

Figure 49-28 Typical findings in a child with subluxation of the right radial head (nursemaid's elbow). It may be difficult to determine exactly where the pathology exists, and the wrist is often thought to be the area of injury. This child will not use the injured right arm but has minimal discomfort as long as the elbow is not manipulated. **A,** The affected arm hangs down at the side, slightly flexed and pronated. **B,** Once the subluxation is reduced, full activity is generally regained in a matter of minutes.

been reported in infants younger than 6 months[82,83] and in older children up to the preteen years.[84] There is a slight predilection for this injury to occur in girls and in the left arm.[83,85] The classic mechanism of injury is longitudinal traction on the arm with the wrist in pronation, as occurs when the child is lifted up by the wrist (Fig. 49-27A).[83] There is no support for the common assumption that the relatively small head of the radius in relation to the neck of the radius predisposes the young to this injury.[86] The pathologic lesion is generally a tear in the attachment of the annular ligament to the periosteum of the radial neck, with the detached portion becoming trapped between the head of the radius and the capitellum (see Fig. 49-27B).[86]

Clinical Assessment

The history offered by the caretaker may not be that of the classic pulling-type mechanism. Schunk,[83] in a series of 83 patients, reported that only 51% described such a mechanism whereas 22% reported a fall. In patients younger than 6 months, the mechanism in the majority is simply rolling over in bed.[82] Therefore, isolated radial head subluxation in children younger than 6 months does not automatically necessitate a child abuse investigation. The typical patient with a nursemaid's elbow is in no distress and the arm is held slightly flexed and pronated at the side (Fig. 49-28). This has been termed the *nursemaid's position*.[87] The exact area of pain is often difficult to locate. The child will refuse to use the arm, and this may be the chief complaint.[84] An older child will usually point to the dorsal aspect of the distal end of the forearm when asked where it hurts, which may mislead the clinician to suspect a distal radial buckle fracture.

Although tenderness about the elbow has been reported occasionally, there is often little tenderness or swelling in the elbow region.[83,84] In a cooperative child, the arm and shoulder are carefully palpated to discern any tenderness. Areas of focus on palpation should include the clavicle and distal end of the radius because these are common sites for pediatric fractures. When patient anxiety interferes with reliable assessment of tenderness in a child whose arm is in the classic nursemaid's position, the examiner can stand at a distance and have the parent or caretaker palpate the extremity to ascertain tenderness. This may also be done with a cooperative patient to reassure a doubtful parent regarding the absence of a fracture. If no tenderness is noted on palpation, it is appropriate to attempt reduction without prior radiographs.[88]

Although resistance to or pain with supination is a frequent finding in patients with radial head subluxation,[83] one need not test for this finding until the time of reduction.

Radiographic Examination

Radiographs are not generally needed with the classic finding: a child with an arm in the nursemaid's position that is not tender (or minimally tender in the radial head area) on palpation and an appropriate history.[88] In these cases, findings on radiographs are generally normal, and if obtained, the positioning of the child's arm by the x-ray technician often effects reduction.[83] However, Frumkin[86] described three cases of nursemaid's elbow in which a line drawn through the longitudinal axis of the radius did not normally bisect the capitellum on prereduction radiographs but did so after reduction. Radiographs are sometimes recommended if the child is not moving the arm normally 15 minutes after reduction.[87] However, this time frame may be too short because reuse can be delayed for more than 30 minutes, particularly in children initially seen some time after the injury. Quan and Marcuse[84] recommended an approach in which no radiographs are obtained on the first visit, including in children released from the ED before regaining full use of the arm. At the time of a 24-hour follow-up visit, radiographs are obtained only if repeat attempts at manipulation are not successful.

Even though this condition does not generally require radiographs, they can be valuable if external signs of trauma are present (e.g., swelling, abrasions, ecchymoses) or if the child does not use the arm normally within 24 hours after the subluxation is thought to be reduced. Other less common

NURSEMAID'S ELBOW REDUCTION

1

Grasp the elbow with one hand and place your thumb over the region of the radial head.

2

Grasp the wrist with your other hand and supinate the extended forearm in a steady and deliberate manner. Apply slight traction to the arm.

3

Once supinated, flex the arm. An audible or palpable click signifies successful reduction but is not always noted.

Figure 49-29 Nursemaid's elbow (radial head subluxation) reduction. *(From Fleisher GR, Ludwig S, eds.* Textbook of Pediatric Emergency Medicine. *Baltimore: Williams & Wilkins; 1988:1322. Reproduced by permission.)*

conditions that can have similar findings are fractures, joint infections, tumors, and osteomyelitis.

Reduction Techniques

Supination Method

Reduction of nursemaid's elbow (Fig. 49-29) is generally performed without premedication. If the subluxation has been present for hours, oral or nasal midazolam can be a useful adjunct to overcome the child's anxiety related to manipulation. It is important to explain to the caretaker that the reduction will probably cause the child discomfort but that this is transient and a clue to the diagnosis. Position the child seated on the lap of an assistant (often a parent) who stabilizes the arm by holding the humerus adducted to the side. Grasp the elbow with one hand and place the thumb over the region of the radial head. Although it has been stated that the thumb can apply pressure on the radial head, this positioning is mainly useful for palpation of the reduction "click." Grasp the child's wrist with the other hand and supinate the extended forearm in a steady, deliberate manner. Slight traction before supination is generally recommended, but it is unclear whether this increases the likelihood of successful reduction. Once supinated, flex or extend the arm; however, flexion is the most common maneuver and may actually be somewhat more successful than extension.[83] An audible or palpable click signifies successful reduction but is not always noted. Once the reduction has been performed, the child usually cries for a few minutes. Generally, the operator should leave the room and then return in 10 to 15 minutes to repeat the examination. Full use of the arm should be evident (see Fig. 49-28*B*).

Pronation Method

This technique is performed with the child positioned as for the supination method. However, the forearm is not supinated. Instead, the forearm is rapidly hyperpronated and flexed. A recent study by McDonald and colleagues[85] reported equal success rates with this technique and the supination technique.

After Attempted Reduction

If a click is detected, the child will generally regain use of the affected arm quickly (almost always by 30 minutes).[84] Therefore, if a definite click is detected, it is reasonable to observe the child for up to 30 minutes before further intervention. If there is still no use at 30 minutes, the operator may try to determine whether supination is still painful, which would suggest the need to repeat the attempt. In children in whom a click is not detected, the majority will not use the arm by 30 minutes.[84] Therefore, a repeated attempt at reduction is recommended after 10 to 15 minutes of nonuse in children who do not initially have an initial click during the primary reduction. In these children, two or more attempts are required to produce the click in up to 30% of patients.[84]

If the child has not regained use of the arm after a few attempts and a reasonable period of time, some authors recommend that radiographs be obtained.[87] X-ray films may also help relieve parental anxiety. Alternatively, instructions may be given for 24-hour follow-up if normal function is not restored, with consideration of radiographs at the time of follow-up.[84] In two series of patients with nursemaid's elbow, 6 of 10 patients released without normal arm use had spontaneous restoration of function, whereas the other 4 required remanipulation (which successfully restored function).[83,84] Delayed use of radiographs may decrease overall radiation exposure in a child with a radial head subluxation.

The use of a posterior splint to protect the elbow of a child who refuses to use the affected arm after a presumed reduction is of uncertain value. However, some form of immobilization (e.g., splint, sling, or both) may be valuable in a child with significant residual discomfort after a prolonged period

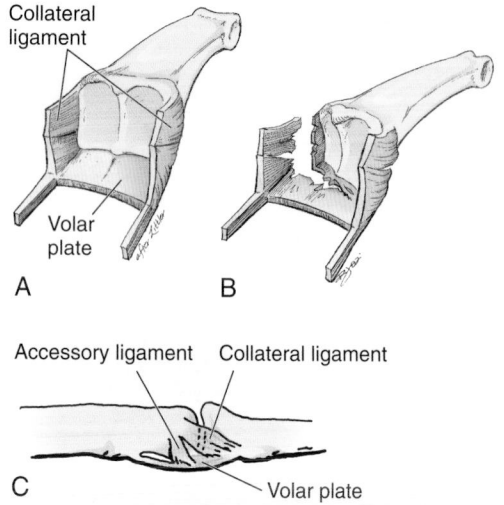

Figure 49-30 A and **B,** The collateral ligament–volar plate relationship. The metacarpophalangeal and interphalangeal joints derive their strength from a combination of the two collateral ligaments and the volar plate. Dislocations of these joints require tearing of at least two parts of this three-part structure. **C,** Lateral view demonstrating the collateral ligament–volar plate relationship. (*A and B, From Carter P, ed.* Common Hand Injuries and Infections. *Philadelphia: Saunders; 1983:114. Reproduced by permission; C, redrawn from Eaton RG.* Joint Injuries of the Hand. *Springfield, IL: Charles C Thomas; 1972.*)

Figure 49-31 Phalangeal dislocations. **A,** Dorsal dislocation of the metacarpophalangeal (MCP) joint of the thumb. **B,** Dorsal dislocation of the proximal interphalangeal (PIP) joint of the middle finger. Note the presence of a small volar plate fracture (*arrow*). **C,** Dorsal dislocation of the distal interphalangeal (DIP) joint of the little finger. Dorsal dislocations are much more common than volar ones.

of subluxation or in whom recurrent subluxations have taken place.

On occasion, a successful reduction painfully resubluxates with movement; in this case, immobilization and referral may be necessary.[86] If reduction has been achieved clinically and maintained in the ED, analgesics or a follow-up visit is unnecessary. Because other pathology can rarely mimic this condition (e.g., occult fracture, osteomyelitis, joint infection, tumor), full, unrestricted, and painless use of the arm must be evident by 24 hours. If not, further workup is warranted.

The emergency clinician should consider parental education regarding prevention of radial head subluxation. Parents or caregivers should be instructed to lift toddlers who are at an age most at risk for these injuries from beneath their axilla, as opposed to forcibly lifting or pulling them by the wrist or hand.

HAND INJURIES

The hand is extremely susceptible to dislocation injuries because of its frequent use and exposed nature. Proper motion and function of the hand are intimately related to normal anatomic alignment.[89] The emergency clinician must therefore be skilled in the diagnosis and management of dislocations about the hand. An improperly managed hand injury can result in significant disability in the patient.

Anatomically, the joints of the digits are quite similar and consist of a hinged joint with a tongue-in-groove–type arrangement.[89] The soft tissue support includes two collateral ligaments attached to a volar plate (Fig. 49-30). The volar plate is composed of dense fibrous connective tissue that is thickened at its distal attachment and thinner at its proximal attachment to allow folding with joint flexion.[89,90] Dorsal

dislocation of a digit requires failure of the volar plate, whereas lateral dislocation disrupts a collateral ligament and induces at least a partial tear in the volar plate.

Radiographic examination of all hand injuries is relatively straightforward and includes at least two views (AP and lateral) of the injured area (Fig. 49-31). The most important radiographic error in evaluating joint injuries in the hand is failing to get a true lateral view of the injured joint.[90] This may lead to missing a fracture or a loose body in the joint.

Anesthesia is generally required for proper management of dislocations about the hand. It is most often accomplished with a finger or wrist block (see Chapter 31), although a more proximal regional or Bier block may be used on occasion (see Chapter 32). Getting a secure grip on the digits may be difficult and could complicate the reduction. Wearing rubber gloves or wrapping gauze around the fingers may be useful.

PHALANGEAL JOINT DISLOCATION REDUCTION

A. Traction Method

Dorsal PIP dislocation

Apply axial traction to the finger, and then push anteriorly on the base of the dislocated phalynx.

Flex the finger while continuing to apply traction and anterior pressure.

After reduction, test for range of motion and stability. Obtain a postreduction x-ray and apply a splint.

B. Exaggeration Method

Dorsal PIP dislocation

Exaggerate the dislocation to distract the phalanges, and then apply pressure to the base of the dislocated phalynx.

Flex the finger while continuing to apply traction and anterior pressure.

After reduction, test for range of motion and stability. Obtain a postreduction x-ray and apply a splint.

C. Thumb MCP Dislocation

If a simple thumb MCP dislocation is treated with traction alone, the forces will often interpose the volar plate and result in an irreducible complex dislocation. To reduce the joint properly, (*1*) firmly grasp the thumb, (*2*) exaggerate the dislocation by hyperextending the thumb, and (*3*) apply pressure to the base of the dislocated phalynx.

To complete the reduction, flex the thumb forward. Postreduction, check the stability of the joint by putting it through the full range of motion, and assess the integrity of the collateral ligaments (see text). Apply a thumb spica splint with the thumb held in flexion.

Figure 49-32 Phalangeal dislocation reduction.

Thumb Dislocations

The opposable thumb is an essential structure for countless activities. Despite its strong ligamentous and capsular support, the exposed positioning of the thumb makes it a frequent site of dislocations and subluxations. The metacarpophalangeal (MCP) joint in the thumb is similar to the MCP joints in the fingers but has a stronger volar plate and collateral ligaments.[90]

IP Joint Dislocation of the Thumb
The single interphalangeal (IP) joint of the thumb has strong cutaneous-periosteal attachments, and dislocations of this type are therefore frequently open.[90] The dislocations are generally dorsal and can be reduced in a manner similar to that for IP dislocations of the finger (Fig. 49-32*A* and *B*). The mechanism of injury is recreated by longitudinal traction and hyperextension to distract the phalanges. Reduction is accomplished by flexing the IP joint with continued traction and by applying direct pressure on the base of the distal phalanx.[90]

After reduction, range of motion is tested and the stability of the reduction is ascertained. An adequate reduction documented on postreduction films is then splinted in slight flexion for 3 weeks.[90] Orthopedic or hand specialist referral is advisable.

MCP Joint Injury of the Thumb
Dorsal Dislocation
The MCP joint of the thumb can be dislocated dorsally by a hyperextension injury. The proximal phalanx will come to rest in a position dorsal to the first metacarpal (Fig. 49-33; also see Fig. 49-31*A*). There are two basic types of MCP dislocation (this applies to the fingers also): simple and complex. In a complex MCP dislocation, the volar plate becomes entrapped

Figure 49-33 Dorsal dislocation of the metacarpophalangeal joint of the thumb.

Figure 49-35 Irreducible metacarpophalangeal joint dislocation of the thumb. Note the sesamoid bone (*arrow*), which indicates interposition of the volar plate between the two ends of the bone and may prevent closed reduction. (*From Carter P, ed.* Common Hand Injuries and Infections. *Philadelphia: Saunders; 1983:115. Reproduced by permission.*)

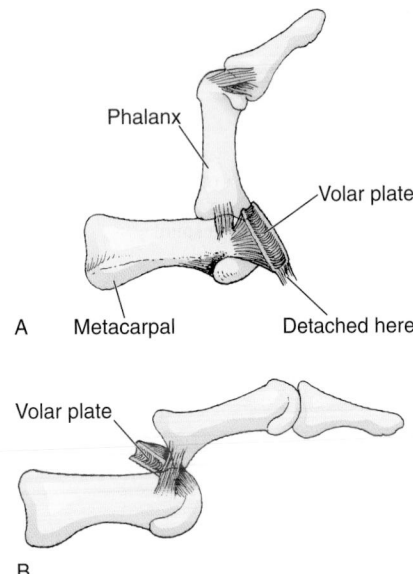

Figure 49-34 A, In a simple dorsal metacarpophalangeal joint dislocation (note the right angle between the phalanx and the metacarpal), the volar plate remains in front of the metacarpal head, although it is detached from its weaker metacarpal insertion. **B,** In a complex dislocation (note the more parallel alignment between the phalanx and the metacarpal), the volar plate becomes entrapped in the joint, and this makes reduction by closed methods impossible. (*A and B, From DePalma AF.* Management of Fractures and Dislocations: An Atlas. *Philadelphia: Saunders; 1970:1177. Reproduced by permission.*)

dorsal to the metacarpal head (Fig. 49-34), with the flexor tendons and lumbricals acting to completely entrap the metacarpal head.[90] The simple type is amenable to closed reduction, whereas the complex type requires operative reduction because of interposed soft tissue.[89,90] It is important to note that a simple MCP dislocation can be converted into a complex one during reduction.[89]

Clinical features that suggest a complex MCP dislocation include a proximal phalanx that is less acutely angulated than with a simple dislocation (i.e., <60 degrees).[90] Dimpling may also be noted over the thenar eminence as a result of pressure from the entrapped metacarpal head.[89] On radiographic studies of simple dislocations, the joint surfaces are in close contact, whereas they are separated in complex dislocations.

The presence of a sesamoid bone in the joint space is diagnostic of a complex MCP dislocation (Fig. 49-35).[89]

To reduce a simple MCP dislocation, hyperextend the joint as far as possible with the wrist in flexion to relax the tendons (see Fig. 49-32C). Once maximal hyperextension is achieved, push the base of the proximal phalanx distally while bringing the joint back into flexion.[89] Applying simple traction alone as an initial maneuver risks trapping the volar plate and creating a complex dislocation.[89] After reduction, test the stability of the joint by putting it through a full range of motion. Assess the integrity of the collateral ligaments with the MCP joint in flexion (see later). Simple MCP dislocation injuries generally require casting for 3 weeks with the joints in moderate flexion.[90]

Volar Dislocation

Volar dislocations are rare and generally associated with collateral ligament ruptures. They are commonly irreducible because of interposition of one or both extensor tendons and the dorsal capsule.[89] Orthopedic consultation is required.

Ulnar Collateral Ligament Rupture

Also known as *gamekeeper's* or *skier's thumb*, this injury results from a laterally directed force at the thumb MCP joint causing rupture of the ulnar collateral ligament (Fig. 49-36). The usual mechanisms include falling with a ski pole in the hand or having the thumb alone draped over the steering wheel in an auto crash. These injuries are most often initially seen in the reduced state with just a complaint of pain in the area. Early recognition of this injury is essential to prevent further disability because this ligament is important for the grasping function of the thumb. A strain or partial tear probably cannot be diagnosed in the ED. It is therefore prudent to immobilize all significantly "sprained thumbs" in a thumb spica splint for a few days and reexamine those with significant injuries. A complete or severe ligamentous tear is generally diagnosed by stress testing of the MCP joint (Fig. 49-37). Radiographs occasionally demonstrate an avulsion-type fracture. The exact positioning of the thumb for stress testing is debatable, but the metacarpal should be stabilized with the thumb and index finger of one hand while applying stress with the other hand. Louis and associates[91] recommended stressing the joint in full

Figure 49-36 Rupture of the ulnar collateral ligament (gamekeeper's thumb). *1,* This injury is caused by forcible abduction. If unrecognized and untreated, progressive metacarpophalangeal (MCP) subluxation may occur (*2*), which interferes with grasping and causes significant permanent disability. Suspect this injury when there is a complaint of pain in this region. Look for tenderness on the medial side of the MCP joint. (*Modified from McRae R.* Practical Fracture Treatment. *Edinburgh: Churchill Livingstone; 1981:162. Reproduced by permission.*)

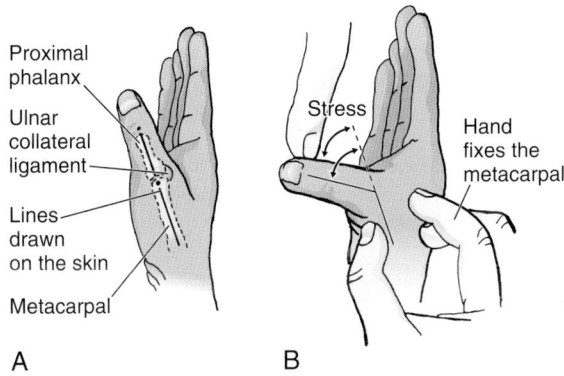

Figure 49-37 Stress testing of the ulnar collateral ligament of the thumb. This is done both clinically and with an anteroposterior radiograph. **A,** A line is drawn on the skin with a pen. The line is along the long axis of the metacarpal and the proximal phalanx. **B,** Deviation of the straight line during stress indicates instability. The metacarpal is fixed with the operator's other hand. *Note:* With acute injuries of the thumb, a simple sprain may be diagnosed when an ulnar collateral ligament injury is partial or severe and stress tests are negative because of swelling and spasm. Therefore, it is prudent to splint all significantly sprained thumbs and reexamine them in a few days if the symptoms persist.

flexion because virtually no lateral movement of the MCP joint should be noted in this position. Instability in full flexion of greater than 35 degrees is indicative of a complete rupture. Hossfeld and Uehara[90] suggested testing the MCP joint in 20 to 30 degrees of flexion to lessen the stabilizing effects of the volar plate; the results should be compared with stability on the other side.

Figure 49-38 Carpometacarpal (CMC) dislocation of the thumb (*arrows* in **A** and **B**). **A,** Anteroposterior (AP) and lateral (LAT) radiographs of a CMC dislocation of the thumb, which is an uncommon injury. The patient sustained this injury when an air bag deployed during a motor vehicle collision. These dislocations are not generally amenable to closed reduction and usually require Kirschner wires. **B,** Prereduction and postreduction films of a CMC dislocation.

Cast partial injuries to the ulnar collateral ligament for 3 weeks; complete rupture usually requires operative repair.[91] An associated nondisplaced fracture may be treated in closed fashion, whereas a displaced fracture is an indication for operative repair.[91]

CMC Dislocations of the Thumb
Carpometacarpal (CMC) dislocations of the thumb are uncommon (Fig. 49-38); when present, they often occur with an associated fracture. Because closed reduction is generally unstable, operative stabilization by percutaneous placement of Kirschner wires (K-wires) is usually required.[90]

Finger Dislocations
The basic anatomic structure of the fingers is similar to that of the thumb with the exception that the fingers have more lateral support from the MCP joints, which makes collateral ligament injury here much less common than in the thumb. The treatment principles are also similar. It is advisable to order radiographs for a specific finger (not just "hand" films). Complete views of the finger will include an AP view, a true lateral view, and an oblique view. A true lateral view is

Figure 49-39 Fracture-dislocations of the proximal (PIP) and distal interphalangeal (DIP) joints. True lateral radiographs are required to maximize sensitivity for small avulsion fractures. **A,** A volar avulsion fracture (*arrow*) is readily seen on this dorsal DIP dislocation. **B,** The fractures are more difficult to appreciate on this unfortunate patient who sustained dislocations of both the DIP and PIP joints in a fall (*arrows*).

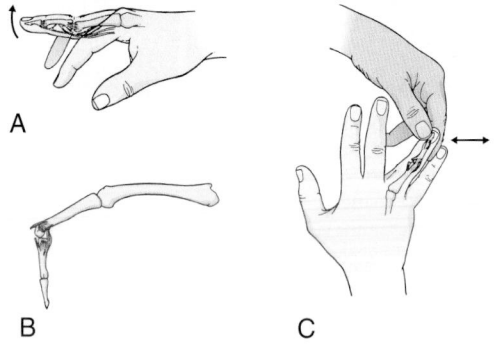

Figure 49-40 Postreduction stress applied to a dislocated proximal interphalangeal (PIP) joint. **A,** If the volar plate has been completely disrupted, the PIP joint will hyperextend with both passive and active motion. **B,** Inability to actively extend the PIP joint indicates rupture of the central slip of the extensor tendon. **C,** Passive lateral stress is applied to check the integrity of the collateral ligaments. (*A-C, From DePalma AF.* Management of Fractures and Dislocations: An Atlas. *Philadelphia: Saunders; 1970:1203-1204. Reproduced by permission.*)

extremely important for detection of subtle dislocations or small avulsion fractures on the volar surface (Fig. 49-39).

PIP Joint Dislocations
The proximal interphalangeal (PIP) joint is extremely important, and any loss of motion in this joint may severely restrict normal function.[89] This joint is also prone to stiffness, so careful treatment of injuries in this area is essential. Injuries to the PIP joint are generally slow to heal and often result in an increase in joint size as a result of scar tissue formation.[89] Because of this propensity for a less-than-perfect outcome, it is advisable to refer PIP injuries after emergency care.

Proper examination of the PIP joint (Fig. 49-40) includes the application of ulnar and radial stress to test the integrity

Figure 49-41 Dorsal proximal interphalangeal joint dislocation.

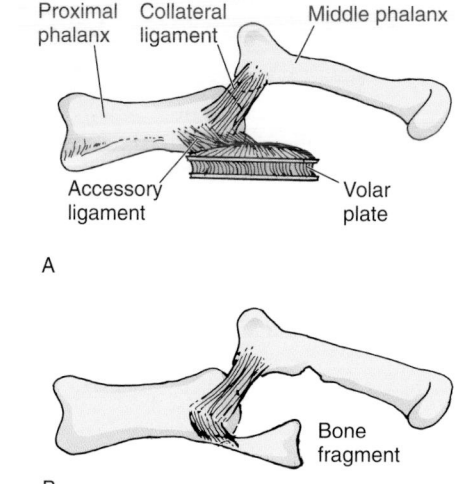

Figure 49-42 A dorsal proximal interphalangeal joint dislocation may involve rupture of the volar plate itself (**A**) or may involve avulsion of varying amounts of bone from the middle phalanx (**B**). If a large fragment of bone is avulsed from the base of the phalanx, the dislocation is unstable after reduction. The collateral ligaments will tear in varying degrees and should be assessed with stress testing after reduction.

of the collateral ligaments and hyperextension to determine the integrity of the volar plate. Inability to actively extend the flexed PIP joint against resistance suggests a central slip rupture, which may progress to a boutonnière deformity (see Chapter 48).[89] Such an examination should be carried out *after* any successful joint reduction. This examination should also be conducted on a painful PIP joint that is radiographically normal to detect soft tissue injury in a spontaneously or field-reduced dislocation. This is extremely important in athletes because coaches often reduce these injuries.[89]

Dorsal PIP Dislocations
Dorsal PIP dislocations are among the most common types encountered in the ED (Fig. 49-41; also see Fig. 49-31*B*). The mechanism is usually a blow to the end of the finger, such as from a thrown ball, that creates an axial load and hyperextends the finger.[90] The middle phalanx comes to rest dorsal to the proximal phalanx (Fig. 49-42). An associated disruption of the volar plate is generally present.[89,90] The deformity is obvious on clinical examination, and radiographs clearly demonstrate the injury. An associated fracture of the volar lip may be

detected. If this fracture affects greater than 33% of the joint surface, closed reduction will be unstable because the collateral ligament is attached to the bony fragment. In these cases, operative repair will be necessary.[90]

A dorsal PIP dislocation can be reduced after a digital block. The usual method (see Fig. 49-32A and B) is to exaggerate the injury by slight traction and hyperextension, thereby distracting the middle phalanx. Apply pressure to the base of the middle phalanx as the finger is brought into flexion. These injuries usually reduce fairly easily, and failure of routine attempts should raise suspicion of interposed soft tissue, for which orthopedic consultation should be sought.

After reduction is completed, place the joint through a range of motion to ensure stability of the reduction. If stable, splint the joint in 20 to 30 degrees of flexion for 3 weeks.[89,90] Alternatively, buddy taping to an adjacent finger for 3 to 6 weeks allows early active motion and prevents hyperextension, which should be avoided.[90] Because PIP injuries can be slow to heal and are complicated by stiffness, it is advisable to refer these patients for orthopedic follow-up.

Volar PIP Dislocations

Volar PIP dislocations are uncommon injuries and virtually always accompanied by injury to the central slip of the extensor tendons. If the dislocation is reduced before the ED visit and there is no indication that the dislocation was volar, this injury may be incorrectly treated by splinting in mild flexion as though it were the more common dorsal dislocation. However, with disruption of the central slip of the extensor tendons, immobilization in flexion will lead to the development of a boutonnière deformity.[89,92] Even when this is recognized and treated properly, some impairment of mobility may occur. It is generally best to seek early orthopedic consultation for these injuries because some require operative repair. If the emergency clinician accomplishes a closed reduction, postreduction films must demonstrate normal congruity of the joint surfaces, and a central slip attachment fracture must be excluded.[92] If so, splinting of only the PIP joint in full extension should be undertaken for 3 weeks and early orthopedic follow-up ensured.[89]

Lateral PIP Dislocations

Lateral PIP dislocations are fairly common and often reduced in the field. The patient will frequently describe dramatically how the finger was pointing in an unnatural manner (Fig. 49-43). The injury can be detected by applying ulnar and radial stress to the PIP joint. If still dislocated, re-create the injury and then apply longitudinal traction to reduce the dislocation. Treat partial tears of the collateral ligaments by buddy-taping the finger for 3 to 6 weeks.[89] Management of complete tears is controversial, with some advocating operative therapy for all such injuries and others using varying durations of immobilization or buddy taping.[89] Referral is suggested for all but the mildest of PIP collateral ligament injuries.

DIP Dislocations

As in the thumb, the distal phalanx is attached firmly to skin and subcutaneous tissue by osteocutaneous fibers. For this reason, dislocations of the distal interphalangeal (DIP) joint are frequently open.[89] A DIP dislocation is usually dorsal, and the mechanism is a blow to the end of the finger. Despite the dislocation, the DIP joint may retain some range of motion,

Figure 49-43 Lateral proximal interphalangeal dislocation. These injuries are fairly common and will have dramatic and obvious clinical findings. The dislocation is often reduced in the field, before emergency department evaluation.

so it is important to not overlook these injuries.[93] Lateral radiographs are diagnostic.

Management of a dorsal DIP dislocation involves reduction in a fashion similar to that described for other IP joint injuries (see Fig. 49-32). Hyperextend the finger and apply traction to distract the joint, and then apply pressure on the base of the distal phalanx during flexion. Following reduction, check the joint for stability and place the finger in a dorsal splint for 10 to 12 days.[89]

An injury to the DIP joint that may be confused with a dislocation is the mallet finger (Fig. 49-44). This injury is often caused by forced flexion of an extended finger (e.g., struck by a baseball). The patient is unable to extend the fingertip, but the joint appears normal on passive extension by the examiner. The injury is a rupture of the extensor tendon, with or without avulsion of a small piece of bone. Unless the injury is properly splinted or surgically immobilized, permanent deformity will occur (see Chapter 48).

MCP Dislocations

The pathology and management of finger MCP dislocations are identical to those of the thumb, as discussed earlier. The same classification of simple and complex applies; the complex type requires operative repair. Dimpling on the palmar surface suggests the presence of a complex dislocation. It is important to remember that application of traction alone for a simple MCP dislocation may convert it to a complex dislocation. For dorsal dislocations, flex the wrist to relax the tendons and hyperextend the joint as far as possible. Then apply pressure on the base of the proximal phalanx to effect reduction. After reduction of a simple dorsal MCP dislocation, buddy taping is generally sufficient to secure the reduction.[89] Volar dislocations are rare and require orthopedic consultation.

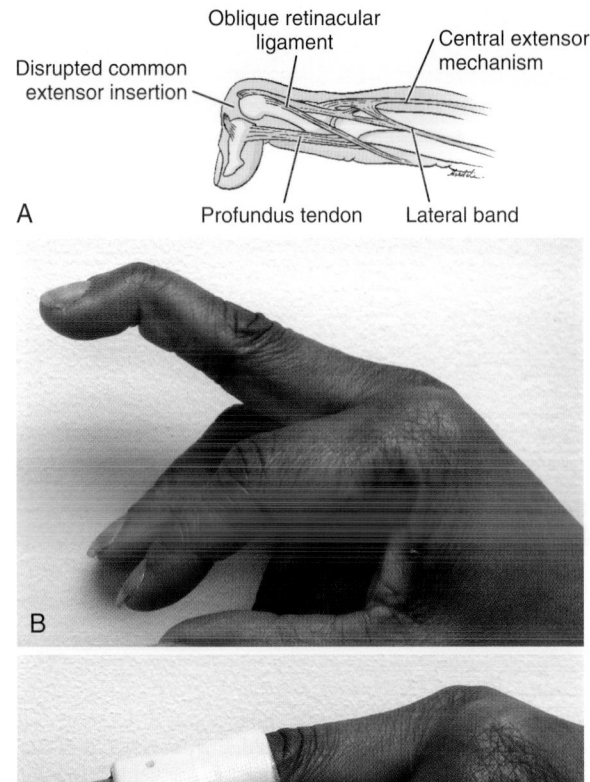

Oblique retinacular ligament

Central extensor mechanism

Disrupted common extensor insertion

A

Profundus tendon

Lateral band

B

C

Figure 49-44 A, A mallet finger injury is not a dislocation; it is a rupture of the extensor tendon to the distal phalanx. It can occur with or without (demonstrated here) an avulsion fracture after seemingly minor trauma. **B,** This mallet deformity was caused by a baseball striking the fingertip end on and producing acute flexion of the joint. **C,** A stack splint, *with the proximal interphalangeal joint left free to allow relaxation of the distal interphalangeal joint*, is kept in place for 6 to 8 weeks. Caution the patient to avoid flexing the joint to "test it out" during splint changes. Wire fixation may be required.

CMC Dislocations

CMC dislocations are rare injuries that are frequently misdiagnosed. The usual site of injury is the fifth CMC joint, which is dorsally dislocated.[90] The injury is generally the result of a high-energy mechanism, such as a motor vehicle crash or a fall. The diagnosis can be quite difficult to make because the appearance may be subtle even on a lateral radiograph. Associated fractures and other injuries are frequently present, and percutaneous fixation is usually required.[90]

Carpal Dislocation/Dissociation

Dislocation and dissociation of the carpal bones are significant injuries that require identification in the ED and expeditious immobilization and reduction to ensure the best ultimate outcome. Nonetheless, these injuries often produce significant long-term disability, such as chronic pain and weakness,

Figure 49-45 With this much soft tissue swelling 2 days after a fall on an outstretched hand, something more than a sprain or bruise is likely. If no fracture is seen on radiographs, consider carpal bone dislocation or dissociation as the culprit. Computed tomography or magnetic resonance imaging may be required to define the exact pathology.

premature arthritis, and avascular necrosis. Specific intervention to establish anatomic alignment is usually undertaken on diagnosis or within a few days of the injury, so identification in the ED, initial splinting, and proper referral are paramount. Definitive treatment is beyond the scope of this chapter and is performed by a consultant, often a hand surgeon.

The most common carpal injuries are scapholunate dissociation and lunate and perilunate dislocation, although a number of variations exist. These injuries are often sustained by a fall on an outstretched hand. Carpal dislocations and dissociations produce pain, weakness, decreased range of motion, and often significant soft tissue swelling, with many symptoms seemingly out of proportion to the radiographic findings. Specific radiographic diagnosis is frequently difficult, and it is not uncommon for definitive diagnosis to be missed on initial ED evaluation. CT or magnetic resonance imaging may be required to delineate the specifics of the injury. Marked swelling on the dorsal surface of the hand or wrist, in the absence of a definitive fracture on plain radiographs, is a common scenario, and such findings should prompt consideration of carpal dislocation or dissociation (Fig. 49-45). If a diagnosis is not forthcoming, splinting and reevaluation of a markedly swollen and painful hand or wrist in 2 to 3 days is prudent.

Scapholunate dissociation is characterized by a widened space (>3 mm) between the scaphoid and lunate bones on a plain radiograph. This is best visualized on a posteroanterior view with the hand closed in a fist and the wrist in ulnar deviation (Fig. 49-46). It is indicative of disruption of ligaments stabilizing the two carpal bones. Even though the symptoms and swelling may be impressive, the radiographic findings are subtle and often overlooked, with initial and subsequent complaints being attributed to a severe bruise or sprain. When identified, the hand and wrist are immobilized in the ED by a splint in neutral position or in 10 to 15 degrees of wrist dorsiflexion. Referral should also be initiated.

Lunate dislocation and perilunate dislocation (Figs. 49-47 and 49-48) can also occur as a result trauma and produce pain, swelling, and disability. Plain radiographs will usually delineate the pathology. Identification, splinting, and referral are the mainstays of ED treatment. These injuries may be reduced on initial diagnosis. The hand and wrist are immobilized in a

Figure 49-46 Scapholunate disassociation. **A,** A posteroanterior view of the wrist demonstrates a widened space between the scaphoid (S) and the lunate (L) (*arrow*) because of ligamentous disruption from an impaction injury. **B,** A normal wrist shows that the typical distance between the scaphoid and lunate should be about the same as that between the scaphoid and the radius.

Figure 49-47 Perilunate dislocation. **A,** A posteroanterior view of the wrist does not show the normal two crescentic rows of carpal bones but rather shows significant overlap of the hamate (H) and the lunate (L), as well as the capitate (C) with the scaphoid (S). **B,** A lateral view shows that the lunate remains in alignment with the end of the radius (R) but the remainder of the carpal bones have been dislocated.

splint in neutral position or in 10 to 15 degrees of wrist dorsiflexion.

HIP DISLOCATIONS

The hip is generally a stable ball-and-socket joint. The head of the femur is deeply situated in the acetabulum, and ligamentous and muscular support is very strong. Therefore, hip dislocations are usually the result of significant force, and a careful search for other limb- or life-threatening injuries must be undertaken. Common mechanisms of hip dislocation include motorcycle or car accidents, vehicles striking pedestrians, and falls.[94]

Associated fractures are quite common with hip dislocations. In fact, up to 88% of hip dislocations are accompanied by an associated fracture.[95] If a fracture complicates the dislocation, orthopedic consultation is generally indicated. However, the emergency clinician should be able to reduce simple hip dislocations, which are dislocations without an associated fracture or with a very minor fracture.[96] Hip dislocations may occasionally be missed in the setting of severe trauma because other injuries garner more attention. A missed diagnosis can also occur when a fracture of the femur obscures the clinical picture of hip dislocation.[96] Common complications of hip dislocation include sciatic nerve injuries and avascular necrosis of the femoral head. Sciatic nerve injuries are seen with 10% to 14% of posterior hip dislocations.[96]

Figure 49-48 Lunate dislocation. **A,** On a posteroanterior view of the wrist, significant overlap is seen of the capitate (*C*) and scaphoid (*S*), as well as the hamate (*H*) and lunate (*L*). Furthermore, clear overlap appears between the scaphoid and the radial styloid. All these findings suggest dislocation. **B,** On the lateral view, the carpal bones remain in alignment with the distal end of the radius, but the lunate has rotated and dislocated in the palmar direction (*arrow*). (*From Mettler FA, ed.* Essentials of Radiology. *2nd ed. Philadelphia: Saunders; 2005.*)

Avascular necrosis of the femoral head is one of the more disabling complications associated with hip dislocation. Although it is generally stated that early reduction will reduce the frequency of this complication, evidence for this statement is hard to find. Dreinhofer and coworkers[95] noted poor outcomes despite early (i.e., <6 hours) reduction of type I hip dislocations (dislocation without a significant associated fracture). Yang and colleagues[94] found that reduction beyond 24 hours was associated with a worse prognosis, but they could not find a significant time factor for those reduced in less than 24 hours. Nevertheless, it is still advisable to reduce hip dislocations as soon as feasible to decrease soft tissue distortion. If evidence of nerve injury exists, the dislocation should be treated as an emergency and be reduced as early as possible.

Radiographic Examination

Dislocation of the hip is generally obvious on the standard AP pelvic film that is often taken during trauma resuscitation (Fig. 49-49). A lateral or oblique view may help clarify the type of dislocation and allow detection of associated fractures.

Analgesia and Anesthesia

Dislocation of a prosthetic hip can usually be managed with moderate amounts of IV premedication in the ED. Premedication recommendations for other acute traumatic dislocations run the gamut from general anesthesia for all reductions[95] to IV sedation only.[97] Most clinicians would agree that some type of IV premedication is necessary, and patients often require deep sedation if the procedure is to be successful in the ED. One should not hesitate to opt for spinal or general anesthesia if reasonable attempts at reduction in the ED fail.

Figure 49-49 This patient was in a motor vehicle accident and has both an anterior and a posterior dislocation of the hips. Posterior dislocation occurs 90% of the time and is seen here on the *left*, with the femoral head displaced superior and lateral to the acetabulum. On the *right* is an anterior dislocation with the femoral head displaced inferiorly and medially. This patient also has a fracture of the pelvis and possibly the left acetabulum and will require a computed tomography scan to unravel the extent of all injuries. (*From Mettler FA, ed.* Essentials of Radiology. *2nd ed. Philadelphia: Saunders; 2005.*)

Posterior Hip Dislocation

Posterior dislocation is the most common type of hip dislocation. Posterior dislocations generally occur secondary to a blow to the flexed knee with the hip in varying degrees of flexion (e.g., a knee striking the dashboard in a head-on motor vehicle collision). The greater the amount of flexion of the hip at the time of the injury, the less the chance of an

POSTERIOR DISLOCATION   ANTERIOR DISLOCATION

Figure 49-50 A, Posterior hip dislocation in a patient with a hip prosthesis. The right leg is adducted, flexed at the knee, shortened, and internally rotated. **B,** The much less common anterior dislocation. The left leg is shortened, abducted, flexed at the knee, and externally rotated, similar to the appearance of a hip fracture.

associated fracture.[96] The femoral head is forced out of the acetabulum and rests behind it. The sciatic nerve is located just behind the hip joint and may be injured with a posterior hip dislocation. The clinical picture includes a shortened, internally rotated, and adducted leg (Fig. 49-50*A*).

Reduction Techniques
Several basic methods of hip reduction have been reported. Some techniques involve placing the patient in the prone position (e.g., the Stimson technique), whereas others require that the patient be supine with downward stabilization of the pelvis performed by an assistant. The supine position may be preferable in multiply injured patients because of the difficulty involved in closely monitoring a critically ill patient in the prone position.

Stimson Technique (Fig. 49-51*A*)
In the prone or gravity method described by Stimson, the patient is placed so that the distal portion of the pelvis overhangs the edge of the stretcher. Flex the hip, knee, and ankle to 90 degrees and apply downward pressure on the posterior aspect of the proximal end of the tibia.[96] Gently rotate the hip internally and externally to facilitate reduction. If needed, an assistant may apply direct downward pressure on the femoral head. An alternative and more comfortable way to provide downward pressure on the tibia is to grasp the patient's ankle, place your knee on the patient's calf, and use your body weight to apply pressure.[97] This method is believed to be the least traumatic; however, associated thoracoabdominal injuries or a need for deep sedation, which may pose an airway risk, may make the prone position risky for the patient.[96]

Allis Technique (see Fig. 49-51*B*)
For the Allis technique, place the patient supine and have an assistant stabilize the pelvis by applying downward pressure at the anterior superior iliac spines. Exert upward traction in line with the deformity and flex the hip to 90 degrees. Gently rotate the hip internally and externally until it is reduced.[96] Some prefer to stand on the patient's stretcher so that body weight can be used for leverage. Howard[98] suggested

modifying this technique by applying lateral traction on the flexed upper part of the femur to disengage the head of the femur from the outer lip of the acetabulum.

Whistler Technique (see Fig. 49-51*C*)
Another method known as the Whistler technique was described by Walden and Hamer.[99] Place the patient in the supine position with both knees flexed to 130 degrees. While an assistant stabilizes the pelvis, stand beside the affected limb. Place an arm under the affected knee and grab the unaffected knee. With the other hand, anchor the ankle of the affected leg firmly against the stretcher. Using the arm placed under the knee as a lever, raise your shoulder to elevate the affected knee. This allows the femoral head to move anteriorly around the acetabular rim and relocate.[99] Although experience with this technique is limited, it appears to be a promising, gentle reduction method.

Captain Morgan Technique (see Fig. 49-51*D*)
Another gentle method for reducing posterior hip dislocations is similar to the Whistler technique but uses the clinician's knee as opposed to the arm. For the Captain Morgan technique, place the patient supine with the affected knee flexed. Stand on the affected side and place your flexed knee underneath the patient's flexed knee. Apply force with your leg in an upward direction. Internal or external rotation can be added as needed. One case series described an extremely high success rate with this method of reduction, with only one failed attempt secondary to bony fragments in the joint space, which required open reduction.[100]

Once reduction is achieved, the legs are immobilized in slight abduction by placing an abduction pillow or another object between the knees. Radiographs should be repeated to confirm reduction, and the patient should be admitted to the hospital.

Dislocations of Hip Prostheses

Dislocation of a hip prosthesis is a separate issue (Fig. 49-52). Unlike primary dislocations, which require significant trauma, a prosthetic hip may dislocate with minimal force, such as rolling over in bed or trying to get out of a chair. Most dislocations occur in the first 3 to 4 months after surgery, but recurrent dislocation may take place much later. The majority of dislocations are posterior. The emergency physician should consider consultation with the orthopedic surgeon who placed the prosthesis.

The three major causes of prosthetic hip dislocations include (1) assumption of a position that exceeds the stability of the prosthesis, (2) soft tissue imbalances, and (3) component malposition.[101]

Emergency clinicians have been shown to be highly successful in reducing prosthetic hip dislocations.[102] Reduction techniques are similar to those described earlier; however, the urgency is not as paramount because problems with bone necrosis do not exist. Although complications are occasionally unavoidable, the clinician must be aware that forceful reduction of a dislocated hip prosthesis may dislodge the acetabular cup, fracture underlying osteoporotic bone, or loosen the prosthesis. Unlike other hip dislocations, patients with prosthetic hip dislocations often will not require hospital admission and may be discharged after discussion with the consulting orthopedic surgeon. The most common way to reduce such dislocations is shown in Figure 49-53.

POSTERIOR HIP DISLOCATION REDUCTION

A. Stimson Technique

Place the patient prone with the distal part of the pelvis overhanging the edge of the stretcher. Flex the hip, knee, and ankle to 90°. Apply downward pressure on the posterior aspect of the proximal end of the tibia. Internally and externally rotate the hip to facilitate reduction. Instruct an assistant to apply downward pressure on the femoral head.

C. Whistler Technique

Position the patient supine with the knees flexed to 130°. Instruct an assistant to stabilize the pelvis, and place your arm under the affected knee and grab the other knee. Anchor the ankle to the bed with your other hand. Using your arm under the knee as a lever, raise your shoulder and elevate the affected knee.

B. Allis Technique

Instruct an assistant to apply downward pressure on the anterior superior iliac spines. Exert upward in-line traction on the femur and flex the hip to 90°. Gently rotate the hip internally and externally until it is reduced. Standing on the bed helps increase your leverage.

D. Captian Morgan Technique

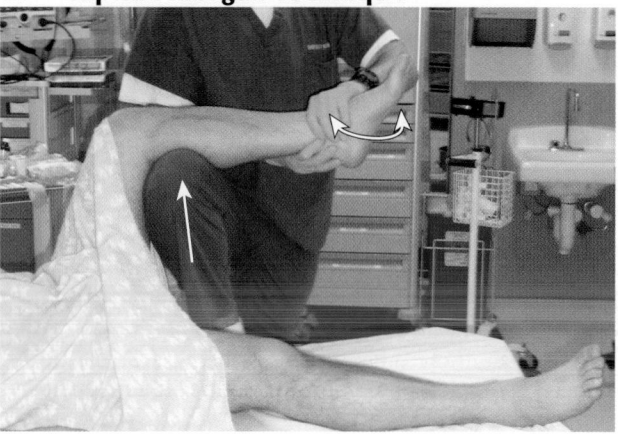

Place the patient supine with the knee flexed. Place your flexed knee under the patient's knee. Apply force with your leg in an upward direction. Internally and externally rotate the hip as needed to facilitate reduction.

Figure 49-51 Posterior hip dislocation reduction methods. (*A, From DeLee JC. Fractures and dislocations of the hip. In: Rockwood CA, Green DP, eds.* Fractures in Adults. *Vol 2. Philadelphia: Lippincott; 1991:1588. Reproduced by permission.*)

Anterior Hip Dislocation

Anterior hip dislocations are less common than posterior dislocations and account for 10% to 15% of all hip dislocations.[96] There are three general types of anterior hip dislocation that are defined by the place where the femoral head comes to rest (Fig. 49-54): iliac or subspinous, pubic, and inferior or obturator dislocation. Anterior hip dislocations generally result from forced abduction of the thigh, which may occur with a fall or motor vehicle crash.[96] The clinical picture varies with the type of dislocation. With the obturator (inferior) type, the leg is abducted and externally rotated with varying degrees of flexion. In the other types, the hip is usually extended and externally rotated.[96]

Reduction Techniques (Fig. 49-55)

The Stimson gravity method may work for anterior hip dislocation, although it is not recommended for the pubic type.[96] Alternatively, the Allis maneuver can be applied in a modified fashion. Place the patient in a supine position and have an assistant stabilize the pelvis while applying lateral countertraction on the thigh. Flex the hip slightly and apply traction along the long axis of the femur. Gently adduct and internally rotate the leg to effect reduction.[96]

For the reverse Bigelow technique, place the hip in partial flexion and abduction. Apply traction in the line of the deformity, and adduct, sharply internally rotate, and extend the hip. Caution should be exercised when using this technique because the sharp internal rotation may result in fracture of

Figure 49-52 Prosthetic hip dislocation. **A,** This patient has bilateral hip replacements. This posteroanterior radiograph shows left-sided dislocation, with the femoral component displaced in a superior direction. **B,** A cross-table lateral view demonstrates that this is a posterior dislocation (posterior is at the *bottom* of the image, anterior at the *top*). The majority of prosthetic dislocations are posterior.

Figure 49-53 A, A common method of reducing a posterior hip dislocation is to stand on the bed as shown. Apply traction with external rotation to move the femoral head away from the metallic cup. Assistants protect the operator and provide countertraction. **B,** After reduction, a knee immobilizer prevents dislocation again since hip motion is hampered.

Figure 49-54 Anterior dislocations of the hip: obturator, pubic, and iliac. *(From Simon R, Koenigsknecht S. Orthopedics in Emergency Medicine. New York: Appleton-Century-Crofts; 1982:367. Reproduced by permission.)*

the femoral neck in patients with osteoporotic bone.[96] As with posterior dislocations, admission to the hospital is required for patients with these injuries.

KNEE (FEMUR, TIBIA) DISLOCATIONS

Although the knee is a simple hinge joint, dislocations are quite rare because of its strong ligamentous support. The major ligaments include the anterior and posterior cruciate and the collateral ligaments. The usual mechanism of a knee dislocation involves a great deal of force, such as a motor vehicle crash or a sporting injury. However, knee dislocation has been reported after minor mechanisms, such as stepping off a curb or into a hole, usually in association with a twisting action.[103] Obese patients may be more likely to dislocate a knee with surprisingly minor trauma, commonly when stepping into a hole causes a twisting motion (Fig. 49-56). As with other joint dislocations, knee dislocations are described with respect to the position of the distal bone in relation to the proximal one (i.e., tibia in relation to the femur).[104] The more common types are shown in Figure 49-57. There are five general types of knee dislocation, including anterior (Fig. 49-58), posterior, lateral, and the less common medial and

rotatory. Rotatory dislocations may be anteromedial, anterolateral, posterolateral, or posteromedial.[105]

Clinical Assessment

Knee dislocations are usually clinically obvious; however, in some cases the dislocation may have spontaneously reduced before evaluation in the ED and be manifested only as severe

ANTERIOR HIP DISLOCATION REDUCTION

Modified Allis Technique

Place the patient supine and instruct an assistant to stabilize the pelvis. Flex the hip slightly and apply traction along the long axis of the femur.

Gently adduct and internally rotate the leg to reduce the dislocation.

Figure 49-55 Anterior hip dislocation reduction.

Figure 49-56 A, In an obese patient, a dislocated knee may not be obvious on initial inspection. This patient stated that she stepped into a hole and twisted her knee (a classic mechanism for dislocation), which caused the clinician to suspect only ligamentous injury or a sprain with a hemarthrosis. **B,** A radiograph demonstrated the seriousness of this seemingly benign injury. If spontaneous reduction occurs before evaluation in the emergency department, this diagnosis may not even be considered. Note the equipment for Doppler pulse evaluation in **A.** An arteriogram is the gold standard for evaluation of arterial injuries, which can initially be subtle or delayed.

Figure 49-57 The three most common types of knee dislocations: anterior (1), posterior (2), and lateral (3). (*From DePalma AF. Management of Fractures and Dislocations: An Atlas. Philadelphia: Saunders; 1970:1621. Reproduced by permission.*)

Figure 49-58 Anterior knee dislocation seen on a lateral radiograph. The patient sustained this injury when he was struck by a vehicle.

knee pain with hemarthrosis. When a spontaneously reduced knee dislocation is associated with other major trauma, the diagnosis can be missed. Obese patients may have a seemingly normal appearance of their knee, but an obvious deformity will be visible on the initial radiographs (see Fig. 49-56). A grossly unstable knee that does not appear to be dislocated is probably a reduced dislocation and carries the same risk for vascular and other complications as a dislocated knee.[106] A severely unstable knee can be defined as one that has greater than 30 degrees of recurvatum (hyperextension) on lifting the leg off the stretcher by the heel[106] or one that exhibits gross instability after reduction.[104] Because pain and muscle spasm may limit the physical examination for stability, a knee hemarthrosis, usually a large one with signs of posterior or calf hemorrhage, is a potential tip-off to a reduced dislocation.

An impressive effusion may not be present with a knee dislocation because the joint capsule is often disrupted and extravasation occurs into the surrounding tissue, usually posteriorly. The most important part of the clinical assessment is the vascular status of the extremity (see the next section). Nerve injury is less common, but peroneal nerve injury is a recognized complication, particularly with a posterolateral dislocation.[104] Peroneal nerve injury should be suspected if the patient is unable to dorsiflex the ankle (footdrop) or has decreased sensation on the dorsum of the foot. Posterolateral dislocations may be irreducible because the medial femoral condyle buttonholes through the joint capsule.[104] A clue to this injury is the presence of a dimple sign at the medial joint line.

Vascular Injury

The most feared complication of a knee dislocation is severance or internal injury of the popliteal artery (Fig. 49-59). Injury to the popliteal artery may complicate both anterior and posterior knee dislocations and occurs because the artery is relatively fixed both proximally and distally.[104] If popliteal artery injury occurs, it is often due to transection with posterior dislocations or traction (producing intimal tears) during anterior dislocations.[105] In addition, Varnell and associates[106] noted that vascular injury was as common in a severely unstable knee (e.g., field reduced) as in an acutely dislocated knee. The incidence of popliteal artery injury in a dislocated knee is around 20% in most series.[106,107] The seriousness of this complication is largely due to the fact that the collateral circulation about the knee is poor,[48] and the end result of injury to the popliteal artery (or vein) may be amputation, particularly if recognition of vascular injury is delayed.[108,109] It should also be noted that nerve injuries are more common in patients with a vascular injury.[110,111]

It has previously been stated that popliteal artery disruption may be present despite a normal pulse.[112] Such statements have led to recommendations to perform arteriography or exploration of all knee dislocations.[104] However, some studies question this perspective. Varnell and associates[106] reported a pulse deficit or absent pulse in all patients with vascular injury. Kendall and coworkers[107] also reported clear clinical evidence of all popliteal artery injuries in knee dislocations. This group recommended exploration for obvious ischemia, angiography for patients with ischemia whose pulse is restored after relocation, and observation for all others.[107] Dennis and colleagues[113] reported that physical examination alone had 100% accuracy in predicting the need for surgical intervention in patients

Figure 49-59 Complete occlusion of the popliteal artery after posterior knee dislocation. *(From Valji K, ed.* Vascular and Interventional Radiology. *2nd ed. Philadelphia: Saunders; 2006).*

with posterior knee dislocations. Miranda and associates[114] reported that popliteal artery injury can be safely and reliably predicted by a physical examination that includes specific evaluation for active posterior hemorrhage, expanding hematoma, absent pulse, or the presence of a thrill or bruit. However, it is noted that the hard physical signs of arterial injury might be delayed for 24 to 48 hours. Thus, although focused clinician examination may be quite accurate in the vast majority of cases, any dislocated knee should prompt serious concern about the vascular integrity of the leg given the sometimes subtle or delayed manifestation of vascular injuries.

Simple palpation of the artery may not be sensitive enough to detect a decreased pulse. An ankle-brachial arterial pressure index (ABI) should be considered to compare blood pressure in the ankle with that in the arm. Also, consider digit pulse oximetry to compare the uninjured leg with the injured one. Mills and coworkers[111] 91reported the results of a prospective study of 38 patients with knee dislocation to evaluate the accuracy of ABI in identifying vascular injury. Patients with an ABI of less than 0.90 underwent arteriography, whereas those with an ABI of 0.90 or greater underwent serial examination and delayed arterial duplex evaluation. Eleven (29%) of the patients had an ABI of less than 0.90, and all of them had arterial injuries requiring surgical intervention. Of the remaining 27 patients with an ABI of 0.90 or greater, none had a vascular injury noted on serial

KNEE DISLOCATION REDUCTION

Apply (1) countertraction and (2) traction on the extremity. Often this maneuver alone will reduce the joint because of the severe ligamentous disruption associated with the dislocation.

Additional maneuvers may be required, depending on the type of dislocation. Apply posteriorly directed pressure on the tibia for anterior dislocations.

For a medial dislocation, apply a lateral force to the medial side of the tibia. Adjust the reducing force according to the type of dislocation present.

Figure 49-60 Knee dislocation reduction.

examination or duplex ultrasonography. No patient in this group was found to have vascular compromise at follow-up (range, 4 to 36 months).[111]

Knee dislocations are usually clinically obvious or easily visible on plain radiographs. Therefore, it is occult knee dislocations (i.e., dislocated and spontaneously reduced) that are problematic for the emergency clinician to diagnose. Internal derangement with a knee hemarthrosis (often of the size noted with a torn anterior cruciate ligament) is a common first sign that the knee had previously been dislocated and spontaneously reduced. Therefore, all knee injuries with significant swelling, hemarthrosis, or a dislocating mechanism of injury should be evaluated with the specific intent of ruling out vascular injury.

If vascular compromise is detected on clinical assessment, it is appropriate to reduce the knee dislocation without obtaining radiographs, although a few minutes to obtain portable radiographs and to administer IV medication would be unlikely to make a difference in the final outcome.[104] Use of Doppler ultrasound for pulse checks and ABI should also be considered with these injuries (see Chapter 1). Early consultation should be sought for knee dislocations because of the high incidence of complications and the frequent need for operative intervention. The decision to pursue angiography in a patient with a dislocated knee is best made in consultation with the patient's orthopedic surgeon.

Reduction Technique (Fig. 49-60)

The need for IV sedation and analgesia depends on the clinical situation, but it should be considered whenever possible (see Chapter 33). The basic initial approach for all types of knee dislocation is to apply traction to the extremity. This alone is often all that is required for reduction because of severe disruption of the ligamentous support of the knee.[78] For anterior dislocations, lift the distal end of the femur to effect reduction. For posterior dislocations, lift the proximal end of the tibia to complete the reduction.[48] For medial, lateral, and rotatory dislocations, a similar approach is acceptable, with pressure exerted in the medial or lateral direction as needed.

After reduction, splint the extremity in 15 degrees of flexion. A posterolateral dislocation may be irreducible, and

operative intervention should be considered if reduction is not easily accomplished.[48]

Postreduction Care

Appropriate aftercare for knee dislocations requires serial reassessment of the neurovascular status of the extremity, postreduction films, and admission to the hospital. Use a knee immobilizer to provide stabilization and comfort. These injuries cause severe ligamentous and other derangements in the knee and generally require operative stabilization with a long period of recovery and physical therapy.

DISLOCATIONS OF THE FIBULAR HEAD

The fibula can be dislocated at its proximal articulation in the knee joint. This is most commonly an anterolateral dislocation.[104] The fibular head is normally nestled in a stable manner behind the lateral tibial condyle with two supporting tibiofibular ligaments.[115] The tibiofibular joint has a separate synovial cavity, and therefore a typical knee joint effusion will not be seen with this dislocation. When the knee is flexed, the stability of this joint is decreased because of relaxation of the fibular collateral ligament.[115] The typical mechanism of injury is a fall on a flexed, adducted leg, often combined with ankle inversion. This mechanism is seen in sports and parachute landings.[115] Posterior dislocations can result from a twisting mechanism or a direct blow to the area while the knee is flexed.[104]

Anterolateral dislocation is the most common type. It is accompanied by obvious prominence of the fibular head anteriorly; no associated neurovascular problems are noted. The less common posterior dislocation may be accompanied by peroneal nerve injury.[104] Patients have varying degrees of disability, and some may walk on the leg with only mild discomfort.[115] On radiographic examination the three cardinal signs of anterolateral dislocation are lateral displacement of the fibula on an AP film, a widened proximal interosseous space, and anterior displacement of the fibular head on a lateral view (Fig. 49-61).[95] If high clinical suspicion exists for fibular head dislocation and radiographs are nondiagnostic, CT is the next study of choice.[116,117]

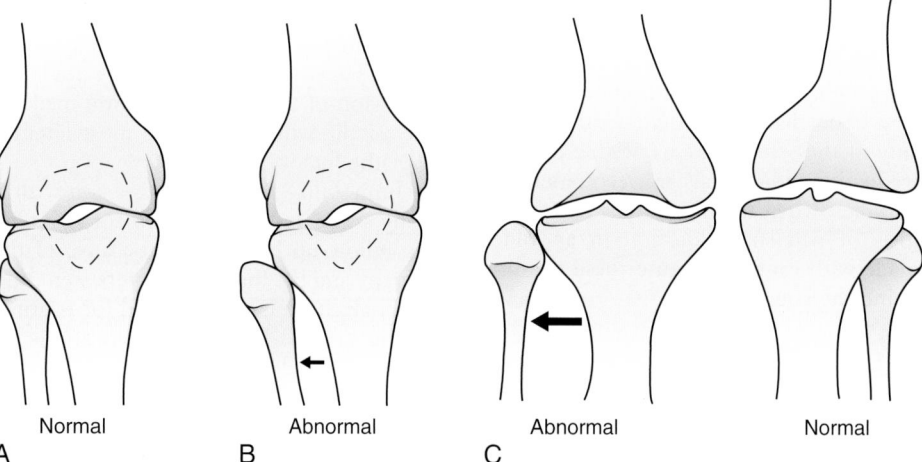

Figure 49-61 Anterolateral fibular head dislocation compared with a normal knee. The interosseous distance is widened and the proximal end of the fibula is displaced laterally. **A,** Normal anteroposterior projection of the knee. **B,** Lateral displacement of the proximal end of the fibula. **C,** Use of bilateral comparison views to highlight the fibular displacement.

Reduction Technique

To reduce an anterior fibular head dislocation, place the patient supine and flex the affected knee to 90 degrees to relax the biceps femoris tendon. Dorsiflex and externally rotate the foot and apply direct pressure to the fibular head; reduction is usually signified by a snap.[104] The method for reduction of a posterior dislocation is the same except that direct pressure is applied in a forward direction. Patients should not bear weight for 2 weeks and should receive orthopedic referral. Immobilization is probably unnecessary.[104]

PATELLAR DISLOCATION

Patellar dislocations are fairly common, especially in adolescents. The usual mechanism is a powerful quadriceps contraction combined with a strong valgus and external rotation component.[118] This may be seen in activities such as making a "cut" in sports or with dancing. The patella may also dislocate with a direct blow to the flexed knee.[48] Factors predisposing to patellar dislocation include chronic patellofemoral abnormalities such as genu valgum and femoral anteversion.[118] Patellar dislocation is described by the relationship of the patella to the knee joint. Lateral dislocations are the most common by far. Other types include superior, medial, and intercondylar (Fig. 49-62).

Clinical Assessment

Lateral dislocation of the patella is generally clinically obvious (Fig. 49-63). The knee is held in some degree of flexion and the patella can easily be seen and palpated on the lateral side of the knee. Tenting of the patella is often detectable unless significant soft tissue swelling is present.

The patella may be spontaneously reduced in the field with simple leg straightening. The patient will report that the leg "went out" and may describe actually seeing the lateral deformity caused by the displaced patella. Clinical clues to a spontaneously reduced patella include the presence of a knee effusion and tenderness along the medial edge of the patella. Fairbank's test or the patellar "apprehension" sign is elicited when the

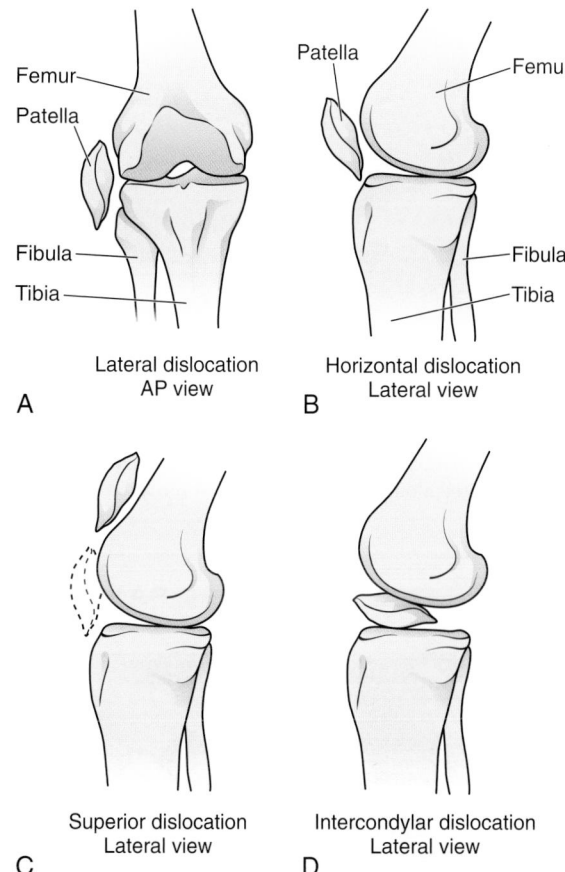

Figure 49-62 A-D, Various types of patellar dislocation. Lateral dislocation is the most common. *AP,* anteroposterior.

patella is pushed laterally and the patient grabs for the knee, a response indicative of the sensation of repeated injury.[48]

Radiographs

Prereduction films are difficult to obtain because the patient is usually in flexion. Some recommend prereduction films when possible in all patients[48]; however, it is easy to reduce these injuries before radiographs are obtained. The diagnosis is usually obvious, and there are no reports in the literature of complications from gentle reduction. Osteochondral fractures are detectable in about half the patients with patellar dislocations, but many of these fractures are visible only on arthroscopy.[118] Postreduction radiographs are recommended, as are prereduction studies, when the diagnosis is uncertain. The clinical diagnosis of patellar dislocation in an older patient should be made with caution because these are primarily injuries involving the young.

Reduction Technique and Postreduction Care
(Fig. 49-64)

Reduction of a lateral patellar dislocation is usually quite simple. Premedication is often not required if the patient can

Figure 49-63 Lateral patellar dislocations are usually clinically obvious. The knee is held in flexion, and the patella (*arrow*) can be seen and palpated along the lateral aspect of the knee.

be verbally reassured. If the patient is anxious or in great discomfort, premedication should be considered (see Chapter 33). The two basic maneuvers for patellar relocation are extension of the knee and gentle medial pressure applied to the patella while lifting the most lateral edge of the patella over the femoral condyle.[48]

Immobilize the leg in extension with a splint or commercially available knee immobilizer (see Chapter 50). Orthopedic follow-up is necessary because of the need for physical therapy and the high rate of persistent instability.[118] However, hospitalization is not required for routine lateral dislocations of the patella. Recurrent dislocations and those associated with an osteochondral fracture might require operative repair.

Patellar dislocations in other locations are often irreducible, and orthopedic consultation should be sought. Intracondylar and superior dislocations are extremely rare and require operative reduction. The rare horizontal dislocation may relocate with closed reduction, but surgical reduction is often necessary.

ANKLE DISLOCATIONS

The ankle joint is a modified saddle joint in which the talus is nestled in the mortise formed by the distal ends of the tibia and fibula.[48] The ligamentous support of the ankle is quite strong, and pure dislocations are uncommon. Usually, there are associated fractures of the ankle joint (Fig. 49-65). Ankle dislocations are described by the relationship of the talus to the tibia. Posterior dislocations of the ankle are more common than anterior dislocations, and they usually result from a fall on a plantarflexed foot. Patients with posterior dislocations often have an associated fracture of one or more of the malleoli,[48] occasionally seen only after reduction (Fig. 49-66). The clinical picture usually consists of significant deformity and disability.

Anterior dislocations generally result from forced dorsiflexion or a blow directed posteriorly onto the distal end of the tibia while the foot is fixed. The talus is prominent

LATERAL PATELLAR DISLOCATION REDUCTION

Gently extend the knee (*white arrow*) and apply medial pressure on the patella (*black arrow*) while lifting up the most lateral edge of the patella over the femoral condyle.

Reduction is usually quite simple and the knee will regain a normal appearance. Immobilize the leg in extension with a splint or knee immobilizer. Arrange for orthopedic follow-up.

Figure 49-64 Lateral patellar dislocation reduction.

| Anterior | Posterior | Lateral | Superior ("diastasis") |

Figure 49-65 Types of ankle dislocation. Note that there are usually associated fractures of the tibia, fibula, or both.

Figure 49-66 Isolated posterior tibial lip fracture (*arrow*), seen only after reduction of a posterior ankle dislocation. (*From Harris JH Jr, Harris WH. Radiology of Emergency Medicine. 2nd ed. Baltimore: Williams & Wilkins; 1981:629. Reproduced by permission.*)

anteriorly, and the dorsalis pedis pulse may be lost secondary to pressure from the talus. Superior dislocations are uncommon and result in diastasis of the tibiofibular joint. These injuries are usually the result of a significant axial force, such as a fall from a significant height. Therefore, clinicians should search for concomitant calcaneal or low spine fractures. Lateral dislocations of the ankle are always associated with fractures of the malleoli or distal end of the fibula.

Radiographic Examination

Because of the high rate of associated fractures and the clinical difficulty in assessing for the presence or the exact nature of a dislocation, it is recommended that prereduction radiographs be obtained for all suspected ankle dislocations (see Figs. 49-2 and 49-65). It is acceptable to reduce the dislocation without a radiograph if severe vascular compromise is present, but for the vast majority of cases, the few minutes taken to obtain bedside radiographs and administer IV medications rarely affects the final outcome. It may be impossible to accurately determine the exact type of dislocation unless prereduction films are obtained. AP and lateral views usually suffice for emergency management; other views can be ordered if necessary after the joint is relocated.

Reduction Techniques (Fig. 49-67)

Unless a strong contraindication is present, it is advisable to administer IV sedation and analgesia to patients with an ankle dislocation early in their care, preferably before conducting any manipulations or radiologic studies. Reduction is always painful in an awake patient, and sufficient premedication must be administered. For posterior dislocations, place the patient supine and flex the *knee slightly* to relax the Achilles tendon. An assistant can do this, or the patient can be positioned such that the knee hangs over the end of the bed. Grasp the foot with both hands; place one hand on the heel and the other on the forefoot. Apply traction on the slightly plantar-flexed foot. Have a second assistant apply downward pressure on the distal end of the tibia and move the heel anteriorly to effect reduction.[119]

For anterior dislocations, the initial steps and positioning are the same as those for posterior dislocation. However, instead of plantar flexion, dorsiflex the foot to free the talus. The second assistant applies upward pressure on the distal end of the tibia while the operator applies traction and pushes the foot in a posterior direction.[48]

Lateral dislocations are really fracture-dislocations, and orthopedic consultation is generally required as part of the

ANKLE DISLOCATION REDUCTION

A. Posterior Dislocations

(1) Slightly flex the knee. (2) Instruct an assistant to provide countertraction on the leg. (3) Grasp the heel with one hand and the dorsal metatarsals with the other. (4) Slightly plantar-flex the foot and apply straight downward counterpressure on the foot.

(5) Pull the foot forward with longitudinal traction on the heel. (6) Dorsiflex the foot. (7) Instruct a second assistant to provide counterpressure on the front of the lower part of the leg.

B. Anterior Dislocations

(1) Flex the knee. (2) Grasp the forefoot with one hand and the heel with the other. (3) Dorsiflex the foot to disengage the talus. (4) Instruct an assistant to provide countertraction on the leg.

(5) Apply straight longitudinal traction. (6) Push the foot directly backward. (7) Instruct a second assistant to apply countertraction on the back of the lower part of the leg.

Figure 49-67 Ankle dislocation reduction.

ED course. The emergency clinician will often need to reduce these injuries because of the extreme lateral deformity and occasional compromise of the dorsalis pedis artery by stretch. Open dislocations (in the absence of vascular compromise) may be better handled by operating room washout before attempting reduction (Fig. 49-68). If a lateral fracture-dislocation is to be reduced in the ED, the approach is quite similar to that for posterior ankle dislocations. However, instead of pressure in the AP direction, the foot is moved medially after the application of traction.[48]

Postreduction Care

After reduction, splint the ankle at 90 degrees with a long leg posterior splint. Application of a stirrup splint in addition to the posterior splint may provide additional stability (see Chapter 50). The necessity of admission to the hospital must be determined in consultation with an orthopedic surgeon. Many patients with these injuries have associated fractures that require surgical intervention.

DISLOCATIONS OF THE FOOT

The importance of the foot is recognized by anyone who has had to spend time ambulating with an injury in this area. For purposes of this discussion, dislocation injuries of the foot can

Figure 49-68 A seemingly minor laceration is evidence of the fractured bone previously protruding through the skin (*arrow*). Compound fractures such as this require antibiotics and open débridement.

be divided into those of the hindfoot and those of the forefoot.

Hindfoot Injuries

Injuries to this area are uncommon and usually result from high-energy transfer. The major dislocations are subtalar and

Figure 49-69 A, A Lisfranc fracture-dislocation is a serious and debilitating injury that is easily missed. This patient complained of extremely severe pain in the foot and was unable to walk after falling down the steps while intoxicated, so the mechanism was unclear. Drug seeking was suspected; however; *note the significant soft tissue swelling* suggestive of internal injury. **B,** This radiograph was initially read as a minor avulsion fracture around the base of the second metatarsal, but a closer review shows widening of the space between the first and second metatarsals and *lateral displacement of the rest of the metatarsals (arrows).* This injury often requires operative repair, and permanent disability is common in the best of circumstances.

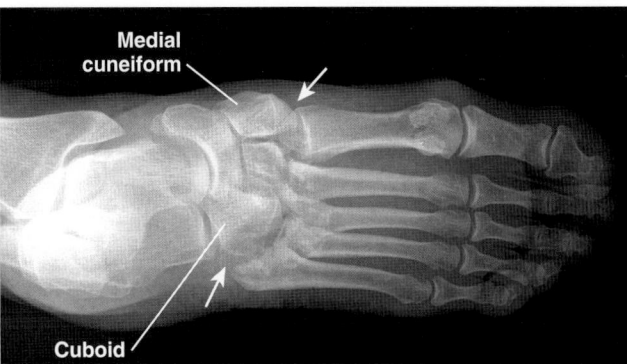

Figure 49-70 Lisfranc fracture-dislocation. Note that the first through fifth metatarsals are shifted laterally with respect to the tarsal bones. This is termed a homolateral dislocation. Poor alignment between the first metatarsal and medial cuneiform and between the fifth metatarsal and cuboid is a clue that this substantial injury is present (*arrows*). Also note the irregularities at the bases of the second through fifth metatarsals, which may represent fractures in this region. Computed tomography or magnetic resonance imaging may be needed to fully assess this subtle, yet complex injury.

Figure 49-71 Medial subtalar dislocation. Note that the tibia, talus, and fibula retain a normal anatomic relationship but that the calcaneus, navicular, and forefoot are displaced medially.

talar dislocations and midtarsal fracture-dislocations (Lisfranc injury). Although x-ray findings are often subtle and easily overlooked, a Lisfranc injury is complex and always a fracture-dislocation because of the rigid nature of the region (Figs. 49-69 and 49-70). These injuries require orthopedic management and are not discussed here.

Subtalar Dislocation

This uncommon injury generally occurs secondary to sports, falls from heights, or motor vehicle crashes. The calcaneus, navicular, and forefoot are displaced from the talus (Fig. 49-71).[119] The primary mechanisms are severe inversion causing medial dislocation or severe eversion resulting in lateral dislocation. The medial type occurs so commonly during basketball that it has been termed *basketball foot.*[120] This injury is usually seen in young adult males. Medial dislocations constitute the majority (85%) of these injuries, with lateral dislocations making up the rest.[120]

The diagnosis is usually obvious because the talus is prominent and often tents the skin of the proximal part of the foot.

The medial type has been termed an *acquired clubfoot*; the lateral type appears as an *acquired flatfoot.*[120]

Some authors recommend spinal or general anesthesia for all such injuries[120]; however, it is usually possible to reduce these injuries with IV premedication. Position the patient in a supine fashion and flex the hip and knee much as for reduction of a posterior ankle dislocation. Place one hand on the forefoot and grasp the heel with the other hand. Apply firm longitudinal traction to effect reduction. Dangling the leg over the end of the bed allows the operator to use body weight to assist in traction. Once traction is applied, the deformity is initially increased (inversion for medial; eversion for lateral) and then reversed to effect reduction.[120]

Dislocation of the Talus

In this extremely rare injury, the talus is essentially extruded from its normal position and comes to lie anteriorly. This injury is generally open,[120] is not amenable to closed reduction, and virtually always progresses to avascular necrosis.[121]

Figure 49-72 Toe dislocations. **A,** Dorsal dislocation of the first metatarsophalangeal joint. **B,** Lateral dislocation of the fourth proximal interphalangeal joint. Reduction of toe dislocations follows the same technique as described for finger dislocations (see Fig. 49-32).

Talectomy and arthrodesis are often required,[120] and orthopedic referral should be undertaken on an emergency basis if vascular compromise of the foot is present.

Forefoot Dislocations

Much of what is pertinent to the diagnosis and management of forefoot dislocations has already been discussed in the management of dislocations of the finger and hand MCP joints. Anatomically, the joints are quite similar.

MTP Dislocations

These uncommon injuries are generally the result of hyperextension resulting in dorsal dislocation of the great toe metatarsophalangeal (MTP) joint (Fig. 49-72A).[122] Among the lesser toe MTP joints, lateral or medial displacement of the digit on the metatarsal head is more common and usually the result of jamming the toe on a piece of furniture.[120] As with MCP dislocations, they can be simple or complex. Complex dislocations of the first toe can be suspected by the presence of sesamoid bones in the joint space on prereduction radiographs.[120] Complex MTP dislocations are often irreducible.

For simple MTP dislocations, reduction is accomplished by increasing the deformity through hyperextension and then applying traction while exerting thumb pressure over the base of the dislocated proximal phalanx. Plantar flexion of the foot may be used to relax the flexor tendons.[119] Operative intervention is required after reduction if crepitus is present on motion, the joint is unstable, or an intraarticular loose body is noted on postreduction radiographs.[120]

IP Dislocations

In the foot, IP dislocations result from an axial load on the toe, such as from kicking a wall (see Fig. 49-72B). These dislocations are generally dorsal and can be reduced as in the hand. Specifically, the toe should be dorsiflexed to exaggerate the deformity and then undergo traction followed by plantar flexion. Dislocations of the first toe IP joint are usually buddy-taped to the second toe for 2 to 3 weeks, whereas those of lesser toes can be taped for 10 to 14 days.[120] Reduction of dorsal dislocations may be difficult because of entrapment of the plantar plate inside the joint.[123] As in the hand, complex dislocations or those failing closed reduction may occur. Such dislocations require open reduction and internal fixation.[123]

CONCLUSION

The following points are important regarding the assessment and management of dislocations:

1. A search for other more serious injuries should be undertaken when there is a high-energy mechanism of injury.
2. Neurovascular assessment should be performed early in the evaluation and appropriately documented.
3. Radiographs and IV premedication are generally indicated before attempts at reduction.
4. Reduction attempts should involve gentle, gradual application of force and patience on the operator's part.
5. After completing reduction, the operator should recheck the patient's neurovascular status, request postreduction radiographs (except with radial head subluxations), and in certain circumstances, assess the stability and range of motion of the joint.
6. A definite percentage of dislocations are irreducible, and the need for multiple attempts should halt prolonged and forceful attempts in the ED and prompt orthopedic consultation.
7. Dislocations accompanied by neurologic injury should be reduced by the most expeditious and least traumatic method.

References are available at www.expertconsult.com

CHAPTER 50

Splinting Techniques

Carl R. Chudnofsky

Splints are used frequently in the emergency department (ED) for temporary immobilization of fractures and dislocations and for definitive treatment of soft tissue injuries.[1,2] Patients with a variety of nontraumatic musculoskeletal disorders (e.g., gout, inflammatory joint diseases, infections, burns) also benefit from short-term immobilization. Immobilization is the mainstay of fracture therapy, but though intuitively beneficial, it is difficult to find firm scientific data that support the use of splinting for soft tissue injuries.[3,4] Although the general principle of immobilizing sprains and contusions is strongly supported by custom and personal preference, its exact influence on healing, number of complications, and ultimate return to normal activity is not known. In most studies of ankle sprains, for example, the function and pain of the injured joint are similar at 6 weeks' follow-up, regardless of whether treatment consisted of ad lib walking, a simple elastic bandage, a posterior splint, or a formal cast.[5,6] A systematic review of 22 clinical trials comparing various treatments of acute lateral ankle sprains (cast, splint, or early mobilization with support) found no favorable effect of immobilization.[7] The current data support functional management for most acute ankle sprains.[7]

Patients are routinely seen in the ED with injuries that are amenable to splinting to relieve pain and augment healing (see Review Box 50-1). Although a strict standard of care cannot be promulgated, the use of short-term splinting in the ED for

Splinting Techniques

Indications

Immobilization of a variety of clinical conditions:
- Fractures and dislocations
- Deep lacerations that cross joints
- Tendon lacerations
- Inflammatory disorders (e.g., gout, tenosynovitis)
- Deep space infections of the hands or feet
- Cellulitis overlying a joint
- Selected puncture or bite wounds

Contraindications

No absolute contraindications

Complications

Ischemia
Heat injury
Pressure sores
Infection
Dermatitis
Pruritis
Joint stiffness
Cast pain
Compartment syndrome

Equipment

Equipment for plaster splints

Equipment for preformed fiberglass splints

Review Box 50-1   Splinting techniques: indications, contraindications, complications, and equipment.

acutely painful conditions remains a common practice. Emergency clinicians have virtually abandoned the use of circumferential casts in favor of premade commercial immobilizing devices or splints constructed of plaster of paris or fiberglass. The impetus for this change is primarily related to the complications occasionally associated with circumferential casts, liability issues, and ease of application brought about by new technology. In most instances, properly applied splints provide short-term immobilization equal to that of casts while allowing continued swelling and thus reducing the risk for ischemic injury. Other obvious advantages of splints are that patients can take them off when immobilization is no longer needed or can remove them temporarily to bathe, exercise the injured part, or perform wound care.

Most splinting techniques are handed down from house staff or experienced clinicians, but the procedure is often suboptimal and haphazard.[8] This chapter presents guidelines for adequate immobilization of injuries commonly encountered by emergency clinicians. Details of the construction and application of commonly used custom-made plaster splints are provided.

INDICATIONS AND CONTRAINDICATIONS

Theoretically, immobilization facilitates the healing process by decreasing pain and protecting the extremity from further injury. Other benefits of splinting are specific to the particular injury or problem being treated (Fig. 50-1). For example, in the treatment of fractures, splinting helps maintain bony alignment. Splinting deep lacerations that cross joints reduces tension on the wound and helps prevent wound dehiscence. Immobilizing tendon lacerations may facilitate the healing process by relieving stress on the repaired tendon. The discomfort of inflammatory disorders such as tenosynovitis or acute gout is greatly reduced by immobilization. Deep space infections of the hands or feet, as well as cellulitis over any joint, should similarly be immobilized for comfort. Limiting early motion may also reduce edema and theoretically improve the immune system's ability to combat infection. Hence, selected puncture wounds and mammalian or human bites of the hands and feet may be immobilized until the risk for infection has passed. Splinting large abrasions that cross joint surfaces prevents movement of the injured extremity and reduces the pain produced when the injured skin is stretched. Finally, victims of multiple trauma should have fractures and reduced dislocations adequately splinted while other diagnostic and therapeutic procedures (e.g., fluid resuscitation, airway control, computed tomography scans, tube thoracostomy) are completed. Immobilization decreases blood loss, minimizes the potential for further neurovascular injury, reduces the need for opioid analgesia, and may decrease the risk for fat emboli from long-bone fractures.

Figure 50-1 Indications for splinting. Splinting is traditionally thought of as a treatment of fractures, such as the comminuted distal radius fracture depicted in **A.** However, splinting is also beneficial in a wide variety of other conditions, such as acute gout (**B**), human and mammalian bites of the hand (**C**), and tendon injuries (**D**). Other indications include inflammatory disorders such as tenosynovitis, deep lacerations that cross joints, and deep space infections of the hands and feet.

EQUIPMENT (see Review Box 50-1)

Support Materials

Plaster of Paris

Plaster of paris is the most widely used material for ED splinting.[9] Its name originated from the fact that it was first prepared from the gypsum of Paris, France. When gypsum is heated to approximately 128°C, most of the water of crystallization is driven off and a fine white powder is left behind—plaster of paris. When water is added to the plaster, the reaction is reversed, and the plaster recrystallizes or "sets" by incorporating water molecules into the crystalline lattice of the calcium sulfate dehydrate molecules.

Today, plaster is impregnated into strips or rolls of a crinoline-type material. The crinoline allows easy application, helps keep the plaster molded to the proper form during the setting process, and adds support to the finished splint. Plaster rolls and sheets are available in a variety of setting times and widths (2-, 3-, 4-, or 6-inch widths). The distinct advantage of plaster over commercially available premade splints is that plaster can more easily be molded and tailored to the individual's anatomy, thereby negating the "one-size-fits-all" approach. Also, plaster rolls and strips are generally less expensive than premade splints.

Prefabricated Splint Rolls

The use of plaster splints in the form of prefabricated splint rolls (e.g., OCL, BSN Medical) is very popular among emergency clinicians. These splint rolls have 10 to 20 sheets of plaster enclosed between a thick layer of protective foam padding on one side and a thin layer of cloth on the other. Like custom-constructed splints, they are secured to the extremity with an elastic bandage. The major advantage of prefabricated splint rolls is that significant time is saved because the splint and padding come ready to apply. In addition, prefabricated splint rolls are ideal for intermittent splinting and can be removed and reapplied by the patient as needed. However, prefabricated plaster splint rolls are more expensive than simple plaster rolls, and they lack some of the versatility and custom-fit qualities of self-made plaster splints.

Prefabricated splint rolls composed of layers of fiberglass between polypropylene padding (e.g., Ortho-Glass, 3M Scotchcast One-Step) are now commonplace in many EDs. Fiberglass splint rolls offer the same time-saving aspect as prefabricated plaster splint rolls but require only 3 minutes to set, thus making application faster. In addition, splints made of prefabricated fiberglass rolls cure more rapidly (20 minutes),

have no messy residue (i.e., they can be hydrated in a conventional sink without a special trap), can be washed and reapplied, and are stronger and lighter than splints constructed of prefabricated plaster rolls. Another advantage is the polypropylene padding, which wicks moisture away from the skin better than polyester, nylon, or cotton padding does.[10] Prefabricated fiberglass splint rolls are more expensive than both simple plaster rolls and prefabricated plaster splint rolls and, like prefabricated plaster splints, lack some of the versatility and custom-fit qualities of self-made plaster splints.

Protective and Miscellaneous Equipment

Stockinette

A single layer of stockinette is commonly used under cotton (Webril) padding, circumferential casts, and splints. It protects the skin and, when folded back over the ends of the plaster, creates a smooth, professional-looking, padded rim. Stockinette is available in 2-, 3-, 4-, 8-, 10-, and 12-inch widths.

Padding

Padding under the splint protects the skin and bony prominences and accommodates swelling of the injured extremity. Most commercially available splints contain adequate padding in the premade product, but in some instances, additional padding is prudent. In general, the older thin cotton padding known as sheet wadding has been replaced by newer material such as Webril (Curity) and Specialist (Johnson & Johnson) cast padding. Webril is soft cotton with a much coarser weave than sheet wadding; consequently, it has greater tensile strength, adheres better, and can be applied more evenly. Specialist padding uses micropleated cotton fibers that relax when moistened. This results in uniform, feltlike padding that conforms to the surface being wrapped. Felt (0.5 inch thick) may also be used to pad bony prominences.

Elastic Bandages

Elastic bandages are used to secure the splint in place. Elastic bandages are available in 2-, 3-, 4-, and 6-inch widths. Some bandages use metal clips, whereas others use a Velcro-type mechanism to secure the bandage in place. Metal clips should be taped in place to avoid inadvertent removal.

Patients often use or request an elastic bandage for many soft tissue injuries. Although applying an elastic bandage to an injured part is popular, it is of minimal benefit alone. The downside is that the bandage may be wrapped too tightly and cause additional injury or distal swelling (Fig. 50-2).

Figure 50-2 Elastic bandages. **A,** An elastic bandage is a popular home treatment of many painful conditions, such as sprains and contusions. An actual medical benefit is unproven. **B,** Wrapping an extremity too tightly may cause additional injury or distal swelling. This patient complained of a swollen hand after an elbow injury. Note the grooves in the skin (*arrows*) indicating that the wrap was the culprit causing the hand swelling. **C,** Markedly swollen foot after application of a useless elastic bandage on the lower part of the leg.

Adhesive Tape

Use adhesive tape to prevent slippage of the elastic bandages, to line the cut edges of a bivalved cast, and to buddy-tape digits. Coban tape can be used in a similar manner and has the advantage of adhering only to itself.

Utility Knife, Scalpel, and Plaster or Trauma Scissors

Use a utility knife, a No. 10 scalpel blade, or plaster or trauma scissors to cut and shape dry plaster.

Bucket

Use a large bucket (preferably stainless steel) for wetting plaster. Do not prepare the plaster in the sink unless it is equipped with a special drain designed to accept plaster residue without clogging. A bucket is not required for the minimal amount of water used to soften premade fiberglass splints. They can be placed directly under the faucet.

Protective Gear

Use gowns or sheets to prevent soilage of both the patient's and the clinician's clothing. Use gloves (vinyl or latex) and safety glasses to prevent skin or eye damage from plaster dust, wet plaster, or uncured fiberglass polymer. Wearing gloves also decreases clean-up time for the clinician.

GENERAL PROCEDURE OF CUSTOM SPLINT APPLICATION

This following text refers to the application of custom-made plaster splints unless otherwise stated (Figs. 50-3 and 50-4). If periodic wound care is required, apply a more easily removable splint (e.g., OCL, Ortho-Glass, Velcro-type splint described below) in lieu of the standard splint (Fig. 50-5). Address the issue of removability before the splint is applied. In addition, use of Webril (Curity) cast padding is described, but other suitable cast padding may be substituted. Caveats for proper ED splinting are listed in Box 50-1.

Patient Preparation

If the clinical situation permits, cover the patient with a sheet or gown to protect clothing and the surrounding area from water and plaster. Nursing staff and housekeeping also appreciate this courtesy. Properly drape hallway patients if areas of the body are exposed. Carefully inspect and examine the involved extremity before splinting, and clearly document the presence of all skin lesions and soft tissue injuries. Clean, repair, and dress all wounds in the usual manner. When open fractures or joints are to be immobilized, cover the soft tissue defect with saline-moistened sterile gauze.

Padding

When the splint involves the digits, place padding between the fingers and toes to prevent maceration of the skin. This can be done with pieces of Webril or gauze cut to the appropriate length.

Following placement of padding between the fingers and toes in self-made splints, use a stockinette over the skin as the first protective layer (see Fig. 50-3, *step 2*). Extend the stockinette at least 10 to 15 cm beyond the area to be splinted at both ends of the extremity. Later, after the plaster has been applied, fold the stockinette back over the ends of the splint to create smooth, padded rims and to help hold the splint in place when applying elastic bandages (see Fig. 50-3, *step 7*). To avoid pressure damage, do not pull the stockinette too tightly over bony prominences such as the heel. In addition, prevent wrinkling over flexion creases by slitting and overlapping the stockinette at bony prominences. One may also use two separate pieces of stockinette (one at each end of the splint) to produce the smooth padded rims. As a general rule, use 3-inch-wide stockinette for the upper extremity and 4-inch-wide stockinette for the lower extremity.

After the stockinette has been properly positioned, wrap Webril around the entire area that will be exposed to plaster. Apply at least two or three layers of Webril, with each turn overlapping the previous turn by 25% to 50% of its width (see Fig. 50-3, *step 3*). Make sure that the Webril extends 2.5 to 5.0 cm beyond the ends of the splint so that it, too, can be folded back over the splint to help create smooth, well-padded edges. Place extra padding over areas of bony prominence, such as the radial condyle or the malleoli (Box 50-2). Although this can be done with Webril, Mother's Cotton adds an additional measure of protection without the worry of wrinkling or ischemic injury. If significant swelling is anticipated, use three or four layers of Webril. Be careful to avoid wrinkling because this can result in significant skin pressure when a tight splint is worn for a long period. Prevent wrinkles by proportionately stretching or even tearing the side of the Webril that must wrap around the larger portion of an extremity. Joints that must be immobilized in a 90-degree position, such as the ankle, make continuous Webril wrapping difficult. To avoid wrinkles around the ankle, place the joint in the proper position before padding. Wrap the Webril around the malleolar and midtarsal regions first, and then cover the bare calcaneal region with overlapping vertical and horizontal Webril strips until the entire heel region is evenly padded. Use the same approach in similar areas such as the elbow. Choose a width of Webril appropriate for the extremity to be splinted. In general, use the 2-inch width for the hands and feet, the 3- or 4-inch width for the upper extremity, and the 4- or 6-inch width for the lower extremity.

A final caveat when using Webril is to be aware of the potential for ischemic injury. This rare complication is most likely to occur in an extremity that continues to have significant swelling after the patient is released from the ED. Ischemia may result because the concentrically placed Webril can become a constricting band. If this situation is anticipated, it can easily be prevented. Cut through the Webril along the side of the extremity that is opposite the plaster splint. Then, secure the splint to the extremity in the usual manner. Alternatively, place two or three layers of Webril (the same diameter as the plaster) directly over the wet plaster (see Fig. 50-4). Position the Webril-lined splint over the area to be immobilized and secure it in place with an elastic bandage.

Plaster Preparation

The choice of plaster setting time depends on the nature of the injury and the expertise of the clinician. Use extra-fast–setting plaster when rapid hardening is desired to help maintain alignment of an acutely reduced fracture. However, for the majority of ED splints, plaster with slower setting times

PLASTER SPLINT APPLICATION: STANDARD METHOD

 Measure the length of plaster to be used against the area to be splinted. Roll out the appropriate layers of plaster (roughly 8 layers for upper extremities, 12–15 for the lower).

Place a single layer of stockinette over the extremity. The stockinette should extend 10–15 cm beyond both ends of the area to be splinted. Generally, use a 3-inch stockinette for the arm, and a 4-inch for the leg.

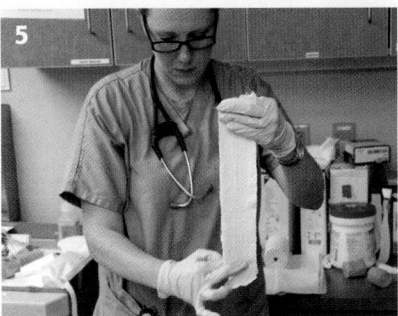 Wrap 2 to 3 layers of Webril around the entire area to be splinted, overlapping each pass by 25 to 50%. Avoid wrinkling, which may cause pressure sores. See text for precautions regarding potential ischemic injury.

Submerge the plaster strips in a bucket of water until the bubbling stops. Do not use water hotter than 24°C (75°F). Using warmer water may cause thermal injury, because the plaster releases heat when activated.

Smooth the plaster between your fingers and remove all excess water. Lay the plaster out on a table and smooth further to remove all wrinkles and ensure uniform lamination of all layers.

Apply the plaster over the Webril and smooth it over the extremity. Avoid using your fingertips, which may leave indentations in the plaster. A layer of Webril may be placed over the plaster to prevent it from sticking to the elastic wrap.

Fold the stockinette over the edge of the plaster and Webril. This helps to hold the splint in place, and provides a smooth padded edge.

Secure the splint to the extremity with an elastic wrap by proceeding in a distal-to-proximal fashion. Do not wrap the elastic bandage too tightly.

If metal clips are used to secure the elastic wrap, cover them with tape to prevent them from falling off. Alternatively, the wrap can simply be secured with tape.

Place the extremity in the desired position, and use the palms of your hands to mold the splint to the contour of the extremity. Again, avoid using your fingertips, which may leave indentations that result in pressure sores.

Figure 50-3 Plaster splint application: standard method (volar wrist splint depicted here).

PLASTER SPLINT APPLICATION: ALTERNATIVE METHOD

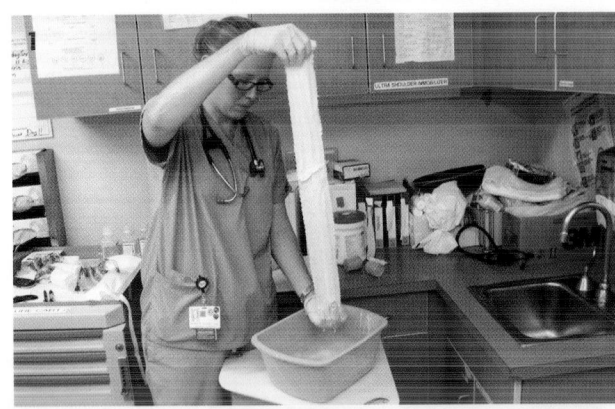

Measure the splint and apply stockinette as depicted in steps 1 and 2 of Figure 50-3. Additionally, premeasure 5 to 6 layers of Webril of the same length as the plaster. Soak and prepare the plaster.

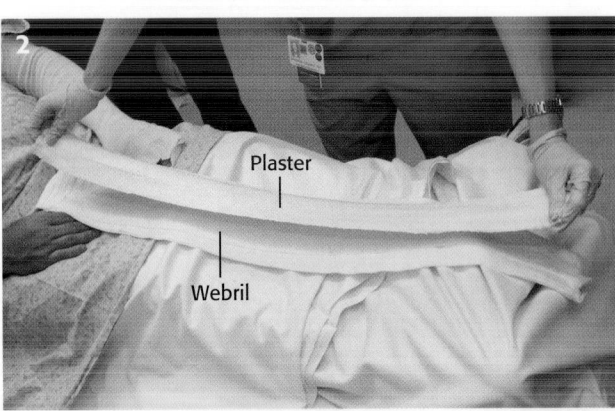

Lay out 3 to 4 layers of Webril, which will serve as padding for the splint. Place the plaster (which has already been smoothed) on top of these layers of Webril.

Place an additional layer of Webril on top of the plaster, which will prevent it from sticking to the elastic wrap. Essentially, you are sandwiching the plaster between layers of Webril.

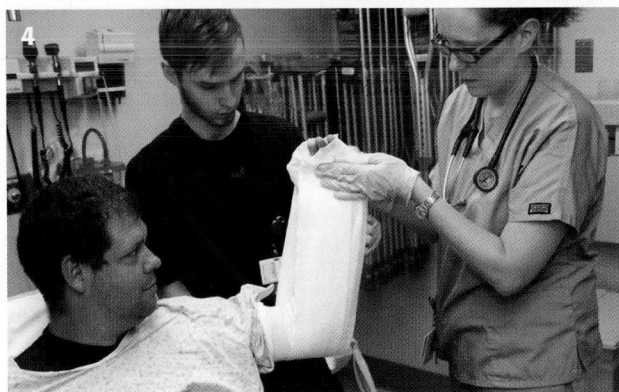

Apply the splint to the extremity. Enlist the help of an assistant to hold the splint in place.

Secure the splint to the extremity with elastic bandages by wrapping in a distal-to-proximal fashion. Remember to fold the stockinette over the edges of the plaster and Webril.

Position the extremity as desired, and then gently mold the splint using the palms of your hands.

Figure 50-4 Plaster splint application: alternative method (sugar-tong splint depicted here). This technique may be used if significant swelling is anticipated since Webril (the same diameter as the plaster) is placed directly over the wet plaster rather than wrapped circumferentially around the extremity.

PREFABRICATED FIBERGLASS SPLINT APPLICATION

Measure the length of splint to be used against the area to be splinted. These splints are available in a variety of lengths and widths.

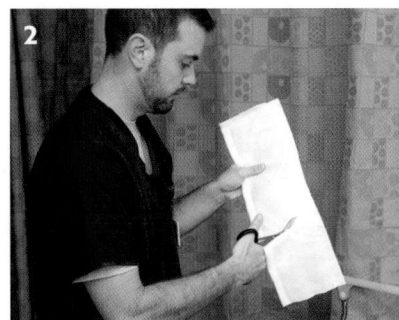

Cut the splint to length using a pair of trauma shears. Round the corners of the cuts to avoid sharp edges of fiberglass.

Padding

Fiberglass

Stretch the cotton padding several inches beyond the edge of the fiberglass on both ends of the splint to assure that there will be no fiberglass in contact with the skin.

Prefabricated fiberglass splints require minimal wetting. Simply open one end of the pouch and run tap water over the fiberglass. When water exits the bottom, it is ready to apply. Excess water may be wrung out.

Apply the splint to the extremity. If stockinette is used (optional though recommended), fold the edges of the stockinette over the splint. This provides comfort and also holds the splint in place during application.

Secure the splint to the extremity using elastic bandages wrapped in a distal-to-proximal fashion.

For splints that involve the hand, cut a hole in the center of the elastic bandage, in the loop that is in the region of the thumb.

Bring the thumb through the hole. This provides a perfect fit, reduces bunching of the elastic in the web space, and allows for more thumb mobility.

Place the extremity in the desired position, and mold the splint with your palms to the contours of the body. Avoid using fingertips, which may leave indentations in the fiberglass.

After splint application, observe for vascular compromise or increased patient discomfort. If either occur, loosen the elastic wrap. Never discharge a patient with increasing pain after splint application.

Figure 50-5 Prefabricated fiberglass splint application (volar wrist splint depicted here).

- Always use cool, clean water.
- Do not oversaturate the plaster splint. Minimal water is required for fiberglass splints.
- Make the splint *smooth* when placing it on the patient to avoid bumps and pressure points.
- Smooth and mold the splint without squeezing. Use the palms of the hands, not the fingers, to mold the splint to fit the contour of the body part.
- Place padded side against the skin. Extra cotton padding is optimal.
- Simply roll elastic bandages over the extremity without undue tension.
- Protect or pad the edges.
- Leave the fingertips exposed to check for circulation and sensation.
- Keep the patient still until the splint has dried and hardened.
- The postsplint check includes function, arterial pulse, capillary refill, temperature of the skin, and sensation (FACTS).
- Emphasize and demonstrate splint elevation to the patient.
- Tape over metal clips used to fasten the elastic bandage to keep it in place and avoid ingestion by a child.

ED, *emergency department.*

BOX 50-2 **Areas of the Upper and Lower Extremity That Require Additional Padding**

UPPER EXTREMITY
Olecranon
Radial styloid
Ulnar styloid

LOWER EXTREMITY
Upper portion of the inner aspect of the thigh
Patella
Fibular head
Achilles tendon
Medial and lateral malleoli

TABLE 50-1 Setting Times of Fast- and Extra-Fast–Drying Plaster

PLASTER	SETTING TIME (min)
Fast drying	5-8
Extra-fast drying	2-4

BOX 50-3 **Effect of Water Temperature and Different Additives on the Setting Time of Plaster**

ACCELERATES SETTING TIME	SLOWS SETTING TIME
Reusing the dip water	Cool dip water
Higher dip water temperature	Glue
Salicylic acid	Gum
Zinc	Borax
Magnesium	
Copper	
Iron	
Aluminum	
Salt	
Alum	

(e.g., Specialist Plaster Bandage Fast Setting) is recommended.[11] Plaster that sets more slowly is easier for some clinicians to use because it affords more leeway in applying and molding the splint. Furthermore, plaster with a longer setting time produces less heat, thus reducing both patient discomfort and the risk for serious burns.[12] Table 50-1 lists the setting times for commonly used plaster. These setting times can be adjusted by adding different substances to the plaster during the production process (Box 50-3). Given plaster with equal setting times, the most important variable affecting the rate of crystallization is water temperature. Warm water hardens a splint faster than cold water does and should not be used when extra time is needed for splint application.

The ideal length and width of plaster depend on the body part to be splinted and the degree of immobilization required. The best way to estimate length is to lay the dry splint next to the area to be splinted. It is best to use a generous length because wet plaster shrinks slightly from its dry length. Also, if the wet splint is too long, the ends can be folded back easily. Plaster width varies according to the type of splint being made and the body part that is injured, but generally, it should be slightly greater than the diameter of the limb to be splinted. Specific recommendations regarding splint length and width are discussed in the sections describing individual splints.

The thickness of a splint depends on the size of the patient, the extremity that is injured, and the desired strength of the final product. An ankle splint may crack quickly and become useless if only eight layers are used, but this thickness may be ideal for a wrist splint. In general, it is best to use the minimum number of layers necessary to achieve adequate strength. Thicker splints are heavier and more uncomfortable. It is also important to note that plaster thickness is a major determinant of the amount of heat given off during the setting process. More than 12 sheets of plaster create an increased risk for significant burns, especially when using extra-fast–drying plaster, when using dipping water with a temperature higher than 24°C, or when a pillow is placed under or around the extremity for support during the setting process (Box 50-4). For an average-sized adult, splint the upper extremities with 8 sheets of plaster and the lower extremities with 12 to 15 sheets. Such layering usually provides the strength necessary for adequate immobilization while reducing the patient's discomfort and the risk for significant burns. In a 136-kg (300-lb) patient, however, up to 20 layers may be required to make a durable ankle splint.

Keep the dipping water clean and fresh. Reusing water that has been used previously for wetting plaster increases the amount of heat given off during crystallization and causes the plaster to set more quickly. As a rule of thumb, keep the temperature of the water around 24°C. This temperature allows a workable setting time and has not been associated with increased risk for significant burns. As the temperature of the dipping water approaches 40°C, the potential for serious burns increases, even with splint thicknesses consisting of fewer than 12 plies. It is interesting to note that water temperature has been shown to be only a minor consideration in heat production in some studies (see Box 50-4).

Splint Application (see Fig. 50-3)

Completely submerge the dry splint in the water bucket until the bubbling stops. Remove the splint and gently squeeze out excess water until the plaster has a wet and sloppy consistency. Place the splint on a hard table or countertop (a protective covering is recommended to prevent water or plaster damage) and smooth out the splint (with gloved hands) to remove any wrinkles and ensure uniform lamination of all layers. Lamination helps increase the final strength of the splint. Position the splint over the Webril and gently smooth it over the extremity. Plaster is usually somewhat adherent to Webril, but an assistant may be required to hold the splint in place during positioning. Once the splint has been properly positioned over the extremity, fold back the underlying stockinette and Webril to help hold it in place. Secure the splint with an appropriately sized elastic bandage by wrapping in a distal-to-proximal direction. Finally, place the extremity in the desired position and mold the wet plaster to the contour of the extremity with only the palms of the hand. Finger indentations may cause ridges, which can produce pressure points.

Molding the wet splint to conform to the body's anatomy is probably the most important, yet the most frequently overlooked step to ensure adequate immobilization. The act of molding may cause some pain, so be sure to forewarn the patient. Mold with the palm or flat side of the fingers to avoid putting ridges or indentations in the underlying plaster. Complete all manipulation of the wet plaster before it reaches a thick, creamy consistency. Any movement after this time, which is known as the critical period, results in an imperfect crystalline network of calcium sulfate molecules and greatly weakens the ultimate strength of the splint. *While the plaster is setting, do not wrap a pillow or blanket around the extremity for support*. This leads to inadequate ventilation around the splint and greatly increases the amount of heat produced (see Box 50-4).

If an elastic bandage is applied directly over wet plaster, it may be incorporated into the drying plaster, thus making subsequent removal of the bandage difficult. To make it easier for patients to remove and reapply the splint, wrap a single layer of Webril or roll gauze around the wet plaster loosely before applying the elastic bandage. This prevents the wet plaster from becoming stuck to the elastic bandage. Use only one layer of Webril over the plaster because multiple layers are associated with high drying temperatures.

Before the patient is released from the ED, check the extremity for adequate immobilization and evaluate the patient for any evidence of vascular compromise or significant discomfort. If either occurs, loosen the elastic bandage. If the discomfort persists, place additional padding over the painful areas. If this measure, too, is unsuccessful, make a new splint while paying special attention to proper molding so that the wet plaster does not become indented. By resting tender tissue, splinting usually relieves the discomfort quickly, and patients generally say that they feel better soon after the splint has been applied. In general, a splint should decrease the patient's pain, not increase it; hence, *do not readily release a patient who complains of increased pain after a splint has been placed*. Such complaints may be due to manipulation during splinting, but increased pain should be further addressed or explained.

After a properly fitting, comfortable splint has been applied, place two strips of tape along each side of the splint to prevent the elastic bandage from slipping. It is also prudent to place tape over any metal fasteners used to secure the elastic bandages because these objects can fall off and be swallowed or aspirated by infants and small children. Use enough tape to include the entire circumference of the area under the fasteners, not just small pieces of tape that may not adhere to the moist splint. Finally, provide a sling for patients with upper extremity injuries and, if required, crutches (and instructions for their proper use) for those with lower extremity injuries.

Patient Instructions

Give patients both verbal and written instructions on splint care and precautions. Stress the importance of elevation in helping to decrease pain and swelling. Demonstrate this as well because most patients do not understand the medical definition of elevation. At night, wrap and secure a pillow around the injured extremity to help the patient keep it satisfactorily elevated. If the injury is less than 24 hours old, encourage the application of ice bags or cold packs. It is useless to apply cold packs over plaster, but it can be beneficial to apply them over Webril or an elastic bandage directly over an injury. It may be necessary to remove the splint to ice the injury. In theory, cold therapy stiffens collagen and thus reduces the tendency for ligaments and tendons to deform. Cold therapy also decreases muscle spasm and excitability, reduces blood flow (thereby limiting hemorrhage and edema), raises the pain threshold, and decreases inflammation. Because the thermal conductivity of subcutaneous tissue is poor, apply cold packs for at least 30 minutes at a time. This guideline is in contrast to the popular recommendation of "ice 20 minutes on, 20 minutes off," which often does nothing more than cool the skin. Do not use cold packs for more than the first 24 to 48 hours because cold can interfere with long-term healing. Instruct the patient to not stress the splint for at least 24 hours because plaster does not approach optimal strength until evaporation has reduced the water content of the plaster to approximately 21% of its initial hydrated level. This process of removing excess water by evaporation is called *curing*, and it generally takes several days to be completed. However, by 24 hours the water content of the plaster has usually been reduced enough to produce a strong, resilient splint. In addition, because the chemical process involved in the formation of plaster is reversible, the patient should avoid getting the splint wet. If the injury permits, the splint can be removed for showering and then reapplied. Alternatively, one or more plastic bags may be placed over a splint before showering.

Splints may crack, break, or disintegrate with wear, and such a useless splint should be removed or replaced. Give patients general guidelines for length of immobilization and appropriate follow-up care. Avoid long-term immobilization, particularly in the elderly, because this can produce permanent disability. It is extremely important for the patient to continue to check for signs of vascular compromise. If the patient experiences a significant increase in pain, numbness or tingling of the digits, pallor of the distal end of the extremity, decreased capillary refill, or weakness, instruct the patient to return to the ED or to see his or her primary clinician without delay. As with casting, increased pain after splinting is a warning sign that should prompt a return visit—not telephone advice. Avoid giving excessive doses of opioids during the first 2 to 3 days after splinting to allow pain to prompt a follow-up visit.

UPPER EXTREMITY SPLINTS

Long Arm Splints

Long Arm Posterior Splint
Indications. Use a long arm posterior splint (Figs. 50-6 and 50-7) to immobilize injuries to the elbow and proximal end of the forearm. It completely eliminates flexion and extension of the elbow but does not entirely prevent pronation and supination of the forearm. Therefore, it is not recommended for immobilization of complex or unstable distal forearm fractures unless used in conjunction with a long arm anterior splint (see later in this section). Alternatively, a double "sugartong" splint can be applied (see later in this section).

Construction. Construct a long arm posterior splint with 8 to 10 layers of 4- or 6-inch-wide plaster. Start the splint on the posterior aspect of the proximal end of the arm. Extend it down the arm to the elbow and then along the ulnar aspect of the forearm and hand to the level of the metacarpophalangeal (MCP) joints.

Application. Apply a stockinette and Webril as described previously. Cut a hole in the stockinette to expose the thumb, and place extra padding over the olecranon to prevent pressure injury. Position the arm with the elbow flexed to 90

degrees, the forearm neutral (thumb upward), and the wrist neutral or slightly extended (10 to 20 degrees). Ask an assistant to hold the wet splint in place, particularly when applying both a posterior and an anterior splint. Once the splint has been properly positioned, fold the ends of the stockinette and Webril back and secure the splint in place with 2-, 3-, or 4-inch elastic bandages. Finally, fold the sides of the splint up to create a gutter configuration and carefully mold the plaster around the extremity with the palms of the hand. The fingers and thumb should remain free to prevent stiffness from unnecessary immobilization.

Long Arm Anterior Splint
Indications. A long arm anterior splint is never used alone but, rather, as an adjunct to a long arm posterior splint to improve immobilization by increasing stability and preventing pronation and supination of the forearm (see Fig. 50-6B).

Construction. Construct a long arm anterior splint in the same manner as described for a long arm posterior splint. It mirrors the posterior splint by running down the anterior aspect of the arm to the antecubital fossa, where it continues along the radial aspect of the forearm to the distal end of the radius.

Application. Use stockinette, Webril, and positioning similar to the way it was described for application of a long arm posterior splint. When using both an anterior and a posterior long arm splint, have an assistant available to hold the wet splint in place. Place the anterior splint first and then position the posterior splint. Once both splints have been properly positioned, fold the ends of the stockinette and Webril back and secure the splint in place with 2-, 3-, or 4-inch elastic bandages. Finally, fold up the sides of the splint to create a gutter configuration and carefully mold the plaster around the extremity with the palms of the hands. Keep the patient's fingers and thumb free to prevent stiffness from unnecessary immobilization.

Double Sugar-Tong Splint
Indications. Use a double sugar-tong splint (Fig. 50-8) like a long arm posterior splint to immobilize injuries to the elbow and forearm. However, because it prevents pronation and supination of the forearm, it is preferable for some distal forearm and elbow fractures.

Construction. The splint consists of two separate pieces of plaster, a forearm splint and an arm splint. Construct each piece with eight layers of 3- or 4-inch plaster. The forearm portion of the splint runs from the metacarpal heads on the dorsum of the hand along the dorsal surface of the forearm around the elbow. It continues along the volar surface of the forearm to the palm of the hand and stops at the level of the MCP joints. The arm portion of the splint begins on the anterior aspect of the proximal end of the humerus. It runs down the arm over the forearm splint and around the elbow. It then continues up the posterior aspect of the arm, once again going over the forearm splint, until it reaches the starting point.

Application. Use a stockinette, Webril, and positioning similar to the way it was described for the application of a long arm posterior splint. Secure the two splints in place with 2-, 3-, or 4-inch elastic bandages starting with the forearm splint at the hand. Once the forearm splint is secured in place,

LONG ARM POSTERIOR SPLINT

Application

A, Extend the splint from the posterior aspect of the humerus to the elbow and then along the ulnar aspect of the forearm to the distal metacarpals. Flex the elbow to 90°, maintain the forearm in the neutral (thumb-up) position, and place the wrist in a neutral or slightly extended (10° to 20°) position.
B, An anterior splint that mirrors the posterior splint may be used to increase stability and prevent supination and pronation. An anterior splint is never used alone.

Indications

Injuries of the elbow and distal end of the forearm, including:
Distal humerus fractures (shown above)
Supracondylar fractures
Olecranon fractures
Elbow dislocations

Figure 50-6 Long arm posterior splint.

Figure 50-7 When preparing a splint (such as a long arm splint) that involves a right angle, cut out a notch (*arrow*) to allow a smooth bend. Note that padding needs to be applied before splinting.

wrap the arm portion of the splint beginning at its proximal end. Keep the patient's fingers and thumb free to prevent stiffness.

Forearm and Hand Splints

Volar Splint

Indications. Use a volar splint (Fig. 50-9) to immobilize a variety of soft tissue injuries to the hand and wrist. It is also used for temporary immobilization of triquetral fractures,

lunate and perilunate dislocations, and second through fifth metacarpal head fractures. For these more serious injuries, some clinicians prefer to add a dorsal splint to create a more stable bivalve effect (see Fig. 50-9*B*). Because a volar splint does not completely eliminate pronation and supination of the forearm, it may not be ideal for distal radial and ulnar fractures, although many clinicians use this splint for nondisplaced or minimally displaced distal ulnar and radial fractures.

Construction. Construct the splint with 8 to 10 layers of 3- or 4-inch-wide plaster. The splint begins in the palm at the metacarpal heads and extends along the volar surface of the forearm to just proximal to the elbow. If there is an injury to any of the fingers, extend the splint to incorporate the involved digit or digits.

Application. Apply a stockinette and Webril as described previously. Cut a hole in the stockinette to expose the thumb. If the splint is going to incorporate one or more digits, insert a piece of Webril or gauze between the digits to prevent skin maceration. Place the forearm in the neutral position (thumb upward) with the wrist extended slightly (10 to 20 degrees). Avoid wrist flexion. After properly positioning the wet plaster, fold back the ends of the stockinette and Webril and use a 3- or 4-inch elastic bandage to secure the splint in place. Fold the sides of the splint up around the forearm to create a gutter effect, and carefully mold the plaster to conform to the contours of the palm and wrist. Some clinicians prefer to extend the splint to the fingertips and then fold the wet plaster back

DOUBLE SUGAR-TONG SPLINT

Olecranon
fracture

Application

Apply the forearm portion of the double sugar-tong splint first. Begin the splint at the metacarpal heads on the dorsum of the hand, and then extend it along the dorsal surface of the forearm and around the elbow. Continue along the volar surface of the forearm and stop at the level of the metacarpophalangeal joints.

Begin the arm portion on the medial aspect of the proximal part of the arm, and then run it down over the forearm splint and around the elbow. Continue up the lateral aspect of the arm (once again going over the forearm splint) until it reaches the starting point.

Keep the elbow flexed at 90°, the forearm in the neutral (thumb-up) position, and the wrist in a neutral or slightly extended (10° to 20°) position. Allow the fingers and thumb to remain free to avoid stiffness.

Indications

Injuries of the elbow and distal part of the forearm, including:
 Distal humerus fractures
 Supracondylar fractures
 Olecranon fractures (shown above)
 Elbow dislocations

Indications are similar to the those for the long arm splint. Since the double sugar-tong splint prevents supination and pronation, it may be preferable for some fractures of the distal humerus and of the forearm and elbow.

Figure 50-8 Double sugar-tong splint.

toward the palm, which allows the fingers to "grasp" the rounded distal end when at rest. With either method, keep the thumb and fingers free to move unless they are injured and are being intentionally immobilized by the splint.

Sugar-Tong Splint
Indications. Use a sugar-tong splint (Fig. 50-10) for fractures of the distal end of the radius and ulna. The advantage of this splint over a volar splint is prevention of pronation and supination of the forearm. In addition, it immobilizes the elbow, which is desirable for the first few days after a distal forearm fracture.

Construction and Application. Construct and apply this splint in the same manner as the forearm portion of the double sugar-tong splint described earlier.

Thumb Spica Splint
Indications. Use a thumb spica splint (Fig. 50-11) to immobilize injuries and fractures of the scaphoid, lunate, thumb, and first metacarpal. It is also used for the treatment of de Quervain's tenosynovitis. Traditionally, a thumb spica splint or cast was thought to be a requirement for properly

immobilizing scaphoid fractures; however, there is no totally agreed standard. Clay and coworkers[13] stated that the optimal method of casting scaphoid fractures has not been definitively established. They were unable to prove a difference in patient comfort, recovery of function, or incidence of nonunion between a Colles cast and a traditional scaphoid cast that included the thumb.

The incidence of nonunion of scaphoid fractures is about 10%, regardless of the type of immobilization in the ED, but it is greatest with unstable proximal pole fractures. Because some scaphoid fractures heal poorly under the best of circumstances, it seems prudent to provide thumb immobilization in the initial splinting. Failure to do so, such as when a "sprained wrist" is suspected, should not be construed as being beneath the accepted standard of care. Most volar splints will at least partly immobilize the base of the thumb, so the discussion may be moot.

Construction. Construct the splint with eight layers of 3-inch-wide plaster. Extend the splint from just distal to the interphalangeal joint of the thumb to the midforearm level.

Application. Place the forearm in the neutral position with the wrist extended 25 degrees and the thumb in the wineglass

VOLAR SPLINT

Triquetral fracture

Application

A, Begin the splint in the palm at the metacarpal heads and extend it along the volar surface of the forearm to a point just proximal to the elbow. If any of the fingers are injured, extend the splint to incorporate the involved digits. Place the forearm in the neutral (thumb-up) position with the wrist slightly extended (10° to 20°). Wrist flexion should be avoided.

B, For more serious injuries, add an additional dorsal slab to create a bivalve splint.

Indications

Soft tissue injuries of the hand and wrist
Orthopedic injuries of the hand and wrist, including:
   Triquetral fractures (shown above)
   Lunate and perilunate dislocations
   Second through fifth metacarpal head fractures
   Minimally displaced distal radius and ulna fractures

The volar splint does not eliminate supination and pronation of the forearm and therefore is not ideal for more complicated distal radius and ulna fractures.

Figure 50-9 Volar splint.

FOREARM SUGAR-TONG SPLINT

Distal radiu fracture

Application

Begin the splint at the metacarpal heads on the dorsum of the hand, extend it along the dorsal surface of the forearm, and then around the elbow. Continue along the volar surface of the forearm and stop at the level of the metacarpophalangeal joints.

Keep the elbow flexed at a 90° angle, the forearm in the neutral (thumb-up) position, and the wrist in a neutral position or slightly extended (10° to 20°).

Indications

Distal radius and ulna fractures (shown above)
Distal forearm fractures

The forearm sugar-tong splint, unlike the volar wrist splint, prevents supination and pronation of the forearm. Additionally, it immobilizes the elbow, which is desirable for the first few days after a distal forearm fracture.

Figure 50-10 Forearm sugar-tong splint.

THUMB SPICA SPLINT

Scaphoid
fracture

Application

Extend the splint from just distal to the interphalangeal joint of the thumb to the midforearm level.

Place the forearm in the neutral position with the wrist extended 25° and the thumb in the wineglass position (see Fig. 50-12).

Inset: Make a small (1- to 2-cm) perpendicular cut 1 cm distal to the first metacarpophalangeal joint on each edge of the plaster to allow molding of the splint around the thumb without creating a buckle in the plaster.

Indications

Scaphoid fractures (shown above)
Lunate, thumb, and first metacarpal fractures
de Quervain tenosynovitis

Figure 50-11 Thumb spica splint.

position (Fig. 50-12). Apply a stockinette and Webril from the base of the palm to the midforearm level. It is difficult to place a stockinette around the thumb. Instead, cut a hole in the stockinette to expose the thumb, and then pad the exposed thumb with small vertical strips of Webril or wrap it with 2-inch Webril. Place the dry plaster over the radial aspect of the forearm from just beyond the thumb interphalangeal joint to the midforearm level. Once in position, mark the location of the first MCP joint and make a small (1- to 2-cm) perpendicular cut 1 cm distal to the mark on each edge of the plaster (see Fig. 50-11 *inset*). This allows the splint to be molded around the thumb without creating a buckle in the plaster. If the plaster distal to the cut notches is too wide to mold around the thumb without overlapping, trim the edges to the desired width. Wet the plaster and secure it in place with a 2- or 3-inch elastic bandage. It is important to carefully mold the wet plaster around the thumb and palm and to maintain the thumb in the wineglass position while the plaster is drying.

Ulnar Collateral Ligament Injury (Gamekeeper's or Skier's Thumb)

Forced abduction with hyperextension of the thumb is the usual mechanism for injury to the ulnar collateral ligament. This is a rather disabling injury that requires early recognition since improper treatment can result in chronic pain, pinch weakness, and loss of stability of the thumb. Characterized by MCP joint pain, tenderness of the ulnar side, and laxity of this joint with valgus stressing, this is not a simple sprain. Although

immobilization with a thumb spica splint or figure-of-eight thumb splint may suffice as definitive treatment (Fig. 50-13), surgery is often recommended for more advanced injuries. Splinting in the ED with referral to a consultant is prudent for all significant thumb soft tissue injuries consistent with an ulnar collateral ligament injury.

Ulnar Gutter Splint

Indications. Use an ulnar gutter splint (Fig. 50-14) to immobilize fractures and serious soft tissue injuries of the little and ring fingers and fractures of the neck, shaft, and base of the fourth and fifth metacarpals.

Construction. Make the splint with six to eight layers of 3- or 4-inch plaster. It incorporates both the little and the ring fingers. It runs along the ulnar aspect of the forearm from just beyond the distal interphalangeal joint of the little finger to the midforearm level.

Application. Apply a stockinette and Webril as usual. Place additional Webril or gauze between the little and ring fingers to prevent maceration of the skin. Position the forearm in the neutral position with the wrist in slight extension (10 to 20 degrees), the MCP joints in 50 degrees of flexion, and the proximal and distal interphalangeal joints in slight flexion (10 to 15 degrees). When immobilizing a metacarpal neck fracture (i.e., boxer's fracture), flex the MCP joint to 90 degrees. Once in proper position, fold the sides of the splint up to form a gutter. Finally, fold the ends of the stockinette and Webril

Figure 50-12 A, The wineglass position, also termed the position of function, is a safe splint position for the hand and fingers for short-term splinting (7 to 14 days). The wrist should allow alignment of the thumb with the forearm, the metacarpophalangeal (MCP) joint should be moderately flexed, and the interphalangeal joints should be only slightly flexed. The thumb should be abducted away from the palm. **B,** For longer splinting, the fingers should be extended to prevent flexion contractures. This is referred to as the intrinsic position. The MCP joint is flexed at 90 degrees. Either **A** or **B** is an acceptable position for initial splinting in the emergency department.

back to help hold the splint in place while it is secured to the extremity with a 2- or 3-inch elastic bandage.

Radial Gutter Splint
Indications. Use a radial gutter splint (Fig. 50-15) to immobilize fractures and serious soft tissue injuries of the index and long fingers and fractures of the neck, shaft, and base of the second and third metacarpals.

Construction. Make the splint with six to eight layers of 3- or 4-inch plaster. It runs along the radial aspect of the forearm from just beyond the distal interphalangeal joint of the index finger to the midforearm level.

Application. Apply a stockinette (with a hole cut to expose the thumb) and Webril as described previously. Insert an additional piece of Webril or gauze between the index and long fingers to prevent maceration of the skin. Place the hand and fingers in the *position of function* or in the *intrinsic position* (see Fig. 50-12). Neither position has been proved to be superior for the first few weeks of splinting, which makes them both acceptable for initial immobilization in the ED. In the position of function, the forearm is in the neutral position with the wrist in slight extension (10 to 20 degrees), the MCP joints in 50 to 60 degrees of flexion, and the proximal and distal interphalangeal joints in slight flexion (5 to 10 degrees) (see Fig. 50-12*A*). When immobilizing a metacarpal neck fracture, the intrinsic position is often used, with the MCP joint flexed to 90 degrees and the fingers extended (see Fig. 50-12*B*).

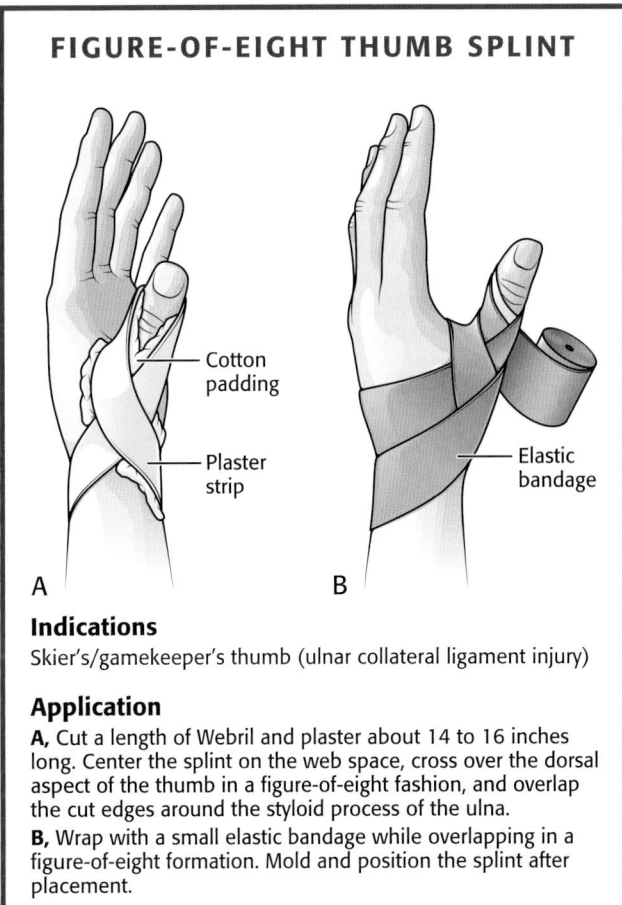

FIGURE-OF-EIGHT THUMB SPLINT

Indications
Skier's/gamekeeper's thumb (ulnar collateral ligament injury)

Application
A, Cut a length of Webril and plaster about 14 to 16 inches long. Center the splint on the web space, cross over the dorsal aspect of the thumb in a figure-of-eight fashion, and overlap the cut edges around the styloid process of the ulna.
B, Wrap with a small elastic bandage while overlapping in a figure-of-eight formation. Mold and position the splint after placement.

Figure 50-13 Figure-of-eight thumb splint.

Place the dry plaster over the extremity and mark the location of the thumb. Cut a hole in the dry plaster to expose the thumb. Dip the plaster and position the wet splint over the extremity. Fold back the ends of the stockinette and Webril to help hold the splint in place and secure it to the extremity with a 2- or 3-inch elastic bandage.

Finger Splints
Use finger splints for sprains, fractures, tendon repairs, or infections. Minor finger sprains can often be managed with dynamic splinting (e.g., buddy taping) (Fig. 50-16*A*) or a commercially available foam splint with aluminum backing (one-surface splint) (see Fig. 50-16*B*), but fractures, tendon repairs, and some soft tissue injuries benefit from formal splinting (e.g., thumb spica and ulnar and radial gutter splints). Specific conditions, such as mallet finger, require a specialized splint (plaster or Stack splint) (see Fig. 50-16*C*). When complete immobilization of a finger is required (e.g., unstable phalangeal fractures), an "outrigger" finger splint that incorporates the wrist may be used (see Fig. 50-16*D*). Both the position of function and the intrinsic position are acceptable for initial splinting.

Pitfalls of Hand Dressings and Splints
The two most common problems with hand dressings and splints are putting them on too tightly and leaving them on too long (Table 50-2). One must be especially careful to avoid wrapping elastic bandages too snugly. Before discharge from the ED, instruct patients to loosen an elastic bandage if it feels

ULNAR GUTTER SPLINT

Fifth metacarpal
(boxer's) fracture

Application

The ulnar gutter splint incorporates both the little and the ring fingers. Therefore, place Webril or gauze between the digits to prevent maceration of the skin. Run the splint along the ulnar aspect of the forearm from just beyond the distal interphalangeal joint of the little finger to the midforearm level.

Maintain the forearm in the neutral position with the wrist in slight extension (10° to 20°), the metacarpophalangeal (MCP) joint in 50° of flexion, and the proximal and distal interphalangeal joints in slight flexion (10° to 15°). When immobilizing a metacarpal neck fracture, flex the MCP joint to 90°.

Indications

Injuries of the ulnar side of the hand, including:
    Fourth and fifth metacarpal fractures (shown above)
    Serious injuries of the ring and little fingers

Figure 50-14 Ulnar gutter splint.

too tight, and be sure that they have access to emergency follow-up care. It is often advisable to start patients on a regimen of early protected motion. This means that the patient removes the splint for a specified period, performs a prescribed exercise, and then replaces the splint. A splint is not an all-or-none device, and the patient is generally weaned from it slowly before it is discarded entirely. A stiff hand is a nonfunctional one, and stiffness is often a consequence of prolonged immobilization. It is important for patients to be made aware of their responsibility for the injured hand.

Sling, Swathe and Sling, and Shoulder Immobilizer

Sling

Use a sling to maintain elevation and provide immobilization of the hand, forearm, and elbow (Fig. 50-17). It is most often used in conjunction with a plaster splint or cast. A number of commercial slings are available to choose from. Many of them are fairly economical and simple to use, whereas others are more expensive and do not allow the versatility of a simple, inexpensive triangular muslin bandage. When applying a sling, make it long enough to adequately support the wrist and hand. A sling that is too short will allow the wrist and hand to hang down (ulnar deviate) and can result in ulnar nerve injury.

Swathe and Sling

Use of a swathe and sling is the treatment of choice for most proximal humeral fractures and shoulder injuries, such as reduced dislocations. The sling supports the weight of the arm, and the swathe immobilizes the arm against the chest wall to minimize shoulder motion.

Shoulder Immobilizer

In most EDs the swathe and sling have been replaced by commercially available shoulder immobilizers. Its advantage is that it may be removed for showering and range-of-motion exercises and is easily reapplied by the patient (a desirable option in the care of a shoulder dislocation). If the shoulder immobilizer is used for more than a few days, pad the axilla to absorb moisture and decrease skin chafing.

A Velpeau bandage is a sling and swathe device that positions the forearm diagonally rather than horizontally across the chest with the hand elevated to the level of the shoulder. It offers no particular advantage over a standard sling and swathe, is difficult to apply, cannot be removed easily, and is not well tolerated with prolonged immobilization.

Figure-of-Eight Clavicle Strap

In the past, clavicle fractures were often treated with an uncomfortable and complex figure-of-eight bandage. Despite

RADIAL GUTTER SPLINT

Second metacarpal fracture

Application

The radial gutter splint incorporates both the index and the long fingers. Therefore, Webril or gauze should be placed between the digits to prevent maceration of the skin. Run the splint along the radial aspect of the forearm from just beyond the distal interphalangeal joint of the index finger to the midforearm.

Maintain the forearm in the neutral position with the wrist in slight extension (10°–20°), the MCP joint in 50° of flexion, and the proximal and distal interphalangeal joints in slight flexion (10°–15°). When immobilizing a metacarpal neck fracture, flex the MCP joint to 90°.

Indications

Injuries on the radial side of the hand, including:
  Second and third metacarpal fractures (shown above)
  Serious injuries to the index and middle fingers

Figure 50-15 Radial gutter splint.

its early popularity, this device never proved to be superior to a simple sling (in terms of cosmesis, functional outcome, or pain relief).[14,15] Moreover, use of a figure-of-eight clavicle strap may actually promote nonunion or increase the deformity at the fracture site. When compared with a simple sling, a figure-of-eight clavicle strap is very uncomfortable, prohibits bathing, often causes chafing and discomfort in the axilla, and may predispose to axillary vein thrombosis.[4] Thus, most emergency clinicians have abandoned the figure-of-eight dressing in favor of a simple sling, which is sufficient to treat most clavicular fractures.

LOWER EXTREMITY SPLINTS

Knee Splints

Knee Immobilizer

Indications.   A knee immobilizer (Fig. 50-18) is commonly used for mild to moderate ligamentous and soft tissue injuries involving the knee. It is removable and extremely easy to apply, which makes it popular among patients and clinicians alike. In most EDs it has replaced the more bulky plaster splint. Its use should be restricted to injuries that do not require immediate surgical intervention, traction, or casting. For these injuries, in which temporary but more complete immobilization is needed, use a plaster knee splint because it

provides better stabilization and costs much less than a knee immobilizer. The exact scientific benefit of a knee immobilizer is poorly studied and difficult to document. However, it clearly helps relieve pain and, at least theoretically, hastens healing.

Application.   Knee immobilizers are available in small, medium, large, and extra-large sizes. To choose the appropriate size, place the knee immobilizer next to the injured leg so that the tapered end lies distal to the patient's knee; if present, the cutout patellar area on the anterior aspect of the splint lies adjacent to the knee joint. In this position, the splint should extend distally to within a few inches of the malleoli and proximally to just below the buttocks crease. To apply the knee immobilizer, slide the open splint under the injured leg, wrap it around the extremity, and secure it in place with the Velcro straps. A knee immobilizer can be applied directly over clothing, thus obviating the need to remove or cut the patient's pants.

Posterior Knee Splint

Indications.   In many EDs the knee immobilizer has virtually replaced the plaster knee splint for mild to moderate injuries to the knee. However, a plaster knee splint can be particularly useful in patients whose extremities are too large for a knee immobilizer, in the treatment of angulated fractures, or for temporarily immobilizing injuries that require

FINGER SPLINTING TECHNIQUES

A. Buddy Taping

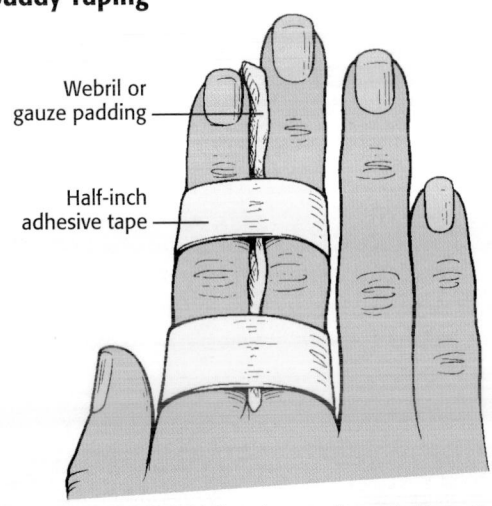

Webril or gauze padding

Half-inch adhesive tape

Taping between the digital joints (toes or fingers) allows the normal adjacent finger to protect the collateral ligament of its injured neighbor. Place Webril between the digits to prevent maceration of the skin.

B. Dorsal Aluminum Foam Splint

The bone is subcutaneous dorsally, and splints here afford better immobilization of the digit. The dorsal splint also allows preservation and use of tactile sense, which encourages function and better splint acceptance on the part of the patient.

C. Mallet Finger Splints

D. "Outrigger" Finger Splint

Foam finger splint with aluminum backing

Finger splint sandwiched between layers of plaster

Top: The dorsal splint immobilizes only the distal interphalangeal joint, which allows use of the finger. Hyperextension of this joint predisposes to skin sloughing and should be avoided. The patient should be advised to not flex the joint during splint changes.

Bottom: A Stack splint is designed especially to treat a mallet finger. Long-term immobilization (8 weeks) or surgical fixation is required for this injury.

A padded aluminum splint is incorporated into the middle of a plaster splint to form an outrigger configuration. The plaster splint is applied to the dorsum of the hand and wrist with an elastic bandage; the finger is then taped to the aluminum splint. This provides complete immobilization of the finger.

Figure 50-16 Finger splinting techniques

TABLE 50-2 Useful Estimates of Splint Times for Various Hand Problems

INJURY	SPLINT TYPE	IMMOBILIZATION TIME*
Mallet finger	FIN	8 wk
Boutonnière deformity	FIN	6 wk
Distal phalanx—soft tissue	FIN	1-2 wk
Extensor tendon	DHWF	3 wk
Sprain-strain† Interphalangeal joint Wrist	FIN DHWF	1-2 wk 1-2 wk
Hand burn	DHWF	5-7 wk
Infection Digit Hand	DHWF DHWF	5-7 day 5-7 day
Severe hand contusion	DHWF	5-7 day
Fracture Distal phalanx Middle phalanx	FIN FIN	2-3 wk 2-3 wk
Proximal phalanx Metacarpal	DHWF DHWF	2-3 wk 2-3 wk
Carpal tunnel	DHWF	Night only
de Quervain's disease	DHWF	2-3 wk
Trigger finger	FIN	Night only

DHWF, digit-hand-wrist-forearm; *FIN*, finger.

*These are average times only. Every patient is treated as an individual when a splint is used. Clinical judgment is critical.

†Diagnosis of a sprain should be made only after a thorough effort has been made to rule out a fracture or dislocation. This is particularly true in the wrist.

immediate operative intervention or orthopedic referral. The posterior (gutter) knee splint (Fig. 50-19) is the type most commonly applied, but as alternatives, two parallel splints can be placed along each side of the leg and foreleg to create a bivalve effect (see Fig. 50-19B), or a long leg U-splint can be applied (see later). A bilateral knee splint is slightly more difficult to apply than a posterior knee splint, but it may provide better immobilization of the lateral and medial collateral ligaments and can be used for injuries to these structures.

Construction. Construct a posterior knee splint with 12 to 15 layers of 6-inch plaster. It should run from just below the buttocks crease to approximately 5 to 8 cm above the malleoli. The sides of the splint are folded upward to form a gutter configuration.

Application. Apply a stockinette in the usual manner, and wrap the leg with 4- or 6-inch Webril. Have an assistant elevate the leg and hold the splint in place while securing it to the extremity with 4- or 6-inch elastic bandages. If no aide is available, place the patient in the prone position and have him use his toes to elevate the lower part of the leg off the bed to allow sufficient room to wrap the Webril and elastic bandages around the injured extremity. Lay the splint along the posterior surface of the extremity, and secure it in place with 4- or 6-inch elastic bandages.

Jones Compression Dressing

Indications. A Jones compression dressing is commonly used for short-term immobilization of soft tissue injuries of the knee. It immobilizes and compresses the knee, thereby reducing both pain and swelling. However, because it does allow slight flexion and extension of the knee, it should not be used for injuries that require strict immobilization. In addition, it is difficult to maintain the splint for more than a few days.

Construction. A Jones dressing is fashioned from 6-inch Webril and elastic bandages.

Application. To apply a Jones dressing, place the patient supine on the stretcher. If available, ask an assistant to elevate the patient's leg to facilitate wrapping. If no help is available, place a pillow under the patient's heel to lift the extremity off the stretcher. Wrap Webril around the extremity from the groin to a few inches above the malleoli. Use two or three layers of Webril and overlap the previous turn by 25% to 50%. Complete the dressing by wrapping 6-inch elastic bandages (two are usually required) around the Webril. If more support is required, repeat the process with another two or three layers of Webril held in place by additional elastic bandages.

Ankle Splints

Posterior Splint

Indications. A posterior ankle splint (Fig. 50-20) is one of the most common splints applied in the ED. As noted in the introductory section, the entire concept of splinting an acutely sprained ankle has been questioned, with no firm evidence to support better outcomes with splinting or casting versus functional management (early mobilization with an external support). Nonetheless, an acutely sprained ankle is painful, and if nothing else, splinting for a few days helps alleviate the pain.

Use a posterior splint primarily to immobilize severe ankle sprains, fractures of the distal ends of the fibula and tibia, and reduced ankle dislocations. It can also be used for fractures of the tarsal and metatarsal bones or for other foot conditions that require immobilization. With particularly severe or unstable injuries, an additional anterior splint may be used to provide extra immobilization resembling that of a formal cast (Fig. 50-21). For severe lateral or bilateral ligamentous injuries, add a U-splint or stirrup splint (see later) to the posterior splint for increased immobilization. With minor soft tissue injuries, patients may have partial weight bearing on ankle splints after 24 hours. If the patient will be bearing weight, wearing a cast shoe over the splint makes it easier to walk and increases the longevity of the splint. Generally, though, walking on the splint is prohibited if immobilization for more than 2 or 3 days is desired.

Construction. Make the posterior splint with 4- or 6-inch-wide plaster strips. It should extend from the plantar surface of the great toe or metatarsal heads along the posterior surface of the foreleg to the level of the fibular head. If it hurts to move the toes, incorporate them into the splint (after padding is placed between the digits). It is a common mistake to apply

SHOULDER SLINGS

The shoulder immobilizer is used for most proximal humerus fractures and shoulder injuries. It may be removed for showering and range-of-motion exercises and is easily reapplied by the patient.

Proximal humerus fracture

Proximal humerus fractures are common injuries in the elderly, especially after a fall. A shoulder sling is the immobilization device of choice.

An elastic bandage and sling provide similar shoulder immobilization. Note that the wrist is supported by the slings.

A, Stepwise application of a triangular muslin sling. (1) Place tip X over the uninjured shoulder. (2) Bring tip Y over the injured shoulder to enclose the arm. (3) Draw tip Z around the front and pin. **B,** Completed triangular muslin sling. (*Note:* When applying a sling it is important to have adequate support of the wrist and hand. A sling that is too short will allow the wrist and hand to hang down [ulnar deviate] and can result in hand edema and ulnar nerve injury).

Figure 50-17 Shoulder slings.

KNEE IMMOBILIZER

Application

Choose the appropriate-size knee immobilizer for the patient. The tapered end should be distal to the knee. The splints simply wrap around the leg (and can be applied over clothing) and are secured with Velcro straps.

Indications

Ligamentous and soft tissue injuries of the knee.

Above, a *Segond fracture* is demonstrated. Note the small bony avulsion fracture on the lateral aspect of the tibial plateau. Although at first glance this appears to be a rather innocuous injury, a Segond fracture is highly associated with tears of the anterior cruciate ligament. This patient should be treated with a knee immobilizer until orthopedic follow-up can be arranged.

Segond fracture

Figure 50-18 Knee immobilizer.

POSTERIOR KNEE SPLINT

A   B

Periprosthetic distal femur fracture

Application

A, Extend the posterior knee splint from just below the buttocks crease to approximately 2 to 3 cm above the malleoli.

B, Alternatively, place two parallel splints along each side of the leg and foreleg to create a bivalve effect. Although this variation is more difficult to apply, it may provide better immobilization of the lateral and medial collateral ligaments.

Indications

Angulated fractures around the knee (shown above)
Tempory immobilization of injuries prior to operative repair
Knee injuries in patients with extremities too large for a knee immobilizer

The knee immobilizer has largely replaced the posterior knee splint in modern emergercy department practice.

Figure 50-19 Posterior knee splint.

POSTERIOR ANKLE SPLINT

Distal fibula fracture

Application

Extend the splint from the plantar surface of the great toe (or metatarsal heads) along the posterior surface of the foreleg to the level of the fibular head. The ankle should be at a 90° angle.

Indications

Fractures of the distal ends of the fibula and tibia (shown above)
Severe ankle sprains
Reduced ankle dislocations

A, Apply the splint with the patient prone and the knee bent to 90°, thereby relaxing the calf muscles. Position the ankle at 90° so that the foot is flat for partial weight bearing. **B,** This is an unacceptable fiberglass splint. Note the very sharp frayed fiberglass edges (*arrows*) and the multiple internal ridges and folds that will produce soft tissue trauma when worn. **C,** Three things are wrong with this posterior ankle splint: (1) It does not extend distally enough to support the entire foot. (2) The ankle is not maintained at a 90° angle. (3) The edges and ankle area are not molded or protected. Overall, the splint is sloppy and ineffective.

Figure 50-20 Posterior lower leg splint.

a posterior splint that does not extend far enough to support the ball of the foot. Use 15 to 20 layers if partial weight bearing is allowed because this splint frequently breaks or cracks when walked on.[16]

Application. The easiest way to apply a posterior splint is to place the patient in the prone position with the knee and ankle flexed at a 90-degree angle. Failure to place the ankle in a 90-degree angle results in a plantar-flexed splint. A supine patient may help maintain the ankle in a 90-degree angle by pulling up on the foot with a wide stockinette stirrup. Flexing the knee to a 90-degree angle relaxes the gastrocnemius muscle and facilitates ankle motion. With the knee and ankle in the proper position, apply a stockinette and pad the foot and leg with Webril as described earlier. Use extra padding over bony prominences, particularly the malleoli. To prevent skin maceration, place pieces of Webril or gauze between the toes if they are to be included in the splint. Lay the wet plaster

ANTERIOR-POSTERIOR ANKLE SPLINT

Severely comminuted distal tibia and fibula fracture

Application

Apply the posterior splint as described in Figure 50-20.

For the anterior portion, begin on the dorsal surface of the foot at the level of the metatarsophalangeal joints. Extend the splint along the anterior portion of the foreleg, to the same height as the posterior splint. Maintain the ankle at a 90° angle.

Indications

Serious fractures and soft tissue injuries of the ankle.

The anterior portion of the splint is never used by itself; it is always used to augment the immobilization provided by the posterior ankle splint.

Figure 50-21 Anterior-posterior ankle splint.

over the plantar surface of the foot and secure it in place by folding back the ends of the stockinette and Webril and wrapping with one or two 4-inch-wide elastic bandages. Carefully mold the wet plaster around the malleoli and instep to ensure maximum comfort and immobilization. Leave the toes partially exposed for later examination of color and capillary refill.

Anterior-Posterior Splint

Indications.   An anterior splint is never used by itself, but it can augment a posterior splint to create a bivalve effect (see Fig. 50-21). Use it for serious fractures and soft tissue injuries of the ankle.

Construction.   Cut a piece of plaster several centimeters shorter than the one used for the posterior splint, but since this splint does not bear weight, only 8 to 10 layers are required.

Application.   Position the patient and apply padding as described for a posterior splint. After the wet posterior splint has been applied, place the anterior splint over the anterior aspect of the ankle and foreleg parallel to the posterior splint. Hold the two in place with elastic bandages as described earlier for a posterior splint alone. An assistant is needed to apply an anterior-posterior splint because it is extremely difficult to hold both splints in place while wrapping the elastic bandages. Once secured, carefully mold both splints over the instep and ankle joint.

U-Splint (Stirrup Splint)

Indications.   Use a U-splint or stirrup splint (Fig. 50-22) primarily for injuries to the ankle. It functions like a posterior splint, and either one provides satisfactory ankle immobilization. In one study that compared these splints in normal volunteers, the U-splint allowed less plantar flexion and broke less often with plantar flexion than did the posterior splint.[16] Also, because it actually covers the malleoli, a U-splint may protect the medial and lateral ligaments from further injury better than a posterior splint can.

Construction.   Construct a U-splint of 4- or 6-inch-wide plaster strips. The splint passes under the plantar surface of the foot from the calcaneus to the metatarsal heads and extends up the medial and lateral sides of the foreleg to just below the level of the fibular head.

Application.   Position the patient and pad the extremity as described for a posterior splint. Lay the wet plaster across the plantar surface of the foot between the calcaneus and the metatarsal heads with the sides extending up the lateral and medial aspects of the foreleg. Secure it in place with 4-inch elastic bandages. Wrap the elastic bandage around the extremity starting at the metatarsal heads and continuing around the ankle in a figure-of-eight configuration. Once the ankle has been wrapped, use another 4- or 6-inch elastic bandage to secure the remainder of the splint in place. Carefully mold the splint around the malleoli. The plaster may overlap on the anterior aspect of the ankle; this overlap does not interfere

U-SPLINT (OR STIRRUP/SUGAR-TONG SPLINT)

PREREDUCTION   POSTREDUCTION

Application

Apply the splint under the plantar surface of the foot and extend it up the medial and lateral sides of the foreleg to just below the level of the fibular head. Keep the ankle at a 90° angle.

For immobilization of the knee, extend the sides of the splint proximally to the groin to create a long leg splint.

Indications

Injuries of the ankle, including:
Fractures of the distal tibia and fibula
Postreduction stabilization of ankle dislocations (above)

The U-splint can be combined with the posterior ankle splint to provide both anterior-posterior and medial-lateral stability.

Figure 50-22 U-splint (also referred to as a stirrup or sugar-tong splint).

with the splint's ability to accommodate further swelling. Note that if a U-splint is combined with a posterior splint, apply the posterior splint first.

Walking Boots

Indications. Use a walking boot (e.g., Cam Walker Boot) for the treatment of moderate to severe soft tissue injuries of the ankle, including second- and third-degree sprains (Fig. 50-23*A*).[17] In addition, many orthopedic surgeons use it for isolated, nondisplaced lateral malleolar fractures.[18] A walking boot provides a degree of immobilization similar to that of a U-splint but is easier to remove for bathing and dressing, and the Velcro straps allow adjustment for edema.

Refer patients in a walking boot for follow-up with an appropriate specialist. Advise them of the importance of partial or non–weight bearing as indicated by the type and degree of injury. When cleared by the follow-up physician, a walking boot allows easy transition to full weight bearing. Studies have shown that rapid mobilization after ankle injuries improves functional outcome and reduces disability time.[7]

Application. Walking boots come in a variety of sizes from extra small to extra large, depending on the manufacturer. The boot should fit comfortably with the patient's calcaneus snugly in the heel of the boot and the patient's toes close to but not extending over the front edge of the boot. Once the appropriate size has been determined, place the patient's bare foot and ankle into the boot, and adjust the Velcro straps for a secure, but comfortable fit.

Semirigid Orthosis

Indications. In patients with lateral ankle sprains associated with a stable joint, a functional brace with early mobilization is frequently more comfortable and results in earlier return to normal function than does complete immobilization in a plaster splint or cast (see Fig. 50-23*B*).[17-25] Consequently, functional bracing with early mobilization has become the treatment of choice in most EDs. However, it should be pointed out that there is no documented difference in long-term outcome between the two methods of treatment.

Application. Most functional ankle braces resemble a U-splint with air bladders (Aircast, Inc., Summit, NJ) or foam padding (DeRoyal, Inc., Powell, TN) for cushioning the malleoli. The braces are secured about the ankle with Velcro straps. The device can be worn within the patient's shoe over a sock and helps eliminate ankle instability.

Hard Shoe (Cast or Reese Shoe)

Indications. Use a hard shoe to help reduce pain on ambulation in patients with fractures or soft tissue injuries of the foot. This device can also be used over a splint or cast to allow partial weight bearing. A hard shoe is commonly used for fractured toes that have been buddy-taped.

Application. If a cast shoe is going to be used for a patient with a fractured toe, first buddy-tape the injured digit to the adjacent toe (Fig. 50-24). After this is done, the patient can

SPLINTS FOR ANKLE SPRAINS

A walking boot can be used for the treatment of moderate to severe soft tissue injuries of the ankle, including second- and third-degree sprains and isolated, nondisplaced lateral malleolar fractures. A walking boot provides a similar degree of immobilization as a U-splint but is easier to remove for bathing and dressing, and the Velcro straps allow adjustment for edema.

Prefabricated semirigid orthoses such as the Aircast (pictured above) are often used for patients with minor ankle sprains. The Aircast can be worn inside the patient's shoe to provide early mobility along with increased ankle stability.

The Unna boot or an Ace wrap provides effective immobilization of an ankle soft tissue injury. The Unna boot is applied from a semisolid paste roll. The wrap is then covered with gauze or an elastic bandage. The entire dressing can be cut off by the patient at home. For similar short-term immobilization without plaster, a modified Jones dressing can be used. Copious Webril is wrapped around the ankle and foot and covered with an elastic bandage. A cast shoe can be used with this dressing.

Figure 50-23 Splints for ankle sprains.

HARD SHOE SPLINT

Cotton or Webril between toes

Indications
Reduction of ambulatory pain in patients with fractures or soft tissue injuries of the foot
Used over a splint to allow partial weight bearing

If the shoe is going to be used for a fractured toe, first buddy-tape the toe to the adjacent digit. Remember to place a piece of cotton or Webril between the toes to prevent skin maceration.

Figure 50-24 Hard shoe splint.

slip the hard shoe on like a sandal. Fasten the shoe with ties or Velcro straps.

Ankle Wraps and Bandages

There are no data supporting the routine use of ankle wraps for simple sprains, but some pain relief may be afforded by a proper wrap. Some type of temporary immobilization is commonly used in the ED and usually requested and expected by patients. For minor ankle injuries, a simple elastic (Ace) bandage can be applied. Use a figure-of-eight configuration (see Fig. 50-23*C*). Apply the wrap to give only lateral support with minimal compression. *It should not be tight enough to impair venous drainage*, a common problem when patients apply their own elastic wraps (see Fig. 50-2).

An Unna boot placed over Webril is an alternative to a simple elastic bandage (see Fig. 50-23*C*). The Unna boot is constructed from a semisolid paste roll that hardens as it dries. Apply an Unna boot in a figure-of-eight configuration, similar to a simple elastic bandage. Once in place, wrap the ankle with roller gauze or an elastic bandage. The entire dressing can be cut off by the patient at home.

Soft Cast

Indications. A soft cast is basically a modified Jones compression dressing for the ankle. Use it for minor ligamentous and soft tissue injuries of the foot and ankle that do not require prolonged or complete immobilization. A soft cast can help reduce the pain and swelling often associated with mild ankle sprains, and it gives support for early weight bearing.

Construction. Make the soft cast of 3- or 4-inch Webril and elastic bandages.

Application. Place the patient in a supine position with the foot and ankle extending off the end of the stretcher. Alternatively, ask an assistant to elevate the leg or place pillows under the knee and foreleg. Wrap the ankle and foot with five to seven layers of Webril starting at the metatarsal heads and continuing around the ankle in a figure-of-eight configuration. Extend the Webril 5 to 7 cm above the malleoli and overlap each turn by 25% to 50% of its width. After the Webril is in place, wrap an elastic bandage around the foot and ankle in a similar fashion. Additional layers of Webril and elastic bandages are seldom required. A cast shoe can be used with this dressing.

COMPLICATIONS OF SPLINTS

Ischemia

A compartment syndrome leading to ischemic injury and ultimately to a Volkmann ischemic contracture is the most worrisome complication of cylindrical casts. Although the risk for ischemia is drastically reduced with splinting, Webril or elastic bandages can cause significant constriction. To reduce the likelihood of constriction occurring, do not pull the elastic bandage excessively tight. If the patient has a high-risk injury, cut the Webril lengthwise before the plaster is applied. Stress the importance of elevation, no weight bearing, and application of cold packs, and carefully review the signs and symptoms of vascular compromise with every patient. All patients whose injuries have the potential for significant swelling or loss of vascular integrity should receive follow-up care in the first 24 to 48 hours. *Never ignore*

Figure 50-25 If a patient complains of a cast being too tight, it probably is. The cast must be removed to inspect the area for infection or other problems. Complaints of pain under this cast were incorrectly met with a phone call to suggest elevation and a call-in prescription for narcotics.

complaints of increasing pain under a splint. Patients with splint-related discomfort must be reevaluated clinically and should not be treated with a telephone prescription for opioid analgesics (Fig. 50-25).

Heat Injury

Fiberglass splints produce minimal heat when drying, but plaster generates considerable heat as it hardens. Many clinicians are unaware of the potential for drying plaster to produce second-degree burns.[26] Thermal injury can occur with both cylindrical casts and plaster splints. Some clinicians have reported a higher incidence of burns with the use of plaster splints, although the reasons for this are unclear.[26,27] Box 50-4 lists factors that can increase the amount of heat produced during plaster recrystallization. Their effects are additive, and this fact should be taken into account when applying a splint. For example, if 15 sheets of plaster are needed for strength in a particular splint, one should not increase the heat production further by using extra-fast–drying plaster or reusing warm dip water. To avoid plaster burns, use only 8 to 12 sheets of plaster when possible, use fresh dip water with a temperature near 24°C, and never wrap the extremity in a sheet or pillow during the setting process. Peak temperatures usually occur between 5 and 15 minutes after plaster wetting.

The patient should be warned that the hardening process produces warmth. The heat of drying may produce pain in patients with hemophilia-related hemarthroses. Splinting these patients may require that the plaster splint be placed only long enough to verify proper fit; the splint is then reapplied after setting (and cooling) of the plaster. If any patient complains of significant burning while the plaster is drying, *do not ignore this complaint!* Immediately remove the splint, and promptly cool the area with cold packs or cool water. Patients with vascular insufficiency or sensory deficits (e.g., diabetic neuropathy, stroke) are at high risk for plaster burns and require close observation during the drying process.

Pressure Sores

Pressure sores are an uncommon complication of short-term splinting (Fig. 50-26).[28] They can result from stockinette

Figure 50-26 The problem with this splint is that it was intended to be used for only a few days, but the patient wore it and walked on it for 3 weeks. Note the resultant full-thickness skin loss. No padding was used under the premade splint. Skin grafting was eventually required.

Figure 50-27 This 9-year-old tried to scratch an itch under his splint with a pencil and the eraser fell off. This resulted in skin irritation and infection, requiring removal of splint.

wrinkles, irregular wadding of Webril, incorrectly padded or unpadded bony prominences, irregular splint ends, plaster ridges, or indentations produced from using the fingers rather than the palms to smooth and mold the wet plaster. Attention to detail during padding and splinting reduces the incidence of pressure sores. However, whenever a patient complains of a persistent pain or burning sensation under any part of a splint, remove the splint and inspect the symptomatic area closely. The padding incorporated in premade plaster and fiberglass splints is generally all that is needed for safe short-term splinting. However, the life of a splint applied in the ED may be longer than intended by the clinician; therefore, it is prudent to err on the side of additional padding when placing splints on patients who may overuse the splint, such as those who will not use crutches, or for those who may not have ready access to follow-up.

Infection

Bacterial and fungal infections can occur under a splint.[29,30] Infection is more common in the presence of an open wound but may occur with intact skin or in a skin lesion produced by prolonged splinting. The moist, warm, and dark environment created by the splint is an excellent nidus for infection. Toxic shock syndrome has been rarely reported from a staphylococcal skin infection that clandestinely developed under a splint or cast. Also, it has been shown that bacteria can multiply in slowly drying plaster. To avoid infection, clean and débride all wounds before splint application, and use clean, fresh tap water for plaster wetting. If necessary, apply a removable splint that allows periodic wound inspection or local wound care.

Dermatitis

Occasionally, a rash develops under a plaster cast or splint.[31-35] Allergy to plaster is exceedingly rare, but there are several reports of contact dermatitis when formaldehyde and melamine resins are added to the plaster.[33,34] The rash is usually pruritic with weeping papular or vesicular lesions. Because these resins are unnecessary for ED splints, their use should be avoided whenever possible. Dermatitis has also been reported with the use of fiberglass splinting material.[36]

Pruritus

Itching under a cast can be problematic. Patients, especially children, use various objects such as a pencil, coat hanger, or fork to get to the itch. This can cause skin maceration and possible infection, or a foreign body can be left under the cast (Fig. 50-27).

Joint Stiffness

Some degree of joint stiffness is an invariable consequence of immobilization (Fig. 50-28). It can range in severity from mild to incapacitating and can result in transient, prolonged, or in some cases, permanent loss of function. Stiffness appears to be worse with prolonged periods of immobilization, in elderly patients, and in patients with preexisting joint diseases such as rheumatoid arthritis or osteoarthritis. Thus, splints should be left on for only the time necessary for adequate healing. Table 50-3 lists several injuries that commonly require splinting, along with some suggestions for length of immobilization. Fractures, dislocations, or other conditions that require prolonged immobilization (>7 days) should have orthopedic follow-up. Tell patients that a splint is only a short-term device and that prolonged immobilization can be detrimental. For minor injuries, suggest that patients use their own judgment about when to remove the splint, but a definite end point should be set.

Cast Pain

Cast-related pain is a common complaint that brings patients to the ED. Because of the potential for ischemia with

Figure 50-28 A, Never splint an injured wrist in flexion even though the patient prefers this position. **B,** When immobilizing an infected human bite, this splint was not held in position until hardened, and the patient reflexively flexed the wrist.

TABLE 50-3 Suggested Length of Immobilization for Conditions That Frequently Require Splinting	
LENGTH OF CONDITION	**IMMOBILIZATION (DAYS)**
Contusions	1-3
Abrasions	1-3
Soft tissue lacerations	5-7
Tendon lacerations	Variable*
Tendinitis	5-7
Puncture wounds and bites	3-4
Deep space infections and cellulitis	3-5
Mild sprains	5-7
Fractures and severe sprains	Variable†

*Considerable controversy surrounds the length of immobilization for tendon lacerations, and duration is therefore best left to the consultant surgeon.
†Usually requires prolonged immobilization, which is best determined by an orthopedic surgeon.

circumferential casts, fully investigate all complaints, and rule out vascular compromise. *If a patient states that a cast is too tight, it probably is* (see Fig. 50-25). Do not prescribe narcotics for cast pain until a properly fitting (i.e., one that is not too tight) cast has been ensured.

Perform a detailed history and physical examination on all patients complaining of cast pain. The nature and onset of the pain are of particular importance. A dull, nonspecific pain that has worsened gradually since the time of injury may be the only clue to an early compartment syndrome (see Chapter 54). A sudden onset of throbbing pain associated with swelling and redness suggests a possible deep venous thrombosis. In both these cases, rapid intervention is the key to decreasing morbidity and mortality. During the physical examination, pay particular attention to areas of tenderness and the effect of active and passive movement on the severity of the pain.

With a compartment syndrome, tenderness over the involved compartment is a common finding, and stretching or contracting ischemic muscle elicits significant pain. Evaluate for the presence and quality of distal pulses, the amount of edema fluid present, distal sensation, capillary refill, and color and temperature of the digits. The five P's (pain, pallor, paresthesias, paralysis, and pulselessness) are pathognomonic for ischemia. Unfortunately, they seldom occur simultaneously, and their presence together is usually a late finding that carries a poor prognosis. Hence, the emergency clinician must maintain a high index of suspicion for possible ischemia and remove the cast if any possibility of vascular compromise exists. Almost any cast can be bivalved and reapplied after inspection without significant loss of short-term immobilization.

To loosen a cast, use an oscillating cast saw to cut along the medial and lateral aspects of the cast (Fig. 50-29). This is called *bivalving the cast*, and it allows the halves to be spread and reapplied in a less constricting manner while still maintaining proper immobilization. To use an oscillating power saw, proceed in a series of downward cutting movements facilitated by wrist supination, and remove the blade between cuts to prevent it from getting hot enough to burn the skin. This is particularly important if synthetic material has been used in the cast. Also, do not allow the blade to slide along the skin, and never use the saw on unpadded plaster. In an apprehensive patient, demonstrate that the cast saw blade only vibrates (it does not turn) and that it does not cut the skin.

After the medial and lateral sides of the cast are completely cut through, separate the two halves with a cast spreader, and cut the padding lengthwise with scissors. This may be sufficient to relieve early ischemia if the problem is simple postinjury swelling, but both the padding and the cast can be totally removed to inspect the injured area if necessary. If ischemia cannot be ruled out, measure compartment pressures (Chapter 54) and obtain an orthopedic consultation.

If vascular integrity is established and no other problems are found, replace the bivalved cast. First, pad the extremity in the usual manner with fresh Webril. Line the cut ends of the bivalved cast with white adhesive tape, and replace the cast around the extremity. Finally, secure the cast in place with elastic bandages.

If plaster sores are causing the patient discomfort, consult the clinician who placed the cast. In some cases, additional padding is all that is needed, but in others, a window should be cut out over the problem area. Because pressure sores can lead to significant tissue necrosis, refer the patient for follow-up care within 24 hours.

If the patient's problem is plaster (or, more likely, resin) dermatitis, administer topical or oral steroids and antihistamines. Provide therapy in concert with an orthopedic surgeon because the patient may require admission for other forms of immobilization until the cast can be replaced. In mild cases, changing the cast or splint and using antihistamines for symptomatic relief may suffice. All patients should receive close follow-up, and if the condition does not improve, the cast must be removed.

CAST REMOVAL

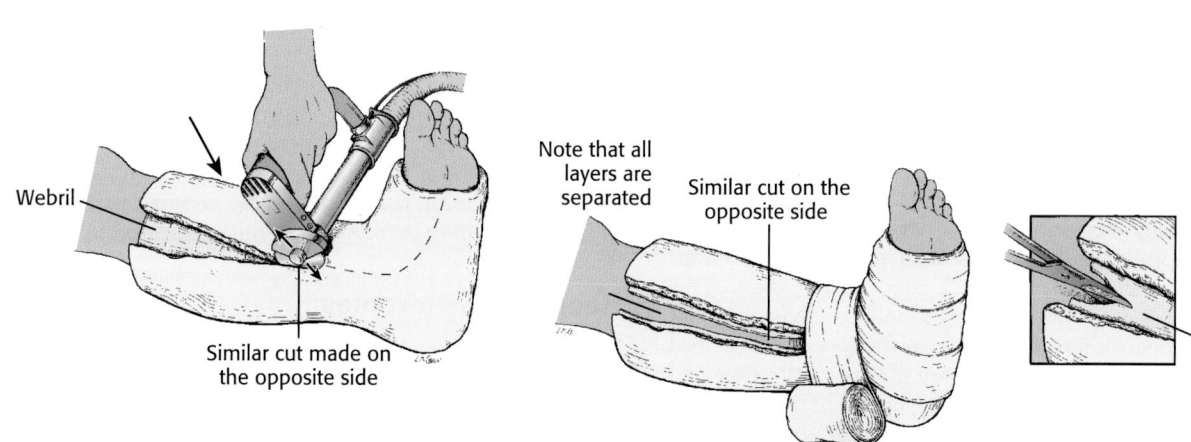

The cast saw vibrates; it does not rotate. It will not cut the patient. Note that the underlying Webril padding is cut to relieve pressure but is not removed.

The blade is controlled by placing the thumb (*arrow*) on the splint and lowering the saw blade to the plaster. The blade is raised and lowered for each cut; it is not drawn across the plaster like a knife.

This cast was too tight, and it was therefore bivalved from calf to forefoot with a cast saw. After separation of the edges of the cut cast, the anterior and posterior components were secured in place with an elastic bandage. A bivalved cast provides temporary immobilization equal to that of an intact cast. Extra padding can be used to protect the skin from the cut edges.

Figure 50-29 Cast removal.

CONCLUSION

Splinting is an important means of temporary fracture immobilization and provides protection and comfort for a variety of soft tissue injuries. The clinician should be aware of potential complications that can occur with improper splint application, including ischemia, thermal injury, and pressure sores. Use proper technique to minimize the risk for these adverse outcomes. When ischemia is suspected, the emergency clinician should also be facile in the release of circumferential cast and splint material.

References are available at www.expertconsult.com

CHAPTER 51

Podiatric Procedures

Douglas L. McGee

Normal daily activities cannot easily be accomplished without walking, so patients with painful or infectious conditions of the feet often seek medical attention. This chapter focuses on procedures performed for common maladies of the foot. Other procedures on the foot are described elsewhere in this text, including anesthesia of the foot and ankle (see Chapters 29 and 31), management of nail bed injuries (see Chapters 35 and 37), incision and drainage of paronychia (see Chapter 37), joint fluid analysis (see Chapter 53), management of common dislocations of the foot (see Chapter 49), and splinting (see Chapter 50).

COMMON NONTRAUMATIC CONDITIONS OF THE FOOT

Many painful conditions of the foot are chronic and do not usually require definitive treatment in the emergency department (ED); however, patients are often seen with common conditions that require evaluation and proper referral. To accomplish this, the clinician must be cognizant of basic podiatric conditions, including painful lesions over bony prominences, heel pain, foot infections, and pain on the plantar surface of the foot.

Footpad Use

Footpads redistribute pressure over an inflamed, tender area of the foot. The particular type of footpad and its placement depend on the condition being treated (Fig. 51-1). Commercially available aperture footpads are recommended for the temporary relief of warts, corns, hyperkeratoses, and bunions. Verruca virus introduced into the plantar surface of the foot may produce a painful hyperkeratotic lesion, commonly referred to as a "plantar wart," on the sole of the foot. A simple callus may be painful and result in the formation of a "hard corn" when formed over the bony prominence of a digit. Once recognized and after other conditions are ruled out, definitive care of these lesions is rarely indicated in the ED.

When tenderness is elicited over more than one metatarsal head, the diagnosis is metatarsalgia. Pain that is progressively worse while walking but relieved by rest, often beneath the second or third metatarsal head, is typical in this case. A pad placed under the first metatarsal head to raise the second and third metatarsals may provide some relief.

A bunion develops when unbalanced forces applied to the first metatarsal cause lateral displacement of the distal end of the hallux. Bunions typically form in women wearing heeled shoes with narrow toe boxes. The patient may complain of numbness over the distal, medial aspect of the first toe as a result of compression of the terminal branch of the medial dorsal cutaneous nerve. The mechanical forces that precipitate bunion formation may also cause other painful conditions, including intermetatarsal neuromas, hammertoes, ingrown toenails, corns, and calluses. Bursitis may develop over the medial bony prominence of the first metatarsophalangeal (MTP) joint. Self-adherent bunion pads placed over the first MTP joint may provide temporary relief (Fig. 51-2). In the ED, treat patients suffering from these common disorders with analgesics and footpads followed by referral for definitive care. Recommend that the patient avoid wearing the offending shoes. Consider gout when evaluating pain over the first MTP joint, particularly in the presence of other signs of inflammation (e.g., redness, swelling, warmth).

Heel Pain Syndromes

Bony spurs on the plantar surface of the calcaneus, retrocalcaneal bursitis, calcaneal apophysitis, and other conditions may cause heel pain. Treat most of these conditions with rest, nonsteroidal antiinflammatory drugs (NSAIDs), modification of physical activities or shoe wear, footpads, and orthoses. Some clinicians also include injection of anesthetics or steroids for these conditions.

Heel spur pain can be quite bothersome and chronic or recurrent. This condition is not easily remedied in the ED, and after other conditions are ruled out, minimal intervention with podiatric referral is often the best course of action. Patients typically have pain over the medial border of the plantar aspect of the calcaneus. The pain gradually worsens over a period of months. A bony prominence that begins as periostitis extends from the medial aspect of the calcaneal tuberosity into the central plantar fascia and may be seen on radiographs. Radiographs of the calcaneus that do not demonstrate a bony spur suggest plantar fasciitis (see the section "Painful Conditions of the Plantar Surface of the Foot" later in this chapter), even though many patients with plantar fasciitis have plantar calcaneal and Achilles spurs. Plantar calcaneal heel spurs are found in nearly 15% of the population, only 30% of whom have heel pain. Although many persons with heel spurs are asymptomatic, 75% of patients with heel pain have heel spurs.[1] However, radiographs have little value in evaluating nontraumatic heel pain because they rarely demonstrate radiographic abnormalities that prompt additional treatment.[2]

Shoe supports with a heel pad or cup or a doughnut-shaped orthotic often help reduce the discomfort by redistributing weight. Few randomized, controlled trials have evaluated steroid therapy; those that have do not provide substantial evidence supporting its long-term efficacy.[3,4] Treatment of the painful site is done with 10 to 20 mg of methylprednisolone injected from the medial aspect of the foot while avoiding the sensitive plantar surface. Some evidence suggests that injecting 25 mg of prednisolone acetate into the medial aspect of the heel provides partial pain relief at 1 month in comparison to lidocaine only, but no advantage can be detected at 3 months.[5] A short-leg walking cast may be effective in some patients with recalcitrant heel pain.[6] There is little evidence to suggest that specific interventions aimed at reducing heel pain are superior to conservative, supportive treatment alone.

Retrocalcaneal Bursitis, Achilles Tendinopathy, and Calcaneal Apophysitis

Although retrocalcaneal bursitis and Achilles tendinopathy, formerly referred to as Achilles tendinitis, are anatomically distinct, the clinical findings are similar. Pain at the insertion

Figure 51-1 Use of aperture pads to redistribute pressure from painful areas to surrounding structures. *(Courtesy of Kenneth R. Walker, DPM.)*

Figure 51-2 Use of an adhesive bunion pad. *(Courtesy of Kenneth R. Walker, DPM.)*

of the Achilles tendon is worsened with prolonged standing or walking and is aggravated by passive or active range of motion in both conditions. Directed palpation can distinguish one entity from the other, but both are treated similarly. Tenderness of the Achilles tendon suggests tendinopathy, whereas tenderness between the tendon and the calcaneus suggests retrocalcaneal bursitis. *Achilles tendinopathy has been noted to develop spontaneously after the use of quinolone antibiotics, occasionally with rupture.* The condition may occur during quinolone use or a few weeks after therapy and prompts immediate discontinuation of use of the drug if recognized. Rest, elevation, ice, NSAIDs, heel pads, and an open-backed shoe provide relief in the majority of patients. A corticosteroid injection is not usually performed, but it may provide some relief, although its superiority over conservative measures is unproved. Repeated steroid injection is associated with Achilles tendon rupture.[7] Injection of platelet-rich plasma (PRP) as treatment of Achilles tendinopathy has gained some support among sports medicine physicians, but recently published studies have failed to demonstrate short- or long-term improvement in pain or function when PRP injection is compared with placebo.[8,9] Osteochondrosis of the posterior calcaneal apophysis may cause pain worsened by activity in children between 7 and 10 years of age. It is thought to represent an overuse syndrome in an athletically active child

with tenderness in the posterior heel region.[7,10] Treat this self-limited condition with rest, ice, and heel pads. Radiographs are not indicated unless other diagnoses are suspected.[11] Activity is resumed when the pain abates.

Painful Conditions of the Plantar Surface of the Foot

Plantar Fasciitis
Repeated microtrauma to the plantar aponeurosis causes pain on the plantar surface of the foot (Fig. 51-3A). Plantar fasciitis is typically unilateral and found in women who wear high-heeled shoes. The pain is maximally severe in the morning or after prolonged sitting and improves after walking, often referred to as "first-step pain." Some patients with plantar fasciitis may also have a calcaneal heel spur, but the presence or absence of this radiographic finding is clinically irrelevant. Pain is elicited with palpation (see Fig. 51-3B), toe walking, or passive stretching of the plantar aponeurosis. Frequently, this annoying condition resolves spontaneously, but resolution is slow, with as long as 6 to 18 months being needed. Conservative therapy, including rest, elevation, ice, and NSAIDs, results in a satisfactory outcome after 6 to 8 weeks in 90% of patients.[12] The pain improves over time in most patients with or without NSAIDs, although the addition of NSAIDs appears to increase pain relief when compared with conservative treatments alone.[13] The emergency clinician can do little to treat this chronic, distressing condition. Stretching exercises each morning and evening can be suggested (see Fig. 51-3D). Night splinting to keep the foot dorsiflexed and custom orthoses made from the patient's foot impression can be very helpful but usually require referral to podiatry for proper fitting (see Fig. 51-3C). Corticosteroid injection is used by some clinicians; its benefit remains unproved, however. A single injection may be warranted as supplemental therapy in resistant cases. Repeated injections of corticosteroids should be avoided and have been associated with rupture of the plantar fascia and fat pad atrophy.[14] In a recent study, 50 units of botulinum toxic type A injected into the plantar fascia decreased pain in comparison to placebo but did not cure the disease.[15]

Forefoot Neuroma
A forefoot neuroma, also known as Morton's neuroma, is a painful condition of the plantar surface of the foot. It most commonly affects women who wear high-heeled shoes. The neuroma forms after chronic irritation to the digital sensory nerve between the metatarsals. A neuroma frequently occurs in the third interspace but may be found in the second space (Fig. 51-4A). Patients report the sensation of a lump or cord in the interspace and describe paresthesia or numbness in the third or fourth toes. Direct compression plus release of the forefoot causes pain and often a "click" (the Mulder sign) (see Fig. 51-4B). Rest, elevation, ice, and NSAIDs may result in some improvement, but surgical excision is often required.[16,17] Few data support the use of corticosteroid injections. In one study, less than 50% of patients with a foot neuroma had any benefit from injected corticosteroids.[16] Another study demonstrated complete or partial relief in 80% of patients injected with corticosteroids.[18] Although this study demonstrated a trend toward improved outcome when injected corticosteroids were compared with footwear modifications, corticosteroid injection therapy alone was not statistically better than footwear modification at 1 year.[18]

Figure 51-3 Plantar fasciitis. **A,** The plantar fascia spans the plantar aspect of the foot. The origin is the *medial* tubercle of the calcaneus, which is the most common site of pain. A heel spur may be seen on radiographs, but inflammation of the plantar fascia, not the spur, is the source of the pain. **B,** Palpation of the tubercle of the calcaneus reproduces the pain of plantar fasciitis. **C,** A posterior lower leg splint may be created for patients in the emergency department, and it is intended to be worn at night to keep the foot in a position of dorsiflexion. Referral to podiatry for custom-fit orthoses may also be beneficial. **D,** Rolling the arch of the foot back and forth over a frozen water bottle will stretch the fascia and, over time, may lessen the pain of plantar fasciitis. A tennis ball can also be used.

Figure 51-4 Morton's neuroma. **A,** Site of Morton's neuroma arising from a digital nerve. **B,** Palpation of the distal metatarsal area may reveal pain from Morton's neuroma. Squeezing and releasing this area (not shown) can elicit pain and a clicking sensation, termed *Mulder's sign*.

Ganglion Cyst of the Foot

A ganglion cyst is histologically similar to the synovial sheath and contains synovial fluid. The diagnosis is easy to make when the cyst is located over a tendon on the dorsum of the foot (Fig. 51-5) but may be difficult when located among the compact structures of the plantar forefoot. A ganglion cyst usually causes edema along the involved tendon sheath. The mass should roll under the examiner's finger; a painless, immovable mass suggests a soft tissue neoplasm. Painful ganglion cysts are treated by aspiration with or without injection of a corticosteroid (see Chapter 52). After local or regional anesthesia (see Chapters 29 and 31), insert a 20-gauge needle

Figure 51-5 Ganglion cysts. A small amount of gel substance was aspirated with a needle, but a cyst of this size is best totally excised surgically.

Figure 51-6 Proper treatment of displaced fractures of the proximal phalanx of the great toe includes reduction, a non–weight-bearing splint that extends beyond the great toe, and referral to a foot and ankle surgeon.

into the cyst and withdraw yellow, thick, synovial fluid. Manually express any remaining synovial fluid after the needle is withdrawn. Corticosteroid injection is often advocated for ganglion cysts, but recurrence is common after aspiration and corticosteroid injection—as high as 57% in one study.[19] Recurrence, chronic pain, neuritis, stiffness, and infection are not uncommon even after surgical excision in many studies.[20] Other authors report improved functional outcome, a 9% occurrence of paresthesia, and only a 5.7% recurrence rate after excision.[21]

TRAUMATIC CONDITIONS OF THE FOOT

Trauma to the feet and toes is common and covers a broad spectrum of injury. Lacerations, fractures, compartment syndromes, and nail bed injuries are described in other chapters of this text. Three specific injuries—toe fractures, sesamoid bone fractures, and puncture wounds to the plantar surface of the foot—are discussed in detail here.

Toe Fractures and Fractures of the Sesamoid Bones

Emergency clinicians often treat toe fractures and can intervene to relieve the pain and encourage healing. As with any other fracture, pay attention to the possibility of disrupted joint cartilage, hypermobility of the fracture segments, and malposition or malunion of the fracture fragments. Fracture displacement greater than 2 mm is uncommon; reduction is rarely needed for most toe fractures.[22] However, aggressive reduction is indicated for fractures of the proximal phalanx of the great toe because it represents the main propulsive segment of the forefoot (Fig. 51-6). A plaster cast alone without anatomic reduction is insufficient treatment. Displacement suggests axial rotation or abnormal biomechanical interaction between the hallux and its own interphalangeal or MTP joint.

In the acute setting, a non–weight-bearing ankle splint that extends beyond the great toe provides protection until the patient with a complicated fracture of the great toe obtains follow-up with a foot and ankle surgeon. Open fractures

require careful cleaning, usually antibiotic therapy, and close follow-up. Fractures of the lesser toes generally result from jamming the toe into a nightstand or bedpost while barefoot. Radiographs of the lesser phalanges confirm the suspected fracture and may occasionally reveal an unsuspected interphalangeal or MTP dislocation. However, radiographs are not typically required, and the injured digit is easily reduced.

Treat closed, lesser phalangeal fractures with "immobilization" for 6 weeks. After the fracture is reduced, splint the injured toe against an adjacent noninjured toe. Place a soft corn pad or other suitable material between the toes to prevent skin maceration, and hold the toes together with adhesive tape or a self-adherent wrap such as Coban (Fig. 51-7). Demonstrate the procedure to the patient or family and dispense or prescribe enough material so that the splint can be changed every 2 to 3 days at home. Have the patient wear a less restrictive, stiff-soled shoe (Fig. 51-8). A postoperative shoe (or similar footwear) may be a comfortable alternative for the first several days.

Jumping from a height can result in a fracture of the first MTP joint sesamoid bone (Fig. 51-9*A*). The great toe sesamoid bones lie in grooves on the bottom of the metatarsal head. Each bone lies within the tendon of its respective flexor hallucis brevis muscle belly. Localized pain on the plantar aspect of the first metatarsal head accompanies a sesamoid bone fracture. Bipartite sesamoids (tibial more frequently than fibular) are common. Comparison radiographs clarify whether the radiographic abnormality represents a fracture.

For a tibial sesamoid injury, an aperture bunion-type pad, reinforced medially with 0.5- to 0.75-cm-thick felt, protects the sesamoid and transfers weight bearing to the surrounding structures (see Fig. 51-9*B*). A hard-soled shoe and NSAIDs are also helpful. Subsequent radiographs rarely show bony consolidation, but the fracture interface appears smoother.

Stress Fractures

A metatarsal stress fracture, commonly of the distal second and third metatarsals, can develop in runners, military recruits, or those with repetitive trauma to the foot (Fig. 51-10). Other

Figure 51-7 Buddy taping. **A,** Displaced fractures of the lesser toes (*arrow*) are often a result of jamming the foot into a bedpost or nightstand while barefoot and are easily reduced with in-line traction. **B,** A pad is placed between the injured toe and an adjacent toe. **C,** The toes are secured together with tape or a self-adherent wrap. (*B and C, Courtesy of Kenneth R. Walker, DPM.*)

Figure 51-8 A stiff-soled "postoperative shoe" prevents flexion of the foot and will provide comfort for patients suffering from toe and sesamoid fractures.

risk factors are listed in Box 51-1.[23] There is pain on walking but minimal to no external findings. A bone scan or magnetic resonance imaging (MRI) may detect the subtle fracture that often eludes a plain radiograph. Occasionally, an occult foreign body (FB) of the foot is the culprit and can mimic a stress fracture. Women are more prone than men to stress fractures. Treatment is usually rest and alleviation of the precipitant causes.

Plantar Puncture Wounds

Plantar puncture wounds present a diagnostic and therapeutic challenge for the clinician. Considerable controversy exists regarding the proper initial management of puncture wounds in the plantar surface of the foot, and no universally accepted standard of care exists. Treatment recommendations range from simple cleaning of the wound to aggressive débridement. No single approach has been demonstrated to be superior. The author supports close inspection for retained foreign material and an initially conservative approach, but an aggressive one is recommended if the patient returns or has an infection or if the pain persists for more than a few days.

Although nails produce many such wounds, various other objects may cause them, including other metal objects, wood, and glass. Patient response to the injury depends on the penetrating material, location and circumstances of the wound, depth of penetration, footwear, time from injury until initial evaluation, and underlying health. Since superficial puncture wounds generally do well, depth of penetration may be a primary determinant of outcome.[24] Because one's reflexes are not fast enough to pull back when stepping on a sharp object, the clinician should assume that the entire length of a

Figure 51-9 Sesamoid fracture. **A,** Jumping from a height can result in a sesamoid fracture (*arrow*). **B,** Bunion shields can be used to redistribute pressure away from fractured sesamoid bones.

Figure 51-10 Metatarsal stress fractures. Repetitive foot trauma can lead to metatarsal stress fractures, most commonly to the second and third metatarsals (*arrows*). These are usually subtle fractures that can be difficult to identify on conventional radiographs. Slight cortical disruptions (**A**) or periosteal reactions indicative of healing (**B**) may be seen, but often a bone scan or magnetic resonance imaging is needed to confirm the diagnosis. Treatment consists of rest and removing the precipitant causes.

protruding nail has entered the foot (minus the thickness of the footwear). Stepping on an unknown object in a field or while walking in a stream requires a more cautious approach than does a simple puncture from a known object, such as a protruding nail.

The vast majority of patients who step on a nail suffer nothing more than transient pain and never seek medical attention. Because most minor puncture wounds are not seen in the ED, the true risk for infection, including osteomyelitis, is unknown. Consequently, reported infection rates vastly overstate the actual incidence. Probably no more than 2% to

---

| BOX 51-1 | **Risk Factors for Stress Fractures** |

Sports involving running and jumping, especially on angled, hard, or irregular surfaces
Rapid increase in a physical training program
Poor physical condition
Female gender
Hormonal or menstrual disturbances
Osteoporosis or decreased bone density
Nutritional deficiencies (including extreme dieting)
Obesity and overweight
Inappropriate footwear
Poor flexibility

Adapted from Sanderlin BW, Raspa RF. Common stress fractures. Am Fam Physician. 2003;68:1527.

8% of puncture wounds become infected, and in only a small percentage of these wounds does osteomyelitis develop.[24,25] A prospective series suggested that only the presence of symptoms (e.g., redness, tenderness, increased swelling) at 48 hours is associated with risk for infection or a potential retained FB.[26] Retained foreign material (e.g., a portion of a tennis shoe sole) in the wound is an important factor in persistent infection. Because no single test detects all possible FBs, tailor the evaluation of a suspected FB to the suspected object.

Evaluation

The approach to the patient depends on several factors, including the time from injury to evaluation, suspicion of an FB, and the presence of infection. The extent to which an FB is pursued depends on the history and findings on physical examination. When the patient clearly states that a needle, pin, or nail was removed intact, radiographs or local wound exploration for a retained metallic FB is not needed. Stepping on an identified intact nail does not always require a radiograph, but if there is any debate regarding a retained metallic object, plain radiographs readily demonstrate their presence. Plain radiographs also demonstrate other radiopaque objects such as glass, gravel, bone, and teeth (Fig. 51-11). Rubber or pieces of a sock will not be visible on a radiograph. If the patient steps on an unknown object, a radiograph is usually indicated unless the entire depth of the wound can be ascertained and inspected. Ultrasonography is noninvasive and does not use radiation, thus making it potentially useful for radiolucent FBs, but soft tissue air or calcifications may suggest a retained FB when none is present. Bedside ultrasound has been used to localize radiolucent FBs for removal.[27,28] Computed tomography (CT) can demonstrate radiopaque and radiolucent objects, but its expense and greater radiation exposure than with plain films make it unsuitable as an initial screening tool. Use CT scanning when other screening tools fail to demonstrate a suspected FB, when infection is present, or when joint penetration is suspected. Fluoroscopy may be used to help localize metallic or radiopaque FBs during exploration and removal. It may be particularly useful for long metallic objects such as needles and pins. MRI provides no additional benefit and cannot be used when metallic objects are retained. Diabetics with unexplained foot pain or infection warrant investigation for a retained FB; diabetic neuropathy may mask the initial puncture injury.

Figure 51-11 Radiographic appearance of foreign bodies in the foot (*arrows*). Conventional radiographs will demonstrate a variety of foreign bodies. Shown above are glass (**A**), pencil graphite (**B**), and a metallic pin (**C**). Some objects, such as rubber or pieces of sock, will not be visible.

Treatment

As a general rule, the plantar surface of the foot should be *examined under good lighting and in a bloodless field*. This is best accomplished with the patient in a prone position, *not in a chair* (Fig. 51-12). Plantar puncture wounds explored for persistent infection often have foreign material in them. Because persistent infection does not develop in most patients, initial deep exploration in the absence of evidence or strong suspicion of retained material cannot be advocated.[24] Routine initial deep wound exploration, including coring of the wound, is not supported by scientific research and is not recommended for simple, noninfected puncture wounds.[24] However, selected wounds may benefit from exploration to facilitate a search for FBs and to promote irrigation, cleansing, and drainage. When the wound is large and retained organic material is suspected, local wound exploration may be warranted. Patients wearing rubber-soled shoes during plantar puncture wounds may retain a portion of the shoe in the wound. Exploration of the wound is most productive after local anesthesia or a regional anesthetic block and excision of the epidermal flap. An incision may be required to facilitate removal of the FB when known, but extensive removal of surrounding tissue has not been proved to increase successful removal of retained material.[24]

Some clinicians favor a coring technique *when an FB is found or suspected*. Although this may be too aggressive for many wounds, it may be the best way to remove particulate matter as a block (Fig. 51-13). To accomplish coring, advance a No. 11 blade to the hilt and excise a 2- to 3-mm core. Use a hemostat to grab the cutout core or to open the tract to better visualize the wound. Alternatively, use a 2- to 3-mm punch biopsy instrument to core out the tract. The tract can be packed with gauze for a few days or be left open. There is no evidence that coring a plantar puncture wound produces better outcomes than conservative or expectant treatment does, and it should be reserved for selected cases. Occasionally, blunt probes may facilitate exploration of the wound. It is generally impossible and probably counterproductive to attempt to probe or visualize the entire length of the puncture tract. Patients initially seen within 24 hours and without signs of infection generally require only simple topical wound care. Although irrigation of all exposed dermal tissue is recommended, high-pressure irrigation of deep tissues with distention of soft tissues is unlikely to be helpful and is not recommended. Schwab and Powers described a case series of uncomplicated puncture wounds in healthy individuals who underwent conservative treatment with cleansing and crutches.[26] Radiographs were obtained at the discretion of the treating clinician, and antibiotics were not given. At the 6-month follow-up, 88% of all patients healed without complication. In the remaining 12% complications developed, including wound infection from retained FBs. *No findings on initial evaluation predicted a subsequent infection.* Initial antibiotic therapy remains controversial, but there is *no evidence to suggest that prophylactic antibiotics reduce the already low rate of infection.* In fact, some cases of *Pseudomonas* osteomyelitis develop despite initial treatment with anti-*Pseudomonas* antibiotics. The author does not suggest routine prophylactic antibiotics for uncomplicated puncture wounds, and such treatment may theoretically select out resistant organisms.

Symptomatic patients who are initially seen later after injury (≥48 hours) are at increased risk for a retained FB because delayed evaluation is often associated with the development of inflammation or infection. Local wound exploration is warranted unless the patient does not have an infection or a clearly superficial cellulitis is expected to respond to simple oral antibiotics. Recurrent infection, deep soft tissue tenderness, and increasing soft tissue swelling suggest a retained FB or deep space infection, such as osteomyelitis. Such patients require prompt specialty referral or additional diagnostic studies in the ED.

Patients with obvious signs of infection within a few days of a puncture wound usually have a simple cellulitis (with or without an FB) with a gram-positive organism (Fig. 51-14). In a patient with persistent pain or swelling days to weeks after a puncture wound, the presence or absence of a deep soft tissue infection or low-grade osteomyelitis cannot be ruled in or ruled out by physical examination, plain radiographs, or laboratory tests (such as a sedimentation rate, complete blood count, or wound cultures). A high index of suspicion, coupled with additional investigation, is the prudent approach to patients with minimal findings on physical examination, normal laboratory test results, and continued pain or swelling after a seemingly simple puncture wound in the bottom of the foot. This usually entails CT, bone scan, or MRI. A study of 80 children with plantar puncture wounds and signs of infection found simple cellulitis in 59, retained FBs in 11, and osteomyelitis or septic arthritis in 10 children. Because a significant number of children in this study had retained FBs or bony infections, a cautious approach is warranted.[29]

Plantar puncture wounds complicated by *Pseudomonas* osteomyelitis and osteochondritis are clinically clandestine and particularly devastating. They have been described for nearly 40 years. Some investigators have cultured *Pseudomonas* from the soles of tennis shoes, thus suggesting that puncture wounds made through athletic footwear may be inoculated with *Pseudomonas* (Fig. 51-15).[30] No evidence suggests that prescribing prophylactic anti-*Pseudomonas* antibiotics on

FOREIGN BODY REMOVAL

The best way to examine a puncture wound of the foot is to place the patient prone on a stretcher, have good lighting, and obtain a bloodless field (blood pressure cuff was used here). First, remove the flap of skin at the puncture site. A local anesthetic injection (lidocaine 1%) is usually required but can be quite painful.

An amateur move is to try to examine the bottom of the foot with the patient in a hallway chair.

This piece of rubber (*arrow*) was introduced into a puncture when a nail went through a sneaker. It was not seen or expected until the skin flap was removed and carefully examined.

After removing the foreign body, the wound can be left open or packed, as depicted here. Packing gauze can be dry or wet with saline or iodine solution.

Figure 51-12 Removal of a foreign body in the plantar surface of the foot.

FOREIGN BODY REMOVAL: CORING TECHNIQUE

A foreign body is difficult to appreciate in this puncture wound of the big toe.

To core out a puncture, use a No. 11 blade and advance it to the hilt.

When the cored-out section is removed with a hemostat, note the present of a piece of rubber deep in the wound.

After coring out a puncture tract, the wound can be left open (as shown here) or packed (as shown in Fig. 51-12).

Figure 51-13 Foreign body removal: coring technique.

Figure 51-14 This 5-day-old inflamed and infected puncture wound tract probably harbors a foreign body. Minor lymphangitis (*arrow*) spread up the ankle, but there were no systemic complaints, adenopathy, or leukocytosis. Excision of a core of the tract found scant pus and a few pieces of the patient's sock embedded in the wound. The wound did well with oral antibiotics and warm soaks.

Figure 51-15 A patient stepped on a nail while wearing this shoe. An initial evaluation in the emergency department 3 weeks earlier found no foreign body or infection. A week previously the patient began taking antibiotics but did not improve. Findings on physical examination were quite benign, but the continued aching pain and minimal swelling suggested a deep infection. The complete blood count, sedimentation rate, and plain film were negative. Magnetic resonance imaging demonstrated osteomyelitis. *Pseudomonas* is often the offending organism in this scenario.

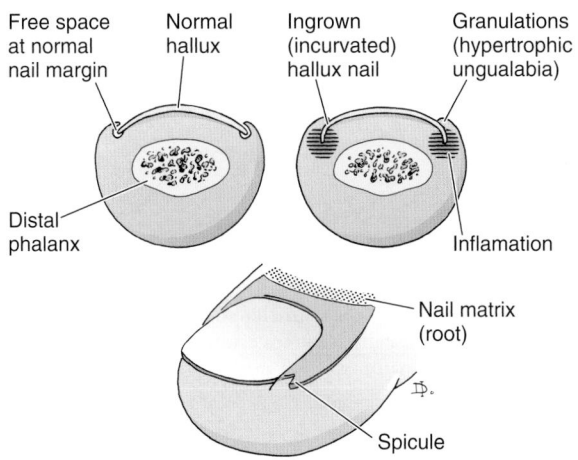

Figure 51-16 Pathology of an ingrown toenail. The normal free space at the nail margin is obliterated by inflammation and granulation tissue, which is caused by improper nail trimming, trauma to the matrix, and faulty footwear. *(From Hill GL II, ed.* Outpatient Surgery. *3rd ed. Philadelphia: Saunders; 1988. Reproduced by permission.)*

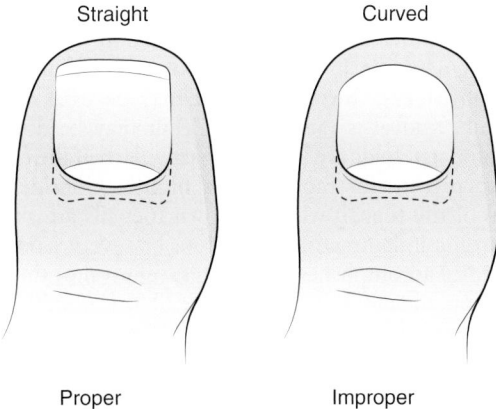

Figure 51-17 The proper way to trim a toenail that is prone to becoming ingrown is to cut the end of the nail *straight across, not at an angle.* This is counterintuitive to a patient who wants the nail to conform to the contour of the toe.

initial evaluation of an uncomplicated wound will prevent infection in patients with subsequent deep space or bone infections.[30] Some argue that prophylactic antibiotics, at the time of puncture, may select out resistant organisms.[30] Surgical débridement and prolonged intravenous antibiotics are often required for established infections.

INGROWN TOENAIL

An ingrown toenail is characterized by progressive curving or excessive widening of the lateral margin of the toenail and impingement of the nail into the periungual soft tissue (Fig. 51-16). The toenail normally grows distally in an unimpeded manner, thereby allowing the nail to pass beyond the lateral nail fold. Nail deformity, tight-fitting shoes, and rotational deformity of the toes increase the friction between the nail and the nail fold (Fig. 51-17). Toenails that have been trimmed in a curve increase the likelihood that the lateral nail margin will impinge on the lateral nail fold. The resulting soft tissue

Figure 51-18 An ingrown toenail of this degree requires removal of a portion of the nail and débridement of inflamed tissue.

injury may lead to hyperkeratosis, edema, and erythema of the nail fold or frank infection (Fig. 51-18). Although an ingrown toenail can be found on any toe, the majority occur on the great toe.

Evaluation

The patient has pain, edema, and erythema of the lateral nail fold. Pressure over the nail margins increases the pain. Because intense pain often precipitates an early visit to the ED, most inflammatory or infectious responses are confined locally. Recurrent ingrown toenails or those in patients with circulatory dysfunction, neuropathy, or diabetes may have underlying osteomyelitis. Cleanse the toe gently to facilitate visualization of the periungual debris. When the free edge of the lateral part of the nail can easily be visualized as separate from the lateral nail fold, consider other painful conditions of the toe such as trauma, gout, paronychia, and cellulitis.

Treatment

Because the toe is exquisitely tender, additional treatment will usually require digital block anesthesia. The decision to treat and what course of action to take in the ED depend on the patient's degree of discomfort. Two general courses of action are often suggested: removal of the offending nail spicule or removal of the spicule and some portion of the nail. Any degree of nail removal is usually followed by ablation of the nail bed.[31] Nail-splinting techniques may also be effective and are less invasive than nail removal techniques.

Removal of the Nail Spicule and Débridement of Hyperkeratosis for Minor Ingrown Toenails

When the amount of inflammation and pain and the degree of nail deformity are both minimal, such as involvement of only the distal toenail area, simple removal of the impacted nail spicule is indicated and usually curative. If the condition is advanced, complete removal of a portion of the nail may be required. All procedures are best done with a tourniquet to produce a bloodless field. After a digital block and thorough cleansing, remove an oblique segment of the nail about one third to one half the way to the proximal nail fold (Fig. 51-19). The ideal instrument is an English anvil nail splitter, which

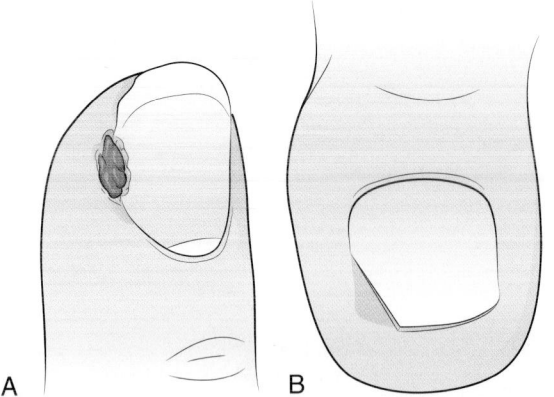

Figure 51-19 A, This minor ingrown toenail can be treated by removal of a portion of the distal end of the nail. **B,** An oblique wedge of nail is trimmed from the lateral margin of the nail to free it from the hyperkeratotic area. (*A and B, Courtesy of Kenneth R. Walker, DPM.*)

Figure 51-20 English nail anvil used to divide the nail. (*Courtesy of Gill Podiatry Supply Company, Middleburg Heights, OH.*)

is designed to cut the nail while minimizing trauma to the underlying nail matrix (Fig. 51-20). Sharp, pointed scissors may be substituted if care is taken to minimize injury to the nail bed by maintaining upward pressure while cutting the nail. Some clinicians use a disposable electric cautery device to cut the nail after softening it by soaking in warm soapy water.

After cutting the nail spicule free from the bulk of the nail, grasp the free edge of the nail with forceps or hemostats and remove it to expose the irritated area. The nail fold typically contains impacted debris that must be removed after the nail fold has been gently retracted away from the nail. Remove debris until the epidermis or dermis is uncovered while taking care to avoid aggressive débridement that causes bleeding. A silver nitrate stick applied to the débrided area may be used to control bleeding. Dress the area with antibiotic ointment and a nonadherent dressing. Soaking the toe in warm water two or three times a day, with home redressing, is explained. Harsh chemicals are avoided in the soaking regimen. The wound should be reinspected for signs of infection at 48 to 72 hours. If the problem has resolved, no further therapy is necessary. If the problem is persistent or recurrent, referral for definitive podiatric care is reasonable. Instruct patients to wear less constricting shoes and to trim the nail straight across. Like most FB reactions, removal of the nail spicule resolves the inflammation and infection. Antibiotics given without removal of the nail spicule will not ensure a satisfactory result or add benefit after removal of the spicule.[32] Topical antibiotics (avoid those containing neomycin) are reasonable, but systemic antibiotics are not required. Diabetics and those

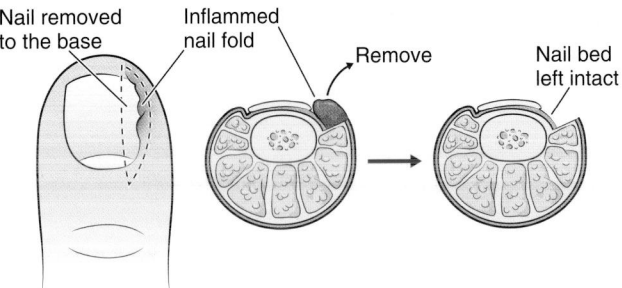

Figure 51-21 Resection of the entire length of a toenail plus removal of inflamed tissue is usually a curative intervention for a complex ingrown toenail. The nail bed is left intact.

with peripheral vascular disease require closer follow-up. When the ingrown toenail is caused by a nail deformity, a podiatrist or primary clinician can perform definitive removal during follow-up evaluation.

Toenail Removal for Complex or Extensive Ingrown Toenails

When irritation, infection, or both are more widespread or include the entire toe, removal of a portion of the nail and débridement of the inflamed tissue may be required (Figs. 51-21 and 51-22). Toenail removal may be total or partial. Total nail removal is rarely needed but may be done when both lateral nail folds are infected, particularly if the condition has been present for more than a month. Consider partial removal of the toenail when ingrown toenails are associated with chronic inflammation, infection, or severe pain. Partial nail removal accomplishes two things: removal of the offending portion of nail and destruction of the underlying nail matrix to prevent regrowth of the nail. Phenol, the most commonly applied chemical, causes neurolysis of the nerve endings and necrosis of the nail matrix in a procedure called *matricectomy*. Several studies have demonstrated that 10% sodium hydroxide solution is as effective as phenol and may be associated with less postprocedure pain and faster recovery.[33-35] Since most EDs do not stock phenol or sodium hydroxide solution, nail bed ablation is usually not pursued on the initial visit.

After a digital block, exsanguinate the toe by squeezing or wrapping, and apply a tourniquet at the base of the toe. Stabilize the toe with the nondominant hand. Separate the lateral third of the nail from the nail bed by advancing and separating scissors held parallel to the nail bed (Fig. 51-23). Split the nail lengthwise toward the cuticle. An English anvil nail splitter is desirable to begin the procedure, but sharp scissors or a No. 11 blade also work. Take care to perform a controlled division along the longitudinal lines of the nail for several millimeters past the proximal nail fold (cuticle). Grasp the end of the cut toenail with a hemostat or forceps. Remove the free piece of nail by twisting it toward the remaining nail. This will pull the nail root out from under the cuticle. Inspect the remnant to be certain that the entire piece of nail has been removed as desired. Sharply remove any remaining or swollen/heaped-up skin and all hyperkeratotic debris. After removal of the nail, most clinicians apply a silver nitrate stick to the nail bed and to granulation tissue for 2 to 3 minutes.[36] When finished, the nail bed is open and the heaped-up tissue is now flat.

INGROWN TOENAIL REMOVAL

1

Cleanse the toe with antiseptic and then administer a digital block. Use of a tourniquet to provide a bloodless field is ideal but is not depicted here.

2 Iris scissors

First separate the nail from the nail bed by advancing and separating scissors held parallel to the nail bed (see Fig. 51-23), and then split the nail lengthwise toward the cuticle as depicted above.

3 Hemostat

Grasp the end of the cut toenail with a hemostat and twist toward the remaining nail.

4 Nail spicule

Exposed nail bed

Nail root

Use the twisting motion to remove the free piece of nail. Sharply remove any remaining skin and hyperkeratotic debris. Silver nitrate may be applied to the nail bed if desired.

5 Spicule

Inspect the remnant to make sure that the entire piece of nail has been removed as desired. Note the prominent spicule present on this ingrown toenail.

6

Cover the wound with antibiotic ointment, a nonadherent dressing, and a dry sterile wrap.

Figure 51-22 Removal of an ingrown toenail.

As an option and if phenol or other ablating solutions are available, the following is suggested to permanently ablate the nail bed so that a new nail will not grow (Fig. 51-24). Apply a 10% sodium hydroxide solution to the nail bed with a cotton-tipped applicator for 1 to 2 minutes to provide effective ablation of the nail matrix.[33-35] Alternatively, apply a 1% solution of aqueous phenol to the nail matrix beneath the involved area of the lateral nail groove and proximal nail fold

with cotton-tipped applicators. A 1% phenol solution can be prepared by diluting a 70% to 90% aqueous phenol solution in an 80:1 ratio (e.g., 8 mL distilled water to 0.1 mL phenol). Remove some of the cotton if the applicator is too bulky to concentrate the solution beneath the proximal nail fold and lateral nail groove. Apply thoroughly moistened (but not saturated) applicators for three 30-second applications. Avoid forcing phenol under the remaining nail by rolling the

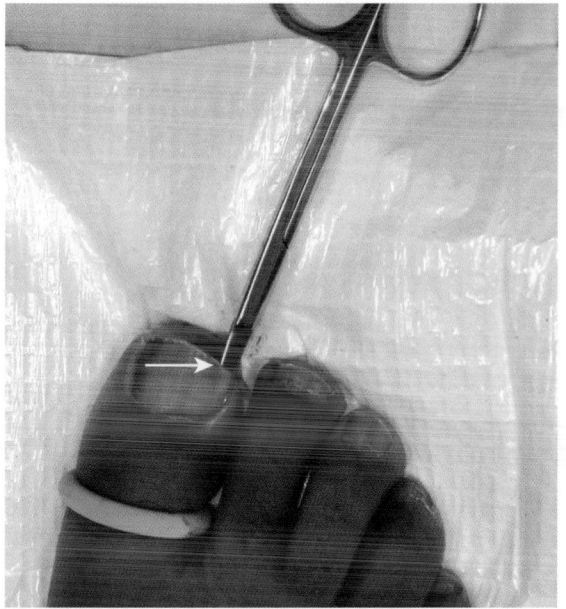

Figure 51-23 Before cutting the nail lengthwise, separate the nail from the nail bed by advancing and spreading iris scissors held parallel to the nail bed. Note the use of a tourniquet to provide a bloodless field.

applicator so that it rolls over the matrix and over the nail surface rather than against the split edge of the nail. Although it is necessary to cover the lateral aspect of the nail bed and lateral nail fold, do not allow excess phenol to contact the exposed nail bed or surrounding healthy tissue. After the third application, the cauterized tissue appears brown tinged or gray. Alternatively, a 1% phenol solution can be applied for 5 minutes. Thoroughly irrigate the cauterized nail bed with water and rub the area with a gloved finger to remove all traces of phenol. Snip away any remaining debris or dead skin with scissors.

Apply antibiotic ointment (not containing neomycin) and a nonadherent dressing to the wound, followed by a dry sterile wrap. *Do not forget to remove the tourniquet after the dressing has been applied.* Instruct the patient to wash the wound twice daily followed by dry dressing changes. Systemic antibiotics do not hasten wound healing and are not necessary in most cases.[31,32] Soaking the open wound in warm water twice a day is soothing and allows the patient to view the healing process. The wound will heal in 2 to 4 weeks and may be accompanied by serous drainage for 2 weeks. The patient should be informed of this possibility. Complications include nail regrowth, infection, growth of an inclusion cyst, or delayed healing. If the condition returns, podiatric referral is recommended for more extensive ablation of the nail bed.

NAIL ABLATION TECHNIQUE FOR INGROWN TOENAIL

Portion of the nail cut to the base and removed

Granulation tissue

Nail plate incision beneath the eponychium and above the matrix

Matrix

A

Granulation tissue curetted

Exposed nail bed

Nail matrix exposed beneath the eponychium

B

Nail bed

Nail

Curetted nail groove

C

Cotton applicator soaked in phenol

Phenol exposure concentrated at the matrix area (beneath the eponychium)

D

Figure 51-24 Nail ablation technique for the treatment of an ingrown toenail. The lateral portion of the nail is cut and removed (**A**) to expose the nail bed. Granulation tissue is curetted (**B** and **C**), and the nail matrix is cauterized with hydrogen peroxide or phenol (**D**) (see text).

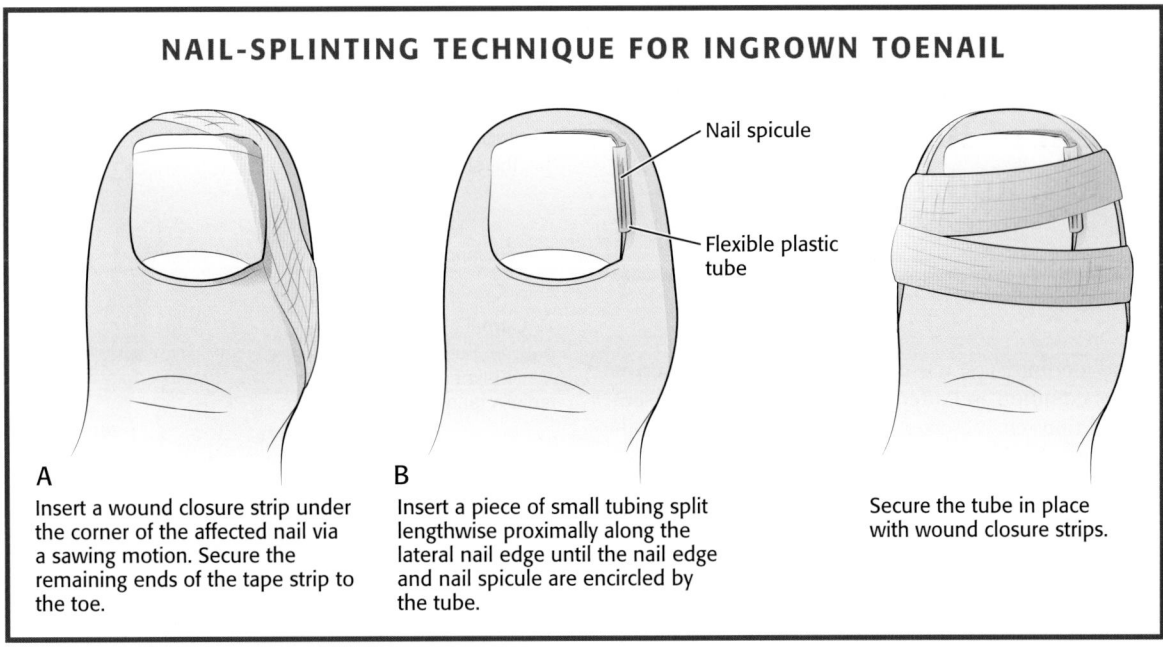

NAIL-SPLINTING TECHNIQUE FOR INGROWN TOENAIL

Nail spicule

Flexible plastic tube

A
Insert a wound closure strip under the corner of the affected nail via a sawing motion. Secure the remaining ends of the tape strip to the toe.

B
Insert a piece of small tubing split lengthwise proximally along the lateral nail edge until the nail edge and nail spicule are encircled by the tube.

Secure the tube in place with wound closure strips.

Figure 51-25 Splinting techniques for ingrown toenails.

Nail-Splinting Technique

Splinting of the nail spicule at the lateral edge of the affected nail may allow the toenail to grow out without affecting the inflamed soft tissue. This technique provides time for the periungual tissue to heal while the nail continues to grow until it can be trimmed straight across. No portion of the nail is removed when the nail is initially splinted. When the degree of inflammation is minimal, elevation of the nail spicule is easily accomplished with forceps or a hemostat. A cotton pledget inserted under the lateral edge to maintain elevation is often sufficient in minor cases. Alternatively, a wound closure strip can be used to elevate the corner of the offending nail.[37] After cleansing the edge of the nail and providing drainage if an abscess is present, insert a wound closure strip obliquely under the corner of the nail with a to-and-fro sawing motion until the corner is sufficiently elevated. Secure the tape closure around the toe (Fig. 51-25*A*). Instruct the patient to soak the toe in warm water daily, remove the tape closure, and reinsert a new tape strip. This procedure is repeated until the corner of the nail or the nail spicule has grown out and cleared the periungual soft tissue, at which time it can be cut straight across. When the degree of inflammation is moderate, nail splinting is accomplished by using the flexible tube procedure.[38,39] Obtain a surgical drain used to perform percutaneous drainage procedures that is 2 to 3 mm in diameter or the small tubing in venipuncture kits. Split a 1-cm piece of the drainage tube lengthwise. Perform a digital block and elevate the lateral edge of the nail with forceps or a hemostat. Insert the split drainage tube along the lateral edge of the nail so that it completely encircles the nail spicule and push it proximately until as much of the lateral nail and nail spicule as possible are covered (see Fig. 51-25*B*). Some authors suggest that the tube be secured with 2-0 suture passed through the nail,[38] but securing the tube with wound closure strips is more easily accomplished.[39] Instruct the patient to wash the affected area daily and replace loosened tape strips when needed. When the inflammation and granulation tissue have subsided and the nail spicule has grown sufficiently to not impinge on the periungual soft tissue, the tube splint is removed by the patient and the nail is cut straight across.

References are available at www.expertconsult.com

CHAPTER 52

Treatment of Bursitis, Tendinitis, and Trigger Points

Jason P. Becker and Joshua E. Markowitz

Bursitis and tendinitis are terms frequently used to describe a variety of common and often ill-defined regional musculoskeletal conditions characterized chiefly by pain and disability at the involved site. They are either periarticular or contained within specific soft tissue structures. Myofascial pain syndromes are characterized by sensory, motor, and autonomic symptoms that are associated with a trigger point, a hyperirritable point in skeletal muscle that reproduces the patient's symptoms. These musculoskeletal conditions largely rely on a clinical diagnosis in that they often cannot be confirmed by objective data such as radiographs or laboratory studies. Use of injection therapy with local anesthetics and corticosteroids for bursitis and tendinitis can relieve pain, reduce inflammation, and improve mobility. Injection therapy may provide definitive treatment of a condition or serve as an adjunct to facilitate rehabilitation therapy. Several invasive and noninvasive techniques can be used for the treatment of trigger points and myofascial pain syndromes. Successful treatment of any these musculoskeletal conditions depends highly on an accurate diagnosis and the use of appropriate techniques.

GENERAL ANATOMIC CONSIDERATIONS

Bursae and Tendon Sheaths

Bursae are potential spaces or sacs, subcutaneous and deep, that develop in relation to friction and facilitate the gliding motion of tendons and muscles. There are approximately 78 bursae on each side of the body as described by Monro and Spalteholz.[1,2] Tendon sheaths are similar in composition to bursae but differ in overall shape. Tendon sheaths are long and tubular, whereas bursae are usually round and flat.

Inflammation of bursae, as in bursitis, can be seen microscopically as a thickening of the normal thin surface of synovial cells lining the bursal wall.[3] *Tendinitis* and *tenosynovitis* are used to describe similar inflammatory reactions in tendons and tendon sheaths, respectively. Because of the adjacent location of bursae and tendons, an inflammatory process in one may also involve the other.[4] Common sites of tendinitis and bursitis in the body are depicted in Figure 52-1.

Bursitis may be caused by trauma, infection, crystal deposition, and chronic friction from overuse. Adventitial bursae may form in response to abnormal shearing stress at sites subjected to chronic pressure, such as a bunion over the metatarsal head of the great toe. Underlying systemic diseases, such as rheumatoid arthritis, ankylosing spondylitis, psoriatic arthropathy, and gout, may also involve the bursae and tendon sheaths.

In addition, some forms of tendinitis may be caused by factors other than overuse, inflammation, trauma, and degenerative disease. Gonococcemia, for example, is one cause of

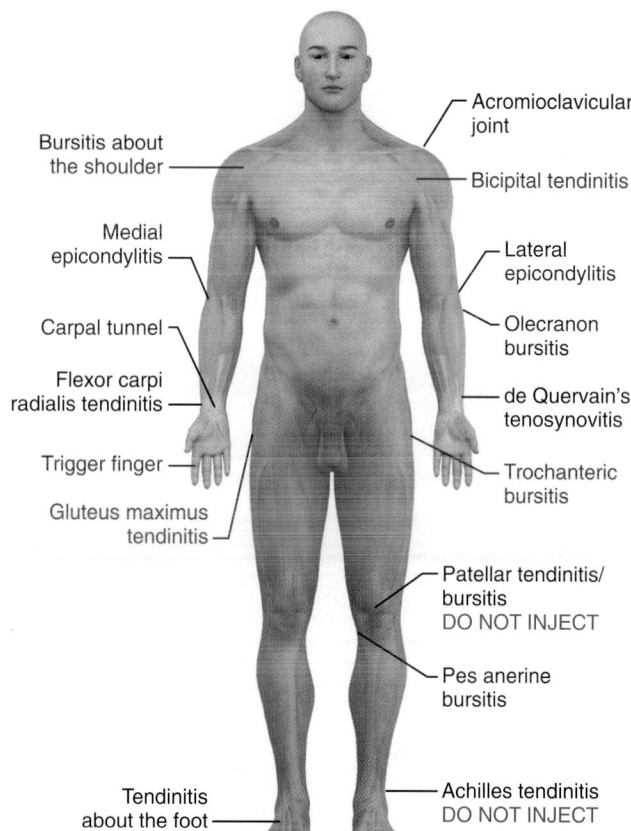

Figure 52-1 Common sites of tendinitis and bursitis. Corticosteroid injection therapy for tendonitis and bursitis is universally accepted and practiced, and the initial relief may be dramatic. However, the actual long-term benefit over other modalities, such as physical therapy, nonsteroidal antiinflammatory drugs, time, and even oral corticosteroids, is somewhat debatable. If the practitioner is reluctant to inject steroids, a course of oral prednisone or methylprednisolone may give similar short-term benefit. In most cases it is prudent to limit the number of injections at a single site to two or three. See Table 52-1. Do not inject areas of Achilles tendinitis or patellar tendinitis since rupture of the weight-bearing tendons can occur. *(Redrawn from Walker LG, Meals RM. Tendinitis: a practical approach to diagnosis and management.* J Musculoskelet Med. *1989;6:24.)*

tenosynovitis that should be considered in the appropriate setting.[5] Another rare cause is hemodialysis.[6] In 2008 the Food and Drug Administration added a black box warning to fluoroquinolone antibiotics highlighting the potential for tendinopathy and tendon rupture (Box 52-1). Clinicians should avoid tendon sheath injections in patients who are taking this class of drugs.[7]

Trigger Points

Myofascial pain related to trigger points is probably omnipresent, but it is vague and ill defined in the literature, the specific syndromes are unknown to many clinicians, and the disorders are difficult to clarify in many patients. Hence, myofascial pain originating from trigger points is often attributed to a plethora of other conditions. Consequently, the true incidence is unknown, and few clinicians practice trigger point injection therapy. Examples of misdiagnosis can include fibromyalgia, overuse syndromes, statin-induced myopathy, and malingering.

BOX 52-1	Information for Health Care Professionals

Fluoroquinolone antimicrobial drugs include ciprofloxacin (marketed as Cipro and generic ciprofloxacin), ciprofloxacin extended release (marketed as Cipro XR and Proquin XR), gemifloxacin (marketed as Factive), levofloxacin (marketed as Levaquin), moxifloxacin (marketed as Avelox), norfloxacin (marketed as Noroxin), and ofloxacin (marketed as Floxin and generic ofloxacin)

FDA ALERT (7/8/2008)

Fluoroquinolones are associated with increased risk for tendinitis and tendon rupture. This risk is further increased in those older than 60 years; in kidney, heart, and lung transplant recipients; and with the use of concomitant steroid therapy. Physicians should advise patients, at the first sign of tendon pain, swelling, or inflammation, to stop taking the fluoroquinolone, to avoid exercise and use of the affected area, and to promptly contact their doctor about changing to a nonfluoroquinolone antimicrobial drug.

Selection of a fluoroquinolone for the treatment or prevention of an infection should be limited to conditions that have been proved or are strongly suspected to be caused by bacteria.

This information reflects the FDA's current analysis of data available to the FDA concerning fluoroquinolone antimicrobials. The FDA intends to update this sheet when additional information or analyses become available.

From MedWatch. The FDA Safety Information and Adverse Reporting Program. *Available at www.fda.gov/medwatch/safety/2008.* FDA, *Food and Drug Administration.*

BOX 52-2	Clinical Characteristics of Myofascial Pain Syndromes

Characteristic distribution pattern of the pain
Restricted range of motion with increased sensitivity to stretching
Weakened muscle because of pain with no muscular atrophy
Compression causing pain similar to the patient's chief complaint
A palpable taught band of muscle correlating with the patient's trigger point
Local twitch response elicited by snapping palpation or rapid insertion of a needle
Reproduction of the referred pain with mechanical stimulation of the trigger point
Associated autonomic phenomena

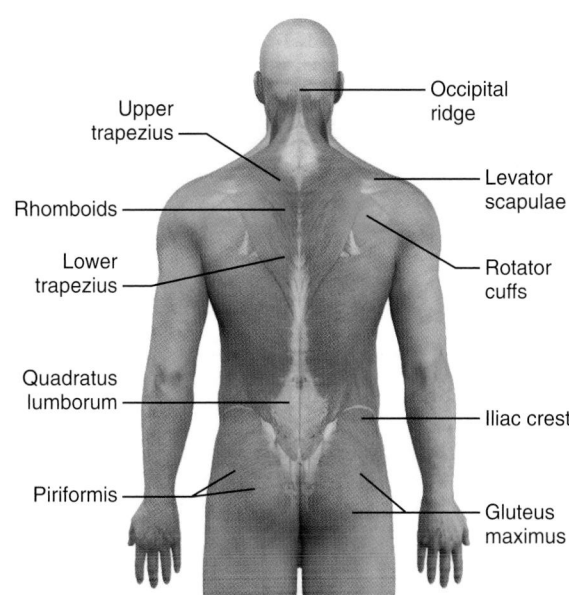

Figure 52-2 Common trigger point clusters. In the upper part of the trunk, a common trigger point cluster involves the muscles of the neck and shoulder area, including the trapezius, levator scapulae, and infraspinatus muscles. The quadratus lumborum, gluteus medius, and tensor fasciae latae are commonly affected lower trunk muscles.

Trigger points are hyperirritable areas, usually within a taut band of skeletal muscle or in the muscle fascia, that are painful on compression and associated with a characteristic pattern of referred pain, motor dysfunction, and autonomic phenomena (Box 52-2).[8] Trigger points can also be identified by the *local twitch response,* a brisk contraction of muscle fibers elicited by snapping palpation or rapid insertion of a needle into the trigger point itself.[9]

Trigger points probably develop in response to muscle fiber injury. The injury may be an acute traumatic event or more subtle repetitive microtrauma. The underlying pathophysiology has not been fully elucidated but probably involves chronic muscle stress, excessive release of acetylcholine, and dysfunctional motor end plates.[10]

Trigger points can occur in any muscle or muscle group; they are generally unilateral, but bilateral trigger points have been reported. Since the stress associated with myofascial pain commonly affects both single muscles and whole muscle groups, trigger points tend to cluster. In the upper part of the trunk, a common trigger point cluster involves the muscles of the neck and shoulder area, including the trapezius, levator scapulae, and infraspinatus muscles (Fig. 52-2). In the lower part of the trunk, the quadratus lumborum, gluteus medius, and tensor fasciae latae are commonly affected. Trigger points often affect other muscles innervated by the same spinal segments, and subsequent treatment is usually directed at all muscles innervated by both the anterior and posterior branch of the same spinal nerve. Table 52-1 lists common trigger points and their associated myofascial pain syndromes.

RATIONALE FOR INJECTION THERAPY

Bursitis and Tendinopathies

Management of the pain resulting from bursitis and tendinitis may be greatly enhanced by the proper selection and administration of local injections. Successful application of local injection and intrasynovial (bursa and tendon sheath) therapy requires an understanding of the diagnosis, accurate localization of the pathologic condition, and appropriate injection techniques. Lidocaine and corticosteroid preparations may be injected separately or together as adjuncts for pain control. The goal of corticosteroid injection therapy is relief of pain so that the patient is able to regain function and participate in a physical rehabilitation program.[5] In many cases a single

TABLE 52-1 Myofascial Pain Syndromes

MUSCLE*	TRIGGER POINT LOCATION	AREA OF PAIN	COMMENTS
Levator scapulae	Superior medial aspect of the scapula along the flat muscle belly; insertion sites on the transverse processes of C1-C4	Posterior cervical region, posterior aspect of the scalp, periauricular area	May cause or contribute to headache syndromes in some patients
Splenius capitis and semispinalis capitis	May occur in any part of these muscles	Over the muscles themselves, head, face	Having the patient point to the area of maximal pain may help localize the trigger point or points; may also cause dizziness
Trapezius	Angle of the neck, occipital insertion sites	Trapezius muscle itself, occiput	Inject neck trigger points carefully to avoid iatrogenic pneumothorax
Sternocleidomastoid	Sternal and clavicular origins, occipital insertion site, upper two thirds of the muscle belly	Sternocleidomastoid muscle itself, periauricular area, frontal area, face	May also cause dizziness, ipsilateral ptosis, lacrimation, and conjunctival injection
Infraspinatus	Anywhere in the infraspinatus muscle	Arm, posterior and lateral aspects of the shoulder	May cause sympathetic hyperactivity; subject to early degeneration
Rectus abdominis	Most common in the upper 3 segments, less often in the lower muscle segments	Anterior abdominal wall (upper segment), back (lower segments)	Often flare after abdominal surgery
Pectoralis major and minor	Most common at the insertion site on the anterior medial aspect of the shoulder and in the inferior muscle belly, but may be found anywhere in the muscle	Over the trigger point, upper most part of the muscle, ipsilateral arm	Because trigger points may be found anywhere in the muscle, it is important to search the entire muscle
Intercostals	Intercostal spaces	Chest (increased during inspiration)	Often flare after chest surgery or trauma; inject carefully to avoid iatrogenic pneumothorax
Tensor fasciae latae	Muscle belly	Lateral thigh pain to the knee	Tensor fasciae latae trigger points are generally easy to locate
Anterior tibialis	Upper third of muscle	Anterior aspect of the foreleg and ankle, dorsal surface of the ankle	
Gastrocnemius and soleus	Medial and lateral muscle margins, along the midline of the muscle	Posterior of the knee, Achilles tendon near the heel	Often flare with vascular insufficiency of the lower extremities
Quadratus lumborum	Along the 12th rib, around the iliac crest, lateral border of the muscle	Area of the 12th rib (especially during deep inspiration), anterior abdominal wall	May accentuate postoperative pain or pain associated with abdominal wall scars
Gluteus medius	Along the iliac shelf; in severe cases, the entire gluteal ridge may be involved (including the gluteus minimus and maximus from the sacroiliac joint to the anterior superior iliac spine)	Most often cause hip, leg, and lower back pain; may cause remote pain in the cervical region and head	Often associated with sympathetic hyperactivity; common in late-stage pregnancy and in patients with unequal leg lengths

*See also Figure 52-30 for diagrams of trigger points for specific muscles.

injection may be all that is required to ameliorate a painful condition. However, injection therapy is best viewed as an adjunct in the management of painful tendinitis and bursitis syndromes. It should not be viewed as a single quick fix, but a method to facilitate other modalities.

The precise mechanisms for the lasting analgesia and beneficial therapeutic effects of local injection therapy have not been clarified. Few clinical trials have adequately measured the efficacy of corticosteroid therapy. Although steroids are known to reduce inflammation, it is unclear whether the anti-inflammatory effect is responsible for the increased range of motion and relief of pain that the patient usually experiences. Histologic studies of chronic tenosynovitis lesions demonstrate degeneration, but not inflammation.[5] It is therefore possible that the pain experienced with tendinitis and bursitis occurs as a result of mechanisms other than inflammation, such as mechanoreceptor stimulation by shearing, traction, or activation of nociceptive receptors by substance P and chondroitin sulfate.[5]

Though often performed in the emergency department (ED) and ubiquitous therapy by orthopedic surgeons, rheumatologists, and family practitioners, injection therapy may not be definitive care. Hence, follow-up and additional evaluations and interventions should be considered. In short, injection therapy should be considered an *adjunct to a variety of treatment modalities*, including pain control, physical therapy, occupational therapy, relative rest, immobilization, and exercise. Additional pain control can be achieved with such options as nonsteroidal antiinflammatory drugs (NSAIDs), acupuncture, ultrasound, ice, heat, and electrical nerve stimulation.[5,11,12] Besides pain relief, early participation in rehabilitative activities and exercises can be an important aspect of patient recovery. Patients receiving only analgesics may have worse outcomes than those who also incorporate exercise as part of their treatment.[4] Any factors that provoke the initial injury should also be identified because failure to eliminate these provoking factors can contribute to the injury developing into a chronic condition.[5]

Although opinions in the literature differ, we recommend that corticosteroid injections not be repeated in the same site unless at least a partial clinical response has occurred. In addition, an injection should not be repeated in the same site more than once every 3 months.[5,11-14] Some limit corticosteroid injections at any given site to two or three injections before alternative therapy is pursued. Despite few data on the outcome of repeated injections, these recommendations are generally accepted and may limit the risk for adverse effects.

Though universally practiced and generally considered safe and effective for short-term therapy, there are sparse scientific data defining a true benefit of corticosteroid injections for musculotendinous conditions. Inflammation is not always the cause of tendinopathy. Although true inflammatory tendonitis may respond quite well to corticosteroid injections, conditions such as posttraumatic shoulder impingement and rotator cuff tears may not be expected to benefit more from local injection than from treatment consisting of rest, time, physical therapy, and NSAIDs.[13,14] Despite appearing to initially be effective for conditions such as olecranon bursitis, lateral epicondylitis, and de Quervain's tenosynovitis, long-term relief of other conditions is often superior with other modalities. In addition, oral corticosteroids can be as effective as local injection and can be an alternative for emergency clinicians reluctant to perform an injection.

BOX 52-3 Modalities for Treating Trigger Point Pain*

NONINVASIVE TECHNIQUES
Spray and stretch
Massage therapy
Ischemic compression

INVASIVE TECHNIQUES
Injection
Dry needling

Physical therapy, transcutaneous electrical stimulation, and ultrasound are adjuncts to both invasive and noninvasive techniques.

Trigger Points

Injection therapy is the most widely accepted and scientifically supported modality for treating trigger point pain.[15] However, because it may place patients at risk for becoming dependent on injection for pain relief, some authors reserve injection therapy for patients who have failed other measures (Box 52-3).[16]

Various substances have been used for trigger point injections, including local anesthetics, botulinum toxin, sterile water, and sterile saline.[16] Dry needling, a technique that involves multiple advances of a needle into the muscle at the region of the trigger point, provides as much pain relief as an injection of lidocaine.[17] In fact, in a recent systematic review on needling therapies for trigger points, Cummings and White[18] concluded that based on current medical evidence, "the nature of the injected substance makes no difference to the outcome and wet needling is not therapeutically superior to dry needling." In support of these findings, it has been proposed that the needle (not the injected substance) reduces trigger point pain by mechanically disrupting dysfunctional activity at the motor end plate.[16] Nevertheless, the addition of a local anesthetic is recommended to reduce the degree of postinjection soreness.[17]

The use of steroids for trigger point injection is controversial and without a clear rationale because there is little evidence to support an inflammatory pathophysiology for trigger point pain.[16] Hence, *the use of steroids for trigger point injection is not recommended.*

INDICATIONS AND CONTRAINDICATIONS
Bursae and Tendon Sheaths

The indications for steroid injection are twofold: therapy and diagnosis. Injection therapy offers not only relief of pain, particularly when a local anesthetic is used concurrently, but also a medium to deliver therapeutic agents. In addition to relieving pain, injection therapy may aid in diagnosis. When injecting a bursa, for example, bursal fluid is sometimes collected for laboratory analysis. Finally, the relief of pain helps differentiate a localized site of injury from referred or visceral pain.[12]

Absolute contraindications to local injection therapy are limited and include specific infections such as bacteremia, infectious arthritis, periarticular cellulitis or ulceration, and

> **BOX 52-4** **Contraindications to Local Injection Therapy**
>
> **ABSOLUTE**
>
> Infection (bacteremia, infectious arthritis, periarticular cellulitis or ulceration, adjacent osteomyelitis)
> Uncontrolled bleeding disorder
> Hypersensitivity to corticosteroid or vehicle
> Osteochondral fracture
>
> **RELATIVE**
>
> Anticoagulant therapy
> Joint instability
> Poorly controlled diabetes (steroids raise blood glucose levels)
> Hemarthrosis
> Decubitus ulcers
> Joint prosthesis
> Adjacent abraded skin
> Chronic foci of infection
> Internal joint derangement
> Partial tendon rupture

adjacent osteomyelitis (Box 52-4). The procedure is also contraindicated in patients with bleeding disorders. A history of hypersensitivity, either to the corticosteroid or to the vehicle by which it is delivered, is an absolute contraindication. Finally, corticosteroid injections should not be performed in a patient who has a documented osteochondral fracture. Relative contraindications depend on both the clinician's experience and the indication for the injection. Violation of the integrity of the skin or chronic foci of infection, either locally or in the vicinity of the site of involvement, is a relative contraindication. The procedure is also relatively contraindicated in patients taking anticoagulants, in patients with poorly controlled diabetes, and in those with internal joint derangements or hemarthroses. Patients with a preexisting tendon injury may be subject to tendon rupture if the corticosteroid injection relieves the pain and full activity is then resumed. Hence, partial tendon rupture is a relative contraindication.

Trigger Points

Consider trigger point injection once a myofascial pain syndrome has been identified (see Box 52-2 and Table 52-1). As mentioned previously, some authors reserve injection for patients who fail noninvasive modalities (Box 52-3). There are few contraindications to trigger point injection. Overlying infection is an absolute contraindication. Relative contraindications include proximity to sensitive structures, bleeding disorders, anticoagulation, an uncooperative patient, and lack of clinician experience. Dry needling is as effective as injection therapy, so in those with allergy to local anesthetics, the clinician may perform dry needling to avoid the problem.

HAZARDS AND COMPLICATIONS

Local anesthetics should be mixed with a corticosteroid preparation to increase volume, decrease postinjection pain, and assess the accuracy of bursae and tendon sheath injections.

Use of corticosteroids alone can be very painful. Local anesthetics may also be used alone, before injecting the corticosteroid. The major hazards with injection of local anesthetics are hypersensitivity and accidental intravenous or intraarterial injection (see Chapter 29). Serious or fatal hypersensitivity to procaine and other regional anesthetic compounds is encountered very rarely. This possibility is usually suggested by a previous history of reactions to these compounds. Ester solutions (e.g., procaine, tetracaine) that produce the metabolite paraaminobenzoic acid (PABA) account for the majority of these reactions. Amide solutions (e.g., lidocaine, bupivacaine) are rarely involved, and usually the preservative methylparaben, which is structurally similar to PABA, is responsible. When a definite history of sensitivity is present, use of any agent from that class of anesthetic agents is absolutely contraindicated.

Although there is evidence of allergic reactions from corticosteroids given orally and parentally, the possibility of an allergic reaction caused by corticosteroid injection is highly unlikely, and such cases occur infrequently.[19] Nevertheless, the clinician should be aware that anaphylaxis after injection of methylprednisolone acetate has been reported.[20] In addition, an unusual rash after an intraarticular methylprednisolone injection, which appears to be consistent with a delayed type of hypersensitivity, has also been documented.[21]

Minor reactions occasionally seen after injection of amide preparations include light-headedness or dizziness, pallor, weakness, sweating, nausea, fainting (rare), and tachycardia. These symptoms usually disappear within a few minutes after the injection and rarely require any treatment except reassurance and application of a cold compress to the patient's forehead. Frequently, it is difficult to determine whether the symptoms are the result of sensitivity to the drug or a fright (vasovagal) reaction to needles and injections. *Always place the patient in a supine, prone, or reclining position during the injection to minimize the effect of a potential vasovagal reaction.*

Be aware of the local anatomy and aspirate after injecting every 1 to 2 mL of solution to help prevent inadvertent vascular injection. Penetration into or striking a nerve may cause sharp pain or paresthesias, and the patient should be warned of this possibility in advance.

Corticosteroid injections have been found to be safe procedures with few complications (Box 52-5).[22] Although the possibility of introducing infection is one of the most serious potential complications, infections occurring as an aftermath of intrasynovial injections are extremely rare. In a study at the Mayo Clinic involving 3000 injections given in 1 year, no infections were reported.[21] Others have found the risk for infection to be 4.6 per 100,000 intraarticular injections.[23]

Although the problem of infection is usually avoided with meticulous attention to aseptic technique, caution the patient to watch for the development of any significant pain, redness, or swelling after local injections. We do not recommend routine prophylactic antibiotic administration after corticosteroid injections.

Local undesirable reactions are usually minor and reversible. After steroid injection, about 2% of patients may experience an acute synovitis otherwise known as "postinjection" flare.[10,16] This may be slightly more common with methylprednisolone acetate (Depo-Medrol) and less common with triamcinolone acetonide (Kenalog). Characterized by an increase in pain and joint swelling, symptoms usually begin a few hours after steroid injection and can last as long as 3 days.

BOX 52-5 Potential Side Effects of Corticosteroid and Local Anesthetic Injection Therapy

SYSTEMIC SIDE EFFECTS

Facial flushing

Nausea

Impaired diabetic control

Menstrual irregularity

Hypothalamic-pituitary axis suppression

Fall in the erythrocyte sedimentation rate and C-reactive protein level

Anaphylaxis

Dysphoria

Pancreatitis

Cataracts

LOCAL SIDE EFFECTS

Postinjection flare of pain

Skin depigmentation, fat atrophy

Bleeding, bruising

Steroid "chalk" calcification

Steroid arthropathy

Tendon rupture and atrophy

Joint and soft tissue infection

Histologically, steroid crystals have been seen within polymorphonuclear leukocytes, which makes it a true synovitis.[13,19] This reaction may be difficult to differentiate from an infection, and infection must be ruled out if the symptoms last longer than 48 hours or are associated with fever, warmth, or other suspicious signs of infection. Postinjection flare appears to be more likely to develop with the more soluble (shorter-acting) steroid solutions and may be related to the carrier in which the steroid is manufactured.[13,21] Limiting activity of the involved area for 2 days after the injection might help reduce the incidence.[19] When it does occur, the reaction is usually mild and can be controlled adequately with the application of ice or cold compresses and analgesics as needed.

Rarely, "afterpain" may occur and last for several hours after an injection. Although the cause is obscure, this phenomenon may result from the trauma of needle insertion, penetration of inflamed tissue, or pressure on adjacent nerves from local swelling or bleeding. Afterpain can usually be relieved by the application of moist or dry heat and analgesics until the pain abates, but it is best prevented by mixing a long-acting anesthetic, such as bupivacaine, with the steroid preparation.

Subcutaneous bleeding may occur occasionally at the site of injection if a venule, an arteriole, or a capillary is penetrated. Warn patients that this may occur and reassure them that the discoloration or hematoma will disappear spontaneously. Advise patients to apply ice packs or cold compresses to the involved area for the first 24 hours.

Another relatively minor complication is localized subcutaneous or cutaneous atrophy at the site of the injection.[13] This problem is chiefly of cosmetic concern and is recognized as a small depression in the skin frequently associated with depigmentation, transparency, and the occasional formation of telangiectases. These changes in the skin occur when injections are made near the surface and some of the injected steroid leaks back along the needle track. The skin depression usually recedes and the skin returns to normal when the crystals of the steroid have been completely absorbed. These changes are usually evident 6 weeks to 3 months after the initial injection and generally resolve within 6 months, although they can be permanent.[11,13] In the *two-syringe technique*, the anesthetic is injected first, the needle is advanced into the bursa/peritendon area, and the syringe is then exchanged for another to inject steroid. This technique helps prevent injection site atrophy by avoiding any leakage of the steroid suspension to the skin's surface.[24] Use a small amount of lidocaine or normal saline to flush the suspension from the needle before removing it. The *Z-tract technique* is a method of creating an indirect route from the skin puncture to the ultimate site of the steroid injection.[24] To perform this technique, insert the needle 0.5 to 1.0 cm from the actual target site. When the needle is halfway through the fat tissue, redirect it to the target site and inject both the anesthetic and the corticosteroid. Injection site atrophy is more likely to occur with preparations that are less soluble and thus longer acting.[11]

Minor skin depigmentation, especially in dark-skinned individuals, may be encountered, particularly with superficial injections. One cause is leakage of the steroid preparation back along the needle track. This complication can be limited by applying pressure to the site during withdrawal of the needle. Hydrocortisone would be the preferable agent for superficial injections to minimize depigmentation.

One of the most serious complications after local steroid injection is tendon rupture. In general, the risk is very low (<1%) and appears to be related to the dose used.[11,13] Some believe that injecting steroids directly into the tendon leads to a decrease in the tendon's tensile strength.[13,19,25,26] Gray and Gottlieb,[13] however, noted no cases of tendon rupture after more than 300 tendon sheath injections. We still advise that one be diligent and careful about injecting into the surrounding area of the tendon sheath and not into the tendon substance. Moreover, by using one size of needle and syringe, the operator is more likely to appreciate the increase in resistance when injecting directly into the tendon. We also suggest limiting the frequency of injections to no more than once every 3 months in the same site.[5,11-13] *Tendon rupture is more likely to occur in major stress-bearing tendons in athletes, such as the Achilles tendon and the patellar tendons. For this reason, injection of corticosteroids in these areas should be avoided in the ED.*[20]

There have been reports of accidental nerve injury after corticosteroid injection, particularly of the ulnar nerve (for treating medial epicondylitis) and the median nerve (for treating carpal tunnel syndrome).[27] In addition, pericapsular calcifications develop in up to 42% of patients undergoing local steroid therapy, although they are generally asymptomatic.[13,24] Finally, within minutes to hours of injection, approximately 1% of patients may experience facial and neck flushing. This reaction may last a few days, but it is usually a benign and self-limited reaction. Facial flushing seems to be more common with triamcinolone preparations.[11,13,19]

Systemic absorption of local corticosteroid injections does occur, though at a slower rate than with oral steroids.[12] As a result, patients are at low risk for systemic complications, but they do occur. Specifically, intrasynovial injections of steroids have been shown to suppress the hypothalamic-pituitary-adrenal axis for 2 to 7 days.[11] This complication is more likely to occur in patients who receive repeated injections in a short period or multiple injections in different sites at one time.[19]

TABLE 52-2 Injectable Corticosteroids

INTRASYNOVIAL PREPARATIONS	POTENCY*	RANGE OF USUAL DOSAGE (mg)	SOLUBILITY
Short Acting			
Hydrocortisone acetate	1	12.5-75	High
Cortisone	0.8	15-25	High
Intermediate Acting			
Prednisone	3.5	2.5-5	Medium
Prednisolone acetate	4	5-30	NA
Methylprednisolone acetate†	5	5-40	Medium
Long Acting‡			
Triamcinolone acetonide‡	5	5-40	Low
Triamcinolone diacetate	5	4-40	Low
Triamcinolone hexacetonide	5	4-25	Low
Betamethasone acetate and disodium phosphate	25	1.5-6	Low
Dexamethasone acetate	25	0.8-6	Low

*Hydrocortisone equivalents (per milligram).
†Preferred for emergency department use.
‡Best used for intraarticular injection.

Corticosteroids can also exacerbate hyperglycemia in diabetics.[12,24] Abnormal uterine bleeding has been reported as well.[11,12,20]

Other potential complications of corticosteroid and local anesthetic injections are outlined in Box 52-5.

CORTICOSTEROID PREPARATIONS

Commonly used corticosteroid repository preparations for the injection of bursae and tendon sheaths are described in Table 52-2. Local anesthetics such as lidocaine or bupivacaine can be mixed with the corticosteroid preparation in the same syringe. All corticosteroid suspensions, with the exception of cortisone and prednisone, can produce a significant and rapid antiinflammatory effect (in the synovial spaces). *Corticosteroids should not be used for trigger point injections.*

Corticosteroid preparations are categorized by their solubility and relative potency. Solutions that are more soluble have a shorter duration of action, primarily because they are absorbed and dispersed more rapidly. The addition of tertiary butyl acetate to the solution causes decreased solubility and therefore a longer duration of action. For example, triamcinolone hexacetonide, the least soluble preparation, has the longest duration of action.[13] Because the long duration of action increases its potential for subcutaneous atrophy, some authors use this preparation only for intraarticular injections.[12,13]

There is little consensus in the literature regarding which corticosteroid to use and what dosage is most appropriate for a given site.[5,21,24] Centeno and Moore[28] noted that the choice of injection agent is most dependent on the institution where the clinician trained. In 1995 a survey of 172 rheumatologists found that opinions differ regarding almost every facet of soft tissue and intraarticular injection, including patient preparation, choice of corticosteroid, and postinjection advice.[29] Some clinicians advocate mixing both shorter- and longer-acting corticosteroids in the same syringe with little consideration for the location or type of condition.[12,13] We do not recommend using longer-acting corticosteroids for soft tissue injections, particularly because of the increased risk for associated atrophy,[5,12] including atrophy of surrounding structures such as ligaments and fascia.[30] In general, use a short- or intermediate-acting agent for an acute or subacute condition such as bursitis or tendinitis; reserve longer-acting agents such as triamcinolone for chronic and prolonged conditions, including arthritis.[11,13] Triamcinolone acetonide and methylprednisolone acetate are reasonable first choices for most ED procedures.

DOSAGE AND ADMINISTRATION

Bursae and Tendon Sheaths

The dose of any corticosteroid suspension used for intrasynovial injection may be selected arbitrarily. Factors that influence the dosage and expected response include the size of the affected area, the presence or absence of synovial fluid or edema, the severity and extent of any synovitis, and the steroid preparation selected (Table 52-3). Dosages may also need to be reduced in the elderly.[31]

A useful guideline for estimating dosage is as follows: for relatively large spaces such as the subacromial, olecranon, and trochanteric bursae, use 40 to 60 mg of methylprednisolone acetate or its equivalent. For medium- or intermediate-sized bursae and ganglia at the wrists, knees, and heels, use 10 to 20 mg. For tendon sheaths, such as flexor tenosynovitis of the digits and the abductor tendon of the thumb (de Quervain's disease), use 5 to 15 mg. Sometimes it may be necessary to give larger doses for an optimal response. Intrabursal treatment of the elbow (olecranon) or the knee (prepatellar) bursae, which contain a considerable amount of fluid, may require 30- to 40-mg doses.

Unlike intraarticular injections for synovitis in patients with chronic joint disease, repeated infiltration for soft tissue conditions such as bursitis and tendinitis is not generally recommended or required. However, if only a partial response occurs or if recurrence develops, a single injection can be repeated as long as one waits at least 12 weeks between injections.[5,11-13,20]

Trigger Points

In contrast to injection of bursae and tendon sheaths, use small volumes of local anesthetic, botulinum toxin, sterile water, or sterile saline for trigger point injection.[15] In most cases, 1 to 2 mL of the chosen agent is sufficient.

TABLE 52-3 A Guide for Needle Size and Dosage for Injection of Common Regional Disorders

DISORDER OR INJECTION SITE	NEEDLE SIZE	USUAL DOSAGE OF METHYLPREDNISOLONE ACETATE (mg)*
Bicipital tendinitis	1.5-2 inches, 22-25 gauge	20-40
Calcareous tendinitis Subacromial bursitis	1.5-2 inches, 22-25 gauge	20-60
Radiohumeral bursitis Epicondylitis	1.5 inches, 22-25 gauge	20-40
Olecranon bursitis	1-1.5 inches, 20 gauge†	15-30
Ganglia on the wrist	1 inch, 22-25 gauge	10-15
de Quervain's disease	⅞ inch, 22-25 gauge	10-20
Carpal tunnel syndrome	1-1.5 inches, 22-25 gauge	20-40
Digital flexor tenosynovitis	⅞ inch, 22-25 gauge	5-10
Trochanteric bursitis	1.5-2 inches, 22-25 gauge	20-40
Prepatellar bursitis	1-1.5 inches, 22-25 gauge	15-20
Anserine bursitis	1-1.5 inches, 22-25 gauge	20-40
Bunion bursitis	1 inch, 22-25 gauge	5-10
Calcaneal bursitis	1 inch, 22-25 gauge	10-20
Superficial trigger point	1.5 inch, 22 gauge	N/A
Deep trigger point	2.0-2.5 inch, 21 gauge	N/A

N/A, not appropriate.
*Empirical dose. A larger or smaller dose may be used, depending on the clinical scenario.
†Allows bursa aspiration and steroid injection without removing the needle.

PREPARATION OF THE SITE

Preparation of the site before injection requires meticulous adherence to aseptic technique. Anatomic landmarks may be outlined with a skin pencil. It is important that the injection site and needle tip remain sterile with use of the "no-touch" technique, although sterile drapes are not generally considered necessary.[5,22] For operator protection, universal precautions should be followed.[12]

TECHNIQUES
General Considerations

Before beginning the injection, inform the patient of the specific indication or indications for treatment. Describe the procedure, including the risks and complications, and obtain informed consent. Subsequently, document the details of the procedure in the medical record. Use of a written consent form is not standard and is best based on institutional or departmental policy.

The material required for local injection procedures includes antiseptic solution, needles, syringes, a hemostat, culture and laboratory tubes, bandages, and sterile gauze (Fig. 52-3). Special trays may be stocked for this purpose. The usual sizes of needles for injection sites and corticosteroid doses are listed in Table 52-3.

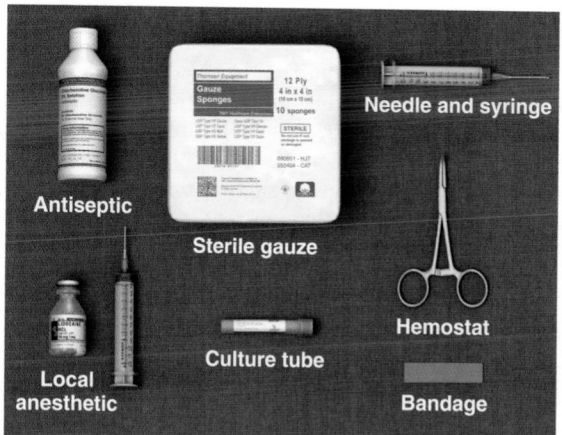

Figure 52-3 Equipment required for injection therapy. Needle sizes and corticosteroid doses are listed in Table 52-3. For those reluctant to inject areas of tendonitis or bursitis, a short course of oral steroids, combined with rest, physical therapy, ice, and nonsteroidal antiinflammatory drugs, is appropriate.

Bursae and Tendon Sheaths

Local skin anesthesia is an option before injection but not universally practiced. For bursae and tendon sheaths, local anesthetics can be injected alone or with corticosteroids mixed together in the same syringe. Use the Z-*tract technique* to limit the risk for a fistulous tract in the soft tissue. Because the steroid may theoretically precipitate or layer in the barrel of the syringe during the injection, agitate the syringe immediately before using it to optimize its distribution. In addition to minimizing the pain associated with the injection, mixing an anesthetic with the corticosteroid also produces a larger volume for delivery.[5]

The duration of action of lidocaine is approximately 1 hour, whereas bupivacaine may last up to 8 hours. Caution the patient that the local anesthetic effect may wear off within a couple of hours and that the beneficial effects of the corticosteroid may be delayed.

The optimum technique for joint and soft tissue injections has not been firmly established. However, one important aspect of a successful technique is accurate positioning of the needle. Injecting an inflamed synovial space, such as a bursa containing fluid, may be as simple as puncturing a balloon. Aspiration of fluid confirms that the needle has correctly entered the sac. Conversely, direct injection into a painful soft tissue lesion requires additional skill that can be acquired only with experience. Sometimes it is advisable to reaspirate and reinject several times within the barrel of the syringe, a procedure called *barbotage*, to obtain heterogeneous mixing and maximal dispersion of the steroid throughout the synovial cavity. Although it is desirable to inject the solution directly into the bursa, direct injection into the tendon itself is best avoided. If the injection requires the application of significant pressure, the needle may be in the tendon and should be withdrawn or advanced a few millimeters. The patient may commonly feel some myofascial radiating pain during the injection, but true paresthesias should not be elicited. "Electric shocks" felt with an injection may signal that the needle is in a nerve and should be repositioned.

Although an accurate injection is desirable, using a generous volume of anesthetic (3 to 6 mL) to dilute and hence disperse the steroid can compensate for less than perfect injections. Asking the patient to use one finger to localize the area of maximum pain and tenderness is the best way to ensure the most accurate positioning of the needle. In general, if the patient cannot localize a specific area of tenderness, the diagnosis should be reconsidered or the expectations of success lowered. Diffuse pain, such as throughout the entire shoulder or knee, is probably not tendinitis or bursitis and is not likely to be relieved with a local injection.

Trigger Points

Successful treatment of a myofascial pain syndrome requires accurate diagnosis (see Box 52-2 and Table 52-1) and precise identification of the trigger point (a taut band of muscle fibers). There are three generally accepted methods for identification of trigger points: *flat palpation, pincer palpation, and deep palpation.*[15]

To perform flat palpation, slide a fingertip across the muscle fibers of the affected muscle group while using the opposite hand to retract the skin to either side until the taut band is identified (Fig. 52-4, *left*). Snap the band like a violin string to precisely identify the trigger point. Pincer palpation involves firmly grasping and rolling the muscle fibers between the thumb and forefinger until the taught band is found (Fig. 52-4, *right*). Use deep palpation when the taut band is obscured by superficial tissue. Place a fingertip over the

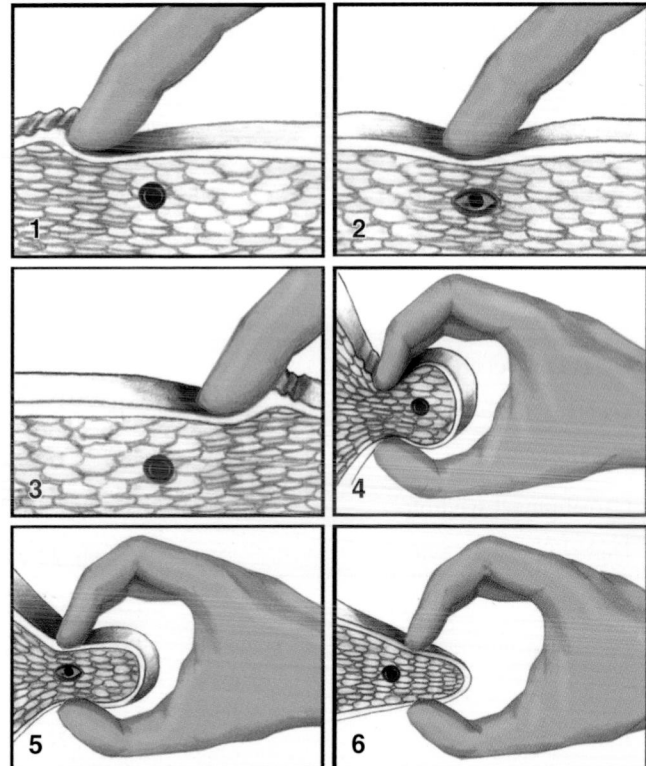

Figure 52-4 Identification of trigger points. *1,* Push the skin to one side to begin palpation. *2,* Slide the fingertip across the muscle fibers to feel the cordlike texture of the taut band rolling beneath it. *3,* Push the skin to the other side at completion of the movement (this same movement performed vigorously is snapping palpation). *4,* Surround the muscle fibers with the thumb and fingers in a pincer grip. *5,* Feel the hardness of the taut band while rolling it between the digits. *6,* Sharply define the palpable edge of the taut band as it escapes from between the fingertips, often with a local twitch response. *(Modified from Sola AE. Myofascial trigger point therapy. Res Staff Physician. 1981;27[8]:44.)*

muscle attachment of the area suspected of housing the trigger point and apply pressure in different directions. Reproduction of the patient's symptoms identifies the trigger point. It may be helpful to mark the trigger point with a skin marker for easy identification before treatment.

Once the trigger point has been found, therapy can be divided into invasive and noninvasive techniques (see Box 52-3). Noninvasive techniques used in the ED include spray and stretch, massage therapy, and ischemic compression therapy.[15] Physical therapy, transcutaneous electrical stimulation, and ultrasound treatments are adjuncts that may be arranged by the patient's primary care physician. Invasive techniques involve injecting the trigger point with local anesthetic or botulinum toxin or dry needling.

Noninvasive Techniques
Spray and Stretch
This technique of spray and stretch was once advocated by some as the single most effective treatment of trigger point pain.[8] Place the patient in a comfortable position and ensure that the target muscle is well supported and under minimal tension and that one end of the trigger point is securely anchored. Anesthetize the skin overlying the trigger point with vapocoolant spray (ethyl chloride,

dichlorodifluoromethane, or trichloromonofluoromethane) over the entire length of the muscle. Apply the spray at a 30-degree angle to the skin. After the first pass of spray, apply immediate pressure on the other end of the muscle to create a passive stretch. Perform multiple slow spray passes over the entire width of the muscle while maintaining passive stretch until the muscle achieves a full range of motion. Do not perform more than three repetitions before rewarming the area with moist warm heat, and do not allow each spray to last more than 6 seconds. Educate patients to not overstretch muscles after each therapy session.

Massage Therapy
This technique, as described by Simons and colleagues, uses "deep stroking" or "stripping" massage to allow the affected muscle group to be lengthened and relaxed as much as possible.[32]

Ischemic Compression Therapy
The principle behind ischemic compression therapy is to use pressure to induce ischemia for ablation of the trigger point. To perform this technique, apply and maintain pressure on the trigger point with increasing resistance until tension in the muscle is relieved. The patient might perceive mild discomfort but not profound pain. Repeat the process for each trigger point encountered.

Invasive Techniques
Injection Therapy
Almost any trigger point is suitable for injection therapy. Those that fail to respond to noninvasive treatments should be strongly considered for injection. Historically, various substances have been used, including local anesthetics, botulinum toxin, sterile water, and sterile saline. Despite the different compositions, durations of action, and mechanisms of action of these substances, a common finding is that the duration of pain relief following the procedure outlasts the duration of action of the injected substance.[15] As noted earlier, the authors of a recent systematic review concluded that based on current medical evidence, the nature of the injected substance makes no difference on the outcome and that wet needling is not therapeutically superior to dry needling.[18] Nevertheless, the addition of a local anesthetic has been shown to reduce the degree of postinjection soreness and is recommended by most authors.[17]

The technique most often recommended for trigger point injection has been referred to as the *universal technique*. Position the patient in a recumbent position to assist in relaxation of the affected muscles, overall comfort, and prevention of syncope. Reidentify the previously marked trigger point of interest, and scrub the overlying skin with a topical antiseptic solution. For superficial trigger points, use a 22-gauge, 1.5-inch needle. Deeper muscles may require a 21-gauge, 2- or 2.5-inch needle (see Table 52-3). Grasp the skin overlying the trigger point between the thumb and index or middle finger of the nondominant hand. Insert the needle approximately 1 to 1.5 cm from the point and advance it into the trigger point at a 30-degree angle. Aspirate to confirm that a blood vessel has not been entered, and inject a small amount of the agent. Withdraw the needle to the skin, redirect it to another area of the trigger point, and inject again. Use a "fast-in, fast-out approach" to elicit a local twitch response, which has been shown to increase the effectiveness of the trigger point injection and allows the entire trigger point area to be treated.[33,34]

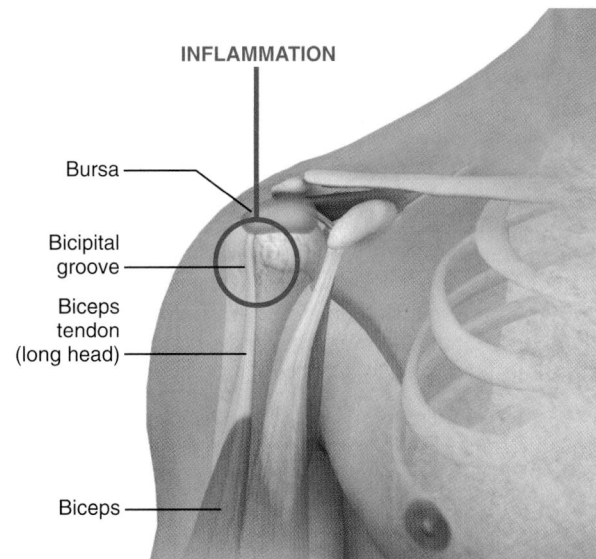

INFLAMMATION

Bursa

Bicipital groove

Biceps tendon (long head)

Biceps

Figure 52-5 Bicipital tendinitis and subacromial bursitis. Pain in the shoulder may be caused by biceps tendinitis or subacromial bursitis, but this is difficult to clinically differentiate from other shoulder conditions. Sudden pain and a distinct soft tissue bulge in this area indicate rupture of the long head of the biceps. Surgical repair is not usually required.

Severe cramping or paresthesias suggest inadvertent nerve entry and mandates withdrawal and redirection of the needle. For best results, it is critical to elicit a local twitch response with every injection. Following the procedure, the muscle group that was injected should undergo a full active stretch.[15]

Specific Regions and Clinical Entities

Bursitis and Tendinitis
Shoulder Region
Pain associated with disability may result from any of the intrinsic shoulder disorders, including bicipital tendinitis, calcareous tendinitis, and subacromial bursitis (Fig. 52-5). Because injection is easy and safe to perform, these areas are frequently injected, especially in patients who have failed more conservative therapy such as ice, rest, and oral antiinflammatory medications. Injections may also offer a diagnostic advantage when evaluating a patient with subacromial pain or a rotator cuff syndrome in differentiating shoulder weakness caused by impingement (shoulder strength improves after injection) and a true rotator cuff tear (no change in strength following injection). A potential long-term complication of untreated persistent inflammation is the development of a "frozen shoulder" (adhesive capsulitis).[35]

Bicipital Tendinitis (Tenosynovitis) (Fig. 52-6). This is a nonspecific low-grade inflammation of the biceps tendon or its sheath (or both) that is more common in those who repeatedly flex the elbow against resistance, such as weight lifters and swimmers.[4,36] The tendon courses through the joint and along the bicipital (intertubercular) groove, which can be appreciated when the elbow is held at 90 degrees of flexion and the arm is internally and externally rotated.[36] Patients may have restricted or normal range of motion and normal strength; however, they usually complain of tenderness on palpation over the bicipital groove.[4] Efforts to elevate the shoulder, reach the hip pocket, or pull a back zipper all aggravate the symptoms. Tenderness over the bicipital groove does not confirm the diagnosis, however, because the supraspinatus tendon is in close proximity to the insertion of the bicipital tendon.[36] Other diagnostic clues include the Lipman test, in which "rolling" the bicipital tendon produces localized tenderness; the Yergason test, which elicits pain along the bicipital groove when the patient attempts supination of the forearm against resistance while holding the elbow flexed at a 90-degree angle against the side of the body; and the Speed test, in which pain is reproduced when the patient resists forward elevation of the humerus against an extended elbow. Radiographic findings are normal and they are not required if the clinical diagnosis is supported.

APPROACH. Locate the point of maximal tenderness along the bicipital tendon. Make entry with a 22- or 25-gauge, 3.9- to 5.0-cm needle through an optional lidocaine skin wheal. *Avoid an intratendinous injection*, which may cause weakening of the tendon and predispose the patient to tendon rupture.

Advance the needle along the side of the tendon at a 30-degree angle and aim at one border of the bicipital groove to perform a *peritendinous infiltration*. Administer one third of the injection at this point. Withdraw the needle slightly but keep it subcutaneous and redirect it upward approximately 2.5 cm for injection of another third of the drug. Withdraw it again and redirect it downward so that it touches the bicipital border gently. Deposit the remainder of the drug at this point. With any of these injections, resistance to injection suggests intratendinous needle placement, which should be avoided.[37] If the two-syringe technique is used, instill 1 to 1.5 mL of an intermediate-acting corticosteroid suspension, such as prednisolone tebutate, at the point of maximum tenderness. Inject the anesthetic (2 to 4 mL of 1% lidocaine or 0.25% bupivacaine) along the upper and lower borders of the tendon.

Calcareous Tendinitis, Supraspinatus Tendinitis, and Subacromial Bursitis. These inflammations are so clinically similar that their symptoms and signs are difficult to

BICIPITAL TENDINITIS

Yergason's test. Yergason's test helps determine the stability of the long head of the biceps tendon in the bicipital groove. This test, which involves resisted supination of the forearm with the elbow flexed to 90°, may accurately reproduce symptoms of bicipital tendinitis.

Speed's test. While the elbow is maintained in extension and the forearm in supination, perform forward flexion of the shoulder against resistance. Patients with bicipital tendinitis may have pain or tenderness in the bicipital groove with this maneuver.

Bicipital groove

Biceps tendon

Insert the needle along the side of the biceps tendon (long head) at a 30° angle, aimed at one border of the bicipital groove.

Make a peritendinous infiltration by injecting around the biceps tendon in a fan-wise distribution. Avoid intratendinous injection. Use a 10- to 20-mg equivalent of Kenalog 40 (triamcinolone acetonide).

Figure 52-6 Bicipital tendinitis.

differentiate. The musculotendinous rotator cuff is composed of the supraspinatus, infraspinatus, teres minor, and subscapularis muscles, which insert as the conjoined tendon into the greater tuberosity of the humerus. The subacromial bursa lies just superior and lateral to the supraspinatus tendon (Fig. 52-7). Both the tendon and the bursa are located in the space between the acromion process and the head of the humerus and are particularly prone to impingement in this "critical zone." Impingement can occur when the shoulder moves forward and compresses the cuff and bursa under the anterior third of the coracoacromial arch. Injections into either the bursa or the tendon sheath area are commonly performed to relieve inflammation and overuse.

Figure 52-7 The "critical zone." Note the close relationship of the supraspinatus tendon and subacromial bursa to the humeral head and acromion, which make an exact clinical diagnosis very difficult.

In *calcareous* (or calcific) tendinitis of the shoulder, a calcific deposit (hydroxyapatite) is located within the substance of one or more of the rotator cuff tendons (commonly the supraspinatus).[38] These calcium crystals can occasionally rupture into the adjacent subacromial bursa and cause acute pain and tenderness in the deltoid area (Fig. 52-8). The bursae in relation to the greater tuberosity and the subdeltoid (subacromial) bursa are the most common sites of calcific deposits.

During the acute or hyperacute stage, the patient holds the arm in a protective fashion against the chest wall. The pain may be incapacitating, and all ranges of motion are disturbed, with internal rotation being markedly limited. Tenderness is often diffuse over the perihumeral region. The patient may also complain of pain at night when lying on the affected side and with abduction of the arm. Supraspinatus tendon impingement is most apparent when the humerus is abducted and internally rotated. The Hawkins test elicits pain with forcible internal rotation while the patient's arm is passively flexed forward at 90 degrees, and the Neer test elicits pain with full forward flexion between 70 and 120 degrees (Fig. 52-9). Both tests are fairly sensitive but not specific for supraspinatus tendon impingement.[39] Constitutional symptoms are rare, but swelling may sometimes be apparent with the hyperacute form, and a fever and accelerated sedimentation rate may even develop in some patients. When shoulder radiographs demonstrate a calcific deposit, the shadow appears "hazy" with lightening of the periphery caused by the pressure of inflammatory edema (see Fig 52-8*B*). Night pain may be intolerable and require opioids for control.

ANTERIOR APPROACH. In calcific tendinitis or supraspinatus tendinitis without calcification, use the anterior (subcoracoid) approach. With the extremity resting on the patient's lap, externally rotate the arm about 15 degrees. The point of insertion is over the depression that is palpable inferior and lateral to the coracoid process and medial to the head of the humerus (see Fig. 52-9).

Figure 52-8 Calcareous tendinitis. **A,** In calcareous tendinitis of the shoulder, calcium hydroxyapatite crystals are deposited in the tendons of the rotator cuff and occasionally rupture into the adjacent bursa. **B,** Abnormal calcific deposits in calcareous tendinitis of the shoulder are usually demonstrated roentgenographically in the suprahumeral region or adjacent to the greater tuberosity. When the bursal calcifications appear to be dense (as on this x-ray film), they are frequently asymptomatic, whereas lightening at the margins of the calcium deposit is compatible with the presence of inflammatory edema in the rotator cuff, which produces pain and tenderness in the shoulder region. The location of the calcific deposit on the radiograph may be a useful guide for the point of entry for aspiration and injection. Direct the needle to the calcareous deposit, aspirate, and deposit a portion of the steroid medication there. The calcium may subsequently disappear. Not infrequently, it does so spontaneously.

CALCAREOUS TENDINITIS, SUPRASPINATUS TENDINITIS, AND SUBACROMIAL BURSITIS

Hawkin's test. With the patient's arm and elbow flexed to 90°, the examiner rotates the forearm internally (i.e., thumb pointed down so that the palm of the hand is directed as far posteriorly as possible). Pain is reproduced if there is impingement of the coracoacromial ligament.

Neer's test. With one hand placed on the patient's scapula, the forearm is slowly flexed forward. The arm should be internally rotated such that the thumb is pointing downward. This test causes pain as the greater tuberosity of the humerus impinges on the acromion. Pain may be reproduced between 70° and 120° of forward flexion.

Anterior Approach

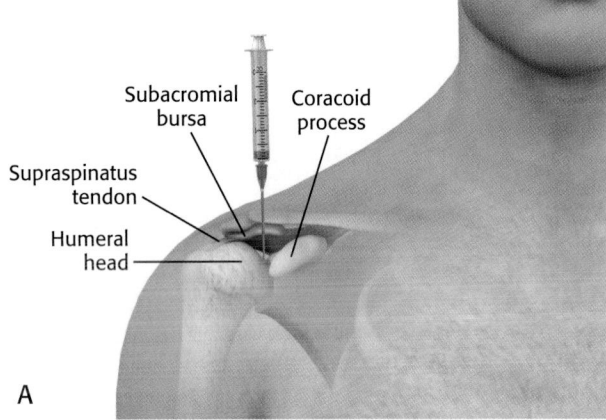

A

Externally rotate the arm to 15°. Insert the needle over the depression that is palpable inferior and lateral to the coracoid process and medial to the head of the humerus.

B

The bursa lies mainly under the acromion, but this is variable. Supraspinatus tendinopathy often occurs with subacromial bursitis.

Posterolateral Approach

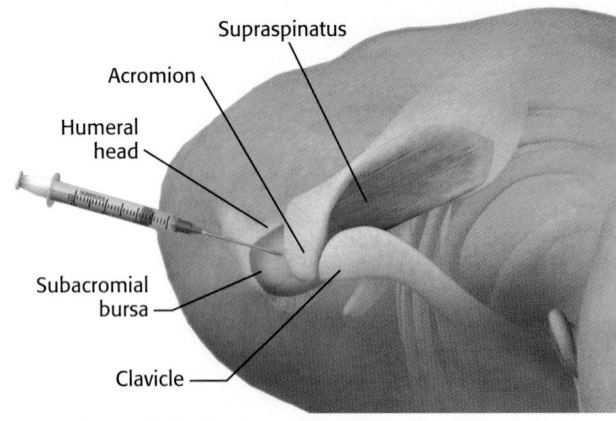

Insert the needle in the depression just inferior to the posterolateral tip of the acromion and superior to the head of the humerus.

Lateral Approach

For the lateral approach, insert the needle over the superior aspect of the humeral head and under the lateral margin of the acromion.

Figure 52-9 Calcareous tendinitis, supraspinatus tendinitis, and subacromial bursitis. Subacromial bursitis pain is quite common and responds well to injection. Recurrent pain can be due to a rotator cuff tear, which requires evaluation with magnetic resonance imaging. Pain is felt in the deltoid area and can radiate down the arm. The bursa lies mainly under the acromion, but this is variable. Supraspinatus tendinopathy often occurs together with subacromial bursitis.

POSTEROLATERAL APPROACH.   With the patient sitting and the lower part of the extremity resting on the lap, make a lidocaine skin wheal at the depression about 1 cm inferior to the posterolateral tip of the acromion, located between the head of the humerus and the acromion. Direct a 3.9- to 5.0-cm, 22- or 25-gauge needle toward the center of the head of the humerus and upward at an angle of approximately 10 degrees. Because the bursa does not extend posteriorly beyond the midportion of the acromion, it is important that the needle be positioned sufficiently anterior and inferior to the acromion (see Fig. 52-9).[40] After the site has been penetrated 2 to 3 cm, aspirate for any fluid or calcific material. Remove the syringe, but leave the needle in position. Attach another syringe containing 20 to 40 mg of methylprednisolone suspension or an equivalent intermediate-acting steroid, and inject the medication. Little resistance should be encountered when injecting the steroid. If resistance is appreciated, reposition the needle because it may be in the tendon substance of the rotator cuff. Follow this injection with 4 to 6 mL of 1% lidocaine (or a similar volume of 0.25% bupivacaine). Alternatively, combine the local anesthetic and steroid in the same syringe. Be generous with the volume of local anesthetic injected to ensure adequate dispersion of the steroid. A single treatment relieves the majority of acute disorders. An injection into the peritendinous space is similar to that described previously except that the needle is advanced deeper than with a subacromial bursal injection.[41]

If calcific tendinitis is suspected, some recommend attempting to aspirate the calcium deposits. After the bursa has been anesthetized, use an 18-gauge needle to penetrate the calcium, which often creates a "gritty" sensation.[36] In addition, consider using barbotage to facilitate cleavage of the calcium deposits and obtain greater dissemination of the injection. Use this method as described previously by aspirating and reinjecting the steroid or anesthetic-steroid combination repeatedly.[38]

Sometimes a painful reaction develops after the analgesic has worn off. Warn the patient about this possibility and give appropriate analgesia. A sling may provide additional relief.

Short-term use of opioids is appropriate. Although some authors claim that patients who do not also undergo physical therapy after corticosteroid injection have satisfactory results, some evidence supports the importance of close patient follow-up, range-of-motion exercises, and physical therapy for total recovery.[36]

AC Joint Inflammation.   Pain arising in the acromioclavicular (AC) joint is frequently an aftermath of an acute injury, such as falling on an outstretched hand or the result of weight lifting. With this injury, all ranges of motion of the shoulder cause pain, and the joint is tender but rarely swollen. Be aware that an obvious deformity or mechanism of injury may suggest AC separation or dislocation. With AC joint inflammation, crepitus is not uncommon.[36] Adduction of the arm across the body with forward elevation to 90 degrees (the cross-arm test) may exacerbate the pain because the AC joint is compressed with this motion.[36] In a study by Jacob and Sallay,[42] injection of corticosteroids provided short-term relief of symptoms but did not alter the long-term course of patients with AC joint arthropathy. Hence, some clinicians believe that AC joint injection should be performed only in patients with persistent pain despite a trial of rest, oral antiinflammatory medications, and modification of activity.[37]

APPROACH.   Make entry through an optional cutaneous lidocaine wheal over the interosseous groove at the point of greatest tenderness (Fig. 52-10). This is usually at the AC joint, which is palpated as a small V-shaped depression posteriorly at the most lateral aspect of the clavicle.[36] In this area the joint line is relatively superficial. Advance a 2.2- to 2.5-cm, 22- or 25-gauge needle approximately 5 mm and inject 1 to 2 mL of lidocaine and 5 to 10 mg of a prednisolone suspension. It is not necessary to advance the needle beyond the proximal margin of the joint surface.

Elbow Region
The elbow is subject to characteristic extraarticular disorders, including radiohumeral bursitis, lateral and medial

ACROMIOCLAVICULAR JOINT

Insert the needle in the interosseous groove at the point of greatest tenderness. This is usually at the AC joint, which is a small V-shaped depression at the most lateral aspect of the clavicle.

The joint is relatively superficial, and the needle will need to be advanced only about 5 mm. It is not necessary to advance the needle beyond the proximal margin of the joint surface.

Figure 52-10 Acromioclavicular (AC) joint inflammation.

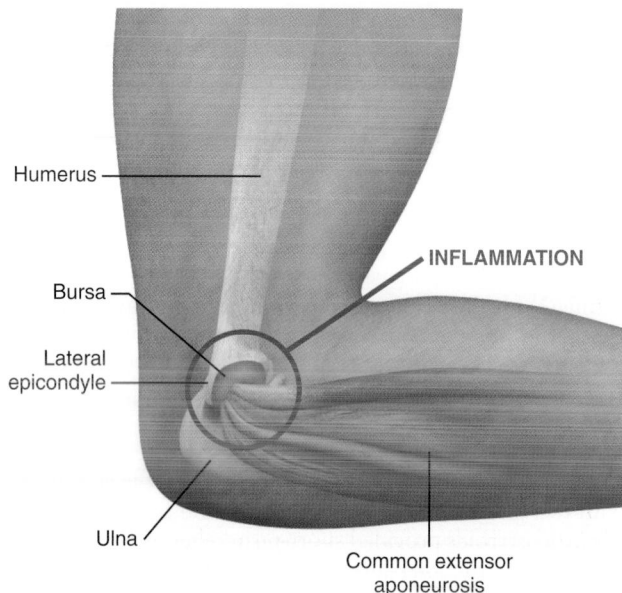

Figure 52-11 Lateral epicondylitis. Commonly known as "tennis elbow," this condition is common and quite painful and the result of microscopic rupture and incomplete tendinous repair of the extensor carpi radialis brevis origin on the lateral epicondyle of the humerus. Pain usually occurs over the lateral humeral epicondyle during work or recreation.

epicondylitis ("tennis elbow" and "golfer's elbow"), and olecranon bursitis ("barfly's elbow").

Radiohumeral Bursitis, Lateral Epicondylitis, and Medial Epicondylitis.
Radiohumeral bursitis occurs at the juncture of the radial head and the lateral epicondyle of the elbow. This condition is commonly found in combination with lateral epicondylitis, which is thought to result from repetitive microtrauma at the insertion of the *extensor carpi radialis* and *extensor digitorum* muscles. The symptoms of the two adjacent problems are indistinguishable, but tenderness overlies the radiohumeral groove with bursitis, whereas tenderness occurs chiefly at the lateral epicondyle with tennis elbow (Fig. 52-11). Although the term *epicondylitis* suggests an inflammatory cause of the pain, some evidence suggests that the injury in lateral epicondylitis results from a degenerative process causing a "tendinosis."[43] Regardless of the exact pathophysiology, there is often a history of repetitive motion of the wrist (flexion, extension, supination, pronation, or any combination thereof), such as while golfing, gardening, or using tools.[4] A clinical sign supporting the diagnosis of tennis elbow is provocation of pain when the patient attempts extension of the middle finger against resistance with the wrist and elbow held in extension. Alternatively, pain is reproduced at the elbow when the patient is asked to extend the wrist against resistance.

Medial epicondylitis (golfer's elbow) is a similar condition, although it occurs on the side opposite that of lateral epicondylitis and is much less common (Fig. 52-12).[4] This condition involves the origin of the *pronator teres* and *flexor carpi radialis* muscles. On physical examination the patient usually complains of pain when the wrist is *flexed* against resistance or when the forearm is pronated. Palpation of the medial epicondyle also elicits tenderness.

There is evidence supporting the short-term efficacy of corticosteroid injection for both lateral and medial

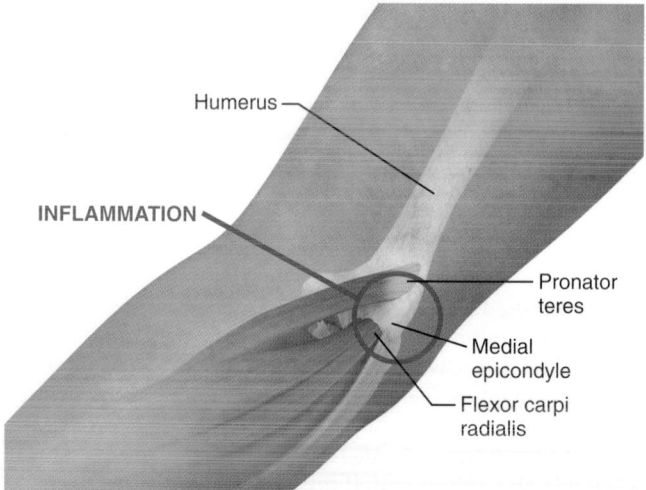

Figure 52-12 Medial epicondylitis. Also known as "golfer's elbow," medial epicondylitis is a flexor tendinitis with pain in the medial aspect of the elbow that is elicited by flexing the wrist. This condition is much less common than the lateral variety.

epicondylitis.[44-52] Successful injection of lateral epicondylitis produces a predictable short-term improvement (less than 6 weeks) in pain that is superior to that with nonsteroidal drug therapy and physical therapy.[45,49-52] However, after 6 weeks, physical therapy reduces symptoms more than corticosteroid injection does.[51] A similar effect was noted with medial epicondylitis: at 6 weeks patients injected with corticosteroids also reported significantly less pain than did those receiving physical therapy, but at 3 months and 1 year there were no significant differences in pain between groups receiving corticosteroids and physical therapy and physical therapy alone.[47]

APPROACH. For lateral epicondylitis, pronate the patient's forearm and flex the elbow to 90 degrees (Fig. 52-13). Palpate the radial head as a bony protrusion just distal to the epicondyle (confirm identification of the radial head by rotating the patient's forearm). The entry site is at the point of maximal tenderness, which is usually found at a location slightly distal to the lateral epicondyle. Using a 3.9-cm, 22-gauge needle, deposit 20 to 30 mg of methylprednisolone or equivalent intermediate-acting steroid mixed with anesthetic through a lidocaine skin wheal. Alternatively, follow the steroid with 1 to 3 mL of local anesthetic. Inject the solution in a fanlike pattern while avoiding direct tendon injection. For radiohumeral bursitis, instill part of the repository preparation into the radiohumeral bursa and part at the lateral epicondyle (see Fig. 52-11). With medial epicondylitis (golfer's elbow), use a similar technique, but take care to avoid the ulnar nerve, which lies in the ulnar groove behind the medial epicondyle (Fig. 52-14). Damage to this nerve during steroid injection has been reported.[53] Subcutaneous injection should also be avoided because it can result in skin depigmentation, atrophy, or both.[48]

Olecranon Bursitis (Aseptic).
Olecranon bursitis is an inflammation of the olecranon bursa of the elbow, located between the skin and the olecranon process (Fig. 52-15). The most common cause of olecranon bursitis is trauma,[54] which is usually minor, or activities that involve chronic leaning or repetitive elbow motion. Olecranon bursitis is also known as "barfly elbow" or "student's elbow," so named because

LATERAL EPICONDYLITIS

Patients often localize the pain with one finger.

Because this is an extensor tendinitis, extending the wrist against resistance or taking a book off a shelf elicits pain with lateral epicondylitis.

Insert the needle at the point of maximum tenderness, which is usually at a point slightly distal to the lateral epicondyle.

Infiltrate the injection in a fanlike distribution while avoiding direct injection of the tendon.

Figure 52-13 Lateral epicondylitis.

MEDIAL EPICONDYLITIS

Enter the skin at the point of maximum tenderness, over the medial epicondyle.

During injection, avoid the ulnar nerve, which lies in the ulnar groove behind the medial epicondyle.

Figure 52-14 Medial epicondylitis.

OLECRANON BURSITIS

Radial head

Humerus

Olecranon bursa

Olecranon (proximal ulna)

The olecranon bursa is found on the posterior aspect of the elbow and is directly superficial to the olecranon process of the ulna. Trauma is the leading cause of olecranon bursitis, but if may also be related to rheumatoid arthritis, lupus, uremia, and gout. Most cases are sterile, although septic bursitis is a clinical possibility and should be considered.

Aspiration and injection are not usually difficult because the bursa is often quite distended with fluid. Insert the needle into the most dependent aspect of the bursal sac. Minimize the risk for persistent drainage and skin contamination by inserting the needle through the skin 2 to 3 cm away from the bursa.

Aspiration and Injection of Olecranon Bursitis

Painless swelling over the posterior aspect of the elbow is characteristic of nonseptic olecranon bursitis. The mass is soft, movable, and fluctuant.

Using sterile preparation, advance a 20-gauge needle on a 10-mL syringe parallel to the forearm.

Aspirate the bursal fluid completely. Compress the bursa during aspiration. Typically, slightly blood-tinged serous fluid is obtained.

Change the aspirating syringe while the needle remains in the bursal sac.

Inject a long-acting steroid preparation (such as 40 mg of methylprednisolone). Use an elastic bandage to compress the site for 12 hours.

Figure 52-15 Olecranon bursitis.

prolonged leaning on the elbow can lead to bursitis. It may also be seen after an AstroTurf rug burn of the elbow during sporting activities. Other patients at risk for olecranon bursitis include gardeners, auto mechanics, carpet layers, gymnasts, and wrestlers.[55] More significant trauma, such as a direct blow to the elbow, can also cause olecranon bursitis. In this case,

hemorrhage into the bursa results in acute hemorrhagic bursitis. Other causes of olecranon bursitis include hemodialysis[56] and systemic diseases such as rheumatoid arthritis, lupus, uremia, and gout.[57]

The olecranon bursa is located superficially and is consequently susceptible to injury. Although most cases of olecranon bursitis are sterile, the olecranon bursa is the most frequent site of septic bursitis.[58] Therefore, it is important to accurately differentiate between the two entities. Steroid injections are absolutely contraindicated in cases of confirmed or suspected septic bursitis. Frequently, the diagnosis will be suggested by the history and physical examination, but it may be necessary to aspirate and analyze the fluid if septic bursitis is suspected.

In aseptic olecranon bursitis, findings on radiographs are usually normal, but soft tissue swelling may be evident. Bony spurs or amorphous calcific deposits may also be seen, especially in older patients.[54] Occasionally with rheumatoid arthritis and gout, nodules or tophi may be palpated within the bursal sac. The bursa and surrounding structures are not typically tender, and there is full and painless range of motion of the involved elbow. Signs of infection such as warmth and erythema of the overlying skin are also usually absent. It should be noted, however, that pain, warmth, tenderness, and erythema might be present in both septic and aseptic olecranon bursitis. If there is any suspicion of septic olecranon bursitis, aspiration should be performed and corticosteroid injection deferred until an infectious cause has been ruled out.[54]

Aseptic olecranon bursitis may be cosmetically bothersome to the patient but does not usually cause discomfort and may resolve spontaneously. In cases of bursal swelling that are nontender and not tense, treatment is symptomatic and includes NSAIDs, compression, and avoidance of further injury.[54] In cases of acute hemorrhagic bursitis, aspiration of the bursa followed by a dressing and ice will decrease the incidence of chronic bursitis.[54] When the bursa is large, tense, and inflamed and infection has been excluded, aspiration with steroid injection has been shown to hasten the resolution of symptoms.[59] Smith and colleagues[60] demonstrated the superiority of intrabursal methylprednisolone acetate over oral naproxen or placebo at 6 months and noted faster resolution and less reaccumulation of fluid with the steroid injection. The addition of a course of an oral NSAID after steroid injection did not affect the outcome.[60] Following steroid injection, application of a compression dressing and a brief period of relative immobilization may be helpful.[54] Repetitive steroid injections for aseptic olecranon bursitis have been associated with triceps rupture and should be avoided.[61]

Septic Bursitis. Septic bursitis is most common in the olecranon, prepatellar, and superficial infrapatellar bursae because of their superficial location and vulnerability to injury.[62] Infection of the other bursae is much less common. The infection is most likely caused by direct percutaneous inoculation of common skin organisms into the bursae as a result of trauma or contiguous spread from an overlying cellulitis.[54,62,63] Septic bursitis secondary to hematogenous spread is rare.[54,62,63] Most cases of septic bursitis are caused by *Staphylococcus aureus* (80%), followed by streptococcal organisms.[64] Other less common organisms include coagulase-negative staphylococci, enterococci, and gram-negative organisms such as *Escherichia coli* and *Pseudomonas aeruginosa*.[62] Isolated cases of bursitis caused by fungi (*Aspergillus terreus, Candida lusitaniae*), *Brucella*, and *Mycobacterium tuberculosis* have also been reported.[54] Such unusual organisms should be considered in cases of septic bursitis that are subacute or chronic and those discovered in an immunocompromised host.[54]

The most common cause of olecranon septic bursitis is trauma. It has been estimated that as many as 70% of cases of septic bursitis are related to trauma, either chronic and caused by repetitive injury or acute and often associated with occupational or recreational activities.[62] Other risk factors for the development of septic bursitis include chronic illnesses (e.g., diabetes mellitus, alcoholism) and previous inflammation of the bursa, as occurs with gout, rheumatoid arthritis, and uremia.[62] Infection may follow an injection of corticosteroids into the bursae in up to 10% of cases.[65]

At times the diagnosis of septic bursitis can be challenging. Acute gouty olecranon bursitis may have a very similar clinical picture and can often be accurately differentiated from septic arthritis only by fluid analysis (Fig. 52-16). Other conditions that may mimic bacterial septic olecranon bursitis include acute rheumatoid bursitis, aseptic bursitis secondary to oxalosis induced by dialysis, or infectious bursitis caused by unusual organisms such as *Mycobacterium, Serratia marcescens*, or fungi. About one third of all cases of olecranon bursitis are septic.[54]

In some cases the diagnosis of septic bursitis is obvious (see Fig. 52-16*A*). The onset of pain and swelling may be quite rapid (over a period of 8 to 24 hours), as opposed to the more gradual onset of aseptic bursitis. The bursa is erythematous, tense, swollen, warm, and very painful. Flexion of the elbow is limited by pain; however, some joint mobility may be present because the bursa does not usually extend into the joint.[62] The patient may report a history of trauma to the area, which may be evident on physical examination. Some patients will also have a fever. Smith and associates found that the infected bursa was generally 2.2°C or more warmer than the unaffected elbow.[66]

Aspiration of infected bursal fluid with culture of bacteria from the aspirate confirms the diagnosis of septic bursitis. Fluid is usually easily obtained from the tense bursa and (in the case of established infection) may be cloudy or grossly purulent. The white blood cell count of the fluid in septic bursitis is usually 5000 to 100,000 cells/mm^3 or greater, and the proportion of polymorphonuclear cells usually exceeds 90%. Neither fever nor systemic leukocytosis is considered sensitive or specific for the disease. However, in immunocompromised patients (e.g., those with diabetes mellitus, alcoholism), the white blood cell count in the bursal fluid tends to be higher.[67] Because of some overlap in the leukocyte count of bursal fluid in septic versus aseptic bursitis, it is important to remember that a low bursal white blood cell count does not exclude a septic cause. Moreover, the sensitivity of Gram stain may be 50% or less.[68] In a large study of 200 patients with olecranon bursitis, cell count and Gram stain were not always helpful in the acute evaluation and treatment of new cases of septic bursitis.[69] Therefore, if clinical suspicion for septic olecranon bursitis is high, even in the presence of a normal or equivocal fluid cell count or Gram stain, *steroid injection should be delayed* and empirical antibiotic therapy started until the results of culture are available.[54]

Treatment of septic bursitis includes the use of antibiotics directed against penicillinase-producing *Staphylococcus*, splinting, warm soaks, and drainage of the bursa. Drainage may be performed by daily needle aspiration until the fluid is sterile.[63] However, open incision and drainage might be required, particularly if the infection is recurrent or refractory.[70] In addition to daily drainage of the bursa as necessary, administer antibiotics for at least 2 weeks.[63] Consider additional antibiotic coverage against methicillin-resistant *S. aureus* based on the patient's risk factors and epidemiology.[62] Outpatient

Figure 52-16 A, Fully developed septic bursitis is usually distinguished from nonseptic bursitis by clinical parameters. In the septic variety, there is diffuse swelling (as opposed to a discrete mass), and the area is red, warm, and quite tender. In addition, bursal fluid leukocytosis is present. **B,** Acute gout can cause painful olecranon bursitis resembling septic bursitis. **C,** Aspiration can yield urate paste. **D,** Tophi in a patient with advanced gout.

therapy with oral antibiotics is generally acceptable, although this approach has been challenged for immunocompromised patients.[67] This decision is generally guided by the clinical appearance of the bursa, as well as associated comorbid conditions, compliance, and other factors regarding patient care. Response to antibiotic therapy might be slow. Thus, it is important to initiate antimicrobial treatment as soon as clinical suspicion of septic bursitis exists. Additional treatment with oral NSAIDs may help reduce the pain. Standard gout medications will generally resolve acute gouty bursitis.

APPROACH.   Insert a 2.5- to 3.9-cm, 20-gauge needle through a lidocaine skin wheal at a dependent aspect of the bursal sac (see Fig. 52-15, *steps 1 to 5*). To minimize the risk for persistent drainage after aspiration and for contamination of the overlying skin, penetrate the skin 2 to 3 cm from the bursa.[54,55] If infected or inspissated fluid is anticipated, use a 16- to 18-gauge needle to aspirate the viscous contents. Aspirate as much fluid as possible, and then inject 15 to 30 mg of methylprednisolone or an equivalent intermediate-acting steroid. With aseptic bursitis, the aspirated fluid may be yellow and clear, but it is often mildly serosanguineous in appearance. The leukocyte count of the aspirated fluid of aseptic bursitis should be less than 1000/mm³. Counts of about 2000 to 10,000/mm³ are associated with a higher incidence of infection or acute gout. After aspiration and injection, wrap the elbow in an elastic compression bandage for 5 to 7 days. *Again, if septic olecranon bursitis is suspected, do not perform corticosteroid injections.*

Wrist and Hand Region

Ganglion Cysts of the Wrist or Hand.   These cystic swellings occur frequently on the hands, especially on the dorsal aspect of the wrist (Fig. 52-17). Ganglion cysts are common and make up approximately 60% of all soft tissue tumors

affecting the wrist and hand. They usually develop spontaneously in adults between 20 and 50 years of age, with a female-to-male ratio of 3:1. Ganglion cysts may also be seen on the foot and ankle, generally on the extensor surface.

The etiology of ganglia remains obscure; there is usually no history of trauma.[71] The word *ganglion* is derived from the Greek word meaning "cystic tumor." The mesothelium- or synovium-lined cystic structures are attached to or may arise from tendon sheaths or near the joint capsule and do not extend into the joint itself.[72] Attachment is often by a pedicle. The wall of a ganglion is smooth, fibrous, and of variable thickness. The cyst is filled with a clear, gelatinous, sticky, or mucoid fluid of great density. The viscous fluid in the cyst may sometimes represent almost pure hyaluronic acid.

The types of ganglia vary with their location. The most common ganglia are located on the dorsal surface of the wrist and arise from the scapholunate joint. These constitute approximately 65% of ganglia. Volar wrist ganglia, which arise over the distal aspect of the radius, constitute another 20% to 25% of ganglia and are often adherent to the radial artery.[73] Flexor tendon sheath ganglia make up the remaining 10% to 15% and are found on the hand and wrist.

Most ganglia are of no great clinical significance and most do not require treatment. Spontaneous regression is common. However, if the appearance of the cyst is disturbing to the patient or if the ganglion is painful or tender (from soft tissue or nerve compression or bone erosion), simple aspiration with or without injection of a corticosteroid suspension is usually an effective approach. Up to three aspirations may be required before the technique is considered a failure. In one study, 69% of 116 patients required only a single aspiration for successful treatment.[74] Two or three aspirations were required in 19%, and only 12% of patients ultimately needed surgical excision.[74] It should be noted, however, that ganglia often recur

Figure 52-17 Typical dorsal ganglion cyst of the wrist (**A**) and dorsum of the foot (**B**).

after aspiration or surgery. In a study by Dias,[75] 42% of palmar wrist ganglia treated by surgical excision and 47% treated by aspiration recurred within 5 years. Because aspiration with or without steroid injection is associated with considerable cost savings and shorter recovery times than with surgery and because there is no difference in recurrence rates, aspiration appears to be the initial treatment of choice.[75] In the event that nonsurgical treatment fails, surgical excision may be indicated. The "old" treatment of attempting to rupture the ganglion with a heavy book is not advised because of the potential for local injury. Aspiration of volar wrist ganglia should also be undertaken with caution because the radial artery often adheres to the cyst and may be at risk for injury.[73]

APPROACH. Following the instillation of 1% lidocaine for local anesthesia, insert a 2.5-cm, relatively large-bore needle (17 to 18 gauge) into the center of the ganglion and aspirate the contents (see Fig. 52-17*A*). Usually, 1 to 2 mL of mucinous fluid can be aspirated. Milk the contents of the cyst toward the aspiration needle to maximize the volume removed, but do not stick yourself with the needle.[76] After the cyst is localized by aspiration, use another smaller needle to

Figure 52-18 de Quervain's disease and intersection syndrome. de Quervain's tenosynovitis occurs in the first dorsal compartment of the wrist secondary to tenosynovitis of the abductor pollicis longus and extensor pollicis brevis tendons. Symptoms, which include pain over the radial styloid, are generally caused by overuse. Intersection syndrome, often confused with de Quervain's disease, produces symptoms 4 to 8 cm more proximally.

administer 10 to 15 mg of methylprednisolone (or an equivalent intermediate-acting steroid). Instillation of steroids into the cyst is a common procedure that has been proved to significantly augment the success of simple aspiration.[77] Following aspiration, a splint is not usually required, and activity need not be restricted. There is no proven role for routine NSAIDs or oral steroid therapy.

de Quervain's Disease and Intersection Syndrome. de Quervain's disease, a relatively common disorder, is a stenosing tenovaginitis of the extensor pollicis brevis (EPB) tendon and the abductor pollicis longus (APL) tendon of the thumb (Fig. 52-18). Though commonly referred to as a tenosynovitis, which denotes inflammation of the synovial sheaths, this condition is more accurately described as a tenovaginitis.[78] *Tenovaginitis* refers to thickening of the fibrous sheath of the first extensor compartment. In 1912, de Quervain described "thickening of the dense fibrous connective tissues without any fresh sign of inflammation, neither round cell inflammation nor increase in numbers of cells."[78] Histologically, the thickening is caused by the accumulation of mucopolysaccharide within the tendon sheath.[79,80]

It is commonly thought that the disorder occurs more often after repetitive use of the wrists, especially with a wringing motion. The syndrome has been called "washerwoman's sprain," and often no specific cause is apparent. Women during pregnancy or within 12 months of childbirth are also frequently affected.[57] However, a study by Kay[78] challenged the association between repetitive motion and de Quervain's disease. In a retrospective study of 100 cases, no strong correlation was found with occupation or history of repetitive activities in patients in whom de Quervain's disease was diagnosed. Thus, it may be possible that repetitive activities exacerbate the pain associated with a condition for which the etiology is unclear.

Tenderness and occasionally palpable crepitation are elicited just distal to the radial styloid process, where both tendons come together in an osseofibrous tunnel. Patients usually have wrist pain and often mistakenly attribute the discomfort to some distant, albeit irrelevant trauma. The condition may be confused with first carpometacarpal arthrosis (osteoarthritis of the thumb) and intersection syndrome. Radiographs will have normal findings in de Quervain's disease but might be appropriate to rule out other pathologic abnormalities. Ultrasound may demonstrate thickening and edema of the synovial sheath[81] but has not yet been routinely used to make or confirm the diagnosis. Rarely, gonococcal tenosynovitis might simulate this inflammatory condition (Fig. 52-19).

A useful clinical maneuver that indicates de Quervain's disease is the Finkelstein test (Fig. 52-20). Abduct the patient's thumb into the palm of the hand, fold the fingers over the thumb, and then apply ulnar deviation at the wrist; severe pain at the site of the affected tendon sheaths indicates a positive test. When performing the Finkelstein test, also palpate the tender area for crepitus. If axial traction or compression (the carpometacarpal grind test) and rotation of the thumb produce pain, the condition is most likely due to degenerative changes in the carpometacarpal joint of the thumb rather than de Quervain's disease. It should be noted that gonococcal tenosynovitis of the wrist may mimic de Quervain's disease, and one should inquire about other symptoms (e.g., sore throat, penile or vaginal discharge, or fever) and carefully look for the characteristic rash of this sexually transmitted disease (see Fig. 52-19).

Local corticosteroid injection as the therapeutic preference for de Quervain's tenovaginitis is well founded in the literature. In a study comparing steroid injection of de Quervain's disease with immobilization and oral NSAID therapy alone, the latter was effective only in a small group of patients with minimal symptoms.[82] In a retrospective study, 84% of 58 patients were effectively managed either with a single injection (60%) or with repeat injections (24%), with only 12% requiring surgical treatment.[83] These data support a metaanalysis of 495 subjects treated for de Quervain's tenovaginitis in which an 83% cure rate was found with injection alone versus 61% for injection and splinting, 14% for splinting alone, and 0% for rest or NSAIDs.[84] The strikingly favorable response to local injection therapy suggests that surgery to release the tendon sheaths is seldom needed. Interestingly, some evidence suggests that failure of steroid injections may be due to an anatomic variant in which the EPB is located in a separate synovial compartment.[84,85] This is supported by a study in which steroids selectively injected into the EPB tenosynovium resulted in the resolution of symptoms in all 50 patients.[86] Clinical suspicion for this anatomic variant should be raised when previous steroid injections have failed and patients have pain with firm resistance to thumb metacarpophalangeal joint extension (the EPB entrapment test).[85] Consider selective injection into the EPB tenosynovium in these patients.

Accurate injection of the corticosteroid has been found to be an important aspect of the patient's response to treatment.[87] Using radiographic dye to verify correct corticosteroid placement, researchers have found that when the corticosteroid and anesthetic injection did not successfully reach either the EPB or the APL compartment, the patient did not experience relief of pain. Conversely, when the medication was injected accurately, most patients reported an improvement in symptoms. If available, ultrasound may help guide the injection. In 2002, Kamel and coworkers[88] used ultrasound to guide steroid injection in 21 patients with the clinical diagnosis of de Quervain's disease. No complications were reported, and all patients had decreased edema and thickening of the tendons at 6 and 12 weeks. A similar study by Jeyapalan and Choudhary used ultrasound as an adjunct for injection in 17 patients in whom de Quervain's disease was diagnosed clinically. One patient was identified as having solitary EPB involvement and 15 of the remaining 16 patients (1 patient was lost to follow-up) had significant relief at a mean of 6.75 weeks with no immediate or delayed complications reported.[89] Larger studies are needed to confirm the benefits of ultrasound.

Intersection syndrome is a condition that may easily be confused with de Quervain's disease. Because the treatment approach and the clinical course of intersection syndrome differ from that of de Quervain's tenovaginitis, it is important that the clinician also be familiar with this entity. First described in 1841 by Velpea, intersection syndrome describes a clinical entity approximately 4 to 8 cm proximal to the location of de Quervain's disease (see Fig. 52-18).[90] Although the cause is not yet clear, intersection syndrome is thought to result from inflammation of the second dorsal compartment of the wrist, which houses the extensor carpi radialis longus (ECRL) and extensor carpi radialis brevis (ECRB) tendons.[91] Other possible causes include inflammation of a bursa that develops between the APL and the ECRB tendons[71] and inflammation of the ECRL and ECRB tenosynovium where they cross the muscle bellies of the APL and EPB.[92]

Intersection syndrome is characterized by pain, tenderness, edema, and occasional crepitus 4 to 8 cm proximal to the radial styloid and may be mistaken for de Quervain's disease. This condition is seen in athletes who play sports that require forceful repetitive wrist flexion and extension, such as rowing, weight lifting, gymnastics, and tennis.[71] Treatment includes rest, NSAIDs, and immobilization with a thumb spica splint in 15 degrees of wrist extension. After a 2- to 3-week trial of splinting, corticosteroid injection therapy is recommended. In contrast, steroid injection is recommended early in the course of de Quervain's disease. Some authors, in fact, recommend corticosteroid injection therapy on initial diagnosis of de Quervain's disease.[93] Most patients with intersection syndrome, on the other hand, respond well to nonoperative treatment, and surgery is generally reserved for refractory cases.[92]

APPROACH. For injection of de Quervain's tenosynovitis, position the patient's hand so that the ulnar side of the wrist is on the table and the radial side is facing upward (see Fig. 52-20). Introduce a 2.2-cm, 25-gauge needle at the most tender point (about 1 cm distal to the radial styloid) through a lidocaine skin wheal, and inject 10 to 20 mg of prednisolone or an equivalent intermediate-acting steroid suspension mixed with 4 to 5 mL of 1% lidocaine adjacent and parallel to the tendon sheath (peritendinous infiltration). The injection should be under the edge of the first dorsal compartment retinaculum within the first extensor compartment. If firm resistance is met or if needle movement is noted when the patient abducts and extends the thumb, the needle may be in the tendon and should be redirected to prevent intratendinous injection.[93] Because many superficial vessels are present in this area, aspirate before injecting to verify that the needle is not in a blood vessel.[87] Be generous with the injection volume because a common reason for failure is the inability to get medication into both tendon sheaths. This may be partially overcome by increasing the volume of steroid-lidocaine injected.

Frequently, edema is visible at the radial aspect of the first metacarpal base and at the thumb metacarpophalangeal joint dorsally after successful injection.[87] A lightweight thumb or wrist splint for support and protection may be used at night for several weeks after the injection, but routine splinting after injection is not required.[90] Oral NSAIDs may be prescribed for analgesia but will probably not effect a cure by themselves. There is no proven role for oral corticosteroids.

Injection for intersection syndrome is similar to that for de Quervain's disease, except that the target site is at the point of maximal tenderness, which is usually 4 to 8 cm proximal to the radial styloid (see Fig. 52-20).

Carpal Tunnel Syndrome. Carpal tunnel syndrome is the most common nerve entrapment neuropathy of the wrist.[94] Caused by median nerve compression in the fibroosseous tunnel of the wrist, carpal tunnel syndrome is characterized by pain at the wrist that sometimes radiates proximally into the forearm and is associated with tingling and paresthesias of the medial aspect of the thumb, palmar side of the index and middle fingers, and radial half of the ring finger. Typically,

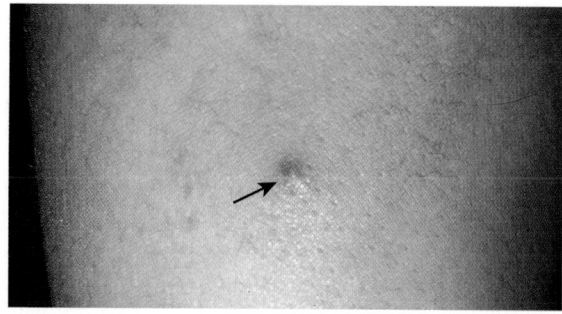

Figure 52-19 This 25-year-old woman had signs and symptoms of tenosynovitis of the wrist that was initially thought to be de Quervain's disease. A single hemorrhagic papule (*arrow*) demonstrating a septic embolus was found on the forearm and is a subtle but classic lesion of gonococcal bacteremia. One aspect of this sexually transmitted disease is tenosynovitis. Cervical cultures were positive for *Neisseria gonorrhoeae* despite the absence of vaginal symptoms.

de QUERVAIN'S DISEASE AND INTERSECTION SYNDROME

Finkelstein's test. The Finkelstein test is positive when pain is reproduced by ulnar deviation of the wrist while the patient grasps the thumb with the fingers.

Occasionally, crepitus may be palpated over the involved area. To elicit this sign, the examiner's fingers are placed over the painful area and the patient's wrist is placed in ulnar deviation, which produces the characteristic sensation.

A, For de Quervain's disease, insert the needle through the most tender point, usually about 1 cm distal to the radial styloid. *B,* For intersection syndrome, the target site is again the site of maximal tenderness, which is usually 4 to 8 cm proximal to the radial styloid. (*APL,* abductor pollicus longus; *EPB,* extensor pollicus brevis).

Injection for de Quervain's tenosynovitis usually produces a good result.

Figure 52-20 de Quervain's disease and intersection syndrome.

the patient wakes during the night with burning or aching pain, numbness, and tingling. Occasionally, the discomfort is extremely severe and causes the patient to seek emergency care. Clinical signs that support this diagnosis include a positive Tinel sign, which is elicited by reproducing the tingling and paresthesias by tapping (with a reflex hammer) over the median nerve at the volar crease of the wrist (Fig. 52-21).[95] In addition, one can perform the Phalen test, described as holding the dorsal sides of the flexed wrists at a 90-degree angle against each other for several minutes to provoke symptoms in the median nerve distribution.[95] Phalen's test is more sensitive than Tinel's sign and is more specific for carpal tunnel syndrome.[94] Severe muscle atrophy of the thenar eminence may develop in advanced or neglected cases. In many cases the disturbance is idiopathic, without a recognizable underlying cause. However, people who participate in repetitive activities of the wrist, such as typing, driving, assembly line work, and racquet sports, are at risk for the development of carpal tunnel syndrome.[57] Other conditions associated with carpal tunnel syndrome include rheumatoid arthritis (sometimes as the initial manifestation), pregnancy, hypothyroidism, diabetes, and acromegaly.

Initial therapy for carpal tunnel syndrome consists of modification of activity and splinting; the latter is particularly helpful at night.[57] Of the medications sometimes used to treat carpal tunnel syndrome, diuretics, NSAIDs, and pyridoxine have been shown to offer little to no relief.[96] In contrast, the benefits, at least in the short term (e.g., 4 to 6 weeks), of local steroid injections for carpal tunnel syndrome have been well proven.[97] In a Cochrane review of randomized trials by Marshall and colleagues,[98] local steroid injection provided greater clinical improvement 1 month after injection than did placebo and up to 3 months after injection than did oral steroid treatment. However, symptoms after local corticosteroid injection were no different from the symptoms after either NSAIDs or splinting at 8 weeks. The benefits of initial steroid injection versus surgical intervention for carpal tunnel syndrome are controversial because there is little scientifically valid information on which to draw any conclusions. In one small study, Hui and associates[99] found that surgery resulted in a better symptomatic outcome (but not grip strength) than did local steroid injection over a 20-week period. It appears that local steroid injection for carpal tunnel syndrome offers improvement in symptoms, but this improvement may not be

CARPAL TUNNEL SYNDROME

Tinel's test. Tap over the median nerve at the volar wrist crease with a reflex hammer; reproduction of tingling and paresthesias supports the diagnosis.

Phalen's test. Instruct the patient to hold the wrists together in a flexed position for several minutes; observe for symptoms in a median nerve distribution.

Prior to needle insertion, identify the palmaris longus tendon (*arrow*) by instructing the patient to oppose the thumb and pinky finger while flexing the wrist.

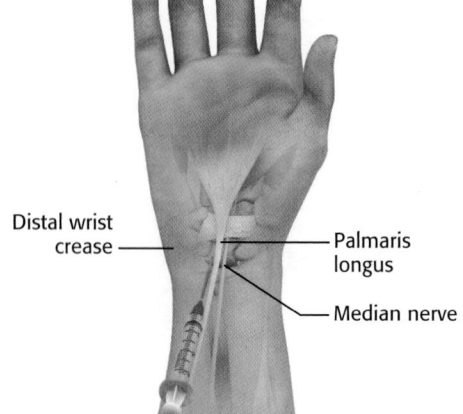

Distal wrist crease — Palmaris longus — Median nerve

Insert the needle on the ulnar side of the palmaris longus tendon about 1 cm proximal to the distal wrist crease.

Hold the needle at a 45° angle, aimed toward the tip of the middle finger. Advance the needle about 1 to 2 cm. If the patient experiences paresthesias, reposition the needle tip because direct nerve injection should be avoided.

Figure 52-21 Carpal tunnel syndrome.

permanent or long term. Current recommendations include a trial of conservative treatment (including possible steroid injection) for patients who have mild to moderate symptoms and lack thenar wasting.[100] Surgery is indicated for patients with persistent symptoms after conservative treatment and for those with severe weakness of the thumb abductors.[94] Nerve compression should be confirmed by nerve conduction studies before surgery.[97]

APPROACH. Insert the needle through a lidocaine skin wheal just ulnar to the palmaris longus tendon and about 1 cm proximal to the distal crease at the wrist. The palmaris longus tendon can be appreciated by having the patient pinch all the fingertips together while holding the wrist in a neutral position (see Fig. 52-21).[101] Injecting medial (ulnar) to the palmaris longus is preferred because it avoids accidental injection of the median nerve and superficial veins. Direct a 2.5- to 3.9-cm, 25-gauge needle at a 45-degree angle to the skin surface toward the tip of the middle finger. Advance the needle 1 to 2 cm and inject 20 to 40 mg of methylprednisolone (or another intermediate-acting steroid equivalent) with

or without lidocaine along the track and into the tissue space. If the patient complains of paresthesias or the needle meets resistance during injection, redirect the needle to avoid injecting directly into a nerve or tendon, respectively.[101] Up to 2 weeks may be required for the paresthesias to abate significantly, although it usually takes only a few days for improvement of nocturnal pain.[102] A lightweight wrist splint may hasten recovery. Repeated injections may be given, but if a response is not elicited or permanent after two or three injections, decompressive surgery should be considered.

Digital Flexor Tenosynovitis ("Trigger Finger"). A "trigger" or "snapping" finger is one of the most common problems of the hand and is characterized by a stenosed tendon sheath at the level of the first annular pulley (A1), which is located on the palmar surface over the base of the metacarpal head (Fig. 52-22).[103] In this condition the A1 pulley becomes inflamed, and a nodule develops on the tendon as it gets "pinched" under the constricted sheath.[103] Locking occurs when the involved digit is in flexion and is especially troublesome when the patient awakens in the morning. This

DIGITAL FLEXOR TENOSYNOVITIS ("TRIGGER FINGER")

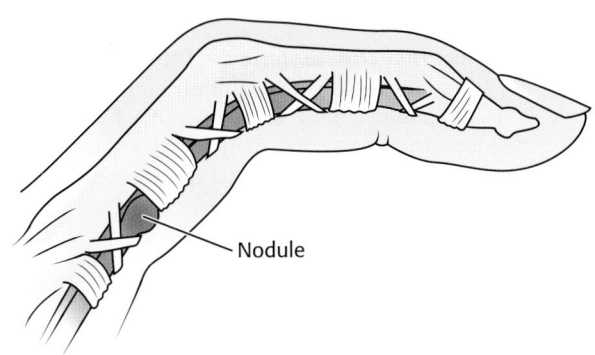

Trigger finger (stenosing tenosynovitis) can affect any digit, including the thumb, but it is most common in the ring and middle fingers. Palpation of the flexor tendon sheath over the metacarpophalangeal joint often reproduces the symptoms. Injection is often very effective, but the nodule may persist.

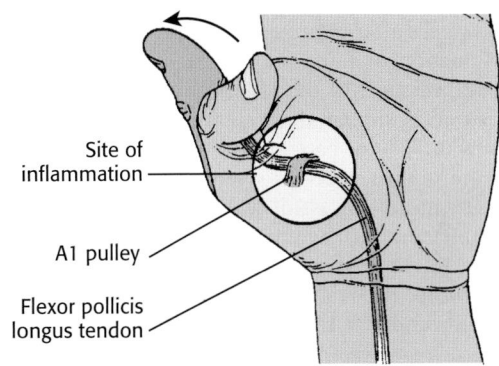

In advanced cases, inflammation at the proximal (A1) pulley of the flexor tendon sheath overlying the metacarpophalangeal joint may hold the digit in either a flexed or an extended position. Generally, the tendon becomes thickened either proximal or distal to the pulley, which causes a snapping or a locking phenomenon with finger flexion or extension.

Locate the tendon point at the base of the finger flexion crease, which is located between the A1 and A2 pulleys.

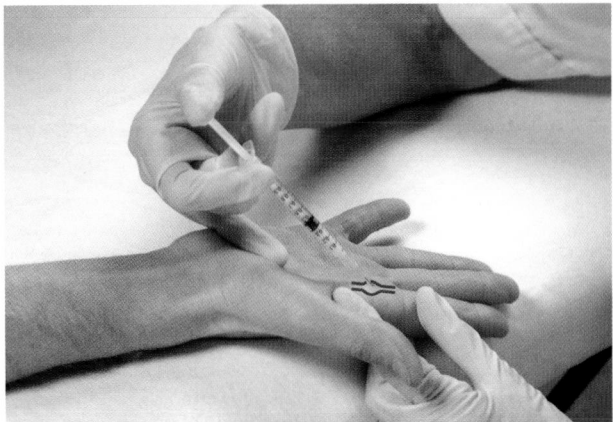

Angle the needle 30° into the involved tendon sheath, parallel to the tendon fibers.

Figure 52-22 Digital flexor tenosynovitis ("trigger finger"). (*Top right, from Walker LG, Meals RA. Tendinitis: a practical approach to diagnosis and management.* J Musculoskelet Med. *1989;6:41. Reproduced with permission.*)

can occur in any finger but is seen most frequently in the ring and middle fingers.

Besides thickening and stenosing of the tendon sheath, a trigger finger may also be characterized by flexor tendon synovitis. The tendon sheaths are long and tubular, and the walls are lined with a thin layer of synovial cells. Symptoms develop when the tendon becomes trapped and is unable to glide within the tendon sheath. A nodule or fibrinous deposit may form at a site in the tendon sheath, usually over or just distal to the metacarpal head of the trigger finger. When the digit is flexed, the nodule moves with the tendon proximally, and on extension it gets "stuck" on the pulley, thereby leading to intermittent catching of the tendon.[103] The nodule may be palpable on physical examination, but this is not necessary for diagnosis.[57] Carpal tunnel syndrome commonly coexists with a trigger finger and may be caused by tenosynovitis. Common causes of tenosynovitis include trauma, diabetes mellitus, and rheumatoid arthritis, although it may also be a primary and idiopathic disorder.[91]

Conservative treatment, including local rest or splinting, application of moist heat, and NSAID therapy, is the usual initial approach for symptomatic tenosynovitis. If these simple measures fail to control the symptoms, corticosteroid injection is indicated. One double-blind, placebo-controlled, randomized study of trigger finger demonstrated that steroid injections were significantly more effective than placebo.[104] At follow-up 3 weeks after treatment, 9 of the 14 patients receiving a combination of lidocaine and steroid injections were asymptomatic versus 2 of the 10 patients receiving lidocaine injections alone. A similar study showed complete resolution of symptoms in 52% of patients who received corticosteroid injections and improvement of symptoms in 47%.[103] Steroid injections are more successful when performed in patients with a palpable nodule or symptoms for less than 6 months.[105] Alternatively, some evidence suggests that the efficacy of steroid injections for trigger fingers diminishes with each subsequent injection at the same site.[106] As a guideline, if treatment fails after three injections (separated by several weeks or months), consider surgery as treatment of the condition.[57] In addition, patients with diabetes mellitus more often require surgical release for trigger finger than do non–insulin-dependent diabetics.[103] Division of the first annular pulley, digital nerve injury, scarring, and recurrence are well-known complications of surgical release.[106]

APPROACH. Preparation of the site before injection requires meticulous adherence to aseptic technique. Rest the patient's hand on a table with the palm facing upward. The injection point is at the base of the finger's flexion crease between the A1 and the A2 tendon pulleys. Using a 2.2-cm, 25-gauge needle, enter the skin at a 30-degree angle and insert the needle into the tendon sheath parallel to the tendon fibers. Inject 0.25 to 0.35 mL of an intermediate-acting corticosteroid suspension mixed with 1.5 to 3 mL of anesthetic (see Fig. 52-22). If resistance is felt on insertion of the needle, an intratendinous location is suggested. Withdraw the needle slightly before injection. Similar injections can be administered in the base of the thumb metacarpal for a "snapping" thumb. Although injection into the tendon sheath is the goal, Taras and coworkers[107] showed that injection of steroid into the subcutaneous tissue surrounding the tendon sheath provided similar improvement as intrasheath injections. If relapses are frequent or the clinical response is not satisfactory, surgical release is indicated.

Carpal/Metacarpal Inflammation. Overuse and aging can lead to pain at the base of the thumb and fingers. This is especially common in elderly women and can be quite painful. The first metacarpal articulates with the trapezium, a common site for this condition. Injection therapy is usually quite successful (Fig. 52-23).

Hip Region
Trochanteric Bursitis. Trochanteric bursitis is the second leading cause of lateral hip pain after osteoarthritis.[108]

CARPAL/METACARPAL INFLAMMATION

Painful and limited motion of the thumb is often caused by inflammation at the trapezium-metacarpal joint. Inject at the apex of the snuffbox while avoiding the radial artery. (*EPB*, extensor pollicis brevis; *EPL*, extensor pollicis longus. The anatomic snuffbox is outlined by these two tendons.)

Injection therapy is usually quite successful for this very painful condition, which is common in older women.

Figure 52-23 Carpal/metacarpal inflammation.

However, trochanteric bursitis can be confused with other conditions at or near the hip, such as sacrolumbar disease, hip or femur pathology, and metastases.[109-111] Patients with trochanteric bursitis, though, usually demonstrate discrete tenderness on deep palpation at or adjacent to the greater trochanter; relief of symptoms with a proper corticosteroid injection can help confirm the diagnosis.[109]

The principal bursae associated with this condition are the subgluteus maximus bursa, the subgluteus minimus bursa, and the gluteus minimus bursa, although other bursae of the hip may be affected (Fig. 52-24). The pain may be acute but is more often subacute or chronic; frequently, patients have already tried NSAIDs without success and have been assigned a number of incorrect diagnoses. The chief locus of the pathologic condition is in the abductor mechanism of the hip. Pain occurs near the greater trochanter and may radiate down the lateral or posterolateral aspect of the thigh and, rarely, into the knee.[112] The pain is described as "deep," "dull," and "aching," and it often interferes with sleep.

Lying on the affected hip, stepping from curbs, and descending steps provoke pain. Tenderness may be elicited over and adjacent to the greater trochanter. In contrast to true hip joint involvement, the Patrick FABERE sign (*f*lexion, *ab*duction, *e*xternal *r*otation, and *e*xtension) may be negative, and complete passive range of motion is relatively painless. Active abduction when the patient lies on the opposite side typically intensifies the discomfort, and sharp external rotation may accentuate the symptoms. Internal rotation does not usually affect the level of pain.[109] Hip radiographs may demonstrate a calcific deposit adjacent to the trochanter; however, the incidence of this finding is low.[110]

Corticosteroid injection for trochanteric bursitis is often an effective therapy.[110] In one study, 77% of patients reported improvement of their pain after an injection of betamethasone mixed with lidocaine.[113] In addition, 61% of the patients reported improvement in their pain 26 weeks after receiving the injection. Failure of corticosteroid therapy should prompt the clinician to seek alternative diagnoses, such as true hip joint disease, which can easily be confused with trochanteric bursitis.[114] In addition, though rare, there have been case reports of septic trochanteric bursitis caused by tuberculosis.[115]

APPROACH.   Place the patient in a supine or lateral recumbent position and identify the site of maximum tenderness for needle entry. Advance a 3.9- to 5.0-cm, 20- or 21-gauge needle perpendicular to the skin until the tip of the needle reaches the trochanter (Fig. 52-25). Withdraw the needle slightly, and widely infiltrate the site with 3 to 10 mL of

Gluteus medius
Gluteus minimus
Subgluteus medius bursa
Greater trochanter
Subgluteus maximus bursa
Fascia lata
Femur

Figure 52-24   Trochanteric bursitis. The principal bursa lies between the gluteus maximus and the greater trochanter, although other bursae may also be involved.

TROCHANTERIC BURSITIS

Greater trochanter
Tensor fasciae latae

Place the patient in the lateral recumbent or supine position. Insert the needle at the area of maximum tenderness, and advance perpendicular to the skin until the needle tip reaches the greater trochanter.

After the trochanter is reached, withdraw the needle slightly, and infiltrate the site widely with 3 to 10 mL of lidocaine and 20 to 40 mg of methylprednisolone (or the equivalent).

Figure 52-25   Trochanteric bursitis.

lidocaine and 20 to 40 mg of methylprednisolone or an equivalent steroid.

Ischiogluteal Bursitis. "Weaver's bottom" is a painful disorder characterized by pain over the center of the buttocks with radiation down the back of the leg.[110] This condition is rarely diagnosed initially and is often mistaken for lumbosacral strain, a herniated disk, or a spinal cord tumor. When it is recognized, a skillful intrabursal injection, coupled with a few days' rest, usually relieves the extreme pain. The ischial or ischiogluteal bursa is adjacent to the ischial tuberosity and overlies the sciatic and posterior femoral cutaneous nerves. Sitting on hard surfaces, bending forward, and standing on tiptoes may all provoke the pain. Tenderness is present over the ischial tuberosity. At times, a soft tissue mass may also be felt in this area.[116]

APPROACH. Place the patient in a prone position and insert a 5.0-cm, 20- to 22-gauge needle through a lidocaine skin wheal. Advance the needle cautiously to avoid the sciatic nerve, which lies at a depth of approximately 6.5 to 7.5 cm. If paresthesias occur (indicating contact with a nerve), withdraw and redirect the needle. Inject 5 to 10 mL of lidocaine and 20 to 40 mg of methylprednisolone into the bursa.

Knee Region

Prepatellar Bursitis. "Housemaid's knee" or "nun's knee" is characterized by swelling with effusion of the superficial bursa overlying the lower pole of the patella (Fig. 52-26). In contrast to intraarticular pathology, passive motion of the knee is fully preserved and the pain is generally mild, except during extreme knee flexion or direct pressure. Although the disorder is usually caused by pressure from repetitive kneeling on a firm surface ("rug cutter's knee"), it can also develop after direct trauma, and occasionally it is a manifestation of rheumatoid arthritis or gout.[117] Though uncommon, the

Figure 52-26 Bursae of the knee (medial view). The prepatellar bursa lies superior to the patella, and the pes anserine bursa lies deep to the insertion of the sartorius, gracilis, and semitendinosus tendons. Prepatellar bursitis is common in carpet layers, and pes anserine bursitis is seen in dancers and runners. Infrapatellar bursitis is common in long-distance runners and can be mistaken for patellar tendinitis. Pain is felt below the patella at the midpoint of the patellar tendon and is elicited by knee extension. Note that there are two infrapatellar bursae. Osgood-Schlatter disease is similar in adolescents, a condition that should not be injected.

prepatellar bursa is one of the most frequent sites of septic bursitis.[4] Moreover, patients with septic prepatellar bursitis may not have the classic signs of infection such as erythema, warmth, or fever, and this makes it difficult to differentiate from aseptic bursitis.[118] The bursal aspirate should therefore always be sent for laboratory analysis.[4]

APPROACH. Place the patient supine with the affected leg extended (Fig. 52-27). The bursa is located superficially, between the skin and the patella, and can often be "milked" during the procedure to facilitate aspiration. Use a 2.5-cm, 20- to 21-gauge needle to enter the bursa and aspirate as much fluid as possible. Aspiration often yields a surprisingly scant amount of clear, serous fluid because the prepatellar bursa is multilocular rather than the usual single cavity. Once aspiration is complete, instill 1 to 2 mL of lidocaine with 15 to 20 mg of a prednisolone (or an equivalent steroid) suspension. In some cases the procedure may need to be repeated more than once (in 6-to 8-week intervals) to obtain a lasting result. The provocative activity should be discontinued.

Suprapatellar Bursitis. Suprapatellar bursitis is usually associated with synovitis of the knees. On occasion the bursa is largely separated from the synovial cavity with only a very minor communication, and the swelling and effusion are chiefly confined to the suprapatellar area. This may be traumatic in origin or a manifestation of an inflammatory arthropathy.

APPROACH. The procedure for aspiration and injection of the suprapatellar area is similar to that for the knee.

Anserine Bursitis. "Cavalryman's disease" now mainly occurs in heavy women with disproportionately large thighs in association with osteoarthritis of the knee, although this entity is also seen in athletes involved in running, baseball, and racquet sports.[110] The bursa is on the anteromedial side of the knee, inferior to the joint line at the site of insertion of the conjoined tendons of the sartorius, semitendinous, and gracilis muscles and superficial to the medial collateral ligament. The entity is characterized by a relatively abrupt onset of knee pain along with localized tenderness and a sense of fullness in the vicinity of the anserine bursa about 4 to 5 cm below the anteromedial aspect of the tibial plateau. Pain is exacerbated by flexion of the knee. Corticosteroid injection for anserine bursitis has been shown in clinical trials to be an effective treatment.[119]

APPROACH. Position the patient with the knee flexed 90 degrees (Fig. 52-28). Using an anterior or medial approach with a 2.5- to 3.9-cm, 22-gauge needle, identify the point of greatest tenderness and gently advance the needle until the tibia is reached; withdraw the needle 2 to 3 mm and inject 2 to 4 mL of lidocaine along with or followed by approximately 20 to 40 mg of a corticosteroid suspension. Prompt symptomatic relief is frequently obtained, but the duration of benefit is variable and probably correlates with the patient's weight-bearing activities. It is important to avoid direct injection of the corticosteroid suspension into the nearby tendons.

Medial Collateral Ligament Bursa. This bursa is located anterior to the tibia and posterior to the medial collateral ligament. Injury to this bursa often occurs when the patient undergoes a twisting motion with concurrent external rotation of the tibia. Tenderness may be appreciated along the anteroinferior aspect of the medial collateral ligament, and

The labels on Figure 52-26:
- Patella
- Prepatellar bursa
- Deep infrapatellar bursa
- Superficial infrapatellar bursa
- Tibia
- Sartorius
- Gracilis
- Semitendinosus
- Anserine bursa

PREPATELLAR BURSITIS ASPIRATION

This patient has had anterior knee swelling for 6 weeks after falling directly onto his knee. This collection is confined to the prepatellar space, and passive range of motion of the knee is preserved.

After careful antiseptic preparation, infiltrate the entry site and the anticipated trajectory of the needle with lidocaine.

Keep the knee extended during the procedure. Insert the needle into the fluctuant area in the space between the skin and the patella; either a medial or a lateral approach may be used.

Once in the bursa, aspirate the fluid. Occasionally, a substantial volume of fluid may be obtained, so use a large syringe.

"Milk" the bursa during aspiration to facilitate fluid removal. The needle may be repositioned if needed because the prepatellar bursa is a multiloculated structure (as opposed to a single cavity).

Note that this patient's aspirate was grossly hemorrhagic, consistent with his history of knee trauma.

Remove as much fluid as possible. This patient's knee regained a normal appearance after the procedure.

At the end of the procedure, apply a compressive dressing to reduce recurrence.

Figure 52-27 Prepatellar bursitis aspiration.

ANSERINE BURSITIS

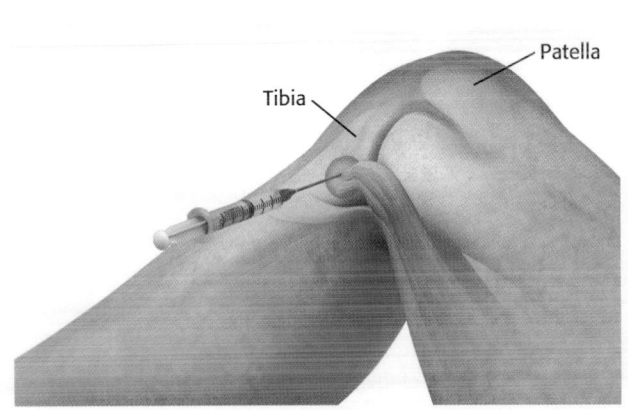

Patella

Tibia

Insert the needle at the point of maximum tenderness. This will be inferior to the patella and medial to the tibial tuberosity.

Advance the needle until the tibia is reached, and then slightly withdraw the needle and inject the steroid. Avoid direct injection into the nearby tendons.

Figure 52-28 Anserine bursitis.

the pain is exacerbated with extension of the knee. This condition may sometimes be confused with a medial meniscus tear, and magnetic resonance imaging might be necessary to differentiate the two conditions. Treatment is usually successful with conservative measures, including relative rest, compression, and NSAIDs.[110]

Popliteal Cyst. "Baker's cysts" are herniated fluid-filled sacs of the articular synovial membrane that extend into the popliteal fossa, sometimes through the natural communication between the bursa in the posterior of the knee and the joint itself. These cysts may also be due to swelling of the medial gastrocnemius or semimembranosus bursae alone. Baker's cysts can occur secondary to trauma, although they are also seen in patients with rheumatoid arthritis, gout, and osteoarthritis.[110] Patients will often complain of *popliteal fossa* tenderness and swelling that may extend into the calf. Activities that involve active flexion of the knee, such as walking or jumping, exacerbate the symptoms.

The clinical manifestation of Baker's cysts can mimic that of deep venous thrombosis (DVT), and it is important to take great care in differentiating the two. For this reason, symptomatic Baker's cysts are also known as pseudothrombophlebitis syndrome.[120] In most studies, 2% to 6% of patients suspected of having DVT actually have a popliteal cyst as the cause of their knee or calf pain. Ultrasound is an important tool in this diagnosis.

Many cases of Baker's cyst resolve spontaneously over a few weeks. However, treatment of Baker's cysts may require surgery to correct any articular injury or to remove the cyst. Steroid injections are not usually performed because of the risk for neurovascular injury.

Ankle, Foot, and Heel Region

Ankle Tendinitis. This is a relatively uncommon condition that may result from unusual repetitive activity or, rarely, from acute trauma. The disorder is differentiated from ankle joint involvement by the lack of pain or restricted motion during passive flexion and extension of the ankle. Active flexion and

extension of the toes produce pain. Local tenderness is elicited along the involved tendons. Initial treatment consists of rest, NSAIDs, and immobilization, sometimes for several weeks. Some patients may eventually need operative intervention for prolonged symptoms.[121] Local steroid injections have been used successfully in patients who do not respond to conservative measures; however, the risk for tendon rupture is well documented. As a result, tendon sheath injections should be reserved for patients with persistent symptoms despite an adequate trial of conservative therapy and should be done in consultation with a foot and ankle specialist.

APPROACH. Enter the tendon sheath tangentially with a 2.5- to 3.9-cm, 22- or 25-gauge needle and inject approximately 2 to 4 mL of a mixture of corticosteroid (20 to 40 mg of methylprednisolone) and lidocaine.

Bunion Bursitis. It is common for bunion bursitis to overlie the first metatarsophalangeal joint at its medial surface on the great toe. On occasion, tense swelling occurs, and decompression is required. Aspiration with culture of the fluid should be performed.

APPROACH. If no infection is present, the bursa is injected with 5 to 10 mg of methylprednisolone via a 2.5-cm, 20-gauge needle. Special shoes or an orthopedic correction will be needed if the swelling recurs.

Heel Pain. *Talalgia* may be caused by many different conditions, including Achilles tendinitis, retrocalcaneal bursitis, and plantar fasciitis (Fig. 52-29). Additional discussion may be found in Chapter 51. The bursae of clinical significance around the heel include the retro-Achilles bursa (located in the space between the skin and the Achilles tendon), the retrocalcaneal bursa (located between the Achilles tendon and the calcaneus), and the subcalcaneal bursa. Achilles tendinitis or bursitis may be traumatic in origin but is more apt to be part of a systemic disease, such as rheumatoid or gouty arthritis. Although a normal Achilles tendon is thick and strong, when affected by an inflammatory arthropathy, it is

HEEL PAIN

Achilles tendon

Retrocalcaneal bursa

Retro-Achilles bursa

Flexor hallicis longus

Flexor digitorum longus

Heel pain. Talalgia may involve the tendons, bursae, or fasciae around the heel. Do not inject Achilles tendinitis since tendon rupture may occur. Fluoroquinolones can cause significant Achilles tendinopathy (see Box 52-1).

Injection of calcaneal bursitis with a heel spur. A lateral injection is preferred (see Chapter 51).

Figure 52-29 Heel pain.

predisposed to degeneration, and because the Achilles tendon is not invested by a full synovial sheath, it is more vulnerable to intratendon instillation. Because of the potential hazard of tendon rupture after local steroid injection, it is wise to avoid infiltration of steroids into this area. In a double-blind, randomized, controlled trial it was shown that injection of methylprednisolone and bupivacaine (Marcaine) had no benefit over injecting bupivacaine alone.[5] It is preferable to treat Achilles tendinitis with rest, splinting, and oral NSAIDs and to avoid injection therapy.

Retrocalcaneal bursitis is often seen in association with Haglund's deformity, a bony ridge on the posterosuperior aspect of the calcaneus. The bursa lies anterior to the Achilles tendon and posterior to the calcaneus. Local swelling and tenderness at the posterior aspect of the heel, proximal (and sometimes lateral) to the insertion of the Achilles tendon, characterize this bursitis. Treatment is focused on minimizing pressure on the bony ridge, which includes the use of open-heeled shoes (clogs), bare feet, sandals, or a heel lift. Conservative measures such as ice, oral NSAIDs, and rest are other common treatment modalities. Corticosteroid injections are not recommended because of the risk for Achilles tendon rupture.[122,123]

The condition in this region that is most amenable to injection therapy is plantar fasciitis, which is also the most common cause of heel pain in adults.[124] The plantar fascia is located deep to the fat layer of the foot and extends from the calcaneus to the base of the digits. It is responsible for support of the medial longitudinal arch of the foot.[125] Signs of this condition include pain on the plantar medial aspect of the heel, which is often worse in the morning, after long periods of rest, and with passive dorsiflexion of the toes.[124] The pain may be relieved with activity. Although patients may have a heel spur, many symptomatic patients do not, and the presence of a heel spur should not be considered pathognomonic for the condition. Though still debated, the pathology is generally thought to originate from microtears in the fascia, often

as a result of overuse.[122,123] Obesity may also increase the risk for plantar fasciitis because of the excessive load on the fascia.[124]

Most cases of plantar fasciitis eventually resolve with nonsurgical management.[126] Treatment begins with elimination of any precipitating activity, relative rest, strength and stretching exercises, arch supports, and night splints. If these conservative measures are not effective, injection of the painful heel will usually provide short-term improvement. In a recent Cochrane review, steroid injections for plantar fasciitis resulted in significant improvement at 1 month but not at 3 or 6 months when compared with control groups.[127] In addition, there is a risk for rupture of the plantar fascia and fat pad atrophy with corticosteroid injections.[122] One study reported a rupture rate of close to 10%.[128] Therefore, caution should be exercised when injecting steroids into a painful heel. In addition, because this condition tends to be chronic or recurring, referral to an appropriate specialist is recommended.

APPROACH.   Insert a 2.5-cm, 22- to 24-gauge needle at the spot of maximal tenderness on the medial aspect of the heel (see Fig. 52-29). Enter the plantar surface at 90 degrees by sliding into the space at the midpoint of the calcaneus. The tip of the needle should lie in the aponeurosis of the attachment to the os calcis. Inject 1 mL of lidocaine and 10 to 20 mg of methylprednisolone. Injection through the more superficial aspect of the base of the foot should be avoided because it may result in dispersion of medications into the fat pad and produce fat pad atrophy.[125]

Trigger Points
The technique for trigger point injection (*universal technique*) is the same regardless of location and is described in detail earlier in the chapter (see "Invasive Techniques").

Myofascial Headache Syndromes
Trigger points commonly contribute to the muscle component of many headache syndromes, so it is important

to carefully examine the muscles of the face, scalp, neck, shoulders, and back for hypersensitive areas when evaluating patients with headaches. Trigger points are often found in the sternocleidomastoid, levator scapulae, and trapezius muscles and less frequently in the scalp and facial muscles. The posterior strap muscles, including the splenius and semispinalis muscles, are also commonly involved. Trigger points in the thoracic paraspinal muscles are frequently associated with both migraine and tension headaches, whereas trigger points in the quadratus lumborum and gluteus medius have been associated with unilateral headaches. Exercise caution when injecting the trapezius muscle to avoid puncture of the apical pleura, which rises higher in some individuals.

Torticollis. Myofascial causes of torticollis usually involve the trapezius, sternocleidomastoid, and levator scapulae muscles, either alone or in a synergistic manner. The splenius and semispinalis muscles may also be involved. As mentioned earlier, carefully inject trigger points in the trapezius muscle to avoid puncture of a high-rising apical pleura.

Levator Scapulae Muscle Syndrome. Painful sensitive foci may occur at the origin of the levator scapulae muscle on the superior medial aspect of the scapula, along the flat muscle belly, or at the insertion on the transverse processes of the first four cervical vertebrae (Fig. 52-30*A*). Pain is usually referred to the posterior cervical region, the posterior aspect of the scalp, and the periauricular area.

Splenius Capitis and Semispinalis Capitis Muscle Syndrome. Pain resulting from trigger points in the splenius capitis and semispinalis capitis muscles may be located over the muscles themselves or be perceived in the head and face and give rise to headache syndromes (see Fig. 52-30*B*). Some patients may also experience dizziness. Trigger points in the splenius capitis and semispinalis capitis muscles may be difficult to pinpoint, so having the patient point to the area of maximal tenderness is extremely helpful.

Trapezius Muscle Syndrome. The trapezius muscle is a frequent source of muscle pain and headache, especially at the angle of the neck or at the occipital insertions, where trigger points are most commonly located (see Fig. 52-30*C*). When injecting trigger points at the angle of the neck be careful to not puncture the apical pleura.

Sternocleidomastoid Muscle Syndrome. The sternocleidomastoid muscle is also a frequent source of neck pain and headache. Trigger points are most often found at its sternal and clavicular origins and occipital insertion, as well as in the upper two thirds of the muscle belly (see Fig. 52-30*C*). Dizziness, ipsilateral ptosis, lacrimation, and conjunctival injection may accompany trigger points located in the sternocleidomastoid muscle.[129] Pain may involve the muscle itself or be referred to the periauricular, facial, or frontal areas.

Myofascial Shoulder Disorders

Myofascial shoulder pain is frequently misdiagnosed as bursitis. Thus, it is important to remember that a painful shoulder may be due to trigger points, which are most often located in the posterior scapular muscles. Other common sites include the supraspinatus, infraspinatus, and pectoralis major muscles. The teres, deltoid, and triceps muscles are rarely involved. Occasionally, trigger points located in the splenius, semispinalis, and gluteal muscles contribute to shoulder pain syndromes and should be treated if found.

Scapula Muscles. When injecting trigger points in the lateral scapular and periscapular muscles, place the patient prone with a pillow under the chest to round the shoulders and facilitate injection. Note the anatomy and boundaries of the shoulder before injection, and warn the patient to not move the shoulder. Stabilize the scapula with the nondominant thumb and fingers to prevent movement of the lower portion of the scapula, which could result in inadvertent puncture of the pleura.

Myofascial pain is also commonly associated with a number of muscle beds at the medial border of the scapula, including the rhomboids, the serratus anterior, the subscapular muscles, and the levator scapulae. To inject trigger points in these medially situated muscles, have the patient place the ipsilateral hand behind the back. This will cause "winging of the scapula" and a safer approach. Direct the needle tangentially for easy access to the serratus anterior and subscapularis muscles. As with the lower portion of the scapula, care should be taken to inject the levator scapulae at an oblique angle that is nearly parallel to the thorax to help reduce the chance of accidentally inducing pneumothorax.

Infraspinatus Muscle Syndrome. Because of its multiple functions, this muscle is subject to earlier degeneration than other muscles of the rotator cuff and is more susceptible to trigger points (see Fig. 52-30*D*). Trigger points in the infraspinatus muscle invariably cause sympathetic hyperactivity and often contribute to dystrophy-like syndromes of the upper extremity. To identify trigger points in the infraspinatus muscle, it is important to palpate along the entire length of the muscle bundles, as well as across the "grain" of the muscle (see Fig. 52-4).

Somatic Visceral Reflex Phenomenon

Skeletal muscle trigger points may contribute to visceral pain by either induction or continuation of the spinal reflex arc.[130-135] Visceral sympathetic afferent nerves converge on the same dorsal horn neuron as somatic nociceptive afferent nerves do. Reflex sympathetic efferent nerve activity may result in spasm of the visceral sphincters, as well as cutaneous nociceptors (leading in part to referred cutaneous pain). The rectus abdominis muscle is particularly prone to trigger point development in conjunction with visceral pain. For example, right upper quadrant trigger points are associated with gallbladder disease, left upper quadrant trigger points with esophageal and ulcer disease, right lower quadrant trigger points with dysmenorrhea, and left lower quadrant trigger points with intestinal disorders.

Treatment of abdominal wall trigger points can provide significant relief of somatic and visceral pain in appropriate patients. Consider injecting these trigger points when palpating the trigger point or placing the affected muscle under tension (e.g., performing a sit-up) produces the characteristic visceral discomfort. It should also be noted that abdominal wall trigger points are often accompanied by trigger points in the corresponding posterior paraspinal muscle segment. For example, esophageal spasm is frequently associated with trigger points on the left posterior aspect of the thorax at spinal nerve levels T3 through T6. To provide more effective pain control, treat these trigger points also.

Rectus Abdominis Muscle Syndrome. These muscles are frequent sites of anterior abdominal wall pain. They often flare up after abdominal surgery and may be a major cause of

TRIGGER POINTS

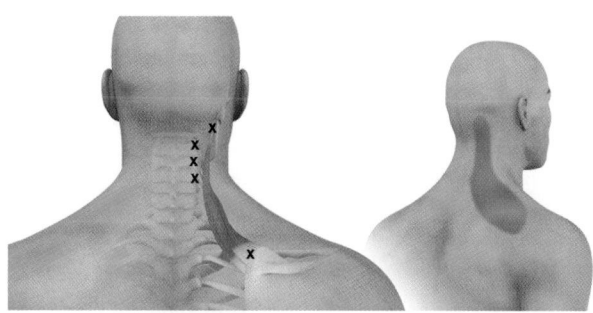

A. Levator scapulae muscle syndrome

B. Splenius capitis and semispinalis capitis muscle syndrome

C. Trapezius and sternocleidomastoid muscle syndromes

D. Infraspinatus muscle syndrome

E. Rectus abdominis and pectoralis muscle syndromes

F. Intercostal muscle syndrome

G. Tensor fasciae latae muscle syndrome

H. Anterior tibialis muscle syndrome

I. Gastrocnemius/soleus muscle syndrome

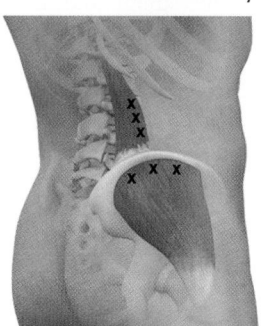

J. Quadratus lumborum/gluteus medius muscle syndromes

Figure 52-30 Trigger points. See text for descriptions of the various syndromes.

postoperative pain in some patients. Abdominal wall trigger points are most commonly found in the upper three segments of the rectus muscle and can more easily be located by placing the patient in a supine position with the head and neck flexed so that the rectus muscles are under tension (see Fig. 52-30*E*). Pain and tenderness are usually localized directly over the trigger point. Trigger points in the lower rectus segments may be a cause of low back pain. Lower segment trigger points may be associated with trigger points in the corresponding posterior lumbar spinal segments (i.e., L4, L5, S1).

Pectoralis Major/Pectoralis Minor Muscle Syndrome. The pectoralis major muscle is a frequent site of myofascial pain, particularly at its insertion on the anterior medial portion of the shoulder (see Fig. 52-30*E*). The inferior belly of the muscle is also a common area for trigger points, so be sure to carefully search the entire muscle to avoid missing a treatable area. Pain is usually located at the trigger point, but patients with trigger points in the clavicular portion of the muscle may have referred pain in the uppermost part of the muscle, whereas others may experience referred pain in the arm.

Intercostal Muscle Syndrome. In patients with musculoskeletal chest pain, palpate the intercostal muscles for areas of tenderness. Pain emanating from the exterior intercostal muscles is usually localized near the site of the trigger point and is emphasized during inspiration (see Fig. 52-30*F*). Intercostal muscle trigger points often flare after chest surgery or trauma. Exercise extreme care when injecting an intercostal muscle trigger point to avoid entry into the pleural space.

Knee Region

Tensor Fasciae Latae Muscle Syndrome. Because the tensor fasciae latae muscle is easy to examine, trigger points located here are easy to identify (see Fig. 52-30*G*). Patients usually complain of pain along the lateral aspect of the thigh as far down as the knee.

Ankle, Foot, and Heel Region

Anterior Tibialis Muscle Syndrome. Trigger points located in the anterior tibialis muscle usually cause pain along the anterior aspect of the ankle, but the entire ankle may be involved in severe cases. Trigger points are most commonly found in the upper third of the muscle and typically cause pain in the anterior portion of the leg and dorsal portion of the ankle (see Fig. 52-30*H*).

Gastrocnemius/Soleus Muscle Syndrome. Myofascial pain related to trigger points in the gastrocnemius and soleus muscles is usually located behind the knee and along the Achilles tendon near the heel (see Fig. 52-30*I*). These trigger points are generally found along the lateral and medial margins of the muscle group or along the midline (or in both areas) and often flare in patients experiencing vascular insufficiency of the lower extremities. One author suggests locating and injecting these trigger points for relief of the pain associated with intermittent claudication.[135]

Myofascial Back Pain

Unilateral back pain is often responsive to trigger point injection. The most common trigger points are found in the quadratus lumborum, gluteus medius, and tensor fasciae latae muscles. Gluteal trigger points may cause hip pain that mimics trochanteric bursitis (common during the latter stages of pregnancy) or back pain indistinguishable from sciatica.

The lumbosacral muscles are also commonly involved in lower back pain. Trigger points may occur secondary to nerve root or vertebral spondylolysis and cause neuropathic pain. In these cases, patients may experience only minimal or temporary relief from trigger point injections. Hence, if the patient is no better after a reasonable trial of trigger point injections, referral should be made to further evaluate for more invasive treatment.

Quadratus Lumborum Muscle Syndrome. The quadratus lumborum is considered a hip hiker and lateral flexor of the spine. It also assists respiratory function by anchoring the 12th rib for the pull of the diaphragm. Trigger points may be found along the 12th rib, around the iliac crest, and along the lateral border of the muscle (see Fig. 52-30*J*) and are often associated with distress on deep inspiration and 12th rib pain. Pain can be local or referred to the anterior abdominal wall. In addition, these trigger points may accentuate postoperative pain or painful abdominal scars over the lower quadrant.

Gluteus Medius Muscle Syndrome. Trigger points located in the gluteus medius may be the most critical trigger points in the lower extremities (see Fig. 52-30*J*). They are most commonly found along the iliac shelf and, with extensive involvement, along the entire gluteal ridge, including the gluteus minimus and the gluteus maximus muscles from the sacroiliac joint to the anterior superior iliac spine. It is estimated the 10% of people have legs that differ in length by at least 1 cm. This discrepancy in length may cause unilateral back pain and trigger points of the gluteus, erector spinae, and quadratus lumborum muscles.

Similar to the infraspinatus muscle syndrome, trigger points in the gluteus medius muscle are frequently associated with sympathetic hyperactivity. In addition, when these trigger points flare, they often recruit trigger points in the quadratus lumborum, tensor fasciae latae, and other gluteal muscles, where they induce diffuse lower back pain, or in the cervical muscles and cause neck pain and headaches. Though less common, isolated gluteus medius pain may also occur and usually projects along the iliac crest into the posterior of the hip, thigh, and calf.

Acknowledgment

The editors and author wish to acknowledge the significant contributions of Brenda Foley, Theodore A. Christopher, and Anders E. Sola to this chapter in previous editions.

References are available at www.expertconsult.com

Arthrocentesis

Stewart O. Sanford

BACKGROUND

Arthrocentesis, the puncture and aspiration of a joint, is an acknowledged, useful procedure that is easily performed in the emergency department (ED).[1] It has been established as both a diagnostic and therapeutic tool for various clinical situations. When performed properly, the procedure offers a wealth of clinical information and is associated with few complications. In the ED it is difficult to make an accurate assessment of an acutely painful, hot, and swollen joint without performing arthrocentesis.

INDICATIONS AND CONTRAINDICATIONS

The indications for arthrocentesis are listed in Review Box 53-1.

Infection in the tissues overlying the site to be punctured is generally considered an absolute contraindication to arthrocentesis. However, inflammation with warmth, swelling, and tenderness may overlie an acutely arthritic joint, and this condition may mimic a soft tissue infection. Once convinced that cellulitis does not exist, the clinician should not hesitate to obtain the necessary diagnostic joint fluid. Known bacteremia is a theoretical relative contraindication because infection can spread to the joint; however, this complication should be weighed against the useful information and culture results

gained by fluid analysis. A unique indication—or a serendipitous finding during arthrocentesis—is identification of fat globules in joint blood (lipohemarthrosis), which signifies an occult fracture.

Bleeding diatheses are rarely a relative contraindication, and arthrocentesis to relieve a tense hemarthrosis in bleeding disorders such as hemophilia is an accepted practice after infusion of the appropriate clotting factors. There are few data regarding the safety or dangers of arthrocentesis in patients taking anticoagulants or platelet inhibitors. Studies have demonstrated that the risk for iatrogenic hemarthrosis in patients treated with oral anticoagulants is extremely low, even in those who have international normalized ratios as high as 4.5.[2] One prospective trial of 32 patients taking warfarin found no complications after athrocentesis.[3] Hence, when necessary, arthrocentesis should be performed in patients taking anticoagulants. The value of reversing a coagulopathy with blood components before the procedure is not proved, and clinical judgment should prevail. Prosthetic joints are at high risk for infection, and arthrocentesis should be avoided whenever possible in this situation. However, if an infected prosthesis is suspected, arthrocentesis should be performed.

Articular versus Periarticular Disease

Periarticular conditions such as trauma, tendinitis, bursitis, contusion, cellulitis, or phlebitis may mimic articular disease and suggest the need for arthrocentesis. Therefore, evaluation of acute joint disease requires that the clinician first determine whether the patient's constellation of signs and symptoms derives from the joint itself or from some other musculoskeletal or periarticular structure. Such a distinction, however, may be difficult, if not impossible to make without analysis of synovial fluid. No specific test or physical finding has high specificity for solving this dilemma; however, some physical findings may prove helpful. A common periarticular structure

Arthrocentesis

Indications
Diagnosis of septic or crystal-induced arthritis
Diagnosis of traumatic bony or ligamentous injury
Instillation of medications for acute or chronic arthritis
Relief of the pain of acute hemarthrosis
Determination of communication between the laceration and joint space

Contraindications
Absolute:
  Overlying cellulitis
Relative:
  Bleeding diathesis

Complications
Introduction of infection
Bleeding
Allergy to local anesthetic
Pain

Equipment

Chlorhexidine or Betadine solution

Sterile gauze

Sterile drape

18- or 20-gauge needle

3-way stopcock

Lidocaine

Syringes

Review Box 53-1 Arthrocentesis: indications, contraindications, complications, and equipment.

Figure 53-1 Periarticular problems may mimic an intraarticular process. This patient suffered trauma to the knee, and anterior soft tissue swelling and fluctuance developed, which represents a hematoma of the prepatellar bursa, not a hemarthrosis. Pressure applied to the edge of the swelling aids in the aspiration of all blood from the bursa (*arrow*).

that can be associated with a joint effusion is a Baker cyst (popliteal cyst).

If the swelling is secondary to joint effusion or inflammation, the entire articular capsule will be inflamed and distended and fluid can often be palpated within the joint. In the knee, this condition must be differentiated from effusion into the prepatellar bursa, where swelling distends the bursa that lies mainly over the lower portion of the patella, between it and the skin. Effusion into the joint occurs posterior to the patella, whereas bursal swelling occurs anterior to it (Fig. 53-1). When considerable articular effusion of the knee is present, the capsule of the joint is distended and an inverted U-shaped swelling of the joint develops. This characteristic shape occurs because the dense patellar ligament prevents distention of the capsule along its inferior border. Also, with the knee extended a large effusion causes the patella to "float" or lift away from the femoral condyles. Complete extension and flexion are often impossible because of the joint tension produced by the effusion.

Joint effusion causes limited movement of the joint in all directions, with active and passive motion producing pain. The pain arising from a pathologic condition involving a joint may be diffuse or clearly localized to the joint, or it may radiate. Hip pain, for example, frequently radiates into the groin or down the front of the thigh into the knee. Shoulder joint pain commonly radiates into the elbow or the neck. Therefore, complete examination of contiguous structures is essential for adequate diagnosis.

In contrast, pain from a periarticular process is often more localized, and tenderness can be elicited only with certain specific movements or at specific points around the joint. In periarticular inflammation, one can often passively lead a joint through a range of motion with minimal discomfort, yet pain is significant when the patient attempts active motion. *Crepitus* may be elicited with tendinitis, or the pain may be traced along the course of a specific tendon.

Septic Arthritis

Acute monarticular arthritis is a common problem in emergency medicine. Although acute monarticular arthritis has

many causes, septic arthritis is the one requiring most urgent diagnosis and treatment. Infectious arthritis is still relatively frequent, and suspicion of a septic process in the joint is the first step in appropriate management; confirmation requires arthrocentesis and culture of synovial fluid. In the ED, synovial fluid analysis is the diagnostic test most heavily relied on in making the diagnosis of an acute intraarticular infection. Culture remains the most definitive study, although it is not 100% sensitive.[4] Gram stain may be helpful, but a negative Gram stain does not exclude the presence of a joint infection because not all infected joints have a positive Gram stain. Therapeutic arthrocentesis might be need to be repeated when treating a septic joint. Such therapy is usually performed on an inpatient basis.[5]

Infection of a joint occurs by one of several mechanisms: hematogenous spread (bacteremia, infective endocarditis, intravenous drug use), spread from a contiguous source of infection, direct implantation, postoperative contamination, or trauma.[4] Septic arthritis is typically monarticular with a swollen, erythematous, and painful joint. The noninfectious differential diagnosis includes crystal-induced arthritis, fracture, hemarthrosis, foreign body, osteoarthritis, ischemic necrosis, and monarticular rheumatoid arthritis. In addition, osteomyelitis may mimic septic arthritis because of the close proximity of the infected metaphysis to the joint space.[6] In many instances an acutely inflamed joint from gout or other arthritides simply cannot be distinguished from infection clinically. Nonetheless, early diagnosis is essential to prevent complications such as impairment of growth, articular destruction with ankylosis, osteomyelitis, and soft tissue extension.[7]

Because an acutely swollen joint may be indicative of a number of disease entities, a thorough history and physical examination are the cornerstones of evaluation, followed by arthrocentesis (Fig. 53-2). Laboratory findings can be useful in making a diagnosis, as can response to therapy (e.g., the response to empirical antibiotics in gonococcal arthritis is often the only criterion for diagnosis because the organism is difficult to culture). Blood cultures may be positive since joint infections may be due to hematogenous spread. Patients with malignancy (especially leukemia) or those who are immunosuppressed or otherwise debilitated are at particular risk for a septic cause. Infectious arthritis should be considered primarily in these patients, as well as in those with preexisting joint diseases such as rheumatoid arthritis. In general, a swollen joint is not usually injected with corticosteroids until the possibility of infection has been eliminated.[8]

Neisseria gonorrhoeae, *Staphylococcus* (including methicillin resistant), and *Streptococcus* are the most frequently identified etiologic agents. *N. gonorrhoeae* is the most common organism causing septic arthritis in adolescents and young adults. Patients older than 40 years and those with other medical illnesses are more likely to have *Staphylococcus* joint infections. In children, *Staphylococcus*, *Streptococcus*, and *Escherichia coli* predominate. *Haemophilus influenzae* was a common cause of pediatric septic arthritis in the past, but widespread use of the conjugate vaccine has reduced *H. influenzae* infection rates to nearly zero.[8-10] In neonates, staphylococci, Enterobacteriaceae, group B streptococci, and *N. gonorrhoeae* are the most likely organisms. Staphylococcal or pseudomonal infections commonly develop in injection drug abusers. *Salmonella* arthritis is more prevalent in patients with sickle cell disease than in the general population; however, more common

Figure 53-2 A and **B,** Tophaceous gout. These nodules are painless and full of uric acid crystals. **C,** The acutely swollen and painful wrist joint in this patient is most likely due to acute gouty arthritis, which can produce fever and leukocytosis. In some cases, joint fluid analysis is the only way to differentiate gout from a septic joint. **D,** Aspiration of a tophus yields a precipitated, waxy, soft uric acid conglomeration.

organisms still predominate. Prosthetic joints or postoperative infections have high rates of *Staphylococcus aureus, Streptococcus epidermidis,* Enterobacteriaceae, and *Pseudomonas* infection.[11]

The prevalence of community-acquired methicillin-resistant *S. aureus* (CA-MRSA) mandates special attention. Epidemiologic data on the incidence of CA-MRSA septic arthritis are sparse; however, one recent study noted that 50% of synovial fluid cultures in suspected septic arthritis ultimately grew MRSA.[12] It would be prudent to consider empirical therapy for MRSA in those suspected of having septic arthritis until the results of culture become available. MRSA-infected joints can be multiple, progress rapidly, and be very destructive of joint tissue and adjacent bone.

Although precise incidence data for nongonococcal septic arthritis have not been established, predisposing factors have been described and include age 80 years or older, diabetes mellitus, rheumatoid arthritis, hip or knee prosthesis, joint surgery, and skin infection.[13] The simultaneous occurrence of gout and septic arthritis is possible, and one should not allow the establishment of a diagnosis of crystal-induced disease to stop a thorough search for infection.[14]

Because *N. gonorrhoeae* is the most common organism causing septic arthritis, gonococcal arthritis deserves special mention. Disseminated gonococcal infection occurs in 0.5% to 3% of cases of mucosal infection. Gonococcal septic arthritis is more common in women, especially during pregnancy or after menstruation, because women with sexually transmitted gonorrhea infections are more likely to be asymptomatic. The time needed for local infection to disseminate can vary from several days to weeks. Patients will often experience systemic symptoms, including fevers, chills, and malaise, as well as migratory polyarthralgia. Gonococcal

tenosynovitis without joint involvement occurs in two thirds of patients. Dermatitis is also present in two thirds of patients (Fig. 53-3). The most common rash consists of scattered painless, nonpruritic 0.5- to 0.75-cm macules or papules with necrotic or pustular centers distributed on the extremities and trunk. Eventually, the infection settles into one or two large joints to yield a purulent arthritis.[9,15] Overt urethritis and vaginitis may be absent or overlooked because of concentration solely on the obvious joint pathology. Hence, it is important to realize that disseminated gonococcal infections can be associated with surprisingly minimal or even absent signs and symptoms of a genital infection source. Some joints may become inoculated through hematogenous spread from anal and oral sites of infection. Even though *N. gonorrhoeae*–infected joint fluid is usually "septic" in character, the yield of positive synovial fluid cultures has ranged from 25% to 50%. Blood cultures appear to be less helpful since they are positive in only 20% to 30% of cases. Because blood and joint fluid culture has a low yield, it would be prudent to culture all possible sites of gonococcal infection, including anal and pharyngeal sites. The organism can often be identified in asymptomatic genitourinary sites,[9] with cultures from the primary mucosal site being positive in up to 80% of infected patients.[15]

A positive Gram stain is immediately diagnostic of septic arthritis. However, Gram stains are positive in only 71% of gram-positive infections, 40% to 50% of gram-negative infections, and 25% of gonococcal infections.[16,17] An elevated synovial white blood cell (WBC) count and a reduction in synovial fluid glucose may give confirmatory data. However, the synovial fluid WBC count in gonococcal arthritis is often between 10,000 and 20,000 cells/mm.[3,4] Although mild leukocytosis and an elevated erythrocyte sedimentation rate

Figure 53-3 A, Often mistaken for insect or spider bites, these multiple embolic skin lesions, ranging from single or multiple petechiae to pustules, may be seen in patients with acutely swollen joints infected with *Neisseria gonorrhoeae*. Skin lesions are usually found on the extremities, especially the feet and hands, and may be present before a large joint effusion accumulates or with gonococcal tenosynovitis. **B,** A genital manifestation of urethritis or vaginitis may be seen but can be rather clinically silent. **C,** Maculopapular rash associated with *N. gonorrhoeae.*

may occur, normal laboratory values do not exclude infection.[16,18]

Hemarthrosis

Isolated nontraumatic hemarthrosis may occasionally be seen by the emergency clinician. An inflammatory reaction may follow intracapsular bleeding, and the proliferative reaction and the hyperplastic synovium formed might predispose patients to recurrent hemorrhage in that joint, especially those with bleeding diatheses. The knee is the most commonly affected joint, followed by the ankle, elbow, shoulder, and hip.[1]

The most common cause of intraarticular hemorrhage in the setting of no or minor trauma is a hereditary clotting factor deficiency such as hemophilia. Hemarthrosis is an infrequent complication of oral anticoagulant therapy but might occur even with prothrombin times within the normal range.[19] Cessation of anticoagulant therapy in these patients must be weighed against the risk for adverse clot formation (e.g., acute cerebrovascular accident). Chronic arthritis does not appear to be a long-term complication in patients with intraarticular bleeding from oral anticoagulant therapy. Hemarthrosis may also be a complication of sickle cell anemia, pseudogout, amyloidosis, pigmented villonodular synovitis, synovial hemangioma, rheumatoid arthritis, and infection.[18,20]

Management of acute hemarthrosis depends on the cause. Hemarthrosis associated with oral anticoagulant therapy improves only after use of the oral anticoagulant is discontinued and the prothrombin time returns to normal. Hemarthrosis after trauma is a frequent occurrence. It is most common in the knee and often denotes significant internal damage. A massively swollen knee after trauma is frequently seen with knee dislocation (*occasionally with spontaneous relocation*) and a tear of the anterior cruciate ligament. Intraarticular fractures can cause a significant hemarthrosis.

Distension of the joint by effusion or hemorrhage causes considerable pain and disability. If the fluid is not removed, it is partially absorbed, but part of it may undergo organization and result in the formation of adhesions or bands in the joint. This is one argument for drainage of the joint.[2] Some believe that in an otherwise healthy joint that is subjected to a single traumatic event, even a relatively large hemarthrosis will be spontaneously reabsorbed without significant sequelae and therefore presents no pressing need for drainage. Unfortunately, no literature exists to guide the best approach; hence, there is no universal standard of care regarding the need or lack thereof of draining blood from a traumatic joint.

Nonetheless, a large, tense, traumatic effusion is quite painful, and its presence precludes proper evaluation of an injured joint. Therapeutic arthrocentesis to drain a symptomatic traumatic effusion is a common and well-accepted practice.[2,19,21,22] The source of blood after trauma is frequently a tear in a ligamentous structure, capsule, or synovium or a fracture. Cruciate (especially anterior) ligament injury is the most common cause of significant hemarthrosis after trauma to the knee.[20] A joint effusion that develops 1 to 5 days after trauma may be secondary to a slow hemorrhage or reinjury, but the swelling is often caused by a nonhemorrhagic irritative synovial effusion.

Figure 53-4 Blood aspirated from a traumatized joint is placed in an emesis basis and put under a bright light to search for lipohemarthrosis, which is clinical evidence of an intraarticular fracture. Note the characteristic greasy sheen of floating fat. Do not throw away this blood before assessing for lipohemarthrosis.

TABLE 53-1 Intrasynovial Corticosteroid Preparations*

PREPARATION	LARGE-JOINT DOSE (mg)	SMALL-JOINT DOSE (mg)[†]
Triamcinolone hexacetonide	20	2-6
Triamcinolone acetonide	20	2-6
Methylprednisolone acetate	40	3.5-10.5
Triamcinolone diacetate	20	2-6
Dexamethasone acetate	5	0.5-1.5

From Gray RG, Gottlieb NL. Corticosteroid injections in RA: appraisal of a neglected therapy. *J Musculoskelet Med.* 1990;7:53. Reproduced by permission.
*Listed in approximate descending order of duration of action.
[†]The dose will depend on joint size, capsular distensibility, and degree of inflammation.

Occasionally, one will diagnose an occult fracture by the presence of lipohemarthrosis, or fat globules in the arthrocentesis specimen (Fig. 53-4). This may be appreciated when the bloody effusion is placed in a clear container (e.g., emesis basin) and held to a light. If the history of trauma is vague, arthrocentesis may be required to differentiate hemorrhage from other causes of joint effusion. *An occult tibial plateau fracture is an example in which evaluating for lipohemarthrosis may be of particular value.* Following therapeutic arthrocentesis for a hemarthrosis, it may be desirable to inject 2 to 15 mL, depending on joint size, of a long-acting local anesthetic (see Chapter 29) into the joint to facilitate examination or provide temporary relief of the symptoms.

Intraarticular Corticosteroid Injections

In 1951 Hollander and coworkers[23] first demonstrated that intraarticular corticosteroid injections are useful for relief of symptoms in patients with severe rheumatoid arthritis. The use of steroids has proved to be a dependable method for providing rapid relief of pain and swelling of inflamed joints, although it is strictly local, usually temporary, and rarely curative.[2,24,25] It is easily performed in the emergency setting. Acute gout responds well to joint injection, and this may be preferable in patients who cannot tolerate indomethacin or colchicine.

Corticosteroid injections are most helpful when only a small number of joints are actively inflamed. The most frequently used corticosteroids for intraarticular injection are shown in Table 53-1.[2] Diminution of joint pain, swelling, effusion, and warmth is usually evident within 6 to 12 hours after injection.

Though very rare, the most serious complication of this practice is intraarticular infection.[2] Therefore, steroids should not be injected into a joint if a joint space infection is suspected. Repeated injections into one joint pose a risk for necrosis of juxtaarticular bone with subsequent joint destruction and instability and suppression of the hypothalamic-pituitary axis from systemic absorption. Other complications include local soft tissue atrophy and calcification, tendon rupture, intraarticular bleeding, and transient nerve palsy.[2,25] Transient elevations in blood glucose, as well as erythema, warmth, and diaphoresis of the face and torso, may also occur after intraarticular steroid injections. Acute pain, redness, and swelling 12 to 24 hours after steroid injection can mimic infection, but with this timing it is most likely an inflammatory reaction (steroid flare) to crystal-containing steroid preparation (often methylprednisolone). Deposition of steroid crystals on the synovium might give rise to a transient, self-limited flare-up of synovitis.[2,26]

It is always important to determine whether local corticosteroid therapy has been used previously, not only to consider the array of clinical conditions associated with steroid use but also because crystalline corticosteroid material can hinder proper interpretation of crystals found in synovial fluid.[26]

EQUIPMENT

The material needed for arthrocentesis includes skin preparation solutions (e.g., chlorhexidine); sterile gloves and drapes (optional in some cases); local anesthetic; syringes for injecting local anesthetic and aspirating joint fluid; a three-way stopcock for draining large amounts of fluid; lavender-, red-, and green-topped blood tubes; and various sizes of needles and intravenous catheters (see Review Box 53-1).

Depending on the size of the effusion to be drained, a 10-, 20-, or 30-mL Luer-Lok syringe can be used. If a large effusion is suspected, a three-way stopcock between the needle and the syringe allows complete drainage with a single joint penetration. Fluid for cell count should be collected in a lavender-topped tube; however, viscosity, protein, and glucose determinations do not require anticoagulants, and fluid should be placed in a red-topped tube. Though still common practice in many institutions, recent evidence suggests that synovial fluid protein and glucose levels are poor differentiators of noninflammatory and inflammatory effusions and are no longer recommended (see "Synovial Fluid Interpretation," later).[2,27-29] Immediately examine fresh synovial fluid in its unadulterated form for crystals. Calcium oxalate and lithium heparin anticoagulants have been reported to introduce artifactual crystals into the fluid. Joint fluid to be analyzed for crystals should be collected in a green-topped tube containing sodium heparin. If culturing for *N. gonorrhoeae*, the fluid should be immediately placed on proper medium and stored in a low-oxygen environment in the ED.

Text continued on p. 1084

ULTRASOUND: Arthrocentesis

by Christine Butts, MD

Ultrasound offers a significant advantage when evaluating a patient with a complaint of joint pain. Patients with obesity or significant pain limiting physical examination make the diagnosis of joint effusion difficult. Attempting blind aspiration in these patients may cause significant pain in the patient and frustration in the clinician. Ultrasound allows the physician to thoroughly evaluate the joint space for the presence of effusion and to plan the best approach for aspiration. The initial evaluation of the major joints is discussed below, followed by a general approach to aspiration.

Knee

Although effusions of the knee are frequently diagnosed on physical examination alone and aspirated blindly, ultrasound allows the clinician to distinguish effusion from other conditions that may cause generalized swelling (such as bursitis).

A high-frequency transducer (7.5 to 10 mHz) should be used to allow the greatest resolution. Begin with the indicator pointing toward the patient's head (in longitudinal orientation) over the anterior aspect of the knee and attempt to locate the patella (Fig. 53-US1). The patella can be seen as a brightly echogenic (white) object with posterior shadowing (Fig. 53-US2). Locating the patella is key to distinguishing prepatellar bursitis, which will appear as a dark, fluid-filled collection superficial to the patella, and a joint effusion, which will appear as a dark, fluid-filled collection deep to the patella. Once the patella has been identified, the transducer should be moved medially or laterally to "look under" the patella into the joint space (Fig. 53-US3). Fluid will appear as a dark gray or black collection between the articular surface of the femur and fibula or tibia (Fig. 53-US4). Once this area has been evaluated, the transducer should be moved superiorly to evaluate the suprapatellar bursa, which lies superior to the patella and deep to the quadriceps tendon. The suprapatellar bursa communicates with the joint space and frequently houses a large amount of fluid (Fig. 53-US5).

Shoulder

Either an anterior or posterior approach can be used to evaluate the shoulder. In the anterior approach, the patient should first be placed in a seated position with the elbow adducted and the palm facing up. The high-frequency transducer can then be placed in a transverse orientation over the approximate location of the biceps tendon (Fig. 53-US6). The biceps tendon is an extracapsular extension of the joint and will be seen

Figure 53-US1 Placement of the ultrasound transducer in a longitudinal orientation over the patella. Such placement will enable localization of the patella and serves to orient the sonographer.

Figure 53-US2 Ultrasound image of a normal patella. The patella is seen as a brightly echogenic (*white*) arcing line just beneath the surface (*arrow*). Prepatellar fluid collections, such as bursitis, will be seen superficial to this area.

Figure 53-US3 Placement of the ultrasound transducer to "look under" the patella into the joint space.

Figure 53-US4 Ultrasound image of the junction of the femur (at the *left* of the image) and the tibia (at the *right* of the image) (*arrow*). When an effusion is suspected, the suprapatellar recess should be evaluated in addition to this space because fluid frequently collects in the potential space superior to this junction.

ULTRASOUND: Arthrocentesis, cont'd

Figure 53-US5 Ultrasound image of a joint effusion within the suprapatellar recess of the knee joint. The recess is distended with anechoic (*black*) fluid and the femur can be seen as the hyperechoic (*white*) line at the bottom of the image.

Figure 53-US6 Placement of the ultrasound transducer over the anterior aspect of the shoulder to evaluate the biceps tendon. To obtain the best view, the patient's arm should be flexed at the elbow, supinated, and slightly abducted.

Figure 53-US7 Ultrasound image of a normal-appearing biceps tendon. The tendon will appear as a hyperechoic (*white*) bundle within the groove of the humerus as indicated by the *arrow*.

Figure 53-US8 The biceps tendon is surrounded by anechoic (*black*) fluid. (*Courtesy of Verena Valley, MD.*)

to distend with fluid when a joint effusion is present. A normal tendon can be seen to lie within the biceps groove of the humerus (Fig. 53-US7). When surrounded by fluid, the tendon will be seen to "float" within an anechoic (black) area (Fig. 53-US8).

To evaluate the joint from the posterior approach, place the patient in a seated position with the affected hand on the opposite shoulder to open the joint space. The transducer can then be placed at the approximate location of the articulation of the humeral head with the glenoid (Fig. 53-US9). In a normal joint, the humerus can be seen to articulate with the glenoid without any intervening fluid (Fig. 53-US10). When an effusion is present, a dark gray or black collection can be seen medial to the glenoid (Fig. 53-US11).

Ankle

The ankle joint is best evaluated in the longitudinal axis with the transducer placed over the space between the posterior edge of the tibia and the talus (Fig. 53-US12). Slightly plantar-flexing the foot will enable the transducer to "fit" in this space. In a normal joint, the distal edge of the tibia can be seen to articulate with the talus without any intervening fluid (Fig. 53-US13). When an effusion is present, it is seen as a triangular, dark gray to black pocket between the tibia and talus (Fig. 53-US14). Ultrasound can also be used to identify the location of the dorsalis pedis artery before aspiration.

Figure 53-US9 Placement of the ultrasound transducer over the posterior aspect of the shoulder to evaluate the glenohumeral joint. This joint line can typically be palpated to approximate the best initial position.

Continued

ULTRASOUND: Arthrocentesis, cont'd

Figure 53-US10 Ultrasound of a normal-appearing shoulder joint. Deep to the overlying musculature, the glenoid can be seen at the left of the image (*arrowhead*). The humeral head is seen to the right of the glenoid (*arrow*).

Figure 53-US11 Shoulder effusion as viewed from a posterior approach. Free fluid will appear as an anechoic collection medial to the glenoid rim. (*Courtesy of Verena Valley, MD.*)

Figure 53-US12 Placement of the ultrasound transducer over the anterior aspect of the ankle to evaluate for an ankle effusion.

Figure 53-US13 Ultrasound image of a normal ankle joint. At the *left* of the image is the tibia, with the talus seen at the *right*. The intervening area is free of fluid, and the extensor hallucis longus can be seen superficial to this area.

Figure 53-US14 Ultrasound image of an ankle effusion. As with the normal image, the tibia and talus can be seen on either side of the image. However, in the intervening area, an anechoic (*black*) fluid collection can be seen.

Elbow

The elbow is easily evaluated from the posterior approach. With this approach the transducer is placed over the olecranon fossa with the elbow flexed and the lower part of the arm supported (Fig. 53-US15). In a normal elbow the olecranon fossa can be seen as a slight "divot" between the olecranon of the ulna and the humerus (Fig. 53-US16). When an effusion is present, dark gray or black fluid can be seen to distend this space (Fig. 53-US17).

Hip

The hip joint is unique in that physical examination may suggest the presence of an effusion, but direct confirmation is difficult with traditional examination techniques. Ultrasound will easily confirm the presence of an effusion. To evaluate the hip joint, a low-frequency transducer (3 to 5 mHz) should initially be selected because of the depth of the joint. In very thin patients, the distance from the skin to the joint may be small enough to allow the use of a high-frequency transducer. The transducer should be aligned in a slightly oblique axis (mimicking the orientation of the femoral neck) along the inguinal area. It may be helpful to aim toward the umbilicus. The femoral neck and head should be sought. They will appear as brightly echogenic outlines in the expected shape of the bones

ULTRASOUND: Arthrocentesis, cont'd

Figure 53-US15 Placement of the transducer in the transverse plane over the area of the olecranon fossa. For best resolution, a high-frequency transducer should be used.

Figure 53-US16 Ultrasound image of a normal elbow joint. The olecranon fossa can be identified as the echogenic (*white*) crescent at the bottom of the image (*arrow*). The area just above the fossa should be evaluated for the presence of fluid indicative of an effusion.

Figure 53-US17 Elbow joint distended by anechoic fluid (*arrow*) superficial to the olecranon fossa. (*From Allan PL, Baxter GM, Weston MJ, eds. Clinical Ultrasound. 3rd ed. Philadelphia; Elsevier; 2011.*)

(Fig. 53-US18). Once the femur has been identified, the joint capsule should be sought. It will appear as an arcing, hyperechoic line superficial to the bones (Fig. 53-US19). In a normal hip there will be very little tissue between these two structures. There may be a small amount of anechoic or hypoechoic fluid present in this space in a normal hip, and correlation with the unaffected side will aid in evaluation. In the presence of a significant effusion, a large anechoic or hypoechoic fluid collection will be seen between the femoral neck and the capsule (Fig. 53-US20).

Figure 53-US18 Normal ultrasound of the hip. The femoral head can be seen as the hyperechoic (*white*) line highlighted by the arrow. The area immediately superficial to the femur is devoid of any significant fluid collection.

Figure 53-US19 Ultrasound image of the hip with demonstration of the joint capsule. The joint capsule can be seen as the hyperechoic (*white*) arcing structure marked by the *arrow*.

Figure 53-US20 Ultrasound image of a hip effusion. As in a normal hip, the femur can be seen at the bottom of the image. Immediately superficial to the femur, an anechoic (*black*) fluid collection is highlighted by the *arrow*.

Continued

ULTRASOUND: Arthrocentesis, cont'd

Aspiration

Once the joint in question has been evaluated, the optimal site for aspiration can be planned. In contrast to the traditional, blind aspiration technique, the use of ultrasound may suggest an alternative approach. Ultrasound will enable the clinician to map the best approach to the effusion. Once this approach has been clarified, one of two techniques can be applied. The site can be marked and the aspiration can then proceed blindly under sterile conditions. In other cases it may be preferable to perform the tap under direct ultrasound guidance. In these circumstances the needle is inserted either from the transverse or from the long-axis approach and guided directly into the joint space.

GENERAL ARTHROCENTESIS TECHNIQUE

Joint fluid may be obtained even when there is little clinical evidence of an effusion. Although one may aspirate successfully at the point where the joint bulges maximally, certain landmarks are important. The most crucial part of arthrocentesis is defining the joint anatomy by palpating the bony landmarks as a guide. A puncture site and an approach to the joint should be selected; tendons, major vessels, and major nerve branches should be avoided. In most instances the approach is via the *extensor surfaces of joints* because most major vessels and nerves are found beneath the flexor surfaces. Also, the synovial pouch is usually more superficial on the extensor side of a joint. Ultrasound may be particularly helpful in locating small effusions.

Aseptic technique, including the use of sterile gloves and instruments, is essential to avoid infection. Arthrocentesis should not be attempted if there is a definite or suspected infection overlying the joint. Antiseptic preparation solution should be allowed to dry for several minutes because the bactericidal effects of iodine are both concentration and time dependent. Iodine solution is then removed with an alcohol sponge to prevent transference of iodine into the joint space, which can lead to an inflammatory process. Although the utility of draping is unproved and it may obscure the site, a sterile perforated drape may be placed over the joint.

With appropriate local anesthesia, arthrocentesis should be a relatively painless procedure; without anesthesia, it may be quite painful and distressing to the patient. The synovial membrane itself has pain fibers associated with blood vessels, and the articular capsule and periosteum are richly supplied with nerve fibers and are very sensitive. The articular cartilage has no intrinsic pain fibers. It is important to have the patient relax during the procedure. Tense muscles narrow the joint space and make the procedure more difficult, often necessitating repeated attempts or resulting in inadequate drainage. Distraction of the joint may enhance the target area, especially in areas such as the wrist and finger joints. Traction not only increases the chance of entering the joint but also lessens the chance of scoring the articular cartilage with the needle.

Anesthesia is best accomplished by infiltrating the skin *down to the area of the joint capsule along the entire route of needle penetration* with a local anesthetic agent such as 1% or 2% lidocaine (Xylocaine) via a 25- to 27-gauge needle. For extremely painful joints, a regional nerve block is appropriate.

The landmarks described in "Specific Arthrocentesis Techniques" later in this chapter should be used and care taken to not bounce the needle off bony structures as a means of finding the joint space because this may cause unnecessary pain. However, in contrast to earlier beliefs, striking bone with the arthrocentesis needle is unlikely to damage articular cartilage.[2] An 18- to 22-gauge needle or intravenous catheter and needle set of suitable length attached to an appropriately sized syringe is inserted at the desired anatomic point through the skin and subcutaneous tissue into the joint space. The largest needle that is practical is used to avoid obstructing the lumen with debris or clot. In large joints such as the knee, which can accommodate large effusions, it is suggested that one use a 30- to 60-mL syringe because it may be difficult to change a syringe when the needle is within the joint cavity (Fig. 53-5). A three-way stopcock placed between the needle and the syringe is an option for draining large effusions (Fig. 53-6). If the syringe must be changed during the procedure, the hub of the needle should be grasped with a hemostat and held tightly while the syringe is removed. The authors prefer to use only a rigid needle and not a flexible catheter to perform arthrocentesis; however, a sturdy catheter is used by some clinicians. If an intravenous catheter and needle set is used, the needle is removed while leaving the outer atraumatic plastic catheter in the joint space. The syringe is then attached to the catheter for aspiration. Manipulation of the joint or catheter can now occur with little threat of tissue injury.

Aspiration of synovial fluid and easy injection and return of fluid indicate intraarticular placement of the needle tip. As a general rule, *one should try to remove as much fluid or blood as possible.* If the fluid stops flowing, it indicates that the joint has been drained completely, the tip of the needle has become dislodged, or debris or clot is obstructing the needle. One should slightly advance or retract the tip of the needle, rotate the bevel, or lessen the force of aspiration. One should never *reintroduce* a needle through a plastic catheter that has been left in the joint. Occasionally, reinjecting a small amount of fluid into the joint space confirms placement of the needle and may clear the needle. If fluid flows freely back into the joint and is easily reaspirated, one has probably removed all the fluid. If resistance is met, the needle has probably been jarred from the joint space and is lodged in soft tissue. In some instances, minor changes in position produced by flexion or extension of the joint may allow the fluid to flow more freely. Scraping or shearing the articular cartilage with the needle should be avoided. One should enter the joint in a straight line and avoid unnecessary side-to-side motion of the needle.

Synovial fluid should be sent for studies as indicated by the clinical situation. Studies usually obtained include cell count with differential, crystal analysis, Gram staining, and bacterial culture and sensitivity analysis. Synovial protein, glucose, and lactate dehydrogenase determinations have been shown to be

GENERAL ARTHROCENTESIS TECHNIQUE

Position the patient and identify all landmarks.

Cleanse the skin with antiseptic; use of a sterile drape is optional.

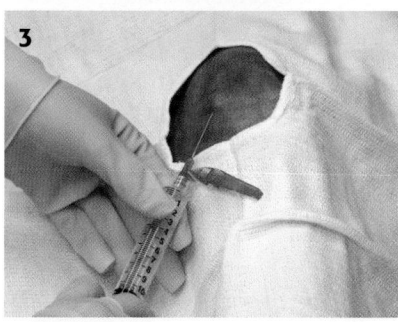
Raise a wheal with local anesthetic.

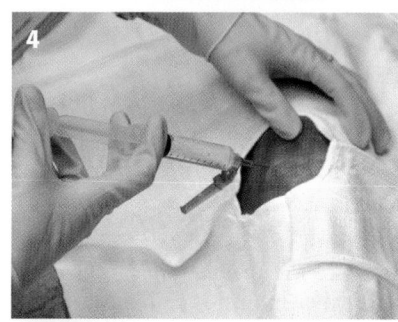
Inject anesthetic along the entire track of the aspiration needle.

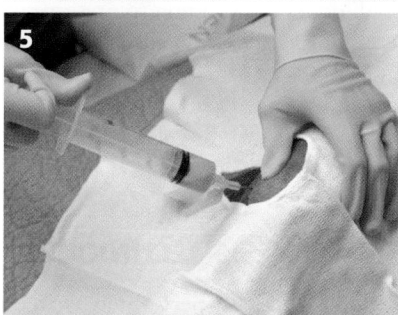
Aspirate as the needle is advanced; always use a large syringe if there is a potential for a large effusion.

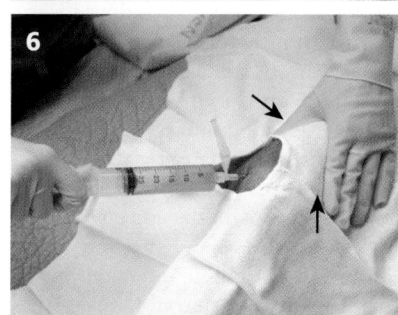
"Milk" the effusion if necessary; always remove as much fluid as possible.

Grasp the needle hub with a hemostat (to maintain correct position) if a syringe change is needed.

Place fluid into appropriate tubes and submit to the laboratory.

Figure 53-5 General arthrocentesis technique.

unreliable in distinguishing noninflammatory from inflammatory and infectious causes and are no longer recommended.[2,29-33] Less frequently obtained studies include rheumatoid factor analysis, lupus erythematosus cell preparation, viscosity analysis, mucin clot, fibrin clot, fungal and acid-fast stains, Lyme titer, fungal and tuberculous culture, and synovial fluid complement analysis. If the arthrocentesis is performed for the relief of hemarthrosis, the fluid need not be sent for analysis. One should be selective in ordering tests.

There is no need to order a large battery of tests routinely on all fluids. If the volume of fluid collected is low, Gram stain, culture, and examination of the "wet preparation" under regular and polarizing microscopy have the highest priority. Prompt examination of specimens should be performed to avoid misdiagnosing borderline inflammatory fluids, missing crystals that dissolve with time, or overinterpreting the findings because of new artifactual crystals that appear over a prolonged time.[34]

Figure 53-6 Use of a stopcock will negate the need to change the syringe during arthrocentesis. Turn the stopcock to collect and then expel fluid, or inject lidocaine or steroid without moving the needle.

Figure 53-7 Landmarks for arthrocentesis of the first carpometacarpal joint. All small joints pose a difficult aspiration. When aspirating small joints, apply continuous suction to the syringe, and walk the tip of the needle along the bones until the joint is entered or fluid is obtained. Apply longitudinal traction to facilitate entry into a small joint. *MCP*, metacarpophalangeal.

COMPLICATIONS

Significant complications are rare with arthrocentesis but include the following:

1. *Infection.* Skin bacteria may be introduced into the joint space during needle puncture. Nevertheless, infection occurs rarely because the bacteria are either quickly cleared or not viable.[2] One can further limit this complication by maintaining rigorous sterile technique and avoiding insertion of the needle through obviously (or possibly) infected skin or subcutaneous tissue. Various studies report the incidence of infection after routine arthrocentesis to be in the range of 1 in 10,000.[34] However, in immunocompromised patients, particularly those with rheumatoid arthritis, the incidence is higher (1 in 2000 to 10,000 aspirations).[35,36] Joint aspiration in the presence of bacteremia was discussed previously. Acute pain, redness, and swelling 12 to 24 hours after steroid injection can mimic infection but is most likely an inflammatory reaction (steroid flare) to the steroid preparation (often methylprednisolone).

2. *Bleeding.* Bleeding with subsequent hemarthrosis is rarely a complication, except in patients with a bleeding diathesis. In those with a bleeding diathesis such as hemophilia, arthrocentesis should be delayed until clotting competence has been enhanced by infusing specific clotting factors. In general, spontaneous bleeding into a hemophiliac's joint is an indication for replacement of clotting factors. Occasionally, a small quantity of blood may be aspirated along with synovial fluid. This happens most often when the joint is nearly emptied. A small amount of blood-tinged fluid is generally the result of nicking a small synovial blood vessel; it is usually inconsequential.

   Arthrocentesis and joint injections in patients receiving chronic warfarin therapy, with a therapeutic INR, were shown to be safe by Ahmed and Gertner,[37] without an increased risk of bleeding complications. In this study of 456 procedures in patients on chronic warfarin therapy, there was no statistically significant difference in the overall complication rate between patients with an international normalized ratio 2.0 or greater and patients with an international normalized ratio less than 2.0. Of note, 103 of 456 procedures (22.5%) were safely performed in patients with an international normalized ratio greater than 3, with the highest international normalized ratio being 7.8.

3. *Allergic reaction.* Hypersensitivity to the local anesthetic can usually be prevented by thorough history taking. Facial and torso flushing associated with corticosteroid injection may represent an idiosyncratic reaction to preservatives in the steroid preparation.[2] Fainting during the procedure is not uncommon and most often the result of vasovagal influences.

4. *Corticosteroid-induced complications.* See "Intraarticular Corticosteroid Injections," earlier.

SPECIFIC ARTHROCENTESIS TECHNIQUES

Arthrocentesis of the hip is generally performed by an orthopedic surgeon under fluoroscopic, ultrasound, magnetic resonance imaging, or computed tomography guidance and is not discussed here. If available, fluoroscopy or ultrasound can also be used to guide aspiration of other joints, but these imaging adjuncts are not generally required. For small joints, *application of traction* is often very helpful in obtaining fluid. While applying continuous suction to the aspirating syringe, walk the needle over palpated bone until the joint is entered or fluid is obtained. However, *it may be quite difficult to obtain fluid from small joints in the hand and foot, and the clinician must often treat empirically. If only one drop of fluid is obtained from small joints, it is best to send it for culture.*

First Carpometacarpal Joint (Fig. 53-7)

Landmarks. The radial aspect of the proximal end of the first metacarpal is the arthrocentesis landmark for this joint. The abductor pollicis longus (APL) tendon is located by active extension of the tendon.

Position. Oppose the thumb against the little finger so that the proximal end of the first metacarpal is palpable. *Apply traction to the thumb* to widen the joint space between the first metacarpal and the greater multangular bone.

Needle Insertion. Insert a 22- to 23-gauge needle at a point proximal to the prominence at the base of the first metacarpal on the palmar side of the APL tendon.

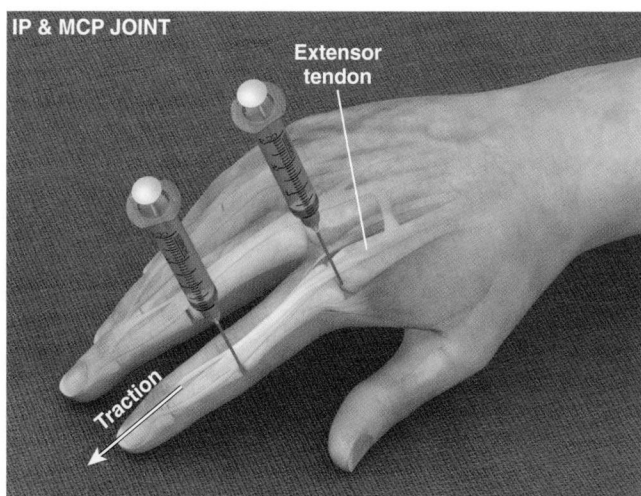

Figure 53-8 Landmarks for arthrocentesis of the interphalangeal (IP) and metacarpophalangeal (MCP) joints.

Comments. Degenerative joint disease commonly affects this joint. Arthrocentesis is moderately difficult. The anatomic "snuffbox" (located more proximally and on the dorsal side of the APL tendon) should be avoided because it contains the radial artery and superficial radial nerve. A more dorsal approach may also be used.

Interphalangeal and Metacarpophalangeal Joints (Fig. 53-8)

Landmarks. The landmarks are located on the dorsal surface. For the metacarpophalangeal joints, palpate for the prominence at the proximal end of the proximal phalanx. For the interphalangeal joints, palpate for the prominence at the proximal end of the middle or distal phalanx. The extensor tendon runs down the midline.

Position. Flex the fingers to approximately 15 to 20 degrees and *apply traction*.

Needle Insertion. Insert a 22- to 25-gauge needle into the joint space dorsally, just medial or lateral to the central slip of the extensor tendon.

Comments. Synovitis causes these joints to bulge dorsally. Normally, it is unusual to obtain fluid in the absence of a significant pathologic condition.

Radiocarpal Joint (Wrist) (Fig. 53-9)

Landmarks. The dorsal radial tubercle (Lister's tubercle) is an elevation found in the center of the dorsal aspect of the distal end of the radius. The extensor pollicis longus tendon runs in a groove on the radial side of the tubercle. The tendon can be palpated by active extension of the wrist and thumb.

Position. Position the wrist in approximately 20 to 30 degrees of flexion with accompanying ulnar deviation. *Apply traction to the hand.*

Needle Insertion. Insert a 22-gauge needle dorsally, just distal to the dorsal tubercle on the ulnar side of the extensor pollicis longus tendon. The anatomic snuffbox, located more radially, should be avoided to prevent injury to the radial artery or superficial radial nerve.

Figure 53-9 A, Landmarks for arthrocentesis of the radiocarpal (wrist) joint. **B,** Acute joint effusion of the right wrist. *EPL,* extensor pollicis longus.

Radiohumeral Joint (Elbow) (Fig. 53-10)

Landmarks. The lateral epicondyle of the humerus and the head of the radius are the arthrocentesis landmarks for the radiohumeral joint. With the elbow extended, palpate the depression between the radial head and the lateral epicondyle of the humerus.

Position. With the palpating finger still touching the radial head, flex the elbow to 90 degrees. Pronate the forearm, and place the palm flat on a table.

Needle Insertion. Insert a 20-gauge needle from the lateral aspect just distal to the lateral epicondyle and directed medially.

Comments. Elevation of the anterior fat pad or the presence of a posterior fat pad on a lateral soft tissue elbow radiograph signifies blood, pus, or fluid in the elbow joint (see Fig. 53-10*B*). Effusions in the elbow joint may bulge and be readily palpated (see Fig. 53-10*C*). Frequently, the effusion appears inferior to the lateral epicondyle. The bulge can then be aspirated from a posterior approach on the lateral side (see Fig. 53-10*D*). A medial approach is not recommended because the ulnar nerve and superior ulnar collateral artery may be

Figure 53-10 A, Landmarks for arthrocentesis of the radiohumeral (elbow) joint. **B,** On a lateral elbow radiograph, displacement of the anterior fat pad (*arrows*) or the presence of a posterior fat pad (*arrows*) indicates blood, pus, or fluid in the joint. **C,** An effusion in the elbow joint can usually be readily palpated. A palpating finger is placed over the lateral epicondyle (*asterisk*) and slid posteriorly and inferiorly toward the olecranon (*arrow*). Usually, a depression is felt as the finger leaves the epicondyle, but a bulge is appreciated if a joint effusion is present. **D,** Removal of only a few milliliters of blood will reduce pain and hasten recovery of range of motion. The most common pathology after trauma with a radiograph negative for fracture but positive for hemarthrosis is a nondisplaced radial head fracture.

damaged. Gout and septic arthritis commonly affect this joint. The most common cause of elbow hemarthrosis after trauma with no obvious fracture is a nondisplaced radial head fracture. A small hemarthrosis need not be aspirated, but removal of blood from a tense elbow joint will significantly hasten recovery and facilitate range of motion in patients with a radial head fracture.

Glenohumeral Joint (Shoulder), Anterior Approach (Fig. 53-11)

Landmarks. Anteriorly palpate the coracoid process medially and the proximal end of the humerus laterally.

Position. The patient should sit upright with the arm at the side and hand in the lap.

Needle Insertion. Insert a 20-gauge needle at a point inferior and lateral to the coracoid process and direct it posteriorly toward the glenoid rim.

Comments. Arthrocentesis of this joint is moderately difficult. Other approaches have been suggested but are less well accepted.

Knee Joint, Anteromedial Approach
(Fig. 53-12)

Landmarks. The medial surface of the patella at the middle or superior portion of the patella is the landmark for the knee joint.

Position. It is usually recommended that the knee be extended as far as possible. Alternatively, some practitioners prefer to flex the knee 15 to 20 degrees by placing a towel under the popliteal region to open the joint space up. Relaxation of the quadriceps muscle greatly facilitates needle placement. Keep the foot perpendicular to the floor.

Needle Insertion. Insert an 18-gauge needle or catheter and needle set at the midpoint or superior portion of the patella

SHOULDER JOINT

Coracoid process

Humerus

Figure 53-11 Landmarks for arthrocentesis of the glenohumeral (shoulder) joint.

KNEE JOINT

Patella

Femur

Intercondylar femoral notch

A

B

Figure 53-12 A, Landmarks for arthrocentesis of the knee joint. **B,** Note the use of a stopcock on the syringe to allow complete drainage without repositioning the needle. Note that the syringe is held parallel to the table. Compression of the suprapatellar region by the operator or an assistant will facilitate complete aspiration. For the knee, a 60-mL syringe and an 18-gauge needle should be used to drain large effusions. Note that the red streaks of blood denote a traumatic tap rather than hemarthrosis. The blood streaks started after clear fluid had been withdrawn.

approximately 1 cm medial to the anteromedial patellar edge. Direct the needle between the posterior surface of the patella and the intercondylar femoral notch. The patella may be grasped with the hand and elevated to aid entry of the needle into the joint. *Keeping the needle/syringe parallel to the bed limits internal injury.*

Comments. If the patient is tense, contraction of the quadriceps will greatly hinder entering the joint. However, the knee is probably the easiest joint to enter, and removal of a tense hemarthrosis will relieve pain and facilitate examination for ligamentous injury. If fluid stops flowing, the operator or assistant should squeeze the soft tissue area of the suprapatellar region to "milk" the suprapatellar pouch of fluid. Alternatively, wrap the patient's thigh with a 6-inch elastic bandage from the groin to the suprapatellar area before beginning the procedure. The knee can easily accommodate 50 to 70 mL of fluid, and the clinician should therefore use a large syringe. Holding or securing the hub of the needle with a hemostat allows the clinician to remove the syringe without changing the position of the intraarticular needle. Alternatively, a stopcock on the needle will allow complete removal of fluid without changing the position of the needle (see Fig. 53-12*B*). The knee is a common site for septic arthritis (especially gonococcal) and various inflammatory or degenerative diseases. An anterolateral approach can be accomplished in a similar manner.

Tibiotalar Joint (Ankle) (Fig. 53-13)

Landmarks. The medial malleolar sulcus is bordered medially by the medial malleolus and laterally by the anterior tibial tendon. The tendon can easily be identified with active dorsiflexion of the foot.

Position. With the patient lying supine, plantar-flex the foot.

Needle Insertion. Insert a 20- to 22-gauge needle at a point just medial to the anterior tibial tendon and directed into the hollow at the anterior edge of the medial malleolus. The needle must be inserted 2 to 3 cm to penetrate the joint space.

Comments. If the joint bulges medially, one may use an approach that is more medial than anterior and enter at a point just anterior to the medial malleolus. The needle may have to be advanced 2 to 4 cm with this approach.

Metatarsophalangeal and Interphalangeal Joints (Fig. 53-14)

Landmarks. For the first digit, landmarks are the distal metatarsal head and the proximal base of the first phalanx. For the other toes, the landmarks are the prominences at the proximal interphalangeal and distal interphalangeal joints. The extensor tendon of the great toe can be located by active extension of the toe.

Position. With the patient supine, flex the toes 15 to 20 degrees. *Then apply traction.*

Needle Insertion. Insert a 22-gauge needle on the dorsal surface at a point just medial or lateral to the central slip of the extensor tendon.

Figure 53-13 A, Landmarks for arthrocentesis of the tibiotalar joint. **B,** Acute gout of the ankle is common but can mimic an infected joint, an uncommon condition. Arthrocentesis was unsuccessful, but a previous history of gout and the clinical features allowed empirical treatment of gout.

Figure 53-14 A, Landmarks for arthrocentesis of the first metatarsophalangeal joint. **B,** Acute gout can be mistaken for cellulitis, but this is classic podagra. Aspiration of small joints may be difficult. One can treat gout empirically with close follow-up to be certain that infection or coinfection is not present. **C,** The red, warm, swollen, and painful condition of the dorsum of the foot is a common finding with gout but may suggest cellulitis. Clinical acumen may diagnose gout (e.g., woke up with sudden acute pain, diuretic use, previous gout, elevated uric acid level), but arthrocentesis is often helpful, especially if this is the first manifestation of gout.

SYNOVIAL FLUID INTERPRETATION

Synovial fluid examination is essential for the diagnosis of septic arthritis, gout, and pseudogout.[38-40] Inflammatory joint disease of previously unknown etiology can often be diagnosed precisely by synovial fluid analysis. Joint fluid is a dialysate of plasma that contains protein and hyaluronic acid. Normal fluid is clear enough to read newsprint through and will not clot. It is straw colored, flows freely, and has the consistency of machine oil. Normal fluid produces a good mucin clot and yields a positive "string sign" (see the next section). The uric acid level of joint fluid approaches that of serum, and the glucose concentration is normally at least 80% of that in serum. Clarity of fluid reflects the leukocyte count. High leukocyte counts result in opacity, the degree of which generally correlates with the degree of elevated synovial fluid leukocytes. However, the degree of opacity cannot be used to reliably determine the synovial fluid leukocyte count and should not be used as a surrogate for laboratory cell count measurements.

String Sign

Viscosity correlates with the concentration of hyaluronate in synovial fluid. Any inflammation degrades hyaluronate, which characteristically results in low-viscosity synovial fluid. The string sign is a simple test for assessing viscosity. The practitioner measures the length of the "string" formed by a falling drop of synovial fluid extruded from a syringe or stretched between the thumb and the index finger of a gloved hand. Normal joint fluid produces a string 5 to 10 cm long (Fig. 53-15). If viscosity is reduced, as with inflammatory conditions, synovial fluid forms a shorter string or falls in drops.

Mucin Clot Test

The mucin clot test also corresponds to viscosity and inflammation. The greater the inflammatory response, the poorer the mucin clot and the lower the viscosity. This test may be useful to define the degree of polymerization of hyaluronate. Mucin clots are produced by mixing one part joint fluid with four parts 2% acetic acid. A good clot indicates a high degree of polymerization and correlates with normal high viscosity. In inflammatory synovial fluid, such as that seen with

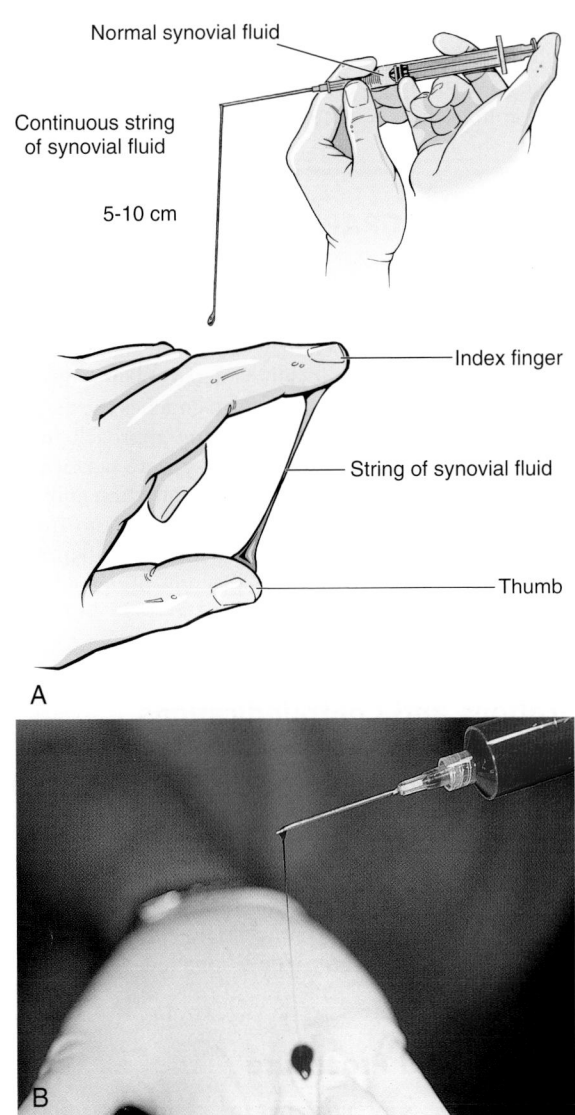

Normal synovial fluid

Continuous string of synovial fluid

5-10 cm

Index finger

String of synovial fluid

Thumb

A

B

Figure 53-15 A, Ability of normal synovial fluid to form a long tenacious string. Inflammatory fluid will not produce this finding. **B,** Bloody joint fluid from recent trauma forms a normal string sign.

osteoarthritis- and rheumatoid arthritis–related effusions, the mucin clot is poor. This test is rarely performed.

Cell Count

A leukocytosis consisting predominantly of neutrophils is usually seen with inflammatory arthritides; a WBC count greater than 50,000/mm³ (i.e., >50,000/μL) is highly suggestive of a septic joint. Shmerling and colleagues[38] found a WBC count of greater than 2000/mm³ to be 84% sensitive and 84% specific for *all* inflammatory arthritides. Of their septic arthritis patients, 37% had a synovial WBC count lower than 50,000/mm³. However, 89% of their patients with a synovial WBC count greater than 50,000/mm³ had a septic joint.[38]

Glucose and Protein

Current literature suggests that synovial protein and glucose are highly inaccurate markers of inflammation.[2,28] In one study of 100 consecutive patients undergoing diagnostic arthrocentesis, the sensitivity of synovial protein and glucose was found to be 0.52 and 0.20, respectively.[36] The authors of this study recommended that ordering chemistry studies on synovial fluid should be discouraged because such studies are likely to provide misleading or redundant information.

Serology

Though available, most serologic tests are not likely to be useful in the emergency setting. Polymerase chain reaction (PCR) is an effective means of identifying septic arthritis, even in the setting of a negative fluid culture or when antibiotics have been administered previously. PCR can also help isolate slowly growing microorganisms. Gas-liquid chromatography, a rapid and sensitive method for detection of short-chain fatty acids, may complement the currently available methods used to diagnose septic arthritis.[39]

Counterimmunoelectrophoresis and latex agglutination are also useful and available in some centers on an emergency basis. Other immunologic markers such as complement, rheumatoid factor, and antinuclear antibodies have little diagnostic value in the acute setting but may be useful to the clinician providing follow-up care when compared with serum levels.

Fluid Processing

Proper collection of joint fluid is essential for examination and testing. Tests for viscosity, serology, and chemistries are done on fluid collected in a red-topped (clot) tube, whereas cytology samples are collected in tubes with an anticoagulant (purple top). One should always transfer the fluid for crystal examination into a tube with liquid heparin (green top) because undissolved heparin crystals from powdered anticoagulant tubes can be seen on microscopy. Early transfer of synovial fluid to this green-topped tube is essential to prevent clotting. Culture requirements for transport and processing should be accessed before the procedure to ensure appropriate processing or plating of specimens.

Polarizing Microscope

No synovial fluid analysis is complete until the fluid has been examined under a polarizing light microscope for crystals. The polarizing microscope used for crystal identification differs from the ordinary light microscope in that it contains two identical polarizing prisms or filters. One filter, called the *polarizer*, is positioned below the condenser. The other filter is called the *analyzer* and is inserted at some point above the objective. Examination for crystals is performed by most hospital laboratories.

Polarization Physics

The polarizer allows passage of light in only one specific orientation. The analyzer acts as a crossed filter by removing all light in the light path unless the material being examined rotates the beam from the polarizer into the plane of the analyzer. The compensator functions by imparting color of a certain wavelength (red at about 550 nm). Birefringent materials change the wavelength to blue or yellow, depending on the direction (negative or positive) of refringence.

Microscopic Analysis

When examining crystals under polarized microscopy, the technician orients crystals on a stage according to two axes, referred to as x and z. If the long axis of the crystals is blue when parallel to the z-axis and yellow when perpendicular to it, it is calcium pyrophosphate and termed *positively birefringent*. If the long axis of the crystal is yellow when parallel to the z-axis and blue when perpendicular to it, it is monosodium urate and termed *negatively birefringent*. Urate crystals are 2 to 10 μm and usually needle shaped (Fig. 53-16). Calcium pyrophosphate crystals range from 10 μm down to tiny crystals that have to be examined with the oil objective; they appear as rods, rhomboids, plates, or needle-like forms and are weakly birefringent (Fig. 53-17). Cholesterol crystals are sometimes seen and are large, very bright square or rectangular plates with broken corners.[40,41]

Items found in synovial fluid that can be confused with sodium urate or calcium pyrophosphate crystals include collagen fibrils, cartilage fragments, cholesterol crystals, metallic fragments from prosthetic arthroplasty, and corticosteroid esters.[40] One may also identify fat globules (Fig. 53-18). Note that rare cases of uric acid spherulites in gouty synovia have been reported.[40] The spherulites are birefringent and do not take up fat stains.

Table 53-2 summarizes synovial fluid features for the joint diseases commonly encountered and studies commonly performed in the ED.

JOINT ARTHROGRAPHY

Background

Wounds near joints raise concern regarding joint penetration. Treatment and interventions may be altered significantly if a joint space has been traumatically violated. Plain radiographs may demonstrate air in the joint, which clinches the diagnosis, but in questionable cases the diagnostic approach includes injection arthrograms. Historically, these were performed by injecting methylene blue into the joint in question and assessing leakage from the joint. However, the dye can interfere with arthroscopic evaluation and produce an inflammatory reaction, so saline arthrography (SA) is now preferred. SA, or a "saline load test," was first described in 1975 but became more popular in the 1990s.[42,43]

Indications and Contraindications

SA should be performed in patients with penetrating injuries near a joint in which violation of the joint itself is unclear (Fig. 53-19). Smaller joints such as those in the hand are inspected visually. However, for larger joints, SA is the preferred test.

Contraindications to performing SA are essentially the same as for performing arthrocentesis. When indicated, underlying fracture of the joint should first be ruled out. An obvious open fracture would preclude the need to perform SA.

Equipment and Procedure

Aseptic technique is essential, but the equipment and procedure are essentially the same as for performing arthrocentesis, with minor differences. First, a source of sterile saline is required (e.g., a small bag of intravenous fluid). Second, larger joints require more saline infusion, and this is most easily performed if a stopcock is used to allow refill of the syringe (Fig. 53-20).

Because saline is not as viscous as joint fluid, a 20-gauge needle is sufficient. Once the joint space has been reliably entered, a variable amount of saline to "load" that joint is slowly injected. The amount of saline injected varies with the size of the joint. In general, *a sufficient volume should be injected to visibly distend the joint or create resistance to injection and cause the patient discomfort.* The sensitivity of the test in detecting small traumatic joint injuries is proportional to the volume injected. Specifically, for knee injuries, injecting 50 mL of saline was 46% sensitive and injecting 100 mL, 75% sensitive; to achieve 95% sensitivity required an average of 194 mL of saline.[43] The following is the recommended volume of injection per joint:

- Knee—100 to 200 mL
- Elbow—20 to 30 mL
- Ankle—20 to 30 mL
- Wrist—5 mL
- Shoulder—40 to 60 mL

Figure 53-16 Monosodium urate (MSU) crystals under a polarizing light microscope. MSU crystals are positively birefringent and usually needle shaped. *(From Hochberg MC, Silman AJ, Smolen JS, eds. Rheumatology. 5th ed. St Louis: Elsevier; 2011.)*

Figure 53-17 Calcium pyrophosphate dihydrate (CPPD) crystals under a polarizing light microscope. CPPD crystals are negatively birefringent and rhomboid shaped. *(From Hochberg MC, Silman AJ, Smolen JS, eds. Rheumatology. 5th ed. St Louis: Elsevier; 2011.)*

Figure 53-18 A, Blood aspirated from a traumatized joint is placed in an emesis basin and put under a bright light to search for lipohemarthrosis, which is clinical evidence of an intraarticular fracture. Note the characteristic greasy sheen of floating fat. Do not throw away this blood before assessing for lipohemarthrosis. **B,** A fibular head fracture (*arrow*) was initially thought to be responsible for a large knee hemarthrosis, but anatomically it is extraarticular. A tibial plateau fracture is not appreciated on this radiograph. Such injuries are often occult. **C,** On this view one might appreciate the radiolucent lines suggestive of a lateral tibial plateau fracture (*arrows*), but such subtle findings are easily missed, as was the case with this patient. Therapeutic arthrocentesis was performed to alleviate pain, and an obvious lipohemarthrosis was noted. **D,** Magnetic resonance imaging demonstrates an obvious lateral tibial plateau fracture (*arrows*), which was searched for only after lipohemarthrosis was noted. Computed tomography could also be used.

TABLE 53-2 Characteristics of Synovial Fluid

	APPEARANCE	VISCOSITY	CELLS PER mm³	PMN (%)	CRYSTALS
Normal	Transparent	High	<180	<10	Negative
Osteoarthritis	Transparent	High	200-2000	<10	Occasional calcium pyrophosphate and hydroxyapatite crystals
Rheumatoid arthritis	Translucent	Low	2000-50,000	Variable	Negative
Psoriatic arthritis	Translucent	Low	2000-50,000	Variable	Negative
Reactive arthritis	Translucent	Low	2000-50,000	Variable	Negative
Spondyloarthropathy	Translucent	Low	2000-50,000	Variable	Negative
Gout	Translucent to cloudy	Low	200 to >50,000	>90	Needle-shaped, positive birefringent monosodium urate monohydrate crystals
Pseudogout	Translucent to cloudy	Low	200-50,000	>90	Rhomboid, negative birefringent calcium pyrophosphate crystals
Bacterial arthritis	Cloudy	Variable	2000 to >50,000	>90	Negative
PVNS	Hemorrhagic or brown	Low			Negative
Hemarthrosis	Hemorrhagic	Low			Negative

Adapted from Harris ED, Budd RC, Genovese MC, et al, eds. *Kelley's Textbook of Rheumatology.* 7th ed. Philadelphia: Elsevier; 2005.
PMN, polymorphic nuclear cell; *PVNS,* pigmented villonodular synovitis.

Figure 53-19 This periarticular laceration raises the question of knee joint penetration. A plain radiograph may demonstrate air in the joint space, but a saline arthrogram may also be used. Methylene blue alone is not generally required and it can cause an inflammatory reaction and obscure arthroscopy. A small amount of methylene blue may be added to color the saline.

Figure 53-20 Saline arthrography. Using a stopcock and an 18-gauge needle, enter the joint in a manner identical to that for arthrocentesis. Note that a bag of intravenous saline (or additional vials of saline) introduced into the syringe may be required to provide enough saline to distend the joint properly. Unless the joint is markedly distended, a false-negative test may result. When completed, drain the injected saline via the original needle. A positive test is egress of saline into the original wound or slow loss of saline from the joint. A small amount of methylene blue may be added to the saline.

Once the injection is complete, do not remove the needle but close the stopcock to avoid backflow. Examine the joint for evidence of leakage of fluid from the wound. This is performed in a static position but, if negative, also with some gentle passive movement of the joint. Visible leakage of fluid into the laceration confirms the diagnosis of joint space violation. A negative test is defined as absence of evidence of leakage after an appropriate amount of saline has been injected. A slow loss of fluid may indicate a small insult to the joint, and saline can be left in the joint for a few minutes to observe for this. After completion, the fluid should be evacuated for patient comfort. This is generally performed by leaving the original needle in place with a closed stopcock attached, which is then used to aspirate the saline in the joint.

Complications

Complications associated with performing SA are essentially the same as those for performing arthrocentesis. In addition, some temporary patient discomfort because of joint distention should be assumed.

Conclusion

Small traumatic joint penetration can be difficult to diagnose clinically. SA can help confirm the diagnosis. To be a sensitive test, it must be performed with an adequate amount of saline infusion to truly "load" the joint. If the test is positive, orthopedic consultation is indicated.

Acknowledgment

The editors would like to thank Drs. Steven J. Parrillo, Daniel S. Morrison, and Edward A. Panacek for their work in the previous edition.

References are available at www.expertconsult.com

CHAPTER 54

Compartment Syndrome Evaluation

Merle A. Carter

Open fractures, dislocations, and exposed joints are true orthopedic emergencies that must be managed aggressively to prevent morbidity and mortality. Even when managed appropriately, these injuries may be further complicated by compartment syndrome, a condition of increased pressure within a limited space that results in compromised tissue perfusion and, ultimately, dysfunction of the neural and muscular structures contained within that space.[1] The magnitude of the trauma is usually significant, but compartment syndrome may also develop after seemingly minor injuries, prolonged proximal arterial occlusion, or prolonged external pressure in the absence of acute injury or fracture. In addition, compartment syndrome can develop without direct trauma, such as from muscular exertion, from the toxic effects of drugs, and following intramuscular hemorrhage in those with a bleeding diathesis.

Causes of compartment syndrome are categorized into those that decrease compartment volume capacity, those that increase the contents of a compartment, and those that create externally applied pressure (Box 54-1).[1] Subtleties in the early signs and symptoms of compartment syndrome or other clinical priorities render some cases *simply impossible to recognize and treat early enough to thwart the ultimate disability*. About 10% of cases of acute compartment syndrome secondary to fractures will have muscle necrosis requiring débridement at the time of surgery. About 20% of cases of compartment syndrome in non–fracture-associated cases will have muscular necrosis at the time of surgery, thus indicating that even with diligent clinical care, it is not standard to identify all cases before injury to muscles occurs,[2] particularly in uncooperative, unconscious, or critically injured patients who are unable to report symptoms. Unfortunately, the vagaries of the clinical scenario that result in failure to recognize the early signs and symptoms of compartment syndrome may have severe and irreversible limb- or life-threatening consequences.

Numerous drugs and toxins have been reported to cause rhabdomyolysis, possibly because of a direct effect or secondary to agitation and exertion, with the *theoretical potential* for the development of compartment syndrome (Fig. 54-1). This list is exhaustive but includes heroin, various hydrocarbons, cocaine, amphetamines, antidepressants, antipsychotics, salicylates, propoxyphene, nonsteroidal antiinflammatory drugs, succinylcholine, human immunodeficiency virus medications, antimetabolites and cancer drugs, antimalarials, diphenhydramine, baclofen, ecstasy, ethanol, anticoagulants and thrombolytics, strychnine, statins, and phenothiazines.[3]

Although compartment syndrome is essentially a clinical diagnosis, objective measurement of compartment tissue pressure may assist in confirming the diagnosis and determining if operative management is required. This chapter discusses the indications, complications, and interpretation of compartment pressure monitoring, as well as the equipment and techniques required to monitor compartment pressure.

Compartment Syndrome Evaluation

Indications

Suspected compartment syndrome with clinical findings that are equivocal or difficult to interpret:
- Unresponsive patients
- Uncooperative patients
- Children
- Patients with multiple or distracting injuries
- Patients with peripheral nerve deficits attributable to other causes (fracture-associated nerve injury, diabetic peripheral neuropathy

Contraindications

Absolute
  None
Relative
  Coagulation disorders
  Overlying infection, cellulitis, or burns

Complications

Pain from needle insertion, fluid injection, or bleeding
Inaccurate readings due to poor technique, improper needle position, injected fluid or anesthetic, or external compression
Injury to underlying tissue, nerves, or blood vessels
Local or systemic infection

Equipment

Stryker pressure monitor

3-mL syringe prefilled with saline

Side-port 18-gauge needle

Diaphragm chamber

Equipment shown is for the Stryker method. The side-port needle, prefilled syringe, and diaphragm chamber are packaged together in the Stryker 295-2 Quick Pressure Monitor Set *(Stryker, Kalamazoo, MI)*.

Review Box 54-1 Compartment syndrome evaluation: indications, contraindications, complications, and equipment.

BOX 54-1 Causes of Compartment Syndrome

DECREASED COMPARTMENTAL VOLUME
Closure of fascial defects
Application of excessive traction to fractured limbs
Compressive devices (casts, splints, circumferential dressings)

INCREASED COMPARTMENTAL CONTENTS
Bleeding
Major vascular injury
Coagulation disorders
    Bleeding disorder
    Anticoagulation therapy
    Thrombolytic therapy
After placement of an arterial line

INCREASED CAPILLARY FILTRATION
Reperfusion after ischemia
    Arterial bypass grafting
    Embolectomy
    Ergotamine ingestion
    Cardiac catheterization
    Lying on the limb
Trauma
    Fracture
    Contusion
Intensive use of muscles
    Exercise or severe exertion
    Seizures
    Eclampsia
    Tetany
Burns
    Thermal
    Electric

Intraarterial drug injection
Cold
Orthopedic surgery
    Tibial osteotomy
    Hauser's procedure
    Reduction and internal fixation of fractures
Snakebite

INCREASED CAPILLARY PRESSURE
Intensive use of muscles
Venous obstruction
    Phlegmasia cerulea dolens
    Ill-fitting leg brace
    Venous ligation

DIMINISHED SERUM OSMOLARITY, NEPHROTIC SYNDROME

OTHER CAUSES OF INCREASED COMPARTMENTAL CONTENTS
Infiltrated infusion
Pressure transfusion
Leaky dialysis cannula
Muscle hypertrophy
Popliteal cyst
Carbon monoxide poisoning

EXTERNALLY APPLIED PRESSURE
Tight casts, dressings, or air splints
Lying on the limb
Pneumatic antishock garment
Congenital bands

Modified from Matsen FA. Compartmental Syndromes. *New York: Grune & Stratton, 1980.*

BACKGROUND

Though recognized as a clinical syndrome in the mid-19th century, the pathophysiology of ischemia in extremities was not fully described until more than a century later. Postischemic myoneural dysfunction and its associated contractures were first described in the 1870s by the German surgeon Richard von Volkmann, who recognized the effects of increased pressure causing vascular compromise of the limb.[4]

Various needles and equipment have been developed to measure compartment pressure (Fig. 54-2).[5-11] The wick catheter, originally developed to measure subcutaneous and brain tissue pressure, was modified during the mid-1970s to provide continuous compartment pressure measurements. This catheter is rarely used today because of the fear of catheter breakdown leading to errors in measurement and retained foreign bodies. This prompted development of the slit catheter in 1980.[10,11] This catheter has slits at its distal end that prevent the catheter from clogging. The proximal end of the catheter is connected to a transducer and infusion system, which permits continuous monitoring. Both the wick and slit catheters have been shown to offer similar accuracy and reproducibility as long as patency of the catheter is ensured.[11-13] A newer approach to predicting the onset of compartment syndrome involves measuring compartment pH as a marker of compromised circulation and decreased tissue perfusion.[14] A rise in lactic acid from ischemic tissue lowers the pH of the compartment and has promise as an early predictor of compartment syndrome.

The Stryker Intracompartmental Compartment Pressure Monitoring System (Kalamazoo, MI) has become the most commonly used commercially available device to measure compartment pressure in the emergency department (see Review Box 54-1). This device uses a fluid-filled pressure measurement catheter, a pressure monitor, and a fluid infusion mechanism that maintains catheter patency and ensures accurate measurement. In contrast to earlier devices in which relatively large volumes of fluid were injected into the compartment to measure pressure, the Stryker system uses a minimal amount of saline (<0.3 mL). This helps ensure accurate measurements while reducing the chance of further increases in compartment pressure. The Stryker system also has the ability to record a single measurement or provide continuous compartment pressure recordings when required.

Noninfusion systems such as the transducer-tipped fiberoptic system offer a distinct advantage over conventional

Figure 54-1 The diagnosis of compartment syndrome is not always straightforward. **A,** This man was initially seen while in a coma from a heroin overdose and had been lying on his arm for a number of hours. He was hypotensive, in renal failure, comatose, and on a ventilator. The entire arm was swollen and rhabdomyolysis was correctly suspected. **B,** Clear urine, a strongly positive dipstick for blood (*arrow*), and no red blood cells by microscopy equate to myoglobinuria. Because of the coma, he was unable to voice any complaint of pain. **C,** When he awakened 20 hours later, the pain was severe, and compartment pressures indicated the need for fasciotomy. Heroin can cause rhabdomyolysis, and hypotension/reperfusion and certainly prolonged pressure on the muscles may have exacerbated the condition. **D,** The classic wringer washer injury predisposes to compartment syndrome, but industrial rollers are now usually the culprit.

Transducer tips

Figure 54-2 **A,** An 18-gauge straight needle. **B,** An 18-gauge side-port needle. **C,** A slit catheter. (*A–C, from Boody AR, Wongworawat MD. Accuracy in the measurement of compartment pressures: a comparison of three commonly used devices.* J Bone Joint Surg Am. *2005;87:2415.*)

fluid-filled systems in that they do not produce hydrostatic pressure artifacts or require the injection of fluid for long-term or continuous measurements. However, the fiberoptic transducer is relatively large, must be attached to a sheath approximately 2.0 mm in diameter, and is likely to cause pain during measurements.[15] In recent years, noninvasive, less painful methods of measuring compartment pressure have been studied in patients with both acute and chronic exertional compartment syndrome. Investigations using magnetic resonance imaging (MRI), single-photon emission computed tomography (SPECT), myotonometry, electromyography, ultrasound, near-infrared spectroscopy, and microwave tomography have provided encouraging results in the evaluation of compartment syndrome.[16-33] In addition, externally applied devices that measure muscle tissue "hardness" are under investigation as an economic alternative to these modalities, although support of their use has been mixed.[34-36]

Though promising, these evolving noninvasive methods have not yet replaced needle-driven techniques as the standard for measuring intracompartmental pressure. The remainder of this chapter describes the most commonly used devices and techniques for measuring compartment pressure in the acute setting. Each method provides rapid measurements with reasonable accuracy. The method chosen will depend on the availability of the supplies and equipment necessary for a particular procedure and the experience of the operator.

PATHOPHYSIOLOGY

Several theories have been proposed to account for the tissue ischemia associated with compartment syndrome, including the "arteriovenous (AV) gradient" theory, which suggests that reduced AV pressure-perfusion gradients prevent adequate blood supply[37]; the "critical closure" theory, in which blood flow is arrested well before the AV perfusion gradient declines to zero[38,39]; and the "venous occlusion" theory,[40] which states that externally applied pressure, thrombotic events, and reperfusion contribute to the increased compartment pressure and, ultimately, tissue ischemia. Although the exact mechanism has not been agreed on, inherent in each of these theories is a decrease in blood flow to levels below those required to meet the metabolic demands of the tissue. Hence, the final common pathway is cellular hypoxia and muscle necrosis.

Adequate blood flow to tissues is a function of AV gradients across capillary beds. Once blood flow falls below a critical level, delivery of oxygen to these structures is impaired and aerobic cellular metabolism is no longer possible. Anaerobic metabolism then ensues until energy stores become depleted. Muscles become ischemic, and a reduction in venous and lymphatic drainage creates increased pressure within this confined space. It is important to note that ischemia and necrosis of the musculature can occur despite an arterial pressure *high enough to produce pulses*, so merely assessing distal pulses is insufficient.[41]

A drop in blood pressure, an increase in compartment pressure, or a combination of the two can reduce AV gradients and lead to insufficient blood flow to tissues. Hypotension can occur in a variety of settings, including hypovolemia, acute blood loss, cardiac disease states (e.g., ischemia), and sepsis. An increase in the contents of a compartment, a decrease in its volume capacity, and external constriction of a compartment can all lead to increases in compartment pressure. Thus, the relationship between intracompartmental pressure and the circulatory status of the extremity is an important factor in the development of compartment syndrome.[42] Compartment syndrome may also develop in an extremity in the absence of direct trauma. This is most often due to prolonged ischemia associated with acute arterial occlusion by thrombi or proximal arterial injury.

At rest, normal adult compartment pressure is typically below 10 mm Hg. However, deviations of 2 to 6 mm Hg have been reported.[1,8-10,12] Recent data suggest that normal compartment pressures in the lower extremity at rest are higher in children.[43] The *perfusion pressure* of a compartment, also known as the compartment *delta pressure* (ΔP), is defined as the difference between diastolic blood pressure and intracompartmental pressure.[44] A model using legs of normal volunteers has shown that a progression of neuromuscular deficits occurs when intracompartmental pressure rises to within 35 to 40 mm Hg of diastolic blood pressure.[45] Above this level, tissue perfusion is interrupted. Studies of neuromuscular tissue ischemia have demonstrated that inflammatory necrosis can occur at pressures between 40 and 60 mm Hg.[46,47]

Whitesides and colleagues demonstrated that when tissue pressure within a closed compartment rises to within 10 to 30 mm Hg of the patient's diastolic blood pressure, inadequate perfusion ensues and results in relative ischemia of the involved limb.[6] Heppenstall and associates further clarified this relationship by demonstrating that the difference (ΔP) between mean arterial pressure (MAP) and the measured compartment pressure is directly related to blood flow to the tissue.[48] They noted that as compartment pressure approaches MAP, ΔP decreases. Once ΔP falls below 30 mm Hg, tissue ischemia becomes more likely. In normal musculature, a ΔP of less than 30 mm Hg results in loss of normal aerobic cellular metabolism.[48] In traumatized muscle, a ΔP of less than 40 mm Hg is associated with abnormal cellular function, thus highlighting the importance of maintaining adequate systemic blood pressure in the setting of neuromuscular injury.[48]

For years, conventional wisdom maintained that immediate reperfusion of traumatized tissue would provide improved motor and neurologic function after injury. In the last decade, research suggests that muscle tissue may remain viable even after prolonged periods of ischemia and that a substantial proportion of the injury is generated on reperfusion.[49,50] Tissue acidosis, intracellular and extracellular edema, free radical–mediated injury, loss of adenine nucleotide precursors, and interruption of mitochondrial oxidative rephosphorylation by increased intracellular calcium have been implicated in the development of reperfusion-associated compartment syndrome.[49-54] A recent study has identified the potential role of *N*-acetylcysteine in the attenuation of tissue injury in compartment syndrome.[55] Even in the absence of local trauma, ischemia followed by reperfusion has been shown to increase compartment pressure in canine models of hypovolemic shock.[56]

Evidence also suggests that elevated compartment pressure itself (in addition to causing ischemia) plays a role in the cellular deterioration seen with compartment syndrome.[57] In a study by Heppenstall and associates,[57] muscle ischemia caused by placement of a tourniquet was compared with an experimentally derived high-pressure compartment syndrome. The authors found no difference in the degree to which phosphocreatine levels fell between groups. However, levels of adenosine triphosphate (ATP) diminished rapidly in the compartment syndrome group in comparison to the tourniquet group. Moreover, phosphocreatine levels, ATP, and tissue pH normalized within 15 minutes of releasing the tourniquet. In the group with compartment syndrome, these levels remained low even after fasciotomy. These results suggest that elevated tissue pressure plays a synergistic role with ischemia in cellular deterioration.

CLINICAL FEATURES

Any compartment limited by fascial planes is potentially at risk for compartment syndrome. However, because of their propensity for injury and the presence of several low-volume compartments, the lower extremities are most commonly affected. In the leg, the anterior compartment is involved most often,[58] whereas the posterior compartment is a site frequently missed. The hands, feet, forearms, upper part of the arms, thighs, abdomen, gluteal musculature, and back are other locations where compartment syndrome is known to occur.[1] Increased compartment pressure may be caused by a variety of conditions (see Box 54-1). Risk factors for the development of compartment syndrome include recent trauma to an extremity (including acupuncture, venipuncture, intravenous infusions, or intravenous drug use), bleeding within a compartment, a restrictive cast or splint, a crush or compression injury, a prolonged lithotomy position, placement of a tourniquet during an operative procedure, and circumferential burns.[59-63]

Long-bone fractures account for about 75% of traumatic compartment syndromes, and the absence of a fracture in a traumatized extremity is a factor in delayed diagnosis. The tibia is most often involved, followed by bones of the forearm. Supracondylar fractures in children are at risk for compartment syndrome. Comminuted fractures increase the risk. Closed fractures are of greatest concern, but an open fracture does not necessarily decompress elevated compartment pressure. Treatment of fractures, by both open and closed reduction, can increase compartment pressure. Compartment pressure may peak *immediately after reduction*. In addition, some evidence suggests that compartment syndrome may occur in the setting of chronic exertion and muscle overuse.[64,65] Although the exact etiology remains elusive, studies have demonstrated elevated lactate and water levels in the tibialis anterior muscle after exercise with a reduction in these levels after fasciotomy.[66,67] Increases in muscle mass (related to a rise in blood volume during exertion) and hypertrophy of muscle and fascia with chronic use and exertion have also been reported.[68-72]

Clinical hallmarks of compartment syndrome include *pallor* of the extremity, a *pulse deficit* with respect to the opposite limb, *paresis or paralysis* of the involved extremity, *paresthesias* in the distribution of the involved nerves, and *pain on passive stretch* of the involved musculature (the "5 P's" of compartment syndrome). Paresthesias are secondary to ischemic nerve dysfunction. These signs and symptoms may be unreliable in pediatric populations.[73,74] In addition, though commonly seen, pain and paralysis are late findings. Early, more subtle signs of compartment syndrome include a burning sensation over the involved compartment, nonspecific sensory deficits, or poorly localized deep muscular pain. *Pain that seems out of proportion to the apparent injury and clinical examination* and pain that intensifies when the musculature is passively stretched are common features.

The period between the injury and the onset of symptoms can be as short as 2 hours and as long as 6 days.[75] The peak interval appears to be 15 to 30 hours. Frequently, the first symptom described by patients is pain greater than expected given the clinical scenario. Although pain out of proportion to the visible injury may raise the question of drug-seeking behavior, a focused evaluation for the possibility of limb-threatening disorders must precede this diagnosis of exclusion. Physical examination may reveal muscles that are weak and tense with hypoesthesia in the distribution of the involved nerves. Sensory deficits, including loss of two-point discrimination and decreased vibratory sensation, are frequently present.[76-78] The presence or absence of a palpable arterial pulse is not an accurate indicator of relative tissue pressure or the risk for compartment syndrome. Pulses may be present in a severely compromised extremity.[79] Table 54-1 lists the signs and symptoms of compartment syndrome specific to each compartment.

DIAGNOSIS

Even experienced clinicians find it difficult to evaluate a potential compartment syndrome, and no specific standard of care exists with regard to a time interval from injury to definitive treatment. In an unconscious patient or in those with other life-threatening conditions that mandate other priorities, the clinical scenario simply does not allow a diagnosis to be made in timely fashion. In cases without trauma or in patients who are unable to voice pain or cooperate with an examination, compartment syndrome is often not considered and the diagnosis is delayed. Regional nerve blocks or epidural anesthesia may also obscure the signs and symptoms of increased compartment pressure and cause further delays in diagnosis.

The difficulty in diagnosing acute compartment syndrome was highlighted in a report by Vaillancourt and coworkers.[80]

TABLE 54-1   Compartment Syndromes and Associated Physical Signs

COMPARTMENT	SENSORY LOSS	MUSCLES WEAKENED	PAINFUL PASSIVE MOTION	LOCATION OF TENSENESS
Foot	Digital nerves	Foot intrinsics	Toe flexion, extension	Dorsal or plantar surface of the foot
Lumbar	—	Erector spinae	Lumbar flexion	Paraspinous
Forearm				
Dorsal	—	Digital extensors	Digital flexion	Dorsal surface of the forearm
Volar	Ulnar, median nerves	Digital flexors	Digital extension	Volar surface of the forearm
Hand				
Interosseus	—	Interosseus	Abduction/adduction (metacarpophalangeal joints)	Dorsum of the hand between the metacarpals
Leg				
Anterior	Deep peroneal nerve	Toe extensors Tibialis anterior	Toe flexion	Anterior aspect of the leg
Superficial posterior	—	Soleus and gastrocnemius	Foot dorsiflexion	Calf
Deep posterior	Posterior tibial nerve	Toe flexors Tibialis posterior	Toe extension	Distal medial part of the leg between the Achilles tendon and tibia
Gluteal	(Rarely sciatic)	Gluteals, piriformis, or tensor fasciae latae	Hip flexion	Buttock
Upper Part of Arm				
Flexor	Ulnar and median nerves	Biceps and distal flexors	Elbow extension	Anterior aspect of the upper part of the arm
Extensor	Radial nerves	Triceps and forearm extensors	Elbow flexion	Posterior aspect of the upper part of the arm

In a retrospective review of 76 patients who underwent fasciotomy at major university trauma centers or teaching hospitals, the interval from initial patient assessment to diagnosis of compartment syndrome was up to 8 hours. Delay in diagnosis was most common in nontraumatic cases. The interval from the precipitating event to definitive surgery was up to 35 hours, thus reflecting the difficulty in suspecting this diagnosis and instituting definitive therapy in clinical practice. Such statistics describe actual care, which may be less than ideal when compared with theoretical benchmarks.

Notwithstanding the difficulty just described, the diagnosis of compartment syndrome is primarily a clinical one that may be supplemented by direct measurement of compartment pressure. In a study evaluating the utility of clinical findings in making the diagnosis of compartment syndrome, Ulmer noted that the sensitivity and positive predictive value of clinical findings are low whereas the specificity and negative predictive value of these findings are high.[81] Nevertheless, the study found that although the sensitivity of an individual clinical finding may be low, the probability of compartment syndrome rises considerably when more than one clinical hallmark is present.[81] However, other studies have suggested that the absence of clinical evidence is more useful in excluding compartment syndrome than its presence is in confirming the diagnosis.[82-84] All things considered, compartment syndrome remains largely a clinical diagnosis, and a high index of suspicion is paramount.

The differential diagnosis of compartment syndrome is extensive and includes primary vascular, nerve, and muscle injuries that produce similar findings. Acute arterial occlusion, cellulitis, osteomyelitis, neurapraxia, reflex sympathetic dystrophy, synovitis, tenosynovitis, stress fractures, envenomations, necrotizing fasciitis, deep vein thrombosis, and thrombophlebitis are additional diseases that should be considered. Differentiating compartment syndrome from these and other orthopedic disorders requires a detailed history and thorough physical examination, often supplemented by measurement of compartment pressure (Table 54-2).

ANCILLARY STUDIES

In general, laboratory and radiographic studies are not helpful in confirming the diagnosis of compartment syndrome.

TABLE 54-2   Clinical Findings in Patients with Compartment Syndrome, Arterial Occlusion, and Neurapraxia

	COMPARTMENTAL SYNDROME	ARTERIAL OCCLUSION	NEUROPRAXIA
Pressure increased in the compartment	+	−	−
Pain with stretch	+	+	−
Paresthesia or anesthesia	+	+	+
Paresis or paralysis	+	+	+
Pulses intact	+	−	+

From Mubarak S, Carroll N. Volkman's contracture in children: etiology and prevention. *J Bone Joint Surg Br.* 1979;61:290.

BOX 54-2   **Ancillary Studies That May Be Helpful in Identifying Other Diagnoses, Associated Conditions, and Complications in Patients Suspected of Having Compartment Syndrome**

LABORATORY STUDIES

- Complete metabolic profile (including electrolytes and renal function testing)
- Complete blood count with differential
- Serum and urine myoglobin
- Creatine phosphokinase
- Urinalysis to evaluate for concurrent rhabdomyolysis
- Coagulation studies

IMAGING STUDIES

- Radiography of the affected limb to evaluate for a fracture or foreign body
- Ultrasonography to rule out deep vein thrombosis or Doppler ultrasonography to evaluate blood flow to the extremity

However, they might be useful in identifying other diagnoses, associated conditions, and complications. Box 54-2 lists useful studies for patients in whom compartment syndrome is suspected.

INVASIVE COMPARTMENT PRESSURE MONITORING

Indications and Contraindications

The earliest objective manifestation of acute compartment syndrome is an elevation in the tissue pressure of one or more compartments. However, signs and symptoms do not generally develop until tissue pressure has reached a critical level (see "Pathophysiology"). In some patients the diagnosis of compartment syndrome is clinically obvious, and one can proceed directly to fasciotomy. When the clinical findings are equivocal or difficult to interpret, measurement of tissue pressure may help guide treatment (Fig. 54-3). However, even though pressure measurements may suggest the presence of compartment syndrome, *the interpretation of such measurements always requires clinical judgment.*

There are several groups of patients in whom clinical findings are difficult to obtain or interpret and who would benefit from measurement of compartment pressure. These groups include unresponsive patients, uncooperative patients, children, patients with multiple or distracting injuries, those with peripheral nerve deficits attributable to other causes (e.g., fracture-associated nerve injury, diabetic peripheral neuropathy), and those whose clinical findings are equivocal.

There are no absolute contraindications to measuring or continuous monitoring of compartment pressure. Caution should be taken when performing these procedures on patients with platelet dysfunction or other coagulation disorders. If possible, avoid inserting needles through overlying areas of infection, cellulitis, or burns.

Patient Preparation and Positioning

Explain the procedure to the patient or surrogate. Written informed consent is not a universal standard. Positioning of the patient and extremity for measurement of compartment pressure depends on the extremity and the compartment being studied, coexisting injuries, and the clinical status of the patient. In general, patients should be in the supine position.[85-87] The exceptions to supine positioning are discussed in subsequent sections related to the extremity of interest.

For most patients, measurement of compartment pressure is a painful procedure that requires adequate local anesthesia (see Chapter 29), systemic analgesia, or procedural sedation (see Chapter 33). Anesthetize the skin with a small amount of local anesthetic while avoiding the underlying muscle and fascia. Inadvertent injection into the underlying structures may falsely elevate compartment pressure. Patient movement (as a result of inadequate analgesia or improper positioning) may also falsely elevate compartment pressure, particularly if the patient requires limb restraint. To minimize the discomfort of multiple attempts at localizing the correct compartment, some have advocated the use of ultrasound guidance to improve the accuracy of needle insertion.[88] However, there is currently no consensus regarding the use of ultrasound guidance in this setting.[89-90]

Place the extremity being studied at the level of the heart and in a position that permits insertion of the needle perpendicular to the compartment being measured. This may require

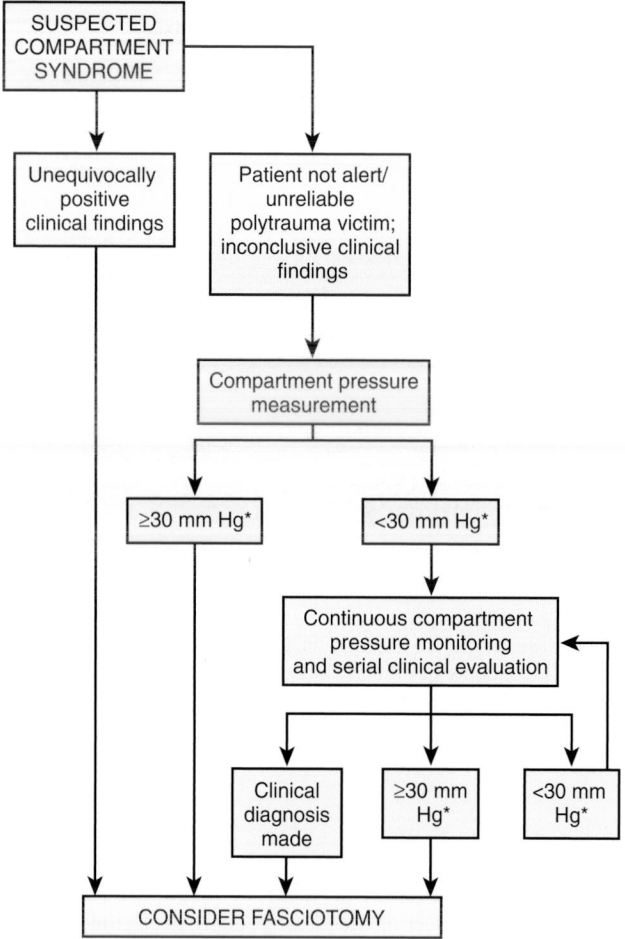

Figure 54-3 Algorithm for the management of a patient with suspected compartment syndrome. Pressure thresholds (*asterisks*) are based on published case series. Compartment pressures alone can be misleading, are not pathognomonic, and do not always mandate fasciotomy. Clinical correlation is paramount for proper interpretation of compartment pressure measurements. Normal tissue compartment pressure is between 0 and 18 mm Hg. Pain usually develops when tissue pressure reaches 20 to 30 mm Hg. Relying solely on a single measured compartment pressure may result in unnecessary fasciotomy. Trends in pressure are more indicative of the need for fasciotomy. Higher compartment pressure may be necessary to produce ischemic injury in those with systemic hypertension. The difference between diastolic blood pressure and compartment pressure is the compartment *delta pressure*. A delta pressure of less than 20 to 30 mm Hg, which signifies compartment pressure approaching diastolic blood pressure, may be a more accurate way to determine the need for fasciotomy. (*From Rorabeck CH. Compartment syndromes. In: Browner BD, Jupiter JB, Levine AM, et al, eds. Skeletal Trauma: Fractures, Dislocations, Ligamentous Injuries. Vol 1. 2nd ed. Philadelphia: Saunders; 1992:290.*)

that an assistant hold the extremity above the stretcher. Remove any obstruction to entry of the needle and all objects that may constrict or exert pressure on the compartment.

Perform compartment pressure measurements with sterile technique, including standard skin preparation and draping at the planned insertion site (see Chapter 34). Avoid placing the needle through areas of overlying burn or infection. If a circumferential cast is present, bivalve the cast or, if necessary, create a window overlying the desired area with a cast saw.

Equipment

Needles commonly used for measurement of compartment pressure include a simple 18-gauge needle, an 18-gauge spinal needle (for deep compartments), and a side-port needle (Stryker Instruments, Kalamazoo, MI). The side-port needle and slit catheter have comparable efficacy when used for measurement of compartment pressure and may be more accurate than simple 18-gauge needles.[42] Simple 18-gauge needles are more readily available and more commonly used. The wick catheter and slit catheter methods described previously generally require specialized, cumbersome equipment not often available in most emergency departments and are therefore not described.

In an effort to reduce the pain associated with insertion of larger-gauge needles, Mars and colleagues evaluated the accuracy and reliability of measuring compartment pressure with smaller-gauge needles.[91] The authors compared compartment pressures measured with 18- to 25-gauge needles and found that smaller-gauged needles provided results similar to or better than the more traditional 18-gauge needles did. Furthermore, the addition of a side port did not improve accuracy.[91] Unfortunately, no additional studies have been done to corroborate these findings. As a result, most clinicians continue to use 18-gauge needles.

Pressure Measurement Systems

Mercury Manometer System (Fig. 54-4)
Equipment
- Two 18-gauge simple or spinal needles
- Two plastic extension tubes
- One 20-mL syringe
- One three-way stopcock
- One vial of sterile normal saline
- One mercury manometer

Setup and Procedure

1. Position the patient. Prepare and anesthetize the needle insertion site according to the guidelines described earlier.
2. Assemble the syringe, tubing, extension tubing, and needle as shown in Figure 54-4*A*.
3. Insert the needle into a vented vial of sterile saline. Aspirate a column of saline into the tubing halfway to the stopcock; care should be taken to avoid the formation of bubbles. Close the three-way stopcock to the tube to prevent the loss of saline during insertion of the needle.
4. Insert the needle into the muscle of the compartment being measured (see "Needle Placement Techniques" later in this chapter).
5. Attach the second extension tubing to the monitor and to the third port of the three-way stopcock. Turn the stopcock so that the syringe is open to both extension tubes (see Fig. 54-4*B*). This closed system has equal pressure in both extension tubes.
6. Increase the pressure in the system gradually by *slowly* depressing the syringe plunger while simultaneously watching the column of saline. The mercury manometer will rise as pressure in the system increases. When the pressure in the system exceeds that in the tissue, inject saline into the compartment, which causes the saline column to move. Read the manometer at the moment that

Figure 54-4 A and **B,** Mercury monitor technique for monitoring compartmental pressure. This system is not usually applicable to use in the emergency department. *IV,* intravenous. (*A and B, From Whitesides TE, Haney TC, Morimoto K, et al. Tissue pressure measurements as a determinant for the need of fasciotomy. Clin Orthop. 1975;113:43.*)

the saline is noted to move. This reading corresponds to the tissue pressure in millimeters of mercury.

7. To obtain a second reading, completely remove the needle and repeat steps 4 through 6. A third measurement might be necessary to achieve two readings in agreement. Check the needle for tissue plugs and blood clots between readings.

Procedural Caveats

The most common error with this system is depressing the syringe plunger too quickly. Only when saline is injected slowly into the compartment will the mercury column (which has greater inertia) accurately reflect compartment pressure. Another source of error is obstruction of the needle with a plug of tissue (or blood clot) if the plunger of the syringe is pulled back. Finally, aneroid manometers are prone to inaccuracy, are not well calibrated at lower pressure ranges, and should not be substituted for the more accurate mercury manometers for this procedure.

Arterial Line System (Fig. 54-5)
Equipment

- One 18-gauge simple or spinal needle
- High-pressure tubing
- Pressure transducer with cable
- Pressure monitor
- Sterile saline
- Transducer stand that allows variable adjustments in height
- Two three-way stopcocks
- One 20-mL syringe

Setup and Procedure

1. Position the patient and prepare and anesthetize the needle insertion site according to the guidelines described earlier.
2. Connect the transducer cable to the pressure monitor.
3. Assemble the stopcocks, transducer, transducer cable, syringe, high-pressure tubing, and needle as shown in Figure 54-5.

Figure 54-5 Arterial line system for measurement of compartmental pressure. This system is not usually applicable to use in the emergency department. *(From Rorabeck CH. Compartment syndromes. In: Browner BD, Jupiter JB, Levine AM, et al, eds. Skeletal Trauma: Fractures, Dislocations, Ligamentous Injuries. Vol 1. 2nd ed. Philadelphia: Saunders; 1992:290.)*

4. Fill the syringe with 15 mL of sterile saline and place one of the stopcocks on the syringe. Turn the stopcocks to allow filling of the transducer, high-pressure tubing, and needle. Once filled, close the stopcock to the high-pressure tubing.
5. Open the top stopcock to air and place the transducer at the height of the compartment being measured. Calibrate the transducer to zero and then close the top stopcock.
6. Open the lower stopcock that is attached to the high-pressure tubing.

7. Insert the needle into the desired muscle compartment (see "Needle Placement Techniques" later in this chapter for details). If the needle is in the proper location, applying slight external pressure to the compartment or passively moving the muscles within the compartment should cause a pressure spike on the monitor. Allow the compartment to equilibrate for several seconds after this maneuver, and then measure the mean compartment pressure.

8. To obtain a second reading, completely remove the needle and repeat steps 4 through 7. A third measurement might be necessary to achieve two readings in agreement. Check the needle for tissue plugs and blood clots between readings.

Stryker Intracompartmental Pressure Measurement (Fig. 54-6)
Equipment
- Stryker Quick Pressure Monitor System
- Stryker handheld pressure monitoring unit (included)
- One side-port 18-gauge needle (included)
- One diaphragm chamber (included)
- One syringe prefilled with 3 mL of saline (included)

Setup and Procedure (see Fig. 54-6)

1. Position the patient and prepare and anesthetize the needle insertion site according to the guidelines described earlier.
2. Open the Quick Pressure Monitor Set and remove the contents while maintaining sterile conditions.
3. Place the needle firmly on the tapered chamber stem.
4. Remove the cap on the prefilled syringe and screw the syringe onto the remaining chamber stem. Take care to avoid contaminating the fluid pathway.
5. Open the monitor cover and inspect the device for damage or contamination. Place the chamber into the device well (black surface down) and push gently until it seats.
6. Snap the cover closed—DO NOT FORCE IT. The latch must have "snapped" in place.
7. Hold the needle at approximately 45 degrees from the horizontal plane and slowly force fluid through the disposable system to purge it of air. *Caution:* DO NOT allow saline to roll down the needle into the transducer well.
8. Turn on the unit; it should read between 0 and 9 mm Hg.
9. Hold the device at the intended angle of insertion and press the "ZERO" button to calibrate it. After a few seconds, the display should read "00." Failure to calibrate the device while in the intended angle of insertion may result in inaccurate readings. *Note:* The display must read "00" before continuing. If it does not, follow the troubleshooting instructions provided by the manufacturer before proceeding.
10. Now insert the needle into the compartment being measured (see "Needle Placement Techniques" for anatomic details). Slowly inject no more than 0.3 mL of saline into the compartment to equilibrate with the interstitial fluid.
11. Wait for the display to reach equilibrium and record the resulting pressure.
12. *For additional measurements*, turn the unit off and repeat steps 8 through 11. Recalibrate the unit to zero before each measurement.

13. For continuous monitoring with an indwelling slit catheter, refer to the instructions accompanying the system.

NEEDLE PLACEMENT TECHNIQUES FOR SPECIFIC COMPARTMENTS
General Principles

Accurate pressure measurements depend on careful needle insertion and confirmation of correct placement. Proper needle insertion requires (1) reliable placement in the compartment being measured, (2) avoidance of important neurovascular structures, (3) simplicity and reproducibility, and (4) minimal patient discomfort.[92] Most compartments are superficial and easily accessible. Only the deep posterior compartment in the lower part of the leg and the gluteal compartment may require a spinal needle to reach the required depth. Most approaches require that the needle enter the tissue perpendicular to the skin.

Lower Extremity

Because of its high vulnerability to injury and limited fascial compliance, the lower part of the leg is predisposed to compartment syndrome. The foreleg traditionally has four compartments: anterior, lateral, deep posterior, and superficial posterior (Fig. 54-7).[1] The anterior compartment is the most frequent site of compartment syndrome.[45] In some patients the tibialis posterior muscle may occupy its own compartment, separate from the rest of the deep posterior compartment.[93-95] Keep this possibility in mind when measuring compartment pressure in this area.

The easiest cross-sectional level for placement of the needle in any foreleg compartment is approximately 3 cm on either side of a transverse line drawn at the junction of the proximal and middle thirds of the lower part of the leg (see Fig 54-7). When measuring compartment pressure in the foreleg, place the patient in the supine position with the leg at the level of the heart. An exception occurs when measuring the superficial posterior compartment. In this case, place the patient in the prone position. Prepare and anesthetize the needle insertion site as described previously in this chapter.

Anterior Compartment (Fig. 54-8*A*)
With the patient supine, palpate the anterior border of the tibia at the junction of the proximal and middle thirds of the lower part of the leg. Insert the needle perpendicular to the skin 1 cm *lateral* to the anterior border of the tibia to a depth of approximately 1 to 3 cm. A severalfold rise in pressure during (1) external compression of the anterior compartment just proximal or distal to the needle insertion site, (2) plantar flexion of the foot, or (3) dorsiflexion of the foot confirms proper needle depth.

Deep Posterior Compartment (see Fig. 54-8*B*)
With the patient supine, have an assistant elevate the leg slightly off the stretcher (if the clinical situation permits). Palpate the medial border of the tibia at the junction of the proximal and middle thirds of the lower part of the leg while simultaneously palpating the posterior border of the fibula on the lateral aspect of the leg at the same level. Insert the needle perpendicular to the skin just posterior to the medial border of the tibia and direct it toward the palpated posterior border

COMPARTMENT PRESSURE EVALUATION: STRYKER METHOD

Place the 18-gauge needle with a side pont on the tapered stem of the diaphragm chamber.

Screw syringe prefilled with 3 mL of saline onto the back of the diaphragm chamber.

Place the diaphragm chamber assembly into the pressure monitor, black side down. Gently push the chamber until it is well seated in the device.

Snap the cover closed-- *do not force it!* Listen for the latch to snap into place.

Hold the needle at a 45° angle up from horizontal and depress the plunger to force fluid through system and purge it of air.

Turn the pressure monitor on. It should read between 0 and 9 mm Hg.

Hold the pressure monitor at the intended angle of insertion and press the "ZERO" button to calibrate the unit. The device display should read "00."

Insert the device into the compartment being measured (after skin cleansing and administration of anesthetic). Slowly inject no more than 0.3 mL into the compartment and wait for the device to record and display the pressure.

Figure 54-6 Measuring compartment pressure with the Stryker 295-2 pressure monitor. Normal tissue compartment pressure is between 0 and 8 mm Hg.

Figure 54-7 Fascial compartments of the lower part of the leg with enclosed muscle groups (*insert, upper left*): (*1*) anterior, (*2*) lateral, (*3*) superficial posterior, and (*4*) deep posterior compartments.

of the fibula to a depth of 2 to 4 cm (the final depth depends on the amount of subcutaneous adipose tissue.). Confirm proper needle depth by observing a rise in pressure during (1) toe extension or (2) ankle eversion.

Lateral Compartment (see Fig. 54-8*C*)

With the patient supine and the leg at heart level, have an assistant elevate the leg slightly off the stretcher (if the clinical situation permits). Palpate the posterior border of the fibula at the junction of the proximal and middle thirds of the lower part of the leg. Insert the needle into the skin just anterior to the posterior border of the fibula and direct it toward the fibula to a depth of 1 to 1.5 cm. If the needle contacts bone, withdraw it approximately 0.5 cm. Confirm proper needle depth by observing a rise in pressure during (1) external compression of the lateral compartment just inferior or superior to the needle's entrance or (2) inversion of the foot and ankle.

Superficial Posterior Compartment (see Fig. 54-8*D*)

With the patient in the prone position and the leg at heart level, identify an imaginary transverse line (or draw one with a marking pen) between the proximal and middle thirds of the lower part of the leg. Insert the needle perpendicular to the skin at this level, 3 to 5 cm on either side of a vertical line drawn down the middle of the calf. Direct the needle toward the center of the leg to a depth of 2 to 4 cm. Confirm proper needle depth by observing a rise in pressure during (1) digital external compression of the posterior compartment just

inferior or superior to the needle insertion point or (2) dorsiflexion of the foot.

Forearm

Traditionally, the forearm has been considered a two-compartment limb.[1] However, some authors place the *extensor carpi radialis brevis*, the *extensor carpi radialis longus*, and the *brachioradialis* muscles in a third compartment called the "mobile wad."[96-98] The forearm compartments (particularly the volar compartment) are predisposed to compartment syndrome because of their use during vigorous exercise, accessibility for drug use, intravenous infiltration of fluid or medication, and vulnerability to injury and burns.[1,99-102]

The junction of the proximal and middle thirds of the forearm is the cross-sectional level for insertion of the needle.[96] When measuring forearm compartment pressure, place the patient in the supine position with the arm at the level of the heart. Prepare and anesthetize the needle insertion site as previously described.

Volar Compartment (Fig. 54-9*A*)

Hold the forearm in supination. Identify the *palmaris longus* tendon by having the patient oppose the thumb and small finger with the wrist flexed against resistance. Follow the tendon to the junction of the proximal and middle thirds of the forearm. Palpate the posterior border of the ulna and insert the needle perpendicular to the skin just medial to the

LOWER EXTREMITY COMPARTMENTS

A. Anterior

Place the patient in the supine position. Insert the needle at the junction of the proximal and middle thirds of the lower part of the leg, 1 cm *lateral* to anterior border of the tibia. Direct the needle perpendicular to the skin to a depth of 1 to 3 cm.

B. Deep Posterior

Place patient in the supine position with the leg slightly elevated. Insert the needle at the junction of the proximal and middle thirds of the lower part of the leg, just posterior to the medial border of the tibia. Direct the needle perpendicular to the skin and toward the posterior border of the fibula to a depth of 2 to 4 cm.

C. Lateral

Place patient in the supine position with leg slightly elevated off the stretcher. Insert the needle at the junction of the proximal and middle thirds of the lower part of the leg, just anterior to the posterior border of the fibula. Direct the needle toward the fibula to a depth of 1 to 1.5 cm.

D. Superficial Posterior

Place the patient in the prone position. Insert the needle at the junction of the proximal and middle thirds of the lower part of the leg, 3 to 5 cm on either side of the anatomic midline. Direct the needle perpendicular to the skin toward the center of the leg to a depth of 2 to 4 cm.

Figure 54-8 Lower extremity needle placement techniques. *(From Custalow CB. Color Atlas of Emergency Department Procedures. Philadelphia: Saunders; 2005.)*

palmaris longus tendon. Direct the needle toward the palpated posterior border of the ulna to a depth of 1 to 2 cm. Confirm proper needle depth by observing a rise in pressure during (1) external compression of the volar compartment just proximal or distal to the needle insertion point or (2) extension of the fingers or wrist.

Dorsal Compartment (see Fig. 54–9B)
Hold the forearm in pronation with the elbow flexed and the dorsum of the forearm facing upward. Palpate the posterior aspect of the ulna at the junction of the proximal and middle

thirds of the forearm. Insert the needle perpendicular to the skin 1 to 2 cm lateral to the posterior aspect of the ulna to a depth of 1 to 2 cm. Confirm proper needle placement by observing a rise in pressure during (1) digital external compression of the dorsal compartment just proximal or distal to the needle insertion point or (2) flexion of the wrist or fingers.

Mobile Wad (see Fig. 54–9C)
Hold the forearm in supination. Identify the most lateral (radial) portion of the forearm at the junction of its proximal

UPPER EXTREMITY COMPARTMENTS

A. Volar

Hold the forearm in supination. Insert the needle at the junction of the proximal and middle thirds of the forearm, just medial to the palmaris longus tendon. Direct the needle perpendicular to the skin, toward the posterior border of the ulna, to a depth of 1 to 2 cm.

B. Dorsal

Hold the forearm in pronation with the elbow flexed and the dorsum of the forearm facing up. Insert the needle at the junction of the proximal and middle thirds of the forearm, 1 to 2 cm lateral to the posterior aspect of the ulna. Direct the needle perpendicular to the skin to a depth of 1 to 2 cm.

C. Mobile Wad

Hold the forearm in supination. Insert the needle at the junction of the proximal and middle thirds of the forearm, at the most lateral (radial) portion of the forearm. Direct the needle perpendicular to the skin to a depth of 1 to 1.5 cm.

Figure 54-9 Upper extremity needle placement techniques. (*From Custalow CB. Color Atlas of Emergency Department Procedures. Philadelphia: Saunders; 2005.*)

and middle thirds. Insert the needle into the muscle tissue lateral to the radius perpendicular to the skin to a depth of 1 to 1.5 cm. Confirm proper needle placement by observing a rise in pressure during (1) digital external compression of the mobile wad just proximal or distal to the needle entry point or (2) deviation of the wrist.

Gluteal Musculature

A two-layer fascia encases the muscle bellies of the tensor fasciae latae anteriorly and the gluteus maximus posteriorly.

This fascia divides the musculature into three distinct compartments: maximus, tensor, and medius/minimus (Fig. 54-10*A*). The sciatic nerve is deep to the fascia but lies between the pelvis–external rotator complex and the gluteus maximus, which makes it vulnerable to injury when compartment syndrome occurs here. Gluteal compartment syndrome is very rare and unknown to many clinicians. Most reported cases of gluteal compartment syndrome result from prolonged immobilization and local compression in association with drug or alcohol intoxication.[103-107] Prolonged pressure from a toilet seat or significant soft tissue contusions (whipping,

GLUTEAL COMPARTMENTS

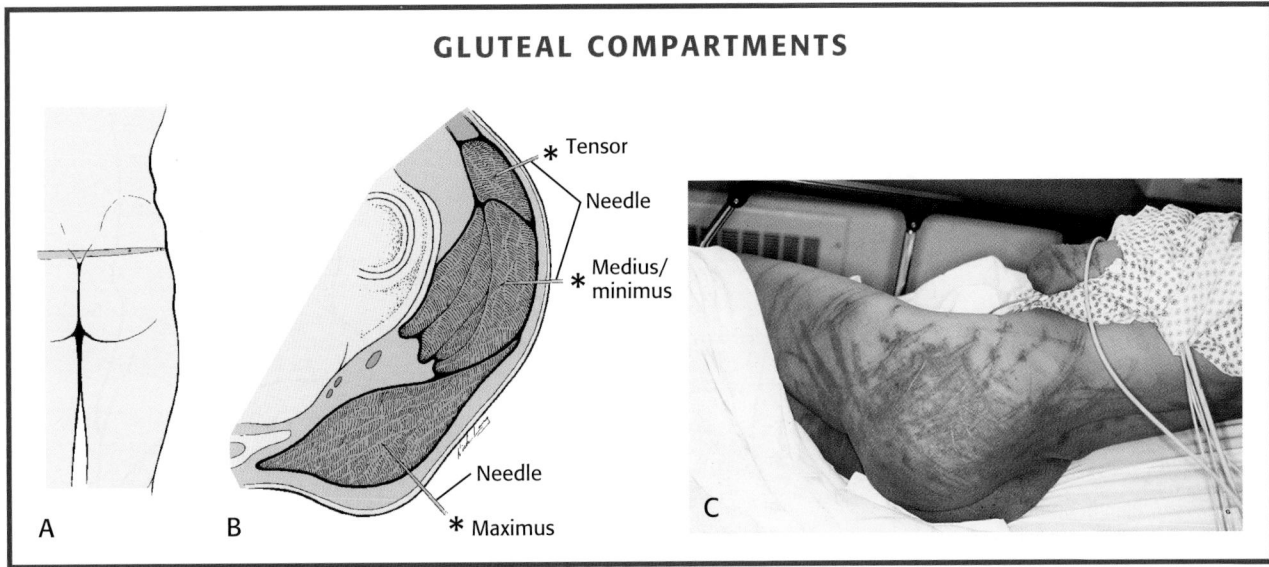

Figure 54-10 Gluteal compartment syndrome. **A,** Suggested entry points are indicated along the blue line. The needle should be inserted to a depth of 4 to 8 cm, depending on which compartment is being measured. **B,** Needle tips (*asterisks*) are shown entering the muscle compartments. **C,** This patient suffered extensive soft tissue trauma to the buttocks as a result of repeated blows from a stick (domestic abuse) and is at risk for rhabdomyolysis and gluteal compartment syndrome. (*A and B, Modified with permission from Owen CA, Moody PR, Mubarak SJ, et al. Gluteal compartment syndromes. Clin Orthop. 1978;132:57.*)

paddling) may predispose to this condition. Patients typically have gluteal tenderness that is often attributed to contusion or hematoma. This, combined with the rarity of a compartment syndrome in this area, frequently results in a delayed or missed diagnosis. Rhabdomyolysis should be considered in patients with gluteal compartment syndrome given the large muscle mass involved.

Gluteal Compartments

To measure gluteal compartment pressure, place the patient in the prone position with the gluteal structures at the level of the heart. Prepare and anesthetize the needle insertion site as described previously. Cutaneous landmarks for the three compartments are not consistent from patient to patient. Therefore, in cases of suspected gluteal compartment syndrome, insertion of the needle at the point of maximal tenderness is considered sufficient to provide adequate pressure measurements.[103] Insert an 18-gauge spinal needle perpendicular to the skin and direct it toward the point of maximal tenderness to a depth of 4 to 8 cm (see Fig. 54-10B). Confirm proper needle placement by observing a rise in pressure during external compression of the gluteal musculature.

Foot

Crush injuries account for the majority of reported cases of compartment syndrome in the foot,[108-110] but it may also be seen after vascular injuries, fractures, and other high-energy injuries. Although compartment syndrome of the foot is rare, it is being reported with increasing frequency as clinicians become more aware of this entity. Despite a lack of universal agreement on the number or exact location of the anatomic compartments in the foot,[111-115] it is generally accepted that there are at least nine compartments separated into four

groups: the central/calcaneal, intrinsic/interosseous, medial, and lateral (Fig. 54–11A).

For measurement of pressure in any of the foot compartments, place the patient in the supine position with the foot at the level of the heart and prepare and anesthetize the needle insertion site as described previously. Note that pedal edema has been shown to increase resting tissue pressure in the foot.[116,117]

Medial Compartment (see Fig. 54-11B)

The medial compartment contains the *abductor hallucis* and *flexor hallucis brevis muscles*. The compartment is bounded medially and inferiorly by an extension of the plantar aponeurosis, laterally by an intramuscular septum, and dorsally by the first metatarsal. To measure pressure in this compartment, insert the needle perpendicular to the skin at the medial aspect of the foot just inferior to the base of the first metatarsal into the *abductor hallucis* muscle, which is approximately 1 to 1.5 cm deep.[118] Confirm proper needle depth by observing a rise in pressure during external compression of the medial compartment of the foot.

Central (Calcaneal) Compartment (see Fig. 54-11B)

The central compartment contains the *flexor digitorum brevis*, the *quadratus plantae*, the *lumbricals*, and the *abductor hallucis* muscles. Its boundaries are the plantar aponeurosis inferiorly, the osteofascial tarsometatarsal structures dorsally, and the intermuscular septa medially and laterally. To measure pressure in this compartment, insert the needle perpendicular to the skin at the medial aspect of the foot just inferior to the base of the first metatarsal. Advance the needle through the *abductor hallucis* muscle to a depth of 3 cm.[118] Confirm proper needle depth by observing a rise in pressure during external compression of the central compartment of the foot.

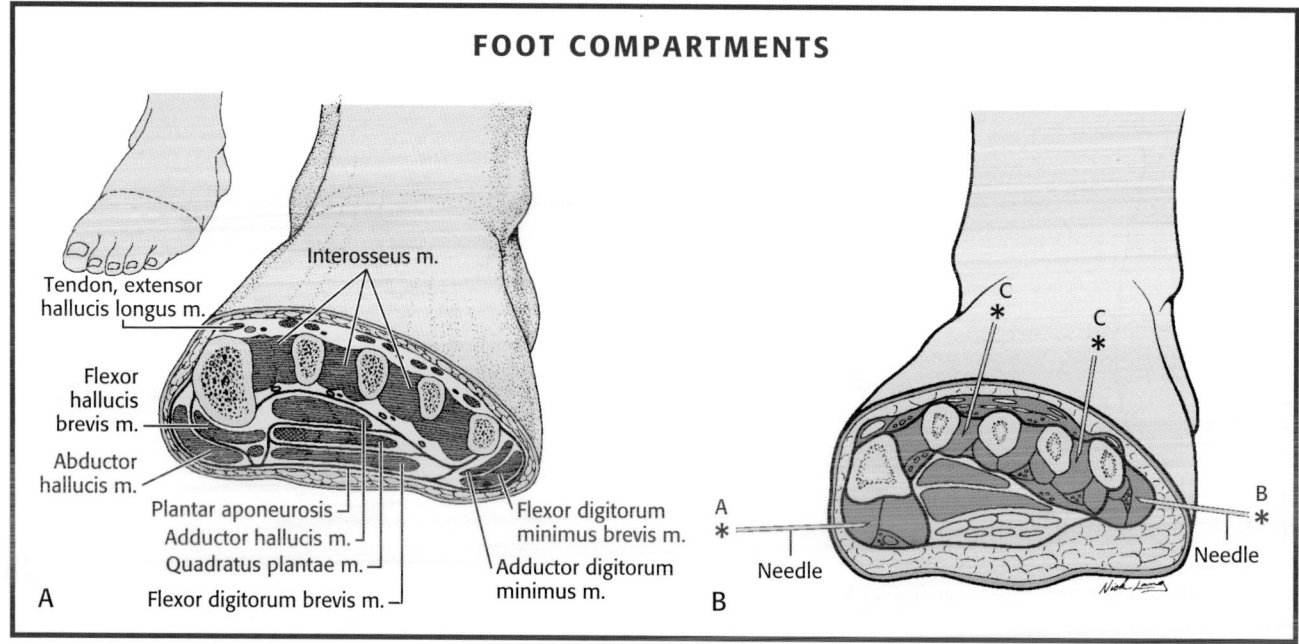

Figure 54-11 *A,* Compartments of the foot. *B,* Suggested needle pathways (*asterisks*) to measure intracompartmental pressure: *A,* medial; *B,* lateral; *C,* interosseous. The central compartment is surrounded by these compartments. (*A, From Mubarak SJ, Hargens AR. Compartment Syndromes and Volkmann's Contracture. Philadelphia: Saunders; 1981; B, modified from Myerson M. Acute compartment syndromes of the foot. Bull Hosp Jt Dis. 1987;47:251.*)

Lateral Compartment (see Fig. 54-11*B*)

The lateral compartment contains the *abductor, flexor,* and *opponens* muscles of the fifth toe. The boundaries are the fifth metatarsal dorsally, the plantar aponeurosis inferiorly and laterally, and an intermuscular septum medially.[118] To measure pressure in this compartment, insert the needle parallel to the plantar aspect of the foot just inferior to the base of the fifth metatarsal. Advance the needle to a depth of 1 to 1.5 cm. Confirm proper needle depth by observing a rise in pressure during external compression of the lateral compartment of the foot.

Intrinsic (Interosseous) Compartment

(see Fig. 54-11*B*)

The intrinsic compartment contains the seven interossei muscles and is bounded by the metatarsals and the interosseous fascia. Pressure in this compartment is measured in two areas, the second and fourth web spaces. Avoid the first web space to prevent inadvertent puncture or disruption of the *dorsalis pedis* artery or the *deep peroneal* nerve.[118] Insert the needle perpendicular to the skin at the dorsum of the second and fourth web spaces at the base of the metatarsals, and advance the needle to a depth of 1 cm.[118] Confirm proper needle depth by observing a rise in pressure during external compression of the intrinsic compartment adjacent to the needle insertion site.

INTERPRETATION OF COMPARTMENT PRESSURE MEASUREMENTS

Compartment pressures must be interpreted within the context of the clinical picture. Inaccurate measurements are far worse than no measurement at all, and *clinical evaluation is more telling*

than pressure measurements alone. To be most accurate, compartment pressures should be measured in the area of highest pressure and greatest tissue damage.[79,119] Inaccurate measurements may result from placement of the needle into tendon or fascia, plugged needles, defective or poorly calibrated devices, injection of fluid into the compartment, and movement during the procedure. Whitesides and colleagues found a 1–mm Hg increase in compartment pressure for every 1 mL of saline infused into the anterior compartment of the lower extremity.[6] It is difficult to assess the relevance of this finding, but recognition of the potential for its occurrence is important.

Reports of normal human compartment pressure vary in the literature. In comparing several techniques, Shakespeare and associates found an average normal pressure of 8.5 mm Hg with slightly higher resting pressure in individuals who were physically fit.[12] Willy and coworkers found a mean of 15 mm Hg (±8 mm Hg) when using an electronic transducer-tipped probe in healthy volunteers.[15] Although the generally accepted range of normal is between 0 and 10 mm Hg, others have noted pressures in normal subjects ranging from 0 to as high as 18 mm Hg.[1,8,78,120] Even though compartment pressure measurements have not been studied extensively in pediatric populations, one study reported higher resting compartment pressure in children than in adults.[43]

When properly performed, each method has acceptable accuracy in the clinical setting. Studies have found standard deviations of between 2 and 6 mm Hg with all the techniques described earlier.[1,8-10,12] It is generally agreed that the mercury manometer method of measuring compartment pressure is the least accurate. The arterial line system used with a simple (straight) or side-port needle provides a higher degree of accuracy for simple, episodic readings. The Stryker Intracompartmental Pressure Monitoring System provides consistent, accurate readings for both episodic and continuous pressure monitoring. The development of miniature transducer-tipped devices is ongoing.[121] Noninvasive modalities, including MRI, SPECT, myotonometry, electromyography, near-infrared spectroscopy, and ultrasound, continue to be investigated as painless alternatives to needle-driven compartment pressure measurements, and although the early results are promising, they are not currently in widespread use.[16-33]

Mubarak and coworkers[9,122] and Hargens and colleagues suggested that an absolute compartment pressure of 30 mm Hg is the "critical pressure" requiring fasciotomy.[123] Others have corroborated these findings.[119,124] Despite the fact that this tissue pressure is abnormally high and corresponds to the onset of pain and paresthesias,[9] it does not necessarily precipitate compartment syndrome in the absence of other factors and must be interpreted within the context of the clinical scenario. Although compartment syndrome may develop in some patients at this pressure, in others it will not because tolerance to increasing pressure appears to be variable.[1,8,12,78]

Despite a body of literature addressing measurement of compartment pressure, there continues to be *no consensus regarding a specific compartment pressure threshold at which fasciotomy should be performed.* Obviously, no measured compartment pressure, by itself, is an indication for fasciotomy, but it may guide consultation and further observation. A single pressure reading can be misleading, and trends in pressure provide more information to the clinician. Some argue that an absolute compartment pressure of 30 mg Hg or greater should be the threshold for fasciotomy.[9,122-124] Matsen found that no patients with a pressure lower than 45 mm Hg had symptoms of compartment syndrome[1] whereas all patients with a pressure higher than 60 mm Hg had symptoms. Whitesides and colleagues found that fasciotomy was required when intracompartmental pressure approaches 20 mm Hg below diastolic pressure,[6] whereas McQueen and associates recommended using a differential pressure (diastolic minus compartment pressure) of less than 30 mm Hg as a criterion for fasciotomy.[125] Heppenstall and coworkers concluded that use of either the Whitesides or McQueen criteria would produce similar results and recommended using a ΔP (MAP minus the measured compartment pressure) of 30 mm Hg or less in nontraumatized muscle and a ΔP of 40 mm Hg or less in traumatized muscle as a guide for fasciotomy.[48,57]

In summary, absolute compartment pressures of 30 mm Hg or higher garner concern for consultation or intervention for compartment syndrome. Based on pathophysiology, it appears quite reasonable to consider the difference between diastolic blood pressure and the measured compartment pressure (ΔP) as a guide for diagnosing compartment syndrome and a strong consideration for fasciotomy. A compartment pressure within 30 mm Hg of the patient's diastolic blood pressure, essentially a ΔP of less than 30 mm Hg, is generally considered the threshold for consideration of fasciotomy.[47,119,126]

Factors other than compartment pressure alone are important in the development of compartment syndrome and the need for fasciotomy. In patients with chronic systemic hypertension, higher compartment pressure may be necessary before nerve injury or muscle ischemia occurs. Situations in which MAP is low (e.g., hypovolemia, peripheral vascular disease) might interfere with the patient's ability to tolerate even mildly elevated compartment pressure. Moreover, the duration of increased compartment pressure is also an important factor in the development and severity of compartment syndrome.

COMPLICATIONS

All invasive monitoring systems are associated with some degree of pain during insertion of the needle or catheter. Adequate analgesia and, when necessary, procedural sedation are often necessary to gain the patient's cooperation and prevent movement during pressure measurements. When using local anesthetics, avoid injections into the compartment because this can increase pain and result in inaccurate (higher) readings.

Failure to properly use pressure measurement devices may result in inaccurate results and a delay in the diagnosis of compartment syndrome. As with any invasive procedure, care must be taken to minimize bleeding and additional damage to underlying tissue, nerves, or blood vessels. The risk for both local and systemic infection is similar for all the measurement procedures described in this chapter. Strict adherence to aseptic technique and universal precautions is mandatory. This includes sterilization of catheters and the use of sterile solutions in addition to sterile gloves and supplies whenever possible.

Acknowledgment

The author recognizes the original contributions of Neal R. Frankel, DO, and L. Albert Villarin, Jr., MD, to a previous edition of this text.

References are available at www.expertconsult.com

Genitourinary, Obstetric, and Gynecologic Procedures

CHAPTER 55

Urologic Procedures

Jonathan E. Davis and Michael A. Silverman

INTRODUCTION

This chapter addresses urologic conditions that are either initially or eventually associated with an emergency procedure and that may need to be performed in the absence of a urologic surgeon.

TESTICULAR TORSION

Although acute scrotal pain accounts for less than 1% of overall emergency department (ED) visits, it may provoke great anxiety in the patient or caretaker given its highly sensitive nature.[1] One of the most challenging aspects of scrotal complaints is that a wide variety of clinical conditions may have similar signs and symptoms: a male patient complaining of an acute, painful, swollen, and tender hemiscrotum. The most common urologic emergencies manifested as acute scrotal pain include testicular torsion, severe infectious epididymitis, and Fournier's necrotizing fasciitis. Other painful conditions include torsion of the appendix testis, inguinal hernia, trauma, testicular cancer, referred pain (such as ureterolithiasis and diverticulitis), Henoch-Schönlein purpura, and orchitis (mumps, brucellosis, coxsackievirus disease, etc.). Hydrocele, varicocele, spermatocele, and testicular cancer tend to be characterized by painless, isolated swelling. Although the differential diagnosis is extensive, testicular torsion is the principal threat to fertility that needs to be ruled out. Definitive management of testicular torsion involves surgical exploration and orchiopexy. Manual detorsion, with or without spermatic cord anesthesia, can be attempted while simultaneously preparing for operative intervention.

Testicular torsion is a scrotal emergency that can be challenging to diagnose under the best clinical circumstances. Although surgical exploration is the only definitive diagnostic and therapeutic procedure, many urologists prefer an initial diagnostic imaging study before surgical exploration, but only if imaging can be obtained expediently while simultaneously preparing for operative intervention.

Background

An *acute scrotum* is defined as an acute painful swelling of the scrotum or its contents, accompanied by local signs or general symptoms.[2] Acute epididymitis is commonly the cause of acute scrotal pain in adolescents and adults. Torsion of testicular (or epididymal) appendages is another frequent cause of acute scrotal pain in prepubertal boys.

Differentiating testicular torsion from alternative conditions takes precedence over definitive diagnosis. The presence of an intact cremasteric reflex and testicular sonography are frequently used, yet imperfect diagnostic tools in assessing for testicular torsion. The cremasteric reflex is assessed by stroking the upper part of the thigh while observing the ipsilateral testis. A normal response is cremasteric contraction with elevation of the testis. The reflex is present in the majority of healthy boys between the ages of 30 months and 12 years; it may be less consistently present in infants and teenagers. The reflex may be absent in patients with testicular torsion, which may help distinguish this condition from other causes of scrotal pain.

Anatomy and Physiology

A congenital anomaly of fixation of the testis, termed the *bell-clapper deformity*, is associated with the development of testicular torsion.[3] It occurs when the intrascrotal portion of the spermatic cord lacks firm posterior adhesion to the scrotal wall and remains surrounded by the tunica vaginalis (Fig. 55-1A). As a result of the abnormal attachment, the testis may be suspended horizontally.[4] These anatomic features predispose the affected testis to rotation.

Pathophysiology

Testicular salvage rates decrease with time. A metaanalysis of 1140 patients in 22 series demonstrated a greater than 90% salvage rate when surgery was performed within 6 hours of the onset of pain.[5] Testicular atrophy may lead to decreased fertility. Furthermore, testicular loss may result in dysfunction of the contralateral testis through immune-mediated or other mechanisms.[5]

MANUAL TESTICULAR DETORSION

A. Anatomy of testicular torsion. Testicular torsion occurs when the testis twists within the tunica vaginalis. Patients with the bell-clapper deformity (i.e., incomplete fusion of the tunica along the epididymis, which results in incomplete attachment of the testicle to the scrotum) are at higher risk.

B. Spermatic cord block. Grasp the spermatic cord between your thumb and index finger. Use a 30-gauge needle to infiltrate the entire cross section of the spermatic cord and its surrounding rim with anesthetic. This will cause visual ballooning of the grasped segment of the cord. Gently massage this bulge to disperse the anesthetic. Usually about 10 mL is required.

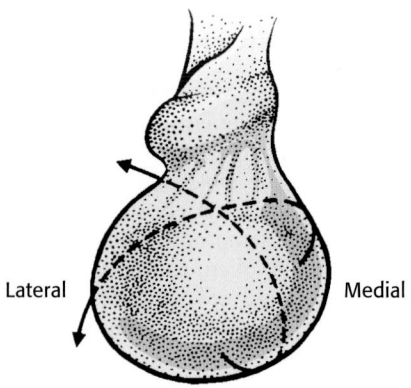

C. Testicular torsion more commonly occurs in a medial direction. Initially attempt detorsion by rotating the testis outward toward the thigh. This is most successful if attempted within the first few hours of torsion, before the onset of significant scrotal swelling. Intravenous narcotics (such as fentanyl) can be administered or a cord block performed before attempting detorsion.

D. Detorsion maneuver. Detorsion of the testicle may require testicular rotation through two planes. To release the cremasteric muscle, rotate the testis in a caudal-to-cranial direction simultaneously with medial-to-lateral rotation. The right testis is shown.

Figure 55-1 A, Anatomy of testicular torsion. **B,** Achieve anesthesia of the spermatic cord by injecting lidocaine at the superficial inguinal ring. (*A, From Snyder HM III. Urologic emergencies. In: Fleisher GR, Ludwig S, eds. Textbook of Pediatric Emergency Medicine. 4th ed. Philadelphia: Lippincott, Williams & Wilkins; 2000:1585-1593; B, from Issa MM, Hsiao K, Bassel YS, et al. Spermatic cord anesthesia block for scrotal procedures in outpatient clinic setting. J Urol. 2004;172:2358-2361; D, from Freeman S, Chapman J. Urologic procedures. Emerg Med Clin North Am. 1986;4:543.*)

Figure 55-2 Ischemic necrosis of the right testicle secondary to testicular torsion. This patient was evaluated in the emergency department 9 days after the onset of intermittent testicular pain. **A,** Transverse view of the scrotum showing the right testicle to be in a horizontal lie. Also note the cobblestoning of surrounding tissue (*arrow*), indicative of localized edema. **B,** Sagittal view of the right testicle revealing diffuse, round, complex hypoechoic foci (*arrows*), indicative of ischemic necrosis. **C** and **D,** Color flow Doppler imaging revealing no flow in the right testicle and normal flow in the left. Right orchiectomy was required.

Intermittent testicular torsion should be considered in all boys with a history of scrotal pain without other identifiable causes. Intermittent torsion is characterized by acute and intermittent sharp testicular pain and scrotal swelling, with rapid resolution (within seconds to a few minutes) and long intervals without symptoms. It is often associated with nausea or vomiting and pain that awakens them from sleep. Although findings on physical examination may include a horizontal or very mobile testis, anterior epididymis, or bulkiness of the spermatic cord from partial twisting, the clinical and radiographic evaluation of some boys with intermittent torsion may be normal at the time of ED evaluation, with no clinical clues to its prior presence. If intermittent torsion is suspected, ED consultation or close outpatient follow-up with a urologist is prudent.

Since the testes are subject to torsion, detorsion, and retorsion, clinicians should be cautious about assigning an exact time of onset. If urologic consultation is deferred because of an erroneous assumption, the testis may not be salvageable. The "gold standard" for determining testicular viability is intraoperative visualization of the affected testis, which

dictates early urologic involvement. Although all clinicians recognize the need for expedient surgery in the setting of known torsion, not all consultants agree on surgical exploration without adjunctive testing. It is generally agreed, however, that scrotal exploration is necessary for diagnosis in cases in which clinical examination and imaging cannot exclude testicular torsion.

When used in the appropriate clinical setting, ultrasound remains the most useful diagnostic modality in the evaluation of genitourinary (GU) complaints (Fig. 55-2). A patient with compelling findings of testicular torsion on the history and physical examination does not require any preoperative diagnostic tests. Color flow Doppler ultrasonography (CDUS) may be very helpful in all other cases. The classic sonographic finding of testicular torsion is diminished intratesticular blood flow. In addition, examination of the spermatic cord with high-resolution gray-scale ultrasonography may reveal "coiling" or "kinking" of the cord at the site of torsion.[6-8]

Sonography is used not only to exclude testicular torsion but also to search for alternative causes of acute scrotal pain.[9] With epididymitis, perfusion may be normal (or increased) because of the effects of inflammatory mediators on local vascular beds, although this is a nonspecific finding.[10,11] An infarcted appendage may be visualized on ultrasound as well.[12] Emergency physicians with appropriate training may be able to accurately assess intratesticular blood flow with bedside sonography in patients with acute scrotal pain.[13]

CDUS has long been regarded as the diagnostic modality of choice in assessing for testicular torsion. However, false-negative ultrasound results have been reported.[14-20] Many of these studies are case reports or case series limited by small numbers and retrospective design. Two larger series reported documented intratesticular blood flow with CDUS in 6 of 23 (26%) and 50 of 208 cases (24%), respectively, of confirmed testicular torsion.[6,21] Unfortunately, Doppler ultrasound may reveal seemingly adequate intratesticular blood flow in those with partial torsion, which can mislead the practitioner.[22]

Radionuclide scintigraphy and CDUS have similar sensitivity, as well as false-negative rates, for the diagnosis of testicular torsion.[23] However, given the widespread availability of and expertise in ultrasound technology, combined with the risks associated with exposure to radioactive isotopes, radionuclide procedures have fallen out of favor. The use of magnetic resonance imaging has been explored, but limitations include speed of imaging and availability.[24,25]

Intravaginal testicular torsion is a congenital *bilateral* abnormality. The ischemic testis must undergo detorsion and be fixated with nonabsorbable (e.g., nylon, polypropylene) rather than absorbable (e.g., chromic, Vicryl) suture. A torsed testis that is fixated with absorbable suture remains at risk for subsequent postoperative torsion. Given the bilateral nature of the congenital abnormality, orchiopexy of the nonischemic contralateral testis is mandatory to ensure prevention of future torsion.

Once the diagnosis of testicular torsion is suspected, immediately place a call to notify a urologist of the suspected diagnosis, the perceived need for surgical exploration, and the fact that you will be attempting testicular detorsion (and perhaps bedside ultrasound) while awaiting transport of the patient to the operating room. At some point during the ED course, chart meticulously and document the time, suspected diagnosis, notification of the urologist, and any manipulation of the affected testis.

Indications

Testicular torsion can be relieved by manual detorsion. A study of 162 cases of testicular torsion revealed that the anticipated lateral-to-medial rotation occurred in 67% of cases, with medial-to-lateral rotation seen in the remaining 33%.[26] This challenges the standard dogma of medial-to-lateral rotation, or "opening the book," as the standard method of detorsion. As noted, there may be a cranial-caudal component to the torsion as well. The end point of manual detorsion is relief of pain or return of intratesticular blood flow as seen on ultrasound imaging.[27] Although manual detorsion may allow reperfusion of the testis, a lesser degree of residual torsion may remain. Given that infarction can occur with as little as 180 degrees of torsion, immediate surgical exploration is still advocated after what is thought to successful manual detorsion.[26] The bottom line is that specialty consultation and plans for possible immediate surgical exploration need to occur regardless of the outcome of the detorsion procedure.

Contraindications

The detorsion procedure is relatively contraindicated in the presence of an alternative cause of acute scrotal pain; however, precise diagnosis may be impossible before definitive surgical exploration. A nonanomalous, appropriately fixated testicle should not be adversely affected by an initial trial (e.g., 180 degrees) of manual detorsion if the circumstances are highly suggestive of spermatic cord torsion.

Procedure

Manual Detorsion and Spermatic Cord Anesthesia

Manual detorsion is performed in the following manner. Advise the patient that the procedure will be painful and offer systemic analgesia or light sedation if appropriate and necessary. Spermatic cord anesthesia is not advised during attempted detorsion because it takes away an important subjective end point: the patient will not be able to feel relief after successful detorsion of the testis. However, many authors do advocate spermatic cord anesthesia before detorsion, and if anesthesia of the spermatic cord is elected, it can be done in the following manner.

Spermatic Cord Anesthesia

Local anesthesia of the spermatic cord can be induced with 1% plain lidocaine injected at the external or superficial inguinal ring (Fig. 55-1*B*).[28] First prepare the skin with an antiseptic solution. Grasp the cord between the thumb and index finger, and inject 10 mL of 1% plain lidocaine (in an adult) directly into the cord. If the cord is swollen, which is frequently the case with testicular torsion, or if the testicle is lying very high in the hemiscrotum because of spermatic cord torsion (thus precluding grasping), palpate the cord at the pubic tubercle as it passes over the pubis and inject the lidocaine at this landmark. Lee and colleagues[29] were able to perform manual detorsion with local spermatic cord anesthesia in 70% of their cases of torsion in adults. Kresling and associates[30] had success in 15 of 16 patients and noted a fair amount of associated cremasteric muscle spasm, which must also be relieved.

Manual Detorsion

The goal of manual detorsion is to reestablish or increase blood flow to a previously ischemic testis. This should be done while the operating suite is being prepared. It should never delay operative intervention.

Before initiating detorsion, ensure that the patient is as comfortable as possible in a reclining or supine position. The lithotomy position gives the examiner the most access to the patient's genitalia and prevents the patient from retreating during the procedure. Administer light analgesia and sedation at this time if indicated.

Begin manual detorsion with the clinician standing comfortably at the side of the bed or stretcher, preferably on the patient's right side if the clinician is right handed or on the left side if left handed. Begin detorsion just as one would open a book (i.e., an initial 180-degree detorsion of the patient's right testis is done in a counterclockwise fashion) (see Fig. 55-1*C* and *D*). The patient's left testis is detorsed 180 degrees in a clockwise fashion. Ask the patient whether there was any relief of pain after the maneuver. If one rotation relieves some but not all of the pain, continue with another rotation of the testis. The degree of torsion may range from 180 to 1080 degrees, with medians of 360 to 540 degrees.[26] Many patients will require two or three rotations to fully alleviate their pain. If the initial detorsion is mechanically difficult (which it will be if detorsion is done in the wrong direction) or makes the pain worse, detorse the testis in the opposite direction and observe the result. Approximately one third of testicular torsions occur in the lateral, or unexpected, direction.[26] The objective success or failure of testicular manipulation can be further substantiated by an increase in Doppler signal and symptomatic relief of pain.

With successful detorsion, the testicle returns to its normal anatomic position. Resolution of induration and swelling of the spermatic cord, testis, and epididymis depends on the degree and duration of ischemia. Thus, the more severe the torsion and the longer it has been present, the longer it will take for the edema and induration to resolve. With significant ischemia, the entire epididymis often becomes enlarged like a link sausage and the testis becomes quite firm, like a testicular tumor. This is uncommon with epididymitis, except in severe cases or those that are initially misdiagnosed or seen late in the clinical course. In many cases these reversible changes resolve over a 3- to 4-hour period.

Aftercare

Provide systemic analgesics as needed for discomfort. Importantly, even though manual detorsion will save an ischemic testicle, it should not be substituted for definitive scrotal exploration.

Complications

In a proportion of cases the testis will torse in the opposite direction (medial to lateral) or have multiple twists. This may become apparent as the clinician assesses the results of the detorsion procedure by palpation, relief of edema, and return of or increase in the Doppler signal.

Conclusion

Spermatic cord torsion may be relieved by manual detorsion. In two thirds of cases it is accomplished by medial-to-lateral rotation of the affected testicle. However, in the remaining third of cases, lateral-to-medial rotation is necessary to untwist the spermatic cord. In all cases, manual detorsion, even when successful, serves only as a temporizing bridge to definitive surgical management.

PRIAPISM

Priapism is defined as a prolonged erection of the penis, generally for more than 4 hours, in the absence of sexual desire or stimulation (Fig. 55-3). This medical condition was named after Priapus, an ancient Greek god of fertility and horticulture who was endowed with oversized genitalia.[31]

Priapism can be divided into two main categories. Ischemic priapism, also known as low-flow priapism, is the most common variant and is due to painful venous engorgement of the corpora cavernosa. It requires emergency treatment. Nonischemic (high-flow) priapism is quite rare and is often painless. It is caused by increased arterial inflow to the penis

Figure 55-3 Typical appearance of priapism. It has many causes, is painful, often recurrent, and can lead to impotence. Many cases can be effectively treated in the ED, but definitive ED intervention is not a mandated standard of care.

as a result of traumatic arterial-cavernosal fistulas and does not require urgent treatment.

Ischemic priapism can be thought of as a compartment syndrome of the penis.[32] The corpora cavernosa become engorged with stagnant, oxygen-depleted venous blood because of either intraluminal obstruction of venous blood flow or an inability of the penile muscle tissue to adequately contract and augment venous outflow.[33]

Background

Priapism is manifested as a persistent, usually painful penile erection, unrelated to sexual stimulation and not relieved by ejaculation.

More than a third of patients with severe priapism may suffer permanent erectile dysfunction despite treatment, with obvious functional and emotional sequelae.[33]

Anatomy and Physiology

Priapism is characterized clinically by a soft glans penis and spongy urethra in the presence of two erect penile bodies (corpora cavernosa) (Fig. 55-4). Two important concepts are worthy of mention. First, there is communication of blood flow between the corpora cavernosa; therefore, in most cases the operator needs to access only one of the corpora. Second, the introduction of vasoactive or other agents into the corpora is akin to an intravenous injection and may precipitate systemic effects, particularly when partial detumescence is achieved.

Pathophysiology

The pathophysiology of priapism is complex. The pharmacologic basis of treatment involves manipulation of blood flow via α and β receptors. Priapism is believed to result from increased arterial inflow of blood into the corpora cavernosa secondary to dilation of the cavernosal arteries. Relaxation of the cavernosal tissue occurs and secondary compression of the emissary veins leads to engorgement of both corpora cavernosa during an erection. When cavernosal pressure approaches arterial pressure, blood flow is markedly reduced. Ischemic or low-flow priapism results after several hours of a continuous painful erection. It can lead to intracavernosal acidosis, sludging of blood, thrombosis of the cavernosal arteries, fibrosis of corporal tissue, and even irreversible impotence.

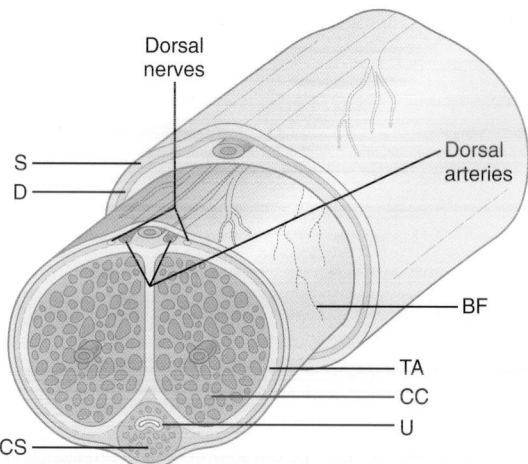

Figure 55-4 Anatomy of the penile shaft: skin (S), dartos (D), Buck's fascia (BF), tunica albuginea (TA), corpora cavernosa (CC), corpus spongiosum (CS), and urethra (U). The corpora cavernosa communicate with each other, and thus unilateral injections/aspirations suffice in the treatment of acute priapism. (*From Bostwick DG, Cheng L, eds.* Urologic Surgical Pathology. *2nd ed. St. Louis: Mosby; 2008.*)

High-flow priapism is less common than low-flow priapism and usually results from the production of an arterial-cavernosal fistula as a result of trauma. It is not associated with intracavernosal ischemia or acidosis, so it is painless. It may be treated electively rather than on an emergency basis.

In the past, priapism was most often encountered as a complication of a number of medical conditions, such as hematologic, neoplastic, or drug-related conditions. Today, many cases are iatrogenic and result from the current practice of using vasoactive substances (e.g., papaverine and phentolamine). Another cause is the newer erectile dysfunction medications used to induce penile erections in impotent men. Sickle cell disease continues to be a leading cause of priapism. Sickle cell patients may experience such a high rate of recurrence that home self-injection of vasoactive drugs into the penis has been advocated. Cocaine use is one cause that is likely to be underreported.[34] A drug screen may unravel some discrepancies between the clinical findings and history. As an end result, vasoactive drugs promote engorgement of the corpora cavernosa and reduction in venous outflow, which may result in low-flow or ischemic priapism.[35-37] Several phosphodiesterase inhibitors and prostaglandin E_1 are the drug treatments of impotence approved by the U.S. Food and Drug Administration. These medications act by increasing penile blood flow by enhancing smooth muscle relaxation. The incidence of priapism with these medications is quite low, particularly with the phosphodiesterase inhibitors. Penile rigidity secondary to a nondeflating penile prosthesis (pseudopriapism) or malignant replacement of the corpora in patients with bladder or prostate cancer should not be confused with true priapism.

Selected causes of ischemic priapism are listed in Table 55-1.

Indications

Attempt to identify reversible causes of low-flow priapism and initiate specific corrective therapy as soon as possible. Low-flow priapism in children and young adults may be due

TABLE 55-1 Selected Causes of Ischemic Priapism

CATEGORY	EXAMPLES
Medications	
Impotence agents	Intracavernosal therapies (prostaglandin E_1, papaverine, phentolamine)
	Oral agents (sildenafil)
Anticoagulants	Heparin, warfarin
Antihypertensives	Hydralazine, prazosin, doxazosin
Antidepressants	Trazodone, fluoxetine, sertraline, citalopram
Antipsychotics	Phenothiazines, atypical antipsychotics
Hormones	Gonadotropin-releasing hormones, testosterone
Illicit substances	Cocaine, marijuana, alcohol
Miscellaneous	Hydroxyzine, metoclopramide, omeprazole, total parenteral nutrition, general anesthetics
Hematologic/Oncologic Disorders	
Sickle cell disease	
Hematologic malignancies	Leukemia, myeloma
Other malignancies	Prostate, bladder, metastatic cancer
Central Nervous System	
Brain	Cerebrovascular accident
Brainstem	Medulla injury
Spinal cord	Spinal stenosis, spinal cord injury, lumbar disk herniation
Others	
Genitourinary trauma	Straddle injury
Infections	Malaria, rabies
Toxins	Black widow, scorpion, carbon monoxide
Metabolic	Amyloidosis, gout, hypertriglyceridemia
Idiopathic	

to sickle cell disease, and such cases may respond to noninvasive standard antisickling measures. However, the role of transfusion therapy in patients with priapism caused by sickle cell anemia is uncertain.[38]

Regardless of the etiology, treat this distressing condition first with adequate analgesia, such as parenteral opiates or benzodiazepines.

Treatment of ischemic priapism is frequently initiated in the ED. The classic teaching is that the initial treatment—oral or subcutaneous terbutaline—is the same regardless of the cause, but its utility is debated.[39-41] It is thought that terbutaline, a β_2-adrenergic agonist, increases venous outflow from the engorged corpora by relaxing venous sinusoidal smooth muscle. Terbutaline is of unproven benefit and is often ineffective; however, given its limited propensity for adverse effects, it is reasonable to initiate a trial in selected circumstances.[42]

If sedation, analgesia, and terbutaline fail to work rapidly, the next step in the treatment of priapism is intracorporal instillation of an α-adrenergic receptor agonist such as dilute phenylephrine or epinephrine. If this fails, one can proceed to penile blood aspiration and irrigation of the corpora cavernosa.

Contraindications

A subtype of ischemic priapism is known as *stuttering priapism*. This entity is typically observed in patients with sickle cell disease. Patients experience recurrent episodes of priapism that often last less than 3 hours and frequently do not require emergency treatment unless the symptoms become markedly prolonged.[43] High-flow (non-ischemic) priapism is treated surgically (nonurgent). Although perhaps intuitive treatment, transfusion therapy for acute priapism of sickle cell disease is controversial. *Exchange transfusion* has been associated with acute neurological events (headache, seizures, obtundation) that are thought to be due to a rapid elevation of hemoglobin (greater than 12 g/dL) and a release of procoagulant and vasoactive factors from the corpus carvernosa (ASPEN syndrome). *Partial exchange transfusion* (target hemoglobin less than 10 g/dL) has not been associated with these condition.

Procedure

A suggested algorithm for the initial treatment of acute nonischemic priapism in the emergency setting is presented in Box 55-1.

Minimally Invasive Technique—Simple Injection

Relief of priapism by simple injection of vasoactive solutions into the corpus cavernosum is a procedure that has been reported.[44] Intercavernous injection therapy for the management of priapism is simple to perform, less traumatic, and less invasive than aspiration and irrigation. This minimally invasive procedure may be attempted as an initial approach. The same procedure may be used as a self-injection technique for home treatment of recurrent priapism. With this technique, a 25- to 27-gauge needle (tuberculin or insulin syringe) is used to inject vasoactive substances into the corpus at the proximal end of the penis (2 to 4 cm distal to the origin of the shaft), with the goal of pharmacologically reversing the priapism (Fig. 55-5A). The principle is sympathomimetic-initiated contraction of the cavernous smooth muscle to permit venous outflow. Frequently, this small needle injection can be accomplished without anesthesia and is usually barely perceived by the patient. The most recommended technique is to inject 0.2 to 0.5 mg of phenylephrine into the corpus every 10 to 15 minutes to a maximum of four to five doses, although more frequent dosing has also been advocated. Use the lower dose in patients with cardiovascular pathology. Phenylephrine is

---

BOX 55-1 Suggested Algorithm for the Initial Treatment of Acute Priapism in the Emergency Department

Proceed with treatment of acute priapism in the following order until detumescence is achieved:

1. Parenteral narcotic analgesia/sedation.
2. Terbutaline, 0.25 to 0.5 mg subcutaneously (may be repeated in 15 minutes), or terbutaline, 5 mg orally (one dose only).
3. Intracorporal injection of adrenergic agents. May repeat every 20 minutes for a total of three doses.
4. If unsuccessful, perform corporal aspiration of 30 to 60 mL of blood, followed by observation. If detumescence is not achieved, irrigate (inject and remove 10- to 20-mL aliquots) with a diluted α-agonist solution (e.g., phenylephrine, 10 mg in 500 mL of normal saline, or 1 mg epinephrine in 1 L of normal saline). Multiple irrigations may be required. The initial aspiration removes venous blood (dark red), and return of arterial blood (bright red) may serve as a marker of success.
5. For persistent erections, consult urology for possible corpus cavernosum-spongiosum shunt placement.
6. If treatment is successful in the emergency department, discharge is possible. A 3-day course of an oral α-adrenergic agent such as pseudoephedrine to promote continued vasoconstriction is recommended. The value of this intervention is unproven, however.
7. For patients with recurrent priapism secondary to sickle cell disease, consider intramuscular injections of leuprolide (Lupron) (consult a hematologist for recommended doses).

---

available as a 1% solution (10 mg/mL), which *must be diluted for this procedure*. If 1 mL (10 mg) of the 1% solution of phenylephrine is added to 9 mL of saline, the final phenylephrine concentration is 1 mg/mL. Then withdraw 0.2 mL (0.2 mg) or 0.5 mL (0.5 mg) of this diluted solution with a tuberculin or insulin syringe and add saline to increase the final volume for injection to 1 mL. Phenylephrine is preferred by the American Urologic Society because of minimal cardiovascular side effects. An alternative, readily available injection solution is a mixture of epinephrine and saline. Draw up 0.1 mg of epinephrine (0.1 mL of 1:1000) in a tuberculin or insulin syringe and dilute it with 0.9 mL of saline (total volume of 1 mL). *Systemic effects, such as hypertension, headache, tremors, and cardiac arrhythmias, are potential side effects of any sympathomimetic injection, so caution is advised, especially if multiple injections are used in a semi-erectile state.*

Puncture the corpus with the needle at the 10- or 2-o'clock position at the base of the penis (with 12 o'clock being the dorsal vein of the penis). Aspirate blood to confirm the correct position, and then inject the solution. If not successful in 20 to 30 minutes, repeat the injection up to a total of three injections. In one small study, successful detumescence was achieved in eight of nine patients by simple intracorporal injection of phenylephrine via this regimen, and three or fewer injections were required.[45] Only one side needs to be injected. Two or three injections might be necessary. Wait at least 20 minutes after each injection before trying additional interventions. *Note that this is essentially an intravenous injection and systemic effects may occur, especially if partial detumescence has been achieved. Accordingly, proceed with caution in patients*

MANAGEMENT OF ACUTE PRIAPISM

A. Minimally Invasive Method

10-o'clock approach   2-o'clock approach

- Anesthesia is not required. Use a small-gauge needle to inject a small aliquot of an adrenergic agent into the corpus at 10 or 2 o'clock at the proximal end of the penile shaft. (Only one side need be injected.)
- Aspirate blood *(2)* to confirm placement prior to injection.
- Consider a repeated injection after 20 minutes if unsuccessful, but be wary of the systemic effects of adrenergic agents (especially if repeated doses or injections are given during partial detumescence).
  Maximum: 3 to 5 doses, 10 to 30 minutes apart

ADRENERGIC AGENTS
- 0.2 to 0.5 mg of phenylephrine per dose (refer to text for instructions on dilution)
- 0.1 mg of epinephrine (0.1 mL of a 1:1000 solution) mixed with 0.9 mL of saline

(Use a 1-mL tuberculin syringe to draw up these small volumes.)

B. Aspiration and Irrigation Method

This patient experienced 18 hours of priapism after penile self-injection of papaverine as therapy for impotence.

For corpus irrigation the irrigation needle can be placed through a simple skin wheal, or peform a penile dorsal nerve block by injecting 1% plain lidocaine at the base of the dorsal aspect of the penis. The dorsal nerves are relatively superficial and deep injections are not required.

Insert no smaller than a 19-gauge butterfly needle into the corpus via the proximal penile shaft at either the 2-o'clock or the 10-o'clock position and aspirate. Only one side need be punctured. Slow steady suction will be most successful, whereas excessive suction may halt the aspiration. Do not puncture the corpus via the glans (see text). After initial aspiration, irrigate (slowly inject and withdraw) 10 to 20-mL aliquots of vasoactive solution until detumescence persists.

After detumescence with the first aspiration or with aspiration-irrigation-aspiration of a vasoactive medication (see text), wrap the penis with an elastic bandage to discourage reengorgement and to compress the puncture site. *Note*: Acceptable procedures include aspiration alone followed by instillation of a small aliquot of epinephrine (0.1 mg) and combined multiple aspirations and irrigations with a vasoactive solution. The end point is the appearance of bright red arterial blood and/or persistent detumescence.

Figure 55-5 Management of acute priapism. The minimally invasive technique (**A**) is often successful and can be used at home by a motivated patient with recurrent problems (such as sickle cell disease).

Table 55-2 Adrenergic Agents Used for Intracavernous Injections

AGENT	DOSE	VOLUME
Phenylephrine*	0.2-0.5 mg	Dilute with saline; final volume, 1 mL*
Epinephrine (1:1000)	0.1 mg (0.1 mL)	Dilute with 0.9 mL saline; final volume, 1 mL
Lidocaine (2%) with epinephrine (1:100,000) (local anesthetic solution)	40 mg lidocaine 0.02 mg epinephrine (2 mL)	1 mL injected into each side of the corpus cavernosum; final volume, 2 mL†

From Roberts JR, Price C, Mazzeo T. Intracavernous epinephrine: a minimally invasive treatment for priapism in the emergency department. *J Emerg Med.* 2009;36:3:285-289.
*Single side injected with the entire amount. See text for preparation of the phenylephrine injection solution.
†Total amount divided into two doses. Inject each side with half the total volume (1 mL) or inject the total volume (2 mL) into one side.

BOX 55-2 **Equipment Needed for Aspiration of the Corpus Cavernosum for Low-Flow Priapism**

27-gauge needle (for penile block)
1-mL syringe (for local anesthetic)
1% lidocaine without epinephrine (for penile block)
Sterile drapes
Gauze sponges
Chlorhexidine preparation solution
19-gauge butterfly needles (for aspiration)
Two 10-mL to 30-mL syringes (for aspiration)
Sterile basin for aspirated blood
Blood gas syringe with cap
Irrigation fluid (one of the following vasoactive agents* is diluted with 500 mL of normal saline and up to 20 to 30 mL is administered in small aliquots; 5000 units of heparin added to the solution is optional)
Phenylephrine, 10 mg/500 mL of saline
Norepinephrine, 1 mg/500 mL of saline
Epinephrine, 0.5 mg/500 mL of saline

Systemic absorption of vasoactive agents may occur and result in adverse cardiovascular effects.

Figure 55-6 An 18-gauge dialysis access catheter can be used for irrigation of the corpora if simple aspiration or injections of medication are unsuccessful. Using needles smaller than 19-gauge is usually counterproductive.

with cardiovascular disease. Success has also been noted by injecting the corpus cavernosum with 1 mL of the local anesthetic lidocaine (2%) with epinephrine (1:100,000) into each side or 2 mL into one side.[44]

Table 55-2 lists adrenergic agents used for intracavernosal injections.

Aspiration/Irrigation Technique

If injection is unsuccessful or if the erection has persisted for more than 4 to 6 hours, aspiration of blood from the corpus cavernosum, with or without irrigation, is performed. This is usually combined with an intracavernosal injection of a sympathomimetic drug. Box 55-2 lists the equipment needed for aspiration and irrigation of the corpus cavernosum. This procedure entails drainage of blood from the erect penis, irrigation with saline if necessary (i.e., inadequate return of blood with lack of detumescence), and finally, instillation of a vasoactive medication. As an alternative to instillation of a sympathomimetic drug, irrigation with aliquots of a *dilute* vasoactive solution (1 mg of epinephrine added to 1 L of saline) may be effective (aspirate-infuse-aspirate cycle as needed).

Place the patient in the supine position. Use parenteral analgesia and sedation. Local anesthesia is recommended and may be achieved with a generous local wheal of lidocaine injected at the puncture site but is best obtained with a penile nerve block (Fig. 55-5B, *step 2*). Perform the block by injecting 1% plain lidocaine at the base of the dorsal and ventral surface of the penis for a dorsal penile nerve block, or place a circumferential penile block. The nerves are relatively superficial and deep injections are not required. Prepare and drape the penis in sterile fashion. Grasp the shaft of the penis with the nondominant thumb and index finger. Palpate the engorged corpus cavernosum laterally (2- and 10-o'clock positions), and insert a 19-gauge butterfly needle into the corpus cavernosum (see Fig. 55-5B, *step 3*).[46] A dialysis access butterfly needle may also be used (Fig. 55-6). Small butterfly needles and standard intravenous catheters are not ideally suited for the procedure but may be used. If palpation fails to identify the corpus, blindly insert the needle at either 10 or 2 o'clock to gain access to this large vascular structure. Because there is communication of blood flow between both sides, only one of the corpora needs to be aspirated or irrigated. Either side may be punctured. The site of needle placement is typically anywhere from the base to the proximal end of the shaft, approximately 2 to 4 cm distal to its origin. *Do not use the glans as a puncture site.*

Advance the needle at a 45-degree angle while suctioning constantly. *Blood is usually readily aspirated.* Once blood is obtained, do not advance the needle further, but stabilize it. Avoid deep penetration to minimize the risk for injury to the cavernosal artery during the procedure.

Aspirate corporal blood while milking the corpus with the nondominant hand. Do not apply excessive suction because this often halts the aspiration. A common error is to use too much suction when aspirating with a 60-mL syringe. Preferably, use a 10-mL syringe and change it when it fills with blood. Using a butterfly needle reduces the danger of dislodging the needle during syringe changes.

Continue aspirating until the original egress of dark blood ceases and bright red arterial blood returns or until complete detumescence is achieved and remains that way. Because multiple anastomoses exist between the two corpora cavernosa, there is no need to aspirate bilaterally. If return of blood is inadequate with lack of detumescence, consider irrigating with 20- to 30-mL aliquots of saline, with or without a sympathomimetic agent.

If detumescence is achieved and maintained after initial aspiration, no further treatment may be necessary. Even if this is successful, some advise instilling an aliquot of a vasoactive substance. Phenylephrine is recommended as the agent of choice because it may minimize the risk for cardiovascular side effects that are caused by the more common sympathomimetic agents.[41] Inject 0.2 to 0.5 mg of phenylephrine (diluted in 1 mL of normal saline). The concentration recommended for instillation is similar to that suggested for the *minimally invasive technique* detailed earlier. Use lower concentrations in smaller volumes for patients with cardiovascular risk factors or for children. *If irrigation has been performed with a dilute vasoactive substance as delineated below, additional instillation of medication is not suggested.*

If aspiration alone does not result in detumescence, irrigation with a dilute vasoactive substance is another option. A number of dilute irrigation solutions have been suggested, but none has proved to be superior. Some suggest injecting 20 to 30 mL of a phenylephrine and normal saline solution (10 mg of phenylephrine in 500 mL of normal saline) as the exchange for 20 to 30 mL of aspirated corporal blood. Some clinicians add 2500 to 5000 units of heparin to the solution, but the use of heparin is of unproven value. Alternatively, 1 mg of epinephrine can be added to 1 L of saline, with irrigation performed with 20- to 30-mL aliquots. It is important to note that corporal irrigation is performed with a much less concentrated solution (phenylephrine, 20 μg/mL) than that used for the *minimally invasive technique.*

Note that the corpus cavernosum has ready access to the systemic circulation and that injecting a drug into it is essentially the same as an intravenous injection. When detumescence occurs, the unmetabolized drug enters the systemic circulation, so vasoactive drug dosages should be monitored carefully.

Aftercare

Observe the patient in the ED for recurrence. Although the ideal observation period is unknown, 2 hours has been suggested.[44] Figure 55-5*B*, *step 4*, demonstrates the entire penis loosely wrapped with an elastic (Ace) bandage to prevent hematoma formation at the injection site or sites. Provide strict return precautions for recurrence of priapism, and ensure that urgent urology follow-up is possible. A short course of an oral α-adrenergic agent, such as pseudoephed-

rine for 3 days, is often recommended.[44] However, this intervention is of questionable value and unproven benefit.

Complications

Although hematoma and infection can occur after properly performed aspiration, these complications are infrequent. Injected or instilled vasoactive agents can be absorbed systemically, with potential toxic effects.[47] Therefore, the intracavernosal use of vasoactive agents is relatively contraindicated in patients with conditions that are sensitive to these agents (e.g., severe hypertension, dysrhythmias, monoamine oxidase inhibitor use). Monitor blood pressure and cardiac rhythm throughout the procedure if the patient is at risk. Failure to aspirate blood is a potential complication, usually because of a misplaced needle, application of excessive suction, or clotted blood. Because impotence is a well-recognized complication of priapism regardless of the cause or promptness of therapeutic intervention, advise the patient regarding this potential complication.

If patients do not respond to repeated cavernous aspiration and α-agonist therapy, shunt surgery is the next treatment option. Regardless of the intervention, prolonged priapism or recurrent priapism may lead to permanent erectile dysfunction. The exact parameters under which permanent dysfunction occurs have not been proved or characterized.

Conclusion

Because prolonged priapism increases the risk for subsequent erectile dysfunction, an aggressive management strategy is advised. After 4 hours of persistent priapism there is heightened release of inflammatory cytokines in the acidotic and hypoxic corpora cavernosa. Inflammation may result in changes in smooth muscle, including cell death and fibrosis, which may cause permanent erectile dysfunction.[48] Recurrence is not uncommon, and some patients require multiple procedures on a recurring basis. Surgical shunting procedures might be required if these other measures are not met with success.

PARAPHIMOSIS

Paraphimosis is the inability to completely reduce the penile foreskin distally, back to its natural position overlying the glans penis. This condition occurs exclusively in uncircumcised males and is a urologic emergency.

Paraphimosis may occur at any age but is often seen in the extremes of life (Fig. 55-7). The condition can be quite subtle and may be either unrecognized or misdiagnosed as an allergic reaction, penile trauma, infection, or edema resulting from systemic volume overload (i.e., congestive heart failure, nephrotic syndrome) (Fig. 55-8).

Iatrogenic paraphimosis may occur following urinary catheterization or medical examination if the foreskin is not returned to its native location overlying the glans. Poor hygiene or balanoposthitis is also associated with the development of paraphimosis. Inflammation can result in contracture of the distal part of the foreskin. Later, when the foreskin is retracted proximally over the compressible glans, the retracted foreskin forms a constrictive band and gets stuck in the retracted position.

Figure 55-7 Paraphimosis often occurs in the extremes of life. **A,** Uncircumcised boy with paraphimosis. This may be mistaken for infection or localized trauma, especially if it is unclear whether circumcision has been performed. Always seek this history. **B,** Paraphimosis, pictured here, may be mistaken for penile trauma, angioedema, or infection. Note that the swollen tissue is proximal to the coronal sulcus (*asterisk*). The cause of paraphimosis in this case was failure to replace the foreskin after a catheter change in an uncircumcised nursing home patient. Before reduction, the catheter is usually removed. When the edema is minimal, the catheter may be left in place during reduction. **C,** Appearance of the penis after catheter removal and foreskin reduction.

Figure 55-8 A, This edematous foreskin may have numerous causes, from benign edema to paraphimosis, and at first glance the cause might not be obvious. This patient has paraphimosis that is appreciated by careful inspection to identify the normal coronal sulcus (**B**) and a phimotic foreskin band proximal to the glans (**C**).

Background

Paraphimosis is a urologic emergency that must be treated promptly to prevent necrosis of the glans. It can frequently be managed in the ED without the need for emergency specialty consultation. Many methods for successful reduction of paraphimosis have been reported; however, the most commonly used initial maneuver involves manual compression of the distal end of the glans penis to decrease edema, followed by reduction of the glans penis back through the proximal constricting band of foreskin.[49]

Anatomy and Physiology

The penis consists of the paired corpora cavernosa, or erectile bodies, which lie dorsal to the corpus spongiosum (see Fig. 55-4). The corpus spongiosum surrounds the penile urethra. The corpora cavernosa and the corpus spongiosum are wrapped in a thin connective tissue layer called the tunica albuginea. The glans is the distal head of the penis. The distal foreskin, or prepuce, in uncircumcised males lies over the

glans and can be retracted proximally to expose the glans. The coronal sulcus distinguishes the glans penis from the penile shaft (see Figs. 55-7*B* and 55-8*B*).

Pathophysiology

Patients will have a red, painful, and swollen glans penis associated with an edematous, proximally retracted foreskin that forms a circumferential constricting band. The normal anatomy and identification of the foreskin may be obfuscated by edema, and the condition can be asymmetric and rather bizarre appearing (Fig. 55-9, *step 1*). The penile shaft proximal to the constricting band is typically soft. The entrapped foreskin forms a constricting band on the penile shaft. Compression inhibits venous drainage of the glans, sulcus, and distal part of the foreskin itself and results in a vicious circle of progressive glans and foreskin edema that may further prevent reduction of the foreskin to its natural position. The edema may become so severe that arterial flow is compromised, which can result in necrosis and gangrene of the glans penis.

PARAPHIMOSIS REDUCTION

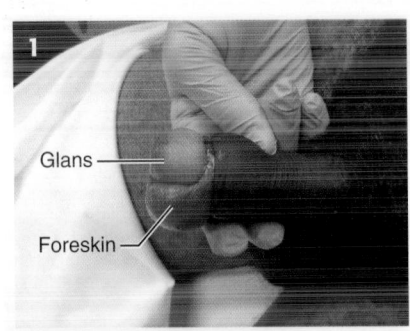

This patient had asymmetric paraphimosis. Note that the glans is edematous, as is the foreskin. A circumferential constricting band is found proximal to the glans and foreskin.

Perform a penile block in cases that will require significant manipulation. First, block the dorsal penile nerves by depositing anesthetic at the 2- and 10-o'clock positions on the dorsal aspect of the shaft of the penis.

Complete a ring block of the penis by depositing anesthetic circumferentially around the proximal part of the shaft.

Compress the foreskin and glans by grasping it with the palm of your hand and applying pressure for several minutes.

Alternatively, wrap an elastic bandage around the distal end of the penis for several minutes. This step is often omitted, which makes the procedure unnecessarily difficult.

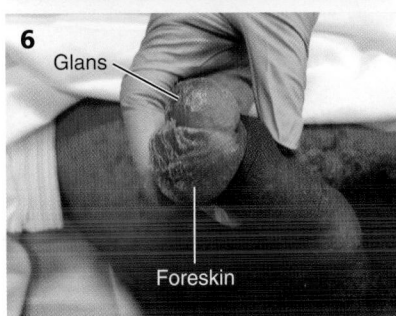

Note that manual compression substantially reduced the amount of swelling (compare with *step 1*; the foreskin and glans were taut prior to compression).

Grasp the shaft of the penis with one hand and apply force onto the urethral meatus with the thumb of your other hand. Push the glans forward while sliding the foreskin distally.

Alternatively, grasp the penis with the fingers of both hands just proximal to the phimotic ring, and use your thumbs to apply constant pressure on the glans.

The key to success is the application of slow, steady pressure. Note that the glans has retracted into its normal position and only the edematous foreskin is visible.

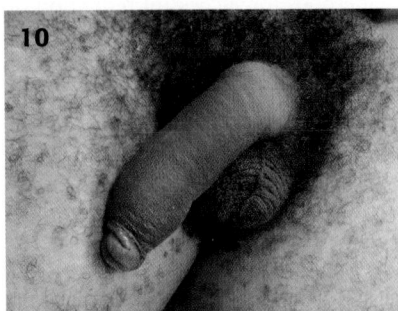

Successful reduction results in the appearance of an uncircumcised penis with a phimotic foreskin.

Figure 55-9 Paraphimosis reduction. (*Step 8, from Neuwirth H, Frasier B, Cochran ST. Genitourinary imaging and procedures by the emergency clinician.* Emerg Med Clin North Am. *1989;7:1.)*

Indications

Emergency reduction of a paraphimotic foreskin is indicated whenever the condition exists.

Contraindications

There are no contraindications.

Procedure

Manual Reduction Technique

The current standard for reducing paraphimosis is manual reduction. It can be facilitated by applying a nonirritating topical anesthetic lubricant onto the inner surface of the foreskin (not the shaft of the penis) and the glans to reduce friction and decrease the discomfort of the procedure. A dorsal and ventral penile block should be performed in cases that require significant manipulation (see Fig. 55-9, *steps 2 and 3*). If significant discomfort or patient apprehension is present, systemic analgesia or procedural sedation may be useful adjuncts. For young children, general anesthesia may be necessary.[50]

Compress the foreskin and glans by snugly grasping it with the palm of the hand and apply pressure for several minutes, or wrap an elastic bandage around the distal end of the penis to reduce as much edema fluid as possible (see Fig. 55-9, *steps 4 and 5*).[51] Compression is often omitted and makes the procedure more difficult. A significant amount of edema can be alleviated with simple compression (see Fig. 55-9, *step 6*). Place the index and long fingers of both hands in apposition just proximal to the phimotic ring. Align both thumbs on the urethral meatus and apply constant force. Use the thumbs to invert the glans penis proximally, and use the index and long fingers to attempt to reduce the phimotic ring distally over the glans penis into its normal anatomic position (see Fig. 55-9, *step 8*). Successful reduction results in the appearance of an uncircumcised penis with a phimotic foreskin (see Fig. 55-9, *steps 9 and 10*). Alternatively, use the thumb to push the glans through the foreskin that is encircled by the entire palm (see Fig. 55-9, *step 7*). The key to success in both these maneuvers is the application of slow, steady pressure.

Adjunctive Techniques to Assist in Manual Reduction

Several alternative methods for reducing the edema before attempting manual reduction or if simple manual reduction fails have been described in the literature.

Use Babcock clamps (noncrushing tissue clamps) to reduce the paraphimotic foreskin (Fig. 55-10*A*).[52] Apply six to eight Babcock clamps spaced evenly around the foreskin and straddling the phimotic ring (one edge just proximal and the other edge just distal to the phimotic ring). Grasp all the clamps and apply simultaneous distal traction to pull the phimotic ring over the glans. After reduction, remove the clamps. It is important to inspect the foreskin afterward for injury.

Other techniques focus on reduction of glans or foreskin edema (or both), followed by reduction of the paraphimosis. Diminished glans edema may allow the edematous foreskin to be reduced distally to its natural position. A suggested maneuver involves the application of an ice pack. In the "iced-glove" method, cold compression is used to reduce foreskin swelling and induce vasoconstriction in the glans penis (see Fig. 55-10*B*).[53] Fill a large glove halfway with crushed ice and

water, and tie the cuff end securely. Invaginate the thumb of the glove and then draw it over the lubricated paraphimotic penis. Hold the thumb of the glove securely in place over the glans for 5 to 10 minutes. The combination of cooling and compression usually decreases the edema sufficiently to permit manual reduction of the foreskin. Wrapping the glans (and penis) in a compressive bandage is another option.[51]

Alternatively, techniques focusing on reduction of foreskin edema have been advocated (Box 55-3). Though not usually pursued in the ED, they will be included for completeness. The Dundee technique involves making multiple micropunctures in the edematous foreskin and then squeezing out the edema fluid.[54] Hyaluronidase has been reported to result in rapid reduction of prepuce edema to facilitate manual reduction of the foreskin. This enzyme, when injected into the swollen retracted foreskin, causes hydrolysis of hyaluronic acid, which in turn increases tissue permeability so that the edema in the foreskin is diffused out into the surrounding tissue of the penis.[55] There have even been advocates of a noninvasive way to reduce the foreskin edema via the application of granulated sugar to the penis. Sugar forms an osmotic gradient that draws out the fluid with reduction of the edema, but this may take several hours.[56] Publications on these alternative procedures are generally observational in design with very small numbers. To date, there have not been any large studies of comparative effectiveness; consequently, it is difficult to recommend any one method as being superior to the others.[57]

If the aforementioned methods are unsuccessful, it may be necessary to incise the constricting phimotic tissue to permit reduction of the foreskin over the glans (dorsal slit procedure).[58,59] In adults, this can generally be carried out under penile block anesthesia, but procedural sedation or general anesthesia may be necessary for young children.

Aftercare

Observe the patient to ensure adequate local hemostasis, ability to void spontaneously, and recovery from analgesia or sedation, if administered. Replacing the foreskin to its native position following examination, catheter placement, sexual activity, or any other manipulation is essential to prevent recurrent episodes. Patients should be referred to a urologist for evaluation of possible surgical options, including circumcision.

Complications

Penile shaft laceration or simple tearing of compromised penile skin may occur during manual or surgical paraphimotic reduction. Simple suturing will resolve most injuries. If reduction of paraphimosis cannot be achieved with other means, surgical intervention should be considered, including the dorsal slit procedure.

Conclusion

Emergency manual or surgical reduction of the edematous foreskin is mandatory to restore proper circulation, relieve discomfort, and permit resolution of potential serious sequelae: skin ulceration and gangrene. It must be done as soon as paraphimosis is recognized. Once the foreskin is successfully reduced, urgent referral for a dorsal slit procedure or definitive circumcision is necessary.

PARAPHIMOSIS REDUCTION: ALTERNATIVE TECHNIQUES

A. Babcock Clamps

Babcock clamps will not crush tissue. *1,* Place 6 to 8 clamps so that they are evenly spaced on the distal edge of the foreskin and straddling the phimotic ring. *2,* Grasp all clamps and apply simultaneous distal traction to pull the phimotic ring over the glans.

B. Iced-Glove Method

Fill a large glove halfway with crushed ice and water.

Securely tie the cuff end, and invaginate the thumb of the glove.

Draw the invagination over the lubricated paraphimotic penis, and hold it in place for 5 to 10 minutes. The combination of cooling and compression decreases edema and facilitates foreskin reduction.

Figure 55-10 Paraphimosis reduction: alternative techniques.

BOX 55-3 | **Adjunctive Methods to Reduce Foreskin Edema**

Dundee micropuncture technique: Make approximately 20 puncture holes in the edematous foreskin tissue with a 26-gauge (or similar) needle and express the fluid.[54]

Hyaluronidase technique: Inject 1 mL of hyaluronidase (150 U/mL) by tuberculin syringe into one or two sites in the edematous foreskin to reduce edema fluid immediately.[55]

Sugar technique: Granulated sugar has been studied, but a better alternative for patients in the emergency department is to soak a swab in 50 mL of 50% dextrose solution and leave it wrapped around the paraphimotic foreskin for 1 hour.[56]

Iced-glove technique: see Figure 55-10*B*.

PHIMOSIS

Phimosis is constriction of the foreskin (or prepuce) that limits its retraction proximally over the glans (Fig. 55-11). Uncircumcised infants and young children often have physiologic phimosis secondary to adhesions between the prepuce and glans. This is in contrast to pathologic phimosis,

where failure to retract results from distal scarring of the prepuce.

Circumcision, or removal of the foreskin that renders phimosis and paraphimosis (described earlier) anatomically impossible, is commonplace in America. However, circumcision rates vary depending on socioeconomic status, religious affiliation, and racial and ethnic group.

Phimosis does not ordinarily require any treatment, but it may be seen acutely in the ED when a patient is unable to void spontaneously as a result of distal urethral obstruction. It may prevent or make urethral catheterization more challenging. In such situations the phimotic opening may need to be dilated. An alternative strategy is to crush a portion of the foreskin followed by an incision (dorsal slit) under local anesthesia (with or without parenteral analgesia or sedation) to allow access to the urethral meatus. This minor operative procedure can readily be performed in the acute care setting when necessary.

Anatomy and Physiology

Physiologic phimosis consists of a pliant, unscarred preputial orifice on physical examination. The foreskin gradually becomes retractile over time as a result of intermittent

Figure 55-11 Phimosis is constriction of the foreskin that inhibits retraction over the glans. Ordinarily, treatment is not required; however, dilation of the phimotic opening may be required if the patient is unable to void or if urethral catheterization must be performed. *(From Studdiford JS, Altshuler M, Salzman B, et al, eds.* Images from the Wards: Diagnosis and Treatment. *Philadelphia: Saunders; 2009.)*

erections and keratinization of the inner epithelium. By 3 years of age, 90% of glans can easily be retracted, with nearly all becoming retractile by late adolescence.[60,61]

Pathophysiology

Pathologic phimosis exists when failure to retract results from distal scarring of the prepuce. This is typically a subacute condition that may be encountered acutely in the ED when a patient is unable to void spontaneously as a result of distal urethral obstruction. Pathologic phimosis is caused by local trauma, infection, chemical irritation, complications of circumcision (insufficient removal of tissue), or poor hygiene.

Patients with acute phimosis complain of penile pain lasting hours to days. On physical examination the physician will discover a tender foreskin that is not easily retracted. Even though the prepuce may be gently manipulated to allow a better examination, do not attempt forced retraction. Forceful retraction contributes to future adhesion and stricture formation.

Indications

Dorsal slit of the foreskin is performed in any emergency situation either to gain access to the urethral meatus for urethral catheterization or as definitive treatment after simple foreskin reduction or incision of the phimotic ring and reduction of the foreskin in a patient with paraphimosis. Elective circumcision rather than dorsal slit of the foreskin is the definitive procedure of choice in nonemergency situations.

Contraindications

There are no contraindications.

Procedure

Box 55-4 lists the equipment needed to perform a dorsal slit of the foreskin. With the patient in the supine position, clean and drape the penis with sterile towels. Clipping of pubic hair is unnecessary. Then infiltrate 1% *plain lidocaine without epinephrine* into the dorsal midline of the foreskin just beneath the superficial fascia throughout the course of the proposed incision, starting proximally at the level of the coronal sulcus

---

BOX 55-4   Equipment Necessary for the Dorsal Slit Procedure

1% lidocaine without epinephrine
5-mL syringe
27-gauge needle
1 straight Crile clamp
1 straight scissors
1 needle holder
4-0 absorbable suture

---

and proceeding distally to the tip of the foreskin (Fig. 55-12, *step 1*). Consider mixing equal volumes of 1% lidocaine with 0.5% bupivacaine. After 3 to 5 minutes, grasp the foreskin with toothed forceps to test for anesthesia. Be certain that the inner surface of the foreskin is also anesthetized. If this area is not numb, use a dorsal nerve block or "ring block" at the base of the penis (Fig. 55-13).[62]

After achieving both adequate local anesthesia and systemic analgesia (or procedural sedation if needed), take a straight hemostat and carefully advance both jaws of the hemostat proximally to the area of the coronal sulcus between the inner layer of the foreskin and the smooth glans penis and carefully separate any existing preputial adhesions (see Fig. 55-12, *step 2*). Take care to visualize or palpate the meatus and urethra at all times to avoid inadvertent injury during this maneuver. Once release of adhesions is complete, open the hemostat and place one jaw in the recently developed plane between the glans penis, opened to tent the skin and ensure proper placement, and the superior overlying inner layer of foreskin. Advance the hemostat to the level of the coronal sulcus and then close it, thereby effectively crushing the interposed anesthetized foreskin. Leave the closed hemostat in place for 3 to 5 minutes, and then remove it and cut the resultant serrated crushed foreskin longitudinally with straight scissors throughout the extent of the crushed tissue.

Normally, the incised, anatomically approximated skin edges bleed and ooze. Not infrequently, these skin edges of the foreskin separate into two layers, the outer foreskin and the inner foreskin (see Fig. 55-12, *step 3*). Two absorbable chromic or Vicryl (4-0 to 5-0 for children and 3-0 to 4-0 for adults) running hemostatic sutures may be placed, each beginning proximally at the apex of the dorsal slit and carried distally, to reapproximate the two leaves of foreskin. Standard antibiotic ointment may be used to lubricate the suture material and facilitate passage of suture through the delicate skin tissue.

After successful dorsal slit of the foreskin, the prepuce is easily retracted for cleansing the glans penis or exposure of the urethral meatus. To avoid iatrogenic paraphimosis, reduce the foreskin to its normal anatomic position after any distal penile procedure.

If reduction of *paraphimosis* cannot be achieved with other means, consider surgical interventions. Figure 55-14 describes the dorsal slit procedure, which involves carefully sterilizing the field, anesthetizing the penis on the dorsal aspect, and then making a linear incision.

Aftercare

Ideally, definitive elective circumcision is recommended after a dorsal slit procedure. Some patients complain about the

DORSAL SLIT (PHIMOSIS TREATMENT)

— Skin wheal at the sulcus; then infiltration along the proposed dorsal slit to the phimotic opening (*arrow*)

— Foreskin over the coronal dorsal slit

— Line of the proposed dorsal slit

— Phimotic opening in the foreskin

1. Infiltrate plain lidocaine without epinephrine into the dorsal midline of the foreskin just beneath the superficial fascia throughout the course of the planned incision. Begin at the coronal sulcus and proceed distally to the tip of the foreskin. Alternatively, consider a dorsal nerve block or ring block of the penis (see Fig. 55-13).

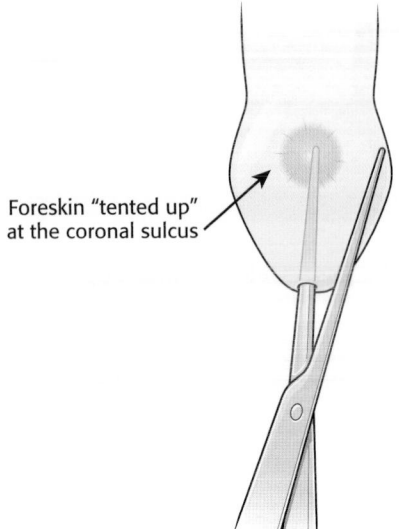

Foreskin "tented up" at the coronal sulcus

2. Insert both jaws of the hemostat proximally to the level of the coronal sulcus and carefully separate any adhesions. Remove the hemostat, then reinsert only one jaw, and advance again to the coronal sulcus. Close the instrument and crush the foreskin. Leave the hemostat in place for 3 to 5 minutes. Remove the hemostat then use straight scissors to cut along the crushed tissue.

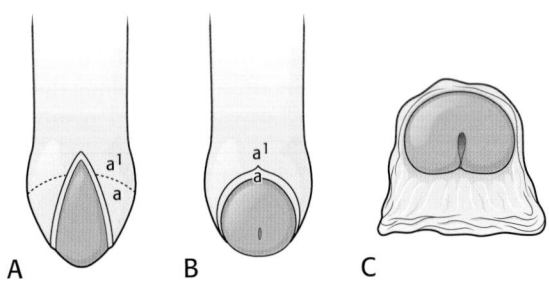

3. *A,* Use straight scissors to cut along the crushed tissue. The exposed glans is shaded. (*a¹,* outer layer of the foreskin; *a,* inner layer of the foreskin). *B,* Retract the cut edges of the foreskin drawn back around the glans penis. If hemostasis is required, first suture *a¹* to *a* and then sew the remainder of the cut edges together. *C,* The ventral transposed foreskin will assume a "beagle-ear" deformity after the dorsal slit procedure has been completed.

4. Postoperative appearance of the dorsal slit showing the "beagle ear." A formal, complete circumcision can be performed after the inflammation has resolved, if desired.

Figure 55-12 Dorsal slit treatment of phimosis.

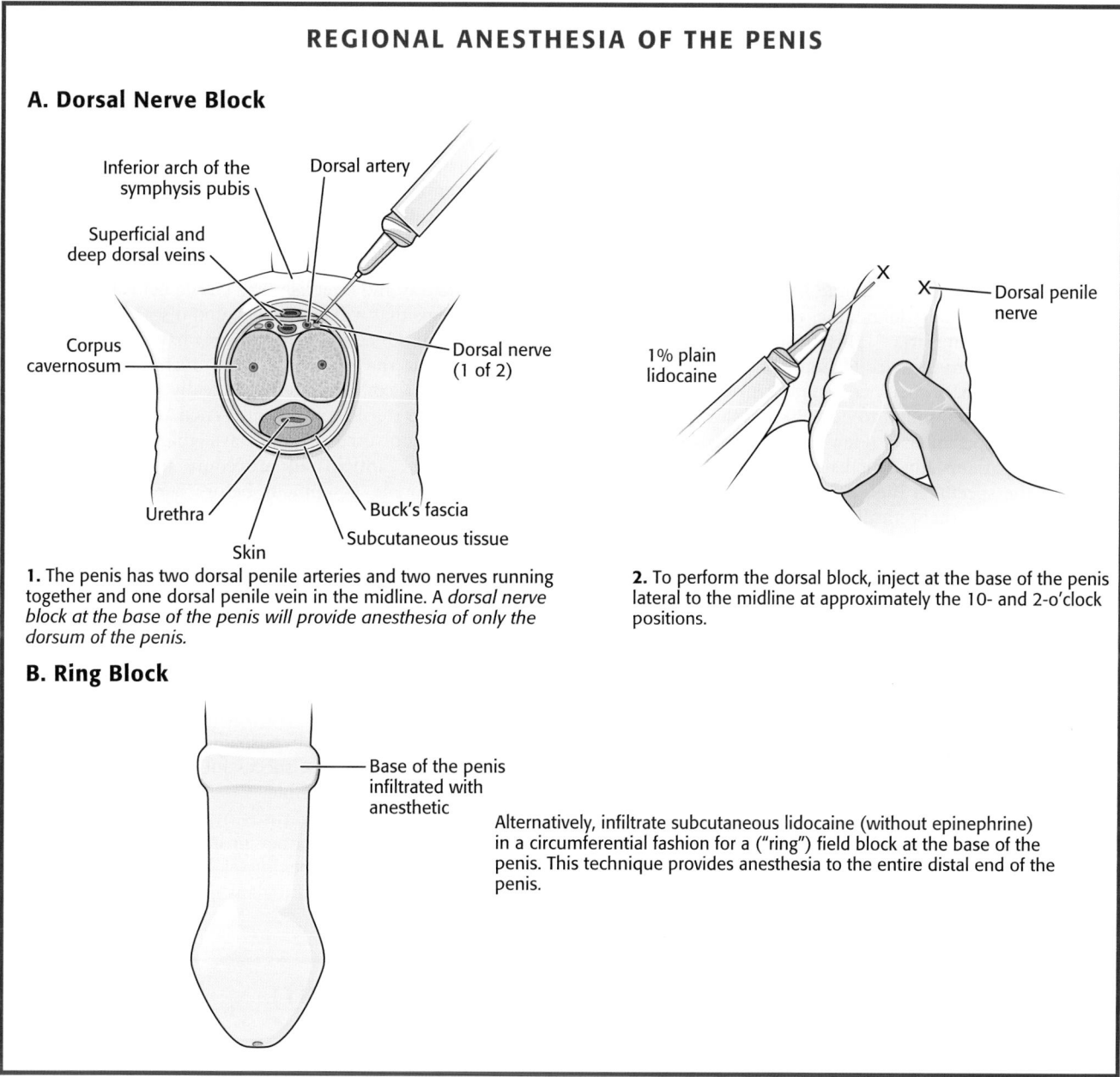

REGIONAL ANESTHESIA OF THE PENIS

A. Dorsal Nerve Block

Inferior arch of the symphysis pubis
Dorsal artery
Superficial and deep dorsal veins
Corpus cavernosum
Dorsal nerve (1 of 2)
Urethra
Buck's fascia
Subcutaneous tissue
Skin

1% plain lidocaine
Dorsal penile nerve

1. The penis has two dorsal penile arteries and two nerves running together and one dorsal penile vein in the midline. A *dorsal nerve block at the base of the penis will provide anesthesia of only the dorsum of the penis.*

2. To perform the dorsal block, inject at the base of the penis lateral to the midline at approximately the 10- and 2-o'clock positions.

B. Ring Block

Base of the penis infiltrated with anesthetic

Alternatively, infiltrate subcutaneous lidocaine (without epinephrine) in a circumferential fashion for a ("ring") field block at the base of the penis. This technique provides anesthesia to the entire distal end of the penis.

Figure 55-13 Regional anesthesia of the penis. Consider the use of supplemental intravenous analgesia or procedural sedation, or both, based on the clinical scenario. (*A1, From Soliman MG, Tremblay NA. Nerve block of the penis for postoperative pain relief in children. Anesth Analg. 1978;57:495. Reproduced by permission.*)

appearance of their incised foreskin ("dog-ears") and the relative inconvenience during urination, whereas others are pleased that they no longer have their phimosis and decline further operative intervention.

Complications

The urethral meatus and glans penis may be injured if the hemostat or straight scissors are blindly and unknowingly introduced into the urethra. Bleeding may occur if the hemostat has not adequately crushed the foreskin or the scissors incision is made lateral to the serrated crushed tissue. The latter two problems are easily resolved with the previously described running hemostatic suture.

Conclusion

Dorsal slit of the foreskin is performed in any emergency situation either to gain access to the urethral meatus for urethral catheterization or as definitive treatment after simple foreskin reduction or incision of the phimotic ring and reduction of the foreskin in a patient with paraphimosis. This minor operative procedure can readily be performed in the acute care setting when necessary.

URETHRAL CATHETERIZATION

Urethral catheterization seems to be a simple task—insertion of one tube into a larger tube. Nonetheless, many difficulties arise. Patients often remember catheterization as either painful or uneventful, depending on the operator's expertise, confidence, and gentleness.

The merits of various approaches to collection of urine specimens depend on the patient's age and the clinical setting.

Urethral catheterization is definitive and routinely used to collect urine for analysis and culture in infants and young children who are not yet potty-trained. For older children who can follow directions, midstream urine collection is a reasonable alternative approach to urethral catheterization for collection of specimens.

In adult men without anatomic lesions, first-voided midstream specimens can define the presence or absence of culture-proven bacteriuria.[63] This certainly represents a user-friendly approach to urine collection in a busy ED setting.

In adult women, properly collected clean-catch midstream specimens have been found to be as bacteriologically reliable as catheterized specimens.[64] A few caveats are worth mentioning. Ideally, patients must sit backward on the toilet when collecting the specimen (i.e., patient facing the wall behind the toilet, which theoretically promotes spreading of the labia). Of more concern is the fact that such studies excluded patients with vaginitis, urologic abnormalities, pregnancy, and vaginal bleeding. These conditions represent the clinical circumstances for which urine is commonly examined in young women visiting the ED. In this at-risk population, catheterized urine specimens are optimal. However, this needs to be balanced with the view that catheterization may introduce unnecessary patient discomfort and resource utilization, as well as the risk of introducing bacteria into the bladder.[65]

Background

Patients are often apprehensive about catheterization. Frequently, if the clinician shows concern regarding positioning and exposure, the patient is reassured. Although adequate exposure may be obtained with the frog-leg position, use of an examination table with stirrups (lithotomy position) is ideal, especially for female catheterization.

Anticipation and preparation of all the material necessary for urethral catheterization beforehand are reassuring to the patient. It is frustrating for the health care provider and upsetting to the patient when the patient is told "not to move or touch anything" while a search is made for additional equipment. Most catheterizations are performed with the use of a standard catheterization tray. Frequently, these trays contain more equipment than is truly needed. This necessitates opening the tray and establishing a sterile field at the bedside, selecting items that will be needed, and discarding the rest of the equipment. Once the penis or labia have been touched in preparation for the procedure, the touching hand (usually nondominant) is contaminated and ideally should not be handling any of the sterile equipment. When a standard catheterization tray is not used or is not available, providers should go through the anticipated procedure mentally to secure all the appropriate equipment before actually starting the procedure.

Anatomy and Physiology

Female Catheterization

The female urethra is a short (4 cm) straight tube, usually of wide caliber, that lies on top of the vagina. It must be approached between the double labia, and the urethral meatus is occasionally hidden and not obvious (in contrast to most males, except those with hypospadias). If a female patient nervously adducts her legs, successful catheterization will be very difficult, if not impossible.

The female urethral meatus is oval but may appear as an anteroposterior slit with rather prominent margins situated directly superior to the opening of the vagina and approximately 2.5 cm inferior to the glans clitoris (Fig. 55-15). It is

DORSAL SLIT (PARAPHIMOSIS TREATMENT)

Line of infiltration and incision

Constricting ring

Paraphimosis

Glans

1. Infiltrate local anesthetic from the constricting band of the paraphimosis proximally along the dorsal aspect of the penis. Make an incision along this line.

Extending the incision too far here will foreshorten and tether the penis

2. A diamond-shaped defect will result from the linear incision of the foreskin. Approximate the two apices of the dorsal slit (*a* and *b*) after the foreskin is reduced.

Figure 55-14 Dorsal slit treatment of paraphimosis. This procedure may be necessary if manual reduction of paraphimosis (see Fig. 55-9) is unsuccessful.

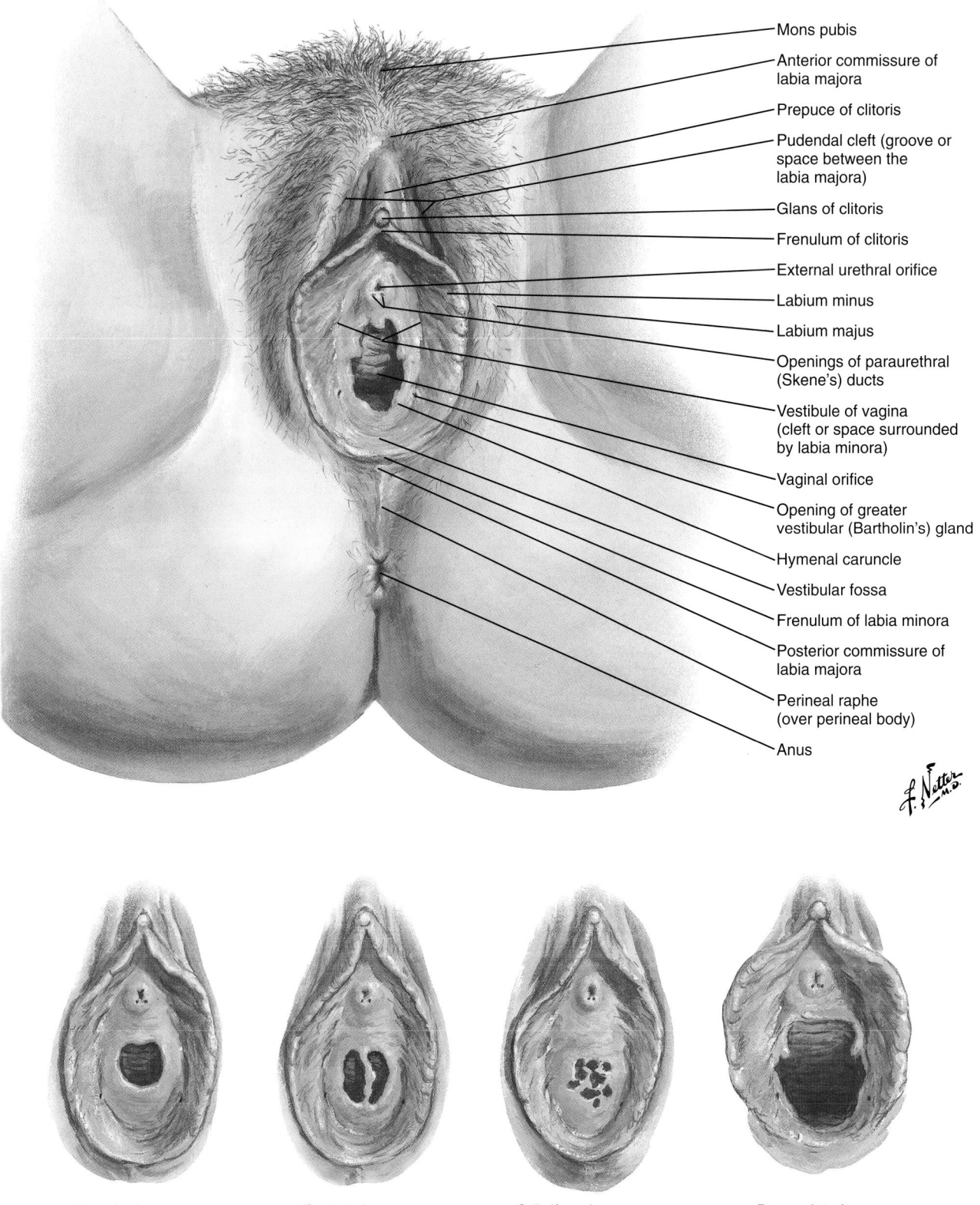

- Mons pubis
- Anterior commissure of labia majora
- Prepuce of clitoris
- Pudendal cleft (groove or space between the labia majora)
- Glans of clitoris
- Frenulum of clitoris
- External urethral orifice
- Labium minus
- Labium majus
- Openings of paraurethral (Skene's) ducts
- Vestibule of vagina (cleft or space surrounded by labia minora)
- Vaginal orifice
- Opening of greater vestibular (Bartholin's) gland
- Hymenal caruncle
- Vestibular fossa
- Frenulum of labia minora
- Posterior commissure of labia majora
- Perineal raphe (over perineal body)
- Anus

Annular hymen   Septate hymen   Cribriform hymen   Parous introitus

Figure 55-15 External female genitalia. The urethral meatus is directly superior to the vaginal introitus and approximately 2.5 cm inferior to the clitoris. *(Netter illustration from* www.netterimages.com. © *Elsevier, Inc. All rights reserved.)*

A

B

Figure 55-16 Female urethra. **A,** Normal sagittal anatomy of the female urethra (*arrow*). **B,** In a patient with a cystocele/urethrocele or prolapsed bladder, the normal anatomy may have to be re-created for passage of a catheter. Insert two fingers into the vagina and lift upward while passing the catheter.

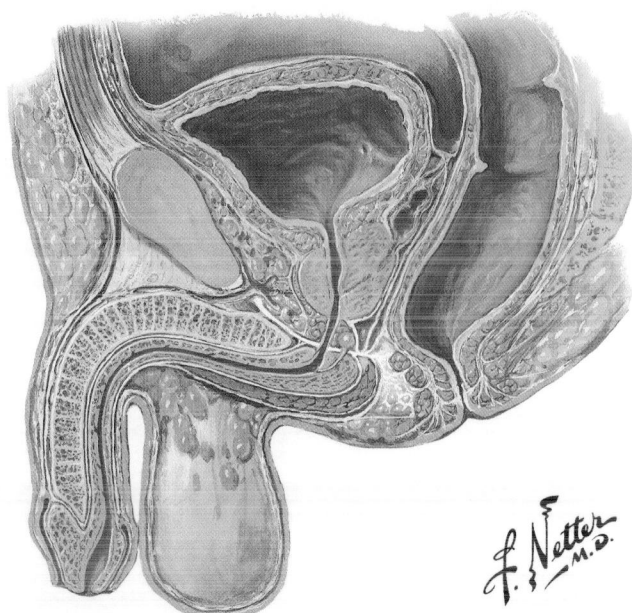

Figure 55-17 Male urethra. The male urethra is approximately 20 cm long from the meatus to the neck of the bladder. The prostatic urethra and membranous urethra can be up to 7 cm combined. Thus, it is essential to advance the urethral catheter to the hilt before balloon inflation to avoid urethral injury. (*Netter illustration from www.netterimages.com. © Elsevier, Inc. All rights reserved.*)

the first of three orifices encountered when examining the female genitalia from cephalad to caudad in the lithotomy position. The urethral meatus might be especially difficult to find in very young infants and in older, postmenopausal women. Anticipation of this problem and knowledge of anatomic variations will help mollify any patient discomfort associated with needless catheter tip probing, which is an unsettling experience for both the patient and the person performing the catheterization.

Occasionally, the urethral meatus recedes superiorly into the vagina and is not immediately visible because of either previous surgical procedures or atrophic postmenopausal changes. Anticipation of such cases will allow the examiner to gently advance a nondominant index finger into the vagina in the superior midline. The urethral meatus can usually be palpated and then visualized as a soft mound surrounded by a firmer ring of supporting periurethral tissue. Rarely, the meatus will have receded so far superiorly and intravaginally that it cannot be visualized at all, and catheterization must be carried out by palpation alone. From the meatus (if the patient assumes a supine position), the urethra proceeds straight back to slightly downward as it advances into the bladder just behind the symphysis pubis (Fig. 55-16*A*).

In women with a urethrocele or cystourethrocele in whom the urethra or the bladder falls into the vagina, the "normal"

urethral course might be considerably more posterior. The normal anatomic relationships in these situations may be re-created by spreading the index and long fingers, placing them along the superior vaginal wall, and gently applying upward support (see Fig. 55-16*B*). This reconstitutes the normal anatomic relationships and permits straight, rapid urethral catheterization. Because the female urethra is so short, only half the total length of the catheter has to be inserted before it is safe to inflate the Foley balloon.

Male Catheterization

Because the urethral meatus is usually evident in most males, it might seem a simple matter to insert a urethral catheter.[66] Yet catheterization can be quite difficult. The normal male urethra is approximately 20 cm long from the external urethral meatus to the neck of the bladder (Fig. 55-17). The posterior prostatic urethra is approximately 3.5 cm long, and the contiguous external sphincter or urogenital diaphragm that encompasses the membranous urethra is located 4 cm from the neck of the bladder. In males, *any catheter must be fully inserted to the balloon-inflating side arm channel before it is safe to inflate the balloon*. At the first egress of urine from the catheter, the balloon is just passing through the membranous urethra. *The catheter balloon still has about 3 cm to go before clearing the neck of the bladder.* Inflation of the Foley balloon at any point before full insertion of the catheter might result in iatrogenic urethral injury.

The male urethra is relatively fixed at the level of the urogenital diaphragm and symphysis pubis; traction downward on the penis kinks and promotes urethral folding at the level of the penile suspensory ligament, which creates a level of spurious obstruction (Fig. 55-18*A*). For this reason, always hold the penis taut and upright during any urethral instrumentation, including catheterization. The catheter then needs

Urethral Catheterization

Indications
Acute urinary retention
Obstructive uropathy
Urine output monitoring in any critically ill or injured patient
Collection of a sterile urine specimen for diagnostic purposes
Intermittent bladder catheterization in patients with neurogenic bladder dysfunction
Urologic study of the lower urinary tract

Contraindications
Situations in which a less invasive procedure is sufficient
Trauma patient with suspected urethral injury

Complications
Urethral trauma and hemorrhage
Paraphimosis (if the foreskin is not reduced after the procedure)
Infection
Undesirable catheter retention (nondeflating balloon)

Equipment

Review Box 55-1 Urethral catheterization: indications, contraindications, complications, and equipment.

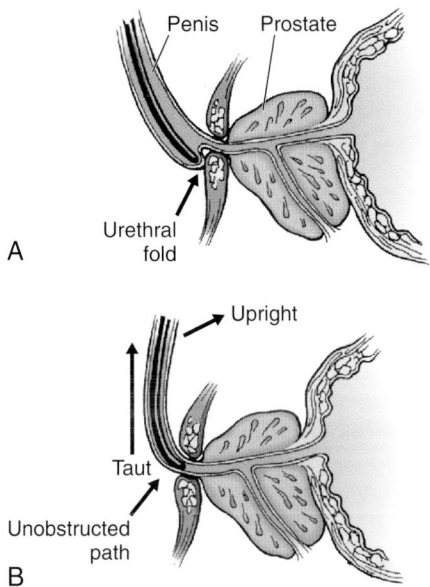

Figure 55-18 A, The urethra may fold and kink if the penis is not held taut and upright. This will halt the advancement of a catheter, even though there is no other anatomic blockage. **B,** The taut and upright position allows an unobstructed path for the catheter.

to make only a single curve rather than a complex S curve as it traverses into the bladder (see Fig. 55-18*B*).

Indications

Urinary catheterization and instrumentation are rarely a primary cause of urinary infection in otherwise healthy patients who urinate normally and carry small amounts of postvoid residual urine. As with any procedure, limit catheterization to clinical situations in which the benefits outweigh the risks. The following are indications for urethral catheterization:

1. Acute urinary retention
2. Urethral or prostatic obstruction leading to compromised renal function
3. Monitoring of urine output in any critically ill or injured patient
4. Collection of a sterile urine specimen for diagnostic purposes
5. Intermittent bladder catheterization in patients with neurogenic bladder dysfunction
6. Urologic study of the lower urinary tract

Contraindications

Avoid urethral catheterization when other less invasive procedures are equally effective and informative. A traditional, albeit currently relative contraindication to urethral catheterization (see the following discussion) is a trauma patient with suspected urethral injury who has blood at the urethral meatus; an abnormal-feeling or high-riding prostate on rectal examination; penile, scrotal, or perineal hematoma; or radiographic evidence of urethral or bladder trauma. In the setting of a severely fractured pelvis or diastasis of the pubic symphysis, urethrography should always precede attempts at catheterization. Although some authors[67] and more liberal clinical protocols allow gentle attempts at passage of the catheter in the presence of the previously discussed traditional contraindications, these findings dictate a selective approach or the need for retrograde urethrography (RUG), or both, to define the integrity of the urethra before any attempted urethral catheterization.[68]

Procedure

Equipment

The equipment shown in Review Box 55-1 is included in most standard catheterization trays and must be at hand before attempting urethral catheterization. Check the list of contents

Figure 55-19 Urethral catheters. A wide variety of types and sizes of catheters are available. For most adult catheterizations, a 14- or 16-Fr Foley catheter is sufficient. For male patients with prostatic enlargement, a 14- to 18-Fr coudé catheter may be used (see Fig. 55-20). For patients with gross hematuria, a large (20 Fr and up) "three-way" catheter is ideal because it allows continuous bladder irrigation and its large diameter allows the passage of blood clots.

Figure 55-20 Coudé catheter. A coudé catheter is used for men with prostatic enlargement. It features a semirigid curved tip that helps the catheter traverse the median lobe of the prostate gland. When inserting the coudé, the curved tip should be pointing upward toward 12 o'clock, that is, pointing toward the dorsal aspect of the penis.

TABLE 55-3	Pediatric Urethral Catheter Size
AGE GROUP	**PEDIATRIC CATHETER SIZE***
Infants	5- to 8-Fr feeding tube
1-3 yr	8-Fr feeding tube
4-6 yr	10-Fr feeding tube
7-12 yr	10- to 12-Fr red rubber catheter (Robinson)
>12 yr	14-Fr red rubber catheter (Robinson)

*Sizes are approximate; 6 Fr is the smallest balloon catheter and is quite flimsy, and therefore 8 Fr is recommended; 12 Fr is the smallest coudé catheter.

before opening the tray because some trays do not include everything that is needed. For most routine adult in-and-out catheterizations, a 14-Fr red rubber catheter or Foley balloon catheter is adequate (Fig. 55-19). In neonates or infants, a 2- or 5-Fr feeding tube taped in place produces the least amount of urethral trauma. In older boys, a 5- to 12-Fr red rubber catheter or Foley balloon catheter may be used. Table 55-3 lists appropriately sized catheters and feeding tubes for urethral catheterization in patients of all ages.[69]

Consider using a 14- to 18-Fr coudé catheter after unsuccessful passage of a straight Foley balloon catheter or in a male patient with known enlargement of the prostate (Fig. 55-20). If a coudé catheter is not available, attempt catheterization with a larger 18- to 22-Fr Foley balloon catheter. In a male patient with a urethral stricture in whom attempts at catheterization with a straight Foley or coudé catheter have failed, the next step is retrograde cystoscopy, passage of a guidewire, or passage of filiforms or followers under the direction of a urologist. If immediate bladder access is required in an emergency, suprapubic placement of a peel-away sheath and Foley balloon catheter via the Seldinger technique will be needed (as described in the suprapubic cystostomy section of this chapter).[70]

General Procedure (Figs. 55-21 and 55-22)

As stated previously, always use sterile technique during urethral catheterization. Both male and female patients have special urethral meatal considerations. In an uncircumcised or partially circumcised male, absolute total control of the penile foreskin is paramount to ensure success. Before establishing a sterile field, retract the available foreskin to its fullest extent proximal to the glans penis (Fig. 55-23A). Unfold a standard 4 × 4 gauze pad, refold it in its longest dimension, and carefully wrap it around the retracted foreskin at the level of the coronal sulcus (see Fig. 55-23B). This will prevent the tendency for lubricated foreskin to reduce during catheterization and thus provides a continuously dry and sterile field. Secure the folded 4 × 4 gauze around the foreskin between the nondominant long and ring fingers at the beginning the procedure and do not release it until the procedure is completed. This position leaves the nondominant index finger and thumb available for manipulating the catheter. After catheterization, remove the 4 × 4 pad and *reduce the penile foreskin to its normal anatomic position to prevent the development of iatrogenic paraphimosis.*

After exposing the urethral meatus in females and the glans penis and urethral meatus in males, use cotton balls or oversized cotton-tipped applicators soaked in an antiseptic solution (e.g., povidone-iodine) to cleanse the exposed meatus and surrounding tissue. This is best done by hand but can also be done with the plastic forceps in the catheterization tray. Begin the cleansing circular motion on the urethral meatus and proceed outward to move any debris toward the periphery and thus create a sterile field.

Lubricate an appropriately sized catheter (10 Fr is adequate for small children, whereas 14 to 16 Fr is commonly used in adults) with viscous rather than inspissated lubricating jelly. Pass the catheter gently by hand or with the aid of a hemostat or plastic forceps. Insert it into the urethra and then upward into the bladder. Inject the male urethra with 5 mL of 2% viscous lidocaine or a similar syringe filled with anesthetic lubricant to help in urethral distention and topical anesthesia. Regardless, advise the patient of mild urethral discomfort and the potential urge to void. Pass the catheter slowly and gently while remaining aware of the anatomic

MALE URETHRAL CATHETERIZATION AND BLADDER IRRIGATION

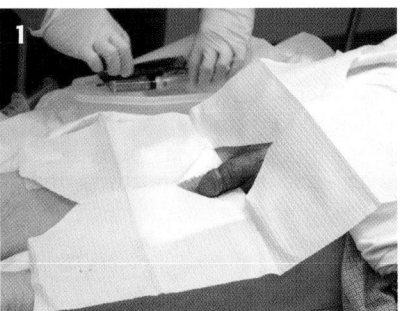

Prepare your equipment and place a sterile fenestrated drape around the penis. If the patient is uncircumcised, retract the foreskin prior to the procedure (see Fig. 55-23).

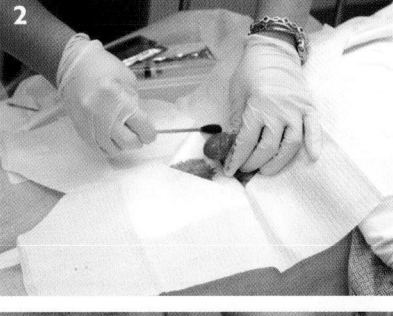

Use your nondominant hand to hold the penis, and cleanse the meatus and surrounding tissue with antiseptic. Your nondominant hand is now contaminated and should not let go of the penis or handle sterile equipment until the insertion has been completed.

Viscous lidocaine ("Urojet")

Inject the urethra with 5 to 10 mL of 2% viscous lidocaine to distend the urethra and provide topical anesthesia. A commercially available Urojet syringe (depicted here) is ideal. If possible, wait 5 to 10 minutes for maximum anesthetic effect.

Hold the penis taut and upright with your nondominant hand while you pass the catheter into the urethra. (See Fig. 55-18.)

Catheter advanced to the hilt before balloon inflation

Advance the catheter to the hilt before inflating the balloon with the recommended amount of air or water. If there is obvious resistance or patient discomfort, immediately deflate and reevaluate the position of the catheter.

After balloon inflation, slowly withdraw the catheter until the balloon is against the bladder neck and precluding further withdrawal. Connect to a drainage system if one is not preattached.

Affix the catheter to the thigh with tape or a catheter-specific attachment device. Note that a "three-way" catheter was placed in this patient with gross hematuria.

Drainage port

Inflation port

Irrigation port

To irrigate the bladder, attach the irrigation port to a 2- to 4-L bag of saline irrigation fluid. (Hand irrigation with a 60-mL catheter-tipped syringe is an alternative.) Attach the drainage port to a large-volume collection bag.

Irrigation fluid

Continuously infuse the irrigant into the bladder. Rates of 1 to 2 L/hr are acceptable, provided that the amount of irrigant drained equals the amount infused.

Monitor output carefully during the procedure. The goal of irrigation is to obtain clear urinary effluent.

Figure 55-21 Male urethral catheterization and bladder irrigation.

considerations discussed previously. Discard the catheter if it inadvertently enters the vagina.

After passing the catheter "to the hilt" in a male patient, slowly inflate the balloon with 10 mL of air or tap water. Sterile water or saline is not necessary. Most 5-mL balloons will easily accommodate up to 30 to 50 mL of air or water without bursting. If there is obvious resistance or patient discomfort during inflation of the balloon, erroneous urethral positioning may have occurred and mandates reevaluation. In this case, immediately deflate the Foley balloon and reposition or slightly withdraw the catheter. Then pass it to the hilt again

before reinflating the balloon. If the second time is unsuccessful, remove the catheter and evaluate the urethra for a potential obstructive problem or false passage. RUG is recommended (see the section "RUG" later in this chapter). It may be difficult or impossible to pass a Foley catheter in a male with a markedly edematous penis (Fig. 55-24). If it cannot be accomplished, a suprapubic catheter may be required.

After successful passage of the catheter and inflation of the Foley balloon, slowly withdraw the catheter until the balloon is close to the bladder neck and precludes further withdrawal. Connect the catheter to either a sterile leg bag or a

FEMALE URETHRAL CATHETERIZATION

Place the patient in the "frog-leg" position: the hips externally rotated and slightly flexed and the knees bent.

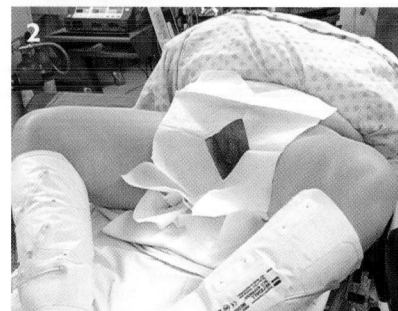

Place a sterile fenestrated drape over the area. Strict attention to sterile technique is required.

Use your nondominant hand to spread the labia and identify the urethral meatus. This hand is now considered contaminated and should not release the labia or handle sterile equipment throughout the procedure.

Cleanse the urethral meatus with antiseptic in progressively increasing concentric circles.

Insert the catheter into the meatus under direct vision. If the catheter accidentally enters the vagina, it should be discarded and a new one used (to prevent iatrogenic infection).

Once the catheter is in the bladder and urine returns in the tubing, advance the catheter several centimeters further and inflate the balloon with the recommended amount of water or air.

Gently retract the catheter until the balloon encounters the bladder neck and resistance is felt.

Attach the catheter to a collection device (if not already preconnected), and affix the catheter to the patient's thigh with tape or a connection device.

Figure 55-22 Female urethral catheterization.

closed-system bedside drainage bag. If the patient will be released with an indwelling Foley catheter in place, connect it to a leg bag, and fasten it comfortably to the lower thigh and upper calf region. Instruct the patient and family regarding proper care of the catheter and drainage device. In most other cases, secure the catheter to either the thigh or the lower part of the abdomen (preferred in males) with adhesive tape, or simply place it under the knee and let it drain dependently into the bedside drainage bag.

Bladder Irrigation

After prostate surgery (transurethral resection), blood clots may form in the bladder and cause acute urinary retention. Blood loss can be significant. This condition can frequently be easily relieved by using a large three-way irrigation catheter. A Bardex 22- to 26-Fr Foley catheter is preferred. Infuse saline irrigation fluid continuously into the bladder while allowing the egress of fluid and blood clots. Continue the procedure until the bladder remains decompressed or the bleeding stops (see Fig. 55-21, *steps 8 to 10*). Gravity alone usually provides adequate ingress and egress of fluid, but gentle syringe irrigation with 60-mL aliquots of saline may also be used. Irrigation can be brisk, 1 to 2 L/hr or greater, as long as the *volume of drained saline is equal to the volume infused*. Use only saline (supplied in 2- or 4-L bags) and infuse it *via gravity*. Syringe irrigation of a Foley catheter with 60- to 100-mL aliquots is an alternative. The goal is to obtain clear urine.

DUC

Difficult urethral catheterization (DUC) is a common urologic problem. In females DUC is due primarily to vaginal atrophy with retraction of the meatus into the vagina. This

Figure 55-23 A, In this uncircumcised male, the foreskin has been fully retracted for placement of a catheter. **B,** A gauze pad allows a firm grasp on the foreskin to prevent movement during catheterization. Reduce the foreskin to its original position once the catheter is in place.

Figure 55-24 A, The urethral meatus cannot be found in the markedly edematous penis in this patient with massive anasarca. **B,** Wrap the penis in an elastic bandage for 8 to 10 minutes. **C,** The edema is reduced with compression alone. **D,** An assistant stabilizes the penile shaft with the thumb and index finger (*arrow*) while the operator (*asterisk*) spreads the redundant tissue with forceps to visualize the meatus deep within the swollen tissue and advances the catheter.

problem can typically be overcome by placing the patient in the lithotomy position, using a speculum, or guiding the catheter blindly with the provider's index and middle fingers. However, DUC in males may present greater challenges. Common causes in males include urethral strictures, contracture of the neck of the bladder, false passage, and prostate disease. A trial of a coudé catheter is generally the first-line approach to DUC. Alternatives used by urologists include flexible cystoscopy, passage of a guidewire, or use of filiforms/ followers.[71] Consider suprapubic cystostomy an option of last resort given its inherent complications. Various causes and approaches to DUC in the emergency care setting are presented in Table 55-4.

Aftercare

Systemic antimicrobial prophylaxis should not be used routinely in patients with short-term (or long-term) catheterization to reduce catheter-associated bacteriuria or urinary tract infection because of concern about selection of antimicrobial resistance.[72]

Complications

Although urethral catheterization performed by skilled personnel in appropriate circumstances has an acceptable complication rate, untoward sequelae of catheterization are not unusual.

Mechanical
False passages might be established in any area of the urethra when force is exerted on the catheter. In an uncircumcised patient, negligence in reducing the retracted foreskin to its normal anatomic position after urethral catheterization or instrumentation might lead to painful paraphimosis and associated complications.

Bleeding
Hematuria has long been thought to be common after even atraumatic catheterization. Careful monitoring of symptoms is prudent since most often postprocedural hematuria resolves rapidly and spontaneously.

Infection
The incidence of bacteriuria associated with indwelling catheterization is 3% to 8% per day, and the duration of catheterization is the most important risk factor for the development of catheter-associated bacteriuria.[71] However, in hospitalized, elderly, debilitated, or postpartum patients, the rate might be considerably higher. Urinary catheterization is the leading cause of nosocomial infection.[71]

Long-Term Catheter Use
By 1 month, nearly all patients with an indwelling catheter will be bacteriuric.[72] Other less frequent complications of long-term indwelling urethral catheterization include bladder stones, recurring bladder spasm, periurethral abscesses, urethral stricture formation, bladder perforation,[73] and urethral erosion.[74]

Undesirable Catheter Retention
Catheters may be retained because of balloons that do not deflate (see the next section) or, very rarely, because of a knot that spontaneously developed in the catheter.

Removal of a Nondeflating Catheter
Occasionally, an indwelling catheter balloon fails to deflate, thereby leading to undesired retention of the Foley catheter in the bladder. This problem has challenged and frustrated many clinicians and has produced a number of ingenious solutions.[75-77] Unfortunately, pretesting Foley catheter balloons by trial inflation and deflation before insertion does not eliminate the potential for a nondeflating Foley catheter balloon.

A common cause of a nondeflating catheter balloon is malfunction of the flap-type valve in the balloon lumen of the catheter, which normally allows fluid to fill the balloon of the catheter but prevents passive egress (Fig. 55-25, *step 1*).[75] The ideal solution is one that resolves the problem—deflating the balloon—without creating another problem, such as unnecessary bladder irritation or balloon fragmentation. Of the methods recommended to decompress nondeflating catheter balloons, the only technique that approaches the ideal directly attacks this flap valve deformity.

The inflate-deflate channel normally prevents passive egress of inflating fluid or air. Occasionally, cutting off the inflation port will deflate the balloon, but usually, the problematic area is further along the catheter, closer to the bladder. Once the port has been removed, use a needle/syringe in the inflation channel to suck out the fluid in the balloon (see Fig. 55-25, *step 4*). Cutting the catheter closer to the bladder may fortuitously cut off the offending area, but be careful to not cut off an excessive length of exposed catheter. More often, the inflation channel may have a valve defect or be filled with debris (see Fig. 55-25, *step 2*). When presented with this situation, insert a thin, rigid wire into the balloon port lumen in an attempt to deflate the valve flap defect sufficiently and to promote escape of fluid from the balloon (see Fig. 55-25, *step 3*). Occasionally, the balloon itself may be punctured by this wire. The wire stylets from a central venous or angiographic catheter, guidewires from ureteral catheters, and very small well-lubricated ureteral catheters themselves have all been reported to be successful. When a ureteral catheter guidewire was used in one series, 34 of 39 balloons were deflated without fragmentation.[76]

Once a malfunctioning balloon has been deflated, inspect the balloon itself for missing fragments. If a piece of the balloon is missing, arrange for subsequent cystoscopy to look for and remove the fragments.

Alternative methods for removal of a nondeflating catheter are presented in Table 55-5.

A variation of the nondeflating balloon is "cuffing," essentially an *asymmetric deflation* in which the balloon does not deflate flush with the catheter. The irregularity becomes more pronounced as the catheter is withdrawn into the urethra and thus prevents easy withdrawal. It occurs more often when the balloon fluid is aspirated quickly and less often with more gradual withdrawal of the fluid. Inflate the balloon again and try to deflate it slowly if this occurs. Reinflating the balloon to a smooth surface with 0.5 to 1 mL of saline during withdrawal may also obviate this problem. An example of cuffing is shown in Figure 55-25, *step 6*, and this is more common with suprapubic tubes.

Traumatic Foley Catheter Removal
Occasionally, uncooperative or demented patients will pull out their Foley catheter with the balloon still inflated (Fig. 55-26). One would intuit that urethral injury is possible; however, there are no prospective data on the incidence or type of injury from this maneuver or how to deal with this

TABLE 55-4   Approach to Difficulties in Male Catheterization

CONDITION	ISSUE	WORK-AROUND STRATEGY
Phimosis	Inability to identify the urethral meatus because of a tight phimotic opening	Dilate the phimotic opening sufficiently to identify the urethral meatus and blindly pass the catheter Dorsal slit of the foreskin to expose the glans and urethral meatus in extreme cases
Foreskin edema	Edema may obscure the glans penis and urethral meatus	Attempt to identify the cause of the edema; exclude paraphimosis and foreign body strangulation Manually compress the swollen foreskin by hand or between opposing cold packs If unsuccessful, snugly wrap the distal penis in a compressive dressing for 10 min
Meatal stenosis	The urethral meatus may be either congenitally or secondarily narrowed by scarring	Trial of a smaller-caliber catheter If a larger-caliber catheter is necessary, meatal dilation or meatotomy might be necessary under the direction of a urologist
Urethral stricture	May develop as a result of trauma, infection (especially STDs), lower urinary tract instrumentation, or long-term indwelling catheter drainage	Trial with a coudé catheter However, manual force should not be used to negotiate or to dilate urethral strictures because it may lead to false passages, bleeding, and future increased scarring Consideration of urethral dilation with the use of filiforms and followers under the direction of a urologist
External urethral sphincter spasm	Voluntary or involuntary contraction of the urogenital diaphragm (external sphincter) produces spurious urethral resistance at approximately 16 cm from the meatus	Encourage the patient to lay supine and take slow, deep breaths while consciously trying to relax the perineum and rectum Plantar flexion of the toes and ankles may also aid in relaxation of the pelvic floor Gentle but steady pressure exerted on the syringe or the catheter along with the aforementioned steps may aid in passage The external sphincter is composed of striated muscle and fatigues within a few minutes If continued resistance, assume an anatomic abnormality and consider RUG before further instrumentation
High bladder neck	Enlarged intravesical portion of the prostate with a secondary high-riding bladder neck Typically resistance encountered after the catheter has been passed 16-20 cm into the urethra	Slow instillation or injection of 20-30 mL of sterile lubricating jelly If unsuccessful, consider a trial with a coudé catheter; may be enhanced by digital compression of the prostate during digital rectal examination
Pelvic trauma, straddle injury	Partial or complete urethral injury might occur Injudicious catheterization has the potential for conversion of a partial injury (may heal with little or no scarring) to a complete urethral injury (often requires surgical repair and usually results in some degree of postoperative morbidity) Blood at the urethral meatus, a "high-riding" or abnormal-feeling prostate on rectal examination, and penile, scrotal, or perineal ecchymoses might be evidence of potential urethral or bladder injury but have poor sensitivity[66]	Consider precatheterization RUG in suspected cases Maintain a low threshold for urologic consultation Suprapubic catheter placement may be necessary in certain cases

RUG, retrograde urethrography; *STDs*, sexually transmitted diseases.

REMOVAL OF A NONDEFLATING CATHETER

1

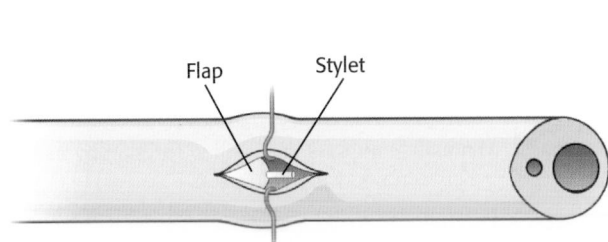

A flaplike defect in the inflating channel of a balloon catheter may prevent balloon deflation. A wire stylet (from a central venous catheter kit) can be passed down the inflating channel to raise the flap and deflate the balloon.

2

Note that the entire inflation channel is filled with debris (arrow), thus preventing egress of fluid from the retaining balloon.

3

Cut the catheter, remove the inflation port, and advance the stiff end of a guidewire through the inflation channel. The wire may puncture the balloon or clear the channel so that fluid escapes.

4

Once the channel has been cleared, insert a 20-gauge needle gently into the inflation channel to aspirate the balloon fluid.

5

In the case of a nondeflating suprapubic balloon, you can try to insert a 25-gauge spinal needle parallel to the catheter to puncture the balloon. Maintain traction on the catheter to stabilize the balloon during the procedure.

6

This balloon demonstrates "cuffing" where the balloon deflated asymmetrically and got caught up during withdrawal.

Figure 55-25 Removal of a nondeflating catheter. (*A, From Eichenberg HA, Amin M, Clark J. Nondeflating Foley catheters. Int Urol Nephrol. 1976;8:171. Reproduced by permission.*)

TABLE 55-5 Alternative Methods of Removing Nondeflating Catheters

METHOD	COMMENTS
Needle puncture of the balloon (see Fig. 55-25, *step 5*)	Overinflate the balloon (50-100 mL of saline) Draw the balloon against the bladder neck Use local anesthesia for the suprapubic approach Use a 25- to 27-gauge spinal needle to puncture the balloon Ultrasound guidance may be helpful
Hyperinflation of the balloon	High rate of balloon fragmentation: 100 of 100 in one report[74] Postprocedure cystoscopic inspection of the bladder essential Consider adding 50-100 mL of saline into the *bladder* to cushion the effects of subsequent balloon rupture if no urinary retention is present Inject up to 200 mL of air into a 5-mL balloon to induce rupture
Injection of an erosive substance into the balloon port (e.g., mineral oil)	This technique has fallen out of favor High rate of balloon fragmentation: 95 of 100 in one report[74] Associated with chemical cystitis

Figure 55-26 Traumatic Foley catheter removal. **A,** This patient pulled out his Foley catheter with the balloon inflated. Blood appeared at the meatus. His mental status prevented assessment of his ability to void spontaneously. Given the large volume of the inflated balloon and gross blood, it was decided to perform retrograde urethrography, although some would simply try to gently pass a new catheter. **B,** Place a balloon-tipped catheter into the meatus and inflate with 1 to 2 mL of air or water. **C,** Squeeze the glans while an assistant slowly injects contrast material. **D,** Overzealous injection resulted in venous uptake of the dye and spillage on the patient's leg. The urethra is intact. A new catheter was easily passed.

situation. Usually, blood is apparent at the meatus, and it may be difficult to know whether the patient can urinate spontaneously. If the patient can urinate spontaneously, it would seem reasonable to gently pass another Foley catheter to avoid urethral obstruction by tears or clots and to allow healing of the urethral trauma with a new catheter in place. Most of the time, however, the clinician has minimal data yet is faced with the decision on how to approach this conundrum.

Surprisingly, such incidents do not usually result in massive urethral injury. It is assumed that a new catheter will be required, either to continue the original indication for the catheter or to provide a stent while any urethral injury heals. In the absence of available urologic consultation, gently attempt to pass another Foley catheter without routinely performing RUG (described later in this chapter). If the catheter does not pass easily, stop and perform RUG to assess the extent of the pathology. Most of the time, simply replacing the catheter will be the most prudent approach. Prophylactic antibiotics are reasonable under these circumstances. Complete eversion and prolapse of the bladder have been associated rarely with this misadventure.[78]

Conclusion

Access to and subsequent evaluation of bladder urine are clinically important to all emergency practitioners. The merits of various approaches to collection of urine specimens depend on the patient's age and clinical setting. Urethral catheterization generally provides a relatively safe and effective means of bladder access.

SUPRAPUBIC ASPIRATION

Introduction

Suprapubic aspiration of the bladder, first reported as a method of collecting urine for bacteriologic study in 1956,[79] is a relatively simple means of obtaining uncontaminated bladder urine. It is used primarily in young children, although there are limited indications for this procedure in adults as well.

It has been demonstrated that with proper technique, suprapubic aspiration consistently provides an uncontaminated urine specimen on which true bacteriuria can be distinguished from contamination.[80,81] However, the perception of increased discomfort and the procedural failure rate have led to a precipitous decline in its use, particularly outside the neonatal intensive care unit.[81-83] Nevertheless, suprapubic aspiration continues to be considered the gold standard method of urine collection.[84]

Despite the lack of experience by most currently practicing clinicians, the procedure may still be necessary in girls with labial adhesions and in boys with phimosis. The introduction of ultrasound technology has led to a significant improvement in success rates and probably in the comfort of the clinician performing the procedure.[85-87]

Indications

In a neonate or young child, suprapubic aspiration or urethral catheterization can provide the clinician with a sample that is reliable for bacteriologic interpretation. Though disconcerting to some parents (they may wish to leave the room or look away during the procedure), suprapubic aspiration is not a dangerous procedure, and the sensitivity of urinalysis of this urine for bacteriuria approaches 100%. However, for many young children, urine can generally be more readily collected by urethral catheterization.

In adult patients, the indications for suprapubic aspiration are more limited because these patients can usually cooperate with the clinician. Men with condom catheters or phimosis, however, may require suprapubic aspiration to minimize urethral contamination. Aspirated rather than catheterized specimens may help rule out contamination in patients with asymptomatic bacteriuria on routine urine collection. With infections caused by organisms that in other circumstances are often discounted as contaminants (e.g., *Staphylococcus epidermidis* or *Candida albicans*), suprapubic aspiration or a catheterized specimen is required to confirm the presence of such pathogens.

In patients in whom the possibility of infravesical infection is a concern (e.g., those with chronic infections of the urethra or the periurethral glands), suprapubic aspiration may help differentiate a bladder from a urethral source.

Contraindications

Skin or soft tissue infection in the area of the proposed anterior abdominal wall puncture site is a contraindication.

Procedure

Place the child supine in a frog-leg position and restrained as necessary (Fig. 55-27, *A1*). First locate the bladder. A full, palpable, or percussible bladder should be readily apparent, but this can be difficult to discern in all but the thinnest patients. If there is any question about the location or the amount of bladder urine, a quick ultrasound examination is informative. The point of entry in the skin should be 1 to 2 cm above the superior edge of the symphysis pubis. The syringe and needle are passed perpendicular to the abdominal wall toward the bladder, usually at a 10- to 20-degree angle from the true vertical, somewhat *cephalad* in children (see Fig. 55-27, *A2*) and somewhat *caudad* in adults (see Fig. 55-27*B*). Note that the bladder of a newborn is an abdominal organ and will be missed if the needle is inserted too close to the pubis or angled toward the feet.

After preparing and draping the skin, choose the point of entry. Raise a skin wheal of local anesthetic to reduce discomfort. After anesthetizing the skin, advance a longer, larger-caliber needle (usually 22 gauge, 3.75 to 8.75 cm in length) in the midline through the skin and quickly into the bladder. The authors prefer to advance the needle while it is attached to a syringe and to aspirate actively during advancement. As soon as the bladder is entered, urine will appear in the syringe. A short needle is adequate for virtually all pediatric patients. After collecting the urine, withdraw the syringe and needle. Microscopic hematuria always follows the procedure, but gross hematuria is uncommon.

If urine is not obtained, do not remove the needle but withdraw it to a subcutaneous position and redirect it at a different angle. Frequently, a child may spontaneously start to void after any type of invasive stimulus (e.g., bladder irritation by a probing needle, venipuncture, or lumbar puncture). Hence, make preparations to collect a spontaneously voided specimen should that option arise. Anticipate this before beginning blood or spinal fluid collection during the bacteremic workup of a febrile neonate.

In most patients, an acceptable urine sample can be obtained on the first needle pass. If the needle is pointed too far caudad in an effort to avoid entering the peritoneum, it is possible to enter the retropubic space by skimming the bladder muscle and never penetrating the bladder mucosa.

Aftercare

Following withdrawal of the needed, place a bandage over the puncture site.

Complications

Bacteremia does not typically result from this procedure.[88] Bowel penetration has occurred in children with distended

SUPRAPUBIC ASPIRATION

A. Pediatric

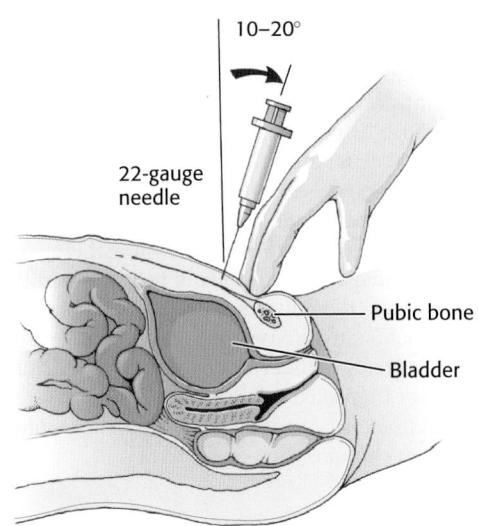

10–20°

22-gauge
needle

Pubic bone

Bladder

1. Restrain the infant and place her in a frog-leg position. Prepare and drape the skin, and raise a skin wheal with local anesthetic to reduce discomfort. Despite the safety of this procedure, it may be disconcerting for worried parents, and they may wish to leave the room during the aspiration.

2. Puncture the abdominal wall with a 22-gauge needle in the midline approximately 1 to 2 cm cephalad to the superior border of the pubic bone. Keep the syringe perpendicular to the plane of the abdominal wall (usually 10° to 20° from the true vertical). The bladder is an abdominal organ in infants, and placing the needle too close to the pubic bone or angling toward the feet might cause the needle to miss the bladder. Localizing the bladder with bedside ultrasound facilitates this procedure.

B. Adult

Peritoneum

In adults, the peritoneum is pushed cephalad by the filled bladder during suprapubic aspiration. Direct the needle slightly caudad.

Figure 55-27 Suprapubic aspiration.

abdomens from gastrointestinal disturbances.[89] The combination of gaseous bowel distention and relative hypovolemia might displace and flatten the relatively empty bladder against the pelvic floor. Even when the large bowel has been penetrated, patients recover uneventfully. Simple penetration of the bowel with a needle is considered an innocuous event and requires no specific treatment.

Conclusion

Although it can be performed in a patient of any age, suprapubic aspiration is occasionally used for urine collection in young children. It consistently provides a urine specimen on which true bacteriuria can be distinguished from contamination. However, in many cases, alternative methods of urine collection are preferred instead of this procedure.

SUPRAPUBIC CYSTOSTOMY

Introduction

In general, patients who require a urethral catheter but in whom a catheter cannot be safely passed are candidates for suprapubic cystostomy tubes. In emergency situations, the majority of patients requiring suprapubic cystostomy are trauma patients with urethral disruption or men with severe urethral stricture or complex prostatic disease.

Among the user-friendliest devices for suprapubic bladder access is the Cook peel-away sheath unit.[90] It uses the Seldinger (guidewire) technique to gain bladder access and allows suprapubic placement of a Foley balloon catheter for definitive bladder drainage. This device is readily suitable for ED use when compared with other suprapubic bladder access approaches, such as trocar-type devices.

When emergency bladder drainage is required and a Foley catheter cannot be placed transurethrally, any device suitable for central venous access can be inserted suprapubically via the Seldinger technique (Fig. 55-28).

Indications

If time allows, discussion with a urologist is prudent to explore alternative methods of bladder access and urine drainage before the initiation of suprapubic cystostomy. Even with

Figure 55-28 Suprapubic cystostomy. **A,** Any catheter that can be used as a central venous catheter can be inserted suprapubically via the Seldinger technique. **B,** The more traditional and more permanent suprapubic cystostomy with a Foley catheter inserted through a Cook peel-away sheath introducer.

major trauma, many affected patients might require laparotomy for associated injuries, and suprapubic catheter placement can be achieved intraoperatively.

Contraindications

Because placement of a suprapubic tube involves some risk, patient selection is important. The procedure should not be performed on a patient whose bladder is not definable. Although no absolute reported minimum bladder volume has ever been established, there must be enough urine in the bladder to allow the needle to fully penetrate the dome of the bladder without immediately exiting through the base. There must also be enough urine in the bladder to displace the bowel away from the anterosuperior surface of the bladder and the entrance of the needle. Ultrasound may be helpful in defining bladder anatomy.

In individuals with a history of previous lower abdominal surgery, intraperitoneal surgery, or irradiation, adhesions or adherence of the bowel to the anterior bladder wall may have developed. Such patients are potentially at greater risk for bowel injury during percutaneous suprapubic cystostomy tube placement than those without previous abdominal surgery. Blind suprapubic cystostomy tube placement should be avoided in these patients. Absence of any of these risk factors does not totally exclude the risk for bowel or intraperitoneal injury, but it reduces their incidence significantly.

Patients with bleeding diatheses are at greater risk for postinsertion bleeding, either into the bladder or into the retropubic space.

Procedure

The following comments describe placement of the Cook peel-away sheath, as reported by Chiou and colleagues.[91] With modifications, the same principles apply to any type of suprapubic catheter placement.

If necessary, shave the lower part of the abdomen and apply topical antiseptic. Fill a 6-mL syringe with 1% lidocaine and attach a 22-gauge, 7.75-cm spinal needle. Raise a skin wheal in the proposed site (2 to 3 cm above the pubic symphysis), and infiltrate the subcutaneous tissue and rectus abdominis muscle fascia at a 10- to 20-degree angle toward the pelvis.

Locate the bladder by advancing the needle in the prescribed direction while aspirating the syringe. Urine is easily aspirated when the bladder is entered (Fig. 55-29, *step 1*).

Once the bladder has been located, remove the syringe from the needle and advance a guidewire through the needle into the bladder (see Fig. 55-29, *step 2*). Withdraw the needle while leaving only the guidewire traversing the anterior abdominal wall and positioned inside the bladder. Use a No. 15 scalpel blade to make a stab incision directly posterior to the wire through the skin, subcutaneous tissue, and superficial anterior abdominal wall fascia. Then pass the peel-away sheath and indwelling fascial dilator together over the wire into the bladder (see Fig. 55-29, *step 3*). Remove the guidewire and fascial dilator and leave only the peel-away sheath inside the bladder (see Fig. 55-29, *step 4*). Then pass a preselected Foley balloon catheter through the indwelling intravesical sheath into the bladder (see Fig. 55-29, *step 5*). Aspirate urine to confirm proper placement. Inflate the Foley balloon with a minimum of 10 mL of air, water, or saline (see Fig. 55-29, *step 6*). Withdraw the peel-away sheath from the bladder and

SUPRAPUBIC CYSTOSTOMY (PEEL-AWAY SHEATH TECHNIQUE)

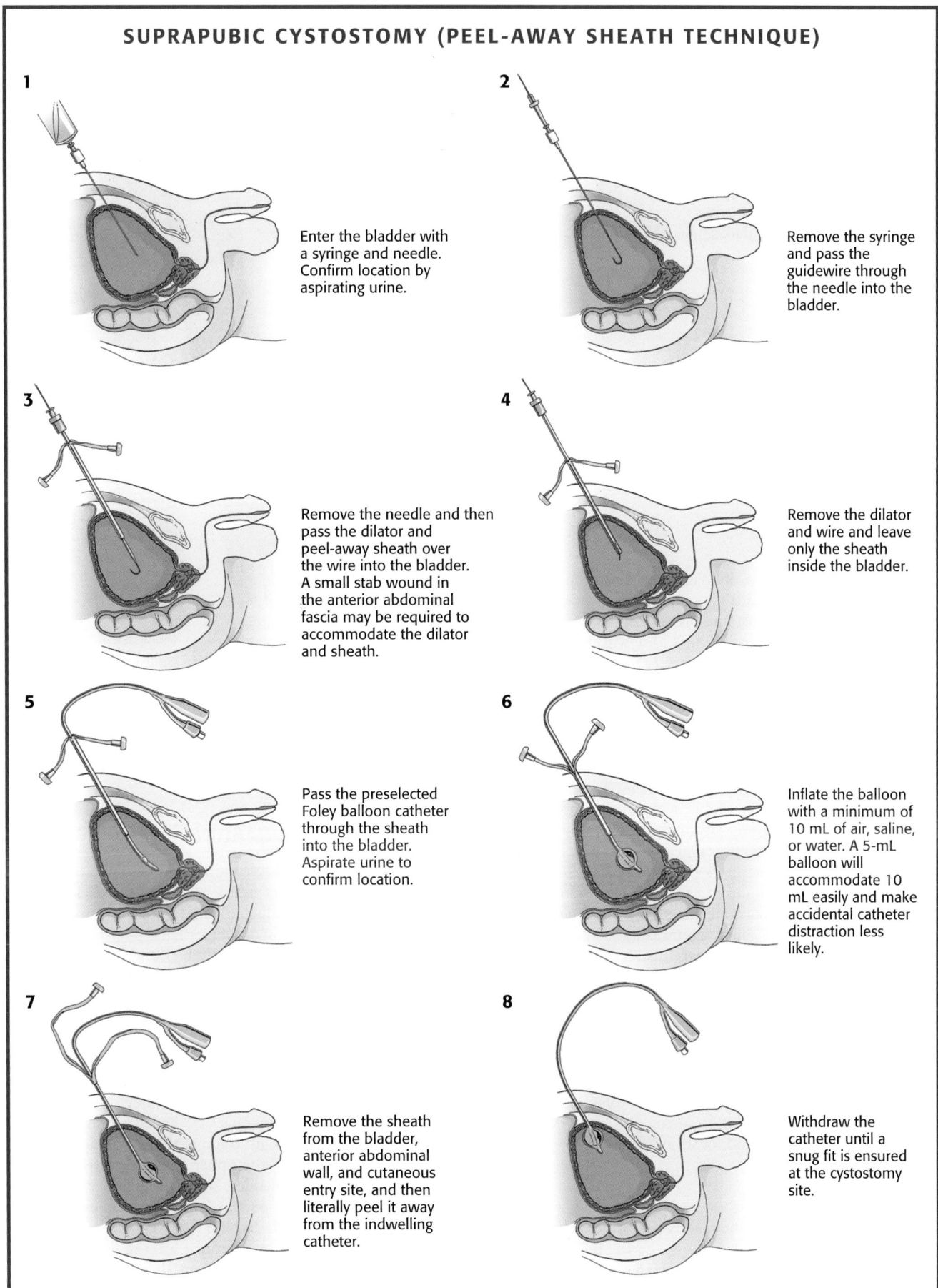

1 Enter the bladder with a syringe and needle. Confirm location by aspirating urine.

2 Remove the syringe and pass the guidewire through the needle into the bladder.

3 Remove the needle and then pass the dilator and peel-away sheath over the wire into the bladder. A small stab wound in the anterior abdominal fascia may be required to accommodate the dilator and sheath.

4 Remove the dilator and wire and leave only the sheath inside the bladder.

5 Pass the preselected Foley balloon catheter through the sheath into the bladder. Aspirate urine to confirm location.

6 Inflate the balloon with a minimum of 10 mL of air, saline, or water. A 5-mL balloon will accommodate 10 mL easily and make accidental catheter distraction less likely.

7 Remove the sheath from the bladder, anterior abdominal wall, and cutaneous entry site, and then literally peel it away from the indwelling catheter.

8 Withdraw the catheter until a snug fit is ensured at the cystostomy site.

Figure 55-29 Suprapubic cystostomy using a peel-away sheath. If this equipment is not available, an analogous procedure using any catheter suitable for central venous catheterization may be performed.

anterior abdominal wall and literally peel it away from the catheter, with only the indwelling suprapubic Foley catheter left in place (see Fig. 55-29, *step 7*). Withdraw the catheter slowly until the inflated balloon approximates the cystostomy site (see Fig. 55-29, *step 8*).

Aftercare

Connect the catheter to a drainage bag, and then dress the wound with 4×4 gauze pads to complete the procedure. The major difficulty with cystostomy tubes of all designs has been securing them to the patient's skin. Those with retention balloons, such as the standard Foley urethral catheter, are most secure and need only tape to secure them to the anterior abdominal wall.

Complications

A wide variety of complications have been reported, which serve as reminders that suprapubic cystostomy is not innocuous. Occasionally, despite the best intentions, the suprapubic tube or catheter cannot be positioned or maintained successfully without untoward sequelae (Box 55-5).

The most serious complications involve perforation of the peritoneum or the intraperitoneal contents. Although finding the bladder with a small-gauge scout needle may help reduce bowel injury, even in the most apparently successful of bladder punctures a complication might result.

Occasionally, the clinician is tempted to proceed with suprapubic cystostomy when the bladder is not palpable and has not been located with a syringe and needle. Injury to adjacent organs is much more frequent in these circumstances. If clinicians remind themselves that the bladder eventually refills, they will find waiting much more tolerable. If faced with an emergency, ultrasound guidance may be helpful in determining bladder size and location.

Conclusion

Suprapubic cystostomy can be readily performed when emergency bladder access is needed. However, the procedure may be associated with significant risks to the patient. Accordingly, when time affords, discussion with a urologist is prudent to explore alternative methods of bladder access and urine drainage.

3. Kidneys/ureters

2. Bladder

1. Urethra

Figure 55-30 Diagnostic approach to genitourinary (GU) tract trauma. The GU tract is studied in a retrograde fashion, proceeding from the urethra (retrograde urethrography) to the bladder (conventional or computed tomographic [CT] cystography) to the kidneys and ureters (CT urography with delayed/excretory images). These studies must be carried out in the proper sequence and in a retrograde fashion to avoid missing potential injuries.

LOWER GU TRACT IMAGING

Although the signs of GU trauma in general can be quite subtle, lower urinary tract injury can often be quickly identified and thoroughly evaluated radiographically in the ED. Radiologic imaging of the upper urinary tract is generally a less urgent matter and can usually be done in the radiology suite or, when important for emergency operative decision making, as single-shot intravenous pyelography (IVP) in the operating room.

The timing of any radiologic evaluation can be challenging in the emergency setting, especially when faced with a critically ill, multiply injured patient. The trauma team of clinicians involved in each resuscitation must determine the priority and extent of such an evaluation on a case-by-case basis.

In patients with urologic trauma, the lower urinary tract should be studied before the upper urinary tract (e.g., study the urethra before the bladder; study the bladder before the kidneys). Consequently, specific diagnostic studies should be conducted in a retrograde fashion (Fig. 55-30).

RUG and retrograde cystography are the diagnostic procedures of choice to evaluate potential injury to the lower urinary tract. These studies must be carried out in the proper sequence and in a retrograde fashion to avoid missing potential injuries. *Retrograde* refers to the technique of instilling

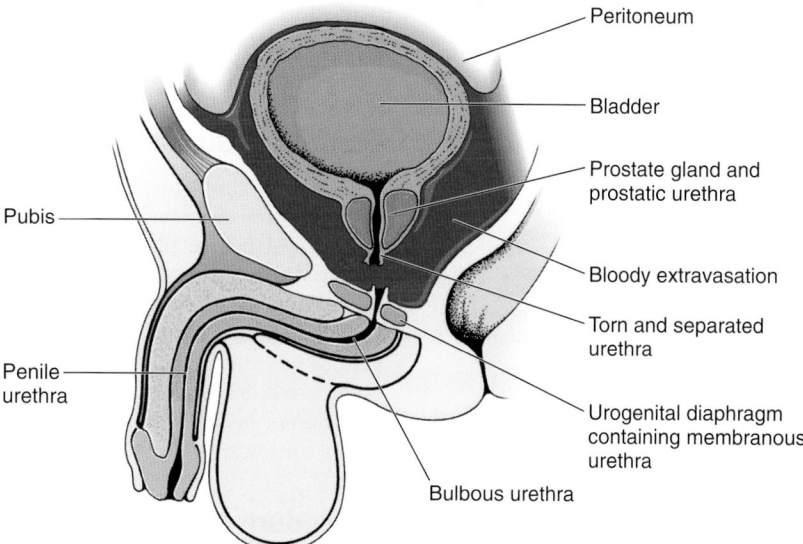

Figure 55-31 Posterior urethral injury. A common posterior urethral injury is disruption of the membranous urethra. In this case, a distended bladder and attached prostate gland are sheared from the fixed membranous urethra. Note the development of a perivesical hematoma and the presence of a "high-riding" prostate gland.

contrast material retrograde through the urethra or by gravity filling of the bladder. It must be distinguished from antegrade filling, in which intravenous contrast for IVP or abdominal computed tomography (CT) is excreted from the kidneys and allowed to fill the bladder passively over time.

Background

In the resuscitation of any trauma patient, placement of a Foley catheter has become the standard method for monitoring urinary output. Blood at the urethral meatus, however, may indicate a potential partial or complete urethral disruption and dictates the need for RUG to delineate urethral integrity. This study can be done by the resuscitating clinician in the ED or on the operating room table by the trauma surgeon or urologist if the patient requires immediate surgical intervention for life-threatening injuries. RUG is a quick, technically easy study to perform and should be part of every emergency clinician's armamentarium. Similarly, RUG allows evaluation of bladder integrity.

Anatomy and Physiology

The anatomy of the male urethra is demonstrated Figure 55-17. The male urethra varies from around 17.5 to 20 cm in length in adults and consists of anterior and posterior portions, each of which is subdivided into two parts (pendulous and bulbous for the anterior portion, membranous and prostatic for the posterior portion). The female urethra is approximately 4 cm long and extends from the neck of the bladder at the urethrovesical junction to the vaginal vestibule, where it forms the external meatus between the labia minora (see Figs. 55-15 and 55-16).

Pathophysiology

The male posterior urethra, which includes the membranous and prostatic urethra, is injured more frequently than the anterior urethra. The urogenital diaphragm encloses and fixes the membranous urethra; the prostate and prostatic urethra are firmly attached to the posterior surface of the symphysis pubis by the puboprostatic ligaments. Blunt trauma and pelvic fractures, especially in the presence of a full bladder, may result in shearing forces that partially or completely avulse portions of the firmly attached posterior urethra. Usually, the bladder and prostate gland are sheared from the membranous urethra, which results in complete urethral disruption (Fig. 55-31). The female urethra, in contrast, is short and relatively mobile and generally escapes injury with blunt trauma. Occasionally, a significant pelvic fracture will result in a laceration or avulsion of the female urethra at the bladder neck. Direct injuries to the female urethra may also occur secondary to penetrating trauma to the vagina or perineum. These injuries are often disclosed by blood at the introitus or abnormal findings on vaginal examination in a female patient with a pelvic fracture.[92]

Contusions or lacerations of the male anterior urethra occur when the bulbous urethra is compressed against the inferior surface of the symphysis pubis. This happens most commonly as a result of straddle injuries in males but may be caused by any blunt perineal trauma. Significant trauma to the penile urethra is rare without penetrating injuries or urethral instrumentation. Anterior urethral injuries may result in extravasation of blood or urine into the penis, scrotum, or perineum or along the anterior abdominal wall, depending on whether Buck's fascia has been violated (Fig. 55-32).[93] This is in contrast to posterior urethral injuries, in which blood and urine extravasate into the pelvis.

Indications

RUG is indicated whenever uncertainty exists about the integrity of the urethra. RUG is an anatomic rather than a physiologic examination but is critical in identifying a possible urethral injury before insertion of a urinary catheter to preclude a potentially devastating complication.[94]

The traditional physical indications to perform RUG in the trauma setting include blood at the urethral meatus, a nonpalpable or high-riding prostate, or urethral trauma. However, the value of these findings to the emergency clinician has been called into question given their low sensitivity.[95,96]

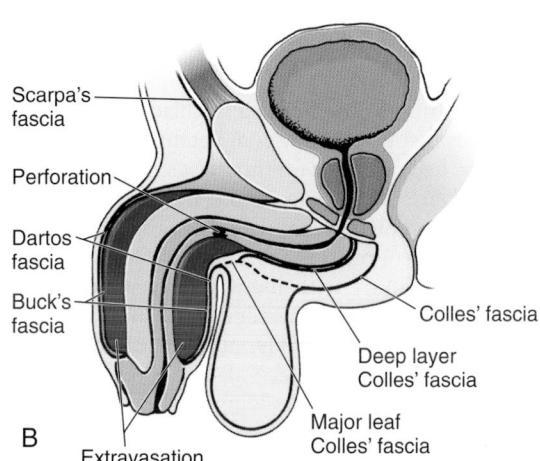

Figure 55-32 Anterior urethral injury. **A,** Disruption of the anterior urethra (bulbous urethra) occurs with straddle-type injuries in a male. Extravasation of urine and blood may occur in the perineum or scrotum or along the anterior abdominal wall. Note that in this diagram Buck's fascia has been penetrated. **B,** Anterior urethral injury in which Buck's fascia remains intact. In this situation, extravasation is confirmed and results in a swollen and ecchymotic penis. Such an injury usually results from instrumentation of the anterior urethra.

Perform RUG any time that a bladder injury is suspected. It is assumed that the urethra is normal before passing the Foley catheter required for retrograde cystography.

Contraindications

Uncertainty about urethral integrity is a contraindication to blind urethral catheterization. Hence, urethral integrity must be ensured before placement of a Foley catheter, which is essential for retrograde cystography. A history of a reaction to radiographic contrast material is a relative contraindication, depending on the route of administration selected. Intravenous administration for antegrade imaging carries a much greater risk for serious adverse events than does retrograde injection or instillation of the iodinated contrast material necessary for lower GU tract imaging, which has negligible risks.

Procedure

Several different iodinated contrast agents are suitable for retrograde studies (urethrography, cystography). Common agents, dosages, and methods of administration are listed in Table 55-6.

Retrograde cystography and urethrography should ideally be performed under fluoroscopic guidance to provide real-time imaging, but plain films are an acceptable and frequently used alternative.

RUG

In cases associated with pelvic fracture, the patient should remain supine throughout the entire radiographic examination. In cases of suspected urethral injury not associated with pelvic fracture, it is acceptable to obtain oblique films (supine 45-degree oblique position) during the study, which may complement the findings on examination.

First, take a plain film (kidney, ureter, bladder [KUB]) for reference before injecting any contrast material.[98] Retract and secure the penile foreskin with a folded 4 × 4 gauze sponge. Second, hold the penis between the long and ring fingers of the nondominant hand to allow a snug fit of the contrast-filled syringe or catheter inside the urethra. The penis should be stretched laterally over the proximal part of the thigh with moderate traction to prevent folding of the urethra (i.e., the double image of the proximal penile and bulbous urethra superimposed on one another) and allow high-quality RUG (Fig. 55-33, *step 3*).

TABLE 55-6 Common Agents, Dosages, and Administration Information for Contrast-Enhanced Retrograde Urologic Imaging

AGENTS[97]	USE	PROCEDURE
Diatrizoate (Cystografin) Iohexol (Omnipaque) Iodixanol (Visipaque)	Use a stock concentration of solution* *or* Use a one-half stock concentration of solution *or* Dilute the stock solution with saline in a ratio of 1 part contrast to 10 parts saline (resulting in a <10% solution)	**Urethrography**: 10-15 mL of dilute solution injected slowly through the urethral meatus for adults (children: 0.2 mL/kg) **Cystography**: after a plain film and with the Foley catheter in place, fill the bladder of adults with 400 mL of dilute contrast material introduced under gravity (children: 5 mL/kg)

*A higher concentration may allow improved image quality; however, extravasation of contrast material into periurethral or perivesical tissues may cause a considerable inflammatory reaction at higher concentrations.

RETROGRADE URETHROGRAPHY

1

Insert the balloon portion of a Foley catheter (8 Fr) into the urethra, and slowly inflate the balloon with 2 mL of air or water to create a snug fit. Then slowly inject 10 to 60 mL of a 10% solution of contrast material through the catheter lumen. Usually only 10 to 20 mL is required.

2

Alternatively, use a plain-tipped (non–Luer-Lok) syringe or a catheter-tipped ("Toomey") syringe in the urethra. Squeeze the glans around the syringe to prevent spillage of the contrast material. Inject slowly.

3

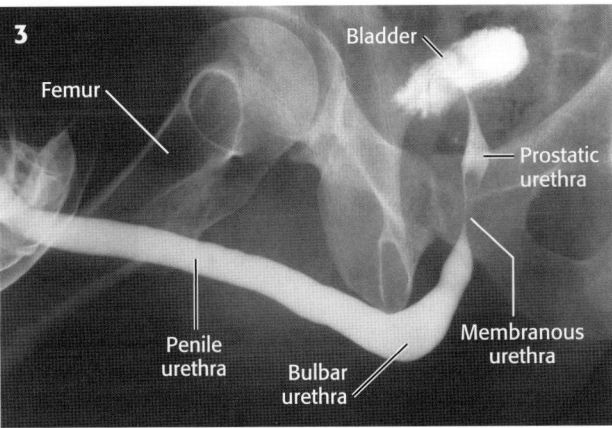

Normal retrograde urethrogram. Note that penis is pulled taut over the proximal part of the thigh to prevent urethral folding. After injection of contrast material, the entire urethra can be visualized and inspected for injury.

4

Inject the contrast material slowly. Injecting too fast causes venous intravasation (*arrows*). This may mimic urethral extravasation but it clears immediately, as opposed to actual extravasation, which remains indefinitely. If unsure, take another film in 10 minutes. The presence of intravasation is benign but can confuse the clinician.

5

Penile urethra disruption. Extravasation of contrast material (*arrow*) is seen in the corpus cavernosum.

6

Bulbar urethral disruption. Extravasation of contrast material (*white arrows*) is seen in the scrotum.

7

Supramembranous urethral disruption. Extravasation of contrast material (*arrow*) is noted superiorly.

Figure 55-33 Retrograde urethrography. (**Step 4,** *From Richter MW, Lytton B, Myerson D, et al. Radiology of genitourinary trauma.* Radiol Clin North Am. *1973;11:626; step **7,** from Morehouse DD, MacKinnon KJ. Posterior urethral injury: etiology, diagnosis, initial management.* Urol Clin North Am. *1977;4:74.)*

After sterile penile preparation, prepare to inject the dye. A small Foley catheter may be used (see Fig. 55-33, *step 1*). Seat the balloon portion of the catheter in the fossa navicularis of the penile urethra, and delicately inflate it with 1.0 to 1.5 mL of saline solution to ensure a snug fit.[99] Lubrication is not recommended because it may prevent the balloon from remaining in place. Steady manual pressure of the balloon against the external urethral meatus (distal to the fossa navicularis) is an alternative strategy. Another option is to gently advance a catheter-tipped Toomey irrigating syringe or a regular 60-mL syringe with an attached Christmas tree adapter or a non–Luer-Lok syringe inside the urethral meatus until a snug fit is ensured (see Fig. 55-33, *step 2*). Always gently squeeze the meatus over the injecting device to prevent leakage.

Inject contrast material through the catheter or syringe. If not done carefully, this technique often results in spillage and deposition of contrast agent outside the urethra and onto the patient and the examination table, thereby yielding a spurious result. For this reason, *slowly* inject anywhere from 10 to 60 mL of contrast material (typically 10 to 20 mL is all that is needed) under constant pressure into the urethra. Not uncommonly, spasm of the external urethral sphincter will be encountered and prevent filling of the posterior urethra. Slow, gentle pressure is usually needed to overcome this resistance.[100] Overly forceful injection of contrast material may cause intravasation of contrast material into the venous plexus of the urethra and simulate an injury (see Fig. 55-33, *step 4*). Finally, during injection of the last 10 mL of contrast material, a film (the urethrogram) is taken (see Fig. 55-33, *step 3*). Alternatively, the urethrogram can be viewed in real time with use of fluoroscopy.

Extravasation of contrast material from a urethral disruption usually appears as a flamelike density outside the urethral contour (see Fig. 55-33, *plates 5 to 7*). If any contrast material is seen within the bladder in conjunction with urethral extravasation, a partial rather than complete urethral disruption is more likely. With complete urethral disruption, urethral extravasation will be present without evidence of contrast material within the bladder. The examiner needs to be certain that the lack of bladder contrast is not secondary to voluntary contraction of the external sphincter. Occasionally, as mentioned previously, intravasated contrast material is seen in the periurethral penile venous plexus (see Fig. 55-33, *step 4*). It is of no clinical significance and should not be mistaken for urethral extravasation. As expected, penile venous intravasation (venous plexus opacification) is noted to clear spontaneously on any postvoid films, unlike urethral extravasation, which remains.

If a Foley catheter has been successfully placed into the bladder and a partial urethral injury is suspected later, such an injury can easily be demonstrated without removing the catheter. Place the lubricated end of a pediatric feeding tube into the penile urethra alongside the existing Foley catheter (Fig. 55-34). Obtain a seal by compressing the glans penis with the nondominant thumb and index finger and gently inject contrast material via a Luer-Lok syringe with the dominant hand. In this way, extravasation can be demonstrated. It should be noted, however, that successful placement of the Foley catheter obviates the need for further treatment of a partial urethral tear in the emergency setting because an indwelling catheter alone is appropriate initial management of this type of injury. The finding of an associated urethral

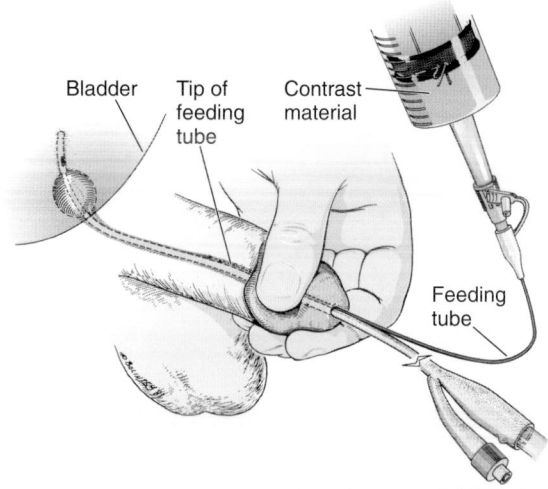

Figure 55-34 Evaluation of a urethral injury with a Foley catheter in place. A lubricated pediatric feeding tube has been advanced into the urethra beside the indwelling Foley catheter.

injury must be conveyed to a urologist because it will dictate the duration of definitive Foley catheter drainage.

Retrograde Cystography

As noted, it is assumed that the urethra is normal before passing the Foley catheter required for retrograde cystography.

Obtain a preliminary KUB film, which will serve as reference for the entire examination. Next, fill the bladder under direct operator supervision by gravity instillation of contrast material. After removing the central piston from a 60-mL catheter-tipped syringe, attach the catheter-tipped end of the syringe to the Foley catheter and hold it above the level of the patient's bladder. Pour the contrast material into the syringe and allow it to fill the bladder by gravity instillation to one of three end points: (1) 100 mL with evidence of gross extravasation on fluoroscopy or on plain film (if the examiner elects to check at this point); (2) 400 mL in an adult or any child 11 years or older; in children younger than 11 years, bladder capacity and therefore appropriate contrast volumes are estimated from the formula[101] (age in years + 2) × 30; or (3) the point of initiating a bladder contraction (see later). Then add an additional 50 mL by hand injection under pressure.

Obtain anteroposterior (AP) and complementary oblique projections as long as no evidence of a pelvic fracture is present (Fig. 55-35, *A1*). In the presence of a pelvic fracture, obtain all films with the patient in the supine position for the same reasons that were elucidated for RUG. A lateral film may be informative when oblique films are not possible (see Fig. 55-35, *A2*). Obtain an AP *postevacuation film in all cases after bladder drainage to disclose posterior perforation in selected cases, especially those associated with penetrating trauma* (see Fig. 55-35, *A3*). Again, a dilute solution of contrast material (see Table 55-6) may be used rather than full-strength contrast. Some authors recommend a dilute solution of contrast material (≤10%) because extravasation into periurethral or perivesical tissue may cause a considerable inflammatory reaction at higher concentrations. Dilute solutions do not appear to compromise the quality of the study, but this must be a consideration. Retrograde cystography done by any technique

RETROGRADE CYSTOGRAPHY

A. Normal Examination

AP view. Fill the bladder with at least 400 mL (see text for details). The normal bladder has a smooth outer contour and no extravasation of contrast material is seen.

Lateral view. Obtain a lateral or oblique view to assess for posterior extravasation because the opacified bladder would prevent visualization of this injury on the AP view.

Postvoid film. Always perform a postvoid film to assess for subtle posterior perforation, especially in the case of penetrating trauma.

B. Abnormal Examinations

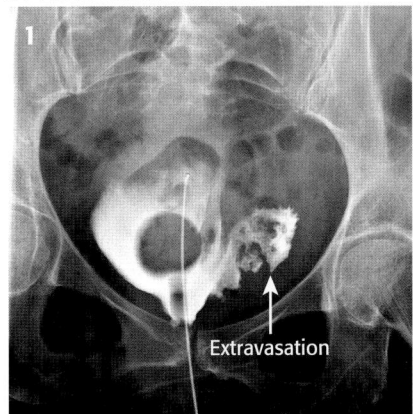

Extravasation

Extraperitoneal bladder perforation. Contrast material is seen adjacent to the bladder neck. The bladder itself is displaced rightward by an adjacent hematoma.

Posterior injury. On this AP film, the bladder appears normal, and no extravasation of contrast material is noted. However, postvoid films are required to rule out posterior injury.

Postvoid

The postvoid film demonstrates substantial posterior extravasation of contrast material. This injury would have been missed if only the AP study were performed.

Extraperitoneal bladder rupture. Extravasated contrast material is seen surrounding the bladder (*arrows*) but no loops of bowel are outlined. This injury can typically be treated conservatively with a Foley catheter.

Intraperitoneal bladder rupture. Note the contrast material outling the paravesical space, tracking up the right paracolic gutter and outlying loops of bowel (*arrows*). This typically requires operative repair.

Pelvic hematoma. Note the "open-book" pelvic fracture (*arrows*). No extravasation of contrast material is seen, however, the pear-shaped bladder indicates the presence of a pelvic hematoma.

Figure 55-35 Retrograde cystography. *AP*, anteroposterior.

RETROGRADE CT CYSTOGRAPHY

Extraperitoneal bladder perforation. Retrograde cystography may be performed in conjuction with abdominal CT scanning. Fill the bladder in the same fashion as for conventional cystography (obtaining delayed images with IV contrast material collected in the bladder is not sufficient). Above, extravasation of contrast material is noted adjacent to the left side of the bladder.

Intraperitoneal bladder perforation. This patient complained of abdominal pain after routine cystoscopy. Standard IV and oral contrast-enhanced CT imaging of the pelvis revealed nonspecific inflammatory changes in the right pelvis. CT cystography was required to diagnose the bladder perforation, as evidenced by extravasation of contrast material into the peritoneal cavity (*arrow*).

Figure 55-36 Retrograde computed tomographic (CT) cystography. *IV,* intravenous.

other than hand-poured gravity instillation is subject to inadequate bladder filling or disconnection of the connector tubing from the catheter. Both conditions will result in spurious examination results, which may adversely affect important patient management decisions.

It must be stressed that in the absence of initial gross extravasation, the bladder must be filled to 400 mL in an adult and to an appropriate capacity in a child and the catheter clamped with a Kelly clamp. Volumes less than 400 mL have been associated with false-negative findings, especially with penetrating bladder injuries.[102] At times the patient may have difficulty cooperating with bladder filling because of a head injury or associated pain, and in the case of severe injury, the patient may have involuntary bladder contractions that cause contrast material to back up into the Toomey syringe. If this occurs, refill the bladder to the point of initiating a bladder contraction, clamp the Foley catheter, remove the initial syringe, replace it with a 60-mL contrast-filled syringe, unclamp the catheter, hand-inject the additional 50 mL under pressure, and reclamp the catheter. The goal is to overdistend the bladder. Once the filled-bladder films have been obtained and reviewed, unclamp the Foley catheter and allow the contrast material to drain into a bedside drainage bag. Then obtain an AP postevacuation film to visualize any posterior extravasation that may have been hidden by the distended bladder during the AP filled-bladder film (see Fig. 55-35, *B2 and B3*). Once again, take care to ensure that contrast material is not spilled onto the patient or the examination table during the procedure. Spilled contrast can lead to spurious examination results.

Extravasation from an injured bladder may be intraperitoneal, extraperitoneal, or both. Extraperitoneal extravasation

is usually seen as flamelike areas of contrast material confined to the pelvis and projecting laterally to the bladder (see Fig. 55-35, *B1 and B4*). If contrast material extravasates intraperitoneally, it tends to fill the paracolic gutters and outline the intraperitoneal structures, particularly the bowel, spleen, or liver (see Fig. 55-35, *B5*). It is important to distinguish extraperitoneal from intraperitoneal injury because the treatment options are totally different: surgical repair for all intraperitoneal injuries and for extraperitoneal injuries that extend into or primarily involve the neck of the bladder, especially in women. Most other extraperitoneal injuries can be managed confidently by Foley catheter drainage alone.

Retrograde cystography may be done in conjunction with contrast-enhanced abdominal CT scanning (Fig. 55-36). The bladder must be filled just as though conventional retrograde cystography were being performed. Clamp the catheter and seek evidence of contrast-enhanced ascites on the CT scan. When this is encountered, bladder injury with extravasation must be searched for with selective images of the pelvis.

Aftercare

A Foley catheter is placed following demonstration of urethral integrity by RUG. Consult urology to aid in decision making in any case of urethral or bladder injury.

Complications

Extravasation of contrast material into periurethral or perivesical tissue in the case of urethral or bladder injury, respectively, may cause a considerable inflammatory reaction, particularly with higher concentrations of contrast material.

UPPER GENITOURINARY TRACT IMAGING

Grade 3 renal laceration. This contrast-enhanced CT scan reveals a renal laceration >1 cm in depth without urinary extravasation (*arrow*) and hence a grade 3 injury.

Grade 4 renal injury. This laceration extends through the renal parenchyma and into the collecting system. Extravasation of contrast material is seen (*long arrow*), thus making this a grade 4 injury. Note the large perinephric hematoma (*short arrows*).

Urethral transection. This intraoperative excretory urogram reveals extravasation (*arrow*) in the upper part of the right ureter consequent to a stab wound. No contrast material is seen in the ureter below the site of injury a finding indicative of complete transection.

Normal CT urogram. A coronal projection of a CT urogram in the excretory phase demonstrates opacification of the proximal and middle section of the ureters (*arrows*) without evidence of extravasation of contrast material.

Distal ureter injury. This patient suffered a gunshot wound to his abdomen. After emergentcy laparotomy and bowel resection, abdominal pain worsened. The initial arterial phase CT demonstrated a large fluid collection in the inferior recesses of the peritoneum (*arrow*).

Delayed images revealed extravasation of contrast material from the distal end of the ureter (*arrow*) into the fluid collection. This part of the ureter was not explored during the initial operation.

Figure 55-37 Upper genitourinary tract imaging. *CT,* computed tomography. (Step 3, *from Wein AJ, Kavoussi LR, Novick AC, et al, eds.* Campbell-Walsh Urology. *10th ed. Philadelphia: Saunders; 2011;* step 4, *from Haaga JR, Dogra VS, Forsting M, et al, eds.* CT and MRI of the Whole Body. *5th ed. St. Louis: Mosby; 2008;* steps 5 and 6, *from Jankowski JT, Spirnak JP. Current recommendations for imaging in the management of urologic traumas.* Urol Clin North Am. *2006;33:365-376.)*

BOX 55-6 American Association for the Surgery of Trauma Classification System for Renal Injuries

GRADE 1 INJURIES

Hematuria with normal imaging

Contusions

Subcapsular, nonexpanding hematoma without parenchymal laceration

GRADE 2 INJURIES

Nonexpanding perinephric hematomas confined to the retroperitoneum

Renal cortical lacerations less than 1 cm in depth without urinary extravasation

GRADE 3 INJURIES

Renal cortical lacerations greater than 1 cm in depth without urinary extravasation

GRADE 4 INJURIES

Parenchymal laceration extending through the renal cortex/medulla and into the collecting system

Main renal artery or vein injury with contained hemorrhage

Segmental infarction without associated laceration

GRADE 5 INJURIES

Shattered or devascularized kidney

Complete avulsion or thrombosis of the main renal artery or vein

Avulsion of the ureteropelvic junction

From Moore EE, Shackford SR, Pachter HL, et al. Organ injury scaling: spleen, liver, and kidney. J Trauma. *1989;29:1664-1666.*

Conclusion

RUG and retrograde cystography are the diagnostic procedures of choice to evaluate potential injury to the lower urinary tract. These studies must be carried out in the proper sequence and in a retrograde fashion to avoid missing potential injuries.

UPPER GU TRACT IMAGING

Once the lower GU tract has been exonerated with retrograde urethrography and cystography, the upper tract (kidneys and ureters) should be evaluated. For adult blunt trauma patients with gross hematuria or hypotension (systolic pressure lower than 90 mm Hg), upper tract imaging is indicated.[103] Data show that 12.5% of such patients will have a major renal injury as compared with only 0.2% of adults with microscopic hematuria and normal blood pressure.[104] In the presence of a major mechanism of injury or other extenuating circumstances, inclusion criteria for upper tract imaging may be broadened. It should be noted that these criteria are not intended for use in pediatric populations, and opinions regarding diagnostic strategies in children remain controversial.

Contrast-enhanced CT is the gold standard for evaluating patients with suspected renal trauma.[103] Parenchymal injuries, vascular injuries, and urinary extravasation can all be readily identified on CT (Fig. 55-37, *plates 1 and 2*). Traumatic renal injuries are graded on a 5-point scale (Box 55-6). For patients with a mandate for emergency laparotomy, upper tract imaging can be performed in the operating room with an excretory urogram (see Fig. 55-37, *plate 3*).

Ureteral injuries can also be identified on contrast-enhanced CT imaging; however, it is *essential to obtain delayed images* (i.e., about 10 minutes after the initial intravenous contrast bolus) (see Fig. 55-37, *plates 4 to 6*). This delay allows the contrast material to become concentrated in the kidneys and excreted through the ureters. Ureteral injury can then be identified by extravasation of contrast material into adjacent tissues.

Acknowledgment

The authors and editors acknowledge the contributions made to previous editions by Robert E. Schneider, MD, Ivan Zbaraschuk, MD, Richard E. Berger, MD, Jerris R. Hedges, MD, Martin Schiff, Jr., MD, Morton G. Glickman, MD, and Geoffrey E. Herter, MD. In addition, the authors wish to acknowledge Dr. Robert E. Schneider, who trained and practiced in both emergency medicine and urology, for his guidance and mentorship.

References are available at www.expertconsult.com

Emergency Childbirth

George H. Lew and Michael S. Pulia

BACKGROUND

Of the more than 4.1 million births in the United States in 2009, 99% were delivered in a hospital setting. The percentage of these births that occur in the emergency department (ED) setting is unknown.[1] Childbirth is a relatively rare occurrence in the ED and is not identified as a specific diagnosis by the Centers for Disease Control and Prevention. It is instead categorized in the "supplemental classification," along with other miscellaneous and noncodable diagnoses.[2] Emergency delivery of an infant continues to be one of the most challenging and stress-inducing procedures facing emergency physicians (EPs). The clinician needs to assess the mother and fetus, prepare for delivery, and anticipate potential difficulties or complications during and after the birthing process.

In institutions where on-site and timely obstetric services are available, the primary duty of the EP may be only to determine that labor is active and delivery imminent. However, in the case of unavailable obstetrics, precipitous delivery, or delayed arrival, the EP may be required to solely manage a patient in active labor. This role includes handling neonatal and maternal resuscitation.

ANATOMY AND PHYSIOLOGY

Labor is the process by which the fetus is expelled from the uterus. It begins with a sequence of regular and effective uterine contractions that result in effacement and dilation of the cervix.[3] Identification of true labor versus false labor is best determined in a dedicated obstetric unit, often with external uterine monitoring. Labor can also be divided into *phases*. The latent phase of labor is the period between its onset and when labor becomes active, which generally requires 80% effacement and cervical dilation of greater than 4 cm.[4] Active labor is normally divided into three generally progressive stages. The first stage begins with cervical effacement and dilation and ends when the cervix is completed dilated. In multiparous women this stage of labor typically lasts about 5 to 8 hours, as opposed to 7 to 13 hours in nulliparous women, but with much individual variation.[3,4] The second stage of labor begins when dilation of the cervix is complete and ends with delivery of the infant. The duration of this stage is also variable, with a median of 50 to 60 minutes in nulliparas and 15 to 20 minutes in multiparas.[3,4] The third stage of labor begins after delivery of the infant and ends with delivery of the placenta. The fourth stage of labor refers to the 1 hour immediately after delivery, the period in which postpartum hemorrhage is most likely to occur.[3] It is recommended that maternal blood pressure and pulse be recorded immediately after delivery and every 15 minutes for the first hour to rapidly detect any ongoing hemorrhage.[3]

IDENTIFICATION OF LABOR

It is not uncommon for women to have contractions late in pregnancy, although not all are true or effective labor contractions. Irregular, brief Braxton-Hicks contractions of the uterus, usually with discomfort and confined to the lower abdominal region and groin, are typically irregular in timing and strength. These pains do not cause any change in the cervix or result in descent of the fetus. Although these pains usually stop spontaneously, they can rapidly convert to true labor contractions; if they occur, a period of observation may be necessary.

True labor is characterized by a regular sequence of uterine contractions with progressively increasing intensity and decreasing intervals between contractions. The interval between contractions gradually diminishes from 10 minutes at the onset of labor to as short as 1 minute or less in the second stage of labor. This should be accompanied by effacement and dilation of the cervix, along with descent of the presenting part into the pelvis. The onset of true labor can be difficult to identify given that patients are far more likely to be at home than in a hospital when labor begins.

Show or *bloody show* is a sign of approaching labor. The normal mucous plug sealing the cervix discharges as the cervix dilates. Show consists of a small amount of blood-tinged mucus discharged from the vagina and indicates that labor is already in progress or will probably occur during the next several hours to a few days. The coloring of the mucus can become pink or brown tinged as a result of minor bleeding. However, if more than a small amount of blood escapes with the mucous plug, an abnormal cause such as abruption of the placenta or placenta previa should be considered. Digital vaginal examination under these circumstances is generally contraindicated.[3]

Spontaneous rupture of membranes can occur during the course of active labor, typically evident by a sudden gush or continuous leakage of a variable amount of clear or slightly turbid vaginal fluid. Rupture of membranes before the onset of labor at any stage of gestation is referred to as *premature rupture of membranes* (PROM). Term PROM, which occurs before the onset of labor, complicates approximately 8% of pregnancies.[5] In the majority of cases it is followed by the onset of labor and delivery within 5 hours.[5] The most significant maternal risk associated with term PROM is intrauterine infection. Fetal risks associated with PROM include umbilical cord compression and ascending infection.[5] The ideal management of PROM should be deferred to the consulting obstetrician.[6]

Membrane rupture occurring before 37 weeks of gestation is called *preterm premature rupture of membranes* (pPROM). Birth within 1 week generally occurs regardless of management or the clinical findings. The most significant maternal risk related to pPROM is intrauterine infection. The most significant risks to the fetus are complications related to prematurity. Preterm delivery occurs in approximately 12% of all births in the United States.[5]

Accurate diagnosis of PROM will be helpful in further management. Suspected PROM should be confirmed by an examination that minimizes the risk of introducing infection. Avoid digital cervical examination unless the patient is in active labor or delivery is imminent.[5] A sterile speculum examination can be performed to look for amniotic fluid extruding from the cervical os or pooling in the posterior fornix, as well as to inspect for fetal or umbilical cord prolapse and assess cervical effacement and dilation.[3,5]

Amniotic fluid may be differentiated from vaginal fluid by testing the pH of the fluid with Nitrazine paper or similar swab devices (Fig. 56-1). The pH of vaginal fluid is generally 4.5 to 6.0, whereas amniotic fluid has a pH of 7.0 to 7.5. The yellow testing paper turns blue-green to deep blue in the presence of amniotic fluid. With vaginal secretions the Nitrazine paper remains yellow.[3,5] False-positive results may occur with blood, semen, bacterial vaginosis, or alkaline urine. If rupture of membranes is documented in the ED, notify the patient's obstetrician and plan for hospital admission or possible transfer.

EVALUATION OF LABOR

When a woman is initially seen with contractions, the general condition of both the fetus and mother should be assessed quickly. Under the federal Emergency Medical Treatment and Labor Act (EMTALA), hospitals with an ED must conduct an appropriate screening examination to rule out true labor. In addition, under EMTALA, a woman in labor is considered unstable for interhospital transfer unless done so at the direction of the patient or a physician who certifies that the benefits outweigh the risks of transfer.[3] A brief obstetric history, including the onset and frequency of contractions, the presence or absence of bleeding, possible loss of amniotic fluid, previous prenatal care, and due date, should be obtained. In the absence of active vaginal bleeding, a sterile vaginal examination should be performed in addition to maternal abdominal palpation to determine the stage of labor, as well as the position, presentation, and lie of the fetus. Monitor

fetal well-being by evaluation of the fetal heart rate, particularly immediately after a uterine contraction. In an ED setting, fetal assessment is increasingly done via bedside ultrasonography, which can assess fetal movement and heart rate (Fig. 56-2). The traditional approaches of using external Doppler or auscultation are also acceptable. The normal baseline fetal heart rate is 110 to 160 beats per minute.

Lie refers to the relationship of the long axis of the fetus to the long axis of the uterus. It is either longitudinal, transverse, or oblique (Fig. 56-3). Oblique lies are unstable and will convert to a longitudinal or transverse lie during labor. Longitudinal lies occur in more than 99% of pregnancies at term.[3] Transverse lies generally cannot be safely delivered vaginally.[4]

The presentation, or presenting part, refers to the portion of the body of the fetus nearest to or foremost in the birth canal. The presenting part can be felt through the cervix on sterile vaginal examination. In longitudinal lies, the presenting part is the fetal head, the buttocks (breech), or the feet (footling breech). With a transverse lie, the presenting part is the shoulder. The presentation can be cephalic, breech, shoulder, or compound. All presentations except cephalic are considered malpresentations.[7]

Cephalic presentations are classified by the bony leading landmark of the fetal skull. Ordinarily, the head is sharply flexed so that the occipital fontanelle is the presenting part.

Figure 56-2 Assessment of fetal heart rate. **A,** Fetal assessment is often done via bedside ultrasonography in the emergency department. **B,** Traditional methods, such as external Doppler, are also acceptable. The normal baseline fetal heart rate is 110 to 160 beats/min.

Figure 56-1 Amniotic fluid has an alkaline pH, whereas normal vaginal secretions are acidic. Both Nitrazine or pH paper (**A**) and an indicator swab (**B**) (Amnicator device/Amnicator.com) will turn yellow in the absence of amniotic fluid and dark blue in the presence of amniotic fluid within a few seconds.

This is referred to as a *vertex* or *occiput presentation*. Less commonly, the neck is fully extended and the face is foremost in the birth canal; this is termed *face presentation*. A partially flexed or partially extended neck position results in *sinciput* and *brow presentations*, respectively. Sinciput and brow presentations associated with preterm infants are almost always unstable and convert to either an occiput or face presentation as labor progresses.

Breech presentations are classified as frank, complete, or incomplete (Fig. 56-4). A fetus presenting with the buttocks and hips flexed and the legs extended is termed a *frank breech*. *Presentation of the buttocks with flexion of the fetal hips and knees* results in *a complete breech* presentation. When one or both of the feet or knees are lowermost in the canal, an *incomplete or footling breech* results.

At or near term, 97% of fetuses will be vertex and 3% will be breech.[3] The incidence of breech delivery is approximately 25% at 28 weeks, 17% at 30 weeks, and 11% at 32 weeks.[3,8,9]

Position refers to the relationship of the presenting part to the maternal pelvis and may be either left or right. The occiput is the reference point in cephalic presentations, whereas the sacrum is the determining part in breech presentations. The vertex occiput anterior position is the most common and considered normal. The other position is occiput posterior.

LABOR MOVEMENTS: VERTEX

Full dilation of the cervix signifies the second stage of labor and heralds delivery of the infant. Typically, the patient begins to bear down, which coincides with descent of the presenting part. Uterine contractions may last 1.5 minutes and recur after a resting phase of less than 1 minute. Delivery of a vertex-presenting infant usually occurs spontaneously. The role of the clinician or attendant is principally to provide control of the birth process by preventing forceful, sudden expulsion or extraction of the infant with resultant fetal or maternal injury.

The mechanism of labor in vertex presentations consists of engagement of the presenting part, flexion, descent, internal rotation, extension, external rotation or restitution, and expulsion (Fig. 56-5).[3] These are often referred to as *cardinal movements*. The mechanism of labor is determined by the pelvic dimensions and configuration, the size of the fetus, and the strength of the uterine contractions. Essentially, the fetus will follow the path of least resistance by adaptation of the smallest achievable diameter of the presenting part to the most favorable dimensions and contours of the birth canal.

The sequence of movements in vertex presentations is as follows:

1. *Engagement* refers to the mechanism by which the greatest transverse diameter of the head, the biparietal diameter in occiput presentations, passes through the pelvic inlet. A fetus is engaged when the presenting part is at 0 station. In a primiparous patient, it usually occurs in the last 2 weeks of pregnancy; in a multiparous patient, it can occur at the onset of labor.
2. *Flexion* of the head is necessary to minimize the presenting cross-sectional diameter of the head during passage through the smallest diameter of the bony pelvis. In most cases, flexion is necessary for both engagement and descent and occurs passively.
3. *Descent* is the downward passage of the fetal presenting part. It is gradually progressive but is not necessarily

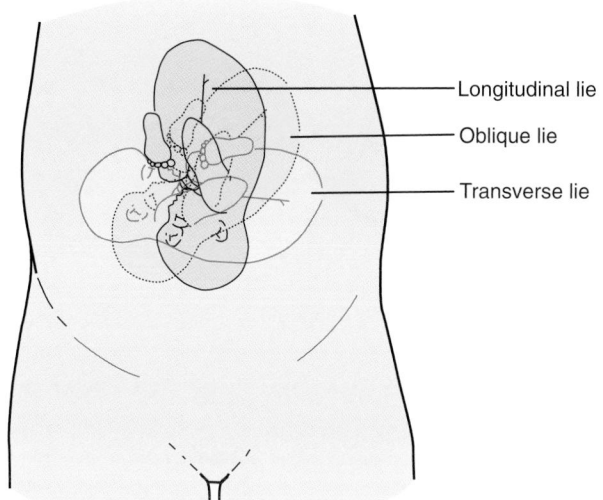

Figure 56-3 Examples of different fetal lie. *(From Gabbe SG, Niebyl JR, Simpson JL, eds. Obstetrics: Normal and Problem Pregnancies. Philadelphia: Churchill Livingstone; 2007.)*

Longitudinal lie

Oblique lie

Transverse lie

Complete breech   Incomplete breech   Frank breech

Figure 56-4 A fetus in a complete breech presentation is flexed at the hips and at the knees. An incomplete breech shows incomplete deflexion of one or both knees or hips. With a frank breech presentation the fetus is flexed at the hips and extended at the knees.

continuous. Descent is affected by uterine and abdominal contractions, as well as by straightening and extension of the fetal body.

4. *Internal rotation* occurs with descent and is necessary for the head or presenting part to traverse the ischial spines. This movement essentially turns the head such that the occiput gradually moves from its original, more transverse position anteriorly toward the symphysis pubis or, less commonly, posteriorly toward the hollow of the sacrum. This is known as occiput anterior or occiput posterior, respectively.

5. *Extension* occurs as the flexed head reaches the anteriorly directed vaginal introitus. The occiput reaches the inferior aspect of the pubic symphysis. The head is born by further extension as it rotates around the pubic symphysis and the occiput, bregma, forehead, nose, mouth, and finally, the chin pass successively over the anterior margin of the perineum. Immediately after its birth, the head drops downward such that the chin lies over the maternal anal region.

6. *External rotation* or restitution is return of the head to the correct anatomic position with respect to the fetal torso.

It follows delivery of the head as it rotates to the transverse position that it occupied at engagement. This is also a passive movement.

7. *Expulsion* of the remainder of the fetal body then occurs. The shoulders descend in a path similar to that traced by the head (i.e., rotating anteroposteriorly for delivery). First, the anterior shoulder is delivered beneath the symphysis pubis followed by the posterior shoulder across the perineum.

LABOR MOVEMENTS: BREECH

The mechanism of labor for breech presentations varies (see Fig. 56-4). The widest diameter that is engaged is the bitrochanteric diameter. Usually, the hips engage in one of the oblique diameters of the pelvic inlet. As descent occurs, the anterior hip generally descends more rapidly than the posterior hip. Internal rotation occurs as the bitrochanteric diameter assumes the anteroposterior (AP) position. Lateral flexion takes place as the anterior hip catches beneath the symphysis pubis, which allows the posterior hip to be born first. The

A Before engagement

B Engagement, flexion, descent

C Descent, rotation

D Complete rotation, early extension

E Complete extension

F Restitution

G Anterior shoulder delivery

H Posterior shoulder delivery

Figure 56-5 A-H, Cardinal movements of labor. *(From Gabbe SG, Niebyl JR, Simpson JL, eds.* Obstetrics: Normal and Problem Pregnancies. *5th ed. Philadelphia: Churchill Livingstone; 2007.)*

infant's body then rotates to allow engagement of the shoulders in an oblique orientation. Gradual descent occurs, with the anterior shoulder rotating to bring the shoulders into the AP diameter of the outlet. The anterior shoulder follows lateral flexion to appear beneath the symphysis, with the posterior shoulder being delivered first as the body is supported. The head tends to engage in the same diameter as the shoulders. Subsequent flexion, descent, and rotation of the head occur to bring the posterior portion of the neck under the symphysis pubis. The head is then born in flexion. Breech delivery is associated with a greater incidence of prematurity, prolapsed cord, and increased perinatal morbidity and mortality.[3,10-12]

The increased use of cesarean section has greatly decreased the morbidity and mortality associated with breech delivery. Although cesarean is the preferred method of delivery, vaginal delivery may be the method of choice in carefully selected cases.[10,13,14] The emergency clinician should be cognizant of the imminent vaginal delivery of a breech infant in any presentation, frank, complete, or footling. However, a breech presentation is always problematic for any clinician, even under the best of circumstances. It is not expected that the EP will always be able to successfully deliver a breech presentation.

Types

There are three types of vaginal breech deliveries. *Spontaneous breech* is a breech delivery in which the infant is delivered spontaneously without any manipulation or traction other than supporting the infant. This form of delivery is rare with term infants, and there is little associated traumatic morbidity. *Partial breech extraction* occurs when the infant is delivered spontaneously as far as the umbilicus and the remainder of the body is extracted. *Total breech extraction* occurs when the entire body of the infant is extracted by the clinician.

Similar to cephalic presentations, the role of the clinician is to assist the mother in the birthing process and allow maternal expulsive efforts to effect delivery of the infant. Premature or aggressive assistance or traction can significantly increase the risk for fetal or maternal morbidity.

To perform any vaginal breech delivery, the birth canal must be sufficiently large to allow passage of the fetus without trauma and the cervix must be completely effaced and dilated. If these conditions do not exist, cesarean section is indicated. To ensure full cervical dilation in a footling or complete breech, it is important that the feet, legs, and buttocks advance through the introitus to the level of the fetal umbilicus before the clinician intervenes and further delivery is attempted. The mere appearance of the feet through the vulva is not in itself an indication to proceed with delivery. This may be a footling presentation through a cervix that is not completely dilated. In this case there may be time to transfer the patient to the labor and delivery suite, preferably in the knee-chest position to minimize the risk for cord compression.[15] Similarly, if the breech is frank, cervical dilation and outcome are improved if the infant is allowed to deliver to the level of the umbilicus. Before this, as with complete and footling presentations, there may be time to safely transfer the mother to the labor and delivery area. Tocolytics such as subcutaneous terbutaline may be used to inhibit labor until such patients can be safely transferred.[15]

VAGINAL EXAMINATION

Cleanse the perineum with an antiseptic and use a sterile lubricant to decrease potential contamination. A sterile vaginal (not speculum) examination is performed to identify the fetal presentation and position and assess the progress of labor, except in cases of suspected bleeding. Take care to avoid the anal region and potential fecal contamination during the digital examination. Assess cervical effacement and dilation, as well as fetal station, presentation, and position.[3] The finger should not be withdrawn from the vagina until the examination is complete. The number of vaginal examinations during labor correlates with infectious morbidity, especially in cases of early membrane rupture.[3]

Cervical effacement refers to the process of cervical thinning that occurs before and during the first stage of labor as the cervical canal shortens from a length of about 2 cm to a circular opening with almost no length remaining (Fig. 56-6). Effacement is expressed as a percentage from 0% (uneffaced and thick) to 100% (completely effaced). Assess the degree of cervical effacement by palpation and determine the palpated length of the cervical canal in comparison to that of an uneffaced, or normal, cervical canal.

Determine *cervical dilation* by estimating the average diameter of the internal cervical os. Sweep the examining finger from the cervical margin on one side across the cervical os to the opposite margin. Express the diameter in centimeters. Ten centimeters constitutes full cervical dilation. A diameter of less than 6 cm can be measured directly. A cervix that accommodates one index finger is 1 cm, and one that accommodates two fingers is dilated approximately 3 cm. For a diameter greater than 6 cm, it is frequently easier to determine the width of the remaining cervical rim and subtract twice that measurement from 10 cm. For example, if a 1-cm rim is felt, dilation is 8 cm.

Station refers to the level of the presenting fetal part in the birth canal relative to the ischial spines, which lie halfway between the pelvic inlet and the pelvic outlet (Fig. 56-7). Zero station is used to denote that the presenting part is at the level of the ischial spines. When the presenting part lies above the

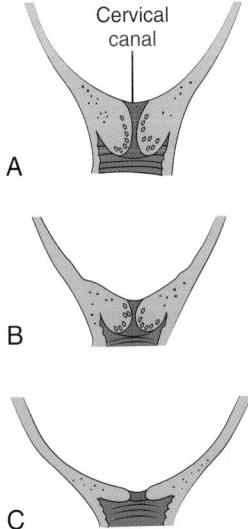

Figure 56-6 Effacement of the cervix. **A,** None. **B,** Partial. **C,** Complete. (*A-C, From Romney S, Gray MK, Little AB, et al, eds.* Gynecology and Obstetrics: The Health Care of Women. *New York: McGraw-Hill; 1975.*)

OLD CLASSIFICATION
(Subjective)

NEW CLASSIFICATION
(Estimated distance in
centimeters from the
ischial spines)

Figure 56-7 The relationship of the leading edge of the presenting part of the fetus to the plane of the maternal ischial spines determines the station. Old and new classification are included. *(From Gabbe SG, Niebyl JR, Simpson JL, eds.* Obstetrics: Normal and Problem Pregnancies. *5th ed. Philadelphia: Churchill Livingstone; 2007.)*

spines, the distance, estimated in centimeters ranging from 1 to 5, is stated in negative figures (−5, −4, −3, −2, −1). Below the ischial spines, the presenting fetal part passes +1, +2, +3, +4, and +5 stations to delivery. This measurement is made by simple palpation.[3] The ischial spines can be palpated at roughly the 8- and 4-o'clock positions on the vaginal examination.

Three maneuvers are used to determine fetal presentation and position. In the first, introduce two fingers into the vagina and advance them to the presenting part to differentiate face, vertex, and breech presentations. In vertex presentations, move your fingers up behind the symphysis pubis and then sweep them posteriorly over the fetal head toward the maternal sacrum to identify the course of the sagittal suture. Define the positions of the two fontanelles, which are located at opposite ends of the sagittal sutures, by palpation. The anterior fontanelle is diamond shaped; the posterior fontanel is triangular. In breech presentations the fetal sacrum is the point of reference, whereas in face presentations the fetal chin is used.

FETAL WELL-BEING

Auscultation

Make the initial determination of fetal well-being by assessing the fetal heart rate with a fetoscope, bedside ultrasound, or a fetal Doppler ultrasound device placed firmly on the maternal abdominal wall overlying the fetal thorax and reposition it until fetal heart tones are heard. When a Doppler device is used, apply a conducting gel to the abdominal wall to interface with the Doppler receiver. To avoid confusion of the maternal and fetal heart sounds, palpate the maternal pulse as the fetal heart rate is auscultated.

The normal baseline fetal heart rate is 110 to 160 beats/min and varies considerably from a baseline measured for a minimum of 2 minutes in a 10-minute segment of time.[16] Rates above or below this range may indicate fetal distress. Accelerations in the fetal heart rate lasting longer than 10 seconds and less than 2 minutes commonly occur during labor and are probably a physiologic response to fetal movement.[3,16,17] Persistent fetal tachycardia occurs most frequently in response to maternal fever or amnionitis but may also indicate fetal compromise.[3,16]

As with brief accelerations in the fetal heart rate, a gradual decrease in the fetal heart rate in association with a uterine contraction with an onset to nadir of 30 seconds or more (with the nadir coinciding with the peak of contraction) is termed an *early deceleration*. Decelerations are physiologic and probably the result of vagal nerve stimulation secondary to compression of the fetal head. Decelerations that occur independently of uterine contractions, are abrupt, or last between 15 seconds and 2 minutes are known as *variable decelerations*. *Late decelerations* are those that are delayed in timing with respect to a contraction, with the nadir of the deceleration occurring after the peak of the contraction. Variable decelerations are relatively common and can be further classified according to their severity. Variable decelerations may be temporarily corrected by maternal repositioning. Late decelerations can be an ominous sign and may represent cord compression and uteroplacental insufficiency.[3,16,17] It may necessitate emergency delivery.

Changes in the fetal heart rate indicating fetal distress are usually evident immediately after a uterine contraction, and therefore the fetal heart rate is optimally assessed at this time. Formal monitoring of labor should be performed in an obstetrics unit. Fetal monitoring is not performed in the ED, but examples of various fetal heart rate patterns are included for completeness in Figure 56-8.[3,16]

Management of Fetal Distress

Definitive evaluation of fetal distress should be performed in the obstetric unit by the delivery team. There is no role for sophisticated fetal monitoring in the ED. In the absence of a dedicated obstetric unit, transfer to another hospital is the only option, albeit a less than ideal one. An EP working in an ED without adequate obstetric backup can do little to effect a positive outcome in high-risk situations. Eclampsia, bleeding, and abnormal fetal presentation may be identified, but the EP needs to focus attention on maternal well-being while expediting transfer, referral, or both. The EP has limited options for managing fetal distress.

If fetal distress is suspected on the basis of the resting fetal heart rate or changes after contractions, change the maternal position, typically into the *left lateral decubitus position*, and reevaluate. Administer *supplemental oxygen* to the mother to optimize fetal oxygenation. In the absence of bleeding, perform a vaginal examination to rule out the possibility of umbilical cord prolapse.[16,18] *Cord prolapse* usually occurs at the same time as rupture of the membranes and is diagnosed by palpation of the umbilical cord on vaginal examination or by visualization of the cord protruding through the introitus.

61181   61182

Onset at beginning
of contraction

Early onset

FHR
Uniform shape

Early deceleration

Recovery at end of contraction

Head compression (HC)
Early deceleration

A

61183

Late recovery

FHR
Uniform shape

Late deceleration

Late onset

Uteroplacental insufficiency
(UPI)
Late deceleration

B

61180

FHR
Variable shape

Rapid return

Sudden drop

Variable deceleration

Variable time relationship to contractions

Umbilical
cord compression
(CC)
Variable deceleration

C

Figure 56-8 Deceleration patterns of the fetal heart rate (FHR). **A,** Early deceleration caused by head compression. **B,** Late deceleration caused by uteroplacental insufficiency. **C,** Variable deceleration caused by cord compression. *Note: fetal monitoring is not done in the emergency department; this figure is supplied for completeness. (Modified from Lowdermilk DL, Perry SE, Bobak IM.* Maternity and Women's Health Care. *6th ed. St. Louis: Mosby; 1997.)*

Cord prolapse is frequently encountered with breech presentations, multiple pregnancies, and prematurity.[19-21]

Management of cord prolapse is directed at sustaining fetal life until delivery is accomplished. Unless immediate delivery is feasible or the fetus is known to be dead, prepare for an emergency cesarean section. If immediate obstetric services are not available, four temporizing measures can be undertaken. (1) Place the patient in the knee-chest or deep Trendelenburg position, and keep the patient in this position until delivery.[18,21,22] (2) Minimize compression of the umbilical cord by inserting a sterile gloved hand and exerting manual pressure in the vagina *to lift and maintain the presenting part away from the prolapsed cord.* (3) After manual elevation of the presenting part, instill 500 to 700 mL of saline into the bladder to raise the presenting part and maintain cord decompression. Once the bladder is filled, remove the vaginal hand.[22,23] (4) Tocolytic therapy can be administered to decrease uterine contractions and improve fetoplacental perfusion.[22,23] Unfortunately and realistically speaking, outcomes of true obstetric emergencies managed solely in the ED are often bleak and essentially out of the hands of the EP.

Tocolytic Therapy

Tocolytic therapy is rarely instituted in the ED, and there is no standard mandating its use by the EP. However, under dire circumstances and preferably under obstetric guidance, this intervention may be initiated in the ED. Before instituting pharmacologic tocolytic therapy for either preterm labor or fetal distress, initiate basic maneuvers to improve maternal and fetal status. Because uterine hypoxia may induce uterine contractions, administer supplemental oxygen and infuse 500 mL of crystalloid intravenously. Place the mother in the left lateral decubitus position to improve uterine perfusion.[3,18,24] Because uterine, cervical, or urinary tract infections account for 20% to 40% of cases of preterm labor, search for a specific cause and treat infections appropriately.[18,25,26] If the contractions persist and cervical changes are documented despite these basic interventions, consider pharmacologic therapy.[3,18,24] Although tocolytic agents are commonly used and have been shown to prolong pregnancy by 2 to 7 days, there are few data to suggest that tocolysis improves long-term perinatal or neonatal outcome.[3,24,27,28] In addition, none of the commonly used tocolytic medications are approved for use by the U.S. Food and Drug Administration (FDA) as a tocolytic agent. The principal benefit of pharmacologic therapy may be only to prolong pregnancy to allow maternal transfer to a tertiary care facility or to delay delivery sufficiently to improve fetal maturation with corticosteroids.[3,24-26,29] General contraindications to tocolytic therapy include severe preeclampsia, placental abruption, intrauterine infection, advanced cervical dilation, and evidence of fetal compromise or placental insufficiency.[24]

There are no clear "first-line" tocolytic agents to manage preterm labor (Table 56-1). Clinical circumstances and preferences should dictate treatment. Agents such as calcium channel blockers and the prostaglandin inhibitor indomethacin have shown varying efficacy in clinical trials.[3,16,24,25,27] The most commonly used tocolytic agents in the United States are the calcium channel blocker nifedipine, magnesium sulfate, and the β₂-receptor agonist terbutaline. Calcium channel blockers are the preferred tocolytics by the World Health Organization.[30]

TABLE 56-1 Tocolytics for the Emergency Management of Preterm Labor

DRUG	DOSE	END POINT
Indomethacin	50-100 mg PO or 50 mg PR	May repeat 25-50 mg PO q6h for a maximum of 48 hr
Terbutaline	0.25 mg SC	May repeat q20-60min Cessation of uterine contractions Intolerable maternal side effects
Magnesium sulfate	4-6 g IV over 20 min followed by an infusion at 1-3 g/hr IV	Cessation of uterine contractions Signs of magnesium toxicity (e.g., respiratory depression, hypotension, somnolence)
Nifedipine*	10 mg PO	May repeat q15-20min Cessation of uterine contractions Harmful maternal side effects, e.g., hypotension Maximum dose, 40 mg

IV, intravenously; *PO,* orally; *PR,* per rectum.
*Variable doses have been used. Data on effects, particularly uteroplacental blood flow, are limited.

β₂-Receptor Agonists

The most commonly used β₂-adrenergic tocolytic agent is terbutaline. The β-mimetic agents react with adrenergic receptors to reduce intracellular ionized calcium levels and prevent the activation of myometrial contractile proteins.[3] Although terbutaline stimulates β₂-receptors primarily, it has some β₁-activity, which is responsible for its cardiovascular side effects. Another β-mimetic agent, ritodrine, was the only agent approved for tocolysis in the United States but has been withdrawn from the market.

Terbutaline is commonly used for the treatment of preterm labor.[3,25,31] When given subcutaneously, administer terbutaline in a 0.25-mg dose and repeat it every 20 to 60 minutes until contractions cease or intolerable maternal side effects occur.[18,24,32,33] In 2011 the FDA required the addition of a *Boxed Warning and Contraindication* ("black box warning") against the use of injectable terbutaline for the prevention or prolonged treatment of preterm labor beyond 48 to 72 hours because of adverse effects, including maternal death.[34] Use terbutaline with caution in patients with cardiovascular disease, hypertension, hyperthyroidism, diabetes, and seizures and in those taking other sympathomimetic amines.[24,35] The general clinical side effects of arrhythmias, myocardial ischemia, and pulmonary edema are related to its inherent activity as a β-mimetic drug. Treatment of the majority of side effects is supportive; severe cardiovascular effects may be treated with β-blocking agents.[32,35]

Magnesium Sulfate

Magnesium sulfate (MgSO$_4$) is not approved in the United States for use as a tocolytic agent. Nevertheless, some perinatal centers prefer MgSO$_4$ over the β-mimetic agents because of its lower incidence of side effects.[18,36,37] Even though the use of MgSO$_4$ as a tocolytic has fallen out of favor, findings of fetal neuroprotective effects have resulted in its ongoing use.[38-41] Although its mechanism of action is not fully understood, magnesium probably decreases myometrial contractility through its role as a calcium antagonist.[3] Its fetoprotective effects probably result from noncompetitive antagonism of the N-methyl-D-aspartate receptor or through antiapoptosis and prevention of neuronal cell loss.[42]

MgSO$_4$ is generally administered at a dose of 4 to 6 g intravenously over a period of 20 to 30 minutes, followed by a maintenance intravenous infusion beginning at 1 to 3 g/hr.[24,43] Infusion of MgSO$_4$ often produces sweating, warmth, and flushing. Rapid parenteral administration may cause transient nausea, vomiting, headache, or palpitations.[24,25,37] The major side effect of magnesium therapy is impairment of the muscles of respiration with subsequent respiratory arrest, an effect not usually seen until the serum magnesium level exceeds 10 mEq/L. At levels of 12 mEq/L or greater, respiratory arrest may occur.[35]

The first sign of magnesium toxicity, a decrease in the patellar reflex, typically occurs as serum magnesium levels exceed 4 mEq/L, with loss of the reflex as levels increase further. The dosing and ongoing maintenance of magnesium therapy should be guided by the clinical status of the patient rather than by laboratory values. Monitor the patellar reflex throughout therapy. Because magnesium is almost totally excreted by the kidney, it is contraindicated in the presence of renal failure. Monitor urinary output and renal function throughout therapy. If respiratory depression develops, inject 10 mL of a 10% solution of calcium gluconate or calcium chloride over a 3-minute period as an antidote. For severe respiratory depression or arrest, prompt endotracheal intubation may be lifesaving.[3]

Calcium Channel Blockers

Calcium antagonists inhibit the influx of calcium ions through the muscle cell membrane and reduce uterine vascular resistance. The decrease in intracellular calcium also results in decreased myometrial activity. Although dosing regimens vary, nifedipine is frequently given as an initial loading dose of 30 mg orally and then 10 to 20 mg every 4 to 6 hours.[24,32] When oral nicardipine (Cardene) was compared with MgSO$_4$, less time was required to achieve tocolysis, 3.3 versus 5.3 hours, respectively. Preterm labor also recurred less frequently with nicardipine.[44] The calcium channel blocker–induced decreased vascular resistance can lead to maternal hypotension and thus decreased uteroplacental perfusion.

Prostaglandin Inhibitors

Prostaglandins are smooth muscle stimulants. Prostaglandin synthetase inhibitors inhibit cyclooxygenase and thereby prevent the conversion of free arachidonic acid to prostaglandin. Because the prostaglandin E and F series are mediators of uterine contractions, a decrease in production results in decreased contractile activity.[32] Indomethacin is administered as an initial oral or rectal dose of 50 to 100 mg followed by 25- to 50-mg doses every 6 hours for a total of 48 hours.[24] Ketorolac can be used as an alternative with a 60-mg intramuscular loading dose, followed by 30 mg intramuscularly every 6 hours for 48 hours.[24] Side effects include oligohydramnios and premature closure of the ductus arteriosus.

Steroids

In addition to tocolytics, patients in preterm labor and less than 34 weeks' gestation are candidates for antenatal steroid administration. This may reduce the incidence of neonatal respiratory distress syndrome, intraventricular hemorrhage, and necrotizing enterocolitis.[24] Appropriate patients should receive betamethasone, 12 mg intramuscularly every 24 hours for a total of two doses, or dexamethasone, 6 mg intramuscularly every 12 hours for a total of four doses.

VAGINAL BLEEDING DURING THE THIRD TRIMESTER

Bleeding during the third trimester should always be considered an emergency because shock may occur within minutes. Prepare for the most typical causes of bleeding in late gestation, placenta previa and placental abruption (Fig. 56-9). *Placenta previa* refers to implantation of the placenta in the lower uterine segment with varying degrees of encroachment on the cervical os. Placenta previa is classically characterized by vaginal bleeding with little or no abdominal or pelvic pain. Premature separation of the placenta, or *abruptio placentae*, refers to separation of the placenta from its site of implantation in the uterus before delivery of the fetus. Although the clinical signs and symptoms with placental abruption can vary considerably, abruptio placentae is typically associated with varying degrees of abdominal pain and uterine irritability or contractions.[3]

Stabilization of a patient with third-trimester bleeding should be initiated with large-bore intravenous access. Blood should be drawn for a complete blood count with platelets and a type and crossmatch. If abruption is suspected, clotting studies, including a fibrinogen level and a toxicology screen for cocaine, may be indicated because of the association of abruption with disseminated intravascular coagulation and cocaine abuse, respectively. Until the diagnosis of placenta previa is excluded, digital vaginal examination is *contraindicated* because of the possibility of tearing or dislodging a placenta previa, which may result in profuse, potentially fatal hemorrhage.[3] The simplest and most precise method of placental localization is by transabdominal ultrasound, which has an accuracy in locating placenta previa of about 96%. In contrast, ultrasonography has limited sensitivity in detecting abruptio placenta, with a reported negative predictive value of between 63% and 88%.[3] Therefore, negative findings on ultrasound should not be used to exclude placental abruption. Immediately transfer the patient to the care of an obstetrician for further evaluation.

PROCEDURE

Technique for Uncomplicated Delivery

Although complete sterility is not a priority, when time permits, use sterile technique and equipment. Wear sterile

Abnormalities of Placental Implantation

Marginal placenta previa

Partial placenta previa

Total (central) placenta previa

A

Figure 56-9 A, Placenta previa.

Placental Abruption

External bleeding

Internal
(concealed)
bleeding

Obstruction of
cervix by
presenting part

Section through placenta
in premature separation
showing nodular ischemia
and infarction above clots.

B

Figure 56-9, cont'd B, Abruptio placentae. *(Netter illustrations from* www.netterimages.com. *© Elsevier Inc. All rights reserved.)*

gloves, a gown, mask, and eye protection. Clean the perineum and vulva as for a vaginal examination and drape with sterile towels so that only the immediate area about the vulva is exposed. Be careful to avoid fecal contamination of the infant or perineum.

Ideally, place the patient on a delivery table in the dorsal lithotomy position to increase the diameter of the pelvic outlet (Fig. 56-10, *step 1*). Alternatively, position the patient on a stretcher with her hips and knees partially flexed, her thighs abducted, and the soles of her feet placed firmly on the stretcher. Additional personnel may assist in keeping the patient in this position. If the foot of the bed cannot be removed, enhance the delivery position by placing the underside of a bedpan under the patient's buttocks to provide additional space between the bed and the perineum.

Spontaneous Vertex Delivery

Spontaneous delivery of a vertex-presenting infant is divided into three phases: delivery of the head, delivery of the shoulders, and delivery of the body and legs.

Delivery of the Head

Anticipate delivery when the presenting part reaches the pelvic floor. With each contraction, the perineum bulges further and the vulvovaginal opening becomes more and more dilated by the fetal head. Just before delivery, *crowning* occurs, which is when the head is visible at the vaginal introitus and the widest portion, or the biparietal diameter of the head, distends the vulva.

Gentle, gradual, controlled delivery is desirable. Avoid explosive delivery of the head. Once the fetal head distends the vaginal introitus to 5 cm or more during a contraction, place the palm of one hand over the occipital area and provide gentle pressure to control delivery of the head (see Fig. 56-10, *step 2*). With the other hand, preferably draped with a sterile towel to prevent contamination from the anus, exert upward pressure on the chin of the fetus through the perineum just in front of the coccyx in a modified Ritgen maneuver (Fig. 56-11). This maneuver extends the neck at the proper time such that the smallest diameter of the head passes through the introitus and over the perineum to protect the maternal perineal musculature. It is not uncommon for the vagina and perineum to tear with expulsive maternal effort during delivery of the head. If maternal expulsive efforts are insufficient to allow delivery of the head, an episiotomy should be considered at this time.[3]

Gently support the head during subsequent delivery of the forehead, face, chin, and neck. With delivery of the neck, pass a finger around the infant's neck to determine whether it is encircled by one or more coils of the umbilical cord. If a loop of cord is felt, loosen it carefully and gently slip it over the infant's head (Fig. 56-12). If this cannot be done easily, clamp the cord doubly, cut the cord between the clamps and promptly deliver the infant.

Delivery of the Shoulders

Just before external rotation the head usually falls posteriorly, almost bringing it into contact with the mother's anus. If maternal defecation occurs, avoid fecal contamination of the fetus. As rotation takes place, the head assumes a transverse position and the transverse diameter of the thorax rotates into the AP diameter of the pelvis. In most cases the shoulders are born spontaneously. Aid delivery by grasping the sides of the head and exerting *gentle* downward (posterior) traction until the anterior shoulder appears beneath the symphysis pubis (see Fig. 56-10, *step 3*). Gently lift the head upward to aid in delivery of the posterior shoulder (see Fig. 56-10, *step 4*). The remainder of the body usually follows without difficulty.

If delivery of the body is delayed after the shoulders have been freed, assist by providing *moderate* traction on the exposed fetal body. To avoid injury to the brachial plexus, do not hook the fingers in the axilla during delivery. Always exert traction in the direction of the long axis of the infant. If traction is applied obliquely, bending of the neck and excessive stretching of the brachial plexus may occur.[3,15]

Clearing the Airway

Once the head has been delivered, quickly wipe the infant's face and mouth. Routine suctioning is not indicated for vigorous newborns. Current recommendations also no longer advise routine oropharyngeal and nasopharyngeal suctioning of infants with meconium staining by amniotic fluid. Studies have shown that this practice offers no benefit if the infant is vigorous. A vigorous infant is one who has strong respiratory effort, good muscle tone, and a heart rate greater than 100 beats/min.[45] Perform endotracheal suctioning immediately after birth for infants with meconium staining who are not vigorous.[45] The benefit of the routine use of 100% oxygen, rather than room air, for infant resuscitation has also recently been questioned by the American Heart Association, but this area of research is ongoing and not yet fully elucidated. For a more complete discussion of the possible harm of excessive supplemental oxygen for infant resuscitation, see Chapter 3.

Clamping the Cord

The infant should be positioned at or slightly below the level of the vaginal introitus during clamping of the cord.[15] Cut the umbilical cord with scissors between two Kelly clamps placed 4 to 5 cm from the infant's abdomen (see Fig. 56-10, *step 6*). Delayed clamping of the umbilical cord for at least 2 minutes after birth consistently improves the short- and long-term hematologic and iron status of full-term infants.[46] Later, apply an umbilical cord clamp 2 to 3 cm from the infant's abdomen. Collect blood samples from the placental end of the cord for infant serology, including Rh determination.[15]

After cutting the umbilical cord, evaluate the infant and, if necessary, initiate resuscitation as described in the later section "The Newborn." Rapidly assess the infant by determining the following:

● Was the baby born after a full-term gestation?
● Is the baby breathing or crying spontaneously?
● Does the baby have good muscle tone?

If the answer to these questions is "yes," the baby will probably not need resuscitation.[45]

Delivery of the Placenta

Placental separation usually occurs within about 5 minutes after delivery of the infant, although it may take longer. It can be recognized by the following signs:

1. The uterus becomes globular and firmer as it contracts.
2. There is a sudden gush of blood as the placenta separates from the uterine wall.
3. The umbilical cord lengthens and protrudes further out of the vagina.

SPONTANEOUS VERTEX DELIVERY

1 Place the patient in the dorsal lithotomy position. Anticipate delivery when *crowning* occurs; the fetal head will be visible at the vaginal introitus.

2 Place one hand over the occiput and provide gentle pressure to control delivery of the head. Use your other hand to exert pressure on the chin of the fetus through the perineum (the modified Ritgen maneuver).

3 Apply gentle downward (posterior) traction until the anterior shoulder appears beneath the symphysis pubis.

4 Gently lift the head upward to aid in delivery of the posterior shoulder.

5 The remainder of the body usually delivers spontaneously without difficulty. Routine suctioning is not indicated for vigorous newborns.

6 Position the infant at or slightly below the level of the vaginal introitus during clamping of the cord. Cut the cord with scissors between two Kelly clamps placed 4 to 5 cm from the infant's abdomen.

7 Deliver the placenta (placental separation usually occurs within 5 minutes after delivery). Ask the mother to bear down to aid in delivery.

Figure 56-10 Spontaneous vertex delivery. (*Adapted from* Ferri's Clinical Advisor 2013. *St. Louis: Mosby; 2013.*)

Figure 56-11 For controlled and gentle delivery of the head, use the modified Ritgen maneuver. *(From Seils A, Noujaim S, Davis K, et al, eds.* Williams Obstetrics. *22nd ed. New York: McGraw-Hill Medical; 2005.)*

Figure 56-12 As the head is delivered, use a finger to determine whether the umbilical cord is encircling the neck. If a loop of cord is felt, loosen it carefully and gently slip it over the infant's head.

Figure 56-13 Delivery of the placenta and fetal membranes by exerting controlled *traction on the cord and suprapubic pressure with the abdominal hand to prevent uterine inversion.* Care should be taken to avoid avulsion of the cord. Active management with uterotonic agents such as oxytocin administered at delivery hastens delivery of the placenta and may reduce the incidence of postpartum hemorrhage and total blood loss. *(From Gabbe SG, Niebyl JR, Simpson JL, eds.* Obstetrics: Normal and Problem Pregnancies. *5th ed. Philadelphia: Churchill Livingstone; 2007.)*

Ask the mother to bear down; the increased intraabdominal pressure produced by this maneuver may be enough to effect complete expulsion of the placenta (see Fig. 56-10, *step 7*). If maternal force alone is insufficient, aid in delivery of the placenta. After ensuring that the uterus is firmly contracted and placental separation has occurred, use one hand to exert gentle pressure through the abdominal wall to lift the uterine fundus cephalad while keeping the umbilical cord slightly taut with the other hand (Fig. 56-13). Repeat this maneuver until the placenta reaches the introitus. At this time, stop uterine pressure and gently lift the placenta upward and out of the vagina. Never force expulsion of the placenta before placental separation has occurred, and never use forceful traction to pull the placenta out of the uterus. Such maneuvers may result in separation of the cord from the placenta or uterine inversion with potentially catastrophic hemodynamic consequences. The placenta should be examined for completeness and saved for later evaluation by the obstetrician.[3,15,18]

Examine the vulva, vagina, and cervix for traumatic lacerations. Cervical lacerations most typically occur at the 9- or 3-o'clock position; vaginal lacerations typically occur at the point of the ischial spines. The most common areas for lacerations are the vagina, hymen, and perineum. Based on the availability of resources and the clinical setting, definitive repair of uncomplicated or minor obstetric lacerations may be performed in the ED by the EP, but this is often done by a consultant obstetrician.

After delivery of the placenta, the primary mechanism by which hemostasis is achieved at the placental site is through myometrial contraction. Agents such as oxytocin, methylergonovine, and ergonovine may be used to stimulate myometrial contraction. In an effort to prevent uterine atony and subsequent bleeding, oxytocin is often administered after delivery of the placenta.

Oxytocin (Pitocin, Syntocinon) is the most commonly used oxytocic drug and is usually given by continuous intravenous infusion. Add 20 units of oxytocin to 1 L of normal saline and administer the solution at a rate of 10 mL/min for several minutes until the uterus remains firmly contracted and bleeding is controlled. At this point, reduce the infusion rate to 1 to 2 mL/min.[3,15,18] Alternatively, ergot derivatives such as methylergonovine maleate (Methergine), 0.2 mg, or ergonovine maleate (Ergotrate), 0.2 mg, may be given intramuscularly.[3,18] Because of their vasoconstrictive properties, ergot preparations are relatively contraindicated in patients with hypertension, including pregnancy-associated hypertension or preeclampsia.[3] The synthetic prostaglandin misoprostol (Cytotec) can also be given as an 800- to 1000-μg rectal dose. In the United States, oxytocic agents are not generally administered before delivery of the placenta because of concerns that the resultant uterine contraction may entrap the placenta or trap an undiagnosed twin within the uterus.[3,15] Even when oxytocics are administered, the hour after delivery of the placenta is the time during which postpartum hemorrhage secondary to uterine atony is most likely to occur. For this reason, palpate the uterus frequently to ensure that it is well contracted. A normally contracted uterus will feel firm with its upper margin just below the maternal umbilicus. If the uterus is flaccid or bleeding, gently massage the uterus through the abdominal wall. Occasionally, the placenta may fail to separate completely and result in a retained placenta or placental fragments with persistent uterine bleeding. Support the patient with intravenous fluids and blood transfusions as indicated until definitive therapy is available. Constant firm uterine massage can lessen hemorrhage and may be lifesaving.

COMPLICATIONS

Complex Deliveries

Shoulder Dystocia

Shoulder dystocia refers to impaction of the fetal shoulders in the pelvic outlet after delivery of the head and occurs in 0.6% to 1.4% of deliveries (Fig. 56-14).[47] Shoulder dystocia is associated with several risk factors, including fetal macrosomia, maternal diabetes, obesity, multiparity, and postterm pregnancy.

Impaction of the fetal shoulders and thorax in the maternal pelvis prohibits adequate respiration, and compression of the umbilical cord frequently compromises the fetal circulation. For these reasons, shoulder dystocia is a serious and potentially fatal complication of delivery.[15,48] Fetal complications include brachial plexus injury, clavicular and humeral fractures, and rarely, death.[44-49]

Management

The techniques used to treat shoulder dystocia frequently require an assistant, and delivery can result in fetal injury or hypoxia, as well as increased rates of postpartum hemorrhage.[51] Call for emergency assistance from a pediatrician, an obstetrician, and an anesthesiologist. An episiotomy may be performed to reduce the incidence of major perineal lacerations and provide additional space for manipulation. A fetal fracture or nerve injury is not unusual with shoulder dystocia during any delivery technique.

Although a variety of techniques have been described to free the anterior shoulder from its impacted position beneath the symphysis pubis, the initial technique of choice is the McRoberts maneuver because of its ease and potential for success (Fig. 56-15A). In one study, approximately 40% of shoulder dystocias were relieved with the McRoberts maneuver alone.[50] To perform the McRoberts maneuver, place the mother in the extreme lithotomy position with her hips completely flexed so that her knees rest alongside her chest. This causes a flattening of the lumbar lordosis, rotates the maternal pelvis cephalad, and frequently frees the impacted anterior fetal shoulder.[3,47-51] If the McRoberts maneuver fails to effect delivery, ask an assistant to apply moderate suprapubic, not fundal, pressure to the maternal abdomen while providing gentle downward traction on the fetal head (see Fig. 56-16B).[47-49]

If these initial maneuvers fail to effect delivery, several other techniques exist, the choice of which will depend on clinician preference and experience. In the first maneuver, place two fingers in the vagina and exert pressure on the fetal scapula to rotate the *posterior* shoulder 180 degrees in a clockwise or counterclockwise fashion, depending on the orientation of the torso ("reverse Wood's screw"), to free the entrapped anterior shoulder (see Fig. 56-15C). Other maneuvers include the Rubin maneuver, in which rotation is achieved by applying pressure on the posterior aspect of the anterior shoulder, or the Wood's screw maneuver, in which pressure is placed on the anterior aspect of the posterior shoulder. This may cause release of the impacted anterior shoulder and result in progression of delivery.[48,52] Alternatively, attempt to deliver the posterior arm (see Fig. 56-15D). In this maneuver, insert the hand along the hollow of the maternal sacrum to the level of the fetus' posterior elbow. Exert pressure at the antecubital fossa, flex the posterior forearm of the fetus, and grasp the hand or forearm. Next, carefully sweep the posterior arm of

Figure 56-14 Shoulder dystocia. When delivery of the fetal head is not followed by delivery of the shoulders, the anterior shoulder has often become caught behind the symphysis.

the fetus across its chest to effect delivery of the posterior arm and shoulder. Rotate the shoulder girdle into one of the oblique diameters of the pelvis and subsequently deliver the anterior shoulder.[3,49] If all these strategies fail, it may be necessary to perform a controlled destructive procedure, such as fracture of the fetal clavicle, or the cephalic replacement maneuver (Zavanelli) with subsequent cesarean delivery.[3,15] The Zavanelli maneuver should be a last resort.

Breech Delivery

Technique

If a breech delivery becomes necessary in the ED, an episiotomy may need to be performed, especially with a term gestation, unless there is considerable perineal relaxation. As the breech progressively distends the perineum, the posterior hip will be delivered, usually from the 6-o'clock position (Fig. 56-16, *step 1*). The anterior hip will then be delivered, followed by external rotation to the sacrum-anterior position. Ideally, two attendants should be available for a breech delivery.

Delivery of the Presenting Part and Body. Continued descent of the fetus will allow delivery of the legs, which may be aided by splinting the medial part of the thighs of the fetus with the fingers positioned parallel to the femur and exerting pressure laterally to sweep the legs away from the midline (see Fig. 56-16, *steps 2 to 4*). After delivery of the legs, grasp the fetal bony pelvis with both hands with the fingers resting on the anterior superior iliac crests and the thumbs on the sacrum. Because the fetal body is slippery and difficult to hold, wrap it in a towel to assist delivery. Use the maternal expulsive efforts in conjunction with gentle downward traction. Rotate the fetal pelvis to bring the fetal sacrum into the transverse position to effect delivery of the scapulae. Two methods of shoulder delivery are commonly used (see Fig. 56-16, *steps 5 to 7*). In the first, with the scapulae visible, rotate the trunk so that the anterior arm and shoulder appear at the vulva and can easily be released and delivered. Next, rotate the body of the fetus in the reverse direction to deliver the other shoulder and arm beneath the symphysis pubis. In the second method, if trunk rotation is unsuccessful, deliver the posterior shoulder. Grasp the feet in one hand and draw them upward over

MANAGEMENT OF SHOULDER DYSTOCIA

The McRoberts maneuver is the least invasive maneuver to disimpact the shoulders in shoulder dystocia. Position the patient in the extreme lithotomy position with the hips completely flexed (knee-chest position); this may free the anterior fetal shoulder.

Moderate suprapubic pressure will often disimpact the anterior shoulder. Desperate traction on the fetal head is not likely to facilitate delivery and might lead to trauma. Delivery of an infant with shoulder dystocia often results in fracture of the clavicle or humerus to accomplish delivery.

Rubin or reverse Wood's screw maneuver. *1*, Rotate the posterior shoulder. *2*, Deliver the rotated shoulder.

Posterior shoulder delivery. Insert a hand and sweep the posterior arm across the chest and over the perineum. Take care to distribute the pressure evenly across the humerus to avoid unnecessary fracture.

Figure 56-15 Management of shoulder dystocia. (*A, B, and D, From Gabbe SG, Niebyl JR, Simpson JL. eds. Obstetrics: Normal and Problem Pregnancies. 5th ed. Philadelphia: Churchill Livingstone; 2007.)*

BREECH DELIVERY

1 As the fetus begins to emerge, the posterior hip will deliver, usually from the 6-o'clock position.

2 Avoid premature aggressive traction, which increases the risk for head entrapment or nuchal arm entrapment.

3 After spontaneous expulsion of the umbilicus, rotate the thigh externally and rotate the pelvis in the opposite direction.

4 As the knees flex during the rotational maneuvers, the legs can be delivered.

5 When the scapulae appear under the symphysis, reach over the left shoulder and sweep the arm across the chest.

6 Deliver the left arm.

7 Gently rotate the shoulder girdle to facilitate delivery of the right arm.

8 Rest the fetal body on your palm and forearm.

Place your index and middle fingers over the infant's maxilla to maintain head flexion. Apply downward traction on the shoulders, and then elevate the body of the fetus to deliver the head.

Figure 56-16 Breech delivery.

the mother's groin. Exert leverage on the posterior shoulder, which will slide out over the perineal margin, usually followed by the arm and hand. Deliver the anterior shoulder, arm, and hand beneath the symphysis pubis by downward traction on the fetal body.

Occasionally, spontaneous delivery of the arm and hand does not follow delivery of the shoulder. If this occurs, provide upward traction on the fetal body after delivery of the posterior shoulder. Pass two fingers along the fetal humerus until the fetal elbow is reached. Using the fingers to splint the fetal arm, sweep it downward and deliver it. Deliver the anterior arm by depression of the fetal body alone. In some cases it may be necessary to sweep the anterior arm down over the thorax by using two fingers as a splint.

Delivery of the Head. After the shoulders appear, the head usually occupies one of the oblique diameters of the pelvis, with the chin directed posteriorly. Extract the head by using the Mauriceau maneuver as follows. With the fetal body resting on the clinician's palm and forearm, place the index and middle fingers of one hand over the infant's maxilla, not the mandible, to maintain flexion of the fetal head (see Fig. 56-16, *step 8*). Hook two fingers of the other hand over the fetal neck and, while grasping the shoulders, apply downward traction until the suboccipital region appears under the symphysis pubis. Elevate the body of the fetus toward the mother's abdomen, and the fetal mouth, nose, brow, and eventually the occiput will emerge over the perineum. Avoid excessive elevation of the fetal torso to prevent hyperextension of the neck. If available, have an assistant apply suprapubic pressure to help in delivery of the head. If delivery of the head is not affected by the Mauriceau maneuver, forceps delivery may be necessary but is beyond the scope of this text and most ED practitioners. Once the breech baby is delivered, further management proceeds as for a normal vertex delivery.

Rarely, *breech extraction* of an infant becomes necessary and is indicated only if there is a definite diagnosis of fetal distress unresponsive to routine maneuvers, if obstetric services are unavailable, and if cesarean section cannot be performed promptly. To perform the extraction, introduce the hand into the vagina and grasp both feet of the fetus, with the index finger placed between the fetal ankles. Apply gentle traction until the feet are pulled through the vulva. Continue gentle downward traction while grasping successively higher portions of both legs and thighs. When the breech appears at the vulva, apply gentle traction until the hips are delivered. As the buttocks emerge, rotate the fetal back anteriorly. Place the thumbs over the sacrum and the fingers over the hips and deliver the remainder of the breech as described earlier. At times, delivery of a frank breech may be necessary. Facilitated by an episiotomy, allow the breech to deliver spontaneously as far as possible. Place a finger on each side of the fetal groin and exert moderate traction. Once the knees appear outside the birth canal, flex the legs slowly to assist in delivery, and proceed with delivery as described earlier.

Episiotomy

Routine use of episiotomy is no longer recommended, but it is still performed with some frequency.[53] Selected indications include breech delivery, shoulder dystocia, occiput-posterior presentations, and imminent perineal tear (Box 56-1). It may also be necessary to expedite delivery in situations of fetal

BOX 56-1 **Traditional Indications for Episiotomy**

Fetal macrosomia	Risk for major perineal
Shoulder dystocia	laceration
Breech delivery	Nonreassuring fetal heart rate
Occiput-posterior presentation	tracing
Operative vaginal delivery	

distress. Two types of episiotomy are used: median (midline) and mediolateral (Fig. 56-17). The median approach is the easiest type to perform and repair, results in the least amount of blood loss, heals more rapidly with minimal discomfort, and is generally more common in the United States. A major complication of median episiotomy is potential inadvertent extension of the incision into the anal sphincter or rectum, which results in third- and fourth-degree lacerations, respectively.[3,15,54,55] A mediolateral episiotomy seldom results in extension into the anal sphincter, but blood loss is greater, repair is more difficult, and healing may be more painful.[3,15]

Technique

With vertex presentations, perform the episiotomy during the second stage of labor, when the fetal head begins to distend the perineum and becomes visible to a diameter of 3 to 4 cm during a contraction.[3] Anesthesia for episiotomy in the ED is usually limited to local infiltration of the perineum with 1% or 2% lidocaine.

The incision is made with Mayo scissors through the skin and subcutaneous tissue, the vaginal mucosa, the urogenital septum, and the superior fascia of the pelvic diaphragm (see Fig. 56-17). Make the incision up to one half the length of the perineum, and extend it 2 to 3 cm upward into the vaginal mucosa. If the incision is in the midline, extend the incision through the lowermost fibers of the puborectalis portion of the levator ani muscles. As the head crowns, place the index and middle fingers inside the vaginal introitus to expose the mucosa, posterior fourchette, and perineal body. Use tissue scissors to incise the median raphe of the perineum halfway to the anal sphincter. For a mediolateral episiotomy, direct the incision downward and outward in the direction of the lateral margin of the anal sphincter either to the right or to the left.

The episiotomy should be repaired after delivery of the infant and placenta. Repairs are usually performed by the obstetric consultant in the delivery suite but can be done by an EP experienced in the procedure (Fig. 56-17). The goals of episiotomy repair are to restore both anatomy and hemostasis with a minimal amount of suture material. Perform the closure after delivery of the placenta and following inspection and repair of the cervix and upper vaginal canal if indicated. The principles of repair are the same regardless of the type of episiotomy.

Because there is minimal tension on the closed wound, use 2-0 or 3-0 absorbable suture, such as chromic catgut or polyglycolic acid, on a large atraumatic needle. The first step is to close the vaginal mucosa with a continuous suture from just above the apex of the incision to the mucocutaneous junction to reapproximate the margins of the hymenal ring (see Fig. 56-17, *step 1*). Ligate large actively bleeding vessels during closure with separate absorbable sutures. Next, reapproximate the perineal musculature with three or four interrupted

EPISIOTOMY AND REPAIR

Midline Episiotomy

Make the incision through the lowermost fibers of the puborectalis portion of the levator ani muscles. Incise the median raphe of the perineum halfway to the anal sphincter.

A major complication of midline episiotomy is incision of the anal sphincter or rectum, which leads to third- and fourth-degree lacerations.

Mediolateral Episiotomy

Make the incision through the lowermost fibers of the puborectalis portion of the levator ani muscles. Direct the incision downward and outward in the direction of the lateral margin of the anal sphincter.

The mediolateral approach rarely extends into the anal sphincter but may be associated with greater blood loss and more difficult repair.

Episiotomy Repair

1 Place a taped sponge in the upper part of the vagina. Expose the full extent of the episiotomy with the left hand. Place the first suture 1 cm cephalad to the most superior margin of the episiotomy or laceration to ensure hemostasis of the repair. Use continuous locked absorbable suture to close the vaginal epithelium from the apex of the laceration to the hymenal ring.

2 Use simple interrupted (absorbable) suture to close the deep perineal fascia and underlying levator ani muscles (*black arrows*).

Bring the vaginal epithelial suture below the skin into the subcutaneous tissue (*white arrow*).

3 Use the vaginal epithelial suture to close the superficial fascia down to the edge of the episiotomy.

4 Use the same suture again as a subcuticular stitch coming back to the hymenal ring, where it is tied off.

Remove the vaginal sponge.

Figure 56-17 Episiotomy and repair. Routine episiotomy is no longer advised, but the procedure is often performed. Simple repairs may be done in the emergency department (ED), but this is often performed by the obstetrician or in the delivery room after an ED birth. (*From Hacker NF, Gambone JC, Hobel CK. Hacker & Moore's Essentials of Obstetrics and Gynecology. 5th ed. Philadelphia: Saunders; 2009.*)

TABLE 56-2 Drugs for the Management of Immediate Postpartum Hemorrhage

DRUG	DOSE	COMMENTS
Oxytocin*	20-40 units in 1 L of crystalloid initially infused at 200-500 mL/hr and then titrate to sustain uterine contractions and control hemorrhage	Do not administer as an IV bolus. First-line therapy. If IV access is unavailable, may use 10 units IM
Methylergonovine maleate or ergonovine maleate	0.2 mg IM	Avoid in patients with hypertensive disease, including preeclampsia
Carboprost tromethamine	0.25 mg IM Repeat q15min until uterine hemorrhage is controlled or a maximum dose of 2 mg	Concurrent use of antiemetics and antidiarrheals recommended to control side effects
Misoprostol (Cytotec)	800-1000 μg PR	Single dose; can give PO. May cause tachycardia

IM, intramuscularly; *IV*, intravenous; *PO*, orally.
*Note the increased concentration of oxytocin when used for the treatment of postpartum hemorrhage versus that given to stimulate uterine contractions after uncomplicated delivery.

sutures (see Fig. 56-17, *step 2*). Close the superficial layers by one of two methods. In the first method, use a continuous suture to close the superficial mucosa from the mucocutaneous junction outward and then continue it upward as a subcuticular skin closure, with the suture returning to and ending at the mucocutaneous junction (see Fig. 56-17, *steps 3 and 4*). Alternatively, place several interrupted sutures through the skin and subcutaneous fascia and tie them loosely. This last method of skin closure avoids burying two layers of suture in the more superficial layers of the perineum.[3,15]

The most common complication of episiotomy is hematoma formation, which requires evacuation and drainage. Infection is an infrequent complication that usually responds to sitz baths, good hygiene, and antibiotic therapy.

Immediate Postpartum Hemorrhage

The average blood loss with a vaginal delivery is estimated to be approximately 500 mL.[56] There is no exact definition of postpartum hemorrhage, but a general guide is maternal blood loss greater than 500 mL or bleeding that exceeds a clinician's estimate of "normal."[4] Postpartum hemorrhage is divided into early hemorrhage, which occurs within 24 hours of delivery, and late hemorrhage, which occurs more than 24 hours and up to 6 weeks after delivery.

Postpartum hemorrhage is not necessarily sudden and massive. It is frequently characterized by persistent moderate bleeding until serious hypovolemia develops. Observe carefully for blood loss, including evaluation of uterine size and consistency, during the early postpartum period. The most common cause of early postpartum hemorrhage is uterine atony, which is involved in up to 80% of cases.[57] Less common causes include lacerations of the lower genital tract, retained placenta or placental fragments, coagulation disorders, uterine rupture, uterine inversion, and placental site bleeding.[4]

Management

Management of postpartum hemorrhage is similar to management of acute blood loss. It consists of replacement of intravascular volume with crystalloid and blood products as needed in addition to correction of the underlying cause of the hemorrhage. The diagnosis of uterine atony, the most

Figure 56-18 Use uterine massage to control postpartum bleeding. Insert one hand into the vagina to compress the anterior uterine wall while massaging the posterior aspect of the uterus through the abdominal wall with the other hand.

common cause of bleeding, is made when uterine palpation reveals a soft "boggy" uterus. The diagnosis may be suspected on the basis of abdominal examination with confirmation made on bimanual examination.

Uterine atony is initially managed with firm manual massage of the uterine fundus through the abdominal wall in conjunction with the administration of oxytocic agents (Table 56-2). If bleeding persists, bimanual uterine compression is indicated. Use one hand to compress and massage the uterus through the abdominal wall while using the fist of the other hand to gently massage the anterior aspect of the uterus through the vagina (Fig. 56-18). Avoid vigorous downward massage, which can result in acute uterine inversion or can injure the blood vessels in the broad ligament.

Oxytocics

Oxytocin (Pitocin) is the usual first-line drug for postpartum hemorrhage secondary to uterine atony. Administer oxytocin as an intravenous infusion. A typical initial dose is 20 to 40 units in 1 L of crystalloid infused at a rate of 200 to 500 mL/hr, although higher doses of up to 80 units have been used. Titrate to sustain uterine contractions and control uterine hemorrhage. Slowing of hemorrhage should be

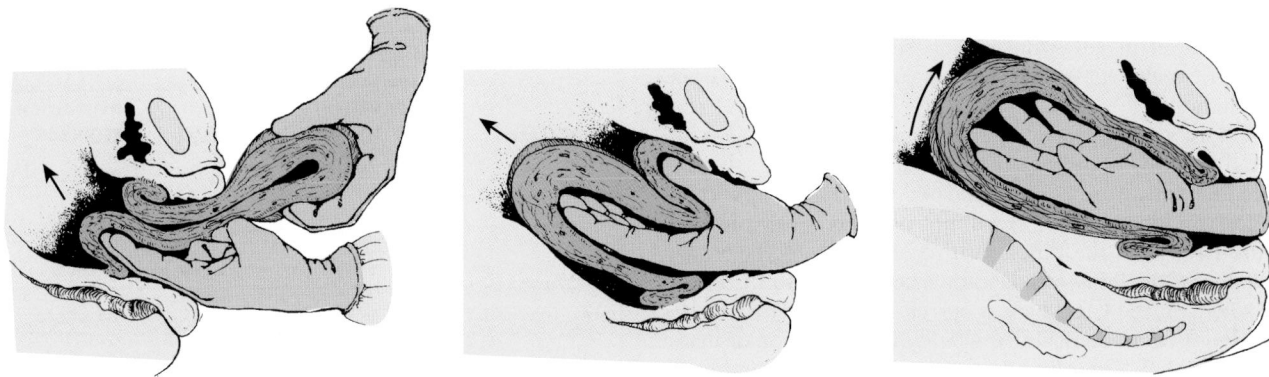

Figure 56-19 Manual replacement of an inverted uterus. Uterine inversion should be suspected with the sudden onset of brisk vaginal bleeding in association with an absent palpable fundus abdominally and maternal hemodynamic instability. It may occur before or after placental detachment. The diagnosis is made clinically with bimanual examination, during which the uterine fundus is palpated in the lower uterine segment or within the vagina. Use sonography to confirm the diagnosis if the findings on clinical examination are unclear.

observed within minutes of administration. If an intravenous line is not available, administer 10 units of intramuscular or intrauterine oxytocin.[35] Because severe hypotension may occur if oxytocin is administered as an intravenous bolus, this should generally be avoided.[58]

If bleeding and poor uterine tone persist despite oxytocin therapy, consider additional therapy. Second-line therapy includes ergot derivatives such as methylergonovine or a prostaglandin. Give methylergonovine (Methergine) as a 0.2-mg dose intramuscularly every 2 to 4 hours, with uterine contractions occurring within 2 to 5 minutes of administration and lasting regularly for several hours.[59] Though not the route of choice, methylergonovine can also be given via the oral route. Because of their tendency to cause severe hypertension, avoid administering ergot preparations to women with hypertensive disease, including preeclampsia.[59,60] Alternatively, give 15-methylprostaglandin $F_{2\alpha}$ (carboprost tromethamine [Hemabate]) to stimulate uterine contractions.[59-61] Administer carboprost at a dose of 0.25 mg intramuscularly repeated at 15 to 90-minute intervals as determined by the clinical course, but not to exceed 2 mg.[59,62] Misoprostol (Cytotec), a synthetic prostaglandin E_1 analogue, can also be given as an 800- to 1000-µg rectal dose.

If bleeding continues despite these measures, consider uterine tamponade with sterile gauze packing or insertion of a Foley catheter into the atonic uterine cavity until surgical intervention or arterial embolization can be performed.[59]

If vaginal bleeding persists despite a firmly contracted uterus, search for additional causes of bleeding. The lower genital tract should be inspected for lacerations. Control bleeding by direct pressure or by the gentle application of ring forceps to bleeding cervical lacerations. Use absorbable suture to control bleeding from accessible lacerations. Adequate visualization of the upper part of the vagina and cervix can be difficult, and repair of lacerations may require general anesthesia and obstetric intervention regardless of the location. Genital tract hematomas may also be a significant cause of hemorrhage but are not generally recognized until several hours after delivery.[47] Also consider retained placental fragments and coagulopathy.

Rarely, postpartum hemorrhage is due to uterine inversion, with an estimated incidence of one in several thousand deliveries.[63] Uterine inversion should be especially considered when there is severe pelvic pain, absence of a palpable fundus,

brisk excessive postpartum hemorrhage, and maternal hemodynamic instability. Shock develops in up to 40% of patients.[60,64-66] The diagnosis is made by visualization or palpation of the uterine fundus in the vaginal vault or protruding through the introitus. On abdominal examination, no mass representing the uterus may be palpated, or when palpated, the uterus may have a cuplike dimpling of the fundus.[60,62,65,66] Treat with crystalloid intravenous fluids to maintain cardiovascular stability. Reposition the uterus immediately (Fig. 56-19). Conscious sedation and general anesthesia may be necessary. Use tocolytic agents such as terbutaline or magnesium sulfate for uterine relaxation and repositioning.[3,59,60,66]

To reposition the uterus, insert one hand into the vagina with the tips of the fingers at the uterocervical junction and hold the uterine fundus firmly in the palm of the hand. Gently apply pressure to the uterine fundus in the direction of the umbilicus. Do not initially exert pressure centrally on the fundus because this will cause the uterus to become compressed and force more "layers" of the uterus to lie within the relatively tight cervical ring.[64-66] General anesthesia and laparotomy may be necessary for uterine positioning.

PCS

Perimortem cesarean section (PCS) is a dramatic surgical procedure with the potential to save the fetus from an otherwise certain demise.[67] Its origin can be traced to antiquity when King Numa Pompilius of Rome decreed that the child be excised from the womb of any woman who died late in pregnancy. When enforced by the emperors of Rome, it became known as *Lex Caesare*, hence the name cesarean section.[68]

Fortunately, the need to perform this procedure is rare because maternal cardiac arrest is reported to occur in only 1 in 30,000 pregnancies.[69] From 1879 until 1985 there were 188 reports of PCS resulting in delivery of a live infant.[70] An updated review through 2004 found only an additional 38 cases with an overall survival rate of 89%.[71] Before this review, reported infant survival rates ranged from 11% to 70%.[68,70,72] Because of the small numbers of cases in the literature and probably underreporting of those with unfavorable outcomes, definitive conclusions about the incidence and success of this procedure cannot be made. However, given that the anecdotal potential for survival of a normal infant exists, PCS may be considered in any woman who suffers a cardiac arrest after 24 weeks' gestation and is unresponsive to brief resuscitation.[70,73]

PCS is a complicated and emotional procedure, with limited success. Similar to ED thoracotomy, it is a heroic procedure whose use is not mandated but can be supported. In most circumstances PCS will not be aggressively pursued by the EP. Given the time-sensitive nature of any favorable outcome for the fetus, the decision to proceed with PCS may rest solely on the EP. There is currently no standard of care regarding PCS in the ED that would mandate action or inaction by the EP. Regarding medicolegal concerns, there have been no reported judgments against a physician for performing PCS.[74]

Indications

Although the lower limit of fetal viability varies among institutions, performance of PCS before approximately 24 weeks is not generally indicated.[18] If the duration of gestation is not known from the history, estimate fetal maturity quickly by calculating gestational age on the basis of the date of the patient's last normal menstrual period or by measuring the height of the uterine fundus. Between 18 and 30 weeks' gestation, the age of the fetus in weeks will correspond to the distance in centimeters from the uterine fundus to the symphysis pubis (e.g., at 28 weeks' gestation the fundus lies approximately 28 cm above the symphysis pubis or halfway between the umbilicus and the costal margin).[75] Establish criteria for intervention prospectively at each institution in accordance with the institution's neonatal care policies.[18,75]

Survival of the infant is directly related to the time elapsed from maternal cardiac arrest to delivery, prompt performance of cardiopulmonary resuscitation (CPR) on the mother, the maturity of the fetus, pre-arrest health status of the mother, and in certain circumstances, the availability of neonatal intensive care facilities.[68,70,73] In accordance with advanced cardiac life support guidelines, initiate CPR immediately on recognition of maternal arrest and continue it until the infant has been delivered. The anatomic and physiologic changes of pregnancy will inhibit the effectiveness of CPR on the mother. Aortocaval occlusion by the gravid uterus may occur after 20 weeks' gestation. It can reduce venous return and compromise maternal cardiac output, especially in the supine position. For this reason, it is advisable to perform CPR in the left lateral, head-down position or to have an assistant manually displace the uterus away from the inferior vena cava.[71] In addition, the decreased functional residual capacity of the lungs may impede ventilation efforts. Under these conditions, CPR generates only 30% to 40% of normal cardiac output, which severely compromises placental perfusion. The potential for infant survival decreases and the chance of neurologic damage increases as the time from maternal cardiac arrest to PCS rises (Table 56-3). When PCS is performed within 5 minutes, neonatal outcome is best, but not guaranteed; from 5 to 10 minutes, good; from 10 to 15 minutes, fair; and from 15 to 20 minutes, poor. Make every attempt to begin PCS within 4 minutes of cardiopulmonary arrest and complete the procedure within 5 minutes of arrest.[18,70,73,75] Fetal prognosis is generally better in the later stages of pregnancy and after the sudden death of a previously healthy mother rather than death secondary to chronic illness.[68,70,75]

TABLE 56-3 Outcome of Infants Who Survived PCS as a Function of Time from Maternal Death to Delivery

TIME (min)	NO. OF PATIENTS (%)	NORMAL	NEUROLOGIC SEQUELAE
0-5	42 (69)	42	0
6-10	8 (13)	7	1 (mild)
11-15	7 (11)	6	1 (severe)
16-20	1 (2)	0	1 (severe)
21-25	3 (5)	1	2 (severe)

From Katz VL, Dotters DJ, Droegemueller W. Perimortem cesarean delivery. *Obstet Gynecol.* 1986;68:571.
PCS, postmortem cesarean section.
Note: Although PCS can be supported in the emergency department, it is not a standard of care for emergency physicians. Even though some heroic interventions have been successful, optimistic outcomes cannot be expected in the general population. The incidence of severe neurologic sequelae may sway individual clinical decisions.

In addition to fetal benefits, PCS may improve maternal outcome. Emptying the uterus by PCS removes the aortocaval compression, thereby resulting in a 30% increase in cardiac output, which increases the likelihood of maternal survival.[76,77] CPR should continue during and after the procedure. PCS in itself may represent the most important variable for successful maternal resuscitation.[68,70,78]

Limited resources often place the EP in the difficult situation of deciding whether to continue efforts to resuscitate the mother or to attempt to deliver the fetus under less than ideal conditions. The decision to perform this procedure may be one of the most challenging that an EP will encounter. In the absence of immediate obstetric backup, it is reasonable to proceed with PCS if initial maternal resuscitation efforts are unsuccessful. Prolonged attempts to resuscitate the mother are unlikely to benefit either the mother or the fetus.

Technique

The most experienced person present should perform the PCS, preferably an obstetrician. Under ideal circumstances a neonatologist should also be in attendance, so contact them as soon as possible. However, do not delay the procedure to allow time for their arrival. Also, time should not be wasted searching for fetal heart tones or attempting to evaluate fetal viability with ultrasonography.

Extract the infant rapidly while avoiding fetal and maternal injury (Fig. 56-20). Hence, do not waste time preparing a sterile operating field or transporting the patient to an operating suite outside the ED. Use a large (e.g., No. 10) blade and make a midline vertical incision through the abdominal wall that extends from the symphysis pubis to the umbilicus. Carry the incision through all abdominal layers and into the peritoneal cavity. In most gravid women the hyperpigmented "linea nigra" is apparent, and when present, use this as a guide for the incision. If available, place retractors in the abdominal wound and draw them laterally to expose the anterior surface of the uterus. Reflect the bladder inferiorly. If full, aspirate the bladder to evacuate it and permit better access to the uterus. While avoiding injury to fetal parts, make a small

PERIMORTEM CESAREAN DELIVERY

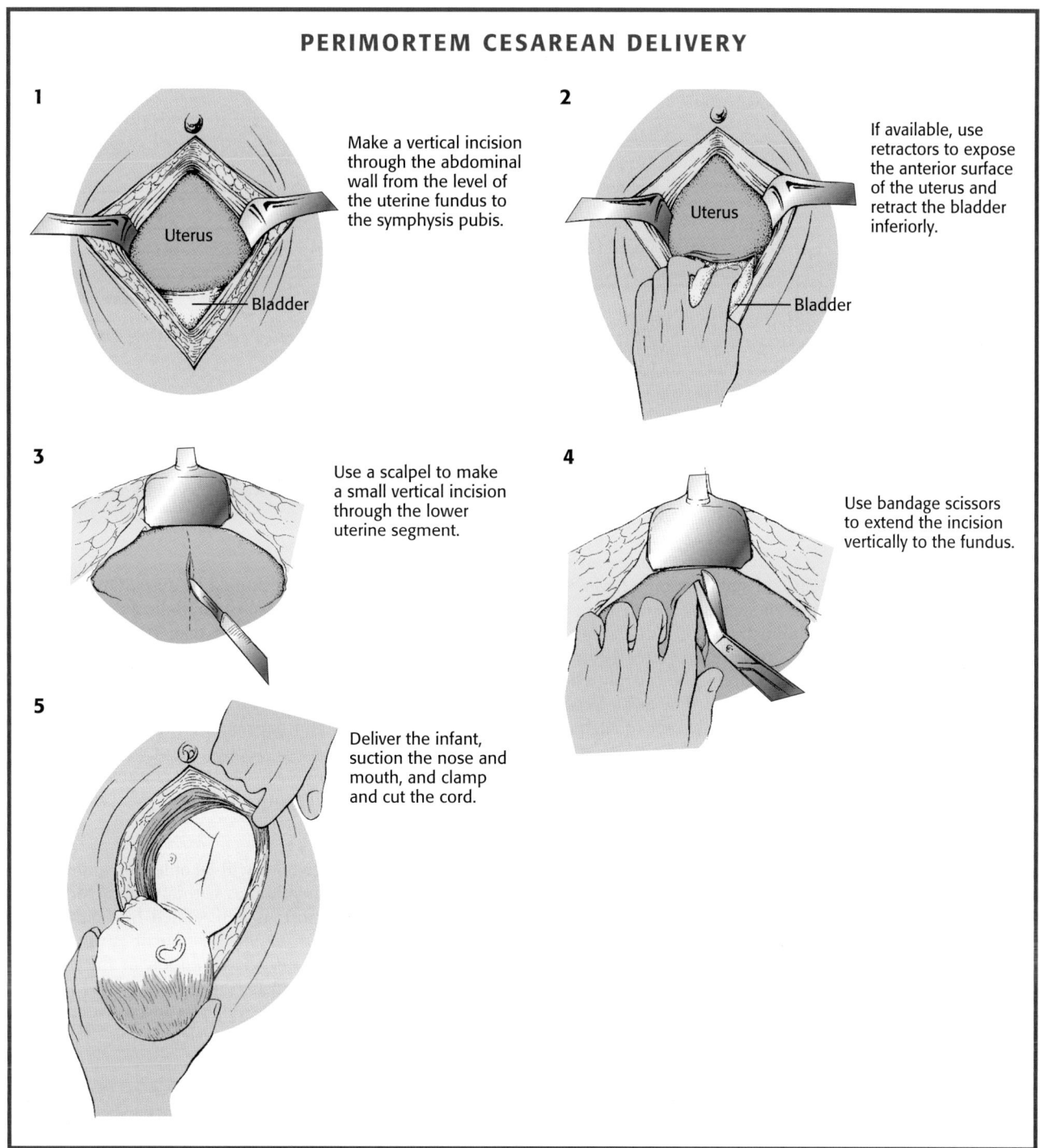

1 Make a vertical incision through the abdominal wall from the level of the uterine fundus to the symphysis pubis.

Uterus

Bladder

2 If available, use retractors to expose the anterior surface of the uterus and retract the bladder inferiorly.

Uterus

Bladder

3 Use a scalpel to make a small vertical incision through the lower uterine segment.

4 Use bandage scissors to extend the incision vertically to the fundus.

5 Deliver the infant, suction the nose and mouth, and clamp and cut the cord.

Figure 56-20 Perimortem cesarean delivery.

(≈5-cm) vertical incision through the uterus until amniotic fluid is obtained or the uterine cavity is clearly entered. Insert the index and long fingers into the incision and use them to lift the uterine wall away from the fetus. Use bandage scissors to extend the incision vertically to the fundus until a wide exposure is obtained. Gently deliver the infant, suction the mouth and nose, and clamp and cut the cord. Because the incision is relatively high in the uterus, the infant's head may not be readily accessible to the clinician. In this case, grasp the infant's feet and deliver the infant through maneuvers similar to those used for a breech delivery.

THE NEWBORN

Approximately 10% of newborns require some degree of assistance to begin breathing at birth (e.g., some sort of stimulation to breathe), but less than 1% require extensive resuscitation.[45] Evaluation of the newborn begins before delivery with assessment of maternal well-being and identification of risk factors for fetal distress: multiple pregnancy of less than 35 weeks, maternal infection or hypertension, oligohydramnios, preterm delivery at less than 36 weeks, breech presentation, meconium-stained amniotic fluid, nonreassuring fetal

TABLE 56-4 Apgar Scoring System

SIGN	0	1	2
Heart rate (beats/min)	Absent	Slow (<100)	>100
Respiratory effort	Absent	Slow, irregular	Good, crying
Muscle tone	Flaccid	Some flexion of extremities	Active motion
Reflex irritability	No response	Grimace	Vigorous cry
Color	Blue, pale	Body pink, extremities blue	Completely pink

Table 56-5 Targeted Preductal SpO$_2$ After Birth

1 min	60-65%
2 min	65-70%
3 min	70-75%
4 min	75-80%
5 min	80-85%
10 min	85-95%

From Kattwinkel J, Perlman JM, Aziz K, et al. Neonatal resuscitation: 2010 American Heart Association Guidelines for Cardiopulmonary Resuscitation and Emergency Cardiovascular Care. *Pediatrics*. 2010;126:e1400-e1413.

heart rate, emergency caesarean section, shoulder dystocia, and opiate use in normal labor.[79]

Newborn resuscitation can be divided into four categories of action: (1) initial assessment and stabilization; (2) ventilation, including bag-valve-mask or bag-tube ventilation; (3) chest compressions; and (4) administration of medications or fluids. Although most newborns require no resuscitation or only basic steps such as warming, drying, and stimulation, others will require further intervention. The most crucial action of neonatal resuscitation is establishment of adequate ventilation.[45]

Evaluation

Traditionally, the Apgar scoring system, applied at 1 and 5 minutes after birth, has been the standard of newborn evaluation (Table 56-4).[3,80] In general, the higher the score, the better the condition of the infant. Waiting for the traditional 1-minute Apgar score to indicate the need for resuscitation has been replaced by the concept of "the golden minute." Begin basic resuscitation maneuvers, reevaluation, and positive pressure ventilation (PPV), if required, by the first 60 seconds after birth. Use the heart rate and respiratory effort to guide resuscitation efforts because skin color does not reliably predict oxygenation status in the newborn period.[45]

Respiration

Normally, the newborn begins to breath and cry almost immediately after birth.[3] After initial respiratory efforts, the newborn should be able to establish regular respirations sufficient to improve color and should be able to maintain a heart rate higher than 100 beats/min. Generally, drying and stimulation (rubbing the back or flicking the soles of the feet) are enough to induce effective respirations in the newborn.[81] Gasping and apnea after 30 seconds of stimulation are signs indicating the need for assisted ventilation and continuous pulse oximetry monitoring.[45,80] It is important to note that even in healthy newborns, blood oxygen saturation does not reach extrauterine levels until 10 minutes after birth. Recent studies have demonstrated potential harmful effects from both excessive and insufficient supplemental oxygen versus room air during neonatal resuscitation. This is an area of

ongoing research, and controversy exists (see Chapter 3 for current recommendation by the American Heart Association). Therefore, the application of supplemental oxygen should be guided by normal newborn oxygen saturation ranges (Table 56-5). Establishing adequate ventilation and oxygenation will restore vital signs in the vast majority of newborns.[45]

Heart Rate

The heart rate may be determined by auscultation or palpation of the pulse at the base of the umbilical cord. The heart rate should consistently be greater than 100 beats/min in an uncompromised newborn. If after 30 seconds the heart rate is less than 100 beats/min, initiate PPV with supplemental oxygen. If the heart rate is less than 60 beats/min despite adequate ventilation and oxygenation for 30 seconds, commence chest compressions. Because chest compressions may diminish the effectiveness of ventilation, do not initiate them until lung inflation and ventilation have been established.[81]

Color

An uncompromised newborn will be able to maintain a pink color of the mucous membranes without supplemental oxygenation. Central cyanosis is determined by examining the face, trunk, and mucous membranes, but it is not a reliable method of determining oxygen saturation in the immediate neonatal period. Acrocyanosis is usually a normal finding in the newborn and not a reliable indicator of hypoxemia. It may, however, indicate other conditions such as cold stress.[80,81]

Stabilization Technique

Following delivery of the infant and cutting of the umbilical cord, place the newborn on the side in the sniffing position and the neck in a neutral or slightly extended position.[81] Place a rolled blanket or towel under the back and shoulders of the supine infant to elevate the torso 2 to 2.5 cm because this may help maintain head position.[80,81] Prevent heat loss in the newborn because cold stress can increase oxygen consumption and impede effective resuscitation.[81] Avoid hyperthermia, however, because it is associated with perinatal respiratory depression.[81,82] Place the infant under a radiant warmer, rapidly dry the skin, and wrap the infant in warmed blankets to reduce heat loss.[45,80,81] Alternatively, use the mother's body as a heat source for the newborn. If initial evaluation indicates that the infant is stable, dry and place the infant skin to skin on the mother's chest or abdomen, and cover both with blankets.[80,81]

TABLE 56-6   Medications Commonly Used in Neonatal Resuscitation

DRUG	DOSE	INDICATIONS	COMMENTS
Epinephrine*	0.01-0.03 mg/kg (0.1-0.3 mL/kg of a 1:10,000 solution)	Bradycardia, asystole	May be repeated every 3-5 min as indicated High-dose epinephrine in newborns is contraindicated
Volume expanders (normal saline or Ringer's solution)	10 mL/kg IV over 5-10 min	Suspected hypovolemia, shock, or blood loss	May be repeated after determination of clinical response
Bicarbonate	1-2 mEq/kg of a 0.5-mEq/mL solution given over at least 2 min	Prolonged arrests unresponsive to other therapy	Not indicated during brief periods of CPR Should be used only after adequate ventilation and perfusion are established

From Kattwinkel J, Perlman JM, Aziz K, et al. Neonatal resuscitation: 2010 American Heart Association Guidelines for Cardiopulmonary Resuscitation and Emergency Cardiovascular Care. *Pediatrics*. 2010;126(5):e1400-e1413; and Pediatric Working Group of the International Liaison Committee on Resuscitation. Neonatal resuscitation. *Circulation*. 2000;102:343.

CPR, cardiopulmonary resuscitation.

*The intravenous route is now strongly preferred, but one can consider administering epinephrine via an endotracheal tube in doses of 0.05 to 0.1 mg/kg while obtaining intravenous access.

Vigorous newborns should not be routinely suctioned after delivery, even those delivered through meconium-stained fluid.[45,83] Reserve suctioning (including suctioning with a bulb syringe) immediately after birth for babies who exhibit obvious obstruction to spontaneous breathing or require PPV. Despite a paucity of data to support the practice, endotracheal suctioning is still recommended for nonvigorous babies born through meconium-stained amniotic fluid.[45] If suctioning is necessary, first clear secretions from the mouth and nose with a bulb syringe or suction catheter (8 or 10 Fr). Aggressive pharyngeal suctioning can cause laryngeal spasm and vagal bradycardia, so limit the depth and duration of suctioning and do not exceed a negative pressure of 100 mm Hg.[81]

For newborns who do not quickly respond to conservative measures, PPV is indicated. Most newborns who require PPV can be adequately ventilated with a bag and mask. Perform assisted ventilations at a rate of 40 to 60/min (30 breaths/min if mechanical compressions are being performed). Typically, higher inflation pressures (≥30 to 40 cm H_2O) and longer inflation times are required for the first several breaths than for subsequent breaths. Visible chest expansion is a more reliable indicator of appropriate inflation pressure than a specific manometer reading.[80,81] Because bag-valve-mask ventilation can produce gastric distention and impede respiration, insert an orogastric tube (8 Fr) in infants undergoing prolonged PPV.[81]

Endotracheal intubation may be indicated when bag-valve-mask ventilation is ineffective, when tracheal suctioning for meconium is required, when chest compressions are performed, or when prolonged PPV is required.[45,80] Alternatively, a neonatal laryngeal mask airway may provide effective airway management, especially in the case of ineffective bag-valve-mask ventilation or failed endotracheal intubation.[45] Use of the laryngeal mask airway, however, has not been adequately studied in preterm infants and those with deliveries complicated by meconium-stained fluid. Its use, therefore, cannot be recommended in these situations.[45]

Monitor the heart rate during the course of neonatal evaluation and stabilization by either direct auscultation over the chest or palpation of the pulse at the base of the umbilical cord. A readily discernible heartbeat of 100 beats/min or greater is acceptable. If the heart rate is less than 60 beats/min despite adequate ventilation and oxygenation for 30 seconds, institute chest compressions while continuing to ventilate.[45] Deliver chest compressions on the lower third of the sternum and not over the xiphoid to avoid damage to the liver.[80] There are two techniques for performing chest compressions in the newborn. In the preferred method, two thumbs of the resuscitator's hands are positioned side by side over the lower third of the sternum just below the nipple line. If the infant is large or the resuscitator's hands are too small to encircle the chest, two-finger compressions with the ring and middle fingers may be used.[45,80] The depth of compression should be approximately one third to one half the AP diameter of the newborn's chest such that a palpable pulse is generated.[45] Coordinate compressions and ventilations to avoid simultaneous delivery, which may compromise the efficacy of ventilation. The compression-to-ventilation ratio should be 3:1 with 90 compressions and 30 breaths to achieve approximately 120 events/min.[45] If the heart rate remains less than 60 beats/min despite these interventions,[45] establish an umbilical or intravenous line and initiate appropriate drug therapy. Alternatively, use intraosseous access, but this may not be as effective in a preterm infant.[81] The medications most commonly used during neonatal resuscitation are listed in Table 56-6.[45,81]

Selected Readings

Delke I. Delivery in the emergency department. In: Benrubi GI, ed. *Handbook of Obstetric and Gynecologic Emergencies*. 4th ed. Baltimore: Lippincott, Williams & Wilkins; 2010:160.

Stallard TC, Burns B. Emergency delivery and perimortem C-section. *Emerg Med Clin North Am*. 2003;21:679.

CHAPTER 57

Culdocentesis

G. Richard Braen

Culdocentesis is a procedure in which a hollow needle is inserted through the posterior vaginal wall into the peritoneal space to obtain peritoneal fluid for analysis and culture. This procedure is simple, rapid, and safe. The technique is used primarily to diagnose ruptured ectopic pregnancies and ruptured ovarian cysts and, rarely, to obtain material for culture to aid in the diagnosis of pelvic inflammatory disease (PID). The availability of bedside ultrasound, high-resolution transvaginal ultrasound, and highly sensitive β-human chorionic gonadotropin (β-hCG) assays has led to a decline in the use of this procedure. Despite this change, culdocentesis is still valuable in patients in whom a ruptured ectopic pregnancy is suspected but who are too unstable to transport for a formal sonographic examination.[1]

ANATOMY

Before attempting culdocentesis, the clinician must be familiar with the anatomy of the vagina and the rectouterine pouch (pouch of Douglas) (Fig. 57-1). In adult women, the vagina is approximately 9 cm long. From its inferior to its superior aspect, the posterior wall of the vagina is related to the anal canal by way of the perineal body, the rectum, and the peritoneum of the rectouterine pouch.[2] The uterus lies at nearly a right angle to the vagina. The rectouterine pouch and the posterior wall of the vagina are adjacent only at the upper quarter (≈2 cm) of the posterior vaginal wall. The vaginal wall in this area is less than 5 mm thick.

The blood supply to the upper part of the vagina comes from the uterine and vaginal arteries, which are branches of the internal iliac artery. This area is drained by a vaginal venous plexus that communicates with the uterine plexuses. The vagina has its greatest sensation near the introitus and little sensation in the area adjacent to the rectouterine pouch.

The rectouterine pouch is formed by reflections of the peritoneum, and it is the most dependent intraperitoneal space in both the upright and the supine positions. Blood, pus, and other free fluids in the peritoneal cavity pool in the pouch because of its dependent location. This pouch separates the upper portion of the rectum from the uterus and the upper part of the vagina. The pouch often contains small intestine and, normally, a small amount of peritoneal fluid.

INDICATIONS

Culdocentesis is indicated in any adult woman in whom aspiration of fluid from the rectouterine pouch will help confirm the clinical diagnosis. If ultrasound examination is not readily available in the emergency department (ED) or if the patient is too hemodynamically unstable to be transported to an off-site location for ultrasound, culdocentesis may be the fastest and most accurate diagnostic technique available to the emergency clinician.[3] Analysis of peritoneal fluid is also a reliable method of differentiating inflammatory from hemorrhagic pelvic pathologic conditions. Conditions in which culdocentesis may be of diagnostic value include a ruptured viscus (particularly an ectopic pregnancy or a corpus luteum cyst), PID and other intraabdominal infections (particularly

Culdocentesis

Indications
Diagnosis of acute pelvic conditions when ultrasound is not available or clinically feasible, including:
  Ruptured viscus (ectopic pregnancy or corpus luteum cyst)
  Pelvic inflammatory disease
  Other intraabdominal infections
  Splenic or liver injuries
  Ruptured aortic aneurysm

Contraindications
Uncooperative patient
Pelvic mass detected on bimanual examination
Nonmobile retroverted uterus
Coagulopathies

Complications
Rupture of unsuspected tuboovarian abscess
Bowel perforation
Pelvic kidney perforation
Bleeding

Equipment

Lidocaine with epinephrine

19-gauge butterfly needle

Bivalve vaginal speculum

Ring forceps

Uterine cervical tenaculum

18-gauge spinal needle

Review Box 57-1 Culdocentesis: indications, contraindications, complications, and equipment. Not shown is optional prepuncture topical anesthetic, such as a cocaine (4%)-soaked cotton ball.

appendicitis with rupture or diverticulitis with perforation), intraabdominal injuries to the liver or spleen, and ruptured aortic aneurysms.[4]

Ectopic Pregnancy

Ectopic pregnancy is often one of the most difficult gynecologic lesions to diagnose.[5] The incidence of ectopic pregnancy is on the rise, and it accounts for 1.6% of all pregnancies. Ectopic pregnancy is the most common obstetric cause of maternal death in the first trimester.[5] In a series of 300 consecutive cases of ectopic pregnancy, 50% of patients received medical evaluation at least twice before the correct diagnosis was made.[6] In 11% of patients in this series, the diagnosis was not made until the third medical visit.

The clinical picture of ectopic pregnancy may include vascular collapse, pelvic pain, isolated rectal or back pain, amenorrhea, abnormal menses, shoulder pain, syncope, cervical or adnexal tenderness, adnexal mass, anemia, and leukocytosis. It is important to note that blood in the peritoneal cavity does not consistently correlate with peritoneal irritation, blood pressure, or pulse rate.[7] In fact, bradycardia in the presence of significant intraperitoneal bleeding from a ruptured ectopic pregnancy is not unusual (Tables 57-1 and 57-2).

Risk factors for an ectopic pregnancy include a history of salpingitis, use of an intrauterine contraceptive device, or tubal ligation; however, no combination of these signs, symptoms, or historical data is diagnostic of an ectopic pregnancy. To confuse the diagnosis further, a normal menstrual history is reported in approximately 50% of patients with an ectopic pregnancy. A urine pregnancy test is occasionally negative.[8] Though rarely seen, the combination of a uterine decidual cast (Fig. 57-2) and a positive pregnancy test is virtually pathognomonic of an ectopic pregnancy. A uterine cast is decidua that has been hormonally stimulated by the ectopic pregnancy but is passed vaginally when the tissue can no longer be supported. The cast is an outline of the uterine cavity, but it can be mistaken for products of conception if not inspected carefully. Therefore, all tissue passed vaginally should be carefully inspected before being sent to the laboratory for analysis for products of conception. An ectopic pregnancy can occasionally occur in conjunction with an intrauterine pregnancy. Patients who have undergone a therapeutic abortion may actually have had an unrecognized ectopic pregnancy, hence the need for pathologic evaluation of any tissue obtained by uterine evacuation procedures.

The greater sensitivity of the serum and urine β-hCG assay, coupled with the increased availability of emergency medicine physicians trained to perform pelvic ultrasound, has greatly increased the chance of early diagnosis of unruptured and ruptured ectopic pregnancy.[9] Urinary β-hCG tests provide a sensitivity to 20 to 50 mIU/mL and are positive in

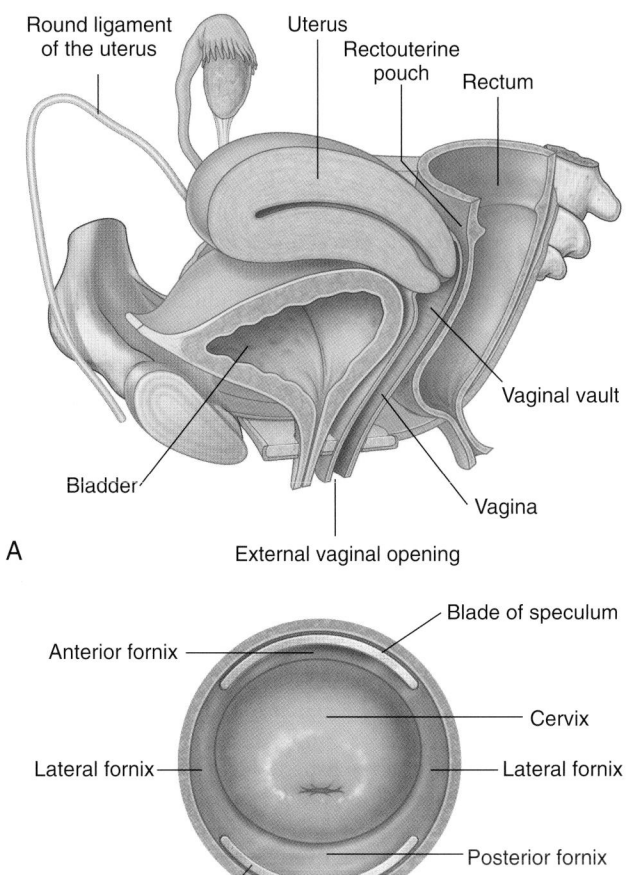

Figure 57-1 Anatomy of the vagina and rectouterine pouch (pouch of Douglas). *(Modified from Drake RL: Gray's Anatomy for Students. 2nd ed. Philadelphia: Elsevier; 2010, Fig 5.56.)*

TABLE 57-1 Correlation between the Results of Culdocenteses Performed on 77 Patients with Ectopic Gestation and Various Clinical Parameters									
	CLASSIC TRIAD			Peritoneal Signs	Pulse ≥100 Beats/min	Blood Pressure <90/40 mm Hg	Mean Hematocrit (%)	Hemoperitoneum ≥100 mL	Ruptured Tube	Total
	Bleeding	Pain	Adnexal Mass							
Positive	37	54	10	26	19	9	35	52	30	54
Negative	8	8	3	1	1	0	39	0	0	8
Inadequate	13	15	6	5	4	1	38	13	7	15
Total patients	58	77	19	32	24	10		65	37	77

From Cartwright PS, Vaughn B, Tuttle D. Culdocentesis and ectopic pregnancy. *J Reprod Med.* 1984;29:88.
Note: There is a lack of correlation between positive culdocentesis and peritoneal signs and changes in vital signs. Patients are grouped by the result of culdocentesis (i.e., positive, negative, or inadequate). Note that only 10 patients were hypotensive and only 24 experienced tachycardia.

TABLE 57-2 Correlation between Tubal Status and Hypotension, Tachycardia, Hematocrit, Signs of Peritoneal Irritation, and Hemoperitoneum in 77 Patients with Ectopic Gestation

CULDOCENTESIS	CULDOCENTESIS POSITIVE	PERITONEAL SIGNS	BLOOD PRESSURE <90/40 mm Hg	PULSE ≥ 100 BEATS/MIN	HEMOPERITONEUM ≥100 mL	AVERAGE HEMATOCRIT (%)
Ruptured (*n* = 37)	30	25	8	19	37	33.6
Intact (*n* = 40)	24	7	2	5	28	37.3
Total patients	54	32	10	24	65	

From Cartwright PS, Vaughn B, Tuttle D. Culdocentesis and ectopic pregnancy. *J Reprod Med.* 1984;29:88.
Note: Culdocentesis is frequently positive in the absence of rupture. Patients are grouped by the presence (i.e., "ruptured") or absence (i.e., "intact") of hemoperitoneum. Note that only about half the patients with "ruptured" status had tachycardia.

Figure 57-2 This decidual cast, a perfect outline of the uterine cavity, was initially thought to be a product of conception when found in the vaginal vault of a pregnant woman treated for abdominal pain and vaginal bleeding. The initial diagnosis was a spontaneous abortion, but this cast is *virtually diagnostic of an ectopic pregnancy.* Hypotension developed later and the woman was found to have a ruptured tubal pregnancy.

the first few weeks of pregnancy. However, ectopic pregnancy is often associated with very low production of this hormone.

Quantification of the serum test adds additional information since it is sensitive to 5 mIU/mL. Therefore, a negative *urine* β-hCG test rules out pregnancy in greater than 98% of cases, and pregnancy in any site can be ruled out in virtually all patients with a negative *serum* β-hCG test.[10] A single quantitative β-hCG level is a poor predictor of the size of the pregnancy or the risk for ectopic pregnancy, but serial testing

is quite helpful. It is expected that the quantitative serum β-hCG level should double approximately every 2 days in the first trimester.

Serum progesterone determinations are not standardly used in the ED, but they may also help identify a normal or abnormal pregnancy. Though not infallible, a serum progesterone level of less than 10 ng/mL is usually associated with a nonviable intrauterine pregnancy or ectopic pregnancy, and a level greater than 25 ng/mL is usually associated with a viable intrauterine pregnancy.

To increase the accuracy of diagnosis, it is helpful to combine quantitative β-hCG testing with ultrasound examination (Fig. 57-3). An empty uterus by transvaginal or abdominal ultrasound combined with certain quantitative serum β-hCG results can be quite helpful to the clinician. The quantitative range in which the ultrasonographer should detect an intrauterine pregnancy varies, but an intrauterine pregnancy should be detected if the serum β-hCG level is in the range of 1200 to 1500 mIU/mL when using a *transvaginal probe* and greater than 6000 mIU/mL when using a *transabdominal probe.* Endovaginal ultrasonic scanning consistently identifies a 4-week gestational sac if the β-hCG level is 2000 mIU/mL or greater. The presence of a fetal pole and cardiac activity are detectable with endovaginal ultrasound scanning at approximately 6 and 7 weeks, respectively.[11] *Note that a heartbeat can occasionally be detected in an ectopic pregnancy* or in an extrauterine pregnancy and may be mistakenly deemed intrauterine. It is important to note that the absence of an intrauterine pregnancy by ultrasound, when the β-hCG level is *below the discriminatory zone (defined as the hCG level at which a normal intrauterine pregnancy can be detected by ultrasound),* is *nondiagnostic* and could represent an early viable normal pregnancy, a nonviable intrauterine pregnancy, a completed abortion, or an ectopic pregnancy. When no intrauterine pregnancy is detected by ultrasound and the serum β-hCG level *exceeds the discriminatory zone,* the chance of an ectopic pregnancy ranges from 86% to 100%.[12]

Culdocentesis may play an important role in some patients in the diagnosis of ectopic pregnancy. The test has an accuracy rate of 85% to 95%.[3,13,14] Romero and coworkers[15] reported that an ectopic pregnancy was found in 99% of patients with a positive pregnancy test and positive results on culdocentesis. Although culdocentesis is most often positive in the presence of a frankly ruptured ectopic pregnancy, it may be diagnostic even in a nonruptured case when bleeding has been slow or intermittent. Note that many ectopic pregnancies leak varying amounts of blood for days or weeks before rupture. Hemoperitoneum has been found in 45% to

Figure 57-3 A, Pelvic ultrasound showing an empty uterus. The endometrial stripe (*arrow*) is clearly visible, and there is no evidence of a gestational sac. If the β human chorionic gonadotropin (β-hCG) level is below the discriminatory zone (see text), this could represent an early viable intrauterine pregnancy, a nonviable intrauterine pregnancy, completed abortion, or an ectopic pregnancy. If β-hCG exceeds the discriminatory zone, the chance of an ectopic pregnancy exceeds 85%. **B,** Pelvic ultrasound showing the presence of a yolk sac (*arrow*) within a gestational sac in the uterus. This patient was 5 weeks pregnant by dates.

60% of cases of *unruptured* ectopic pregnancy, as proved at surgery.[7,16]

Hence, culdocentesis may be helpful in a stable patient whose ultrasound examination does not demonstrate an intrauterine pregnancy despite a quantitative serum β-hCG level in the appropriate range. Although some clinicians opt for outpatient monitoring of serial β-hCG levels in this setting, patients in whom the clinician has high suspicion for an ectopic pregnancy (e.g., a patient who has or had significant discomfort) or in whom close follow-up cannot be ensured may be candidates for culdocentesis.[3] Even though a negative finding on culdocentesis does not rule out an early ectopic pregnancy, patients with a nondiagnostic ultrasound and a negative culdocentesis generally represent those at lower risk for "rupture" of an ectopic pregnancy during outpatient serum β-hCG monitoring. Patients with a nondiagnostic ultrasound examination and a serum β-hCG level below the threshold at which an intrauterine pregnancy should be visible on the ultrasound examination must be individualized. These patients, especially those with significant pain, an unexplained low hematocrit, or postural changes in vital signs (or near syncope), might be candidates for culdocentesis.

Blunt Abdominal Trauma

Historically, diagnostic peritoneal lavage (DPL) and computed tomography (CT) have been used to identify hemoperitoneum in blunt trauma patients. The use of culdocentesis has also been advocated to aid in this diagnosis.[4,17] In the ED, two factors have largely obviated the need to perform invasive procedures for diagnosis of hemoperitoneum: (1) the increasing availability of high-resolution CT and (2) emergency clinicians trained to perform the bedside ultrasound FAST (focused assessment with sonography for trauma) examination. However, because small amounts of blood tend to collect in the rectouterine pouch, aspiration of clear peritoneal fluid is of great potential value in excluding a diagnosis of hemoperitoneum. This is especially helpful in situations in which ultrasound is unavailable or the patient is too unstable to leave the ED for a CT scan. In fact, culdocentesis may be more advantageous than DPL in some instances because there is less risk for urinary bladder perforation or bowel injury. In addition, previous abdominal surgery is not a relative contraindication to culdocentesis, as it is with DPL.[18]

CONTRAINDICATIONS

Contraindications to culdocentesis are relatively few and include an uncooperative patient, a pelvic mass detected on bimanual pelvic examination, a nonmobile retroverted uterus, and coagulopathies. Pelvic masses may include tuboovarian abscesses, appendiceal abscesses, ovarian masses, and pelvic kidneys. It has been suggested that the only major risk with the procedure is rupture of an unsuspected tuboovarian abscess into the peritoneal cavity. This can be avoided by careful bimanual pelvic examination to exclude patients with large masses in the cul-de-sac.[19] Although no data are available to guide the age at which culdocentesis may be performed safely, the procedure is generally limited to patients beyond puberty. This limitation is suggested on the basis of anatomy and with the consideration that the procedure is difficult to perform through a small prepubertal vagina.

EQUIPMENT

The equipment required for culdocentesis is depicted in Review Box 57-1. Either an 18-gauge spinal needle or a 19-gauge butterfly needle held by ring forceps is acceptable. It may be helpful to anesthetize the posterior vaginal wall at the site of the puncture with 1% to 2% lidocaine with epinephrine administered through a 27-or 25-gauge needle. Some physicians use a topical anesthetic (eutectic mixture of local anesthetics [EMLA], benzocaine) or a cocaine-soaked cotton ball to anesthetize the mucosa before infiltration with a local anesthetic. Although local anesthesia is often unnecessary (because *puncture of the posterior vaginal wall at the upper fourth of the vagina is generally no more painful than a venipuncture*), there is some advantage to using a local anesthetic if multiple attempts at culdocentesis are required, as is sometimes the case. In addition, the epinephrine may produce vasoconstriction and reduce bleeding associated with the needle puncture. Culdocentesis is often stressful to the patient, and all attempts should be made to render the procedure as painless as possible. Parenteral analgesia and sedation should also be considered when the patient is uncomfortable or anxious.

TECHNIQUE

Preparation

Culdocentesis is an invasive procedure that requires a written, witnessed, and signed consent form from the patient, parent, or guardian when the patient's condition permits. If verbal consent is obtained, this action should be witnessed and a notation made in the medical record documenting that the procedure was described, complications were discussed, and any alternatives (e.g., CT, sonography, or immediate laparoscopy) were offered when appropriate.

Once written or verbal consent is obtained, place the patient in a lithotomy position with the head of the table slightly elevated (reverse Trendelenburg position) so that intraperitoneal fluid gravitates toward the rectouterine pouch. Place the patient's feet in stirrups. Premedicate with intravenous opioids or sedatives if appropriate. Administration of nitrous oxide analgesia is also an accepted practice. Procedural sedation with propofol, etomidate, or benzodiazepines can be considered. Although the pain associated with passage of the culdocentesis needle is generally minor, judicious use of analgesia and sedation makes the procedure easier for both the clinician and patient.

If radiographs are indicated, take them before culdocentesis to avoid confusion with procedure-induced pneumoperitoneum.

Exposure

Perform a bimanual pelvic examination before culdocentesis to rule out a fixed pelvic mass and to assess the position of the uterus. It is possible to palpate an adnexal mass if the mass exceeds 3 cm in diameter. Insert a bivalve vaginal speculum and open it widely by adjusting both the height and the angle thumbscrews (Fig. 57-4, *step 1*). Grasp the posterior lip of the cervix with the toothed uterine cervical tenaculum and elevate the cervix. Warn the patient in advance that she may feel a sharp pain when the cervix is grasped with the tenaculum. Inform the patient also that bleeding from the tenaculum puncture site or culdocentesis site, or both, may produce postprocedural spotting.

Use the tenaculum to elevate a retroverted uterus from the pouch, to expose the puncture site, and to stabilize the posterior wall during puncture with the needle. Some clinicians prefer to use longitudinal traction on the cervix to produce the same result. The vaginal wall adjacent to the rectouterine pouch will be tightened somewhat between the inferior blade of the bivalve speculum and the elevated posterior lip of the cervix. Such tightening of the vaginal wall exposes the puncture site and keeps it from moving away from the needle when the wall is punctured.

After the tenaculum is applied and the posterior lip of the cervix is elevated or traction is applied, swab the vaginal wall in the area of the rectouterine pouch with an antiseptic, followed by a small amount of sterile water. Administer a local anesthetic (1% lidocaine with epinephrine) at this point. Anesthetic may be injected through a separate 27- or 25-gauge needle or with the spinal needle that will be used for the culdocentesis. Use a cotton ball soaked in 4% cocaine or 20%

benzocaine solution for topical anesthesia of the posterior vaginal wall approximately 15 minutes before infiltration with a local anesthetic. This combination will make the needle puncture nearly painless. Attach the needle to a 20-mL syringe. *A smaller syringe might not be long enough to allow adequate control of the needle*, and the clinician's hand may block the view of the puncture site if a smaller syringe is used.

Aspiration

Following local anesthesia, advance the syringe and the spinal needle parallel to the lower blade of the speculum (Fig. 57-4, *step 2*). Fill the syringe with 2 to 3 mL of saline (nonbacteriostatic) before puncture. After needle puncture, the free flow of fluid from the syringe will expel tissue that may have clogged the needle and will confirm that the tip of the needle is in the proper position and not lodged in the uterine wall or the intestinal wall. Use saline rather than air because if air is used, it may be difficult to interpret the presence of free peritoneal air on subsequent radiographs. To avoid the need to change the syringe during the procedure, use 1% lidocaine for both anesthesia and confirmation of proper needle placement; however, the bacteriostatic property of this agent precludes its use if the procedure is performed to obtain fluid for culture.

Penetrate the vaginal wall in the midline 1 to 1.5 cm posterior (inferior) to the point at which the vaginal wall joins the cervix (Fig. 57–4, *step 2*).[20] Pass the needle a total of 2 to 2.5 cm.[20,21] Apply gentle suction with the syringe while slowly withdrawing the needle. Avoid aspirating any blood that has accumulated in the vagina from previous needle punctures or from cervical bleeding because this may give the false impression of a positive tap. Bleeding from the puncture site in the vaginal wall can be minimized by adding epinephrine to the local anesthetic.

Blood or fluid may be obtained immediately but may also be obtained when the needle is withdrawn from the peritoneal cavity. Therefore, it is important to aspirate continuously while *gradually* withdrawing the needle. If no fluid is aspirated, reintroduce the needle and direct it only slightly to the left or right of the midline. Directing the needle too far laterally may result in puncture of the mesenteric or pelvic vessels. If no fluid is obtained on the first attempt, *repeat the procedure*.

Some physicians prefer the use of a 19-gauge butterfly needle held with ring forceps (Fig. 57-4, *step 3*, and Fig. 57-5).[20] This technique offers a built-in guide to needle depth and allows good control of the needle during puncture. An assistant must aspirate the tubing while the physician controls positioning and withdrawal of the needle.

Fluid that is aspirated may be old nonclotting blood, bright red blood, pus, exudate, or a straw-colored serous liquid. Any fluid that is not blood should be submitted for Gram stain, aerobic and anaerobic culture, and cell count. Blood should be observed for clotting. Blood should also be sent for determination of the hematocrit.

INTERPRETATION OF RESULTS

Interpretation of the results of culdocentesis depends primarily on whether any fluid was obtained. It should be noted that in the absence of a pathologic condition, 2 to 3 mL of clear yellowish peritoneal fluid can be aspirated. When there

CULDOCENTESIS

1

Urethra

Cervix

Tenaculum to
elevate the
cervix

B

x

A

Place the patient in the lithotomy position with the head of the bed slightly elevated so that intraperitoneal fluid gravitates toward the rectouterine pouch. Premedicate with sedatives or intravenous opiates as clinically indicated. Perform a bimanual pelvic examination to exclude the presence of a pelvic mass.

Insert a bivalve pelvic speculum and open it widely by using both the height (*A*) and angle (*B*) thumbscrews. Grasp the posterior lip of the cervix with a tenaculum and elevate the cervix.

Swab the vaginal wall in the area of the rectouterine pouch with antiseptic followed by a small amount of sterile water.

Administer a local anesthetic with a separate 25- or 27-gauge needle or with the needle that will be used for culdocentesis. The site of needle entry is 1 cm posterior to the point at which the vaginal wall joins the cervix (*x*). (*Optional:* before injecting the local anesthetic, place a cocaine [4%]- or benzocaine [20%]-soaked cotton ball on the area to be punctured for 15 minutes.)

2

Bladder

Pubis

Cervix

Blood

Rectum

Fill the syringe with 2 to 3 mL of saline prior to puncture. Advance the spinal needle parallel to the lower blade of the speculum. Gently depress the plunger during advancement of the needle. Free flow of fluid will confirm proper needle placement in the rectouterine pouch. Pass the needle 2 to 2.5 cm. Apply gentle suction while slowly withdrawing the syringe.

3

Alternatively, use a 19-gauge butterfly needle held with ring forceps. This technique offers a built-in guide to needle depth and allows good control of the needle during puncture. Use the help of an assistant to aspirate while you control needle position and withdrawal.

Figure 57-4 Culdocentesis. (*1 and 2, from Vander Salm TJ, Cutler BS, Wheeler HB.* Atlas of Bedside Procedures. *Boston: Little, Brown; 1979; 3, from Webb MJ. Culdocentesis.* JACEP. *1978;7:452.*)

is no return of fluid of any type (a so-called dry tap), the procedure has *no diagnostic value*. Because a dry tap is nondiagnostic, it should not be equated with normal peritoneal fluid. In addition, when less than 2 mL of clotting blood is obtained, this is also considered to be a nondiagnostic tap because the source of this small amount of blood may be the puncture site on the vaginal wall. Such blood will usually clot. More than 2 mL of *nonclotting blood* is certainly suggestive of hemoperitoneum. However, some researchers interpret as little as 0.3 mL of *nonclotting* blood as a positive tap.[7] There is no particular significance of larger amounts of blood because absolute volume may be related to the position of the needle or the rate of bleeding. Brenner and colleagues[6] reported no blood from culdocentesis in 5% of patients with proven ectopic pregnancies even when rupture had occurred. In the series of 61 patients with surgically proven ectopic

pregnancy reported by Cartwright and associates,[7] culdocentesis performed within 4 hours of surgery was positive in 70%, negative in 10%, and inadequate in 20%. "Positive" in their series was defined as obtaining at least 0.3 mL of nonclotting blood with a hematocrit of greater than 3%. "Negative" was defined as obtaining 0.3 mL of fluid with a hematocrit of less than 3%. An "inadequate" tap was one in which no fluid was obtained. In the 252 patients reported by Vermesh and coworkers[16] who had surgically proven ectopic pregnancies and underwent culdocentesis, 83% had a positive tap. They defined a positive tap as nonclotting blood with a hematocrit of greater than 15%.

When culdocentesis is used to diagnose a ruptured ectopic pregnancy, a "negative tap" is one that yields pus or clear, straw-colored peritoneal or cystic fluid. A large amount of clear fluid (>10 mL) indicates a probable ruptured ovarian cyst, aspiration of an intact corpus luteal cyst, ascites, or possibly carcinoma. The significance of this fluid and interpretation of the results are outlined in Table 57-3 and Box 57-1. Elliot and colleagues[22] cautioned that obtaining greater than 10 mL of clear fluid should not automatically rule out an ectopic pregnancy because the latter may coexist with other pathologic conditions.

A "positive tap" is one in which nonclotting blood is obtained, although the presence of nonclotted blood does not confirm a tubal pregnancy. Intraperitoneal blood from any source (ectopic pregnancy, ovarian cyst, ruptured spleen) may remain unclotted after aspiration for days in the syringe as a

Figure 57-5 Variations in culdocentesis technique. **A,** An 18-gauge spinal needle attached to a syringe. The operator applies continuous suction during withdrawal of the needle. **B,** A 19-gauge butterfly needle attached to a syringe and held with ring forceps. An assistant is required to aspirate the syringe while the operator controls the needle with the forceps.

TABLE 57-3   Interpretation of Culdocentesis Fluid

ASPIRATED FLUID	CONDITION AND SUGGESTED DIFFERENTIAL DIAGNOSIS
Clear, serous, straw colored (usually only a few milliliters)	Normal peritoneal fluid
Large amount of clear fluid	Ruptured or large ovarian cyst (fluid may be serosanguineous); pregnancy may be coexistent Ascites Carcinoma
Exudate with polymorphonuclear leukocytes	Pelvic inflammatory disease Gonococcal salpingitis Chronic salpingitis
Purulent fluid	Bacterial infection Tuboovarian abscess with rupture Appendicitis with rupture Diverticulitis with perforation
Bright red blood*	Ruptured viscus or vascular injury Recently bleeding ectopic pregnancy* (ruptured or unruptured) Bleeding corpus luteum Intraabdominal injury Liver Spleen Other organs Ruptured aortic aneurysm
Old, brown, nonclotting blood	Ruptured viscus Ectopic pregnancy with intraperitoneal bleeding over a few days or weeks Old (days) intraabdominal injury (e.g., delayed splenic rupture)

Note: The hematocrit of blood from a ruptured ectopic pregnancy is usually 15% or greater (97.5% of cases), but some authors use greater than 3% as positive.

BOX 57-1   **Interpretation of Culdocentesis**

POSITIVE

>0.5 mL nonclotting, bloody fluid (hematocrit >12%)
Indicates hemoperitoneum
    When β-hCG is also positive, ectopic pregnancy is found in greater than 95%
    Nonspecific—can occur in intrauterine pregnancies and nonpregnant women (e.g., ruptured cyst, retrograde bleeding)
Does not necessarily indicate tubal rupture
    50% to 62% of ectopic pregnancies with peritoneal blood may be unruptured

NEGATIVE

Serous fluid
    Excludes hemoperitoneum and tubal rupture
    Falsely negative in 10% to 15% of ectopic pregnancies (generally unruptured)

NONDIAGNOSTIC

Dry tap or clotting blood
    Excludes neither ectopic pregnancy nor hemoperitoneum
    15% of procedures are nondiagnostic
    16% of ectopic pregnancies have nondiagnostic study results

From Brennan DF. Ectopic pregnancy: II. Diagnostic procedures and imaging. Acad Emerg Med. 1995;2:1090.
β-hCG, β subunit of human chorionic gonadotropin.

result of the defibrination activity of the peritoneum. Return of serosanguineous fluid also suggests a ruptured ovarian cyst. The hematocrit of blood from active intraperitoneal bleeding is greater than 10%. In one series, the hematocrit of blood from a ruptured ectopic pregnancy was 15% or greater in 97% of cases.[6]

It should be emphasized that a positive finding on culdocentesis in the presence of a positive pregnancy test does not always prove an ectopic pregnancy.[16] A ruptured corpus luteum cyst in the presence of an intrauterine pregnancy test is probably the most common cause of a false-positive scenario. Whenever possible, ultrasound can help corroborate the findings on culdocentesis.

COMPLICATIONS

Culdocentesis is one of the safest procedures performed in the emergency setting, and there are probably fewer complications with this technique than with peripheral venous cannulation. Complications have been reported, however, the most serious being rupture of an unsuspected tuboovarian abscess.[20] Other complications include perforation of the bowel, perforation of a pelvic kidney, and bleeding from the puncture site in patients with clotting disorders. Because the most common complications result from puncture of a pelvic mass, careful bimanual examination of the patient should help prevent this problem. Puncture of the bowel and the uterine wall occurs relatively frequently but does not generally result in serious morbidity. Obviously, penetration of a gravid uterus has greater potential for harm. Occasionally, one will aspirate air or fecal matter, thereby confirming inadvertent puncture of the rectum.

References are available at www.expertconsult.com

Examination of the Sexual Assault Victim

Carolyn Joy Sachs and Malinda Wheeler

The majority of sexually assaulted individuals never report the crime to anyone, and only one third of sexual assaults are reported to law enforcement. In many cases, after contact with law enforcement, sexual assault victims are taken to the emergency department (ED) for evaluation, examination, and treatment. Sexual assault victims may also go to the ED without prior contact with law enforcement. In 2009, sexually assaulted patients accounted for approximately one tenth of all assault-related visits to the ED by female patients.[1]

Some sexual assault victims will cooperate with police investigations, but others will not. Federal legislation guarantees all victims the right to a forensic examination and treatment of sexual assault regardless of their cooperation with legal investigation or their desire to initially pursue prosecution.[2] Some states require medical personnel treating sexual assault victims to report the assault to local law enforcement, whereas others forbid such reporting without patient consent. Clinicians must know their own state laws regarding such reports.

DEFINITIONS

Sexual assault refers to any sexual contact between one person and another without appropriate legal consent.[3] Physical force may be used to overcome the victim's lack of consent, but this is not mandatory to prove assault. Coercion into sexual contact by intimidation, threats, or fear also defines sexual assault. State laws differ slightly on the definition of exact acts that constitute sexual contact and on which populations are unable to give legal consent. In general, persons under the influence of drugs or alcohol, minors, and those who are mentally incapacitated are considered unable to give consent for sexual contact.

Clinicians who treat sexual assault victims have a professional, ethical, and moral responsibility to provide the best medical and psychological care possible. At the same time, they must collect and preserve the proper medicolegal evidence that is unique to the evaluation of sexual assault cases.

Many hospitals and jurisdictions affiliate with designated sexual assault examination teams to provide specialized evaluation and treatment of victims. These sexual assault response teams (SARTs) provide clear advantages outlined near the end of the chapter. However, victims may be brought to an ED that does not routinely provide specialized care for sexual assault. This chapter is designed to aid clinicians in such a general care location. Prepared emergency personnel can help attenuate the psychological and physical impact of sexual assault. Through proper care of the victim and careful acquisition of evidence, ED staff can help the victim recover from the assault and aid society in improving the prosecution and conviction of sexual predators.

EVALUATION AND TREATMENT OF PATIENTS SUFFERING FROM SEXUAL ASSAULT

Preparation

Most often local jurisdictions or hospitals provide clinicians with detailed forms and instructions for examination and documentation of sexual assault. This chapter is meant to supplement such instructions and forms. Clinicians should be familiar with local documents before performing a sexual assault examination. Careful step-by-step planning and the use of written protocols ensure the best care for victims and aids in the prosecution and conviction of assailants.

ED personnel must secure patient privacy and designate a separate area for the care of sexually assaulted patients. If medically and logistically possible, interviews should be conducted in a private room separate from the examination room. EDs often have such an area, frequently called the "grieving room" or the "family room." Law enforcement or other governmental agencies may provide examination kits for the collection of forensic evidence from victims (Fig. 58-1). These kits should be available in the ED and the staff should be familiar with them. If such kits are not provided by local sources, hospital staff may need to assemble their own kits from material found in most EDs. Alternatively, private companies assemble and sell such kits (www.lynnpeavey.com or The Lynn Peavey Company, PO Box 14100, Lenexa, KS 66285-4100). Prepared kits save a tremendous amount of nursing and clinician time when a victim comes to the ED. A checklist of local requirements for sexual assault examination should be included in the kits and serves as a reminder for all the medicolegal procedures to be completed.

Although this chapter is devoted primarily to the evaluation of adult female sexual assault victims, guidelines for the evaluation of adult male sexual assault victims, female child victims, male child victims, and accused assailants are provided in separate sections of this chapter. The same examiners designated to perform adult female examinations may easily perform male victim and assailant examinations; however, examination of a child sexual assault victim often requires considerable expertise and training. When possible, medical staff with extra training in the examination of child sexual assault victims should perform these examinations. If this is not possible, the section "Child Sexual Assault Examinations" should provide emergency medical personnel with a framework to perform an initial examination.

Consent

Consent for the evaluation and treatment of a sexual assault victim is mandatory. The victim has undergone an experience in which her right to grant or deny consent was taken from her, and obtaining consent for medical treatment and gathering evidence has important psychological and legal implications. The victim has the right to decline medicolegal examination and even medical treatment. Before beginning evaluation and treatment, obtain witnessed, written, informed consent. If no local forensic examination forms are available, use the standard ED "consent to treat" forms, but ensure that the patient is well informed and gives verbal consent to each step of the examination. Although a few states mandate that medical personnel report sexual assaults to law enforcement, victims may choose to not discuss the event with police. If the

Figure 58-1 Sexual assault evidence collection kit. Law enforcement or other governmental agencies may provide examination kits for collection of forensic evidence from sexual assault victims. Emergency department staff should be familiar with the kits used in their institution.

TABLE 58-1   Maximal Reported Time Intervals for Sperm Recovery

BODY CAVITY	MOTILE SPERM	NONMOTILE SPERM
Vagina	6-28 hr	14 hr-10 days
Cervix	3-7 days	7.5-19 days
Mouth	—	2-31 hr
Rectum	—	4-113 hr
Anus	—	2-44 hr

From Marx J, ed. *Rosen's Emergency Medicine: Concepts and Clinical Practice.* 6th ed. Philadelphia: Elsevier; 2006.

victim cannot give consent for a forensic examination because of a reversible process (e.g., intoxication, an acute psychological reaction), wait several hours for the victim's mental status to improve to a reasonable level before consent is obtained. When victims cannot give consent because of minor status or a developmental disability, the person authorized to give medical consent for the patient may give consent for the examination unless that person is a suspect in the assault. Many states allow an adolescent victim of a certain age (e.g., >12 to 14 years old) to consent to an examination for conditions related to sexually transmitted diseases (STDs), sexual assault, and pregnancy. State laws also differ in examiners' requirements to make an attempt to contact the legal guardian (unless the guardian is a suspected perpetrator). Clearly, emergency personnel must be informed regarding their local laws concerning these requirements. In the rare case that a victim cannot give consent as a result of a potentially irreversible medical condition, such as severe head trauma and coma, seek the advice of institutional legal council before proceeding with a forensic examination. In some cases, the next of kin may provide the needed consent, whereas in other cases, it may be necessary to obtain a court order to proceed.

History

The history of the event should include only the elements necessary to complete the required forms, to perform a focused physical examination, and to collect evidence. Questions beyond this, such as the details leading up to the assault, should be left to police investigators. Avoid the urge to "help" the alleged victim by unduly embellishing or detailing uncorroborated or nonmedical information supplied during the examination. Limiting the history not only shortens the evaluation in the ED but also helps prevent discrepancies between the ED history and the official police investigation report, which could weaken the victim's case in court. Document the pertinent medical history, including the last menstrual period, current contraception, recent anal-genital injuries or surgeries, and preexisting injuries.

The history of the event required by legal forms or protocol usually includes the time, date, and place of the alleged assault and a description of the use of force, threats of force, and the type of assault. Elements of force may include the type of violence used (e.g., grabbing, hitting, kicking, strangling, weapon use), threats of violence, the use of restraints, the number of assailants, the use of alcohol or drugs (forcibly or willingly) by the victim, and any loss of consciousness experienced by the victim. Sexually assaultive acts may include fondling (of breasts, genitalia, or both); vaginal, oral, or anal penetration or attempted penetration (with fingers, penis, or other objects); ejaculation on or in the body; and the use of a condom. Use of physical force or violence is partly a police matter, but from a medical standpoint, it is desirable to correlate positive findings on the physical examination (e.g., abrasions, ecchymoses, and scratches) with a description of any force, restraint, or violence.

Document the postassault activity commonly requested on forms, including douching, bathing, urinating, defecating, gargling, and brushing teeth. These activities can alter the recovery of seminal specimens and other sexual assault evidence. However, hygiene activities should not deter the clinician from the collection of evidence since DNA has been recovered from the victim's skin after multiple showers. In addition, question victims about potential injuries from any body trauma before the assault.

Elements of the victim's history should help in deciding which potential samples to collect. For example, sperm may be recovered from the cervix for up to 12 days after intercourse and from the vagina for up to 5 days (Table 58-1).[4] If the victim had voluntary intercourse 48 hours before the examination and was sexually assaulted 3 hours before the examination, obtain samples from both the vagina and the cervix and keep the two types of specimens separate. Taking a careful history makes it possible to perform an appropriate examination given these two separate events. In general, cervical swabs should be collected in addition to the usual vaginal swabs if the time between assault and examination is longer than 48 hours or if intercourse with a different person took place within a few days of the assault. Some experts advocate cervical samples in all cases that will involve speculum examination because of greater forensic yield.

Obtain a gynecologic history in preparation for documentation of injuries and treatment plans. From a medicolegal standpoint, question victims about any recent gynecologic surgical procedures or unintentional genital trauma that might alter the expected normal genital appearance. The history should also include the use of any method of birth control before the attack (with information regarding any missed birth control pills), last normal menstrual period, last voluntary intercourse, gravidity and parity, and recent STDs. As with all assaulted patients, the medical history should include current medications, tetanus immunization status, and allergies.

While taking the history, observe the patient's ability to understand and respond appropriately to questions. Victims of sexual assault may not possess the capacity to consent to intercourse because of a developmental disability, young age, or intoxication with drugs or alcohol. Consider obtaining blood, urine, or both and testing for drugs or alcohol when the history suggests lapses of (or impaired) consciousness. Victims who lack consenting capacity because of a developmental disability may have sufficient prior documentation of the condition. In the rare instance in which an examiner suspects a previously undocumented developmental disability, formal examination of the patient's mental capacity can be performed at a later time by request of the district attorney.

Physical Examination

Physical examination of a sexual assault victim differs from most other ED examinations in that examiners are not only caring for a patient's physical and mental well-being but also investigating a crime scene and collecting specific evidence. Explain every step of the examination to the victim. Remind the victim to communicate any discomfort or questions during the examination and to ask for a break from the examination if needed. In addition, remind the victim of her right to decline any portion of the examination and the ability to stop at any point. Each victim should have the opportunity to have a family member, friend, victim advocate, or any combination of such individuals in the room during all parts of the examination.

Collection of Clothing

If not already collected by law enforcement, collect the clothes that the victim wore during the assault for potential evidence. The victim should disrobe by dropping her clothes onto a clean sheet or a large clean piece of paper. Using gloved hands, place each item of clothing in a separate paper bag. Label all collected material meticulously and describe it in the chart. Bundle the sheet or paper and any material that might have fallen during the victim's disrobing and place it in a separate paper bag. When a victim's clothing must be collected, be sure to provide suitable clothing for the victim to wear home after release from the ED.

General Body Examination

After the patient disrobes and is placed in a gown, examine her body for signs of trauma and foreign material. Uncover one part of the body at a time to examine and then carefully re-cover it. This allows the victim to retain some modesty

during the examination. Important areas for evaluation are the back, thighs, breasts, wrists, and ankles (particularly if restraints were used). Even in the absence of ecchymosis, note tender areas during the examination. Evidence from the physical surroundings of the assault can occasionally be found in the hair or on the skin. Retain such material as evidence. Document areas of trauma and evaluate further (e.g., with radiographs) as indicated by the type and extent of injury. Approximately 10% to 67% of sexual assault victims display bodily injuries.[3] Document these injuries because they correlate significantly with successful prosecution of perpetrators.[5] Bodily evidence may range from abrasions to major blunt and penetrating trauma. If the victim has not bathed, bodily evidence in the form of dried semen stains may be visible on the hair or the skin of the victim. In a darkened room, dried semen (and, unfortunately, many other substances) on skin may fluoresce under examination with short-wave light, such as that produced by a Wood lamp or an alternative light source, but may also be noticed equally well by its reflective appearance under regular room lighting.[6,7] Use moistened swabs to collect potential dried secretions; then air-dry them thoroughly and preserve as evidence. Fragments of the assailant's skin, blood, facial hair, or other foreign material from the assault site may be trapped beneath a victim's fingernails. Obtain fingernail scrapings by cleaning under a victim's nails with a toothpick or small swab or by cutting the nails closely over a clean piece of paper. Fold the toothpick and debris into the paper, place it in an envelope, and package it with the other specimens.

Imaging

Photographs can be a valuable addition to the documentation of bodily injury. Medical institutions may employ professional-quality photographic teams; others must rely on law enforcement for photo documentation. Most institutions require patient consent for photographs taken by hospital personnel. Optimally, institutions should have a prearranged plan to handle film or digital media according to a written "chain of custody." Alternatively, self-developing film (Polaroid) or instant digital prints that can be permanently labeled (e.g., subject, date, details of the pictured injury) may be used but will provide inferior resolution in most cases. The photographs should be labeled immediately and may be added to the legal evidence. In some jurisdictions, photographs of physical injuries will be taken and retained by an accompanying law officer. These photographs may serve as evidence or may simply refresh the examiner's memory at the time of the trial.

Oral Evaluation

If indicated by the history, inspect the oral cavity closely for signs of trauma and collect evidence if indicated. Mouth injuries from forced oral copulation include lacerations of the labial or lingual frenulum, mucosal lacerations, and abrasions. Injury to the lips is often produced by the victim's own teeth as her lips are forced inward by forced oral penetration with the perpetrator's penis. Potential injuries to the posterior pharyngeal wall and soft palate include petechiae, contusions, and lacerations (Fig. 58-2). Document these injuries at the initial examination because mucosal injuries heal quickly and may not be present hours or days later. Collect potential evidence with swabs rubbed between the teeth and the buccal mucosa on both the upper and lower gingival surfaces bilaterally.

Figure 58-2 Mucosal labial injury after forced oral copulation.

Figure 58-3 The hymen in a prepubertal female as seen with inferior labial traction.

Spermatozoa have been identified in oral smears for hours after the attack despite brushing the teeth, using mouthwash, or drinking various fluids and may provide valuable evidence up to 12 hours after examination.[8,9] Collect any foreign material (e.g., hair) to include as potential evidence. During the oral inspection, local law enforcement may request that examiners collect buccal cell swabs to provide the crime laboratory with a sample for victim DNA reference.

Genital Examination

Once the victim is in the lithotomy position, inspect the thighs and perineum for signs of trauma and for foreign material such as seminal stains. Use an ultraviolet light again to look at suspicious dried secretions. Many jurisdictions recommend routine collection of swabs from the external genital area because of the high likelihood of evidence being present and the inconsistent fluorescence of seminal fluid with a Wood lamp.

Pubic Hair Samples

If local crime laboratories request pubic hair samples, proceed with the following protocol. Before the pelvic examination, comb the victim's pubic hair for foreign material (particularly pubic hair belonging to the assailant). Place clean paper below the victim's buttocks with the victim in the lithotomy position and comb the pubic hair onto the paper. Fold these hairs and the comb into the paper and place them directly in a large paper envelope to be given to law enforcement. Foreign pubic hairs can often provide enough cellular DNA material from the root to enable the crime laboratory to perform DNA analysis. In addition, specialized laboratories possess the capability of performing mitochondrial DNA analysis from the hair shaft in many cases.

Significant hair transfer occurs in less than 5% of assaults.[10] For the small minority of cases in which foreign suspect hairs must be compared with the victim's hair, a sample pulled from the victim may be desired. Although pulling the patient's hair from the roots may provide the best sample, this collection method is painful, considered insensitive, and not recommended by these authors during the initial evaluation. These hairs will rarely be needed because the vast majority of cases are never adjudicated and those that are rarely concern this type of evidence. A victim can provide the hairs at a later time, if needed, and frequently the victim is willing to pluck the hairs herself at that time.

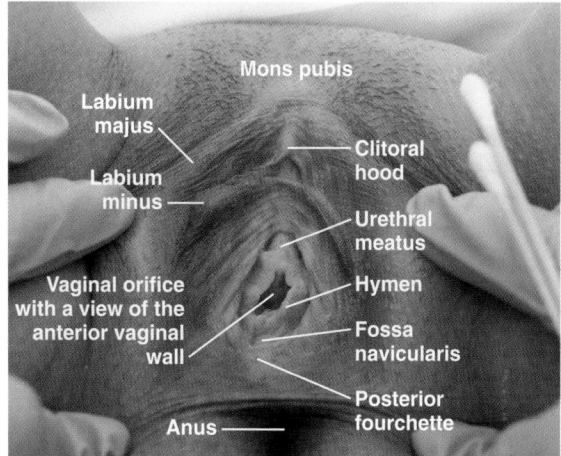

Figure 58-4 Female anatomy.

Genital examination of a sexual assault victim differs considerably from most ED pelvic examinations. First, perform a careful evaluation of the vulva and vaginal introitus for signs of trauma. The techniques of separation and traction move the tissues most likely to suffer injury into view. In performing separation, examiners use both hands to separate the labia laterally in each direction and inspect the posterior fourchette and vaginal introitus. Similarly, in performing traction, examiners use both hands to hold each labium majus and apply gentle inferior labial traction (i.e., toward the examiner); this gives a much-improved view of the hymen, especially in prepubertal females (Fig. 58-3). If the examiner fails to perform these maneuvers, traumatic genital injuries may be missed.

Familiarity with female (Fig. 58-4) and male (Fig. 58-5) genital anatomy, including all terms, is important for accurate descriptions. Although most novice examiners concern themselves with detecting injuries to the hymen, the majority of *sexual assault–related vaginal injuries occur to the posterior fourchette* (Fig. 58-6).[11] In fact, hymenal injuries are rare in sexually active adult women and are more commonly observed in sexually inexperienced adolescents[12,13] (Fig. 58-7). More uncommon injuries to the vaginal walls and cervix may be discovered during the speculum examination. Reported rates of genital injury in forensically examined victims range from 6% to 20% without colposcopy to 53% to 87% with colposcopy.[11-13] Most importantly, examiners must be

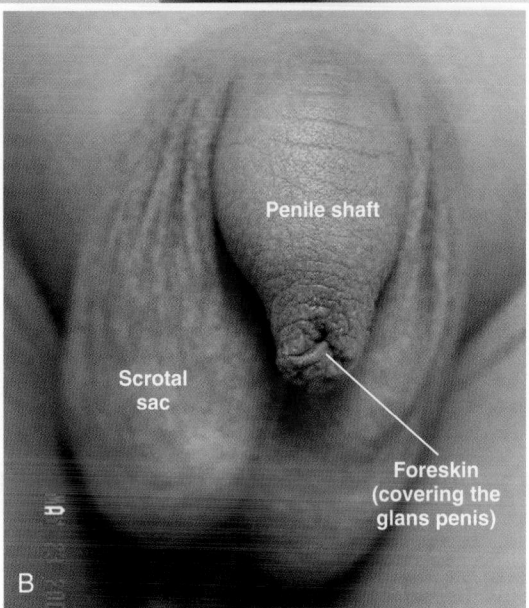

Figure 58-5 Male anatomy. **A,** Circumcised. **B,** Uncircumcised.

Figure 58-6 The posterior fourchette is the most common site of injury in adult victims of sexual assault. **A,** Before application of toluidine blue. **B,** After application of toluidine blue.

Figure 58-7 Hymenal injury at the 6-o'clock position, usually found in adolescent girls. Such injuries are uncommon in adults.

cognizant of the fact that completely normal findings on genital examination remain consistent with forced sexual assault. In fact, a study of more than 1000 sexual assault victims found that almost half of all victims with forensic evidence positive for sperm had no genital injury.[14]

Colposcopy

Teixeira first described the use of colposcopy for documentation of sexual assault in 1981.[15] Although it is not readily available nor a standard of care in most EDs, the use of colposcopy has revolutionized the documentation of injury. The colposcope provides magnification, a bright light source, and usually permanent documentation of injuries in the form of still images or video (mainly in digital format but occasionally traditional film). In one small study the colposcope increased the rate of detection of genital injury from 6% to 53%.[16] Colposcopes with photo or video attachments provide excellent photographic documentation for the court and allow review by expert practitioners for court testimony without subjecting the victim to reexamination (Fig. 58-8).

Experienced sexual assault examiner programs are increasingly using high-quality digital single-lens reflex cameras mounted on a tripod to obtain excellent images that are indistinguishable from those obtained with colposcopy. ED practitioners may have access to such equipment. Colposcopically visible injuries have also been described in adolescent women after the first consensual intercourse; hence, genital injury does not always correlate with nonconsensual vaginal penetration.[17] Conversely, totally normal findings on genital examination by colposcopy are often found after sexual assault.

Figure 58-8 Colposcope (**A**) and method of examination (**B**). This technique is not a standard intervention by an emergency physician.

Even in sexually inexperienced adolescents, forced penetration can occur without leaving discernible genital injury.[17] Although previous sexual experience by the victim decreases the likelihood of finding genital injury, experts cannot fully explain the reasons why some rape victims sustain measurable genital injury whereas others do not.

Forensic Evidence Collection

Protocols for collection of evidence vary by legal jurisdiction. Many sexual assault evaluation centers have abandoned the cumbersome kits used in the past and substituted simple collection methods that concentrate on important and usable legal evidence. The following discussion draws from the model protocol suggested by the state of California and the American College of Emergency Physicians manual.[3]

Obtain standard specimens during inspection of the external genitalia, rectum, vagina, and cervix. Lubricate the speculum with warm water rather than other lubricants because of the potential spermicidal activity of lubricants. However, if lubricants are inadvertently used, the potential for corruption of DNA evidence should be negligible.[18] Generally, the specimens collected will be determined by victim's history and local protocol, but they may include any of the items listed in Box 58-1 and shown in Figure 58-9. Some protocols recommend that examiners make a wet mount of one swab from the vaginal pool and look at it under the microscope for the presence of motile sperm. Because of rapid cell death, studies have shown a negligible chance of finding motile sperm from a vaginal wet mount more than 8 hours after intercourse.[19] Furthermore, in complying with the Clinical Laboratory Improvement Amendments of 1988, ED practitioners in the United States rarely have sufficient access or experience with microscopy to make this step a routine recommendation. Several swabs from the vaginal pool (including the one used to make the wet mount, if done) and the external genitalia should be obtained and then applied over clean slides for a

BOX 58-1 Potential Evidence Collected

Clothing (list and describe all clothing collected on the chart and checklist form)
Debris
Dried secretions, swabs, and slides
External genital swabs and slides
Pubic hair combings
Oral mucosal swabs and slides
Anal swabs and slides
Vaginal pool swabs and slides
Vaginal lavage fluid in a test tube or urine container
Cervical swabs and slides
Tampon or condom present in the vagina (dried or frozen)
Urine or blood toxicology sample (timed collection)
Reference blood, buccal mucosa, and/or hair sample
Collect all evidence with gloved hands to avoid DNA contamination
Change gloves when necessary to avoid interlocation contamination

dry mount. These slides should be allowed to air-dry and then labeled; all swabs and slides should be packaged in paper envelopes for the local crime laboratory. Some EDs maintain specific equipment (i.e., a Dry Box) to aid in the drying of specimens; in others, the swabs and slides must be left out until completely dried.

Crime laboratories may also request collection of a vaginal washing. For this procedure, insert 5 mL of sterile (but not bacteriostatic) water or saline into the vagina and then remove it. Place the washing in a sealed container (such as those used for urine collection or a red-topped blood tube). In addition, collect cervical swabs if the time from assault to examination (the postcoital interval) is longer than 48 hours or if there is a history of recent consensual intercourse as well. The crime laboratory may recover sperm from cervical specimens up to 12 days after coitus.[3]

Figure 58-9 Sample contents of a sexual assault evidence kit. Note that an instruction booklet is provided, along with labels, swabs, glass slides, blood tubes, collection envelopes, and other necessary equipment.

Each sample should be labeled separately and the area from which the specimen was collected should be recorded in the chart.

Genital Testing for STDs

Guidelines from the Centers for Disease Control and Prevention (CDC) suggest obtaining a cervical, rectal, or oral specimen for culture or polymerase chain reaction (PCR), or both, for *Chlamydia trachomatis* and *Neisseria gonorrhoeae*. However, the majority of SART programs in the United States do not routinely perform these tests.[20] STD testing during sexual assault examination can detect only infection before the assault and provides no meaningful information for the crime laboratory. In addition, routine prophylactic treatment with antibiotics effective against *N. gonorrhoeae* and *C. trachomatis* makes detection of these preexisting infections superfluous; however, clinicians might want to consider obtaining samples for culture from child victims, in whom the presence of an STD would be indicative of previous sexual contact.

Perineal Toluidine Blue Dye Staining

Toluidine blue dye is a nuclear stain, also used for cancer detection and mast cell staining, that highlights areas of injury. It adheres to areas denuded by abrasions and lacerations where the epidermal layer of nonnucleated cells has been removed (Fig. 58-10). The underlying nucleated cells take up the dye. Although it is not a uniform standard of care and unavailable in many EDs, the dye can enhance the examiner's ability to visualize and photographically document more subtle genital injuries (see Fig. 58-6). Genital lacerations may provide corroborating evidence of nonconsensual intercourse, or at least sexual activity. To outline injuries, apply a 1% aqueous solution of toluidine blue dye to the perineum and wipe the excess dye off with a cotton ball moistened with lubricating jelly. A swab containing the dye is commercially available. After the excess dye is removed, any areas that retain the stain signify a disruption in the epidermis, most likely injury. Separate any folds of the area and carefully examine them to avoid missing injuries. Ideally, apply the dye before speculum examination to eliminate the possibility of iatrogenic injury. The procedure is described in Figure 58-10 and Box 58-2. In one study, use of toluidine blue dye increased the injury detection rate from 16% to 40% in women without the use of colposcopy[21]; however, injuries detected with the aid of toluidine blue dye are not 100% specific for sexual assault because such injuries have also been found after consensual intercourse, especially in adolescents.[22]

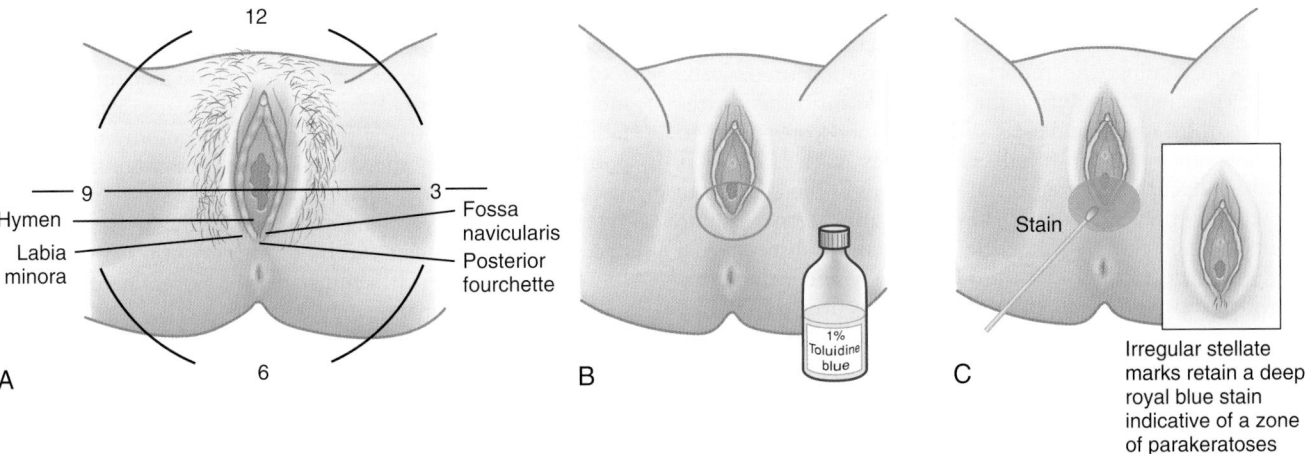

Figure 58-10 A, During a sexual assault, injuries are often multiple and typically occur between the 3-, 6-, and 9-o'clock positions. **B** and **C,** Traumatic skin injuries can be highlighted by applying toluidine blue to the perineum and vaginal area and then wiping it off to show the lesions. (**A,** From Marx J. Rosen's Emergency Medicine: Concepts and Clinical Practice. 6th ed. Philadelphia: Elsevier; 2006.)

BOX 58-2 Toluidine Blue* Staining of the Perineum to Detect Microabrasion†

1. Collect all external genital specimens as indicated by examination before application of the dye.‡
2. Before speculum examination or anoscopy, apply 1% toluidine blue to the entire vulva (labia majora, labia minora, posterior fourchette, perineal body, and perianal area). The anus may also be stained. Do not use dye in the vaginal vault or mucous membranes.
3. Allow it to dry for approximately 1 minute.
4. Remove excess dye with water-soluble lubricant by gently blotting the area until the excess dye is removed.
5. DO NOT rub the area.
6. Photograph the area if indicated.
7. The dye will fade in 1 to 2 days.

*A prefilled swab (T-Blue Swab/TBS, Tri-Tech, Inc.) is available through the National Forensic Nursing Institute).
†See Figure 58-10.
‡This does not interfere with DNA or semen testing. Modified from The National Forensic Nursing Institute (NFNI.org/t-blueswab.html). This testing is not usually performed in the emergency department without a special assault team.

Collect external genital samples before the application of toluidine blue to avoid washing away potential DNA evidence. The use of toluidine blue dye itself does not interfere with DNA evidence from vaginal specimens, and it has proved safe for mucosal application.[23-25]

Anal Evaluation

The anal examination follows the genital examination in most cases (Fig. 58-11). Documentation of anal penetration holds significant value because it is a separate crime in addition to vaginal penetration and may increase criminal penalties against convicted sexual predators. Separate the anal folds to look for lacerations and abrasions, and if desired, apply toluidine blue as outlined in the genital section. Collect two external anal swabs before applying the dye. Clean the dye off thoroughly. If anoscopy is not planned, collect the internal

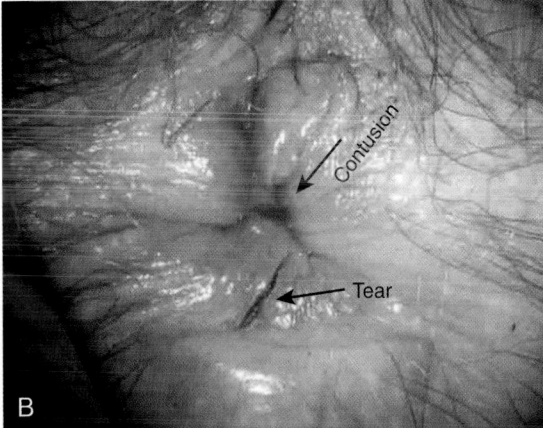

Figure 58-11 Anal injury is best seen with separation of the perianal tissues. **A,** Anal tear in a 13-year-old boy after forced penile-anal penetration. **B,** Anal contusion and tear (*arrows*) in an adult man after forced penile-anal penetration.

rectal sample as follows: separate the anal folds as much as possible and insert swabs approximately 2 cm into the anus. Gently move them in a circular motion and then remove them. Use the swabs to make slides, air-dry them, and include them in the evidence sent to the crime laboratory. Use toluidine blue dye, as described earlier, to better visualize injuries. Anoscopy is indicated to document potential rectal injuries in victims who report anal penetration or describe loss of consciousness during the assault. Perform this procedure in the same manner as diagnostic anoscopy done to evaluate other anal or rectal emergencies in the ED. It is best to collect the internal rectal specimens at the end of the anoscope to prevent contamination from any external sample being dragged internally. In one retrospective observational study of male victims, the use of anoscopy and colposcopy provided superior documentation of injuries over colposcopy alone.[26] The location of anoscopically detected injuries may be recorded geographically on an imaginary clock face as with vaginal injuries.

Reference Samples

Crime laboratories may request reference samples from various locations on the victim's body to use in comparison testing with potential evidence from the perpetrator. These reference samples include blind swabs on the victim's skin in a location complementary to suspicious skin samples. For example, if a suspicious discharge is swabbed from the victim's right shoulder, take a control swab from the victim's left shoulder as well. Crime laboratories may also request other control samples for reference to the victim's DNA, such as blood, buccal mucosa cells, head hairs, or pubic hairs. The need for such samples will be determined by local protocol.

Blood Tests

Some crime laboratories request blood samples for DNA reference, toxicology analysis, or both. Include these samples with the material sent to law enforcement. When collecting blood for toxicology testing, record the exact date and time of collection on the specimen so that the criminologist may estimate the dose and timing of substances used by perpetrators to facilitate the assault.

Urine Tests

Perform bedside urine β-human chorionic gonadotropin (β-hCG) testing in all women victims of childbearing age to exclude preexisting pregnancy before instituting pregnancy and STD prophylaxis. Collect the victim's first available voided urine as requested by local crime laboratories to optimize recovery of potential toxicology evidence.

Spermatozoa, Semen, and DNA Testing

Motile and immotile sperm may be found microscopically in wet mounts of vaginal aspirates and in vaginal, oral, and rectal swabs. If formally trained, evaluate the slide microscopically immediately after the physical examination. Examiners find sperm in 13% to 26% of vaginal wet mount specimens.[13,27] Early discovery of sperm may be helpful to law enforcement investigations. However, most ED examiners lack formal training in this process and crime laboratories possess much higher sensitivity for detection of sperm, thus making a negative initial wet mount unhelpful. For these reasons, many examiners do not routinely perform the wet mount examination.[13] After consensual intercourse with a normal ejaculate, laboratory testing of vaginal secretions detects sperm in 50%

of specimens 4 days after coitus.[27] However, despite penile penetration during sexual assault, crime laboratories may fail to detect sperm. Reasons for failure include inadequate specimen collection, degradation of the ejaculate, azoospermia, failure of the perpetrator to ejaculate, vasectomy in the perpetrator, washing by the victim, or use of a condom.

A crime laboratory analyst initially looks for semen in a given sample by searching microscopically for sperm on a concentrated specimen and by testing for other components found in semen. Such seminal plasma components include p30 and acid phosphatase. p30 is a glycoprotein specific to the prostate and is regarded as conclusive evidence of semen (i.e., ejaculation within 48 hours), whereas acid phosphatase is presumptive evidence only because it can occur in other body fluids, such as vaginal secretions.[28] Although this was a main component of crime laboratory investigation in the past, many laboratories have abandoned the acid phosphatase test in favor of the more specific p30 test.[28,29] Despite negative testing for seminal plasma components, laboratories may be able to detect valuable DNA evidence from persistent sperm cells or the perpetrator's epithelial cells.[30,31] As DNA testing technology rapidly changes, the ability of crime laboratories to perform a specific forensic test varies by location and over time. Most crime laboratories look for unique short tandem repeats in perpetrator DNA with PCR amplification testing, which requires minimal material.

Chain of Custody

Give samples and other evidence to the police, a crime laboratory, or a forensic pathologist. Label each sample with the patient's name, hospital number, date, time of collection, area from which the specimen was collected, and collector's name. Package these specimens according to local crime laboratory specifications and transfer them to the next appropriate official (police officer, pathologist, or other individual) along with a written chain of custody, including a list of the specimens, the signature of each person who collected them, and the signature of each person who received them. If this chain is broken, important evidence might be deemed inadmissible in court.

TREATMENT
STD Prophylaxis

The approach to prophylaxis for potential diseases transmitted by sexual assault vary by region, disease prevalence, and local practice and is often influenced by the emotional state of the victim and personal and religious viewpoints. We present an overview that may serve as a general guideline, with the understanding that many issues are vague, unsettled, and not totally adopted by all clinicians (Box 58-3).

It is advisable to address the issues of STD, pregnancy, psychological distress, and follow-up in the treatment of a sexual assault victim. Because infection rates before the assault are not known, the risk of contracting an STD as a consequence of a sexual assault has been difficult to determine, and estimates vary widely (Table 58-2).[32] Jenny and colleagues found the postassault incidence of STDs to be 2% for *Chlamydia* and 4% for gonorrhea.[33] The reported rates of 12% for *Trichomonas* and 19% for bacterial vaginosis seem high and may reflect a preexposure infection because male transmission of these infections, especially bacterial vaginosis, is uncommon. We lack specific data on risk for the development of herpes, hepatitis B, or human immunodeficiency virus (HIV) infection from sexual assault. However, HIV transmission has been noted.[34]

Because victims tend to have relatively low compliance with keeping follow-up visits, most examiners offer, at the

---

BOX 58-3 Recommended Empirical ED Testing and Pharmacologic Treatment after Sexual Assault

- NO routine STD cultures of the victim unless symptomatic for an STD or the victim is a child (a positive test in a child is indicative of abuse).
- Treat empirically for GC,* Chlamydia, Trichomonas (optional), and bacterial vaginosis (optional) (see Box 58-4).
- Administer a tetanus booster vaccine if indicated.
- If not immunized for hepatitis B or unsure of the victim's vaccination status, give first dose of vaccine empirically and follow with subsequent vaccination at 1 to 2 and 4 to 6 months. If previously vaccinated, offer hepatitis surface antibody testing with follow-up vaccination if the test result is negative. In addition to vaccination, consider HBIG in nonimmune patients after high-risk exposure to a known hepatitis B–positive perpetrator, followed by a full vaccination schedule.
- If the suspect is known or suspected to be HIV positive, treat with medications recommended by local ID experts or provided in occupational exposure kits or consider either of the following: Combivir (2 times a day) or Truvada (once a day) for 28 days.
- If the suspect is not known to be HIV positive, there is no consensus on recommendations for treatment, and clinicians must consider each patient individually.[†] This is an area of uncertainty. HIV prophylaxis may be given after a discussion of the risks and benefits with the patient.
- Obtain a pregnancy test and administer pregnancy prevention if not already pregnant and physically able to conceive (see Table 58-3).

GC, gonococci; HBIG, hepatitis B immune globulin; HIV, human immunodeficiency virus; ID, infectious disease; STD, sexually transmitted disease.
Note: Treatment regimens are subject to change based on sensitivities and local patterns.
*Treatment of GC will treat incubating syphilis. Prophylaxis for herpes is not recommended.
†There are no published data on the effectiveness of HIV postexposure prophylaxis after sexual assault.

TABLE 58-2 Risk for STDs after Sexual Assault

DISEASE	RISK (%)
Gonorrhea	6-18
Chlamydia	4-17
Syphilis	0.5-3
Human immunodeficiency virus	<1

From Marx J, ed. Rosen's Emergency Medicine: Concepts and Clinical Practice. 6th ed. Philadelphia: Elsevier; 2006.
STDs, sexually transmitted diseases.

---

least, treatment of gonorrhea and Chlamydia at the time of the initial examination.[21] Though most often termed *prophylaxis*, technically this antibiotic administration is considered "treatment" given so early that the disease is subclinical. The need for routine administration of medication to combat *Trichomonas* is unclear, and many clinicians do not recommend it as a routine intervention. Prophylaxis for bacterial vaginosis is rarely suggested.

With the increasing prevalence of antibiotic-resistant *N. gonorrhoeae*, ceftriaxone and cefixime have become the CDC's recommended antibiotics of choice in targeting gonorrhea after sexual assault. Ceftriaxone also treats incubating syphilis. (The World Health Organization [WHO] also considers a 2-g dose of azithromycin to be effective against incubating syphilis.) No single-dose regimen for gonorrhea is effective against coexisting *C. trachomatis* infection. Therefore, give patients either a single dose of azithromycin (1 g orally) or a 7-day course of doxycycline (100 mg orally twice a day) or tetracycline (500 mg orally four times a day). A negative pregnancy test is a prerequisite for using either of the latter two antibiotics. Erythromycin may be used as a second alternative for *Chlamydia* prophylaxis in a pregnant patient. Some examiners administer prophylaxis for *Trichomonas* with a single 2-g oral dose of metronidazole; although effective and recommended by the CDC,[35] this dose of metronidazole may cause significant nausea, vomiting, and diarrhea, which can interfere with the efficacy of pregnancy prophylaxis. Box 58-4 provides several options for STD prophylaxis.

Prevention of Hepatitis B

Most sexual assaults involve perpetrators whose hepatitis B status is unknown. In these cases, the CDC recommends hepatitis B vaccination at the time of examination, followed by two more vaccines at the age-appropriate vaccine dose and schedule for previously unvaccinated victims.[35] Give the vaccine to victims as soon as possible after the assault. The CDC recommends that it be given within 24 hours, but this

---

BOX 58-4 CDC Recommended Regimens for Prevention of STDs after Sexual Assault*

Ceftriaxone, 250 mg intramuscularly in a single dose (for prevention of *Neisseria gonorrhoeae* infection)
or
Cefixime, 400 mg orally in a single dose[†]
plus
Metronidazole, 2 g orally in a single dose (optional for prevention of *Trichomonas* infection and bacterial vaginosis)
plus
Azithromycin, 1 g orally in a single dose (for prevention of *Chlamydia* infection)
or
Doxycycline, 100 mg orally twice a day for 7 days

STDs, sexually transmitted diseases.
*Because of widespread resistance, fluoroquinolones are no longer recommended. Prophylaxis for hepatitis B (vaccination without hepatitis B immune globulin) is also suggested.
†Current recommendation for the treatment of uncomplicated infection that may intuitively substitute for prophylaxis.

may not be possible in all cases. When a perpetrator is known to be hepatitis B antigen positive and the victim is known to be hepatitis B antigen negative and has not been adequately vaccinated, the CDC recommends the administration of hepatitis B immune globulin (HBIG) in addition to vaccination. HBIG is not recommended if the patient is first seen by medical providers 14 days or more after the sexual exposure. Hepatitis B vaccine should be administered simultaneously with HBIG in a separate injection site, and the vaccine series should be completed at subsequent visits. Complete CDC recommendations for treatment of hepatitis B and other sexually transmitted infections in sexual assault victims can be found at http://www.cdc.gov/std/treatment/2010/sexual-assault.htm.

Prevention of HIV Infection

In a non–assault-related scenario, the risk for transmission of HIV from one episode of unprotected consensual receptive vaginal intercourse with an infected individual is approximately 1 in 1000. The incidence with unprotected receptive anal intercourse is significantly higher at 8 to 32 per 1000.[36] However, sexual assault victims often sustain tissue injury because of the violent nature of the act, which may increase the rate of transmission of the virus. Although postexposure prophylaxis (PEP) for parenteral occupational exposure to infected body fluids (i.e., needlestick) is believed to be effective based on case-control studies, there is no proof that PEP for human sexual exposure prevents transmission of the virus.[37] Furthermore, victims of sexual assault frequently arrive for treatment much later than those who have occupational exposures.

However, 40% of sexual assault victims fear contracting HIV after assault and should, at a minimum, receive counseling and, some argue, the option of taking anti-HIV medications because they may be effective.[38,39] Unfortunately, immediate testing of the perpetrator remains a remote option. The majority of cases lack a perpetrator in custody for testing, and few state laws provide for legal preconviction HIV testing of alleged perpetrators.[40] In 2005 the U.S. Department of Health and Human Services Working Group on Nonoccupational Postexposure Prophylaxis recommended administering PEP to sexual assault victims only in cases in which the perpetrator is known to be HIV positive.[41] This recommendation specifies a 28-day medication course for sexual assault victims who arrive for care less than 72 hours after the event with an HIV-positive perpetrator when that exposure represents a substantial risk for transmission (i.e., mucosal contact with genital secretions). As with occupational exposure, antiretroviral medications should be initiated as soon as possible after exposure. For sexual assault exposure with a perpetrator of unknown HIV status, the working group declined to offer a recommendation concerning antiretroviral administration; this must be addressed by practitioners on an individual case-by-case basis.[42] Given the extreme negative outcome, the relative safety of treatment, and the lack of conclusive scientific evidence, at least two states have written policies to guide examiners in this complex issue. One such policy is shown in Table 58-3.

Pregnancy Prophylaxis

Pregnancy occurs in up to 4.7% of sexual assault victims.[43] An estimated 22,000 annual rape-related pregnancies could be avoided if all victims received pregnancy prophylaxis within 72 hours.[44] Perform a urine pregnancy test before administering postcoital contraception (PCC). Modern urine pregnancy tests possess a detection threshold approaching 20 to 25 mIU/mL and will usually be positive 1 to 2 weeks after conception, often before a menstrual period is missed.

Offer pregnancy prevention with available oral PCC to all sexual assault victims. Several methods can be used to prevent pregnancy after assault (Table 58-4). The drug of choice for PCC is levonorgestrel, which is available in the United States in a commercial kit called "Plan B," "Plan B One-Step," or "Next Choice." The U.S. Food and Drug Administration (FDA) approved the sale of Plan B without a prescription for individuals 17 years or older. Although the original Plan B kit included two pills containing 0.75 mg of levonorgestrel, each approved for administration 12 hours apart, a large WHO trial demonstrated that both pills may be taken at once with the same efficacy as the divided dose and the potential for increased compliance.[45] The newer Plan B One-Step is a single 1.5-mg pill to be taken as outlined in the WHO study. In the rare instance in which levonorgestrel is unavailable, there are several combined oral contraceptive pills, known as the *Yuzpe regimen*, that may be used for PCC (see Table 58-4).[45] The Yuzpe method is somewhat less effective but prevents approximately 75% of pregnancies that would otherwise have occurred.[45] Plan B prevents 89% of pregnancies that would otherwise have occurred and causes fewer side effects. Potential adverse side effects of both methods include nausea, vomiting, and breast tenderness. If the patient vomits within 1 hour of taking a dose, repeat the dose. Some practitioners routinely offer prophylactic antiemetic therapy; others reserve such treatment for patients who vomit. In 2010 the FDA approved a third option for pharmacologic emergency contraception, ulipristal acetate (brand name ella). This selective progesterone receptor modulator has been demonstrated to be as effective as levonorgestrel for prevention of pregnancy 72 hours after intercourse and more effective for longer postcoital use. Ulipristal requires a prescription and is approved for use up to 120 hours after intercourse.[46]

All available evidence demonstrates no untoward effects on the fetus should pregnancy occur despite PCC.[47] The common practice of obtaining written patient consent for these medications seems unwarranted.

Unfortunately, religious preferences may deter some hospital EDs from providing PCC.[48] In these instances, the website and number listed at the end of this paragraph provide practitioners information to give referral for easy access to PCC for patients who cannot obtain Plan B (i.e., those younger than 17 or lacking funds to pay for the medication). In addition, given the ever-increasing availability of new methods and drugs for PCC, examiners may want to obtain up-to-date information from this site (www.not-2-late.com; telephone: 1-800-not-2-late).

Psychological Support

Sexual assault precipitates a psychological crisis for the patient, and psychological care should begin when the patient first arrives in the ED.[49,50] Reassure the victim that she will be in control of the examination, that she may ask questions at any point, and that she should notify the examiner if anything hurts or if she needs a break. Giving the victim control over her body and the examination is the first step toward

TABLE 58-3 Empirical Guide to Offering Postexposure Prophylaxis for HIV

Has less than 72 hours passed since the assault occurred?
If less than 72 hours has passed, continue risk analysis.
If more than 72 hours after the assault, PEP is not recommend; refer for follow-up HIV antibody testing.

Is the victim 12 years or older?
If yes, continue risk analysis.
If no, consult a pediatric HIV specialist.

What is the risk for transmission of HIV from the assault?
Was the assault one with a measurable risk for transmission of HIV, such as an assault with anal penetration, vaginal penetration, or injection?
Was the assault one with a possible risk for HIV transmission, such as oral penetration with ejaculation, an assault involving other mucous membranes (e.g., eyes), an unknown assault, an assault in which the victim bit the assailant or the assailant (with a bloody mouth) bit the victim?
Was the assault one with no risk for HIV transmission, such as kissing, object or digital penetration, ejaculation on intact skin, or an assault in which a condom was used?
What other risk factors were present in the assault, including the presence of blood, survivor or perpetrator with an STD, significant trauma to the survivor; ejaculation by the assailant, or multiple penetrations of the survivor?

Is the assailant's HIV status known?
If known to be HIV negative, do not offer PEP.
If known to be HIV positive:
 Recommend PEP if an assault with a measurable risk for transmission of HIV has occurred.
 Recommend PEP if an assault with a possible risk for transmission of HIV has occurred and at least one additional risk cofactor was present in the assault.
 Offer PEP if an assault with a possible risk for transmission of HIV has occurred and no additional risk cofactors are present.
 Do not offer PEP for exposures carrying no risk.

Does the assailant engage in behavior that put him or her at risk for contracting HIV?
High-risk groups include men who have sex with men, past or present injection drug users, commercial sex workers, individuals with multiple sex partners, individuals with previous convictions for sexual assault, and individuals with a history of prison incarceration.
If known or suspected risk factors exist:
 Recommend PEP if an assault with a measurable risk for transmission of HIV has occurred.
 Recommend PEP if an assault with a possible risk for transmission of HIV has occurred and more than one additional risk cofactor was present in the assault.
 Recommend or offer PEP if an assault with a possible risk for transmission of HIV has occurred and only one additional risk cofactor was present in the assault.
 Offer PEP if assault with possible risk for transmission of HIV has occurred with no additional risk cofactors present.
 Do not offer PEP for exposures carrying no risk.
If the assailant is not known or if assailant's risk factors are unknown:
 Offer PEP if an assault with a measurable risk for transmission of HIV has occurred.
 Offer PEP if an assault with a possible risk for transmission of HIV has occurred and more than one additional risk cofactor was present in the assault.
 Offer PEP if an assault with a possible risk for transmission of HIV has occurred and only one additional risk cofactor was present in the assault.
 Offer or do not offer PEP if an assault with a possible risk for transmission of HIV has occurred with no additional risk cofactors present.
 Do not offer PEP for exposures carrying no risk.

Offering PEP after sexual assault

| | SOURCE | | |
EXPOSURE RISK	Known HIV*	Known or Suspected Risk Factors	Unknown Risk Factors or Unknown Assailant
Measurable risk[†]	R	R	O
Possible risk plus more than 1 cofactor*	R	R	O
Possible risk plus 1 cofactor*	R	R/O	O
Possible risk plus 0 cofactors	O	O	O/N
No risk[‡]	N	N	N

HIV, human immunodeficiency virus; N, do not offer; O, offer; PEP, postexposure prophylaxis; R, recommend; STD, sexually transmitted disease.
*Acts with a possible risk for transmission of HIV, including oral penetration with ejaculation, unknown act, contact with other mucous membranes, victim biting the assailant, and an assailant with a bloody mouth biting the victim.
[†]Acts with a measurable risk for transmission of HIV, including anal penetration, vaginal penetration, and injection with a contaminated needle.
[‡]Acts with no risk for HIV transmission, including kissing; penetration of the vagina, mouth, or anus with digits or objects; and ejaculation on intact skin.

TABLE 58-4 Emergency Contraception*

BRAND	MANUFACTURER	PILLS†
Progestin-Only Emergency Contraception Oral Therapy: Recommended		
Plan B One-Step	WCC	1 pill (levonorgestrel, 1.5 mg) immediately
or		
Progesterone Receptor Agonist/Antagonist		
Ulipristal (ella)	Watson	One 30-mg pill immediately

Note: For the most up-to-date and alternative recommendations and general information, call 1-800-not-2-late or view www.not-2-late.com.

* Some regimens cause nausea and an antiemetic may be used. If vomiting occurs, repeat the dose of antiemetic.

†Alternatively, the older Yuzpe method may be used. Examples include Lo/Ovral or Ogestrel oral contraceptive, two pills immediately and two pills in 12 hours.

psychological support. Unfortunately, if this is not made a priority, full recovery may be impaired. Posttraumatic stress disorder (PTSD), manifested as numbed responsiveness to the external world, disturbances in sleep, feelings of guilt, memory impairment, avoidance of activities, and other symptoms, often develops in sexual assault victims.[51] *Rape trauma syndrome* is the specific label for PTSD in this population.[52] Rape trauma syndrome stems from the following characteristics of sexual assault: (1) it is sudden and the victim is unable to develop adequate defenses, (2) it involves intentional cruelty or inhumanity, (3) it makes the victim feel trapped and unable to fight back, and (4) it often involves physical injury. Attention to the initial psychological care of a rape victim in the ED is fundamental and can reduce distress during forensic examination.[53]

Many areas have a local sexual assault crisis agency that can dispatch an advocate to be with victims during the interview and examination. This same agency may then provide the follow-up psychological support that must be offered to all victims. It is critical that all examiners maintain current contact information with these agencies and use their services. The importance of this contact is emphasized in some areas by the fact that state law dictates that medical personnel contact a local sexual assault crisis agency when a victim arrives for examination (California penal code 264.2, Notification of a Counseling Center). In the absence of immediate local crisis services, a hospital social worker may fill this role.

Postexamination Follow-Up

Medical and psychological follow-up of sexual assault victims is essential. Unfortunately, less than one third of victims complete follow-up medical care.[54] Many protocols recommend a 2-week follow-up to reexamine any injuries and to repeat testing for STDs and pregnancy. The timing of this follow-up seems to be less important given the widespread use of prophylactic medication to prevent STDs and pregnancy. However, because of the measurable failure rate of PCC, repeated pregnancy testing is critical for a victim who does not experience an expected menses. Further follow-up evaluations may be performed at 4 or 6 weeks and 4 to 6 months to repeat serologic tests for HIV, hepatitis B, hepatitis C, and

syphilis. In addition, local volunteer support groups can be of immense assistance to a sexual assault victim; contact with such a group should be offered to each victim.

SPECIFIC POPULATIONS
Male Evidentiary Examinations

Male evidentiary examinations include all of the same forensic evidence collection as for female victims except vaginal and cervical specimens. As with all victims, the forensic examination is guided by the history of events related by the victim. Most male victims suffer from anal penetration, or sodomy, by a perpetrator. In addition to rape trauma syndrome, heterosexual male victims may suffer psychological trauma and wonder whether the assault dictates a change in their sexual orientation. Examiners should inform such victims that forced sodomy does not indicate subsequent sexual orientation as a victim may believe that suffering sodomy makes one a homosexual. The increased risk for transmission of HIV with anal intercourse has been noted (see "Prevention of Human Immunodeficiency Virus Infection" earlier in this chapter). Because of the extreme emotional reaction that men often feel after a sexual assault, they report the crime even more sporadically than female victims do.[54,55] Male victims deserve the same unhurried, nonjudgmental manner that female victims do. Penile samples from the shaft, glans, corona, and scrotum may be obtained if there is oral or anal contact with the perpetrator.

Child Sexual Assault Examinations

In general, the care and treatment of a pediatric sexual assault patient requires expert knowledge and experience. Frequently, ED practitioners are the first professionals to examine a child victim, and based on the history provided, the presence of obvious genital injury and trauma may speak for itself. However, in less obvious cases, the subtle variations in developmental changes and congenital anomalies may leave many clinicians ill equipped to render an opinion concerning findings indicative of sexual assault. The lives of children and families may be disrupted or severely affected, depending on the practitioner's opinion of the presence of genital penetration–type findings.

A well-known study by Adams and associates demonstrated that the majority of children reporting sexual abuse have normal or nonspecific genital findings.[56] As these authors succinctly stated regarding child sexual assault, it is "normal to be normal." Despite expert physical examination, the vast majority of sexually abused children cannot be differentiated from nonabused children.[57] Discovery of one of the rare examination markers of injury should be confirmed by experts, and a discussion of these findings, though beyond the scope of this chapter, is covered extensively in other resources.[58] The potential sexual assault history provided by the child or caretaker should therefore remain the primary indicator that inappropriate genital contact has occurred. At the very least, the history warrants an investigation of the possibility of sexual abuse.

It cannot be emphasized enough that the examiner's responsibility in the care of a child victim of sexual abuse remains within the realm of experts. However, in EDs lacking timely availability of local experts, inspect the genitalia carefully in an

Figure 58-12 "Frog leg" position to examine children.

Figure 58-13 Child in the knee-chest position to facilitate examination of the hymen.

unhurried, child-friendly manner, and if indicated, collect forensic specimens. For a very young child with small genital orifices, the aid of a magnification source may be extremely helpful. Ask a parent to assist in the calming, reassurance, and positioning of the child for careful inspection. However, when the parent is a suspect, the practitioner must exclude that parent from the examination. Whereas the basic lithotomy position may be used for an older, more mature child or an adolescent patient, use of alternative positioning of a pediatric female patient is essential for inspection. The frog leg position (the feet together and the knees spread widely apart) with the use of labial or gluteal (or both) separation and traction is often beneficial in children (Fig. 58-12). Take care to gently separate the labia to avoid superficial examiner-induced injuries. In addition, to get a better look at the hymenal perimeter in prepubertal girls and the anus in girls and boys, ask them to turn over into the knee-chest position (Fig. 58-13). Genital findings that are deemed definitive of sexual abuse or penetration or are nonspecific are included in Box 58-5. However, many normal hymenal differences exist from one child to the next, and the definitive diagnosis of "abnormal" is often difficult even for experts. When any doubt exists in the ED, describe the findings and refer the child for later examination by experts. The availability of a colposcope or alternative photographic equipment with magnification clearly aids in the documentation of any injuries that may heal before examination by an expert can be performed.

When disclosure or genital injuries confirm possible penetration of the child, collect specimens for potential evidence. On all conscious prepubertal children, collect the specimens without inserting a pediatric speculum. If there is no bleeding or significant trauma, procedural sedation is rarely indicated.

BOX 58-5 **Acute Findings on Examination Diagnostic of Sexual Contact in Children***

ACUTE TRAUMA TO EXTERNAL GENITAL/ANAL TISSUES

Acute lacerations or extensive bruising of the labia, penis, scrotum, perianal tissues, perineum, posterior fourchette, or hymen

Ecchymosis (bruising) on the hymen (in the absence of a known infectious process or coagulopathy)

Perianal lacerations extending deep to the external anal sphincter (not to be confused with partial failure of midline fusion)

PRESENCE CONFIRMS CONTACT WITH INFECTIVE BODY SECRETIONS LIKELY TO HAVE BEEN SEXUAL IN NATURE

Positive confirmed culture for gonorrhea from the genital area, anus, or throat in a child outside the neonatal period

Confirmed diagnosis of syphilis, excluding perinatal transmission

Trichomonas vaginalis infection in a child older than 1 year with organisms identified by culture or in vaginal secretions by examination of wet mounts by an experienced technician

Positive culture for *Chlamydia* from genital or anal tissue if the child is older than 3 years at the time of diagnosis with the use of cell culture or a comparable method approved by the Centers for Disease Control and Prevention

Positive serology for human immunodeficiency virus, exclusive of perinatal transmission, transmission from blood products, and needle contamination

DIAGNOSTIC OF SEXUAL CONTACT

Pregnancy

Sperm identified in specimens taken directly from a child's body

Adapted from Adams JA, Harper K, Starling SP, et al. Guidelines for medical care of children who may have been sexually abused. J Pediatr Adolesc Gynecol. 2007;20:163-172.
*The findings support a disclosure of sexual assault if one is given and are highly suggestive of assault even in the absence of disclosure, unless the child or caretaker provides a clear, timely, plausible description of the accidental injury.

If a child proves to be too uncooperative for an ED examination, refer the patient to a child sexual assault expert for examination the next day. For the rare cases involving severe vaginal trauma or suspected internal genital injury (active bleeding) that will possibly require surgical repair, conduct the examination under deep procedural sedation or general anesthesia. External anal and vulvar swabs are usually collected without difficulty on a child of any age. Because of lack of estrogen, contact with the prepubertal hymen generates much pain, thus making vaginal samples difficult to obtain. The samples should remain the very last evidence collected. Make every effort possible to avoid swab contact with hymenal tissue during collection. Vaginal aspirates obtained with a feeding tube or plastic angiocatheter may provide an alternative to vaginal swabs.

Genital specimens to screen for STDs remain a controversial issue in the realm of child abuse experts. For *N. gonorrhoeae*, at least, the literature supports the notion that all infected children will display an abnormal discharge.[59] With very young children, the practitioner may have only one opportunity to collect vaginal specimens without causing agitation prohibiting further examination. Forcing specimen collection under physical restraint is considered a second assault on the child. Because the child is being evaluated for possible sexual abuse, the primary specimens collected should be for forensic DNA analysis. STD detection and treatment can be performed at a later time. Clinicians should consult local child abuse centers for protocols regarding immediate STD specimen collection, referral, and follow-up services.

Suspect Examinations

As forensic evidence collection in the form of DNA retrieval continues to evolve, EDs may see more requests from local law enforcement for collection of evidence from suspects. EDs should be familiar with local and state protocols, especially regarding consent. Some jurisdictions permit examination of suspects without consent given the imminent degradation of potential biologic evidence. Other jurisdictions require that suspects give consent or, at the very least, that police obtain a search warrant from the court. The sooner that a suspect is apprehended and brought in for a medical-forensic examination, the better the quality of forensic biologic evidence.

Performing a medical-forensic examination on a suspect can give important corroborating information for the investigation of a crime. It can also help exonerate the innocent. Law enforcement should always be in attendance during the examination of any suspect to ensure the safety of the examiner. The suspect and victim should never encounter one another in the hospital setting during the examination period, and care should be taken to examine the victim and suspect in separate locations within the ED or clinical setting. It is extremely beneficial to conduct the examination and history of the victim before the suspect's examination to search for physical findings on the suspect indicated by the victim's history. For example, if during the victim's history she relates that she scratched the suspect's left shoulder in defense, the examiner can be certain to examine, document, and preferably photograph the presence (or absence) of an injury on the suspect's left shoulder.

The physical and evidentiary examination of the suspect is similar to that of the victim. The primary differences lie in history taking, reference samples, and more "blind" samples. During the examination of a suspect, law enforcement officers rather than the suspect provide the history of the event. Collect reference samples of head and pubic hairs, as well as blood, saliva, and urine, if possible. Apply special attention not only to nail scrapings but also to swabbing all the fingers for possible vaginal epithelial cells from digital penetration. The shaft and corona of the glans penis should be swabbed along with separate swabs of the scrotum for vaginal secretions. With an unwashed penis, swabs almost uniformly show evidence of female cells up to 24 hours after coitus.[30]

Examining suspects requires the same amount of professional sensitivity and respect that any patient receives within the ED. It is not within the realm of the clinician's expertise to determine whether the suspect is guilty or innocent.

The Unconscious Victim and "Drug-Facilitated Sexual Assault"

Alcohol and other drugs play an important role in many sexual assaults. Half of all sexual assaults involve drug or alcohol

BOX 58-6 Possible Date Rape Drugs*	
Alprazolam	Ketamine[†]
Amphetamines	Lorazepam
Barbiturates	Meprobamate[†]
1,4-Butanediol (BD)[†]	Methamphetamine
γ-Butyrolactone (GBL)[†]	Midazolam (Versed)[†]
Cannabis	Oxazepam
Cocaine	Phencyclidine (PCP)
Chloral hydrate[†]	Propoxyphene[†]
Clonazepam[†]	Scopolamine[†]
Clonidine[†]	Secobarbital
Diazepam	Temazepam
Ethanol	Triazolam
Flunitrazepam (Rohypnol)[†]	Zolpidem[†]
γ-Hydroxybutyrate (GHB)[†]	

*Frequently, more than one drug is found. Most common are alcohol, marijuana, cocaine, and benzodiazepines; others account for less than 5% of positive tests.
[†]Will not be detected on a routine immunoassay drug screen. A more detailed analysis will be required.
After Slaughter L. Involvement of drugs in sexual assault. J Reprod Med. 2000;45:425; and Schwartz RH, Milteer R, LeBeau M. Drug-facilitated sexual assault ("date rape"). South Med J. 2000;93:558.

ingestion.[60] In many cases it is unclear whether a drug was taken voluntarily or whether it was surreptitiously given to the assaulted victim.

Popular media has raised public awareness of drugs used to facilitate sexual assault under the term *date-rape drugs* (Box 58-6).[61] Although date-rape drugs are of significant concern, extensive forensic testing in the United States shows that a minority of sexual assault cases involve the scenario in which a victim's drink is covertly spiked with a tablet, capsule, powder, or liquid containing mind-altering drugs.[62] However, laboratory testing may be inadequately sensitive to test for all substances used during drug-facilitated sexual assault. The drugs most commonly associated with drug-facilitated sexual assault are ethanol, marijuana, cocaine, and benzodiazepines. Frequently, more than one drug is found. Although any type of sedative or hypnotic drug, or a combination of both, may be used to facilitate sexual assault, the most publicized drugs include flunitrazepam (Rohypnol), γ-hydroxybutyrate (GHB), and most recently, beverages containing high amounts of alcohol and caffeine (for example, Four Loko).[62,63] In previous decades, laboratory testing implicated flunitrazepam and GHB in drug-facilitated sexual assault in approximately 3% to 5% of cases.[61] Flunitrazepam is a benzodiazepine unavailable in the United States but available in Mexico. It can be detected in urine up to 3 weeks after ingestion.[64] In the United States, GHB is a schedule 1, federally banned central nervous system depressant. Legally, it is available only by prescription as the drug Xyrem for narcolepsy with a schedule 3 exception, but it can easily be manufactured illegally by users. It can be detected in drinking material residue by crime laboratories as well in the victim's urine up to 4 hours after a sufficiently large ingestion. Drugs similar to GHB are 1,4 butanediol and γ-butyrolactone.

Often, the victim's last memory is of using drugs or alcohol and then passing out. A common scenario is for the victim to have one glass of wine (or other usual drink), suddenly feel nauseated, and then wake up hours later in a different location and lacking intervening memory. Some remember short segments of activity that may indicate some type of sexual acts. Victims may lack any memory at all but desire to be "checked" for intercourse. A comprehensive medical-forensic examination should be conducted on these individuals. Without a history from the victim, examiners must collect samples from every potential oral or genital contact, including the neck, breasts, and vulva and from all orifices (oral, vaginal, and anal). Obtain samples of both blood and urine, if possible, for toxicology (including ethanol), with exact times of collection documented. Remember to collect the first voided urine to optimize potential recovery. Many of the drugs used to facilitate sexual assault are not found on routine hospital laboratory testing. Some forensic laboratories offer a "date-rape panel" that tests for a variety of commonly used substances. Obviously, a positive drug test does not prove date rape, and it may be impossible to distinguish self-administration from clandestine ingestion.

Extreme sensitivity must be used when discussing positive genital findings with a victim who has no memory of any sexual activity. Many times the imagined sexual acts can create just as severe a traumatic response as an actual remembered sexual assault. For the unconscious victim, there is no memory of events to fill in the blanks, only her terrifying imagination of what could have happened.

LEGAL ISSUES

When the local government decides to proceed with a sex crime case against an alleged perpetrator, the district attorney will commonly contact the examiner to give legal testimony. A well-documented chart often negates the need for a clinician to appear in court. When required for this task, it is best for the examiner to work with the prosecuting attorney to prepare testimony. As is the case for all ED patients, chart notes should be written carefully in the expectation that the ED evaluation and evidence collection may be presented in court. In some jurisdictions it is possible to minimize the time spent away from work by arranging to be called to the courtroom just before the time of testimony or by giving a deposition before the court date. Once on the witness stand, the examining clinician is most often considered a percipient witness and not necessarily an expert in the area of sexual assault. The law requires that one testify only to one's best recollection and to what is indicated in the chart. Factual information in answer to questions should be given only if one knows the facts; assumptions should be avoided. One should not be afraid to acknowledge the limits of one's knowledge or expertise. Statements such as "there were marks on the body that were consistent with bite marks" are preferable to statements such as "there were bite marks." The court decides if a person was sexually assaulted, and the clinician is there to give information about the patient's findings and statements, what was found, and what was done for treatment.

SEXUAL ASSAULT RESPONSE TEAMS

Before the 1990s, sexual assault examinations were mostly the responsibility of emergency clinicians. However, since the early 1990s, nurses or nurse clinicians have been performing an increasing number of sexual assault examinations. Called sexual assault nurse examiners (SANEs), these nurses are the core members of SARTs. Other members of SARTs include law enforcement individuals, victim advocates, prosecutors, and forensic laboratory personnel.

Most examinations still take place in the ED but may be done in a space near the ED or an affiliated clinic. To establish SARTs, extra funding by government or a charitable organization is often needed because many local police jurisdictions do not adequately reimburse for the evidentiary examination to support a program. However, law enforcement is increasingly willing to pay more for a SANE-performed forensic examination because they believe that it provides superior documentation for legal proceedings. Nurse examiners have formed the International Association of Forensic Nurses. This group has drafted standards of practice for sexual assault examiners' education and the examinations themselves. Advantages of SARTs using SANEs include the following:

1. The practitioner performing the examination is specifically dedicated to treating the victim, not tending to multiple patients in a busy ED.
2. The clinician has usually completed more extensive training on sexual assault examination (mean of 80 hours) and evidence collection and, accordingly, may perform a more comprehensive examination with better collection of evidence.[21,65]
3. Many involved feel that designated clinicians consider the emotional needs of the victim more fully because of their extra specialty training.

Useful guidelines and resources for establishing SANE programs are currently available.[2,3,63,66]

Acknowledgment

The editors and author wish to acknowledge the contributions of G. Richard Braen to this chapter in previous editions; Dean Gialamas, Director of the Los Angeles County Sheriff's Department Crime Laboratory; Mary Hong of the Orange County Crime Laboratory; and Elizabeth Swanson of the LAPD crime laboratory for their technical advice.

References are available at www.expertconsult.com

Neurologic Procedures

CHAPTER 59

Management of Increased Intracranial Pressure and Intracranial Shunts

Jessica L. Osterman and Megan L. Rischall

Headache and head injury are encountered commonly in the emergency department (ED). If either is accompanied by vomiting, decreased level of consciousness, or abnormal vital signs, the possibility of increased intracranial pressure (ICP) should be considered. Acutely increased ICP is a neurologic emergency that must be managed quickly before further brain damage and death ensue. In some cases the accompanying clinical symptoms may be vague or subtle and make diagnosis difficult. Familiarity with the pathophysiology of increased ICP facilitates its diagnosis and management.

PATHOPHYSIOLOGY OF ICP

Alexander Monro, an anatomist in the 18th century, described the intracranial contents as containing a fixed volume. The fixed-volume theory was supported by George Kellie a few years later and became known as the Monro-Kellie doctrine. This doctrine has since guided our understanding of intracranial dynamics and the principles of autoregulation.

The components of the calvaria are the brain parenchyma, cerebrospinal fluid (CSF), the venous blood supply, and the arterial blood supply (Fig. 59-1). CSF and the venous blood supply have the greatest ability to change their volume to compensate for increases in pressure. These dynamic changes in the relative proportion of the cranial content may not affect the patient if ICP is not excessive. However, if a pathologic process overwhelms the compensatory mechanisms, the result will be a nearly exponentially increase in ICP (Fig. 59-2).

Normal supine ICP ranges from 5 to 15 mm Hg. Transient increases in ICP as high as 80 to 100 mm Hg occur with coughing or straining. Other factors that can transiently increase ICP are movement, pain, and fever. A space-occupying lesion such as a tumor, hematoma, abscess, or foreign body can also raise ICP. Figure 59-3 demonstrates that the area and cause of the increased ICP will determine where shifts occur to result in brain herniation.

Brain

Brain volume can be increased by edema, idiopathic intracranial hypertension (IIH), tumor, or bleeding. The three types of edema are vasogenic, cytotoxic, and interstitial. Vasogenic edema results from increased permeability of the capillaries, which leads to passage of excess fluid into the extracellular space. Cytotoxic edema is due to accumulation of intracellular fluid in brain tissue (neurons and glia) secondary to dysfunction of the adenosine triphosphatase pump. Interstitial edema occurs when fluid accumulates as a result of blockage of CSF absorption.

IIH, formerly known as pseudotumor cerebri, is a chronic condition characterized by increased CSF pressure not caused by a tumor, edema, hydrocephalus, or change in CSF composition. It occurs most frequently in obese women. Symptoms may include headache, nausea, and blurry vision. The headache is typically worse on waking or with exertion. In general, patients with IIH have normal findings on neurologic examination except for the frequent presence of papilledema. Although the precise pathophysiology remains unclear, severe cases can lead to permanent loss of vision. Commonly associated conditions are listed in Box 59-1. IIH is a diagnosis of exclusion. Because of its often subtle symptoms and normal findings on computed tomography (CT), it is often not suspected or diagnosed on initial clinical evaluation.

Brain tumors encompass neoplasms that originate in the brain itself (primary brain tumors) or involve the brain as a metastatic site (secondary brain tumors). *Primary brain tumors* include tumors of the brain parenchyma, meninges, cranial nerves, and other intracranial structures (the pituitary and pineal glands). Primary central nervous system (CNS) lymphoma refers to non-Hodgkin's lymphoma confined to the CNS. The site of origin of this type of tumor remains unknown. *Secondary brain tumors*, the most common type, originate elsewhere in the body and metastasize to the intracranial compartment.

Bleeding in the brain can occur spontaneously (as in the case of hemorrhagic stroke or spontaneous subarachnoid hemorrhage) or can be a result of trauma. In addition to the mass effect of the blood itself, the associated edema in both instances contributes to further increases in ICP. Diffuse axonal injury (DAI) may occur in isolation or in conjunction with intracerebral bleeding. With DAI it is believed that the axons are not actually torn, but instead suffer significant injury that may lead to edema (shearing effect).[1]

CSF

CSF is produced by the choroid plexus at a daily rate of 500 mL. It flows from the ventricles into the cisternae of the subarachnoid space and is drained by the arachnoid villi of the dural sinuses to maintain a constant volume of 100 to 150 mL. *Obstructive hydrocephalus* occurs when flow is blocked at any point in the ventricular system by clotted blood, tumor, colloid cyst, edema, or primary stenosis. *Communicating hydrocephalus* is due to impedance of flow beyond the ventricular system at the level of the basal cisternae or lack of absorption by the arachnoid villi. Communicating hydrocephalus can occur with both infection and subarachnoid hemorrhage (Fig. 59-4).

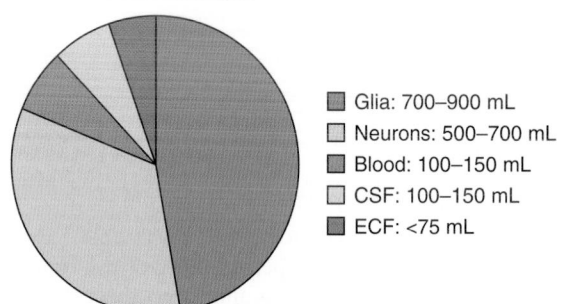

Glia: 700–900 mL
Neurons: 500–700 mL
Blood: 100–150 mL
CSF: 100–150 mL
ECF: <75 mL

Figure 59-1 Intracranial contents and their volumes in healthy adults. *CSF,* cerebrospinal fluid; *ECF,* extracellular fluid.

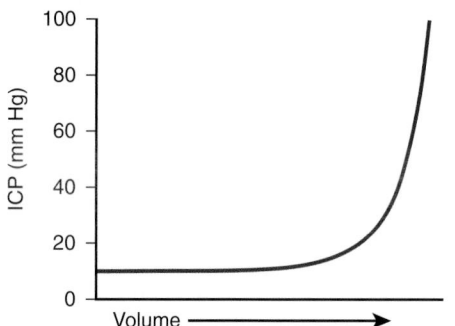

Figure 59-2 The intracranial volume-pressure relationship demonstrates the limits of compensatory mechanisms. *ICP,* intracranial pressure.

Blood

Up to a certain range, cerebral blood flow (CBF) is maintained by an autoregulatory mechanism despite fluctuations in cerebral perfusion pressure (CPP) (Fig. 59-5). Constant CBF can typically be maintained at any CPP between 60 and 160 mm Hg. Once CPP is out of the autoregulatory zone, CBF is linearly related to CPP. CPP lower than 60 mm Hg can lead to ischemia, whereas CPP higher 160 mm Hg can result in hypertensive encephalopathy.

SIGNS AND SYMPTOMS

Findings on neurologic examination can be normal in a patient with a mild increase in ICP because of the brain's compensatory mechanisms. Patients with a complaint of headache or head injury may not initially manifest the more dramatic and worrisome symptoms of increased ICP such as vomiting, syncope, altered mentation, or Cushing's reflex (bradycardia, increased blood pressure, and irregular respirations). ICP

Figure 59-3 Intracranial shifts as a result of supratentorial lesions. **A,** Relationships of the various supratentorial compartments as seen in a coronal section. **B,** Herniation of the cingulate gyrus under the falx (*1*); herniation of the temporal lobe into the tentorial notch (*2*); compression of the opposite cerebral peduncle against the unyielding tentorium, which produces Kernohan's notch (*3*); and downward displacement of the brainstem through the tentorial notch (*4*). (*A and B, From Plum F, Posner JB.* The Diagnosis of Stupor and Coma. *2nd ed. Philadelphia: Davis; 1972. Reproduced by permission.*)

BOX 59-1 **Clinical Conditions and Factors Associated with Idiopathic or Benign Intracranial Hypertension (Pseudotumor Cerebri)**

HEMATOLOGIC DISORDERS
Iron deficiency anemia
Pernicious anemia
Polycythemia vera
Thrombocytopenia
Lupus
Cushing's disease
Hypoparathyroidism
Hypothyroidism

ENDOCRINE CONDITIONS AND DISORDERS
Addison's disease
Menstrual irregularities, menstrual cycle
Pregnancy

MEDICAL/SURGICAL CONDITIONS WITH IMPAIRED CEREBRAL VENOUS DRAINAGE
Otitis media, mastoiditis
Idiopathic dural sinus thrombosis
Radical neck surgery
Chronic pulmonary disease with venous hypertension
Heart failure with venous hypertension
Congenital heart disease
Renal failure
High-flow arteriovenous malformation

Chronic obstructive pulmonary disease
Sleep apnea
Growth hormone
Cimetidine

COMMON DRUGS
Systemic steroid withdrawal
Topical steroid withdrawal (infants)
Oral contraceptives
Tetracycline/minocycline
Nitrofurantoin
Sulfamethoxazole
Vitamin A excess

Glucocorticoids
Nalidixic acid
Levothyroxine
Lithium
Isotretinoin (Accutane)
Nonsteroidal antiinflammatory drugs
Tamoxifen
Cyclosporine

DIETARY CONSIDERATIONS
Hypervitaminosis A
Hypovitaminosis A
Obesity
Malnutrition

correlates poorly with clinical symptomatology. One of the earliest clinical signs is decreased venous pulsation on funduscopic examination, but this may be difficult to appreciate in an acutely ill patient in a busy ED. Moreover, the initial findings on head CT might not reveal the true extent of injury, especially with early stroke or when DAI is involved. However, as compensatory mechanisms fail, CT findings, as well as clinical symptoms, will become more obvious.

Signs and symptoms of severely increased ICP include a decreasing level of consciousness, papilledema, cranial nerve palsies, and lateralizing neurologic deficits. When any of these are noted, particularly when CT confirms the presence of a mass effect such as hydrocephalus or a midline shift, urgent intervention is necessary (Fig. 59-6). Neurosurgical consultation for possible invasive means of reducing ICP and monitoring is indicated. Medical management of increased ICP should also proceed without delay.

MEDICAL TREATMENT OF INCREASED ICP

Oxygenation

Management of the airway and breathing is paramount in patients with brain injury. If the patient is hypoxic, supplemental oxygen is necessary to prevent further ischemia. Patients with a Glasgow Coma Scale (GCS) score of 9 or

lower or with impending signs of inadequate respiratory status should undergo rapid-sequence intubation (RSI) to protect the airway and better control blood levels of oxygen and carbon dioxide (Po_2 and Pco_2).

Sedation and Paralytics

Rapid assessment of findings on the patient's neurologic examination should be performed before sedation and paralysis (RSI). If time allows, premedicate the patient with lidocaine, 1 to 1.5 mg/kg, 3 minutes before intubation while preoxygenating the patient. Lidocaine has been reported to blunt the rise in ICP associated with laryngoscopy and may protect against some hypoxia-related dysrhythmias; however, its true value is unproven (see Chapters 4 and 5). Fentanyl is an excellent drug for control of pain, which if untreated, can lead to increased ICP. Fentanyl can also be given during the pretreatment phase of RSI (3 minutes before administration of the paralytic agent) if time allows. Caution should be exercised, however, to avoid precipitous drops in blood pressure, which can actually threaten CBF and exacerbate the brain injury. It is for this reason that we recommend titrating fentanyl up to the target dose rather than giving a full dose (typically 3 µg/kg) up front. We also recommend caution in brain-injured patients with concomitant trauma, who may have exaggerated episodes of hypotension with narcotics and sedatives. A defasciculating dose $\frac{1}{10}$ of the intubating dose of a nondepolarizing neuromuscular blocking agent may also be administered as pretreatment. If given 3 minutes before a paralyzing dose of succinylcholine, it counteracts the transient fasciculations and increase in ICP that occur with the administration of succinylcholine. *It is important to note, however, that practice variations are common, and though theoretically attractive, none of these pretreatment options have been demonstrated to improve patient-oriented outcomes.*[2]

Induction (sedation) may be achieved with drugs that block the rise in ICP, such as etomidate (0.3 mg/kg intravenously

Figure 59-4 Cerebrospinal fluid production and flow. (*From Rengachary SS, Wilkins RH, eds.* Principles of Neurosurgery. *Philadelphia: Mosby; 1994.*)

CPP = Blood pressure − ICP

Figure 59-5 Cerebral autoregulation. *CPP,* cerebral perfusion pressure; *ICP,* intracranial pressure.

Figure 59-6 Acute subdural hematoma. The large hyperdense (i.e., white) collection on the right side of the brain is an acute subdural hematoma. The finding of hypodense areas (*black arrow*) within the subdural is referred to as the "swirl" sign, which suggests active bleeding. Also seen is about 3 cm of midline shift (*white arrow*), which indicates subfalcine herniation. Immediate reduction of intracranial pressure and surgical intervention are required.

[IV]), thiopental (50 to 100 mg IV or 3 to 5 mg/kg IV), or propofol (1 mg/kg IV).[3-5] Etomidate is preferred over thiopental in patients with unstable hemodynamic status. Etomidate has two significant benefits—it has minimal effect on systemic blood pressure and does not appear to increase ICP.[3,4] Propofol has gained acceptance as a sedative in patients with increased ICP because of its short duration of action and depression of cerebral metabolism and oxygen consumption. This may have a neuroprotective effect. However, propofol can cause profound decreases in systemic blood pressure and with higher doses and extended periods of use can be associated with significant morbidity.[5]

The paralytic agent of choice is succinylcholine (1.5 mg/kg in adults and up to 2.5 mg/kg in pediatric patients). Nondepolarizing agents are appropriate when contraindications to succinylcholine exist (see Chapter 5). Sedatives and paralytics should be short acting to facilitate close monitoring of the patient's neurologic status.

Oxygenation and Hyperventilation

As the airway is secured, adequate supplemental oxygen should be provided, with titration down rapidly from the initial FIO_2 of 1.0 used for RSI to ensure oxygen saturation greater than 90%.[1]

In general, avoid hyperventilation in patients with brain injury because low PCO_2 levels cause cerebral vasoconstriction, which results in decreased CBF in the critical hours following injury.[1,6] Hyperventilation is also associated with poor survival and neurologic outcomes.[6,7] For the majority of brain-injured patients, the target is thus eucapnia with a PCO_2 of 35 to 40 mm Hg.[6] Nevertheless, if a patient displays evolving signs of brain herniation (e.g., anisocoria, hemiparesis, asymmetric posturing, Cushing's reflex, or rapid deterioration in GCS score), hyperventilation may be necessary to arrest the process. Current recommendations target a PCO_2 of 28 to 35 mm Hg in these scenarios as a temporizing measure until surgical intervention to lower ICP can occur.[6]

Head Position

If not in shock, elevate the patient's head to decrease ICP. This position allows drainage of cerebral veins. Feldman,[8] Ng,[9] and their colleagues demonstrated that elevation of the head to 30 degrees significantly reduces ICP in most patients without impairing CBF, CPP, or cerebral metabolism. Raising the head of a patient with hypotension, however, exacerbates any decrease in the patient's mean arterial pressure (MAP) and hence lowers CPP. If head elevation is to be used, MAP must be maintained above 90 mm Hg to facilitate a CPP of approximately 60 mm Hg.[10] It is also important to avoid neck rotation and flexion or any other intervention that could result in compression of the jugular vein. If the jugular veins are compressed, venous outflow from the head can be further compromised.

Fluid Management

The goal in fluid management is to maintain euvolemia; head-injured patients with hypotension have double the mortality of normotensive patients. Patients with increased ICP may be hypovolemic from profuse vomiting, decreased fluid intake, or hemorrhage. Distributive shock may also be present and occurs as a result of loss of vasomotor sympathetic tone,

especially in patients with concomitant cervical spine injury. Only isotonic or hypertonic fluids should be used (normal or hypertonic saline) to avoid worsening the brain edema. Vasopressors may also be necessary. A target CPP of 60 mm Hg and MAP of greater than 90 mm Hg are recommended.[11]

Diuresis

Mannitol effectively reduces ICP. Mannitol can be given at doses of 0.25 to 1 g/kg infused every 2 to 6 hours. Current recommendations favor bolus therapy over continuous infusion. Mannitol can cause a precipitous drop in blood pressure (and hence CPP) in patients who are hypovolemic. Thus, mannitol is contraindicated in those with preexisting hypotension (typically defined as blood pressure lower than 90 mm Hg systolic). The effect of mannitol on ICP is transient; repeated doses lose their ability to decrease ICP over time. It also may cause renal damage as serum osmolarity increases. Similar to hyperventilation, mannitol should be viewed as a bridge to definitive neurosurgical intervention and reserve its use for patients with signs of impending transtentorial herniation.

Mannitol has two properties—it initially acts as a volume expander and then serves as an osmotic agent. On administration of mannitol, intravascular volume expands and blood viscosity decreases, which results in augmentation of CBF. Once volume expansion has occurred, osmotic movement of fluid from the cellular compartment to the intravascular compartment begins and results in a decrease in ICP. The osmotic effect usually occurs within 15 minutes. The half-life of mannitol ranges from 90 minutes to 6 hours.[11] Its effect is most pronounced in patients with CPP lower than 70 mm Hg.[11]

Hypertonic saline is an alternative to mannitol in patients who are hypotensive. Theoretically, hypertonic saline is an ideal resuscitation fluid for patients with concomitant head injury and hemorrhagic shock because it can effectively expand intravascular volume while causing osmotic diuresis of the brain. However, its efficacy in human studies remains uncertain, so its use should be reserved for patients with contraindications to mannitol. Although hypertonic saline is generally administered in boluses of 100 to 250 mL of 3% to 7% saline, there is no consensus on the preferred concentration and volume of administration.[11,12]

Seizure Prophylaxis

Controlling seizure activity is important in the early stages of traumatic brain injury to avoid hypoxia and aspiration, as well as elevation of ICP and possible herniation. In the absence of a seizure, it is currently controversial whether or not *prophylactic* anticonvulsant medication should be routinely administered after *spontaneous intracranial hemorrhage*. If a seizure occurs, anticonvulsant therapy is warranted. However, current literature supports the use of prophylactic anticonvulsant therapy for the first week following *traumatic brain injury*, with the recognition that this has no effect on the occurrence of late seizures.[13] Rapidly acting benzodiazepines such as lorazepam and diazepam are first-line therapy, followed by anticonvulsant agents such as pentobarbital or phenytoin. Fosphenytoin can be given more rapidly (up to 150 mg/min IV by infusion) than phenytoin, which can be administered no faster than 50 mg/min IV. Phenytoin can induce hypotension and lower CPP, even at rates below 50 mg/min. Levetiracetam has also been used in cases of severe head injury and stroke. Although beneficial effects of prophylactic anticonvulsants on outcomes have not been established, in the ED setting the risks associated with the administration of anticonvulsants are probably small in comparison to the potentially devastating secondary injury that results from uncontrolled seizure activity.

Patients who are paralyzed, either chemically or by their neurologic disease, are difficult to monitor for seizure activity without the use of electroencephalography (EEG). These patients may manifest seizures by subtle rhythmic movements of the extremities, tonic gaze deviation, an elevation in heart rate or blood pressure, or spikes on an ICP monitor (if one is placed by the neurosurgeon). Whenever possible, avoid giving paralytic agents so that seizure activity can be monitored. If seizures are not controlled despite upward titration of benzodiazepines, phenytoin, or other agents, endotracheal intubation and induction of a barbiturate or propofol coma may be necessary. Pentobarbital has been used to treat uncontrolled elevations in ICP when other medical and surgical treatments have failed. It decreases CBF, metabolism, oxygen consumption, and cerebral edema. It also scavenges free radicals.[14] Pentobarbital is given at a loading dose of 10 mg/kg over a 30-minute period followed by infusion at 1 to 3 mg/kg/hr with an EEG monitor available for burst suppression. Intensive monitoring of the patient's hemodynamic status is necessary because of pentobarbital's hypotensive effect.

Steroids

Steroids have been shown to be beneficial in patients with vasogenic edema—edema associated with brain tumors. Steroids decrease CSF production, stabilize membranes, and restore normal membrane permeability.[15-17] Dexamethasone is usually administered at 10 to 20 mg IV as a loading dose, followed by 4 to 10 mg every 6 hours. No studies support the use of steroids in head-injured patients; in fact, steroid use in this population was found to increase mortality in a recent randomized trial.[18,19]

Glucose Control

Head-injured patients tend to be hyperglycemic in response to stress or steroid administration. Optimization of blood glucose levels is currently undertaken in the management of these patients to avoid cellular edema in brain tissue. Hypoglycemic states can exacerbate brain injury and therefore should be scrupulously avoided. However, the long-term value of tight glycemic control in the management of acute brain injury with increased ICP is unclear.

Hypothermia

Lower body temperatures have been associated with a decrease in blood flow, ICP, and metabolism. The previous method of keeping core temperatures lower than 30°C has been abandoned. It fell out of favor because of the complications of cardiac arrhythmias and difficulty maintaining such profound hypothermia. More recently, mild therapeutic hypothermia (32°C to 34°C) has become popular in the management of post–cardiac arrest victims who do not regain consciousness. Although one study has shown a benefit in survival and decreased ICP with mild hypothermia (32°C to 34°C),[20] in the setting of traumatic brain injury and stroke it is not currently recommended.[21] Hyperthermia increases ICP and must be avoided.

Skull Trephination

Skull trephination or burr hole placement is a technique that has been traced back to the Neolithic age.[22] Though rarely performed by nonsurgeons, it can be a lifesaving procedure for severely head-injured patients. In a patient with an *acute epidural hematoma* and deteriorating findings on neurologic examination (decreasing level of consciousness, anisocoria, or hemiparesis), skull trephination has been shown to improve both short- and long-term neurologic outcomes.[23,24] Trephination is an appropriate treatment of acute subdural hematoma as well, but this requires incision through the dura mater and is less realistic for non-neurosurgeons (Figs. 59-7 and 59-8). Trephination may be lifesaving if performed before transport in selected patients from remote practice environments without neurosurgical capability. This heroic procedure is not standard nor is it an expected skill for most emergency clinicians; nonetheless, it may be attempted when the situation is dire.

Trephination in the ED should be performed only in the temporal regions. Trephination in the parietal and occipital regions is associated with a much higher risk for hemorrhage and air embolism because of their proximity to the dural venous sinuses. These approaches should generally be performed only after the results of CT are available for guidance.[23]

In practice environments without access to CT, it is not unreasonable to attempt this procedure before transport of the patient when all other measures to lower ICP have failed and signs of evolving brain herniation are present. The blind approach for temporal trephination is depicted in Figure 59-9 and involves locating an area 2 cm anterior and 2 cm superior to the tragus on the side of the suspected hematoma.[23] In the

Figure 59-7 Epidural hematoma (*left*): rupture of a meningeal artery (usually associated with a skull fracture) leads to accumulation of arterial blood between the dura and skull. Subdural hematoma (*right*): damage to bridging veins between the brain and superior sagittal sinus leads to accumulation of blood between the dura and the arachnoid. (*From Mitchell R, Kumar V, Fausto N, et al. Pocket Companion to Robbins & Cotran Pathological Basis of Disease. 8th ed. Philadelphia: Saunders; 2011.*)

Emergency Skull Trephination

Indications
Acute epidural hematoma and *both* of the following:
1. Deteriorating finding on neurologic examination (e.g., decreasing level of consciousness, anisocoria, hemiparesis)
2. Delay in obtaining definitive neurosurgical care (e.g., remote practice environments)

Contraindications
Parietal or occipital epidural hematomas (high risk for hemorrhage and air embolism because of dural venous sinuses)
Subdural hematomas (requires an incision through the dura mater and is less realistic for the nonneurosurgeon)

Complications
Bleeding
Infection
Brain parenchymal injury

Equipment

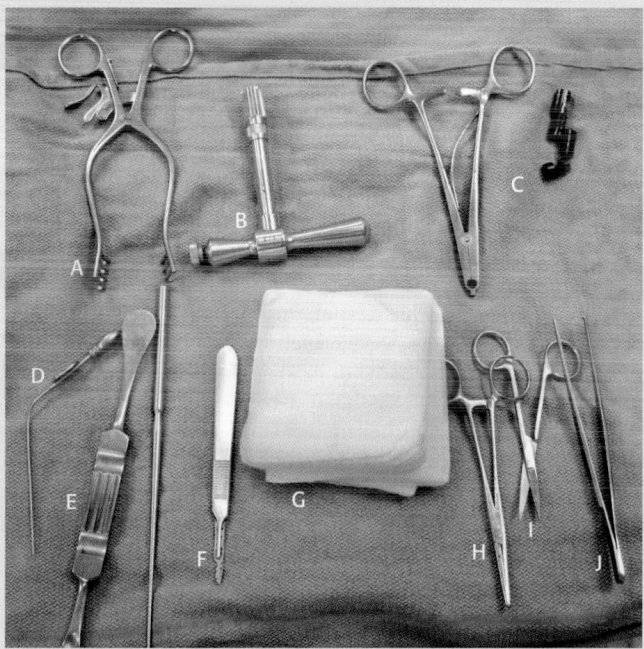

A. Self-retaining scalp retractor
B. ¹/₂-inch Galt trepine
C. Raney clips and applier
D. Suction
E. Periosteal elevator
F. Scalpel
G. Gauze 4 × 4 pads
H. Kelly clamp
I. Scissors
J. Adson (toothed) forceps

Review Box 59-1 Emergency skull trephination: indications, contraindications, complications, and equipment.

Figure 59-8 Epidural and subdural hematomas. **A,** Acute epidural hematoma. The hyperdense (*white*) appearance of this lesion indicates that it is acute. The inner margins of epidurals (*arrows*) have a convex appearance, which results in a lens-shaped hematoma. Note that the hematoma does not cross the suture lines (temporal-sphenoid anteriorly, temporal-parietal posteriorly.) **B,** Acute-on-chronic subdural hematoma. The heterogeneous density of this lesion (hypodense anteriorly [*double asterisk*], hyperdense posteriorly [*asterisk*]) suggests an acute-on-chronic hemorrhage. The inner margins of subdurals (*arrows*) are concave, which results in a crescent-shaped hematoma. Subdural hematomas may cross suture lines (note that this hematoma extends from the frontal to the parietal regions). Both these examples demonstrate effacement of the lateral ventricles and midline shift, which are indicators of increased intracranial pressure.

EMERGENCY SKULL TREPHINATION

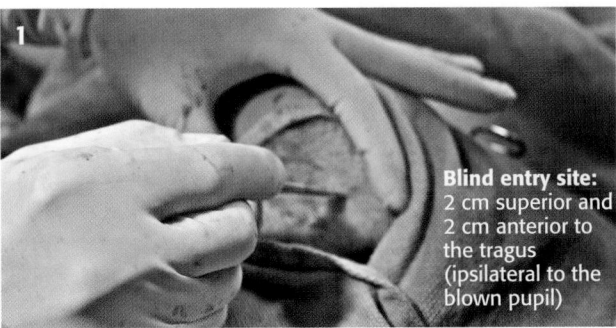

Blind entry site: 2 cm superior and 2 cm anterior to the tragus (ipsilateral to the blown pupil)

Shave, prepare, and drape the entry site. Use CT to guide the location of the burr hole placement. If CT is not available, choose a site 2 cm anterior and 2 cm superior to the tragus.

Make a 4-cm vertical incision extending down to the periosteum. Optionally apply Raney clips to the skin edges to control bleeding.

Insert a self-retaining scalp retractor to provide exposure. The exposed area should be about 2.5 cm in diameter.

Use the periosteal elevator to elevate the periosteum off the skull.

Adjust the centering point of the trephine so that it protrudes 1/8 inch. With the trephine at a 90° angle to the skull, apply gentle pressure with a clockwise-counterclockwise rotating motion.

Stop sawing into the skull when you feel a slight give, which indicates that you have penetrated the full thickness of the skull. Remove the trephine.

Bone fragment

If the bone fragment does not come out in the trephine, use toothed forceps or a hooked instrument to remove it. Preserve the bone fragment in sterile saline.

Allow the clot and blood to extrude from the burr hole. Apply gentle suction as needed to assist evacuation of the clot. A small suction catheter can be left in place during transport if needed.

Figure 59-9 Emergency skull trephination. This technique is for patients with epidural hematomas in the temporal region. It should not be used for parietal or occipital hematomas. If a subdural hematoma is present, the dura must be opened. If no blood is encountered on a blind procedure done on the same side as a blown pupil, repeat it on the opposite side. *CT,* computed tomography.

majority of cases the appropriate side for trephination is ipsilateral to pupillary dilation and contralateral to motor paresis.

The temporal area (between the ear and the orbit) should be shaved and prepared with chlorhexidine or Betadine via sterile technique. Local anesthetic can be used to infiltrate the area of the planned incision; however, this is not necessary in an unconsciousness patient and adds time to the procedure.

Once the proper location is identified, either with a blind approach or by using the results of CT, make a 4-cm vertical incision through the skin and temporalis fascia. Divide the temporalis muscle. Once the periosteum is identified, incise it. Expose the skull by elevating the periosteum (with a periosteal elevator if available). Insert a trephine or hand drill into the area underneath the periosteum.[23] While holding the drill perpendicular to the skull, apply continuous gentle downward pressure and rotate the drill in an alternating clockwise-counterclockwise motion. As progress is made with the hand drill, gradually reduce pressure to avoid inadvertent "plunging" into the brain parenchyma. The operator will know when penetration through both the outer and inner tables of the skull has been accomplished once resistance against the drill is no longer felt. After skull penetration has been accomplished, remove the round piece of bone that has been cored out (with the diameter of the drill) and place it in saline.

In many cases, epidural blood and clots under pressure will extrude from the site on full penetration of the skull. Insertion of a suction catheter into the trephinated space may be necessary, however, for full evacuation of the clotted material. If easily identified, the bleeding artery (usually the middle meningeal artery) may be clamped.[23] After successful trephination, the patient's status should immediately be reassessed for signs of improvement. In a significant minority of patients, false localizing signs may lead the clinician to suspect a hematoma on the wrong side. Thus, if no improvement is noted with trephination on the side of the suspected hematoma, the procedure may be repeated on the opposite side. However, in all cases the delay in definitive neurosurgical care caused by attempts at trephination must be weighed against the possible benefits of the procedure. Moreover, trephination should ideally be performed after consultation with the accepting neurosurgeon.[24]

Complications of the procedure include bleeding, infection, and injury to the brain parenchyma.

Operative Management

Operative management is the definitive treatment of increased ICP secondary to a space-occupying lesion. This entails either craniotomy or ventriculostomy with drainage of blood and CSF.

INTRACRANIAL SHUNTS

Intracranial shunts are used for the long-term management of increased ICP. A recurrent elevation in ICP because of shunt malfunction can occur days to years after shunt placement.

Intracranial shunt malfunctions are often diagnosed in the ED. In many cases the patient's significant other or caretaker provides the subtle clues that lead to the diagnosis. Depending on the age of the patient, recurrent symptoms of increased ICP may include changes in behavior, headache, nausea, vomiting, and visual disturbances. In children, lethargy, poor feeding, vomiting, ataxia, decreased or increased activity level,

fever, diaphoresis, and fussiness can all be indications of shunt malfunction. Accordingly, in children, lethargy and shunt site swelling are the most predictive signs of shunt malfunction.[25] Failure of upward gaze is another sensitive sign of nonacute shunt malfunction (sunset eyes). Cranial nerve and visual field examination should be routine in the assessment of older, cooperative patients with intracranial shunts.

The essential elements of any shunt system include the proximal and distal catheters, a valve, and a reservoir. A wide array of valves, catheters, and other devices are available for use in shunt systems. The valve allows unidirectional flow, incorporates a pumping chamber, and regulates the pressure at which flow will occur across it. The reservoir is usually located between two valves. The proximal valve allows flow from the ventricles to the reservoir, whereas the distal valve allows flow from the reservoir to the distal catheter (Fig. 59-10). Many different types of shunt systems incorporating a variety of designs are available (Fig. 59-11). Some have unique characteristics, such as a double dome, whereas in others, valves are absent altogether.

In most cases the reservoir gives access to the system for measurement of pressure, testing of patency, fluid sampling, and injection of medication or contrast material. In rare cases, other equipment is incorporated into the shunt system for specific purposes, including an on-off switch, a telemetric pressure sensor, and an antisiphon device.

In the ventriculoperitoneal (VP) shunt system, a ventricular catheter is placed in the right frontal horn of the lateral ventricle (nondominant hemisphere) and connected to a subcutaneous valve traversing the temporal aspect (Fig. 59-12). This valve is then connected to a distal catheter threaded subcutaneously into the neck and finally into the peritoneum or another body compartment (Fig. 59-13). Ventricular catheters can be either straight or angled, with the latter having the option of a reservoir component attachment. Valves come in four different types (ball, diaphragm, miter, slit), each with unique flow characteristics. The distal catheter has either an open or closed end. Identifying the type of shunt in place is

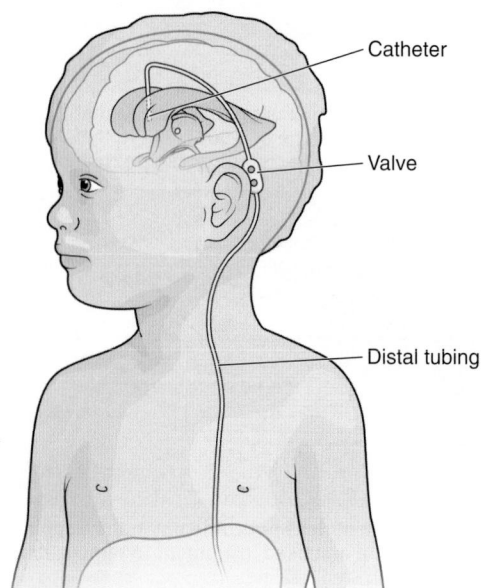

Figure 59-10 The basic tripartite ventricular shunt system is composed of a ventricular catheter, valve mechanism, and distal tubing. A slit valve may be used in the far end of the distal tubing instead of a more proximally placed valve, as shown.

often difficult unless the patient or caretaker has the information available. Moreover, the skin overlying the subcutaneous component of the shunt in the temporal regions can scar, thus rendering palpation of the shunt type impossible.

The principle of any extracranial shunting technique is to divert CSF into a body cavity from which it can readily be eliminated and drained. VP shunts are at present the mainstay for treatment of hydrocephalus in infants and children because of their ease of insertion and reliable long-term function.

Other types of extracranial shunts include ventriculovenous, ventriculoatrial, ventriculopleural, and lumboperitoneal. These other shunts are usually reserved for circumstances in which VP shunting has failed or when the patient has a history of multiple abdominal surgeries or peritoneal infections.

Shunt Assessment

The usual cause of shunt malfunction is catheter obstruction. Proximal blockage may be due to tissue debris or choroid

Figure 59-11 Shunt components. (*From Rengachary SS, Wilkins RH, eds.* Principles of Neurosurgery. *Philadelphia: Mosby; 1994.*)

Figure 59-12 Cross-section of a Pudenz flushing valve (American Heyer-Schulte, Santa Barbara, CA) illustrating the diaphragm valve. The proximal inlet tube and silicone base are placed in the burr hole so that only the reservoir (silicon dome) protrudes above the skull. (*Courtesy of PS Medical, Goleta, CA.*)

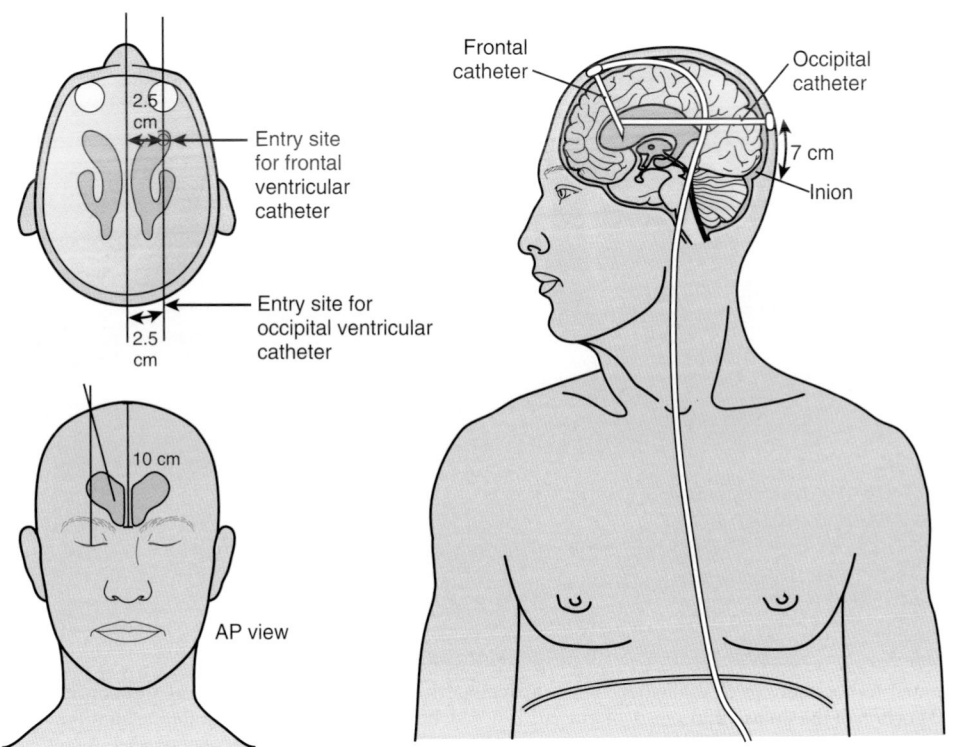

Figure 59-13 Ventriculoperitoneal shunt and alternative occipital placement. *AP*, anteroposterior. (*From Rengachary SS, Wilkins RH, eds.* Principles of Neurosurgery. *Philadelphia: Mosby; 1994.*)

plexus within the ventricular catheter. Distal obstruction of venous shunts may result from thrombus or venous occlusion (such as in a ventriculovenous shunt). Peritoneal shunts may be associated with infection (peritonitis) or mechanical obstruction (e.g., omental blockade). Some evidence suggests that delayed hypersensitivity to the shunt material is also an occasional cause of obstruction. Symptoms of shunt malfunction may be difficult to interpret, particularly if the symptoms are atypical or nonspecific or if they occur in young children. Likewise, asymptomatic shunt obstruction can take place in children in whom shunt independence has developed. Clinical evaluation of a child may not always be diagnostic of a shunt malfunction.

The characteristics of valve pumping may be useful in diagnosing shunt malfunction in some cases.[26] Partial shunt valve compression should be done because full depression and release may lead to suction of the choroid plexus. If the CT scan shows narrow (slit) ventricles, indicative of overdrainage, further valve compression may cause blockage of the shunt by suction of the choroid plexus. When palpating the shunt, a normal refill time of 15 to 30 seconds should be observed. If the valve fills more slowly than this but can be compressed easily, the obstruction is proximal to the valve. If the valve is not compressible, the blockage is either at the valve or distal to it. Proximal obstruction is more common than distal obstruction. Other sources of proximal blockage include blood clots or debris related to the surgical procedure. Sources of distal occlusion include malposition, infection, shunt disconnection, and pseudocyst formation. The entire shunt tract

and surgical incisions should be examined for signs of wound infection, disruption of the tubing, or CSF leakage around the tract. Definitive treatment usually requires shunt revision.

Infection is usually due to skin organisms overlying the valve that may ulcerate the skin and colonize the shunt.[27] Typical organisms include *Staphylococcus epidermidis* and *Staphylococcus aureus*, as well as gram-negative bacilli, which are thought to be introduced into the system during manipulation of the site.[28] Approximately 70% of these infections are seen within 2 months of shunt placement (see later under "Special Considerations—Postoperative Shunt Complications"). Other risk factors associated with shunt infection include perioperative infection and dental or urologic instrumentation. Two studies have shown that approximately 8% of neurosurgical patients with implanted shunts acquire infections.[29,30]

Radiographic evaluation of shunt function in the ED begins with a non–contrast-enhanced head CT scan and shunt series radiographs. Shunt series radiographs consist of anteroposterior (AP) and lateral skull, AP chest, and AP abdominal radiographs (Figs. 59-14 and 59-15). These films may reveal kinking, breakage, or disconnection of the catheter (Fig. 59-16). Head CT has a sensitivity of 83% in detecting shunt obstruction and a negative predictive value of 93%. Shunt series radiographs have a sensitivity of 20% and a negative predictive value of 22%. When combined, the two tests have a sensitivity of 88% and a negative predictive value of 95%. Because they are complementary, it is important to obtain both studies.[31-33] It should be noted, however, that the finding of enlarged ventricles on CT reveals little about shunt

Figure 59-14 Computed tomography (CT) evaluation of a ventriculoperitoneal shunt. Axial (*top row*) and coronal (*middle row*) CT images reveal the intracranial portion of the shunt. Mild ventriculomegaly is noted; however, this reveals little about shunt function without comparison to previous scans. The shunt (*arrows*) can also be visualized on the CT scout images (*bottom row, left and middle*). A companion chest radiograph (*bottom row, right*) demonstrates continuity of the shunt (*arrows*) through to the peritoneal cavity.

function unless comparison with previous images or serial scans show progressive ventricular expansion.

If the distal catheter is in the peritoneum and a distal obstruction is suspected or if the patient complains of abdominal pain, abdominal ultrasound should be obtained. Ultrasound may reveal a pseudocyst at the distal portion of the catheter or an abnormal fluid collection.

Finally, CSF analysis is important whenever an assessment of infection or shunt function is undertaken. Shunt evaluation should include tapping the reservoir proximal to the distal valve to allow percutaneous testing of proximal shunt patency. Although this is useful in most instances, it can be difficult to assess the rate of inflow or runoff adequately with a small-bore needle, particularly if the patient is a child or is unable to cooperate. The potential for infection is a disadvantage of percutaneous tapping. Other invasive techniques include injection of either radionuclide or contrast material into the shunt as a marker of flow. If ventricular fluid pressure is low,

there may be little evidence of flow, thus giving a false indication of shunt malfunction.

Various noninvasive techniques have been devised for assessing shunt function. Changes in visual evoked potentials associated with elevated ICP have been suggested as a means of determining function. Thermographic and Doppler detection of shunt flow is also possible. Magnetic resonance imaging techniques can likewise assess CSF flow and shunt patency.

Shunt Tapping

Clip the scalp hair over and around the reservoir, prepare the skin with a surgical scrub brush for 10 minutes, followed by the application of a povidone-iodine solution, and then allow it to fully dry. After appropriate draping, infiltrate the skin with 1% plain lidocaine to a level of adequate local anesthesia. Use a 25-gauge butterfly needle with tubing and enter the reservoir percutaneously at a 20- to 30-degree angle (Fig.

Figure 59-15 Conventional radiography standard shunt series. A standard shunt series includes skull, chest, and abdominal radiographs. **A,** This anteroposterior (AP) skull radiograph reveals the proximal intracranial portion of the shunt and a Rickham reservoir (*arrow*) over the burr hole. A companion non–contrast-enhanced head CT scan (see Fig. 59-14) is usually performed to further evaluate shunt function. **B,** The lateral skull radiograph better reveals a cylindrical Holter valve (*long arrow*) several centimeters distal to the Rickham reservoir (*short arrow*). **C,** This AP chest and abdominal radiograph reveals the distal portion of the shunt (*arrow*). Note the length of the catheter to allow patient growth. **D,** The lateral chest and abdominal view redemonstrates the course of the shunt.

Figure 59-16 Before and after series of a shunt malfunction. The left column (**A-C**) demonstrates a malfunctioning shunt. The right column (**D-F**) is the same patient after shunt revision. **A,** The shunt has become disconnected at the valve; no efferent catheter tubing is seen coming from the inferior portion of the valve (*arrow*). **B,** The catheter has migrated inferiorly and has coiled in the pelvis (*arrow*). **C,** Head computed tomography (CT) scan showing ventriculomegaly (*arrow*), a direct result of the shunt malfunction. **D,** After shunt revision, the lateral skull radiograph shows that a catheter is now connected to the valve (*arrows,* difficult to appreciate on this film). **E,** The catheter is seen coursing through the abdomen (*arrows*). **F,** Repeated head CT shows resolution of the ventriculomegaly.

59-17). Lack of CSF flow from the reservoir indicates a proximal obstruction unless the ventricles are completely deflated (slit ventricles syndrome). Even so, a small amount of CSF should be obtained within the tubing, thus ensuring that entry into the lumen of the reservoir has been accomplished. If the ventricles are deflated and only a small amount of CSF is aspirated, hold the end of the tubing 5 to 10 cm below the level of the reservoir to see whether CSF will fill the tubing and eventually begin to drip at the rate of 2 to 3 drops/min. If CSF is readily aspirated from the reservoir, hold the tubing vertically to obtain an indication of intraventricular pressure. This pressure reading, as well as the ease with which CSF is aspirated, will give some indication of proximal obstruction. To assess runoff or patency of the distal end, apply pressure

Figure 59-17 Tapping a ventriculoperitoneal shunt. Use a 25-gauge butterfly needle to puncture the reservoir. To avoid damage to the reservoir, the angle should be approximately 20 to 30 degrees. Note that the dome reservoir is under the skin. Before passing the butterfly needle, the skin is anesthetized, sterilized with povidone-iodine, and nicked with a No. 11 scalpel blade or a larger needle. Fluid is not aspirated but is allowed to drain passively.

to the tubing proximal to the reservoir and then deflate the reservoir without any resistance. If any resistance is encountered when deflating the reservoir, suspect a distal obstruction.

It is essential to send any aspirated CSF for laboratory analysis, including a cell count, protein, glucose, and most importantly, Gram stain and culture to evaluate the system for infection.

Special Considerations—Postoperative Shunt Complications

Major complications in the immediate postoperative period include hemorrhage, overdrainage, migration, obstruction, malpositioning, fractured tubing, infection, radiculopathy, and seizures.

Hemorrhage
Bleeding can occur after placement of a shunt. Both intracerebral and subdural hemorrhages have been noted. Intracerebral hemorrhage is due to trauma to the brain parenchyma as the catheter is passed through the ventricles. Subdural hematoma is due to sudden decompression of the ventricles, which leads to tearing of the bridging veins as the brain pulls away from the dura. Acute or chronic subdural bleeding can also be encountered in shunts with overdrainage problems.

Shunt Malfunction
The ventricles usually begin to diminish in size within a week after shunt placement in patients with high-pressure hydrocephalus, so continued enlargement suggests (but does not confirm) shunt malfunction. The shunt series images confirm the continuity of the drainage system from the insertion site

through the proximal catheter, reservoir, and distal catheter to the receiving draining cavity, most commonly the peritoneum. It is important to know that with normal-pressure hydrocephalus, the ventricles may remain large despite good functional shunting. The timing and indications for shunt placement are important factors for the neurosurgeon when assessing the urgency of management.

Seizures
Seizures are an infrequent complication of shunt placement and occur in about 5% of patients. Technically, occipital catheter placement may lessen the incidence of seizures because this location is far from the motor cortex. In patients thought to be at risk for a seizure, antiepileptic medication may be indicated.

Shunt Infection—Treatment and Prevention
Of all the potential complications associated with shunting procedures, infection is the most notorious and occurs in 2% to 10% of cases.[26] Most shunt infections appear within the first 2 months after surgery. The diagnosis may be obvious in patients with variable systematic signs, wound infection, meningitis, peritonitis, or septicemia. It is also possible that the shunt may harbor an indolent infection without symptoms or signs. Culture of CSF obtained from a shunt tap may be negative even when the shunt is ultimately shown to be infected.[34,35]

Most shunt infections are caused by otherwise nonvirulent bacteria such as *S. epidermidis*. In the presence of the shunt, these organisms exhibit unusual virulence. This reflects a variety of factors, including the ability to adhere to shunt surfaces, as well as production of mucoid substances that protect the bacteria from host defenses. The Silastic shunt material itself has an adverse effect on the immune system. Specifically, leukocytes cannot adhere to such surfaces as well as bacteria can. Controversy exists over the need for shunt removal in the treatment of infection. Although systemic antibiotics alone are of uncertain benefit, the addition of intraventricular drugs has allowed successful treatment without removal of a functioning shunt. Nevertheless, many neurosurgeons still recommend replacement of the entire shunt after the infection is eradicated.

If a shunt infection is suspected, systemic antibiotics should be given as soon as possible in the ED. Consultation with a neurosurgeon and infectious disease specialist is recommended before administering antibiotics directly into the CSF.

Acknowledgment
The author thanks Frederick K. Korley, MD, Khosrow Tabassi, MD, and Cecile G. Silvestre, MD, for their contributions to this chapter in previous editions, as well as special thanks to Stuart P. Swadron, MD.

References are available at www.expertconsult.com

CHAPTER 60

Spinal Puncture and Cerebrospinal Fluid Examination

Brian D. Euerle

Cerebrospinal fluid (CSF) examination is performed in the emergency department (ED) to obtain information relevant to the diagnosis and treatment of specific disease entities. Many urgent and life-threatening conditions require immediate and accurate knowledge of the nature of the CSF. However, on rare occasions, certain harmful consequences may result from a spinal puncture. Perform a careful neurologic examination before the procedure, and give special thought to the risks and merits of the procedure in each situation.

HISTORICAL PERSPECTIVE

In 1885, Corning punctured the subarachnoid space to induce cocaine anesthesia in a living patient.[1] In 1891, Quincke first removed CSF in a diagnostic study and introduced the use of a stylet.[2] He studied the cellular contents and measured protein and glucose levels. Quincke was also the first to record CSF pressure with a manometer. Subsequently, increasingly sophisticated bacteriologic, biochemical, cytologic, and serologic techniques were introduced. In 1919 Dandy reported on replacing CSF with air to determine normal brain anatomy and to identify pathologic changes.[3] Water-soluble contrast media have since been used to delineate the spinal subarachnoid space and cerebral cisterns. Other uses of spinal dural puncture include drainage of fluids and injection of anesthetic agents, chemotherapeutic agents, and antibiotics.

ANATOMY AND PHYSIOLOGY

In adults, CSF occupies approximately 140 mL of the spinal and cranial cavities, with approximately 30 mL in the spinal canal. This volume is the result of a balance between continuous secretion (primarily by the ventricular choroid plexus) and absorption into the venous system (mainly by way of the arachnoid villi). After formation, the fluid passes out of the ventricles via the midline dorsal foramen of Luschka and the lateral ventral foramina of Magendie. The fluid then flows into the spinal subarachnoid space, the basilar cisterns, and the cerebral subarachnoid space. The rate of production is approximately 0.35 mL/min, and ventricular production of CSF is such that there is a net flow out of the ventricles of 50 to 100 mL/day. The usual volume of CSF (15 to 20 mL) removed at lumbar puncture is commonly regenerated in about 1 hour.

CSF may have an embryologic nutritive function; at maturity, CSF most likely acts as a mechanical barrier between the soft brain and the rigid fibroosseous dura, skull, and vertebral column. It also appears to support the weight of the brain.[4] When buoyed by CSF, the functional weight of the brain is reduced from 1400 to 50 g. Contraction and expansion of CSF accommodates changes in brain volume.

Spinal Puncture

Indications
Suspected central nervous system infection (meningitis)
Suspected spontaneous subarachnoid hemorrhage
Suspected central nervous system syphilis
Suspected idiopathic intracranial hypertension

Contraindications
Absolute:
  Presence of infection near the puncture site
Relative:
  Coagulopathy
  Presence of increased intracranial pressure caused by
    a space-occupying lesion
  Severe thrombocytopenia

Complications
Brain herniation	Meningitis
Cauda equina syndrome	Minor backache
Cranial nerve VI palsy	Postdural puncture headache
Epidermoid tumor	Retroperitoneal abscess
Epidural cerebrospinal fluid collection	Subarachnoid hemorrhage
Epidural hematoma	Subdural hematoma

Equipment

The equipment for spinal puncture is most commonly found in a prepackaged kit.

Review Box 60-1   Spinal puncture: indications, contraindications, complications, and equipment.

INDICATIONS FOR SPINAL PUNCTURE

General Indications

The indications for spinal puncture have been reduced with the introduction of noninvasive diagnostic procedures—magnetic resonance imaging (MRI) and computed tomography (CT). A few clinical situations require early or even emergency spinal puncture. The primary indication for an emergency spinal tap is the possibility of central nervous system (CNS) infection (meningitis), with the exception of a suspected brain abscess or a parameningeal process. The need for early detection of meningitis results in the performance of many more lumbar punctures than ultimate diagnoses of infection.[5] No other method can be used to completely exclude meningitis.

The mere presence of a fever does not mandate lumbar puncture. However, CSF should generally be examined for evidence of infection in patients with a fever of unknown origin, especially if consciousness is altered or the immune system is impaired, even in the absence of meningeal irritation. Meningeal signs may not be present in patients who are old, debilitated, or immunosuppressed; are receiving antiinflammatory drugs; or have had partial treatment with antibiotics.[6,7] In a newborn, even a fever is not a dependable sign because temperatures may be normal or even subnormal. For infants younger than 1 year, a high index of suspicion is required to make the diagnosis of meningitis.

Approximately 25% of infants with meningitis will not have nuchal rigidity, but many appear toxic or moribund. A tense and bulging fontanelle is somewhat more reliable, although this sign may be absent in a dehydrated child. Neonatal meningitis occurs in 25% of sepsis cases. In addition, 15% to 20% of infants with meningitis have negative blood cultures.[8,9] In a child between the ages of 1 month and 3 years, fever, irritability, and vomiting are the most common signs of meningitis. Typically, handling is painful for the child, and the child cannot be comforted. In addition, an older child may complain of a headache. At all ages, patients generally appear ill and drowsy with a dulled sensorium. Physical signs become more useful in diagnosing meningitis in children older than 3 years[10] and include nuchal rigidity, Kernig's sign (effort to extend the knee is resisted), and Brudzinski's sign (passive flexion of one hip causes the other leg to rise, and effort to flex the neck makes the knees come up). The jolt accentuation test is a more sensitive sign of meningeal irritation.[11] This test is considered positive when the patient's pain is exacerbated by lateral rotation of the head to either side. A petechial rash in a febrile patient should also raise suspicion for *Neisseria* meningitis.[12] Previous use of antimicrobial agents may modify the clinical and CSF findings; partially treated children are less likely to be febrile or exhibit an altered mental status. In addition, patients in the early stages of meningitis may lack the classic features associated with advanced disease.

The second indication for emergency spinal puncture is suspected spontaneous subarachnoid hemorrhage (SAH). The diagnosis is usually made by imaging (head CT) or by the direct finding of blood in CSF obtained by spinal puncture.[13,14] The sensitivity of CT has been estimated to be as high as 95% soon after hemorrhage, but it drops in patients evaluated later than 24 hours after the event to 76% after 48 hours and to about 50% at 1 week. Before a major hemorrhage, 20% to 60% of patients with aneurysmal SAH have had a "sentinel thunderclap" or "warning leak" headache (i.e., an unusual sudden headache caused by a "minor" leak of blood from the aneurysm). The headache may precede a major rupture by hours to months. The goal of early clinical recognition is surgical or other interventional therapy before a recurrent major hemorrhage. After a warning leak, head CT is more likely to be negative, thus giving added importance to the performance of a lumbar puncture. Migraine or "vascular" headache is a common misdiagnosis in patients with SAH who initially have negative findings on head CT.

The usual clinical picture of SAH is an instantaneous excruciating headache. Patients generally recall the exact moment that the headache occurred. The location of the headache is variable and does not necessarily indicate the site of hemorrhage. Nausea, vomiting, and prostration are common symptoms, with approximately one third of patients becoming unconscious at the onset. Examination reveals an acutely ill patient with irritability or overt altered mental status. Meningeal signs are commonly present at the time of initial examination and usually develop within 2 to 3 days. The meningeal signs may become more severe during the first week after hemorrhage and correspond to the breakdown of blood in CSF. During the first week many patients are febrile, a reflection of chemical hemic meningitis.[15] Failure to detect blood radiographically in an awake patient may indicate a small hemorrhage or a predominant basal accumulation of blood. If a patient is initially seen several days after the hemorrhage, the blood may have become isodense with brain tissue and may no longer be visible on CT. The proper diagnosis would then require spinal puncture.

Newer CT scanners detect recent SAH quite accurately.[16] However, because acute SAH is not detected by the initial CT scan in at least 2% to 5% of all patients, lumbar puncture is appropriate to rule out the diagnosis with certainty.[17-19] If the neurologic picture demonstrates localizing findings, the presence of a large intracranial hematoma should be suspected, and spinal puncture is contraindicated until imaging studies delineate the nature of the lesion.

Other nonemergent reasons for examination of CSF include evaluation for CNS syphilis or unexplained seizures, instillation of chemotherapy and contrast agents, assessment for a suspected demyelinating or inflammatory CNS process, and treatment of headache from SAH. Carcinomatous meningitis and suspected spinal cord compression from metastatic disease may require spinal puncture for myelography and cytologic examination. MRI is a suitable alternative for identifying compressive myelopathy and has largely replaced contrast-enhanced myelography in developed countries.

IIH (Pseudotumor Cerebri)

Idiopathic intracranial hypertension (IIH) is a rare condition of unclear etiology. Patients with IIH have a marked elevation in intracranial pressure (ICP; usually to 250 to 450 cm H_2O) without hydrocephalus or mass lesions in the setting of normal CSF composition. Findings on neuroimaging studies are typically normal, and most cases are idiopathic. Because of the nonspecific signs and symptoms, many cases initially escape detection by clinicians. IIH has been associated with hypervitaminosis A, tetracycline, estrogen therapy, and a plethora of other conditions such as sarcoidosis, tuberculosis, and carcinomatosis. Because of the nonspecific findings, many cases initially escape detection by clinicians. IIH is most common in obese adolescent girls and young women, but it can also occur in children and men. Patients suffer from chronic headaches, typically worse with maneuvers that increase ICP (e.g., Valsalva maneuver, squatting, bending, coughing). Papilledema is frequently present. Cranial nerve palsies, particularly of the sixth cranial nerve, are due to increased ICP alone and may be falsely localizing.[20]

IIH may regress spontaneously after a few months. The major concern is visual loss, which may be permanent. The diagnosis can be made only by lumbar puncture performed after neuroimaging. This condition underscores the need to measure opening pressure during lumbar puncture whenever possible. Many cases can be controlled with medication, but occasionally, lumbar puncture is required to lower ICP. One way to lower ICP in the ED is to drain CSF via lumbar puncture by removing 5- to 10-mL aliquots of CSF and checking ICP after each removal until a pressure lower than 200 mm H_2O is achieved. Herniation does not occur despite the elevated pressure in IIH, probably because ICP is uniform in all CNS compartments. Since spinal fluid is regenerated rapidly, the procedure may need to be repeated every few days to keep CSF pressure at this level. Analysis of CSF should demonstrate all parameters to be normal. Drug therapy, in the form of acetazolamide, glycerol, diuretics, or corticosteroids, has been advocated and may negate the need for repeated lumbar puncture. Resistant cases may require shunting procedures.

Figure 60-1 This computed tomography scan demonstrates a low-density mass lesion with an enhancing rim and surrounding edema in an immunosuppressed patient with an *Aspergillus* abscess. Lumbar puncture in such a patient would be contraindicated. *(From Zitelli BJ and Davis HW: Atlas of Pediatric Physical Diagnosis. 5th ed. Philadelphia: Saunders; 2007.)*

CONTRAINDICATIONS TO SPINAL PUNCTURE

Spinal puncture is absolutely contraindicated in patients with infection in the tissues near the puncture site.[4,21] Spinal puncture is relatively contraindicated in the *presence of increased ICP caused by a space-occupying lesion.* Caution is particularly advised when lateralizing signs (hemiparesis) or signs of uncal herniation (unilateral third-nerve palsy with an altered level of consciousness) are present. In such cases, a tentorial or cerebellar pressure cone may be precipitated or aggravated by the spinal puncture. Cardiorespiratory collapse, stupor, seizures, and sudden death may occur when pressure is reduced in the spinal canal.[22]

The risk for herniation seems to be particularly pronounced in patients with brain abscesses.[23,24] Brain abscesses are frequently manifested as expanding intracranial lesions that induce headache, mental disturbances, and focal neurologic signs rather than as an infectious process with signs of meningeal irritation. Fever is often absent. In 75% of cases, a primary source of chronic suppuration is present. Common predisposing factors for brain abscess include craniofacial trauma; craniocerebral trauma; penetrating injuries that push bone fragments into the brain; large animal bites of infants' skulls; neurosurgical procedures; cardiovascular disorders treated with right-to-left shunts; bacterial endocarditis; gram-negative sepsis in neonates; dental infections; chronic sinusitis; otitis; mastoiditis; chronic abdominal, pulmonary, or pelvic infection; bacterial meningitis; and immunosuppression. Abscesses may also develop in infarcted brain tissue in septic patients if the blood-brain barrier is compromised.[25] Although the CSF is usually abnormal (elevated pressure, elevated white blood cell [WBC] count, and elevated protein concentration), spinal puncture in patients with a known or suspected abscess is contraindicated. Brain herniation markedly reduces the patient's likelihood of survival. If the history

suggests abscess, CT can rapidly diagnose and localize the lesion (Fig. 60-1).[26] Because the appearance of brain abscesses on CT is similar to that of neoplastic and vascular lesions, false-positive reports of brain abscess are possible.[26]

Spinal epidural hematomas are very rare but may occur in certain subpopulations of patients undergoing lumbar puncture. Those most at risk are individuals with a bleeding diathesis, including those treated with anticoagulants either before or immediately after lumbar puncture and those with abnormal clotting mechanisms, especially thrombocytopenia. The condition can rarely occur even with a nontraumatic tap and in the absence of a coagulation defect.[27] Spinal subdural hematomas after lumbar puncture are even rarer.[28,29] Lumbar puncture can injure the dural or arachnoid vessels, which may result in minor hemorrhage into the CSF. This is generally of little consequence. However, the number of patients with hemophilia and human immunodeficiency virus (HIV) infection who require lumbar puncture has increased since the late 1990s.

In a coagulopathic patient, attempt to correct the clotting deficiency if clinically feasible and time permits. The procedure should be performed by experienced clinicians, who are less likely to traumatize the dura. After the procedure, monitor the patient carefully for progressive back pain, lower extremity motor and sensory deficits, and sphincter impairment. Thoroughly investigate any complaints of motor weakness, sensory loss, or incontinence after lumbar puncture. Lumbar puncture may be performed in patients with a coagulation defect if the procedure is expected to provide essential information such as in the diagnosis of meningitis and the pathogen responsible. In cases of severe thrombocytopenia, infusion of platelets before the puncture may be desirable. Correct warfarin-induced coagulopathy with fresh frozen plasma (FFP) or prothrombin complex concentrate together with vitamin K. However, the vitamin K–FFP protocol may take

12 to 24 hours to totally reverse the effect of warfarin. Correct the coagulopathy before a puncture if the clinical situation permits such delay. Lumbar puncture can be performed safely in patients with hemophilia A or B whose deficient clotting factor is replenished before the procedure.[30] Additional replacement of the clotting factor after the procedure is of unknown value.

Performance of lumbar puncture in patients with leukemia and low platelet counts has also been studied. Howard and coworkers reported on 5223 lumbar punctures performed on 958 children with newly diagnosed acute lymphoblastic leukemia.[31] The platelet count was 10×10^9/L or lower in 29 children, 11 to 20×10^9/L in 170 children, and 21 to 50×10^9/L in 742 children. No serious complications were reported in any group. The overall rate of traumatic taps was 10.5%, but such taps were not associated with adverse sequelae. The authors concluded that in children with acute lymphoblastic leukemia, prophylactic platelet transfusion for lumbar puncture is not required if the platelet count is higher than 10×10^9/L. The number of patients with platelet counts lower than 10×10^9/L was too small to allow any conclusion about this group. A more recent review concluded that in the absence of additional risk factors, a platelet count of 40×10^9/L is "safe" for lumbar puncture. Lower counts are probably safe as well, but there was insufficient evidence to make recommendations.[32]

Aspirin and nonsteroidal antiinflammatory agents have not been shown to increase the risk for bleeding following lumbar puncture. Subcutaneous heparin administration is not believed to pose a substantial risk for bleeding after lumbar puncture if the total daily dose is less than 10,000 units. The risk for bleeding in patients taking clopidogrel, ticlopidine, or a glycoprotein (GP) IIb/IIIa receptor antagonist is not known but is probably small; however, use of these agents should cause the clinician to proceed with caution. In such cases, performing the procedure under fluoroscopy may be prudent if the test is needed on an emergency basis. One scenario is the need to diagnose meningitis because of an unusual or difficult-to-treat pathogen. It is necessary to withhold clopidogrel and ticlopidine 1 to 2 weeks before their anticoagulant effect has fully dissipated, thus making the decision for emergency lumbar puncture in such patients a risk-benefit scenario, with no firm guidelines. Pharmacologic data suggest that cessation of the GP IIb/IIIa receptor antagonist tirofiban may allow lumbar puncture after 8 hours and cessation of abciximab after 24 to 48 hours. Spinal hematoma may develop in 1% to 2% of patients who receive full anticoagulant therapy *after* undergoing lumbar puncture.

The clinician should proceed with caution in a patient with prior lumbar fusion or laminectomy. It is technically difficult to enter the subarachnoid space in the presence of significant postoperative changes. It would be acceptable to perform the puncture in an applicable space above or below the surgical scar; otherwise, opting for fluoroscopic guidance is prudent.

Some cases of bacterial meningitis have been related to performing lumbar puncture in a bacteremic patient. Presumably, the procedure introduces bacteria into the CSF. This phenomenon is rare, difficult to substantiate, and not supported by clinical data. Though of theoretical concern, bacteremia should not be used as a criterion to forego lumbar puncture if meningitis is suspected.

If the history and physical examination suggest a treatable illness such as meningitis or SAH, the clinician may perform a spinal puncture after careful consideration of the entire clinical picture. In all cases, undertake the study after careful thought regarding how the results will contribute to evaluation and treatment of the patient. It is unlikely that spinal puncture will beneficially alter management in patients with neoplastic disease, intracranial hematoma, abscess, a completed nonembolic infarction, or cranial trauma. Moreover, even when acute life-threatening emergencies such as SAH or meningitis are suspected, delaying CSF examination temporarily while empirical treatment proceeds is an important management option when there are concerns about the safety of the procedure.

EQUIPMENT

Assemble the standard equipment for a spinal puncture before starting the procedure. Place it where the operator can easily access it. A standard-point Quincke cutting needle is most often used and supplied with the kit. Some operators prefer to use a Sprotte needle (Havel's, Inc., Cincinnati, OH) or a Whitacre needle (Becton Dickinson and Company, Rutherford, NJ) to minimize any dural injury associated with passage of the needle (Fig. 60-2). These styletted needles have a side port for withdrawal of fluid and, theoretically, are more likely to separate than cut the dural tissue.

Although commercial kits provide most of the items needed for lumbar puncture, the operator should bring additional supplies, including supplemental spinal needles, specimen tubes, gauze, antiseptic solution, additional local anesthetic, needles and syringes, and extra sterile gloves of the appropriate size (see Review Box 60-1).

PROCEDURE

Lumbar puncture is commonly carried out with the patient in the lateral recumbent position (Fig. 60-3). A line connecting the posterior superior iliac crests intersects the midline at approximately the L4 spinous process (Fig. 60-4). Spinal needles entering the subarachnoid space at this point are well below the termination of the spinal cord, and the only important neurologic structure is the cauda equina. Generally, the needle pushes isolated nerves to the side during advancement. The adjacent interspace above or below may be used, depending on which area appears to be most accessible to palpation. The space between the lumbar vertebrae is relatively wide. In the thoracic region, the spinous processes overlap and are directed caudally; therefore, there is no midline area free of overlying bone. In adults, the spinal cord extends to the lower level of L1 or the body of L2 in 31% of persons, thus eliminating higher levels as sites for puncture. Puncture in adults and older children may be performed from the L2-L3 interspace to the L5-S1 interspace.

Developmentally, the spinal canal and the spinal cord are of equal length in the fetus. Growth of the cord does not keep pace with the longitudinal growth of the spinal canal. At birth, the cord ends at the level of the L3 vertebra. Consequently, in infants the needle should be placed at the L4-L5 or L5-S1 interspace. The subarachnoid space extends to the S2 vertebral level; however, the overlying bony mass prevents entry into this lowermost portion of the subarachnoid space.

Figure 60-2 A, Various spinal needles. **B,** Penetration of the dura by Whitacre (pencil-point) and Quincke (cutting) needles. The Whitacre needle separates the fibers of the dura without cutting them, whereas the Quincke needle cuts the fibers. The Quincke needle leaves a hole in the dura through which cerebrospinal fluid can leak until the hole heals several days or weeks later. Use of the Whitacre needle has been associated with a lower incidence of post–lumbar puncture headache. (*A, From Thomsen T, Setnik G, eds. Procedures Consult—Emergency Medicine Module. Copyright 2008 Elsevier Inc. All rights reserved.*)

When performed with parenteral sedation and proper local anesthesia, a spinal tap is neither overly distressing nor very painful to most patients. Almost all patients are likely to have some anxiety about a spinal puncture for several reasons, including the stories commonly told of severe complications. Explain the procedure in advance and discuss each step during the course of the test to reduce the patient's anxiety. Inquire about any history of allergies to local anesthetic agents and topical antiseptics. Obtain written informed consent whenever possible. In all cases, include a detailed procedural note that documents the process of patient or guardian education regarding the indications, procedural techniques, risks and benefits, alternatives to the procedure, and the patient's or guardian's consent for the procedure. Abridge this step when the patient is critically ill or eliminate it when the patient is mentally incapacitated and no guardian is present. Many

patients greatly fear lumbar puncture, and hence some clinicians provide routine preprocedure sedation or analgesia if not clinically contraindicated. Intravenous midazolam and fentanyl are useful adjuncts, but practices vary and there is no consensus on standards with regard to the use or nonuse of preprocedure medications. In anxious patients it is reasonable to give a benzodiazepine agent parenterally (e.g., midazolam, 0.1 to 2.5 mg intravenously for a healthy adult younger than 60 years of age) to facilitate the procedure. Fentanyl at a dose of 0.5 to 1.5 µg/kg (adults) is a reasonable alternative.

The next important step is positioning the patient. Generally, place older children and adults in the lateral decubitus position for the procedure. Give the patient a pillow to keep the head in line with the vertebral axis. Position the shoulders and hips perpendicular to the stretcher or table. Use a firm table or bed when available. Because flexion of the neck does not facilitate the procedure to any great extent and severe flexion may add to the patient's discomfort, this step may be omitted. Severe flexion of the neck in an infant may cause airway compromise. Pull the knees up to the chest and arch the lower part of the patient's back toward the clinician by having the patient's knees drawn toward the chest.

Some clinicians place the patient in an upright sitting position because the midline is more easily identified. This position can be used in both adults and infants (Fig. 60-5). The higher CSF hydrostatic pressure while sitting may aid flow of CSF in a dehydrated patient. Observe caution regarding orthostatic changes in blood pressure and airway maintenance. Generally, allow a sitting patient to lean onto a bedside stand and use a pillow to rest the head and arms. Have an assistant support the patient during the procedure. Radiographic studies by Fisher and colleagues have demonstrated the advantages of hip flexion when the sitting position is used.[33] To accomplish hip flexion, use a stool to support the patient's feet, which pulls the knees up toward the chest. This increases lumbar interspinous width, which may increase the success and ease of needle passage.

Iatrogenic infection after lumbar puncture is extremely rare. Use sterile gloves during the procedure, but the need for face masks is debatable.[34-36] Apply the same guidelines for control of central line infection (caps, gowns, gloves, and masks) to lumbar puncture.[37] Wash the patient's back with an antiseptic solution applied in a circular motion and increase the circumference of the cleansed area with each motion. Place a sterile towel or drape between the patient's hip and the bed. Commercial trays have a second sterile drape with a hole that may be centered over the site selected for the procedure.

Infiltrate the skin and deeper subcutaneous tissue generously with local anesthetic. Buffered or warmed 1% lidocaine is preferred. Warn the patient about transient discomfort from the anesthetic. Anesthetizing the deeper subcutaneous tissue significantly reduces procedural discomfort. Merely raising a skin wheal is insufficient anesthesia. Some operators not only anesthetize the interspinous ligament but also apply local anesthetic in a vertically fanning distribution on both sides of the spinous processes near the lamina. Such a field block on each side of the spinous processes anesthetizes the recurrent spinal nerves that innervate the interspinous ligaments and muscles.

While waiting for the anesthetic to take effect, connect the stopcock and manometer and ensure that the valve is working. Commonly, a 3.5-inch, 20-gauge needle is used in adults, and

SPINAL PUNCTURE

1 Position the patient in the bed. Generally, the lateral decubitus position is preferred. Arch the patient's back towards you.

Consider mild sedation or analgesia when clinically appropriate.

2 Identify and mark anatomic landmarks. The L4 spinous process is at the level of the posterior-superior iliac crests.

— Level of iliac crest

— Anatomic midline

3 Prepare the skin with antiseptic solution. Apply in a circular motion with a gradually increasing circumference.

4 Apply a sterile drape.

5 Create a wheal with anesthetic in the skin overlying the entry site. Then, infiltrate and anesthetize the deeper tissues.

6 Insert the needle in the midline. Hold the needle parallel to the bed, and advance it toward the umbilicus. Remove the stylet periodically to check for CSF.

7 CSF will flow from the needle hub when the subarachnoid space has been penetrated.

8 Attach the manometer and measure the opening pressure.

9 Collect the CSF sample in sequential, numbered vials.

10 Replace the stylet before removing the needle.

Figure 60-3 Spinal puncture. *CSF,* cerebrospinal fluid.

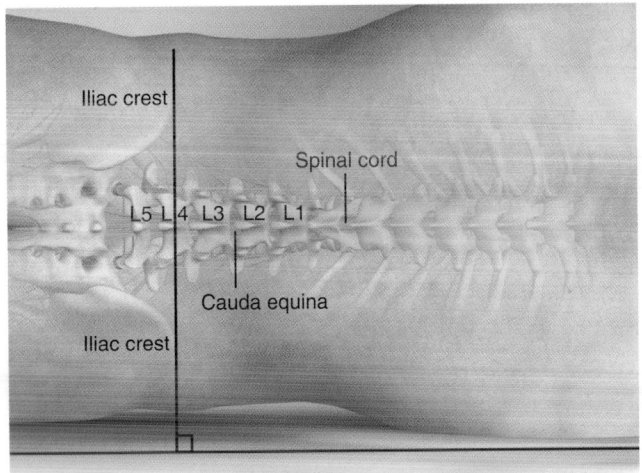

Figure 60-4 The L4 spinous process is at the level of the posterior superior iliac crest. The spinal cord ends approximately at the level of L1 or L2 in adults; fibers of the cauda equina extend inferiorly from there. When the patient is positioned correctly for lumbar puncture, an imaginary line connecting the iliac crests will be exactly perpendicular to the bed, and the spine will be parallel to the bed.

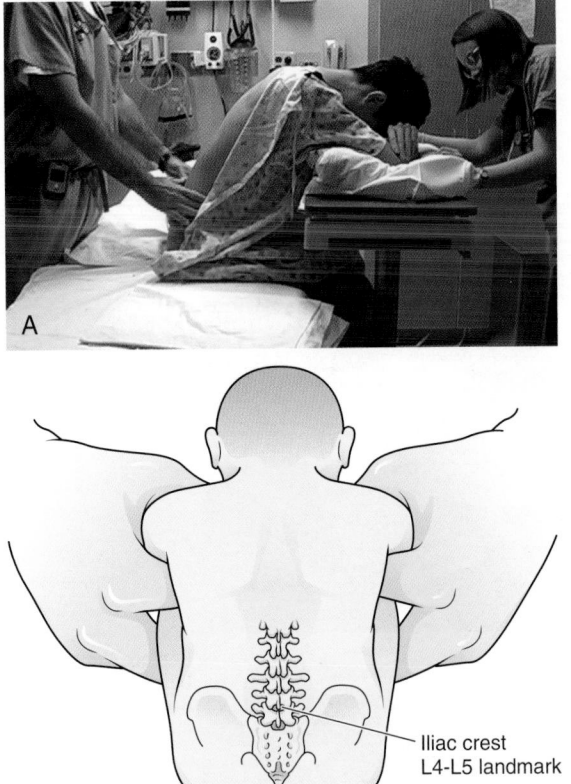

Figure 60-5 A, Many clinicians prefer the sitting position for lumbar puncture because of the ease of entering the dural space. However, the opening pressure obtained in this position is not accurate. If possible, place the patient in the lateral decubitus position for measurement of pressure, usually after fluid has been collected. **B,** Upright positioning in an infant. (**A,** *From Thomsen T, Setnik G, eds.* Procedures Consult—Emergency Medicine Module. *Copyright 2008 Elsevier Inc. All rights reserved.* **B,** *from Dieckmann R, Selbst S, eds.* Pediatric Emergency and Critical Care Procedures. *St. Louis: Mosby; 1997.)*

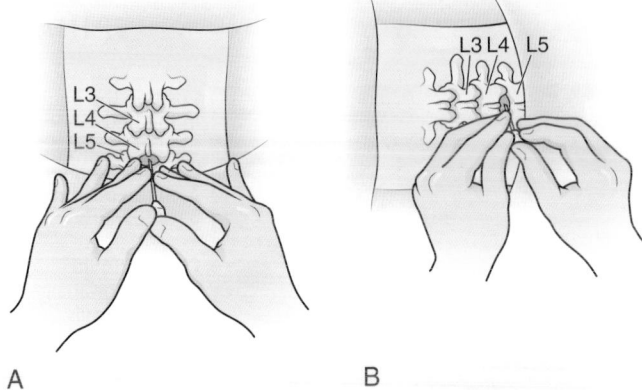

Figure 60-6 Various ways to hold the spinal needle.

a 2.5-inch, 22-gauge needle is used in children (a 1.5-inch, 22-gauge needle is available for infants). Needles of these sizes have enough rigidity to allow the procedure to be accomplished easily but make less of a dural tear than larger needles do. Patients should be told to report any pain and be informed that they will feel some pressure.

With the patient in the lateral decubitus position, place the needle into the skin in the midline, parallel to the bed. Hold the needle between both thumbs and index fingers (Fig. 60-6). After the subcutaneous tissue has been penetrated, angle the needle toward the umbilicus. The bevel of the needle should be facing straight up toward the ceiling.

The supraspinal ligament connects the spinous processes, and the interspinal ligaments join the inferior and superior borders of adjacent spinous processes. The ligamentum flavum is a strong, elastic membrane that may reach a thickness of 1 cm in the lumbar region. The ligamentum flavum covers the interlaminar space between the vertebrae and assists the paraspinous muscles in maintaining an upright posture (Fig. 60-7). The ligaments are stretched in a flexed position and are more easily crossed by the needle. The ligaments offer resistance to the needle, and a "pop" is often felt as they are penetrated. Hold the stylet in place during advancement but remove it frequently to see whether the subarachnoid space has been reached. The pop may not be felt with the very sharp needles contained in disposable trays.

If bone is encountered, partially withdraw the needle to subcutaneous tissue. Repalpate the back and ascertain that the needle is in the midline. Directing the tip of the needle toward the navel often enhances navigation of the interspinal space. If bone is encountered again, slightly withdraw and reangle the needle so that the point is placed at a more sharply cephalad angle (Fig. 60-8). This approach should avoid the inferior spinous process.

Normal CSF is a clear fluid and will flow from the needle when the subarachnoid space has been penetrated and the stylet is removed. In normal patients, the dura will be penetrated when the needle is advanced about one half to three fourths of its length. In obese patients, the entire length of the needle may be required to reach the subdural space (Fig. 60-9).

If feasible, attach the manometer and record the opening pressure (Fig. 60-10). This step is commonly omitted in critically ill patients. Pressure readings from a struggling patient may be inaccurate. Readings are valid only if taken with the patient relaxed and in the lateral decubitus position (not the sitting position). A three-way stopcock, supplied in disposable

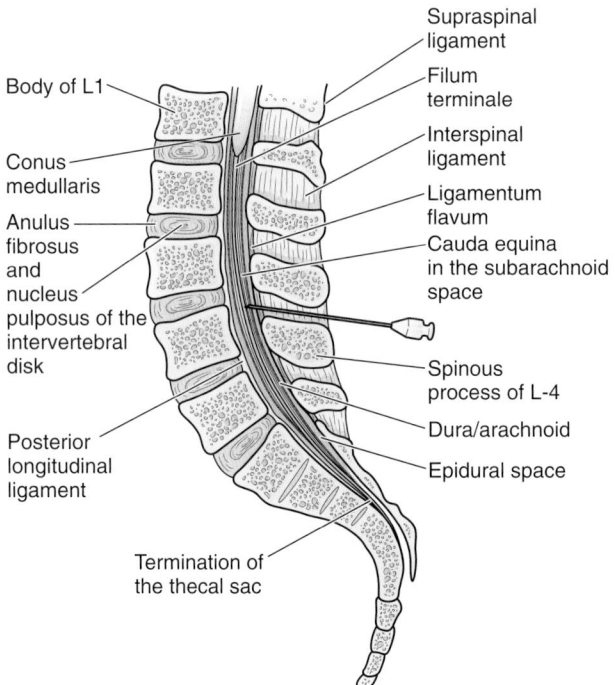

Figure 60-7 Midsagittal section through the lumbar spinal column with a spinal puncture needle in place between the spinous processes of L3 and L4. Note the slightly ascending direction of the needle. The needle has pierced three ligaments and the dura/arachnoid and is in the subarachnoid space. (*From Lachman E. Anatomy as applied to clinical medicine.* New Physician. *1968;17:145.*)

Figure 60-8 A, This 22-gauge spinal needle has struck bone during advancement (notice the bend in the needle) and needs to be repositioned. **B,** If bone is encountered, it is usually the inferior spinous process (red spinal needle). The needle must be partially withdrawn into subcutaneous tissue and then readvanced in a more cephalad direction (*green needle*).

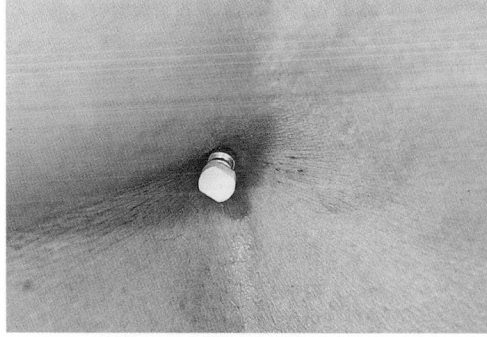

Figure 60-9 The spinal needle is usually advanced one half to three fourths of its length before the spinal canal is reached. In this obese patient, the needle was advanced all the way to the hub of the needle before spinal fluid was returned.

trays, allows both collection of CSF and measurement of opening pressure with a single needle. Positioning of the manometer is often more convenient if an extension tube (provided with most disposable trays) connects the needle hub to the stopcock, which in turn is attached to the manometer. Position the manometer so that the "zero" mark is at the level of the spinal needle. Then ask the patient to relax. Extending the legs after needle placement does not meaningfully decrease opening CSF pressure.[38] The observation of phasic changes in the fluid column with respirations and arterial pulsations confirms needle placement in the subarachnoid space. If the needle is against a nerve root or is only partially within the dura, the pressure may be falsely low, and respiratory excursions will not be reflected in the manometer. Minor rotation of the needle may solve these problems. Hyperventilation will reduce the pressure readings because of hypocapnia and the resultant cerebral vasoconstriction.

After measuring the pressure, turn the stopcock and collect enough fluid to perform all the studies desired. The first sample of fluid exits from the manometer if pressure has been measured, and then additional fluid flows from the spinal canal. Even if the pressure is elevated, remove sufficient fluid for performance of all indicated studies because the risk associated with the procedure involves the dural rent, not only the amount of fluid initially removed. Presumably, more fluid will subsequently be lost through the hole in the dura. Replace the stylet into the needle before withdrawing it.

Commercial trays generally supply four specimen tubes. One tube is commonly used for determining protein and glucose levels and for electrophoretic studies, another is used for microbiologic and cytologic studies, and a third is used for serologic tests. Cell counts should be performed in the first

and third tubes to help differentiate traumatic taps from true SAH. Depending on the clinical scenario, additional tests may be indicated. Use special stains, such as India ink for suspected *Cryptococcus* infection in patients with acquired immunodeficiency syndrome (AIDS), acid-fast stain in patients with possible tuberculous meningitis, and viral studies in patients with suspected encephalitis. The fourth tube can be stored under refrigeration in the laboratory for any additional studies that may be required after the initial assessment.

Traumatic taps are common and usually clinically inconsequential. Nevertheless, they can be minimized by proper patient and needle positioning. A traumatic tap most commonly occurs when the subarachnoid space is transfixed at the entrance of the ventral epidural space, where the venous plexus is heavier. A plexus of veins forms a ring around the cord, and these veins may be entered if the needle is advanced too far ventrally or is directed laterally (Fig. 60-11). If blood is encountered and the fluid does not clear, repeat the procedure at a higher interspace with a fresh needle. A traumatic tap, per se, is not a particularly dangerous problem in a patient with normal coagulation, and no specific precautions are needed if blood-tinged fluid is obtained. However, observe for signs of cord or spinal nerve compression from a hematoma developing within the first several hours in patients with a coagulopathy.

Lateral Approach for Lumbar Puncture

The supraspinal ligament might be calcified in older persons, thus making a midline perforation difficult. A calcified ligament may deflect the needle. In this case, use a slightly lateral approach. Because the lower lamina rises upward from the midline, direct the needle slightly cephalad to miss the lamina and slightly medially to compensate for the lateral approach. The needle passes through the skin, superficial fascia, fat, the dense posterior layer of the thoracolumbar fascia, and the erector spinae muscles. The needle then penetrates the ligamentum flavum (bypassing the supraspinal and interspinal ligaments), the epidural space, and the dura before CSF is obtained (Fig. 60-12). Lateral cervical puncture is an alternative approach that can be performed utilizing an insertion site 1 cm inferior and 1 cm dorsal to the mastoid process.[39]

Lumbar Puncture in Infants

Lumbar puncture in infants is usually performed to exclude meningitis or encephalitis. The sitting position may allow the midline to be identified more easily. Use of a needle without a stylet has been suggested for small infants because this device allows the pressure to be estimated as the needle

punctures the dura.[40] However, failure to use a stylet may cause the subsequent development of an intraspinal epidermoid tumor.[41] Use of a butterfly infusion set needle simplifies the procedure, which is helpful when managing a squirming or hyperactive patient.[40] In general, a stylet is recommended primarily at the time of skin penetration and on needle withdrawal, although many operators use the stylet during any advancement of the needle.

Figure 60-11 The spinal contents at L4 and L5 show the relationship of a lumbar puncture needle to the major vessels at this level. The major radiculomedullary vein, shown accompanying the L5 nerve root, is situated far lateral to a needle correctly positioned in the midline of the dural sac. Note the avascular subdural space. *(From Edelson RN, Chernik IVL, Rosner JB. Spinal subdural hematomas.* Arch Neurol. *1974;31:134. Illustration by Lynn McDowell. Reproduced by permission. Copyright 1974, American Medical Association.)*

Figure 60-10 To measure the opening pressure, attach the manometer to the needle hub with a 3-way stopcock. The "zero" mark of the manometer should be level with the site of needle entry.

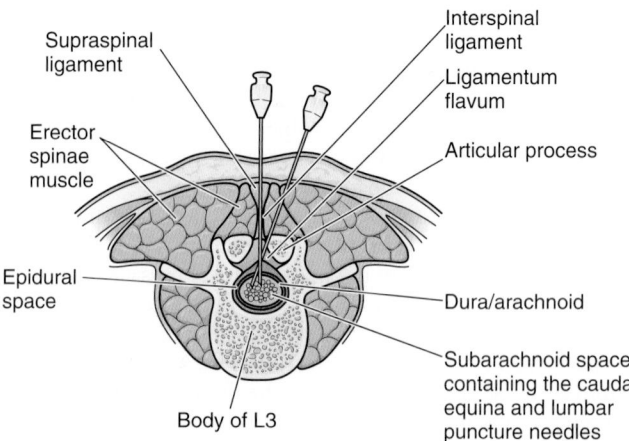

Figure 60-12 Horizontal section through the body of L3. Note the two puncture needles in the subarachnoid space. The medial needle is in the midline. The lateral needle exemplifies the lateral approach, which avoids the occasionally calcified supraspinal ligament. Note the lateral needle piercing the intrinsic musculature of the back and only one ligament, the ligamentum flavum. *(From Lachman E. Anatomy as applied to clinical medicine.* New Physician. *1968;17:745.)*

If the child's neck is very tightly flexed, CSF might not be obtained. However, if the head is held in midflexion, CSF usually flows briskly. If CSF fails to flow, gently suction with a 1.0-mL syringe to exclude a low-pressure syndrome. Because pressure readings are inaccurate in a struggling child, measurement of pressure is not commonly attempted in infants and young children.[42]

Avoid prolonged severe flexion of the neck in an infant because it may produce dangerous airway obstruction. If the infant suddenly stops crying, check the airway immediately.[43] Proper positioning is best accomplished by an assistant, who maintains the spine maximally flexed by partially overlying the child and using the chest and body weight to immobilize the thorax and hips while holding the child behind the shoulders and knees.[44] Infants have poor neck control; therefore, the assistant must also ensure that the child maintains an open airway. Pay particular attention to avoiding marked neck and trunk flexion. Incorrect positioning usually results in multiple punctures and a bloody tap.

Newborn and preterm infants may experience significant hypoxia and clinical deterioration during lumbar puncture; a sitting position appears to be preferable.[45] Lumbar puncture in infants with respiratory distress syndrome may pose greater risk than benefit.[46] This is a problem primarily in neonates but may also apply to younger infants with sepsis. Closely monitor all infants with serious cardiopulmonary disease during the procedure. Preoxygenation with or without monitoring oxygen saturation may be used as a precaution.

Although local anesthesia or sedation has not been a routine practice during lumbar puncture in an infant or child, it is being reconsidered.[47,48] Neonates perceive pain, and local anesthesia neither produces physiologic instability nor makes the procedure more difficult.[49,50] The use of topically applied EMLA (eutectic mixture of local anesthetics) (AstraZeneca) reduces the pain associated with needle insertion in newborns.[51] Sedation of an anxious child may be considered, but sedatives are relatively contraindicated in an obtunded patient without a protected airway and in the setting of hemodynamic instability.

The Difficult Lumbar Puncture

The traditional approach to lumbar puncture depends on palpation of bony landmarks to determine the correct location for insertion of the needle. However, landmarks are difficult to palpate in overweight and obese patients.[52] When lumbar puncture fails, the usual alternative has been fluoroscopic guidance, which necessitates movement of the patient out of

---

ULTRASOUND: Lumbar Puncture   *by Christine Butts, MD*

When ultrasound is used to guide lumbar puncture, it is generally done in a static manner: the ultrasound probe is used to determine the site of skin entry, the skin is marked, and the probe is then set aside.

Equipment

A linear probe is preferred, although for patients with an extremely high body mass index, a curvilinear probe may be required because of the distance between the skin and the spine.

Image Interpretation

The bony spinous process will appear as a hyperechoic crescent-shaped structure with posterior acoustic shadowing. In the transverse view, acquisition of a perfectly symmetric image will provide assurance that the probe is in the anatomic midline (Fig. 60-US1). In the longitudinal view, multiple spinous processes can be visualized, along with the interspaces between them (Fig. 60-US2).

Figure 60-US1 Transverse image of the lumbar spine. The crescent-shaped hyperechoic structure (*arrow*) is a spinous process. Note the presence of posterior acoustic shadowing. Align the probe so that the spinous process is directly centered in the image. The general symmetry of the image provides additional assurance that the probe is centered correctly.

Figure 60-US2 Longitudinal image of the lumbar spine. Again visible are the spinous processes (*small arrows*), which appear as crescent-shaped hyperechoic structures with acoustic shadowing. In between each spinous process is the interspinous space (*large arrow*). Note how this space is bordered on either side by the acoustic shadow of the spinous process. Note also how the probe is centered directly over the interspace.

Continued

ULTRASOUND: Lumbar Puncture, cont'd

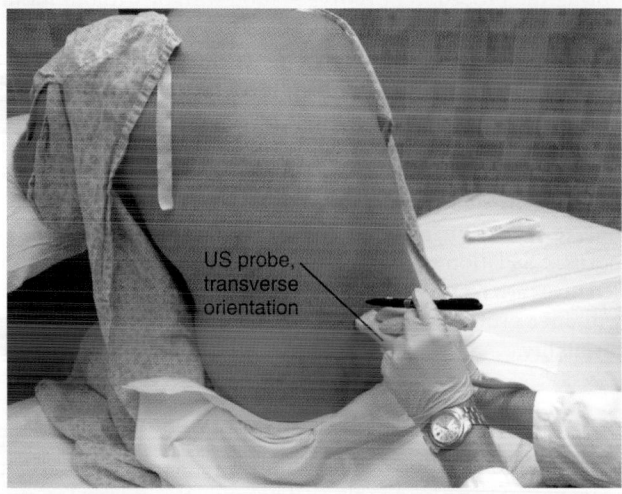

Figure 60-US3 First use the ultrasound (US) probe in the transverse orientation at the level of the iliac crests, and obtain an image with the shadow of the spinous process centered on the screen (as in Fig. 60-US1). Mark the skin at the exact midpoint of the transducer. This represents the anatomic midline.

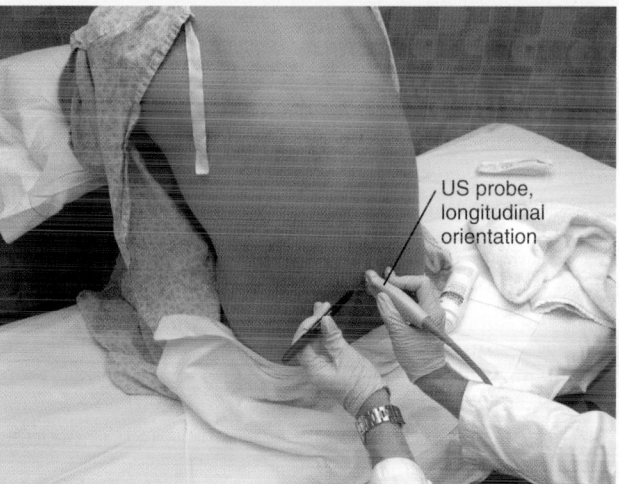

Figure 60-US4 Rotate the ultrasound (US) probe 90 degrees and obtain a midline longitudinal view. Position the probe so that the interspace is centered on the screen (as in Fig. 60-US2). Mark the skin at the midpoint of the transducer. This represents the level of needle entry.

Procedure and Technique

To perform ultrasound-guided lumbar puncture, position the patient in the usual manner. Place the ultrasound probe over the spine in a transverse orientation at the level of the iliac crests such that the shadow caused by the spinous process is centered on the screen. Use a pen to mark the skin on each side of the transducer, exactly at the midpoints (Fig. 60-US3). These two marks can then be connected to mark the midline of the spine. Next, rotate the transducer 90 degrees to obtain a midline longitudinal view and position it until the gap between two spinal processes is in the center of the screen. Mark the skin at the midpoint of each side of the transducer and then connect the marks to form a single line (Fig. 60-US4). The intersection of the two lines is the site for entry of the needle (Fig. 60-US5). Cleanse the skin with antiseptic solution and perform the remainder of the procedure in the usual fashion.

Figure 60-US5 The intersection of the anatomic midline and the level of the interspinous space is the site of needle entry.

the ED, as well as the availability of an appropriately trained radiologist.[52] Bedside ultrasound is increasing being used in emergency and critical care medicine, and its scope of practice has expanded to include guidance for a number of procedures, including lumbar puncture (see Ultrasound Box).[53-56] Ultrasound can be used in adults, as well as in neonates and infants.[57]

COMPLICATIONS

Headache after Lumbar Puncture

A number of complications from lumbar puncture have been reported.[58] One of the most common is headache, which occurs after 1% to 70% of spinal taps.[59-66] In general, the development of postpuncture headache can be neither prognosticated nor prevented. The syndrome most commonly starts within the first 48 hours after the procedure (although a case occurring 12 days after the procedure has been reported)[67] and usually lasts for 1 to 2 days (occasionally as long as 14 days). Cases lasting months have been described. The headache usually begins within minutes after the patient arises and characteristically ceases as soon as the patient lies down. The pain is mild to incapacitating and is generally cervical and suboccipital in location but might involve the shoulders and the entire cranium. Exceptional cases include nausea, vomiting, vertigo, blurred vision, ear pressure, tinnitus, and stiff neck. The headache may change to a positional backache or neck ache.

The technique of spinal puncture probably has little to do with the development of a postprocedure headache. The syndrome is widely thought to be caused by leakage of fluid through the dural puncture site. This results in a reduction in CSF volume below the cisterna magna and downward movement of brain tissue, along with displacement and stretching of pain-sensitive structures such as the meninges and vessels, and causes a traction headache. The recumbent position brings relief because the weight of the brain is shifted cephalad. Another proposed mechanism is cerebral vasodilation. A more recent hypothesis suggests that the headache is caused by an altered distribution of craniospinal elasticity and acute intracranial venous dilation.[68] Some authors have commented on the incidence and severity of post–dural puncture headache as being related to the orientation of the spinal needle bevel and its type and size.[69-79] It is clear that the incidence of post–dural puncture headache is lower when the bevel of the needle is oriented parallel to the longitudinal axis of the spine. Until relatively recently the explanation for this was that the parallel bevel would separate rather than cut the longitudinal dural fibers and thus produce a smaller dural hole and less CSF leakage. However, it is now known that the dural fibers are oriented randomly, not longitudinally.[80] Even with random fiber orientation, back flexion is more likely to close a dural hole in the longitudinal plane than a hole in the horizontal plane.

The two basic types of spinal needles are cutting (Quincke) and noncutting or pencil point (Sprotte and Whitacre). Noncutting needles cause a lower incidence of headache after dural puncture, perhaps because the tip of the needle tends to separate rather than cut the dural fibers. It has traditionally been thought that the dural hole resulting from puncture with a noncutting needle is smaller than that created by puncture with a cutting needle; however, this may not be true. The important difference may be that the cutting needle causes a clean-cut opening in the dura whereas the noncutting needle produces a jagged opening with rough edges.[81] The jagged opening may produce a more intense inflammatory response that results in edema and more complete closure of the hole. The use of atraumatic spinal needles is not routine.[82] As more spinal kit manufacturers include them in kits, their use might increase.[83] A single-institution study suggested that routine use of noncutting needles yields a potential cost savings.[84] However, in thick-skinned individuals, passage of a thin, noncutting needle may be technically difficult. Making the initial pass with a thicker cutting needle to the level of the interspinal ligament, followed by removal and advancement of a noncutting needle in the same soft tissue tract, can be helpful.

Use of a smaller-diameter needle is one intervention that will probably cause a lower incidence of postpuncture headache because it creates a smaller dural hole. If diameter were the only consideration, as small a needle as possible would be used. However, a needle must provide adequate CSF flow rates to allow timely CSF collection and pressure measurement. With a very small needle, a syringe may be needed to withdraw fluid, and pressure cannot be recorded easily. In addition, technically, a small needle such as a 26 gauge is difficult to place and manipulate into a position in which it does not become intermittently obstructed by nerve roots. When these characteristics are considered, a 20- to 22-gauge

atraumatic needle seems to be the best overall choice for diagnostic lumbar puncture.[72]

Despite common beliefs about techniques and postprocedure interventions, lumbar puncture headaches may not be completely preventable. Studies of the influence of directives such as strict bed rest on postpuncture headache have yielded contradictory results, with no consensus on any specific preventive intervention forthcoming concerning the worsening of, improvement in, or effect on the incidence. Brocker reported a reduction in the incidence of headache from 36.5% to 0.5% when patients lie prone instead of supine for 3 hours after puncture with an 18-gauge needle.[85] He postulated that the prone position caused hyperextension of the spine and disrupted alignment of the holes in the dura and the arachnoid, thus making leakage less likely. Thoennissen and coworkers concluded that there was no evidence that longer bed rest after lumbar puncture was better than immediate mobilization or short bed rest in reducing the incidence of headache.[86] There appears to be no reason to enforce bed rest following lumbar puncture.

Other factors that might influence the incidence of a post–spinal puncture headache were reviewed by Fishman and by Lin and Giederman.[21,87] The incidence is higher in young patients than in older patients and is also increased in females and individuals with a history of headache. Many medications have been advocated for the treatment of headache after lumbar puncture: barbiturates, codeine, neostigmine, ergots, diphenhydramine (Benadryl), dimenhydrinate (Dramamine), caffeine, amphetamine sulfate (Benzedrine), ephedrine, intravenous fluids (normal saline, lactated Ringer's solution), magnesium sulfate, and vitamins.[21,88-90]

Caffeine is a traditional common initial intervention for postpuncture headache, and it appears to be of benefit.[90] Caffeine can be administered in the ED, and pain relief can be seen within a few hours and is thought to result from caffeine's vasoconstrictive effect on the cerebral vasculature. One suggested regimen is 500 mg of caffeine (sodium benzoate) diluted in 1000 mL of normal saline infused over a 1- to 2-hour period. A second dose can be given if the headache is not relieved. If successful, consumption of caffeinated beverages may be continued as an outpatient.

Most postpuncture headaches can be managed by bed rest with the head in the horizontal position. Avoid dehydration because it lowers CSF pressure and might aggravate the headache. Although dehydration should be avoided, the role of fluid supplementation in the prevention of post–dural puncture headache remains uncertain.

Simple analgesics are commonly prescribed, but they have no apparent advantage over bed rest and fluid intake. A patient with a prolonged headache after spinal puncture should be reassessed to rule out structural causes. Because a spinal headache has classic signs and symptoms, if the headache is not postural, consider other causes.

In summary, because most post–lumbar puncture headaches are mild and self-limited, conservative therapy for the first 24 to 48 hours is recommended. Bed rest and oral analgesics, including opioids, are usually effective, as well as perhaps oral caffeine drinks, but for those refractory to conservative measures, an epidural blood patch is recommended.

For patients with a prolonged low-pressure headache, placement of an epidural blood patch by experienced operators is highly successful and often provides dramatic relief.[91-95] Consider a blood patch for all patients with seriously symptomatic spinal headaches. Perform an epidural tap at the level of the previous lumbar puncture. Use the loss-of-resistance technique with sterile saline to locate the epidural space.[96] Draw 10 to 20 mL of autologous blood into a syringe aseptically and slowly inject it (1 to 2 mL every 10 seconds) into the epidural space at the site of the dural puncture.[97] Slow or discontinue the injection if back pain or paresthesia develops. Keep the patient supine for 1 hour while hydration is administered intravenously. Relief usually occurs within 20 to 30 minutes after the procedure. Epidural patches are less likely to be effective if symptoms have been present for more than 2 weeks. Pain is relieved when the blood patch forms a gelatinous tamponade that stops the CSF leak and immediately elevates CSF pressure. Patch failures (15% to 20%) are believed to be caused by improper needle placement, injection of an inadequate quantity of blood (after which a second patch is usually successful), or an incorrect diagnosis.

Complications reported after placement of an epidural patch include back stiffness, paresthesia, radicular pain, subdural hematoma, adhesive arachnoiditis, and bacterial meningitis.[98] The procedure should be used in patients with refractory headaches that do not respond to conservative therapy, and it should be performed by clinicians trained in the procedure.

Infection

Spinal puncture is contraindicated in the presence of local infection at the puncture site (cellulitis, suspected epidural abscess, or furunculosis) because of the danger of inducing meningitis. A large concentration of bacteria in the bloodstream at the time of CSF examination is associated with meningitis. The meningitis could be coincidental ("spontaneous") or could result from leakage of blood containing bacteria into the subarachnoid space after lumbar puncture ("induced"). It is likely that many cases of puncture-induced meningitis emerge after a cautious clinician performs a lumbar puncture early in the course of meningitis, before the infection has had time to be reflected in CSF. A recent review concluded that the majority of cases of postpuncture meningitis are probably caused by contamination of the site with aerosolized bacteria from medical personnel, contamination from skin flora, or least commonly, direct or hematogenous spread from an endogenous infectious site.[37] Suspected bacteremia is not a contraindication to lumbar puncture. Delay in diagnosis because of concern regarding the risks associated with lumbar puncture is probably more serious than the risk of causing meningitis with the procedure.[99,100]

Herniation Syndromes after Lumbar Puncture

Lumbar puncture is of value in confirming a diagnosis of meningitis, encephalitis, or SAH. Generally, when the patient has symptoms consistent with bacterial meningitis but not increased ICP, it is safe to perform lumbar puncture before a head CT scan. Lumbar puncture may also be the best initial procedure to diagnose SAH, thus reducing the need for routine CT scanning in certain low-risk patients with acute sudden headache.[101] However, in patients with focal findings, papilledema, or a suspected intracranial mass lesion, one should perform a CT scan before lumbar puncture. When meningitis remains in the differential diagnosis, antibiotics are best administered after blood is obtained for culture and before the CT scan.

Particularly in patients with supratentorial masses, there may be a large pressure gradient between the cranial and lumbar compartments. When brain volume is increased because of a mass or edema, rostrocaudal displacement may occur after lumbar puncture if the skull is intact.

The question of whether lumbar puncture precipitates brain herniation in cases in which herniation would not have occurred spontaneously cannot be answered with certainty. Controversy still exists regarding the risk for brain herniation from lumbar puncture in patients with acute bacterial meningitis, and data continue to be sparse.[102] Herniation may occur in the absence of lumbar puncture in the setting of acute bacterial meningitis and has been temporally related to the procedure. Brain herniation occurs in about 5% of patients with acute bacterial meningitis and accounts for about 30% of the deaths associated with the disease.[102] Although CT imaging may reveal contraindications to lumbar puncture, normal findings on CT do not eliminate the risk for herniation and do not necessarily mean that a lumbar puncture is safe.

Lowering pressure in the lumbar spinal canal by removing CSF can increase the gradient between the cranial and lumbar compartments and thereby theoretically promote both transtentorial and foramen magnum (cerebellar) herniation. The frequency with which lumbar puncture causes or accelerates transtentorial herniation is unknown because herniation might have developed spontaneously in a seriously ill patient without the procedure. With the current use of small-caliber spinal needles, herniation appears to be extremely rare; nonetheless, it is fully predictable neither by CT nor by opening CSF pressure readings.

A careful neurologic examination should precede all spinal punctures. When the patient has a history of headache and fever with progressive deterioration in mental status and localizing neurologic signs, spinal puncture should not be performed as the initial diagnostic procedure. Gopal and colleagues identified three statistically significant predictors of new intracranial masses: papilledema, focal abnormalities on neurologic examination, and altered mental status.[103] Greig and Goroszeniuk made similar recommendations.[104] Hasbun and associates demonstrated that in adults with suspected meningitis, the presence of any of 13 clinical features is predictive of abnormal findings on CT (Box 60-1).[105] Theoretically, the presence of abnormal findings on CT portends potential herniation, with or without lumbar puncture. The absence of abnormal findings suggests the patient is a good candidate for immediate lumbar puncture because the risk for brain herniation as a result of the procedure is low (see Box 60-1). Joffe argues that clinical signs of impending herniation are the most appropriate criteria on which to base decision making regarding the timing of lumbar puncture in patients with acute bacterial meningitis.[102] Such signs include a significantly decreased level of consciousness (Glasgow Coma Scale score ≤11), brainstem findings (pupillary changes, posturing, irregular respirations), and a very recent seizure.[102] It is recommended that these patients undergo neuroimaging (CT or MRI) and receive antibiotics empirically while awaiting the results of imaging, which will help in assessment of the safety of a subsequent lumbar puncture. Measures to lower ICP before spinal puncture may also be considered. Appropriate cultures of blood and more easily accessible body fluids should be obtained before the administration of antibiotics. Blood cultures are positive in 80% of infants with meningitis.

Critically ill patients with acute bacterial meningitis often deteriorate rapidly and experience fatal brain herniation, both shortly after lumbar puncture and in the absence of the procedure. A direct cause-and-effect relationship between lumbar puncture and brain herniation in the setting of suspected meningitis is obscure and probably cannot be defined prospectively in the ED when clinical decisions must be made. A recent review identified 22 case reports of rapid deterioration and herniation after lumbar puncture in adults and children with acute bacterial meningitis.[102] The general consensus is that less ill patients (clearly a subjective clinical judgment) with a clinical scenario that includes meningitis as a possibility can be evaluated safely with lumbar puncture. In critically ill patients, especially those with localizing neurologic signs, severely depressed level of consciousness, or papilledema, diagnostic lumbar puncture may be delayed until the risk for herniation is lower, and aggressive and empirical treatment with meningitis doses of antibiotics should proceed.

Head CT can identify hemorrhagic lesions and most neoplasms. Its results should contribute to the decision regarding the need for and the risk involved with spinal puncture. Head CT can identify patients with unequal pressure between intracranial compartments, who are at greater risk for cerebral herniation. Findings that suggest unequal pressure include (1) lateral shift of midline structures, (2) loss of the suprachiasmatic and perimesencephalic cisterns, (3) shift or obliteration of the fourth ventricle, and (4) failure to visualize the superior cerebellar and quadrigeminal plate cisterns with sparing of the ambient cisterns.[106] The presence of a mass in the posterior fossa is a strong contraindication to lumbar puncture. Unfortunately, because of bone and motion artifact, the posterior fossa may be a difficult area to visualize on CT.

Although there is no clear standard with respect to the use of CT before lumbar puncture, a reasonable and logical approach is to avoid initial lumbar puncture and first perform head CT when a mass lesion is suspected or if the patient has signs and symptoms of increased ICP (see Box 60-1). This approach correlates with the clinical policy promulgated by the American College of Emergency Physicians in 2002.[107]

Epidermoid Tumor

An epidermoid tumor or cyst is a mass of desquamated cells containing keratin within a capsule of well-differentiated stratified squamous epithelium. Congenital lesions arise from epithelial tissue that becomes sequestered at the time of closure of the neural groove between the third and the fifth weeks of embryonic life, but such lesions are rare. Acquired intraspinal epidermoid tumors result from the implantation of epidermoid tissue into the spinal canal at the time of lumbar puncture performed with needles without stylets or with ill-fitting stylets. The clinical syndrome consists of pain in the back and lower extremities developing years after spinal puncture. Failure to use a stylet on needle withdrawal might also result in aspiration of a nerve root into the epidural space.

Backache and Radicular Symptoms

Minor backache from the trauma of the spinal needle occurs in 90% of patients. Frank disk herniation has been reported from passage of the needle beyond the subarachnoid space into the anulus fibrosus. Transient sensory symptoms from irritation of the cauda equina are also common.

Other reported complications include transient unilateral or bilateral sixth-nerve palsies caused by stretching or displacement of the abducens nerve as it crosses the petrous ridge of the temporal bone, SAH, subdural and epidural hematoma, epidural CSF collection, cauda equina syndrome, anaphylactoid reactions to local anesthetics, settling of cord tumors, and retroperitoneal abscess produced by laceration of the dura in patients with meningitis.[108-114] Most of these complications are rare and seldom encountered; however, they should be considered if a patient returns after a lumbar puncture with worsening back pain or abnormal findings on neurologic examination.

The complications associated with lateral cervical and cisternal puncture are similar to those encountered with lumbar puncture. Perforation of a large vessel with resultant cisterna magna hematoma or obstruction of vertebral artery flow has been described. Puncture of the medulla oblongata may cause vomiting or apnea, and puncture of the cord may be associated with pain. Long-lasting side effects of cord puncture seem to be rare. A traumatic tap and postpuncture headache may occur.

Spinal Epidural Hemorrhage

Rarely, serious bleeding leading to spinal hematoma secondary to lumbar puncture can produce spinal cord compromise and permanent significant neurologic deficits, such as cauda equina syndrome.[27] This may occur more frequently in coagulopathic patients but can occur in those with a normal coagulation profile and a seemingly atraumatic tap. The bleeding is concealed and may be suspected only by persistent severe backache or neurologic findings. Weakness, numbness, and incontinence after spinal puncture must be investigated, usually with MRI for a possible spinal hematoma. Surgical intervention, including laminectomy and evacuation of blood, may be required and must occur in a timely manner to avoid permanent loss of neurologic function. Those with mild symptoms and progressive recovery may be managed conservatively with close monitoring.

INTERPRETATION

Pressure

CSF pressure is clinically important.[115] Measure it accurately whenever feasible. Unfortunately, in some cases it will be logistically impossible to obtain. If the lumbar puncture is being performed with the patient in a seated position, place the patient in the lateral decubitus position before a measurement is obtained. This may be done initially, before fluid is collected, or after fluid collection, in which case a closing pressure is obtained. By repositioning the patient and measuring the pressure after fluid is collected, the likelihood of the needle being displaced as a result of the repositioning is minimized.[13,17] Accurate measurement depends on cooperation of the patient. Measurements from struggling or agitated patients will probably be inaccurate; in such cases, sedation may allow more accurate readings to be obtained.

Normal CSF pressure is between 7 and 20 cm H_2O. Obese patients may have a CSF pressure of up to 25 cm H_2O. Elevated pressure is abnormal. Opening pressure is taken promptly, thereby avoiding falsely low values caused by leakage through and around the needle. Herniating cerebellar tonsils may occlude the foramen magnum and prevent increased ICP from being reflected in the lumbar pressure reading. Increased ICP can result from expansion of the brain (edema, hemorrhage, or neoplasm), overproduction of CSF (choroid plexus papilloma), a defect in absorption, or obstruction of flow of CSF through the ventricles. Cerebral edema may be associated with meningitis, CO_2 retention, SAH, anoxia, congestive heart failure, or superior vena cava obstruction. Pressure may be falsely elevated in a tense patient when the head is elevated above the plane of the needle and, possibly, in markedly obese patients and those experiencing muscle contraction.[21] Pressure is not usually measured in neonates because a struggling or crying child will have a falsely elevated pressure. Avery and colleagues concluded that for most children (1 to 18 years of age), an opening pressure above 28 cm H_2O should be considered elevated.[116]

Low pressure suggests obstruction of the needle by the meninges. Low pressure can also be seen with a spinal block. Rarely, a primary low-pressure syndrome occurs in a setting of trauma, after neurosurgical procedures, secondary to subdural hematoma in elderly patients, with barbiturate intoxication, and in cases of CSF leakage through holes in the arachnoid.[117,118]

The Queckenstedt test is useful for demonstrating obstruction in the spinal subarachnoid space,[4,21] but this test is seldom performed today because myelographic techniques have been refined and the availability of MRI has reduced the number of myelograms and associated lumbar puncture studies. However, because situations might arise when this simple and reliable test is important diagnostically, the technique is described here.

With the patient in the lateral recumbent position, compression of the jugular vein causes decreased venous return to the heart. This distends the cerebral veins and causes a rise in ICP, which is transmitted throughout the system and measured in the manometer. After 10 seconds of bilateral compression, CSF pressure usually rises to 15 cm H_2O over the initial reading and returns to baseline 10 to 20 seconds after release. If there is no change in lumbar pressure or if the rise and fall are delayed, one may conclude that the spinal subarachnoid space does not communicate with the cranial subarachnoid space. In this situation, to facilitate subsequent myelography, consider injecting Pantopaque before removing the needle. This is necessary because the lumbar dural sac may collapse and thus make it impossible to reenter the canal. If cervical cord disease is suspected, repeat the test with the neck in the neutral position, hyperextended, and flexed. When lateral sinus obstruction is suspected, use unilateral jugular venous compression (Tobey-Ayer test).

Appearance

If CSF is not crystal clear and colorless, a pathologic condition of the CNS should be suspected. The examiner should compare the fluid with water and view down the long axis of the tube or by holding both tubes against a white background. A glass tube is preferred because plastic tubes are frequently not clear. CSF will appear grossly bloody if more than 6000 red blood cells (RBCs)/μL are present. Note that the fluid may appear clear with as many as 400 RBCs/μL and 200 WBCs/μL.[21] Xanthochromia, a yellow-orange discoloration of the supernate of centrifuged CSF, is generally considered to be the result of SAH of at least a few hours' duration and has been used to differentiate prior bleeding from a traumatic tap. A traumatic tap does not usually exhibit xanthochromia (see the later section "The Traumatic Tap"). Xanthochromia is produced by red cell lysis and is caused by one or more of the following pigments: oxyhemoglobin, bilirubin, or methemoglobin

Traditionally, CSF samples have been assessed for xanthochromia by visual inspection by a laboratory technician after centrifugation of a sample of CSF. Most hospitals still use this method.[119] Recently, spectrophotometry, designed to demonstrate both oxyhemoglobin and bilirubin, has been advocated as a more precise way of determining xanthochromia. Oxyhemoglobin alone without bilirubin in a CSF sample is thought to be artifactual (traumatic). Visually, bilirubin and oxyhemoglobin cannot be differentiated. Therefore, detection of bilirubin by spectrophotometry should define xanthochromia and prompt additional investigation for SAH. Relying on spectrophotometry to identify xanthochromia without pigment differentiation will cause a high false-positive interpretation. The absence of both oxyhemoglobin and bilirubin by spectrophotometry does not support the diagnosis of SAH. Oxyhemoglobin causes red coloration; bilirubin, yellow; and methemoglobin, brown. Oxyhemoglobin is seen within 2 hours after subarachnoid bleeding and red cell lysis, but it may be detected immediately if the bleeding is profuse. Formation of oxyhemoglobin peaks 24 to 48 hours after hemorrhage, and the discoloration disappears in 3 to 30 days.[4]

Blood must be present in CSF (in vivo) for a number of hours for bilirubin to appear; it will not appear spontaneously once CSF is in the collection tube. The appearance of bilirubin in CSF involves the conversion of oxyhemoglobin by the enzyme heme oxygenase. The enzyme is found in the choroid plexus, the arachnoid, and the meninges. Enzyme activity appears approximately 12 hours after the hemorrhage.[4] Bilirubin may persist in CSF for 2 to 4 weeks. Moreover, bilirubin in CSF caused by hepatic or hemolytic disease does not appear until a serum level of 10 to 15 mg of total bilirubin per 100 mL is reached, unless underlying disease associated with high CSF protein levels is present. Xanthochromia may also be seen with CSF protein values above 150 mg/dL. CSF may clot in patients with a complete spinal block and very high CSF protein.

Graves and Sidman noted that an RBC concentration of 5000/µL, created by adding RBCs to acellular CSF, will produce xanthochromia evident on spectrophotometry by 2 hours.[120] The addition of RBCs to achieve RBC concentrations of 20,000/µL and 30,000/µL will produce xanthochromia by 1 hour or immediately, respectively. Therefore, xanthochromia may occur with a traumatic tap and does not always indicate SAH.

Methemoglobin is a reduction product of oxyhemoglobin that is characteristically found in encapsulated subdural hematomas and in old intracerebral hematomas.

Cells

In adults, WBC counts higher than 5 cells/µL indicate the presence of a pathologic condition. A recent large study by Kestenbaum and colleagues determined 95th percentile WBC reference values in normal infants: 19 cells/µL for infants 28 days of age or younger and 9 cells/µL for those between the ages of 29 and 56 days.[121] A median CSF WBC count of 271 WBCs/µL has been reported in infants with group B *Streptococcus* in the era of intrapartum antibiotic prophylaxis. The CSF WBC count in infants is higher with gram-negative meningitis than with gram-positive CNS infections. In general, polymorphonuclear leukocytes are never seen in normal adults. However, with use of the cytocentrifuge, an occasional specimen from an otherwise normal individual may show one to two neutrophils.[122] More than three neutrophils is always abnormal in an adult. Moreover, as many as 30% of patients exhibit CSF pleocytosis after a generalized or focal seizure. Nonetheless, such a finding should prompt culture of CSF because the presence of neutrophilic pleocytosis is commonly associated with bacterial meningitis or the early stages of viral or tuberculous meningitis. Small lymphocytes may be seen in normal individuals. Small and large immunocompetent cells are found with a variety of bacterial, fungal, viral, granulomatous, and spirochetal diseases.

Eosinophils always indicate an abnormal condition, most commonly a parasitic infestation of the CNS. They may also be seen after myelography and pneumoencephalography and, to a minor degree, with other inflammatory diseases, including tuberculous meningitis and neurosyphilis. Normal CSF RBC counts are lower than 10 cells/µL. Herpes simplex virus (HSV) encephalitis may elevate the RBC count. Finally, myeloid and RBC precursors may contaminate CSF with bone marrow cells from an adjacent vertebral body.[123]

Glucose

Glucose enters CSF by way of the choroid plexus, as well as by transcapillary movement into the extracellular space of the brain and the cord via carrier-mediated transport. It then

BOX 60-2 Low CSF Glucose Syndromes

Bacterial meningitis
Tuberculous meningitis
Fungal meningitis
Sarcoidosis
Meningeal carcinomatosis
Amebic meningitis
Cysticercosis
Trichinosis
Syphilis
Chemical meningitis
Subarachnoid hemorrhage
Mumps meningitis
Herpes simplex encephalitis
Hypoglycemia

CSF, cerebrospinal fluid.

equilibrates freely within the CSF subarachnoid space. Once in CSF, glucose undergoes glycolysis and there is an invariable rise in CSF lactate levels. Glucose levels remain subnormal for 1 to 2 weeks after effective treatment of bacterial meningitis.

The normal range of CSF glucose is 50 to 80 mg/dL, which is 60% to 70% of the glucose concentration in blood. Ventricular fluid glucose levels are 6 to 8 mg/dL higher than in lumbar fluid. A ratio of CSF glucose to blood glucose of less than 0.5 or a CSF glucose level below 40 mg/dL is invariably abnormal. The ratio is higher in infants, in whom a ratio of less than 0.6 is considered abnormal. Hyperglycemia may mask a depressed CSF glucose level; when present, the ratio of CSF glucose to blood glucose should be measured routinely. With extreme hyperglycemia, a ratio of less than 0.3 is abnormal.[124] Between 90 and 120 minutes is required before CSF glucose reaches a steady state with changes in blood glucose (e.g., after an intravenous injection of glucose). When CSF glucose is of diagnostic importance, obtain CSF and blood samples, ideally after a 4-hour fast.

Low CSF glucose levels may be associated with several diseases of the nervous system (Box 60-2). Only low concentrations of glucose are of diagnostic value; elevated CSF glucose levels generally have little significance and usually reflect hyperglycemia. A rapid estimate of the CSF glucose level can be obtained by using bedside reagent strip testing with a commercial autoanalyzer. Formal laboratory testing is recommended for confirmation of the bedside levels.

Protein

The normal range of lumbar CSF protein is 15 to 45 mg/dL. Infants normally have a lower level than adults do, and protein levels may drop after lumbar puncture. The concentration is lower in the ventricles (5 to 15 mg/dL) and the basilar cisterns (10 to 25 mg/dL) as a result of a gradient in the permeability of capillary endothelial cells to proteins in blood. Levels of CSF protein in premature infants and full-term neonates are higher than in adults, with a mean of 90 mg/dL; protein levels decline by the age of 8 weeks because of maturation of the blood-brain barrier.

Most of the proteins in CSF come from blood, which normally has a protein concentration of up to 8000 mg/dL.

Protein entry is determined by its molecular size and the relative impermeability of the blood-CSF barrier. A full range of serum proteins is found in CSF at a several hundred–fold dilution.

An increase in the total CSF protein level is a nonspecific abnormality associated with many disease states. Levels higher than 500 mg/dL are uncommon and seen mainly with meningitis, subarachnoid hemorrhage, and spinal tumors. The high levels that occur with cord tumors result from an increase in local capillary permeability. With high levels (generally 1000 mg/dL), CSF may clot (Froin's syndrome).

Hemorrhage into CSF or the introduction of blood by a traumatic tap increases CSF protein levels. If the serum protein concentration is normal, the CSF protein level should theoretically rise by 1 mg/dL for every 1000 RBCs, but this relationship varies. The inflammatory effect of hemolyzed RBCs may also significantly increase CSF protein.

Selective measurement of immunoglobulin fractions in CSF has proved to be of diagnostic value in suspected cases of multiple sclerosis. Elevated CSF immunoglobulin levels may reflect disruption of the blood-brain barrier or a local antibody response to a CNS immune response.[125] Stimuli may be infectious or antigenic and produce an inflammatory response. Elevated immunoglobulin levels have been found in many conditions, including syphilis, viral encephalitis, subacute sclerosing panencephalitis, progressive rubella encephalitis, tuberculous meningitis, sarcoidosis, cysticercosis, and acute inflammatory demyelinating polyneuropathy (Guillain-Barré syndrome).

The Traumatic Tap

The incidence of a traumatic tap is 10% to 30%, depending on the criteria used to define the condition.[126-128] Currently, there is no consensus on what constitutes a traumatic tap. Traditionally, the number of RBCs in CSF, the rate of clearance of RBCs from tube 1 to tube 3 or 4, and the presence or absence of xanthochromia have guided clinicians in attempts to define the need for further investigation for SAH when blood is detected during lumbar puncture.

Absolute Number of RBCs

The current literature makes no firm recommendations regarding the absolute CSF RBC count that can be used as a cutoff to differentiate SAH from a traumatic tap. However, SAH consistently produces more RBCs in CSF than a traumatic tap does. In tube 3 or 4, an absolute RBC value of 400 to 500 RBCs/μL or less is very suggestive of a traumatic tap, and this value has been traditionally used by clinicians.[13] In a retrospective study of 300 patients, Gorchynski and coworkers reported a 100% negative predictive value for SAH with an RBC count in tube 4 of 500 RBCs/μL or less, with a sensitivity of 100% for SAH.[129] No radiographically normal subject had an RBC count of greater than 10,000 RBCs/μL, thus suggesting that results above this number are suspicious for radiographically detectable SAH. When the RBC count in tube 4 ranged between 500 and 10,000 RBCs/μL, SAH could not be ruled out without further study. Any attempt to define precisely how low an RBC count must be to eliminate the possibility of SAH would result in an arbitrary threshold. As the foregoing discussion suggests, SAH is exceedingly unlikely with RBC counts lower than 500 and becomes progressively less likely as this number decreases.

RBC Clearance from First to Last Tubes

In traumatic punctures, the fluid generally clears of RBCs between tubes 1 and tubes 3 or 4 as the needle is washed by CSF. In fact, a decrease in the RBC count between the first and last tubes of at least 25% to 30% has traditionally been considered strong evidence of a traumatic tap.[2,130] However, it must be remembered that a traumatic tap may also occur in a patient with true SAH. Thus, regardless of the change in RBC count from the first to last tubes, SAH cannot be excluded unless the RBC count approaches zero in either tube. If this is not the case and xanthochromia is not present (see below), it may be most prudent to repeat the puncture at a different interspace or site. To help avoid this situation, when a clinician encounters what is suspected to be a traumatic tap (e.g., a streak of blood flowing into an otherwise clear-appearing stream of CSF), wasting the first 2 or 3 mL of CSF while positioning the needle to obtain the clearest possible sample will increase the odds of an RBC count approaching zero.

Xanthochromia

RBCs undergo hemolysis in CSF after a few hours and xanthochromia is produced. Xanthochromia persists for up to 4 weeks, depending on the number of RBCs originally present. Xanthochromia is suggestive of but not pathognomonic for SAH.[131] An early CSF examination may show clear fluid before the development of hemolysis, even after spontaneous subarachnoid bleeding. However, xanthochromia may be detected immediately after a traumatic tap if the RBC count exceeds 30,000/μL.[120] The presence of a clot in one of the tubes strongly favors a traumatic tap. With SAH, clotting does not occur because blood is defibrinated at the site of the hemorrhage. Lumbar puncture performed several days after a traumatic tap may also yield stained fluid. Collection of clear CSF from an immediately repeated puncture at a higher interspace also indicates a traumatic tap. The fluid from a traumatic tap should contain about 1 WBC per 700 RBCs if the complete blood cell count is normal, but this ratio is highly variable. All blood-contaminated CSF should be cultured, especially samples from uncooperative infants and children being evaluated for sepsis.

A D-dimer test on CSF can be used to determine SAH by identifying local fibrinolysis.[132] Other conditions such as disseminated intravascular coagulation, a previous traumatic tap, or prior thrombolytic therapy may produce false-positive results.

Fluoroscopically guided lumbar puncture in patients with suspected SAH and negative findings on CT is another option that may reduce the frequency of traumatic punctures, but it requires specific expertise and is frequently performed in the radiology suite.[133]

CSF Analysis with Infections

Bacterial Infections

The CSF findings are essential to establish a provisional diagnosis of acute bacterial meningitis.[134] CSF analysis establishes not only the diagnosis but also the causative organism and therefore the choice of antibiotics (Table 60-1). CSF must be transported to the laboratory immediately and be examined at once. CSF cells begin to lyse within 1 hour after collection; this process can be slowed by refrigeration. In cases of meningococcal infection, a delay in processing may cause the

TABLE 60-1 CSF Analysis in Bacterial and Viral Meningitis*

	BACTERIAL MENINGITIS	VIRAL MENINGITIS
Opening pressure	Usually elevated	Usually normal
White blood cell count (per mm³)	Elevated, 500-10,000+	Elevated, 6-1000
Differential count	Polymorphonuclear predominance	Lymphocytic predominance
Glucose level	Decreased, 0-40 mg/dL	Usually normal
Protein level	Elevated, >50 mg/dL	Normal or slightly elevated

Adapted from Fong B, Van Bendegem J. Lumbar puncture. In: Reichman E, Simon R, eds. *Emergency Medical Procedures*. New York: McGraw-Hill; 2004:875.
CSF, cerebrospinal fluid.
*This is only a guide. Care must be taken when interpreting these parameters, especially early in the clinical course.

diagnosis to be missed because the organism tends to autolyze rapidly. For other organisms, speed is somewhat less important but still warranted.

Gram stain is of great importance because the results direct antibiotic therapy. Gram-negative intracellular or extracellular diplococci are indicative of *Neisseria meningitidis*. Small gram-negative bacilli may indicate *Haemophilus influenzae*, especially in children. The presence of gram-positive cocci indicates *Streptococcus pneumoniae*, other *Streptococcus* species, or *Staphylococcus*. Twenty percent of Gram stains are falsely negative because too few organisms are present. The Gram stain smear is more likely to be positive in patients who have not received prior antibiotic therapy. Acridine orange stain may improve the yield with gram-negative organisms.[135]

For culture, blood and chocolate agar are required. *N. meningitidis* and *H. influenzae* grow best on chocolate agar. The plates are incubated under 10% CO_2. Thioglycolate medium is used for possible anaerobic organisms. Cultures are examined at 24 and 48 hours, but the plates should be kept for at least 7 days. Large volumes of CSF may improve yields.

While the culture results are pending, bacterial infection should be suspected in patients with an elevated opening pressure and marked pleocytosis ranging between 500 and 20,000 WBCs/μL. The differential count with bacterial infections is usually neutrophil predominant. A count higher than 1000 cells/μL seldom occurs with viral infections. Occasionally, acellular fluid may be collected from a severely immunosuppressed patient. Moreover, repeated lumbar puncture may be required in febrile patients whose clinical features remain compatible with meningitis.[124,136,137] In such scenarios, broad-spectrum empirical antibiotics should be continued until the results of repeated testing or bacterial culture are available.

CSF glucose levels of 40 mg/dL or lower or less than 50% of a simultaneous blood glucose level should raise the question of bacterial meningitis, even in the presence of a negative Gram stain and a low cell count. Glucose levels with bacterial meningitis are occasionally below 10 mg/dL but are normal in a small percentage of patients.[124] The CSF protein content with bacterial meningitis ranges from 500 to 1500 mg/dL and usually returns to normal by the end of therapy. Of note, previous antibiotic therapy may adversely affect the sensitivity of cultures and Gram stain for bacterial meningitis but does not significantly affect WBC counts, the ratio of CSF glucose to blood glucose, or CSF protein values.[138] Spanos and colleagues developed a useful nomogram to help distinguish bacterial from viral infections[139]; however, no technique is

perfect in this regard, and in general the clinician should err on the side of diagnosing bacterial meningitis until the results of culture are available.

Microbial Antigens and PCR

In 50% to 80% of cases of bacterial meningitis, blood cultures are positive for the etiologic agent.[140] In addition to Gram stain and cultures, several tests are available to establish a bacterial cause of meningitis, including CSF counterimmunoelectrophoresis (CIE), CSF latex agglutination, and coagglutination CIE.[6] In general, these ancillary tests have low sensitivity for bacterial meningitis, thus limiting their use.

CIE uses wells in two rows of agarose gel. A different antiserum is placed in each well. A current is passed through the gel, which causes the reactants to move toward each other by electrophoretic mobilization of the antigen. The appearance of a line of precipitation in 1 to 4 hours represents a positive reaction between antiserum and antigen.[141] Commercial kits are available to detect *S. pneumoniae*; *Listeria monocytogenes*; *H. influenzae*; *N. meningitidis* A, B, C, and W135; group B streptococci; K1 strains of *Escherichia coli*; *Klebsiella*; and *Pseudomonas* species.[142]

Particle agglutination involves staphylococcal coagglutination and latex agglutination. Antibody on the surface of a colloid combines with antigen-binding sites to cross-link the colloid-forming antigen bridges. A matrix forms and appears as a macroscopic agglutination. Agglutination tests can detect levels of antigen that are approximately 10 times lower than CIE is capable of detecting. False-positive results can occur in the presence of rheumatoid factor, serum complement components, and possibly other serum proteins. The technique may be used for infections with *H. influenzae*, *S. pneumoniae*, *N. meningitidis*, and group B streptococci.

Another technique that has some potential use for identification of bacterial meningitis is the enzyme-linked immunosorbent assay. This technique may detect levels of antigen 100 to 1000 times lower than agglutination tests can but is technically more difficult and requires 4 hours to perform.

A positive CSF antigen test may be expected in 70% to 90% of patients with *Neisseria* meningitis. This compares with a positive Gram stain in approximately 70% of patients. Positive latex antigen tests have been reported in approximately 60% of *S. pneumoniae* meningitis cases, with a positive Gram stain in 80%. A positive latex test and Gram stain are reported in approximately 85% of *H. influenzae* meningitis cases.[140,141]

Group B streptococci can be detected with 60% to 90% sensitivity.

Bacterial antigens may persist in CSF for several days after antibiotic therapy. With appropriate antimicrobial therapy, 25% to 33% of positive tests convert to negative per day. A negative test, however, does not rule out bacterial meningitis.[142] In addition, blood and urine can be examined for antigen. Frequently, antigen is found only in urine. Urine needs to be concentrated and may have the disadvantage of reflecting urinary tract infections. Moreover, the particle agglutination test for *H. influenzae* type B may be positive up to 10 days after children have received *H. influenzae* polysaccharide vaccine. Antigen tests are not useful in diagnosing gram-negative bacillary, staphylococcal, and *Listeria* meningitis. In addition, although antigen tests may identify the bacterial pathogen, they do not provide information about the antibiotic susceptibility of the organism.

Polymerase chain reaction (PCR) may aid in the rapid diagnosis of CNS infection when results of the aforementioned common techniques are suboptimal. PCR amplifies target nucleic acid in CSF by the use of repeated cycles of DNA synthesis. PCR requires the use of flanking DNA sequences at the opposite ends of the target DNA. Synthetic primers anneal to their respective recognition sequences at the opposite end of the target sequence; they serve as primers for new DNA synthesis. PCR allows detection and quantification of organisms whose genetic material is DNA or messenger RNA. PCR permits the diagnosis of infectious disease with a high degree of sensitivity and specificity and allows rapid reliable detection of microbes present in small numbers. Nonetheless, false-negative and false-positive laboratory results may occur.

Empirical Antibiotic Use before Lumbar Puncture

Many patients are transported within a facility or to a referral center for a CT to rule out an intracranial mass after clinical concern for meningitis is raised. In such instances, CSF examination might not be performed before transport because of technical problems (an uncooperative or a large patient) or concerns regarding the safety of lumbar puncture in an obtunded patient with possible increased ICP.[124,143] The initial clinician may have to decide whether to initiate empirical antibiotic therapy. Antibiotic administration could obscure the bacterial source, whereas a delay in initiating therapy increases morbidity and mortality. It may be difficult to identify individuals at risk for a fulminant course, and bacterial meningitis cannot always be diagnosed with confidence; some cases may be misdiagnosed as SAH or metabolic encephalopathy.

After administration of parenteral antibiotics, CSF cultures are not adversely affected for 2 to 3 hours. Twenty-four hours after treatment, as many as 38% of patients with meningitis may still have positive CSF cultures. Kanegaye and associates demonstrated that CSF sterilization may depend on the infecting organism.[144] They reported CSF sterilization after antibiotic administration within the following time frames: meningococcal, less than 2 hours; pneumococcal, less than 4.3 hours; and group B streptococcal, longer than 8 hours.

Blood should be obtained for culture immediately before the administration of antibiotics whenever possible. When CSF is cultured more than a few hours after parenteral antibiotics are administered, antigen tests may be helpful.

Occasionally, lymphocytic pleocytosis may develop in response to antibiotic therapy, but in most cases, the cell count, differential, and glucose and protein concentrations are unchanged in the first 2 to 3 days of antibiotic therapy.[124] It is thus is reasonable to initiate therapy on the premise that a delay might be deleterious. If a lumbar puncture cannot be performed, consultation with clinicians at a referral center seems appropriate. If a lumbar puncture is performed before transfer, a portion of the CSF (chilled on ice) should be sent with the patient or held in the referring hospital laboratory.

Bacterial meningitis in children younger than 10 years has historically been caused by *H. influenzae*. Fortunately, this organism is easy to grow in early postantibiotic cultures and is likely to be associated with positive blood cultures and antigen tests. In the pediatric population, a single dose of an antibiotic before transport is unlikely to prevent identification of bacteria. In neonates, adults, and immunosuppressed patients, the sensitivity of blood cultures and immunologic tests is less reliable. CSF examination as early as possible in the course of treatment is preferred.

For suspected or confirmed cases of acute bacterial meningitis, antimicrobial therapy can be started and be based on the most likely causative organism with respect to the age of the subject, associated diseases, and renal function. Tables 60-2 through 60-4 offer guidelines for emergency antibiotic therapy. For immunocompromised patients and after neurosurgery, a third-generation cephalosporin (cefotaxime, ceftizoxime, ceftazidime, or ceftriaxone) plus ampicillin and vancomycin should be used for coverage against staphylococci, *L. monocytogenes*, and gram-negative organisms.[6] The third-generation cephalosporins are efficacious in many

TABLE 60-2 Empirical Therapy for Purulent Meningitis*

PREDISPOSING FACTOR	ANTIMICROBIAL THERAPY†
Age	
0-4 wk	Ampicillin plus cefotaxime or ampicillin plus an aminoglycoside
4-12 wk	Ampicillin plus a third-generation cephalosporin‡
3 mo-18 yr	Third-generation cephalosporin‡ or ampicillin plus chloramphenicol
18-50 yr	Third-generation cephalosporin‡§
>50 yr	Ampicillin plus a third-generation cephalosporin‡
Immunocompromised state	Vancomycin plus ampicillin plus ceftazidime
Basilar skull fracture	Third-generation cephalosporin‡
Head trauma; post neurosurgery	Vancomycin plus ceftazidime
Cerebrospinal fluid shunt	Vancomycin plus ceftazidime

*Consider corticosteroids before administration of antibiotics (see text).
†Vancomycin should be added to all empirical therapeutic regimens when strains of *Streptococcus pneumoniae* that are highly resistant to penicillin or cephalosporin are suspected.
‡Cefotaxime or ceftriaxone.
§Add ampicillin if meningitis caused by *Listeria monocytogenes* is suspected.

empirical regimens or situations in which the organism is known. Reliance on third-generation cephalosporins alone for all cases of bacterial meningitis would result in treatment failure for all *Listeria* species and increasing numbers of *Enterobacter*, *Serratia*, and *Pseudomonas* groups.

Dexamethasone Therapy for Bacterial Meningitis

In acute bacterial meningitis, bacterial cell wall components, including lipopolysaccharides and teichoic acid, initiate and exacerbate the host response. These substances stimulate the production of cytokines, including interleukin-1 and tumor necrosis factor, from macrophages and monocytes. Cytokines may injure vessels, diminish cerebral perfusion, and stimulate cerebral swelling.[143] The outcome of acute bacterial meningitis has been related to the severity of the inflammatory process in the subarachnoid space.

Studies have suggested benefit from adjunctive dexamethasone therapy in reducing neurologic sequelae, especially hearing loss, in children with *H. influenzae* meningitis and in lowering the mortality rate and providing a better overall outcome in adults with community-acquired acute bacterial meningitis caused by *S. pneumoniae*.[145] There appear to be few adverse sequelae from steroid therapy. The adjunctive benefit of corticosteroids during treatment of meningitis caused by other viral, fungal, or parasitic organisms is unknown. A recent Cochrane review concluded that "the corticosteroid dexamethasone leads to a major reduction in hearing loss and death in both children and adults with bacterial meningitis,

TABLE 60-3 Recommended TOTAL DAILY DOSE (with Divided Dosing Intervals in Hours) of Antimicrobial Agents for Meningitis in Adults with Normal Renal and Hepatic Function*

ANTIMICROBIAL AGENT	TOTAL DAILY DOSE (INTRAVENOUS)	DOSING INTERVAL (hr)
Ampicillin	12 g/day	4
Cefotaxime	8-12 g/day	4-6
Ceftazidime	6 g/day	8
Ceftriaxone	6 g/day	12-24
Chloramphenicol[†]	4 g/day	6
Gentamicin[‡]	2 mg/kg IV load, then 1.7 mg/kg q8h	8
Tobramycin[‡]	2 mg/kg IV load, then 1.7 mg/kg IV q8h	8
Vancomycin[‡]	2-3 g/day	8-12

*Consider corticosteroids before the administration of antibiotics (see text).
[†]High dose recommended for pneumococcal meningitis.
[‡]Peak and trough serum concentrations must be monitored.

TABLE 60-4 Recommended Total Daily Doses with Divided Dosing Intervals in Hours of Antimicrobial Agents for Meningitis in Neonates, Infants, and Children with Normal Renal and Hepatic Function

ANTIMICROBIAL AGENT*	NEONATES (0-7 DAYS)[†]	NEONATES (8-28 DAYS)[†]	INFANTS AND CHILDREN
Amikacin[‡]	15-20 mg/kg/day IV divided q12h	30 mg/kg/day IV divided q8h	15-22.5 mg/kg/day IV divided q8h (max dose 1.5 g/day)
Ampicillin	200-300 mg/kg/day IV divided q8h	400 mg/kg/day IV divided q6h	300-400 mg/kg/day IV divided q3-4h (max dose 10-12 g/day)
Cefotaxime	100-150 mg/kg/day IV divided q8-12h	200 mg/kg/day IV divided q6h	200-300 mg/kg/day IV divided q6-8h (max 12 g/day)
Ceftazidime	100-150 mg/kg/day IV divided q8-12h	100 mg/kg/day IV divided q12h	150 mg/kg/day IV divided q8h (max 6 g/day)
Ceftriaxone	—	—	100 mg/kg/day IV divided q12h
Chloramphenicol	25 mg/kg/day IV q24h (initial loading 20 mg/kg, then first maintenance dose 12 h later)	25-50 mg/kg/day IV divided q12-24h (initial loading 20 mg/kg, then first maintenance dose 12 h later)	75-100 mg/kg/day IV divided q6h (max 2-4 g/day)
Gentamicin[‡]	2.5 mg/kg/day IV divided q8h*	4-5 mg/kg/day IV divided q12-48h*	7.5 mg/kg/day IV divided q8h*
Tobramycin[‡]	4-5 mg/kg/day q24-48h*	4-5 mg/kg/day IV divided q12-48h*	5-7.5 mg/kg/day IV divided q8h*
Vancomycin[‡]	10-15 mg/kg/day IV divided q8-12h	45-60 mg/kg/day IV divided q8-12h	60 mg/kg/day IV divided q8h

*Consider corticosteroids before the administration of antibiotics (see text).
[†]Smaller dosages and longer intervals of administration may be advisable for very-low-birth-weight neonates (<2000 g).
[‡]Peak and trough serum concentrations must be monitored.

without major adverse effects."[146] Interestingly, in children in low-income countries, the use of corticosteroids was associated with neither benefit nor harmful effects.

The dosage of dexamethasone is 0.15 mg/kg (10 mg intravenously in adults) every 6 hours for 4 days. It is recommended that the corticosteroid be given before or simultaneously with antibiotic use, but the exact timing and specific benefits are unclear. It has been suggested that caution be exercised when administering corticosteroids to immunocompromised and leukopenic patients with bacterial meningitis, but no specific recommendations have been published.

A moderate inflammatory response in the meninges is required for penetration of the CNS by many antibiotics. Reducing meningeal inflammation reduces the concentration of antibiotics in CSF. Corticosteroids should be discontinued after approximately 4 days of treatment, at which time the meningeal inflammation should have been reduced.[147,148]

Neurosyphilis

The true incidence of neurosyphilis is unknown. Approximately 5000 new cases of this disease occur in the United States each year.[149] Its natural history and clinical manifestations have been modified in the antibiotic era. The widespread use of oral antibiotics has changed neurosyphilis into chronic, partially treated meningitis. Partial therapy may clear peripheral infection and attenuate the immune response. Therapy may be sufficient to minimize symptoms but insufficient to eradicate organisms in the CNS and eye, which may then multiply.

CSF findings suggestive of neurosyphilis include more than 5 WBCs/μL, an elevated protein concentration, an elevated γ-globulin concentration, and a positive serologic test for syphilis. The glucose concentration is usually normal. Cell and protein values are higher in early neurosyphilis than in late neurosyphilis.

Diagnostic certainty remains difficult. The diagnostic criterion standard is darkfield microscopy to identify the morphology and flexing "corkscrew" motility of spirochetes. Serologic tests for syphilis are either treponemal or nontreponemal. Nontreponemal tests detect a nonspecific globulin complex called reagin. Reagin tests, such as the Venereal Disease Research Laboratory (VDRL) flocculation test, lack sensitivity and should not be used to exclude the diagnosis of neurosyphilis. One third to one half of patients with neurosyphilis have a negative VDRL test on serum, and more than one third have a negative VDRL test on CSF.[149] CSF VDRL is quite specific, with false-positive results seen primarily after traumatic taps.

Treponemal tests provide evidence of a specific immune response to *Treponema pallidum*. These tests include serum fluorescent treponemal antibody absorption (FTA-ABS), microhemagglutination tests for *T. pallidum*, and the *T. pallidum* hemagglutination assay. A positive serum treponemal test indicates past infection with syphilis and may be reactive indefinitely, even after treatment. Therefore, CSF is used as a guide to the presence and activity of neurosyphilis. The VDRL test is commonly used on CSF and, when positive, is strong evidence of neurosyphilis. False-positive CSF VDRL tests are rare. The FTA-ABS test can be used on CSF; the false-positive rate is between 4% and 6% and is believed to represent antibodies that have entered passively from serum.[150] The FTA-ABS test measures immunoglobulin G (IgG) antibody and cannot differentiate active from past infection. The

CSF VDRL may be reactive as a result of contamination with seropositive blood (traumatic tap, SAH) or because of entry of serum reagin into CSF during meningitis. In summary, CSF VDRL and CSF FTA-ABS are complementary tests in the diagnosis of neurosyphilis; CSF VDRL is highly specific but not sensitive, whereas CSF FTA-ABS is less specific but more sensitive.

There is some concern that many patients with parenchymal neurosyphilis have normal CSF. This finding has led to the recommendation that a patient with signs of progressive neurosyphilis and a positive treponemal serologic test be treated with antibiotics regardless of the CSF findings. CSF pleocytosis may be provoked after 1 week of therapy and may provide supportive evidence for a diagnosis of neurosyphilis. PCR may have future applications for the diagnosis of neurosyphilis (see "Neurosyphilis in Patients Infected with Human Immunodeficiency Virus" later in this chapter).

Viral Meningitis

The organisms most commonly isolated in viral meningitis are the enteroviruses (coxsackieviruses, echoviruses) and mumps virus. Enteroviruses are most commonly seen in the summer and fall, and mumps appears most frequently in the winter and spring. Viral cultures in most hospitals are not available and play little role in acute decisions regarding diagnosis and treatment. A serial rise in CSF antibody titers may be helpful but are difficult to obtain in patients who have recovered clinically. Intrathecal production of organ-specific antibodies (IgM, IgG, and IgA isotopes) may be diagnostic of neurologic infection if there is no history of infection. Serum and CSF antibody titers must be measured in a specialized laboratory. Viral meningitis is diagnosed when bacterial culture and Gram stain are negative. A tentative diagnosis may be based on analysis of CSF.

The WBC count in viral meningitis and encephalitis is characteristically 10 to 1000 cells/μL. The differential cell count is predominantly lymphocytic and mononuclear in type. In the early stages of meningoencephalitis, however, polymorphonuclear cells may predominate, thus making the distinction between viral and bacterial infection difficult. In such cases, a tap repeated in 12 to 24 hours will assist in clarifying the diagnosis. Protein levels are usually mildly elevated, but normal levels may be seen. Antibiotic coverage pending the results of culture may be reasonably initiated if the diagnosis of viral meningitis is in doubt.[124] The CSF glucose concentration is characteristically normal; notable exceptions include some cases of mumps meningoencephalitis and HSV encephalitis. CSF pleocytosis and elevated protein levels have also been found in asymptomatic HIV-seropositive individuals.[151]

If CSF cannot be delivered to the viral laboratory in 24 to 48 hours, it should be refrigerated at 4°C. Members of the enterovirus group are occasionally isolated from CSF. Herpesviruses and arboviruses are also found in CSF. PCR is the diagnostic test of choice for HSV meningoencephalitis and will be used increasingly for the diagnosis of other CNS viral infections. Although the majority of cases of viral meningitis are self-limited and have a good outcome, HSV encephalitis is a rapidly progressive and life-threatening emergency that responds to treatment with intravenous acyclovir. Thus, in an acutely ill patient in whom the diagnosis of acute meningoencephalitis is being considered, a negative Gram stain and pleocytosis are sufficient grounds to initiate empirical acyclovir therapy until the results of more definitive diagnostic data from PCR are available.[152]

CSF Analysis in Immunocompromised Patients

The number of immunocompromised individuals is increasing because of the HIV epidemic and the increased survival of patients with cancer and autoimmune disorders. The nervous system is a major target of the HIV virus: neurologic disease develops in 40% to 60% of infected individuals during their lifetime. One third of HIV-infected patients have neurologic complaints as the initial manifestations of AIDS, and an even higher incidence of nervous system involvement is found at autopsy.[153] The risk for CNS infection depends on the underlying disease, treatment, duration, and type of immune abnormality. Abnormalities include defects in T-lymphocyte and macrophage cellular immune function, defects in humoral immunity, defects in the number and function of neutrophils, and loss of splenic function with an inability to remove encapsulated bacteria.[154] The major neurologic manifestations of HIV infection, including clinical characteristics, are summarized in Table 60-5.

Patients with defective cell-mediated immunity include those with lymphoma, organ transplants recipients, those taking corticosteroids daily, and patients with AIDS. These individuals are vulnerable to infections with microorganisms that are intracellular parasites. A common source of acute bacterial meningitis in such patients is *L. monocytogenes*. Clinical findings include fever, headache, seizures, focal neurologic deficits, and brainstem encephalitis.

Patients with defective humoral immunity include those with chronic lymphocytic leukemia, multiple myeloma, and Hodgkin's disease after radiotherapy or chemotherapy. These patients have difficulty controlling infection by encapsulated bacteria. A fulminant meningitis caused by *S. pneumoniae*, *H. influenzae* type B, or *N. meningitidis* may develop. After splenectomy, patients are at risk for the development of meningitis for the same reason. Neutropenic patients are at risk for meningitis caused by *Pseudomonas aeruginosa* and the Enterobacteriaceae.

Establishing a specific diagnosis in HIV and organ transplant patients may be difficult or impossible because of overlapping clinical and radiographic findings, the presence of simultaneous infections with more than one organism, and changes in CSF that may be nonspecific. The immune response may be altered, with absence of the usual signs of meningeal irritation. Patients may have diffuse encephalopathy or focal neurologic deficits. CSF is abnormal in 60% of asymptomatic HIV-infected individuals, thus complicating correlation of the CSF and clinical findings.[153]

Neurosyphilis in Patients Infected with HIV

Syphilis and HIV infection may both be transmitted sexually, and patients with syphilis are at increased risk for HIV infection. CNS invasion is probably no more common in patients with HIV than in those not infected with the virus.[155] Both diseases may cause an elevation in CSF WBC counts, protein levels, and γ-globulin levels. The incidence of syphilitic meningitis, meningovascular syphilis, and ocular syphilis seems to be increasing. HIV-infected patients treated for syphilis may have viable organisms in CSF after therapy or have persistent CSF VDRL titers. Treatment failures are more likely to occur with single-dose benzathine penicillin therapy.

Neurosyphilis may be more difficult to diagnose in HIV-infected patients. A small number of patients with secondary or ocular syphilis have negative serum reagin tests. Positive treponemal tests may revert to nonreactivity after treatment, particularly in individuals with advanced symptomatic HIV disease and a low VDRL titer at the time of diagnosis. CSF pleocytosis and increased γ-globulin levels may not help distinguish between HIV infection and CNS syphilis.

HIV-infected patients should undergo serum treponemal and nontreponemal tests early in their illness to minimize the likelihood of false-negative results.[155] Infected patients should undergo a CSF examination. Previously treated patients who did not have a CSF examination at the time of initial syphilis treatment should undergo lumbar puncture because of a probable increased risk for neurosyphilis even with a decline in serum nontreponemal titers.

Cryptococcal Meningitis

The most common cause of CNS fungal infection is *Cryptococcus neoformans*. Infection with this fungus develops in approximately 5% of AIDS patients. Clinical findings in AIDS and non-AIDS patients include nonspecific symptoms of headache and altered mental status with or without meningeal signs. Most patients have increased ICP. Immunocompetent patients show a lymphocytic pleocytosis with CSF WBC counts lower than 500/μL. Glucose levels are depressed, with elevation of CSF protein. India ink preparations are positive in 50% of cases. CSF is less likely to have abnormal cell counts and chemistries in patients infected with HIV. However, CSF cultures and cryptococcal polysaccharide capsular antigens are almost always positive. False-positive antigen tests are rare but may be seen in the presence of rheumatoid factor. Blood cultures are frequently positive in AIDS patients. Cisternal puncture for fluid analysis may be helpful in undiagnosed cases of lymphocytic meningitis in which multiple lumbar punctures have not established a diagnosis.[153]

Toxoplasmosis

Toxoplasma gondii, an intracellular protozoan, is associated with CNS infection in up to 30% of AIDS patients who have antibodies to this organism. Most adults have antibodies against this organism; infection is believed to represent reactivation of latent primary infection. *Toxoplasma* encephalitis usually develops within the first 2 years after the diagnosis of AIDS. Cerebral toxoplasmosis is usually accompanied by the acute or subacute development of focal disease, including seizures. MRI or CT scanning often reveals multiple abscesses that may represent multiple pathogens. Toxoplasmosis and lymphoma may be difficult to distinguish clinically. Less commonly, the manifestation is one of chronic meningitis with confusion, memory loss, and lethargy similar to the AIDS-dementia complex. CSF in these patients is nonspecific with increased protein, mononuclear pleocytosis (<100 cells/μL), and rarely, a reduced glucose concentration. Serum and CSF serology may be either positive or negative and does not help make a diagnosis, although most patients with encephalitis have detectable IgG antibodies. The diagnosis is usually based on clinical and imaging responses to antibiotics (pyrimethamine or sulfadiazine) or on brain biopsy. Treatment failures with relapse occur in 50% of AIDS patients and in 15% to 25% of non-AIDS patients and necessitate life-long treatment.

TABLE 60-5 Major Neurologic Manifestations of HIV Infection

	CD4+ COUNT (CELLS/mm³)	INITIAL SYMPTOMS	NEUROLOGIC SIGNS	DIAGNOSTIC STUDIES	THERAPY
HIV dementia	<200	Memory loss, gait disorder, behavioral change	Dementia, spasticity, psychosis	CT/MRI: brain atrophy, white matter abnormalities CSF: increased β₂-microglobulin	High-dose zidovudine, clinical trial
Toxoplasma encephalitis	<200	Headache, fever, confusion, lethargy, seizures	Dementia, ataxia, hemiparesis	Serum *Toxoplasma* antibodies CT/MRI: multiple enhancing lesions, edema	Pyrimethamine, sulfadiazine, clindamycin
CNS lymphoma	<100	Headache, confusion, lethargy, memory loss, seizures	Dementia, hemiparesis, aphasia	CT/MRI: enhancing lesions (especially if single) Stereotactic biopsy	Radiotherapy
Progressive multifocal leukoencephalopathy	<100	Lethargy, confusion, weakness	Hemiparesis, ataxia, visual disturbance	CT/MRI: multiple hypodense, nonenhancing white matter lesions Stereotactic biopsy	High-dose zidovudine, ara-C (IV, IT); clinical trial
CMV encephalitis	<50	Rapidly progressive confusion, apathy, weakness	Dementia, cranial neuropathies, spasticity	CT/MRI: periventricular and meningeal abnormalities CSF: CMV culture, PCR Electrolyte abnormalities	Ganciclovir, foscarnet
Vacuolar myelopathy	<200	Gait dysfunction, lower extremity weakness and stiffness, urinary dysfunction	Spastic paraparesis, Babinski's signs, sensory abnormalities	MRI/CSF: normal or nonspecific abnormalities	Baclofen, physical therapy
Cryptococcus neoformans meningitis	<200	Fever, headache, neck stiffness, memory loss	Lethargy, confusion, meningeal signs, cranial nerve palsies	CSF India ink Serum and CSF *Cryptococcus neoformans* antigen and culture	Amphotericin B (plus or minus flucytosine), fluconazole

	CD4 count	Clinical features	Diagnostic findings	Treatment
Neurosyphilis	Any	Dementia, stroke, meningeal or myelopathic signs, cranial nerve palsies	CSF: increased leukocyte count, increased protein Serum and CSF VDRL	Penicillin IV (plus probenecid)
Distal symmetric polyneuropathy	<200	Distal numbness, paresthesias, pain	Stocking-glove sensory loss, decreased ankle reflexes	EMG: distal axonopathy	Neurotoxin withdrawal, analgesics, tricyclic antidepressants, anticonvulsants, capsaicin
Inflammatory demyelinating polyneuropathy	>500 (early), <50 (late)	Progressive weakness, paresthesias	Weakness, areflexia, mild sensory loss	CSF: increased leukocyte count, elevated protein EMG: demyelination	Early (increased CD4+ count): plasmapheresis, IVIG, steroids Late (decreased CD4 count): ganciclovir
Mononeuropathy multiplex	>500 (early), <50 (late)	Facial weakness, footdrop, wristdrop	Multifocal cranial and peripheral neuropathies	EMG: multifocal axonal neuropathy Nerve biopsy: inflammation, vasculitis, CMV inclusions	Early: none Late: ganciclovir
Progressive polyradiculopathy	<50	Lower extremity weakness, paresthesias, urinary dysfunction	Flaccid paraparesis, saddle anesthesia, decreased reflexes, urinary retention	CSF: increased leukocytes (PMNs), CMV culture, PCR EMG: polyradiculopathy	Ganciclovir, foscarnet
Myopathy	Any	Muscle weakness, myalgia, weight loss	Proximal muscle weakness	Increased creatine kinase EMG: irritative myopathy Muscle biopsy: myofiber degeneration, inflammation, inclusions	Zidovudine reduction or withdrawal, corticosteroids

From Simpson DM, Tagliati M. Neurologic manifestations of HIV infection. *Ann Intern Med.* 1994;121:770.
CMV, cytomegalovirus; *CNS,* central nervous system; *CSF,* cerebrospinal fluid; *CT,* computed tomography; *EMG,* electromyography; *HIV,* human immunodeficiency virus; *IT,* intrathecal; *IV,* intravenous; *IVIG,* intravenous immunoglobulin; *MRI,* magnetic resonance imaging; *PCR,* polymerase chain reaction; *PMNs,* polymorphonuclear leukocytes; *VDRL,* Venereal Disease Research Laboratory.

Mycobacterial Tuberculosis

CNS mycobacterial infection is almost always the result of infection with *Mycobacterium tuberculosis*. Infection typically occurs in the setting of disseminated tuberculosis. Atypical *Mycobacterium* infection in HIV-infected individuals uncommonly affects the CNS.

The clinical manifestation is meningitis (particularly meningitis involving the basal cisterns), encephalitis, or abscess formation. If tuberculosis is suspected, a large volume of CSF (10 mL) is required for adequate culture. The cell count varies from 100 to 400 cells/μL, with a lymphocytic predominance; 30% may show predominantly neutrophils early in the course of infection. Protein levels are elevated (100 to 500 mg/dL), and the CSF glucose level may be depressed. Acid-fast stains should be examined by experienced technicians. Fluid is inoculated onto Löwenstein-Jensen medium, and the absence of visible growth on the medium should not be considered negative until 8 weeks has elapsed. CSF cultures are more sensitive than stains.

Primary CNS Lymphoma

CNS lymphoma develops in 2% of AIDS patients. The signs and symptoms resemble those of diffuse encephalopathy, although focal neurologic deficits occur occasionally. Leptomeningeal spread of malignancy is reflected in a modest lymphocytic pleocytosis with slightly elevated protein and decreased glucose levels. Cytologic yield is improved by repeated lumbar punctures and submitting large quantities of CSF or fluid obtained by cisternal puncture.[153]

Progressive Multifocal Leukoencephalopathy

Progressive multifocal leukoencephalopathy is an uncommon disorder in individuals with impaired cell-mediated immunity and is caused by reactivation of JC papovavirus in the kidney. Progressive demyelination is manifested as dementia, blindness, aphasia, hemiparesis, and seizures, which progress until death. MRI and CT demonstrate nonenhancing white matter lesions without a mass effect. Definitive diagnosis is made by brain biopsy, but CSF may show the presence of myelin basic protein, increased IgG, and an acellular or a mild CSF pleocytosis (<50 WBCs/μL). Average survival is 4 months.[154]

Cytomegalovirus Infection

Cytomegalovirus is detected in the brains of 30% of HIV-infected persons at autopsy. A distinct CNS disorder has not been defined. CSF pleocytosis may be minimal. Retinitis and painful polyradiculopathies are recognized, with a prominent CSF pleocytosis found in the latter condition.[153]

Acknowledgment

The editors and author acknowledge the contributions of Jon Kooiker to this chapter in previous editions. The author would like to thank Linda J. Kesselring, MS, ELS, for copy-editing the manuscript and incorporating revisions into the final document.

References are available at www.expertconsult.com

CHAPTER 61

Special Neurologic Tests and Procedures

J. Stephen Huff

Neuro-otologic tests and procedures are used in a variety of clinical scenarios ranging from evaluation of a dizzy patient to diagnosing brain death. Some of these procedures have become less common with the advent of advanced neuroimaging and electrophysiologic testing; nonetheless, their simplicity and effectiveness give them continued relevance, especially in practice environments with limited resources.[1]

CALORIC TESTING

Accurate assessment of a comatose patient requires a thorough neurologic examination, including careful evaluation of the patient's responses to a variety of external stimuli. In a comatose individual with normal brainstem and cranial nerve function, stimulation of the vestibular labyrinth results in well-described and reproducible extraocular movements. This response is known as the vestibulo-ocular reflex (VOR) and forms the physiologic basis for caloric testing. Caloric testing (calor from Latin, meaning heat) involves delivering a thermal stimulus to the external auditory canal to activate the labyrinth. Pathologic conditions involving either the vestibular or the oculomotor reflex pathways will alter or abolish the usual response to caloric stimulation.

Caloric tests may be performed in either conscious or unconscious patients, depending on the diagnostic circumstances. Quantitative caloric examination is conducted in awake ambulatory patients for evaluation of possible vestibular dysfunction. This type of testing requires precisely controlled irrigation temperatures and specialized recording devices and is best undertaken in a properly equipped laboratory under the supervision of an experienced neuro-otologist. However, a neurologist, neurosurgeon, or emergency clinician may perform *qualitative* caloric testing in a comatose patient to detect gross disruption of the VOR pathways that may indicate structural lesions or metabolic abnormalities affecting the labyrinth, vestibulocochlear nerve, or brainstem. In this clinical setting, ice water is used to provide stimulation of the vestibular system. Such testing needs no special expertise and can be done at the bedside with equipment readily available in the emergency department (ED). This simple procedure can provide valuable diagnostic and prognostic information necessary for the management of a comatose patient.

Historical Perspective

Brown-Séquard[2] first described the effects of introducing cold water into the ear canal in the mid-19th century. The clinical importance of the phenomenon was first realized in 1906 by Bárány,[3] who developed a caloric procedure involving an ice water stimulus. He postulated, correctly, that caloric stimulation of the auditory canal induces the formation of convection currents within the semicircular canals of the vestibular labyrinth.

Standardization of the procedure awaited introduction of the Fitzgerald-Hallpike technique in 1942. This technique used both warm and cool water stimuli under rigidly specified conditions, which permitted quantification of normal and abnormal caloric responses. Today, most formal caloric testing of conscious patients is based on variations of the original Fitzgerald-Hallpike procedure.[4]

The value of caloric testing in the assessment of comatose patients was emphasized by the work of Klingon[5] and Bender and associates.[6] Electronystagmography (ENG) can provide a graphic record of reflex eye movements and permit precise determination of the intensity of the caloric response.

Physiology and Functional Anatomy

Proper performance and interpretation of a caloric test requires a basic understanding of the structure and function of both the vestibular and oculomotor systems. The anatomic pathways underlying the VOR begin in the posterior portion of the labyrinth of the inner ear. The peripheral vestibular apparatus is located within the temporal bone and consists of the utricle, the saccule, and the lateral, anterior, and posterior semicircular canals. Because of its proximity to the external ear canal, the lateral or horizontal canal is of principal interest in caloric testing. The lateral canal is oriented at a 30-degree angle to the horizontal plane. Deflections of the cupola because of movement of endolymphatic fluid within the canal result in changes in polarization in the underlying hair cells, which in turn are relayed to the afferent limb of the primary vestibular neuron.

Impulses of the primary neuron travel via Scarpa's ganglion and cranial nerve VIII to the brainstem and synapse with secondary vestibular neurons in the superior and medial vestibular nuclei of the upper medulla and lower pons (Fig. 61-1). Although the connections between the vestibular and oculomotor nuclei in the brainstem are quite complex, two main pathways exist. The direct projection runs from the vestibular complex to the nuclei of cranial nerves III and VI via the medial longitudinal fasciculus (MLF) and involves only three neurons: (1) primary vestibular, (2) secondary vestibular, and (3) oculomotor. The indirect projection between these nuclei occurs over multisynaptic circuits in the tegmental reticular formation. Another brainstem structure that contributes to the vestibulo-ocular interaction is the paramedian pontine reticular formation (PPRF), a poorly characterized group of pontine neurons that coordinate both voluntary and involuntary lateral gaze. The PPRF receives multiple inputs. Including projections from the vestibular system and the contralateral frontal cortex, and sends output to oculomotor neurons through both direct and indirect pathways. Excitatory impulses originating in the lateral canal finally travel via the oculomotor and abducens nerves to the ipsilateral medial rectus and contralateral lateral rectus muscles.[7]

Rotation of the head generates flow of endolymphatic fluid within the semicircular canals. The firing rate of the primary vestibular neuron is dependent on the direction of flow. For example, in the lateral canal, flow toward the ampulla (ampullopetal) increases the firing rate, whereas flow away

THE VESTIBULO-OCULAR REFLEX AND ITS
CONTRIBUTION TO OCULAR MOVEMENTS

Figure 61-1 Vestibulo-ocular reflex and its contribution to horizontal eye movements. The semicircular canals respond to rotational acceleration of the head by driving the vestibulo-ocular reflex to maintain the eyes in the same direction in space during head movement. Fibers from the horizontal semicircular canal travel first to the vestibular nuclei and then to each paramedian pontine reticular formation. Excitatory projections that travel to the contralateral sixth cranial nerve nucleus and, via the medial longitudinal fasciculus, to the ipsilateral medial rectus subnucleus cause gaze to the left. In a similar manner, inhibitory projections are sent to the antagonist ipsilateral lateral rectus and contralateral medial rectus. *(Adapted from Lavin PJ, Donahue SP. Disorders of supranuclear control of ocular motility. In: Yanoff M, Duker JS, eds.* Ophthalmology. *3rd ed. St. Louis: Mosby; 2008.)*

AMPULLOPETAL DEVIATION OF CUPULA

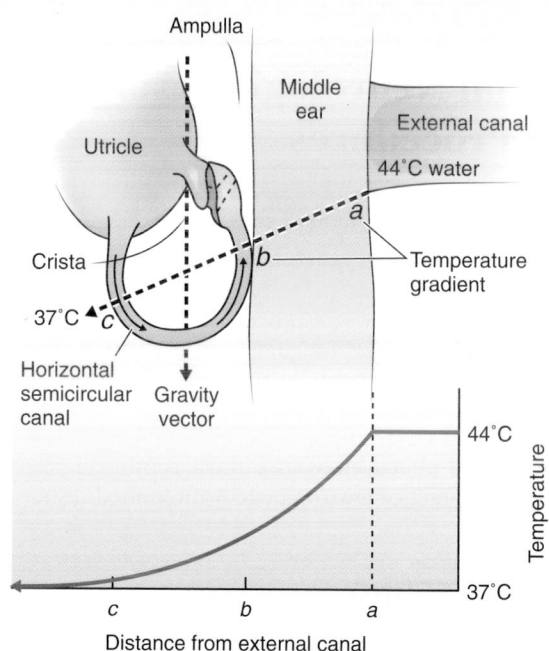

Figure 61-2 Convective flow mechanism of the caloric response. Irrigation with warm or cold water (or air) results in a temperature gradient across the horizontal semicircular canal. With the horizontal canal oriented in the earth-vertical plane, gravity induces convective flow of endolymph from the cooler area of the canal, in which endolymph is more dense, into the warmer area of the canal, in which endolymph is less dense. For the warm caloric irrigation shown in this diagram, an ampullopetal deflection of the cupula results from this flow of endolymph. Vestibular nerve afferents innervating the horizontal semicircular canal are excited, and a horizontal nystagmus with slow-phase components directed toward the opposite ear is produced. A cold caloric stimulus results in an oppositely directed response, with ampullofugal deflection of the cupula, inhibition of horizontal canal afferents, and nystagmus with slow-phase components directed toward the ear to which the cold caloric stimulus is applied. *(Adapted from Baloh RW, Honorubia V, eds.* Clinical Neurophysiology of the Vestibular System. *3rd ed. Philadelphia: Davis; 2001.)*

from the ampulla (ampullofugal) decreases the firing rate. Increased firing on one side results in conjugate deviation of the eyes toward the opposite side, whereas decreased firing causes deviation to the same side. This principle forms the physiologic basis of caloric testing. When the lateral canal is in the vertical position (patient placed supine) and ice water is infused into the ear, the endolymph nearest the canal cools and sinks, which results in ampullofugal flow (Fig. 61-2). As the firing rate decreases, the eyes deviate conjugately toward the side of irrigation. When warm water is used in the same position or when the canal is inverted 180 degrees, the opposite occurs.

The eye movements induced by caloric stimulation in conscious, neurologically normal individuals are more complex. Ice water infusion induces a rhythmic jerking of the eyes that includes a slow deviation toward the irrigated side followed by a quick compensatory saccade toward the midline. This is known as *caloric nystagmus*. By convention, caloric nystagmus is named for the fast component, thus the popular mnemonic "fast COWS" (Cold irrigation—Opposite beating nystagmus; Warm irrigation—Same-sided beating nystagmus). Most sources attribute the slow phase of nystagmus to vestibular activity transmitted over the direct pathway, whereas the fast phase is believed to be generated by the PPRF in conjunction with cortical activity and carried over indirect pathways within the reticular formation. Numerous factors, including physiologic, pharmacologic, and pathologic, can alter caloric-induced eye movements.

Indications and Contraindications

Caloric testing of a comatose patient is indicated when the clinician needs information on the functional integrity of the brainstem. When the cause of the coma is initially unknown, qualitative caloric testing at the bedside may assist in differentiation among structural, metabolic, or psychogenic causes of unresponsiveness. Even when the cause of the coma is clear, caloric testing may provide an indication of the depth of the coma and possibly the prognosis for eventual recovery.

Few contraindications exist to caloric testing of an unresponsive patient. An absolute contraindication is the presence of a basilar skull fracture, either documented radiologically or suspected by clinical signs, because of the risk of introducing infection into the central nervous system (CNS) through an associated dural tear. If a basilar skull fracture is discovered to be unilateral, testing of the intact ear with warm water and then cold water will yield results similar to those of the standard bilateral examination with cold water stimulation.

Relative contraindications to caloric testing with water include perforation of the tympanic membrane (including perforations not caused by temporal bone fractures), otitis media and externa, and the presence of previous otologic surgery (e.g., mastoidectomy). Although the risk of causing otitis media is probably small, performing the caloric test on a comatose patient under these conditions remains a matter of clinical judgment.

Equipment

The equipment needed for performance of the caloric test is minimal and readily available in the ED. Although almost any size of syringe will suffice, a 30- or 50-mL plastic syringe is ideal for irrigation. The syringe may be used as is or a short length of soft plastic tubing may be attached. A good source of tubing is a butterfly catheter with the needle cut or pulled off. At least 100 mL of ice water should be available, although larger quantities of cool tap water (<25°C) can be used with similar results if ice is unavailable. Sterile or bacteriostatic saline may be used, but no advantage over tap water has been demonstrated. A small, curved plastic emesis basin is useful to collect water as it drains from the ear canal. Other equipment required includes an otoscope, several sizes of ear specula, and equipment for removal of cerumen. Towels and a thermometer that reads from 0°C to 50°C may be helpful.

Procedure

Defer VOR testing until the patient's condition has been stabilized, with attention to the airway and evaluation of the cervical spine in trauma patients. Perform a thorough neurologic assessment before caloric testing, with special attention directed to the ocular examination. Observe pupillary responses, spontaneous ocular movements, and the resting position of the eyes. Inspect the ears before inserting the otoscope. If active bleeding or cerebrospinal fluid otorrhea or rhinorrhea is noted in the trauma victim, defer caloric testing and evaluate the patient for a potential basilar skull fracture. If the external ear canal appears to be normal, conduct the remainder of the otoscopic examination. Signs of active ear infection and perforation of the tympanic membrane are contraindications to caloric testing. Tympanic rupture, hemotympanum, or step-off deformities of the canal may indicate fracture of the temporal bone. Caloric testing is contraindicated in this situation. Remove excess cerumen and foreign material. Clearly visualize the tympanic membrane. Leave the ear speculum in the canal as a guide for irrigation.

Perform the test with the patient in the supine position and the head and upper part of the body raised to 30 degrees if possible. This amount of elevation places the lateral canal in the vertical plane and ensures a maximal response. Drape the patient with a towel and position a small emesis basin below the ear to collect the outflow of water from the ear. Fill a container with ice water and place it near the bedside.

Fill a syringe and catheter system (minus the needle) with 10 mL of ice water and direct the irrigation stream toward the tympanic membrane. Because the goal of qualitative caloric testing is to induce a maximum response, the amount and rate of infusion are not critical. As a general guide, infuse 5 to 10 mL of ice water initially over a period of 5 to 10 seconds. Amounts less than 5 mL may be advisable in suspected cases of light coma or psychogenic unresponsiveness. If no response is noted within a moment, infuse at least 100 mL before declaring that there is no response. Begin testing the contralateral ear 5 or 10 minutes after the eyes have returned to their original position. Ask an assistant to hold the patient's eyelids open, which makes it easier to observe for eye deviation. Movement usually occurs after a latency of 10 to 40 seconds, with the response persisting for as long as 4 to 5 minutes. Focusing on a small scleral vessel makes small deviations easier to detect. Alternatively, use a dermographic pencil to mark the initial position of the pupil with respect to the eyelid.

Variations of the caloric technique may be useful in certain situations. If there is no response to bilateral ice water caloric testing or in cases in which only one ear can be tested, perform warm water caloric testing. Keep the water temperature below 50°C. The response elicited will be the opposite of that obtained with ice water. In patients who fail to respond to ice water caloric testing alone, additional stimulation may be provided by combining irrigation with repeated head turning away from the irrigated side (doll's-eye maneuver). This should not be performed in trauma patients unless cervical injury has definitely been ruled out. This combination of techniques may produce eye movements in patients who do not respond to caloric testing alone.[8] Eviatar and Goodhill[9] described a technique for caloric testing in patients with tympanic perforations that involves placing a small latex finger cot in the ear canal to prevent water from entering the middle ear.

Complications

The few complications that are possible with caloric testing can be avoided by carefully selecting both the patients to be tested and the equipment and technique to be used. Using needles or other sharp objects to irrigate the ear may result in laceration or perforation of the tympanic membrane or canal wall if the patient moves unexpectedly. The use of plastic syringes and soft catheter tubing aids in reducing such occurrences.

Other potential complications of caloric testing include otitis media, meningitis, and induction of vomiting and subsequent aspiration. Although meningitis may follow basilar skull fractures with meningeal tears, the additional risk associated with caloric testing in such situations is not known. Therefore, omit caloric testing in a head-injured patient if there is any suspicion of temporal bone fracture. Although ice water irrigation might produce nausea and emesis in awake patients, vomiting with aspiration has not been reported as a complication of caloric testing in comatose patients. Nevertheless, some operators may prefer to delay testing until the patient's airway is protected.

Interpretation

First Phase of Interpretation

Analyze initial eye position and spontaneous movements before irrigation. A description of eye movement abnormalities in comatose patients is beyond the scope of this chapter and is only briefly summarized here. The eyes of comatose patients with intact oculomotor pathways are usually directed straight ahead or are slightly divergent. Unilateral destructive lesions of the cerebral hemisphere can cause conjugate deviation of the eyes toward the side of the lesion, whereas irritative foci, as might be seen with status epilepticus, can cause conjugate deviation away from the affected side. Deviations of

1. Normal nystagmus
   - - - → Fast component
   → Slow component

Cold H₂O   Cold H₂O   Cold H₂O   Hot H₂O

2. Conjugate deviation

Cold H₂O   Cold H₂O   Cold H₂O   Hot H₂O

3. Dysconjugate deviation (with MLF lesion)

Cold H₂O   Cold H₂O   Cold H₂O   Hot H₂O

4. Absent responses

A

Cold H₂O   Cold H₂O   Cold H₂O   Hot H₂O

	OCULOCEPHALIC TESTING		OCULOCEPHALIC TESTING			
	Horizontal head rotation	Vertical head rotation	Cold water in one ear	Warm water in one ear	Cold water in both ears	Warm water in both ears
Physiologic response in a comatose patient with intact brainstem funtion	Doll's-eyes movements do not occur in alert persons	Conjugate downwrd eye movement when head is moved backward	Conjugate eye movement toward stimulated ear	Conjugate eye movement away from stimulated ear	Conjugate downward eye movement	Conjugate upward eye movement
Pseudocoma	Doll's-eyes movements are not present. Often, eyes remain straight ahead or turn in same direction as head	No consistent movement	Nystagmus in pseudocoma, stupor, or (occasionally) light coma. Slow ocular movement toward stimulated ear with fast jerk back to midline	In pseudocoma, stupor, and (occasionally) light coma, slow movement away from stimulus; jerky fast componenet in other direction	In pseudocoma, the slow component is downward movement. Fast component is upward movement	In pseudocoma, slow component is upward movement; fast component is downward movement
Brainstem abnormality at pontomedullary junction with eighth cranial nerve involvement	No movement	No movement	No movement	No movement	No movement	No movement
Brainstem abnormality at midbrain level with bilateral third cranial nerve involvement	Dysconjugate movement. Right eye does not move medially	No movement	Dysconjugate movement. Right eye does not move medially	Dysconjugate movement. Left eye does not move medially	No movement	No movement
Brainstem abnormality at pontine level with bilateral sixth cranial nerve and PPRF* involvement	No horizontal movement	Eyes move downward by third cranial nerve action	No horizontal movement	No horizontal movement	Eyes move downward; third cranial nerve at midbrain is still functioning	Eyes move upward; third cranial nerve at midbrain is still functioning

*Pontine paramedian reticular formation

B

Illustrations by Charles H. Boyer

this type can usually be overcome by caloric stimulation, although combined irrigation and head turning may be required in the first hours after the insult. Lesions in or near the PPRF in the brainstem cause conjugate deviation away from the side of the lesion. This finding cannot usually be overcome by caloric stimulation. Conjugate downward deviation can be seen with structural lesions of the brainstem or in the deeper phases of metabolic coma. Dysconjugate gaze might indicate damage at the level of the oculomotor nuclei or below or might reflect disruption of the ocular muscles themselves.[10] Dysconjugate gaze may also be seen with drug-induced coma in the presence of a structurally intact brainstem. In the very late stages of brainstem dysfunction, the eyes usually return to the central position. Spontaneous roving movements of the eyes, either conjugate or dysconjugate, may be seen with supratentorial insults, but these, too, disappear with brainstem involvement.[11] Ocular "bobbing" is an intermittent, spontaneous downward jerking of the eyes that may occur with massive pontine lesions. Ocular "dipping" is a more prolonged, downward conjugate deviation of the eyes that has been reported in cases of severe anoxic encephalopathy (e.g., carbon monoxide poisoning).[11] The pathophysiologic basis of these eye movements is poorly understood.[12]

Second Phase of Interpretation

After irrigation, ocular movements should be observed for any response to the stimulus. Again, typically there is a latency of response of 10 to 40 seconds. Reactions to ice water irrigation may be divided into four categories: (1) caloric nystagmus, (2) conjugate deviation, (3) dysconjugate deviation, and (4) absent responses (Fig. 61-3). The first reaction, caloric nystagmus with the fast component beating away from the side of ice water irrigation, is seen in normal, alert individuals, in cases of psychogenic unresponsiveness, and in those who have very mild organic disturbances in consciousness. The intensity of nystagmus is highly variable in conscious subjects and depends on the degree of visual fixation and the level of mental alertness. The response is present in more than 90% of children by 6 months of age and declines in magnitude only after the seventh decade of life.[13]

Caloric-induced nystagmus after cold water irritation in an apparently comatose individual usually occurs when testing individuals with psychogenic unresponsiveness as a result of catatonia, conversion reactions, schizophrenia, or feigned coma. Hyperactive caloric responses may result from testing in the presence of tympanic perforation or mastoid disease. Hypoactive caloric responses are recorded in patients with a wide variety of vestibular and neurologic disorders.

Hypoactive or abnormal caloric responses may be further evaluated with quantitative caloric testing, ENG, or other techniques such as auditory evoked responses. Caloric-induced nystagmus may be inverted (beating to the wrong side) or perverted (beating in the wrong plane); both responses may be seen with brainstem lesions. Pseudocaloric nystagmus is a preexisting latent nystagmus that is brought out by the general arousal of ice water irrigation; it can be distinguished from true nystagmus by its failure to reverse direction with warm water irrigation.

As the level of coma deepens, the fast phase of nystagmus becomes intermittent and then disappears, probably because of decreased activity in the cerebral cortex.

In the second type of response to cold caloric stimulation, the eyes deviate conjugately toward the side of ice water stimulation (they "look" toward the source of irritation). When present, this reaction indicates intact brainstem function, as well as intact afferent and efferent limbs of the reflex. This is seen during general anesthesia, in supratentorial lesions without brainstem compression, and with many metabolic and drug-induced comas. In such situations, bilateral simultaneous irrigation with ice water might result in conjugate downward deviation, thus implying that the brainstem centers for vertical gaze are functional.

Dysconjugate reactions constitute the third type of caloric response to ice water stimuli. The most common dysconjugate reaction is internuclear ophthalmoplegia, in which a lesion of the MLF causes weakness or paralysis of the adducting eye after caloric irrigation. Internuclear ophthalmoplegia might be due to acute damage to the rostral pons or could be seen as a manifestation of multiple sclerosis or stroke.

With acute supratentorial lesions, the development of dysconjugate caloric responses is a significant sign that may indicate compression of the brainstem and impending herniation. Caloric responses of this type are less common with metabolic and drug-induced coma; when present in metabolic coma, their significance is less ominous. Reversible internuclear ophthalmoplegia has been reported in patients with hepatic coma and may occur during toxic responses to phenytoin, barbiturates, or amitriptyline. Forced downward deviation of the eyes, either conjugate or dysconjugate, may be seen in sedative-hypnotic drug–induced coma when unilateral caloric testing is performed.[14]

Palsies of the oculomotor nerves are another cause of dysconjugate reactions, although most should be apparent before irrigation. Causes include diabetic neuropathy, increased intracranial pressure, and Wernicke's encephalopathy. Finally, Plum and Posner[10] reported that unusual and poorly characterized caloric responses may be obtained when testing comatose patients with long-standing severe brain injury.

Absent caloric response is the fourth category of reactions to ice water stimuli. As a general rule, the VOR is preserved more than other brainstem reflexes; however, the oculocephalic, or doll's eye, response may persist in the absence of caloric responses. Loss of caloric responses in comatose patients with structural lesions is usually a sign of brainstem damage. With supratentorial lesions, progressive loss of caloric responses may be seen in the final stages of transtentorial herniation. The VOR may also be transiently absent or decreased on the side opposite massive supratentorial damage during the first hours after injury.[15] Absent caloric responses may occur with any subtentorial lesion that affects the vestibular reflex pathways, including pontine hemorrhage, basilar artery occlusion, cerebellar hemorrhage, or infarction with encroachment on the brainstem, and with any expanding mass lesion within the posterior fossa. Caloric responses may disappear in patients with deep coma resulting from subarachnoid hemorrhage, perhaps because of pressure on the brainstem.

Figure 61-3 A, The four types of caloric responses seen with unilateral and bilateral irrigation. *1,* Normal nystagmus. *2,* Conjugate deviation. *3,* Disconjugate deviation. The most common type, internuclear ophthalmoplegia, is shown here. Vertical eye movements usually remain intact in this lesion. *4,* Absent caloric responses. MLF, medial longitudinal fasciculus. **B,** Oculocephalic and oculovestibular testing in patients with selected clinical conditions. (*A, Modified from Plum F, Posner JB, eds.* The Diagnosis of Stupor and Coma. *3rd ed. Philadelphia: Davis; 1980:55; B, from Smith M, Bleck T. Techniques for evaluating the cause of coma.* J Crit Illness. *1987;2:51.*)

The VOR is usually retained until the late stages of metabolic coma. Nevertheless, caloric responses may be transiently absent in certain types of drug-induced coma, with eventual complete recovery of the patient. The VOR seems to be particularly sensitive to the effects of sedative-hypnotic drugs, antidepressants (e.g., amitriptyline, doxepin), and anticonvulsants (e.g., phenytoin, carbamazepine).[16,17] As one would expect, neuromuscular blocking agents (e.g., succinylcholine) will abolish caloric-induced ocular movements.

Finally, the caloric response may be absent for reasons other than the neurologic causes responsible for the coma. Inadequate irrigation because of excessive cerumen or poor technique and unilateral or bilateral dysfunction of the peripheral vestibular apparatus must be considered. Bilateral loss of the caloric response (areflexia vestibularis) is uncommon in conscious patients, constituting 1.7% and 0.2% of the ENG clinical population in two large series of patients.[18,19]

The VOR has prognostic as well as diagnostic significance in comatose patients. In a study of 100 patients who were comatose as a result of head trauma, absence of caloric responses 1 to 3 days after injury was associated with extremely high mortality.[20] Testing in the immediate posttraumatic period may yield inconsistent responses and is of considerably less prognostic value. Levy and coworkers[21] studied 500 cases of nontraumatic, non–drug-induced coma in a large multicenter study. Absence of the VOR correlated with less than a 5% chance of achieving functional recovery within 1 year when tested within 6 to 24 hours of the onset of coma. In one study of comatose patients, the combination of absent VOR and absent pupillary light reflex at 24 hours was associated with 100% mortality.[22] Complete loss of caloric responses is part of the criteria for the diagnosis of brain death and correlates with irreversible cessation of cerebral function at least as well as an isoelectric electroencephalogram (EEG) does.[23] Excessive reliance on a single clinical sign must be avoided during consideration of brain death and in decisions regarding neurologic prognosis, and therapy should be based on complete evaluation of all the evidence available (see the later section "Brain Death Testing").

Summary

Caloric testing is a simple, easily performed bedside procedure that may enhance the neurologic assessment of comatose patients. When reliably interpreted, caloric testing may furnish valuable diagnostic and prognostic information. Even if the cause of the coma is known, the test may provide a baseline for the evaluation of changes in the patient's status. In the ED this test should be reserved for stable patients undergoing secondary assessment. The examination requires minimal equipment and can be conducted in a few minutes while awaiting the results of laboratory testing or neuroimaging. Complications are few if patients are properly selected and correct technique is used.

DIX-HALLPIKE TEST FOR THE DIAGNOSIS OF POSITIONAL VERTIGO

Vertigo occurring only and repeatedly with change in position is probably benign paroxysmal positional vertigo (BPPV); the head-hanging positioning maneuver (Dix-Hallpike test, sometimes referred to as the Nylen-Báràny maneuver) is useful in confirming clinical suspicion of BPPV because the abnormal nystagmus provoked is characteristic of the disorder.[24,25] In BPPV, it is thought that calcium crystal material displaced from the vestibule floats within the endolymph of the posterior semicircular canal. Head movement induces bidirectional forces in the fluid acting on the cupula that trigger the attack of BPPV.[26-29] The posterior semicircular canal is most commonly affected,[25,28] but at times the horizontal canal is thought to be involved, thereby leading to variants of typical BPPV.[30-32]

Background

BPPV is a common mechanical disorder of the inner ear in which vertigo is precipitated by certain head movements; nystagmus and autonomic symptoms such as nausea and vomiting commonly accompany the vertigo. Although patients may have quite dramatic findings with severe autonomic symptoms, the actual episodes of vertigo are extremely brief and typically last less than 1 minute. Syndromes of positional vertigo and provocative maneuvers have been described by clinicians for more than 100 years; the description of BPPV has been attributed to Adler, Bárány, Nylèn, Bruns, Borries, Dix, and Hallpike.[33] Dix and Hallpike most fully defined the disorder, and the provocative technique that they described is superior; thus it most accurately should bear the eponym *Dix-Hallpike positioning test* or the *Dix-Hallpike test*.[25-33] Rarely, paroxysmal positional vertigo from a central cause has also been described in patients with small cerebellar hemorrhages.[34]

Indications and Contraindications

The Dix-Hallpike test may be a useful diagnostic test in confirming BPPV by provoking a specific type of nystagmus and in selecting patients suitable for positional therapy (discussed later). The maneuver should not be performed on patients with severe cervical spine disease, unstable spinal injury, high-grade carotid stenosis, or unstable heart disease.[25] Patient discomfort and physical infirmity are relative contraindications; some elderly patients or those with ongoing nausea or vertigo may not tolerate the changes in body position necessary for performance of the procedure. If nystagmus is present at rest without any provocation or if associated neurologic signs or symptoms exist, the diagnosis of BPPV is probably excluded and the maneuver is not clinically indicated.

Procedure

The Dix-Hallpike maneuver is illustrated in Figure 61-4. Place the patient initially in the seated position on the stretcher with the head turned 45 degrees to one side. With the patient instructed to keep the eyes open and focused on the examiner, quickly lay the patient down flat with the head hanging over the edge of the bed and observe the eyes for induced nystagmus. Repeat the entire maneuver with the head turned 45 degrees toward the opposite side.[25]

Interpretation

The Dix-Hallpike head-hanging positioning maneuver produces vertigo in patients with positional vertigo that is most commonly characterized as BPPV. The stereotypic positive

DIX-HALLPIKE MANEUVER

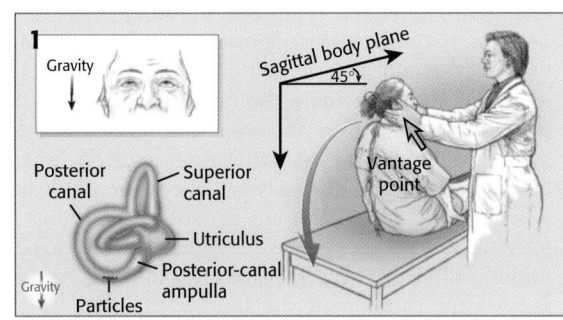

The examiner stands at the patient's head, 45° to the right, to align the right posterior semicircular canal with the sagittal plane of the body.

The examiner moves the patient, whose eyes are open, from the seated to the supine, right-ear-down position and then extends the patient's neck slightly so that the chin is pointed slightly upward. The latency, duration, and direction of nystagmus, if present, and the latency and duration of vertigo, if present, should be noted. *Inset:* The arrows over the eyes depict the direction of nystagmus in patients with typical BPPV. The presumed location in the labyrinth of the free-floating debris thought to cause the disorder is also shown.

Figure 61-4 The Dix-Hallpike test for evaluating a patient complaining of dizziness for benign paroxysmal positional vertigo (BPPV) affecting the right ear. (*Adapted from Furman C. Benign paroxysmal positional vertigo. N Engl J Med. 1999;341:1590.*)

response in BPPV is provoked vertigo developing after a brief delay (1 to 10 seconds), lasting less than a minute, and with direction-fixed rotary nystagmus. Nausea or other systemic symptoms are often present.[24,25] The eye movements are mixed torsional and vertical nystagmus of both eyes with the upper pole of the eye beating toward the dependent ear and the vertical nystagmus beating toward the forehead. The side with the ear in the downward position during the Dix-Hallpike test that elicits greater nystagmus usually identifies the affected ear. After the patient is returned to the sitting position, the nystagmus may again be transiently observed in a reverse direction. If the positional nystagmus is atypical or if the maneuver fails to elicit nystagmus in a patient with ongoing symptoms of vertigo, another diagnostic possibility should be considered.[25,35]

Complications

The maneuver may precipitate brief vertigo and nausea in patients with BPPV.

Summary

The Dix-Hallpike test may be useful in confirming the diagnosis of BPPV and in localizing the abnormality to one ear. Accurate identification of BPPV is of interest because of the possibility of canalith-repositioning maneuvers, as described next.

CANALITH-REPOSITIONING MANEUVERS

If the clinical evaluation of a patient with vertigo is consistent with the diagnosis of BPPV and the Dix-Hallpike test is supportive of the diagnosis and lateralizes to one ear, the patient may be a candidate for attempted canalith-repositioning maneuvers. These techniques have largely been described in the otologic and neurologic literature and have recently been described in the ED setting. Success rates of 44% to 100% are reported.[25] One small ED-based study concluded that the Epley maneuver was more efficacious than a placebo maneuver.[36]

Background

With theory suggesting that stray material in the posterior semicircular canal causes the symptoms of BPPV, maneuvers were designed that involved sequential head movements to reposition the debris to the vestibule.[25,29,37,38] Manipulation of head position theoretically allows the debris ("canaliths") to sequentially fall from the problematic location in the semicircular canal to the vestibule of the labyrinth, where they presumably adhere. The currently recommended maneuver was introduced by Epley.[29] Other maneuvers are described but require repeated trials or are more difficult to perform and perhaps more uncomfortable for the patient.[25,37,39] The Semont maneuver is also described because it may be performed at the bedside. In theory, the Semont maneuver would be effective primarily in patients in whom the displaced canaliths were adhering to the cupola of the posterior semicircular canal (Schuknecht cupolith theory), although it might be effective as well when the debris are free floating in the long arm of the semicircular canal; the Epley maneuver would be effective only in patients with debris floating in the long arm of the posterior semicircular canal (canalith theory).[40] In one small trial comparing the efficacy of either the Semont or the Epley maneuver in a carefully selected outpatient otolaryngology population, the maneuvers were found to be of roughly the same effectiveness (90%) in relieving or improving symptoms of BPPV.[40]

Indications and Contraindications

The indication for any canal-clearing or "liberatory" procedure is the clinical diagnosis of BPPV as confirmed by the history and physical examination, including the Dix-Hallpike maneuver. Careful patient selection is probably a key point in the success of any of these maneuvers, as well as correct identification of the impaired ear, which will govern the initial position and movement of the patient. Contraindications are the same as for the Dix-Hallpike maneuver, as noted earlier.

Procedure

The Epley procedure is illustrated in Figure 61-5. Briefly, as in the Dix-Hallpike maneuver, place the patient initially in the seated position on the stretcher with the head turned 45 degrees toward the affected side. Lay the patient down flat with the head hanging over the edge of the bed. After 20 seconds or after the symptoms subside, rotate the patient's head so that it faces the opposite shoulder while maintaining the head-hanging orientation. Roll the patient further onto the side and rotate the head further into a face-down position. Again, after 20 seconds or after any symptoms subside, return the patient to a seated position.[26,35,39] Some authors suggest keeping the patient's head in each position long enough for any provoked symptoms of nystagmus or vertigo to resolve.[25] Others suggest a period of 4 minutes after the head is placed in the hanging position and again after rotation of the head ("modified Epley maneuver").[40] The maneuver may be repeated a few times until some

EPLEY PROCEDURE

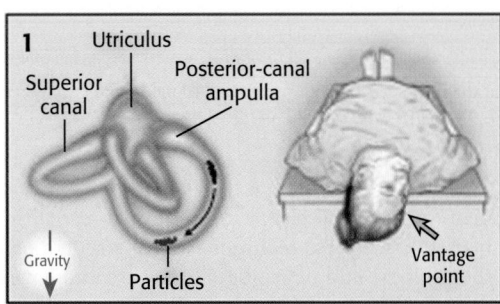

1

First, a Dix-Hallpike test is performed with the patient's head rotated 45° toward the right ear and the neck slightly extended with the chin pointed slightly upward. This position results in the patient's head hanging to the right.

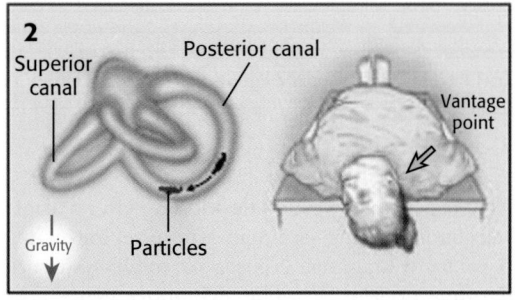

2

Once the vertigo and nystagmus provoked by the Dix-Hallpike test cease, the patient's head is rotated about the rostral-caudal body axis until the left ear is down.

3

Then the head and body are further rotated until the head is face down. The vertex of the head is kept tilted downward throughout rotation. The manuever usually provokes brief vertigo. The patient should be kept in the final, face-down position for about 10 to 15 seconds.

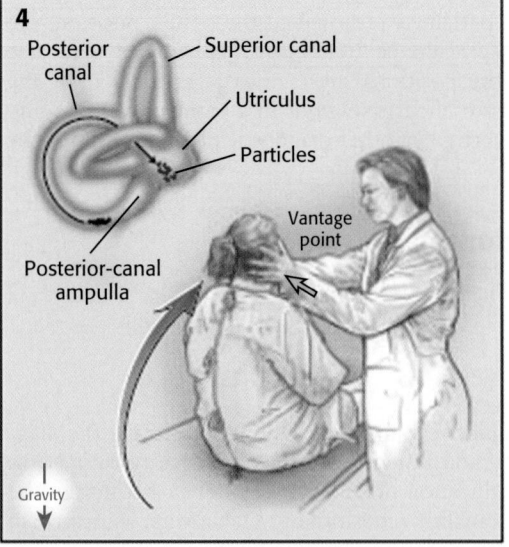

4

With the head kept turned toward the left shoulder, the patient is brought into the seated position. Once the patient is upright, the head is tilted so that the chin is pointed slightly downward.

Figure 61-5 The Epley procedure, a bedside maneuver for the treatment of a patient with benign paroxysmal positional vertigo affecting the right ear. The presumed position of debris within the labyrinth during the maneuver is shown in each panel. (*Adapted from Furman C. Benign paroxysmal positional vertigo.* N Engl J Med. *1999;341:1590.*)

improvement in symptoms occurs, although this is not typically described in the literature.[40] After a successful procedure, advise the patient to remain in a head-upright position for 24 hours.

The Semont maneuver involves larger and more abrupt body movements. Identify the affected ear by the Dix-Hallpike maneuver. With the patient seated on the side of an examination table or bed, turn the patient's head toward the unaffected side. Quickly lay the patient down into a side-lying position (Fig. 61-6) and keep the patient there until the symptoms subside. Move the patient abruptly through the sitting position to the opposite side-lying position and keep the patient there until the symptoms subside. Return the patient to the upright position.[39,40] Advise the patient to remain in a head-upright position for 24 hours after a successful procedure.

Complications

Exacerbation of vertigo occurs occasionally and is thought to result from displacement or dislodgment of canal debris. Repeating the procedure is recommended for relief. Similar symptoms may recur in as many as 50% of patients and in up to 20% in the first 2 weeks.[26]

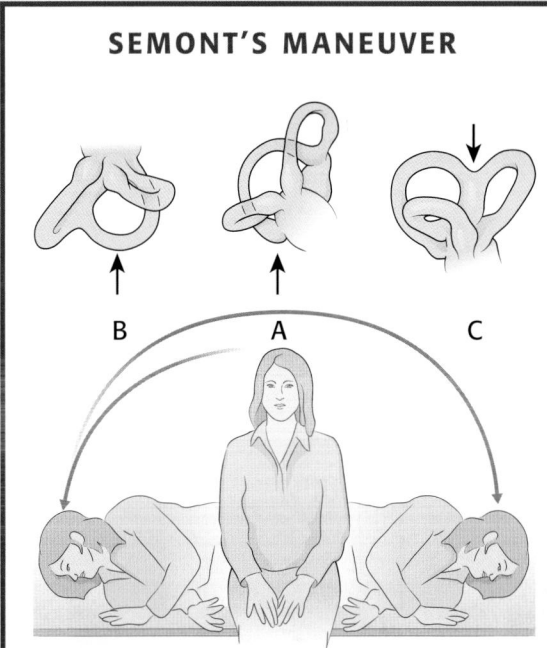

SEMONT'S MANEUVER

The patient is moved quickly into the position that provokes the vertigo and remains in that position for 4 minutes. The patient is then turned rapidly to the opposite side, ear down, and remains in this second position for 4 minutes before slowly sitting up (for detailed description of the technique, see text). *Insets:* The right labyrinth as it would be viewed from the front of the patient. The orientation of the labyrinth is shown when the patient is sitting (*A*), lying on the affected side (*B*), and lying on the opposite side (*C*). The *arrows* indicate the location of the relative position of free-floating debris within the canal during the different stages of this manuever.

Figure 61-6 Semont's maneuver.

Summary

In patients with correctly identified BPPV, canalith repositioning may bring immediate relief or improvement of symptoms. Experience in the ED setting is limited but growing.[36]

TESTS TO DISTINGUISH CENTRAL FROM PERIPHERAL LESIONS IN PATIENTS WITH AVS

Background

Vertigo that is not limited to very brief episodes and triggered by a change in position is not BPPV. Acute vestibular syndrome (AVS) refers to another group of disorders characterized by an acute onset of vertigo, nausea, vomiting, and gait instability that lasts for days to weeks. The majority of these conditions are the result of a peripheral neuropathy, either acute labyrinthitis or vestibular neuritis. Auditory function is preserved in pure vestibular neuritis. The condition is called labyrinthitis when this syndrome is combined with unilateral hearing loss. Both are often preceded by a viral illness.

Unfortunately, a certain percentage of patients with AVS (as many as 25% in some series) harbor a more sinister central pathology such as a brainstem or cerebellar stroke.[41] Moreover, unlike BPPV, which tends to be very specific in its findings, it can be very difficult to distinguish a peripheral from a central process in patients with AVS. Traditional teaching has emphasized a careful neurologic examination in an attempt to find other cranial nerve, cerebellar, or long-tract (descending motor or sensory) findings to corroborate the presence of a central lesion. However, in some patients with stroke involving the posterior circulation, the vertigo is isolated and routine neurologic examination will reveal none of these findings. Magnetic resonance imaging (MRI) may help unravel such cases, but it is not standard to routinely perform MRI in patients with AVS simply because of the rare incidence of occult stroke. Stroke mimicking AVS is rare in young healthy patients, but a stroke causing AVS symptoms may be considered in the elderly or in patients with hypertension, diabetes, previous stroke, atherosclerotic vascular disease, or other vasculopathies.

In 1988, Halmagyi and Curthoys[42] described the horizontal head impulse test (h-HIT), a test of the VOR, as a bedside evaluation to detect peripheral vestibular disease. Subsequent studies have revealed that although a normal finding on the h-HIT is able to reliably identify patients with a central cause of vertigo, it is not as reliable in ruling out central pathology; a positive (abnormal) h-HIT may also occur in patients with lateral pontine and cerebellar stroke syndromes.[43]

The ability of the h-HIT to exclude stroke may be enhanced by the addition of two bedside maneuvers, an examination of nystagmus and a test of skew. The nystagmus that results from a peripheral lesion is unidirectional; its fast or corrective phase beats away from the affected side when the head is rapidly rotated toward that side. Nystagmus that changes its direction (the fast beating phase) with horizontal gaze to either side is highly predictive of a central lesion, as is spontaneous vertical and multidirectional nystagmus.[44] Skew deviation refers to a misalignment of the eyes in the vertical plane; it is usually associated with a central lesion. Although skew deviation can be quite subtle, it can be unmasked by alternately covering each eye in rapid succession while the patient fixes his gaze on the examiner.[45]

Using the h-HIT, Newman-Toker and colleagues[43] were able to distinguish central vertigo from peripheral vertigo in most cases. However, the test is far from perfect; in one study of 43 patients with AVS, 3 patients with stroke (9%) had a positive result on the h-HIT. In a more recent study, when an examination for bidirectional nystagmus and test of skew were added, diagnostic accuracy improved.[46] In 108 patients with chronic risk factors for cerebrovascular disease and a new onset of AVS, the presence of either a normal h-HIT result, direction-changing nystagmus on eccentric gaze, or skew deviation was 100% sensitive and 96% specific for stroke. In this series, 25 peripheral and 76 central lesions were diagnosed by using a combination of MRI and clinical follow-up. Consistent with previous studies, the h-HIT erroneously suggested a peripheral lesion in a small minority (two) of cases. Interestingly, initial diffusion-weighted MRI was falsely negative in 12% of patients in whom a central lesion was ultimately diagnosed.

Indications and Contraindications

Like the Dix-Hallpike maneuver, the h-HIT should not be performed in patients with severe cervical spine disease, unstable spinal injury, high-grade carotid stenosis, or unstable heart disease. Patient discomfort is also a relative contraindication. If nystagmus is present at rest without any provocation (especially if it is vertical or bidirectional), if vertical skew is present, or if any other associated neurologic signs or symptoms exist, a central origin of the vertigo should be suspected and the maneuver is not clinically indicated. There are no absolute contraindications to examination for bidirectional nystagmus or testing for skew.

Procedure

Have the patient seated in a comfortable position. Ask the patient to gaze directly on the examiner's eyes at all times. Quickly rotate the patient's head to each side while carefully observing the eyes for nystagmus. A negative and positive h-HIT maneuver is simulated in Figure 61-7. Next, note any spontaneous vertical nystagmus or nystagmus that is bidirectional with horizontal gaze to both sides. To test for skew, alternately cover each eye in rapid succession while the patient looks directly ahead—note any vertical misalignment that occurs.

HORIZONTAL HEAD IMPULSE TEST (h-HIT)

Normal h-HIT Is Suggestive of Central Lesion (e.g., Cerebellar Stroke)

Instruct the patient to fix his gaze directly on your eyes at all times.

Quickly rotate the head to each side while observing for nystagmus. If the vestibular apparatus is intact, the patient will be able to keep his eyes fixated on you throughout the motion.

Note that the patient's eyes remained fixed on the examiner. A normal test such as this is strongly suggestive of a central origin.

Abnormal h-HIT Is Suggestive of Peripheral Lesion (e.g., Vestibular Neuritis)

Patients with a peripheral vestibular lesion will not be able to keep their eyes fixated on you during the maneuver.

As the head is rapidly turned toward the abnormal side, their eyes cannot maintain fixation.

A corrective saccade (fast jerking movement) will be noted at the end of the maneuver as the patient tries to regain fixation on the examiner.

Figure 61-7 The horizontal head impulse test (h-HIT). In the setting of a sudden onset of isolated vertigo, a normal h-HIT result strongly suggests a central origin (e.g., brainstem or cerebellar stroke). *Top row,* The intact vestibular-ocular reflex causes the subject's eyes to smoothly track the examiner as his head is quickly turned to one side. *Bottom row,* A patient with a peripheral vestibular lesion does not track the examiner when the head is turned to the affected side and requires a quick, corrective saccade back to the examiner.

Interpretation

A positive h-HIT occurs when the head is rotated toward the side of a peripheral vestibular lesion; loss of afferent input from the affected side results in an inability to maintain fixation during head rotation. This requires a corrective saccade (fast jerking movement) back toward the examiner. A negative or normal h-HIT result in the setting of AVS is strongly suggestive of a central origin. A positive h-HIT is consistent with but not diagnostic of a peripheral vestibular lesion. In patients with a positive h-HIT result, diagnostic confidence of a peripheral lesion may be increased if there is an absence of bidirectional nystagmus on lateral gaze and a negative test of skew.

Complications

The h-HIT may exacerbate injury in improperly selected patients with unstable cervical spinal injury or, theoretically, with severe carotid atherosclerotic disease, although no reports of such complications have been reported.

Summary

The h-HIT, along with examination for vertical and bidirectional nystagmus and a test of skew, may be useful in identifying patients with a central cause of vertigo. Although early investigations appear to confirm their role in differentiating central from peripheral vertigo, they should be used with caution and in conjunction with other diagnostic data until further studies confirm their reliability in the ED setting.

BRAIN DEATH TESTING

A textbook of emergency medicine from 1988 once stated that because emergency medicine is a life support–oriented specialty, determination of brain death was outside the practice of the emergency clinician.[47] The date of publication reflects practice at that time; neuroimaging was not often performed while patients were in the ED, and delays for inpatient beds were less common. With increased use of neuroimaging in the ED and general trends toward increased ED length of stay, the occasion may arise for emergency clinicians to be involved in the assessment of brain death. The duty to identify potential organ and tissue donors is another consideration in identifying patients with irreversible loss of brain function. Local practices, policies, regulations, and laws differ, and these remarks are general; the clinician is urged to be familiar with local practices and administrative policies regarding the issue of brain death. Brain death determination has been considered in court cases in the United States, and court rulings have upheld the medical practice of determination of brain death.[48]

For purposes of this discussion, brain death is defined as irreversible loss of functioning of the cerebral hemispheres and brainstem consistent with definitions in the literature.[49-52] The cause of the brain injury should be known or identified because some toxicologic syndromes, notably barbiturate toxicity, exactly duplicate the clinical syndrome of brain death. This section focuses on clinical procedures commonly used to delineate brain death. Radiologic, electrophysiologic, and other tests that are sometimes used are not covered in detail. It should also be noted that in most cases a determination of brain death is not necessary for withdrawal of life-supporting measures. If a cause of coma or severe neurologic injury is identified and a poor prognosis is shared with the family, the option of withholding or withdrawing life support is often exercised. This is entirely within the realm of the patient, family, and clinician, and formal determination of brain death need not occur in these circumstances.

Background

With the advancement of intensive care techniques, patients were identified with continuing spontaneous cardiovascular function while on ventilatory support but without evidence of CNS activity. Observation of these patients revealed that cardiovascular function would eventually fail, although rare prolonged survival has been reported.[53,54] Criteria to reliably identify these patients have been sought for multiple reasons, including to help in family counseling, improve resource allocation, and identify potential organ donors. Part of the impetus for a reliable set of criteria for brain death was legal; a legal pronouncement of death allows discontinuation of advanced life support in cases in which disagreement about continued life support measures may exist.

Death had long been defined as cessation of cardiac function; deeply comatose patients with persistent cardiac activity but without demonstrable brain function challenged the traditional definition of death. The concept of brain death has been entangled in continuing ethical, legal, and policy discussions roughly since the advent of the clinical application of mechanical ventilation in the 1960s.[49,55,56]

Indications and Contraindications

Evaluation for brain death implies that severe CNS dysfunction has been identified, that the cause of the CNS dysfunction is known, and that reversible causes of profound coma have been confidently excluded.[50,52] Formal assessment of brain death is made in preparation for pronouncement of death to allow organ harvest or in uncommon cases of disparate family or caregiver convictions regarding prognosis of the patient. Complex medical issues that may confound the assessment should be considered and ruled out, including severe electrolyte disturbances, hypothermia (defined as a core temperature < 32°C), hypotension, drug intoxication or poisoning, and pharmacologic neuromuscular blockade.[52] Neuroimaging studies should be carefully reviewed.

Procedure

Establishment of Coma and Cortical Assessment

By definition, a patient under evaluation for brain death will be in a coma without spontaneous respirations. Certain examination techniques are used to establish loss of function of the cerebral cortex and brainstem; clinical neurologic examination remains the standard for determination of brain death.[52] It typically involves assessment for cortical function and brainstem reflexes, including respiratory drive.

While holding the patient's eyes open, give loud verbal commands such as "Look up!" and assess for voluntary eye movements, particularly important for patients with the locked-in syndrome. Additionally, deliver a strong painful stimulus by forcefully pressing on the brow, sternum, or nail bed. Should any cerebral or brainstem function be discovered, the patient is not by definition brain-dead even if severe brain injury is present. Some institutions require evaluation by two clinicians with particular specialty training or repeated examinations several hours apart. The need for a second brain death determination has recently been questioned.[57,58] The clinician must be familiar with local practices and policies, which may also require an ancillary EEG, nuclear angiography, or other techniques. Brain death in the pediatric population is more complex, with varying recommendations for repeated examinations and ancillary tests; such discussion is outside the scope of this chapter but is summarized elsewhere.[52,59]

Brainstem Reflex Testing

Pupillary Response

The pupils in brain-dead patients are unreactive and midposition to dilated. Shine a bright light into the pupil and observe for a reaction; none will be seen in a brain-dead patient. Should any reactivity be noted, the patient is not brain-dead.

Auditory Reflex

Deliver a loud handclap into each ear. Observe for eye blink or other reaction. Any reaction establishes that some brainstem function remains and excludes brain death.

Caloric Testing

Perform cold water irrigation of the external auditory canals with large volumes ($\geq$100 mL) to elicit any eye movements through the VOR (described in detail earlier in this chapter). In a brain-dead patient, there will be no movement of the eyes in response to irrigation. Any eye movement excludes brain death.

Corneal Reflex

Stimulate the cornea with a cotton wisp or applicator. Observe for any eye closure, which indicates that the cranial nerve V to VII reflex arc remains intact and excludes the diagnosis of brain death.

Cough Reflex

Stimulate the trachea or main stem bronchi by deep suctioning and observe for coughing. A cough excludes brain death.

Apneic Oxygenation Test

CNS control of respiratory drive resides in the medulla. Establishing apnea is necessary to confirm medullary failure. Mechanical hyperventilation may artificially depress respiratory effort. It is hypercapnia, not hypoxia, that triggers respiratory effort. Simply disconnecting the ventilator to allow the development of hypercapnia for apnea testing may lead to hypoxia.[60] A variety of techniques have been described that allow adequate hypercapnia for medullary stimulation to develop but ensure that oxygenation is adequate during the test. The most commonly described technique is to disconnect the patient from the ventilator and deliver oxygen at 10 to 15 L/min through a catheter inserted into the trachea and then observe for respiratory effort for 8 minutes. Any observed excursion of the abdomen or chest sufficient to produce a tidal volume suggests that brain death is not present. If no respiratory excursions are observed, arterial blood gas analysis is obtained and the patient is reconnected to the ventilator pending results. An arterial partial carbon dioxide pressure (Pco_2) of 60 mm Hg or higher and the absence of respiratory excursions are the criteria for a positive apnea test.[51] Others

suggest that a possibly safer technique is to simply set the ventilator rate to zero while allowing continuous oxygen flow to continue and maintaining any necessary continuous positive pressure through the ventilator.[61]

Declaration of Death

If the criteria for brain death are satisfied, the family and all clinicians involved in patient care should be informed to allow further management decisions. At some institutions the patient is declared dead at the time that the criteria are met, and further care is assumed by the transplant services if that is the anticipated course. Per institutional protocol, confirmation of brain death by two clinicians may be required. Families are generally given the option of being present at the bedside while mechanical ventilation is discontinued, although some advise against this policy because spontaneous reflex movements such as the Lazarus sign (discussed below) may occur and disturb the family.[8] For patients 18 years of age or younger, particularly infants, repeated examinations and confirmatory tests are generally recommended.[52,56,59] A model for direct family conversation in this sensitive interaction has been described and includes a sample script and procedure.[62]

Complications

Carefully following the physical examination protocol reliably identifies the majority of patients with irreversible loss of brain function. Two basic types of error are possible: either erroneously declaring a patient brain-dead when in fact some CNS function is retained or failing to correctly identify brain death.

Profound barbiturate intoxication may simulate the picture of brain death at times. To guard against the error of failing to detect surreptitious pharmacologic coma, some protocols include toxicologic screening tests for barbiturates as part of the process of assessment for brain death. Ancillary techniques for assessing intracranial blood flow would also prevent this error. Two examinations both confirming brain death performed several hours apart have been part of some protocols with the idea that toxicologic coma might improve during this period of observation. Again, familiarity with local policies and practices is necessary.

A variety of movements have been observed in brain-dead patients; at times these spinal level–mediated reflexes may be dramatic and erroneously lead observers to believe that the brain-dead patient is demonstrating voluntary movements or brain-mediated reflex movements. Finger jerks and facial myokymia (spontaneous, fine fascicular muscular contractions) have been reported to be spontaneously present in brain-dead patients. Decerebrate-like extensor posturing, the Lazarus sign (flexion of the arms at the elbows, shoulder adduction, lifting the arms, dystonic posturing of the hands with crossing of the hands), undulating toe flexion, triple-flexion response in the lower extremities, and flexion of the trunk (giving the appearance of sitting up) are among the signs described during apnea testing and after the termination of ventilation or triggered by tactile stimuli.[11,63-67]

Summary

The emergency clinician may become involved in the assessment of patients for brain death in the course of current practice. The cause of irreversible coma should be known. The clinician is urged to be familiar with local practices and regulations in this sometimes complex medicolegal process.

MG TESTING

Background

Myasthenia gravis (MG) is the most common disease of neuromuscular transmission, but the incidence is just 1 in 20,000 in the general population. Patients with MG may be grouped into two major categories. The first group shows weakness in the proximal muscles that increases with activity and improves with rest. The other group has ocular complaints of diplopia or ptosis. Patients in the ocular weakness group may or may not have generalized symptoms as well. Fatigue is the hallmark of the disease; the symptoms typically wax and wane. Patients often see a number of clinicians before a correct diagnosis is made.[68,69]

MG results from immune-mediated destruction of postsynaptic acetylcholine (ACh) receptors, with variable failure of neuromuscular transmission.[68,69] ACh is the transmitter at the neuromuscular junction. When the nerve terminal is stimulated, ACh is released in a quantity far in excess of that needed for effective activation of the ACh receptor. ACh diffuses across the synaptic cleft to transiently interact with the ACh receptor, and an electrical potential is generated at the myoneural end plate. If of sufficient magnitude, the end plate potential initiates an action potential that is propagated along the muscle membrane, and muscle fiber contraction follows. The ACh is rapidly hydrolyzed by acetylcholinesterase in the synaptic cleft. Figure 61-8 summarizes neurotransmitter action at the neuromuscular junction. Of the millions of receptors at each myoneural junction, only a fraction must depolarize to stimulate muscle fiber contraction. Any factor that decreases the interaction of ACh with ACh receptors decreases the probability of an action potential being generated and may lead to failure of neuromuscular transmission with resulting weakness. Acetylcholinesterase inhibitors (anticholinesterases) have been the mainstay of therapy for

MG for years, but they have been supplemented by immunosuppressive regimens and thymectomy. Failure of neuromuscular transmission may also occur with excessive inhibition of acetylcholinesterase; persistence of ACh in the synaptic cleft leads to continuous depolarization of the receptor.

Bedside diagnostic testing for MG has been described in patients seen in the ED with two different clinical pictures. The first involves a known patient with MG and increased weakness who is being treated with cholinesterase inhibitor therapy; pharmacologic testing in this setting is controversial. The second involves a previously undiagnosed patient in whom the diagnosis of MG is suspected because of ptosis, diplopia, or fluctuating muscular weakness; bedside testing may be helpful in selected patients in this group.

A battery of tests can be used for the assessment of a patient with suspected MG, but only a few are available to the emergency clinician.[70,71] ACh receptor antibody assay is positive in more than 80% of patients with MG but has a turnaround time of several days.[72,73] Repetitive nerve stimulation and single-fiber electromyography tests are available in the electrophysiology laboratory.[74] Several pharmacologic tests have been used to aid in the diagnosis of suspected MG, including parenteral administration of edrophonium chloride (Tensilon), neostigmine, or curare. Administration of edrophonium chloride for the diagnosis of MG (Tensilon test) is described in detail because of the drug's rapid onset, short duration of action, and widespread acceptance for this diagnostic challenge; the emergency clinician may find occasion to use this test. The ice pack test is discussed because of favorable reports of its utility and noninvasive nature.[71,75,76] Other noninvasive tests such as the "sleep test" (improvement in ptosis after 30 minutes of rest) and the "peek sign" (failure of the patient to maintain gentle eye closure) have been described.[71] Both systemic and regional administration of curare has also been reported to aid in the diagnosis of MG. A technique is described for administration of curare into an ischemic arm; this modification is known as the *regional curare test*.[74] The use of curare in this setting is outside the realm of practice of the emergency clinician.

Edrophonium (Tensilon) Test

Background

Edrophonium chloride (Tensilon) is an acetylcholinesterase inhibitor that has been used for the diagnosis of MG since the 1960s. The short duration of action of edrophonium that made it unsatisfactory as a therapeutic agent for MG makes it useful as a diagnostic agent. The drug's onset of action is rapid, and the duration of maximal effect is short, usually less than 2 minutes. Any effect resolves within 5 to 10 minutes.[77]

Edrophonium administration has also been recommended in the past to monitor acetylcholinesterase inhibitor therapy.[78,79] However, edrophonium is not sufficiently reliable for titrating the effect of anticholinesterase medication.[80] Use of the Tensilon test in a patient with known MG is controversial and should be done only in consultation with or in the presence of the treating neurologist, if at all.

Myasthenic crisis may be defined as respiratory distress in a patient with MG. In a myasthenic patient with respiratory distress, airway management and assisted ventilation are top priorities. Administration of edrophonium should not be viewed as a possible alternative to intubation and mechanical ventilation.

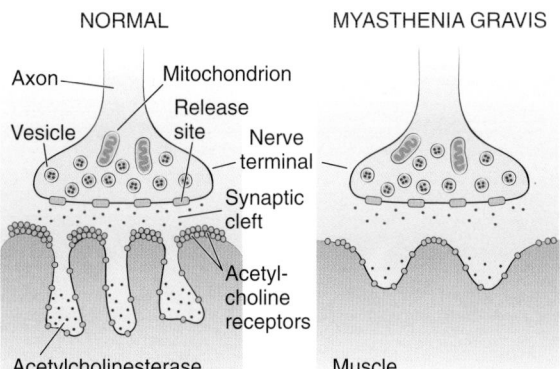

NEUROMUSCULAR JUNCTIONS

NORMAL   MYASTHENIA GRAVIS

Axon
Mitochondrion
Release site
Vesicle
Nerve terminal
Synaptic cleft
Acetylcholine receptors
Acetylcholinesterase   Muscle

Figure 61-8 Neuromuscular junctions. In myasthenia gravis, acetylcholine is released from presynaptic vesicles and diffuses across the synaptic cleft to the postsynaptic receptors. Acetylcholinesterase, located deep within the synaptic folds, hydrolyzes acetylcholine. There is also a simplification of the postsynaptic site with a reduced number of receptors.

Earlier types of crises described included "myasthenic" crisis from insufficient drug administration, "cholinergic" crisis from overdosage of a cholinesterase inhibitor, and the "brittle" patient with rapidly changing drug requirements,[81,82] but terminology in this setting remains controversial.[83] Even the clinical existence of the different types of crises has been debated.[80] Several authorities advocate withdrawing all cholinesterase inhibitors in patients with worsening symptoms because most patients show increased responsiveness to cholinesterase inhibitors after several days without taking the drug.[80,83] Others advocate a trial of edrophonium chloride at reduced dosage (1 to 2 mg) only after ventilator support.[81,84]

Indications and Contraindications

The bedside Tensilon test is indicated for the diagnosis of patients with suspected MG when there is a clinical need to make this diagnosis immediately. If other bedside tests such as the ice pack test (discussed later) are conclusive or if eyelid fatigue on prolonged upgaze can be demonstrated, there is no need to administer edrophonium.[85] If the tempo of the clinical scenario is such that consultation or admission and performing specialized electromyelograms or serologic testing are feasible, deferring the Tensilon test in the ED may be preferred in recognition of the fact that serologic and neurophysiologic testing will not be completed for several days.

Administration of edrophonium is commonly performed in office settings by neuro-ophthalmologists, and occasionally complications of bradycardia occur that at times may be symptomatic with hypotension and loss of consciousness.[86,87] One study reported the complication rate in office settings to be 0.16%.[86] A history of asthma or cardiac dysrhythmias is a relative contraindication to the administration of cholinesterase inhibitors. Complications reported in the literature from edrophonium testing largely date from the era when it was used in cardiology to differentiate supraventricular rhythms.[85] Reported complications include disturbances in cardiac rhythm and even death; several of these patients were taking digoxin or β-blockers.[88-91] One report noted transient asystole after the administration of edrophonium in a patient with suspected MG; the patient was critically ill and had been receiving intravenous labetalol.[85] Hence, caution is advised in administering edrophonium to patients receiving β-blocking agents, digoxin, or other drugs with atrioventricular-blocking properties.

Administration of edrophonium to a patient with MG being treated with cholinesterase inhibitors is controversial. Many investigators consider myasthenic crisis to be a contraindication to edrophonium administration, although in series of patients with myasthenic crisis, its use continues to be reported.[81,84]

A muscle that is clearly weak must be identified to monitor during Tensilon testing; ptosis is a commonly monitored sign. If a specific muscle cannot be isolated for objective testing, administration of edrophonium should be deferred and other approaches to diagnosis pursued.

Equipment

The following material is needed for testing an adult. Intravenous access should be secured with a saline lock. Ten milligrams of edrophonium chloride should be drawn up in a tuberculin syringe. Edrophonium chloride is supplied in 1- and 10-mL vials at a concentration of 10 mg/mL. A second syringe of normal saline should be available to administer as placebo,

although some clinicians have recommended nicotine, calcium chloride, or atropine for this purpose.[79] Atropine and other cardiovascular drugs and resuscitative equipment should be readily available. Cardiac monitoring is generally recommended. Photographic recording equipment is desirable to objectively document any improvement in motor function.

Procedure

Identify a muscle that is clearly weak. A clinically evident extraocular muscle weakness or the presence of ptosis allows direct observation of a single weak muscle becoming stronger in response to the drug. Simple grip dynamometry does not aid in evaluation; a repetitive measure of grip strength (ergogram) is necessary. Ideally, one person is available to administer the edrophonium or placebo and a second person is free to observe the effect of medication on the patient. It is best if both the observer and the patient do not know which syringe contains edrophonium and which contains saline, thus creating a double-blind testing situation.

Again, ptosis is an easy sign to test and is generally used if present (Fig. 61-9). The principles involved in assessing the effect of edrophonium on ptosis may be extended to testing other muscles. Ask the patient to look upward for several moments to fatigue the levator muscles. Note the degree of ptosis and document it by measurements or photographs. After a moment's rest, ask the patient to look straight ahead. Inject 0.2 mL of the test substance in one syringe (2 mg of edrophonium or saline). If no response is seen within 1 minute, inject further increments of 2 mg up to a maximum of 10 mg. Note any increase in strength as reflected by an increase in size of the palpebral fissure. Repeat the procedure

Figure 61-9 Tensilon test. **A,** Bilateral asymmetric ptosis and defective upgaze. **B,** Improvement of ptosis and left upgaze following the intravenous injection of Tensilon. (*From Kanski JJ. Clinical Diagnosis in Ophthalmology. St. Louis: Mosby; 2006.*)

with the other test substance. Any improvement should occur within 30 seconds and disappear in 5 minutes.

Complications

A small percentage of individuals are hypersensitive to even the initial small dose of edrophonium and exhibit the cholinergic side effects of salivation, lacrimation, and miosis. These effects are transient. Atropine, 0.5 mg, may be given intravenously if necessary to counteract these symptoms. A smaller number of patients may experience symptomatic bradycardia that responds to atropine. As described earlier, rare cardiac arrhythmias and death have been reported, usually in patients taking digoxin or β-blockers.

Interpretation

The key to the procedure is its interpretation. If a clearly paretic muscle has been identified, objective signs of improvement in the strength of that muscle within a moment of administration of edrophonium and fading of that improvement over the next 5 minutes are the criteria for a positive test result. Up to 90% of patients with MG have a positive test result under ideal circumstances.[78,79] False-negative results do occur consistently, however.

For evaluating the effect of edrophonium on ptosis, a positive test consists of the patient having increased ability to elevate the eyelids after the administration of 5 to 10 mg of edrophonium. The ptosis returns within 5 minutes. Subjective increases in general strength or relief of fatigue do not constitute a positive test. Fasciculations, or brief twitches of muscles, are not usually observed in a patient with MG who has received edrophonium, in contrast to normal subjects. The Tensilon test may be repeated in 30 minutes if desired.

Normal subjects have no change in muscle strength. They may transiently experience the side effects of salivation, lacrimation, and diaphoresis. Perioral, periocular, or lingual fasciculations are almost always noted in normal patients after edrophonium administration.

Reproducible and unequivocal reversal of weakness in a specific muscle is extremely specific for MG.[92,93] False-positive test results have been reported in patients with Eaton-Lambert syndrome and rarely in patients with intracranial lesions.[94-96] Other rare reports of positive test results involve patients with amyotrophic lateral sclerosis. A "perverse" reaction in which a paretic extraocular muscle, weak from other causes, becomes even weaker with edrophonium administration has been noted rarely.[97]

Ice Pack Test

Background

It has been observed clinically that myasthenic patients have exacerbations of weakness with environmental heat and improvement in strength with cold temperatures. A simple bedside test uses these observations to evaluate ptosis.[71,75,76] Ice placed in a surgical glove or wrapped in a towel is placed lightly over the eyelid of the patient. Cooling of the eyelid below 29°C is accomplished within 2 minutes. Ptosis has been noted to improve in 80% or more of patients tested and may be more sensitive than the edrophonium test in detecting ocular MG. Although the reported number of patients evaluated by this method continues to be small, the test is included here because of its potential application in the ED, its lack of side effects, and its noninvasive nature.

Indications

Unilateral or bilateral ptosis of uncertain etiology in which MG is a diagnostic possibility is the sole indication for this test. Use of the ice pack test for evaluating diplopia possibly related to MG has also been described, but this role has yet to be established and its utility is unclear.[98,99]

Procedure

Ice and a surgical glove or towel are the only material required. A camera to record any response is optional. Measure or photograph the degree of the patient's ptosis. Ask the patient to look upward, which often provokes the ptosis. If bilateral ptosis is present, use the more affected eye for evaluation. Cool the eyelid by lightly holding the wrapped ice to the patient's eyelid for 2 minutes or until patient discomfort limits application. Compare the width of the palpebral fissure with the pretest width (Fig. 61-10; see p. 1258).

Complications

Patient discomfort from ice pack application may limit cold exposure time to less than 2 minutes but may still allow a test to be successfully performed.

Interpretation

A clear improvement in ptosis in the cooled eye is the criterion for a positive test. The effect should be reproducible. In small clinical studies, the ice pack test was found to be at least as sensitive as administration of edrophonium in improving ptosis in patients with ocular MG. False-negative results do occur, probably at about the same frequency as with Tensilon testing. One individual has been reported to have a negative ice pack test result with a positive Tensilon test result. Negative or equivocal Tensilon tests have been reported in other individuals who had clearly positive ice pack test results. Normal individuals showed no change in width of the palpebral fissure after cold exposure. False-positive results are rare.[75,76,100]

Summary

The bedside Tensilon test has a long history of utility in diagnosing MG but it has largely been replaced by acetylcholinesterase receptor assay and electrodiagnostic studies in the ambulatory setting.[72,74,85,93] On occasion, when rapid diagnosis is desired or MG is suspected in the presence of a normal ACh receptor titer, a carefully performed Tensilon test is still clinically valuable. Use of the Tensilon test in the setting of myasthenic crisis is controversial and is discouraged.

The ice pack test is so simple and noninvasive that it should be the initial procedure of choice in the ED for evaluating the possibility of ptosis from ocular MG. A positive ice pack test result strongly suggests ocular MG and obviates the need for the Tensilon test. False-negative results do occur, and additional testing should be performed if clinical suspicion for MG is strong.

It is often the case with neuromuscular diseases, given the broad diagnostic possibilities, that the emergency clinician is unable to establish a confident diagnosis at a single patient encounter.[101] Appropriate consultation and referral are necessary.

References are available at www.expertconsult.com

Figure 61-10 The ice pack test for myasthenia gravis. **A,** Before placement of an ice pack. **B,** Ice pack placed over the eyelid for about 2 minutes. **C,** After placement of an ice pack, improvement is noted in ptosis of the right eye. (For details, see Sethi and colleagues.[76])

Ophthalmologic, Otolaryngologic, and Dental Procedures

CHAPTER 62

Ophthalmologic Procedures

Kevin J. Knoop and William R. Dennis

The following discussion focuses on procedures performed by emergency clinicians during the evaluation and treatment of injuries and diseases of the eye. Emphasis is placed on practical application of the techniques; cautions to be heeded by the emergency clinician are included.

ASSESSMENT OF VISUAL ACUITY

Evaluation of visual acuity may initially be deferred with simple, obvious, or straightforward cases, such as a stye, periorbital laceration, or minor eye irritation; however, assessment of visual acuity should be the first procedure performed in the majority of patients seen in the emergency department (ED) with an eye complaint. Even though it may initially be deferred in the triage or trauma room setting or under other relevant scenarios, it is incumbent on the emergency clinician to ensure that visual acuity or function is ultimately assessed adequately.

Indications

Visual acuity should be assessed as soon as practicable and before the patient is examined with bright lights. In the event of blepharospasm from an injury (e.g., abrasion, chemical exposure), a topical anesthetic may facilitate the examination. Patients are often encountered in the context of an eye complaint and say that they "can't see." In these instances, emergency visual acuity assessment should be performed first, beginning with evaluation of light perception, then hand motion, and finally counting fingers at 3 ft (Fig. 62-1). If the patient succeeds in performing these assessments, a near vision card may then be used or distant visual acuity assessed. In emergency circumstances, detailed formal vision testing is not essential; however, some form of visual acuity assessment is needed. In this situation, the ability to count fingers or read newsprint gives some indication of gross visual function. Formal visual acuity testing should never delay important therapeutic interventions such as eye irrigation.[1]

Distant Visual Acuity Procedure

For formal vision testing, ask the patient to face a well-lit standard Snellen or similar eye chart from a premeasured distance of 20 ft. Use a card or the palm of the hand to occlude one eye at a time. If possible, examine all patients while wearing their current lens correction to obtain the best corrected distant visual acuity. If not available, measure visual acuity first without correction and then with a pinhole device, and note any improvement in visual acuity. This device functions as a corrective lens by reducing corneal refractive error. In general, visual acuity is improved with the pinhole device. Decreased visual acuity that is not improved with this device suggests that corneal refractive error is not the cause. Construct a pinhole device by punching one to several holes in the center of a card (3- × 5-inch index card) with an 18-gauge needle. Devices with one or more pinholes drilled into an eye cover are available commercially (Fig. 62-2A and B) or can be constructed from readily available material in the ED, such as the index card with holes just mentioned. Figure 62-2C presents a chart for testing visual acuity while the patient is on a stretcher or in a chair. The chart can be used directly from this text if held 14 inches from the eye. Begin by testing the affected eye or the one presumed to have the worst visual acuity. First, instruct the patient to read the smallest letters on the chart that can easily be seen. Then ask the patient to read letters that can just barely be made out (i.e., they do not have to be clear). If the patient is unable to read the largest letter on the chart, move the patient to half the distance from the chart (10 ft), or if using the figure in this text, move it 7 inches closer to the eye and repeat the procedure. Record the

Figure 62-1 The "routine" progression for assessing visual acuity is reversed in the emergency situation. Assessment of an intact visual pathway begins with quickly discerning whether the patient has light perception (LP), can see hand motion (HM), and can count fingers at 3 ft (CF). Subsequent progression to assess vision at 10 and then 20 ft from a standard eye chart ensues.

Figure 62-2 A commercial pinhole device reveals refractive error caused by corneal aberration (excessive tearing or nearsightedness). **A,** First measure visual acuity without the device. **B,** Then measure with the pinhole cover lowered. Document the acuity with and without the pinhole device. **C,** If the patient cannot stand or a formal eye chart is not available, ask the patient to read this "distance equivalent" chart by holding the card 14 inches away from the patient.

results reflecting the change in distance (e.g., 10/200). The numerator in the vision ratio is the distance of the patient from the chart and the denominator is the distance at which a patient with normal vision can read the line of letters. For patients who still cannot read the letters on the chart, test vision progressively as follows: the ability to count fingers, detect hand motion, and perceive light (with or without projection—the ability to perceive the direction of light), and finally, the inability to perceive light.[2]

Near Visual Acuity Procedure

Perform near visual acuity assessment in the ED at the bedside or at triage. Hold a pocket near vision card (see Fig. 62-2C) or any printed material in good light at a distance of approximately 14 inches in front of the patient and occlude each eye alternately as described earlier. When using available printed material in lieu of a near vision card, measure the size of the letters that are discerned by the patient. At a later time compare these letters with the size of the letters

Figure 62-3 Optokinetic nystagmus (OKN) testing will determine whether the visual pathway is intact. Induce OKN by passing a regularly sequenced pattern in front of the eye such as this commercially available drum. Hold the drum in front of the patient. Direct the patient to look at the drum as you rotate it slowly. Alternatively, draw a tape measure across the line of sight while asking the patient to look directly at it as it passes.

on the near vision card to deduce the patient's actual visual acuity. When near vision is decreased, it is usually caused by either loss of visual function or poor accommodation as a result of advancing age (presbyopia). Less commonly, it is caused by traumatic mydriasis. Thus, examine patients with presbyopia with their reading correction in place to obtain the best corrected near visual acuity.

For patients who cannot communicate or in whom factitious blindness or malingering is suspected, check for optokinetic nystagmus (OKN) to determine whether the visual pathway is intact. To test for OKN, pass a regularly sequenced pattern in front of the eyes. If an optokinetic drum is available, rotate the drum in front of the patient (Fig. 62-3). This is not available in many EDs, however. In place of the drum, substitute a printed piece of paper such as newsprint (without photographs or large areas with no print) or a standard tape measure. Pass it in front of the patient's eye at reading distance while instructing the patient to look at it as it moves rapidly by. Evaluate for tracking as demonstrated by nystagmus-like eye movements seen when the test object is moved from side to side in front of the patient. Such movement indicates an intact visual pathway. Finally, another effective method is to hold a mirror in front of the patient and slowly rotate the mirror to either side of the patient. Patients with an intact visual pathway will maintain eye contact with themselves as demonstrated by eye movement as the mirror is moved. A large mirror that reflects the patient's entire face is most effective for this purpose.

All patients with decreased visual acuity from baseline require routine referral for further ophthalmologic follow-up; however, patients with moderately or severely decreased visual acuity not explained by refractive error require ophthalmologic consultation in the ED.

DILATING THE EYE

Dilating the eye is useful for both diagnostic and therapeutic purposes. Be advised, however, that an attack of narrow-angle (angle-closure) glaucoma may be precipitated by dilating the pupil. The most common form of glaucoma, however, is

open-angle glaucoma, and this type is not precipitated by dilating the pupil. Some patients may have a "mixed mechanism" glaucoma with both open-angle and narrow-angle components. Systemic reactions, such as bradycardia or even heart block from β-blocker eyedrops, can be induced by mucosal absorption of dilating medications.

There are two types of dilators: sympathomimetic agents, which stimulate the dilator muscle of the iris, and cycloplegic agents, which block the parasympathetic stimulus that constricts the iris sphincter. Cycloplegic agents also block contraction of the ciliary muscles, which control focusing of the lens of the eye. This second effect of cycloplegic agents is beneficial in the therapeutic use of dilators for iritis.

Cycloplegic agents were used cosmetically as early as Galen's time. Beginning in the early 1800s, extracts from the plants *Hyoscyamus* and belladonna were used in ophthalmology. Atropine was first isolated in 1833. Epinephrine was used on eyes in 1900 as the first sympathomimetic agent.[3]

Indications and Contraindications

There are several diagnostic and therapeutic indications for dilating the pupil. Dilation is indicated for diagnosis when the fundus cannot be examined adequately through an undilated pupil. An elderly patient with miotic pupils and cataracts is an example of a patient in whom dilation may facilitate funduscopic examination. Dilation is therapeutically useful for many ophthalmic conditions, including inflammation of the eye. In the emergency setting, corneal injury with secondary traumatic iritis is a common example. Dilation helps the inflamed eye in two ways. First, it may hinder adhesions (synechiae) from forming between the iris and other ocular structures. Such adhesions eventually limit movement of the pupil and may precipitate glaucoma. Second, cycloplegic dilating agents relax the ciliary muscle spasm that often accompanies an inflamed eye and thus may reduce the pain associated with inflammation. Though traditionally used for these purposes, both benefits are largely theoretical with little formal evidence to support or refute their use in the ED.

Dilation is discouraged in patients with head injury who are at risk for herniation when it is necessary to monitor pupil findings. Dilation is contraindicated in the presence of narrow anterior chamber angles. Patients predisposed to having narrow angles may be unaware of this condition. Evaluate the depth of the anterior chamber before this procedure, and do not dilate the eye if there is any question of a narrow angle. To estimate the depth of the anterior chamber, shine a penlight tangentially from the lateral side of the eye. When the depth of the anterior chamber is normal, uniform illumination of the iris is seen. However, when the iris has a forward convexity as in the case of a narrow anterior chamber, only a sector of iris is illuminated and there will be a shadow on the medial (nasal) side of the iris (Fig. 62-4). With a slit lamp, the depth of the anterior chamber angle can be assessed directly. The definitive test for assessing the anterior chamber angle is gonioscopy, in which the anterior chamber angle structures are viewed directly by means of a special mirrored contact lens and a slit lamp. Gonioscopy is not a technique normally performed by emergency clinicians.

Systemic effects can develop after the application of eyedrops.[4-10] Review the following sections on agents and complications before using these drugs in patients with compromised cardiovascular function.

Figure 62-4 **A,** *Left:* The normal eye. Aqueous humor, produced in the posterior chamber, flows through the pupil into the anterior chamber. The major pathway for the egress of aqueous humor is through the trabecular meshwork into Schlemm's canal. *Right:* Primary angle-closure glaucoma. In anatomically predisposed eyes, transient apposition of the iris at the pupillary margin to the lens during pupil dilation blocks the passage of aqueous humor from the posterior chamber to the anterior chamber. Buildup of pressure in the posterior chamber bows the iris forward and occludes the trabecular meshwork. **B,** *Left:* Normal anterior chamber with a negative transillumination test. Note that the entire iris is illuminated. *Right:* Shallow anterior chamber with a positive transillumination test. Note the shadow on the outer half of the iris. **C,** *Left:* Clinical use of the penlight examination to assess the depth of the anterior chamber of the right eye. The examiner sits face to face with the patient to ensure that the light source is perfectly perpendicular to the line of vision. *Right:* The axial anterior chamber depth of the right eye is less than normal. This can be demonstrated by shining a light across the eye from the temporal side. Because of the convexity of the iris-lens diaphragm, the nasal iris manifests a crescentic shadow (eclipse sign). (*A, From Kumar V, Abbas AK, Fausto N, et al, eds. Robbins and Cotran Pathologic Basis of Disease, Professional Edition. 8th ed. Philadelphia: Saunders; 2009; B, from Swartz MH. Textbook of Physical Diagnosis. 6th ed. Philadelphia: Saunders: 2009. C, from Kanski JJ. Clinical Diagnosis in Ophthalmology. St. Louis: Mosby; 2006.*)

Agents

Only two dilating agents are really needed in the ED. Phenylephrine (Neo-Synephrine) 2.5%, a potent sympathomimetic, is used for diagnostic dilation of the pupil and visualization of the fundus. The drug is short acting, and because accommodation is not affected, the patient's vision is not altered. Phenylephrine 10% should *not* be used routinely because it can be absorbed systemically and, in rare cases, has caused hypertensive crisis, myocardial infarction, and death.[8,9]

For therapeutic cycloplegia in patients with iritis, 5% homatropine works well. Even though Table 62-1 indicates a maximum duration of 3 days, 24 hours is more common. Therefore, 5% homatropine is a useful therapeutic agent for traumatic iritis. Atropine should not be used for traumatic

TABLE 62-1   Mydriatic Agents

AGENT	MAXIMUM MYDRIASIS	DURATION OF MYDRIASIS*	COMMON TRADE NAME
Sympathomimetics			
Phenylephrine,[†] 2.5%[‡]	20 min	3 hr	Neo-Synephrine
Cocaine, 5% or 4%	20 min	2 hr	—
Parasympatholytics (Cycloplegics)			
Atropine, 1%	40 min	12 days	—
Scopolamine, 0.25%	30 min	7 days	—
Homatropine, 5%[§]	30 min	1-3 days	—
Cyclopentolate, 1%	30 min	6-24 hr	Cyclogyl
Tropicamide, 1%	30 min	4 hr	Mydriacyl

*The duration of effect shows considerable individual variation. These are general estimates.
[†]Preferred for funduscopic examination.
[‡]A 10% solution may produce cardiovascular reaction and hence should not be used.
[§]Preferred for iritis or corneal abrasion therapy.

iritis because the undesirable effects of pupillary dilation and blurred vision persist for a week or longer after the associated corneal abrasions have healed. Atropine drops may be prescribed as part of the therapy for nontraumatic iritis after appropriate ophthalmologic consultation. Individuals with lightly pigmented irides tend to have greater sensitivity to cycloplegic agents than do individuals with greater pigmentation; the cycloplegic effect might therefore be more prolonged in people with light eyes. It might be difficult to dilate some patients with deeply pigmented irides, however, and numerous applications of drops might be required.

Malingerers may use mydriatic agents to dilate a pupil unilaterally for the purpose of feigning neurologic disease. Normally, the pupillary dilation caused by intracranial compression of the third cranial nerve will constrict with 2% pilocarpine eyedrops. A mydriatic-treated eye can be identified by full motor function of the third cranial nerve and absence of miosis after the instillation of pilocarpine. A fixed and dilated pupil in an awake and alert patient cannot be secondary to brain herniation. Although other neurologic problems may be present, in a normal-appearing patient with a fixed and dilated pupil, a pharmacologic cause is highly likely. It should be noted that legitimate patients may not recall the name of an eye medicine that they used but will usually recall whether the bottle had a red cap, as is found on all cycloplegic solutions. An unexpected mydriasis in a trusted patient may be the result of such an agent. Medications that constrict the pupil, such as pilocarpine, have a green cap. Pressure-lowering drops for glaucoma may be yellow or blue topped (β-blockers), purple topped (adrenergic agents), or orange topped (topical carbonic anhydrase inhibitors).

A fixed and dilated pupil from a pharmacologic cause may be encountered after both nasotracheal and orotracheal intubation (Fig. 62-5). In such ill or injured patients, cerebral herniation must be considered. When phenylephrine is used to constrict the nasal mucosa before nasal intubation (endotracheal tube, nasogastric tube), inadvertent spread to the eye can result in a fixed and dilated pupil. The same scenario may occur during resuscitation when endotracheal epinephrine has been instilled into the lungs and cardiopulmonary resuscitation has expelled epinephrine into the eye. In such scenarios, the affected pupil will not constrict after intraocular pilocarpine administration. Finally, a fixed and dilated pupil might occur as a result of inadvertent contamination of the eye with scopolamine after the application of a scopolamine patch.

Procedure

Instillation of mydriatic agents is similar to the administration of other eye solutions. For medicolegal purposes, note the patient's visual acuity before instillation of the medicine. This documents that any decreased vision is not the result of the mydriatic agent. Whenever dilation is performed, note on the patient's chart the dose and time that agents have been given to avoid confusion during subsequent neurologic evaluation.

Place the patient in a supine or a comfortable semirecumbent position. Instruct the patient to gaze at an object in the upper visual field, such as a fixture on the ceiling. Gently depress the lower lid with a finger on the epidermis. Instill a single drop of the solution into the lower lid fornix, and ask the patient to blink to spread the medication. Do not use more than a single drop because it produces reflex tearing and reduces the concentration in contact with the conjunctiva. Forewarn the patient that the medication is uncomfortable when it goes into the eyes. After the medication has been instilled, the patient may blot the eye when it is closed but should not rub it with a tissue. If the desired effect is not noted in 15 to 20 minutes, repeat the dose, but this is seldom required.

Complications

Any dilator can precipitate an attack of angle-closure glaucoma in susceptible patients.[10] In the case of angle-closure glaucoma, it may take several hours before symptoms become evident. The patient often complains of smoky vision with "halos" around lights, as well as an aching pain that is sometimes severe. Nausea and vomiting may occur. If the affected

Figure 62-5 A, After phenylephrine (Neo-Synephrine) drops were instilled in the nose to facilitate passage of a tube, this comatose patient was nasotracheally intubated for his drug overdose. **B,** On a subsequent examination a unilateral fixed and dilated pupil was noted. The pupil dilation resulted from Neo-Synephrine nose drops that were snorted from the nose into the eye during intubation and simulated cerebral herniation. Other unusual causes of a fixed and dilated pupil are endotracheal epinephrine expelled from the lungs and splashed onto the eye during cardiopulmonary resuscitation and inadvertent contamination of the eye after the application of a scopolamine patch behind the ear.

eye becomes injected in association with a hazy cornea, elevated pressure on tonometry, and an oval, fixed pupil, consult an ophthalmologist immediately. Place the patient supine and administer analgesics and antiemetics. Treatment usually includes the agents suggested in Box 62-1, and later, definitive laser or surgical procedures.

Be aware that if contaminated, an eye medication can introduce infection. Most solutions contain bactericidal ingredients, but contamination of the tips of droppers can still occur (Fig. 62-6A).[11] Use only newly opened bottles of eye medication or single-use vials, particularly if the patient has a deep corneal injury or has recently undergone eye surgery. Promptly discard out-of-date drops and those in which crust or other material is found around the nozzle.

BOX 62-1 Treatment Options for Acute Angle-Closure Glaucoma*

Place patient supine; administer analgesics (such as IV morphine titrated to effect) and antiemetics (such as ondansetron 8 mv IV):
1. Beta blocker[†]: Timolol 0.5% (Timoptic), 1 drop to the affected eye, wait 1 minute, and then
2. Alpha agonist: Apraclonidine 1% (Lopidine), 1 drop to the affected eye, wait 1 minute, and then
3. Miotic agent: Pilocarpine 2% (Isopto Carpine), 1 drop to the affected eye every 15 minutes for 2 total doses; wait 1 minute after first dose, and then
4. Prednisolone acetate 1 percent, 1 drop to the affected eye every 15 minutes for 4 total doses
5. Acetazolamide 500 mg IV (may give by mouth, two 250-mg tablets, if IV medication not available)

Modified from Shields SR. Managing eye disease in primary care. Part 3. When to refer for ophthalmologic care. Postgrad Med. 2000;108(5):99-106.
Empiric therapy, no controlled trials, based on clinical experience.
†*Relative contraindications: severe bronchospasm, second to third degree heart block, uncompensated congestive heart failure.*

Forewarn the patient that any cycloplegic (in contrast to a sympathomimetic) will blur a patient's near vision. Vision will be less blurred in adults older than 45 years, who generally have a reduced ability to focus for near vision. Although most adults will be able to drive safely, even with both eyes affected, it is advisable to have someone else drive whenever feasible. Light sensitivity caused by pupillary dilation may also be bothersome; sunglasses are sufficient for this problem.

Systemic reactions may rarely be induced by sympathomimetic and cycloplegic eyedrops.[4-10] In one report of 33 cases of adverse reactions associated with 10% phenylephrine, there were 15 myocardial infarctions (11 deaths), 7 cases of precipitation of angle-closure glaucoma, and a variety of systemic cardiovascular or neurologic reactions.[9]

After instillation of eyedrops into the conjunctival sac, systemic absorption can occur through the conjunctival capillaries, as well as by way of the nasal mucosa, the oral pharynx, and the gastrointestinal tract after passage through the lacrimal drainage system. Mucosal hyperemia enhances absorption. Symptoms can often be avoided by maintaining digital pressure on the nasal canthus to occlude the puncta for several minutes after administration (Fig. 62-6B).[4]

THE FLUORESCEIN EXAMINATION

Perform fluorescein staining of the eye as part of the evaluation of all patients with eye trauma and infection. It is a quick and easy technique that is crucial for the proper diagnosis and management of common eye emergencies. View the fluorescein-stained cornea and conjunctiva under a "blue" light and ideally in conjunction with slit lamp magnification (see "Slit Lamp Examination," later in this chapter).

Sodium fluorescein is a water-soluble chemical that fluoresces. It absorbs light in the blue wavelengths and emits the energy in the longer green wavelengths. It fluoresces in an alkaline environment (such as in Bowman's membrane, which is located below the corneal epithelium) but not in an acidic

Figure 62-6 A, Administration of eye drops. Position the patient with the head tilted back. Direct the patient's gaze upward. Pull the lower lid downward and instill a single drop of medicine in the lower conjunctival fornix. Ensure that the tip of the dropper does not touch the lid or lashes. Instruct the patient to close the eyelids for 1 minute to increase contact of the medicine with the globe and to decrease outflow of medication down the tear duct and over the lid margin. **B,** If administering large amounts of eye drops that have systemic effects, such as β-blocker drops, place the operator's index finger under the inferior eyelid along the nasal borders of the eye and firmly compress the nasolacrimal duct against the globe for a few minutes, thereby preventing migration of the drops into the nose and reducing systemic absorption.

environment (such as in the tear film over intact corneal epithelium).[12] Thus it is useful in revealing even minute abrasions on the cornea.

Fluorescein was initially used in ophthalmology in the 1880s.[13] It was first used as a drop, but when the danger of contamination by bacteria (especially *Pseudomonas*) was recognized in the 1950s,[14] paper strips impregnated with fluorescein were developed. These strips are now supplied in individual sterile wrappers and should be used instead of the premixed solution.

Indications and Contraindications

Fluorescein staining is indicated for the evaluation of suspected abrasions, foreign bodies (FBs), and infections of the eye,[15] including "simple" cases of conjunctivitis, which may actually be herpetic keratitis. Exposure of the face to pepper spray has been associated with corneal abrasions, and such

patients should undergo fluorescein staining and be evaluated with a slit lamp or Wood's lamp.[16] Corneal defects may be seen after even a few seconds of unprotected viewing of a welder's arc flame.

Fluorescein permanently stains soft contact lenses. Therefore, when fluorescein is used, remove soft contact lenses before instilling the fluorescein and caution the patient to not put the lenses back into the eye for several hours. Topically administered fluorescein is considered nontoxic, although reactions to a fluorescein-containing solution (not impregnated strips) have been described.[17] These reports, which consist of vagal reactions[18] and generalized convulsions,[19] are rare, not rigorously supported, and believed to be caused by agents other than fluorescein in the solution. If using one of these fluorescein-containing solutions rather than the fluorescein-impregnated strips, be aware of these potential, yet scientifically suspect idiosyncratic reactions.

Also be aware that fluorescein dye may enter the anterior chamber of the eye in patients with deep corneal defects. This form of intraocular fluorescein accumulation is nontoxic. When the anterior chamber is viewed under the blue filter of the slit lamp, a fluorescein "flare" is visible and should not be confused with the flare reaction noted with iritis.

Procedure

Theoretically, one should not use topical anesthetics before fluorescein staining because a superficial punctate keratitis may develop in some patients from the anesthetic,[12] which can confuse the diagnosis. However, in patients who are tearing profusely and squeezing their eyes shut from an abrasion or an FB, the examination is often impossible if a topical anesthetic is not first used. Theoretical downsides notwithstanding, it is common practice to apply a local anesthetic before instilling fluorescein.

Grasp the fluorescein strip by the nonorange end and wet the orange end with 1 drop of saline. Several convenient forms are available, including a small bottle of artificial tears or a 5-mL "bullet" or "fish" of normal saline commonly used for nebulizer treatments. Alternatively, wet the strip with tap water or the recently used local anesthetic drops. Once the strip is moistened, place it gently on the inside of the patient's lower lid (Fig. 62-7, *step 1*). Withdraw the strip and ask the patient to blink, which spreads the fluorescein over the surface of the eye. The key to a good examination is to have a thin layer of fluorescein over the corneal and conjunctival surfaces. If the strip is too heavily moistened before placing it in the lower fornix, the eye may become flooded with the solution, which makes evaluation difficult. If too much dye accumulates, the patient can remove the excess dye by blotting the closed eye with a tissue. Conversely, placing a dry strip in an unanesthetized eye may be irritating. Next, use a Wood lamp (4× magnification), the blue filter of a slit lamp, or simply a penlight with a blue filter to examine the eye in a darkened room (see Fig. 62-7, *step 2*). Check for areas of bright green fluorescence on the corneal and conjunctival surfaces. The naked eye may not be able to see small defects. Ideally, use a slit lamp with 10× or 25× magnification to examine the stained cornea before ruling out a pathologic process. A new handheld magnification device, the Eidolon Bluminator ophthalmic illuminator, produces an intense blue light from a light-emitting diode with 7× magnification (see Fig. 62-7, *step 3*). After completion of the fluorescein examination, irrigate

THE FLUORESCEIN EXAMINATION

Moisten the fluorescein strip with 1 drop of saline or topical anesthetic. Depress the lower lid and gently place a wetted strip onto the inside of the patient's lower lid so that only the smallest amount is instilled.

Examine the eye with a Wood lamp or a slit lamp with a cobalt blue filter (shown). Check for areas of bright green fluorescence on the corneal and conjunctival surfaces. Because the naked eyes may not be able to appreciate small defects, magnification should be used.

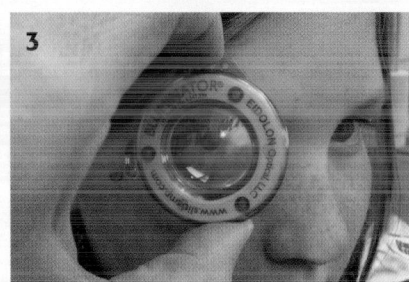

The Eidolon Bluminator ophthalmic illuminator provides an intense blue LED light with 7× magnification. *(Courtesy of Michael W. Ohlson, OD, FAAO, and Victor J. Doherty, Eidolon Optical, LLC.)*

Positive Seidel test. Fluorescein seen streaming down the cornea indicates an open-globe injury. *(From Krachmer JH, Mannis M, Holland E, eds. Cornea. 3rd ed. St. Louis; Mosby; 2010.)*

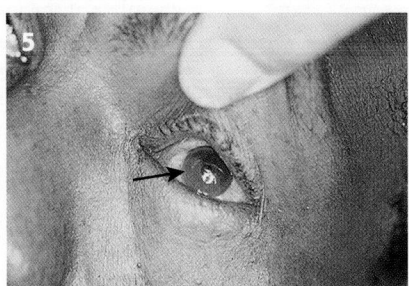

Large corneal abrasion seen with the naked eye. Smaller abrasions or corneal injuries produced by keratitis or a welder's arc flash require slit lamp evaluation to identify minor corneal defects.

Corneal abrasion as seen via a slit lamp. A moderate-sized abrasion *(arrow)* is revealed by fluorescein staining and blue light. *(From Friedman NJ, Raiser PK, Pineda R. Massachusetts Ear & Eye Infirmary Illustrated Manual of Ophthalmology. 3rd ed. Philadelphia Saunders; 2009.)*

Vertical linear abrasions. These types of abrasions are typically caused by a foreign body trapped under the upper eyelid. *(From Kliegman R, Stanton B, Behrman R, et al, eds. Nelson Textbook of Pediatrics. 19th ed. Philadelphia: Saunders; 2011.)*

Superficial punctate keratitis. These diffuse, shallow corneal irregularities are caused by chemical irritation, viral illnesses, exposure to bright light, and many other conditions.

Herpes simplex keratitis. A classic herpetic epithelial dendritic lesion is seen on this fluorescein examination. *(From Palay DA, Krachmer JH, eds. Primary Care Ophthalmology: Concepts and Clinical Practice. 2nd ed. St. Louis: Mosby; 2005.)*

Figure 62-7 The fluorescein examination. Excessive fluorescein may obscure subtle findings and thus should be avoided. Fluorescein will permanently stain contact lenses if they are not removed. LED, light-emitting diode.

excess dye from the eye to minimize damage to the patient's clothing from dye-stained tears.

The Seidel test uses fluorescein to detect perforation of the eye.[20] To perform this test, instill a large amount of fluorescein onto the eye by profusely wetting the strip. Examine the eye for a small stream of fluid leaking from the globe (see Fig. 62-7, *plate 4*). This stream will fluoresce blue or green, in contrast to the orange appearance of the rest of the globe flooded with fluorescein.[12]

Interpretation

Fluorescein is used mainly for evaluation of corneal injuries. Although conjunctival abrasions pick up the stain, most of the staining on the conjunctiva represents patches of mucus rather than a real pathologic condition. Corneal staining is more specific for injury, and the pattern of injury often reflects the original insult.

Corneal staining patterns are illustrated in Figures 62-7 and 62-8. Abrasions usually occur in the central part of the

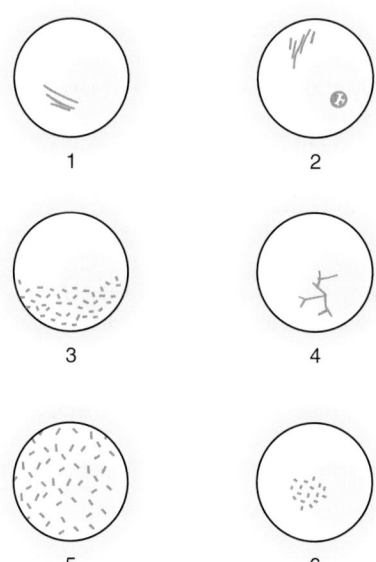

Figure 62-8 Patterns of acute corneal injury. *1*, Traumatic abrasion, usually with linear features and sharp borders when seen early (<24 hours), occurs more in the central part of the cornea. *2*, Abrasion from a foreign body (FB). Vertical abrasions on the upper part of the cornea are seen when an FB is embedded in the upper lid. Also shown is a rust ring with a metallic FB. *3*, Exposure pattern seen with prolonged exposure to ultraviolet light (e.g., welding flash, sunlamp exposure). A bandlike keratitis is produced over the lower half of the cornea. Squinting in the setting of the bright light protected the upper corneal surface. *4*, Herpes simplex keratitis, classic dendritic pattern. *5*, Adenovirus keratitis. Diffuse minute corneal staining is seen in patients with epidemic keratoconjunctivitis about 7 days after the onset of symptoms. *6*, Contact lens overuse, central punctate staining. *(From Knoop K, Trott A. Ophthalmologic procedures in the emergency department—part III: slit lamp use and foreign bodies. Acad Emerg Med. 1995;2:227. Reproduced by permission.)*

cornea because of the limited protection of closure of the patient's eyelids. The margins of the abrasions are usually sharp and linear if seen in the first 24 hours (see Fig. 62-7, *plate 6*). Circular defects are seen about embedded FBs and may persist for up to 48 hours after removal of a superficial foreign object. Deeply embedded objects may be associated with defects persisting for longer than 48 hours. Objects under the upper lid (including some chalazia) often produce vertical linear lesions on the upper surface of the cornea (see Fig. 62-7, *plate 7*). *When vertical lesions are noted, search diligently for a retained FB under the upper lid.* Overuse of hard contact lenses diminishes the nutrient supply to the cornea. The central part of the cornea sustains the most injury and thus fluoresces brightly when stained. Excessive exposure to ultraviolet light as a result of sunlamp abuse, snow blindness, or welding flashes produces a superficial punctate keratitis, which in its mildest form may not be visible without a slit lamp (see Fig. 62-7, *plate 8*). The central part of the cornea is the least protected by the lids, and a central, horizontal band–like keratitis can result. Herpetic lesions may develop anywhere on the cornea. Classically, these lesions are dendritic, although ulcers may also be punctate or stellate (see Fig. 62-7, *plate 9*).[21,22]

Any area of corneal staining with an infiltrate or opacification beneath or around the lesion should alert the practitioner to the possibility of a viral,[21,22] bacterial,[23] or fungal[24] keratitis.

Obtain urgent ophthalmologic consultation so that cultures of the possible etiologic agents can be procured and appropriate treatment initiated.

Many *Pseudomonas* organisms fluoresce when exposed to ultraviolet light[25]; therefore, the presence of fluorescence before the instillation of fluorescein in a red eye should suggest the possibility of infection with this organism.

Summary

Fluorescein staining is a quick and easy diagnostic procedure that should be part of every eye evaluation. The extra minute that the examination takes provides a wealth of diagnostic information on patients with eye trauma or infection. No complications are associated with the procedure with the exception of the reactions noted with the fluorescein solution, possible discoloration of soft contact lenses, and the potential for infection when premixed solutions rather than fluorescein-impregnated paper strips are used.

EYE IRRIGATION

The crucial first step in the treatment of chemical injuries to the eye is irrigation. Irrigate as clinically appropriate for the severity, length of exposure, and causative agent. Serious chemical injury to the eye requires irrigation at the site of the injury, even before the patient is brought to the ED.[15] Corneal injury can occur within seconds of contact with an alkaline substance. Continue eye irrigation in the ED.

This section discusses methods of irrigation. Although it is best to irrigate liberally, copious irrigation is not needed when the patient has just a small amount of a noncaustic, nonalkaline compound in the eye.

Indications and Contraindications

Irrigation is indicated for all acute chemical injuries involving the eyes. Irrigation may also be therapeutic in patients with an FB sensation but no visible FB. Small, unseen foreign material in the conjunctival tissues may be flushed out with irrigation. There is no contraindication to eye irrigation, but in patients with a possible perforating injury, perform the irrigation especially gently and carefully.

Equipment

The following equipment is necessary for eye irrigation:

Topical anesthetic, such as 0.5% proparacaine
Sterile irrigating solution (warmed intravenous saline or lactated Ringer's [LR] solution in a bag with tubing)*
A basin to catch the fluid
Cotton-tipped applicators
Gauze pads to help hold the patient's lids open
Lid retractors
Irrigating device (e.g., Morgan Therapeutic Lens, modified central venous catheter, or Eye Irrigator) for prolonged irrigation

---

*A balanced salt solution designed for eye irrigation is preferred by some (when available) and may produce less corneal edema with chemical injuries. Readily available normal saline and lactated Ringer's solution are equally well tolerated.

Optimal: 10 mL of 1% lidocaine added to a liter of irrigating fluid

Procedure

Basic Technique

First, instill a topical anesthetic into the eye (Fig. 62-9, *step 1*). Evert the eyelid and sweep out any particulate matter in the conjunctival fornices with a moistened, cotton-tipped applicator[15] (see "Ocular FB Removal," later in this chapter, and Fig. 62-9, *step 2*). Hold the eyelids open during irrigation (see Fig. 62-9, *step 3*). The easiest method is to use gauze pads to grasp the wet, slippery lids and hold them open. If the patient has severe blepharospasm, consider using lid retractors (Desmarres or paper clip retractors; Fig. 62-10). When lid retractors are used, be certain that the eye is well anesthetized, that the retractors do not injure the globe or the lids, and that chemicals are not harbored under the retractors. Be aware that simple retractors fashioned from metal paper clips (especially those that are nickel plated and shiny) may have surface chipping, which can create an ocular FB.[26] Exercise caution to avoid ocular injury when using such a makeshift retractor.

Deutsch and Feller[15] recommended an ipsilateral facial nerve block for severe blepharospasm (Fig. 62-11). To avoid swelling of periorbital tissue, block the facial nerve just anterior to the condyloid process of the ipsilateral mandible. Place a subcutaneous line of anesthetic (2% lidocaine) to temporarily paralyze the orbicularis muscle.

Irrigate with normal saline or LR solution directed over the globe and into the upper and lower fornices (see Fig. 62-9, *step 4*). The choice of fluid initially is less important than initiating irrigation as rapidly as possible. If tap water is

IRRIGATION OF THE EYE

Instill a topical anesthetic such as tetracaine HCl 0.5%.

Evert the eyelid and use a moistened cotton-tipped applicator to sweep out any particulate matter in the fornices.

Hold the eyelids open during irrigation. Consider the use of lid retractors if the patient has severe blepharospasm (see Fig. 62-10).

Irrigate with normal saline or lactated Ringer's solution directed over the globe and into the upper and lower fornices.

Be careful to direct the fluid onto the conjunctiva and then across the cornea (without letting the stream directly hit the cornea) because the solution may cause mechanical corneal injury.

In the case of acid/alkali exposure, measure the pH of the conjunctival fornices with litmus paper to check the effectiveness of the irrigation. Normal tear film pH is 7.4.

Figure 62-9 Irrigation of the eye. Intravenous tubing is connected to a liter bag of saline or Ringer's solution, and irrigation occurs at a wide-open rate.

available at the scene of the injury, begin irrigation immediately with copious amounts of fluid before transporting the patient to the hospital. Teach out-of-hospital care providers to irrigate all acid injuries of the eye for at least 5 minutes at the scene and to irrigate all alkali injuries for at least 15 minutes.[27,28] LR or normal saline solution is preferred over tap water or 5% dextrose in water for eye irrigation because these solutions are isotonic and do not contain dextrose. Dextrose can be quite sticky if spilled and might serve as a nutrient for an opportunistic bacterial infection. Although one clinical trial found a balanced salt solution less painful in patients with a chemical eye injury,[29] another volunteer study on uninjured eyes found that LR solution is better tolerated than normal saline and balanced saline solution when used with a Morgan lens.[30] Warmed fluids are also better tolerated than fluids at room temperature.[31] Warmed LR solution should be considered when both it and normal saline are available for eye irrigation.

Be careful to direct the irrigating stream onto the conjunctiva and then across the cornea without letting the stream splash directly onto the cornea because striking the eye with the solution can in itself be harmful and cause mechanical injury (see Fig. 62-9, step 5). Direct irrigation of the cornea can result in the development of a superficial punctate epithelial keratopathy.

Before irrigation, instill anesthetic eyedrops, such as 0.5% tetracaine. Adding 10 mL of 1% lidocaine to a liter of irrigating fluid can decrease patients' discomfort during prolonged irrigation.

Duration of Irrigation

Although Deutsch and Feller[15] recommended that a full liter of irrigating solution be used in every case of caustic injury, the duration of irrigation is best determined by the extent of the exposure and the causative agent. Acids are quickly neutralized by proteins in the surface tissues of the eye and, once irrigated out, cause no further damage. The only exceptions are hydrofluoric and heavy metal acids, which can penetrate through the cornea. Alkalis can penetrate rapidly and, if not removed, will continue to produce damage for days because of slow dissociation of the cation from combination with proteins.[15] Therefore, prolonged irrigation is indicated and at least 2 L of solution should be used. Although rapid flushing with the first 500 mL is prudent, slow continuous irrigation, as discussed later, at a rate sufficient to generate a continuous trickle is often more effective and better tolerated than continued high-volume flushing. If the nature of the offending agent is unknown or in question, use prolonged irrigation.

Consult ophthalmology for all alkaline, hydrofluoric acid, and heavy metal acid injuries. Irrigation on an inpatient basis may be required for a period of 24 hours or longer, especially when the cornea is hazy or obviously thickened. Note that the magnesium contained in sparklers combines with water from tears to produce magnesium hydroxide.[32]

Figure 62-10 Devices for separating eyelids. **A,** A Desmarres retractor, lid specula, or retractor improvised from a paper clip allows active manipulation of the lids. Free-standing specula may require a seventh nerve block to reduce the blepharospasm. **B,** Lid retractor in place. (*A, From Fogle JA, Spyker DA. Management of chemical and drug injury to the eye. In: Haddad LM, Winchester JF, eds.* Clinical Management of Poisoning and Drug Overdose. *2nd ed. Philadelphia: Saunders; 1990. Reproduced by permission.*)

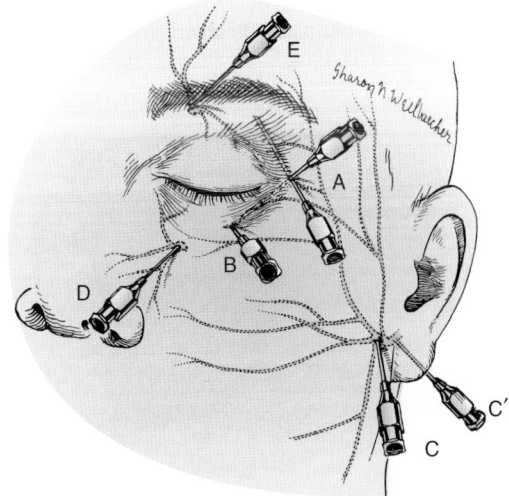

Figure 62-11 Injection points for facial and orbital anesthesia and akinesia. *A,* Van Lint technique for infiltration of the orbicularis. *B,* Retrobulbar injection site. *C,* O'Brien facial nerve block. *C′,* Alternative facial nerve block by injection into the tympanomastoid fissure. *D,* Infraorbital sensory block. *E,* Supraorbital sensory block. Injection of the orbicularis (*A*) or facial nerve (*C* or *C′*) permits examination and treatment of the eye in the setting of severe blepharospasm. Anesthetic is placed within several millimeters of the nerves. (*From Deutsch TA, Feller DB, eds.* Paton and Goldberg's Management of Ocular Injuries. *2nd ed. Philadelphia: Saunders, 1985:17.*)

Treat such fireworks injuries as alkaline injuries rather than as thermal injuries. Treat eye damage from hair straighteners,[33] phosphate-free detergents,[34] and automobile air bags[35] as alkaline injuries also.

Measure the pH of the conjunctival fornices with a pH paper strip to check the effectiveness of irrigation (see Fig. 62-9, *step 6*). In addition to litmus paper, the pH indicator on urine multi-indicator sticks can be used. The pH indicator on urine dipsticks is conveniently closest to the handle; all the distal indicator squares can be cut off with scissors. Normal tear film pH is 7.4. Use the noninjured eye as a control if the results are equivocal. If the pH measured in the conjunctival fornices is still abnormal after the initial irrigation, continue to irrigate. If the pH is normal after irrigation, wait 20 minutes and check it again to make sure

that it remains normal, especially if alkaline contamination has occurred. Delayed changes in pH are usually the result of incomplete irrigation and inadequate swabbing of the fornices. In anticipation of this deficiency, measure the pH deep in the fornices. Consider double-lid eversion with a lid elevator to expose the upper fornix for swabbing, irrigation, and pH testing.

Prolonged Irrigation

Alkaline burns may require prolonged irrigation, and it is essential to consult ophthalmology in such cases. The Morgan Therapeutic Lens is a contact lens–type irrigation device that can provide slow, continuous irrigation once the more vigorous initial irrigation has been completed (Fig. 62-12). First, anesthetize the eye with topical anesthetic drops. Then place

---

MORGAN LENS IRRIGATION

1

The Morgan therapeutic lens is a contact lens–type irrigation device that can provide slow, continuous irrigation once the more vigorous initial irrigation has been done.

2

Prior to insertion, anesthetize the eyes with topical anesthetic drops such as tetracaine HCl 0.5%. The anesthetic will wash out during the irrigation process, so reapply frequently for patient comfort.

3

Carefully place the device on the surface of the eye with the lids closed around the intravenous tubing adaptor.

4

Attach the adaptor to intravenous tubing and provide continuous flow through the device onto the cornea and into the fornices. Bilateral irrigation is easily achieved with this technique.

Figure 62-12 Morgan lens irrigation. A liter bag of saline or Ringer's solution is connected to the Morgan lens with intravenous tubing and irrigated at a wide-open rate.

the device carefully on the surface of the eye with the lids closed around the intravenous tubing adaptor. Attach the intravenous tubing to the adaptor and provide continuous flow through the device onto the cornea and into the fornices. As the local anesthetic agents wash out during the irrigation process, the device can become uncomfortable, so reapply the anesthetic drops frequently during irrigation for patient comfort. Such short-term use of local anesthetics will not inhibit healing of the cornea.

Complications

The only significant complication from irrigation is abrasion of the cornea or the conjunctiva. This can be a mechanical injury from trying to keep the lids open in an uncooperative patient, a small corneal epithelial defect from a Morgan irrigating lens, or fine punctate keratitis from the irrigation itself.[36] For this reason, do not direct the stream directly onto the cornea. If a superficial corneal defect occurs, treat it in the usual manner. Deep or penetrating corneal injuries are likely to be a result of the caustic chemical and require emergency ophthalmologic consultation. Continue to provide slow continuous irrigation pending arrival of the ophthalmologist. Some experimental evidence suggests that massive parenteral or oral ascorbic acid supplementation may prevent the development of deep corneal injury,[37] but such treatment has not gained universal acceptance.

Summary

Eye irrigation is easy, and complications associated with the technique are usually minimal. At times the clinician may be unsure whether a chemical injury is toxic enough to warrant irrigation. If any doubt exists, err on the side of irrigating the eye rather than omitting this vital procedure and risking progression of the eye injury.

OCULAR FB REMOVAL

Patients with an external FB in the eye are frequently seen in EDs. They are often in pain and desperate for help. Maintain a high degree of suspicion for FB injuries and perforation of the eye because such injuries may be occult and not readily detected. Not all FB injuries are associated with pain. Glass embedded in the cornea may be particularly difficult to detect. This section reviews procedures for locating and removing extraocular FBs and appropriate postprocedural care. Finally, a brief discussion covering evaluation of the eye for potential perforation of the globe and detection of the presence of an intraocular FB is provided.

Indications and Contraindications

Extraocular FBs must always be removed. The timing of removal and the technique required vary according to the patient's clinical status and the type of injury. For the most part the emergency clinician can proceed directly to removal of the object via the techniques described in this section. When the patient is extremely uncooperative (e.g., an intoxicated patient, a mentally deficient patient, or a young child) or when the injury is complicated (e.g., deeply embedded object, multiple foreign objects from a blast injury, or possible

globe penetration), consult ophthalmology immediately. A patient with a suspected FB or abrasion after exposure to a projectile (e.g., grinding wheel, hammering, metal objects colliding) should be rigorously evaluated for the presence of a deep intraocular FB. See further discussion later in this chapter. A penetrating injury of the cornea is of particular concern because the iris tissue may prolapse and have an appearance similar to a corneal FB (Fig. 62-13). Hence, in addition to the history of projectile exposure, an irregular pupil, especially a pear-shaped pupil, should alert the clinician that a penetrating injury might have occurred.

Globe Protection

In the evaluation of a patient in whom a penetrating injury to the globe is suspected, perform a careful expeditious examination of the eye, preferably with a slit lamp. Avoid any pressure on the eye or rapid eye movements. If perforation is obvious (e.g., teardrop pupil, flaccid globe, flat anterior chamber, prolapsed iris) or confirmed by slit lamp (positive Seidel test; see Fig. 62-7, *plate 4*), do not perform any procedures (except perhaps irrigation) and consult ophthalmology early for definitive diagnosis and care. Until the ophthalmologist arrives, protect the eye from further harm by keeping the patient quiet, elevating the head of the bed, and placing a protective shield over the eye. Commercial shields are available for this purpose. When a metal shield is not available, construct a makeshift protective shield with the material available (e.g., paper, plastic, or Styrofoam cups; Fig. 62-14). The protective shield helps avoid pressure on the globe and overlying tissue and assists in preventing extrusion of vitreous and other ocular contents. Extend the edges of the shield up to or beyond the bony orbital rim for this purpose. Apply adhesive tape over the shield from the forehead to the cheek to secure the shield in position.

If a patient has a globe perforation, treat with systemic antibiotics (a combination of cefazolin and gentamicin is a good initial choice), tetanus toxoid, and antiemetics in doses aggressive enough to halt vomiting.

Equipment

The following equipment is necessary for removal of an extraocular FB:

Topical anesthetic, such as 0.5% proparacaine
Sterile cotton-tipped applicators
Fluorescein strips
Magnification: loupes plus a Wood lamp, Eidolon Bluminator ophthalmic illuminator, or slit lamp
Eye spud or 25-gauge needle attached to a 1- or 3-mL syringe or to the tip of a cotton-tipped applicator
Dilator drops, such as 5% homatropine
Antibiotic ointment, such as erythromycin

Consideration of an Intraocular FB

When examining a patient with an ocular "FB" sensation, always remain cognizant of the potential for an intraorbital or intraocular FB. Penetrating injuries represent a greater threat to visual loss than an extraocular FB does and can be disastrous if overlooked. Note that an intraocular FB can be deceptively subtle on initial evaluation. Bedside ED

Figure 62-13 Serious eye injuries. **A,** Corneal laceration with prolapse of the iris. The extruded iris is dark and mimics a corneal foreign body (*arrow*). Frequently, the only clue is an abnormal pupil, and the extruded iris may not be appreciated as intraocular tissue. The pupil is irregular (often pear or teardrop shaped) and points toward the laceration. **B,** A pear-shaped pupil without protrusion of the lens is a more subtle, yet characteristic indication of a perforated globe (*arrow*). **C,** Another indication of a penetrating globe injury is periorbital fat protruding from an upper eyelid laceration (*arrow*). This patient was stabbed with a knife. **D,** This patient has an obviously cloudy lens soon after trauma. A projectile entered the temporal portion of the globe and produced a seemingly minor scleral hemorrhage. Patients with penetrating injuries to the globe should be treated with systemic antibiotics (such as a combination of cefazolin and gentamicin), tetanus toxoid if indicated, and antiemetics to control vomiting (which raises intraocular pressure). (**A,** *Courtesy of Lawrence B. Stack, MD.*)

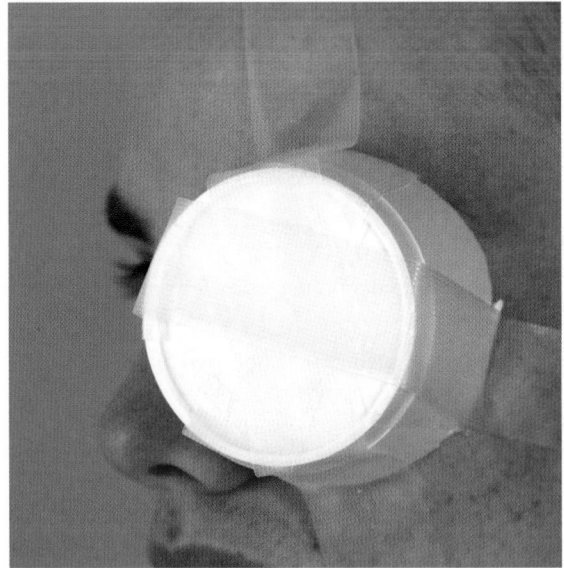

Figure 62-14 When a penetrating globe injury is suspected and a metal shield is not available in the emergency department or prehospital setting, a makeshift shield can be fashioned with available material. A paper cup was used to fashion this shield.

Figure 62-15 Metallic intraocular foreign body. Ultrasound shows a foreign body on the surface of the retina (*short arrow*). Note the marked shadowing just posterior to the foreign body (*long arrow*). (*From Ryan SJ, Hinton DR, Schachat AP, et al, eds.* Retina. *4th ed. St. Louis: Mosby; 2005.*)

ultrasound is a useful adjunct for identification of intraocular FBs (Fig. 62-15).

The clinical findings are most helpful in determining which patients are at risk for a penetrating injury to the globe. An individual who complains of an FB sensation in the absence of trauma or one whose history is simply that something "fell" or "blew" into the eye is at low risk for perforation of the globe. Conversely, there is a greater probability of globe penetration in an individual who has sustained a high-velocity wound to the eye (e.g., drilling, hammering, grinding metal, blasting rock). The presence of any of the following findings on physical examination should alert the clinician to a probable intraocular FB: irregular pupil, shallow anterior chamber on slit lamp examination, prolapsed iris, positive Seidel test (see "The Fluorescein Examination," earlier in this chapter),

Figure 62-16 Computed tomography scan showing a right intraocular foreign body (a BB pellet, *arrow*). *(From Marx JA, Hockberger RS, Walls RM, eds.* Rosen's Emergency Medicine: Concepts and Clinical Practice. *7th ed. St. Louis: Mosby; 2009.)*

focal conjunctival swelling, hemorrhage, hyphema, lens opacification, and reduced intraocular pressure (IOP). Do not perform tonometry if penetrating injury to the globe is suspected. Be aware that a penetrating injury may not be associated with eye pain. If there is strong historical evidence and physical findings to support a diagnosis of globe penetration, obtain emergency ophthalmologic consultation.

An intraocular FB is often not visible on direct ophthalmoscopy. Although orbital radiography for radiopaque objects and ultrasonography of the globe have been used for indirect FB localization,[15,38] computed tomography of the orbit is now considered the most useful technique (Fig. 62-16).[39,40] When plain orbital radiography is performed to look for an intraocular FB, be aware that an eyelid FB may mimic an intraocular FB.[41] Patients with a suspected metallic FB should not undergo magnetic resonance imaging if the FB may be intraocular. Therapy for intraocular and intraorbital FBs must be individualized. Frequently, an ophthalmologist can localize an intraocular FB (if the vitreous is clear) with indirect ophthalmoscopy. The role of the emergency clinician is to suspect the diagnosis, protect the eye from further harm, and obtain ophthalmologic consultation. The remainder of this section addresses the problem of extraocular FBs.

Procedure

FB Location

The first step is to locate the FB. Apply a drop of topical anesthetic to the inside of the lower lid (see Fig. 62-6*A*). The presence of vertical corneal abrasions from FBs under the lids is helpful in localizing these hidden foreign objects (see Fig. 62-7, *plate 7*). Use a penlight and loupes or a slit lamp to examine the bulbar conjunctiva by having the patient look in all directions. Examine the inside of the lower lid by pulling it down with the thumb while asking the patient to look up. Evert the upper lid by asking the patient to look down as the end of an applicator stick is pressed against the superior edge of the tarsal plate of the upper lid. Meanwhile, grasp the lashes and pull down, out, and then up to flip the eyelid over (Fig. 62-17).

Minute FBs under the lid may be missed with simple visual inspection. Ideally, examine the everted lid under magnification with loupes or a slit lamp. With simple lid eversion it is still not possible to see the far recesses of the upper conjunctival fornix. Although double eversion of the upper lid is helpful, the best way to rule out an FB in the upper fornix is to sweep the anesthetized fornix with a moistened applicator as the upper lid is held everted. Examine the tip of the applicator for removed foreign material. Small conjunctival FBs not hidden by the lids are often best removed with a moistened nasopharyngeal swab (e.g., nasopharyngeal Calgiswab).

Reexamine the cornea. Most corneal FBs have an area of fluorescein staining around them. Use a slit lamp or other magnification device such as the Bluminator to make the examination easier. If the clinician is limited to loupes and a penlight, shine the light diagonally on the cornea to locate the FB. With a history of a high-speed projectile hitting the eye, rule out an intraocular FB. In the case of a blast injury, multiple FBs may penetrate the eye. If an FB cannot be found on the surface despite a suggestive history, examine the eye for physical evidence of penetration, as discussed earlier. Dilate the pupil and examine the fundus. Though not foolproof, bedside ultrasonography may identify the presence of a metallic FB (sensitivity of 87.5%, specificity of 95.8%, and positive and negative predictive values of 96.5% and 85.2%, respectively).[42] If in doubt regarding an intraocular FB, consider computed tomography and ophthalmologic consultation.

FB Removal

Once an extraocular FB is located, the technique for removal depends on whether it is embedded. If the FB is lying on the surface, eject a stream of water from a syringe through a plastic catheter, which will usually wash the object onto the bulbar conjunctiva. Once the FB is on the inner lid or bulbar conjunctiva, gently touch a wetted cotton-tipped applicator to the conjunctiva and the object will adhere to the tip of the applicator. Be aware that overzealous use of an applicator for removing corneal FBs can lead to extensive corneal epithelial injury. A spud device is required for removal of objects that cannot be irrigated off the cornea.

To remove embedded corneal FBs (Fig. 62-18), use a commercial spud device, a bur drill, a short 25- or 27-gauge needle on a small-diameter syringe (e.g., insulin or tuberculin syringe), or a cotton-tipped applicator. Use the applicator or syringe as a handle for the attached needle. Contrary to what one might expect, it is difficult to penetrate the sclera or the cornea with a needle, especially when it is applied tangentially to the cornea.[31] As with removal of conjunctival FBs, anesthetize the eye. Position the patient so that the head is well secured (preferably in a slit lamp frame). At this point, provide a simple explanation of the procedure, which usually ensures excellent compliance on the part of the patient. *Rest your hand on the patient's cheek so that unexpected movements by the patient will not result in large movements of the removal device.* Instruct the patient to gaze at an object in the distance (e.g., the practitioner's ear when a slit lamp is used) to further stabilize the eye. Bring the removal device close to the eye under direct vision; then while it is in focus, manipulate it under the magnification device (e.g., Wood's lamp, Eidolon Bluminator ophthalmic illuminator [see Fig. 62-7], or slit lamp) to remove the FB. Hold the device tangential to the globe, and pick up or scoop out the foreign object. If a bur drill is used, press the side of the drill against the FB until removal is accomplished.

LID EVERSION AND FOREIGN BODY REMOVAL

To evert the upper eyelid, place a cotton-tipped applicator against the superior edge of the tarsal plate.

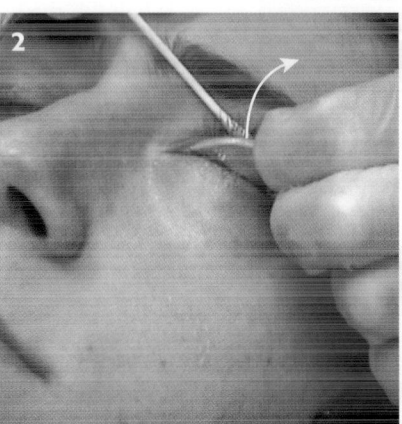

Grasp the eyelashes and pull them down, then out, and then up and over the applicator.

Hold the everted lid in place with the applicator. Use a second applicator to sweep the interior surface of the lid.

This patient complained of an FB in the eye despite irrigation. Lid eversion revealed a small speck (*arrow*) under the upper lid. This could cause a cornea abrasion characterized by vertical striations (see Fig. 62-7, *plate 7*).

The foreign body was easily removed (*arrow*) by touching it with a moistened cotton-tipped applicator.

This patient had a swollen and tender upper eyelid thought to be secondary to a stye. With lid eversion, a small pustule (*arrow*) was found under the upper eyelid.

With a 27-gauge needle, the pustule was incised and a drop of pus was expressed; she made a rapid and uneventful recovery.

Figure 62-17 Lid eversion and foreign body (FB) removal.

CORNEAL FOREIGN BODY REMOVAL

This embedded corneal FB is readily seen under slit lamp examination. A removal device (needle, spud, or bur drill) should be used for careful removal. A rust ring will remain if the FB has been there for only a few hours.

Rust rings (*arrow*) are retained FBs and are removed in a similar manner. Most rust rings should be removed, but there is no urgency. Small ones out of the line of sight may remain. A bur drill can be used for attempted removal, which if unsuccessful, can be reattempted in 24 hours. Alternatively, a small needle can be used to loosen the edges and then the ring scooped out. Both procedures will leave a corneal abrasion.

Under direct vision (not looking through the slit lamp), bring the syringe close to the eye while resting the hand on the patient's cheek. Be sure that the patient's forehead maintains continual contact with the crossbar on the slit lamp.

While looking through the slit lamp, bring the needle to the cornea and remove the FB.

Hold the side of the instrument (drill bit or beveled edge of the needle) tangential to the cornea.

A variety of instruments may be used for FB removal, including an eye spud (*A*), a cotton-tipped applicator (*B*), and a 25- or 27-gauge needle on a tuberculin syringe (*C*).

Figure 62-18 Corneal foreign body (FB) removal.

During removal, rest your hand against the patient's face. It may also be helpful to brace the elbow with a pad or half-full tissue box to provide further support for the arm while removing the FB. If right-handed, place the lower part of your hand against the left maxillary bone when removing a foreign object from the patient's left eye and against the bridge of the patient's nose or infranasal area when removing an object from the right eye. If left-handed, reverse these positions. Using loupes or a slit lamp for magnification is highly recommended to minimize further injury during removal. In particular, corneal contact with the spud device is more readily discerned when magnification is used. Only topical anesthesia is required to remove FBs from the cornea. Although patients may feel pressure during removal of FBs, pain should not be felt after the eye is anesthetized.

Rust Rings

A common problem with metallic FBs is that rust rings can develop (see Fig. 62-18, *plate 2*). *They can develop within hours* because of oxidation of the iron in the FB. There are two preferred techniques for removal of a rust ring. The most direct technique is to remove the ring at the same time as the FB, either with repeated picking away with a spud device or with a rotating bur. The second approach is to let the iron of the rust ring oxidize and kill the surrounding epithelial cells during a 24- to 48-hour period. After that, the rust ring will be soft and often comes out in one solid plug.[43] Generally, a small rust ring produces little visual difficulty unless it is directly in the line of sight. If large, a rust ring may delay corneal healing. Close follow-up is important to ensure healing of the cornea and total removal of the rust ring and FB.

Multiple FBs

If multiple FBs are present in the eye, such as from an explosion, refer the patient to an ophthalmologist. One technique that may be chosen by the ophthalmologist is to denude the entire epithelium with alcohol and remove the superficial FBs. The deeper ones gradually work their way to the surface, sometimes years later.

Aftercare

After removing the FB, an antibiotic ointment is frequently instilled. Though commonly used, the value of the ointment for superficial corneal defects after removal of an FB is unproved, and no specific standard of care is supported by

scientific evidence. Conjunctival and corneal abrasions do not need patching. Data suggest that eye patching offers no benefit in healing corneal abrasions secondary to FBs.[44] If a superficial injury is sustained from the FB, instruct the patient to return only if the eye does not feel completely normal or if there is any blurred vision. The majority of superficial injuries heal without difficulty. The patient should be warned that the FB sensation might return temporarily when the anesthetic agent wears off. One animal study involving direct ocular exposure to *Clostridium tetani* organisms suggested that nonpenetrating ocular injuries are unlikely to lead to tetanus.[45] Tetanus prophylaxis after corneal FB removal is not standard, but it should be considered. However, tetanus prophylaxis appears to be essential for injuries that penetrate through the cornea or sclera.

Use of Ophthalmic Anesthetic Agents

Application of topical anesthetic agents can be both diagnostic and therapeutic. Relief of discomfort with a topical anesthetic often suggests, but does not ensure a conjunctival or corneal injury. An ocular irritant may also be masked by the use of these agents. Classic teaching is that patients should not self-administer anesthetic preparations. It is thought that they delay wound healing by disrupting surface microvilli and causing a decrease in the tear film layer and tear break-up time.[46] Although self-administered topical anesthetic agents are now routinely used after photorefractive keratectomy for the first 3 or 4 postoperative days, this has not become a part of ED practice.[47] The absence of protective reflexes while the patient is under the effect of the medication may encourage use of the eye and result in further corneal injury from the FB or corneal infection. Though not advised for outpatient use, topical anesthetic drops can be used safely for a few days without documented adverse effects.

Bartfield and coworkers[48] found that pain with the instillation of 0.5% proparacaine was significantly less than that with 0.5% tetracaine. As evident from Table 62-2, the anesthetic solutions commonly used have a duration of action of less than 20 minutes. Patients with a large corneal lesion may need a more extended period of pain relief. The discomfort associated with a large healing corneal lesion is usually made tolerable by bed rest, opioid analgesics, and appropriate sedatives. Even in the absence of infection or a retained FB, long-term repeated use of ophthalmic anesthetic ointments might be detrimental to corneal healing.[49]

A final word of caution should be added regarding the use of ophthalmic solutions. Guaiac solutions are commonly supplied in dropper bottles similar in size and appearance to those

TABLE 62-2 Ophthalmic Anesthetic Agents

GENERIC NAME	TRADE NAME	CONCENTRATION (%)	ONSET OF ANESTHESIA	DURATION OF ANESTHESIA (min)	COMMENTS
Tetracaine	Pontocaine	0.5-1.0	<1 min	15-20	Marked stinging; also available as an ointment
Proparacaine	Ophthaine, Ophthetic	0.5	<20 sec	10-15	Least irritating; no cross-sensitization with other agents
Benoxinate	Dorsacaine	0.4	1-2 min	10-15	Only anesthetic compatible with fluorescein in solution

containing ophthalmic solutions. Well-intentioned ED personnel may store the guaiac reagent bottles with the ophthalmic bottles. One should encourage both color coding of the bottles and examination of them and their labels before each use to avoid corneal injury from inadvertently instilling guaiac reagent into the eye.

Use of Ophthalmic NSAIDs

Ophthalmic nonsteroidal antiinflammatory drugs (NSAIDs) have been evaluated for their effectiveness in the treatment of traumatic corneal abrasions. Examples include ketorolac tromethamine, diclofenac, and flurbiprofen. These agents are safe to use and effective for the relief of pain associated with corneal abrasions.[50-53] Topical ophthalmic NSAIDs have also been shown to be safe and effective when used for the treatment of corneal abrasions in conjunction with bandage contact lenses.[54]

Complications

Complications associated with ocular FB removal are rare. The most frequent problem is incomplete removal of the FB. In such cases the epithelium has difficulty healing over the affected area, and thus the eye stays inflamed. Eventually, the diseased epithelium either sloughs off and heals or heals over the FB remnants, which are gradually absorbed. In either case, adverse effects on the eye are minimal; a minute scar on the cornea, even directly in the center, will rarely affect vision. Nonetheless, incomplete removal of a corneal foreign object warrants ophthalmologic follow-up.

Conjunctivitis may develop after removal of an extraocular FB. In most cases the bacteria producing the infection are introduced by the patient rubbing the irritated eye.

Although perforation of the globe by the clinician's spud device is theoretically possible, this complication is exceedingly rare. Treatment of this type of corneal puncture wound consists of antibiotics, placement of an eye shield, and ophthalmologic consultation. In the absence of resultant endophthalmitis, permanent sequelae are unlikely to develop.

Epithelial injury can occur when cotton-tipped applicators are used to vigorously remove corneal FBs. Indeed, the use of cotton-tipped applicators for embedded corneal FB removal is condemned.

Summary

Ocular FBs are one of the most common eye emergencies. Searching for and removing the FB are usually straightforward. The only real trap is missing an intraocular FB. This must be ruled out if there is a history of a high-speed projectile hitting the eye or if the findings on physical examination suggest globe penetration.

EYE PATCHING

Patching the lids shut has traditionally been the last step in the treatment of a number of common eye emergencies; however, multiple studies have shown that eye patching offers no benefit in pain relief or healing rates in patients with conjunctival or corneal abrasions.[44,55-57] A metaanalysis of studies on eye patching and corneal abrasions or ulcers showed that patching might actually slow healing rates and patients might actually have worsening of their pain. This was found to be true in children as well.[58-60] Patching is also contraindicated in contact lens wearers and in situations in which the abrasion or ulcer may be infected.[56] In summary, eye patching is no longer indicated and might actually worsen the ophthalmologic process that it once was thought to help. Application of a therapeutic bandage contact lens directly to the cornea has been recommended as a possible treatment of corneal epithelial defects. Evidence from several small studies suggests that a bandage contact lens is safe, effective, and well tolerated and allows a significant number of patients to immediately resume their regular activities while maintaining baseline visual acuity. Further study on the application of this modality in the ED setting is needed.[54,61-63]

CONTACT LENS PROCEDURES

An estimated 24 million Americans wear a form of contact lenses.[64] Removal of these lenses in the ED may be required to permit further evaluation of the eye or to prevent injury from prolonged wear. Emergency clinicians also evaluate patients for "lost" contact lenses, which may be trapped under the upper lid. At times patients may request that the clinician remove a lens that they have failed to extract from the cornea. Corneal ulcers can occur in patients who wear contact lenses and may require prompt treatment. This section on contact lens procedures addresses these concerns and discusses injuries associated with attempts at removal, the mechanism of injury from prolonged wear, and instructions to be given to patients at discharge. Furthermore, this section introduces the use of bandage contact lenses for the treatment of acute corneal abrasions.

The first contact lenses were scleral lenses made of glass. These lenses, which covered the cornea as well as much of the surrounding sclera, are reported to have been in use from 1888 to 1948.[65] Glass corneal lenses (sitting entirely on the cornea) made by the Carl Zeiss Optical Works of Jena were first described in 1912. A practical synthetic scleral lens using methylmethacrylate rather than glass was discussed by Obrig and Mullen in 1938.[66,67] In 1947, Tuohy redeveloped the corneal lens with methylmethacrylate.[68] This was the forerunner of the current hard contact lens.[68] The development of lenses made of soft gas-permeable polymers was reported in Czechoslovakia in 1960.[69] These hydrogel (hydrophilic gelatinous–like) lenses have evolved into today's soft contact lenses. Soft contact lenses now come in a variety of types, including extended and daily wear. The majority of soft contact lenses in use are now disposable. Soft contact lenses have been used therapeutically by ophthalmologists for decades.[70]

Mechanism of Corneal Injury from Contact Lens Wear

Hard Contact Lenses

Oxygenation of the cornea is dependent on the movement of oxygen-rich tears under hard contact lenses during blinking. During the "adaptation" phase of early wear, a wearer of hard contact lenses produces hypotonic tears as a result of mechanical irritation from the lens.[66] This results in corneal edema, which reduces subsequent tear flow under the lens during blinking. Overwearing a lens at this time leads to corneal ischemia, with superficial epithelial defects found predominantly in the central corneal area (see Fig. 62-8), where the least tear flow occurs. With adaptation, the tears become isotonic and the blinking rate normalizes, thus permitting increased wearing time. During early adaptation, blinking is more rapid than normal and then slows to a subnormal rate during late adaptation. Mucus delivery to the cornea in the tear film may also play an important role in maintaining corneal lubrication. Tight-fitting contact lenses may never permit good tear flow despite an adaptation phase; individuals with tightly fitted lenses may never be able to wear their original contact lenses for longer than 6 to 8 hours. Lenses that are excessively loose can also cause irritation by moving during blinking. Rough or cracked edges can cause corneal abrasions.

In the ED, a patient with irritation caused by prolonged wear may be either a new or an adapted wearer. An adapted wearer may have been exposed to chemical irritants (e.g., smoke), which reduces the tonicity of tears and leads to corneal edema and decreased tear flow. Alternatively, an adapted wearer with irritation may have ingested sedatives (e.g., alcohol) or may have fallen asleep wearing the contact lenses, thus decreasing blinking and tear flow. Another possibility is that the patient may actually be wearing tight-fitting contact lenses that have never allowed true adaptation despite many months of wear.

A patient with overwear syndrome usually awakens a few hours after removing the lenses. The patient experiences intense pain and tearing similar to that caused by an FB. The delay in onset of the symptoms until after removal of the lenses is caused by a temporary corneal anesthesia produced by the anoxic metabolic by-products that build up during extended lens wear.[71] A second factor is the slow passage of microcysts of edema, which are pushed up to the corneal surface by mitosis of the underlying cells. When the cysts break open on the surface, the corneal nerve endings are exposed.[72]

Most patients with overwear syndrome can be managed with reassurance, frequent administration of artificial tears, oral analgesics, and advice to "wait it out" in a darkened room. Some patients require patching for comfort. A patient who has experienced no problems with contact lenses before an overwear episode can return to using the lenses after 2 or 3 days of wearing glasses but should be advised to build up wearing time gradually. A patient who was having chronic problems with lens comfort before the episode should check with an ophthalmologist before using the contact lenses again.

Soft Contact Lenses

Although the cornea is also oxygenated by way of the tear film with soft contact lenses, only approximately one tenth of the flow behind the lens that occurs with a hard lens is present during soft contact wear.[65] The high degree of lens gas permeability permits the majority of oxygenation to occur directly through the lens. A hydrogel lens is more comfortable than a hard contact lens because lid motion over the lens is smooth. The minimization of lid and corneal irritation allows a more rapid adaptation phase because the initial reflex-induced changes in tearing and blinking are reduced. Nonetheless, the lenses may still lead to corneal edema and secondary hypoxic epithelial changes if worn for an excessive period when blinking is inhibited. Some individuals can tolerate the lenses for extended periods and may on occasion sleep with the contact lenses in place, although this practice is not encouraged. Newer extended-wear hydrogel lenses permit wear for up to 1 week without injury. These lenses are not discernible from standard soft lenses on examination.

Although the acute overwear syndrome that occurs with hard contact lenses can also occur with soft lenses, it is infrequent. More commonly, ocular damage from soft contact lenses falls into one of three categories:

1. Corneal neovascularization (Fig. 62-19A). Frequently, the patient is asymptomatic, but on slit lamp examination, fine vessels are seen invading the periphery of the cornea. Refer the patient to an ophthalmologist for refitting with looser or thinner lenses or with contact lenses that are more gas permeable.

Figure 62-19 Complications from contact lenses. **A,** Corneal neovascularization. **B,** Giant papillary conjunctivitis. **C,** Corneal ulcer. See text for details. (*A, From Friedman NJ, Kaiser PK, Pineda A. Massachusetts Ear & Eye Infirmary Illustrated Manual of Ophthalmology. 3rd ed. Philadelphia: Saunders; 2009. B, from Krachmer JH, Mannis M, Holland E, eds. Cornea. 3rd ed. St. Louis: Mosby; 2010. C, from Yanoff M, Duker JS, eds. Ophthalmology. 3rd ed. St. Louis: Mosby; 2008.*)

2. Giant papillary conjunctivitis (see Fig. 62-19*B*).[73] The patient notes decreased lens tolerance and increased mucus production. On examination of the tarsal conjunctiva (best seen with eversion of the upper lid), large papillae are seen. These papillae appear grossly as a cobblestoned surface. Instruct the patient to discontinue wearing the lenses until the process reverses and to see an ophthalmologist to have the lenses refitted.

3. Sensitivity reaction to contact lens solutions (usually thimerosal or chlorhexidine).[74,75] Diffuse conjunctival injection and sometimes superficial keratitis develop. Advise the patient to switch to preservative-free saline with the use of heat sterilization. Frequently, the contact lenses will need to be replaced before lens wear can be resumed.

All these problems with soft lenses have a bilateral, subacute onset and do not require emergency treatment. The only form of ocular damage associated with soft contact lenses that is a true emergency is a bacterial or fungal corneal ulcer (often *Pseudomonas* or *Acanthamoeba* with soft contact lenses) (see Fig. 62-19*C*).[76-78] Because the nature of soft contact lenses is to absorb water, they can also absorb pathogens, which then can invade the cornea, especially if the soft lens is worn continuously for extended periods. The patient has a painful, red eye with associated discharge and a white infiltrate on the cornea. Immediately consult an ophthalmologist for appropriate culturing and antimicrobial treatment. These infections can permanently affect the patient's visual acuity.

Indications for Removal

Remove a contact lens in the following situations:

1. Contact lens wearer with an altered state of consciousness. The emergency clinician should always be aware that a patient with a depressed or acutely agitated sensorium might be unable to express the need to have the contact lenses removed. Furthermore, it is likely that patients with a depressed sensorium will have decreased lid motion. During the secondary survey of these patients, identify the presence of the lenses and arrange for their removal and storage to prevent harm from excessive wear or possible accidental dislodgment at a later time. Without magnification, soft contact lenses may be difficult to see. Examine the eye with an obliquely directed penlight to reveal the edge of the soft lens 1 to 2 mm from the limbus on the bulbar conjunctiva.

2. Eye trauma with lenses in place. After measurement of visual acuity with the patient's lenses in place, remove them and perform a more detailed examination of the cornea. Fluorescein may discolor hydrogel lenses; when possible, remove extended-wear lenses before using this chemical. After the dye is instilled, flush the eyes with normal saline. Advise the patient to wait at least 1 hour before reinserting the lenses.[54] The availability of single-use droppers of 0.35% fluorexon (Fluoresoft) has permitted safe staining of eyes when soft lenses are to be worn immediately after the examination. Limited eye irrigation after the use of fluorexon drops is still recommended before the reinsertion of soft contact lenses.

3. Inability of the patient to remove the contact lens. A patient may have a hard contact lens that cannot be removed because of corneal edema from prolonged wear. Alternatively, the patient may have a "lost" contact lens

believed to be located behind the upper lid. Because there is no urgency for removal of the contact lens in the out-of-hospital setting, it can wait until the patient has been evaluated by a clinician.

Contraindication to Removal

The only major problem with contact lens removal occurs when the cornea may be perforated. In this case the suction cup technique of removal, described later, is preferred.

Procedure

Hard Contact Lens Removal

A number of maneuvers have been devised for removal of a corneal lens. One technique is to first lean the patient's face over a table or a collecting cloth. Pull the lids temporally from the lateral palpebral margin to lock the lids against the edges of the contact lens. Ask the patient to look toward the nose and then downward toward the chin. This movement works the lower eyelid under the lower edge of the lens and flips the lens off the eye. The technique requires a cooperative patient because the clinician must pull the patient's lids tightly against the edge of the contact lens. The movement of the patient's eye then flips the contact free.

In a unresponsive patient in the supine position, modify the technique. Take a more active role in lid movement by using the following procedure (Fig 62-20*A*). Place one thumb on the upper eyelid and the other on the lower eyelid near the margin of each lid. With the lens centered over the cornea, open the eyelids until the margins of the lid are beyond the edges of the lens. Then press both eyelids gently but firmly on the globe of the eye and move the lids so that they are barely touching the edges of the lens. Press slightly harder on the lower lid to move it under the bottom edge of the lens. As the lower edge of the lens begins to tip away from the eye, move the lids together, which allows the lens to slide out sufficiently so that it can be grasped. Remember to use clean hands (and preferably wear examination gloves that have been rinsed in tap water or saline) when removing the lens.

Alternatively, move the lens gently off the cornea with a cotton-tipped applicator to guide the lens onto the sclera. Force the tip of the applicator under an edge of the lens and flip the contact loose. Apply topical anesthetic when using an applicator if the patient is awake. Take care with this technique to avoid contact of the applicator with the cornea when the lens is moved off the eye. Perhaps the easiest technique is to use a moistened suction-tipped device and simply lift the lens off the cornea (Fig. 62-20*B*).

Scleral lenses (hard contact lenses that cover both the cornea and an amount of the sclera) can be removed by an exaggeration of the manual technique described earlier (Fig. 62-20*C*). Elevation of the lens with a cotton-tipped applicator or a suction-tipped device is also an effective technique. Soft contact lenses should not be removed with a suction-tipped device because tearing or splitting of the lens might occur.

Soft Contact Lens Removal

With clean hands (preferably using gloves rinsed in saline or tap water), pull down the lower eyelid with the middle finger. Place the tip of the index finger on the lower edge of the lens.

CONTACT LENS REMOVAL

A. Manual Removal of Hard Contact Lens

1. Separate the eyelids.

2. Entrap the lens edges with the eyelids.

3. Expel the lens by forcing the lower lid under the inferior edge of the lens.

C. Removal of a Hard Scleral Lens

1. Separate the eyelids.

2. Force the lower lid beneath the edge of the scleral lens by temporal traction on the lower lid.

3. Lift the lens off the eye.

B. Suction Cup Removal of Hard Contact Lens

Use a moistened suction cup to remove a hard contact lens.

D. Removal of a Soft Contact Lens

1. Separate the eyelids and then move the contact onto the sclera with the index finger.

2. Pinch the lens between the thumb and index finger.

Figure 62-20 Contact lens removal. (*A, C, and D, From Grant HD, Murray RH, Bergeron JF, eds.* Brady Emergency Care. *5th ed. Englewood Cliffs, NJ: Prentice Hall; 1990:338. Reproduced by permission.*)

Slide the lens down onto the sclera and compress it slightly between the thumb and index finger. This pinching motion folds the lens so it can be removed from the eye (Fig. 62-20D). Alternatively, use a cotton-tipped applicator (e.g., Q-Tip) instead of a gloved hand. Occasionally, a tight-fitting lens will be difficult to remove. One potential method is the use of topical anesthetic drops, lubricating eyedrops (e.g., Refresh Celluvisc lubricant eye drops), and a cotton-tipped applicator to lift the edge of the lens from the limbus. This breaks the seal of the lens on the cornea and allows removal.

Lens Storage

After a contact lens is removed, store it in sterile normal saline solution. Use the patient's own storage container and lens solution if available. A variety of alternative sterile containers are available for use in the ED. Be certain to keep the right and left lenses separate and in appropriately labeled containers. The containers should be kept with the patient until a friend or family member can procure them, or they should be locked up with the patient's valuables.

Evaluation of a "Lost" Contact Lens

A patient may request examination for a "lost" contact lens. The patient may be unsure whether the lens is hidden under a lid, remains on the cornea, or is truly outside the eye. Evaluation of a patient with a "lost" contact should begin, as should all eye examinations, with measurement of visual acuity. Measure visual acuity preferably with a 20-ft eye chart. Diminished visual acuity in the eye with the lost contact is convincing evidence that the lens is missing. Though transparent, soft contact lenses in proper position are usually seen when viewed closely with loupes or a slit lamp. The lens forms a fine line at the point where it ends on the sclera several millimeters peripheral to the limbus. Hard contact lenses are even more evident as they change in position on the cornea.

If the contact lens is not evident on initial inspection, evert the lids as discussed in the section "Ocular FB Removal" (double eversion of the upper lid). If the lens is still not visible, place a drop of topical anesthetic in the eye. Gently sweep the upper fornix with a moistened cotton-tipped applicator while the patient looks toward the chin. If the lens is still not evident even though the patient remains insistent that it is in the eye, perform a fluorescein examination after explaining that the dye will color the lens (permanently). Evert the upper lid again and examine with an ultraviolet light source.

If the lens remains elusive, reassure the patient that a thorough examination was performed and that no object was located under the eyelids or on the cornea. Next, examine the cornea for defects that warrant antibiotic ointment and placement of a pressure patch over the eye (as discussed in "Eye Patching"). Follow-up with the patient's eye specialist for a replacement lens and to provide further reassurance is advised. Ask the patient to retrace his movements at the time that the contact began to give trouble or was missed. Check the clothing being worn at that time and look for the lens there. A final possibility is that the patient may have accidentally placed the two lenses together in the same side of the carrying case, thereby causing them to stick together. Hence, take a methodical approach, as outlined earlier, to ensure that no lens remains hidden in the eye.

Complications of Lens Removal

A corneal abrasion can occur during lens removal. It is difficult at times to determine whether the injury was produced by the patient or was a result of removal by the clinician. Fortunately, the corneal injury is generally of a superficial nature and responds well to symptomatic care.

Summary

Contact lens removal is usually simple. Challenging situations include identifying patients at risk for corneal injury from overuse, helping patients who have lost a contact lens in the eye, and providing aftercare instructions for patients with contact lens–related problems.

BANDAGE CONTACT LENSES FOR TREATMENT OF CORNEAL ABRASIONS

Acute corneal abrasions can cause significant pain, limit function, and result in lost days of work. Several studies have shown that bandage contact lenses are very effective in reducing pain without a requirement for narcotic analgesia, in decreasing time away from work, and in returning to baseline functioning when used for uncomplicated acute corneal abrasions.[79-81] Yet bandage contact lenses are seldom used in the ED. An immediate benefit is gained when the emergency practitioner selectively uses this treatment modality.

Indications and Contraindications

Bandage contact lenses may be used appropriately as an adjunct for the treatment of acute corneal abrasions resulting from minor trauma when symptomatic relief or rapid return of functionality is desired. Obtain a clear history of an acute traumatic abrasion and a fluorescein stain pattern consistent with this diagnosis.

Bandage contact lenses are contraindicated when the cause of the corneal epithelial defect is suspected to be due to infection. Ensure that a corneal ulcer is not present. The hallmark fluorescein stain pattern consistent with a corneal ulcer is a round stain with blurred margins, commonly in the central visual axis (midpupil region) (see Fig. 62-19C). Pain is disproportionate to the findings. An intense ciliary flush and anterior chamber reaction (cells and flare) may also be present. Avoid the use of bandage contact lenses in patients with a history of soft contact lens use and a nontraumatic abrasion in the central part of the cornea. Follow-up for removal of the bandage contact lenses and reevaluation of the eye are required to confirm improvement and identify complications. Unreliable patients who are not likely to be compliant with follow-up are at increased risk for infection and thus not good candidates for this modality.

Equipment

Hydrophilic bandage contact lenses are available and include, but are not limited to, Biomedics 55, Ocular Sciences, Inc., San Francisco, –0.50 dioptric power, 8.6 posterior curvature, and 14.2 diameter of the lens, and Acuvue Oasys BC, zero power (plano) or –0.50 diopter, 8.4 posterior curvature, and 14.0 diameter. Acuvue Oasys has been approved by the Food and Drug Administration for up to 1 week of continuous wear.

Procedure

Assess and document the pain. Instill 1 drop of a fluoroquinolone ophthalmic solution in the affected eye as prophylaxis against infection at the time of lens placement. Use of topical anesthetics is not required, but they have often been used in the evaluation of abrasions. Use a gloved hand that has been rinsed with water to remove the talc. Orient the contact lens on the tip of the examiner's index finger. Ensure that the lens is not inverted. The normal configuration of the lens resembles a cup, whereas an inverted lens resembles a saucer with its edges flaring outward. Another method to determine orientation of the lens is to try to close the edges or have them meet together with your fingers. If the edges curve away from each other, the lens is inverted. Direct the patient's gaze upward and then pull the lower lid slightly downward while inserting the lens over the cornea. Ask the patient to gently blink and assess for placement. After a few minutes, reassess and again document whether pain is present. Instruct the patient to return for follow-up in 1 day. On return, remove the soft lens as described earlier, assess vision, document pain, and reevaluate the eye.

Complications

Because of the hypoxic microenvironment of the cornea, covering the cornea with a bandage contact lens could increase the opportunity for an infection to occur. Patients who do not disclose the use of soft contact lenses are at increased risk for corneal ulcers. Some patients may experience "tight lens syndrome" because of a lens that does not fit well or from drying out as the lens is exposed to the elements. Bandage contact lenses are usually of a generic size and thus do not offer a precise fit, but they are in place only for a short duration. Signs and symptoms may include redness, eye irritation, burning, a dry sensation, blurry vision, halos around objects, and lack of mobility of the contact lens over the cornea. Lack of mobility can reduce oxygen tension and thereby cause corneal edema and an even tighter lens. Rewetting solutions can improve hydration. Removal of a tight fitting lens was described earlier.

Summary

Bandage contact lenses have been shown to be safe, effective, and comfortable in the treatment of corneal abrasions. Careful patient selection and proper technique will optimize this treatment modality when appropriately indicated for routine ED use. Patients will experience significantly decreased pain without the use of narcotic analgesics, significantly increased functionality, and decreased time away from work.

INFECTIOUS KERATITIS

Infectious keratitis with corneal ulceration can have a variety of causes, including overwear of contact lenses. Diagnosis of a corneal ulcer requires the use of a slit lamp and accurate determination of the patient's history. Infectious keratitis is a frequent problem in ophthalmic practice. Herpes simplex is a common corneal pathogen. *Acanthamoeba* is another pathogen particularly associated with contact lens use and exposure to organism-tainted environments. When a patient is seen in the ED with a corneal ulcer, promptly refer the patient to an ophthalmologist. When immediate referral is not possible, obtain telephone guidance from an ophthalmologist for initiation of therapy, and arrange for ophthalmology follow-up within 24 hours.

Patients with herpes simplex keratitis often give a history of previous episodes of the disease. Patients who undergo almost any form of corneal stress may sustain an activation of preexisting corneal disease. Herpes simplex keratitis is classically recognized by its dendritic pattern on fluorescein staining (see Fig. 62-7, *plate 9*).

Acanthamoeba keratitis is a disease with potentially devastating consequences. Its frequency seems to be increasing, particularly in contact lens wearers, and its pathophysiology is not completely understood. Patients often have a red eye in which the initial bacterial culture results are negative.

Bacterial keratitis occurs in a variety of settings. Organisms range from the relatively common *Staphylococcus* (including methicillin-resistant *Staphylococcus aureus*) or *Streptococcus* to *Mycobacterium*, which can be difficult to identify. A variety of antibiotics are used against bacterial agents. Ciprofloxacin is a quinolone that has demonstrated efficacy against most of the common causative agents. Bacterial organisms in the cornea can develop resistance to any antibiotic, and resistance to fluoroquinolones has also been observed.[82] Ideally, treatment follows acquisition of material from the ulcer for culture.

In instances in which a cellular infiltrate is seen on slit lamp examination and there will be a delay of hours before an ophthalmologic consultant can perform the culture, it is prudent to initiate therapy with topical fluoroquinolones such as ciprofloxacin. In such circumstances, obtain corneal samples for culture under the telephone guidance of the consultant before starting the antibiotic. One approach is to lightly touch a culture medium–moistened cotton-tipped swab against the ulcer and then streak standard culture media. If the ulcer is chronic or the patient is immunocompromised, a fungal organism may be the causative agent. Finally, a saline-moistened cotton-tipped swab may be used to obtain a Gram stain of the ulcer. Initiation of therapy before obtaining specimens for culture makes subsequent identification of an organism difficult. For this reason, consider the circumstances of the individual case before initiating treatment.

TONOMETRY

Tonometry is the estimation of IOP. It is obtained by measuring the resistance of the eyeball to indentation by an applied force. Prolonged elevated IOP is associated with visual field loss and blindness. A sudden elevation in IOP can result from trauma or primary angle-closure glaucoma. Patients with primary angle-closure glaucoma are often seen in the ED with systemic complaints, including nausea, vomiting, and headache. Occasionally, these patients are surprisingly free of pain in or about the eye. The emergency clinician must determine the IOP and its relationship to the systemic symptoms.

Ophthalmologists depended on tactile estimation of eye pressure until the 1860s, when von Graefe developed the first mechanical tonometer.[3,13] Applanation tonometry was introduced in 1885 by Maklakoff[83] but was not popularized until Goldmann[84] improved the instrument. Schiøtz[85] developed an impression tonometer in 1905 and modified it in the 1920s; this form is still in use today. Aside from modifications in configuration, current tonometers closely resemble the devices popularized by Schiøtz[85] and Goldmann.[84] The most dramatic variations are the Mackay-Marg tonometer,[86] which permits a continuous tonographic recording, and the noncontact tonometer, a pneumatic applanation tonometer.[87] Pocket-sized tonometers using the principle of the MacKay-Marg tonometer are available. One such device is the Tono-Pen XL (Reichert, Inc, Depew, NY).[88] These devices are portable, lightweight, and relatively accurate, with built-in provisions for calibration. They have the advantage of a one-time-use replaceable cover that eliminates concern about the possible transmission of an infectious agent. Although numerous devices are available, the Schiøtz and Tono-Pen XL tonometers are the standard devices for measuring IOP in the ED.

Tonometric Techniques

Three tonometric techniques are reliable and clinically useful for estimating IOP:

1. The impression method uses a plunger (3 mm in diameter) to deform the cornea, and the "indentation" is then measured. This technique was popularized by Schiøtz[85] and commonly bears his name.
2. The MacKay-Marg method[86] is a refined version of the impression technique in which smaller amounts of cornea are indented.
3. In the applanation method, a planar surface is pressed against the cornea.

The Schiøtz tonometer actually measures total IOP (initial pressure plus the pressure added by the weight of the tonometer and the plunger). Friedenwald[89] empirically found that a "rigidity coefficient" could be introduced to allow an estimation of the true IOP. One must be aware, however, that calculated conversion tables for Schiøtz tonometers use an average estimate of the rigidity coefficient and hence are not accurate when eye rigidity is altered (e.g., after scleral buckle procedures for retinal detachment or with extreme myopia).

Measurement of IOP in the ED by tonometry is a technique available to most emergency clinicians. Tonometry is not a standard procedure for many eye-related complaints, but in the following special situations tonometry it may be particularly helpful:

- Confirmation of a clinical diagnosis of acute angle-closure glaucoma. A middle-aged or elderly patient with acute aching pain in one eye, blurred vision (including "halos" around lights), and a red eye with a smoky cornea and a fixed midposition pupil obviously needs a pressure reading (Fig. 62-21A). Sometimes the findings are less dramatic, and sometimes the patient complains mostly of nausea and vomiting, which suggests "flu" rather than an eye disorder.
- Determination of a baseline ocular pressure after blunt ocular injury. Patients with hyphema often have acute rises in IOP because of blood obstructing the trabecular meshwork (see Fig. 62-21B).[90] Later, angle recession can cause a permanent form of open-angle glaucoma. Arts and colleagues[91] suggested that an IOP greater than 22 mm Hg or

Figure 62-21 Indications for tonometry. **A,** This patient complained of severe headache, nausea, and blurry vision. The eye was obviously inflamed, with corneal edema (note the fragmented light reflex) and a mid-dilated pupil. This is acute angle-closure glaucoma. **B,** Hyphema (layering of red blood cells in the anterior chamber) (*arrow*) in a patient who was struck in the eye with a racquetball. (*From Palay DA, Krachmer JH, eds.* Primary Care Ophthalmology. *2nd ed. St. Louis: Mosby; 2005.*)

a difference of 3 mm Hg or greater between the eyes is a good marker of "ocular injury" in the setting of an orbital fracture.

Tonometry may also be considered in the following scenarios:

- Determination of a baseline ocular pressure in a patient with iritis. Both open- and closed-angle glaucoma, as well as corticosteroid-induced glaucoma, can develop in patients with iritis. Because most cases of iritis are referred, tonometry may also be deferred unless signs of increased IOP are present.

- Documentation of ocular pressure in a patient at risk for open-angle glaucoma. All patients older than 40 years with a family history of open-angle glaucoma, optic disc changes, visual field defects, and pressure of 21 mm Hg or higher should be referred to an ophthalmologist for further workup. Referral should also be made for patients with suspiciously cupped discs who have normal pressure; some of these patients may have "low-pressure" glaucoma associated with visual field defects. This is usually part of an ophthalmologist's examination.

Contraindications to Tonometry

Tonometry is relatively contraindicated in eyes that are infected unless one is using a device such as the Tono-Pen XL, which uses a sterilized cover.[2] Sterilize a tonometer before and after applying it to a potentially infected eye. Measure infected eyes with either a noncontact tonometer or a device with a covered tip (e.g., Tono-Pen). Swab the contact portions of any device with alcohol and allow it to dry before use on another eye. Not all viruses are destroyed by cleansing with alcohol. Hydrogen peroxide is effective in deactivating the human immunodeficiency virus responsible for acquired immunodeficiency syndrome (AIDS). Ultraviolet sterilization, cold sterilizer bathing of the footplate and plunger, and ethylene oxide sterilization have all been advocated as alternatives to sterilizing the tip of the Schiøtz tonometer. The Schiøtz tonometer may also be used with sterile disposable coverings (marketed as Tonofilm). Nonetheless, defer measurement of IOP in an obviously infected eye until a subsequent visit to the ED or private clinician unless the red eye demands an immediate determination of IOP.

Examples of indications for immediate tonometry in the setting of a red eye are suspected angle-closure glaucoma (acute onset of redness and pain in the eye with smoky vision, a cloudy cornea, and a fixed pupil in mid-dilation, often with headache and nausea) and iritis (ciliary injection with photophobia), in which secondary angle-closure glaucoma or corticosteroid-induced changes in pressure may occur. Reported cases of conjunctivitis spread by tonometry predominantly tend to be viral infections. Particular effort should be made to avoid use of the instrument on patients with active facial or ocular herpetic lesions or those who may have AIDS.

The presence of corneal defects also represents a relative contraindication to tonometry.[3,13] Use of a tonometer on an abraded cornea may lead to further injury and is commonly deferred until a subsequent visit. Patients who cannot maintain a relaxed position (e.g., because of significant apprehension, blepharospasm, uncontrolled coughing, nystagmus, or uncontrolled hiccups) are unlikely to permit an adequate examination and can sustain a corneal injury when sudden movements occur during an examination. Furthermore, tonometric examination, with the exception of the palpation technique (through the lids) and the noncontact method, should not be performed on a cornea without complete anesthesia.

Tonometry should not be performed on a patient with a suspected penetrating ocular injury.[2] Globe perforation may be exacerbated by pressure on the globe with resultant extrusion of intraocular contents. Slit lamp examination can be used for detection of a possible perforation.

Procedure

Palpation Technique

All forms of tonometry are essentially ways of determining the ease of deforming the eye; an eye that is easily deformed has low pressure. The most direct way to do this is simply to press on the sclera through the lids and grossly compare one eye with the other. One can easily distinguish the rock-hard eye of acute glaucoma from the normal opposite eye by this method. Direct the patient to look down without closing the lids. Rest both hands on the patient's forehead and apply just enough digital pressure on the involved eye to indent it slightly with one index finger. With the other index finger,

alternately feel and compare the compliance of the other eye (Fig. 62-22, *plate 1*). An experienced examiner is able to estimate IOP within 3 to 5 mm Hg of the actual IOP with the palpation technique, but most emergency clinicians do not have enough experience to trust this method.[31]

Another method is to anesthetize the eyes topically and press a wetted applicator on the sclera of each eye. Again, eye deformation is inversely related to ocular pressure. Rigidity of the globe is also a factor in this crude method of tonometry.

Impression (Schiøtz) Technique

Use of the Schiøtz tonometer requires relaxation on the part of the patient and steadiness on the part of the clinician. After placing the patient in either a supine or a semirecumbent position, instruct the patient to gaze at a spot directly above the eyes. A spot on the ceiling should suffice; alternatively, patients can stretch their arm up over their head and gaze at their thumb. Place a drop of topical anesthetic in each eye. After the irritation of the drop passes, allow the patient to blink while blotting the tears away with a tissue. Rubbing the eyes lowers IOP. Reassure the patient that further discomfort will not occur during the procedure.

Ask the patient to keep both eyes wide open and fixed on an object. Separate the eyelids on the side that you are standing. Test the tonometer on a flat surface to confirm smooth movement of the device (see Fig. 62-22, *plate 2*). Take care to direct pressure onto the orbital rims rather than the orbit because pressure directed into the orbit falsely raises the reading. Hold the tonometer momentarily over the open eye, and inform the patient that the instrument will block vision in the one eye. Instruct the patient to continue to gaze at the fixation point as though the instrument were not there. After the patient relaxes the involuntary muscle contraction that occurs when the instrument is first placed in the line of sight, gently lower the instrument onto the middle portion of the cornea (see Fig. 62-22, *plate 3*). This is a painless experience for patients with an anesthetized cornea. Vertically align the instrument with the footplate resting on the cornea; the reading should be in midscale. Should the reading be on the low end of the scale (<5 units), place additional weight on the plunger after the instrument has been removed. Repeat the process as before with the additional weight.

Measure the opposite eye in the same fashion. Use the chart provided to determine the converted reading based on the reading and amount of weight on the scale. Refer to ophthalmology if the converted scale reading is higher than 21 mm Hg (see Fig. 62-22, *plate 4*). Patients with elevations in IOP of 30 mm Hg or greater require more urgent consultation and initiation of therapy. Associated symptoms or signs of angle-closure glaucoma (primary or secondary) represent an ophthalmologic emergency.[92]

Errors with Impression Tonometry

Inaccurate readings can occur with the Schiøtz tonometer for a variety of reasons. Falsely low readings may occur if the plunger is sticky. Check plunger motion and the zero point of the tonometer on a firm test button before use. If the plunger is sticky, clean it with isopropyl alcohol and dry it with a tissue. Inadvertently directing pressure onto the orbit when the lids are held open may elevate IOP and provide a falsely elevated reading. The following eye movements have been found to elevate IOP: closing the lids (increases by

TONOMETRY: PALPATION AND SCHIØTZ TECHNIQUES

A relatively unskilled examiner can detect the very high intraocular pressure of acute angle-closure glaucoma with tactile tonometry. The examiner rests both hands on the patient's forehead and alternately applies just enough digital pressure on the globe to indent it slightly with one index finger while feeling the compliance of the globe with the other.

Before using the Schiøtz tonometer, test it on a flat surface to ensure smooth motion of the device and that the zero line is achieved.

Apply lid separation pressure to the bony orbital rims. An assistant may separate the lids while you concentrate on proper placement of the tonometer. Hold the tonometer vertically during use, and rest your hand against the patient's facial bones. After anesthetic drops are instilled, the patient will not experience any pain from this procedure. It is important to have a relaxed patient because squinting and blepharospasm may interfere with the reading. Note: Gloves should be worn.

4 Schiøtz Tonometry*

Tonometer Scale	Tonometer Weights (g)		
Reading (Units)	5.5 (mm Hg)	7.5 (mm Hg)	10 (mm Hg)
2.50	27	39	55
3.00	24	36	51
3.50	22	33	47
4.00	21	30	43
4.50	19	28	40
5.00	17	26	37
5.50	16	24	34
6.00	15	22	32
6.50	13	20	29
7.00	12	18	27
7.50	11	17	25
8.00	10	16	23
8.50	9	14	21
9.00	8	13	20
9.50	8	12	18
10.00	7	11	16

* The table porvides estimates of intraocular pressure to the nearest mm Hg for the different weight of the Schiøtz tonometer. Accuracy is most dependable with scale readings greater than 5. If the scale reading is less than 5, use the nest highest weight that will give a reading of 5 or more.

Use the above chart to determine the converted reading based on the reading and the amount of weight on the scale.

Figure 62-22 Tonometry: palpation and Schiøtz techniques.

TONOMETRY: TONO-PEN TECHNIQUE

1 Spray the probe tip with compressed gas prior to use to clean debris away from the tip.

2 Cover the Tono-Pen probe tip with a new Ocu-Film tip cover.

3 Hold the Tono-Pen vertically with the tip pointing down, and press the switch twice in rapid succession.

4 After pressing the switch, 2 beeps will sound and "CAL" will appear on the screen.

5 Wait (up to 20 seconds) until a beep sounds and "-UP-" appears on the screen.

6 Quickly turn the probe so that the tip is pointing straight up.

Figure 62-23 Tonometry: Tono-Pen technique.

5 mm Hg), blinking (increases by 5 to 10 mm Hg), accommodation (increases by 2 mm Hg), and looking toward the nose (increases by 5 to 10 mm Hg).[93] Repeated or prolonged measurements have been found to lower IOP approximately 2 mm Hg and may also lower pressure in the opposite eye.[94] As mentioned in the introduction to this section, calibration of the Schiøtz tonometer is based on a mean rigidity coefficient. Factors that produce a reduction in ocular rigidity falsely lower the measured pressure. Such factors include high myopia, anticholinesterase drugs, overhydration (e.g., four large cups of coffee or six cans of beer), and scleral buckle operations.[95,96]

Ocular pressure measurements can vary with ocular perfusion. When measured after a premature ventricular contraction, IOP may be reduced as much as 8 mm Hg.[93] Similarly, decreased venous return as produced by breath holding, the Valsalva maneuver, or a tight collar can increase IOP.[93]

Impression (Tono-Pen XL) Technique (Fig. 62-23)

When using this device, the preparations for testing are similar to those for the Schiøtz device. Encourage the patient

to relax, and apply a topical anesthetic to numb the cornea. Ask the patient to stare with both eyes at a distant object during testing. As noted previously, help separate the eyelids but do not apply direct pressure on the globe. One major advantage of using the Tono-Pen XL is that the patient may be evaluated in any position as long as the device is applied perpendicular to the corneal surface. Another advantage is that the device can be used in patients with irregular or high corneal astigmatism.

Ideally, the complete instructions provided with the device should be consulted before each use; however, the following synopsis is provided to help in circumstances in which instructions are unavailable (Box 62-2).

First, spray the tip of the probe with compressed gas to clean the mechanism and ensure free movement. Place an Ocu-Film (latex) cover snugly (but without tension) over the probe tip.

Perform calibration before use at least once each day (see Box 62-2). Depress and release the activation switch momentarily. The liquid crystal display (LCD) should show "—." If the device beeps and "====" appears on the LCD, push the

TONOMETRY: TONO-PEN TECHNIQUE

Wait a few seconds. If the calibration was successful, a beep will sound and "Good" will appear on the LCD screen.

Instill a drop of topical anesthetic (e.g., tetracaine 0.5%) into both eyes.

Hold the Tono-Pen as you would hold a pencil, and brace your hand against the patient's cheek for stability.

Activate the Tono-Pen by pressing the switch. A beep will sound and "====" will appear on the LCD screen.

Touch the Tono-Pen against the cornea lightly and briefly. Repeat several times; a click will sound every time that a pressure is measured. After four valid readings, a final beep will sound, and the averaged measurement will appear on the LCD.

Check the reading on the screen. The number represents IOP in mm Hg. The bar below the number represents the statistical reliability. (A reading >20% reflects an unreliable reading and should be repeated.)

Figure 62-23, cont'd *IOP*, intraocular pressure.

activation switch again so that "—" reappears. If the previous calibration shows "bAd" on the LCD, a long beep sounds, followed by "CAL" on the LCD. A short beep follows and then the desired "—" is displayed. Once "—" is displayed, hold the probe vertically with the tip pointing straight down. Press and release the activation switch twice in rapid succession. Two beeps will then sound and "CAL" will appear on the LCD. Hold the probe in this position (up to 20 seconds) until a beep sounds and "-UP-" appears on the LCD. Immediately turn the probe 180 degrees so that the tip points straight up. In a few seconds another beep occurs and the LCD changes. If the LCD reads "Good," the calibration was successful. If the LCD reads "bAd," the calibration was unsuccessful.

With an unsuccessful calibration, repeat the calibration steps described earlier until two consecutive "Good" readings are obtained. If further attempts are unsuccessful, loosen the Ocu-Film tip cover and repeat the calibration process. If

attempts are still unsuccessful, press the reset button and repeat the process. If still unsuccessful, use compressed air to clean the tip of the probe and repeat the process. If still unsuccessful, the battery should be replaced and the process repeated. Continued failure warrants a call to Reichert Technical Support (http://www.reicherttonopen.com/ss.html) at 1-888-849-8955.

Proceed to measurement once the device is calibrated and the patient is prepared as outlined earlier. Depress and release the activation switch to obtain "====" on the LCD. A beep will occur when ready. If the switch is not depressed long enough, the LCD will be blank. If a blank screen is seen, press and release the activation switch again to obtain "====" on the LCD. Hold the probe like a pen and touch it to the cornea briefly and lightly. Touch the cornea four times. A click will sound and a reading will appear on the LCD each time that a valid reading is obtained. After four valid readings, a final beep will sound and the averaged measurement will appear

| BOX 62-2 | Steps in Setting up the Tono-Pen |

1. Remove the Ocu-Film tip cover from the probe.
2. To help prevent buildup of debris around the post of the probe, spray the tip of the probe with compressed gas before the first use of the day.
3. Cover the Tono-Pen XL probe tip with a new Ocu-Film tip cover.
4. Check calibration only before the first use of each day.
   a. Depress the activation switch momentarily and then release it.
   b. If the previous calibration check was good, the LCD will briefly show "—" followed by "====," accompanied by a beep.
   c. If the previous calibration was bad, a long beep sounds, after which "CAL" appears and a short beep sounds. The display then changes to "—" and another short beep sounds.
5. Hold the Tono-Pen vertically with the tip of the probe pointing straight down.
6. Press and release the activation switch twice in rapid succession. Two beeps will sound and "CAL" appears.

7. Wait (up to 20 seconds) until a beep sounds and "-UP-" appears.
8. Quickly turn the probe straight up.
9. Wait a few seconds. A second beep will sound and indicates the end of the calibration check.
10. Instill a drop of topical anesthetic (proparacaine) into both eyes.
11. Instruct the patient to look straight ahead at the fixation target with the eyes fully open.
12. Brace the heel of your hand on the patient's cheek for stability.
13. Activate the Tono-Pen by pressing the activation switch.
14. The LCD will display "=====" and a beep will sound.
15. Once activated, touch the Tono-Pen probe against the patient's cornea lightly and briefly. *Repeat several times.*
16. A click will sound and a digital intraocular pressure measurement is displayed.
17. Proceed to the other eye. Repeat steps 12 through 15.

Adapted from Auerbach PA. Wilderness Medicine. *5th ed. St. Louis: Elsevier Mosby; 2007. Copyright © 2007 Mosby, an Imprint of Elsevier.*
LCD, *liquid crystal display.*

on the LCD. The number represents IOP in millimeters of mercury. The associated bar reflects statistical reliability (a reading >20% reflects an unreliable measurement and should be repeated).

If four dashes ("----") appear on the LCD after the final beep, too few valid readings were obtained. In such a case, reactivate the probe (without recalibration) and repeat the measurement procedure. If the probe is not reactivated within 20 seconds, the LCD will clear, but the device can be activated as noted previously without recalibration.

The values are interpreted as outlined earlier for the Schiøtz device. Readings may be affected by the same features noted as causes of error with impression tonometry via the Schiøtz device. Store the device with an unused Ocu-Film cover protecting the tip of the probe.

Complications

When tonometric instruments are used properly and reasonable precautions are taken, complications are unusual. An eye with preexisting corneal injury should be spared the additional trauma of tonometer placement. Corneal abrasions can be produced by ocular movement during testing. In particular, patients with uncontrollable nystagmus, hiccups, or coughing or those who are extremely apprehensive should not be subjected to tonometry. Infection can be transmitted by use of the instrument. Careful cleansing of the device and avoidance of tonometry in patients with obvious conjunctivitis, corneal ulcers, or active herpetic lesions should minimize the risk of spreading the infection to the unaffected eye or to subsequent patients. Although protective coverings can be placed over the tonometer contact, tonometry can usually be postponed in the aforementioned individuals until the risk for infection is minimal. Extrusion of ocular contents with penetrating injuries is a potential, but rare complication.

SLIT LAMP EXAMINATION

The slit lamp is an extremely useful instrument for examination of the anterior segment of the eye. The instrument can reveal pathologic conditions that would otherwise be invisible, such as minor corneal defects, anterior chamber hemorrhage, and inflammation.

Indications and Contraindications

The slit lamp can be used in the majority of eye examinations. It is especially useful in the ED for the diagnosis of corneal abrasions, FBs, and iritis.[31] The slit lamp facilitates FB removal and is also used in conjunction with most applanation tonometers. Portable slit lamp instruments are readily available (Fig. 62-24) but seldom used in the ED; thus emergency practitioners generally have access only to a stationary, upright device. Therefore, in the absence of a portable device, a slit lamp examination is contraindicated in patients who cannot tolerate an upright sitting position (e.g., those with orthostatic syncope).

Equipment

The slit lamp has three essential components: a binocular microscope mounted horizontally, a light source that can create a beam of variable width, and a mechanical assembly to immobilize the patient's head and manipulate the microscope and light source. The location and arrangement of the knobs that control these components vary in devices made by different manufacturers. Usually, by simply turning each knob and watching the results, one can quickly master a new machine. Figure 62-25 illustrates the location of the functional controls on one particular instrument.

First, locate the on/off switch for the instrument. Frequently, this switch incorporates or is adjacent to a rheostat

Figure 62-24 A portable slit lamp can be used to evaluate patients who cannot tolerate an upright sitting position or cannot be easily moved to the examination chair.

that provides two or three different power settings. The lowest setting is adequate for routine examination and will preserve bulb life. One can use a high-intensity setting when examining the anterior chamber with a narrow slit beam. Often, these controls are located on a transformer placed beneath the table to which the slit lamp has been attached. The second knob that one should find is the locking nut for the mechanical assembly. Loosen the nut so that the assembly can be moved.

Make adjustments so that the patient is comfortable while sitting with the head in the device. Ask the patient to press the forehead firmly against the head rest with the chin in the chin rest. By varying the height of the table and height of the chin rest, one should be able to maximize comfort of the patient's neck and back. Adjust the chin rest to align the patient's eye level with the mark on the head rest support rods.

The binocular microscope has a control for varying the magnification. Usually, low powers such as 10× or 16× are the most useful. Use a higher power to examine the anterior chamber for cells and flare and when the cornea is examined in minute detail. Adjust the binocular interpupillary distance to match that of the examiner. Focus the eyepieces by moving the instrument forward and backward until the narrowed vertical beam is sharpest on the patient's cornea when viewed with the unaided eye. Then, while viewing through each eyepiece individually, adjust the focus of each to produce a sharp image of the anterior surface of the cornea.

Notice that the light source is mounted on a swinging arm. Find the knobs that adjust the width and the height of the light beam. Click various filters in as needed, usually white and blue filters for standard examination. Alter the angle of the slit lamp beam from vertical to horizontal. The vertical alignment is preferred for routine examinations in the ED.

Both the microscope and the light source are mounted on swivel arms linked at their base to a movable table. Change the position of this table by pushing on any part of it. Use the joystick on the table for finer movements. Vary the height of the microscope and the light source by twisting either the joystick or a separate knob at the base, depending on the design of the instrument.

Procedure

There are three setups that every slit lamp operator must know.[97] The first is for an overall screening of the anterior segment of the eye. *For examination of the patient's right eye, swing the light source to your left at a 45-degree angle while the microscope is directly in front of the patient's eye.* Set the slit beam to the maximum height and the minimum width using the white light. To scan across the patient's cornea, first focus the beam on the cornea by moving the entire base of the slit lamp forward and backward. Then move the whole base left and right to scan across the cornea. The 45-degree angle between the microscope and the light source is the default position. The most common mistake is to try to scan by swinging the arm of the light source in an arc; this does not work because the light beam will remain centered on the same point of the patient's eye. Scan across at the level of the conjunctiva and the cornea and then push slightly forward on the base or joystick and scan at the level of the iris. The depth of the anterior chamber is easily appreciated with this low-magnification setup (Fig. 62-26). When the depth of the anterior chamber is reduced, suspect a corneal perforation or a predisposition to angle-closure glaucoma.

Use this basic setup to examine the conjunctiva for traumatic lesions, inflammation, and FBs. Examine the eyelids for hordeolum, blepharitis, or trichiasis. Completely evert the lids (as described earlier in the section "Ocular FB Removal") in conjunction with the slit lamp examination to permit evaluation of the undersurface of the upper lid for FB retention.

Corneal FB removal can be enhanced by use of the slit lamp. In particular, the instrument allows stabilization of the patient's head. Magnification also minimizes corneal injury during FB or rust ring removal. The upper eyelid may be immobilized with a cotton-tipped applicator, as discussed previously. The clinician's hand can be steadied against the patient's nose, cheek, or forehead or against the support rods of the head rest. The patient should be instructed to stare straight ahead at a fixed light or at the clinician's ear during removal of the FB.

The second setup is essentially the same as the first but uses the blue filter. The purpose is to identify any areas of fluorescein staining. After fluorescein is applied, "click" the blue filter into position and widen the beam to 3 or 4 mm. A patient can tolerate a wider beam without photophobia if it is blue. Search for corneal defects (as discussed earlier in "The Fluorescein Examination") with this setup. The blue filter may also be used with applanation tonometry, as discussed earlier in "Tonometry."

The purpose of the third setup is to search for cells in the anterior chamber—either the white cells of iritis or the red cells of a microscopic hyphema. Shorten the height of the beam to 3 or 4 mm and make it as narrow as possible. Switch the microscope to high power. Focus the beam on the center of the cornea and then push forward slightly so that it is focused on the anterior surface of the lens. Pull the joystick back again to a focus point midway between the cornea and the lens, where it will be focused on the anterior chamber (Fig. 62-27). Keep the beam centered over the pupil so that there is a black background. Normally, the aqueous humor of the anterior chamber is totally clear. Small particles seen floating up or down through the beam are usually circulating cells. If the beam lights up the aqueous like a searchlight in the fog, the examiner has found the protein flare that

Figure 62-25 Slit lamp (BM 900, Haag-Streit, Mason, OH).

Figure 62-26 Slit lamp photograph of a normal left eye under low power. The curved slit of light on the right is reflected off the cornea and the slit on the left is reflected off the iris. The depth of the anterior chamber can easily be appreciated under this low-magnification setup. Note that the light source is on the patient's left side to examine the left eye, with the path of the light going in a temporal-to-nasal direction. *(Courtesy of D. Price.)*

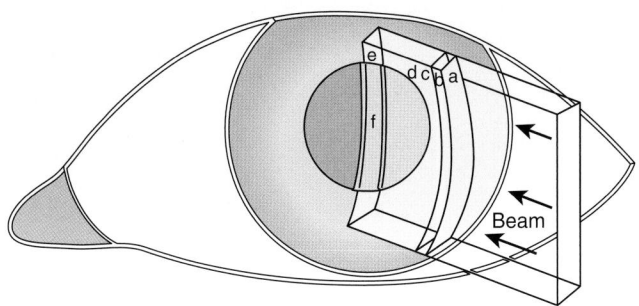

Figure 62-27 Appearance of the left eye during examination of the anterior chamber under low power: *a*, corneal epithelium; *b*, corneal stroma; *c*, corneal endothelium; *d*, anterior chamber (potential location of cells or flare); *e*, iris; *f*, lens reflection. The slit of light shines in the temporal-to-nasal direction at a 45-degree angle to the anterior surface of the cornea. The depth of the cornea and anterior chamber examinations are best done under high power in a dark room.

accompanies iritis. Note that fluorescein can penetrate an abraded cornea and produce a fluorescein flare on slit lamp evaluation. To avoid confusion, some clinicians prefer to examine for anterior chamber flare before the stain is used. A variety of conditions evaluated by the slit lamp are pictured in Figure 62-28.

UNILATERAL LOSS OF VISION

There are a variety of reasons why an individual may sustain complete loss of vision in one eye, but most commonly, such loss is caused by occlusion of the central retinal vein, occlusion of the central retinal artery, or optic nerve damage. Less commonly, pressure on the orbit from a retroorbital hemorrhage may compromise the ophthalmic artery.

Although discussion of all the potential causes of unilateral loss of vision is beyond the scope of this text, amaurosis fugax deserves special mention. Amaurosis fugax is a transient loss of vision that is most commonly due to cholesterol or platelet emboli from atherosclerotic carotid occlusive disease. When plaques are visualized in the retinal vasculature, auscultate the neck for carotid bruits and refer the patient for ultrasound examination of the carotid artery.[98,99]

Central Renal Artery Occlusion

A patient with central retinal artery occlusion (CRAO) has generally experienced a recent sudden painless (complete or nearly complete) unilateral loss of vision. On examination there is an afferent pupillary defect (i.e., sluggish or nonreactive pupil in the affected eye with direct illumination and a normal consensual response) and reduced visual acuity. Immediately after the event the fundus may appear nearly normal; however, it soon becomes pale and a classic "cherry-red spot" in the macula may be evident as a result of patent choroidal vessels showing through the transparent fovea (Fig. 62-29).

Therapy

Visual recovery has been noted to occur up to 3 days after CRAO. Start treatment if the patient is seen within 24 hours after the onset of symptoms.[100] Consult ophthalmology while initiating therapy. In many centers, CRAO is considered an ischemic event and neurology as well as ophthalmology are often involved in acute management. In some stroke centers, patients with CRAO are admitted to neurology on confirmation of the diagnosis.

Most of the emergency techniques suggested for treating vascular insults to the eye in the ED are theoretically sound but are not supported or refuted by rigorous scientific data. No specific standard of care has been promulgated for these interventions by emergency clinicians. Techniques discussed later are probably safe and possibly useful and may be attempted in an emergency situation. It is unknown whether these interventions will be vision saving.

Slow rebreathing into a paper bag is believed to increase the arterial carbon dioxide level, thus aiding vasodilation, permitting the occlusion to move more peripherally, and possibly reducing the ischemic area. At the same time, initiate digital globe massage. With the patient lying supine, apply firm steady pressure with the thumbs to the affected globe through the patient's closed lids. Apply pressure for 5 seconds and then abruptly release it (Fig. 62-30). Immediately repeat this maneuver several more times for up to 20 minutes. The objective of this technique is to help break up the occlusion and encourage movement of it more peripherally.

A more aggressive therapy, generally performed only by ophthalmologists, is anterior chamber paracentesis. In the absence of available consultation, consider this technique when CRAO is recent and unresponsive to the previously described therapeutic approaches. For this procedure, keep the patient supine with the head and eyelids secured. Anesthetize the cornea with topical anesthetic drops (e.g., 0.5% proparacaine drops). Inject the conjunctiva adjacent to the limbus with a 27- or 30-gauge needle until the entire perilimbal area is infiltrated and has the appearance of chemosis in all quadrants. During the remainder of the procedure, ask an assistant to firmly grasp the conjunctiva with toothless forceps at the 3- and 9-o'clock positions to stabilize the eye. Insert a 30-gauge needle on a tuberculin syringe obliquely just adjacent to the limbus at either the 4:30- or the 7:30-o'clock position, and direct it toward the 6-o'clock position to avoid

Staphylococcal blepharitis   External stye (hordeolum)   Chalazion

Subconjunctival hemorrhage   Allergic conjunctivitis and chemosis   Bacterial conjunctivitis

Herpes simplex keratitis   Bacterial corneal ulcer with hypopyon   Pterygium

Anterior uveitis with hypopyon   Acute angle-closure glaucoma   Hyphema

Figure 62-28 Various ocular pathologies. *(From Palay DA, Krachmer JH, eds. Primary Care Ophthalmology. 2nd ed. St. Louis: Mosby; 2005.)*

the lens (Fig. 62-31). Apply gentle pressure on the globe and, after 1 to 2 drops of aqueous are expressed, withdraw the needle.[101,102]

One study described a systematic approach in which ocular massage, sublingual isosorbide dinitrate, 10 mg, acetazolamide, 500 mg intravenously, 20% mannitol (1 mg/kg) or oral 50% glycerol (1 mg/kg), anterior chamber paracentesis, methylprednisolone, 500 mg intravenously, streptokinase, 750 kIU, and retrobulbar tolazoline, 50 mg, were given until the visual symptoms improved or all steps were complete.[103] Of the 11 patients in this arm of the study, 8 had improved visual acuity. In those who improved, all had their symptoms improved in 12 hours or less. The presumed cause was either

a platelet-derived or cholesterol embolus from atheroma or glaucoma.[96] Although this study is small, it supports emergency ophthalmology consultation and aggressive treatment of patients seen within 12 to 24 hours of the onset of symptoms.

Complications

Overzealous globe massage has the potential to produce intraocular trauma, including retinal detachment and intraocular hemorrhage. Anterior chamber paracentesis may produce hemorrhage, infection, or mechanical injury to the cornea, iris, or lens.[104] Although these complications are rare, ophthalmologic consultation for assistance with the underlying

Figure 62-29 Central retinal artery occlusion with a cherry-red spot in the fovea (*arrow*). (*From Friedman NJ, Kaiser PK, Pineda A. Massachusetts Ear & Eye Infirmary Illustrated Manual of Ophthalmology. 3rd ed. Philadelphia: Saunders; 2009.*)

Figure 62-31 Anterior chamber paracentesis. After topical and subconjunctival anesthesia (see text), a 30-gauge needle is directed obliquely from the 4:30- or 7:30-o'clock position toward the 6-o'clock position to avoid the lens. An assistant stabilizes the globe with forceps and grasps the conjunctiva (see text). *Top*, anteroposterior projection; *bottom*, tangential projection. (*Top and bottom, From Knoop K, Trott A. Ophthalmologic procedures in the emergency department: I. Immediate sight-saving procedures. Acad Emerg Med. 1994;1:408.*)

Figure 62-30 To perform digital globe massage, apply firm steady pressure with the thumb on the globe for approximately 5 seconds and then abruptly release the pressure for 5 to 10 seconds. Repeat the process for up to 20 minutes or until improvement in vision is observed.

CRAO and surveillance for these potential complications should be initiated on an emergency basis.

Orbital Compartment Syndrome

Acute facial trauma or recent retrobulbar anesthesia may produce retrobulbar hemorrhage with sufficient pressure to compromise the ophthalmic artery and result in an orbital compartment syndrome (Fig. 62-32). A form of posttraumatic glaucoma may also occur when the retrobulbar hematoma forces the globe against the eyelids. In this case, IOP rises precipitously because the globe is in a relatively closed space as a result of the firm attachment of the eyelids to the orbital rim by the medial and lateral canthal ligaments. The optic nerve and its vascular supply and the central retinal artery are compressed, which can result in ischemia and subsequent visual loss. In this situation, emergency lateral canthotomy may be considered for relief of the pressure on the eye. It

would not be considered a standard of care for most emergency clinicians to possess the skills for this procedure, but in the proper scenario, it may be a prudent intervention.

In this situation, ophthalmoscopic evaluation reveals a blanched ophthalmic artery in the presence of obvious retrobulbar pressure and ecchymosis around the eye. The patient exhibits decreased visual acuity, and an afferent pupil defect is often seen. IOP is markedly elevated but may be relieved by emergency lateral canthotomy and cantholysis. Such a procedure needs to be performed quickly because the ischemic retina will not retain function if it is deprived of blood for a long period.

Technique: Lateral Canthotomy and Cantholysis
(Fig. 62-33)
The goals of the procedure are to release pressure on the globe and decrease IOP sufficiently to reinstitute retinal artery blood flow. Because retinal recovery is unlikely to occur if rapid relief of ischemia is not accomplished, taking time to clean the eye beyond simple saline cleansing of the lids and lateral canthus is ill advised. Stabilize the patient's head and lids and anesthetize the lateral canthus by injecting 1% to 2% lidocaine with epinephrine. Before incising, crush the lateral canthus with a small hemostat for 1 to 2 minutes to minimize bleeding. Incise the canthus with iris or Steven's scissors. Take precautions to avoid injury to the protruding globe. Begin the incision at the lateral canthus and extend it toward the orbital rim. Find the superior and inferior crura of the lateral canthal tendon and release them from the orbital rim. Some operators prefer to release the inferior crus and reassess IOP before

Figure 62-32 A, Retrobulbar hemorrhage of the left eye demonstrating proptosis, lid swelling (*short arrow*), chemosis (*long arrow*), and restricted extraocular motility on upgaze. **B,** Computed tomography scan demonstrating significant proptosis and radiodensity posterior to the left eye (retrobulbar hemorrhage indicated by the *arrow*). The intraocular pressure was measured to be 40 mm Hg and was rapidly lowered to 20 with a lateral canthotomy and cantholysis. Indications for lateral canthotomy and cantholysis include decreased visual acuity, ocular pressure greater than 40 mm Hg, proptosis, afferent papillary defect (Marcus Gunn pupil), cherry-red macula, ophthalmoplegia, optic nerve pallor, and severe eye pain. A ruptured globe is a contraindication.

considering release of the superior crus. An instructional video of the procedure can be found at www.brown.edu/Administration/Emergency_Medicine/eye.htm.[105]

Complications

Although hemorrhage, infection, and mechanical injury might result from the procedure, these complications generally respond to therapy better than retinal injury from prolonged ischemia does. Emergency ophthalmologic consultation should be obtained, although when the procedure is indicated, it may be considered by the emergency clinician. Lateral canthotomy incisions generally heal without suturing or significant scarring.

REDUCTION OF GLOBE LUXATION

Although luxation of the globe is uncommon, the emergency clinician should be aware of the condition and its mechanisms, know how to reduce the globe, and know when to prioritize ophthalmologic consultation. With luxation of the globe there is extreme proptosis, which permits the lids to slip behind the globe equator (Fig. 62-34). Subsequent spasm of the orbicularis oculi muscles sustains the luxation and limits extraocular movement. Traction on the optic nerve and retinal vessels may produce direct or indirect injury to the optic nerve and retina.

Luxation may be spontaneous, voluntary, or traumatic. A variety of conditions (e.g., orbital neoplasms, Graves' disease, histiocytosis X, cerebral gumma, and craniofacial dysostoses) may predispose the patient to luxation. Triggering events include maneuvers that increase IOP (e.g., the Valsalva maneuver), trauma to the orbit or forehead, or eyelid manipulation.

Indications and Contraindications

Early globe reduction is indicated to relieve symptoms and minimize visual impairment. Attempts at reduction in the ED are relatively contraindicated when there is obvious rupture of the globe.

Technique

Before globe reduction, perform a rapid eye examination to document visual acuity, range of eye motion, pupillary reactivity, and any evidence of globe rupture (see earlier discussion).[106] Place the patient in a recumbent position and administer a topical ocular anesthetic agent (e.g., 0.5% proparacaine). When the lashes are visible, ask an assistant to apply steady outward and upward traction while the globe is gently pushed behind the lids. Use gloved fingers to apply steady scleral pressure and to manipulate the globe back into the orbit. When the lashes cannot be grasped, introduce a lid retractor behind the lid to provide countertraction. Others recommend placing a suture through the anesthetized skin of each lid to provide countertraction.

After the procedure, repeat the eye examination to document visual acuity and extraocular movement. It is not uncommon for return of full visual function to be delayed for several days or occasionally longer.

Complications

It is common with this procedure for lashes to be retained in the conjunctival fornices. Evaluate for and remove any free lashes to prevent corneal injury. Edema, retrobulbar hemorrhage, or orbital deformity may prevent outpatient reduction. When reduction is not possible in the ED, saline drops should be applied to the globe and a noncontact eye shield used.

Aftercare

Patients with spontaneous luxation and no visual impairment in whom the globe is easily reduced warrant follow-up within 24 to 48 hours. Instructions to avoid potential triggering maneuvers should be given. Recurrent luxation may warrant

LATERAL CANTHOTOMY AND CANTHOLYSIS

Identify the lateral canthus (*arrow*). Cleanse the area with antiseptic and anesthetize with 1% lidocaine with epinephrine. (The left eye is depicted in this image sequence.)

Crush the lateral canthus with a hemostat for 1 to 2 minutes to reduce incisional bleeding (not shown). Then, cut through the crushed tissue with iris scissors (as depicted above) to perform the canthotomy.

Pull the lower eyelid away from the globe with toothed forceps (*arrow*).

Inferior crus of the lateral canthal ligament

"Strum" the tissue under the canthotomy with the scissors to identify the inferior crus of the lateral canthal ligament. Cut through this ligament with scissors to perform the inferior cantholysis. Note that the scissors are directed inferiorly during this step, perpendicular to the canthotomy incision.

NOTE:
If intraocular pressure remains elevated after inferior cantholysis, the superior crus of the lateral canthal ligament may be released in a similar fashion.

The eye after canthotomy and cantholysis. This procedure relieves increased intraocular pressure by allowing the globe and orbital contents to move forward.

Figure 62-33 Lateral canthotomy and cantholysis. (*From Eisele OW, Smith RV, eds.* Complications in Head and Neck Surgery. *2nd ed. St. Louis: Mosby; 2008.*)

Figure 62-34 Appearance of a luxated globe. **A,** This globe protruded when the lower eyelid was retracted downward to examine the conjunctiva for anemia. **B,** It was easily reduced with slight manual pressure on the closed upper lid. **C,** Afterward, the patient had no eye or vision complaints. This is a normal variant in some people.

lateral tarsorrhaphy. Further evaluation of potential precipitating factors can be pursued on an outpatient basis.

Patients with traumatic luxation are at greater risk for underlying ophthalmic injury and warrant emergency consultation. A computed tomography scan of the orbit is helpful for evaluating both the soft tissue and the bony structures about the globe.

STYE

A stye, or hordeolum, is an acute purulent inflammation (bacterial infection) of the eyelid characterized by pain, swelling, and redness. It can be quite annoying and painful to the touch. A small nodule or abscess first develops in an eyelid hair follicle or a modified sebaceous gland at the margin of the eyelid. This may be external (pointing at the lid margin) or internal (pointing under the conjunctival lid; Fig. 62-35). An obvious pustule may be seen, and if so, incising it with a small needle and expressing pus produce a faster cure. The lid may be inverted to find a small pustule on the inner surface of the lid that can be nicked with a 25-gauge needle (see Fig. 62-17, *plates 6 and 7*). *S. aureus* is the organism most frequently isolated from the infection.[1] Treat with warm compresses on the eyelid as frequently as possible. One method is to fill a sink with very hot water and alternate wet washcloths for 15 to 20 minutes. Topical ophthalmic antibiotics (drops every 2 hours or ointment five to six times a day) are usually prescribed. Erythromycin ointment is often suggested. Topical treatment is generally sufficient, but antistaphylococcal oral antibiotics (dicloxacillin, cephalosporins) might occasionally be needed, especially if in patients with significant surrounding lid cellulitis. More formal incision and drainage may be necessary if the infection is unresponsive to conservative therapy.[107] Spread of the infection can lead to preseptal cellulitis.

Figure 62-35 Stye (hordeolum). **A,** External hordeolum. An erythematous, tender swelling at the lid margin points externally. **B,** Internal stye. This may form a pustule on the inner surface of the lid that may be incised and pus expressed (see also Fig. 62-28).

APD OR MARCUS GUNN PUPIL

An afferent pupillary defect (APD), or Marcus Gunn pupil, is caused by a variety of diseases of the afferent, or "in-going," pathways of the eye. It is produced by a *unilateral* lesion of the retina or optic nerve. Causes include optic neuritis (as seen

NORMAL   DEFECT

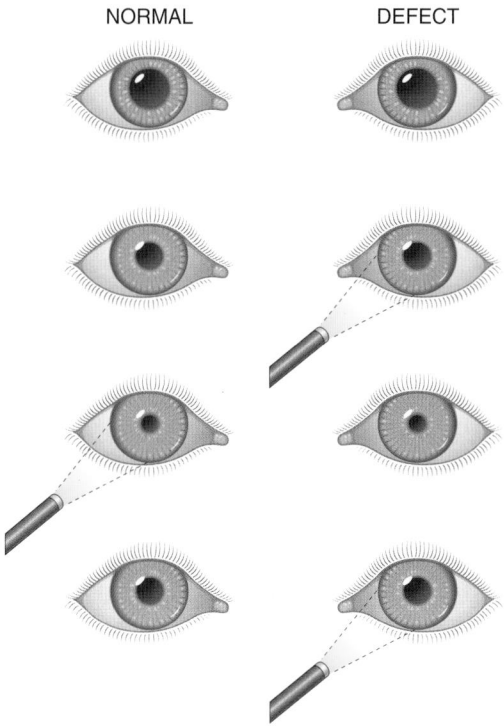

Figure 62-36 Relative afferent pupillary defect (Marcus Gunn pupil). This patient has an abnormal left optic nerve. In ambient light (*top row*), the pupils are equal. As the abnormal eye is illuminated (*second row*), only modest constriction is noted. As the light is swung to the normal eye (*third row*), the pupils constrict briskly. When the light is swung back to the abnormal eye (*bottom row*), paradoxical dilation is noted. (*From Friedman NJ, Kaiser PK, Pineda A. Massachusetts Ear & Eye Infirmary Illustrated Manual of Ophthalmology. 3rd ed. Philadelphia: Saunders; 2009.*)

with multiple sclerosis), ischemic optic neuropathy, optic tumor, and retrobulbar hematoma (an indication for lateral canthotomy). To evaluate for an APD, the swinging flashlight test may be used (Fig. 62-36).[108] *Normally, shining a light in either eye causes bilateral pupil constriction.* To evaluate for an APD (no light reaching the brain via the optic nerve on the affected side), record the pupil size at baseline. Shine a light into the affected eye. Record the direct response (constriction of the illuminated pupil in response to light) and the indirect or consensual response (constriction of the opposite pupil in response to light). Next, shine the light into the other eye and record the direct and indirect responses. Repeat this procedure back and forth until the pattern of response to light is identified. With an APD, there is a *decreased direct response to light along the afferent or "in-going" pathways,* whereas the efferent or "out-going" pathways to the opposite eye are

Figure 62-37 Subconjunctival hemorrhage. A painless bright red hemorrhage of the sclera is noted. The cornea and anterior chamber are unaffected, and there are no visual symptoms. This is a benign condition; no treatment is indicated.

preserved. Thus, light shined into the affected eye will cause neither a direct nor a consensual response, but light shined into the unaffected eye will cause bilateral pupillary constriction.

SUBCONJUNCTIVAL HEMORRHAGE

Subconjunctival hemorrhage may occur spontaneously (often noticed on awakening) or after straining, vomiting, or severe coughing. The patient notices a painless bright red hemorrhage in the eye (sclera). It may be bilateral (Fig. 62-37). Vision is not affected. Although this is concerning to the patient, it is benign. No laboratory evaluation is required unless the patient has taken anticoagulants, in which case clotting studies should be considered. The hemorrhage will disappear spontaneously over a few weeks and turn various colors as it recedes. No treatment will hasten resolution.

Acknowledgment

The authors recognize the many contributions by Jerris R. Hedges, MD, to this chapter through the first five editions of the textbook.

References are available at www.expertconsult.com

Otolaryngologic Procedures

Ralph J. Riviello

The procedures presented in this section are most effectively performed with special equipment and techniques. Some are within the realm of general emergency medicine clinical expertise; others are not. They are reviewed from the perspective of the emergency clinician who must decide whether the patient needs treatment acutely in the emergency department (ED), can be managed with timely referral, or requires urgent consultant expertise.

PHARYNX AND LARYNX

Examination of the Larynx

Visualization of the larynx and pharynx is a critical part of the complete evaluation of patients with complaints of sore throat, hoarseness, foreign body (FB), and stridor.

Anatomy

The pharynx is the part of the throat located posterior to the mouth and the nasal cavity and superior to the esophagus and larynx. It is commonly divided into three sections, the nasopharynx, the oropharynx, and the laryngopharynx (hypopharynx). The nasopharynx is the most cephalad portion and extends from the base of the skull to the upper surface of the soft palate. The oropharynx is behind the oral cavity and extends from the uvula to the level of the hyoid bone. Its anterior wall consists of the base of the tongue and the vallecula; its lateral wall consists of the tonsils, tonsillar fossa, and pillars; and its superior wall is formed by the inferior surface of the soft palate and the uvula. The pharynx is supplied by the pharyngeal branches of the ascending pharyngeal artery, ascending and descending palatine arteries, and pharyngeal branches of the inferior thyroid artery. It is innervated by the pharyngeal plexus and the maxillary and mandibular nerves.

The larynx in adults is located in the anterior part of the neck at the level of the C3-C6 vertebrae. It connects the inferior portion of the pharynx (hypopharynx) with the trachea. The larynx extends vertically from the tip of the epiglottis to the inferior border of the cricoid cartilage. It consists of nine cartilages. The larynx is innervated by branches of the vagus nerve, the superior laryngeal nerve, and the recurrent laryngeal nerve. The relevant anatomy is depicted in Figure 63-1.

Indications and Contraindications

Laryngoscopy is indicated for the evaluation of patients with complaints of dysphagia or odynophagia. More specifically, it should be performed in patients complaining of dysphagia,

hoarseness, FB ingestion or sensation in the throat, and angioedema and in patients who require assessment of their airway status. In general, laryngoscopy can be used to evaluate a problem and to exclude airway compromise, as well as to diagnose several other diseases such as gastroesophageal reflux, cancer, and allergy.[1]

Laryngoscopy has traditionally been discouraged in patients with impending airway compromise; however, it may be performed carefully in stridulous patients as long as a predesignated team (usually consisting of an anesthesiologist, otolaryngologist, or another physician skilled in the management of a difficult airway) is readily available and able to intervene if necessary. Care should be taken to avoid accidental trauma to the laryngopharynx, which may exacerbate the swelling and further compromise the airway.

Equipment

The equipment required depends on the type of laryngoscopic procedure performed. For flexible laryngoscopy you will need a standard flexible nasopharyngolaryngoscope, a light source, gloves, a nasal speculum, surgical lubricant, antifogging solution, decongestant spray, anesthetic spray, and a wall suction setup with a Frazier suction tip catheter (Fig. 63-2, *plate 1*). Many choices of decongestant are available; however, 0.05% oxymetazoline (Afrin) or 0.1% to 1% phenylephrine is commonly used. Lidocaine (4%) is typically used as the anesthetic. A 5% cocaine solution serves as both an anesthetic and decongestant. If nasal spray formulations are not available, medication-soaked cotton pledgets, an atomizer bottle, or a syringe atomizer (Mucosal Atomization Device, MAD Nasal, Wolf Torry Medical, Inc.) may be used.

Mirror laryngoscopy requires a curved dental mirror, an external light source (preferably a head lamp), 4- × 4-inch gauze, and an antifogging solution. If antifogging solution is not available, hot water can be used to prevent fogging of the mirror. Anesthetic solution may be required if the patient cannot tolerate the procedure.

Procedure

Flexible Laryngoscopy

Attach the nasopharyngolaryngoscope to its light source and the suction tubing to its port (if available). Ensure that both are functioning properly before beginning. Before inserting the scope, adjust the eyepiece to your visual acuity; it is helpful to check the focus on newsprint or a small object. Review the scope's directional controls. Examine both nares and choose the more patent one to enter. Anesthetize and vasoconstrict the naris (see Fig. 63-2, *plate 2*). Because this procedure is irritating, allow enough time for these medications to become effective. You may also anesthetize the pharynx to minimize gagging (see Fig. 63-2, *plate 3*). Warm the end of the scope in warm water to help prevent fogging. Place the patient in the seated position with the head placed against a head rest in the sniffing position. Insert the tip of the lubricated scope just inside the naris. (Some authors recommend a series of soft nasal trumpets to gradually dilate the nasal cavity and allow easier passage of the scope.) Movement of the scope against the inside of the nasal passage may be irritating to the patient. *Minimize this sensation by resting your fourth and fifth fingers on the bridge of the patient's nose while stabilizing and guiding the scope between your thumb and index finger* (see Fig. 63-2, *plate 4*).

While looking through the eyepiece, slowly advance the endoscope past the middle turbinate into the nasopharynx or through the lumen of a nasal trumpet. To clear fogging or mucus off the lens, ask the patient to swallow, wipe the lens against the pharyngeal mucosa, or use the suction. Once the scope is in the nasopharynx, direct the tip inferiorly by using the thumb control near the eyepiece. Use the thumb control to accomplish up and down movements of the scope. Rotate the scope about its axis and then apply thumb control to provide lateral movement and visualization. At this point the base of the tongue and the tonsils will come into view. Slide the scope farther caudad to bring the larynx into focus. Once again, systematically view the patient's anatomy and function during both respiration and phonation (see Fig. 63-2, *plate 6*).

If the nasopharyngeal scope will not pass through either naris, pass it through the oropharynx. Properly anesthetize the oropharynx and avoid contacting the posterior portion of the tongue to prevent gagging. A plastic bite block can be used. Alternatively, cut a 10-mL syringe (without the plunger) in half and ask the patient to hold it in the mouth between the incisors (see Fig. 63-2, *plate 5*). Pass the fragile endoscope through this tube into the oropharynx to prevent accidental biting of the scope.

Mirror Laryngoscopy

This traditional method is most commonly used by otolaryngologists, but it can be used in the ED setting if the necessary equipment is readily available. Clinicians unfamiliar with this method should practice frequently because significant eye-to-hand coordination is required to reflect the light beam off the angulated mirror onto the larynx. When this procedure is properly performed, most patients are able to tolerate it without anesthesia of the oropharynx. Fiberoptic nasopharyngoscopy has largely replaced mirror laryngoscopy in the ED when the equipment is available.

Establish rapport with the patient by explaining how the examination will be performed. Have the patient sit erect in the "sniffing position" with the feet flat on the floor and leaning slightly forward. Attach your head lamp and adjust the beam of light (Fig. 63-3). Warm the mirror with warm water to prevent fogging, but check the temperature of the mirror with your hand before placing it into the oropharynx

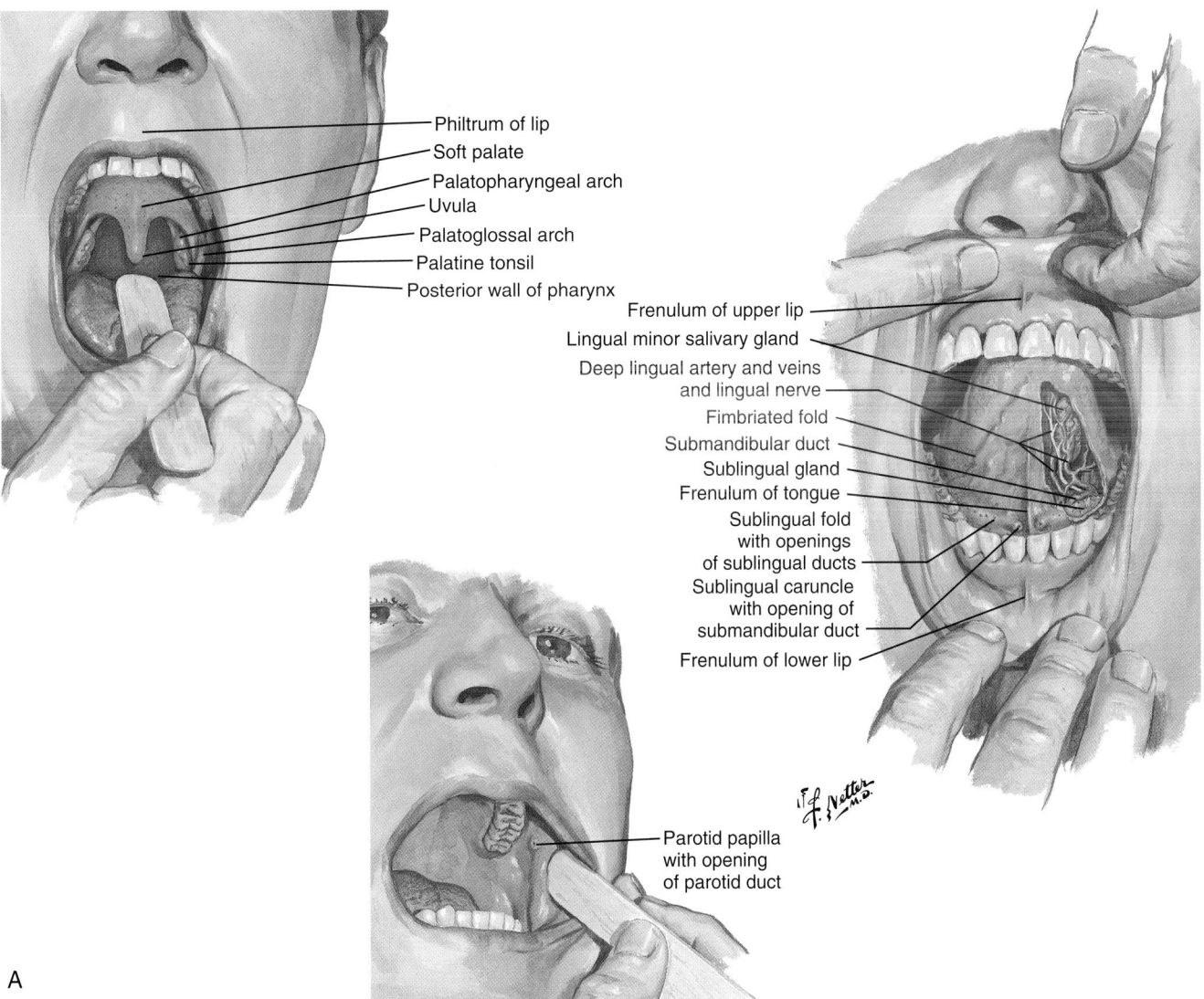

Philtrum of lip
Soft palate
Palatopharyngeal arch
Uvula
Palatoglossal arch
Palatine tonsil
Posterior wall of pharynx

Frenulum of upper lip
Lingual minor salivary gland
Deep lingual artery and veins and lingual nerve
Fimbriated fold
Submandibular duct
Sublingual gland
Frenulum of tongue
Sublingual fold with openings of sublingual ducts
Sublingual caruncle with opening of submandibular duct
Frenulum of lower lip

Parotid papilla with opening of parotid duct

A

Figure 63-1 A, Anatomy of the oropharynx.

Continued

Figure 63-1, cont'd B, Sagittal section of the neck. (*Netter illustration from* www.netterimages.com. © *Elsevier, Inc. All rights reserved.*)

FLEXIBLE LARYNGOSCOPY

Basic equipment required for flexible laryngoscopy. Additional items include anesthetic spray, a nasal speculum, surgical lubricant, and antifogging solution.

Anesthetize and vasoconstrict the naris before inserting the scope. Oxymetazoline (e.g., Afrin) spray is an ideal vasoconstrictor. Atomized 4% lidocaine can be use as an anesthetic.

Anesthetize the oropharynx with benzocaine spray or atomized 4% lidocaine to prevent gagging.

Rest your fingers on the bridge of the patient's nose while stabilizing and guiding the scope between the thumb and middle finger.

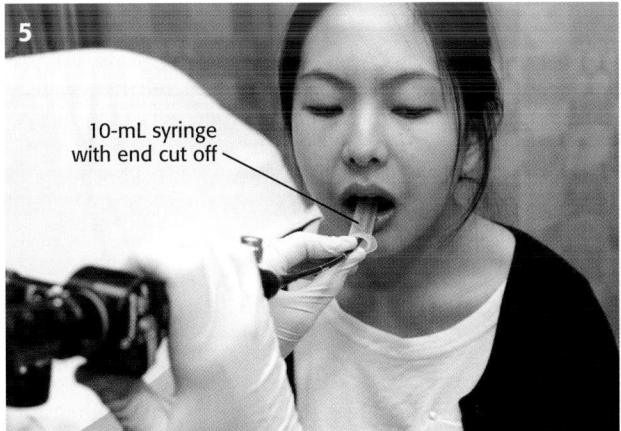

To pass the scope orally, first anesthetize the oropharynx (with atomized 4% lidocaine or benzocaine spray). Use a plungerless 10-mL syringe with the end cut off as a bite block to prevent accidental biting of the scope.

Laryngeal anatomy as seen through the nasopharyngoscope.

Figure 63-2 Flexible laryngoscopy.

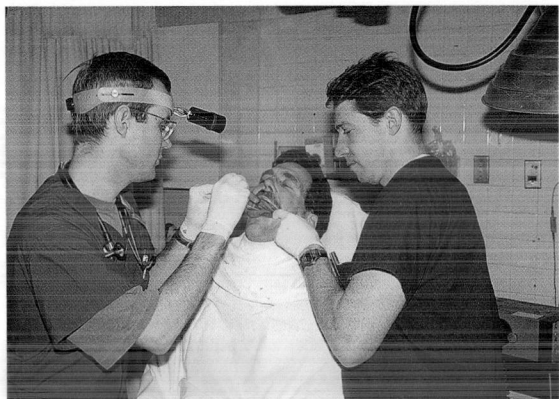

Figure 63-3 A good light source (head lamp) and an assistant facilitate any ear, nose, and throat examination or procedure.

Figure 63-5 Instruct the patient to say "eeeeee" in a high-pitched voice during the examination. This lifts the epiglottis out of your field of view and allows excellent visualization of the glottis. In this picture the vocal cords close with phonation. A paralyzed cord is easily discerned from one that is normal.

Figure 63-4 Indirect mirror evaluation of the oropharynx. Grasp the patient's tongue between the thumb and first finger while using a gauze pad to provide traction. Elevate the upper lip with the middle finger. Advance the warmed (prevents fogging) laryngeal mirror into the posterior of the oropharynx while taking care to not stimulate the posterior part of the tongue or pharynx. Remember that the structures in the mirror will be reversed. Always follow universal precautions.

In patients who cannot tolerate this procedure without gagging, apply topical anesthetic to aid in the examination. Benzocaine (Hurricaine spray or Cetacaine gargle) or aerosolized tetracaine or lidocaine may be used. One or two quick sprays of benzocaine into the posterior aspect of the oropharynx is sufficient. Though rare, prolonged or repeated spraying can result in methemoglobinemia. Reassure the patient beforehand that although this may make the throat feel as though it is swelling or paralyzed, in actuality, it is just the numbness that accounts for the sensation. The tendency to gag can also be minimized by having the patient concentrate on breathing efforts and keep the eyes open and fixed on an object in the distance.

Once the patient is anesthetized, repeat the steps described earlier and position the mirror against the soft palate. Rotate the angle of the mirror and systematically inspect the base of the tongue, valleculae, epiglottis, piriform recess, arytenoids, false and true vocal cords, and if possible, the superior aspect of the trachea (see Fig. 63-2, *plate 6*). Observe for masses, evidence of infection, asymmetry, or FBs. Further evaluate the anterior structure of the larynx and function of the vocal cords by having the patient say "eeee" in a high-pitched voice. This should move the epiglottis away from blocking the view of the larynx and bring the true cords together at the midline (Fig. 63-5).

Complications

There are very few complications with laryngoscopy. Occasionally, the procedure may not be able to be completed because of a prominent gag reflex or patient apprehension and discomfort. Complications include traumatic abrasions and bleeding anywhere along the path of the laryngoscope or on the soft palate or pharynx if a mirror is used. Epistaxis and hemoptysis are uncommon. In patients with head injury, there is always a slight risk of passing the scope intracranially if a basilar skull fracture has occurred; use of a soft nasal trumpet significantly reduces this risk. Laryngospasm and acute airway compromise can be induced in patients with paraglottic infections.

so that the patient is not burned. Alternatively, apply an antifogging solution to the mirrored side. Wrap the patient's tongue with gauze to prevent it from slipping or being injured by the lower incisors and then grasp it with the nondominant hand (Fig. 63-4). Apply gentle traction on the tongue with your thumb and index finger and lift the patient's upper lip with your middle finger. Slide the mirror into the oropharynx with the glass surface parallel to the tongue but not touching it. Place the back of the mirror against the uvula and soft palate and smoothly lift until the larynx is visualized. Although this should not induce gagging, try to make only slight changes in the mirror's position to inspect the appropriate structures.

Peritonsillar Abscess Drainage

Indications

Clinical suspicion of peritonsillar abscess (PTA)

Signs and symptoms of PTA include
  Asymmetric tonsillar bulging
  Uvular deviation (away from the bulging)
  "Hot potato" voice

Contraindications

Severe trismus
Coagulopathy
Uncooperative patient

Complications

Failure to completely drain the abscess
Aspiration of pus and/or blood
Hemorrhage
Carotid artery puncture

Equipment

Tongue depressor

10-mL syringe with 18-gauge needle and covered with a cut cap

Scalpel with a No. 11 blade and tape covering all but 1 cm of the blade

Lidocaine with epinephrine

Topical anesthetic spray

Frazier-tip suction

Kelly clamp

Review Box 63-1   Peritonsillar abscess drainage: indications, contraindications, complications, and equipment. Use a long 25- to 27-gauge needle and a 3- to 5-mL syringe for local anesthesia and a 10-mL syringe for aspiration. Larger syringes obscure the operator's view of the anatomy.

Odontoid

Atlas

Lateral pharyngeal space

Prevertebral space

Retropharyngeal space

Jugular vein

Cartoid sheath

Cartoid artery

Medial pterygoid muscle

Peritonsillar abcess

Peritonsillar space

Parotid gland

Palatine tonsil

Uvula

PATIENT'S RIGHT

PATIENT'S LEFT

Figure 63-6 Anatomy of a peritonsillar abscess. The palatine tonsil and peritonsillar space are identified on the patient's right. A peritonsillar abscess is shown on the patient's left. Note that the abscess can extend medially and displace the uvula. The carotid artery and jugular vein are posterior and lateral to the abscess. Avoid lateral angulation of the aspirating needle and use a needle guard to prevent injury.

TONSIL: PTA

Peritonsillar abscess (PTA), also known as quinsy, is most common during the second and third decades. It is rarely seen in children younger than 6 years and is the most common head and neck abscess in anyone older than 6 years. Treatment of PTA has undergone significant change in the past 100 years and continues to do so at this writing. A myriad of opinions exist on the appropriate treatment method, although most agree that some form of drainage procedure is usually required and should be performed in conjunction with the administration of antibiotics and pain control medication. Three options for surgical drainage include needle aspiration (most common), incision and drainage, and immediate (quinsy) tonsillectomy.

Anatomy

Understanding the relative anatomy before attempting to treat PTA is important (Fig. 63-6). The palatine tonsils are located between the anterior and posterior pillars of the throat, bound in a capsule, and covered by mucosa. The lateral wall of the tonsil is defined by the superior pharyngeal constrictor muscle. Of great importance is the internal carotid artery, which lies approximately 2.5 cm *posterolateral* to the tonsil.

The abscess is defined as a collection of pus between the tonsillar capsule, the superior constrictor muscle, and the palatopharyngeus muscle (Fig. 63-7). *The abscess is not within the tonsil itself.* PTA is believed to arise from spread of infection from the tonsil or from the mucous glands of Weber located in the superior tonsillar pole. The abscess is most commonly initiated from the upper pole of the tonsil. However, it can also spread from the middle or inferior poles.

Pathophysiology and Clinical Findings

PTAs can occur in patients with inadequately treated tonsillitis and in those with recurrent tonsillitis, but in some patients it arises de novo. There are no data proving that antibiotics, even the correct ones in proper doses, invariably prevent the progression of tonsillitis to abscess formation. The abscess is generally unilateral, and bilateral involvement is rare.[2]

Patients with PTA have a sore throat, odynophagia, low-grade fever, and a variable degree of trismus. The trismus develops secondary to irritation of the pterygoid muscle. The patient may also complain of ipsilateral otalgia. As the abscess expands, the patient may experience dysphagia with drooling. Patients may be dehydrated secondary to poor oral intake. Changes in voice are common (hot-potato voice) and caused by transient velopharyngeal insufficiency and muffled oral resonance. Rancid breath is also common. Tender ipsilateral anterior cervical lymphadenopathy is usually present. Although leukocytosis is often present, a complete blood count and other laboratory tests are nonspecific.

The differential diagnosis for this acute process includes unilateral tonsillitis, peritonsillar cellulitis, retropharyngeal abscess, infectious mononucleosis, epiglottitis, herpes simplex tonsillitis, retromolar abscess, neoplasm, FB, and internal carotid artery aneurysm. Chronic conditions include leukemia, carcinoma, and tumor in the parapharyngeal space. Differentiation of PTA from peritonsillar cellulitis may be difficult, especially in the early stages of an abscess. The history and time course of the two disease processes are quite similar. Trismus and uvular deviation are uncommon with peritonsillar cellulitis.[3]

Complications of PTA may include pharyngeal obstruction or extension into the closely approximated neurovascular bundles and parapharyngeal space. Specific complications include airway obstruction, rupture of the abscess with aspiration pneumonia, septicemia, internal jugular vein thrombosis, suppurative thrombophlebitis of the jugular vein (Lemierre's syndrome), carotid artery rupture, mediastinitis, necrotizing fasciitis, and cardiac and renal sequelae of group A streptococcal infection.

Indications and Contraindications

The indication for PTA drainage is usually straightforward, but some advocate that initial medical options exist, especially in children. If obviously present in an adult, the PTA may be drained. However, the difficulty can be in the diagnosis of PTA. As an option to immediate surgical intervention, patients with suspected PTA and no airway symptoms who do not appear to be in a toxic state clinically may be admitted to the hospital without imaging for 24 hours of hydration; for empirical intravenous antibiotics to cover group A streptococci, *Staphylococcus aureus*, and respiratory anaerobes; and for analgesia. If a rapid response to medical therapy is not seen, drainage or tonsillectomy should be performed. About 50% of patients, predominately children rather than adults, will respond to medical therapy alone.

To diagnose PTA, in addition to visualization, place a gloved index finger into the mouth to feel for hardness or fluctuance in the peritonsillar region (Fig. 63-8).

Intraoral sonography may augment diagnostic accuracy and direct localization for drainage (Fig. 63-9; see Chapter 37). It is performed with an intracavitary probe. Blaivis and coworkers[2] found that ED ultrasound was effective in diagnosing and aiding drainage in five cases of PTA. Ultrasound excluded the diagnosis in one. If there is still a question regarding the diagnosis or actual location of the abscess, computed tomography (CT) may be helpful but is not regularly performed and is not standard before a drainage procedure in straightforward cases.

There are very few, if any contraindications to draining a PTA. One contraindication is the absence of a PTA; however, needle aspiration may be performed to confirm the presence of an abscess. Other contraindications can include severe trismus, coagulopathy, and inability of the patient to cooperate with the procedure.

Figure 63-7 Exudative pharyngitis versus peritonsillar abscess. Acute exudative pharyngitis (**A**) is characterized by bilateral tonsillar edema, erythema, and exudate. Note that the edema is for the most part symmetric and that the uvula lies in the midline. A peritonsillar abscess (**B,** *arrow*) is characterized by asymmetric tonsillar bulging, with the uvula deviated away from the side of the abscess.

Figure 63-8 Clinical symptoms and visual inspection may not be sufficient to differentiate a peritonsillar abscess from cellulitis. The clinician's gloved index finger is used to palpate the peritonsillar area to search for fluctuance and localized swelling. Computed tomography or ultrasound will further elucidate the diagnosis, but they are not needed in straightforward cases.

Figure 63-9 Ultrasound, transverse view, of a peritonsillar abscess showing a hypoechoic, heterogeneous abscess (*arrow*) with an intracavitary probe. Color Doppler can be used to delineate the vascular structures. Also see the Ultrasound Box in Chapter 37.

Equipment

The equipment required depends on the technique that is going to be used to drain the PTA. For needle aspiration, you will need a light source, tongue blade, injectable (1% lidocaine with 1 : 100,000 epinephrine) or topical (Cetacaine spray or 4% lidocaine) anesthetic, 3- to 5-mL syringe with a long 25-gauge needle for injection of anesthetic, and a standard or long 18- to 20-gauge needle (spinal needle) on a 10-mL syringe for aspiration (see Review Box 63-1). Long needles and small syringes will not obscure the operator's view of the anatomy. It is also helpful to have wall suction with a Frazier or Yankauer suction tip device available.

For incision and drainage, the same examination, suction, and anesthetizing equipment are required. In addition, a No. 11 or 15 scalpel blade and Kelly forceps will be required.

For either procedure, the patient should be given intravenous pain medication and may require mild sedation or even procedural sedation. One should administer parenteral narcotic analgesia, mild sedation, or both, before attempting aspiration. Fentanyl, 1 to 3 µg/kg administered intravenously a few minutes before the procedure, is often ideal. Midazolam may be used judiciously, but the patient should not be overly sedated. The combination of midazolam, ketamine, and glycopyrrolate is reported to be safe and effective for outpatient peritonsillar drainage in children.[4]

Procedure

Before describing the procedures for drainage of a PTA, one needs to know the clinical circumstances under which to perform the different procedures. A myriad of opinions exist on the appropriate treatment method, although most agree that some form of drainage procedure should be performed in conjunction with the administration of antibiotics and pain control. Three options for surgical drainage include needle aspiration (most common), incision and drainage, and immediate (quinsy) tonsillectomy. Each method is discussed.

Needle aspiration is relatively simple, can be performed by emergency clinicians, does not require special equipment, and is relatively inexpensive. Other benefits of needle aspiration over incision and drainage include decreased pain and trauma. Many believe that this should be the initial surgical drainage procedure for adults and children. The recurrence rate after aspiration is 10%,[3] and its cure rate is 93% to 95%.[5] Approximately 4% to 10% of patients require repeated aspiration.[3,5,6] One drawback is that needle aspiration may miss the PTA and therefore allow misdiagnosis as peritonsillar cellulitis. For this reason, some authors propose admission of patients with negative aspirations and the presumed diagnosis of peritonsillar cellulitis for intravenous antibiotics and observation to prevent further morbidity. Although most studies involved hospitalization and intravenous antibiotics, selected outpatient treatment with oral antibiotics has also been successful and is usually the option chosen unless the patient appears to be in a septic state.[6]

The incision and drainage procedure is commonly done on an outpatient basis under local anesthesia. It is usually performed after pus is obtained by needle aspiration, but occasionally it is the primary procedure. It seems most logical to first attempt aspiration and follow with incision and drainage only if additional pus is suspected or other extenuating circumstances are present. The success rare for incision and drainage is high with a recurrence rate similar to or lower than that with aspiration alone.[5]

Treatment guidelines based on a review of the literature[3,5-7] suggest that patients with PTA should initially be treated by needle aspiration. Incision and drainage and immediate tonsillectomy should be reserved for treatment failures or recurrences. These procedures can be performed in conjunction with hospital admission and administration of intravenous antibiotics or as outpatient treatment with oral antibiotics. One evidence-based review analyzed 42 articles, 5 of which were clinical studies on surgical technique.[5] All three techniques were found to be effective in treating PTA, and the recurrence rate was low (grade C recommendation). The approach depends on the patient's clinical status and medical history. Decisions about the treatment of PTA in the ED are often made by the emergency clinician, but as local protocols dictate, consultation with an otolaryngologist is also appropriate.

The two procedures described here include needle aspiration and incision and drainage. They should be performed only in a cooperative patient without severe trismus. Since the carotid artery is located 2.5 cm behind and lateral to the tonsil, there is minimal room for error, patient movement, or poor anesthesia.

Needle Aspiration

Have the patient sit upright with *a support behind the head*. This is best done as a two-person procedure. Ask an assistant to retract the cheek laterally to maximize visibility. A head lamp provides optimal lighting; a double–tongue blade setup aids in visualization of the operative area (see Fig. 63-3). If required, administer a parenteral narcotic analgesic, a mild sedative, or both before attempting aspiration.

Use manual palpation to locate the fluctuant area of the abscess. Anesthetize the area topically or with local infiltration. Infiltration should be done with 2 to 3 mL of 1% lidocaine with epinephrine via a 25- to 27-gauge needle. Use a 3- to 5-mL syringe with a long needle to be able to visualize the area to be injected (Fig. 63-10, *step 1*). A large syringe can block the operator's view. Displacing the tongue with a finger rather than a tongue blade may provide a better view. Infiltrate the lidocaine intramucosally for the best results, but be careful to not increase the size of the abscess by direct injection into the abscess cavity. The area should blanch. With proper local infiltration, the patient will not feel the penetration of the aspirating needle. If the trismus is so pronounced that it prevents adequate anesthesia, it will probably be too difficult to aspirate or incise the abscess properly.

Novel techniques to assist in the drainage procedure have recently been described. Afarian and Lin described the use of a laryngoscope with a curved blade (Fig. 63-11*A* and *B*).[8] The blade is inserted into the patient's mouth as far posteriorly as the patient can tolerate. The blade shines light from inside the mouth onto the posterior aspect of the pharynx. In addition, the laryngoscope provides better exposure of the area because the handle is below the patient's mouth and the holding hand does not obscure the view. Moreover, the curved blade sweeps the tongue out of the way and the weight of the handle will help overcome trismus. Braude and Shalit described a similar process involving the use of a disassembled disposable vaginal speculum with a fiberoptic light (see Fig 63-11*C*).[9] One advantage of both techniques is that an assistant can hold either light source without getting in the way of the operator. Finally, Chang and Hamilton reported that performing the procedure with the patient in the Trendelenburg position and the operator seated behind the patient's head provides comparable success rates and patient comfort.[10]

For aspiration, attach a long 18- to 20-gauge needle to a 10-mL syringe. Fashion a needle guard by cutting off the distal 1 cm of the plastic needle cover, replace the cover on the needle, and securely attach this guard to the needle and syringe with tape to prevent inadvertent displacement (see Fig. 63-10, *step 2*). Ensure that the needle protrudes only 1 cm beyond the cover to limit the depth of needle penetration and lessen the risk of entering any major vascular structures. If pus is not obtained at a 1-cm depth, deeper penetration is discouraged. Insert the needle into the most fluctuant (or prominent) area as previously determined, which is most commonly the superior pole of the tonsil (see Fig. 63-10, *step 3*). Importantly, *advance the syringe and needle in the sagittal plane only; do not angle to the side toward the carotid artery*. Do not aspirate the

tonsil itself because the abscess develops in the peritonsillar space surrounding the tonsil. Continually aspirate while advancing the needle in the sagittal plane and do not direct it laterally, where it could injure the carotid artery. If the aspirate is positive for pus, remove as much purulent material as possible. If the aspirate is negative, attempt aspiration again in the middle pole of the peritonsillar space, approximately 1 cm caudal to the first aspiration. If still negative, perform a third and final attempt at the inferior pole (see Fig. 63-10, *step 4*). Up to 30% of abscesses will be missed if only the superior pole is aspirated. It must be stressed that a negative aspirate does *not* rule out a PTA.

Usually, 2 to 6 mL of pus is obtained. It is unusual to recover more than 8 to 10 mL (Fig. 63-10, *step 5*). Although culture is recommended, the results rarely alter subsequent therapy. When significant amounts of pus are aspirated, the patient usually feels immediate improvement in pain and dysphagia. After the needle is removed, some bleeding will be noted (see Fig. 63-10, *step 6*). Slight oozing may occur for a few hours, especially if warm water rinses are used. Drainage of pus may continue and is often sensed as a foul taste by the patient. Significant additional drainage of pus may be an indication for repeated aspiration, incision and drainage, or hospital admission.

Some clinicians advise a formal incision and drainage procedure if frank pus is obtained, whereas others now accept needle aspiration (with close follow-up) as the definitive initial treatment. Combined aspiration and formal drainage in the same visit may be indicated if large amounts of pus are obtained (>5 to 6 mL) or if pus continues to drain from the aspiration site. There are no agreed standards regarding the best practice for this issue.

Recently, a new device, the Reciprocating Procedure Device (RPD; AVANCA Medical Devices, Inc.), has been developed that allows one-handed aspiration of the abscess (Fig. 63-12).[11] The RPD consists of two syringe barrels and plungers. The plungers are linked by a pulley system in opposing fashion, which results in a set of reciprocating plungers. When one plunger is pressed with the thumb, the syringe injects; when the accessory plunger is depressed, the syringe aspirates. The RPD allows stable finger positioning and finer control of the needle and syringe. To use the RPD, attach a needle to the RPD. Press the injection plunger with the thumb while advancing the RPD simultaneously in the oral cavity until the needle penetrates the abscess. Once the mucosal surface has been penetrated, depress the aspiration plunger to provide a vacuum for aspiration without moving the needle tip. Studies have shown that the RPD allows enhanced needle control, safer and more accurate aspiration procedures, and decreased complications by 35% to 60%.[12-14]

Incision and Drainage

To incise a PTA, anesthetize the area as described earlier. Prepare a No. 11 or 15 scalpel blade by taping over all but the distal 0.5 cm of the blade to prevent deeper penetration (Fig. 63-13, *step 1*). Incise the area of maximal fluctuance or the area where a preceding aspiration (if one was performed) located pus. *Do not incise the tonsil itself*; instead, incise the peritonsillar area where pus accumulates. Incise the mucosa in an area 0.5 cm long in a posterior-to-anterior direction. A stab incision with a No. 11 blade usually suffices (see Fig. 63-13, *step 2*). Warn the patient that the pus will flow posteriorly and must be expectorated. Expect bleeding because this is a vascular area. Suction the incised area with a No. 9 or 10 Frazier suction tip or a tonsil suction tip to aid in removal of the purulent material. Place a closed Kelly clamp into the opening and gently open it to break up the loculations (see Fig. 63-13, *step 3*). Allow the patient to rinse and gargle with a saline or dilute peroxide-saline solution. Packing is not used in the drainage of this abscess. After aspiration or incision, it is prudent to observe the patient for about an hour to watch for complications (e.g., bleeding) and to ensure that the patient is able to tolerate oral fluids. Most patients can be discharged with

PERITONSILLAR ABSCESS: NEEDLE ASPIRATION

Use a 25- to 27-gauge needle to inject the mucosa with 1–2 mL of lidocaine with epinephrine; observe for blanching. Often, the tongue is best displaced with the finger rather than a tongue blade. Topical anesthetic spray (e.g., Hurricaine) may be used prior to injection.

Use a long 18- to 20-gauge needle for aspiration. As a safeguard to prevent overpenetration of the needle, remove the plastic needle guard and cut off the distal 1 cm. Then, replace the cut-off guard on the needle (*arrow*) and secure it to the hub.

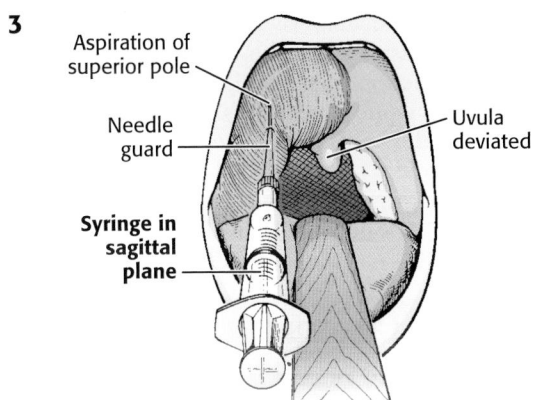

While applying continuous suction, direct the needle *in the sagittal plane only* (directly anterior to posterior), not to the side toward the carotid artery. Aspirate the superior pole initially.

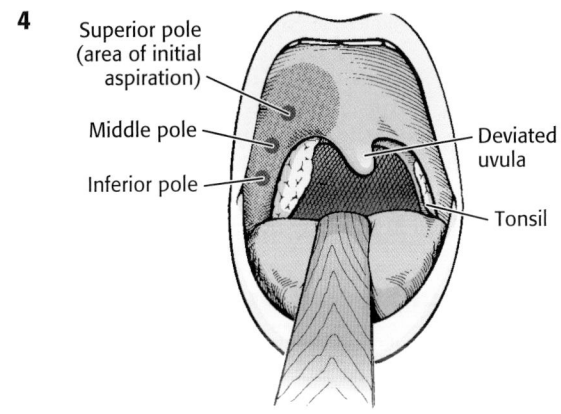

If pus is not obtained from the superior pole, next try the middle pole. The inferior pole may be aspirated last if needed. Note that the tonsil itself is not aspirated.

Usually, 2–6 mL of pus is obtained. It is unusual to recover more than 8–10 mL. If substantial amounts of pus are obtained, the patient usually notices immediate improvement in symptoms.

After needle removal, some bleeding will be noted (*arrow*). Slight oozing of of blood and pus may continue for several hours. Significant additional drainage may be an indication for repeated aspiration, incision and drainage, or hospital admission.

Figure 63-10 Drainage of a peritonsillar abscess: needle aspiration technique.

Figure 63-11 **A** and **B,** Laryngoscope and blade used to illuminate the posterior aspect of the pharynx. **C,** Disassembled disposable plastic speculum with a fiberoptic light source used to illuminate the posterior aspect of the pharynx.

Figure 63-12 The Reciprocating Procedure Device (AVANCA Medical Devices, Inc., Albuquerque NM).

24-hour follow-up. Toxic patients, those with excessive volumes of aspirate, those with persistent bleeding, and those unable to take oral antibiotics are candidates for admission or more prolonged observation. Frequent rinses with warm saline are quite helpful in relieving postaspiration symptoms.

Complications of Surgical Drainage

Needle aspiration is an accepted, safe, and effective technique for treatment of PTA in the ED. There is an approximate 10% failure rate and need for subsequent drainage.[3,5,6] Complications can include aspiration of pus or blood and hemorrhage. If the patient has cellulitis, the aspiration will be of no help, but it will not worsen morbidity. Failure to obtain pus should prompt high-dose antibiotics and follow-up in 24 hours. Many clinicians will opt for admission in such instances. Though often feared, injury to the carotid artery has not been reported as a complication of needle aspiration of PTA. Catastrophic hemorrhage may result from the extremely rare and largely theoretical aspiration of a pseudoaneurysm mimicking a PTA or similarly rare necrosis of the carotid artery. In addition, incisions that are too large or too small may lead to poor healing or an inability to completely evacuate the abscess, respectively.

Antibiotic Therapy

After drainage, empirical oral antibiotics are used in outpatients and intravenous antibiotics are administered to inpatients. PTAs are often polymicrobial, and hence culture of aspirated pus is prudent, although the results rarely affect subsequent treatment. The predominant bacterial species are *Streptococcus pyogenes* (group A streptococcus), *S. aureus* (including in rare cases methicillin-resistant *S. aureus* [MRSA]), and various respiratory anaerobes (including *Bacteroides, Fusobacterium, Prevotella,* and *Veillonella* species). *Haemophilus* species are found occasionally. Aerobes and anaerobes may be recovered simultaneously if appropriate culture techniques are used. Appropriate oral antibiotics for outpatient therapy in areas where *S. aureus* remains susceptible to methicillin include amoxicillin-clavulanate or clindamycin. For inpatients, administer ampicillin-sulbactam or clindamycin. Penicillin plus metronidazole is also a recommended antibiotic regimen. In septic patients it is prudent to also cover for MRSA. Although clindamycin may be adequate for MRSA, some add vancomycin or linezolid to the aforementioned initial antibiotic regimens if MRSA is suspected or predominant in the population. It is prudent to initially cover for MRSA in septic or very toxic patients.

Glucocorticoid Therapy

It is common practice for clinicians to administer short-term corticosteroids, such as intravenous dexamethasone or methylprednisolone, as an adjunct to other therapies in an attempt to provide relief from the symptoms of PTA. Evidence of the benefits of glucocorticoids in the management of PTA is inconsistent, but such intervention may hasten improvement of symptoms in adolescent and adult patients treated with needle aspiration and intravenous antimicrobial therapy. The benefits may be marginal, but since there are no significant complications, it is reasonable to empirically treat adults with short-term corticosteroids. Additional data are necessary before the routine use of glucocorticoids can be recommended in the management of PTA in children.

EAR

Anatomy

The ear consists of three sections, the outer, middle, and inner ear. The outer ear includes the pinna (auricle), the external auditory canal (EAC), and the tympanic membrane (TM) (Fig. 63-14*A*). For the purpose of this chapter, only the parts of the external ear will be discussed. The pinna is

PERITONSILLAR ABSCESS: INCISION AND DRAINAGE

1

Tape prevents scalpel overpenetration ⎯

Place adhesive tape around a No. 11 or 15 scalpel blade so that only the distal 0.5–1 cm is exposed. This prevents overpenetration.

2

Incise the area of maximal fluctuance (or the area where previous aspiration located pus). Expect pus and blood to flow from the incision; have suction ready to remove the purulent material.

3

Use a Kelly clamp to gently break up loculations. Packing is not used. Observe the patient for about an hour to watch for complications such as bleeding.

Figure 63-13 Drainage of a peritonsillar abscess: incision and drainage technique. Aspiration is often the only procedure required to successfully treat a peritonsillar abscess, but it has a 10% failure rate. In some instances the clinician will opt for incision and drainage of a peritonsillar abscess. This procedure may be used initially or after aspiration if copious pus is aspirated or pus continues to drain or reaccumulate.

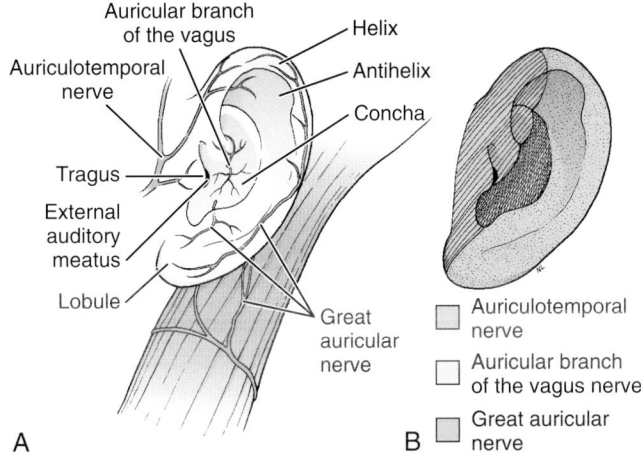

Figure 63-14 A, Anatomy of the ear and innervation of the auricle. **B,** Sensory distribution of nerves of the ear.

flesh-covered cartilage and serves both hearing and cosmetic functions. The EAC extends from the head to the external auditory meatus in the skull and measures approximately 2.5 cm in adults. It is relatively short and straight in early infancy but begins to take on its adult S shape and overall anterocaudal orientation at 2 years of age. Initially, the EAC is almost entirely cartilaginous, but by adulthood its medial two thirds is composed of bony support with an overlying thin, stratified squamous epithelium. The lateral third has a less sensitive, thicker hairy epithelium that produces cerumen and retains its cartilage as support. The arterial supply to the EAC originates from the external carotid artery via the posterior auricular, maxillary, and superficial temporal branches.

The mandibular branch of the fifth cranial nerve (V3) and the vagus nerve innervate the ear.

Other important anatomic considerations include two natural narrowings in the EAC, which are important when considering FBs. One is located at the junction of bone and cartilage and the other lies just lateral to the TM. A blind spot may occur in the tympanic sulcus (inferior and anterior to the TM) because of the oblique orientation of the TM. An examiner using a simple otoscope may not visualize an FB in this sulcus.

Anesthesia of the External Ear

Auricle

Indications for local anesthesia of the auricle include closure of extensive lacerations or performance of other painful procedures such as incision and drainage of hematomas (Fig. 63-15). Four nerve branches supply the external ear; knowledge of their anatomy is required to understand the location for injection of anesthetic (see Fig. 63-14B). The great auricular nerve (branch of the cervical plexus) innervates most of the posteromedial, posterolateral, and inferior aspect of the auricle. A few branches of the lesser occipital nerve may contribute to this area. The auricular branch of the vagus supplies the concha and most of the area around the auditory meatus. The auriculotemporal nerve (from the mandibular branch of the trigeminal nerve) supplies the anterosuperior and anteromedial aspects of the auricle.

Procedure

Fill a 10-mL syringe with either 1% lidocaine or 0.25% bupivacaine. Mix with epinephrine if a regional block is planned in an area without evidence of traumatized vascularity. Attach the syringe to a 25- or 27-gauge needle (5 to 7 cm in length).

Figure 63-15 Closure of extensive lacerations of the ear such as this require a nerve block of the auricle.

One of several methods may be used to induce partial or complete anesthesia, depending on the area of concern. To anesthetize the nerve branches of the great auricular and lesser occipital nerve branches, inject between 3 and 4 mL of anesthetic into the posterior sulcus (Fig. 63-16, *plate 1*). Insert the needle behind the inferior pole of the auricle and gradually aspirate and inject toward the superior pole along the crescent-shaped contour of the posterior aspect of the auricle. Anesthetize the auriculotemporal nerve anteriorly by placing 3 to 4 mL of anesthetic just superior and anterior to the cartilaginous tragus. Provide anesthesia to the auricular branch of the vagus nerve and the more central areas of the auricle by using the technique shown in Figure 63-16, *plates 3 and 4*.

Another and possibly more effective option is the regional block shown in Figure 63-16, *plate 2*. Insert the needle subcutaneously approximately 1 cm above the superior pole of the auricle and direct it to a point just anterior to the tragus. Be sure to inject the skin of the scalp while avoiding the

---

ANESTHESIA OF THE EAR

Auricular Field Blocks

1

Inject anesthetic along the course of the posterior sulcus

One method of auricular block uses approximately 3–4 mL of anesthetic injected both at the posterior sulcus (*red arrow*) and at a point just anterior to the tragus (*blue circle*).

2

Deposit 2–3 mL of anesthetic along each path

An alternative auricular block deposits 2–3 mL of anesthetic in 4 separate injections that encircle the ear. Begin each new injection in a region that is already anesthetized.

External Auditory Canal Blocks

3

Ear speculum

Four-quadrant field block. Inject anesthetic subcutaneously in the four quadrants of the lateral portion of the ear canal. Use the largest speculum that will fit to guide the injections. Withdraw the speculum, tilt it toward each of the four quadrants, and insert the needle subcutaneously (*x*). Inject 0.25–0.50 mL of anesthetic to produce a slight bulge in the soft tissue. A total of 1.5–2.0 mL of anesthetic is usually sufficient to anesthetize the ear canal and permit painless removal of a foreign body. Ketamine procedural sedation may be a better option.

4

Diagram of injection sites for an alternative technique to anesthetize the ear canal and central concha. Inject each site with approximately 0.5 mL of 1% lidocaine. Do not inject if external signs of infection are present.

Figure 63-16 Anesthesia of the ear.

auricular cartilage. Aspirate and then slowly withdraw the needle while injecting anesthetic until the needle is almost to the puncture site. Redirect the needle posteriorly and repeat the process while aiming at the skin just behind the mid-auricular area. Remove the needle and perform the same procedure, but insert the needle just inferior to the insertion of the ear lobule and anesthetize it in a superior direction. Again, block the auricular branch of the vagus as described in Figure 63-16, *plates 3 and 4*, if additional anesthesia of the concha is required.

Use caution if adding epinephrine to the anesthetic solution when performing regional nerve blocks of the ear, especially if the blood supply has already been traumatically reduced. Do not include epinephrine when directly infiltrating wounds of the auricle because restriction of blood flow through the end arteries here may result in tissue necrosis. Other complications related to local anesthesia and regional blocks of the head and neck are reviewed elsewhere in this text.

EAC and TM

The EAC is innervated by the auricular branch of the vagus nerve (inferiorly and posteriorly) and by the auriculotemporal nerve (superiorly, anteriorly, and inferiorly). The primary indication for local anesthesia of the auditory canal is for removal of FBs, including débridement of otitis externa or removal of significant impacted cerumen. *It is very difficult to achieve adequate anesthesia of the inner ear and TM for painful procedures.* Simply stated, no easy and completely effective procedure consistently works well. If total anesthesia is required, general anesthesia, especially in children, is often the only alternative. *Ketamine is an ideal agent for short procedures, especially for children with foreign objects in the ear.* Topical anesthetics are inadequate because of their poor absorption through the rather impermeable and keratinized epithelial surface of the EAC. Though effective for some procedures, injection of local anesthetics into and around the auditory meatus is quite painful and often difficult to perform in a struggling and uncooperative patient. Certain instances warrant adjunctive use of procedural sedation. Auralgan, a combination of benzocaine and other ingredients, may provide analgesia for painful earaches secondary to otitis, but it does little to benefit painful procedures.

Procedure

Local anesthesia is achieved with a 25- or 27-gauge needle (3 to 5 cm in length) attached to a syringe containing 1% lidocaine with epinephrine. A 1:10 mixture of 8.4% sodium bicarbonate to lidocaine helps reduce pain during injection in this sensitive area. Place a speculum just inside the auditory meatus, inject 0.3 to 0.5 mL of the anesthetic into subcutaneous tissue, and stop after a small bulge is raised in the skin. Inject all four quadrants in this manner by moving the speculum after each injection (see Fig. 63-16, *plate 3*). If additional anesthesia is necessary, give two more small injections. Inject the same amount slightly farther into the canal, once along the anterior wall and again at the posterior wall at the bone-cartilage junction.

Another similar technique involves depositing the anesthetic just lateral, or exterior, to the external auditory meatus. Using the same size of needle and type of anesthetic solution as just described, inject approximately 0.5 to 1.0 mL into each of five points around the auditory meatus and tragus (see Fig. 63-16, *plate 4*).

Examination

Several methods can be used to examine the EAC and TM. In all methods, grasp the superior aspect of the pinna and pull cephalad and posterior to straighten the slightly tortuous EAC. Examination is most commonly done with a fiberoptic otoscope (Fig. 63-17). Place a plastic or metal speculum into the auditory meatus for examination and use a head lamp or head mirror/light bulb as a light source. After inspection, the operating hand can be used to pass instruments into the EAC and to maneuver them more easily. Although this technique provides excellent illumination, the use of magnifying loupes can improve visualization during procedures. The ideal setup for removal of cerumen or an FB consists of an operating microscope and a speculum. This provides binocular vision and frees the examiner's hands for instrumentation. Unfortunately, this equipment is seldom found outside the otolaryngology clinic setting. If using a standard otoscope, stabilize the hand holding the otoscope against the temporal part of the patient's skull to prevent inadvertent injury to the canal if the patient moves unexpectedly.

Removal of Impacted Cerumen

Excretions from the ceruminous or apocrine and sebaceous glands together with cells exfoliated from the EAC combine to form cerumen. One study found that cerumen is composed of lipids, complex proteins, and simple sugars.[15] Cerumen repels water, has documented antimicrobial activity, and forms a protective barrier against infection. Cerumen often becomes impacted, which results in complaints of a "blocked" ear, impaired hearing, or dizziness.

Indications and Contraindications

Symptomatic impaction is an indication for removal, although symptoms are rare until complete obstruction is present. Sudden loss of hearing is a common complaint in patients with totally occluding, impacted cerumen. Cerumen obstructs

Figure 63-17 Examination of the ear canal. **A,** Retract the pinna in a superior and posterior direction to straighten out the ear canal (*arrow*). Hold the scope in the other hand and stabilize it against the patient's head. This prevents inadvertent injury if the patient moves unexpectedly. **B,** The pinna can be retracted and the scope held with a single hand that is also resting against the patient's head (*arrow*). This technique is useful if instruments are to be passed through the otoscope.

Cerumen Impaction Removal

Indications
Symptomatic cerumen impaction
Sudden hearing loss in the setting of cerumen impaction
Evaluation of otitis media in the setting of cerumen impaction

Contraindications
Few if any absolute contraindications
Contraindications to irrigation:

Patient aversion to irrigation	Foreign bodies
History of middle ear disease	Uncooperative patient
History of ear surgery	Occluding aural exostoses
Perforated tympanic membrane	Inner ear disturbance
Severe otitis externa	Radiation therapy in the area
Narrow ear canals	

Complications
Otitis externa
Tympanic membrane perforation
Middle ear injury
External auditory canal trauma

Equipment

Syringe and Teflon catheter for irrigation
Ear scoop
Alligator forceps
Otoscope
Ceruminolytic
Frazier-tip suction

Review Box 63-2 Cerumen impaction removal: indications, contraindications, complications, and equipment.

Figure 63-18 A, Extensive contact dermatitis from the use of neomycin-containing eardrops. **B,** Malignant otitis externa in a diabetic patient developed after the patient manually removed cerumen with a cotton swab and a pencil, but it may develop without manipulation of the canal.

visualization of the TM and can be evacuated as a part of the evaluation of a febrile child or a patient complaining of ear pain. However, removal of cerumen in a child is rarely indicated in the ED simply to visualize the TM.

There are few if any true contraindications to removal of impacted cerumen. Cerumen is usually impacted for prolonged periods, and vigorous attempts to remove it may precipitate otitis externa. It is reasonable to instill antiseptics (Vol Sol and others) or antibiotic eardrops for a few days after removal of the cerumen to prevent otitis externa. Neomycin-containing eardrops are best avoided because of precipitation of a contact dermatitis (Fig. 63-18*A*). Caution should be used in removing impacted cerumen in diabetic patients. Diabetics

commonly experience otitis externa after seemingly minor manipulation of the ear canal (see Fig. 63-18*B*).

Contraindications to irrigation include the following[16]:

- Patient aversion to or a history of injury from previous syringe irrigation
- History of middle ear disease
- History of ear surgery
- Known or suspected perforated TM
- Severe otitis externa
- Narrow ear canals
- FBs, especially sharp objects and vegetable matter
- Uncooperative patient
- Occluding aural exostoses
- Known inner ear disturbance, especially if the patient has severe vertigo
- History of radiation therapy encompassing the external or middle ear, base of the skull, or mastoid

Procedure
Removal of cerumen can be accomplished by irrigation, manual extraction, or a combination of both. Generally, the procedures used to remove cerumen are safe; however, otologic injury has occurred after this "minor" procedure and has even resulted in litigation.[17]

Irrigation is an effective approach for removal of cerumen and has the advantage of being painless and simple to perform. It is usually most successful after the instillation of a ceruminolytic (see later). Because the patient does not have to remain completely still, it is ideal for the pediatric population. It is estimated that 150,000 ears are irrigated in the United States each week.[17] Though usually more time-consuming and messy than manual extraction, irrigation is an appropriate initial method to attempt and can be performed by technicians with guidance from the clinician.

A recent evidence-based review concluded that the current evidence suggests little difference in the efficacy of water-based and oil-based preparations for removing cerumen.[18] Non–water-, non–oil-based preparations appear to be most effective in clearing cerumen and improving syringing, but further research is needed.[18] Whichever of the following techniques are used, some tips for successful removal of cerumen include proper lighting, attention to patient comfort, and abrupt cessation when the patient's comfort level is breached.

Ceruminolytics

These products may soften hardened or impacted cerumen. They are used as adjuncts to other procedures—simply instilling ceruminolytics into the canal will not remove enough cerumen to aid the emergency clinician. If irrigation fails, continued outpatient use of ceruminolytics is often prescribed, usually combined with home irrigation via a bulb syringe or a repeated visit in a few days. Although many products are available as ceruminolytics, a 5% or 10% solution of sodium bicarbonate disintegrates cerumen much more quickly and efficiently than do commercially prepared ceruminolytics and other products.[19] Cerumenex, Cerumol, Auralgan, Buro-Sol, alcohol, and oils were all tested and took more than 18 hours to disintegrate cerumen versus approximately 90 minutes for the sodium bicarbonate solutions.[19] Hydrogen peroxide is another commonly used ceruminolytic, but its use has not been systematically studied. One study found that the liquid preparation of the stool softener docusate sodium (Colace) was much more effective than Cerumenex as a ceruminolytic.[20] An evidence-based review of agents found that docusate sodium administered 15 minutes before irrigation was most effective in facilitating removal of cerumen. Triethanolamine (Cerumenex) and olive oil were the next most effective treatments.[21]

Place the patient in the supine position with the affected ear up, instill the solution, and wait at least 15 to 30 minutes before attempts at removal (Fig. 63-19, *step 1*). Repeat the instillation between attempts at manual extraction or irrigation.

Irrigation (Ear Syringing)

After a ceruminolytic has been instilled and left in the canal for 15 to 30 minutes, irrigation of the canal is often effective in flushing out impacted cerumen. Ask the patient to sit upright and hold an emesis or ear irrigation basin flush tightly against the skin just below the earlobe. Insert the irrigation tip into the EAC only as far as the cartilage-bone junction, and direct the stream of water superiorly to wash the impacted cerumen away from the TM (see Fig. 63-19, *step 2*). Warm the water to body temperature to prevent caloric stimulation. Multiple attempts may be necessary, and intermittent attempts at manual removal of loosened cerumen may help hasten the process. During the irrigation, *ask an assistant to apply traction to the pinna to straighten the canal for more efficient irrigation.* Patients usually feel some discomfort with forceful irrigation, but not severe pain.

Attach a 30- to 60-mL syringe to a 19-gauge or larger butterfly device, cut off the needle and wings, and use the resultant tubing for irrigation. A large plastic or Teflon intravenous catheter (16 or 18 gauge with the needle removed) can similarly be affixed to a syringe.

The most common way to irrigate an ear is with a syringe and catheter. The use of oral jet irrigators (Waterpik) is another accepted method, but a syringe-catheter setup is readily found in the ED and unlikely to generate enough pressure to cause injury. After irrigating the EAC, apply several drops of isopropanol to the EAC to facilitate evaporation of residual moisture. Do not use isopropanol if the TM is ruptured. Furthermore, topical steroid-containing suspension drops (ciprofloxacin/hydrocortisone) may be soothing after prolonged irrigation. Because severe otitis externa can develop in diabetics after irrigation, some clinicians routinely prescribe antibiotic eardrops (e.g., fluoroquinolones) for a few days after irrigation in high-risk patients.

Manual Instrumentation

Manual instrumentation is more advantageous because it is usually quicker and the examiner may more easily remove hardened or larger concretions of cerumen under direct visualization. However, it is difficult to manually remove cerumen without causing significant pain, so irrigation is preferred. *Manual removal may be the initial procedure in some cases, followed by irrigation when the cerumen is partially disrupted.* Place the diagnostic or operating head of the fiberoptic otoscope or a speculum as a protective port through which instruments are passed and manipulated (see Fig. 63-19, *step 3*). An operating microscope works best in this situation but, again, is not usually available. To prevent startling or agitating an already anxious patient, allow the patient to experience the sensation of an instrument in the canal by first placing it softly against the wall of the ear canal.

Instruments used for removal of cerumen include flexible plastic or wire loops, right-angle hooks, suction-tipped catheters, or plastic scoops (see Review Box 63-2 and Fig. 63-19, *steps 4 to 6*). The spoonlike instruments and irrigation are both more effective in removing softer cerumen. Firm cerumen is ordinarily more easily withdrawn with loops or right-angle hooks. Gently tease the cerumen off of the canal wall with loops and then pass hooks or loops around the cerumen and withdraw it slowly. Take care to keep both hands in contact with the patient's head because any sudden movement may cause trauma to the canal or the TM.

Complications

Complications from removal of cerumen are rare but can have serious consequences. Although complications from ear syringing are more common with jet irrigators, they may occur with any method of ear irrigation and include otitis externa, TM perforation, or middle ear injury from a preexisting defect in the TM. If the patient is experiencing sudden pain, tinnitus, hearing loss, nausea, or vertigo, stop the irrigation and examine the TM. If the membrane is ruptured, give prophylactic oral antibiotics for otitis media, keep the ear canal perfectly dry with cotton, and refer the patient to an otolaryngologist. This complication is usually benign.

Complications from manual extraction most commonly occur when inadvertent contact is made with the thin, friable skin of the bony canal. Trauma may cause EAC laceration, otitis externa, or perforation of the TM.

Ear Canal Débridement and Wick Placement

Débridement of the ear canal and wick placement are essential components in the management and treatment of otitis

CERUMEN IMPACTION REMOVAL

Instill a ceruminolytic solution into the ear at least 15 minutes before attempts at removal (see text for discussion of various agents). Repeat the instillation between attempts.

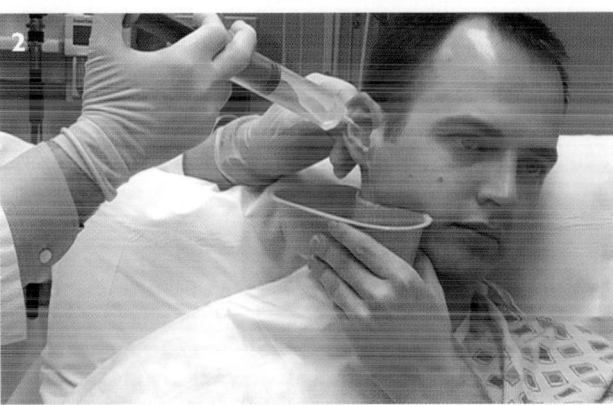

Irrigate with body-temperature water via a syringe with a plastic IV catheter (with the needle removed). Apply traction to the pinna during irrigation to straighten the ear canal. Periodic attempts at manual removal of loosened cerumen may be beneficial.

For manual removal, use the otoscope (with the view piece retracted) as a port for passage of the instrument.

Gently tease the cerumen off the canal wall with a loop or plastic ear scoop. This should be performed only under direct visualization.

Remove dislodged pieces of cerumen from the canal with an instrument such as alligator forceps.

A suction-tip catheter may also be used. However, this should be done under direct visualization only to prevent iatrogenic injury to the fragile ear canal.

Figure 63-19 Cerumen impaction removal. When removal of cerumen is unsuccessful in the emergency department, discharge the patient with a ceruminolytic and attempt irrigation again in 24 to 48 hours.

externa or "swimmer's ear," an acute inflammation of the skin of the EAC. This is essentially a cellulitis of the ear canal. Precipitants of otitis externa include water exposure and trauma. Excessive moisture in the canal raises the pH and removes the cerumen. Keratin cannot absorb water, thereby creating a medium for bacterial growth. Trauma, especially self-manipulation with FBs (e.g., cotton swabs, fingernails), causes abrasions in the ear canal and introduces infection. Removal of cerumen by water irrigation is a well-recognized risk factor for the development of otitis externa.[19]

Diabetics and other immunocompromised patients, especially human immunodeficiency virus–positive patients, are susceptible to malignant (necrotizing) otitis externa, a life-threatening form of otitis externa caused by *Pseudomonas* (see Fig. 63-18*B*). Deep tissue necrosis, osteomyelitis, intracranial extension, and systemic toxicity are hallmark features. Malignant otitis externa is difficult to treat and the mortality rate can be as high as 53%.[19] The diagnosis of malignant otitis externa should be considered in a diabetic or immunocompromised patient with significant symptoms who fails to respond to initial outpatient treatment.

Indications and Contraindications

In patients with suspected otitis externa, attempts should be made to clean debris from the canal to aid in healing. In addition, wick placement will be helpful in delivering antibiotic medications to the swollen canal. It has been touted that the key to successful treatment is adequate removal of canal debris. However, vigorous attempts to remove debris on the first visit are frequently painful, of unproven value, and often eschewed.

Removal of debris is contraindicated in cases of suspected malignant otitis externa, and ear, nose, and throat (ENT) consultation is required.

Procedure

Because of patient discomfort and canal swelling, small swabs (e.g., urethral swabs) should be used to gently remove debris. The canal can be gently irrigated, but realize that *many patients will be cured without extensive débridement.* Irrigation should be performed only in the absence of TM perforation.[16,22] Because the inflamed canal is susceptible to trauma, removal of debris by suctioning under direct visualization with the open or operating otoscope head and a 5- or 7-Fr Frazier suction tip may be a better option (see Fig. 63-19, *step 6*). For more advanced cases with significant exudate and edema, removal of debris is necessary but intensely painful. One approach is to use a local block of the EAC (see Fig. 63-16) as long as the cellulitis has not extended to the tragus or concha. Administer parenteral analgesics if additional control of pain is required.

When edema, debris, and exudate are marked enough to impede antibiotic drops from contacting the skin of the canal, use an ear wick. The wick works as a conduit to deliver the antibiotic solutions to the ear canal. The true benefit of wick implantation is unknown and it is often not performed because it is painful. One approach is to place a 0.25-inch strip of Nu-Gauze dressing covered with an antibiotic and steroid cream (Cortisporin Otic cream) into the external acoustic canal in a fashion similar to the technique used for anterior nasal packing. Using an otoscope and alligator forceps, place the leading edge of the gauze deeply in the canal until it is fully packed. Withdraw the otoscope and finish by also packing the lateral aspect of the canal. Cotton may be used as well (Fig. 63-20*A*).

An easier alternative is to use commercially available ear wicks, such as the Pope Merocel ear wick. Place this dehydrated and trimmed wick into an edematous canal and apply antibiotic/hydrocortisone drops onto it (see Fig. 63-20*B*).

EAR WICK PLACEMENT

Cotton or 0.25-inch Nu-Gauze packing strip can be coated with Cortisporin Otic cream and placed into the external auditory canal with alligator forceps.

An easier solution is to use a Merocel ear wick. Place the dehydrated wick into the canal and apply Cortisporin Otic drops to it. Instruct the patient to place the drops directly on the wick until the follow-up visit.

Figure 63-20 Placement of an ear wick. Ear wicks are used for the treatment of otitis externa and function to deliver antibiotic medications to the swollen external auditory canal.

The wick swells and helps reduce edema by the antimicrobial and antiinflammatory effects of the solution and through pressure exerted against the walls as it expands. Keep the wick moist with drops and leave it in place until the patient is seen again in 24 to 48 hours for removal and further evaluation. Though relatively safe to use, the ear wick is designed for short-term use. Generally, these wicks will fall out of the canal as the edema subsides. However, wicks can harbor bacteria with prolonged retention and cause tissue ingrowth, which results in long-term problems for the patient.[23]

Complications

There are very few complications with canal débridement and ear wick placement. Usually, the wick will fall out as edema in the canal subsides; if not, it may become an FB of the EAC. Care should be taken to not injure the already friable skin of the EAC, which can lead to bleeding and possible infection or cellulitis of the EAC when placing or removing a wick.

FBs in the Ear Canal

Despite its small size, the EAC may play host to numerous types of FBs.[24,25] Living insects account for most FBs found in adults. Children frequently place food (e.g., peas, beans), organic matter (e.g., grass, leaves, flowers), and inorganic objects (e.g., beads, rocks, dirt) into their ear canals during play, and they often fail to admit this to parents. Button batteries may cause significant tissue destruction in a matter of hours, and it is vital to immediately obtain otolaryngologic consultation for removal if the button battery is not easily extracted. Symptoms of FB retention usually consist of ear pain, fullness, or impaired hearing in adults; pediatric patients may not be encountered until an associated otitis externa with a purulent discharge has developed.

As described previously, the anatomy of the EAC predisposes to entrapment of FBs in either a lateral or a deeper position. Removal of more medial objects can be much more painful, and anesthesia is usually required. *Even the most cooperative patient may become difficult after feeling pain during manipulation of the ear canal. It is probably impossible to adequately immobilize the head of an uncooperative awake child and to delicately extract an FB.*

Some authorities claim that local anesthesia makes extracting FBs even more difficult because of soft tissue distortion, although swelling should be minimal if proper amounts of anesthetic are used. Anesthesia of the EAC may be difficult to achieve. Topical anesthetics have a partial effect, and a four-quadrant technique may not produce complete anesthesia, especially of the TM (see Fig. 63-16, *step 3*).[24,25] Procedural sedation (preferably an analgesic-sedative combination or dissociative anesthetic) can aid in the removal of FBs in a distraught child by preventing further struggling and potential canal trauma. *Ketamine is an excellent anesthetic for simple FB removal in the outpatient setting.* The care provider must weigh the inherent risks related to procedural sedation against those of general anesthesia and the cost of hospital admission.

Adequate visualization of the object is needed for successful removal. One study showed that canal lacerations occurred in 48% of patients in whom removal was attempted without a microscope and in 4% when it was used.[25] The otoscope is the traditional ED instrument for viewing FBs in the ear canal. It is less likely to be useful for retrieval because it is difficult to insert the instrument through or around the end of the speculum. A specialized ENT speculum allows more space for instrumentation. A head lamp provides a good light source and leaves both hands free. Magnifying loupes also provide hands-free magnification.

Indications and Contraindications

In the majority of cases, removal of an FB should be attempted in the ED. Before initiating removal, the clinician should set realistic limits on the number of attempts to be made. Even the best clinician can become too aggressive as frustration builds with failed attempts to extract the object. Early consultation with an otolaryngologist should not be considered a failure with difficult FBs. Indeed, with the proper equipment and experience, most objects can be removed atraumatically.

Severely impacted objects and concomitant EAC infection are relative contraindications to removal, and ENT consultation should be obtained. In addition, *patient cooperation is essential for successful removal*. The only other contraindication to removal of FBs from the EAC involves certain circumstances when irrigation will be the technique used. Irrigation should not be performed in cases of known or suspected TM rupture (tinnitus, vertigo, significant hearing loss, or bleeding from behind the object). In addition, irrigation should not be performed if the object is soft or if it is a seed or other vegetable or organic matter because the water may cause the object to swell.

Procedures

Make a judicious effort to remove an ear FB in the ED setting. Avoid prolonged traumatic attempts because this often terrifies the patient, complicates subsequent attempts, and can cause bleeding and swelling, thus making subsequent efforts more difficult. Most approaches to removal of FBs are anecdotal and found in the literature as case reports or case series rather than as prospective clinical trials. Familiarize yourself with several techniques because the most appropriate choice depends on the size, shape, consistency, and depth of impaction of the object.

Irrigation is the least invasive method; the techniques were explained in detail earlier in this chapter (see "Removal of Impacted Cerumen" and Fig. 63-19). Irrigation works particularly well with small rocks, dirt, or sand that lie deep in the canal next to the TM.

Suction-Tipped Catheters

This technique works well with objects that are round and difficult to grasp. Suction is readily available in the ED but should provide 100 to 140 mm Hg of negative pressure to be useful. To avoid iatrogenic injury, inform the patient of the impending noise to prevent sudden movements caused by a startle reflex. Place either the blunt or the soft plastic tip against the object and withdraw it slowly. If using a suction instrument with a thumb-controlled release valve (as with the Frazier suction tip), remember to cover the port to activate the suction.

The Hognose (IQDr, Inc.), a commercially available device designed by an emergency clinician, aids in the removal of FBs in the auditory canal. It is used in combination with an otoscope and suction setup. It is essentially an otoscope speculum with suction attachment and a soft self-molding tip that can attach to objects. The flange comes in three color-coded sizes: 4, 5, and 6 mm. To use, first attach the Hognose to the

Base fits on standard
Welch Allyn otoscopes

Soft suction
cup

Suction entry
port (use low to
medium vacuum)

Figure 63-21 The Hognose device for removal of a foreign body (FB). The Hognose attaches to the otoscope and to wall suction. Occlusion of the open insufflation port (*arrow*) engages suction and removes the FB. The Hognose device is available through IQDr, Inc (iqdr.com).

otoscope and set the standard wall suction at a low to medium vacuum setting (Fig. 63-21). Next, under direct visualization, approach the FB with the otoscope. Finally, engage suction by applying finger pressure on the open insufflation port and withdraw.

Manual Instrumentation

This approach can be attempted with various instruments (Fig. 63-22, *plate 1*). Use the diagnostic or operating head of a fiberoptic otoscope for illumination and magnification. Ask an assistant to hold the pinna back and out so that you can hold the otoscope with one hand and manipulate the instrument with the other. A speculum and either a head lamp or a head mirror/light source can also provide illumination; magnifying loupes are usually required for adequate visualization. Use small alligator forceps to remove objects with edges that can be grasped, but avoid trying to encircle an impacted round FB because this may cause trauma to the canal wall. A small right-angle hook is another choice. Place the tip past the object, rotate it 90 degrees, and then pull the object from the canal. Fine tissue or Adson forceps, curets, and skin hooks are other instruments used occasionally. Use of these instruments is commonly associated with abrasions and bleeding of the ear canal.[24,25] Instruments should be used only on compliant, cooperative patients. Direct visualization of the object is essential.

Fogarty Catheters

Small Fogarty catheters (biliary or vascular) may be used in a manner similar to that described later in this chapter in the section "Nasal FB Removal." Attach the tip of the catheter to a 3-mL syringe. Pass the catheter beyond the FB. Once the tip is past the object, gradually inflate the balloon and drag the FB out along with the balloon. Immediately deflate the balloon if pain suddenly occurs because rupture of the TM is a potential complication.

Cyanoacrylate (Superglue)

The use of glue to remove FBs was first reported in India in 1977.[25,26] Glue is most effective in removing smooth, round objects that are difficult to grasp (see Fig. 63-22, *plate 2*). The FB should be dry and easily visualized. Apply a small amount of glue to the tip of a thin paintbrush, a straightened

paper clip, or the blunt end of a wooden cotton-tipped applicator. Allow the glue to become tacky. Place the tip against the object, allow it to dry, and then carefully withdraw the FB. Minor complications are possible if the tip dries against the canal wall (abrasion, excoriation) or if the glue spills or drips onto the wall (thereby creating a new FB). This technique may be more useful in adults because cooperation is required.[26]

Removal of Insects

Cockroaches are the most commonly found live insects in the ear (Fig. 63-22, *plate 3*). A suggested treatment is to instill various substances into the ear canal to immobilize or kill the insect before removing it. This helps in retrieval by allowing a stationary target and also halts the disturbing and painful movement of the insect. Controversy exists about which agent can most effectively accomplish this task. Mineral oil has traditionally been used, but lidocaine has been reported to paralyze insects and allow easier extraction than with the more viscous mineral oil. An in vitro comparative study showed that immersion in microscope oil versus 2% or 4% lidocaine solution killed roaches in less than 60 seconds (≈27 and 41 seconds, respectively).[27] The roaches struggled less in the viscous oil than in the lidocaine, which did not appear to cause paralysis. Other substances (Auralgan, isopropanol, water, succinylcholine, hydrogen peroxide) were shown to be ineffective in killing the roaches in a reasonable amount of time. Once disabled, insects are removed by mechanical extraction as described previously; pieces can be suctioned out if fragmentation occurs.

If an insect cannot easily be removed or if parts remain, it is quite acceptable to prescribe outpatient antibiotic drops for 24 to 48 hours and try irrigation again or refer to a specialist. As with any FB in the ear canal, prolonged attempts at removal in the ED are counterproductive.

Complications

Hearing should be evaluated before and after removal of an FB, especially in patients with suspected TM or middle ear injuries. Also examine the opposite ear and nose of children to search for the rare but possible second FB. Minor lacerations or excoriations of the canal usually heal quickly with or without antibiotic eardrops, as long as the canal is kept clean and dry. Document preexisting canal trauma or suspected TM rupture before attempts at removal; otherwise, this may be falsely attributed to iatrogenic causes at a later date. Indications for otolaryngologic referral include failed removal of the object in the ED, existent injury to the EAC or TM, TM rupture, EAC infection, object wedged in the medial part of the EAC or up against the TM, glass or other sharp-edged FBs, and special circumstances (disk batteries and putty). Generally, no routine follow-up is necessary except in cases of infection, severe trauma, or perforation of the TM. Parents should be educated to reduce the exposure of children to potential FBs.

Drainage of Auricular Hematomas

Auricular hematomas occur after the application of a shearing force to the ear, most commonly in wrestlers, boxers, and rugby players after fights. A subperichondrial hematoma forms and separates the perichondrium from cartilage. The hematoma may also arise from the cartilage itself. Recurrent

EAR CANAL FOREIGN BODY REMOVAL

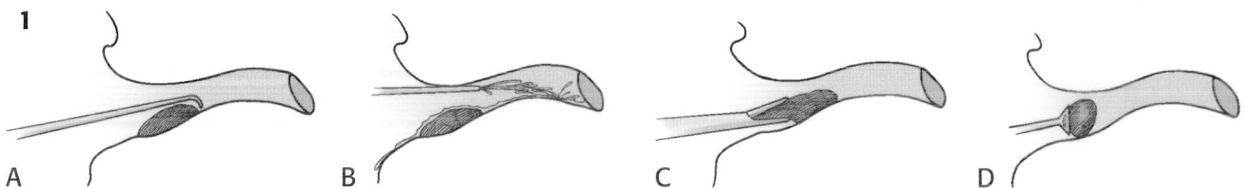

1

A, **B,** **C,** **D,**

Various devices for FB removal from the ear canal. **A,** Right-angle hook. **B,** Irrigation. **C,** Alligator forceps. **D,** Soft-tipped suction. Direct visualization of the canal is mandatory, as is patient cooperation. Abrasions of the ear canal and subsequent bleeding are common.

2

Putting superglue on a stick and allowing it to attach to an FB may be successful. This technique is most effective in removing smooth, round objects that are difficult to grasp. The FB should be dry and easily visualized. A high degree of patient cooperation is required.

3

Removal of an insect can be a disaster or relatively easy. An easy way is to use ketamine anesthesia with careful direct extraction. No patients can cooperate with more than minimal manipulation of the inner ear canal. Instilling mineral oil or lidocaine into the canal to kill the insect before extraction is recommended.

Figure 63-22 Removal of a foreign body (FB) from the ear canal. Avoid excessive and prolonged attempts in the emergency department to remove difficult FBs. For difficult-to-extract insects, it is appropriate to prescribe outpatient antibiotic drops for 24 to 48 hours and again try to irrigate the insect or refer to a specialist. Adequate anesthesia is essential since no patient can fully cooperate with painful deep ear canal manipulation.

or untreated injuries allow the development of new cartilage, which subsequently deforms the auricle (cauliflower ear).

Indications and Contraindications

Diagnosis of an auricular hematoma is based on the history and physical examination (Fig. 63-23). The presence of tender, anterior auricular swelling following trauma that deforms the anatomy of the pinna should prompt drainage of the hematoma. The goal is to prevent cartilage damage and deformation of the pinna.

If the patient is initially seen more than 7 days after injury, drainage may be difficult because of the formation of granulation tissue, and these patients should be referred to an ENT specialist. In addition, patients with concomitant cellulitis, perichondritis, or recurrent and chronic hematomas should be referred to a specialist.

Procedure

Treatment of an auricular hematoma is complete evacuation of the subperichondrial hematoma and reapproximation of the perichondrium to the cartilage.

Needle Aspiration

Though used widely, this technique is no longer recommended by most authorities because of the high risk for reaccumulation of the hematoma. Aspiration is often inadequate

AURICULAR HEMATOMA EVACUATION

Auricular hematomas manifest after trauma with anterior auricular swelling. The hematoma forms between the cartilage and perichondrium and will lead to permanent deformity if not treated.

Anesthetize the pinna via local infiltration of 1% lidocaine without epinephrine or via an auricular block.

Use a scalpel to incise the skin along the natural skin folds at the edge of the hematoma. Follow the natural curve of the pinna.

Gently peel the skin and perichondrium off the hematoma and underlying cartilage. Completely evacuate the hematoma and irrigate the pocket with normal saline.

A compression dressing must be placed to prevent reaccumulation of the hematoma. Place dry cotton into the EAC and fill all external auricular crevices with saline-soaked or Vaseline gauze.

Carefully conform the material into all the convolutions of the auricle. Vaseline gauze, saline-soaked 1/4-inch packing gauze, or saline-soaked cotton may be used. Place gauze behind the ear.

Place 3–4 layers of gauze behind the ear as a posterior pack, and then cover the entire ear with multiple layers of fluffed gauze.

Secure the dressing to the head with Kerlix or an elastic wrap.

Figure 63-23 Evacuation of an auricular hematoma. *EAC,* external auditory canal.

and other management is required. Other sources recommend needle aspiration followed by incision and drainage if reaccumulation occurs.[28]

Aspiration of an auricular hematoma is performed by perforating the hematoma with a 20-gauge needle. "Milk" the hematoma between the thumb and forefinger until the entire hematoma is evacuated. Apply a pressure dressing. Reexamine the ear frequently for reaccumulation of the hematoma. Reaccumulation of blood requires reaspiration. For small hematomas that are acute, needle aspiration alone with a bolster dressing is adequate therapy.[28]

Incision (see Fig. 63-23)

An auricular hematoma may be incised along the natural skin folds. Anesthetize the pinna by local infiltration of 1% lidocaine (without epinephrine) or with an auricular block (described earlier). Incise the skin with a No. 15 blade at the edge of the hematoma, and follow the curvature of the pinna. Gently peel the skin and perichondrium off the hematoma and underlying cartilage. Completely evacuate the hematoma and irrigate the remaining pocket with normal saline.

After removing the hematoma, apply antibiotic ointment and reapproximate the perichondrium to the cartilage with a pressure dressing. A compression dressing, noninvasive or surgical, must be applied because a simple dressing will allow the hematoma to reaccumulate. First, dry cotton should be placed into the EAC. Next, fill all external auricular crevices with mineral oil, saline-soaked gauze, or Vaseline gauze. Then place three to four layers of gauze behind the ear as a posterior pack. Cut a V shape out of the gauze first to allow a snug fit. Cover the packed external ear with multiple layers of fluffed gauze. Bandage the fluffed gauze in place with Kerlix or an elastic wrap.

A surgical compressive dressing involves suturing dental rolls over the area. To accomplish this, pass a 4-0 nylon suture through the entire thickness of the ear and over the hematoma. Wrap the suture around a dental roll on the posterior aspect of the ear and then pass the needle back through the pinna. Wrap and tie the suture around a second dental roll on the anterior aspect of the pinna. A second suture may be placed to secure a third dental roll. The dressing should firmly reapproximate the perichondrium to the cartilage without compromising the vasculature. Remove the dressing in 1 week.

Prescribe antistaphylococcal antibiotics and instruct the patient to inspect the wound frequently for evidence of vascular compromise, infection, or both. Reevaluate the wound in 24 hours for recurrence of the hematoma. Treat infection by removal of the bandage, surgical drainage, and intravenous antibiotics.

Complications

There are a few complications associated with management of auricular hematomas. The first is incomplete evacuation of the hematoma, which can lead to destruction of cartilage (cauliflower ear). The hematoma can reaccumulate. Local site infection can develop and result in the development of chondritis. Finally, scar formation leading to deformity is possible.

NOSE

Anatomy

The nose consists of the vestibule, nasal septum, lateral wall, and nasopharynx. The vestibule is the anteriormost portion

of the nares and is composed of skin and hair follicles. The nasal septum is the midline structure and is composed of cartilage anteriorly and bone posteriorly. The lateral wall of the nose contains the superior, middle, and inferior turbinates, as well as the auditory tube opening.

Three major arteries supply the nose and conjoin via anastomoses. The sphenopalatine artery emerges from the sphenopalatine foramen, which is located at the posterior aspect of the middle turbinate (Fig. 63-24). This is the most common source of posterior epistaxis. This artery supplies the lateral turbinates and the posterior septum. The anterior and posterior ethmoidal arteries branch off the ophthalmic artery and penetrate the cribriform plate to supply the superior nasal mucosa. The superior labial branch of the facial artery completes the triad and supplies the nasal septum and vestibule. The watershed area on the anterior septum, also known as Kiesselbach's plexus, is the most common source of anterior epistaxis (Fig. 63-25).

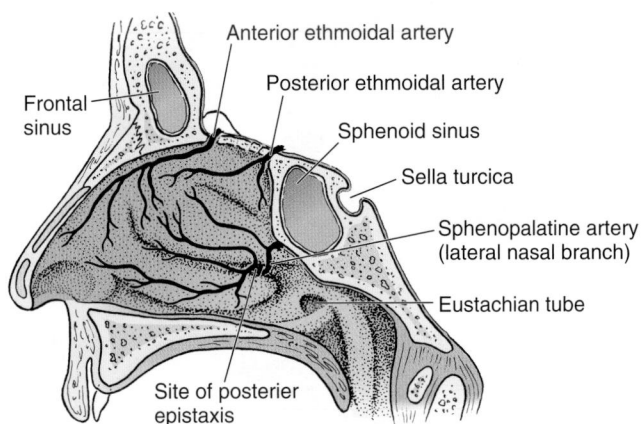

Figure 63-24 Vascular supply to the lateral wall of the nose. The most common site of posterior epistaxis is the sphenopalatine artery as it emerges posterior to the middle turbinate. *(From Maceri DR. Epistaxis and nasal trauma. In: Cummings CW, ed. Otolaryngology—Head and Neck Surgery. 2nd ed. St. Louis: Mosby–Year Book; 1993:728.)*

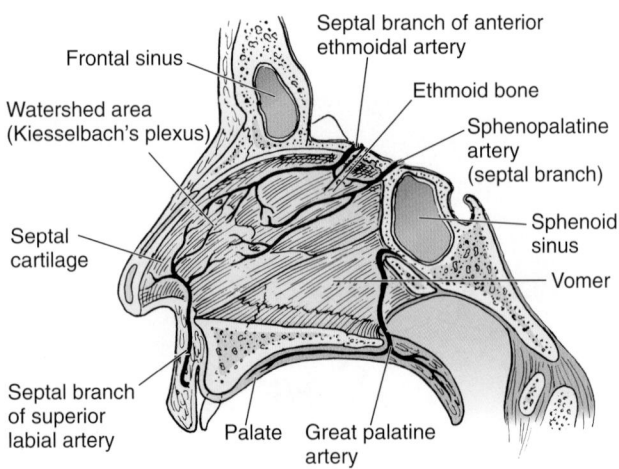

Figure 63-25 Vascular supply to the nasal septum. The most common site of anterior epistaxis is within the area labeled Kiesselbach's plexus. *(From Maceri DR. Epistaxis and nasal trauma. In: Cummings CW, ed. Otolaryngology—Head and Neck Surgery. 2nd ed. St. Louis: Mosby–Year Book; 1993:728.)*

Anesthesia of the Nose

Most nasal anesthesia can be accomplished topically. Numerous preparations are available. *Cocaine (4% solution) is the preferred agent for both vasoconstriction and anesthesia.* Unfortunately, cocaine is not routinely stocked. Alternatively, 2% lidocaine with epinephrine (local anesthetic solution) may be used but is less effective. Be aware of the total amount of cocaine being administered and stay within recommendations for the maximum safe dosage. This is an issue only with elderly patients who have cardiovascular disease. Lidocaine 4% is also quite effective for anesthesia of the nose. A solution of 1% tetracaine and 0.05% oxymetazoline (Afrin) is an effective topical anesthetic and vasoconstrictor.[29]

Apply the local anesthetic and vasoconstrictor to cotton swabs (Fig. 63-26). If a larger area of anesthesia is needed, use cotton pledgets. Figure 63-27 describes the procedure of making pledgets. Soak each pledget in an anesthetic or vasoconstrictor and then squeeze the excess fluid out of the pledget. Place each pledget horizontally on the floor of the nasal cavity and stack the next pledget on top. Three pledgets are usually required to pack the nasal cavity. They can be replaced with new pledgets in 5 minutes if the desired anesthetic effect is not achieved. Benzocaine (Hurricaine) spray may also be used as a topical anesthetic. Remind the patient that excess anesthetic may numb the throat but will not inhibit swallowing.

A local nasal block can be performed for more painful and prolonged procedures. The sensory innervation of the nose is illustrated in Figure 63-28. It begins with topical anesthetic as just described. Next, 1% lidocaine with 1:100,000 epinephrine is injected along the septum, lateral walls, and nasopalatine nerves. A thin 25- or 27-gauge needle should be used. Depending on the procedure, it may be necessary to anesthetize both sides. First, inject along and beneath the soft tissue of the nasal dorsum (infratrochlear nerve). Next, inject in the area of the infraorbital foramen to anesthetize the infraorbital nerve. Finally, inject at the base of the columella (base of the nose between the nasal septa) and along the floor of the nasal cavity. Interestingly, studies have shown that the use of EMLA (eutectic mixture of local anesthetics) cream applied over the

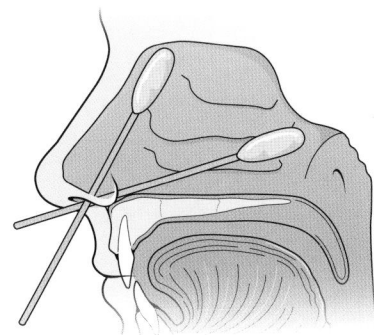

Figure 63-26 Placement of local anesthetic in the nose to block the anterior ethmoidal nerve superiorly and the sphenopalatine ganglion at the posterior end of the middle turbinate before reducing a nasal fracture. Cocaine is the preferred agent. *(From Schuller DE, Schleuning AJ, DeMaria TF, et al, eds. DeWeese and Saunders Otolaryngology: Head and Neck Surgery. 8th ed. St. Louis: Mosby; 1994:152.)*

Figure 63-27 Topical anesthetic and vasoconstrictors are applied on individually made cotton pledgets. The size of the pledget may be changed according to the extent of the nasal cavity to be anesthetized and the size of the patient. **A,** Grasp an appropriately sized cotton pledget with bayonet forceps. **B,** Then grasp the cotton with the opposite hand and rotate the forceps. **C,** The pledget is removed and is ready for insertion. **D,** To completely anesthetize the nasal cavity, three pledgets are necessary. The first is placed on the floor of the nose, the second in the middle meatus between the inferior and the middle turbinates, and the third in the roof of the nasal cavity and the anterior nasal vestibule. *Note:* This pledget technique can be used to make a cotton wick for the treatment of otitis externa.

nose 1 hour before reduction, in combination with topical intranasal anesthetic, provides similar nasal anesthesia for reduction of nasal fractures with less discomfort than occurs with needle infiltration.[30]

Examination

Examination of the nares is relatively straightforward, albeit *often quite stressful to the patient.* When using a nasal speculum,

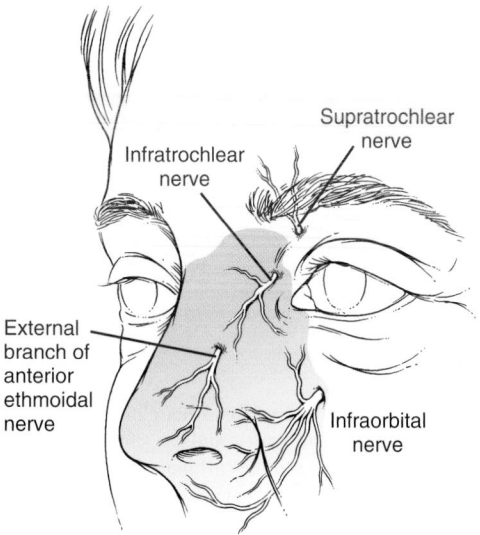

Figure 63-28 Sensory innervation of the nose. (*From Flint PW, Haughey BH, Lund VJ, et al, eds.* Cummings Otolaryngology: Head and Neck Surgery. *5th ed. Philadelphia: Mosby Elsevier; 2010.*)

insert it into the naris with the handle parallel to the floor and slowly open the blades in a *superior-to-inferior direction.* Stabilize your hand on the patient's nose to prevent damage to the mucosa from unexpected movement (Fig. 63-29). When attempting to visualize the nasal passageway, remember to have the patient keep the floor of the nose parallel to the ground. Tilting the head allows a view of only the anterosuperior area. A nasopharyngoscope may be used to view the nasal passageways as well, and its use is described in the previous section on examination of the pharynx.

Management of Epistaxis

Patients with nasal hemorrhage are commonly seen in the ED and account for about 1 in 200 visits.[31] Epistaxis occurs more frequently in the young (<10 years) and old (70 to 79 years). Most cases are traumatic and occur in the winter months. Approximately 6% require hospitalization.[32]

Identification of the source of bleeding and subsequent control are paramount to the treatment of epistaxis. Although this can be frightening to both the clinician and patient, a systematic approach with the proper equipment will lessen the anxiety associated with the situation (Fig 63-30). The goal of the procedure is to tamponade or cauterize the bleeding site. If the source is anterior, this may be the final treatment. For posterior bleeding, temporizing maneuvers are generally used until the process stops or a consultant can complete a definitive hemostatic procedure. The procedures can be performed in the ED with proper lighting and the equipment listed later in this section. Controlling epistaxis may be a time-consuming process without proper equipment or patient cooperation.

Epistaxis Management

Indications
Persistent epistaxis

Contraindications
Massive facial trauma with the possibility of a basilar skull fracture

Complications
Cautery
  Nasal septal injury/perforation
  Rebleeding

Anterior packing
  Sinusitis
  Nasolacrimal bleeding
  Nasal mucosa pressure necrosis

Posterior packing

Infection	Hypoxia
Dysphagia	Hypercapnia
Eustachian tube dysfunction	Aspiration
Tissue necrosis	Hypertension
Dislodgment	Arrhythmias
	Myocardial infarction
	Death

Equipment

Other equipment not depicted: light source/headlight, protective equipment, tongue depressors, kidney basin, gauze, silver nitrate sticks, 12-Fr Foley catheters. See text for details.

Review Box 63-3 Epistaxis management: indications, contraindications, complications, and equipment.

In preparation for any procedure to treat epistaxis, evaluate the patient's hemodynamic status by assessing vital signs and orthostatic symptoms and by quantifying the amount of blood lost. If the patient is symptomatic in any of these areas or if the blood loss is deemed significant, consider starting a

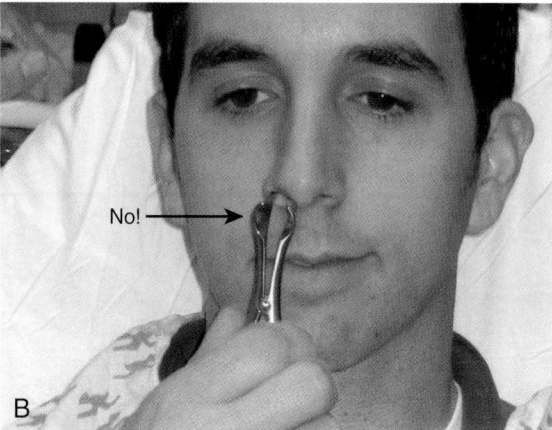

Figure 63-29 To properly examine a nose, use a nasal speculum. **A,** The clinician rests the index finger on the bridge of the nose (*arrow*) and spreads the speculum in an inferior-to-superior direction. **B,** It is incorrect to spread the speculum laterally or to use the instrument in an unsupported manner.

Figure 63-30 A nosebleed is frightening and interventions most unpleasant. Judicious use of parenteral sedation and analgesia, with attention to aesthetics, results in a more rewarding encounter. If required, intravenous morphine is a good choice.

large-bore intravenous line for administration of fluid boluses. Hematologic testing is rarely useful and not required for most patients, but in extenuating circumstances, obtain a complete blood count and consider a type and screen. Coagulation studies are not routinely indicated but should be undertaken in patients taking anticoagulants, those with underlying hematologic abnormalities, or individuals with recurrent or prolonged epistaxis.[32]

Many patients with epistaxis are hypertensive as well, often transiently secondary to stress and anxiety. No direct causal correlation between hypertension and overt epistaxis has been proved. The hypertension that is so often seen with epistaxis is probably a stress response instead of an inciting event. In a hypertensive patient one can administer intravenous opioids (such as morphine) to relieve stress and anxiety, thereby usually lowering blood pressure as well. In most cases, hypertension does not require treatment until evaluation after the bleeding is controlled and the anxiety of the situation has resolved. However, any patient exhibiting other signs of a true hypertensive emergency needs immediate antihypertensive treatment in addition to control of the epistaxis.

Epistaxis is rarely a manifestation of a nasopharyngeal neoplasm, unknown blood dyscrasia, nasal FB, nasal cocaine use, chronic use of nasal corticosteroid sprays, or aneurysm of the carotid artery.

Anticoagulated Patients with Epistaxis

Anticoagulated patients are at high risk for nosebleeds. However, the need for cessation of warfarin, dabigatran, or other anticoagulant or attempts at reversal of the action of warfarin are controversial and not well studied. It is reasonable to continue warfarin when hemostasis is achieved and the international normalized ratio (INR) is in the intended therapeutic range. An excessive INR calls for temporary cessation of warfarin and reversal if markedly abnormal (see Chapter 28). There is no known way to correct the anticoagulation from dabigatran, rivaroxaban, and other newer anticoagulants, but withholding use of the drug is appropriate. Dabigatran levels drop quickly and anticoagulation is almost immediate when reinstituted. Specific factor replacement will be required in patients with hemophilia.

Additional Testing for Epistaxis

Although an evaluation of coagulation parameters (prothrombin time, INR, platelet count) is not standard for patients with epistaxis, these studies should be ordered routinely for anticoagulated patients. Also, if the patient has chronic persistent bleeding, an evaluation of coagulation is prudent. A complete blood count is suggested for those with prolonged or recurrent bleeding to assess for significant blood loss. Though a rare consideration in the ED, epistaxis is a significant problem for patients with hereditary telangiectasia, von Willebrand's disease, and hemophilia. Generally, these conditions are already known. CT or magnetic resonance imaging of the nasopharynx may be considered for elderly patients with recurrent epistaxis to evaluate for neoplasm.

Indications and for Contraindications to Treatment of Epistaxis

Any continuing episode of epistaxis can be treated with the techniques listed in the section "Procedure." Massive facial trauma with the possibility of a basilar skull fracture would preclude the use of an intranasal balloon or packing because it may travel into the skull cavity.

Equipment

Preparation is the key to successful management of a patient with epistaxis. The following list of equipment should be readily available to the emergency clinician (see Review Box 63-3):

- Chair with a head rest or gurney with an inclinable back
- Headlight with a light source and head mirror
- Wall suction with multiple suction catheters
- Gloves, mask, and gown for the clinician
- Gown or drapes for the patient
- Topical anesthetic
- Topical vasoconstrictor
- Nasal speculum
- Tongue depressors
- Small red rubber catheters
- Bayonet forceps
- Scissors
- Kidney basin
- Gauze (4 × 4 inch, 2 × 2 inch), dental rolls or cotton, No. 2 surgical silk ties

- 1.2-cm-wide Vaseline gauze or 0.5-inch-wide Nu-Gauze packing
- Antibiotic ointment
- Silver nitrate sticks or electrocautery
- Pediatric Foley catheters (12 Fr)
- Nasal tampons
- Dual-balloon pack

Procedure

Because most patients are frightened by continued epistaxis and because nasal instrumentation can be annoying or painful, provide reassurance to the patient that the bleeding can be controlled with minimal discomfort. *Judicious use of parenteral sedation or narcotic analgesia is well supported* to make the entire interaction more palatable to the patient and ultimately more successful. Drape the patient with a gown to protect clothing from the bleeding. Have the patient hold an emesis basin to collect any continued bleeding and as a precaution to emesis of swallowed blood. Minor anterior bleeding is usually easily controlled with minimal techniques.

Ask the patient to sit upright in the sniffing position with the neck flexed and the head extended (Fig. 63-31). The base of the nose should remain parallel to the floor. After putting on a face shield, gown, and protective gloves, position yourself in front of the patient, level with the patient's nose. Have the

---

EPISTAXIS MANAGEMENT: INITIAL STEPS

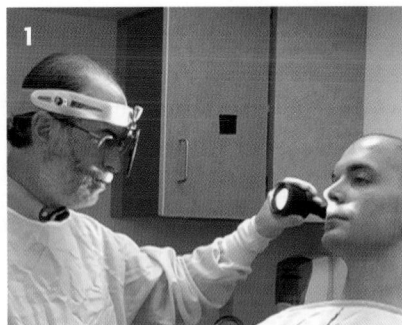

Position the patient sitting upright in the sniffing position with the base of the nose parallel to the floor. Proper lighting with a headlamp or mirror is essential.

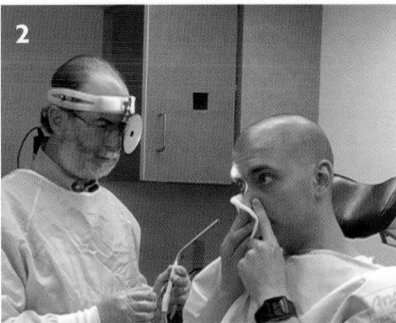

Ask the patient to blow his nose to remove all blood and clots from the nasal passage.

Alternatively, gently suction the nasal cavity. Suction from front to back along the nasal septum and then laterally.

If bleeding is minimal, attempt to locate the specific bleeding source. Use a nasal speculum to maximize visibility.

If bleeding is too profuse for visualization, apply a topical vasoconstrictor such as oxymetazoline.

Alternatively, cotton pledglets soaked in cocaine may be inserted into the nasal cavity with bayonet forceps.

Figure 63-31 Management of epistaxis: initial steps.

patient blow the nose to remove clots or suction the nasal passageway carefully. Suction from front to back along the nasal septum and then laterally. If the bleeding is minimal, *attempt to locate the specific bleeding source.* If the bleeding is too profuse for visualization of the source, administer a topical anesthetic and vasoconstrictor. Ask the patient to clamp the nostrils to limit bleeding and promote contact with the mucosa. If a discrete bleeding site is initially identified, an effective way to provide hemostasis and anesthesia is to inject the mucosa at the base of the bleeder with 2% lidocaine with epinephrine via a tuberculin needle and syringe device.

Insert the nasal speculum into the naris and use the suction catheter to evacuate any blood. Reapply anesthetic or vaso-constrictor if necessary. Because most cases of anterior epistaxis occur in Kiesselbach's plexus, inspect this area closely for areas of bleeding, ulceration, or erosion. After vasoconstriction, the only evidence of the former bleeding site may be a small prominent vessel. Many clinicians will gently stroke the septum with a cotton swab to initiate bleeding so that an exact area of pathology can be identified and then cauterized. If no bleeding source is found and the bleeding has ceased, pack the nose only if the epistaxis is recurrent. Wait 15 to 20 minutes before deciding on further intervention. If no anterior source is found and bleeding continues down the posterior aspect of the pharynx, assume a posterior source and consider packing the nose with anterior and posterior packs.

Cautery

After an anterior source of bleeding is identified, cautery may be used to achieve hemostasis (Fig. 63-32). Silver nitrate sticks may be used to cauterize but will not work on an actively bleeding source; hemostasis must be achieved first. Silver nitrate works well for a small, circumscribed area of bleeding. To apply, hold the tip of the silver nitrate stick against the site for 4 to 5 seconds. Apply again if necessary. Wipe away any excess silver nitrate to prevent inadvertent cautery of other areas of the nose. Most patient will sneeze after the application of silver nitrate, so be careful of blood splatter. If bleeding restarts, the initial cautery was insufficient and should be

applied again. The cauterized area immediately turns white or gray. Electrocautery works in the same manner but will penetrate more quickly than silver nitrate does. With either cautery technique, be careful to not cause septal perforation with overaggressive or repeated cautery. If cautery has not been successful after two attempts, use another technique.

Multiple attempts at cautery can significantly injure the nasal septum, and bilateral cautery should not be performed. If this is the initial bleeding and hemostasis is achieved, no packing is necessary. If it is recurrent bleeding within 72 hours of another or if cautery does not provide hemostasis, pack the anterior cavity. If hemostasis is accomplished, apply petroleum jelly or antibiotic ointment to the area to prevent desiccation. Loughran and coworkers[33] found antimicrobial ointment to be better than petroleum jelly in preventing bleeding. Do not administer aspirin or nonsteroidal antiinflammatory drugs for 4 days after epistaxis. If bleeding recurs at home, instruct the patient to pinch the nostrils closed for 20 minutes. Instruct the patient to return to the ED if this maneuver is unsuccessful or the bleeding is profuse.

Anterior Nasal Packing

Anterior packing achieves hemostasis, prevents desiccation, and protects the area from trauma. However, improperly placed packing may further abrade the area, dislodge prematurely, or migrate into the posterior pharyngeal area. Anterior packing must be placed with adequate analgesia, proper visualization, and deliberate movements. Coating any packing material with antibiotic ointment (if not contraindicated by the manufacturer) aids in placement and theoretically helps prevents infections and toxic shock syndrome (TSS) secondary to nasal packing. *Areas that continue to ooze after cautery are often treated with an anterior pack.*

Traditional petrolatum gauze has largely been supplanted by easier-to-use commercial devices. Packing is applied in an "accordion" fashion so that each layer extends the entire length of the nasal cavity (Fig. 63-33*A*). Place the speculum properly to allow visualization of the floor of the nasal cavity. Lay a strip of petrolatum gauze 1.2 cm across the nasal floor,

---

EPISTAXIS MANAGEMENT: CAUTERY

Cautery is used if an anterior bleeding source is identified. If no bleeding source is seen, brush the septum with a cotton swab *under direct vision* to stimulate the bleeding site. *If there is active bleeding, cautery will not work* and should not be attempted.

Silver nitrate cautery stick

Cautery should be attempted only under direct vision; do not blindly cauterize. To apply, hold the tip of the silver nitrate stick against the site for 4–5 seconds. Most patients will sneeze after the application of silver nitrate.

The cauterized area will turn whitish gray. If bleeding restarts, the initial cautery was insufficient and should be reapplied. Avoid multiple cautery attempts and bilateral cauterization because these practices may lead to septal injury or perforation.

Figure 63-32 Management of epistaxis: cautery.

EPISTAXIS MANAGEMENT: ANTERIOR PACKING

A "Accordion" Petroleum Gauze Pack

1

Place the packing in "accordion" fashion so that part of each layer lies anteriorly, which prevents it from falling posteriorly. Place the first layer on the floor of the nose and then remove the bayonet forceps.

2

Place a second layer on top of the first in an identical manner. After several layers have been placed, use the forceps to push the previous layers down onto the floor of the nose and pack them it tighter.

3

A complete anterior nasal pack can tamponade a bleeding point anywhere in the anterior nasal cavity and will stay in place until the clinician or patient removes it.

B Nasal Tampon (Merocel)

1

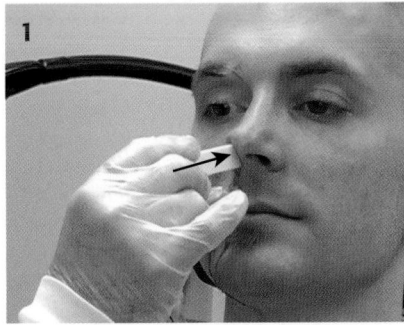

Trim the length and width of the tampon to fit the nose, lubricate with antibiotic ointment, and advance posteriorly, parallel to the nasal floor.

2

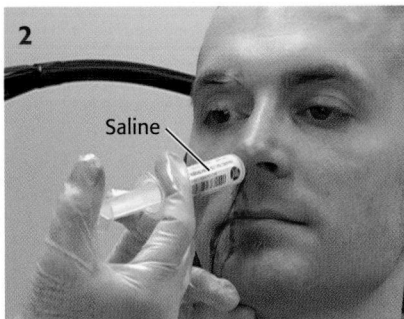

Saline

Once inserted, expand the tampon with 5–10 mL of saline.

3

If the tampon comes with a drawstring, it can be tied around a piece of gauze to prevent posterior displacement.

C Rapid Rhino Device

1

Soak in water for 30 seconds

Soak the device in sterile water for 30 seconds. Do not soak in saline because this can inhibit its gelling characteristics.

2

Insert the Rapid Rhino along the floor of the nasal cavity parallel to the hard palate until the plastic ring is well within the nasal cavity.

3

Fill with air only

Inflate the device with air (do not use water or saline) until the pilot cuff becomes rounded and feels firm to the touch.

Figure 63-33 Management of epistaxis: anterior packing.

with the starting end of the gauze at the naris. Gently pack the gauze strip into the floor of the nose. Measure the gauze so that it is twice the length of the nasal cavity. Grasp the gauze at the midpoint and insert this point all the way back to the posterior aspect of the nasal cavity. Attempt to place this layer of gauze without movement of the underlying layer. Continue this pattern, with replacement of the speculum after each layer, until the cavity is filled.

When compared with gauze packing, compression devices are easier to place, better tolerated, and very successful. Preformed nasal packing products are convenient alternatives to anterior nasal packing (Figs. 63-34 and 63-35). The Merocel packing consists of compressed polyvinyl acetate with or without a drawstring that markedly expands on contact with fluid and thereby exerts pressure on the bleeding site. The pack can be trimmed with scissors or a scalpel before

Figure 63-34 Preformed nasal packing devices. Preformed devices are easier to place and better tolerated than traditional gauze packing. The Rapid Rhino epistaxis device (ArthroCare ENT, Austin, TX) shown here has an air-inflatable balloon covered by a hydrocolloid fabric covering that allows easy insertion and removal. Various lengths and configurations are available. A wide variety of similar products are offered by other vendors. Although insertion techniques for preformed devices follow the same basic steps, review the package inserts of the equipment available at your institution before use.

insertion. The Merocel Doyle nasal pack has an airway tube in the center of the compressed material and a more anatomic shape. Each is available in various sizes, but usually an 8- × 1.5- × 2-cm standard Merocel or 8- × 1.5- × 3-cm Doyle will suffice. The Rapid Rhino Stat Pac (ArthroCare Corporation, Austin, TX; see Fig. 63-34*A*) is a high-volume, low-pressure balloon device with an open lumen air passage, a pilot cuff to check pressure, and a specialized Gel-Knit (carboxymethyl cellulose) covering designed to promote platelet aggregation. Numerous variations for anterior, posterior, and combination packs are available.

The easily applied nasal tampon is a reasonable first choice for most anterior bleeding (see Fig. 63-33*B*). Lubricate the tampon generously with antibiotic ointment and *trim the length and width carefully to minimize trauma to the nose.* Using bayonet forceps, advance the packing carefully along the floor of the nose. Remember to direct it parallel to the floor, not upward toward the top of the nose. Insertion may be painful, so use a single rapid movement. Once the packing is in the nasal cavity, expand it with 5 to 10 mL of saline, although contact with the moisture of the nose will often cause it to swell spontaneously. It is sometimes necessary to place two tampons side by side before inserting them to fill the nasal cavity and provide better pressure on the areas of bleeding.[34,35] Observe for 10 minutes after anterior packing to identify continued bleeding either anteriorly from the naris or running down the posterior aspect of the pharynx. Advantages of the Merocel tampon include rapid insertion, little discomfort, ease of use even by inexperienced personnel, and possible inhibition of bacterial growth.

The Rapid Rhino device is first soaked in sterile water for 30 seconds (see Fig 63-33*C*). Saline should not be used because it can inhibit its gelling characteristics. In addition, lubricants or antibacterial ointments are not needed. The device is then inserted along the nasal septal floor parallel to the hard palate until the plastic ring is well within the nasal cavity. Use a 20-mL syringe to inflate the device with air only.

Figure 63-35 Various packs for epistaxis in a cadaver model. **A,** A posterior Merocel sponge, not inflated, will stop most nosebleeds and is more comfortable than some balloon devices. **B,** Anterior/posterior Rapid Rhino in place. **C,** Double-balloon posterior pack with the balloon inflated.

Stop inflating when the pilot cuff becomes rounded and feels firm to the touch.

Corbridge and colleagues[34] found no significant difference in efficacy, patient tolerance, or complications between commercial products and gauze packing. Singer and associates[36] found that the Rapid Rhino nasal tampon is less painful to insert and easier to remove than the Rhino Rocket and that both were similarly effective in stopping nosebleeds.

Anterior packs are usually left in place for 2 to 5 days. Premature removal may result in rebleeding. A pack or device may stimulate mucus production and act as an impetus for

Figure 63-36 After packing, blood coming from a nosebleed exiting via the nasolacrimal duct gives the appearance that the eye is bleeding. Though benign, it can be alarming to the patient.

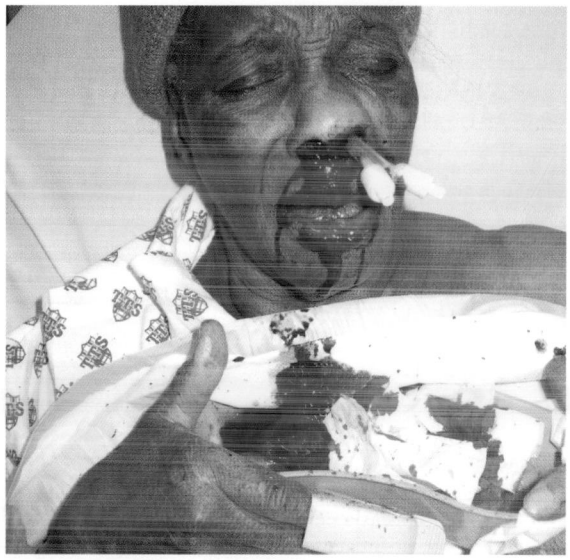

Figure 63-37 Posterior bleeding is usually readily controlled, but blood loss can be significant. Epistaxis is rarely a feature of nasopharyngeal neoplasm, unknown blood dyscrasias, nasal foreign body, cocaine use, or aneurysm of the carotid artery. This elderly patient was very anxious and quite hypertensive, and judicious use of intravenous morphine made the procedure tolerable and reduced blood pressure. Hypertension alone is not a cause of epistaxis.

infection. Oral antibiotics (e.g., cephalexin, amoxicillin, or trimethoprim-sulfamethoxazole) may be prescribed with any nasal packing after emergency treatment because of the minimal risk for sinusitis and TSS. The necessity of antibiotics for short-term anterior packing is unproved. Decongestants are also prescribed to decrease secretions. Practices vary and no common standards exist.

During use and before removal, keep the nasal tampon hydrated with saline. If it contains an airway tube, first remove the tube, irrigate the space once occupied by the tube, and then remove it. To remove the Rapid Rhino, first remove the air and then slide the device out.

Complications

Minor oozing of blood can be expected. Any packing in the anterior nasal cavity may obstruct drainage of the paranasal sinuses or block the nasolacrimal ducts and lead to sinusitis. Occasionally, blood will exit the nasolacrimal duct and be noted in the eye (Fig. 63-36). Other complications can include nasal mucosal pressure necrosis from the packing, balloon migration, and aspiration of the packing. Hollis[37] reported massive pneumocephalus after insertion of a Merocel nasal tampon in an elderly woman, presumably from fracture of the ethmoid plate. There have been case reports of ethmoid fracture after anterior nasal gauze packing and with the use of an intranasal balloon.

Posterior Nasal Packing

If no bleeding source is found anteriorly and the patient continues to hemorrhage down the posterior aspect of the pharynx, the patient most likely has a posterior source of epistaxis (Fig. 63-37). Posterior epistaxis may respond to topical vasoconstrictors. However, anterior nasal packing will not provide hemostasis for posterior bleeding because it will not cover the source of the bleeding. A posterior pack directly compresses the sphenopalatine artery and prevents the passage of blood or anterior packing into the nasopharynx.

Posterior Gauze Pack

A posterior nasal gauze pack is the classic method of treating posterior epistaxis (Fig. 63-38). However, because balloon devices are easier to use and less distressing to the patient, formal posterior nasal packing is less commonly used. To place a formal traditional posterior nasal gauze pack, anesthetize the patient's nares and posterior pharynx with topical

anesthetic. Prepare a roll of gauze with two silk ties (2-0) secured around the middle and extending in opposite directions. One set of ends will be used to place the posterior pack and the second will remain extruding from the oral cavity to remove the pack. Place a No. 10 red rubber catheter through the bleeding nostril. When it is seen in the posterior of the pharynx, grasp it with forceps and guide it out of the mouth. Attach it to one set of the ends of silk ties secured to the gauze pack. Retract the red rubber catheter, thus carrying the No. 2 silk tie through the nasopharynx and out of the nose. Grasp the suture and pull the pack into the nasopharynx. Guide the pack swiftly into the oral cavity and nasopharynx with the other hand. Attach the silk tie that remains in the oropharynx to the patient's cheek to aid in removal or rescue of the posterior pack. Use the silk ties exiting the nostril to maintain the position of the posterior pack. Pack the anterior passage as described for anterior epistaxis. Secure the silk ties over a gauze pad or dental roll. In the past, patients with traditional posterior packing were often admitted to the hospital for the duration of the posterior packing. Administering humidified air or oxygen often makes this pack more comfortable.

Inflatable Balloon Packs

Inflatable balloons come in two varieties. A Foley catheter is often used as a posterior pack because of its availability, ease of use, and successful tamponading effect (Fig. 63-39A). Insert a 12-Fr Foley catheter through the bleeding naris into the posterior aspect of the pharynx. Inflate the balloon halfway with about 5 to 7 mL of normal saline or water. Slowly pull the Foley catheter into the posterior part of the nasopharynx and secure it against the posterior aspect of the middle turbinate. Finish inflating the balloon with another 5 to 7 mL of normal saline or water. If pain or inferior displacement of the soft palate occurs, deflate the balloon until the pain resolves. Ensure proper placement before completely inflating the balloon because the balloon will remain too posterior in the

EPISTAXIS MANAGEMENT: TRADITIONAL POSTERIOR PACKING

1

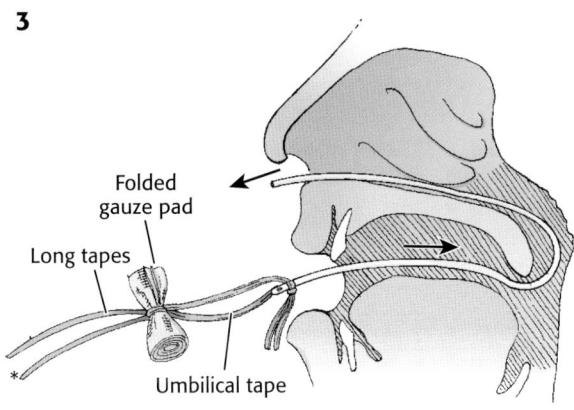

After applying topical anesthetic, pass a red rubber catheter through the nose, carefully grasp it in the oropharynx with ringed forceps, and bring it out through the mouth.

2

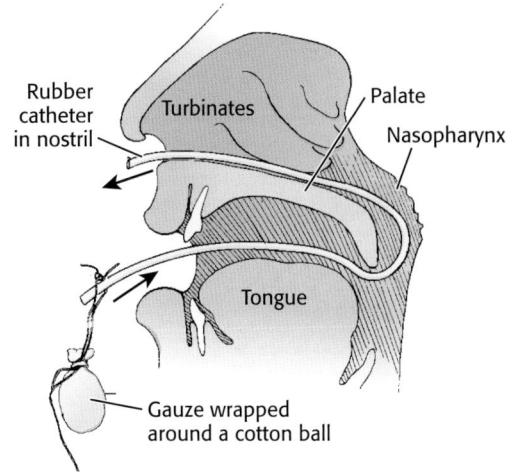

Make a posterior nasal pack by wrapping a cotton ball in a 4 x 4-inch gauze pad and tying two long silk sutures or umbilical tape around the neck of the pack. Leave one tie long so that it can be taped to the cheek until needed for removal of the pack.

3

Alternatively, fold a gauze pad, roll it into a cylinder, and tie it with two strings. Use two of the long strings to tie the pack to the tip of the catheter, and use the other two to remove the pack.

4

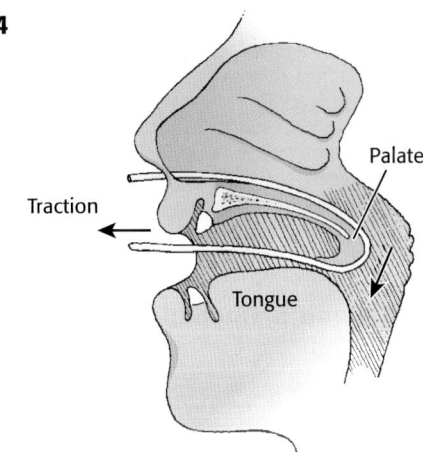

As an option, use a second catheter that has been passed through the nonbleeding side and brought out the mouth to retract the palate forward to aid in placement of the pack.

5

Remove the optional "retraction" catheter after the pack is in the proper position. Digitally guide the pack into the nasopharynx.

6

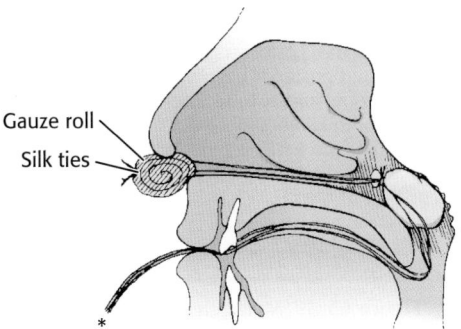

Use a gauze roll to secure the pack to the nose, and tape the rescue ties to the cheek.

Figure 63-38 Management of epistaxis: traditional posterior packing.

EPISTAXIS MANAGEMENT: POSTERIOR PACKING WITH INFLATABLE DEVICES

A   Foley Catheter Technique

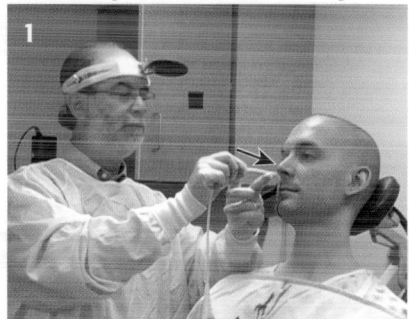

Insert a 12-Fr Foley catheter through the naris and into the posterior pharynx.

Look into the mouth to confirm that the catheter is properly positioned.

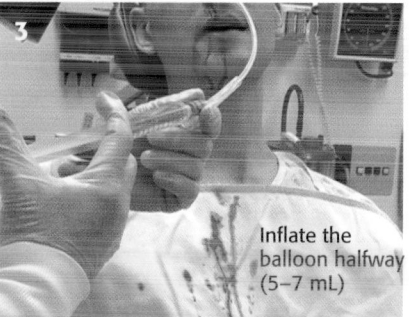

Inflate the balloon halfway (5–7 mL)

Inflate the balloon halfway with about 5–7 mL of water.

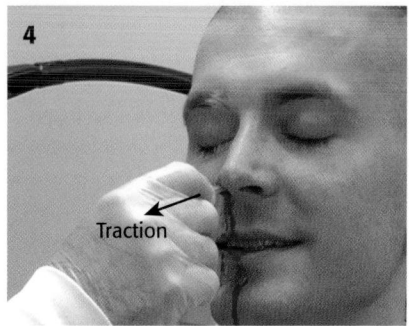

Traction

Slowly pull the catheter into the posterior nasopharynx up against the posterior aspect of the middle turbinate.

Foley catheter in proper position in the posterior nasopharynx. Inflate the balloon with another 5–7 mL of water.

Clamp here

While maintaining traction, place anterior packing with layered gauze. Packing of the opposite side may be required to prevent septal deviation. Place a piece of gauze on the exposed catheter and secure with an umbilical clamp.

B   Dual Balloon Tamponade Catheter

Posterior balloon Anterior balloon Airway tube

Double-balloon epistaxis catheters have both an anterior and posterior balloon, and some have an integral airway tube. These devices serve as both an anterior and a posterior pack. They are easily inserted and are often successful in temporary control of posterior epistaxis in the ED.

Insert the lubricated device along the nasal floor as far back as possible. Inflate the posterior balloon halfway with air, apply traction to pull the balloon up against the middle turbinate, and then complete the inflation. Maintain the position of the balloon and then inflate the anterior balloon with 30 mL of air.

Place gauze here to avoid maceration

This patient with posterior epistaxis was successfully treated in the ED and discharged. Historically, most patients with posterior packs were admitted to the hospital; however, the ease and safety of balloon devices allow selected patients to be treated as outpatients. Consider admission for the elderly, and those with pulmonary or cardiovascular disease.

Figure 63-39 Management of epistaxis: posterior packing with inflatable devices. *ED*, emergency department.

nasopharynx and fail to achieve hemostasis. While maintaining constant gentle anterior tension on the Foley catheter, place anterior nasal packing of layered petrolatum gauze. Pack the opposite nasal cavity to counteract septal deviation. Finally, place a short section of plastic tubing over the catheter and secure it with a nasogastric tube clamp or umbilical clamp. Be careful to not exert undue pressure on the nasal alae to avoid causing necrosis.

The second type of inflatable balloon pack is the premade dual-balloon tamponading system (see Fig. 63-39B). These devices have been a significant advance in the treatment of epistaxis. Several balloon devices are available (Goitschach Nasostat [Sparta Surgical Corp, Hayward, CA], Xomed Epistat [Xomed, Inc., Jacksonville, FL], and Epi-Max Balloon Catheter [Shippert Medical, Centennial, CO]). The dual-balloon pack has a posterior balloon that inflates with about 10 mL of air and an anterior balloon that inflates with about 30 mL of air. Each device may vary slightly. After appropriately anesthetizing the naris, place the lubricated pack along the floor of the affected naris as far back as possible. Inflate the posterior balloon about halfway with air, and then, with traction, pull the balloon into place up against the posterior aspect of the middle turbinate. Complete the inflation of the posterior balloon with air. Some clinicians prefer to inflate all balloons with saline instead of air because air may deflate slowly. *Inflate slowly, and stop if pain is felt. This is usually an uncomfortable sensation to the patient.* If the patient complains of pain or if the posterior soft palate deviates downward, deflate the balloon until the symptoms are relieved. Maintain the position of the balloon and inflate the anterior balloon with up to 30 mL of air. Again, halt inflation if the patient experiences increasing pain or deviation of the nasal septum. Some authors suggest packing the opposite naris to prevent such lateral deviation. Place a small piece of gauze between the nose and the external catheter hub to decrease skin irritation.

Most patients with a posterior pack, especially the elderly and those with pulmonary and cardiovascular diseases, should be admitted to the hospital for sedation and monitoring. This recommendation was common for formal posterior packs, but the ease and safety of balloon devices now allow selected patients to be treated as outpatients despite the presence of posterior packing.

Other Techniques

ENT consultation may be required for posterior nosebleeds that do not respond to the posterior packing techniques. Other treatment options that consultants may consider include ligation or embolization of the internal maxillary artery and posterior endoscopic cautery.

Complications

Posterior nasal packing is uncomfortable and often painful, but serious medical complications from posterior packing are rare. Complications associated with posterior packing include infection, dysphagia, dysfunction of the eustachian tube, tissue necrosis, and dislodgment. Other serious complications rarely and often anecdotally associated with posterior packing are hypoxia, hypercapnia, aspiration, hypertension, bradycardia, arrhythmias, myocardial infarction, and death.[38] It is questionable whether packing alone is the cause of these associated complications. Rebleeding may also be seen with early pack removal; one series found that removal of the packing within 48 hours increased the risk for rebleeding.[39] Most posterior packs are left in place for 72 to 96 hours.

Dysphagia from the packing can lead to poor oral intake and possibly necessitate intravenous fluid hydration.

A decrease in the arterial partial pressure of oxygen (Pao_2; 7.5 to 11 mm Hg) and an increase in the arterial partial pressure of carbon dioxide ($Paco_2$; 7 to 13 mm Hg) can be seen in patients with nasal packing who are *treated with sedation.*[38] However, despite traditional theoretical concerns, such altered pulmonary physiology cannot be attributed to posterior packing alone. Although it has been hypothesized that a posterior pack will cause vagal stimulation and thereby result in varying degrees of bradycardia and bronchoconstriction because of the so-called nasopulmonary reflex, studies have failed to substantiate substantial physiologic changes attributed to posterior packing. Observe patients with significant cardiopulmonary disease and posterior nasal packs in a monitored setting.

Tissue necrosis of the nasal ala, nasal mucosa, and soft palate secondary to improper placement or padding has been described. Protect the skin with gauze placed under the device to reduce skin maceration. The risk for necrosis increases with the duration of the packing, so all packing should be removed in 3 to 5 days.

If the posterior pack becomes dislodged, it will fall into the oropharynx and place the patient at risk for asphyxiation, vomiting, and aspiration. The patient and nursing personnel need to be familiar with the technique for removing the pack. To remove the pack, cut the anterior sutures that exit the naris from the gauze roll if they have not already broken. Grasp the sutures exiting the mouth and guide the packing out of the nasopharynx. It may be necessary to extract the packing with forceps or digits.

Antibiotics Following Nasal Packing

Posterior packing is associated with a risk for infection, including nasopharyngitis, sinusitis, and rarely, TSS.[35,40] Packing blocks the sinus ostia, which prevents proper drainage of the sinuses. TSS has been described rarely with nasal packing and is estimated to occur in about 16 per 100,000 packings. The syndrome is caused by a toxin released by *S. aureus* infection of the packing. A sudden onset of vomiting and diarrhea with high fever, as well as the development of an erythrodermic rash, heralds the onset of the disease. There are no data elucidating the effect of systemic antibiotics for prevention of TSS after nasal packing, and no recommendation can be made. Awareness of the condition is paramount. Antibiotics will not eradicate the carrier state of MRSA or other nasopharyngeal flora. It does not appear reasonable to provide antibiotic prophylaxis for fear of TSS.

Likewise, no data support or refute the routine use of prophylactic antibiotics after nasal packing to reduce the incidence of bacterial sinus infections. Short-term anterior packing is not likely to be a cause of bacterial infection of the nasopharynx and does not call for antibiotic prophylaxis. As with all forms of antibiotic prophylaxis, routine antibiotic use is associated with risks and side effects, including the selection of resistant bacterial strains. Despite the lack of proven efficacy, many clinicians provide prophylaxis against TSS and bacterial infection for patients with *posterior packing* for the duration of the packing. There are, however, no universally accepted standards or mandates regarding this issue. It may be reasonable to provide prophylaxis to patients at greater risk for infection, such as those with diabetes, advanced age, or an immunosuppressed state. If used, an antibiotic with staphylococcal coverage should be selected, such as amoxicillin-clavulanate. Topical mupirocin may also be used on various packing material, but the efficacy of this is unknown.

Patient Disposition following Nasal Packing

After successful cautery or a simple anterior pack, patients can be discharged with follow-up in 48 to 72 hours. The packing is removed at this time and the condition reassessed. Aspirin is avoided. Packs should be left in place. Merocel packs should be moistened three times a day with saline or water. If no packing is used, the patient can coat the cauterized area four times a day with antibiotic ointment or Vaseline and avoid the urge to pick the nose or remove any debris. If minimal bleeding recurs, oxymetazoline spray is usually effective.

Healthy stable patient with various forms of posterior packing or commercial packs can usually be discharged if the bleeding is controlled in the ED for 1 to 2 hours. Minor bleeding may be experienced, but return of significant bleeding requires reevaluation and generally hospitalization. Hospitalization is often appropriate for those with posterior packs, especially the elderly or those with concerning underlying medical conditions. Clinical judgment is the best arbitrator for admission decisions.

Septal Hematoma

Trauma to the anterior portion of the nasal septum may cause a hematoma to form. A buckling stress tears the submucosal blood vessels. If the mucosa remains intact, the blood will accumulate between the mucoperichondrium and the septal cartilage. Stagnant blood is an excellent medium for bacterial growth and the formation of an abscess. Common bacteria include *S. aureus*, *Streptococcus pneumoniae*, and group A β-hemolytic streptococci. Other complications of an untreated hematoma include septal perforation and cartilage destruction with a resultant saddle nose deformity. Septal hematomas may occur immediately after the trauma or, more commonly, in the first 24 to 72 hours after the injury.[41] The hematoma can cause significant destruction of the nasal cartilage and result in a cosmetic deformity.

Indications and Contraindications

The presence of a nasal septal hematoma requires drainage to prevent a cosmetic defect. The most common symptoms of a septal hematoma are nasal obstruction, pain, rhinorrhea, and fever. Most patients will complain of an inability to breathe through the affected side, but the absence of nasal obstruction does not rule out a septal hematoma. It is usually possible to diagnose a septal hematoma by inspecting the nasal septum with a speculum for swelling, pain, and a fluctuant area (Fig. 63-40). The presence of septal asymmetry with a bluish or reddish hue of the mucosa is suggestive of a septal hematoma. Inspect both sides because bilateral hematomas are possible. Direct palpation may be necessary since newly formed hematomas may not yet be ecchymotic. Palpation can further differentiate septal hematoma from septal deviation, which may appear to be similar because of asymmetry. The best way to palpate for a septal hematoma is to insert the gloved small fingers in each side of the nose and palpate the entire septum to feel for swelling, fluctuance, or widening of the septal space.

There are no absolute contraindications to drainage of a nasal septal hematoma. Caution should be used in those

Figure 63-40 Septal hematoma. **A,** Bilateral septal hematoma in a 6-year-old child. Obstruction is present on both sides of the nose (*arrows*). There was no response to vasoconstriction. **B,** If visual inspection of the nose with a speculum does not rule out a septal hematoma, the clinician's gloved fingers, passed posteriorly along both sides of the septum, may feel bulging or fluctuance. A normal septum is thin and smooth. (*A,* Image courtesy of Robert Hickey, MD, Children's Hospital of Pittsburgh, PA; *B,* from Flint PW, Haughey BH, Lund VJ, et al, eds. Cummings Otolaryngology: Head and Neck Surgery. 5th ed. Philadelphia: Mosby Elsevier; 2010.)

with known bleeding diathesis or those who are taking anticoagulants.

Equipment

Very little equipment is required to drain a nasal septal hematoma. A topical or injectable anesthetic should be used. For the procedure itself, a light source, a nasal speculum, a No. 11 scalpel blade, suction apparatus, scissors, nasal saline, small Penrose drain, and some form of nasal packing material are all that is needed.

Procedure

Treatment of a septal hematoma consists of evacuation of the clot with subsequent reapproximation of the perichondrium to the cartilage (Fig. 63-41). To drain the hematoma, incise the mucosa over the hematoma horizontally after adequate anesthesia is achieved. Suction out all of the clot and then irrigate with normal saline. Excise a small amount of mucosa to prevent premature closure of the incision and place a section of a sterile rubber band to act as a drain. Pack the nostril, as for anterior epistaxis, to reapproximate the perichondrium to the cartilage.

SEPTAL HEMATOMA DRAINAGE

1
After application of appropriate topical anesthetic (supplemented by local infiltration if necessary), make a horizontal incision through the mucosa and the perichondrium covering the hematoma.

2
Use small cup forceps or scissors to remove enough mucosa to prevent premature closure of the wound and reaccumulation of the hematoma.

3
Then place a sterile rubber band or gauze as a drain and pack the naris.

Figure 63-41 Drainage of a septal hematoma.

Prescribe broad-spectrum antibiotic therapy. Inspect the septum daily for signs of infection, recurrent hematoma, or necrosis. Evacuate recurrent hematomas. When there is no further hematoma formation over a 24-hour period, remove the drain. Pack the affected naris for 1 more day to complete the apposition of perichondrium to cartilage where the drain had been. If any evidence of infection is present, admit for intravenous antibiotics and surgical débridement.

Complications
Though rare, nasal septal abscess formation is the most common complication of septal hematomas. The infection can spread to the sinus cavities and lead to meningitis, cavernous sinus thrombosis, intracranial abscess, and orbital cellulitis.

A large or rapidly expanding hematoma may cause pressure on the septum and lead to avascular necrosis of the septal cartilage. The nasal septum can collapse and lose its shape, which causes a noticeable cosmetic defect.

After drainage, the hematoma may reoccur and should be treated by repeated drainage to prevent cartilage damage. Reaccumulation can be prevented by incising a piece of mucosa before packing the nasal cavity.

Reduction of Nasal Fractures

A nasal fracture is the most common facial fracture. Nasal fractures are accompanied by a broad range of symptoms, including mild swelling, epistaxis, and periorbital ecchymosis with obvious deformity. As with any trauma involving the head, evaluate for coexistent intracranial injury or neck injury. In the evaluation of nasal trauma, rule out the existence of a septal hematoma or cerebrospinal fluid rhinorrhea. In most cases the swelling and soft tissue deformity prevent adequate evaluation, treatment, or both. Evaluation of a patient with a suspected nasal fracture includes a thorough history, external nasal examination, and internal nasal examination using a nasal speculum with or without the use of a rigid nasal endoscope. Nasal radiographs are not routinely needed because they will not alter the course of treatment or injury.[42] Ask the patient to apply ice to the area and keep the head elevated to reduce soft tissue swelling. Refer the patient to an otolaryngologist or plastic surgeon for reexamination and definitive treatment in 3 to 5 days. Stress the importance of reevaluation within 10 days so that the bones do not set in a malaligned state.

Indications and Contraindications
The indications for reduction of a nasal fracture are first based on the type of deformity and degree of swelling present (timing of reduction). Only simple nasal bone or nasal-septal complex fractures, nasal obstruction or airway compromise from a deviated septum, and fracture of the nasal-septal complex with nasal deviation less than half the nasal bridge should be reduced in the ED. Other indications include less than 3 hours after injury in adults and children if minimal edema is present, reduction 6 to 10 days after injury in adults once the edema has resolved but before setting of the fracture fragments, and reduction 3 to 7 days after injury in children once the edema has resolved. The presence of nasal obstruction or airway compromise from a deviated septum should prompt reduction in the ED.

Contraindications to reduction of nasal fractures in the ED include severe comminution of the nasal bones and septum, associated fractures of the orbital wall or ethmoid bone, deviation of the nasal pyramid greater than half the width of the nasal bridge, caudal septal fracture-dislocation, open septal fractures, and any fracture older than 3 weeks.

Equipment
In addition to the standard equipment of nasal decongestant and anesthetic, nasal speculum, bayonet forceps, Frazier suction tip, anterior nasal packing material, and a good light source, some specialized equipment is needed, including elevators (Goldman, Boies, Salinger, Ballenger), Walsham forceps for grasping the nasal bones, and Asch forceps for reduction of the septum. An external nasal splint is also needed.

NASAL FRACTURE REDUCTION

1

Unilateral
fracture of
the nasal
pyramid

Dislocation
of the septum

2

Nondisplaced and minimally displaced nasal fractures often do not require manipulation, but the true extent of the deformity is difficult to appreciate initially. Note that the septum may also require subsequent intervention. Reduction of a depressed and dislocated nasal bone fracture is usually performed in 3–7 days, after the swelling has subsided and the true deformity is obvious.

Closed nasal reduction. Minor deformities with minimal swelling may be reduced in the ED and mitigate further therapy. After marking the distance of the intercanthal line on the elevator with a thumb, the tip of the instrument is used to reduce the medialized fragment by elevating it. The opposite thumb may simultaneously reduce a contralateral outfractured nasal bone (pyramid). Use the handle of a scalpel if an elevator is unavailable.

3

Asch forceps can be used to reduce a displaced nasal septum. Insert each arm of the instrument on either side of the nasal septum.

4

Use upward and outward force, perpendicular to the plane of the dorsum, to lift the septum until it is no longer overlapping. Then push with the instrument arms until the ends are aligned properly.

Figure 63-42 Reduction of a nasal fracture. *ED,* emergency department. (***Steps 3 and 4,*** *from Flint PW, Haughey BH, Lund VJ, et al, eds. Cummings Otolaryngology: Head and Neck Surgery. 5th ed. Philadelphia: Mosby Elsevier; 2010.*)

Procedure

Most fractures and patients with significant soft tissue swelling should be seen in follow-up for definitive evaluation and possible reduction of the fracture. Complicated fractures and septal injuries are usually referred for follow-up. Simple fractures with minimal local swelling can be treated by closed reduction (Fig. 63-42). Some patients prefer immediate correction, are not concerned with aesthetics, or are unable to comply with follow-up, so ED intervention may be an option. To minimize potential litigation, obtain written consent and take prereduction and postreduction photographs. Inform the patient that the outcome is not guaranteed because impacted fractures may not reduce and greenstick fractures may deform

again after reduction. Acute swelling may obscure the extent of the injury.

If minor manipulation is reasonable, anesthetize the mucosa as described earlier. For more involved manipulation, add a nasal nerve block. Intravenous sedation and analgesia may be necessary.

Most closed reductions can be done with a blunt elevator. A specific nasal elevator (Boies or Joker) or the handle of a metal scalpel can be used. The depth of insertion is determined by placing the instrument against the surface of the skin on the lateral aspect of the nose, with the distal tip at the intercanthal line. Mark the position of the instrument at the alar rim, and then insert the instrument into the nose and stop 1 cm short of the measured depth. Only the tip of the instrument should contact the medial side of the nasal bone. Lift the elevator anteriorly and laterally until the depressed fragment is in proper position. Use the opposite hand to pinch the nasal bones and mold the segments. If reduction with the elevator is unsuccessful, use Walsham forceps to manipulate the nasal bones. Insert one arm of the forceps into the nasal cavity and the other against the surface of the skin. Firmly grasp the displaced bone and disimpact and reposition it into the correct location.

Use Asch forceps to reduce the nasal septum (see Fig 63-42, *plates 3 and 4*). Insert each arm of the instrument on either side of the nasal septum and position it. Use an upward and outward force perpendicular to the plane of the dorsum to lift the septum until it is no longer overlapping. Then push the arms of the instrument until the ends are aligned properly.

Be careful to not perforate the cribriform plate when using surgical instruments. After the maneuvers, assess the reduction for proper alignment or subsequent displacement secondary to a greenstick fracture. If either occurs, refer the patient to an otolaryngologist to see whether open reduction is necessary.

Stabilize the reduction internally with nasal packing and externally with an exterior splint dressing (Thermaplast or Aquaplast). Some authors believe that splinting will mask an incomplete reduction or adversely manipulate the reduction during placement. The packing is removed in 5 days and the splint in 7 to 14 days. Antibiotic coverage is recommended.

Complications

Not all fractures will be reducible and such fractures should be referred for open reduction by a cosmetic facial surgeon (ENT, plastic, or oral and maxillofacial surgeon). Incomplete reduction may result in a poor cosmetic outcome. Reduction may produce a nasal septal hematoma, which if untreated, can lead to cartilage destruction and deformity. Reduction can also cause excessive bleeding. This can be managed with direct pressure and nasal packing. Direct infiltration of anesthetic may result in nerve damage or in dysesthesias or paresthesias after the effects of the anesthetic wear off. Finally, if nasal packing is placed, there is a risk for sinus infection.

Nasal FB Removal

Nasal FBs most frequently occur in pediatric patients, but it is not uncommon to find them in psychiatric or cognitively impaired patients as well. Usually, a family member has witnessed the event or the patient complains of discomfort from the FB. Patients may also have unilateral purulent or bloody nasal discharge, unilateral sinusitis, or recurrent unilateral epistaxis. Retained FBs, especially plastic ones, often initially fail to cause pain or other symptoms.[43] The lack of a history of FB insertion is of little value in children because many will not admit it. Therefore, emergency clinicians need to maintain a high level of suspicion for nasal FBs.

Types of nasal FBs vary widely and include food (e.g., meat, nuts, beans), rubber erasers, paper wads, pebbles, marbles, sponges, beads, jewelry, hardware (e.g., nuts, screws), and even certain living larvae or worms.[43,44]

Alkaline button batteries pose a unique problem because they may cause significant nasal injury within hours to days.[45,46]

They are composed of heavy metals such as mercury, zinc, silver, nickel, cadmium, and lithium. Injuries can occur and include mucosal burns, ulcerations, liquefaction necrosis, septal perforation, synechiae, and stenosis of the nasal cavity.[45,46] It is imperative that these batteries be removed promptly before tissue damage occurs as a result of leakage of the battery contents, electrical currents, or direct pressure. A relatively new and interesting nasal FB is the magnetic nose ring. These small, commercially available earth magnets are usually worn on either side of the alar cartilage and give the appearance of a pierced nasal stud. The magnets can be displaced and become polarized across the nasal septum. The magnetic attraction can be quite strong and may lead to pressure necrosis of the nasal mucosa and possibly septal perforation. This attraction can also make removal difficult, as well as painful for the patient.[46,47] Suggested techniques include using polarized or nonferromagnetic tools.[48]

Many nasal FBs come to rest on the floor of the anterior or middle third of the nose. Metallic or calcified objects may show up on radiographs, but physical examination remains the most reliable means for diagnosis. Maxillary, ethmoid, or sphenoid sinusitis may also accompany FB retention. Plain radiographs or facial CT scanning may be of value in detecting sinusitis, although these studies are not usually necessary with an acutely retained object.

Inability to remove a nasal FB should necessitate ENT consultation and may result in admission for removal under anesthesia; therefore, it behooves emergency clinicians to be skilled in this procedure. Although admission incurs increased cost, has inherent procedural risks, and causes psychological stress in parents and patients, providers should be prepared to call a consultant after several attempts. As with the removal of auricular FBs, removal of nasal FBs can be both frustrating and time-consuming.

Indications and Contraindications

Attempt removal of a nasal FB only if it is likely to be retrieved. ENT consultation is needed if there is any doubt about the ability to successfully retrieve the object. Repeated attempts may result in trauma and displacement of the object into a less favorable location.

Do not attempt mechanical removal if the object appears to be out of range of the instruments. In addition, do not attempt removal in an uncooperative patient unless sedation is provided. Use sedation cautiously because it may increase the risk for aspiration, especially when using agents that blunt the protective airway reflexes.

Equipment

The majority of the equipment used for removing FBs in the ear canal can also be used for nasal FB removal. Topical nasal anesthetic and vasoconstrictor solutions, such as oxymetazoline, can greatly aid in the removal of nasal FBs.

Procedure

A cooperative patient is essential. Weigh the risks and benefits of using simple or procedural sedation. Before attempting removal, anesthetize and vasoconstrict the mucosa of the affected naris topically. Ask an assistant to stabilize the patient's head, and immobilize a younger patient if necessary. Place more cooperative patients in the sniffing position and use a head lamp for proper illumination. Several of the techniques previously mentioned for removing an FB from the EAC can also be used in the management of a nasal FB, including the use of cyanoacrylate glue.

Manual Instrumentation

Use alligator forceps or bayonet forceps to retrieve anteriorly lodged FBs that have edges amenable to grasping (Fig. 63-43, *plate 1*). For harder or larger objects, carefully pass a wire loop, right-angle hook, or even a properly bent paper clip beyond the object and rotate it to allow the FB to be pulled from the naris. Direct mucosal trauma and epistaxis may occur with any of these methods. For a nasal FB with smooth, round edges that are difficult to grasp or get behind, attempt to extract it with a suction-tipped catheter in a manner similar to that described earlier for FBs in the EAC. The Hognose catheter described earlier also works well for nasal FBs (see Fig. 63-21). Local vasoconstriction and anesthesia are helpful, and 2% lidocaine with epinephrine (local anesthetic) may be used.

Balloon Catheter

For an object that cannot be removed with anterior instrumentation, one consideration is to attempt removal with a balloon catheter. A Fogarty catheter can be highly effective in removing a nasal FB (see Fig. 63-43, *plates 2 and 3*). A No. 4 or 5 vascular Fogarty catheter, a 12-Fr Foley catheter, and a No. 6 biliary Fogarty catheter have all been described in the literature for this use. A biliary catheter is reportedly less apt to rupture. Place the patient in the supine position and apply a vasoconstrictor and anesthetic to the nasal mucosa. With a 5-mL syringe attached and the catheter lubricated with lidocaine gel, pass the tip above the object and into the nasopharynx. Inflate the balloon with air or water (≈2 mL in small children and 3 mL in older children) and control the syringe plunger and balloon size with your thumb. Withdraw the catheter until resistance is felt, and then slowly pull the object out. The Katz Extractor otorhinologic FB remover (InHealth Technologies, Carpinteria, CA; Fig. 63-43, *plate 4*) is a disposable, single unit composed of a flexible catheter with a balloon tip attached to a syringe. The procedure is similar to that for the Fogarty catheter. Complications mentioned in the literature include mild posttraumatic bleeding, as well as the theoretical risk for airway obstruction by the balloon or aspiration from further displacement of the object.

NASAL FOREIGN BODY REMOVAL

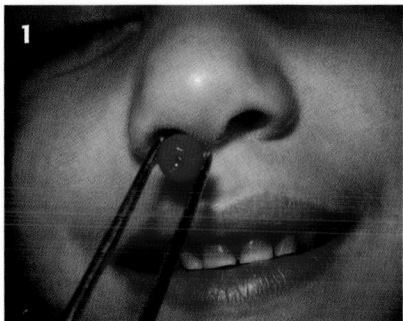

Following vasoconstriction and anesthesia (2% lidocaine with epinephrine was dripped into the nose), some FBs may be easily extracted with forceps.

A Fogarty catheter may be used to extract a nasal FB. Insert the lubricated catheter tip above the FB and then gradually inflate the balloon.

Slowly withdraw until resistance is met and then pull the object out of the naris.

The Katz Extractor *(InHealth Technologies, Carpinteria, CA)*. This device is used in an analogous fashion to the Fogarty catheter.

Bag-valve-mask technique to blow an FB out of the naris. Ensure that the face mask forms a tight seal around the patient's mouth and that the unaffected nostril is completely occluded. Attempt to firmly compress the bag as the patient exhales (an assistant is helpful to hold the mask snugly and to occlude the other nostril). This technique works best with objects that completely occlude the nostril.

To blow an FB out of the nose, have the parent blow into the mouth while occluding the unaffected side with the thumb.

Figure 63-43 Removal of a nasal foreign body (FB).

Positive Pressure

Another approach to a posteriorly placed nasal FB is to blow the object out with positive air pressure. The simplest way is to ask patients to blow their nose while occluding the unaffected nostril. This is really effective only in older children and adults. Alternatively, place a bag-valve-mask device[44,49] over the child's mouth to provide positive pressure (see Fig. 63-43, *plate 5*). Occlude the opposite nostril and apply the Sellick maneuver to prevent passage of air into the esophagus. This technique often requires restraint and can also be threatening to a young child.

The "parent's kiss" technique may be used in children.[44,50,51] First gain the child's cooperation by saying that parent is going to "give them a big kiss." The technique is performed by having the child lie supine. Ask the parent to occlude the child's unaffected nostril with the thumb (see Fig. 63-43, *plate 6*). Next, as in mouth-to-mouth resuscitation, ask the parent to make a firm seal with his or her mouth over the child's open mouth and then give a short, sharp puff of air briskly into the mouth to produce outward pressure behind the object. Keep the opposite nostril occluded throughout the procedure. The object should move within grasping reach of an instrument or pop completely out of the naris. If it fails, the technique can be repeated. Studies of the parent's kiss technique have found it to be highly effective, nontraumatic, and preferable to restraint or instrumentation.[50,51]

A modification of the technique that may be easier for some parents to master uses a drinking straw placed between the parent's mouth and the child's mouth. Instruct the child to make a tight seal, as though drinking, and ask the parent to deliver a quick puff.

Another similar technique may be successful.[52] After a nasal decongestant is instilled into the affected side, place a ¼- or ⅛-inch section of rubber or soft vinyl tubing (6 to 10 inches) into or at the contralateral nostril and hold the tubing in place with the fingers of one hand. Place the free hand gently over the child's mouth, take a good-sized breath, and blow forcefully through the tubing. This step may be repeated up to four times. In one study, success was reported in 40 of 41 cases.[52] Navitsky and colleagues modified this technique to reduce the risk for transmission of disease.[53] Turn a wall oxygen source to a flow of 10 to 15 L/min. Use a male-to-male adapter at the end of oxygen tubing to direct the flow of oxygen into the contralateral (nonobstructed) nostril.

Complications

Most complications are due to the FB itself and include pain, obstruction, rhinorrhea, ulceration of the nasal mucosa, septal perforation, infection, and nasal or choanal stenosis. Bleeding and mucosal laceration are the most commonly reported complications of removal. The bleeding is usually minor and generally resolves with simple pressure. It may occur as a result of the object itself or from trauma during removal. Inadvertent posterior dislodgement of the object may occur and result in ingestion or aspiration of the object.

Theoretically, barotrauma to the lungs and TMs may occur with positive pressure techniques.

MANDIBLE

Dislocation of the Mandible

Mandibular dislocation is more properly known as *temporomandibular joint (TMJ) dislocation*. It is actually the mandibular condyles that dislocate. It may result from trauma but more commonly follows extreme opening of the mouth such as may occur while eating, laughing, or yawning. It may also be seen with dystonic reactions to medications. Patients with a previous history of TMJ dislocation are more prone to repeated dislocations. The condition can be unilateral or bilateral (Fig. 63-44).

TMJ dislocation occurs when the mandibular condyle moves anteriorly along the articular eminence and becomes locked in the anterosuperior aspect of the eminence. Spasm of the masseter, internal pterygoid, and temporalis muscles occurs during an attempt to close the mandible. Trismus then results and the condyle cannot return to its normal position. Predisposing factors include anatomic disharmony between the mandibular fossa and the articular eminence and weakness of the capsule and the temporomandibular ligaments.

Indications and Contraindications

The presence of mandibular dislocation is the indication for reduction. The diagnosis is usually straightforward, but the

Figure 63-44 Mandible dislocations. **A** and **B,** This patient yawned and then could not close his mouth. This was a recurrent bilateral mandible dislocation. **C,** This patient was suspected of having a dystonic reaction because she could not speak and her mandible was misaligned. It was a unilateral mandibular dislocation.

condition can be misinterpreted as an acute dystonic reaction. Patients *cannot close their mouth*, and speech is affected. Pain varies, and patients are often very anxious. With unilateral dislocation, the jaw will deviate to the opposite side. More commonly, bilateral dislocation occurs. With traumatic dislocation, radiographic evaluation should be performed to exclude a fracture. A mandibular series, Panorex, TMJ radiographs, and facial CT are acceptable.

In the absence of a fracture, there are no real contraindications to reduction.

Equipment

Minimal equipment is required. An ENT or dental chair is helpful. Gloves, gauze, and a bite block should be available. Items to protect the operator's fingers such as tongue blades or plastic finger splints can be used.

Procedure

Reduction of a TMJ dislocation is fairly straightforward. Because anterior dislocations are far more common, these techniques will be discussed here. The key to reduction is to direct the mandibular condyle out of its displaced location anterior to the articular eminence[54] (Fig. 63-45A). Procedural sedation is usually required for easy and successful reduction. Local anesthetics can be injected into the TMJ space or directly into the lateral pterygoid muscle. For TMJ injection, prepare the skin anterior to the ear, and introduce the needle into the TMJ space at the palpable depression caused by the dislocated condyle. The needle is directed anteriorly and superiorly onto the inferior surface of the glenoid fossa, where 2 mL of local anesthetic is injected. For the pterygoid muscle, 2 to 3 mL of anesthetic is injected into the muscle posterior to the maxillary tuberosity.

Classic Technique (see Fig 63-45B)

With the patient seated and the head stabilized against the head rest, place a bite block in the mouth to prevent injury to the clinician. Wear gloves to protect your thumbs. Stand and face the patient and place your thumbs on the patient's lower molar teeth. The level of the mandible should not be higher than the operator's elbow. Once the thumbs are positioned on the molars as far posteriorly as possible, curve the fingers and hand around the angle and body of the mandible along the jaw and chin. Then exert steady, constant downward pressure on the lower molar region, and direct the mandible inferiorly and posteriorly back into the temporal fossa. Be careful because once reduced, reflex spasm of the jaw muscles can suddenly snap the mandible shut and injure your thumbs. Alternatively, place the thumbs on the mandibular ridge instead of the molars. For bilateral dislocations, both sides can be reduced simultaneously, but it is easier to do one side at a time.

Recumbent Approach (see Fig 63-45C)

With the patient lying recumbent, stand in front of the patient. Apply caudal and posterior force on the mandible as for the classic technique. Alternatively, stand behind the patient's head and place your thumbs on the molars. Apply downward and backward pressure for reduction.

Posterior Approach

With the patient seated, stand behind the patient. Place your thumbs posterior to the last molar on the retromolar gum and along the ramus of the mandible. Exert downward force in this position. This procedure carries less risk of the fingers being bitten, but proper positioning of the thumbs may be difficult to accomplish.

Ipsilateral Approach (see Fig 63-45C)

The ipsilateral approach involves three routes, extraoral, intraoral, and combined, which are conducted in sequential fashion. With this technique one side at a time is reduced. Stand at the patient's side. Attempt the extraoral route first. Use the thumb of your dominant hand to apply downward pressure on the displaced condyle just inferior to the zygomatic arch. Use the other hand to stabilize the patient's head.

If unsuccessful, attempt the intraoral approach. Exert downward pressure intraorally on the ipsilateral molar teeth. If unsuccessful, use the combined approach. Apply extraoral pressure with one thumb and intraoral pressure with the other thumb on the ipsilateral side.

Alternative Manual Method

This is similar to the extraoral technique described earlier. Place your fingers directly over the preauricular prominence of the dislocated condyle. Massage the condyle in a posterior and inferior direction to induce relaxation of the muscles and guide the condylar head back into the fossa. This pressure on the condyle may be uncomfortable for patients.

Wrist Pivot Method (see Fig. 63-45C)

Face the patient and place your thumbs at the apex of the mentum of the mandible. Wrap the other fingers laterally around the mandible and onto the occlusal surface of the inferior molars. Apply an upward force on the chin with your thumbs, and apply a downward force on the mandible with your fingers. Move the wrists in the direction of ulnar deviation. With these maneuvers, rotate the condyles inferiorly and posteriorly into the fossa.

Gag Reflex Method

The gag reflex method uses a component of jaw relaxation and transient descent of the mandible inferiorly. Induction of the gag reflex has been described as a successful method for reduction of mandibular dislocations. Provide tactile stimulation of the soft palate with a dental mirror or tongue blade in an awake patient. Muscle relaxation occurs and the mandible descends caudally so that the condyle moves inferiorly and relocates back into place.

After relocation and on discharge, advise the patient to avoid extreme mouth opening and to eat soft food for 1 week. Warm compresses, nonsteroidal antiinflammatory agents, and muscle relaxants may be helpful. The patient may be referred to an ENT or oral and maxillofacial surgeon for further care. Patients with chronic dislocation may require surgical fixation.

Complications

Complications include injuries to both the patient and operator. Patient injuries include redislocation, mandibular fracture (rare), joint cartilage injuries, torn ligaments or muscles, and dental or gum injuries as a result of trauma from the attempt at reduction. There may be complications associated with procedural sedation as well.

Operator injuries are usually caused by sudden masseter spasm after reduction. This results in the patient involuntarily biting down on the operator's thumbs. Take measures such as gauze and plastic finger splints to prevent such injuries to the thumbs.

MANDIBLE DISLOCATION REDUCTION

A   Anatomy

In the normally closed position, the mandibular condyle rests in the mandibular fossa behind the articular eminence.

In the maximally open position, the condyle is just under and slightly behind the eminence.

In the dislocated position, the condyle moves forward and upward slightly above the eminence; muscle spasm then occurs.

B   Reduction Maneuver

Sedate the patient or locally inject the TMJ with lidocaine. Wrap your thumbs with gauze and place them in the mouth on the back molars. Apply downward pressure on the lower molar ridge near the angle of the jaw.

Continue to apply downward pressure and push the mandible posteriorly. A rocking motion may be helpful.

C   Alternative Techniques

Recumbent approach with the operator at the head of the patient.

Ipsilateral extraoral approach.

Wrist pivot method.

Figure 63-45 Reduction of mandibular dislocation. *TMJ,* temporomandibular joint. (*C, From Chan TC, Harrigan RA, Ufberg J, et al. Mandibular reduction.* J Emerg Med. *2008;34:435-440.*)

Uvulitis/Angioedema of the Uvula

Most cases of acute angioedema of the uvula (uvula hydrops), also known as Quincke's disease, are spontaneous and no cause can be found. Affected patients wake up with a lump in their throat or a fullness when swallowing, look in the mirror, and see an enlarged uvula (Fig. 63-46). It appears as an edematous, pale, and watery-filled structure.[55] It is not painful. Most patients are young and otherwise healthy.

Although most of the time the cause remains unidentified, there are numerous known precipitants, including smoking of marijuana and cocaine (crack), trauma to the uvula by endotracheal tubes or suction catheters during general anesthesia, and sticking a finger down the throat to induce vomiting. This condition is not to be confused with hereditary angioedema (hereditary angioneurotic edema), which is due to C1 esterase inhibitor deficiency, a recurrent and potentially fatal condition. Uvulitis may rarely be caused by bacterial infection, particularly *Haemophilus influenzae* B, and can coexist with epiglottitis. Angiotensin-converting enzyme inhibitor use does not seem to be related, but nonspecific allergic reactions (food, environmental) have been postulated. This condition, though annoying, is usually benign and self-limited and resolves in 24 to 48 hours. Airway compromise is a theoretical concern but occurs only rarely. Evaluating and maintaining the airway are the most important concerns with uvulitis. The enlarging uvula can cause upper airway obstruction, particularly in children.

There are no controlled studies evaluating therapy, but numerous antiangioedema interventions have been used. Treatment includes topical epinephrine (applied with a cotton swab), subcutaneous epinephrine, intravenous H_1 and H_2 histamine blockers, and parenteral or oral corticosteroids.[56] Inhalation of nebulized vasoconstrictors (such as epinephrine or racemic epinephrine) is an attractive, yet unproven intervention. For severe cases, otolaryngology consultation is warranted, and invasive techniques such as needle decompression (scoring the uvula with a needle to drain fluid has been described) and uvulectomy may be necessary. In an acute airway emergency when intubation is not possible, clamp the base of the uvula with a hemostat and amputate the distal portion.

Posttonsillectomy Bleeding

Hemorrhage is the most serious complication of adenotonsillectomy, with reported rates of 0.5% to 10%, depending on the technique (Fig. 63-47).[57] Bleeding is categorized as intraoperative, primary (within 24 hours), and secondary (between 24 hours and 10 days). Bleeding is serious at all times and must be evaluated and controlled quickly if active. The most common time for patients to be seen in the ED with delayed bleeding is between the fifth and seventh postoperative days. Although some bleeding is minor, sudden severe hemorrhage can be fatal if not managed appropriately. If active bleeding is confirmed by physical examination, consult otolaryngology.

Figure 63-46 A, Very elongated uvula secondary to idiopathic angioedema that measured about 3 cm and reached past the midportion of the tongue. **B,** A globular-shaped enlarged uvula caused the sensation of a lump in the throat. Both cases were treated on an outpatient basis with antihistamines and prednisone after two doses of subcutaneous epinephrine (0.3 mg) in the emergency department. Both resolved over a 48-hour period without sequelae.

Figure 63-47 Typical appearance of the oral cavity 5 to 7 days after bilateral tonsillectomy. This is a common time for bleeding.

Figure 63-48 Posttonsillectomy bleeding is a serious complication that is difficult to control in the emergency department; an ear, nose, and throat surgeon and the resources of the operating room are often required. Massive bleeding can be fatal. This cooperative patient tried to tamponade her bleeding with direct pressure with a 4- × 4-inch pad on a hemostat, without success. She eventually became hypotensive and required urgent tracheal intubation and control of the bleeding in the operating room.

Minor bleeding 5 to 10 days postoperatively secondary to eschar separation may be evaluated and treated in the ED. However, multiple bleeding episodes are common in those who bleed, and minor bleeding may herald more significant subsequent hemorrhage. A severely bleeding patient should be taken to the operating room immediately for hemostasis. Up to 50% of patients who have major postoperative bleeding require control in the operating room. It is difficult and occasionally impossible to even initially control severe hemorrhage in the ED. Do not hesitate to intubate a massively bleeding patient to protect the airway and more easily perform local hemostatic maneuvers. Until the surgeon arrives, apply pressure directly on the bleeding area with a sponge on a long clamp (Fig. 63-48). The sponge may be dipped in epinephrine or thrombin powder if available. The bleeding area can also be infiltrated with lidocaine with epinephrine.

If a patient is seen in the ED with a complaint of posttonsillectomy bleeding but no active bleeding is found on examination and a blood clot is present, do not remove the clot. Definitive treatment and disposition are best made by the surgeon. If bleeding is present, it is prudent to admit the patient for observation. Obtain a sample of blood for a coagulation profile and a complete blood count. Blood transfusions may be required.

References are available at www.expertconsult.com

Emergency Dental Procedures

Kip R. Benko

Complaints pertaining to the teeth and supporting maxillofacial structures are common, and patients frequently go to the emergency department (ED) for evaluation. Complaints may range in scope from a simple chipped tooth to an odontogenic deep space infection or a maxillofacial injury. Treating these patients can be challenging and frustrating for busy emergency clinicians. Many emergency clinicians and other acute care providers do not receive specific training in dental emergencies during their training, yet it is important for them to be able to recognize and treat a wide range of dental problems. Some dental emergencies can lead to significant morbidity such as loss of teeth, chronic pain, infection, and craniofacial abnormality, whereas others can lead to life-threatening airway compromise.

Management of specific dental emergencies requires a thorough understanding of adult and pediatric dentition. The relevant anatomy of both populations is outlined. The techniques described for management of the various traumatic and infectious problems are, in most cases, temporizing until definitive dental or oral and maxillofacial surgery referral can be obtained. Conditions that require emergency consultation are discussed. Topical, local, and regional modes of anesthesia are of particular importance and utility in the management of odontogenic emergencies, so the clinician should be very familiar with these techniques.

Although this chapter describes the diagnosis and treatment of dental injuries that may confront emergency clinicians, no standard of care mandates that complex dental problems (e.g., replacement of avulsed teeth, drainage of infection) be definitively handled in the ED setting. Advances in ED equipment and clinician training, as well as the introduction of dental skills laboratories into the resident curriculum, are gradually raising the existing standard of care. The initial stabilization of fractured, subluxed, luxated, and avulsed teeth is now within the treatment realm of the emergency clinician. It is appropriate to refer all significant dental pathology to a dentist or oral surgeon.

TEETH

The adult dentition normally consists of 32 teeth: 8 incisors, 4 canines, 8 premolars, and 12 molars. From the midline to the back of the mouth on each side, there is a central incisor, a lateral incisor, a canine, two premolars (bicuspids), and three molars, the last of which is the wisdom tooth (Fig. 64-1). The 20 primary or deciduous (baby) teeth include 8 incisors, 4 canines, and 8 molars. From the midline to the back of the mouth, there is a central incisor, a lateral incisor, a canine, and two molars (Fig. 64-2). *Agenesis*, or lack of proper formation of a tooth or teeth, is not uncommon, especially in the maxilla. Likewise, *supernumerary*, or extra, teeth may also

occur. The adult teeth are numbered from 1 to 32, with the first tooth being the right upper third molar and the 16th tooth being the left upper third molar. The left lower third molar is the 17th, and the 32nd tooth is the right lower third molar. Numerous classification and numbering systems of the teeth exist; however, it is probably best for clinicians to simply describe the location and type of tooth in question (e.g., upper left second premolar, lower right canine). This removes any question when discussing a case with a consultant.

A tooth consists of the central pulp, the dentin, and the enamel (Fig. 64-3). The *pulp* contains the neurovascular supply of the tooth, which is responsible for carrying nutrients to the *dentin*, a microporous substance that consists of a system of microtubules. The dentin makes up the majority of the tooth, is a primary determinant of tooth color, and cushions the tooth during mastication. The *enamel* is the relatively translucent, outermost portion of the tooth and the hardest part of the body. The tooth may also be described in terms of the crown (coronal portion) and the root. The *crown* is the portion covered in enamel; the *root* is the part that serves to anchor the tooth in alveolar bone.

The following descriptive terminology is used for the different anatomic surfaces of the tooth. These terms are useful when describing the specific tooth injury to a consultant or colleague:

- *Facial*: The part of the tooth that faces the opening of the mouth. This is the part that you see when somebody smiles. It is a general term applicable to all teeth.
- *Labial*: The facial surface of the incisors and canines.
- *Buccal*: The facial surface of the premolars and molars.
- *Oral*: The part of the tooth that faces the tongue or the palate. This is a general term applicable to all teeth.
- *Lingual*: Toward the tongue; the oral surface of the mandibular (and maxillary) teeth.
- *Palatal*: Toward the palate; the oral surface of the maxillary teeth.
- *Approximal/interproximal*: The contacting surfaces between two adjacent teeth.
- *Mesial*: The interproximal surface facing anteriorly or closest to the midline.
- *Distal*: The interproximal surface facing posteriorly or away from the midline.
- *Occlusal*: Biting or chewing surface of the premolars and molars.
- *Incisal*: Biting or chewing surface of the incisors and canines.
- *Apical*: Toward the tip of the root of the tooth.
- *Coronal*: Toward the crown or the biting surface of the tooth.

THE PERIODONTIUM

The *periodontium*, also known as the attachment apparatus, consists of two major subunits and is necessary for maintaining the integrity of the normal dentoalveolar unit.

The *gingival subunit* consists of the junctional epithelium and gingival tissue. Gingival tissue is composed of keratinized, stratified squamous epithelium; it can be divided into the free gingival margin and the attached gingiva. The free gingiva is the cuff of tissue formed around the neck of the tooth. The

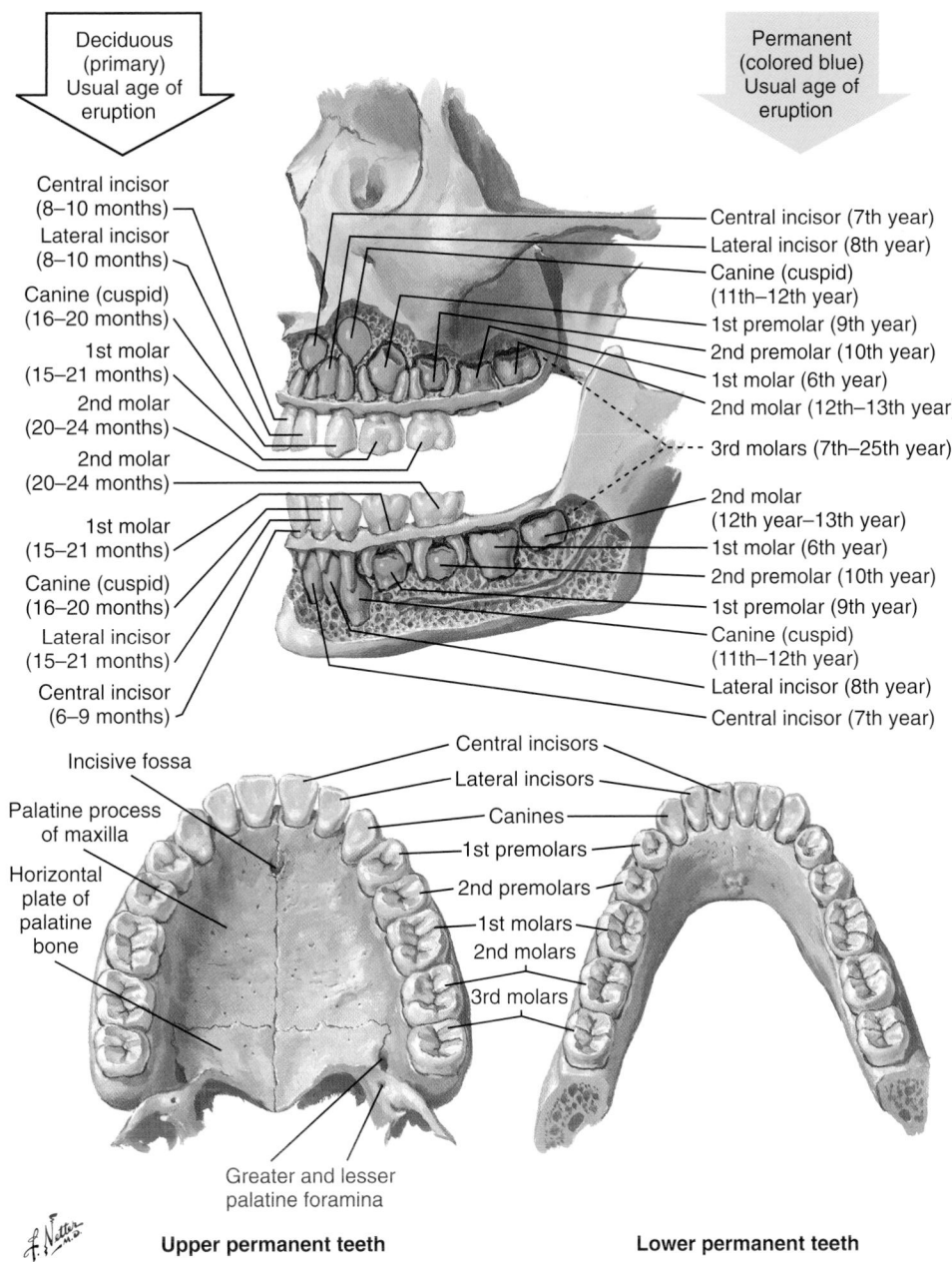

Deciduous
(primary)
Usual age of
eruption

Permanent
(colored blue)
Usual age of
eruption

Central incisor
(8–10 months)
Lateral incisor
(8–10 months)
Canine (cuspid)
(16–20 months)
1st molar
(15–21 months)
2nd molar
(20–24 months)
2nd molar
(20–24 months)
1st molar
(15–21 months)
Canine (cuspid)
(16–20 months)
Lateral incisor
(15–21 months)
Central incisor
(6–9 months)

Central incisor (7th year)
Lateral incisor (8th year)
Canine (cuspid)
(11th–12th year)
1st premolar (9th year)
2nd premolar (10th year)
1st molar (6th year)
2nd molar (12th–13th year)
3rd molars (7th–25th year)
2nd molar
(12th year–13th year)
1st molar (6th year)
2nd premolar (10th year)
1st premolar (9th year)
Canine (cuspid)
(11th–12th year)
Lateral incisor (8th year)
Central incisor (7th year)

Incisive fossa
Palatine process
of maxilla
Horizontal
plate of
palatine
bone

Central incisors
Lateral incisors
Canines
1st premolars
2nd premolars
1st molars
2nd molars
3rd molars

Greater and lesser
palatine foramina

Upper permanent teeth

Lower permanent teeth

Figure 64-1 Anatomy of the teeth, primary and permanent. *Note:* An avulsed primary tooth need not be reimplanted if it is lost traumatically. *(Netter illustrations used with permission of Elsevier, Inc. All rights reserved.)*

gingival sulcus is the space between the free gingiva and the tooth. It is rarely greater than 2 to 3 mm in depth in normal healthy dentition. The attached gingiva is the portion of gingiva attached to alveolar bone and extends apically (away from the tooth) to the mucogingival junction (or the muco-buccal fold). At this point the tissue, loose and nonkeratinized, is called the alveolar mucosa (or buccal mucosa).

The *periodontal subunit* includes the periodontal ligament, alveolar bone, and the cementum of the root of the tooth. The periodontal ligament consists of collagen that extends from the alveolar bone to the root of the tooth. One end of the periodontal ligament inserts into the alveolar bone and the other end into the cementum.

The gingival subunit is primarily responsible for maintaining the integrity of the periodontal subunit. Certain disease

states such as gingivitis weaken the attachment apparatus and can result in loss of a tooth.

ACUTE TOOTHACHE IN THE ED

Patients with an acute toothache (odontalgia) often come to the ED for dental evaluation and relief of symptoms. Although multiple problems can initially cause pain in the area of the teeth, the cause is usually pulpitis or dental trauma. Referral to a dentist is the logical definitive course of action, but pain relief can be initiated in the ED. Dental pain is, however, also a common complaint in drug seekers. Nonsteroidal antiin-flammatory drugs (NSAIDs), acetaminophen, narcotics, and local nerve blocks can provide relief of pain, depending on

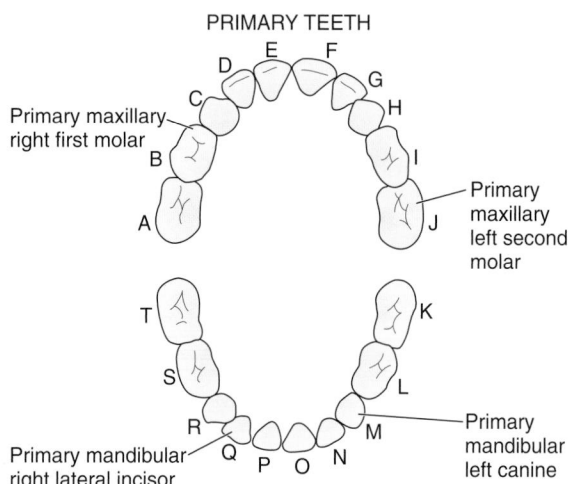

Figure 64-2 Identification of teeth, adult and child. Each tooth has a number assigned to it. By 14 years of age, all primary teeth should normally be lost. Do not reimplant an avulsed primary tooth; rather, refer to a dentist to prevent future misalignment of the permanent teeth.

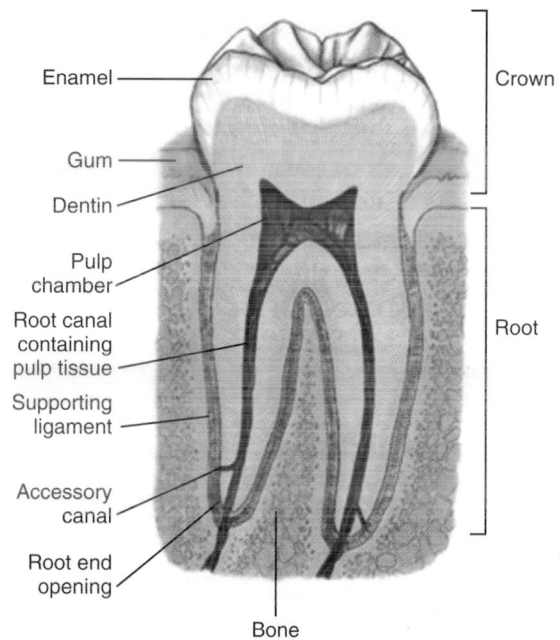

Figure 64-3 The dental anatomic unit.

the scenario. Hile and Linklater[1] recently reported significant pain relief in a fractured tooth by applying 2-octylcyanoacrylate tissue adhesive (Dermabond, Ethicon Products) directly to the tooth. This intervention is currently anecdotal but may also provide temporary pain relief for patients with open decay when air and temperature exacerbate the pain. Dry the tooth thoroughly with gauze, and generously apply a few layers of the product to the affected area. This intervention lasts for a few days only but should not interfere with subsequent dental intervention. Note that the use of skin adhesives has not been approved for intraoral use; they tend to break down quickly in the oral cavity.

Pain in a tooth when exposed to hot liquids usually indicates pulpal inflammation. Sensitivity to cold can signify simple sensitivity or gum recession but can also indicate decay. Pain while biting down can indicate a fractured tooth or decay.

Many fillings can leak and cause pain, and microcracks can occur and not be readily apparent to someone who is not a dentist. One cause of microcracks—or even a totally fractured tooth—is constant trauma from the metal balls implanted with tongue piercing.

For years, clove oil (containing eugenol) has been a popular and reasonably effective short-term home remedy for an acute toothache or inflamed gingiva. For a cavity or gum pain, saturate a piece of cotton in clove oil and place the cotton directly in the cavity or along the gum. This will provide relief for a few hours. Clove oil should not be used more than a few times because of irritation and possible nerve damage. A paste made of water and activated charcoal has also been used. Another simple method of pain management is to apply viscous lidocaine directly onto the tooth or saturate a small cotton ball with the gel and place it in a cavity. This treatment is temporary, and caution should be exercised if reapplication is considered. Do not exceed the total recommended dosage of lidocaine.

Acute dental pain may also be referred pain, so a complete evaluation should be conducted if the area appears to be normal (Fig. 64-4). For example, acute sinusitis can cause tooth pain and vice versa. Obvious dental infection should be treated with antibiotics (e.g., penicillin, clindamycin, erythromycin, metronidazole, amoxicillin-clavulanate [Augmentin]) while awaiting dental evaluation. Chronic acetaminophen overdose is a known complication of overaggressive use of analgesics by patients unable to obtain dental care for an acute toothache.[2] Unfortunately, many patients have irreversible pulpitis by the time that they seek emergency care.[3]

Antibiotics provide no benefit for pain from a simple toothache, dental cavity, or pulpitis, although some clinicians prescribe them because follow-up dental care may be delayed or difficult to obtain.[4]

Individual teeth (except the posterior molars) can be temporarily anesthetized with total pain relief by simply giving a periapical injection of a local anesthetic (see Chapter 30).

Figure 64-4 This physician had severe pain in his jaw thought to be related to a dental problem. Two days after onset of the pain, the rash of herpes zoster appeared, which was the cause of the pain.

Figure 64-5 A chipped front tooth after a punch to the mouth can result in a piece of tooth being aspirated or embedded in the laceration. When this lip laceration was explored, a piece of tooth was found embedded within the laceration. If this foreign body is not removed, an infection is certain to occur within a few days. Note the obvious chipped upper tooth, the source of the piece found in the upper lip laceration.

Bupivacaine has a long duration of action (4 to 12 hours) and has been shown to decrease the narcotic requirement of postoperative oral surgery patients even after the anesthetic properties of the medication have worn off. Molars, which are more difficult to anesthetize with periapical injections, can be blocked via nerve block techniques. Recently, articaine (Septocaine) has been used for this purpose. It is fast acting and penetrates well. Many dentists have replaced lidocaine with articaine for local tooth anesthesia. Note, however, that *this anesthetic is not used for nerve blocks, only local injection, because persistent paresthesias have been associated with nerve blocks.*

DENTOALVEOLAR TRAUMA

Dental Fractures

Dentoalveolar trauma is a common reason for ED visits. Injury to the maxillary central incisors accounts for between 70% and 80% of all fractured teeth.[5-7] Trauma to the teeth is not usually life-threatening; however, the morbidity associated with dental fractures can be significant and includes failure to complete eruption, change in color of the tooth, abscess, loss of space in the dental arch, ankylosis, abnormal exfoliation, and root resorption. Dental injuries are often associated with intraoral lacerations. When a tooth is chipped or missing and there is a concomitant intraoral laceration, it should be noted that the missing portion of the tooth might be embedded in the depths of the laceration (Fig. 64-5).

Some general principles apply to the evaluation and management of dental trauma. First, identify all fracture fragments and mobile teeth. Percuss each tooth surface for mobility and sensitivity. If a tooth is missing, it cannot always be assumed that it has been avulsed. Teeth can be aspirated into the respiratory tract, swallowed into the gastrointestinal tract, or fully intruded into the maxillary sinus, alveolar bone, or nasal cavity. Take radiographs if there is any suspicion of aspiration of tooth fragments or intrusion of fragments into the gingiva or alveolar bone. Second, the dentition is much more easily manipulated if the patient is not in significant discomfort. Tooth infiltration and common dental blocks should be part of the emergency clinician's armamentarium. Third, topical tooth remedies and analgesics, both over the counter and prescribed, should be discouraged because their

use can lead to the development of sterile abscesses and soft tissue irritation. Fourth, administer tetanus vaccine if needed.

Management of fractured teeth depends on the extent of fracture with regard to the pulp, the degree of development of the apex of the tooth, and the age of the patient. Dentoalveolar injuries and, in particular, tooth fractures can be classified in many ways.[8] The Ellis classification is one system often cited in the emergency medicine literature; however, many dentists and maxillofacial surgeons do not use this nomenclature, thus making it less than ideal when discussing these types of injuries (Fig. 64-6).[6] The most easily understood method of classification is one based on a description of the injury.

Crown fractures may be divided into uncomplicated and complicated categories. Uncomplicated crown fractures result from injuries to the enamel alone or to a combination of the enamel and dentin. Complicated crown fractures extend into the pulp.

Ellis Class I Fractures

Uncomplicated crown fractures through only the enamel are known as *Ellis class I fractures* (see Fig. 64-6*B*). They are not usually sensitive to either temperature or forced air. These fractures generally pose minimal threat to the health of the dental pulp. They may feel sharp to the patient's tongue, lips, or buccal mucosa. Immediate treatment is not necessary but may consist of smoothing the sharp edge of the tooth with an emery board or rotary disk sander. The patient should be reassured that a dentist can restore the tooth to its normal appearance with composite resins and bonding material. Follow-up is important with these injuries because pulp necrosis and color change can occur in rare cases (<1%).[6,9,10]

Ellis Class II Fractures

Uncomplicated fractures through the enamel and dentin are called *Ellis class II fractures*. Fractures that extend into the dentin are at higher risk for pulp necrosis and therefore need more aggressive treatment by the emergency clinician (see Fig. 64-6*C*). The risk for pulp necrosis in these patients is less than 10%, but it increases as treatment time extends beyond 24 hours.[6] These patients often complain of sensitivity to

Figure 64-6 A, The Ellis classification for fractured alveolar teeth. The easiest method to classify fractured teeth is by description (e.g., fracture through the dentin of the first upper right molar). **B,** Ellis class I: only the enamel is fractured. These fractures pose no threat to the dental pulp and are not sensitive to temperature or forced air. **C,** Ellis class II: the crown fracture demonstrates involvement of the enamel and dentin, without exposure of the pulp. Immediate dental referral is necessary to prevent contamination of the pulp through the dentinal tubules. **D,** This crown fracture involves enamel, dentin, and the soft tissue of the pulp as well. Immediate dental referral is mandatory to save the tooth. (*C and D, from Zitelli BJ McIntire SC, Nowalk AJ, eds.* Zitelli and Davis' Atlas of Pediatric Physical Diagnosis. *6th ed. St. Louis: Saunders; 2012.*)

heat, cold, or forced air. Physical examination reveals the yellow tint of the dentin in contrast to the white hue of the enamel. With fractures closer to the pulp cavity, the dentin will have a pink tinge. The tooth is usually sensitive to percussion with a tongue blade. The porous nature of dentin allows passage of bacteria from the oral cavity to the pulp, which may result in inflammation and infection of the pulp chamber. This is more likely to occur after 24 hours of dentin exposure but occurs sooner if the fracture site is closer to the pulp. Likewise, patients younger than 12 years have a pulp-to-dentin ratio larger than that in mature adults and are at increased risk for pulp contamination. For this reason, younger patients should be treated aggressively and be seen by a dentist within 24 hours.[10,11]

The goal of treating dentin fractures is twofold: to cover the exposed dentin and thus prevent secondary contamination or infection and to provide relief of the pain. After the tooth is covered, the dentist, using modern composites, can often rebuild the tooth directly over the calcium hydroxide (CaOH) cap that was placed in the ED. Perform supraperiosteal infiltration or a regional tooth block before any manipulation of the tooth. This will make application of the dressing easier because manipulation of the tooth will not cause discomfort. Dressings that may be applied to the surface of the tooth include CaOH, zinc oxide, skin adhesives, and glass ionomer composites. Some literature suggests that glass ionomer may be superior to other coverings; however, the difference is probably slight, and the increased cost of glass ionomer is not

justified for routine use in the ED at this time.[5,12] Certain composites may be cured with a bonding light. This is routinely done in the dentist's office and is beyond the scope of most emergency practice. Bone wax and skin glue such as the cyanoacrylates are not recommended as dressings. Most dressings come as a base and a catalyst, which require mixing. This is easily accomplished with a dental spatula and a mixing pad, which can be obtained from any dental supply house. A commonly used ED dressing is calcium hydroxide (Dycal or other similar products). Mix the catalyst and the base in equal portions, and place a small amount on the exposed area with an applicator such as a dental spatula or another appropriate instrument (Fig. 64-7).

Dry the surface of the tooth before application to ensure adherence of the CaOH. Have the patient bite into gauze pads to accomplish this. Dycal will dry within minutes after being exposed to the moist environment of the mouth. Although placing dental foil over the CaOH dressing is recommended, it is not usually necessary if the patient plans to follow up with a dentist within 24 to 36 hours. To prevent dislodgment of the dressing, instruct the patient to eat only soft foods until seen by a dentist. Begin antibiotic treatment with penicillin or clindamycin until definitive dental treatment can be obtained.[13]

Many patients who sustain a fracture through the dentin will require a root canal or other definitive endodontic treatment. Timely application of an appropriate dressing in the ED, however, may prevent contamination of the pulp and

CALCIUM HYDROXIDE APPLICATION

Calcium hydroxide is used to treat dentin fractures and aids in prevention of infection and pain relief. It is supplied in separate tubes of catalyst and base.

Mix equal portions of catalyst and base on the mixing pad that is supplied with the product. A dental spatula is an ideal tool; however, a simple cotton applicator will suffice.

Dry the tooth surface prior to application by having the patient bite down on a gauze pad. Then place a small amount of the paste onto the exposed surface. It will dry within minutes.

Figure 64-7 Calcium hydroxide application for the treatment of dentin fractures.

make root canal therapy unnecessary. As with any trauma to the anterior teeth, explain to the patient that disruption of the neurovascular supply is possible and that long-term complications such as pulp necrosis, color change, and resorption of the root might occur.

Ellis Class III Fractures

Complicated fractures involving the pulp are also known as *Ellis class III fractures* (see Fig. 64-6D). Complicated fractures of the crown that extend into the pulp of the tooth are true dental emergencies. These fractures result in pulp necrosis in 10% to 30% of cases even with appropriate treatment.[6] They may be distinguished from fractures of the dentin by the pink color of the pulp. Wipe the fractured surface of the tooth with gauze and observe for frank bleeding or a pink blush, which indicates exposure of the pulp. Fractures through the pulp are often excruciatingly painful, but occasionally, there is lack of sensitivity secondary to disruption of the neurovascular supply of the tooth.

Immediate management includes referral to a dentist, oral surgeon, or endodontist. The patient often requires pulpectomy (complete removal of the pulp) or, in the case of primary teeth, pulpotomy (partial removal of the pulp) as definitive treatment.[5,9] The longer the pulp is exposed, the greater the likelihood of contamination and abscess formation. If a dentist cannot see the patient immediately, attempt to relieve the pain and cover the exposed pulp (Fig. 64-8). If significant pain is present, perform a dental block. Subsequently, cover the tooth with one of the dressings described earlier. Sometimes the bleeding is brisk. Control such bleeding by applying a dressing. Ask the patient to bite onto a gauze pad that has been soaked with a topical anesthetic containing a vasoconstrictor such as epinephrine. Alternatively, inject a small amount of anesthetic/vasoconstrictor into the pulp to control bleeding. After the covering is applied, instruct the patient to follow up as soon as possible with a dentist. Antibiotics with coverage

Figure 64-8 Application of periodontal calcium hydroxide paste to the fractured surface of the tooth. The paste hardens quickly in the moist environment of the mouth.

directed at oral flora (e.g., penicillin, clindamycin) should be considered and only soft foods should be eaten. Removal of the pulp with specialized instruments by the emergency clinician is not recommended, although some authors have advocated this in the past. This procedure is the realm of the dental professional and is likely to result in complications if not done properly.

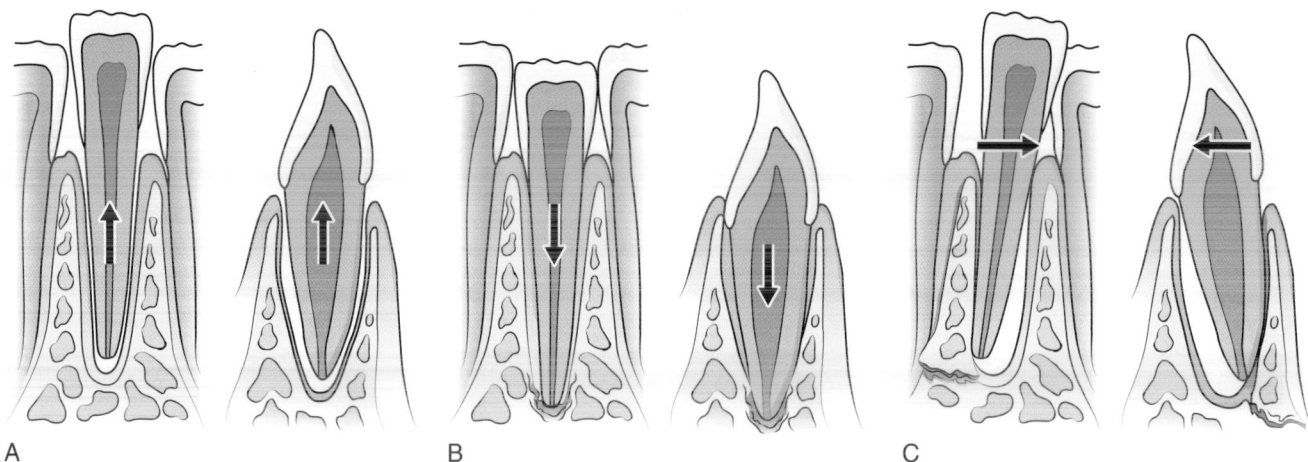

A   B   C

Figure 64-9 Classification of tooth trauma. **A,** Extrusive luxation occurs when the tooth is forced partially out of the socket in an axial direction. **B,** Intrusive luxation of a tooth compresses the periodontal ligament and vascular supply of the pulp. It may even crush the apical bone. **C,** Lateral luxation occurs when the tooth is displaced in a lingual, mesial, distal, or facial direction. Fractures of the alveolus frequently accompany lateral luxation injuries. (*A-C, Adapted from King R. Orofacial infections. In: Montomery MT, Redding SW, eds Oral-Facial Emergencies—Diagnosis and Management. Portland, OR: JBK Publishing; 1994.*)

Luxation, Subluxation, Intrusion, and Avulsion

Luxation and Subluxation

Subluxation refers to teeth that are mobile but not displaced. *Luxation* refers to teeth that are displaced, either partially or completely, from their sockets. Luxation injuries are divided into four types (Fig. 64-9):

1. *Extrusive luxation* is an injury in which the tooth is forced partially out of the socket in an axial direction (see Fig. 64-9*A*).
2. *Intrusive luxation*, or intrusion, occurs when the tooth is forced apically. It may be accompanied by crushing or fracture of the tooth apex (see Fig. 64-9*B*).
3. *Lateral luxation* occurs when the tooth is displaced either facially, lingually, mesially, or distally (see Fig. 64-9*C*). This injury is often associated with injuries to the alveolar wall.
4. *Complete luxation*, also known as complete avulsion, results in loss of the entire tooth from the socket.

Even minor trauma to the oral cavity requires meticulous examination for loose or missing teeth. Examine each tooth for mobility by applying a back-and-forth motion on each side of the tooth surface with either the fingertips or two tongue blades. Any blood in the gingival crevice (area where the gingiva touches the tooth) suggests a traumatized tooth.

Teeth that are minimally mobile and are not displaced do very well with just conservative treatment. The tooth will tighten up in the socket if not retraumatized. Instruct patients to eat only a soft diet for 1 to 2 weeks and see their dentist as soon as possible. Note that a seemingly lost (avulsed) tooth may actually be deeply intruded into the soft tissue (Fig. 64-10).

Grossly mobile teeth require some form of stabilization as soon as possible. It is important to note that in certain patients with poor gingival health, luxated teeth may not be salvageable because of disease of the attachment apparatus. Stabilization is best performed by a dental specialist with enamel bonding material or wire ligation. Although many different

Figure 64-10 Intruded tooth secondary to trauma. **A,** On superficial examination it appears that the tooth was simply knocked out. This missing tooth could be simply lost, fully intruded, or aspirated or swallowed. **B,** In some cases a dental radiograph or computed tomography scan is necessary to determine intrusion or avulsion. Intruded teeth create the potential for infection or cosmetic deformities. Intrusion of an upper tooth into the maxillary sinus can cause recurrent sinusitis. Teeth can also intrude into the nasal cavity and cause infection or bleeding, or they can be aspirated into the airway. The incisors are the teeth most commonly intruded.

DENTAL SPLINT (COE-PAK) APPLICATION

Coe-Pak is a periodontal paste used to splint loosened or avulsed teeth. Like calcium hydroxide, it is supplied as a catalyst and a base.

Mix equal parts of the catalyst and base on the mixing pad supplied with the product.

Roll the claylike mixture between your fingers into an elongated roll. Apply lubricating jelly to your gloves prior to handling the product to prevent it from sticking.

Dry the teeth and gingiva with gauze prior to application. Press the Coe-Pak into the grooves between the teeth, as well as across the adjacent teeth and gingiva. This type of splint works best when applied to both the front and back surfaces of the teeth, although it is usually sufficient to apply it only to the front.

Figure 64-11 Dental splint (Coe-Pak) application.

"home remedies" exist for splinting loosened teeth in the ED, the clinician must be aware of the possibility of aspiration of teeth if the splint fails. Avoid the use of unapproved medications in the mouth. Splinting techniques are suitable for the emergency clinician to perform as temporizing measures until definitive care can be arranged. One simple technique for emergency use is to apply periodontal paste, commercially available as Coe-Pak or other similar commercial products (Fig. 64-11). These products usually consist of a base and a catalyst that when mixed, form a moderately sticky claylike dressing that becomes firm after application. It is applied over the enamel and gingiva, as well as the adjacent teeth, to splint the subluxed tooth into place. Although the splint performs best if placed on the facial and buccal surfaces of the teeth, it is usually sufficient to apply the paste only to the front (facial) surface of the teeth. Make sure that the gingiva and enamel are completely dry. Lubricate your gloves with water or lubricating jelly before applying the dressing. Apply the dressing into the grooves between the teeth, as well as on the adjacent teeth. Remind the patient to eat a soft diet until seen in follow-up within 24 hours. Coe-Pak and other similar products are usually fairly simple for the dentist to remove during formal restoration.

Teeth that are luxated in either the horizontal or the axial plane or are slightly extruded can also be splinted with the techniques described earlier. It is important that the loosened tooth be in perfect alignment when the final adjustments are made at the dentist's office. However, the alignment does not need to be precise when the tooth is splinted in the ED. The important point is that the tooth be splinted adequately and follow-up ensured.

Intrusion and Avulsion

Intruded teeth are those that have been forced apically into the alveolar bone. This often results in disruption of the attachment apparatus or fracture of the supporting alveolar bone, especially in permanent teeth with mature roots.[11,14] These teeth are usually immobile and do not require stabilization in the ED. Intruded teeth frequently require endodontic treatment because of pulp necrosis. It is important to consider the possibility of an intruded tooth anytime there is a space in the dentition (see Fig. 64-10). Undiagnosed intrusion of the teeth can lead to infection and craniofacial abnormalities. Obtain radiographs when it is uncertain whether a tooth is intruded or simply avulsed. Intruded teeth are best managed by a dentist or dental specialist; referral should take place within 24 hours. Permanent teeth often require repositioning and immobilization, but primary teeth are usually given a trial period to erupt on their own before any intervention is taken.

Primary teeth are not replaced after avulsion because they can fuse to the alveolar bone and potentially cause craniofacial abnormalities or infection. Reimplanted primary teeth may also interfere with eruption of the secondary teeth. The parents of these patients need to be reassured that a prosthetic replacement for the avulsed teeth can easily be made and worn until the permanent teeth erupt. See Figures 64-1 and 64-2 as a guide to identifying permanent versus primary teeth.

Avulsed permanent teeth are those that have been completely removed from their ligamentous attachments. These are true dental emergencies. *The majority of patients seen in the ED with an avulsed tooth will lose that tooth*, so patient and physician expectations should not be overly optimistic. Under ideal circumstances, such as arrival at a dentist's office with a properly stored tooth avulsed less than 60 minutes previously, this situation may result in successful reimplantation 80% to 90% of the time but often requires specialized procedures and endodontics (root canal). Emergency clinicians are not expected to save an avulsed tooth, but prompt action may give that replanted tooth some chance for survival.

The first consideration in treating dental avulsions is to ask, "Where is the tooth?" Missing teeth may have been intruded, fractured, aspirated, swallowed, or embedded into the soft tissues of the oral mucosa. Therefore, radiographs should be considered anytime that an avulsed tooth cannot be located. Management of an avulsed tooth in the ED depends on a number of factors, including the age of the patient, the amount of time that has elapsed since the tooth was avulsed, associated trauma to the oral cavity such as alveolar ridge fractures, and the overall health of the periodontium.[14] Time is the other important consideration when deciding whether to replace an avulsed tooth. In general, the longer the tooth is out of the socket, the higher the incidence of necrosis of the periodontal ligament and subsequent failure of reimplantation. Periodontal ligament cells generally die within 60 minutes outside the oral cavity if they are not placed in an appropriate transport medium.[15] A significant amount of research has been conducted on different media used to keep cells of the periodontal ligament alive. Various transport media have been studied, including milk, Hank's Balanced Salt Solution, Save-A-Tooth, saliva, cell culture media, and water. Although certain cell culture media have been developed to stimulate cells of the periodontal ligament to proliferate and remain viable, milk and the commercially available Save-A-Tooth and EMT Toothsaver are the best and easiest for both prehospital care and ED storage (Fig. 64-12).[15,16] Milk will preserve the periodontal ligament for 4 to 8 hours; the commercial products will preserve the ligament for 12 to 24 hours. However, reimplantation should take place at the earliest possible opportunity after the socket has been

Figure 64-12 With the "Save-A-Tooth" (**A**) or "EMT Toothsaver" (**B**) systems, an avulsed permanent tooth is placed into the container and closed. Avulsed primary teeth are not replanted. The preservative will increase the life span of traumatized periodontal ligament cells. Unpreserved teeth replanted after 60 minutes rarely survive; those that do require root canal procedures and close follow-up. This system prolongs the time to successful reimplantation but does not ensure success.

adequately prepared. The key is to get the tooth into the transport medium immediately because even 10 minutes outside some type of storage medium can cause desiccation and death of the periodontal ligament cells. Use saliva at the scene if milk, EMT Toothsaver, or Save-A-Tooth is not available. The patient should reimplant the tooth in the prehospital setting if possible. The principles cited here should be followed when providing instructions to prehospital providers or to a patient who calls for advice. It is always preferable to refer such patients directly to a dentist rather than the ED if this is practical. Patients should be requested do the following:

- Determine whether this is a permanent tooth. By 14 years of age, all primary teeth should have been lost.

- Handle the tooth by the crown only because handling the tooth by the root can damage the alveolar ligament.

- Do not replace the tooth if it is fractured or if significant maxillofacial trauma has occurred such as an alveolar ridge fracture.

- If the tooth can be replaced in the prehospital setting, gently *rinse off* the root first to remove any debris. Do not wipe off the root because this removes the periodontal ligament.

- If the tooth cannot be reimplanted successfully in the field, place it in a transport medium as described earlier. Do not transport the tooth in the oral cavity such as inside the the cheek because it can be aspirated. This location is also not ideal for keeping the periodontal ligament alive because of the bacterial flora and low osmolality of saliva.

Once the patient arrives in the ED, confirm proper placement and alignment. It is not important that the tooth be in perfect position because the dentist can make final adjustments. Splinting the repositioned tooth with periodontal paste or composite as outlined earlier may be necessary if mobility is present.

Should reimplantation not be successful in the prehospital setting, it must be done in the ED according to the following guidelines:

- Store the tooth in an appropriate medium if reimplantation is delayed for any reason.
- Perform supraperiosteal dental infiltration with a local anesthetic before manipulating or replacing teeth to make the procedure more comfortable for the patient and easier to perform.
- Check the oral cavity for trauma. If an alveolar ridge fracture is present or the socket is significantly damaged, do not reimplant the tooth.
- Gently suction the socket first with a Frasier suction tip to remove any accumulated clot. Be careful to not damage the walls of the socket because this can further damage periodontal ligament fibers. Irrigate gently after suctioning. If the clot is not removed, reimplantation and realignment will be difficult. Rinse off any debris on the tooth with saline but do not scrub it. Implant the tooth into the socket with firm, but gentle pressure. Remember to handle the tooth only by the crown.
- Ask the patient to bite down gently on gauze to help align the tooth. The tooth may require splinting after replacement. If significant mobility is present such that temporizing splints are not adequate, consult a dentist to see whether wiring or arch bars are necessary.
- Update the patient's tetanus status as necessary.
- Prescribe a liquid diet until the patient is seen in follow-up.

Antibiotics are controversial in the treatment of fractured and avulsed teeth. Although the American Association of Endodontics does not recommend the routine use of antibiotics for fractures or avulsions, other authors recommend the use of antibiotics effective against mouth flora (e.g., penicillin, clindamycin) to decrease inflammatory resorption of the root.[6,17] It is probably reasonable to use antibiotics if the root or socket is heavily soiled; otherwise, treatment should be tailored to the individual patient and discussed with a knowledgeable and experienced consultant.

Ideally, but rarely possible in real life, the patient is immediately referred to a dentist, and the reimplanted tooth is held in place by biting on gauze. The tooth may be temporarily held in place with Coe-Pak or another similar product (see Fig. 64-11) or the technique described in Figure 64-13.

Prognosis

The prognosis of a reimplanted tooth depends on many things. As discussed earlier, the time until reimplantation is critical. Likewise, the age of the patient, the stage of development of the root (younger is better), and the overall health of the gingiva are also very important. An individual with gingival disease is more likely to have an unsuccessful reimplantation.

The goal in any tooth avulsion or fracture is to keep the native tooth if at all possible. A tooth that has been avulsed and reimplanted usually loses the majority of its neurovascular

Figure 64-13 Temporary suturing to hold a replanted tooth in place. **A,** Use a silk suture. Start by puncturing the gingiva at the border of the replaced tooth (*A*). Bring the suture behind the tooth and then cross over the front of the tooth to the other side. Penetrate the gingiva (*B*), go behind the tooth, cross over the front again, and tie the suture (*A*). **B** and **C,** Multiple teeth can be reimplanted.

supply and undergoes pulp necrosis. However, if the periodontal ligament remains intact, there is a greater chance of a functional tooth. It is important that the patient be aware that some root resorption is always going to occur after reimplantation and that loss of the tooth might occur.

Alveolar Bone Fractures

Trauma involving the anterior teeth may be associated with fracture of the alveolus, which is the tooth-bearing portion of the maxilla or mandible. Alveolus or alveolar ridge fractures often occur in multitooth segments and will vary in the number of teeth involved, the amount of displacement, and

Figure 64-14 Alveolar ridge fracture. Note that a section of teeth is misaligned. Clinically, the section is mobile and malocclusion will be present. *(From Baren JM, Rothrock SG, Brennan J, et al eds.* Pediatric Emergency Medicine. *Philadelphia: Saunders; 2007.)*

Figure 64-15 Facial computed tomography provides a definitive diagnosis of alveolar fracture. Here, axial and reformatted coronal images show a comminuted displaced fracture of the mandible with involvement of the alveolar ridge. *(From Soto JA, Lucey B.* Emergency Radiology: The Requisites. *St. Louis: Mosby; 2009.)*

the mobility of the affected segment. The patient generally complains of pain, as well as malocclusion. The diagnosis is usually clinically apparent and is notable for a section of teeth that are misaligned and variable in mobility (Fig. 64-14). Avulsed teeth, fractured teeth, or displaced teeth may be present within the alveolar segment itself. Dental bite-wing radiographs confirm the diagnosis. In the ED, Panorex or facial x-ray films may show the fracture line just apical to the root of the involved teeth; however, these films are often inconclusive or have normal findings. Facial computed tomography (CT) may provide additional information (Fig. 64-15).

Treatment of alveolar ridge fractures involves rigid splinting after repositioning the involved segment. This is usually beyond the scope of the emergency clinician, and urgent consultation with an oral surgeon or dentist is necessary. The role of the emergency clinician is to identify the injury, as well as any avulsed or fractured teeth, and preserve as much of the alveolar bone and surrounding mucosa as possible. Alveolar bone that is lost, débrided, or missing is difficult to restore properly.[12]

Lacerations and Dentoalveolar Soft Tissue Trauma

Trauma to the face and perioral region is often associated with soft tissue injuries such as abrasions or lacerations. Before any repair can take place, thoroughly inspect all wounds and abrasions to determine the extent of the wound and whether foreign bodies are present. Through-and-through lacerations are easily overlooked, as are small foreign bodies and debris such as tooth fragments. Obtain radiographs if there is any question of tooth fragments. Evaluate the patient for potential airway compromise.

As a general rule, repair injured teeth before undertaking soft tissue repair because manipulating the soft tissue while repairing teeth may damage sutures already in place in the soft tissues. Begin repair in the perioral region with standard wound care. After appropriate local or regional anesthesia, débride devitalized, crushed, or macerated tissue. Irrigate profusely. The role of antibiotics in mucosal trauma has not been conclusively established, and there is no definitive standard of care. Several studies suggest a minimal benefit; however, this remains to be completely proved.[18] A reasonable guideline to follow is to use antibiotics if a significant amount of devitalized or crushed tissue is present or if the wound is a through-and-through laceration. Coverage of oral flora (e.g., penicillin, clindamycin) is fine for mouth lacerations, and additional skin coverage (e.g., clindamycin, dicloxacillin) should be considered for through-and-through lacerations. Dentoalveolar trauma may present the emergency clinician with several different situations that should generally be approached as follows.

Buccal Mucosa

Most small lacerations and abrasions of the buccal mucosa heal quickly and rapidly without repair, but large lacerations (>1 to 2 cm) should be repaired. Use any absorbable suture such as chromic gut or Vicryl in the mouth, but place the sutures so that the knots are buried. Silk is an alternative but has higher reactivity and is nonabsorbable. Avoid using nylon because it is sharp and irritating to tissues.

Through-and-through lacerations of the oral cavity present a special situation. Evaluate for damage to the salivary ducts (Wharton's duct and Stensen's duct) and to the facial nerve. If they are intact, proceed with repair. Guidelines for closure are controversial, but larger lacerations (>1 to 2 cm) should generally be closed. Close the mucosa with absorbable sutures as noted earlier, and close the skin aesthetically with 6-0 nylon, Prolene, or a rapidly absorbable suture. Close the mucosa first so that the skin repair is not disturbed. If the mucosal wound is small or is a puncture wound, it is reasonable to close only the skin layer. Refer very large, gaping, or complicated lacerations to an oral surgeon.

Recheck large or through-and-through lacerations of the oral cavity in 2 to 3 days. Remove nonabsorbable sutures in 7 to 10 days. Advise the patient to rinse four to six times a day with saline solution. Prescribe a soft diet. Apply a topical skin antibiotic for 24 to 48 hours.

Gingiva

Small lacerations of the hard gingiva overlying the maxillary or mandibular alveolus usually heal uneventfully without repair. If the laceration is large, if a flap is present, or if bone is exposed, approximate the gingiva with a 4-0 or 5-0 Vicryl

Figure 64-16 A, Gingival lacerations sometimes leave little tissue for approximation. **B,** The teeth can be used as anchors for sutures and to help approximate the lacerated tissue. **C,** Gingival lacerations usually heal rapidly.

Figure 64-17 Large gingival avulsions should be approximated to an anatomic position with interrupted sutures.

The Tongue

Tongue lacerations are challenging. Although they may be tempting to suture, most large lacerations of the body of the tongue, such as those that occur from a seizure, will heal well without suturing (Fig. 64-19). Tongue lacerations that have the wound edges approximated do not need to be sutured. Repair larger lacerations that gape because the cleft left by the wound will epithelialize and leave a grooved or bifid or lateral flap appearance. Approximate wounds that are bleeding profusely, are flap shaped, involve muscle, or are on the edge of the tongue. Small avulsions (divots) or those in the center of the tongue usually heal without intervention.

Explain the procedure in detail to the patient before repairing these wounds. Ask an assistant to secure the tongue by holding it with gauze. If the tongue cannot be secured in this manner, apply a towel clip to the end of the anesthetized tongue. Children with tongue lacerations that need repair generally require sedation or repair by a specialist in the surgical suite, but many of these lacerations are small and heal uneventfully on their own.

Begin the repair with either local infiltration of an anesthetic or a lingual block (see Chapter 30). To promote hemostasis, infiltrate locally with lidocaine with epinephrine. Use absorbable sutures such as 4-0 chromic, Vicryl, or Dexon. Silk can be used, but it must be removed in 7 to 10 days. Do not use nylon because it is very irritating to the surrounding tissues. *For lacerations extending through muscle, close with one deep stitch penetrating both the mucosa and the muscle.* When possible, bury the knots of absorbable suture because they will often work their way loose. Full-thickness lacerations can be closed in a number of ways. Place a suture through all three layers or close the top mucosa and muscle together and do the same thing on the underside of the tongue. Bleeding from large lacerations is almost always controlled with primary repair. In some instances, hemostasis can be achieved without the use of sutures by using Gelfoam impregnated with topical thrombin (Fig. 64-20).

ORAL HEMORRHAGE

Bleeding from the oral cavity is not unusual and is most commonly associated with dental procedures. It is important to ascertain whether any recent dental work has been performed and what was done. Spontaneous bleeding of the gingiva or oral cavity not associated with dental manipulation or trauma is suggestive of advanced periodontal disease or an underlying

or Dexon suture. As mentioned earlier, silk is another option. It is difficult to suture gingiva because there is little supporting soft tissue underneath. A helpful technique is to wrap the suture around the teeth circumferentially and use the teeth as anchors (Fig. 64-16). Large lacerations should be repaired to approximate the gingiva and cover the base of the teeth (Figs. 64-17 and 64-18).

Frenulum

The maxillary frenulum rarely requires sutures for simple lacerations. If the laceration is extensive or extends significantly into the surrounding mucosa or gingiva, approximate it with chromic Vicryl or Dexon suture. These wounds are often significantly painful. Prescribe analgesic medications even if the wound does not require suturing. The lingual frenulum is very vascular in nature and will often need a suture or two to control hemostasis. Use a local anesthetic with a vasoconstrictor to aid in hemostasis while the wound is repaired.

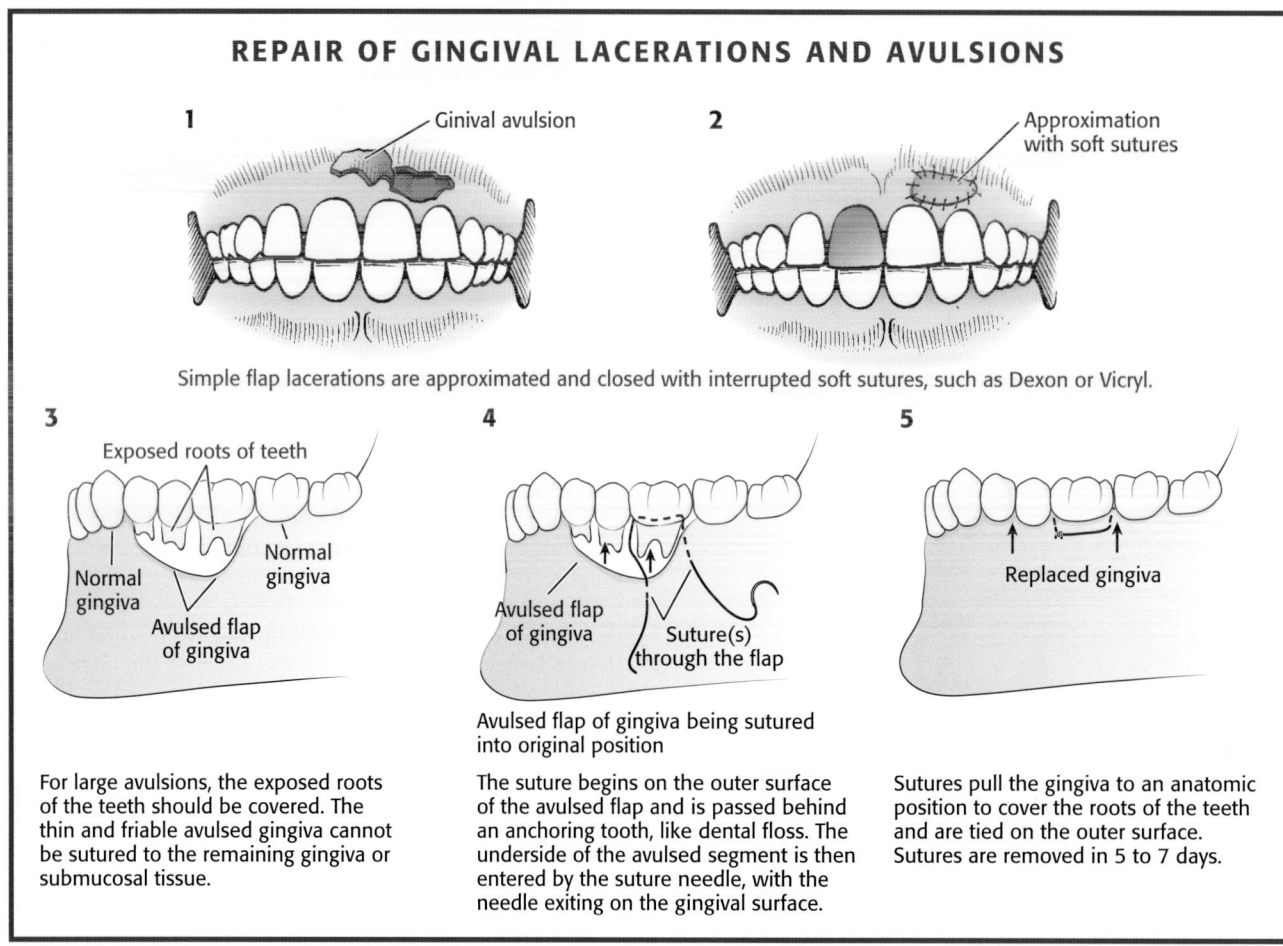

REPAIR OF GINGIVAL LACERATIONS AND AVULSIONS

1 — Ginival avulsion

2 — Approximation with soft sutures

Simple flap lacerations are approximated and closed with interrupted soft sutures, such as Dexon or Vicryl.

3
Exposed roots of teeth
Normal gingiva
Normal gingiva
Avulsed flap of gingiva

4
Avulsed flap of gingiva
Suture(s) through the flap
Avulsed flap of gingiva being sutured into original position

5
Replaced gingiva

For large avulsions, the exposed roots of the teeth should be covered. The thin and friable avulsed gingiva cannot be sutured to the remaining gingiva or submucosal tissue.

The suture begins on the outer surface of the avulsed flap and is passed behind an anchoring tooth, like dental floss. The underside of the avulsed segment is then entered by the suture needle, with the needle exiting on the gingival surface.

Sutures pull the gingiva to an anatomic position to cover the roots of the teeth and are tied on the outer surface. Sutures are removed in 5 to 7 days.

Figure 64-18 Repair of gingival lacerations and avulsions.

systemic process. Ask the patient about other medical conditions that predispose to bleeding (e.g., liver disease, platelet abnormalities), as well as historical factors that may suggest a bleeding abnormality or clotting factor deficiency. Find out whether the patient is taking aspirin or other anticoagulants. Consider laboratory testing if pathologic coagulopathy is a significant concern, but not routinely in a patient seen after dental manipulation.

Control gingival bleeding after scaling or minor dental procedures with direct pressure and saline or hydrogen peroxide rinses. Persistent bleeding from the gingival areas despite pressure and rinses raises suspicion of a bleeding abnormality. A much more common cause of oral hemorrhage seen in the ED is postextraction bleeding. Minor oozing after dental extractions, such as wisdom tooth extraction, is normal for 2 to 4 days after surgery, but many patients get concerned when the bleeding persists despite warnings from the oral surgeon. These patients usually go to the ED when their dentist cannot be contacted and after futile attempts to stop the bleeding at home. The emergency clinician has a number of options to achieve hemostasis of postextraction bleeding.

Direct Pressure

Although the patient may have been using this technique at home, a few simple procedures may make it more effective. If a clot is present inside a recently removed tooth socket,

leave it intact. If excessive clot has built up around the oozing site, remove the excess clot with a suction catheter and then gently irrigate the area. Frequently, this clot is missing or partially missing. Once the clot is removed, place gauze as firmly as possible directly onto the bleeding site. This is best accomplished by using dental roll gauze (see "Dental Material," later in this chapter). Insert it directly over the bleeding site and then cover it with 2- × 2-inch gauze. Dental roll gauze fits more precisely between the teeth and therefore affords more pressure; however, 2- × 2-inch gauze can be substituted. Moisten the roll gauze with a topical vasoconstrictor before placing it over the bleeding site. Instruct the patient to bite down and hold pressure for 15 minutes or so.

If active bleeding persists after 15 minutes, infiltrate the bleeding area and the gingiva surrounding the socket with lidocaine and epinephrine (1 : 100,000) until blanching occurs. Reapply the gauze over the site and instruct the patient to bite down for 15 more minutes. The injection serves two purposes: it causes vasoconstriction, and it anesthetizes the area so that adequate pressure can be generated during biting.

If the bleeding persists, insert a coagulation sponge, such as Gelfoam, into the socket and then loosely close the gingiva surrounding the socket with a 3-0 absorbable figure-of-eight suture. Instruct the patient to bite down on gauze placed over the sutures. Soaking Gelfoam with topical thrombin before placement is a good way to halt minor persistent bleeding (see Fig. 64-20). A new agent showing great promise for oral hemorrhage is the chitosan dental bandage (HemCon), which

Figure 64-19 Tongue lacerations. **A,** A large gaping tongue laceration in a toddler produced by the upper front teeth being forced through the tissue by a fall with the tongue protruded. This type of injury requires suturing. **B,** This small laceration, though gaping slightly, does not require surgical closure. *(From Zitelli BJ, McIntire SC, Nowalk AJ, eds.* Zitelli and Davis' Atlas of Pediatric Physical Diagnosis. *6th ed. St. Louis: Saunders, 2012.)*

Figure 64-20 A, For persistent bleeding of a tongue, mucosa, or dental extraction site, topical thrombin can be used (Thrombin-JM, King Pharmaceuticals). Topical thrombin is available in a spray pump, in a syringe for application, or as a reconstituted powder to saturate absorbable Gelfoam. **B,** A tongue laceration such as this one will heal well without sutures once the bleeding is controlled. Topical thrombin may be an option if hemostasis is problematic, such as in a patient taking warfarin.

is designed specifically for postextraction and oral bleeding. This shrimp-based bandage forms a sticky matrix when it contacts blood, and it quickly forms a seal that stops the bleeding. If these measures fail to control the bleeding, consult a specialist. It is also reasonable to check blood counts and coagulation profiles at this time.

Patients whose bleeding is controlled can be discharged and instructed not to take anything by mouth for 4 hours and then only liquids and soft foods. If silk sutures are used, remove them in 7 days.

ALVEOLAR OSTEITIS (DRY SOCKET)

The pain associated with an extracted tooth is significant but usually manageable with current pharmacologic modalities. The pain associated with a dry socket, however, can be very severe and often requires more definitive treatment. Alveolar osteitis, or dry socket, is a localized inflammation that occurs when the alveolar bone becomes inflamed. This condition usually occurs when the clot that is normally present in the socket after a tooth extraction becomes dislodged or dissolves. It is most common in the 2- to 4-day period after a tooth extraction. The examination is essentially unremarkable with the exception of a missing clot where the tooth was extracted. Signs and symptoms of dry socket include the following:

1. Moderate to severe pain localized to the area or frequently radiating to the ear

2. A foul odor or taste in the absence of purulence or suppuration
3. Symptoms that occur 3 to 5 days after tooth extraction
4. Absence of swelling, purulence, or lymphadenitis
5. Duration of 5 to 40 days

Anything that increases negative intraoral pressure in the mouth (e.g., smoking, excessive rinsing, spitting, drinking from a straw), as well as hormone replacement and periodontal disease, will predispose a patient to a dry socket. In only a small percentage of patients (2% to 5%) will a dry socket develop; however, this number increases with traumatic extractions or impacted third molars.[13,19]

The following contribute to the development of a dry socket:

1. Excessive trauma during extraction
2. Inadequate blood supply to the extraction site
3. Preexisting localized infection
4. Loss of clot from sucking, straw use, rinsing, or smoking
5. Foreign bodies remaining in the socket
6. Use of oral contraceptives
7. Use of corticosteroids
8. Pericoronitis

The pain associated with a dry socket is extremely severe, and if a patient is seen several days after an extraction with relatively normal findings on examination and severe pain, it is probably a dry socket. It must be distinguished from osteomyelitis, which is characterized by fever, leukocytosis, malaise, and nausea. The pain related to a dry socket will not be relieved with traditional pain medications, but a dental block usually provides instant relief. Once the block is performed, the alveolar osteitis can be treated. Irrigate the socket and gently suction out any accumulated debris. Next, fill the socket to prevent recurrence of pain and allow healing to begin. A variety of materials are suitable to fill the socket again.

Gauze (¼ inch) impregnated with eugenol (oil of cloves) or a local anesthetic may be used. Replace the gauze in 24 to 36 hours because it tends to dry out and loosen. The patient should be seen by a dentist the next day if at all possible. The socket may also be packed with a slurry of Gelfoam and eugenol. The Gelfoam acts as a matrix to hold the eugenol in the socket. A commercial product, such as Dry Socket Paste or Dressol-X (Fig. 64-21), can also be applied by itself into the socket or mixed with Gelfoam and placed into the socket. Dry Socket Paste is a very sticky thick paste containing eugenol. It may stay in place longer than gauze and does not dry out. Whichever packing material is used for a dry socket, one or more packings might be necessary before healing is complete.

Although antibiotics may be given to prevent alveolar osteitis, they are not usually necessary once the socket has been packed and should be prescribed at the discretion of the patient's oral surgeon or dentist.[11-13] NSAIDs should also be prescribed because they seem to work better than narcotics for dry socket.[20]

DENTOALVEOLAR INFECTIONS

Infections of the oral cavity run the spectrum from minor, easily managed abscesses to severe, life-threatening, deep space infections that require airway management and operative drainage. Although dental infections of all severity are encountered in the ED, the most common are those related to pulp disease. Others are associated with the attachment structures of the teeth such as the gingiva, periodontal ligament, and alveolar bone. These infections are often chronic conditions, but they can progress to the point where periodontal abscesses form and emergency treatment is required.

Emergency clinicians will be called on to drain abscesses of dental origin that do not extend into the deep spaces and that have well-defined boundaries easily accessible by intraoral or external drainage.

Figure 64-21 Dry Socket Paste.

Disease of the Pulp

Disease of the pulp can occur as a result of trauma, operations, or other unknown causes, but the most frequent cause is invasion of microorganisms after carious destruction of the enamel. As the enamel is destroyed, caries progresses more rapidly through the dentin and into the pulp chamber and causes an inflammatory response referred to as *pulpitis*. If the path of carious destruction through the tooth is adequate for drainage of the developing inflammation, the patient may be only mildly symptomatic or even asymptomatic for a long time. If drainage is blocked, however, the process may progress to rapidly involve the entire pulp cavity and the periapical space. The tooth is usually exquisitely tender at this point. Abscesses in the periapical region are generally picked up on dental x-rays and less commonly on a Panorex film. However, unless extension through the cortex exists, it is not important for the emergency clinician to make the distinction between pulpitis and a periapical abscess. Examination often reveals gross decay of one or many teeth and tenderness of the abscessed tooth to percussion. A periapical abscess will follow the path of least tissue resistance if not treated. This may be through alveolar bone and the gingiva and into the mouth or the deep structures of the neck. If the infection has progressed apically through alveolar bone and localized swelling and tenderness are present, incision and drainage should be performed (discussed subsequently).

In the ED setting it is uncertain whether a periapical abscess or simple pulpitis exists. Dental x-rays are not usually available. In the absence of trauma or recent instrumentation, it is prudent to begin antibiotic coverage for the typical oral flora. Penicillin, amoxicillin, metronidazole, and clindamycin are good choices. Analgesia should be provided as well. In most cases, perform a supraperiosteal infiltration (tooth block) with a long-acting anesthetic such as bupivacaine because this not only provides immediate and long-lasting relief but also decreases the requirement for narcotic analgesics once the anesthetic effect has dissipated. Avoid performing a supraperiosteal injection if the abscess has extended through gingival tissue and is present near the injection site. In this case a regional block away from the infected tissue may be more appropriate.

Disease of the Periodontium

Periodontal disease is also very common and affects practically all adults to some degree. *Periodontal disease* refers to infection of the attachment apparatus of the teeth: the gingiva, periodontal ligament, and alveolar bone. Unlike pulpal disease, periodontal disease is not usually symptomatic and is therefore rarely a primary reason to seek treatment in the ED. *Gingivitis* is an inflammation of the gingiva caused by bacterial plaque. In advanced disease, the gingiva becomes red and inflamed and tends to bleed easily. With chronic periodontal disease, an abscess can form when organisms become trapped in the periodontal pocket. The purulent material usually escapes through the gingival sulcus; however, it occasionally invades the supporting tissues, the alveolar bone, and the periodontal ligament (periodontitis). Periodontal abscesses that are not draining spontaneously through the sulcus can be drained in the ED. Saline rinses are encouraged to promote drainage. Antibiotics should be reserved for severe cases or for abscesses that cannot be drained. If it is uncertain whether the abscess originates from the pulp or the periodontium, prescribe antibiotics even if the abscess has been drained.[13,19]

Pericoronitis is a localized inflammation that occurs when the gingiva overlying erupting teeth becomes traumatized and inflamed. Third molars are especially susceptible; however, any tooth can be affected. The gingiva overlying the crown may entrap bacteria and debris, and infection may subsequently develop. Typical signs of inflammation and infection may develop, including erythema, edema, pus, and foul breath. Examination of the overlying gingiva with a tongue blade or finger will elicit tenderness and may produce drainage from the infection underlying the tissue flap. The pain may be moderate to severe, and referral of the pain to an ear region is common. The localized infection occasionally spreads to deeper areas such as the pterygomandibular or submasseteric spaces. Clinically, patients with significant spread of a pericoronal infection will have trismus secondary to irritation of the masseter and pterygoid muscles.

ED treatment of pericoronitis is directed at detecting regional spread to the deeper spaces. Trismus or other systemic signs of advanced infection require intravenous antibiotics and urgent consultation for drainage procedures, which usually requires extraction of the offending tooth. If pericoronal infection is localized, local or nerve block anesthesia is followed by removal of submucosal debris. Saline rinses and oral antibiotics are prescribed along with dental follow-up in 24 to 48 hours.

Drainage of Dentoalveolar Infections

The important determination for the emergency clinician to make is whether the odontogenic infection is localized, confined, and easily accessible or whether it is complex and involves several potential spaces. Likewise, determine whether the patient appears to be in a toxic state, has trismus, or exhibits any signs of airway compromise. Patients not meeting these criteria require specialist referral. Dental infections are not always obvious and can be mistaken for sinusitis, or vice versa (Figs. 64-22 and 64-23).

Several anesthetic techniques can make the drainage process more comfortable. Nerve blocks and local injections

Figure 64-22 A, This patient had facial swelling up to the right eye. She stated that her sinusitis had returned. She had minor tooth pain but mostly complained of an ache in her face. Radiographs revealed maxillary sinusitis with an air-fluid level. **B,** Intraoral examination revealed a pea-sized pointing abscess (*arrow*) at the base of an upper tooth, the cause of the sinusitis. After a local anesthetic was applied, a No. 11 blade was used to puncture the abscess, and copious pus was drained. **C,** A hemostat was inserted into the abscess cavity and spread open to yield more pus. Intravenous antibiotics (clindamycin) were administered followed by oral antibiotics, and the patient saw her dentist the next day. She recovered fully.

Figure 64-23 Osteomyelitis manifested as a dental infection. **A,** This patient had a chronic toothache for months and got minimally better with antibiotics from numerous emergency departments. No history of trauma was forthcoming. There was diffuse soft tissue swelling with malocclusion. **B,** A Panorex radiograph revealed nonunion of a fractured mandible with osteomyelitis. **C,** In this case a fractured mandible with osteomyelitis produced an obvious abscess. She had been treated for a presumed dental abscess many times in the past and got temporary relief.

Figure 64-24 Apply a dollop of 20% benzocaine gel to dry mucosa before injection of local anesthetic to decrease the pain of infiltration.

work best. Benzocaine 20% gel or a combination of lidocaine, prilocaine, and tetracaine generally provides good topical anesthesia before injection (Fig. 64-24). Application of these medications to the dry mucosa before injection of the local anesthetic decreases the pain associated with injection. After applying the topical anesthetic, slowly infiltrate local anesthetic with a vasoconstrictor until the tissue blanches. Either a short-acting anesthetic (2% lidocaine) or a longer-acting anesthetic (0.5% bupivacaine) may be used, depending on the clinical circumstances. Regional or dental blocks may be performed instead of local infiltration if needle placement would track already infected tissues into healthy areas. Otherwise, consider local infiltration over the site of the abscess. Instruments necessary for drainage of dentoalveolar abscesses are those usually found on a standard incision and drainage tray and include hemostats, scalpel (No. 15 or 11 blade), packing material (¼-inch gauze), and a fenestrated Penrose drain.

Intraoral Technique

Intraoral abscesses do not routinely require any antiseptic mucosa preparation before drainage. After anesthetizing the region, make a small incision (0.5 to 1.0 cm) over the area of fluctuance while keeping the point of the blade directed toward the alveolar bone. Use a hemostat to bluntly dissect the abscess and break up any loculations. Cultures are not necessary unless the patient is immunocompromised. Irrigate the wound profusely with normal saline. If the wound is large enough to place a drain or gauze inside, tack one end to the mucosa with a silk suture to prevent aspiration. Advise the patient to perform salt water rinses hourly and arrange follow-up in 24 to 48 hours with a dentist or oral surgeon to remove the drain and provide continued management. Because the source of the abscess is not always known to the emergency clinician, prescribe antibiotics.

Extraoral Technique

Most simple dental infections can be drained intraorally, but occasionally, an abscess spreads to the face and requires drainage through the skin. It is important to realize that most dental infections should be drained through the mouth, if possible, because any extraoral drainage will cause some scarring. Abscesses on the face, which should be drained in the ED, are usually very localized and fluctuant and have not

spread to any of the deep spaces in the head or neck. It is also important to never make any incisions on the face in direct proximity to important structures such as the facial nerve or the parotid gland and duct. Refer to Chapter 37 for more detail on the incision and drainage technique.

Prepare the patient for incision and drainage with a skin scrub and application of povidone-iodine (Betadine). Drape the face and infiltrate the skin with a local anesthetic containing a vasoconstrictor (1% or 2% lidocaine with epinephrine). Make any incision on healthy skin slightly below the area of fluctuance along dynamic skin tension lines. After making the incision, use blunt dissection in the fluctuant area until adequate drainage is achieved. Irrigate the abscess cavity profusely. Place a drain or packing material in the abscess cavity while being careful to not pack it too tightly. It should be just enough to keep the incision open and draining. Unlike intraoral drainage, suturing the drain in place is not necessary. Instruct the patient to take antibiotics and follow up with an oral surgeon in 24 to 48 hours for packing change and definitive management.

Remember that not all infections about the mouth are the result of a simple dental infection. Osteomyelitis of the mandible, various tumors, and other exotic diseases can simulate a dental infection.

Deep Space Infections of the Head and Neck

It is not unusual for odontogenic infections to spread into the various potential spaces of the face and neck (Fig. 64-25). The signs and symptoms consist of fever, chills, pain, difficulty with speech or swallowing, and trismus. Although infections of certain teeth usually spread to particular contiguous spaces, the rapid spread of these infections often makes localizing the exact space difficult. Any space, including the buccal, temporal, submasseteric, sublingual, submandibular, parapharyngeal, and others, may be involved (Figs. 64-26).

Maxillary extension of periapical abscesses can spread into the infraorbital space and, subsequently, to the cavernous sinus through the ophthalmic veins and result in cavernous sinus thrombosis. Cavernous sinus involvement is associated with periorbital cellulitis, as well as meningeal signs or a decreased level of consciousness. Periapical infections of the anterior mandibular teeth often spread to the buccinator space or the sublingual space, whereas those of the mandibular molars spread into the submandibular space.

The submandibular space connects with the sublingual space. Infection involving both these spaces is known as *Ludwig's angina*, which can be life-threatening. The source is usually a decayed lower tooth, with the tooth itself being relatively asymptomatic (Fig. 64-27). Initially, this infection may be subtle, but it can progress rapidly. As the infection progresses, the submandibular, submental, and sublingual spaces all become edematous, and there may be elevation of the tongue and the soft tissues of the mouth (Fig. 64-28). This is not a simple abscess that can be readily drained. It is considered a true dental emergency. Intervention includes intravenous antibiotics and emergency ear, nose, and throat (ENT) or oral surgery consultation. Patients with established cases of Ludwig's angina cases are admitted to the hospital and undergo operative intervention often involving multiple drains. Minor early cases can be treated and observed for 6 to 8 hours in the ED with close follow-up if the infection is deemed benign. The soft tissues of the posterior aspect of

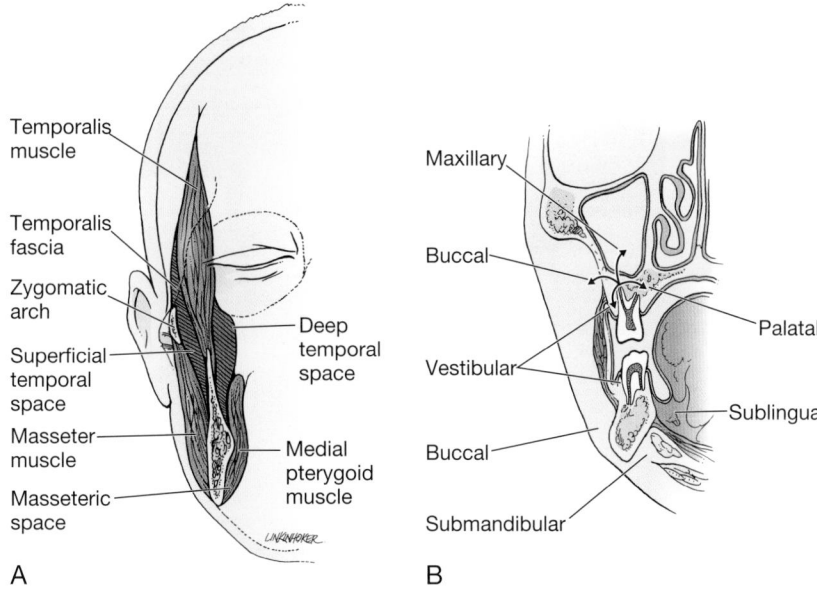

A

B

Figure 64-25 A, Location of temporal space abscesses. **B,** Route of infection into the buccal space, vestibular spaces, submandibular space, sublingual space, and palatal space. *(From Eisele D, McQuone S, eds.* Emergencies of the Head and Neck. *St. Louis: Mosby; 2000.)*

Figure 64-26 A, Advanced dental infection with characteristic facial swelling, probably involving the masseter space. **B,** Local anesthetic (lidocaine with epinephrine) is injected with a 27-gauge needle into an area of obvious fluctuance (shown by the probe). A mandibular nerve block is an alternative to local injection. **C,** After the site is punctured with a No. 11 blade, a hemostat is inserted into the cavity and spread. Copious pus is drained with a suction catheter. Initial intravenous antibiotics (clindamycin), oral antibiotics, and outpatient follow-up yielded good results. The offending tooth was extracted when the infection was controlled.

the pharynx can also become involved. Securing the airway becomes of paramount importance. The suprahyoid region of the neck appears tense and indurated, and landmarks may be obscured. A CT scan can further delineate Ludwig's angina if the diagnosis is in doubt, but in most cases, if the diagnosis is suspected, emergency consultation should be instituted early with careful monitoring for airway compromise.

Treatment of complicated odontogenic head and neck infections centers on airway management, surgical drainage, and antibiotics. If it is uncertain whether the deep spaces are involved, obtain a CT scan to delineate any extension of the infectious process. Perform airway interventions early if there is any question of compromise, and consider tracheostomy. Consult an oral maxillofacial or ENT surgeon because drainage and removal of necrotic tissue might be necessary. Administer antibiotics to slow spread of the infection down and

decrease hematogenous dissemination. The bacteria involved are typically a combination of streptococci and staphylococci, but a mixed aerobic and anaerobic infection is also possible. There has been an emergence of β-lactamase–producing organisms in upward of 40% of isolates from odontogenic neck abscesses.[19] Antimicrobials of choice for complicated odontogenic infections usually include the penicillins. The expanded-spectrum penicillins (ampicillin-sulbactam, ticarcillin–clavulanic acid, piperacillin-tazobactam) are effective against β-lactamase–producing bacteria and also cover the anaerobe *Bacteroides fragilis*. Clindamycin is an effective choice in patients who are allergic to penicillin. It should be used in combination with a cephalosporin, such as cefotetan or cefoxitin, to cover recently emerging resistant organisms. It is important to realize that in many of these infections, antibiotics are an adjunctive therapy and not a substitute for surgical intervention.

Figure 64-27 Ludwig's angina may initially appear to be benign. **A,** This patient's main complaint was dental pain. Tooth No. 27 (*arrow*) was noted to be decayed and a probable source of the infection. **B,** Physical examination revealed erythema and edema of the submandibular space, consistent with early Ludwig's angina. She was admitted to the hospital for intravenous antibiotics (clindamycin.) A high index of suspicion and early treatment are mandated in such patients because this infection can progress rapidly. **C,** This patient had the beginnings of an infection as manifested by elevation of the tongue and swelling of the floor of the mouth, which characteristically raises the openings of the submandibular (Wharton's) ducts (*arrow*). **D,** The cause was a badly decayed lower tooth (*arrow*). **E,** Tenderness and induration can be palpated in the floor of the mouth.

Figure 64-28 Ludwig's angina may progress rapidly and compromise the airway in a few hours. Notice how the massive submandibular edema elevates the tongue in the oral cavity.

DENTAL MATERIAL

As a general rule, EDs should have a well-stocked supply of basic dental material. Many commercially available products can be used interchangeably with many of the items listed here. These products can often be kept with the ENT cart or in another appropriate location. The following is a basic list:

1. Packing gauze
2. Dental roll gauze
3. Calcium hydroxide paste, glass ionomer cement, or zinc oxide cement
4. Dry Socket Paste or eugenol
5. Topical anesthetic gel (20% benzocaine or 5% lidocaine)
6. Topical bactericidal intraoral solution (Ora-5)
7. Periodontal paste (Coe-Pak) or self-cure composite
8. Articaine (Septocaine) cartridges with epinephrine
9. Save-A-Tooth Tooth Preservation System, EMT Toothsaver, or fresh milk
10. Zinc oxide/eugenol temporary cement (Temrex)
11. Ringed injection syringe

Figure 64-29 The Dental Box. This commercially available kit contains most of the items required for dental care in the emergency department. It is available at thedentalbox.com.

12. Stainless steel spatula and mixing pads
13. Oral surgery tray with arch bars and ligature wires
14. Tongue blades and cotton-tipped applicators
15. Gelfoam, HemCom, Surgicel, or topical thrombin

Regional dental supply houses are good sources for these items. The Dental Box is a commercially available kit that contains many of these items and is designed for ED use (Fig. 64-29). It is available at thedentalbox.com.

INTRAORAL PIERCING

Dating back to antiquity, body piercing has been practiced in many countries and cultures as part of ceremonial and

Figure 64-30 Tongue and lip piercing can cause dental and gingival problems. A metal tongue ball and other intraoral piercings can have significant detrimental effects on the teeth and gums. A tongue ball can cause microfractures leading to a suddenly shattered tooth. The longer the post, the greater the tooth damage.

religious rites. In recent years, body and intraoral piercing has gained tremendous popularity throughout the world as a means of self-expression. In the ED, clinicians may see patients with piercings of the lips, tongue, and even uvula. Complications of oral piercing on the gums and teeth include pain, infection, bleeding, increased salivary flow, difficulty swallowing, gingival recession, gingival trauma, and chipped or fractured teeth. Repeated trauma from a metal tongue ball can be quite detrimental to teeth and cause microfractures and a sudden shattered tooth (Fig. 64-30). One study of 400 consecutive patients at a military dental office found that 20% of their patients had at least one type of oral piercing, with the tongue being the most common location.[21] Of these patients, 14% had fractured teeth and 27% had recession of the gums. Another study assessed the impact of time and found that tooth chipping was found on molars and premolars in 47% of patients who had a tongue piercing for longer than 4 years.[22]

Acknowledgments

The contributions of Robert H. Benko, DDS, to this material are greatly appreciated. The editors and author also wish to acknowledge the contributions of James T. Amsterdam to this chapter in previous editions and would like to thank Michael B. Pavel, DMD, for his review of this manuscript.

References are available at www.expertconsult.com

Special Procedures

CHAPTER 65

Procedures Pertaining to Hypothermia and Hyperthermia

Heather M. Prendergast and Timothy B. Erickson

PROCEDURES PERTAINING TO HYPOTHERMIA

With an increase in outdoor activities, changing weather patterns, and the growing epidemic of homelessness in our country, issues pertaining to hypothermia remain in the forefront. Hypothermia is not only a common diagnosis in rural areas but has also become more commonplace in urban centers across the nation secondary to inadequate housing or lack of preparation for cold weather changes.[1] It is also important to note that numerous cases of accidental hypothermia (AH) are reported each year in areas typically considered warm weather locales such as Florida, Texas, California, and Alabama.[2,3] Every year, many recreational and elite athletes participate in outdoor sporting events. The higher the environmental stress, the greater the potential for failure in performance and the development of hypothermia.[4] The high-altitude expeditions on Mt. Everest in 1996, Mt. Denali in 2003, and Mt. Hood in 2006 are reminders that even well-protected, acclimatized individuals can succumb to cold-related fatalities. Optimal treatment of hypothermia remains controversial. It is a well-accepted practice to carry out resuscitation of these individuals for extended periods. The medical literature contains numerous anecdotal reports of profoundly hypothermic individuals who are successfully resuscitated and discharged neurologically intact.[5-8] Despite these spectacular reports of survival, both morbidity and mortality from hypothermia are common. Between 1972 and 2002, 16,555 deaths in the United States were attributed to hypothermia, which equates to 689 deaths per year.[9] Between 1999 and 2002 alone, 4607 death certificates in the United States had hypothermia-related diagnoses listed as the underlying cause of death.[9] The actual number of patients seen in emergency departments (EDs) with hypothermia is unknown. Poverty, homelessness, alcoholism, and psychiatric illnesses are commonly associated conditions. This chapter critically reviews approaches and procedures appropriate to the management of several categories of hypothermic patients. The recommendations combine treatment efficacy with safety. Before describing procedures and making recommendations, essential terms are defined and the pathophysiology of hypothermia is briefly reviewed.

Definitions

Accidental hypothermia has been defined as an unintentional decrease in core (vital organ) temperature to below 35°C (<95°F).[5] Victims of hypothermia can be separated into the following categories: *mild hypothermia*, 35°C to 32°C (95.0°F to 90.0°F); *moderate hypothermia*, lower than 32°C to 30°C (<90.0°F to 86.0°F); and *severe hypothermia*, colder than 30°C (<86.0°F). Other factors that may be useful in separating groups of patients with AH include the presence of underlying illness,[1,10-15] altered neurologic state on arrival at the ED, hypotension, and the need for prehospital cardiopulmonary resuscitation (CPR). A hypothermia outcome score has been developed that incorporates some of these factors and may permit comparison of outcomes in patient groups treated with different modalities.[16]

Risk factors for the development of AH include burn injuries, extremes of age, ethanol intoxication, dehydration, major psychiatric illness, trauma, use of intoxicants, significant blood loss, sleep deprivation, malnutrition, and concomitant medical illnesses.[17,18] Risk factors for the development of hypothermia indoors include advanced age, coexisting medical conditions, being alone at the time of illness, being found on the floor, and abnormal perception or regulation of temperature.[13] Unlike healthy exposed outdoor enthusiasts, such as skiers or mountaineers,[19] hypothermia in urban populations is most often associated with conditions that impair either thermoregulation or the ability to seek shelter. In the majority of studies of urban hypothermia, death has been attributed to the severity of the underlying disease.[1]

Because signs and symptoms may be vague and nonspecific, mild to moderate hypothermia may easily be overlooked in the ED. A common error is failure to routinely obtain an accurate core temperature in all patients at risk. The diagnosis is frequently delayed because of false reliance on standard oral temperatures. Symptoms such as confusion in the elderly and combativeness in intoxicated patients might not initially be recognized as symptoms of hypothermia. *Hypothermic patients frequently will not feel cold or shiver*, particularly the elderly population, who have impaired thermoregulatory responses because of their advanced age.[20-22] Paradoxical undressing, a cold-induced psychiatric dysfunction, has been described in confused patients in whom a sensation of heat

NORMAL BODY TEMPERATURE RANGES

°F	0–2 years	3–10 years	11–65 years	>65 years
Oral	—	95.9 99.5	97.6 99.6	96.4 98.5
Rectal	97.9 100.4	97.9 100.4	98.6 100.6	97.1 99.2
Axillary	94.5 99.1	96.6 98.0	95.3 98.4	96.0 97.4
Ear	97.5 100.4	97.0 100.0	96.6 99.7	96.4 99.5
Core	97.5 100.0	97.5 100.0	98.2 100.2	96.6 98.8

Figure 65-1 Electronic thermometers provide accurate temperatures over various ranges. **A,** The Welch Allyn Model 692/690 SureTemp Plus (oral, axillary, rectal) is accurate from 80°F to 110°F. Note the various ranges for normal temperatures from various sites by age. *It is generally accepted that a rectal temperature higher than 100.3°F represents a fever and that oral readings can be misleading.* **B,** The IVAC electronic thermometer is also commonly used in the emergency department (accurate from 88°F to 108°F). For severe hypothermia or hyperthermia, it is important to know the accuracy of the thermometer being used. **C,** The graph demonstrates variations in normal body temperature by site and age. (*A and B, Images courtesy of WelchAllyn, Inc.*)

develops at lowered body temperatures. It occurs as a result of constricted blood vessels near the surface of the body that suddenly dilate. In many cases these patients are mislabeled as psychotic, thereby leading to further delays in appropriate treatment.[23]

Measurement of Core Temperature

Because of the nonspecific nature of the symptoms of hypothermia, accurate assessment of temperature is a necessity when considering this diagnosis. It is of paramount importance not only for confirmation of the diagnosis but also for guidance in further diagnostic and therapeutic decisions. Any thermometer that does not record temperatures in the hypothermic range is *inappropriate* for evaluating significant hypothermia. Standard glass/mercury thermometers generally cannot record temperatures lower than 34°C (<93.2°F), although some models are available that record temperatures as low as 24°C (75.2°F) (Dynamed, Inc., Carlsbad, CA). An electronic probe with accompanying calibrated thermometer is recommended when monitoring this vital sign. Examples

of thermometers with accompanying accuracy at various temperature ranges are shown in Figure 65-1*A* and *B*.

Core temperature is traditionally estimated with a rectal probe, but rectal temperature often lags behind core temperature because of large gradients within the body.[22] Esophageal probes may be used, although they may be affected by warm humidified air therapy. Other possible sites for measurement of temperature include the tympanic membrane, nasopharyngeal tract, and urinary bladder.[1,24,25] Fresh urine temperature can closely approximate core temperature.[26] "Deep forehead" temperatures measured with a Coretemp thermometer (Teramo, Tokyo) have also demonstrated excellent accuracy and approximation of core temperatures.[27] For continuous monitoring purposes, rectal or bladder probes are preferred. Infrared tympanic temperatures have demonstrated excellent correlation with core temperatures. However, studies show that although easier to use and faster, infrared tympanic temperatures can be inaccurate at extremes of temperature by underestimating higher temperatures and overestimating lower temperatures.[28] When a rectal probe is used, it should be inserted at least 15 cm beyond the anal sphincter and its

TABLE 65-1 Signs and Symptoms of Hypothermia

CORE TEMPERATURE (°C)	CARDIOVASCULAR SYSTEM	RESPIRATORY SYSTEM	CENTRAL NERVOUS SYSTEM
30-34	Tachycardia Increased afterload Increased systemic blood pressure	Tachypnea Increased minute ventilation	Lethargy Mild confusion Loss of fine motor coordination
30-34	Progressive bradycardia Decreased cardiac output Hypotension Lengthening of cardiac conduction Atrial/ventricular dysrhythmias	Increased bronchial secretions Diminished gag reflex Depressed cough response	Delirium Slowed reflexes Muscle rigidity Abnormal EEG findings
<30	Spontaneous ventricular fibrillation Osborne waves at 25°C	Respiratory rate decreased to 5 breaths/min	Areflexia Coma Fixed pupils Rigidity EEG silent at 19°C

EEG, electroencephalogram.

position verified frequently.[6] One should remember that temperature gradients exist in the human body and therefore consistency of monitoring at one or more sites is mandatory. A chart and formula that convert centigrade to Fahrenheit temperatures will assist the clinician in assessing the severity of hypothermia (see Fig. 65-1*C*).

Pathophysiology

AH results from failure of the body's thermoregulatory responses to generate enough heat to compensate for heat losses. These thermoregulatory responses include shivering, tachycardia, tachypnea, increased gluconeogenesis, peripheral vasoconstriction, and shunting of blood to central organs (Fig. 65-2).[29,30] As core temperature drops despite these compensatory mechanisms, the patient becomes poikilothermic and cools to ambient temperature.

Four methods of heat loss affect the body: radiation, conduction, convection, and evaporation. *Radiation* involves transfer of heat from a warmer body to a cooler environment and accounts for approximately 60% of heat loss in a normothermic individual. *Conduction* refers to loss of heat from direct contact with a cooler surface. These losses are most profound with immersion hypothermia. *Convection* occurs when cool air currents pass by the body and accounts for 15% of heat loss, especially with a wind chill factor. *Evaporation* refers to significant loss of heat through sweating and insensible water loss.[21,30] With hypothermia, the enzymatic rate of metabolism decreases twofold to threefold with each 10°C (18°F) drop, and cerebral blood flow decreases 6% to 7% per 1°C (1.8°F) drop. Signs and symptoms of hypothermia vary according to the core temperature. The overall functioning of all organ systems is impaired by the cold.[31] The greatest effects are seen in the cardiovascular, neurologic, and respiratory systems (Table 65-1). As core body temperature drops below 33°C (<91.4°F), the patient becomes confused and ataxic.[32] The initiation of involuntary motor activity (shivering) prevents the reduction in core temperature.[33] Shivering thermogenesis in skeletal muscle operates on acute cold stress. In a malnourished patient, the mechanism may be rendered ineffective secondary to reduced muscle mass.[34] Shivering stops at about 32°C (89.6°F), and shivering artifact on an

electrocardiogram has been associated with increased survival of individuals with severe hypothermia.[35] Atrial fibrillation occurs frequently as the temperature continues to drop and the patient loses consciousness. A J wave on the electrocardiogram often appears before ventricular fibrillation (Fig. 65-3).[36,37] Though classically considered pathognomonic for hypothermia, the J or "Osborne" wave has no prognostic or predictive value in cases of hypothermia. Studies have found that Osborne waves are present in 36% of AH survivors and in 38% of nonsurvivors.[35,38] Ventricular fibrillation may occur below 29°C (<84.2°F) and becomes common as the core temperature drops to 25°C (77°F).[39] The electroencephalogram flattens at 19°C to 20°C (65.2°F to 68°F).[40] Asystole commonly develops at 18°C (64.4°F) but has been seen at higher temperatures. Initial core temperature does not necessarily correlate with patient outcome.[42] The lowest recorded temperature in a survivor of AH is 9.0°C (43.7°F).[30]

Initial Evaluation and Stabilization of Hypothermic Patients

Treatment of hypothermia can be divided into prehospital care and ED management.

Prehospital Care

In the prehospital setting, focus primarily on removing the patient from the current environment to prevent further decreases in core temperature. Studies have shown that oral temperatures are sufficiently accurate for field use[41]; however, infrared tympanic thermometers may not be reliable in the prehospital setting.[42] Handle these patients with special care and anticipate the presence of an irritable myocardium because aggressive measures can inadvertently trigger cardiac dysrhythmias. Hypovolemia and a large temperature gradient often exist between the periphery and the core in a hypothermic patient.[6] Avoid aggressive field management and prolonged transport times.[43,44] After removing the patient's wet clothing, wrap the patient in dry blankets or sleeping bags. "Field rewarming" is a misnomer because adding significant heat to a hypothermic patient in the field is extremely difficult. Studies have shown that for mild hypothermia, resistive heating (e.g., warming blankets) can be used safely in the

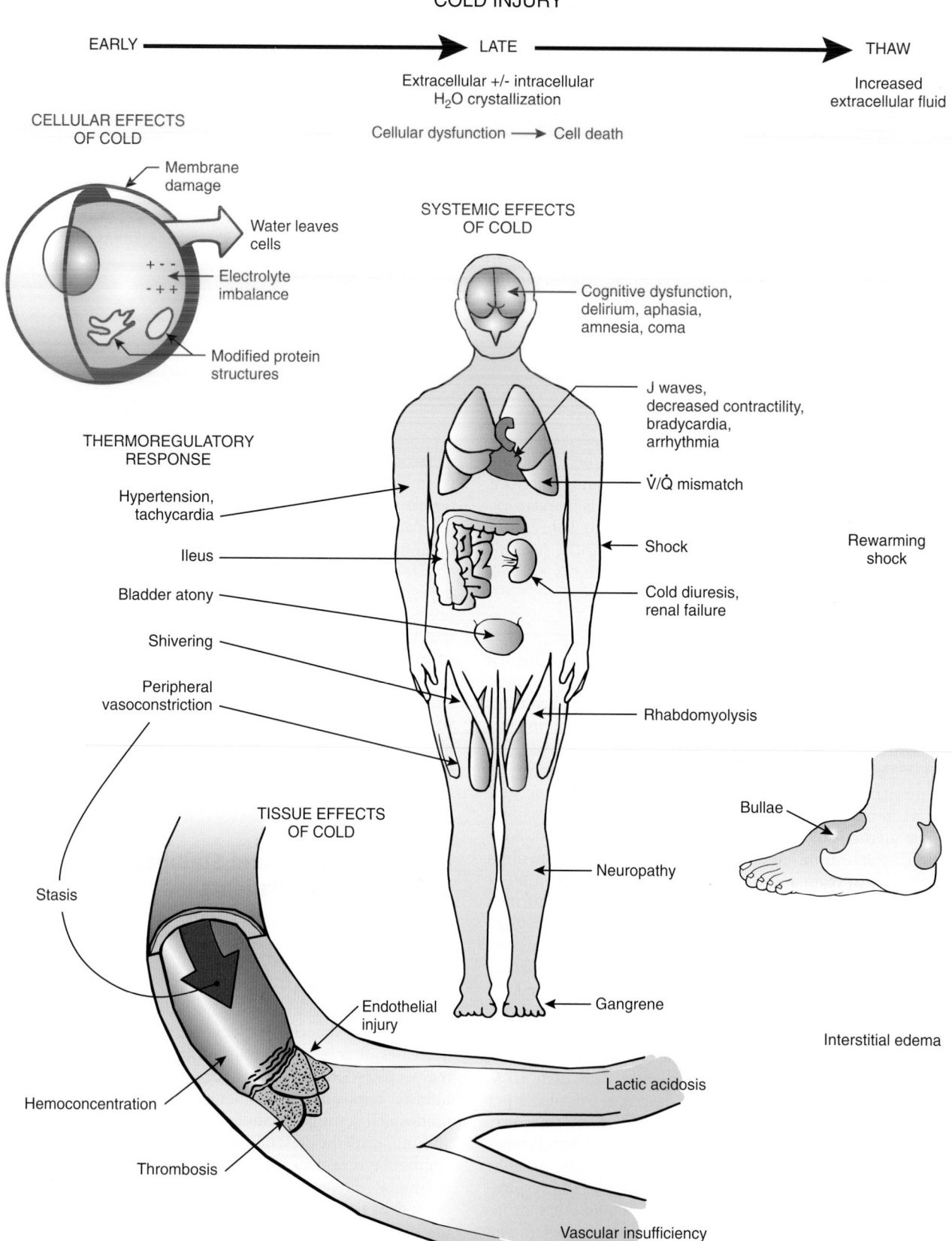

Figure 65-2 Cold-induced injuries such as hypothermia and frostbite lead to a thermoregulatory response (e.g., shivering and increased sympathetic activity), cellular and tissue effects (e.g., membrane damage, electrolyte imbalance, endothelial injury, and thrombosis), and systemic effects (e.g., shock, arrhythmia, and neuromuscular dysfunction). *(From Coughlin MJ, Zumwalt R, Fallico F, eds.* Surgery of the Foot and Ankle. *8th ed. St. Louis: Mosby; 2006.)*

	Admission	One hour	One day
Temperature (°C)	24.1	29.4	36.6
Heart rate (beats/min)	50	70	98
QRS interval (msec)	184	119	71
QTc interval (msec)	516	502	403

Figure 65-3 In severe hypothermia, the electro-cardiogram (ECG) exhibits marked elevation of the J deflection, so-called Osborne waves (*arrow-heads*). The height of the J wave is proportional to the degree of hypothermia, and this finding is usually most marked in the midprecordial leads. This ECG is from a patient with sinus bradycardia, but in approximately half the patients with a temperature below 32°C (89.6°F), slow atrial (*arrows*) fibrillation develops, a rhythm that usually converts spontaneously with rewarming. (*Adapted from Krantz MJ, Lowery CM. Giant Osborne waves in hypothermia. N Engl J Med. 2005;352:184. Used with permission.*)

prehospital setting. Resistive heating augments thermal comfort, increases core temperature by approximately 0.8°C/hr (33.4°F/hr), and reduces patient pain and anxiety during transport.[45] In one study, resistive heating more than doubled the rewarming rate when compared with passive insulation and did not produce an afterdrop.[46] With longer transport times, use active rewarming methods limited to heated inhalation and truncal heat application. Place insulated hot water bottles near the patient's axilla or groin. The Res-Q-Air device (CF Electronics, Inc., Commack, NY) is lightweight and portable and delivers heated humidified air or oxygen at temperatures ranging from 42°C to 44°C (107.6°F to 111.2°F) and down to ambient conditions of −20°C (−4°F). In more remote settings, another option is to use a modified forced-air warming system in the field. The Portable Rigid Forced-Air Cover is heated with a Bair Hugger heater/blower (Augustine Medical, Inc., Eden Prairie, MN). It covers the patient's trunk and thighs and can adapt to various transport vehicle power sources.[6]

Immobilize patients with potential traumatic injuries to the spine or extremities before transport. Pay continuous attention to airway maintenance. Initiate fluid resuscitation with intravenous (IV) crystalloid, preferably 5% dextrose in normal saline (D$_5$NS). Alternatively, give warmed oral glucose-containing drinks to a patient who is awake and alert. Most hypothermic patients are dehydrated because fluid intake is reduced and cold causes diuresis. Avoid using lactated Ringer's solution because it can theoretically decrease the metabolism of lactate by cold-induced hepatic dysfunction. If possible, use warmed IV fluids because they are generally well tolerated.[47,48] If available, use a flameless heater, which is currently being used by military medical units and provides an easy and expedient means of warming fluids in the prehospital setting.[49]

Intubate unresponsive patients, but recognize that there is no universal agreement on when to intubate a hypothermic patient who has detectable vital signs. Pulse oximetry is not usually helpful because vasoconstriction limits blood flow to the periphery and readings may be inaccurate or not possible. Some authors suggest that pulseless victims with core temperatures below 32°C (<89.6°F) should be transported with continuous CPR.[47] Other authors believe that it is unnecessary to perform CPR on a patient who has any perfusing cardiac rhythm because it may precipitate ventricular fibrillation.[50] There is no universally accepted standard for intubation or CPR in hypothermic patients with detectable vital signs.[51]

Definitive prehospital determination of cardiac activity requires a cardiac monitor. Cardiac arrest is a common misdiagnosis because peripheral pulses are difficult to palpate when extreme bradycardia is present along with peripheral vasoconstriction. Some authors report that asystole is a more common rhythm than ventricular fibrillation. In the field, differentiating ventricular fibrillation from asystole may be impractical.

Transport cold, stiff, cyanotic patients with fixed and dilated pupils because the treatment dictum for prehospital personnel remains, "No one is dead until warm and dead." A succinct summary of the prehospital care of a hypothermic patient is rescue, examine, insulate, and transport.[6]

ED Management

There are no universally established standards of care regarding the use of specific techniques for rewarming a hypothermic patient or cooling a hyperthermic patient. This chapter describes all potentially useful modalities. Many are not applicable for general use in the ED, whereas others are safe, beneficial, and easily accomplished in the general ED setting. Some invasive procedures, however, such as cardiopulmonary bypass and irrigation of the peritoneal or thoracic cavity, may be overly aggressive or of anecdotal or theoretical benefit only. Exactly when to institute any given intervention is best determined by the resources available, the initial scenario, and clinical judgement individualized for each patient.

TABLE 65-2 Rewarming Techniques

CORE TEMPERATURE (°C)	METHOD AND TECHNIQUES
>32	PER Dry blankets, clothing Heated intravenous solutions (43°C), D₅NS Warm fluids if fully alert
≤32	AER Heated blankets, heating pads, warm air convection Radiant heat sources Alcohol-circulating blankets ACR Peritoneal dialysis Bladder, gastric, or colonic lavage with warm fluids (43°C) Heated intravenous fluids Heated humidified oxygen Thoracic cavity lavage (43°C) Extracorporeal blood rewarming Hemodialysis Ultrasonic and low-frequency microwave diathermy Arteriovenous anastomoses rewarming

ACR, active core rewarming; *AER*, active external rewarming; *PER*, passive external rewarming.

Treatment priorities in the ED setting are to prevent further decreases in core body temperature; establish a steady, safe rewarming rate; maintain stability of the cardiopulmonary system; and provide sufficient physiologic support. Adjust the rate of rewarming and the techniques used according to the degree of hypothermia and the severity of the patient's clinical condition (Table 65-2). Anticipate and prevent complications.

In a pulseless, apneic patient, initiate CPR and continue until the core temperature is above 34°C (>93.2°F). Profound hypothermia results in coma, hyporeflexia, fixed and dilated pupils, severe bradycardia, and often an unobtainable blood pressure. With severe hypothermia, a pulse might not be palpable and measurement of blood pressure might require the use of a Doppler device. If available, use ultrasound to detect the presence of cardiac wall motion. Follow the heart rate and rhythm with electrocardiographic monitoring. In patients who have anything more than minimal impairment, perform arterial blood gas analysis frequently to determine oxygenation, ventilation, and acid-base status. If feasible, establish large-bore IV lines. Avoid central lines if possible because insertion of such lines may exacerbate the myocardial irritation. Give maintenance IV fluids. Warm all IV fluids to 40°C to 42°C (104°F to 107.6°F), but be aware that the usual volumes administered will not contribute significant heat calories. With long standard IV tubing, the heated IV fluids may actually cool to room temperature before entering the patient's IV site.

With a mild to moderate reduction in core temperature, the level of mentation correlates with the severity of the AH, associated illnesses, or both. Noteworthy exceptions are alcoholics and diabetics, who can be in a coma at higher core temperatures because of concomitant hypoglycemia. Perform

bedside glucose measurements on patients when they arrive in the ED. A high correlation exists between alcohol consumption and the development of hypothermia, especially in colder climates.[1] A review of 68 cases of hypothermic deaths in Jefferson County, Alabama, found that a significant number of cases involved middle-aged men who had consumed alcohol.[3] In the 22 cases of AH reviewed by Fitzgerald,[52] all but 2 patients were alcoholics. The serum glucose level was less than 50 mg/dL in 41% (nine patients). This study noted glycosuria in two patients, even when low serum glucose values were evident, and described a renal tubular glycosuria in patients with AH. Such glycosuria may worsen or cause hypoglycemia. *Glycosuria in AH is no guarantee of an adequate serum glucose concentration.* This supports the routine use of supplemental IV glucose unless a normal serum glucose value can be quickly ensured. Consider administering IV thiamine (100 mg) and a trial dose of 0.4 to 2 mg of IV naloxone (Narcan) in a comatose patient. Although failure to rewarm spontaneously has been noted in victims with hypothyroidism and other endocrine deficiencies, reserve the use of thyroid hormones and corticosteroids for patients with suspected thyroid and adrenal insufficiency, respectively.

The thermoregulatory vasoconstriction caused by hypothermia significantly decreases subcutaneous oxygen tension.[21] Good correlation exists between the incidence of wound infection and subcutaneous oxygen tension. As core temperatures decrease from 41°C to 26°C (105.8°F to 78.8°F), neutrophil function is significantly impaired.[21] In animal models, hypothermia appears to decrease leukocyte sequestration within the brain parenchyma, thus offering some resistance to meningitis.[53] Although antibiotics are not routinely indicated for victims of uncomplicated mild hypothermia, some authors advocate the routine empirical initiation of broad-spectrum antibiotic therapy on admission of severely hypothermic patients. In this setting, detection and treatment of the underlying cause, such as infection, may be more critical than treatment of the hypothermia.[1]

Management Guidelines

Hypothermia affects virtually every organ system because of generalized slowing of the body (see Fig. 65-2). Management goals depend on the severity of the hypothermia, but in all cases the primary goal is to increase core temperature and prevent further loss. In a patient with mild hypothermia, a conservative approach to rewarming is generally advocated. Overly aggressive methods may be more harmful to the patient by causing worsening hypotension, a paradoxical decrease in core temperature, and cardiac dysrhythmias. Other complications may include bleeding and infection of surgical incisions.[21] The optimal rewarming rate remains unclear and varies with each case. Standard rewarming rates are a 0.5°C/hr to 2.0°C/hr (0.9°F/hr to 3.6°F/hr) rise in temperature *in an otherwise stable patient* (Table 65-3). Carefully consider and individualize invasive therapy to the severity of the hypothermia and the condition of the patient. Avoid *overtreating and overusing invasive techniques in an otherwise stable hypothermic patient.* In patients with severe underlying problems such as hypoglycemia, hyperglycemia, sepsis, adrenal crisis, drug overdose, or hypothyroidism, treat these conditions appropriately in addition to treating the hypothermia. Long-term outcome may depend more on treatment of the underlying illness than on treating the hypothermia.[1,55]

TABLE 65-3 Warming Rates (°C/hr)

	PASSIVE EXTERNAL	ACTIVE EXTERNAL	INHALATION OF WARM AIR	PERITONEAL LAVAGE	BLADDER LAVAGE
1st hr	1.4	1.5	1.5	1.5	1.3
2nd hr	1.4	2.4	2.0	2.5	1.7
3rd hr	1.8	2.0	1.9	3.2	1.8

From Danzl D, Pozos RS. Multicenter hypothermia study. *Ann Emerg Med.* 1987;16:1042.
Note: Thoracic lavage had a median rewarming rate of 2.95°C/hr (see Plaisier[54]).

Passive External Rewarming

The cornerstone of the effectiveness of passive external rewarming relies on the body's ability to restore normal body temperature through its own mechanisms for heat production. Stop further heat loss with insulation and manipulation of the environment. Give warm fluids containing glucose to patients who are fully alert. For patients with mild AH, remove wet clothing and then provide passive external rewarming with blankets. The technique is simple, but the patient must be capable of generating enough body heat for this method to be successful. Give warmed IV fluids to counteract the cold-induced diuresis. Internal heat generation is required for rewarming, and this effect will be relatively slow. In an otherwise stable patient, aggressive intervention with drugs and invasive monitoring might be more harmful than beneficial. Patients who cannot shiver, those who are hypotensive, or those who are intoxicated or malnourished may not have this capability. Survival rates with passive external rewarming have ranged from 55% to 100%.[56-59]

For patients in the moderate or severe category of hypothermia, a more aggressive approach may be warranted. The options available are active external rewarming and active core rewarming. Active core rewarming techniques can be further divided into less invasive and more invasive techniques. The aggressiveness of therapy depends more on the patient's underlying health, hemodynamic status, and response to initial therapy than on the initial temperature.

Active External Rewarming

The application of heat to the skin of a hypothermic patient has been termed *active external rewarming*.

Indications

Although there is some suggestion that active external rewarming of profoundly hypothermic patients by immersion may be associated with an increase in mortality over other treatments,[16,60] more recent studies suggest that this technique is highly effective for mild hypothermia.[32,61] Use it selectively and limit it to the trunk. Other forms of active external rewarming are increasingly being used in the ED as adjunctive care of moderately hypothermic, otherwise healthy individuals. Vasoconstriction limits the ability to increase core temperature with techniques that primarily warm the skin.[62]

Active external rewarming is most beneficial when the heat supplied by the external source is greater than the loss of rewarming heat incurred by the cessation of shivering. In more remote wilderness settings where more aggressive warming techniques are precluded because of the lack of equipment or personnel, active external rewarming with body-to-body contact may be the only option. The rewarming contribution of body-to-body contact appears to be limited, however.[63]

Equipment

Traditionally, immersion therapy has used a heated (40°C to 42°C [104.0°F to 107.6°F]) water tank of the type present in most burn units. Generally, immerse a hypothermic patient entirely except for the extremities and head, but immersion of the extremities may hasten rewarming.[64,65] A major drawback is the inability to closely monitor patients undergoing immersion. Alternatively, use a warm water–filled heat exchange blanket (e.g., Blanketrol, Cincinnati Sub-Zero Products, Cincinnati, OH) for conduction warming. Intraoperative studies have demonstrated excellent results.[66] A forced warm air convection system (Bair Hugger, Augustine Medical, Eden Prairie, MN; Snuggle Warm Convective Warming System, Sims Level 1, Inc., Rockland, MA) has been used for postsurgical rewarming.[66,67] This approach has also been used successfully for ED-based AH therapy. Rewarming by warm air convection permits continued monitoring in the ED and is better tolerated than immersion because of the less rapid development of vasodilation in peripheral tissues.

Technique

Because profound fluid shifts can occur with conduction warming, give the patient supplemental IV fluid warmed to 40°C (104.0°F; Hotline Fluid Warmer, Sims Level 1, Inc., Rockland, MA) at a rate sufficient to generate a urinary output of 0.5 to 1.0 mL/kg/hr. Give an initial fluid bolus of 500 mL of D$_5$NS. Note that blood pressure is not an accurate means of gauging fluid resuscitation since serious hypothermia is always accompanied by "physiologic" hypotension. Because patients requiring mechanical ventilation have rarely been subjected to tank immersion, it cannot be recommended for hypothermic patients who require intubation. Rewarming rates ranging from 0.9°C to 8.8°C (1.6°F to 15.8°F) per hour have been reported with immersion therapy.[6,68]

A heat exchange blanket allows the patient to receive other treatments that may be difficult or impossible to carry out in a tub, such as defibrillation, CPR, or more invasive warming techniques. Place the heating blanket and overlying cloth sheet underneath the patient. Set the blanket temperature to 40°C to 42°C (104.0°F to 107.6°F), and initiate the measures described in the section "Passive Rewarming Techniques." Forced-air rewarming (convection) uses a blanket cradle to create an environment through which heated air is blown. Access to the patient is quite good with this system because the overlying blankets can be raised temporarily to evaluate the patient or perform procedures. Experience with mild immersion-induced hypothermia in volunteers suggests that the forced-air technique warms at a rate comparable to that of vigorous shivering, but with less metabolic stress and less afterdrop.[69]

Arteriovenous Anastomoses Rewarming

Arteriovenous anastomoses rewarming (AVR) involves immersion of the distal end of the extremities (hands, forearms, feet, and lower part of the legs). Advantages include rapid rewarming rates. A study of AVR immersion at temperatures of 45°C and 42°C (113.0°F and 107.6°F) in healthy volunteers demonstrated rewarming rates of 9.9°C/hr (±3.2°C/hr) for the former and 6.1°C/hr (±1.2°C/hr) (43.0°F ± 34.2°F/hr) for the latter.[70] There was also a decrease in postcooling afterdrop. AVR is well tolerated by patients because of the rapid rise in core temperature and the shortened period of shivering.[64,71]

Complications

There is concern that surface warming with accompanying vasodilation may produce relative hypovolemia in a hypothermic patient. Other complications described with the active external rewarming method include core temperature afterdrop and rewarming acidosis. In *core temperature afterdrop*, colder peripheral blood is transported to the warmer core organs, thereby further reducing core temperature. In *rewarming acidosis*, colder blood and lactic acid return to the core organs and worsen the acidosis. To limit these complications in patients with moderate hypothermia, some authors advocate using active external warming only after active internal techniques have been initiated.[71]

CPR and other advanced cardiac therapy and monitoring are impossible with immersion rewarming. Until studied further, active external rewarming should be considered only in a clinically monitored setting for mildly hypothermic patients who can protect their airways. When using a heating device, also monitor the potential for burns in areas that have the greatest contact with the heating source.

Active Core Rewarming

There is evidence that active core rewarming may decrease mortality from severe hypothermic exposure when compared with other techniques. In the face of circulatory failure, often the best chance of survival is treatment with extracorporeal circulation (ECC) and warming of the blood.[72] Several methods have been described, including the use of warm humidified air through an endotracheal tube or mask, peritoneal lavage, gastric or bladder lavage with warm fluid, thoracic tube lavage, cardiopulmonary bypass, AVR, peripheral vascular extracorporeal warming, hemodialysis, and thoracotomy with mediastinal lavage. These techniques transfer heat actively to the body core and achieve varying rewarming rates. The specific techniques and some of the advantages and disadvantages for each procedure follow.

Emergency Warming of Saline in a Microwave

Under ideal circumstances, keep saline in a standard warming device. When large amounts of saline are required for such procedures as peritoneal lavage, warm 1-L saline bags rapidly in a standard microwave oven (Fig. 65-4).[73] Although devices vary, a 650-W microwave oven has been demonstrated to warm 1 L of room-temperature non–dextrose-containing saline from 21.1°C to 38.3°C (70°F to 101°F) in 120 seconds on the high setting. At midcycle (i.e., after 60 seconds), interrupt the heating with agitation, and repeat the agitation at the end of the cycle before infusion.

Figure 65-4 A, To rewarm hypothermic patients with intravenous heated saline, a standard 650-W microwave oven, on high for 120 seconds, will raise the temperature of a non–dextrose-containing liter of saline (in a plastic bag) to about 100°F. **B,** Agitate the bag halfway through the warming and again before infusion.

Inhalation of Heated Humidified Oxygen or Air

The use of warm humidified oxygen to treat hypothermia has been well established. Average rates of rewarming of 1°C/hr (33.8°F/hr) via mask and 1.5°C/hr to 2.0°C/hr (34.7°F/hr to 35.6°F/hr) via endotracheal tube with heated aerosol at 40°C (104.0°F) can be obtained.[6,32] Faster rewarming rates may be accomplished with a maximum safe aerosol temperature of 45°C (113°F). Core rewarming with this technique occurs through the following mechanisms. The warmed alveolar blood returns to the heart and warms the myocardium. The heated, humidified air delivered to the alveoli also warms contiguous structures in the mediastinum by conduction. Warming the inhaled air or oxygen eliminates a major source of heat loss.

Indications and Contraindications. The use of heated humidified air or oxygen is a simple technique that *should be used routinely* in all patients with hypothermia, regardless of severity. If the correct equipment is available, it can be used in the field and in the hospital.[44,45] One must address the risk for burns during the inhalation of warm air in the field environment.[74] Mouth-to-tube ventilation in an intubated hypothermic prehospital patient has the theoretical advantage of providing warm humidified air without special equipment. A ventilating rescuer can inhale oxygen before expiring into the patient's endotracheal tube to provide air with increased oxygen content. There are no contraindications to or reported complications from the use of warm humidified air for hypothermia, and there is no afterdrop.[75]

Technique. Use a heated cascade nebulizer with a mask for patients with spontaneous respirations. Use a volume ventilator for intubated patients. Monitor the inspired air to maintain a temperature of approximately 45°C (≈113.0°F).[76] Temperatures higher than 50°C (122°F) may burn the mucosa, and temperatures lower than 45°C (<113°F) do not deliver the maximum heat. Humidify the air or oxygen and note that the heater module may need modification because many units have feedback mechanisms that shut off at a given temperature. It may be difficult to deliver oxygen at the recommended temperature because of equipment limitations. In many cases the air temperature is only 30°C (86°F).

Summary. Inhalation of warm humidified air or oxygen results in gradual rewarming of the core and should be the mainstay of all rewarming therapy. Studies have suggested that the rewarming rate of inhalation therapy is inferior to that of peritoneal lavage, thoracic lavage, and bath rewarming.[6] Inhalation therapy can be combined with any and all other methods of rewarming and is relatively noninvasive and inexpensive. This therapy should be considered as the initial treatment of choice for hypothermic patients.

Peritoneal Dialysis (Lavage)

Peritoneal dialysis (lavage) is an attractive treatment of severe hypothermia because it is available in most hospitals and does not require any unusual equipment or training. Rewarming rates of 2°C to 3°C (3.6°F to 5.4°F) per hour, depending on the dialysis rate, can be achieved without sophisticated equipment that may delay therapy or require transfer of the patient to a tertiary care facility.[77] This technique can also be used to help correct electrolyte imbalances.

Rewarming by peritoneal dialysis was first used successfully in a patient in ventricular fibrillation with a temperature of 21°C (69.8°F).[78] Since that time, there have been reports of successful rewarming with peritoneal lavage in stable, severely hypothermic patients and unstable hypothermic patients in cardiac arrest.[79,80] Peritoneal lavage works via transfer of heat from lavage fluid to the peritoneal cavity. The peritoneal great vessels and abdominal organs provide a large surface area for exchange of heat. The use of warmed peritoneal lavage fluid is an effective approach to rewarming.[81] There have been reports in the literature of success with rapid high-volume peritoneal lavage in pediatric patients. The technique involves the use of an infraumbilical "mini-laparotomy" incision followed by placement of a large silicone peritoneal dialysis catheter. The catheter is connected to a rapid infusion device with delivery of 1 L of warmed normal saline every 90 seconds.[81]

Indications and Contraindications. Peritoneal dialysis is appropriate therapy in a severely hypothermic patient. In practice, it is often omitted if other measures appear to be successful. There are no universally established criteria for performing peritoneal lavage in hypothermic patients who have detectable vital signs. Though theoretically less effective than other techniques that directly warm the thorax in the setting of cardiac arrest, it has been used successfully in that situation. It is theoretically useful in hypothermic patients who have overdosed with a dialyzable toxin. Other less invasive methods, such as gastric or bladder lavage or warm nebulized air or oxygen inhalation, may be preferred in stable patients with temperatures higher than 26°C to 28°C (>78.7°F to 82.4°F). Peritoneal dialysis should not be performed on patients with previous abdominal surgery. It should be used with extreme caution in patients with a coagulopathy.

Equipment. We recommend using the Seldinger technique with a commercially available disposable kit (e.g., Arrow Peritoneal Lavage Kit, product no. AK-09000, Arrow International, Inc., Reading, PA) because of the ease of performance and minimal morbidity associated with this procedure.

Technique. In a noncritical patient, obtain a coagulation profile before the procedure, but in life-threatening situations, initiate the procedure immediately before laboratory studies. Place the patient in the supine position with a Foley catheter and nasogastric tube in place. After infiltrating with lidocaine, make an infraumbilical stab incision with a No. 11 scalpel blade, and place an 18-gauge needle into the peritoneal cavity directed toward the pelvis at a 45-degree angle. Insert a standard flexible J wire through the needle, and then remove the needle. Pass the 8-Fr dialysis catheter over the wire with a twisting motion, and then remove the wire.

Lavage rates of 4 to 12 L/hr can be achieved with two catheters. Warm the fluid with a standard blood warmer to 40°C to 45°C (104.0°F to 113.0°F). Use a standard 1.5% dextrose dialysate solution. Add potassium (4 mmol/L) if the patient becomes hypokalemic. Saline has also been used successfully. The rate should be at least 6 L/hr and preferably 10 L/hr.[80]

Complications. The Seldinger method has a complication rate of less than 1%.[82] A "mini-lap" performed via direct dissection may also be used but might have a higher complication rate.[83] Further discussion of potential complications is provided in Chapter 43.

Summary. Peritoneal dialysis is a useful method because it entails readily available fluid and can be done with a self-contained disposable kit.[83] If a hospital also treats trauma victims, the lavage kit can be the same as that used for evaluation of abdominal trauma. If this technique is combined with warm nebulized inhalation, warming rates of 4°C/hr (7.2°F/hr) can be achieved.[84] Peritoneal lavage rewarms the liver and restores its synthetic and metabolic properties.[85]

Gastrointestinal and Bladder Rewarming

Gastric or bladder irrigation offers some of the same advantages as peritoneal dialysis without invading the peritoneal cavity. Heat is delivered to structures in close proximity to the core. In the Multicenter Hypothermia Study, gastric/bladder/colon lavage had a first-hour rewarming rate of 1.0°C to 1.5°C/hr (33.8°F/hr to 34.7°F/hr) and a second-hour rewarming rate of 1.5°C/hr to 2.0°C/hr (34.7°F/hr to 35.6°F/hr) for severe hypothermia.[83,86] In a multifactorial analysis of the Multicenter Hypothermia Study there was a trend toward improved survival in patients treated in this manner.[16]

Although the amount of heat delivered with gastric lavage appears to be less than that delivered with peritoneal dialysis, it is somewhat easier to use and less invasive. When combined with other methods, gastric or bladder lavage provides significant warming.[83,84] Serum electrolyte levels should be monitored if large volumes of tap water are used because dilutional electrolyte disturbances may occur. Children and geriatric patients might be more susceptible to electrolyte changes with tap water irrigation.[87]

Indications and Contraindications. Warmed gastric or bladder lavage may be used as adjunctive therapy for moderate or severe hypothermia. It can be combined with other warming techniques when rapid rewarming is needed. Patients who are obtunded and lack protective airway reflexes should undergo endotracheal intubation before gastric lavage to prevent aspiration of gastric contents. Refer to the appropriate chapters concerning nasogastric tube placement (see Chapter 40), gastric lavage (see Chapter 42), and urethral catheterization for specific contraindications to these procedures.

Equipment. Use a large-diameter 32- to 40-Fr lavage tube with normal saline solution warmed to 40°C to 45°C (104.0°F to 113.0°F) in a microwave or blood warmer with verification of temperature before use. Although smaller tubes are easily passed nasally, use oral placement of the large lavage tubes. A modified Sengstaken tube with gastric and esophageal balloons may also be used.

Technique. Instill 200- to 300-mL aliquots of fluid into the stomach before removal by gravity drainage. For bladder irrigation the optimal volume is not known, but avoid distention of the bladder (100- to 200-mL aliquots should be sufficient). The amount of time that the irrigant should be left in place before removal is not known, but use of rapid exchanges with a dwell time of 1 to 2 minutes is suggested.

Complications. Complications of lavage include trauma to the nasal turbinates, gastric and esophageal perforation, dilutional hyponatremia, inadvertent placement of the tube in the lungs, and pulmonary aspiration, all of which can be minimized by careful, proper technique. Fluid overload and electrolyte disturbances when using tap water are potential complications in pediatric and geriatric patients.

Summary. Gastrointestinal and bladder lavage with heated fluids is easily performed with equipment and solutions available in any hospital. The stomach, colon, and bladder are poor sites for body cavity lavage as a result of the small surface area for heat exchange.[85] Because of its ease and availability, it can be started early in the resuscitation and be combined with any other rewarming method to significantly add heat,[69] although its specific effect on morbidity and mortality is not known.

Thoracic Cavity Lavage

Thoracic cavity lavage can be performed either by *closed* means, through chest tubes placed in one hemithorax,[88,89] or in *open* fashion, after resuscitative thoracotomy.[90] The former approach offers the advantages of being less invasive and is an effective form of treatment in hospitals not equipped for cardiopulmonary bypass.[89] Furthermore, closed-chest CPR can be continued while this technique is used. The open thorax approach offers the theoretical advantage of direct warming of the heart and the option of open-chest cardiac massage. Rapid warming rates of 6°C to 7°C (42.8°F to 44.6°F) in 20 minutes have been described.[88,89] Pleural irrigation results in cardiac rewarming and might be the method of choice, particularly in patients with an arrhythmia.[85]

Indications and Contraindications. Thoracic cavity lavage should be considered for patients requiring rapid core rewarming in the setting of cardiac arrest or inadequate perfusion (e.g., shock, during CPR) when cardiac bypass is not available. Open thoracic lavage should be considered in patients who will receive open-chest massage or thoracotomy for other reasons (e.g., hypothermic arrest with penetrating trauma). Thoracic lavage is not necessary for patients with mild or moderate hypothermia who can be rewarmed by other less invasive methods. Avoid the technique in patients with a coagulopathy unless required as a lifesaving measure.

Closed Thoracic Lavage. An alternative that is more practical in the ED is pleural rewarming by repeatedly using warmed saline placed intermittently and then withdrawn through a chest tube. Place two large-bore thoracostomy tubes (e.g., 36 to 38 Fr in 70-kg adults) in one hemithorax. Infuse one chest tube with 3-L bags of heated normal saline (40°C to 41°C [104°F to 105.8°F]) via a high-flow fluid infuser (e.g., Level-1 Fluid Warmer, Technologies, Inc., Marshfield, MA). Collect the effluent with an autotransfusion thoracostomy drainage set (e.g., Pleur-evac, Deknatel A-5000-ATS, Fall River, MA). Empty the removable reservoir as needed. Alternatively, use a single–chest tube system with a Y-connector arrangement similar to that used for gastric lavage. Place aliquots of 200 to 300 mL with a 2-minute dwell time followed by suction drainage (at 20 cm H_2O).

Provide closed-chest massage until adequate spontaneous perfusion occurs. Perform closed-chest defibrillation if the patient is warmed to 30°C (86°F) and has persistent ventricular fibrillation. Continue thoracic lavage until the patient's temperature approaches 35°C (95°F).

Open Thoracic Lavage. Perform a left thoracotomy and pour saline warmed to 40°C to 41°C (104.0°F to 105.8°F) continuously into the thoracic cavity to bathe the heart while an assistant suctions the excess fluid from the lateral edge of the thoracotomy. Alternatively, add fluid to the thorax and mediastinum intermittently and suction after several minutes. Follow this with more warmed saline and repeat. This technique also allows direct monitoring of myocardial temperature. Perform direct cardiac massage until adequate spontaneous perfusion occurs. Perform direct cardiac defibrillation in a patient warmed to 30°C (86°F) with persistent ventricular fibrillation. When defibrillation is successful, continue direct myocardial warming until the patient's temperature approaches 35°C (95°F). If defibrillation is unsuccessful at a core temperature of 30°C (86°F), continue warming while oxygenation, perfusion, and other physiologic parameters are optimized before further attempts at defibrillation.

Summary. Thoracic lavage is an effective form of active core rewarming that is usually reserved for hypothermic arrest patients.[54,89,90] Thoracic lavage may be considered when vital signs are inadequate or unstable enough to severely limit perfusion. Precise indications have not been clarified beyond patients in cardiac arrest.

Cardiac Bypass

The use of cardiac bypass or an extracorporeal shunt through either the femoral artery–femoral vein or the aortocaval procedure can result in rapid rewarming but requires surgical expertise, the availability of appropriate equipment, and technical support.[5,50,91] This procedure has not been compared with other rewarming methods in a controlled fashion, and few centers have this modality available in a time frame that would affect survival rates. Its main advantages appear to be the rapid rate of warming that it produces and optimal patient oxygenation and perfusion. Femoral flow rates of 2 to 3 L/min with the warmer set at 38°C to 40°C (100.4°F to 104°F) will raise the core temperature 1°C to 2°C (33.8°F to 35.6°F) every 3 to 5 minutes.[6] Drawbacks include potential delays in assembling the appropriate team and equipment, delays because of the time necessary to complete the operation, complications from the operation, the expense of the procedure and bypass equipment, and the potential for infection. Its use in extreme situations that may include cardiac arrest should be based on individual characteristics of the patient, clinician team, and hospital resources. If readily available, it should be strongly considered in hypothermic patients with asystole or ventricular fibrillation.[41] If oxygenation is not a consideration, venovenous rewarming with an extracorporeal venovenous rewarmer can achieve rapid rewarming rates (2°C/hr to 3°C/hr [3.6°F/hr to 5.4°F/hr]), although they are slower than rates with cardiopulmonary bypass.[71] Such a device is relatively easy to use, involves readily available technology, and probably does not require heparin. This equipment needs to be assembled before patients with hypothermia arrive.[24] In severely hypothermic patients, extracorporeal rewarming using venovenous hemofiltration has also been reported to be successful.[70,71] When compared with adults, children, especially smaller ones, require special consideration with regard to IV cannulation because drainage can be inadequate with femoral-femoral cannulation. In smaller hypothermic children, some sources recommend a more aggressive emergency median sternotomy for cardiopulmonary bypass.[92]

Cardiopulmonary bypass is indicated in the following situations: (1) cardiac arrest or hemodynamic instability with a temperature lower than 32°C (<89.6°F), (2) no response to less invasive techniques, (3) completely frozen extremities, or (4) rhabdomyolysis with severe hyperkalemia.[2] A 47% long-term survival rate was obtained in a Swiss study of 32 young, otherwise healthy individuals, including mountain climbers, hikers, and victims of suicide attempts. Cardiopulmonary bypass is unlikely to confer similar benefit in older, poorly conditioned populations with underlying chronic diseases.[93]

Hemodialysis

Hemodialysis was first described for the management of AH in 1965.[94] It is a rapid and efficient modality for rapid internal rewarming of patients with moderate to severe AH, but it is uncommonly used in clinical practice. One study reported that 26 patients with AH combined with circulatory arrest or severe circulatory failure were rewarmed to normothermia with the use of ECC.[95] Core rewarming by hemodialysis has been achieved after placement of a dialysis catheter or with the use of an existing shunt. Some of the potential advantages and drawbacks of cardiac bypass also apply to this procedure, although slower warming rates have been reported. A range from 0.6°C/hr (33.1°F/hr) to rates as high as 4.5°C/hr (40.1°F/hr) have been achieved with fluid warmed to 40°C (104.0°F).[87] For patients who have ingested a dialyzable toxin (such as barbiturates and toxic alcohols), hemodialysis can be used to both remove the toxin and rewarm the blood.[94] In such cases its use may be appropriate.

Experimental Techniques

Ultrasonic, radiowave, and low-frequency microwave diathermy rewarming appears to be a rapid, safe, noninvasive technique that has shown promise in animal studies.[67,96] Frequencies of 13.6 to 40.7 MHz are typically used. In a volunteer study the technique seemed to be less effective than immersion therapy and equivalent to passive rewarming techniques.[96,97] Total liquid ventilation with warmed oxygenated perfluorocarbon is currently being studied in animals as a method of rapidly rewarming the core. Benefits include shorter rewarming times than with warm humidified oxygen (1.98 ± 0.5 hours versus 8.61 ± 1.6 hours; $P < 0.0001$), no afterdrop phenomenon, and no increase in lactate dehydrogenase and aspartate transaminase.[75]

Very hot IV fluids (65°C [149°F]) have been used in animals with little vascular damage or hemolysis. Trials in humans undergoing burn débridement have been very successful in preventing hypothermia during operative procedures. Saline heated to 60°C (140°F) with modified fluid warmers was infused through central venous access. There was no evidence of intravascular hemolysis or coagulopathy after the infusions.[98] The role of hot IV fluids in the management of AH is currently undefined.

Special Situations

Cardiac Arrest

Cardiac arrest secondary to AH requires immediate treatment for the best chance of a successful outcome. Rapid rewarming and restoration of cardiac rhythm are essential for patients in cardiopulmonary arrest and can best be achieved with a combination of passive and multiple active core rewarming techniques. Because of numerous cases of survival from hypothermic cardiac arrest with prolonged external cardiac compression,[5,41,99] thoracotomy is not mandatory. Thoracotomy does offer some theoretical advantages, however, such as increased cardiac output with open-chest massage,[90] direct observation of cardiac activity, and direct warming of cardiac tissue with thoracic cavity lavage of warm fluid. Cardiopulmonary bypass is an effective technique for rapid rewarming. Blunt trauma and head trauma victims were previously not ideal candidates for cardiac bypass because of the anticoagulation requirement, but some authors have advocated this technique with heparin-bonded tubing even in the setting of known traumatic injury.[5] A review of outcomes after hypothermic cardiac arrest from one institution found that the average time from thoracotomy to the development of a perfusing rhythm was 38 minutes (range, 10 to 90 minutes).[5] The optimal rate of cardiac compressions in hypothermic patients is not known. Because of decreased oxygen consumption by vital organs, the rate required in hypothermic cardiac arrest is less than that recommended for normothermic cardiac arrest. Cardiac compressions should be initiated at half the normal rate in profoundly hypothermic patients. Guidelines developed by the American Heart Association and the Wilderness Medical Society recommend that CPR be initiated in patients with AH unless any of the following conditions exist: a "do-not-resuscitate" status is documented and verified, obvious lethal injuries are present, chest wall depression is impossible, no signs of life are present, or rescuers are endangered by delays in evacuation and altered triage conditions.[6]

The duration of CPR depends on the time required to raise the core temperature to a level at which defibrillation should be successful (i.e., >30°C [>86°F]). Previously, it was recommended that patients not receive a set of three countershocks until a core temperature above 30°C (>86°F) could be attained. There have been reports of successful defibrillation in patients with profound hypothermia with core temperatures of 25.6°C (78.1°F).[86] The decision to terminate resuscitative efforts remains a clinical one, but there are certain poor prognostic factors. Certainly, survival is unlikely in patients who persist in asystole or go from ventricular fibrillation to asystole as they are warmed past 32°C (>89.6°F). Prognostic markers for patients with severe hypothermia and cardiac arrest have been proposed as contraindications to ED thoracotomy and cardiac bypass by some authors.[5] Such markers include potassium levels elevated to above 10 mmol/L (mEq/L) and pH levels below 6.5. Nonetheless, there are reports of survival in patients with higher potassium levels and a pH as low as 6.29.[92] The decision to continue resuscitative efforts should not be based solely on specific laboratory values or the initial core temperature.

Isolated reports of survival of hypothermic patients with prolonged CPR make extended efforts to resuscitate such patients reasonable. Children may be the best candidates for heroic measures.[50] Under ideal conditions, hypothermic cardiac arrest patients may reasonably be admitted to an intensive care unit for a 4- to 5-hour trial of rewarming with CPR in progress. Manual CPR should be replaced by mechanical methods if the equipment is available. The oxygen-powered "thumper" has been successful during prolonged hypothermic resuscitation. Absence of responsiveness to treatment, in conjunction with a highly elevated potassium level, is an indication for termination of resuscitative efforts.

Airway Management
Maintain a secure functioning airway for hypothermic patients, just as in any critically ill patient. With mild hypothermia, deliver heated, humidified oxygen by face mask. Recognize that a hypothermic patient can be combative and uncooperative and may require arm restraints if a mask is used. Intubate patients with decreased sensorium who cannot reliably maintain their airway or hypothermic patients who may be hypoxic. Endotracheal intubation may be performed safely without the added risk of ventricular dysrhythmias.[15] The technique for endotracheal intubation depends on the specific circumstances and the expertise of the operator. Once an endotracheal tube has been placed and secured, use it to provide warm humidified oxygen. There is no evidence that tracheal intubation is detrimental in severely hypothermic patients, and it should be considered if indicated for ventilation, oxygenation, or airway protection.

Acid-Base Disturbances
Acid-base disturbances are variable and can lead to metabolic acidosis from carbon dioxide retention and to lactic acidosis or metabolic alkalosis from decreased carbon dioxide production or hyperventilation. Interpretation of arterial blood gases in a hypothermic patient has been the cause of some confusion. Previously, it was suggested that all blood gases be corrected for temperature with correlation factors. With a decrease in temperature of 1°C (33.8°F), pH rises 0.015, carbon dioxide pressure (Pco_2) drops by 4.4%, and oxygen pressure (Po_2) drops 7.2% relative to values that would be obtained with blood analyzed under normal conditions. Despite the conversion guide, optimal or normal values in

hypothermia have not been well documented.[32] Other recent literature supports the use of uncorrected arterial blood gas values to guide therapy with bicarbonate or hyperventilation.[30] This approach appears appropriate to support optimal enzymatic function. Gradual correction of acid-base imbalance will allow increased efficiency of the bicarbonate buffering system as the body warms. Arterial pH did not correlate with patient death in the Multicenter Hypothermia Study and should not be used as a prognostic guide to resuscitation.[84]

Coagulopathies
Abnormal clotting occurs frequently in hypothermic patients, probably because cold inhibits the enzymatic coagulation cascade.[100-102] Hypothermia-induced coagulopathy does not result from excessive clot lysis, but rather from impaired clot formation.[16,21] Platelet function is also impaired during hypothermia because production of thromboxane B₂ is inhibited. Hypothermia-induced platelet aggregation with or without neutrophil involvement has been associated with neurologic dysfunction in patients undergoing surgical procedures.[91] Hypercoagulability with a risk for thromboembolism may also occur, but the importance of cold-induced coagulopathy mainly involves patients with coincidental trauma. Such victims often have bleeding that is difficult to control. Replace appropriate clotting factors and use warm blood to limit further blood loss and worsening of the hypothermia.

Trauma and Hypothermia
Mortality is increased in trauma patients with temperatures below 32°C (<89.6°F). It is not clear whether this increased mortality is actually a result of the hypothermia or whether the hypothermia is merely an indicator of severe injury and response to a massive transfusion of cold fluid.[21,103] Patients with severe trauma are prone to hypothermia because their injuries often expose them to environmental heat loss. Concurrent alcohol intoxication may add to the heat loss as a result of its vasodilatory effects on cutaneous vasculature and the prolonged cold exposure secondary to altered mental status. Victims of severe injury also lose heat because of exposure during resuscitation and rapid administration of cold fluids.

It is unknown to what degree correcting the hypothermia improves outcome. Nevertheless, devices to rapidly infuse warm fluids such as the Level 1 fluid warmer (Level 1 Technologies, Rockland, MA) and the Thermostat 900 (Arrow International, Reading, PA) are frequently used to warm large-volume fluid transfusions. Use of these devices seems reasonable to prevent the hypothermia associated with massive transfusions (see Chapter 28). Their use for hypothermia not associated with severe trauma is limited by the relatively low fluid requirements of patients with environmental exposure. Another Thermostat device (Aquarius Medical Corp., Phoenix, AZ) is used to accelerate recovery from hypothermia by mechanically distending blood vessels in the hand, thereby increasing transfer of exogenous heat to the body core. One article found that this particular rewarming device was not very effective in accelerating rewarming in hypothermic surgical patients after general anethesia.[104]

Pharmacotherapy and Monitoring
Hypothermia alters the pharmacodynamics of various drugs. It markedly alters drug kinetics, but not enough is known

TABLE 65-4 Commonly Used Medications for Hypothermia

CLINICAL SITUATION	MEDICATION	DOSAGE
Hypoglycemia	$D_{50}W$	1 mg/kg IV
Alcoholic/ malnourished	Thiamine	100 mg IV
Altered mental status	Naloxone	0.4-2 mg IV
Ventricular fibrillation	Bretylium* Magnesium sulfate	5 mg/kg IV 100 mg/kg IV

$D_{50}W$, 50% dextrose in water; *IV*, intravenously.
*The role of more available antidysrhythmics such as amiodarone in patients with hypothermia remains to be determined.

about this phenomenon to define specific therapeutic guidelines. Administer drugs with caution to hypothermic patients (Table 65-4). Because of the negative effects of hypothermia on both hepatic and renal metabolism, toxic levels of medications can accumulate rapidly after repeated use.[105] Avoid certain drugs, such as digitalis. Sinus bradycardia and most atrial arrhythmias do not require pharmacologic treatment because the majority resolve with rewarming. Transient ventricular dysrhythmias also do not require treatment. Bretylium is the preferred agent for patients requiring medication for ventricular dysrhythmias, but lidocaine, magnesium, propranolol, and amiodarone have also been used.[30] For severe acidosis (pH <7.1), IV sodium bicarbonate can be used with extreme caution. Vasopressors should be used with care, perhaps in much smaller doses than usual, because of the arrhythmogenic potential and the delayed metabolism of these agents. A review of intensive care unit admission of hypothermic patients found that treatment with vasoactive drugs was an independent risk factor for mortality, but this phenomenon remains poorly understood.[41] In animal studies, use of epinephrine impaired myocardial efficiency in cases of moderate hypothermia.[106] There was no advantage to repeated doses of epinephrine or high-dose epinephrine in hypothermic cardiac arrest animal models.[107] The use of inamrinone, formerly known as amrinone, has been investigated in cases of deliberate mild hypothermia. Initial results indicate that amrinone accelerates the cooling rate of the core temperature, thereby potentially limiting its usefulness in management of AH.[108]

Administer IV fluids slowly to prevent fluid overload potentiated by the decreased cardiac output. Fluids should be started early because intravascular volume is depleted in most hypothermic patients. D_5NS has been advocated as the ideal initial resuscitation fluid.[61,63,68] Avoid potassium until electrolytes are measured and normal renal function is confirmed. Check serum levels of creatine phosphokinase in hypothermic patients, which may indicate rhabdomyolysis. If elevated, carefully monitor renal function. Replace fluids aggressively because this may help prevent the development of renal failure. In severely hypothermic patients, consider placing a Swan-Ganz catheter and closely monitor urinary output to assist in fluid management. The risk of precipitating ventricular fibrillation should be weighed against the potential benefits of the Swan-Ganz catheter.

It should be emphasized that hypothermic patients exhibit a "classic physiologic response" that may be somewhat protective. This response depends on the severity of the decrease in core temperature and classically consists of hypotension, hypoventilation, depressed mental status, and bradycardia. This prohibits a precise recommendation of the indications and use of medications, intubation, CPR, and other resuscitative interventions, which are better defined in normothermic patients. Hypothermic patients with a blood pressure, respiratory rate, or mental status that would prognosticate certain morbidity in normothermic patients may recover with minimal intervention on their normal pre-hypothermic state. Avoid aggressive therapies or medications aimed at providing hypothermic patients with vital signs that would be desirable in normothermic patients but may be supraphysiologic in hypothermic patients.

Frostbite

Hypothermic patients frequently suffer other forms of cold-related injuries in addition to their systemic hypothermia. The mildest form of frostbite is termed *frostnip*, a condition that involves only the skin and spares subcutaneous tissue. The skin is blanched and numb, but the injury is immediately reversible with no permanent sequelae if the area is quickly rewarmed. Rewarm rapidly in a water bath at 40°C to 42°C (104.0°F to 107.6°F). Frostnip occurs most frequently on the distal ends of the extremities, the nose, and the ears. Nonfreezing temperatures also produce *trench foot*, an intermediate step in the progression to true frostbite. Trench foot is the result of prolonged immersion in cold water. Rewarm patients and apply dry dressings.[109,110]

In frostbite, the body parts most susceptible are those farthest away from the body's core: the hands, feet, earlobes, and nose. Exposure of the fingers to severe cold leads to cold-induced vasodilation.[111,112] Apical structures rich in arteriovenous anastomoses can shunt blood flow away from tissues. Freezing of the corneas has been reported to occur in individuals who keep their eyes open in high–wind chill situations without protective goggles (e.g., snowmobilers and skiers).[97]

The pathophysiology of frostbite includes three pathways of tissue freezing: (1) through the extracellular formation of ice crystals, (2) hypoxia as a result of cold-induced local vasoconstriction, and (3) release of inflammatory mediators. These pathways often occur simultaneously and intensify the tissue damage. At the early stages of frostbite the "hunting reaction" is observed whereby the body alternates between periods of vasoconstriction and periods of vasodilation. As the temperature continues to decrease, the reaction stops and vasoconstriction persists.[109,113] Cold also increases blood viscosity, promotes vasospasm, and precipitates the formation of microthrombi. Release of the inflammatory mediators prostaglandin F_2 and thromboxane A_2 causes further vasoconstriction leading to cell death. Release of these mediators peaks during rewarming, and cycles of recurrent freezing and rewarming only increase their tissue levels. Rewarming must be avoided until refreezing can be prevented.

The clinical signs and symptoms of frostbite vary according to the degree of injury. Though useful clinically, the degree classification does not predict the extent of further tissue damage.[32,92,100] The appearance of the affected extremity depends on the extent of the frostbite. With superficial frostbite, the affected extremity appears pale, waxy, and numb. The limb has poor capillary refill and is very painful on rewarming. With deeper frostbite, the affected extremity is hard, solid, and blanched. Hemorrhagic blisters may be present (Fig. 65-5). Initially, there is no pain or feeling in the frostbitten extremity. After rewarming, severe edema and blistering develop in the affected area, and victims eventually exhibit dry gangrene, mummification, and ultimately tissue sloughing.

Favorable prognostic signs for frostbite include intact sensation, normal color, warm tissues, early appearance of clear blisters, and edema. Early intervention is critical in terms of the ultimate outcome. Delay in seeking medical care for more than 24 hours is associated with an 85% likelihood that surgical intervention will be required. Patients seen within the first 24 hours require surgery less than 30% of the time.[2,110] The predictive value of the initial physical examination is limited, but the presence of nonblanching cyanosis, hemorrhagic blisters, and impaired sensation appears to indicates a poor prognosis.[2]

Based on early bone scans and retrospective studies, researchers from France proposed a new classification for predicting frostbite outcomes on day 0.[114] Four degrees of severity are defined. With *first degree*, there is complete recovery. *Second degree* often leads to soft tissue amputation. With *third degree*, bone amputation is needed, and with *fourth degree*, systemic effects occur.[114]

Rapid rewarming is the treatment of choice for frostbite.[109] The aim is to limit the length of time that the tissue remains in the frozen state. The most practical way to rewarm an extremity is to totally immerse the area in warm water at 40°C to 42°C (104.0°F to 107.6°°F) for 15 to 30 minutes. Carefully protect the affected area to ensure that the tissue is not additionally injured by contact with the sides or rim of the container. After thawing, meticulously protect the area from injury. Elevate the extremity and place cotton or gauze between the toes or fingers to limit maceration. At some point, necrotic tissue should be débrided, most often after the ED encounter has allowed identification of viable tissue; however, the ideal timing and best method or intervention have not been elucidated. A conservative approach is advocated. One method is to débride white or clear blisters. Leave hemorrhagic or dark blisters intact because disruption may theoretically cause damage to the vascular supply and viable tissue.

Use topical aloe vera, a thromboxane inhibitor, and administer systemic antiprostaglandins such as ibuprofen. The use of semiocclusive dressings has shown promising results in the management of deep frostbite injuries of the fingertips.[115] Provide tetanus prophylaxis. Adjuvant therapies involving the use of heparin or low-molecular-weight heparin, warfarin, vasodilators, corticosteroids, or immediate surgical sympathectomy have failed to improve outcomes.

The ideal intervention to ameliorate or limit tissue injury has not been proved, and it is uncertain if any protocol will prove effective. Mixed success has been achieved with the use of hyperbaric oxygen and thrombolytics.[116] In a small study of frostbite victims, Twomey and coworkers suggested the following treatment algorithm for severe frostbite[117]: (1) rapid rewarming; (2) assessment of the patient's clinical appearance; (3) early-phase ^{99m}Tc scintiscan to assess the distal circulation; (4) administration of tissue plasminogen activator (t-PA), 0.15 mg/kg by IV bolus, followed by 0.15 mg/kg/hr to a maximum dose of 100 mg over a 4- to 6-hour period, for patients with digits or limbs showing no flow and an absence of contraindications; (5) therapeutic heparin for 3 to 5 days; (6) administration of warfarin to an international normalized ratio two times control for 4 weeks; (7) pain management as needed; (8) ibuprofen, 400 to 600 mg orally four times daily; (9) light dressings with topical antimicrobials; and (10) no ambulation on frostbitten feet.[117] Bruen and colleagues,[118] in a small retrospective study, reported that administration of t-PA within 24 hours of frostbite injury improved tissue perfusion and reduced amputations. The protocol included t-PA administered at an initial rate of 0.5 to 1.0 mg/hr into the extremity via a femoral or brachial arterial catheter sheath. Heparin was also administered at 500 U/hr into the intraarterial catheter.[118] Thrombolytic therapy for frostbite is encouraging, but the exact parameters for its use are still being investigated.

Agents that can inhibit the formation of free radicals are also promising. Such agents include superoxide dismutase, prostaglandin E_1 analogues, and drugs containing antiplatelet activity such as pentoxifylline.[109,113] The use of antibiotics is controversial, although some authors advocate agents effective against *Staphylococcus* and *Streptococcus* (e.g.,

Figure 65-5 Frostbite. Rapid rewarming is the treatment of choice; immersion in warm water (40°C to 42°C) for 15 to 30 minutes is a practical method. A conservative approach to frostbite debridement is suggested, with many alternatives acceptable. One approach is to débride white or clear blisters and leave hemorrhagic or dark blisters intact.

cephalosporins, penicillins). Avoid débridement of tissue in the ED. Give analgesics (IV opioids) as needed.

Cold Water Immersion and Submersion

One of the leading causes of hypothermia remains cold water immersion or submersion.[119] In a retrospective review of AH cases in a 3-year period, submersion hypothermia accounted for the greatest number of cases.[120] Unlike cases of AH caused by cold exposure, risk factors are harder to identify because of the high mortality from drowning.[100] Studies have shown that at cold water temperatures (8°C [46.4°F]), core cooling occurs at slower rates in persons with increased body mass and subcutaneous fat and at faster rates with increased voluntary activity (e.g., treading water). Risk factors for submersion hypothermia include impaired performance and the initial cardiorespiratory response to immersion. A study in healthy volunteers found that swimming efficiency and length of stroke decreased whereas the rate of stroke and swim angle increased as the water temperature dropped.[121]

The body's response to cold water immersion (head out) has previously been described as occurring in three phases.[67] The initial phase involves the "cold-shock response," which typically occurs within the first 4 to 6 minutes. Signs include peripheral vasoconstriction, gasp reflex, hyperventilation, and tachycardia. At this stage there is a higher incidence of sudden death resulting from hypocapnia, inability to hold one's breath, and increased cardiac output.[67] After the initial cold-shock response, the body undergoes profound cooling of the peripheral tissues. The peripheral cooling tends to be the greatest in the hands, which leads to incoordination and difficulty grasping.[67] With prolonged immersion in cold water, heat is lost from the body quicker than it is produced, with the individual quickly progressing to hypothermia.[122-124]

In cases of cold water submersion, researchers have found that rapid cooling is protective against neurologic impairment and increases the chance of survival.[125] There are numerous reports in the literature of survival in children after cold water submersion but very few reports in adults. There are also reports of survival after up to 65 minutes of cold water submersion.[126] Survival was reported in an elderly male after 22 minutes of submersion.[127] Children tend to have a better prognosis because of the presence of the mammalian dive reflex and a greater body surface area–to-mass ratio, which allows more rapid cooling. A recent case was reported of a 2-year-old boy who suffered from severe hypothermia after falling into ice water.[7] On discovery, cardiac arrest and asystole were present and the first measured temperature was 23.8°C (74.8°F). The patient was rewarmed by ECC with cardiopulmonary bypass and was discharged 9 days later without any sequelae. Orlowski identified five poor prognostic factors for near-drowning in pediatric patients[128]: (1) maximum submersion time longer than 5 minutes, (2) comatose on arrival at the ED, (3) arterial blood gas pH less than 7.10, (4) age younger than 3 years, and (5) resuscitation not attempted for at least 10 minutes after rescue. Adults tend to have higher mortality rates because of the following: (1) lack of the mammalian dive reflex and (2) slower rates of cooling secondary to lower body surface area–to-mass ratios than in children. Recent reports of hypothermia and drowning in commercial fishing deaths in Alaska noted a strong protective association with the use of personal floatation devices, particularly immersion suits, in surviving cold water–related events in adults.[129]

Various mechanisms of brain and body cooling during submersion hypothermia have been described, including the mammalian dive reflex, cold-induced changes in release of neurotransmitters, and water ventilation.[130] The mammalian dive reflex prevents or delays aspiration or ventilation until the body has cooled to a point at which protection against hypothermia occurs. Much attention has focused on the theory of water ventilation as a key component of accelerated brain cooling. Animal studies comparing immersed (head out) and submersed dogs found that cooling rates were faster in submersed dogs than in immersed dogs. The submersed dogs cooled by convective heat exchange in the lungs, whereas the immersed dogs cooled by surface conduction only. Laboratory data obtained after the submersion indicated that there was indeed ventilation exchange in the water.[126] The body also undergoes a relative bradycardia as another protective measure. Bradycardia is inversely proportional to the water temperature, with heart rates reaching 18 beats/min in water at 10°C (50°F).[130] Many authors advocate therapies aimed at symptoms resulting from near-drowning rather than severe hypothermia because in fatal cases of submersion, death occurs too rapidly for hypothermia to be a significant contributor. Complications of near-drowning include pneumonia, lung edema, hemorrhagic pancreatitis, and skin edema.[100]

Conclusion

Mortality rates from AH are decreasing, and this is linked to increased recognition and advanced therapy. Caution should be used when extrapolating published data obtained in adults to children.[56] With the exception of severe hypothermia, the prognosis correlates mostly with the presence or absence of underlying disease states. Studies have shown that the prognosis is excellent in patients in whom no hypoxic event precedes the hypothermia and no serious underlying disease states exist. Previously healthy individuals usually have full recovery with mortality rates lower than 5%, but patients with coexisting medical illnesses reportedly have mortality rates higher than 50%.[55]

As a general guideline, take a conservative approach to rewarming stable hypothermic patients, with avoidance of overtreatment and selective and careful use of invasive monitoring. Evaluate a hypothermic patient's "physiologic" hypotension, hypoventilation, and bradycardia with regard to that expected for the given core temperature.

Because death is related more to underlying illnesses than to hypothermia, some recent sources do not believe that invasive rewarming modalities are useful for poikilothermic patients with severe underlying disease.[1]

With moderate hypothermia, underlying problems should be sought, passive rewarming and basic support started, and less invasive core rewarming begun. This approach should include mask ventilation with warm humidified air or oxygen in conscious patients and intubation and ventilation in unconscious patients. In selected patients, gastric or peritoneal lavage with warm fluid may be considered. For severely hypothermic, *unstable* patients, cardiac bypass and thoracic lavage may offer additional benefits, including rapid warming rates and direct heart warming. The benefits should be weighed against the institutional capabilities, time, expense, and the danger for complications that these procedures entail.

PROCEDURES PERTAINING TO HYPERTHERMIA

As a result of global climate change, it is projected that world-wide there will be a significant increase in the number and intensity of heat waves with resultant deaths from hyperthermia and heat-related illness.[131] Temperature extremes and variability will remain important determinants of overall health, especially in the vulnerable populations of the elderly, children, and those with chronic illness. The mortality associated with heatstroke accounts for more than 200 deaths per year in the United States.[132,133] In the United States from 1999 to 2003, a total of 3442 deaths were attributed to extreme heat exposure.[134] During the heat wave of 2003, France reported 15,000 excess deaths as a result of the heat wave.[135] The morbidity associated with heat-related illness is on the rise. Nationally, an estimated 54,983 patients were evaluated in U.S. EDs for exertional heat-related illness from 1997 to 2006.[136] This represents a 133% increase over the 10-year period.[136] Lack of heat acclimatization during extreme environmental conditions is responsible for the increasing percentage of heat-related illness, particularly in younger populations and agricultural workers.[137]

Other important causes of hyperthermia include malignant hyperthermia (MH) and neuroleptic malignant syndrome (NMS). Both MH and NMS are largely iatrogenic and are mostly triggered by modern pharmacologic therapy.[138] There is evidence that MH involves a dose-dependent response, but the minimum dose is unknown.[138] The incidence of hyperthermic conditions induced by psychostimulant drugs of abuse, such as morphine and amphetamine derivatives, continues to increase.[139]

As with hypothermia, it is important to use the proper thermometer capable of detecting a wide range of body temperatures. Heatstroke remains a common clinical problem with significant morbidity and mortality. A variety of cooling techniques have been advocated since World War II. Although some cooling techniques have been compared in controlled human and animal models of heatstroke, our practice decisions are not based solely on the theoretical rate of cooling. Other important factors include the ease of use, rapidity of initiation, and safety.

Before considering the various cooling techniques, it is essential that the underlying disorders of hyperthermia be clearly understood. Heat illness represents a broad spectrum of disease ranging from mild heat exhaustion to severe heatstroke. The latter includes disorders such as MH and NMS. Treatment of this spectrum of disease requires a discriminating approach, including supportive care only for heat exhaustion and rapid cooling for heatstroke. MH requires specific pharmacologic therapy (e.g., dantrolene), in addition to cooling measures. A brief discussion of hyperthermic disorders is necessary before describing cooling techniques.

Normal Thermoregulation

Body temperature typically follows a diurnal pattern, with an increase from about 36°C (96.8°F) in the early morning to 37.5°C (99.5°F) in the late afternoon, and is normally tightly regulated by an effective thermoregulatory system.[140] Heat is produced as a by-product of metabolic processes and when ambient temperature exceeds body temperature. Body temperature increases when the rate of heat production exceeds the rate of heat dissipation. The brain's thermal center is located in the preoptic nucleus of the anterior hypothalamus. In response to rising core temperature, this thermal center activates efferent fibers of the autonomic nervous system to produce vasodilation and increase the rate of sweating. Vasodilation dissipates heat by convection, and sweat dissipates heat by evaporation.

Hyperthermia occurs when the thermoregulatory mechanisms are overwhelmed by excessive metabolic production of heat, excessive environmental heat, or impaired heat dissipation. Different age-related thermoregulation strategies are used when dealing with heat stress. Children have a greater surface area–to-mass ratio and a lower sweating rate and rely more on "dry" heat exchange to dissipate heat. On the contrary, adults use evaporative heat loss as the primary heat dissipation technique. With primary aging, the reflex cutaneous vasoconstriction and vasodilation capabilities are impaired, thereby allowing increased susceptibility to complications from heat-related exposure.[141] Fever occurs when the hypothalamic set-point is increased by the action of circulating pyrogenic cytokines, which cause peripheral mechanisms to conserve and generate heat until the body temperature rises to the elevated set-point. Hyperthermia and fever cannot be differentiated clinically on the basis of the magnitude of temperature or on the pattern of its changes.[142,143]

Types of Hyperthermia

Mild Heat Illness

Heat cramps and heat exhaustion are induced by a hot environment.[144] The body's heat dissipation mechanisms are generally able to keep up with heat production and absorption in these disorders. Symptoms are largely due to the mechanisms used by the body to dissipate heat, and body temperatures remain at or near normal. Rapid cooling techniques are *not* required, and supportive care and hydration in a cool environment are usually adequate therapy.

Heat cramps are intensely painful but generally benign involuntary skeletal muscle spasms. The pain most often occurs in the calf, hamstring, or quadriceps muscles but may also involve the arms and back. The cramps may be severe and prolonged but only rarely lead to rhabdomyolysis. Heat cramps occur after strenuous exercise or heavy labor in a hot environment. Heat cramps were previously thought to be the result of dehydration associated with significant loss of sodium chloride, but some clinical observations have proved that heat cramps can occur at rest or during exercise under any environmental conditions.[145] Rest in a cool environment plus vigorous oral fluid replacement with isotonic solutions is usually adequate therapy, but in some cases IV saline is required.[145] The benefits of oral rehydration over IV hydration directly relate to oropharyngeal stimulation, which influences the release of antidiuretic hormone (arginine vasopressin), cutaneous vasodilation, thirst sensation, and mean arterial pressure.[146] A common mistake is to rely on thirst to indicate dehydration. The pain of severe cramping may be resistant to narcotics in the absence of adequate fluid replacement.

Heat exhaustion, commonly referred to as heat syncope, is a poorly defined syndrome with nonspecific symptoms that *occur after heat exposure*.[147] Many have suggested replacing the current terminology of heat exhaustion with the term exercise-associated collapse.[148] Malaise, flulike symptoms, orthostasis, dehydration, nausea, headache, and collapse may all occur.

Previously it was believed that heat exhaustion is the result of dehydration-induced heat retention that is not severe enough to cause heatstroke.[149] There is modern evidence that postural hypotension developing after exercise is the result of exercise-induced changes in blood pressure regulation. These changes involve recalibration of the arterial baroreflex to lower pressures after exercise, impaired sympathetic vascular regulation, and H_1 and H_2 receptor–mediated vasodilation.[149] When compared with the more severe heat disorder of heatstroke, mental status is normal and body temperature is normal or mildly elevated with heat exhaustion. There does not appear to be any thermoregulatory failure in persons with heat exhaustion. Rehydration, rest, and supportive care in a cool environment are adequate therapy for heat exhaustion.[144,145,148] Some authors advocate cooling and placing the patient either in the supine position with the legs elevated or seated with the head between the knees to decrease skin blood flow and increase venous blood flow to the heart.[149] Recovery is usually evident within a few minutes to hours. Occasionally, heat exhaustion is accompanied by heat cramps, thus presenting a confusing scenario if the diagnosis is not suspected. Rapid cooling techniques, IV hydration, and advanced therapies are not usually required, but patients should be observed for progression to heatstroke because heat exhaustion and heatstroke are a continuum of one disease process.[146,149]

Heatstroke

When the body's normal heat dissipation mechanisms are overwhelmed, core temperature elevation and heatstroke develop rapidly. Heatstroke is a state of thermoregulatory failure.[133] Previously, the morbidity and mortality associated with heatstroke were attributed to the magnitude of the hyperthermic response.[133] Recent literature has described a more complex interaction between cytokines, coagulation, and the systemic inflammatory response syndrome (SIRS), with endotoxin and cytokines being implicated as key mediators of heat-induced SIRS.[150] Two forms of heatstroke are described in the literature. *Classic (nonexertional) heatstroke* usually occurs during summer heat waves. The poor, urban elderly, infants, homeless, and persons with impaired mobility are at greatest risk.[151,152] Dehydration, lack of air-conditioning, obesity, neurologic disorders, hyperthyroidism, cardiovascular disease, impaired mentation, and medications that interfere with heat dissipation (e.g., phenothiazines, diuretics, and anticholinergics) predispose this population to heatstroke.[151,152] *Exertional heatstroke*, a consequence of strenuous physical activity, usually afflicts a younger segment of the population. Highly motivated, poorly acclimatized, or unconditioned athletes and overweight military recruits are common victims, as are individuals who perform heavy physical labor in hot, humid conditions (Fig. 65-6).[153-155] With exertional heatstroke, the risk appears to be greatest in individuals performing high-intensity exercise for relatively short durations.[155] A retrospective review of long-distance cyclists participating in the California AIDS (acquired immunodeficiency disease) Ride found that as the number of chronic medical illnesses increased, so did the risk for development of an exertional heat-related illness. Human immunodeficiency virus seropositivity alone was not associated with an increased risk for exertional heat-related illness.[155]

The degree of hyperthermia necessary to produce heatstroke in humans is unknown. In tissue culture cells, thermal

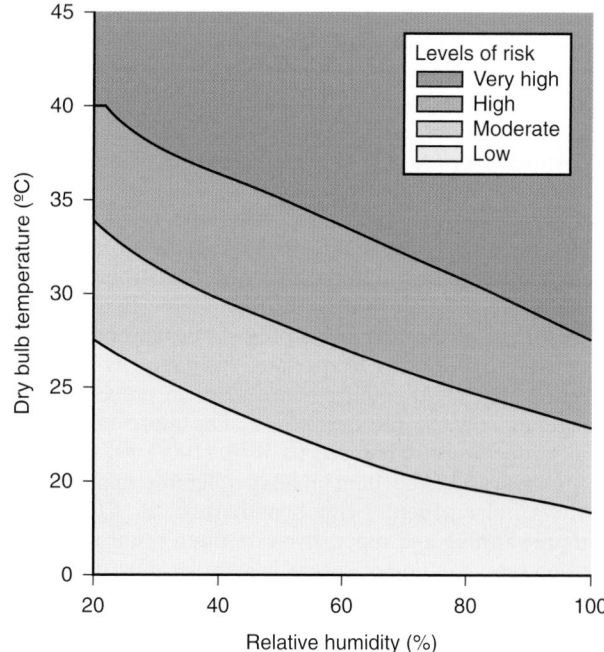

Figure 65-6 Risk for heat exhaustion or heatstroke during intense work in the heat (adjusted to the American College of Sports Medicine position stand: prevention of thermal injuries during distance running[2]). (*Adapted from Epstein Y, Moran D. Environmental aspects of travel medicine. In: Keystone JS, Kozarsky P, Freedman DO, et al, eds. Travel Medicine, ed 3. Philadelphia: Saunders; 2013.*)

injury is observed with temperatures in the range of 40°C to 45°C (104°F to 113°F). Studies of hyperthermia in patients undergoing cancer therapy have revealed that tissue sensitivity to heat is increased by relative hypoxia, ischemia, and acidosis.[156]

The key clinical findings in the diagnosis of heatstroke are (1) a history of heat stress or exposure, (2) a rectal temperature higher than 40°C (>104°F), and (3) central nervous system (CNS) dysfunction (altered mental status, disorientation, stupor, seizures, or coma). The cerebellum is very sensitive to heat, and ataxia may be an early clue. Although anhidrosis is described as a classic sign of heatstroke, investigations have demonstrates that cessation of sweating may be a late finding. Failure to consider the diagnosis of heatstroke in a diaphoretic patient with changes in mental status could prove disastrous.[157]

The sequelae of heatstroke are caused by thermal damage to multiple organ systems.[158] Whole-body hyperthermia decreases pulmonary capillary wedge pressure and cerebral vascular conductance and causes an inotropic shift in the Frank-Starling curve.[159] After a hyperthermic event, tissue injury continues.[157,158] Delirium, seizures, and coma can result from the direct effects of heat on the CNS. Autopsies show profound brain edema after hyperthermic insults. Researchers suggest that in cases of instant death, brain edema from the increased permeability of the blood-brain barrier causes raised intracranial pressure and papilledema, followed by vascular infarction and brain herniation.[160] Cardiovascular collapse results from dehydration, maximal cutaneous vasodilation, and direct heat-induced myocardial depression. Coagulopathies and liver dysfunction (elevated levels of bilirubin and transaminases) occur as a consequence of thermal breakdown, consumption of serum proteins, and direct heat damage to hepatic cells. Children often demonstrate diarrhea. Reduced intestinal blood flow causes barrier dysfunction and endotoxemia.[161,162] Development of an acute abdomen, bloody diarrhea, dilated loops of bowel on radiographic studies, and unexplained shock should raise suspicion for colonic ischemia and pending colonic perforation.[163] Renal failure can result from myoglobinuria (related to rhabdomyolysis) and acute tubular necrosis.[163] Metabolic acidosis is the primary acid-base alteration observed in patients with heatstroke, with the prevalence increasing with the degree of hyperthermia.[164]

Treatment of these sequelae of acute heatstroke does not differ from that of other heat-related disorders, with the sole exception that rapid cooling is necessary to prevent further damage and reverse the heat stress. The more rapidly that rectal temperature is reduced to 38°C (100.4°F), the better the prognosis.[151] The human body tolerates hyperthermia poorly. Unlike patients with hypothermia, in whom slow, gentle rewarming and supportive care often result in a favorable outcome, victims of severe heatstroke must be treated aggressively with measures designed to rapidly lower core temperature. Studies investigating precooling techniques to avoid heatstroke have been relatively unsuccessful in attenuating increases in core body temperature, and such techniques are not recommended.[165] In contrast, whole-body precooling increases overall exercise endurance.[166]

MH

MH is a pharmacogenetic disease attributable to a medication that triggers a life-threatening, hypermetabolic syndrome.[167] It results from a rare inherited autosomal dominant abnormality in the skeletal muscle membrane and has an incidence of 1 in 50,000 in adults.[139] In response to certain stresses or drugs (Box 65-1), patients with this disorder sustain a potentially lethal hypermetabolic reaction with massive efflux of calcium from the skeletal muscle sarcoplasmic reticulum. This results in contraction of the sarcomeres, skeletal muscle rigidity, increased skeletal muscle metabolism, elevated serum creatine kinase levels, heat production, and finally, systemic hyperthermia.[168,169] Hyperthermia is a late development and occurs after rigidity has been present for some time and the body's normal heat dissipation mechanisms are overwhelmed. The earliest signs of MH are increased carbon dioxide production, muscle rigidity, and tachycardia.[170] Cardiac output and cutaneous blood flow also increase to maximize the heat

loss. Diagnosis of MH is based on the clinical triad of (1) exposure to an agent or stress known to trigger the condition, (2) skeletal muscle rigidity, and (3) hyperthermia.

MH is usually encountered in the operating room while patients are undergoing general anesthesia, particularly with halogenated inhalational agents and depolarizing muscle relaxants. Heat production in anesthetized patients can be profound with as much as a fivefold increase in oxygen consumption.[169] Cases of MH may be encountered anywhere that general anesthetics or neuromuscular blocking agents are used.[169,170] A massive increase in creatine kinase is a strong indicator of an MH reaction.[167]

As with heatstroke, treatment of MH requires rapid cooling and supportive care for the sequelae described previously. Unlike heatstroke, MH requires specific pharmacologic therapy to stop excessive heat production by skeletal muscle. Dantrolene sodium induces muscle relaxation in patients with MH by blocking release of calcium from the muscle cell sarcoplasmic reticulum.[171] In all cases of MH, the inciting stimulus (see Table 65-4) should be discontinued immediately and dantrolene therapy administered. A dantrolene bolus of 2.5 mg/kg should started and repeated at 5-min intervals until normalization of the hypermetabolic state is achieved and all MH symptoms disappear.[171] Procainamide has been used successfully when dantrolene is unavailable.[171]

It has been suggested that dantrolene administration speeds cooling of heatstroke victims by reducing skeletal muscle heat production.[171] A randomized, controlled trial of the use of dantrolene for heatstroke found no difference between the treatment and placebo groups in terms of cooling time, complications, or length of stay.[172] In 2005 a metaanalysis concluded that there was no role for the use of dantrolene in the management of heatstroke.[173] Currently, dantrolene administration is best reserved for patients with clinical muscle rigidity or suspected MH. Routine use of this drug in heatstroke patients is not recommended.[173] New and promising treatments of MH are being investigated. Researchers have discovered mutations in the gene coding for the ryanodine receptor calcium release channel (RyRI) in families with MH, which may be the functional basis for MH. Some studies have examined the effects of MH mutations on the sensitivity of the RyRI to drugs and endogenous channel effectors, including Ca^{2+} and calmodulin.[174]

NMS

First described in the late 1960s, NMS is characterized by hyperthermia, muscle rigidity, altered level of consciousness, and autonomic instability.[175] Mortality from NMS is estimated to be 20% in patients in whom the condition develops.[175,176] This idiosyncratic disorder follows the therapeutic use of neuroleptic drugs, including phenothiazines, butyrophenones, thioxanthenes, lithium, and tricyclic antidepressants. The reaction is triggered by blockade of dopaminergic receptors and results in skeletal muscle spasticity, which generates excessive heat and impairs hypothalamic thermoregulation and heat dissipation.[176] Muscle rigidity, described as "lead pipe" rigidity in its most severe form,[176] can be manifested as oculogyric crisis, dyskinesia, akinesia, dysphagia, dysarthria, or opisthotonos. NMS occurs in 0.2% of patients who take neuroleptic agents either chronically or acutely. Haloperidol and depot fluphenazine appear to be the most commonly offending agents.[175] Temperatures can exceed 42°C (107.6°F). The initial agitation often progresses to stupor and coma.

BOX 65-1	**Triggers of MH**

DRUGS	Ketamine
Halothane	Trichloroethylene
Methoxyflurane	Chloroform
Enflurane	Gallamine
Diethyl ether	Nitrous oxide
Cyclopropane	
Succinylcholine	**CONDITIONS**
Tubocurarine	Heat stress
Lidocaine	Vigorous exercise
Mepivacaine	Emotional stress
Isoflurane	

MH, *malignant hyperthermia.*

Catatonia and mutism may also be present. Autonomic instability is manifested as tachycardia, labile blood pressure, sweating, and incontinence. Ventilations are impaired by the chest wall rigidity.

This syndrome is more likely to occur at the initiation of or after an increase in neuroleptic dosage. Researchers suggest that NMS typically occurs over a period of several days (average in patients taking neuroleptic agents). It may also occur if the use of antiparkinsonian drugs is suddenly discontinued.[176-179] NMS resembles MH but usually lasts longer (5 to 10 days) after use of the inciting drug is discontinued. The syndrome may be misinterpreted as worsening of an underlying psychiatric disorder, drug intoxication (e.g., cocaine and amphetamines), a severe dystonic reaction, tetanus, or a variety of CNS infections. In addition to agents with increased dopaminergic blocking activity, other risk factors for NMS include dehydration, previous history of dystonia, catatonia, agitation, and iron deficiency.[175] The mortality rate is high, and respiratory failure, renal failure, cardiovascular collapse, or thromboembolic disease usually causes death.[180]

Treatment of severe NMS (i.e., hypotension, hyperthermia, marked rigidity) closely follows that of MH, except that therapy must be maintained for several days until the symptoms resolve. Therapy for NMS involves discontinuation of the triggering agent; rapid cooling; benzodiazepines; a combination of a central dopamine agonist, bromocriptine, or levodopa; dantrolene; and supportive treatment of the ensuing organ failure.[179] Although the effects are not immediate, pharmaceutical therapy is directed at overriding the dopaminergic blockade caused by the offending neuroleptic agent or the dopamine depletion resulting from the cessation of antiparkinsonian medications. There are reports of successful treatment of NMS with subcutaneous apomorphine monotherapy or high-dose lorazepam and diazepam.[180,181] As with MH, dantrolene (2.5 mg/kg) can be given to treat NMS-induced muscle rigidity.[17] The beneficial response stems not only from effects at the sarcoplasmic reticulum of skeletal muscle but also from central dopamine metabolism of calcium in the CNS. Bromocriptine, a central dopamine agonist, is reported to be efficacious in treating NMS at doses of 2.5 to 10 mg three times a day.[181] Although both these agents have been noted to reduce the duration of hyperthermia, there have been mixed results with the use of bromocriptine and dantrolene.[178,181]

A more recently described disorder often confused with NMS is *serotonin syndrome*.[182] This syndrome involves the newer antidepressants fluoxetine, paroxetine, citalopram, fluvoxamine, venlafaxine, and sertraline,[182] which are selective serotonin reuptake inhibitors. These drugs can adversely react with other stronger serotonin receptor agents such as monoamine oxidase inhibitors and nonselective serotonin reuptake inhibitors (clomipramine and tricyclic antidepressants) to induce a clinical picture similar to that of NMS, only milder. Serotonin syndrome classically occurs when two or more drugs that interfere with serotonin metabolism act synergistically on the 5-HT$_{1A}$ receptor and lead to overstimulation.[178,182] Drugs that act at any of the other serotonin receptors are not likely to produce the syndrome.[182] The range of symptoms varies from mild gastrointestinal upset, insomnia, and agitation to more severe symptoms that include muscle spasms, seizures, ataxia, rhabdomyolysis, and autonomic instability. Treatment is primarily supportive in milder cases and consists of prompt recognition and withdrawal of the offending agent. Most cases resolve spontaneously within 24 hours. For the

most severe cases, aggressive intensive care unit management is warranted to prevent renal failure and death. The drug cyproheptadine (Periactin) has shown promise in managing the agitation often seen in severe cases.[178,182] Cyproheptadine is an antihistamine with antiserotonergic properties. There has been limited success with benzodiazepines and β-blockers in these patients to treat agitation.[182] In cases in which serotonin syndrome and NMS cannot be differentiated, benzodiazepines represent the safest therapeutic option.[178] Further study of the newer antipsychotic drugs, such as ziprasidone, a powerful 5-HT$_{1A}$ receptor blocker, may delineate other possible benefits.[182]

Hyperthermia and Psychostimulant Overdose
As mentioned previously, the recognized incidence of hyperthermia induced by sympathomimetic psychostimulant drugs of abuse is on the rise. The offending agents most commonly described are cocaine, phencyclidine, amphetamine, and amphetamine derivatives such as 3,4-methylenedioxy-N-methamphetamine (MDMA) ("ecstasy") and 3,4-methylenedioxy-N-ethylamphetamine (MDEA) ("Eve").[183,184] A number of studies have looked specifically at the club drug MDMA and its impairment of heat dissipation.[183,184] Animal studies in rats suggest that MDMA-induced hyperthermia results not from MDMA-induced release of 5-HT but from increased release of dopamine acting at D$_1$ receptors, thus suggesting a future role for the use of dopamine antagonists in clinical treatment.[185]

Hyperthermia is a common feature of these potentially severe to lethal poisonings with sympathomimetic psychostimulant drugs and may be the primary cause of fatality or MDMA-induced neurotoxicity.[184] Because of the nonlinear pharmacokinetics of MDMA and γ-hydroxybutyrate, it is difficult to estimate a dose-response relationship.[184] Some have applied a pathophysiologic model of exertional heatstroke or NMS to profound cocaine intoxication.[185] In addition to profound hyperthermia (>42°C [>107.6°F]), acute rhabdomyolysis, disseminated intravascular coagulation, psychiatric and cognitive dysfunction, renal failure, coma, seizures, and death have been described in these patients.[186-189] As demonstrated by Roberts and associates,[188] even a patient with a core temperature of 45.5°C (114°F) because of acute cocaine intoxication may survive with aggressive cooling methods. Treatment requires prompt recognition, maintenance of adequate hydration, rapid cooling, and the aggressive use of sedatives or paralyzing agents (or both) to control agitation. Importantly, the longer that psychostimulant-overdosed patients remain hyperthermic, the higher their morbidity and mortality rates. Agitation and seizures must be chemically controlled because they lead to continued generation of heat and muscle injury. Therefore, liberal doses of benzodiazepines are recommended.[188] Some have advocated the use of bromocriptine and dantrolene as for MH and NMS, but their efficacy in the setting of drug-associated hyperthermia remains controversial.[189,190]

Hemorrhagic Shock and Encephalopathy Syndrome
The condition of hemorrhagic shock and encephalopathy syndrome in children (mainly infants, but some older children also) resembles heatstroke in adults. The full-blown syndrome includes hyperthermia, coagulopathy, encephalopathy, and renal and hepatic dysfunction.[191] Although there may be an association with concurrent viral illness, the condition

TABLE 65-5 Cooling Rates Achieved with Various Cooling Techniques

TECHNIQUE	REFERENCE	MODEL	RATE (°C/min)
Evaporative	Poulton and Walker,[199] 1987	Human	0.10
	Weiner and Khogali,[200] 1980	Human	0.31
	Kielblock et al,[201] 1986	Human	0.09
	Wyndham et al,[202] 1959	Human	0.07
	Daily and Harrison,[203] 1948	Rat	0.93
Immersion (ice water)	Armstrong et al,[204] 1996	Human	0.20
	Weiner and Khogali,[200] 1980	Human	0.11
	Wyndham et al,[202] 1959	Human	0.14
	Magazanik et al,[205] 1980	Dog	0.27
	Daily and Harrison,[203] 1948	Rat	1.86
	Costrini,[206] 1990	Human	0.15
Selective immersion	Clapp et al,[207] 2001	Human	
	Torso immersion		0.16
	Hand/foot immersion		0.11
Ice packing (whole body)	Kielblock et al,[201] 1986	Human	0.034
Strategic ice packs (towels)	Armstrong et al,[204] 1996	Human	0.11
	Kielblock et al,[201] 1986	Human	0.028
Evaporative strategic ice packs	Kielblock et al,[201] 1986	Human	0.036
Cold gastric lavage	Syverud et al,[208] 1985	Dog	0.15
	White et al,[209] 1987	Dog	0.06
Cold peritoneal lavage	Horowitz et al,[210] 1989[I]	Human	0.11
	Bynum et al,[211] 1978[I]	Dog	0.56
	White,[212] 1993	Dog	0.14
Cyclic lung lavage	Harris et al,[213] 2001	Dog	0.5

generally follows an elevation in temperature, which may be triggered by "bundling" of a child with a low-grade fever. Therapy is largely supportive and includes volume replacement with rapid cooling of the hyperthermic child while sources of bacterial infection are sought and treated.

Cooling Techniques

General Considerations

Heatstroke mortality is proportional to the magnitude and duration of thermal stress measured in degree-minutes.[192] *Delay in cooling may be the single most important factor leading to death or residual disability in those who survive.*[144] In addition, advanced age and underlying disease states are significant contributing factors.[144,145,151,152]

Many exertional heatstroke victims are volume-depleted and may exhibit hypotension. Initial stabilization with cooled (room-temperature) IV fluids and correction of electrolyte abnormalities are valuable in hypotensive patients. Traditional sources recommend a rate of 1200 mL over the first 4 hours.[193] Others advise a 2-L bolus over the first hour, with an additional 1 L/hr for the following 3 hours.[194] Seraj and coworkers challenged this more aggressive recommendation.[195] In their study of pilgrims who suffered heatstroke, 65% had normal or above normal central venous pressure (CVP) on arrival. These authors found that an average of 1 L of saline was sufficient to normalize CVP during the cooling period in their patients, who had a mean age of 55

years (range, 31 to 80 years). In older patients, fluid resuscitation should be monitored carefully to avoid pulmonary edema. Regarding antipyretics, *there is no indication for either salicylates or acetaminophen in the setting of heatstroke* because their efficacy depends on a normally functioning hypothalamus. Overzealous use of acetaminophen could potentiate hepatic damage, and salicylates may promote bleeding tendencies.[196] A study comparing acetaminophen and physical cooling methods found that in patients treated with antipyretics only, mean body temperature increased by 0.2°C (32.4°F) on average.[197]

Given that rapid cooling is accepted as the cornerstone of effective heatstroke therapy, the clinician must choose which cooling technique to use. Studies in animal models are based on the assumption that the fastest cooling technique is the best. In clinical patient care, other factors also influence the choice of technique. Patient access, monitoring, safety, ease of use, availability, and speed are all considerations.[198] A technique that may not be the most rapid but allows easy patient access and is readily available may be preferable to more cumbersome (albeit more rapid once established) cooling techniques in some clinical settings.

The cooling rates achieved in various human and animal studies of heatstroke are summarized in Table 65-5.[199-213] The advantages and disadvantages of various cooling techniques are outlined in Table 65-6.

In addition to the cooling procedures outlined, *it is imperative that the clinician institute the judicious use of sedation, muscle*

TABLE 65-6   Advantages and Disadvantages of Various Cooling Techniques

TECHNIQUE	ADVANTAGES	DISADVANTAGES
Evaporative	Simple, readily available Noninvasive Easy monitoring and patient access Relatively fast	Constant moistening of skin required
Immersion	Noninvasive Relatively fast Low mortality rates	Cumbersome Patient access and monitoring difficult Shivering Poorly tolerated by conscious patients
Ice packing	Noninvasive Readily available	Shivering Poorly tolerated by conscious patients
Strategic ice packs	Noninvasive Readily available Can be combined with other techniques	Relatively slower cooling Shivering Poorly tolerated by conscious patients
Cold gastric lavage	Can be combined with other techniques	Relatively slower cooling Invasive Requires airway control Human experience limited
Cold peritoneal lavage	Rapid cooling	Invasive Human experience limited

paralysis, or both to control agitation, suppress shivering, reduce energy expenditure, and make the patient receptive to sometimes unpleasant therapies.[214] In general, IV benzodiazepines are the easiest and safest first-line drugs used for sedation.

Indications for Rapid Cooling

Rapid cooling should be instituted as soon as the diagnosis of heatstroke (rectal temperature >40°C [104°F], altered mental status, history of heat stress or exposure) is made. Rapid cooling is also indicated for the treatment of MH and NMS but should be instituted concurrently with discontinuation of the triggering agent or drug and administration of dantrolene. Because studies show that the degree of organ damage correlates with the degree and duration of temperature elevation above 40°C (>104°F), a reasonable clinical goal is to reduce the temperature to below 40°C (<104°F) within 30 minutes to an hour after the start of therapy.[145,214]

Contraindications to Rapid Cooling

Rapid cooling is never contraindicated in patients with heatstroke. Immersion cooling is relatively contraindicated when cardiac monitoring of an unstable patient is required or when limited personnel make constant patient supervision impossible. Iced gastric lavage is contraindicated in patients with depressed airway reflexes unless the airway is protected by endotracheal intubation. Gastric lavage is also contraindicated by conditions that preclude placement of an orogastric or nasogastric tube. Cold peritoneal lavage is relatively contraindicated when multiple previous abdominal surgeries make placement of a lavage catheter risky.

Evaporative Cooling

Evaporating water is thermodynamically a much more effective cooling medium than melting ice, given an appropriate water-vapor gradient. Evaporating 1 g of water requires 540 kcal. Melting 1 g of ice requires only 80 kcal. In theory, evaporative cooling should be approximately seven times more efficient than ice packing. In practice, evaporative cooling is more efficient. In separate human studies, Wyndham and colleagues and Weiner and Khogali found that evaporative cooling rates were substantially greater than cooling rates with water immersion at 14.4°C (57.9°F).[200,202] Studies in primate models demonstrated faster cooling rates with evaporative cooling as an adjunct to ice bag placement.[215] Methods using convection and evaporation were more effective than those involving conduction for the treatment of hyperthermia. In clinical practice, ice water immersion or ice packing causes heat loss by conduction and heat consumption by the phase change of melting ice. In healthy volunteers, evaporative cooling techniques (e.g., facial fanning) were associated with decreased thermal sensation and improved thermal comfort.[216]

Despite the continued enthusiasm of some clinicians for ice water immersion, *evaporative cooling has been an effective noninvasive cooling technique in human studies.*[214,217] To maximize evaporative cooling rates, several factors must be optimized. Airflow rates must be high and therefore large fans are required. The air must be warm but *not* humid because evaporation is decreased at lower temperatures. The entire body surface must be exposed to airflow and continuously moistened with water. Ideally, the patient is suspended in a mesh sling to expose the back to airflow and moisture. Finally, the temperature of the water used to moisten the skin must be tepid (15°C [59°F]). Warm forced air is essential for effective evaporation. It maintains good peripheral perfusion and prevents shivering by warming the skin.[217] If the water is ice cold, evaporation will be slowed. Conversely, if it is hot, conductive heat gain may occur. Studies conducted in heat-stressed laying hens demonstrated superior cooling rates with ventral cooling regimes over dorsal cooling.[218]

Weiner and Khogali constructed a sophisticated "body cooling unit" (BCU) to maximize evaporative cooling.[200] Patients in the BCU are suspended in a mesh net. High airflow rates (30 m/min) at a temperature of 45°C (113°F) are maintained both anterior and posterior to the mesh net. Atomized water at 15°C (59°F) is continuously sprayed on all body surfaces. For EDs without access to a BCU,[219] temporary units can be set up with shower sprays and fans, provided that the ambient temperature in the ED is relatively cool. An alternative less expensive, portable device developed at King Saud University involves covering the patient with a gauze sheet soaked in water at 20°C (68°F) while two fans direct room air over the patient.[220] Cooling rates obtained with this device (0.087°C/min [32.2°F/min]) were nearly double the cooling rates achieved with the original BCU developed by Weiner and Khogali.[200]

The realities of clinical practice make these conditions hard to reproduce. Half the body surface, the back, will usually be unavailable for evaporative cooling. Airflow rates and temperatures are usually limited by the ambient temperature in the treatment facility and by the size and power of the fan available. These realities are reflected by the slower cooling rates achieved with evaporative cooling in a clinical setting.

Procedure

For evaporative cooling, undress the patient completely. Position a fan at the foot of the bed or stretcher, as close to the patient as possible. Then sponge or mist the patient's skin with tepid water (15°C [59°F]). Spray water continuously over the skin to create a warm microclimate around the skin and to promote water evaporation.[221] A single care provider can continue the technique and monitor the patient once cooling has been initiated. It is important to keep as much of the body surface area as moist as possible and exposed to airflow. Do not cover with sheets or clothing because this will impede skin evaporation and cooling. Studies of evaporative cooling in heatstroke patients show cooling rates of 0.046°C/min to 0.34°C/min (32.1°F/min to 32.6°F/min).[217,221]

Complications

Complications of evaporative cooling are rare and more often a result of the underlying disorder than the cooling technique. Wet skin may interfere with electrocardiographic monitoring, but this can usually be avoided by placing electrodes on the patient's back. Shivering occurs infrequently with this technique when compared with other cooling methods since the water is relatively lukewarm.[222] Because rectal temperature lags behind core (esophageal) temperature, evaporative cooling should be discontinued when rectal temperature reaches 39°C (102.2°F). In cases of mild hyperthermia, tympanic temperature also accurately reflects core temperature and can be useful in this setting.[222] Continued cooling beyond this temperature may lead to subsequent "overshoot hypothermia" as a result of a continued drop in core temperature after active evaporative cooling is discontinued. Shivering indicates that core temperature has decreased to 37°C (89.6°F) or below.[222]

Immersion Cooling

It would seem obvious that the fastest way to cool a heatstroke patient would be immersion in ice water. In a case series of exertional heatstroke patients, iced water immersion cooled patients to lower than 39°C (<102.2°F) within 19.2 minutes.[214]

A recent study found that cold water immersion for 9 minutes in a 2.0°C circulated water bath until a rectal temperature of 38.6°C was achieved avoided any risk associated with overcooling.[223] Some contemporary sources recommend ice water immersion as the cooling technique of choice for heatstroke.[214,224] Plattner and associates demonstrated cooling rates with ice water immersion that were six times faster than rates seen with forced air or circulating water.[225]

Costrini reported no fatalities in 252 consecutive young marine recruits with exertional heatstroke who were treated by ice water immersion within 20 minutes of diagnosis.[206] He regarded ice water immersion as superior to other conventional methods described in the literature in reducing mortality rates.

In clinical trials, cold water immersion remains one of the fastest noninvasive cooling techniques available (see Table 65-5). Cold water immersion takes advantage of the high-conductance property of water, which is 25 times that of air.[224] When an adequate evaporative cooling system is not available, immersion may be the cooling technique of choice. Several factors are important in maximizing the rate of immersion cooling. Conductive heat loss depends on cutaneous blood flow to maintain a heat gradient from skin to water. Theoretically, contact with ice water causes skin and subcutaneous vasoconstriction, which blocks heat exchange and turns these structures into insulators.[226] Intense cutaneous vasoconstriction will impede conductive heat loss. Mekjavic and coworkers reported that motion sickness actually potentiates core cooling during immersion by attenuating the vasoconstrictor response to skin and core cooling, thereby augmenting heat loss and the magnitude of the decrease in deep body temperature.[227] Careful monitoring is required because this may predispose patients to hypothermia.

Researchers have suggested that ice water immersion may be superior to cold water immersion because of the establishment of a steeper thermal gradient between the skin and the environment.[226] A study comparing the cooling capacity of ice water immersion (5.2°C [41.4°F]), tepid water immersion (14°C [57.2°F]), and passive cooling in experienced distance runners with body temperatures of 39.3°C to 39.6°C (102.7°F to 103.3°F) found comparable cooling rates with ice water and cold water immersion. Both techniques were superior to passive cooling techniques.[226] The optimal water temperature for cooling human heatstroke patients has not been defined. Aggressive skin cooling may stimulate shivering and peripheral vasoconstriction, thus hindering cooling efficacy. Investigators suggest the inclusion of skin massage as a crucial component of immersion cooling techniques.[228]

Regardless of the water temperature, it is clear that increasing surface area increases conductive heat loss. Maximizing the body's surface area in contact with water will increase cooling rates with immersion cooling. In clinical practice, this means that complete immersion of the trunk and extremities will cool the patient faster than partial immersion of the trunk (back only) with the extremities extended out of the bath.

Procedure

For immersion cooling, undress the patient completely and transfer the patient to a tub of water with a depth sufficient to cover the torso and extremities. Various water containers may be used. A regular bathtub can be used. Most clinical reports describe tubs that can be moved to the emergency treatment area when needed. A child's plastic wading pool and a decontamination tub or stretcher with waterproof sides and drainage capability are examples of the latter approach. Support the patient's head out of the tub at all times. When tubs are unavailable, place patients on water-impermeable sheets and in a sling apparatus while ice and water are poured into the sling. Securely attach temperature and electrocardiogram leads to the patient if monitoring is to be continued during immersion. Remove the patient from the bath when rectal temperature reaches 39°C (102.2°F) because core temperature will continue to drop for a short period even after the patient is removed. If available, use an electronic temperature monitor with a long flexible rectal probe for continuous monitoring of temperature during immersion. Studies show cooling rates with ice water immersion (1°C–5°C [33.8°F–41.0°F]) in heatstroke patients of 0.15°C/min to 0.23°C/min (32.3°F/min to 32.4°F/min).[206,224,228]

Complications

The common complications of immersion cooling are shivering, cutaneous vasoconstriction, discomfort, and loss of monitoring capability. Shivering generates considerable heat through muscle metabolism. Cutaneous vasoconstriction impedes conductive heat loss. If significant shivering does occur, it can be reduced with benzodiazepines. A recent study found that high-dose IV diazepam facilitates core cooling during cold saline infusion in healthy volunteers. Subjects were randomized to receive high-dose (20 mg) or low-dose (10 mg) diazepam or placebo during cold saline infusion. Administration of high-dose diazepam decreased the shivering threshold without compromising respiratory or cardiovascular status.[229] The use of phenothiazines such as chlorpromazine has been advocated for shivering in the past. They are currently discouraged because administration of these agents may impair heat loss through anticholinergic effects on sweat glands, contribute to hypotension via α-adrenergic blockade, lower the seizure threshold, and cause dystonic reactions. In addition, phenothiazines possess central dopamine-blocking effects, which may exacerbate symptoms of NMS.[175] Benzodiazepines are also valuable if the patient is hyperthermic secondary to sympathomimetic agents such as cocaine. Patient monitoring is a problem under water. Electrodes can be used on the nonimmersed upper part of the shoulders, but electrocardiographic artifact often becomes a major problem during vigorous shivering. Immersion cooling is not recommended for patients with unstable cardiac rhythms or those at risk for the development of these rhythms. A significant change in cardiac rhythm might go undetected during the labor-intensive process of immersion cooling.

Patient access for resuscitative procedures is also a major problem when using this technique. Should ventricular fibrillation develop, the patient must be removed from the bath and dried before defibrillation. Invasive and diagnostic procedures (e.g., IV access and radiography) cannot be performed during the cooling period. Care must be taken to avoid displacement of IV lines during placement into and removal from the bath.

As body temperature drops, mental status will improve in many heatstroke victims. When awake, most people find ice water immersion difficult to tolerate. IV sedation may be required. Finally, this technique is labor-intensive. Several caregivers must be present throughout the process. The patient's head must be maintained out of the bath. If massage is used, one or more individuals will need to immerse their own hands in water to continuously massage the patient. Medications should be given intravenously, and constant attention to temperature and electrocardiogram monitors is also necessary. This cooling technique should be used only if adequate personnel are available.

Whole-Body Ice Packing

Packing a heatstroke victim in ice may enhance conductive heat loss without the attendant logistic problems caused by water immersion (Figs. 65-7 and 65-8). Constant attendance, as required for skin moistening with evaporative cooling and as described for immersion cooling, may not be necessary with ice packing. Kielblock and associates demonstrated in a human study of mild, exercise-induced hyperthermia that whole-body ice packing cooled just as fast as evaporative cooling did (see Table 65-5).[201]

Procedure

For whole-body ice packing, undress the patient completely and then cover the extremities and torso with crushed ice. A

Figure 65-7 It is essential to rapidly lower the core temperature of a severely hyperthermic patient by instituting cooling techniques as soon as possible. Evaporative cooling (see text) is usually quite effective and technically easy. Note the fan for additional cooling. Many such patients require sedation, paralysis, and mechanical ventilation. An alternative aggressive method shown here, in a patient with a rectal temperature of 110°F, is to literally pack the patient in ice. As is often the case, this older patient did not survive.

Figure 65-8 A body bag or plastic sheets may keep water from flooding the floor when packing the patient in ice.

fan blown over the patient may increase cooling. As with any cooling technique, monitor the patient's temperature constantly with an electric thermometer and a long, flexible rectal probe. A large supply of crushed ice will be needed whenever this technique is used. Logistically, ice packing may be problematic. Whole-body ice packing can usually be performed on an ED stretcher without additional equipment. Ideally, the patient is placed in a container that facilitates contact of ice with the skin and prevents water from dripping onto the floor. A body bag makes an ideal device. Iced cooling may also be accomplished by placing the patient in a child's lightweight plastic pool, available in toy stores. Lacking this equipment, plastic cloths or trash bags may be placed under the patient with the edges curled up to form a slinglike apparatus. As with immersion cooling, electrocardiographic monitoring can potentially be difficult because of shivering artifact and displacement of electrodes. If the patient is alert and cannot tolerate the ice packing, use IV sedation or restraint. Treat excessive shivering with benzodiazepines if needed. Once rectal temperature reaches 39°C (102.2°F), remove the ice and dry the patient off. Studies show cooling rates of 0.34°C/min (32.6°F/min) in heatstroke patients with whole-body ice packing.[201,224]

Strategic Ice Packs

Noakes suggested that strategic placement of ice packs over areas of the body where large blood vessels run close to the skin may be an effective cooling technique.[230] Cooling in these areas occurs despite cutaneous vasoconstriction because of direct conductive heat loss from blood within the vessel and across the vessel wall, subcutaneous tissue, and skin to ice. The most common areas used for strategic ice packing are the anterior aspect of the neck (carotid and jugular vessels), the axilla (axillary artery and vein), and the groin (femoral vessels). There have been numerous reports of successful cooling using ice packs as primary or adjunctive therapy (see Table 65-5).[230,231] In addition, application of ice packs, though easier to perform than immersion or total-body ice packing, limits the conductive cooling offered by the latter two procedures. A study in pigtail monkeys demonstrated that a combination of strategic ice packs with evaporative cooling results in faster cooling than either technique alone, although the relative increase achieved by adding ice packs to evaporative cooling was small.[232]

In unconscious patients or in awake patients who can tolerate ice packs without excessive shivering, this technique could be added to evaporative cooling. Kielblock and associates found that the combination of strategic ice packs and evaporative cooling yielded higher cooling rates than did either method individually (0.036°C/min versus 0.027°C/min and 0.034°C/min).[201] The clinical value of strategic ice packs alone or in combination with other techniques remains to be determined. Anecdotally, during the Chicago heat wave of 1995, the majority of heatstroke patients who went to EDs survived after being effectively cooled with the evaporation method accompanied by strategic placement of ice packs.[233]

Procedure

Place large plastic bags filled with crushed ice or an ice and water mixture in both axillae and over both femoral triangles. If the neck is used, place the packs laterally so that they do not compress the trachea or apply excessive weight over the carotid arteries. Do not pack the neck if the patient has carotid bruits or a history of cerebrovascular disease. Some sources advocate rubbing the body surface briskly with plastic bags containing ice after the body has been wet down with water. This is effective, provided that it is combined with evaporation therapy. Studies show ranges of cooling rates of 0.028°C/min to 0.087°C/min (32.0°F/min to 32.2°F/min) in heatstroke patients with strategic ice packs.[234]

Complications

Complications of strategic ice packing are limited to shivering and patient discomfort, as described previously for whole-body ice packing. The ice packs are removed when rectal temperature reaches 39°C (102.2°F) to avoid an excessive drop in core temperature.

External versus Core Cooling

All the external cooling techniques described previously are noninvasive and involve heat loss by evaporation or conduction across the skin as the primary cooling mechanism. With each of these techniques, central temperature will continue to drop even after the technique is discontinued and the skin is dried. This is due to a delay in establishment of an equilibrium between the cold skin and the core. The amount of "core afterdrop" can exceed 2°C (>35.6°F).[217,219,234] For this reason, cooling is discontinued when the core temperature reaches 39°C (102.2°F).

Because the sites of significant cell damage with heatstroke are centrally located (e.g., liver, kidney, heart), central cooling techniques are theoretically preferable to external techniques. Core cooling techniques studied in both animal and human models include iced gastric lavage, intravascular cooling, bladder lavage, and peritoneal lavage.[208-210,212,235,236] Central venous cooling is effective in rapidly decreasing core temperatures.[235] Studies conducted in healthy volunteers have demonstrated that reductions in core temperature vary according to the temperature of the infused fluid. Subjects receiving 30-minute infusions of fluid at 4°C (39.2°F) experienced decreases in core temperature of 2.5°C ± 0.4°C (36.5°F ± 32.7°F). Subjects receiving 30-minute infusions of fluid at 20°C (68°F) experienced decreases of 1.4°C (±0.2°C [34.5°F ± 32.4°F]).[235] Clinical trials investigating this method showed that cooling via the respiratory tract had no significant impact on temperature changes when used exclusively but did demonstrate effectiveness as an adjunctive measure to other external cooling techniques.[224] Cool air (10°C [50°F]) was administered via a hood or mask. Cooling via the respiratory tract has been studied in animals but not investigated clinically.[237-239] Central cooling techniques are necessarily more invasive than external techniques and have the potential for more significant complications.

Cold Gastric Lavage

The stomach lies in close proximity to the liver, great vessels, kidneys, and heart. The gastric mucosa is not subject to the intense vasoconstriction observed on exposure of the skin to ice water.[208] For these reasons, lavage of the stomach might be expected to be an effective central cooling method. Studies of cold gastric lavage in a canine model produced cooling rates five times greater than in controls exposed to ambient air at room temperature (0.15°C/min versus 0.03°C/min).[209] Human heatstroke victims have been cooled successfully with gastric lavage, but only in combination with external techniques.[210] Cold gastric lavage seems to be best suited for use in patients with severe hyperthermia who are cooled at a slow rate with external techniques alone. The presence of an endotracheal tube and passage of a large-bore gastric tube make rapid lavage without aspiration possible. This technique should be reserved for patients whose airway is protected by endotracheal intubation and who do not have a contraindication to gastric tube placement.

Procedure

For cold gastric lavage, instill 10 mL/kg of iced tap water into the stomach as rapidly as possible (usually over a 30- to 60-second period). After a 30- to 60-second dwell time, remove the water by suction or gravity.[213] Cooling will theoretically be faster if a high temperature gradient is maintained in the stomach. A faster lavage rate can be maintained if suction is used to withdraw the instilled fluid. A large container of ice-temperature water maintained 1 to 1.5 m above the patient's body will facilitate the instillation of fluid. Connect this container directly to the lavage tubing and ideally allow passage of water but not ice, which may occlude the tube. Because large volumes of water are needed, it is helpful if additional ice can be added to the container without interrupting the lavage. A large syringe can be used as an alternative to gravity instillation, but this is usually slower.

A simple system that accomplishes this procedure can be devised from equipment readily available in most EDs. Use a standard lavage setup (for use in drug overdoses) and a large-bore gastric tube. Cut the lavage bag open at the top to allow water and ice to be added. Suspend this bag above the patient's body and connect it to the orogastric tube by Y tubing with clamps. Connect the other arm of the Y tubing to suction. Using the clamps, intermittently instill ice water by gravity and withdraw it by suction.

Complications

A major potential complication of cold gastric lavage is pulmonary aspiration. Use of a cuffed endotracheal tube minimizes the incidence of this complication. Because of the large volume of water used and the frequent depression of airway reflexes seen with severe heatstroke, this technique should rarely be used in a patient who is not endotracheally intubated.

If tap water is used, water intoxication, hyponatremia, and other electrolyte disturbances are *potential* complications, particularly in pediatric or geriatric patients. Water is absorbed from the stomach and, with large-volume lavage, may pass the pylorus into the small intestine. In canine studies, large-volume gastric lavage with tap water did not cause electrolyte abnormalities.[208] The actual incidence of these potential complications in human heatstroke has not been determined. Use of normal saline instead of tap water would eliminate this potential problem.

Theoretically, passage of cold water through the esophagus, located directly behind the heart, has the potential to induce cardiac dysrhythmias. Dysrhythmias have not been observed in canine studies or in case reports of human heatstroke victims cooled with this technique.[212,236]

Cold Peritoneal Lavage

The surface area and blood flow of the peritoneum greatly exceed those of the stomach. Peritoneal lavage is expected to exchange heat much faster than possible with gastric lavage. Peritoneal lavage achieves some of the fastest cooling rates ever reported in large animal or human studies (see Table

65-5). A case report of cooling via cold peritoneal lavage for hyperthermia after the ingestion of ecstasy demonstrated rapid cooling.[236] As with gastric lavage, this central cooling technique offers the advantage of directly cooling the core organs that are most susceptible to thermal damage. Unlike gastric lavage, endotracheal intubation is not required. Peritoneal lavage is used extensively to treat hyperthermia under various conditions and typically decreases core temperatures 5°C/hr to 10°C/hr (41°F/hr to 50°F/hr).[210,236]

Peritoneal lavage is a more invasive cooling technique. Because heat exchange is more efficient across the peritoneum, smaller volumes of fluid can be used. Surgical placement of the lavage catheter is necessary. This cooling technique is relatively contraindicated by conditions that preclude placement of a lavage catheter (e.g., multiple abdominal surgical scars).

Peritoneal lavage is the most rapid central cooling technique. It can theoretically be combined with other techniques to speed cooling of heatstroke patients with refractory hyperthermia. As the most invasive cooling technique, it requires time, proper equipment, and surgical expertise to institute. Its use is probably best suited to situations in which heatstroke patients are not responding to external cooling and adequate equipment and personnel are readily available.[217]

Procedure

To institute cooling by peritoneal lavage, immerse 2 to 8 L of sterile saline in an ice water bath to cool while the catheter is being placed. Place a standard peritoneal lavage catheter (as for diagnostic use in trauma patients) via any of the techniques described in Chapter 43. Standard contraindications apply. Use of a larger peritoneal dialysis catheter may speed instillation and withdrawal of fluid. Actual lavage volumes and rates have not been established, however. One approach is to instill and withdraw 500 to 1000 mL every 10 minutes until adequate cooling is achieved. Rectal temperature may be falsely low during lavage because of the presence of cold water around the rectum at the level of the rectal temperature probe. It may be preferable to monitor temperature in the tympanic membrane or esophagus when using this technique. Stop the lavage when core temperature reaches 39°C (102.2°F) to avoid excessive core temperature afterdrop.

Complications

The potential complications of peritoneal lavage cooling are primarily related to placement of the catheter and include bowel or bladder perforation and placement into the rectus sheath rather than the peritoneum.

Other Cooling Techniques

"Rewarming" techniques are used to minimize ongoing heat loss via the respiratory tract in hypothermic patients.[72] Although high-frequency jet ventilation (HFJV) achieves core cooling in critically ill patients,[237] efforts to use the respiratory tract to cool heatstroke victims have been unsuccessful. In a canine model of heatstroke, HFJV was shown to be a relatively ineffective cooling technique.[238] Heat loss by convection (air transfer) is relatively inefficient when compared with the conductive heat loss mechanism used by other cooling techniques. The use of dry, hot air to maximize evaporative heat loss from the lungs might cause respiratory complications.[231]

In human trials, ice water lavage of the bladder (300 mL of iced Ringer's solution every 10 minutes) provided only minimal cooling at rates of 0.8°C/hr (±0.3°C/hr [33.4°F/hr ±

32.5°F/hr]).[201] Iced water lavage of the rectum would theoretically provide faster cooling rates secondary to the increased surface area and better perfusion, but it has not been investigated in human trials.

Hemodialysis or partial cardiopulmonary bypass could theoretically be used to cool heatstroke patients. Before the availability of dantrolene in 1979, partial cardiopulmonary bypass was one of the treatments of MH.[173] Drawbacks include the need for technical expertise and preparation time for the procedure. A recent case report described successful treatment of a heatstroke patient with multiple-organ failure refractory to conventional cooling techniques with cold hemodialysis initially at 30°C (86°F) and later at 35°C (95°F), followed by continuous hemodiafiltration with cold dialysate (35°C [95°F]) at a high flow rate of 18,000 mL/hr. Within 3 hours of starting this particular technique, the patient's body temperature was below 38°C (<100.4°F).[239]

Cyclic lung lavage with cold perfluorochemicals is currently under investigation in animal models. Benefits include rapid cooling rates of 0.5°C/min (32.9°F/min) and minimally invasive nature in already mechanically ventilated subjects.[213,240]

Intravascular cooling catheters have demonstrated efficiency as cooling devices. They circulate temperature-controlled sterile saline placed in the bladder or inferior vena cava. Although these devices have not been used in heatstroke patients, studies have found the cooling catheters to be very effective for neurologic conditions in both human and animal models.[241,242] Another promising cooling technique involves the use of a hypothermic retrograde jugular vein flush (HRJVF) for heatstroke. HRJVF has been studied only in animal models thus far. This technique involves the infusion of 4°C (39.2°F) isotonic sodium chloride solution through the external jugular vein (1.7 mL/100 g of body weight over a 5-minute period). Use of HRJVF was found to increase survival rates during heatstroke by attenuating cerebral oxidative stress, tissue ischemia or injury, systemic inflammation, and activated coagulation.[243]

Pharmacologic agents have demonstrated merit as adjunctive agents in the management of hyperthermia. There are anecdotal reports of enhanced reduction in temperature with IV ketorolac. Cienki and colleagues demonstrated enhanced decreases in temperature with the administration of ketorolac, 30 mg intravenously.[244] All patients received standard hyperthermia treatment (e.g., ice packs, iced lavage, circulating air). Patients were randomized to receive ketorolac versus saline. In the group receiving ketorolac, the average rectal temperature after 90 minutes was two times lower than in those receiving placebo saline (3.7°C versus 1.6°C [38.7°F versus 34.9°F]).

Conclusion

Rapid cooling is the key step in the emergency management of heatstroke patients. Survival rates approach 90% when elevated temperatures are lowered in timely fashion.[157,228] Evaporative cooling appears to be the technique of choice. It combines the advantages of simplicity and noninvasiveness with the most rapid cooling rates achieved with any external technique. It is also logistically easier to institute, maintain, and monitor evaporative cooling measures than with any other cooling technique. If a patient is not cooling rapidly with evaporative cooling, other techniques can be added. Strategic ice packs can be used. If the patient is endotracheally intubated, gastric lavage can be instituted. If facilities and personnel are available, peritoneal lavage cooling can be used as a rapid central cooling technique. If muscle rigidity is present or MH is suspected, dantrolene sodium should be administered. In addition, the clinician should have a heightened index of suspicion for NMS and toxicity from sympathomimetic drugs. Regardless of the cause, a reasonable clinical goal is to reduce rectal temperature to 40°C (104°F) or below within 30 minutes of instituting therapy.[157,228]

Immersion cooling is best limited to centers with the proper equipment and skilled medical personnel experienced in managing hyperthermic patients. This method may also be effective in conditions in which electric power for evaporative cooling is unavailable (e.g., in wilderness settings where bodies of cool water are available nearby and the victim is far from more sophisticated medical care). Central venous cooling with iced saline is a promising technique for rapid cooling of patients with severe hyperthermia. Other cooling techniques require further study before a clear recommendation regarding their efficacy can be made.

Acknowledgments

The authors wish to acknowledge and thank Dwight E. Helmrich, Scott A. Syverud, David Doezema, and David P. Sklar for their contributions and authorship in previous editions.

References are available at www.expertconsult.com

CHAPTER 66

Ultrasound

Christine Butts

Over the past 20 years, bedside ultrasound has become an indispensible tool in the emergency department (ED). It has enabled physicians to make a rapid diagnosis at the bedside and formulate a plan of care. Perhaps most importantly, ultrasound has revolutionized procedures performed in the ED. Use of ultrasound gives the physician the advantage of viewing the anatomy and directly imaging the procedure while it is being performed. Procedures that had previously been performed "blindly" can now be performed with the added assurance of monitoring the procedure while it is in progress. This has resulted in greater safety in both common and uncommon procedures.[1,2]

Ultrasound is now routinely applied to procedures in the ED ranging from the common, such as incision and drainage of an abscess, to the rare, such as drainage of a pericardial effusion. Use of ultrasound to facilitate each procedure is covered in detail in individual chapters. This chapter covers the basic principles of ultrasound that can be applied to any procedure.

PHYSICS

Ultrasound operates on the *pulse echo principle*. Electrical energy created by the ultrasound machine causes crystals in the tip of the transducer to vibrate, also known as the *piezoelectric effect*. This vibration emits high-frequency sound waves that travel into the body. The sound waves are reflected back to the transducer at varying intensities and speeds, depending on the nature of the object that it encounters. The ultrasound machine is able to interpret this information and plot an image on the screen.

Objects in the body that are liquid or water-like, such as a full bladder, reflect very few sound waves and allow most of the energy to pass through them. These objects are presented on-screen as black by ultrasound and are described as *anechoic*, without echoes (Fig. 66-1). Conversely, objects that are dense and have very little water content, such as bones, reflect almost all the sound waves back. These objects are presented on-screen as white by ultrasound and are described as *hyperechoic* (i.e., producing a lot of echoes) (Fig. 66-2). Objects that lie between these two extremes are varying shades of gray, depending on the water content of the object. For example, the liver contains a large amount of blood, a water-like substance, but is not completely liquid and appears on-screen as a dark gray (Fig. 66-3). An object that contains less water but is not completely solid would appear as a lighter shade of gray.

These properties of objects also account for two important artifacts. *Acoustic shadowing* is an artifact that is encountered when dealing with hyperechoic objects. These objects reflect almost all the sound waves back to the transducer. As a result, the ultrasound machine "senses" an absence of information

deep to the hyperechoic object. This absence of information is represented by a strong, dark vertical line emanating deep to the object (Fig. 66-4). This type of shadowing is referred to as a "clean shadow." Although this shadow can be frustrating to the sonographer when attempting to obtain the best image possible, classically, when imaging over the ribs, it can also be helpful in identifying hyperechoic objects, such as gallstones or foreign bodies.

In contrast to a "clean shadow," the presence of air may create a phenomenon known as "dirty shadowing" (Fig. 66-5). Air causes the ultrasound beam to scatter and creates a hazy, gray appearance on the image. This can be an anticipated finding, such as when viewing bowel gas within the abdomen, or an indication of an abnormality, such as when viewing gas within subcutaneous tissue.

Acoustic enhancement, or an *acoustic window*, is the effect created by an anechoic object. As noted earlier, sound waves pass through anechoic objects well and therefore lose less of their energy. This enables more ultrasonic energy to be available when the sound reaches the object on the other side of the fluid. This results in a brighter, clearer image immediately behind the fluid-filled object. As an example, a full bladder enables a clearer image of the pelvic organs (Fig. 66-6).

Figure 66-1 This image demonstrates a fluid-filled bladder, which appears black, or anechoic, when viewed with ultrasound.

Figure 66-2 This image demonstrates the cortex of a bone (*arrow*), which appears white, or hyperechoic, when viewed with ultrasound.

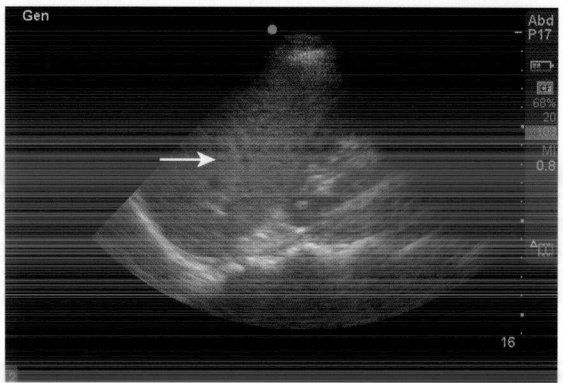

Figure 66-3 The liver (*arrow*) contains a large amount of blood (a water-like substance) but is not completely liquid and appears on-screen as dark gray.

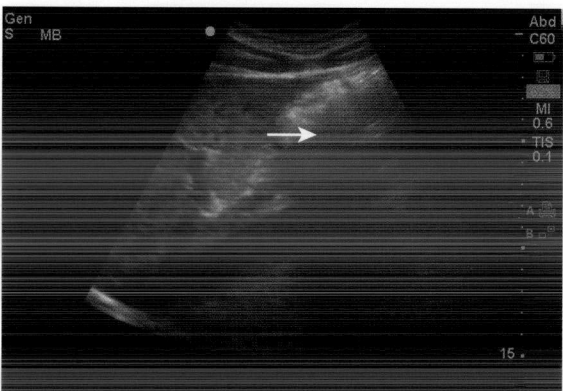

Figure 66-5 In contrast to clean shadowing, the presence of air causes a "dirty" shadow (*arrow*).

Figure 66-4 Acoustic shadowing (*arrow*) occurs when ultrasound encounters a hyperechoic, or hard, object. All the sound waves are returned to the transducer, which results in absence of information behind the hyperechoic object.

Figure 66-6 The presence of a fluid-filled object (in this case a full bladder) creates an "acoustic window" effect (*arrow*). This effect allows objects behind, or deep to, the window to be seen more clearly.

INDICATIONS AND CONTRAINDICATIONS

Although vascular access was one of the first uses of ultrasound in ED procedures, the list of procedures that can be facilitated by ultrasound is growing rapidly and continuously (Box 66-1). Even in cases in which the procedure cannot be directly observed with ultrasound, bedside ultrasound can frequently be used to diagnose the abnormality and to plan the approach for the procedure.

Ultrasound is a very safe modality for imaging at the bedside. It can be used in a variety of populations (pediatrics, pregnancy), without concern for excessive radiation exposure. The only absolute contraindication to using bedside ultrasound for procedural guidance is lack of training or experience in its use. Lack of adequate training or experience may result in an incorrect diagnosis and erroneous evaluation of the anatomy. This may result in harm and unnecessary complications in patients.

EQUIPMENT

The nature of the image obtained depends on the type of transducer used. In general, transducers fall into two categories: high frequency and low frequency, which refers to the type of ultrasound waves generated by the transducer.

High-frequency sound waves do not penetrate very far into the tissue but provide excellent resolution. A linear, or vascular, transducer and an intracavitary transducer are examples of specific types of high-frequency transducers (Figs. 66-7 and 66-8). Examples of types of examinations that are best evaluated with a high-frequency transducer are central or peripheral vascular access, evaluation of the pleura for pneumothorax, and evaluation of soft tissue for an abscess or foreign body. These examinations rely on a high degree of resolution (Fig. 66-9).

Low-frequency sound waves penetrate farther into tissues but do not provide as much resolution as high frequency does. Curvilinear, phased-array, and microconvex transducers are examples of specific types of low-frequency transducers (Figs. 66-10 and 66-11). They are distinguished from each other by the shape of the footprint of the transducer, the part that directly touches the patient, and by the layout of crystals in the tip of the transducer. Examples of the types of examinations that are best evaluated with a low-frequency transducer are evaluation of the pleural or peritoneal cavities for fluid drainage, evaluation of the bladder for aspiration or suprapubic catheter placement, and evaluation of the pericardium for pericardiocentesis. These examinations are not as dependent on resolution but typically require greater penetration (Fig. 66-12).

The growing use of ultrasound for procedures has prompted the development of echogenic needles and needle

BOX 66-1 **Examples of Procedures Performed with Ultrasound Guidance**

Abscess incision and drainage
Arterial line placement
Arterial puncture
Arthrocentesis
Central venous catheter placement
Foreign body localization and removal
Nerve block
Paracentesis
Pericardiocentesis
Suprapubic catheter placement
Thoracentesis
Transvenous pacemaker insertion

Figure 66-9 An example of an image as seen with a high-frequency transducer, in this case soft tissue and tendon (*arrowhead*), can be seen overlying the ankle joint (*arrow*).

Figure 66-7 Linear, or vascular, transducer.

Figure 66-10 Curvilinear transducer.

Figure 66-8 Intracavitary transducer.

Figure 66-11 Phased-array transducer.

guidance systems. Both of these advances are designed to improve the ease and accuracy of ultrasound-guided procedures, but this depends on the operator's familiarity with their properties and correct use.

Additionally, many procedures require sterile conditions. Commercially designed sterile transducer covers are available and allow the operator to completely cover both the transducer and the cord. In the absence of these covers, the transducer can

be placed inside a sterile glove. To further protect the field, a sterile drape can be wrapped around the cord.

GENERAL APPROACH

Although each procedure has unique techniques, there are several general principles that apply when using ultrasound.

Figure 66-12 Example of an image as seen with a low-frequency transducer. In this case the liver and kidney can be seen in the right upper quadrant.

Figure 66-14 Indicator on-screen (*arrow*), which corresponds to the indicator on the side of the transducer.

Figure 66-13 Indicator on the transducer (*arrow*).

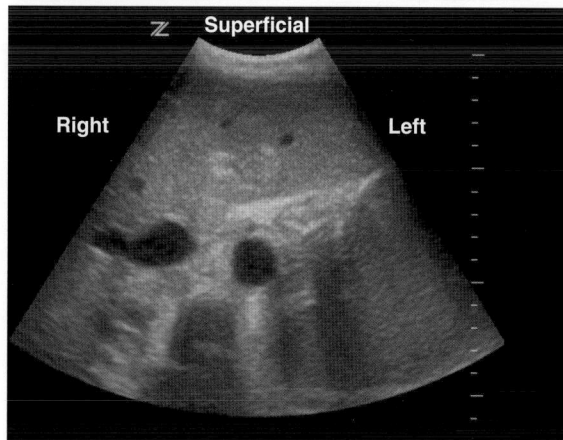

Figure 66-15 Relationships in the transverse orientation. As the indicator points toward the patient's right, objects on the left side of the screen are toward the patient's right (toward the indicator). Objects on the right side of the screen are toward the patient's left (away from the indicator). As in all images, objects closer to the top of the image are closer to the surface, whereas objects at the bottom of the image are deeper in the body.

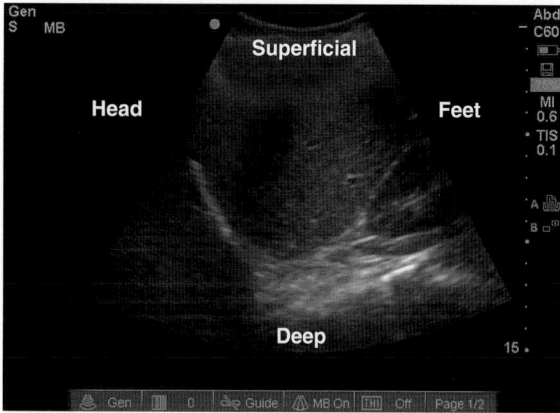

Figure 66-16 Relationships in the longitudinal, or sagittal, orientation. As the indicator on the transducer points toward the patient's head, objects on the left side of the screen are toward the patient's head. Objects on the right side of the screen are toward the patient's feet. As in all images, objects closer to the top of the image are closer to the surface, whereas objects at the bottom of the image are deeper in the body.

Selection of the correct transducer is of the upmost importance for adequate visualization of the anatomy and pathology. This process is described in the preceding section, but in general the degree of resolution and depth of penetration should guide selection of the transducer.

Once the correct transducer has been selected, evaluate the area of interest. This step is key when evaluating the nature of the pathology. For example, understanding the size and position of a subcutaneous abscess and the surrounding anatomy is essential. Determining the correct orientation of objects on the screen can be challenging, but it is crucial for success with ultrasound-guided procedures. All transducers have a dot or mark on one side (Fig. 66-13). This mark corresponds to an indicator on the left-hand side of the screen (Fig. 66-14). When the indicator on the transducer is pointing toward the patient's right side, a transverse image will be generated (Fig. 66-15). Objects on the right of the screen are closer to the patient's left side and objects on the left side, near the on-screen indicator, are closer to the patient's right side. Objects near the top of the screen are closer to the skin and objects near the bottom of the screen are deeper in the body. When the indicator is turned toward the patient's head, a longitudinal image is generated (Fig. 66-16). Objects on the right side of the screen are closer to the patient's feet and objects on the left side of the screen (near the on-screen

Figure 66-17 Inserting a needle in the transverse approach. In this technique the needle is inserted at the midpoint of the transducer. This image is for demonstration purposes only and does not demonstrate sterile technique.

Figure 66-19 Real-time image of the needle as it approaches the vein. The needle (*arrow*) is seen as a hyperechoic object with strong shadowing extending behind it. The portion of the needle seen will correspond to the portion of the needle that is underlying the transducer, as shown in Figure 66-18.

Figure 66-18 As the needle is advanced, the transducer can be seen to transect only a small portion of the needle. The tip of the needle is now away from the transducer and will not appear on-screen.

Figure 66-20 Inserting a needle in the longitudinal approach. In this technique the needle is inserted at the end of the transducer. This image is for demonstration purposes only and does not demonstrate sterile technique.

indicator) are closer to the patient's head. As with the transverse image, objects near the top of the screen are closer to the skin surface and objects at the bottom of the screen are deeper in the body.

Once the initial evaluation has been completed, make a decision whether to use ultrasound to directly guide the procedure or to simply "mark the spot" beforehand. Some procedures, such as paracentesis of large fluid collections, may not require direct guidance. In this case, ultrasound can be used to locate the most optimal puncture site, away from important structures. Once that site has been marked, proceed with the procedure in the usual fashion. For other procedures, such as central line placement, direct visualization throughout the entire procedure may be more important.

When direct visualization is desired, the orientation of the needle to the transducer must be considered. When the needle is introduced at the midpoint of the transducer in the transverse approach, the tip of the needle may be difficult to visualize (Fig. 66-17). In this orientation the operator may have difficulty following the tip of the needle because only a small portion of the needle intersects the ultrasound beam at any given time (Figs. 66-18 and 66-19). Conversely, when the

needle is introduced from either end of the transducer, the needle can be visualized in its entirety (Figs. 66-20 and 66-21). However, slight movement of the transducer may result in "losing" the view of the needle. Consider each potential approach in the context of the particular procedure.

The oblique approach is a combination of the transverse and longitudinal approaches. Primarily, this has been described for central venous access but can also be applied to other procedures as well.[3] In this method, place the transducer on an oblique axis to the target object (Fig. 66-22). This allows an oblique view of the target object while enabling the operator to introduce the needle along the long axis of the transducer (Fig. 66-23).

COMPLICATIONS

In general, the incidence of complications should be reduced with the use of ultrasound, but complications may occur even when performed by an experienced sonographer. Complications may be related to one of several factors. To maximize

Figure 66-21 Real-time image of the needle as it approaches the vein. The needle (*arrow*) can be identified as a hyperechoic object with reverberation artifact. In this orientation it can be seen in its entirety as it progresses toward the vein.

Figure 66-23 Real-time image of the needle approaching the vein. The needle (*arrow*) can be identified as a hyperechoic object with reverberation artifact. It can be seen in its entirety as it advances toward the vein.

Figure 66-22 Inserting a needle in the oblique approach. In this technique the needle is inserted at the end of the transducer. This is similar to the longitudinal approach, with the exception that the vessel is viewed from an oblique angle rather than from a longitudinal orientation. This image is for demonstration purposes only and does not demonstrate sterile technique.

success, obtain an optimal image of the structure in question. Evaluate the anatomic relationships to ensure that the target object (e.g., the femoral vein versus the femoral artery) is correctly identified and pursued. Once the procedure begins, pay constant attention to the orientation and location of the needle. Errors, including inadvertent arterial puncture, can occur when the position of the tip of the needle is not closely followed.[4,5] Techniques to minimize these errors are addressed in the individual chapters.

References are available at www.expertconsult.com

Bedside Laboratory and Microbiologic Procedures

Anthony J. Dean and David C. Lee

ASSESSMENT OF URINE

Obtaining a Urine Specimen

Several methods are available for obtaining a urine specimen. They can be found in Table 67-1 and are listed in order of increasingly precise collection techniques, which comes at the cost of increasing difficulty, patient discomfort, or both.

General Considerations regarding Urine Collection

The advantages and disadvantages of each of the techniques listed in Table 67-1 can be determined only by the purpose of the urine test and the clinical context. The clinical context influences interpretation of the results. For the great majority of clinical scenarios, the basic dichotomy is between specimens obtained for infectious versus noninfectious reasons. With the exception of testing for red blood cells (RBCs) and white blood cells (WBCs), most of the noninfectious tests (e.g., ketones, glucose, bilirubin, protein) are not affected by the collection method. Urine specimens collected to diagnose infection can be contaminated in a number of ways, and the choice and interpretation of tests are intricately influenced by the clinical scenario.

Urinary tract infections (UTIs) are either symptomatic or asymptomatic, and the symptoms determine which collection method is required (Fig. 67-1). With symptomatic UTI, extremely low levels of bacteriuria (10^2 colony-forming units [CFUs]/mL) and pyuria are of clinical significance.[1,2] This may be obscured in some clinicians' minds by an alternative, more widely promulgated fact: in asymptomatic patients the threshold for "significant bacteriuria" is 1000-fold higher at greater than 10^5 CFUs/mL.[3,4] *Symptomatic* patients constitute a clinically distinct group who require a urine test that is much more sensitive and thus will render a false-positive result with much lower levels of contaminants. Although many studies do not show a statistically significant increase in contamination rates with less stringent urine collection techniques, most show increased accuracy with more meticulous or invasive collection methods.[5-8] Because it takes only marginally longer, it makes sense to always strive for the highest-quality urine specimen available, especially in view of the delays, repeated testing, and additional cost entailed by false-positive results. A frequent misconception is that contaminated specimens are characterized by the isolation of multiple pathogens, but in fact, up to 50% of symptomatic women may have polymicrobial infections.[1,9]

The issue of whether a patient is "symptomatic" might appear trivial, but the clinical practice of checking for UTI in most patients with any type of abdominal pain has important implications. Studies of urine collection and testing in symptomatic patients focus on the classic signs and symptoms of UTI (e.g., urgency, frequency, dysuria, flank pain, costovertebral angle tenderness) and do not include patients with nonspecific abdominal pain. Whether undifferentiated abdominal pain or fever constitutes a "symptom" of UTI has never been studied, and how to apply the results of studies done on patients with classic symptoms to those with nonspecific symptoms is unclear.[10] Patients with classic symptoms need the most careful urine collection method because they have the most riding on the outcome of the test. This group of patients should include those with systemic signs of infection (e.g., fever and chills) who are unable to accurately report their symptoms and patients in whom failure to diagnose asymptomatic bacteriuria would be potentially dangerous (e.g., the immunocompromised, neonates and infants, pregnant patients, diabetics) or for whom urine cultures are going to be necessary because of a history of relapsing, recurrent, complicated, or childhood UTI.[9,11]

In cooperative, motivated males and females with symptoms of uncomplicated lower UTI or pyelonephritis who are capable of diligently performing the necessary maneuvers, a midstream clean-catch (MSCC) specimen is as accurate as a catheterized specimen, especially when the possibility of urethral or prostatic trauma and patient discomfort are considered.[12] In patients unable to provide an MSCC specimen, a catheterized specimen is usually warranted.

If no symptoms of UTI are present, the urine examination can be considered a "screening" test. In asymptomatic patients, routine screening for bacteriuria is unwarranted in all but two clinical situations: pregnant women and all patients scheduled for urologic surgery.[13,14] If only a urine culture is to be performed, some would argue that any spontaneously voided specimen would suffice since the diagnosis of asymptomatic bacteriuria depends on 10^5 or more CFUs of a single pathogen per milliliter of urine. With such criteria, contaminants are usually easily identified.[8] Because performing cultures on all such patients is prohibitively costly, dipstick testing, urinalysis (UA), or both are commonly used for screening.[15,16] With these tests, contamination by bacteria, leukocytes, or erythrocytes results in diagnostic confusion. The advantages of a less contaminated specimen are worth the minimal, extra effort of asking the patient to provide an MSCC sample. The approach in Figure 67-1 covers the vast majority of situations. A few circumstances and techniques deserve special mention.

Bladder Percussion and the Midstream Specimen in Infants

The emergency clinician is familiar with how frequently a urine stream is generated in infants confronted by the alarming emergency department (ED) environment and a cold stethoscope. Rather than wasting a potentially perfect MSCC specimen on a laboratory coat with an ensuing delay in obtaining urine, the clinician can exploit the situation by approaching an infant with an open sterile urine container in hand in case the urine stream is spontaneously forthcoming. The process is facilitated by the application of cold povidone-iodine to the genitalia. Such an approach has been shown to generate a urine sample in a median time of 10 minutes.[17] This is less than the typical time needed for straight catheterization or suprapubic aspiration (SPA), and it can be performed concomitantly with the history and physical examination and thereby circumvent an invasive procedure. If the urine specimen is not immediately forthcoming, a parent can

TABLE 67-1 Urine Collection Methods Listed in Order of Increasing Precision

METHOD	DESCRIPTION AND COMMENTS
Random voided	Any specimen provided by the patient
Midstream voided	No skin preparation, container placed in the urinary stream 2-3 sec after initiation of micturition
Clean catch	Same as above, plus antiseptic cleansing of the urethral area. This is performed by retraction of the prepuce in males and the labia in females and then cleansing the meatus in an anterior-to-posterior direction. Use three swabs soaked in povidone-iodine (or some other antiseptic solution). For female patients who are physically capable, the ideal position is sitting astride a toilet, facing backward. This helps separate the labia and position the cup for collection of the specimen
Midstream clean catch	Cleansing as in "clean catch," with midstream collection as in "midstream voided"
Catheterized	Obtained from a newly placed catheter after cleansing of the meatus
Suprapubic aspiration	See Chapter 55

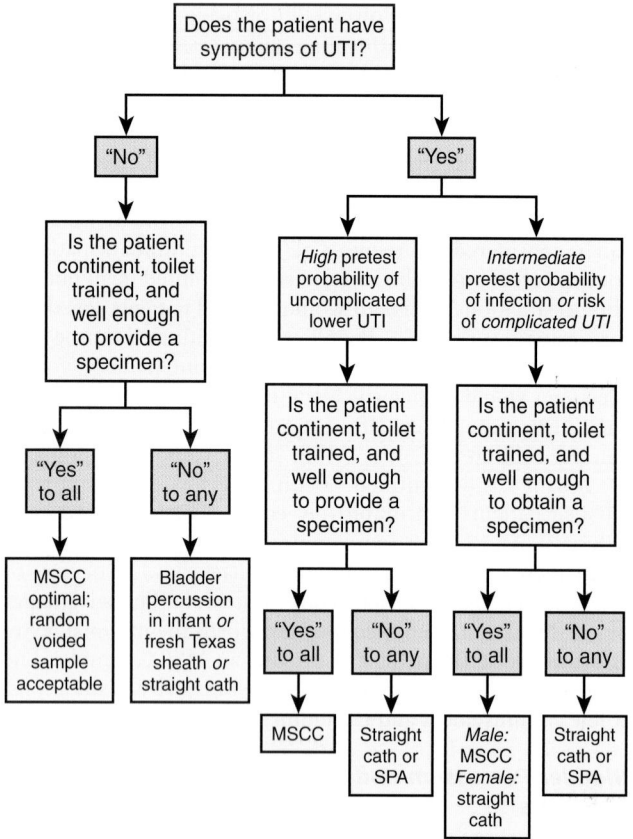

Figure 67-1 Algorithm for deciding the method of obtaining a urine specimen for evaluation of possible urinary tract infection (UTI). *MSCC*, midstream clean catch; *SPA*, suprapubic aspiration.

be equipped with a sterile container and be instructed on collection of an ensuing specimen to free up ED staff for other tasks. Two techniques to actively induce voiding in infants have been described. The first, which is useful in newborns, exploits the Perez reflex.[18] After cleansing the genitalia, hold the infant in one hand while stroking the paraspinal muscles in a cephalad to caudad direction. This causes extension of the back and flexion of the hips and induces micturition in less than 5 minutes in the majority of cases.[18] The second technique is known as "bladder tapping." After urethral

cleansing, if there is still no urine, use two fingers to tap on the suprapubic area at a rate of approximately once per second for a full minute, followed by a minute's rest. Repeat the cycle until urine is produced. The mean time before the production of a urine sample is about 5 minutes. This technique, though not practicable for the staff in a busy ED, can provide an infant's parents with a task that invests them in the clinical process. This clinical pearl may expeditiously furnish a specimen with significantly less investment of staff time than required for more invasive techniques.[19]

Bag Collection in Non–Toilet-Trained Children
The incidence of unsuspected UTI in a febrile neonate or infant is about 5%.[20] A true UTI in an infant or child requires subsequent evaluation for urinary tract pathology, and the disease may produce significant morbidity (e.g., hypertension, renal disease). One must be certain of the presence or absence of infection in this subgroup. Numerous studies have demonstrated the disutility of urine specimens obtained *for culture* from a collection bag stuck to an infant's perineum.[18,19,21-23] Bag specimens may be more sensitive than catheter specimens when used for UA or microscopy to identify infection in children at low or moderate risk for UTI.[24] In this group it is acceptable to perform screening UA, microscopy, or both on a bag specimen.[25,26] If negative, UTI is ruled out. If positive (leukocyte esterase or nitrite present or more than 5 WBCs/high-power field [HPF] on spun urine or bacteria on an unspun Gram-stained specimen), it is followed by catheterization and culture, with treatment usually pending the results of culture.[21,25-27] If a urine specimen is needed solely for chemical analysis (e.g., glucose, ketones, specific gravity), a bag specimen will suffice.

Urine Specimens from Patients with Chronic Urinary Drainage Systems
Urine obtained from any part of a chronic urinary drainage system is highly inaccurate for bacteriologic purposes. If UTI is suspected, insert a new catheter and obtain a fresh bladder urine specimen.[28] A small study advocating replacement of a chronically applied "Texas sheath" catheter with a fresh one was performed on subjects who did not have symptoms of UTI.[29] Such a method might be sufficiently accurate for screening asymptomatic patients, but a Foley catheter should be used to obtain urine from patients with sheath catheters

TABLE 67-2 Overview of Urine Dipstick Tests

	SOURCES OF ERROR AND ARTIFACT	COMMENTS
Glucose	False positive with peroxide, hypochlorite, ketonuria, levodopa, and the dipstick exposed to air False negative with ascorbate, ketones, uric acid, and high specific gravity	Hypothermia may cause glycosuria despite hypoglycemia Glycosuria without hyperglycemia suggests renal tubular dysfunction
Ketones	False positive with ascorbate, low pH urine, high specific gravity, levodopa, valproate, phenazopyridine, *N*-acetylcysteine, high-protein diet, phenylketonuria, phthalein compounds	Very susceptible to deterioration with humidity and delay in analysis, which can cause false-negative results
Nitrites	False positive with phenazopyridine False negative high specific gravity, frequent urination, ascorbate, high urine pH, and urine standing in the specimen cup >2 hr	75% false-negative rate when exposed to air for 15 days Does not detect reductase-negative bacteria
Protein	False positive with pH >7 and chlorhexidine False negative with low pH, very dilute urine	Only reliable for albumin (glomerular proteinuria) Does not detect Bence-Jones protein Positive with pyuria, rarely with hematuria
Blood	False positive with povidone-iodine, certain (peroxidase-producing) bacteria, hypochlorite False negative with high specific gravity and high concentrations of urinary nitrites, ascorbate, or captopril	Positive test with speckles or dots implies nonhemolyzed blood Positive test with a diffuse pattern implies hemolyzed red blood cells or high levels of myoglobin
Bilirubin	False positive with iodine, stool contamination, chlorpromazine, mefenamic acid False negative after prolonged standing	Hard to read with agents causing marked urine discoloration
Urobilinogen	False positive with phenazopyridine, sulfisoxazole, sulfonamides, porphyrin, methyldopa, procaine, aminosalicylic acid, 5-hydroxyindolacetic acid False negative with sulfisoxazole and phenazopyridine	Use a fresh specimen: rapidly broken down by light and in acidic urine
Leukocyte esterase	False positive with vaginal contamination, oxidizing agents, eosinophils in urine, *Trichomonas* False negative with high glucose, ketones, protein (especially albumin), pH, and specific gravity, as well as with cephalexin, tetracycline, oxalates, ascorbic acid, neutropenia	Sterile pyuria seen with tuberculosis, nephrolithiasis, interstitial nephritis
pH	Urea-splitting bacteria elevate pH Run off from the protein strip can falsely lower pH	Use a fresh specimen: standing raises pH by loss of CO_2
Specific gravity	Overestimates specific gravity with low pH, ketoacidosis, and protein Underestimates specific gravity with glucose, urea, or pH >7	Not reliable at specific gravity >1.025 Elevated with use of dextran, intravenous contrast material, proteinuria

who have signs or symptoms of acute UTI and are unable to provide an MSCC specimen.

Catheterization and SPA
The low levels of bacteriuria found in 2% to 8% of patients after straight catheterization are generally below the threshold that defines the presence of UTI.[30] Catheterization can cause minor local injury, as reflected by low-level hematuria in 15% of patients.[30,31] SPA continues to be advocated by some for neonates in cases in which accurate diagnosis is essential and the risk for infection must be minimized. Both SPA (see Chapter 55) and catheterization have an approximately 25% "failure rate" as a result of an empty bladder.[32] This problem and associated complications can be avoided by performing bedside ultrasound before the procedure.[32-34] SPA may

spuriously lower leukocyte or bacterial colony counts because of the necessity of filling the bladder before performing the procedure.[35] A study in infants demonstrated that the discomfort associated with SPA is greater than that with catheterization.[36] Surprisingly, however, older men who underwent both catheterization and SPA strongly preferred SPA.[5]

Urine Dipstick

Urine dipstick tests are available to test 10 separate parameters. The unassuming appearance and commonplace use of the urine dipstick might lead one to mistakenly underestimate its technical sophistication. Each colored square on a urine dipstick involves a biochemically complex assay, and therefore it is essential to *meticulously follow the manufacturer's instructions for storage and use.*[37] Even with optimal storage and testing conditions, the false-negative and false-positive rates of these tests are problematic. In addition, most of the tests are susceptible to interference from a variety of substances (Table 67-2).

Method

Test urine specimens as soon as possible after they are collected. If the urine has been standing, stir or shake the specimen well because cells sink rapidly in a container. Immerse the test strip completely for 1 second or less. Draw the edge of the strip along the rim of the specimen container and lightly tap it to remove excess urine, thus avoiding mixing the reagents between different test patches. Next, hold the strip horizontally or place it on a clean gauze pad until the recommended time has elapsed. Most strips are designed so that all the test results can be read together after 1 to 2 minutes (Fig. 67-2).

Interpretation
Glucose

The urine glucose test is normally negative. Urine glucose testing has limited usefulness in quantitative testing because the serum glucose level at which spillage occurs varies (although in most patients it starts at between 180 and 200 mg/dL).[38] Changes in urine glucose lag behind changes in blood glucose by approximately half the interval between voids.[39] Glycosuria in the absence of hyperglycemia suggests renal tubular dysfunction. Glycosuria may occur in hypothermic patients in the absence of hyperglycemia and indeed may actually occur with hypoglycemia in such patients.[40]

Ketones

Ketones are found in the urine of patients with starvation, inadequate carbohydrate intake, diabetic and alcoholic ketoacidosis, isopropyl alcohol poisoning, or glycogen storage disease. Tests for urine ketones are 5 to 10 times more sensitive to acetoacetate than to acetone, similar to the serum tests. Dipsticks do not detect 5-hydroxybutyrate, which accounts for 80% to 95% of the three "ketone bodies" and is the predominant form in the setting of ketoacidosis. Urine ketone testing is significantly *more* sensitive than serum ketone testing.[41] There is generally no need to obtain "serum acetones" to diagnose or manage diabetic ketoacidosis when urine ketone monitoring is coupled with blood gas and anion gap analysis.

Leukocyte Esterase

This portion of the dipstick test is designed to detect enzymes from the azurophilic granules in neutrophils. Normally the test is negative. Studies report a wide and clinically important range of thresholds for the sensitivity of dipstick testing, from 10 to 100 WBCs/µL urine.[15,16] Studies suggest that the test is between 50% and 96% sensitive in detecting infection.[2,42,43] Its specificity for the presence of WBCs is between 91% and 99%. The most common cause of a false-positive leukocyte test is vaginal contamination.

Nitrites

Normally, urine does not contain nitrites. Nitrites are specific (≈95%), but not sensitive (≈45%) indicators of UTI.[13,44,45] Urinary nitrates are converted to nitrites most strongly by enteric coliform bacteria, thus explaining the nitrite test's 90% sensitivity in detecting UTI caused by *Escherichia coli*.

Figure 67-2 Urine dipstick testing. **A,** Totally immerse the dipstick in urine for a few seconds. **B,** Place it on its side on a paper towel to allow drainage of urine and limit cross-contamination of the individual testing squares. Note that the bottle of test strips should be closed immediately because prolonged exposure to air can produce false results. **C,** Formal reading of the test strip is accomplished electronically rather than only by the naked eye for quality assurance and a permanent record. **D,** Myoglobinuria: strongly positive for blood on the dipstick with no red blood cells (RBCs) on microscopy.

Enterococcus, a moderately frequent urinary pathogen, *Pseudomonas* species, and *Acinetobacter* lack the reductase enzyme and are not detected. False-negative results also occur because of the lack of dietary nitrate, frequent voiding, and diuresis. Early morning–voided specimens are ideal because they allow time for conversion of nitrate to nitrite, but they are rarely available in the ED. If possible, a specimen obtained more than 4 hours after the last voiding is preferred.

Protein

Proteins with a molecular weight below 50,000 to 60,000 daltons can pass through the glomerulus to be reabsorbed in the proximal tubule. Normal passage of protein in urine is less than 150 mg/24 hours, or approximately 10 mg/dL of urine. About 10% to 33% of urinary protein is albumin, 33% is Tamm-Horsfall glycoprotein (secreted by renal tubular cells), and the balance is made up of a variety of immunoglobulins and other proteins. Proteinuria is a finding noted in about 5% of routine urine screens in men.[46] This may represent a normal variant since 3% to 5% of healthy adults have postural proteinuria (proteinuria when standing but not when recumbent).[38] Proteinuria is rarely clinically significant unless 3+ or greater on the dipstick, although lower levels are still indicative of some degree of renal dysfunction (see later). The dipstick detects negatively charged proteins more strongly than positively charged ones; it is therefore most sensitive to albumin. A study of ED patients with severe acute hypertension identified renal dysfunction, defined as elevated serum creatinine, with 100% sensitivity when using urine dipstick detection of 1+ proteinuria or hematuria.[47] Along similar lines, in patients being considered for radiographic contrast-enhanced studies who do not have a serum creatinine measurement, a negative dipstick test for protein or blood combined with the absence of prior renal disease, hypertension, diabetes, congestive heart failure, and age younger than 60 years effectively excludes renal insufficiency.[48] The urine dipstick test is positive for protein with pyuria of greater than 6 WBCs/HPF.[49] This is a false-positive finding for protein but is helpful when the urine dipstick is being used to screen for UTI since the threshold for leukocyte esterase is often significantly higher. Hematuria only slightly elevates urine protein levels.

In assessing a patient with proteinuria, it is helpful to divide the list of causes into those that are and those that are not associated with hematuria. These are listed in Box 67-1. Elevated urinary protein is more commonly due to renal than to systemic causes. The source is either glomerular, with passage of normally unfiltered proteins, or tubular, with failure to reabsorb physiologically filtered, low-molecular-weight globulins. The former condition causes albuminuria. Renal tubular proteinuria is characterized by low levels of urinary albumin and is therefore more likely to be missed.

"Blood"

The blood section of the urine dipstick is positive if exposed to RBCs, hemoglobin (Hb), or myoglobin. Urine in healthy volunteers contains fewer than 7 RBCs/mL. Studies have shown that the urine dipstick is very sensitive to 10 RBCs/mL. False-negative results are confined to clinically insignificant hematuria.[50] The dipstick pad should be inspected for discrete positive "dots," indicative of nonhemolyzed RBCs. Moderate intravascular hemolysis does not cause

---

BOX 67-1 Some Causes of Proteinuria with and without Hematuria

PROTEINURIA USUALLY WITH HEMATURIA

Usually indicates glomerular disease. Most causes in early stages can appear without hematuria

PROTEINURIA USUALLY WITHOUT HEMATURIA

Generally indicates tubular or interstitial disease or high serum levels causing "overflow." In advanced disease, hematuria can develop

INFECTIOUS DISEASES

Post-streptococcal glomerulonephritis, pneumococcal pneumonia, bacterial endocarditis, meningococcemia, secondary syphilis, hepatitis B, severe viral infections, malaria, toxoplasmosis, Guillain-Barré syndrome

MULTISYSTEM DISEASES

Vasculitides: Henoch-Schönlein purpura, polyarteritis nodosa, Wegener's granulomatosis, Kawasaki's disease, etc.
Connective tissue diseases (systemic lupus erythematosus, rheumatoid arthritis, scleroderma)
Neoplasia
Rhabdomyolysis (artifactual hematuria)
Goodpasture's syndrome
Cryoglobulinemias
Toxemia of pregnancy
Serum sickness

PRIMARY GLOMERULAR DISEASES

SYSTEMIC CONDITIONS

Physiologic: after exercise, postural (with standing)
Pathologic: fever, shock states, severe hypovolemia, dehydration, congestive heart failure
Diabetes
Amyloidosis
Sarcoidosis
"Overflow states": multiple myeloma, lymphoma, leukemia, rhabdomyolysis
Renovascular hypertension

MEDICATIONS, DRUGS, AND TOXINS

Nonsteroidal antiinflammatory drugs, gold, penicillamine, probenecid, captopril, lithium, cyclosporine
Heroin
Heavy metal nephropathy: lead, mercury, or cadmium

RENAL DISEASES

Chronic pyelonephritis
Interstitial nephritis
Fanconi's syndrome

TABLE 67-3   Aids in Distinguishing Hematuria, Intravascular Hemolysis, and Myoglobinuria

	HEMATURIA	MYOGLOBINURIA	INTRAVASCULAR HEMOLYSIS
Serum findings	Color: clear	Color: clear Haptoglobin: normal	Color: pink Haptoglobin: low
Urine appearance	Color: clear to brown; clears with centrifugation	Color: clear to red/brown; no clearing with centrifugation	Color: clear to brown; no clearing with centrifugation
Urine microscopy	RBCs, RBC casts, and protein imply as glomerular source No RBC casts, tubular cells, small protein: nephron source Just RBCs: source distal to the nephron (e.g., ureterolithiasis)	Possible occasional RBCs and tubular cells secondary to rhabdomyolysis-induced renal damage	Usually unremarkable

RBC, red blood cell.

TABLE 67-4   Relationship between Urinary Bilirubin, Urobilinogen, and Stool Color in Jaundiced Patients

	HEALTHY NORMAL	COMPLETE BILIARY OBSTRUCTION	INTRAVASCULAR HEMOLYSIS	HEPATOCELLULAR DISEASE
Urinary bilirubin	None	Elevated	None	Elevated
Urinary urobilinogen	None or present	None	Present, sometimes large	Normal early Increased late
Stool color	Normal	Acholic	Normal	Normal

hemoglobinuria because Hb is tightly bound to haptoglobin and is therefore not filtered. Massive intravascular hemolysis gives rise to free plasma Hb with a molecular weight of 32,000 daltons, which easily passes through the glomerulus. Myoglobin has a molecular weight of 17,000 daltons, which also allows easy glomerular passage, but the dipstick has been shown to have a sensitivity of only 14% with heat-induced rhabdomyolysis, as reflected by serum creatine phosphokinase levels of up to 1000 U/L.[51] Guidelines for distinguishing hematuria, hemoglobinuria, and myoglobinuria are outlined in Table 67-3. In asymptomatic men older than 50 years, significant disease can be signaled by intermittent hematuria, thus mandating follow-up of patients with this incidental finding.[52]

Dipsticks are vitiated by humidity and air, which can cause false-negative results after improper storage.[53] Because RBCs may lyse rapidly, delays in performing UA may misleadingly suggest myoglobinuria or hemoglobinuria. Microscopy or dipstick testing of a *freshly* obtained specimen can clarify this issue. Conversely, high specific gravity or low pH can inhibit lysis of erythrocytes, which is necessary for the dipstick chemical reaction to occur, thus causing false-negative results.[53a] A study reproducing clinical conditions has demonstrated that povidone-iodine does not cause false-positive results on the dipstick.[53b] Iatrogenically caused trace positive results may occur after catheterization in 15% of cases.[31]

Urine Bilirubin

Urine bilirubin represents the filtered, soluble, conjugated form of bilirubin. Unconjugated bilirubin is bound to protein and does not pass through the glomerulus. Bilirubinuria is therefore due to intrahepatic or extrahepatic cholestasis. Bilirubinuria will be detected significantly earlier than clinical jaundice. Urinary bilirubin excretion is enhanced by alkalosis.

A fresh sample of urine should be tested because bilirubin glucuronide is hydrolyzed when exposed to light. Ascorbic acid and high levels of urinary nitrites decrease the sensitivity of the test to bilirubin.

Urobilinogen

In a healthy person, conjugated bilirubin is excreted in bile. In the colon it is broken down into a number of compounds, including urobilinogen. Most of these compounds are excreted in stool, which is the source of its characteristic color. A small amount of urobilinogen is absorbed from the colon, and if it is not taken up on the first pass through the liver, it enters the circulation. Ultimately, some of this urobilinogen may enter the urine, so it is normal to have zero to moderate levels of urinary urobilinogen on dipstick testing. Most diseases that cause hepatocyte dysfunction (hepatitis, cirrhosis, passive liver congestion, etc.) increase urinary urobilinogen excretion by impairing hepatic uptake of urobilinogen. As a qualitative test with a wide range of normal values, it is rarely helpful, but in evaluating a patient with jaundice, it can have diagnostic significance (Table 67-4).

pH

The average daily excretion of 50 to 100 mmol of H^+ in urine gives rise to a typical urine pH of around 6 with a range from 4.5 to 8. Dietary protein lowers urinary pH, whereas fruit (especially citrus) and vegetables tend to raise it. The significance of pH testing is in the assessment of normal renal function. In most states of alkalosis and acidosis, healthy kidneys maintain homeostasis by conserving or excreting H^+. Failure to do so suggests renal disease, especially renal tubular acidosis. An exception is the "paradoxical aciduria" of hypokalemic alkalosis secondary to volume contraction, hypercorticism, or diuretics, where the highest priority of the

Figure 67-3 Microscopic urinanalysis. **A,** Neutrophils. **B,** Fine granular cast. **C,** Red blood cell cast (the distinct and uniformly spherical shape of the erythrocyte is visible). **D,** White blood cell cast (seen with intrinsic renal diseases such as pyelonephritis and glomerulonephritis; note the discernible nuclei and cell boundaries). **E,** Uric acid crystals. **F,** Calcium oxalate crystals. **G,** Calcium phosphate crystals. **H,** Cysteine crystal (indicative of cystinuria). **I,** Bacteria and leukocytes. **J,** *Candida,* budding yeast. **K,** *Candida,* pseudohyphae. **L,** *Trichomonas vaginalis.* (*A-K, From McPherson RA, Pincus MR, eds.* Henry's Clinical Diagnosis and Management by Laboratory Methods. *22nd ed. Philadelphia: Saunders; 2011; L, From Bieber EJ, Sanfilippo JS, Horowitz IR, eds.* Clinical Gynecology. *Philadelphia: Churchill Livingstone; 2006.*)

renal tubule is to conserve sodium. pH is elevated by the action of urea-splitting bacteria, especially *Proteus* species. This can occur with "stasis" of urine, either in the bladder or in specimen cups. A persistently alkaline urine is seen in patients with struvite (triple phosphate) urolithiasis.

Specific Gravity

The dipstick test for urine specific gravity assays for the primary urinary cations sodium and potassium. True specific gravity, which is also dependent on anions, albumin, proteins, urea, and glucose, is therefore not measured. Artifactually low specific gravity readings are obtained with alkaline urine, whereas acidic urine and albumin falsely elevate the specific gravity reading. Consequently, some investigators believe that these strips on the dipstick test are of marginal clinical utility.[54] Other clinical indicators of a patient's hydration status are probably more reliable. If necessary, a refractive specific gravitometer or a hygrometer should be used.

Microscopic UA

Microscopic UA is performed to identify cells, bacteria, and other microbes, as well as formed elements such as casts and crystals (Fig. 67-3). The following discussion focuses on the findings of significance in diagnosing UTI: WBCs, bacteria, and WBC casts. The presence of WBCs with bacteria distinguishes infection from colonization (bacteriuria without pyuria). Some authorities state that significant infection without pyuria occurs in less than 5% of cases, thus making pyuria alone a sensitive marker of infection.[53,55] Other studies do not support reliance on pyuria by itself as an indicator of infection.[2,3,5,27] The presence of WBC casts distinguishes pyelonephritis ("upper UTI") from cystitis ("lower UTI").

Microscopic UA is performed by one of five methods. Traditionally, the most common technique has been examination of unstained centrifuged urine. It has the advantage of concentrating formed elements that might otherwise be missed. Its disadvantage is that the presence and quantity of elements in a specimen will depend on many uncontrolled factors: the volume of the specimen, the duration and speed of centrifugation, the fragility of the formed elements, the volume of the "drop" in which the pellet is resuspended, and the size of the microscope's HPF.[14,56,57]

1. **Examination of unspun urine in a hemocytometer counting chamber.** A hemocytometer is a precisely milled slide etched with measured squares, which allows exact enumeration of the cells in each square. Because the distance between the etched surface and the coverslip is known exactly, it is possible to determine the number of cells per unit volume of specimen. Enough fresh unspun urine is placed on the slide to fully cover the counting area, and the cells are counted. There should usually be less than 1 WBC/μL, although more than 10 WBCs/μL and more than 5 RBCs/μL are unequivocally abnormal.[58] The threshold for diagnosing UTI is usually set at 8 or more WBCs/μL.[9,22,56,59,60] Bacteria do not sink to the surface of the hemocytometer, so counting them through the many focal planes of the chamber is not possible, although methods to estimate the bacterial count per unit volume have been described.[57]

   The hemocytometer is accurate, fast (time need not be spent on staining or centrifugation), and relatively easy to master. Its major drawbacks are cost (around $150 for the slide and cover slip) and fragility (easily destroyed if dropped). These characteristics are problematic given the conditions and resources in many EDs, although their use has been advocated by some.[61] Formed elements other than WBCs and RBCs (e.g., casts) occur in such low concentrations that they are encountered in the hemocytometer only by chance, and therefore microscopy of spun urine is needed for their identification.

2. **Examination of unspun, unstained urine placed on a regular microscope slide.** This qualitative method is sometimes used for the diagnosis of UTI. Using 1 organism/HPF as a positive result, the sensitivity and specificity of detecting 10^5 CFUs/mL are between 60% and 90%.[62] This method identifies only 1 WBC/HPF with the highly pyuric state of 250 WBCs/μL,[60] which has led some to advocate the use of more than 1 WBC per *low-power field* as a criterion for infection.[58]

3. **Examination of unstained, centrifuged urine.** With this method, 10 mL of urine is centrifuged at approximately 450*g* (1000 to 4000 rpm) for 3 to 5 minutes. Roughly 9 mL of supernatant is poured off, and the pellet is resuspended in the remaining fluid. This suspension is placed on a slide with a coverslip and examined. The larger formed elements, especially casts, tend to migrate to the edge of the coverslip, and they can be seen with low magnification. One or two casts, depending on the clinical context, may be normal; more are not. The morphology of the more commonly encountered formed elements of urine sediment is shown in Figure 67-3. The significance of each is beyond the scope of this text, but this information can be found in a standard textbook of clinical laboratory procedures and diagnostic testing.[38,39] When examining centrifuged urine, more than 5 WBCs/HPF in the middle of the coverslip has traditionally been taken as being indicative of abnormal pyuria. Most authors have estimated that 10 WBCs/μL is equivalent to approximately 1 WBC/HPF; thus, this oft-cited threshold for diagnosing UTI is actually equivalent to 50 WBCs/μL in unspun urine.[56,58,59] Since the gold standard for the diagnosis of UTI is more than 8 WBCs/μL of unspun urine, many infections will escape detection with this method. Various numbers of bacteria per HPF have been used as criteria for the diagnosis of UTI. A threshold of 10 to 20 organisms/HPF has been recommended to rule out bacteriuria at the 10^5-CFU/mL level.[62] As noted previously, this threshold would not exclude infection in symptomatic patients.

4. **Examination of Gram-stained, uncentrifuged urine.** Also a semiquantitative measurement, it is estimated that 1 bacterium/HPF is equivalent to 10^5 CFUs/mL in bacterial culture.[38,62] A drop of urine is placed on the slide, allowed to air-dry, and then heat-fixed and Gram-stained.

5. **Examination of Gram-stained, centrifuged urine.** This method is probably the optimal technique, short of culture, for the assessment of bacteriuria. It is more than 95% sensitive and more than 60% specific at 10^4 CFUs/mL—an order of magnitude lower concentration of bacteriuria than the previously described methods.[63] Detection of 1 organism per oil-immersion field constitutes a positive result. Specificity is increased to 95% if 5 organisms/HPF are seen.[62]

Summary of Tests Used in the Diagnosis of UTI

The three tests commonly used to evaluate a patient for the presence or absence of UTI are urine dipstick, microscopic UA, and urine culture. Each represents an increasing degree of expense, delay, and resources.[64] A brief discussion of their relative strengths and weaknesses ensues.

Urine Dipstick

Dipstick testing of urine is faster than microscopic UA, is less labor-intensive and cheaper, and circumvents multiple sources of potential and proven error. Is it sufficiently accurate to replace UA, however? If *either* leukocyte esterase *or* nitrites are used to indicate infection, the dipstick is only 50% to 90% sensitive for culture-proven infection.[15,43,44,63,65] This is not adequate to rule out infection in symptomatic patients, in whom the prevalence of disease is high, but may be acceptable in asymptomatic patients, in whom the test has a serviceably high negative predictive value of 95% to 99%. In symptomatic men, sensitivity is enhanced by taking a positive result in *any one* (or more) of *either* leukocyte esterase, nitrites, protein, *or* blood as an indication of UTI.[15,66-68] This process can be augmented by allowing extra time before reading the strip. For women with symptoms of UTI, empirical treatment is recommended because no test can rule out infection.[64] A negative dipstick test in a patient with a high pretest probability of UTI should prompt a search for an alternative source of the patient's symptoms. Maneuvers to enhance dipstick sensitivity diminish its specificity, which may be as low as 26%.[10] This has led some to advocate microscopic UA on all urine specimens that are found to be abnormal by dipstick,[67] but this probably adds little to a carefully performed dipstick test.

Microscopic UA

If the urine dipstick has such poor specificity when it is used as a test with adequate sensitivity, should it be discarded altogether and microscopic UA be relied on instead? Apart from the hemocytometer, the most reliable method for identifying significant bacteriuria is oil-immersion microscopy of Gram-stained, centrifuged urine.[62] Nonetheless, the practice in most hospital laboratories is to examine a resuspended pellet of unstained, centrifuged urine. The problems with this method have been discussed. In various studies a range between 1 and 10 organisms/HPF or 5 WBCs/HPF has been considered a "positive" test (as the threshold number rises, so does specificity, at the price of sensitivity). In aggregate, the accuracy of microscopy in the diagnosis of UTI is similar to that of the dipstick alone, with 22% false-positive and 23% false-negative rates when compared with culture.[53,57,64] Microscopic UA, like the dipstick, cannot rule out infection in symptomatic patients. The specificity of pyuria will be improved when viewed as a marker of all genitourinary infections, including urethritis, prostatitis, epididymitis, vaginitis, and cervicitis. These diagnoses should always be entertained in patients with urinary symptoms, especially those with sterile pyuria.

Urine Culture

Cultures are indicated for any potentially complicated UTI, including infections in children; men; women with recurrences or relapses; immunocompromised individuals; patients with urinary tract pathology, including stones and possible pyelonephritis; and pregnant patients. Cultures are usually recommended around the 16th week of gestation. Every effort should be made to obtain a high-quality specimen because of the difficulty in distinguishing contamination from significant low-count bacteriuria in symptomatic patients and in view of the expense of cultures and treatment if the culture is positive.

The Bottom Line

It is well established that female patients with symptoms of uncomplicated lower UTI can be treated without culture since the prevalence of disease is 50% or greater in women with classic urinary symptoms.[14,45,69,70] Treatment is generally benign, and 95% of urine cultures that are positive will yield a limited number of organisms with predictable antibiotic susceptibilities. Some authors recommend dipstick or microscopic UA (or both) because a negative test might prompt more careful consideration of alternative diagnoses in this group with a high incidence of sexually transmitted disease.[14,45] If none is found, such patients can be treated empirically. Traditionally, trimethoprim-sulfamethoxazole was recommended, although increasing resistance to this drug has lead to levofloxacin (itself with unacceptably high resistance rates in many locations) being the current choice of empirical antibiotics.[71,72]

Urine testing is more likely to influence clinical management in patients with an intermediate pretest probability of infection.[10] Urine microscopy may also help in distinguishing pyelonephritis (WBC casts), vaginitis (absence of pyuria or hematuria in a meticulous MSCC or catheterized specimen), and urethritis (pyuria, rarely hematuria) from cystitis (pyuria and often hematuria).[14,45] In the ED, the ease of performing a dipstick test argues for its use without UA since it is equally sensitive unless formed elements such as casts, crystals, *Trichomonas*, or other parasites are suspected. In patients with pyelonephritis, urine cultures are warranted because they alter therapy in about 5% of cases.[73] In most asymptomatic patients, a negative dipstick or UA result has sufficient negative predictive value to rule out disease unless the patient is pregnant or undergoing urologic surgery. Special clinical considerations in some patients (e.g., the immunocompromised, diabetic females at high risk for UTI) may mandate adjustments to this approach.[15] Recommendations vary regarding infants. Cultures are recommended for all febrile infants younger than 2 months and for children who appear sick or have a high pretest probability of infection.[21,23] In a recent study, combined microscopic and dipstick UA was only 64% sensitive (and 91% specific) for culture-proven UTI in febrile infants younger than 24 months, thus suggesting the use of culture unless an alternative source of infection is clear.[74]

TESTING FOR PREGNANCY

Some investigators have found female patients reliable in determining their own pregnancy status.[75,76] Others have not.[77] With respect to ordering of radiographic studies on women of childbearing age, clinicians should determine from their own practice experience the reliability of patient history in this regard. If in doubt and with the potentially lethal outcome of an ectopic pregnancy, it might be prudent to use an objective test. Pregnancy tests are based on the detection of β-human chorionic gonadotropin (β-hCG) in serum or urine. β-hCG is secreted by trophoblastic cells of the placenta starting from the time of implantation of the blastocyst. Qualitative serum and urine tests can detect β-hCG levels of

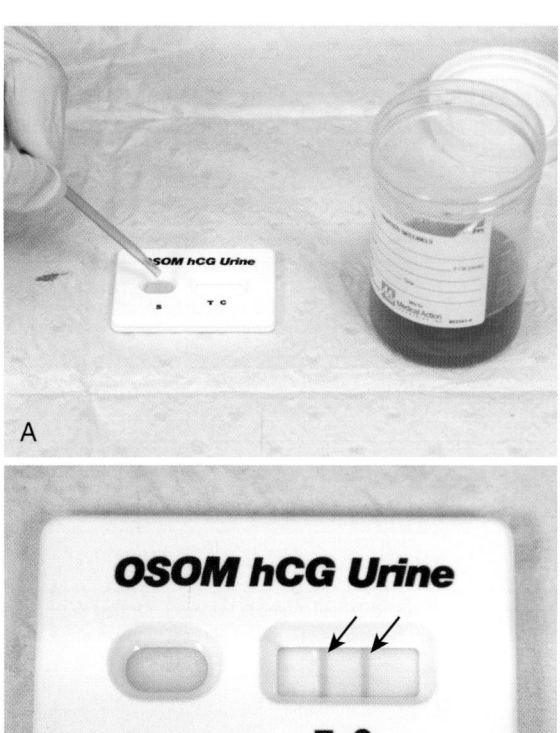

Figure 67-4 Urine β-human chorionic gonadotropin (β-hCG) testing. **A,** Urine β-hCG tests that have a sensitivity of 25 mIU/mL are readily available. The concentration of β-hCG is usually lower in urine than in serum, thus making the urine test slightly less sensitive for the detection of early pregnancy. **B,** This test is positive, as indicated by the dark stripe (*arrows*) in both the test (T) and control (C) positions.

between 15 and 25 mIU/mL (Fig. 67-4).[78] The concentration of β-hCG is usually lower in urine than in serum, which accounts for the slight advantage of serum tests in detecting early pregnancy. Optimal results on urine pregnancy tests are obtained with first-voided, concentrated morning specimens. It has recently been established that whole blood is a reliable specimen for the bedside dipstick tests used in most EDs.[79,80] This alternative may be lifesaving in timely recognition of an ectopic pregnancy in a hypotensive female with pelvic complaints and unknown pregnancy status when a urine specimen is unavailable or results in significant delay.

If fertilization has occurred, β-hCG levels of 5 to 8 mIU/mL (the threshold of the quantitative serum test) correspond to the 9th to 11th day after ovulation (23 to 25 days after the first day of the last normal menstrual period). In a viable intrauterine pregnancy (IUP), the β-hCG level doubles approximately every 2 days during the first 4 weeks of gestation and reaches a serum level of greater than 25 mIU/mL, which is detectable by virtually all pregnancy tests on the first day of the missed menstrual period. The doubling rate declines to every third day thereafter.[81,82] β-hCG reaches a peak of between 100,000 and 200,000 mIU/mL between the 10th and 14th gestational weeks and declines to 10,000 to 20,000 mIU/mL for the rest of the pregnancy (Table 67-5).

TABLE 67-5 Relationship between Gestational Age, Qβ-hCG Levels, and Ultrasound Findings

TIME ELAPSED FROM THE FIRST DAY OF THE LAST NORMAL MENSTRUAL PERIOD	Qβ-hCG LEVEL (mIU/mL) USING THE IRP	ULTRASOUND FINDINGS
<28 days	5-50	
4-5 wk	50-500	From about 4.5 wk and Qβ-hCG level of 1000-1500 EVU can show a nonspecific intrauterine sac
5-6 wk	100-10,000	Definitely abnormal if no DDS seen on TVU with a Qβ-hCG level >2000 or by TAU with a Qβ-hCG level >6500 Abnormal if no YS with an MSD >10 mm
6-7 wk	1000-30,000	FP, cardiac activity 5.5-7 wk, Qβ-hCG level >10,000 Abnormal if no FP with an MSD >18 mm
7-8 wk	3,500-115,000	
8-14 wk	12,000-270,000	
>10 wk	270,000-15,000	

DDS, double decidual sac; *EVU,* endovaginal ultrasound; *FP,* fetal pole; *IRP,* international reference preparation; *MSD,* mean sac diameter; *Qβ-hCG,* quantitative β-human chorionic gonadotropin; *TAU,* transabdominal ultrasound; *TVU,* transvaginal ultrasound; *YS,* yolk sac.

There is a wide range of β-hCG levels in different women at the same stage of gestation, thus making definite clinical determination on the basis of a single quantitative test impossible.[83,84] False-positive test results have been described in association with molar pregnancy, choriocarcinoma, teratoma, occasional malignancies outside the genitourinary tract, and very high levels of proteinuria. There is one report of a positive urine β-hCG finding (but normal serum β-hCG) associated with a tuboovarian abscess.[85]

Although a previous quantitative β-hCG level is rarely available to the emergency clinician, doubling rates are an important part of the assessment of a healthy first-trimester pregnancy. Fetal nonviability, ectopic pregnancy, and intrauterine demise are signaled by abnormalities in the predicted rise in quantitative β-hCG.[86,87] A serum quantitative β-hCG level that does not increase by 66% every 48 hours has a 75% chance of being a nonviable pregnancy.[87,88] β-hCG levels in a healthy IUP and associated sonographic findings are listed in Table 67-5.

The rate of decline in quantitative β-hCG after gestation depends on the reason for the conclusion of the pregnancy. After a term delivery, β-hCG falls to zero in 2 weeks; after surgery for an ectopic pregnancy, the range is 1 to 31 days, with a median of 8.5 days; after a first-trimester spontaneous abortion, the range is 9 to 35 days (median, 19 days); and after a first-trimester elective abortion, the range is 16 to 60 days (median, 30 days).[38]

The association between β-hCG levels and gestational dates has led to the concept of the "discriminatory zone." In a normal pregnancy, a quantitative β-hCG level of 1000 to 2000 mIU/mL should be reflected by the presence of a double decidual sac (at the least) on transvaginal ultrasound (and on transabdominal ultrasound with levels higher than 6500 mIU/mL).[89] The clinician should beware of several potential pitfalls in applying this concept. First, *it applies only to the double decidual sign,* itself subject to interobserver variation among sonographers. The discriminatory zone *cannot* be extrapolated to the expected levels at which any of the more definitive sonographic signs of IUP such as yolk sac, fetal pole, or cardiac motion should be seen. Second, although it is true that if the double decidual sign is absent at these thresholds the pregnancy is almost certainly abnormal with a significant possibility of being ectopic, the converse—that it is pointless to perform ultrasonography if the quantitative β-hCG level is lower than 1000 mIU/mL—is *not* true. This is because the discriminatory zone does not preclude the possibility of identifying an ectopic pregnancy (or an IUP) before the quantitative β-hCG level reaches 1500 mIU/mL. Ectopic gestational sacs are pathological and therefore do not display β-hCG levels according to nomograms established for normal IUPs, and advanced ectopic pregnancies may have low β-hCG levels. One percent of ectopic pregnancies have a quantitative β-hCG level of less than 10 mIU/mL, and approximately a third of ectopic pregnancies are diagnosed in patients with a quantitative β-hCG level lower than 1000.[90-93] Even if no definitive diagnosis can be made, the clinician should be aware that pregnant ED patients with pelvic complaints and a β-hCG level of 1000 mIU/mL or lower have a fourfold *increased* risk for ectopic pregnancy in comparison to those with the same symptoms and a β-hCG level higher than 1000 mIU/mL.[94]

In summary, the "discriminatory zone" provides a basis for *interpreting* the ultrasound image, but not a basis for *deciding whether to perform it.*[89,90,95] Although the percentage of patients below the "discriminatory zone" who will receive a definitive diagnosis by ultrasound is much lower than the percentage in those above the discriminatory zone (25% versus 90%), even a 25% diagnosis rate would seem to merit pursuit for a potentially lethal condition, especially since follow-up for patients whose evaluation is "indeterminate" on their ED visit is time-consuming and resource-intensive.[90,96]

BLOOD CULTURES IN THE ED

Indications

Blood cultures are indicated when the clinical findings suggest an otherwise unidentifiable bacteremic state (Box 67-2).

BOX 67-2 **Summary of Indications for Obtaining Blood Cultures**

PATIENTS WITH FEVER AND ANY OF THE FOLLOWING:

Unexplained alterations in mental status, functional status, or autonomic status in a previously healthy patient between the ages of 5 and 65

No source found and younger than 2 years, older than 65, or immunocompromised

Age younger than 2 months

PATIENTS WITH OR WITHOUT FEVER AND ANY OF THE FOLLOWING:

Rigors

Toxic or "septic" appearance (e.g., unexplained hypotension, altered mental status, shock)

Suspicion of infectious endocarditis

Serious focal infections (e.g., meningitis, septic arthritis, osteomyelitis)

BOX 67-3 **Summary of Arguments for and against the Performance of Outpatient Blood Cultures**

ARGUMENTS *AGAINST* OUTPATIENT BLOOD CULTURES

Low true-positive rates

True positives are rarely clinically significant

False positives are expensive and time-consuming for both the patient and health care system

Unreliability of emergency department follow-up makes positive results a medicolegal liability

ARGUMENTS *FOR* OUTPATIENT BLOOD CULTURES

Permits outpatient evaluation and management of patients with a low probability of disease (especially infectious endocarditis)

Patients: financial, psychological, and nosocomial cost savings from spared admissions

Society: financial and nosocomial cost savings from spared admissions

Allows initiation of antibiotics for possible alternative infectious diagnoses without irrevocable loss of the opportunity for blood cultures

Twenty-five percent of patients with documented bacteremia have periods without fever.[97] In the elderly the proportion is even higher, with 50% of bacteremic patients older than 65 having a temperature between 97.1°F (36.2°C) and 100.9°F (38.3°C) and at least 13% with no documented temperature higher than 99.1°F (37.3°C) at any time.[98-101] In the elderly, increasing age, vomiting, altered mental status, urinary incontinence, presence of a Foley catheter, or greater than 6% band forms is predictive of a positive blood culture.[99,102] The subjective impression of "having fever" in adults is not a reliable indicator of the presence of fever, although the subjective impression of "no fever" is much more likely to be accurate.[103] Prediction models to optimize the use of this costly test have been explored but are cumbersome, add little to educated clinical judgment, and lack widespread validation or acceptance.[104-106] Many studies have shown that blood cultures in patients with uncomplicated pneumonia or pyelonephritis are of very limited clinical value,[107-118] although a recent prospective investigation of patients with upper UTI found that malignancy, an indwelling urinary catheter, and ongoing antimicrobial treatment were clinical conditions that made it significantly more likely that blood cultures would be discordant with urine cultures and that they would reveal clinically important additional information.[119] Blood cultures are obtained during 2.8% of all ED visits in the United States, and in a single recent 3-year period this rate increased by 33%.[120] Since disease prevalence is unlikely to have changed so rapidly, this increase is probably due to changes in practice. These changes have been coincident with regulatory agency–mandated blood cultures in patients being evaluated for pneumonia and have led to calls for more stringent criteria for obtaining blood cultures.

In children, the traditional teaching that blood cultures are indicated for all patients younger than 2 years with fever higher than 38.6°C (>101.5°F) and without an obvious source is being modified by the widespread use of pneumococcal conjugate (PC) and *Haemophilus influenzae* type b (HIB) vaccines.[121,122] In the post-PC and post-HIB vaccine era, the incidence of occult bacteremia in otherwise well-appearing febrile children is probably lower than 1%, thus making the false-positive rate at least four times as high.[121-123] It seems reasonable to withhold blood cultures and empirical antibiotic coverage in otherwise well-appearing febrile children with reliable parents. The risk for bacteremia in a child is positively correlated with the degree of fever, WBC count, and rapidity of onset of the illness. It is inversely proportional to the patient's age.[124-127] In infants younger than 2 months with temperatures higher than 38°C (>100.5°F), some authorities would recommend blood cultures regardless of the presence or absence of a source, although this approach is subject to modification by experienced clinicians based on the patient's age and clinical setting. A child with a normal temperature in the ED and a history from the parents of a tactile fever needs to be approached in the same way as a patient with fever documented on physical examination. Parents' tactile impression of fever is reliable, and bacteremic children, like adults, have intermittent fever, with up to 50% afebrile rates in children with demonstrated bacteremia.[128,129]

The Controversy Regarding "Outpatient Blood Cultures"

There is a long-standing debate regarding the utility of outpatient blood cultures (i.e., blood cultures on patients who are discharged from the ED pending results). Arguments for and against outpatient blood cultures are summarized in Box 67-3. Opponents cite medicolegal issues, problems with follow-up, high contamination rates, low rates of positive cultures, and even lower rates of frequency in patients in whom therapy is changed because of culture results.[130-133] Proponents also cite medicolegal concerns, positive rates similar to those seen with inpatient blood cultures, cost savings, and the benefit of diagnosing significant, yet subtle bacteremic states (such as endocarditis).[134,135] They also point out that the high false-positive rates seen in many ED series should be an indictment of poor technique, not of the test itself.

On the basis of current data, it seems fiscally extravagant to admit all patients in whom a bacteremic state is possible and injudicious to deny blood cultures solely on the basis of a patient not appearing "toxic enough" to warrant admission. Societal and economic pressures to avoid hospital admission buttress these clinical considerations. Outpatient blood cultures, with due attention to collection technique, patient selection, and arrangements for follow-up, have a place in emergency practice. This approach is reflected by the fact that fully half of ED blood cultures are obtained on patients who are not admitted to the hospital.[120]

Technique for Obtaining Blood for Culture

Studies have demonstrated sources of contamination at every stage of the process of performing and processing blood cultures. In addition to obvious sources of contamination from the patient's and phlebotomist's skin, antiseptic agents and gloves have been implicated.[136,137] Some authorities have argued that the primary source of contamination is in the laboratory processing of specimens.[138] The consensus is that the most common source of contamination is the process of phlebotomy and inoculation of blood culture bottles.[139] Obviously, this is the single step over which emergency clinicians have control, either directly or via protocols of technique for blood culture phlebotomy. Contamination rates are typically between 1.5% and 3%,[121,140,141] although many ED series show much higher rates.[132,142]

A high degree of sensitivity is required for blood cultures. Many significant bacteremic illnesses have been documented with as little as 1 CFU/10 mL of blood.[143,144] In a cadaver study, human skin has been shown to have a bacterial concentration of between 10^3 and 10^6 CFUs/mL on the forearm and groin, respectively.[145] Designed to detect vanishingly low concentrations of bacteria, the test is clearly susceptible to false-positive results (impaired specificity) when blood must necessarily be obtained by passing a needle through the skin. Eighty percent of the skin flora is transient, superficial, and removable; 20% inhabit the sebaceous ducts and hair follicles and cannot be removed without destroying the skin.[145,146] The former group consists of predominantly gram-positive and gram-negative aerobes and is the target of skin disinfectants.

The primary agents for skin disinfection are iodine compounds, alcohols, chlorhexidine, and hexachlorophene. Iodine solution remains a gold standard and kills bacteria, fungi, protozoa, and viruses but has been replaced in many institutions because of concern about skin burns and allergic reactions. Reports of the former were probably due to the use of 7% solution. The risk for a burn or an allergic reaction is thought to be negligible with the currently available 2% preparation.[139] The most effective cleansing agent is tincture of iodine, which is a mixture of 2% iodine solution and 70% alcohol.[147,148] Povidone-iodine 10% solution (Betadine) has a much lower free iodine concentration than iodine solution and is therefore less potent. Iodine is superior to hexachlorophene and chlorhexidine in killing gram-negative bacteria. Iodine, like other antiseptic agents, is inhibited by the presence of organic matter and thus requires thorough skin cleansing before the application of any skin disinfectant.

Ethyl or isopropyl alcohol should be used in a 60% to 80% solution. Alcohol prep pads, which generally contain 70%

isopropanol, have solved traditional concerns regarding evaporation of alcohol from cotton balls stored in jars. Alcohol is a less powerful germicide than iodine in vitro and kills only 90% of surface bacteria after a full 2 minutes with reapplication to prevent drying.[149] Alcohol foam applicators can avoid premature drying. Alcohol is inactive against fungi, spores, and viruses, but in vivo studies of blood culture contamination rates have shown it to compare favorably with iodine.[147,150] Because iodine solution is often not available and iodophor solutions are less potent, alcohol still has an important place in skin antisepsis. In addition, alcohol is an excellent solvent, so alcohol pads may assist in skin preparation by removing dirt- and microbe-laden skin oils before the application of iodine compounds.

Chlorhexidine (Hibiclens) and hexachlorophene (pHisoHex) are antiseptics that are more effective against gram-positive than gram-negative bacteria. Both agents are absorbed intradermally, thereby offering prolonged antimicrobial activity, which is the basis of their popularity as surgical scrub and operative site preparations. This also makes them preferable agents when indwelling lines, especially central lines, are being placed.[151] For routine blood culture phlebotomy, they are not as effective as alcohol and iodine combinations, although they are superior to povidone-iodine solution.[141] Most studies show chlorhexidine to be more potent than hexachlorophene, and it has not been associated with induction of seizures in infants.

Box 67-4 presents a skin preparation protocol. Optimal results seem to be obtained with alcohol-iodine mixtures.[145,148,152,153] The most important concept in skin disinfection is that bacteria do not die at the instant of contact with disinfectant agents. Iodine (2%), which is twice as potent as

---

BOX 67-4 Skin Preparation and Technique for Drawing Blood for Culture

Cleanse the skin with alcohol swabs three times or until the swabs appear entirely free of surface dirt.

Allow to dry.

Apply 10% povidone-iodine or (preferably) 2% iodine solution or (ideally) 2% tincture of iodine in 70% alcohol three times in centrifugal circles from the anticipated site of venipuncture.

After the third swab, allow to dry for at least 60 seconds. During this period:
- Remove the covers and sterilize the rubber stoppers of blood culture bottles with iodine, alcohol, or both.
- Lay out sterile gloves.
- Use a paper glove wrapper as a sterile field for the needle and syringe (not necessary if using a Vacutainer system).

Wipe off dry iodine at the venipuncture site with alcohol. Substitute chlorhexidine if placing an indwelling catheter.

Obtain at least 20 mL of blood to place in two bottles.
- If short, use at least 10 mL for an *aerobic* bottle.
- If more than 20 mL, use additional *aerobic* bottles. Place no more than 10 mL of blood per bottle.

Inoculate bottles without changing needles between bottles.

However many bottles are filled, this is *one* "set" of blood cultures. Another "set" *cannot* be obtained from this site, regardless of how many bottles are filled.

10% povidone-iodine, requires at least 90 seconds in contact with the skin to kill 90% of surface bacteria.[149] In many ED patients it will be necessary to use alcohol prep pads to remove gross dirt and debris from phlebotomy sites before initiating the steps of formal skin preparation.

Special Considerations in Obtaining Blood for Culture

"Changing the Needle" after Phlebotomy
In considering this issue it is important to emphasize the distinction between *needle changing* and *needle recapping*.[154] The latter is a well-established risk to health care workers. It contravenes standard recommendations for universal precautions and *should not be performed*. Needle replacement using the standard needle removal device on "sharps" containers is an unquantified risk, but clearly much less dangerous than recapping.

Based on little scientific data it was long considered essential to change the phlebotomy needle before inoculating blood culture bottles. With increasing awareness of the risks associated with needlestick injuries, this practice has come under scrutiny. Studies generally show trends toward lower contamination rates with needle change, but without reaching statistical significance.[155-157] Thus, not changing needles before inoculation of blood culture bottles is acceptable practice for routinely obtaining blood for culture. In situations in which the results of blood cultures are of paramount importance (e.g., suspected infectious endocarditis, where empirical antibiotics are to be started immediately), needles can be changed before inoculation of culture bottles (without recapping).

Special Access Sites
Most studies show that newly placed intravenous (IV) catheters are an acceptable source of blood specimens for culture, provided that the usual measures are taken in skin preparation.[140,157] Chronically placed lines either trend toward or show statistically significant increases in contamination rates.[158-161] An exception can be made for carefully tended central venous access ports in cancer patients. These cultures may have increased sensitivity in identifying bacteremia, possibly because of the fact that the catheters themselves are often a source of bacteremia in these patients.[162]

Heel Stick in Neonates
This technique resulted in recovery rates of bacteria equivalent to those with phlebotomy in two studies.[163,164] Since approximately 25% of bacteremic infants have fewer than 5 CFUs/mL of blood, this proportion (25%) will be missed if less than 0.2 mL is obtained for culture. For this reason, heel stick should be considered a source of last resort for blood culture.

Intraosseous Specimens
This technique may also be used when phlebotomy is impossible.[165]

Timing of Blood Cultures
In most circumstances the timing of blood cultures is moot in the ED. Patients are sick enough to warrant the initiation of empirical antibiotics or are well enough for discharge, so two or more sets of blood need to be drawn immediately. The timing of blood cultures might become a consideration in a patient requiring admission but in whom the diagnosis of bacteremia is in doubt such that empirical antibiotic therapy is withheld. Contrary to medical lore, true-positive blood cultures are more likely if blood is drawn in the 12 hours *before* a fever spike.[166,167] Furthermore, except for infectious endocarditis, most clinically significant bacteremia is thought to be intermittent, so multiple sets of specimens obtained at one time for culture would heighten the risk for missing the period of bacteremia.[168] For patients admitted to the hospital with the tentative diagnosis of sepsis, it is theoretically advantageous to draw the three sets of blood for culture over the first 12 to 24 hours of admission.[169] If immediate administration of antibiotics is indicated, the two or three sets of blood for culture should be obtained before initiation of antibiotic therapy.

Blood Culture Volumes

Volumes in Adults
A large number of studies almost uniformly demonstrate that the sensitivity of blood cultures is directly related to the volume of blood cultured.[170-175] In a representative study, Ilstrup and Washington showed that 20 mL and 30 mL of blood yielded, respectively, 38% and 62% more true-positive results than 10 mL did.[172] Mermel and Maki showed that each additional milliliter of blood yields an average of 3% more true-positive results.[175] This finding is also consistent with the fact that 40% of adults with bacteremia have less than 1 CFU/mL of blood and that 20% have less than 1 CFU/10 mL.[176] Alternatively expressed, if 10 mL of blood is obtained for culture, 20% of patients with continuous bacteremia will be missed. Since most bacteremia is intermittent and endogenous factors in blood will cause some inhibition of bacterial growth even with modern lysis and filtration centrifugation techniques, the false-negative rate in clinical practice will always be significantly higher. On purely mathematical grounds, 10 mL per set of blood cultures is a bare minimum for culture. In adults, most authorities recommend at least 30 mL of blood per culture site or set.[177-179] To ensure dilution of the blood's antibacterial properties (e.g., immunoglobulins, complement, WBCs), culture bottles should contain a concentration of blood of less than 1 part blood to 10 parts medium.[179] If 30 mL of blood is obtained from one site, it should be divided equally into three of the usual 100-mL broth bottles.

Volumes in Children
A blood volume of 30 mL from a 70-kg adult is equivalent to 0.5 mL of blood from a 3.5-kg neonate. Fortunately (for the utility of blood cultures), levels of bacteremia are typically 10-fold higher in neonates than in adults.[180] The sicker the child, the greater the likelihood of a high level of bacteremia.[180,181] As the immune system matures during infancy, levels of bacteremia might be expected to fall toward those seen in adults, so small culture volumes are at increased risk for false-negative results.[182-184] As a rule of thumb, a similar volume of blood with respect to body mass should be drawn from children as is drawn from adults: approximately 1 mL/2.5 kg, or *4 mL blood per 10-kg body mass*.[185,186]

Figure 67-5 These two blood culture bottles (anaerobic and aerobic) represent a *single set* of blood cultures, provided that they are filled with a sample from a single site. Two or more sets of blood culture bottles (each obtained from a different site) represent a *series* of cultures.

TABLE 67-6 Numbers of Blood Culture Sets to Be Obtained in Various Clinical Situations in Adults

NUMBER OF SETS (MINIMUM)	CLINICAL CONTEXT
Two sets	The cause is likely to easily be distinguished from contaminants and the pretest probability of bacteremia is low to moderate
Three sets	Skin contaminants are possible causes of the infectious process, the pretest probability of bacteremia is high, or infectious endocarditis is a consideration, but with a low to moderate pretest probability
Four sets	Infectious endocarditis AND either a moderate to a high pretest probability or the patient has recently been taking antibiotics

How Many Sets of Blood Cultures Are Needed?

A set of blood cultures is the sample obtained from a single site. A 1-mL specimen from a neonate placed in an aerobic bottle and a 30 mL specimen from an adult divided between fungal, aerobic, and anaerobic bottles are both a *single set* of blood cultures (Fig. 67-5). Two or more sets of blood cultures make up a *series*.[169] The information derived from the blood culture sets is pooled in such a way to make both the sensitivity and specificity of the series greater than that of the component sets. Sensitivity is enhanced because as discussed earlier, an individual set is typically not more than 80% sensitive.[187] Specificity is improved for microbes that can act as both pathogens and contaminants by determining whether they appear in all sets (pathogen) or in only some (more likely a contaminant).

Although this conceptual process is applied to all blood culture series, the focus of inquiry depends on the infectious process being ruled in or out. For example, in an elderly patient with sepsis and a chronic indwelling Foley catheter, it is extremely unlikely that the causative organism is a typical skin contaminant. The usual causes of "false-positive" blood cultures will therefore be easily recognized, thus lowering the false-positive rate for the series and yielding a test with intrinsically higher specificity. At the same time, with the typical pathogens in this clinical context being nonfastidious organisms, sensitivity is typically around 99% with two sets consisting of 20 mL of blood per set.[178] Conversely, in a patient with a prosthetic heart valve, fever, and signs of septic emboli, many probable pathogens are also skin contaminants, thereby lowering the specificity of each individual blood culture set. Thus, at least two sets of cultures must be *positive* with such organisms before the overall test (i.e., the *series*) is considered positive. At the same time, this clinical picture makes the pretest probability of disease very high (diminishing the negative predictive value of a negative set), so an extremely sensitive overall test (i.e., series) will be needed to adequately rule out disease. In this setting, most authorities would recommend four sets of blood culture bottles, with good volumes in each.[168,187] Except in infants, single sets of blood for culture are of insufficient sensitivity or specificity to be of any utility and should not be drawn.[167,168,187-189] The recommended numbers of sets of blood cultures as they relate to the pretest probability of disease and causative organism are summarized in Table 67-6.

Aerobic versus Anaerobic (versus Other) Bottles

Anaerobic infections tend to occur in poorly perfused tissues or locations and frequently evolve into abscesses. Both characteristics mean that these infections tend to be isolated from the bloodstream, thereby decreasing the likelihood of bacteremia and detection by blood culture. For these reasons it is not surprising that anaerobic isolates account for 0.5% to 12% of positive blood cultures.[168,190-192] Blood cultures in general have a typical true-positive rate of about 5%; with 5% or less of positive blood cultures being anaerobic, more than 400 patients need to have a complete series of blood drawn for culture to detect one case of anaerobic bacteremia.[193-197] If more than 50% of anaerobic infections are clinically evident before culture, at least 800 blood culture series are needed to generate a single anaerobic result that would alter clinical management. Anaerobic cultures may also have the unintended consequence of compromising the sensitivity of aerobic cultures in situations in which less than the ideal 20 mL of blood is drawn for a blood culture set.[175,192] Allocation of blood to anaerobic bottles will also diminish the likelihood of detecting fungal infections, which are increasingly common in the rising population of immunocompromised patients.[198] In addition to these pathophysiologic considerations, there was a widely reported decrease in the positive anaerobic blood culture rate in the 1980s and 1990s, although some authors have recently suggested a resurgence of anaerobic bacteremia rates.[190-192,194,196,199] At the current time, the arguments for selective use of anaerobic blood cultures are compelling, especially if working in an institution where there is a low rate of anaerobic bacteremia.

TABLE 67-7 Blood Culture Types to Be Used in Various Clinical Settings

CLINICAL SITUATION	BOTTLES TO BE OBTAINED
Children <12 yr	Aerobic bottles only unless the patient has peritonitis or fasciitis (in which case draw blood for standard aerobic and anaerobic culture)
Adults and children >12 yr	Anaerobic infection unlikely, immunocompetent patient: aerobic bottles only Anaerobic infection unlikely, immunocompromised patient: aerobic bottle, one bottle for fungal culture (usually effective in aerobic bottles; consult the laboratory for guidance) Possibility of anaerobic infection: one aerobic and one anaerobic bottle per set

BOX 67-5 Clinical Settings at Higher Risk for Anaerobic Bacteremia

INFECTIOUS FOCI

Abdominal or pelvic infections
Soft tissue or wound infections (e.g., myofasciitis)
Sepsis with decubitus ulcers or necrotic tissue
Aspiration pneumonia
Odontogenic head and neck infections

PREDISPOSING CLINICAL FEATURES

Malignancy
Immunosuppressive medications
Recent abdominal or pelvic surgery
Diabetes

BOX 67-6 Features Suggestive of Contaminant ("False-Positive") Blood Culture Results

Coagulase-negative staphylococci (*Staphylococcus epidermidis*) and *Staphylococcus viridans* in a single bottle in patients not suspected of having infectious endocarditis and without chronic indwelling intravenous access catheters are usually contaminants.

Corynebacteria (preciously known as "diphtheroids"), *Propionibacterium acne*, and *Bacillus* species are usually contaminants but can be pathogenic in the immunocompromised.

Multiple organisms in a series suggest contamination.

Species that grow after prolonged culture have a higher likelihood of being contaminants. Conversely, early-growing bacteria have a much higher likelihood of being pathogens.

The patient's symptoms have resolved or are inconsistent with sepsis (beware with infectious endocarditis, which can have an indolent course).

A primary source (e.g., sputum or urine) has a different pathogen isolated.

Based on a review of this topic, Table 67-7 suggests a possible approach to the allocation of blood specimens to various blood culture media after phlebotomy.[198-202] Clinical features that place a patient at high risk for anaerobic bacteremia are listed in Box 67-5.

Identifying Contaminants

The emergency clinician may receive calls from the laboratory about the results of positive blood cultures obtained on previous shifts. These may be "true positives" as a result of true contamination or may be caused by the intermittent bacteremia that occurs in normal, healthy people. This situation has been complicated by the increasingly common identification of *Staphylococcus epidermidis*, *Streptococcus viridans*, and fungi as real pathogens in blood culture series.[203-206] The expense associated with false-positive blood cultures has been estimated to be $900 per episode for discharged patients and more than $5000 per episode for inpatients. These costs emphasize the importance of good technique in obtaining blood for culture.[207,208] Distinguishing contaminants from clinically significant bacteremia is based on both microbiologic information and the patient's clinical condition. Features of false-positive blood culture results are listed in Box 67-6.[178,187,209] It would probably be prudent to contact discharged patients with positive blood cultures, even when contamination is suspected on a microbiologic basis, to ensure that their condition is improving.

Fungal Cultures

Generally, fungi are difficult to isolate in blood cultures, and it may take 4 to 6 weeks to obtain a positive yield. If fungemia is suspected, it is best to discuss culture media and technique with the laboratory before blood is taken for culture. Cultures of bone marrow are occasionally positive for mycoses when blood cultures are negative.

PRINCIPLES AND PITFALLS IN PHLEBOTOMY FOR BLOOD TESTING

A number of blood tests are ordered as a part of emergency practice, but by far the most common are the complete blood count (CBC) and serum chemistries. Many medications, substances, and diseases have been identified as causes of hematologic abnormalities besides the familiar categories of infectious, inflammatory, stress-related, neoplastic, and hematopoietic processes. These include antibiotics (especially sulfonamides), antineoplastic and therapeutic drugs, immunosuppressives, and toxins (mercury and black widow spider envenomation causing leukocytosis and arsenicals causing leukopenia). There are also substances and disease processes that cause purely artifactual errors by interfering with the equipment or procedures used to perform the tests. Examples include in vivo and in vitro hemolysis, cellular clumping, and markedly elevated platelet, leukocyte, or triglyceride levels, all of which can perturb proper functioning of the machinery used to perform blood assays. The less common causes of

TABLE 67-8 Artifactual Causes of False Values of the CBC*

	ARTIFACTUAL INCREASE	ARTIFACTUAL DECREASE
White blood cell count	Nucleated red blood cells	Multiple myeloma and other monoclonal gammopathies
Hemoglobin and hematocrit	Severe leukocytosis (>30,000), hyperlipemic serum, giant platelets, cryoproteins	Microcytic anemia, in vitro hemolysis

CBC, complete blood count.
*Improper collection techniques are the most common cause of errors in all categories.

Figure 67-6 Phlebotomy using a butterfly needle and Vacutainer system.

Figure 67-7 Phlebotomy via a freshly placed intravenous catheter and Vacutainer system.

laboratory abnormalities (both pathophysiologic and artifactual) are legion. It is necessary for most clinicians, when encountering a confirmed laboratory abnormality, to resort to standard reference texts or online sources to review potential causes or sources of error. Some of the analytical causes of false laboratory values on the CBC are listed in (Table 67-8).

Before checking for obscure or uncommon causes of laboratory abnormalities, one should bear in mind that the most common source of error in laboratory blood tests is in the "preanalytical phase."[210-213] This is the part of the laboratory process that actively involves the practicing clinician. Preanalytical errors have been broken down into problems with specimen loss and handling, clotting, hemolysis, inadequate volume, and patient identity.[212] In one series, more than 90% of these errors related to specimen collection.[214] These key components and their most common pitfalls are as follows:

1. **Preparation of the site.** The importance of aseptic technique in the preparation of a site to draw blood for culture has been discussed. For hematologic and serum analysis, enough time should be allowed for drying of the alcohol since trace amounts can cause hemolysis. Povidone-iodine can cause errors in several chemistry assays. When used, it should be cleaned off with alcohol, as described in the section on blood cultures.
2. **Venous occlusion.** Both intracellular and chemical changes start occurring in blood as soon as a tourniquet is applied, not—as is often thought—only after it has passed through a needle into a specimen container. Serum potassium levels may increase by 6% in a vessel that has been occluded for only 3 minutes.[213] Venous access sites, if visually identifiable, should be prepared before placement of a tourniquet. After tourniquet application, phlebotomy and sample acquisition should proceed as rapidly as possible, ideally within 30 seconds.[215] Pumping the fist should be avoided if possible because it increases serum concentrations of potassium, lactate, and phosphate.[213]
3. **Routine phlebotomy.** Smaller-gauge needles and higher suction pressure are associated with hemolysis. Overexuberant application of suction on a syringe is doubly counterproductive because in addition to causing hemolysis, the needle is likely to be occluded by the wall of the vein. This increases the likelihood of unsuccessful phlebotomy and

iatrogenic injury to the patient. When applying negative or positive pressure to a syringe, a given amount of force on the plunger causes *higher* pressure within the chamber of a *smaller*-diameter syringe (pressure is proportional to $1/radius^2$). Blood drawn into either a standard Vacutainer or a syringe via a butterfly needle and tubing causes similar hemolysis rates (Fig. 67-6).[215] If a phlebotomy site is tenuous, specimens are obtained in order of clinical priority. In most cases, tubes should be filled in the following order to avoid cross-contamination of chemicals: blood cultures, red, blue, speckled red, green, lavender, gray.[213] Consistent with experience, the perception of difficult access or phlebotomy is associated with higher hemolysis rates.[216,217]

4. **Phlebotomy through a freshly placed IV catheter.** Routine phlebotomy typically causes a hemolysis rate of less than 2%.[212] Reported hemolysis rates in ED patients are often 7% to 15%.[217-219] This may be due to any or all of the reasons considered here, but one contributing factor is the number of blood specimens drawn in the ED through a catheter being placed for therapeutic use (Fig. 67-7). Several studies have shown that this arrangement significantly increases rates of hemolysis.[217,219,220] The popularity of this technique in emergency care is most probably due to limitations of personnel and temporal resources and an

---

Hemoglobin	Potassium	Glucose
Hematocrit	Bicarbonate	Creatine phosphokinase
Sodium	Chloride	Troponin I

---

attempt to enhance patient comfort by avoiding an extra needlestick. Since tourniquet times are probably longer with catheter placement than with simple phlebotomy, it is likely that this contributes to hemolysis, although it has never been experimentally verified. Perceived ease of blood aspiration, larger-bore catheters, and small aliquots drawn through the catheter are associated with lower rates of hemolysis.[219,220] Laboratory results of specimens obtained in this manner are accurate within clinically acceptable margins of error.

5. **Phlebotomy through an established IV catheter.** An established IV line appears to be a reliable source of blood for analysis, although success rates are lower and hemolysis rates are higher than for phlebotomy from a fresh site.[221,222] Box 67-7 lists common blood tests that are accurate when drawn through an established IV line.[222,223] As with the use of a freshly placed catheter, results are accurate within clinical tolerances.[221,224] If fluids are being administered through the catheter, it should be turned off for at least 3 minutes *before* the application of a tourniquet for phlebotomy. A typical 18-gauge 30-mm-long plastic IV catheter without a heparin well has a volume of 0.07 mL. The heparin well adds a volume of 0.05 mL to make a combined volume of 0.12 mL. Thus, when using a syringe directly attached to the heparin well (IV tubing detached), just 1 mL of aspirated fluid should have replaced the entire volume of the heparin well at least six times. Most studies have discarded at least three times that volume. Some have suggested a "push-pull" technique (aspirating a small volume into the syringe and reinjecting it before drawing a final 3 mL for discarding) to minimize the likelihood of small sequestered pockets of IV fluid in the heparin well.[225] Use of the standard distal port of the IV tubing (usually 25 cm from the end) is not recommended. The IV tubing has a volume (combined with the heparin well and catheter) of about 1.6 mL, thus making it necessary to discard large volumes of blood, in addition to the risk of contamination from IV fluids entrained in the specimen from the main IV line during aspiration through the port.

6. **Disposition of the specimen after phlebotomy.** If blood has been drawn into a syringe, it should be promptly decanted into the appropriate containers for the laboratory. If it has already started to clot, it should not be forced since this can cause hemolysis of the specimen. Since cells and platelets are fragile, specimens requiring agitation (all except red and speckled red-topped tubes) should be *rocked gently, not shaken.* If specimens are sent to the laboratory in pneumatic tubes, they should be surrounded by shock-absorbing material. Artifactual increases in measured HCO_3^- occur fairly rapidly at room temperature.[221] Progressive hemolysis of blood occurs with prolonged standing, and it is likely that specimens are of little utility after more than 2 to 3 hours of typical ED storage conditions.

One study showed that unrefrigerated, *nonagitated* samples were reliable for up to 8 hours.[226]

BEDSIDE TESTS FOR GI HEMORRHAGE

Detection of Blood in Stool

Bedside fecal blood tests make use of the peroxidase-like activity of Hb. The test card is impregnated with a dye that exhibits a blue color reaction when oxidized. The developer contains 5% hydrogen peroxide and 75% alcohol. The original test used guaiac, but current tests use more sensitive and more reliable quinolone compounds. The addition of hydrogen peroxide developer solution will oxidize the dye to a blue color in the presence of a peroxidase (e.g., Hb).

Testing for occult blood in stool is associated with false-positive and false-negative results, but in its primary role in emergency medical practice the test is usually reliable in detecting significant acute gastrointestinal (GI) hemorrhage (Fig. 67-8).[39] Low pH, heat, dry stools, reducing substances (including antioxidants such as vitamin C), and antacids can cause false-negative findings.[227-229] Slow bleeding in the upper GI tract, during which heme can be converted (denatured) to porphyrin during transit through the gut, may not be identified by stool testing. False-positive results have been attributed to the ingestion of partly cooked or large quantities of meat (dietary sources of myoglobin and Hb) and peroxidase-rich food.[229,230] Most vegetables contain peroxidase, including (in decreasing order) broccoli, turnips, cantaloupe, red radishes, horseradish, cauliflower, parsnips, Jerusalem artichokes, bean sprouts, beans, lemon rind, mushrooms, parsley, and zucchini.[230] A simple in vivo study convincingly called into question the possibility of peroxidase passing through the stomach without being denatured.[231] False-positive test results can also be caused by the presence of povidone-iodine solution at concentrations of less than 0.1% (a 1% dilution of the 10% solutions commonly available at the bedside), but they are uncommon. A positive test should be considered evidence of the presence of blood until proved otherwise. Routine iron supplementation does cause black stool but does *not* a cause a positive Hemoccult test result despite early in vitro studies to the contrary.[232,233]

Normal GI blood loss is limited to less than 2.5 mL/day, which translates to less than 2 mg of Hb per gram of stool (0.2% by weight).[234] The sensitivity of the Hemoccult test varies both with the concentration of Hb present in stool and with the extent of Hb exposure to the proteolytic effects of the digestive tract. The Hemoccult test is 37% sensitive to stool containing 2.5 mg Hb/g of stool but 95% sensitive when the concentration is 20 mg Hb/g of stool, thus indicating that low to moderate levels of blood may be missed.[38] The test is much more likely to detect lower GI hemorrhage than an identical rate of upper GI bleeding because of the 100-fold diminution in the peroxidase activity of blood during

Figure 67-8 A, Hemoccult testing (see text). Test cards contain guaiac resin; the developer contains hydrogen peroxide (5%) and ethyl alcohol (75%). The test is based on the oxidation of guaiac by peroxide in the presence of a hemoglobin catalyst to produce a blue quinolone compound. *Caveats of testing*: Two areas of stool can be tested; use the positive and negative controls; allow the specimen to dry (fix) for 2 minutes, and read within 60 seconds; *any blue color is a positive test*. Positive tests may be due to any source of gastrointestinal bleeding, such as mucosal lesions or drug-induced injury (aspirin, warfarin, heparin, nonsteroidal antiinflammatory drugs). Use of acetaminophen does not alter the results. *False-negative tests* may result from large doses of antioxidants, such as vitamin C (pills, citric juices). **B,** Although Hemoccult will also detect gastric blood, use the Gastroccult card/developer to test gastric contents. **C,** Iron- and bismuth-containing products (such as Pepto-Bismol or Kaopectate) cause a black stool but not a reaction on the Hemoccult test. Do not attribute a positive test for blood in stool to iron therapy.

transition through the GI tract.[71] Impaired detection of Hb may also occur as a result of dilution because of diarrheal illness.[38,39,235] Recent regulatory attempts in the United States to improve quality control in bedside occult blood testing seem to have had the unintended consequence of discouraging digital rectal examination in patients for whom they are indicated.[236,237] In the event of a trace positive Hemoccult test that is not the source of an emergency illness, notification of the patient and advice regarding further outpatient evaluation should not be overlooked.[228]

Method

Smear the stool specimen onto the reagent area on the card and add a drop of developer. Because the reaction must occur in an aqueous medium, add a drop of water to very dry specimens and allow it to moisten the specimen before adding the developer. Adding water increases the false-positive rate.[228,229] Formation of a blue color on the paper anywhere around or under the specimen within 60 seconds should be considered a positive result.

Testing for Gastric Blood

Heme tests designed for use on stool specimens can be unreliable when applied to gastric juices, with increasing inaccuracies being reported as the pH decreases.[238,239] Although a

positive test of gastric contents with a fecal Hemoccult card is likely to be accurate, a negative result with the fecal Hemoccult card does not rule out the presence of blood. The Gastroccult card uses a modified guaiac developer containing buffers to neutralize gastric acid, thereby facilitating accurate detection of Hb. The test works on the same basis as the fecal guaiac test in that it uses the properties of Hb as a peroxidase. In product testing, the Gastroccult card was 100% sensitive in detecting specimens with greater than 500 ppm of blood by volume, equivalent to 0.05% or 0.25 mL of blood in 500 mL of gastric contents.

Method

Apply a drop of gastric aspirate onto the test area and two drops of developer onto the sample. Look for the formation of a blue color within 1 minute. Do *not* use fecal blood test developer. In a specimen that is already a bilious green, the test is considered positive only if new *blue* color is formed. The Gastroccult card also contains a pH testing strip located close to the occult blood testing area, which might be useful in testing emesis after an acidic or alkaline ingestion. Inaccurate results might be anticipated in the presence of the same substances that can confound the Hemoccult test: meats, peroxidase-rich foods, and reducing substances such as ascorbic acid. The accuracy of Gastroccult should not be affected by the presence of cimetidine or sucralfate.

Figure 67-9 Bedside glucose meters analyze capillary blood samples and are generally an excellent substitute for venous blood testing. Errors may occur in patients with poor tissue perfusion or in cases of extreme hypoglycemia or hyperglycemia. Additional errors may be due to the operator, including improper calibration, dirty meters, and improper storage of test strips.

BLOOD GLUCOSE METERS

Bedside testing of capillary blood for glucose levels is a common procedure performed in the ED and is generally an excellent substitute for venous blood testing. A variety of meters are available and they are reasonably accurate (±10%) when a small drop of blood is electronically analyzed (Fig. 67-9). In patients with poor tissue perfusion, the accuracy of determining hypoglycemia is less precise and may vary up to about 5% from venous blood. In the setting of hypoperfusion, bedside measurement of whole blood is preferable. Bedside testing is also less accurate in patients with extreme hypoglycemia or hyperglycemia, but readings are sufficiently accurate to alert the clinician to very high or very low glucose levels. Fingertip capillary blood is the preferred specimen for bedside glucose meter testing. Blood from alternative sites, such as the skin of the forearm, may give slightly lower results than those taken at the fingertips since they may sample venous blood rather than capillary blood. When blood glucose concentrations are rising rapidly or falling rapidly (such as a hypoglycemic response secondary to rapidly acting insulin), blood glucose results from alternative sites may yield significantly delayed results (up to 30 minutes) when compared with finger stick readings, which are generally accurate at all time points.

Older glucose meters reported whole blood glucose values, which made it difficult to compare finger stick results with those from venous blood testing by the laboratory, which measures plasma glucose. Plasma glucose levels are 10% to 15% higher than whole blood glucose levels. The majority of glucose meters now available provide plasma-equivalent values rather than whole blood glucose values, so glucose meters and the results from venous blood analyzed in hospital laboratories should be comparable.

Most errors in bedside glucose testing are, however, due to operator error, including improper calibration, dirty meters, and improperly stored test strips. Meters should be calibrated frequently to ensure quality readings. Glucose strips have batch-to-batch variation. A common error in testing is due to leaving the lid off glucose strips for prolonged periods since inaccuracies on test strips can result from exposure to heat, moisture, and humidity.

DIAGNOSTIC AND THERAPEUTIC TOXICOLOGIC BEDSIDE PROCEDURES

Management of patients with altered mental status can be challenging, especially if the clinician suspects a drug overdose or poisoning. These patients often have no available history or provide an inaccurate history. Clinicians must rely heavily on the findings on physical examination and other sources of information to diagnose or confirm their clinical suspicion of poisoning or overdose. The hospital toxicology laboratory can be valuable in selected cases. Limited screening tests for commonly ingested drugs are available, and ascertaining levels of specific drugs (e.g., acetaminophen, lithium, digoxin, phenytoin) can help guide management. However, hospital laboratories are not equipped to perform timely analytical procedures for the thousands of possible drugs or toxins. In fact, the screening panels for drugs of abuse that most hospitals use have been shown to rarely influence medical management of adult ED patients. Conversely, use of these drug screens in selected pediatric patients may have more of an impact on medical management.

Diagnostic bedside testing for specific poisons or toxins has the advantage of being cost-effective and timely. When applied appropriately, certain bedside tests provide immediate information to the clinician and can significantly influence medical management in a timely manner. Unfortunately, with establishment of the Clinical Laboratory Improvement Amendments of 1988 (CLIA), bedside laboratory testing has undergone stricter oversight. This federal regulation has jurisdiction on any laboratory tests performed on humans and has added a layer of complexity to bedside testing. Tests that are not performed on humans, such as the Meixner test or mothball testing, are not covered by the CLIA act. This section discusses bedside diagnostic and therapeutic toxicologic procedures.

Noninvasive Diagnostic Procedures

Amatoxin: Meixner Test

Ingestion of several types of mushrooms (e.g., *Amanita phalloides*) can be fatal. The most poisonous of these mushrooms contain amatoxins. Patients who have ingested amatoxins often complain of GI symptoms consisting of nausea, vomiting, diarrhea, and abdominal cramping beginning 6 to 8 hours after ingestion. They often bring in specimens of the mushrooms chopped, crushed, cooked, or mixed with stool or gastric contents. Standard hospital laboratories cannot confirm or exclude the diagnosis of amatoxin poisoning; therefore, treatment decisions are based on clinical grounds.

A simple colorimetric test for detecting amatoxins (the Meixner test) has been developed that can be used on gastric

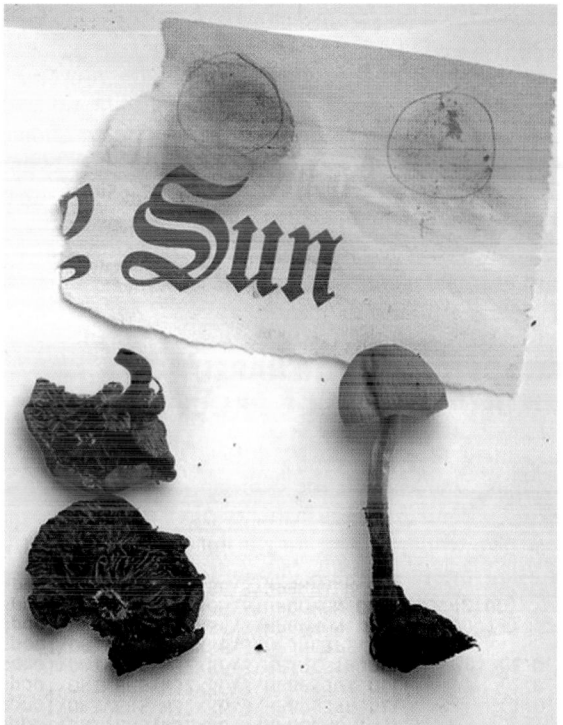

Figure 67-10 The Meixner test is a crude assay for amatoxins. Place portions of the unknown dried mushroom on low-grade newsprint and add 10-N hydrochloric acid. The dried-up mushroom (*left*) is *Galerina marginata*, which yields a blue reaction (positive = probably deadly poisonous); the little brown mushroom (*right*) does not (negative = toxicity uncertain). This test is the only one readily available but has varying accuracy and depends on the paper being used (regular newsprint is shown here). (*Courtesy of Kathie T. Hodge and Kent Loeffler [photographer], Cornell University. Available at* http://blog.mycology.cornell.edu.)

contents, stool, or actual mushroom samples. The basis of this test is the acid-catalyzed color reaction of amatoxins with lignin, a complex organic compound found in wood pulp (Fig. 67-10). Cheaper grades of paper (e.g., newsprint or the whiter pages of a telephone book) contain high amounts of lignin. Although there have been no extensive reports of in vivo studies, in vitro tests have shown this method to be somewhat sensitive and relatively specific for amatoxins, but it should be considered an *adjunctive test only*. Psilocybin-containing mushrooms can cause false-positive results for amatoxin.[240]

The procedure for the qualitative detection of amatoxin consists of squeezing a drop of liquid from a fresh mushroom sample or squashing a piece of fresh mushroom onto a piece of newspaper. If stool or gastric samples are the only specimens available, mix the sample with reagent-grade methanol (99.8%) to extract the amatoxin. If the samples are mixed with methanol, centrifuge and filter them. Then place a drop of the liquid extract on newspaper. Gently air-dry all specimens at room temperature and avoid direct sunlight. Add two to three drops of concentrated hydrochloric acid (37%) to the dried specimen. Use an adjacent area for control. High amounts of amatoxin in the dried samples produce a blue color in 1 to 2 minutes. Small amounts of amatoxin yield a blue color in the sampled area in 10 to 20 minutes. This procedure has *not* been proved to be effective with other bodily secretions, such as blood or urine.[240]

Mothball Identification

At present, commercial mothballs are composed of either nontoxic paradichlorobenzene or possibly toxic naphthalene. Naphthalene can cause a hemolytic reaction in neonates and patients with glucose-6-phosphate dehydrogenase (G6PD) deficiency.[241] In the past, mothballs have also been produced from camphor, which can cause central nervous system depression and seizures. Fortunately, camphor mothballs are no longer commercially available, although they may still exist in older households. Rapid differentiation between these groups of mothballs can expedite patient management and disposition. Several bedside tests have been reported to facilitate this.

1. Paradichlorobenzene is heavier than naphthalene. In turn, naphthalene is heavier than camphor. In lukewarm tap water, camphor will float and naphthalene and paradichlorobenzene will sink. In a solution of 3 tbsp of table salt thoroughly dissolved in 4 oz of lukewarm water, camphor and naphthalene will float and paradichlorobenzene will sink.
2. Paradichlorobenzene has a lower melting point than naphthalene does. Paradichlorobenzene mothballs will melt in a water bath at 53°C, whereas naphthalene requires a water bath hotter than 80°C.
3. Paradichlorobenzene is described as "wet and oily," whereas naphthalene is described as having a "dry" appearance. Paradichlorobenzene is familiar to many people as a cake of disinfectant used in urinals and diaper pails.

Body Secretion Analysis

Careful analysis of bodily secretions, the odor emanating from poisoned patients, and the color of their urine can help identify certain toxins. Some characteristic smells and urine colors are listed in Table 67-9 and Box 67-8.

Bedside Toxicologic Tests on Urine
Ethylene Glycol

Evaluation of the urine of patients who may have ingested ethylene glycol can be helpful. Urine should be tested for fluorescence (an additive in many commercial antifreeze products) under an ultraviolet light and for the presence of calcium oxalate crystals (a metabolic by-product of ethylene glycol metabolism).

The presence of *calcium oxalate crystals* (either envelope-shaped calcium dihydrate or needle-shaped calcium monohydrate) in urine on microscopic inspection is indicative of high oxalate levels in serum (Fig. 67-11; see also Fig. 67-3*F*). Calcium monohydrate crystals can easily be confused with sodium urate crystals; therefore, the presence of the dihydrate crystal tends to be more specific for ethylene glycol ingestion. Lack of these crystals does not rule out significant ethylene glycol ingestion because excretion of these crystals may occur late in the ingestion (>6 hours) and occasionally does not occur at all.[242,243]

Visual inspection of urine under a Wood lamp or ultraviolet light to ascertain *fluorescence* may also be helpful in the diagnosis of ethylene glycol exposure. Antifreeze is the most common source of ingested ethylene glycol. Fluorescein, the actual fluorescing material, is often placed in commercially available antifreeze to enable mechanics to detect radiator leaks with a Wood lamp or other ultraviolet light source. Fluorescein is a

TABLE 67-9 Diagnostic Odors

CHARACTERISTIC ODOR	RESPONSIBLE DRUG OR TOXIN
Acetone (sweet, fruity; pearlike)	Lacquer, ethanol, isopropyl alcohol, chloroform, diabetic ketoacidosis, alcoholic ketoacidosis, trichloroethane, paraldehyde, chloral hydrate, methylbromide, *Pseudomonas* infection
Alcohols	Ethanol (congeners), isopropyl alcohol
Ammonia-like	Uremia
Automobile exhaust	Carbon monoxide (odorless, but associated with exhaust)
Beer (stale)	Scrofula
Bitter almond	Cyanide
Carrots	Cicutoxin (or water hemlock)
Coal gas (stove gas)	Carbon monoxide (odorless, but associated with coal gas)
Disinfectants	Phenol, creosote
Eggs (rotten)	Hydrogen sulfide, carbon disulfide, mercaptans, disulfiram, *N*-acetylcysteine
Feculent	Intestinal obstruction
Fish or raw liver (musty)	Hepatic failure, zinc phosphide, hypermethioninemia, trimethylaminuria
Fruitlike	Nitrites (e.g., amyl, butyl), ethanol (congeners), isopropyl alcohol
Garlic	Phosphorus, tellurium, arsenic, parathion, malathion, selenium, dimethyl sulfoxide, thallium
Halitosis	Acute illness, poor oral hygiene
Hay	Phosgene
Mothballs	Naphthalene, *p*-dichlorobenzene, camphor
Peanuts	*N*-3-pyridyl-methyl-*N*-*p*-nitrophenyl urea (Vacor)
Pepper-like	*O*-chlorobenzylidene malonitrile
Putrid	Anaerobic infections, esophageal diverticulum, lung abscess, scurvy
Rope (burned)	Marijuana, opium
Shoe polish	Nitrobenzene
Sweating feet	Isovaleric acid acidemia
Tobacco	Nicotine
Vinegar	Acetic acid
Vinyl-like	Ethchlorvynol (Placidyl)
Violets	Turpentine (metabolites excreted in urine)
Wintergreen	Methyl salicylate

From Chiang WK. Otolaryngologic principles. In: Goldfrank LR, Flomenbaum NE, Lewin NA, et al, eds. *Goldfrank's Toxicologic Emergencies.* 5th ed. East Norwalk, CT: Appleton & Lange; 1994:374.

nontoxic inert vegetable dye that is eliminated unchanged in urine. Therefore, high levels of fluorescein in urine suggest significant ethylene glycol ingestion. However, lack of fluorescein does not rule out a significant exposure because *not all antifreezes contain fluorescein or high concentrations of fluorescein in relation to ethylene glycol.* False-positive findings can occur if certain plastic urine containers are used.[244]

To perform this procedure, place the test urine sample and control samples into separate glass test tubes. Inspect for fluorescence under a Wood lamp in a dark room. Always perform this test with controls that include urine that does not contain

fluorescein and urine that does contain fluorescein. The use of controls may increase the sensitivity and specificity from 49% and 75%, respectively, to a sensitivity and specificity of 100%.[245] Fluorescein is readily available because fluorescein-containing strips are commonly used in ophthalmologic procedures (see Chapter 62).

Salicylates

Several bedside tests have been developed to qualitatively detect salicylates in urine, including 10% ferric chloride solution, Trinder's solution, and Phenistix reagent strips. All are

BOX 67-8 Drugs That Color Urine

YELLOW

Quinacrine (Atabrine) in acidic urine
Riboflavin (large doses)

YELLOW-GREEN

Methylene blue; see Blue

YELLOW-ORANGE

Fluorescein sodium

YELLOW-PINK

Cascara* in alkaline urine; see Yellow-Brown, Brown, Black
Senna* in alkaline urine; see Yellow-Brown, Brown

YELLOW-BROWN

Cascara* in acidic urine; see Yellow-Pink, Brown, Black
Nitrofurantoin* (Furadantin and others); see Brown

ORANGE

Phenazopyridine* (Pyridium); see Red

ORANGE-RED

Rifampin (Rifadin, Rifamycin, Rimactane)

PINK

Phenothiazines*; see Red, Red-Brown
Phenytoin* (Dilantin); see Red, Red-Brown

RED

Anthraquinone in alkaline urine
Deferoxamine (Desferal)
Methyldopa (Aldomet); see Brown, Black
Phenazopyridine* (Pyridium), see Orange
Phenothiazines*; see Pink, Red-Brown
Phenytoin* (Dilantin); see Pink, Red-Brown

RED-PURPLE

Phenacetin*; see Brown

RED-BROWN

Phenothiazines*; see Pink, Red
Phenytoin* (Dilantin); see Pink, Red

BROWN

Cascara* in alkaline urine; see Yellow-Brown, Yellow-Pink, Black
Levodopa (Dopar)
Methocarbamol* (Robaxin); see Green, Black
Metronidazole (Flagyl)
Methyldopa* (Aldomet); see Red, Black
Nitrofurantoin* (Furadantin and others); see Yellow-Brown
Phenacetin*; see Red-Purple
Quinine*; see Black
Senna* in alkaline urine on standing; see Yellow-Brown, Yellow-Pink

BLUE

Methylene blue*; see Green
Triamterene (Dyrenium), fluorescent

BLUE-GREEN

Amitriptyline (Elavil, Endep)

GREEN

Indomethacin (Indocin) from liver damage
Methocarbamol* (Robaxin); see Brown-Black

BLACK

Cascara* in alkaline urine on standing; see Yellow-Brown, Yellow-Pink, Brown
Iron sorbitex* (Jectofer); see Brown
Methocarbamol* (Robaxin); see Brown, Green
Methyldopa (Aldomet); see Red, Brown
Quinine*; see Brown

From Thoman M. Physicians' primer on the toxicology of adolescent drug use. Vet Hum Toxicol. 1989;31:384.
*The drug imparts more than one color to urine and is listed under each color that it adds.

Figure 67-11 **A,** Monohydrate (needle- or prism-shaped) and dihydrate (envelope- or tent-shaped) calcium oxalate crystals from a patient poisoned with ethylene glycol. The dihydrate form is more specific for ethylene glycol toxicity because the monohydrate form can easily be confused with urate crystals. **B,** Calcium dehydrate crystal (*arrow*) and a pseudocast of a crystal.

Figure 67-12 Adding ferric chloride (10%) to a few milliliters of urine immediately turns it a deep purple color in the presence of very small quantities of aspirin. Beware of other changes in color, such as gray or brown, which is not *a positive test*. This test is also positive in ketoacidotic states such as diabetic ketoacidosis.

rapid, inexpensive, sensitive tests that give a qualitative rather than a quantitative result.

Ferric chloride and Trinder's solution both have sensitivities of 100% with serum salicylate levels of 5 mg/dL. False positives can occur with both tests. Acetoacetic acid, acetone, and phenylpyruvic acid will cause false-positive results. Thus, this test may be falsely positive in patients with diabetic, alcoholic, or starvation ketoacidosis. Phenol-containing drugs such as diflunisal, sulfasalazine, and salicylamide may also produce false positives. Any positive result requires a confirmatory quantitative serum salicylate assay.[246]

The *ferric chloride test* is a commonly used rapid, qualitative, urinary screening procedure. To perform this test, add several drops of 10% ferric chloride to 1 or 2 mL of urine that has been collected in a test tube. The immediate appearance of a bluish purple color signifies that salicylates are present in the urine (Fig. 67-12). This test is very sensitive, and just one aspirin tablet taken within 12 to 24 hours will give a positive result. It will require 60 to 120 minutes from the time of ingestion for this reaction to become positive in patients with normal renal function, so early test results may be misleading.

The *Trinder test* uses a mixture of mercuric chloride and ferric nitrate in deionized water. To perform this test, mix 1 mL of urine with 1 mL of Trinder's solution. A violet or purple color signifies the presence of salicylates. Acetoacetic acid and high levels of phenothiazines may give false-positive results.

Phenistix reagent strips were originally developed to detect phenylketonuria. However, Phenistix strips also turn brown in presence of salicylates. False-positive findings for salicylates can occur if phenothiazines are present.

Bedside Toxicologic Tests on Oral Secretions and Breath: Ethyl Alcohol

Several bedside devices have been developed to measure alcohol concentrations in body fluids. Measurements of the alcohol concentration in expired air or saliva have been shown to correlate well with blood alcohol concentrations in the appropriate settings.

Breath alcohol analyzers have been developed since the 1950s and are currently used in law enforcement. These devices typically use infrared spectral analysis to determine the concentration of alcohol in expired air. Almost all the alcohol found in expired air at the level of the mouth is secondary to alcohol diffused from the bronchial system rather than the alveolar system.[247] Minor alterations in breathing patterns can cause large variations in readings. Thus, uncooperative patients who do not exhale properly will cause an inaccurate reading. Other causes of inaccurate readings include the recent ingestion of alcohol-containing products, belching or vomiting, use of inhalers, poor technique, or restrictive pulmonary pathology.

Alcohol concentrations in saliva have been shown to correlate with serum concentrations. Bedside measurement of salivary alcohol concentrations can also be obtained with a dipstick-like device. These devices use an enzymatic reaction involving alcohol dehydrogenase to measure alcohol concentrations.[248] Patients who are dehydrated (a common occurrence in alcohol-intoxicated patients) are often unable to provide adequate saliva samples, and inaccurate readings have occurred in patients with high blood alcohol concentrations.[249,250]

Bedside Toxicologic Tests on Blood: Methemoglobinemia

Patients with methemoglobinemia will often have a normal partial pressure of oxygen on routine arterial blood gas analysis, a normal *calculated* Hb saturation, a *nondiagnostic pulse oximeter reading*, and a cyanosis that does not clear with O_2 administration. Newer models of co-oximeters are able to reliably measure methemoglobin levels. Bedside visual inspection of venous or arterial blood may be helpful in the diagnosis of methemoglobinemia. Methemoglobinemia occurs when normal Hb is exposed to an oxidant stress (Fe^{2+} converted to Fe^{3+}). If the erythrocytes are not able to handle such stress, such as in the presence of G6PD deficiency, Hb remains in an oxidized state (methemoglobin), which causes a color change in the molecule.

To evaluate for methemoglobinemia, place a drop of sample blood on a white background (a white coffee filter is appropriate) in a well-lit environment. Next to this, place a drop of normal blood as a comparison control sample. Blood with methemoglobinemia appears "darker" or "chocolate brown."[251] This method relies on the ability of the examiner to distinguish changes in color and may therefore have a degree of interobserver variance. Methemoglobin levels of less than 10% may alter the color of blood only slightly and thereby cause a false-negative finding. Methemoglobin levels of between 12% and 14% may cause a false-negative reading 50% of the time. Methemoglobin levels greater than 15% are reported to cause a cyanotic appearance in patients. With levels of 35% or greater, identification of methemoglobinemia by visual inspection of the color of blood is quite accurate.[251] At this level, almost all patients are obviously cyanotic and symptomatic.

Invasive Diagnostic Procedures

Several invasive diagnostic bedside procedures can be useful in the assessment of possible drug overdoses. The basic premise of these procedures is that patients who have been exposed to a certain drug or poison will respond in a particular fashion if given a diagnostic challenge dose of another particular drug or true antidote.

Naloxone

Naloxone hydrochloride (Narcan) is a μ-opioid receptor antagonist. A diagnostic challenge with IV naloxone has been recommended for all patients with central nervous system depression.[252] Certain clinical findings such as miosis, decreased respiratory rate, and evidence of illicit drug use can predict many patients who will respond to a challenge dose of naloxone.[253] If a patient's mental status improves significantly after a dose of naloxone, the patient should be considered to have been exposed to an opioid substance. This is true even if a laboratory drug screen is negative for opioids. Furthermore, many of the synthetic opiates, such as fentanyl, propoxyphene, meperidine, methadone, and pentazocine, may not be detected by the routinely used immunoassay drug screen. Although cases have been reported of patients with nonopioid overdoses (such as alcohol or phencyclidine) responding to naloxone, these single observations have not been confirmed in controlled animal or human studies.

The traditional challenge dose of naloxone in an adult or child is 2 mg every 2 minutes intravenously until a response is achieved or 10 mg is given.[254] Some clinicians prefer to use much smaller doses (0.1 to 0.2 mg) and titrate to effect. This may partially reverse the opioid overdose–related symptoms and confirm the diagnosis without precipitating the opioid withdrawal syndrome seen in patients with opioid dependency. Most patients with an opioid overdose will exhibit some response to 1 to 4 mg of naloxone, but some massive overdoses might require larger amounts. A patient who does not respond at all to 10 mg of naloxone probably does not have a pure opioid overdose. High doses of naloxone may be needed to reverse many synthetic opiates, such as propoxyphene and methadone. Lower doses can be given (0.4 to 0.8 mg in adults or 0.01 mg/kg in children) to reverse known opioid-induced respiratory depression without reversing the analgesia. Because naloxone has a half-life of between 30 and 60 minutes, a continuous drip of naloxone can be used to avoid resedation. A reasonable choice is to use two thirds of the initial bolus dose that achieved the desired reversal effect as the hourly IV dose. For example, a patient who satisfactorily responded to 1.5 mg of naloxone might receive a naloxone solution of 10 mg of naloxone in 500 mL of normal saline at a rate of 1 mg (50 mL) per hour intravenously. Nalmefene, a long-acting opioid receptor antagonist that has a terminal half-life of roughly 11 hours, can also be given to patients with suspected overdose. Theoretically, a single dose of nalmefene will be effective longer than the effects of heroin or most abused opiate substances. The initial recommended dose is 1.0 to 1.5 mg intravenously.

Naloxone and nalmefene have minimal significant side effects, but they can precipitate withdrawal in patients addicted to opioids. Unlike alcohol withdrawal, naloxone-induced opioid withdrawal in adults is short-lived and not usually life-threatening. Withdrawal can be avoided if lower initial doses of naloxone or nalmefene are given and then are slowly titrated upward to the desired effect.

Resedation may occur if the ingested drug (e.g., methadone, oxycodone [OxyContin], morphine sulfate [MS Contin]) has a *clinical effect* longer than that of naloxone. Calculated drug half-lives have minimal clinical validity. If no narcotic effect is evident in 60 to 120 minutes after standard doses of naloxone (common with heroin, for example), no clinically significant resedation is expected. Larger naloxone doses may prolong the expected antidote effect of naloxone, and longer observation is required. All timing and dose recommendations are guidelines, and all clinical decisions with regard to resedation should be individualized.

Flumazenil

Flumazenil (Romazicon) is a competitive benzodiazepine receptor antagonist that has the ability to reverse the central nervous system depression caused by all currently commercially available benzodiazepines. Its routine use in the setting of possible benzodiazepine overdose is controversial but is supported as a diagnostic and therapeutic agent in selected cases. Unlike naloxone, flumazenil can have significant side effects, but only in certain subsets of patients,[253] and its downsides are probably exaggerated in many texts. Complications include precipitation of seizures or a withdrawal syndrome in benzodiazepine-dependent patients. To minimize the chance of seizures, flumazenil should be avoided in known benzodiazepine-dependent patients and those who may have ingested epileptogenic drugs (e.g., cyclic antidepressants, cocaine, theophylline, lithium, carbamazepine, or isoniazid).

In suspected benzodiazepine overdoses in which patients are obtunded and have no history of seizures or suspicion of involvement of epileptogenic agents, flumazenil can be administered intravenously at a dose of 0.2 to 0.5 mg/min. Most benzodiazepine-overdosed patients show improvement in mental status with 1 mg of flumazenil and almost all respond to 3 to 5 mg. Small, escalating doses given slowly (maximally, 0.5 mg/min) have been recommended. Larger doses can be given at one time as a bolus, although this increases such side effects as anxiety, agitation, and emotional lability; it also increases the chances of precipitating withdrawal in benzodiazepine-dependent patients. Fortunately, seizures that occur after flumazenil use are usually transient and can generally be controlled with additional benzodiazepines. In rare cases, higher doses of benzodiazepines, barbiturates, and phenytoin might be required.

If a patient responds to flumazenil with an improvement in depressed mental status, this suggests only that the patient is under the influence of a benzodiazepine. Flumazenil can partially reverse the effects of many of the newer nonbenzodiazepine sleeping agents that affect the γ-aminobutyric acid pathway, such as zolpidem, zopiclone, and eszopiclone. Flumazenil can improve mental status in patients with hepatic encephalopathy.[255-257] It does not have any significant effect on alcohol, barbiturates, and other nonbenzodiazepine sedative-hypnotics.

Resedation is possible if the ingested drug has a *clinical duration* longer than that of flumazenil. Calculated drug half-lives have minimal clinical validity. If no resedation has occurred 60 to 90 minutes after standard doses of flumazenil, clinically significant resedation is not expected. If higher flumazenil doses have been used, additional observation may be warranted. All timing and dose recommendations are guidelines, and all clinical decisions with regard to resedation should be individualized.

Physostigmine

Physostigmine is an acetylcholinesterase inhibitor that can penetrate into the central nervous system and thus can reverse both the central and peripheral effects of anticholinergic agents. In the majority of patients with anticholinergic toxicity, no laboratory tests are available to rapidly confirm the diagnosis, and testing for specific drugs is limited or unavailable. A clinical picture that may consist of mydriasis, dry and flushed skin, dry mucous membranes, urinary incontinence, absent bowel sounds, tachycardia, hyperthermia, hallucinations, agitation, and seizures suggests an anticholinergic syndrome. In some cases (low-dose antihistamines and others), only a central nervous system syndrome characterized by hallucinations, agitation, and confusion exists. A rapid and dramatic response to physostigmine frequently confirms a diagnosis of anticholinergic toxicity. In these patients, physostigmine often decreases the degree of agitation and confusion.[258-260] The use of physostigmine as a diagnostic challenge can be helpful in selected situations, but similar to flumazenil, routine use of physostigmine as a diagnostic bedside challenge in all obtunded patients, especially in those without anticholinergic findings, should be discouraged. In some cases the agitation produced by potent anticholinergics, such as scopolamine, is totally resistant to benzodiazepines, and judicious use of physostigmine is warranted to avoid excessive sedation, chemical paralysis, or impaired ventilation. Physostigmine has recently been used to reverse a curious anticholinergic syndrome precipitated by propofol sedation.

As a diagnostic challenge or therapeutic intervention, physostigmine can be administered intravenously under constant cardiac monitoring at a dose of 1 to 2 mg in adults and 0.02 mg/kg in children over a 3- to 5-minute period. It will take 2 to 4 minutes for the central nervous system effect to become apparent. *Some clinicians empirically pretreat with a benzodiazepine to prevent seizures.* Because the half-life of physostigmine is 30 to 60 minutes, a repeated dose of 0.5 to 2 mg can also be given as clinically indicated.

Similar to flumazenil, physostigmine has been reported to interact detrimentally with cyclic antidepressants and often causes life-threatening dysrhythmias. Physostigmine can also cause an excess of acetylcholine and a resultant cholinergic crisis. This syndrome includes salivation, lacrimation, urination, defecation, bradycardia, bronchorrhea, and seizures. For this reason, 1 mg of atropine intravenously should be readily available to reverse potential cholinergic excess when using physostigmine.

Deferoxamine

Deferoxamine is an organic compound derived from the bacterium *Streptomyces pilosus* and can chelate iron. It can be used as a therapy or as a diagnostic challenge in patients with iron overdoses. Patients who have unstable vital signs or significant GI or central nervous system symptoms usually require therapeutic doses of deferoxamine. *Asymptomatic* patients with a history of iron overdose typically require supportive care only. Patients with persistent but mild symptoms, such as vomiting and diarrhea, may be given a diagnostic challenge dose of deferoxamine. A diagnostic challenge is preferential over ancillary laboratory testing because tests such as iron levels and total iron-binding capacity in the setting of iron overdose can be inaccurate, misleading, and time-consuming.[261]

A diagnostic challenge dose of deferoxamine is administered intramuscularly or intravenously over a 45-minute period at doses of 40 to 90 mg/kg up to a maximum of 1 g in children and 2 g in adults. Deferoxamine can also be administered intravenously as a constant infusion of 15 mg/kg/hr. A positive result occurs when chelated iron in the form of ferrioxamine appears in the urine. This usually causes the urine to turn a reddish orange or "vin rose" color in 2 to 3 hours after the initiation of treatment. The change in color is qualitative only and has no prognostic significance. The color change caused by ferrioxamine is dependent on pH and concentration, and false-negative test results occur.

Chronically administered deferoxamine has been reported to have multiple adverse effects, such as acute respiratory distress syndrome, visual defects, and enhancement of *Yersinia enterocolitica* infection. In the setting of a single challenge dose, flushing, erythema, tachycardia, urticaria, and hypotension caused by rapid administration of deferoxamine are the most serious side effects.

Invasive Therapeutic Procedures

The indications and rationale for the use of certain therapeutic procedures in toxicology are often misunderstood.

Alkalinization of Urine and Blood

Alkalinization of urine consists of manipulating the pH of urine to enhance the excretion of certain drugs (Box 67-9). Weak acids remain in ionic form in a basic milieu. The ionic form often prevents reabsorption of that drug in the proximal tubule, and urinary alkalinization can therefore promote elimination in urine. For certain drugs, this can play a significant role in their elimination. For example, salicylate elimination increases proportionately to the urinary flow rate, but it increases *exponentially* with increases in urinary pH. The increased serum clearance attributed to alkalinization does not correlate well with outcome or length of hospitalization.

Recommendations differ on the actual method or formula to achieve urinary alkalinization. No body of literature supports one method of urinary alkalinization over another. In general, this procedure should be titrated to the patient's fluid and acid-base status to achieve a urinary pH of 7.5 to 8.0. One method uses a constant infusion of a relatively isotonic solution consisting of three ampules of sodium bicarbonate (44 mmol/ampule) added to 1 L of 5% dextrose in water (D_5W). Another formula is to begin with a bolus of two ampules of IV sodium bicarbonate or 1 to 2 mmol/kg of body weight. The bolus is followed with a constant infusion of three ampules of sodium bicarbonate in 1 L of D_5W solution with 20 to 40 mmol of potassium infused at a rate of 100 to 300 mL/hr. These formulas assume that the patient has normal renal function. Repetitive boluses of sodium bicarbonate ampules also can be used, but this may increase the chance of hypernatremia, hypokalemia, relative hypocalcemia, fluid overload, and alkalemia. All of these are potential adverse effects of aggressive urinary alkalinization. The actual amount

---

BOX 67-9 Drugs That Have Increased Elimination with Urinary Alkalinization

Chlorpropamide
2,4-Dichlorophenoxyacetic acid
Formate
Methotrexate
Phenobarbital
Salicylates

TABLE 67-10 Use of Ethanol for Methanol or Ethylene Glycol Poisoning

Intravenous ethanol: Loading dose (using a 10% ethanol solution)* (A 10% volume/volume concentration yields approximately 100 mg/mL)

	VOLUME OF LOADING DOSE (GIVEN OVER 1-2 hr AS TOLERATED)*					
	10 kg	15 kg	30 kg	50 kg	70 kg	100 kg
Loading dose of 1000 mg/kg of 10% ethanol (infused over 1-2 hr as tolerated); *assumes a zero ethanol level to start*. Aim is to produce a serum ethanol level of 100-150 mg/dL	100 mL	150 mL	300 mL	500 mL	700 mL	1000 mL

Oral ethanol: Loading dose (a 20% volume/volume concentration yields approximately 200 mg/mL)

	VOLUME OF LOADING DOSE					
	10 kg	15 kg	30 kg	50 kg	70 kg	100 kg
Loading dose of 1000 mg/kg of 20% ethanol† diluted in juice; may be administered orally or via nasogastric tube; *assumes a zero ethanol level to start*Aim is to produce a serum ethanol level of 100-150 mg/dL	50 mL	75 mL	150 mL	250 mL	350 mL	500 mL

Intravenous ethanol: Maintenance dose (using a 10% ethanol solution)‡ (A 10% volume/volume concentration yields approximately 100 mg/mL; infusion to be started immediately following the loading dose; aim is to maintain a serum ethanol level of 100-150 mg/dL§)

	INFUSION RATE (mL/hr FOR VARIOUS WEIGHTS)‡					
	10 kg	15 kg	30 kg	50 kg	70 kg	100 kg
Normal Maintenance Range (mg/kg/hr)						
80	8	12	24	40	56	80
110	11	16	33	55	77	110
130	13	19	39	65	91	130
Approximate Maintenance Dose for Chronic Alcoholics						
150‖	15	22	45	75	105	150
Range Required during Hemodialysis						
250‖	25	38	75	125	175	250
300‖	30	45	90	150	210	300
350‖	35	53	105	175	245	350

of fluids and bicarbonate administered requires titration to the patient's clinical condition, and careful monitoring of electrolyte, pH, and fluid status is encouraged.

Urinary alkalinization can sometimes be difficult to achieve or maintain. Hypovolemia is probably the leading cause of an inability to achieve alkaline urine. Other theoretical causes are hypokalemia, hypomagnesemia, and hypochloremia. Several authors have suggested that in patients with severe salicylate poisoning, urinary alkalinization may be difficult, if not impossible to achieve.[262] Some will empirically add potassium and magnesium to the diuresis fluid.

Ethanol Infusion

Fomepizole (4-methylpyrazole) has been approved by the U.S. Food and Drug Administration for the treatment of ethylene glycol poisoning. It has also been used successfully in treating methanol poisoning.[263,264] When compared with the traditional treatment of toxic alcohol poisoning, namely, ethanol, fomepizole has the advantages of ease of use, fewer side effects (specifically hypoglycemia), and ability to maintain therapeutic levels.[263,265] Fomepizole is considered the antidote of choice; however, because of the cost and the logistics of stocking this antidote, many hospitals might not have this drug readily available.

Ethanol can be used as a therapeutic intervention in patients with methanol or ethylene glycol poisoning because of ethanol's much greater affinity for alcohol dehydrogenases. These enzymes metabolize methanol and ethylene glycol to toxic by-products. However, with serum ethanol levels of 100 mg/dL, minimal amounts of ethylene glycol or methanol are metabolized by alcohol dehydrogenases.[116,118] Ethanol infusions are not useful in the treatment of isopropyl alcohol poisoning.

Ethanol can be administered orally or intravenously (Table 67-10). IV ethanol has the advantages of achieving therapeutic levels rapidly, ensuring complete absorption,

TABLE 67-10 Use of Ethanol for Methanol or Ethylene Glycol Poisoning—cont'd

Oral ethanol: Maintenance dose (a 20% volume/volume concentration yields approximately 200 mg/mL; infusion to be given each hour immediately following a loading dose; aim is to maintain a serum ethanol level of 100-150 mg/dL§; each dose may be diluted in juice and given orally or via nasogastric tube)

	INFUSION RATE (mL/hr¶ FOR VARIOUS WEIGHTS**)					
	10 kg	15 kg	30 kg	50 kg	70 kg	100 kg
Normal Maintenance Range (mg/kg/hr)						
80	4	6	12	20	28	40
110	6	8	17	27	39	55
130	7	10	20	33	46	66
Approximate Range for Chronic Alcoholics or for Patients Receiving Continuous Oral Activated Charcoal						
150	8	11	22	38	53	75
Range Required during Hemodialysis						
250	13	19	38	63	88	125
300	15	23	46	75	105	150
350	18	26	52	88	123	175

Note: *Concentrations higher than 10% are not recommended for intravenous administration. Concentrations higher than 30% are not recommended for oral administration.* The dose schedule is based on the premise that the patient initially has a *zero* ethanol level. The aim of therapy is to maintain a serum ethanol level of 100 to 150 mg/dL, but constant monitoring of the ethanol level is required because of wide variations in endogenous metabolic capacity. Ethanol is removed by dialysis, and the infusion rate of ethanol must be increased during dialysis. Prolonged ethanol administration may lead to *hypoglycemia.* Note that 10% ethanol for infusion may be difficult to find in the hospital pharmacy. To formulate 10% ethanol for infusion, (1) remove 50 mL from a 1-L bottle of 5% ethanol/5% dextrose in water (D₅W) and replace it with 50 mL of 100% ethanol, or (2) remove 100 mL from a 1-L bottle of D₅W and replace it with 100 mL of 100% ethanol.
*If a 5% ethanol solution is used, *double* the volume of the loading dose.
†Equivalent to a 40-proof solution.
‡If a 5% ethanol solution is used, *double* the volume rate; monitor closely for potential volume overload.
§Serum ethanol levels should be monitored closely.
‖At higher infusion rates, it may be necessary to administer by volume rather than by milliliters per hour.
¶For a 30% concentration, divide the amount by 1.5.
** Rounded off to the nearest milliliter.

limiting the chance of aspiration, and avoiding gastritis. A 5% concentration of ethanol, which can be given in a peripheral vein, requires the use of large fluid volumes. In a 70-kg patient, a loading dose requires 1.4 L of a 5% solution, with a maintenance dose of 700 mL/hr. If IV ethanol is given, maintain careful attention to cardiopulmonary status. In contrast, oral loading can be achieved with much lower volumes. However, oral loading can be difficult in an uncooperative or unconscious patient or if vomiting or GI hemorrhage is present. A therapeutic level is reached more slowly with oral loading.

Ethanol metabolism can vary widely, and ethanol is dialyzable. Therefore, it may be difficult to maintain appropriate ethanol levels during dialysis therapy for ethylene glycol or methanol poisoning. Frequent measurements of ethanol should be obtained and the infusion adjusted accordingly. When patients are given ethanol infusions, central nervous system depression, hypothermia, hypotension, hypoglycemia, and phlebitis are common adverse effects, especially in children. Serial levels of ethanol and glucose should be obtained.

References are available at www.expertconsult.com

CHAPTER 68

Standard Precautions and Infectious Exposure Management

Peter E. Sokolove and Aimee Moulin

Contamination of health care workers with body fluids is a frequent occurrence in the emergency department (ED). A survey of ED staff found that 54% reported contact of intact skin with body fluids and 1.5% reported contact of nonintact skin within the preceding year.[1] These fluids often contain various transmissible infectious diseases because the prevalence of human immunodeficiency virus (HIV) infection, hepatitis, and other communicable diseases is high in ED patient populations.[1,2] In a prospective study of penetrating trauma patients admitted to an urban trauma center, 9% tested positive for anti-HIV, hepatitis B surface antigen (HBsAg), or anti–hepatitis C virus (HCV). Patients were infrequently aware of their seropositive status.[2] In the ED, patient characteristics were found to be poor predictors of hepatitis positivity, thus making it more difficult to identify patients who pose a risk to health care workers.[3] These factors make widespread use of universal precautions in the ED essential.

Compliance with standard precautions, formerly known as universal precautions, is far from universal.[4-6] In a video-taped observational study of 88 ED trauma resuscitations, 33.4% had major breaks in standard precautions. The most common major break was failure to wear a mask (32.2% of procedures), followed by inadequate eyewear (22.2%), no gown (5.6%), and no gloves (3.0%).[6] Henry and colleagues showed that ED personnel significantly overestimate their use of standard precautions.[7]

In 1985, the combination of high-risk illness with low-compliance barrier use prompted the Centers for Disease Control and Prevention (CDC) to recommend guidelines for the protection of health care workers.[8] In 1991, these recommendations were enacted into law by mandate of the Occupational Safety and Health Administration (OSHA).[9] The primary focus of the CDC guidelines is to reduce mucocutaneous exposure to body fluids by encouraging hand washing and barrier protection. These measures do little to protect from percutaneous exposure, which is the most efficient method of transmission of hepatitis and HIV.[10,11] The current strategy for risk reduction in the ED includes immunization against hepatitis B virus (HBV), use of standard precautions (including reengineered safety products), and prompt initiation of postexposure prophylaxis (PEP) when appropriate.

GUIDELINES FOR STANDARD PRECAUTIONS

Appropriate precautions for all patient contact must be viewed as a consistent practice or "way of life" in the ED. The following guidelines, based on CDC recommendations, should be used when there is any possibility of contact with body fluids.

Barrier Precautions

1. Use gloves for any patient contact with a risk for exposure to body fluids (Fig. 68-1). Both cutaneous and percutaneous exposure can be reduced by the use of gloves. Gloves have been shown to reduce disease transmission in needle-stick injuries, with greater reduction seen with double gloving in animal models and in a case crossover study of health care workers.[12] Mansouri and associates compared the biomechanical performance of single and double latex and nitrile examination gloves. Transmission of red blood cells was less with nitrile gloves than with a single layer of latex gloves despite being thinner than the latex examination gloves. A double layer of latex gloves provided the best protection in this study.[13]
2. Wear a mask and protective eyewear when exposure to body fluid aerosols is possible (e.g., wound irrigation, traumatic chest wound) (Fig. 68-2).
3. Wear a gown and shoe covers when there is the risk for large volumes of splashed body fluids (e.g., chest tube, thoracotomy) (Fig. 68-3).

Sharps Precautions

Most importantly, sharps precautions mean no recapping, bending, or breaking of needles. If needle recapping is deemed necessary, use a single-handed technique (Fig. 68-4). A safer alternative is to immediately dispose of the needle in an approved sharps container without recapping. In an observational study of ED employees, the rate of needle recapping was 34%, with most practitioners using a two-handed technique.[14] Various reengineered products are available for use in the ED, including retracting scalpels, auto-capping needles, and needleless intravenous systems (Fig. 68-5). Using such devices decreases percutaneous injury rates among health care workers.[15,16] A survey of infection control professionals at Iowa and Virginia hospitals found that implementation of such devices was the most common action taken to decrease percutaneous injuries.[17] U.S. federal law now requires the use of safety-engineered sharps devices to protect health care workers. In brief, the Needle-stick Safety and Prevention Act of 2000 required the use of safety-engineered sharps devices to protect health care workers from needlestick injuries.[18] A review of data from the Exposure Prevention Information Network (EPINet) sharps injury surveillance program estimated that needlestick injuries have decreased by 34% overall, with a 51% decline in nurses since the implementation of federal legislation.[16]

Respiratory Precautions

During contact with patients who have suspected or confirmed pulmonary tuberculosis (TB), wear a National Institute for Occupational Safety and Health (NIOSH)–approved N-95 particulate respirator (Fig. 68-6). These masks are designed to efficiently filter 1- to 5-μm particles and are less costly and more comfortable than high-efficiency particulate air (HEPA)–filtered masks. In addition, place such patients in a respiratory isolation room with negative pressure, high circulation (optimally at least 12 air changes per hour), and

Figure 68-1 Gloves are mandatory for any patient contact with a risk for exposure to body fluids. "Double gloving" may confer additional protection and should be considered in high-risk situations.

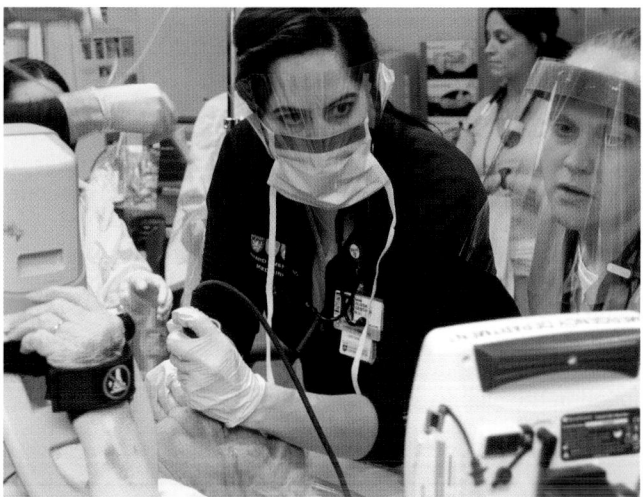

Figure 68-2 A mask and protective eyewear are mandatory when exposure to body fluid aerosols is possible. This patient vomited profusely during intubation, which may have led to an exposure if proper protective gear had not been worn.

external exhaust. While in the ED, avoid procedures resulting in increased release of infectious droplets, such as sputum induction. Make sure that all potentially infectious patients wear a surgical-type mask, especially during transportation outside the respiratory isolation room (e.g., to radiology).[19] Implementation of the CDC guidelines is variable. A study of three California hospitals in which CDC guidelines and hospital procedure were compared with actual practice found that 19% of patients with TB were not in negative pressure rooms. Of the 62 health care workers observed using a respirator for TB, 65% did not use it properly.[20]

Hand Washing

Immediately wash any skin surface coming in contact with body fluids with soap and water. If performed properly, both soap and water and alcohol-based products are generally efficacious in removing bacteria.[21] Soap and water perform better

Figure 68-3 Full protective gear (eye protection, face mask, impervious gown, gloves, and shoe covers) should be worn when there is a risk for large volumes of splashed bodily fluids (e.g., emergency thoracotomy.)

in removing *Clostridium difficile* spores,[22] but alcohol-based products are preferred and may be more viricidal.[21,23] In most health care settings, hand-washing rates remain low.[24-26]

OCCUPATIONAL DISEASE EXPOSURE

Occupationally acquired infections cause considerable morbidity and mortality among health care workers despite OSHA requirements for precautions. Given the often occult manifestation of disease in the ED patient population, emergency health care workers are at high risk for exposure to infectious diseases. There is a high prevalence of HIV, HBV, HCV, and pulmonary TB in ED patients, as well as associated high morbidity and mortality. This chapter focuses on these particular diseases and provider risks.

HBV

Transmission

HBV is a well-recognized occupational risk for health care providers, and multiple studies have documented the high prevalence of hepatitis in ED patients.[3,27-29] An estimated 100 to 200 health care workers have died annually during the past decade because of the chronic consequences of HBV infection.[30] Despite the attention focused on transmission of HIV, the infectivity of HBV is significantly higher. HBV is a more virulent organism and requires a relatively small inoculum for transmission.[31] Percutaneous injuries are the most efficient mode of HBV transmission, but many infected health care workers do not recall a specific injury.[32] Many body fluids

Figure 68-4 A, Recapping a needle by holding the cap in the hand is the most common way to sustain a needle puncture and should never be done! **B,** It is best to discard the needle/syringe without recapping, but if deemed absolutely necessary, use a single-handed technique to partially recap without holding the needle cap. **C,** Make sure that at least 80% of the needle is covered before completing the recapping with the second hand (by holding the base of the needle cap).

Figure 68-5 Using safety systems such as auto-recapping needles and retracting scalpels dramatically reduces percutaneous injuries to health care workers, and their use is now mandated by U.S. federal law.

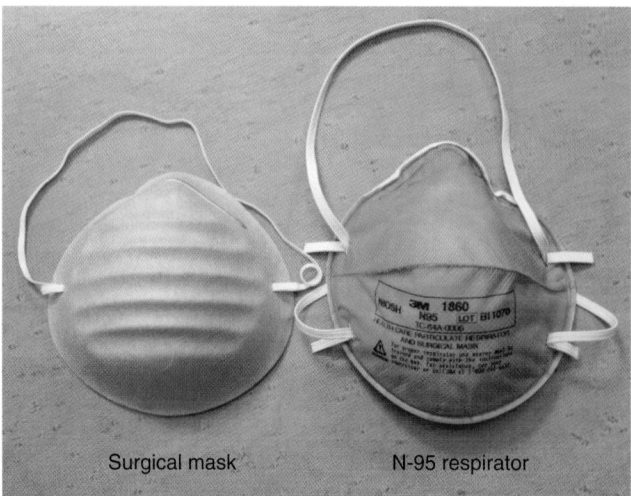

Figure 68-6 Respiratory precautions. Surgical masks are appropriate to protect against pathogens that are larger than 5 μm, such as influenza and *Neisseria meningitidis*. N-95 respirators are required for pathogens smaller than 5 μm, such as tuberculosis.

other than blood contain HBsAg, but levels of infectious HBV particles in blood-free body fluids are 100 to 1000 times lower than in blood itself. Although human saliva alone does not appear to pose a significant risk for transmission of disease, human bites have been associated with transmission of HBV.[33] Implementation of the CDC's standard precautions, along with the OSHA regulations for barrier protection and preexposure vaccination, has led to a decrease in the incidence of HBV transmission.[34]

To understand the risk of HBV transmission resulting from occupational exposure, an understanding of a few key serologic markers for HBV is essential. HBsAg is a marker of active infection in the source patient. From a practical standpoint, HBV can be transmitted when HBsAg is present, and it is not generally transmissible when this marker is absent. Hepatitis B surface antibody (HBsAb) is a protective antibody against HBV. In vaccinating health care workers, the goal is to stimulate the immune system to produce a sufficient quantity of this antibody. Hepatitis B e antigen (HBeAg) can be found in the bloodstream of HBV-infected individuals during times of peak virus replication. When a source patient is positive for HBeAg, the bloodstream contains a much larger number of infectious HBV particles. If a nonimmune individual sustains a needlestick from an HBsAg-positive patient, the risk for HBV transmission depends on the HBeAg status of the source. The risk for clinical hepatitis is approximately 2% (range, 1% to 6%) if HBeAg is absent as opposed to a risk of 22% to 31% if HBeAg is present.[35]

Postexposure Management

PEP following exposure to an HBsAg-positive source may require hepatitis B vaccine, hepatitis B immunoglobulin (HBIG), both, or neither (Table 68-1). This depends on the vaccination and antibody response status of the exposed health care worker. HBIG is derived from pooled human plasma and provides passive immunization for nonimmune exposed individuals. This preparation is very safe and not known to transmit disease.[34,35] When HBIG is used for PEP, give it ideally within 24 hours after exposure, and note that it is of questionable value beyond 7 days.[36] PEP for HBV is remarkably effective, and infection is unlikely to develop in individuals who receive PEP.[30] Hepatitis B vaccine may also be given with PEP. Individuals who have not previously been vaccinated or who have not demonstrated an adequate response should receive the hepatitis B vaccine. Adverse reactions to the hepatitis B vaccine are generally quite mild, and it is safe to give during pregnancy. For primary immunization, give an initial

TABLE 68-1   Recommendations for Hepatitis B Prophylaxis after Percutaneous or Permucosal Exposure

EXPOSED PERSON	SOURCE		
	HBsAg Positive	HBsAg Negative	Source Unknown or Not Available
Unvaccinated	HBIG × 1* and the HB vaccine series	Initiate the HB vaccine series	Initiate the HB vaccine series
Vaccinated			
Known responder	No treatment	No treatment	No treatment
Known nonresponder	HBIG × 2 *or* HBIG × 1 and initiate revaccination†	No treatment	If a known high-risk source, treat as though the source were HBsAg positive
Response unknown	Test the exposed person for anti-HBs 1. If adequate,‡ no treatment 2. If inadequate, HBIG × 1 plus a vaccine booster	No treatment	Test the exposed person for anti-HBs: 1. If adequate, no treatment 2. If inadequate, HB vaccine booster and recheck the titer in 1-2 mo

Adapted from Panlilio AL, Cardo DM, Grohskopf LA, et al. Updated U.S. Public Health Service guidelines for the management of occupational exposures to HIV and recommendations for postexposure prophylaxis. *MMWR Recomm Rep.* 2005;54(RR-9):1-17.
HB, hepatitis B; *HBIG*, hepatitis B immunoglobulin; *HBsAg*, hepatitis B surface antigen.
*HBIG dose = 0.06 mL/kg intramuscularly.
†The option of giving one dose of HBIG and reinitiating the vaccine series is preferred for nonresponders who have not completed a second three-dose vaccine series. For persons who previously completed a second vaccine series but failed to respond, two doses of HBIG are preferred.
‡Adequate anti-HBs = 10 mIU/mL.

intramuscular injection, followed by subsequent intramuscular vaccinations at 1 and 6 months. Check antibody levels (HBsAb) at 4 to 6 weeks after the series is completed to confirm that the desired titer of at least 10 mIU/mL has been attained. Vaccinated individuals who achieve this antibody level are referred to as "responders" and are believed to be immune for life. Although 25% to 50% of vaccine responders demonstrate a decline in HBsAb levels to below 10 mIU/mL within 5 to 7 years, these individuals are still protected against clinical disease because of a robust immune system memory or anamnestic response.[37] There is no need to provide vaccination or to check titers in individuals who have previously had an adequate titer.[30] PEP with these agents is not contraindicated during pregnancy or lactation. Health care workers who have previously been infected with HBV are immune to reinfection, so PEP is not indicated in such individuals.

HCV

Transmission
Approximately 1.6% of Americans (4.1 million) are infected with HCV,[38] and many individuals are unaware of their infection. ED patients have a higher prevalence than the general population. In one study the prevalence of HCV antibody was 4.0% as compared with a prevalence in the overall U.S. population of 1.8%.[27] HCV is often acquired from injection drug use. It was once commonly transmitted by blood transfusion but is fortunately rare now with modern screening. Although HCV can be transmitted sexually, this a minor route. Mucous membrane transmission of HCV is possible but much less common. Percutaneous transmission is the most efficient route. The incidence of seroconversion after an HCV-positive needlestick is about 1.8% (estimates range from 0% to 7%).[35] It is useful to remember that the risk for transmission of HCV after a needlestick is similar to that for transmission of HBV when the source is HBeAg negative. When seroconversion

does occur, 80% of patients will demonstrate antibodies at 15 weeks and 97% at 6 months after exposure. Although the clinical course of HCV is often asymptomatic or mild, chronic hepatitis will develop in approximately 85% of patients, cirrhosis in 10% to 20%, and hepatocellular carcinoma in 1% to 5%.[39-41]

Postexposure Management
Currently, PEP for HCV exposure is not recommended.[41] HCV exhibits a high degree of genetic heterogeneity and a very rapid mutation rate, thus making the development of a vaccine extremely difficult. Work to develop a PEP regimen for HCV is ongoing.[42]

HIV

Transmission
According to the CDC, 57 cases of occupational HIV transmission to health care workers occurred in the United States through 2010. In addition, another 143 health care workers demonstrated HIV seroconversion that may have been occupationally related.[43] The risk for contracting HIV from working in the ED depends on the prevalence of HIV in the local patient population. Wears and coworkers[44] estimated the cumulative career risk of contracting HIV from occupational exposure in a high-prevalence ED to be as high as 1.4%. The overall risk for HIV seroconversion is about 1 in 300 (0.3%) after a needlestick and less than 1 in 1000 for mucous membrane exposure. Cardo and colleagues[45] demonstrated that the risk for HIV seroconversion after needlestick injuries is not uniform. Seroconversion was found to be more likely for deep injuries (odds ratio [OR] = 15), if blood was visible on the device (OR = 6.2), if the needle had been used in a source patient's artery or vein (OR = 4.3), or if the source patient suffered from terminal acquired immunodeficiency syndrome (AIDS; OR = 5.6). It is essential to gather information

regarding the nature of the injury to "risk-stratify" the exposure. Exposure of intact skin to contaminated blood has not been identified as a risk for transmission of HIV.[46,47]

When seroconversion occurs, HIV antibodies can be detected as early as 3 weeks after exposure and are almost always present by 6 months. Seroconversion at 6 to 12 months is rare but has been reported in individuals co-infected with HIV and HCV. Follow-up HIV testing is recommended for 12 months for health care workers who become infected with HCV after dual exposure to both HCV and HIV.[46] Acute retroviral syndrome is a clinical manifestation of HIV seroconversion that occurs in approximately 80% of newly infected individuals at a median of 25 days after exposure. The signs and symptoms of acute retroviral syndrome are similar to those of mononucleosis and consist of fever, lymphadenopathy, and rash.

Postexposure Management[46]
Evidence Supporting PEP
In 1998 the U.S. Public Health Service recommended using PEP for selected HIV exposures.[40] These recommendations were based on a single case-control study.[45] Currently, a large placebo-controlled trial would be considered unethical. The CDC-sponsored case-control study, undertaken in the United States, France, the United Kingdom, and Italy, compared 33 health care workers who seroconverted after exposure to HIV with 665 control health care workers who did not seroconvert after exposure to HIV. About 90% of the patients in this study were exposed via hollow-bore needles.[45] When postexposure zidovudine (azidothymidine [AZT]) was used, the risk for HIV infection was reduced by 81% (95% confidence interval, 48% to 94%). Although the study methodology was limited by its retrospective design and the potential for recall bias, these results strongly support the efficacy of AZT for PEP. In a human study of vertical transmission, the use of antiretroviral agents during pregnancy decreased perinatal HIV transmission by 67%.[48] Of children born to HIV-positive mothers who were given HIV PEP within 48 hours of birth, HIV transmission was also decreased.[49] Although perinatal exposure is different from occupational needlestick, this evidence supports the concept of a "window of opportunity" during which PEP may prevent transmission of HIV to an exposed individual.

Selecting Patients for PEP
In both 2001 and 2005, the U.S. Public Health Service published updated recommendations regarding the use of HIV PEP.[35,46] In general, the decision to use PEP depends on the type of exposure and the source's HIV status. The first step in determining whether PEP is indicated is to assess the severity of exposure. Percutaneous exposure can be categorized as "less severe" or "more severe." A less severe exposure involves a solid needle, a superficial injury, and no blood visible on the device. All other percutaneous injuries are categorized as more severe. Exposure to mucous membranes and nonintact skin is categorized as either "small volume" (a few drops of blood) or "large volume" (a major blood splash). There are no reported cases of HIV seroconversion after exposure of intact skin to blood.[35,46,47] After assessing the severity of exposure, determine the potential infectivity of the source. Consider PEP only for exposure to blood and body fluids from a source known or likely to be HIV positive. Exposure from an HIV-negative source does not require PEP. Do not test sharp instruments for HIV because this is not reliable or recommended. Categorize HIV-positive source patients as either "lower risk" (class 1) or "higher risk" (class 2). Class 1 patients have asymptomatic HIV infection and a low viral load (<1500 RNA copies/mL). Higher-risk patients include those with symptomatic HIV, AIDS, acute seroconversion, or a high viral load. Once the severity of exposure and source HIV status are determined, use Table 68-2 and Table 68-3 to guide the proper PEP regimen. Note that drug development is ongoing and recommendations change rapidly. The clinician is urged to periodically check for updates. The most reliable source is the CDC website or the *Morbidity and Mortality Weekly Report* journals, most easily found via an Internet search under various topics. For exposure of skin and mucous membranes, choose a PEP regimen from three general categories. For small-volume exposure to an HIV class 1 source, consider using the basic regimen (two drugs). If either the exposure is of large volume or the source is HIV class 2, recommend the basic regimen. In cases in which there is both a large-volume exposure and an HIV class 2 source, recommend the expanded regimen (at least three drugs). For most percutaneous exposures, recommend the expanded regimen. For less severe percutaneous exposures from an HIV class 1 source, recommend the basic regimen.

A number of special circumstances may arise when determining the need for HIV PEP. When a source is known but an individual's HIV status is pending, decide about the use of PEP on a case-by-case basis. When the source is high risk, initiate PEP and then stop or modify it later once the HIV status of the source is determined. When a source can be identified but the HIV status of the source is unknown and will not become available, PEP is not generally recommended. If the source has risk factors for HIV, consider using the basic two-drug regimens. Sometimes exposures occur and the source is completely unknown. Although PEP is not generally recommended for such exposures, the basic regimen should be considered if the exposure occurred in an HIV-likely setting (e.g., exposure to a discarded needle on an AIDS ward).

PEP and antiretroviral use are considered safe and recommended during pregnancy[50] and in pediatric patients for occupational and nonoccupational exposure.[51]

Choice of PEP Medications
When HIV PEP is administered, a minimum of two drugs is recommended. Although there is no direct evidence that combination PEP regimens are beneficial, concerns about antiretroviral resistance and the synergistic effects of antiviral medications when treating patients with AIDS support such an approach. As discussed earlier, the U.S. Public Health Service recommends using a basic (two-drug) PEP regimen for lower-risk HIV exposure and an expanded (three- and even four-drug) PEP regimen for higher-risk exposure (Fig. 68-7). The basic PEP regimen consists of either two nucleoside reverse transcriptase inhibitors or a nucleoside reverse transcriptase inhibitor plus a nonnucleoside reverse transcriptase inhibitor. The traditional regimen is zidovudine (ZDV) plus lamivudine (3TC), available as Combivir. Alternative basic regimens include ZDV plus emtricitabine (FTC), tenofovir (TDF) plus 3TC or FTC, and stavudine (d4T) plus 3TC or FTC. When using the expanded PEP regimen, add a protease inhibitor to the basic regimen. In the currently preferred expanded regimen, lopinavir/ritonavir is added to the basic

TABLE 68-2 Recommended HIV PEP for Percutaneous Injuries

Exposure Type	INFECTION STATUS OF SOURCE		SOURCE OF UNKNOWN HIV STATUS[†]	UNKNOWN SOURCE[‡]	HIV NEGATIVE
	HIV Positive, Class 1*	HIV Positive, Class 2*			
Less severe[§]	Recommend a basic two-drug PEP	Recommend an expanded three or more drug PEP	Generally, no PEP is warranted; however, consider basic two-drug PEP‖ for a source with HIV risk factors¶	Generally, no PEP is warranted; however, consider basic two-drug PEP‖ in settings where exposure to HIV-infected persons is likely	No PEP is warranted
More severe**	Recommend an expanded three-drug PEP	Recommend an expanded three or more drug PEP	Generally, no PEP is warranted; however, consider basic two-drug PEP‖ for a source with HIV risk factors¶	Generally, no PEP is warranted; however, consider basic two-drug PEP‖ in settings where exposure to HIV-infected persons is likely	No PEP is warranted

Adapted from Updated U.S. Public Health Service guidelines for the management of occupational exposures to HIV and recommendations for postexposure prophylaxis. *MMWR Recomm Rep.* 2005;54(RR-9):3.

AIDS, acquired immunodeficiency syndrome; *HIV*, human immunodeficiency virus; *PEP*, postexposure prophylaxis.

*HIV positive, class 1: asymptomatic HIV infection or known low viral load (e.g., <1500 RNA copies/mL); *HIV-positive, class 2:* symptomatic HIV infection, AIDS, acute seroconversion, or known high viral load. If drug resistance is a concern, obtain expert consultation. Initiation of PEP should not be delayed pending expert consultation, and because expert consultation alone cannot substitute for face-to-face counseling, resources should be available to provide immediate evaluation and follow-up care for all exposures.

†Source of unknown HIV status (e.g., deceased source person with no samples available for HIV testing).

‡Unknown source (e.g., a needle from a sharps disposal container).

§Less severe (e.g., solid needle or superficial injury).

‖The designation "consider PEP" indicates that PEP is optional and should be based on an individualized discussion between the exposed person and the treating clinician regarding the risks versus benefits of PEP.

¶If PEP is offered and administered and the source is later determined to be HIV negative, PEP should be discontinued.

**More severe (e.g., large-bore hollow needle, deep puncture, blood visible on the device, or needle used in the patient's artery or vein).

TABLE 68-3 Recommended HIV PEP for Mucous Membrane Exposure and Nonintact Skin* Exposure

Exposure Type	INFECTION STATUS OF SOURCE		SOURCE OF UNKNOWN HIV STATUS[‡]	UNKNOWN SOURCE[§]	HIV NEGATIVE
	HIV Positive, Class 1[†]	HIV Positive, Class 2[†]			
Small volume‖	Consider a basic two-drug PEP¶	Recommend a basic three-drug PEP	Generally, no PEP is warranted; however, consider a basic two-drug PEP¶ for a source with HIV risk factors**	Generally, no PEP is warranted; however, consider a basic two-drug PEP¶ in settings where exposure to HIV-infected persons is likely	No PEP is warranted
Large volume‖	Recommend a basic three-drug PEP	Recommend an expanded three-drug PEP	Generally, no PEP warranted; however, consider basic two-drug PEP¶ for a source with HIV risk factors**	Generally, no PEP is warranted; however, consider a basic two-drug PEP¶ in settings where exposure to HIV-infected persons is likely	No PEP is warranted

Adapted from Updated U.S. Public Health service guidelines for the management of occupational exposures to HIV and recommendations for postexposure prophylaxis. *MMWR Recomm Rep.* 2005;54(RR-9):3.

HIV, human immunodeficiency virus; *PEP*, postexposure prophylaxis.

*For skin exposure, follow-up is indicated only if there is evidence of compromised skin integrity (e.g., dermatitis, abrasion, or an open wound).

†*HIV positive, class 1:* asymptomatic HIV infection or known low viral load (e.g., <1500 RNA copies/mL); *HIV-positive, class 2:* symptomatic HIV infection, AIDS, acute seroconversion, or known high viral load. If drug resistance is a concern, obtain expert consultation. Initiation of PEP should not be delayed pending expert consultation, and because expert consultation alone cannot substitute for face-to-face counseling, resources should be available to provide immediate evaluation and follow-up care for all exposures.

‡Source of unknown HIV status (e.g., deceased source person with no samples available for HIV testing).

§unknown source (e.g., splash from inappropriately disposed blood).

‖Small volume (e.g., a few drops); large volume (e.g., major blood splash).

¶The designation "consider PEP" indicates that PEP is optional and should be based on an individualized discussion between the exposed person and the treating clinician regarding the risks versus benefits of PEP.

**If PEP is offered and administered and the source is later determined to be HIV negative, PEP should be discontinued.

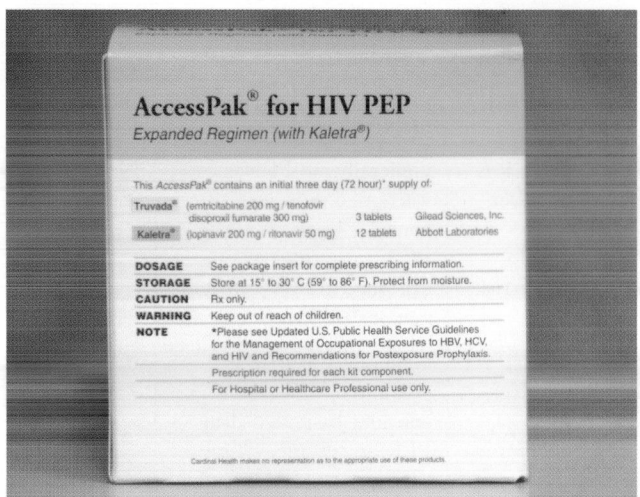

Figure 68-7 Prepackaged human immunodeficiency virus postexposure prophylaxis kits are ideal for use in the emergency department. These kits contain a 3-day supply of medications that can be started immediately while follow-up with an infectious disease specialist is arranged. Both basic and expanded regimens are available. The expanded regimen shown here is a three-drug combination: Truvada (emtricitabine plus tenofovir, which are reverse transcriptase inhibitors) and Kaletra (lopinavir/ritonavir, which is a protease inhibitor). Basic regimens do not include a protease inhibitor. *(Courtesy of Access-Pak, Cardinal Health, Dublin OH.)*

regimen. Acceptable alternative protease inhibitors include atazanavir, fosamprenavir, indinavir, saquinavir, and nelfinavir.

A number of second-line and alternative agents may be chosen for HIV PEP. Regional variation in PEP recommendations exist. New York state guidelines recommend that PEP always consist of three nucleoside analogue transcriptase inhibitors.[52] Expert consultation is recommended, especially if antiretroviral resistance is suspected. An important resource for emergency clinicians is the National Clinicians' Postexposure Prophylaxis Hotline at UCSF/San Francisco General Hospital. Expert consultation can be obtained at www.nccc.ucsf.edu or by calling 888-448-4911

Timing, Duration, and Side Effects of PEP

HIV exposure should be considered a true emergency. Administer PEP as soon as possible after exposure, ideally within 1 hour. Animal studies indicate that the efficacy of PEP diminishes with a delay in initiation.[53] HIV PEP regimens consist of a 4-week course of therapy. In the ED, patients can be prescribed the first 3 days of medications as long as outpatient follow-up is arranged (see Fig. 68-7). Side effects from the medications used for HIV PEP are not insignificant. Side effects are experienced by about 50% of health care workers taking PEP and cause approximately 33% of health care workers to discontinue therapy prematurely.[54] Depending on the choice of PEP medications, patients should also be prescribed antiemetics and antidiarrheal agents when PEP is initiated.

TB

Transmission

During the mid-1980s the United States experienced a resurgence in TB, especially among HIV-positive patients.

Although the incidence of TB cases in the United States has since declined, more than 11,000 cases were reported in 2010.[55] TB continues to pose a serious risk to both public health and health care workers. Baussano and colleagues estimated that the annual risk for TB infection in health care workers, attributable to occupational exposure, is between 3.8% and 8.4%, depending on local prevalence.[56] TB is transmitted by infectious droplets 1 to 5 μm in size. Primary infection occurs when one to three organisms are inhaled into the alveoli, where they begin to replicate. Host defenses usually stop infection within 2 to 10 weeks, and the patient enters the latent period. During this time, patients are asymptomatic and not contagious. Reactivation occurs when cell-mediated immunity wanes, and patients are again contagious. This can be due to advancing age, HIV infection, steroid use, malignancy, malnutrition, or other causes of suppression of the immune system. The lifetime risk for reactivation is 5% to 10%, with about half this risk occurring in the first few years after primary infection. Patients with increased infectivity include those with pulmonary or laryngeal TB, an active cough, positive sputum smears for acid-fast bacilli, cavitary lesions on chest radiographs, and inadequate therapy. Overall, children are less contagious than adults but can still transmit the disease. Extrapulmonary TB is contagious only in cases of an open skin lesion or involvement of the oral cavity.[19]

Depending on the patient population and geographic location, ED personnel can be at high risk for occupational TB infection. In a 1993 study at a county hospital in Los Angeles it was reported that 31% of ED workers became positive for purified protein derivative (PPD) during employment, including 20% of attendings, 32% of nurses, and 33% of residents.[57] The risk for PPD conversion was found to be 6% after 1 year of ED employment, 14% after 2 years, and 27% after 4 years. EDs typically care for higher-risk patients—those who are homeless, foreign born, recently incarcerated, or chronically debilitated. Overcrowding can lead to extended waiting periods and delays in admission. The clinical manifestation of TB in ED patients is often atypical, which can lead to a delay in diagnosis.[58,59] This is especially true for HIV-infected patients, in whom the symptoms may mimic *Pneumocystis jiroveci* pneumonia, skin tests are often negative, findings on chest radiographs are commonly atypical, and sputum tests may be less sensitive.[60-66] In one study of ED patients with TB, the mean time from ED registration to respiratory isolation was 6.5 hours, and 46% of patients were first isolated on the hospital ward.[67] A 14-year review of the U.S. National Tuberculosis Surveillance System showed that rates of advanced pulmonary TB are on the rise, especially in populations without traditional risk factors.[68] These data suggest that substantial delays in diagnosis and misdiagnosis of pulmonary TB may be increasing.

Preventing exposure to TB requires a multifaceted approach.[19] Proper ED ventilation plays a key role; inadequate ventilation has been a contributing factor in many nosocomial outbreaks. Ideally, install single-pass airflow from waiting rooms to the outside. Within the ED, make sure that air flows from clean areas to less clean areas, not vice versa. If patients with TB are seen frequently, provide at least one true respiratory isolation room in the ED. Make sure that such rooms have at least 12 air changes per hour and that they are "negative pressure" rooms in which air flows into the room from other ED areas. Other engineering approaches to

Figure 68-8 N-95 particulate respirators are the preferred mask for health care workers caring for patients who potentially have tuberculosis.

control of TB infection include using HEPA filters and upper room ultraviolet light irradiation.

Familiarize all ED personnel with the appropriate use of respiratory protection against TB. Provide surgical masks (e.g., string-tie masks) for source control. Place these masks on potentially contagious patients to decrease the passage of infectious droplets into the air. Because air can leak around such masks, they are not optimal for protection of health care workers. In late 1995, NIOSH certified a new class of masks known as N-95 particulate respirators.[69] These masks filter particles 1-μm in size with at least 95% efficiency and are generally the preferred mask for health care workers (Fig. 68-8). In some circumstances, such as when patients are undergoing cough-inducing or aerosol-generating procedures, health care workers need better protection. N-95 masks are usually the appropriate choice for ED use, but these masks should be thought of as the minimum required level of respiratory protection against TB.[19]

Initiate early respiratory isolation of patients with suspected pulmonary TB as soon as possible in the ED, ideally at triage. Screening protocols at triage can detect patients with more classic signs and symptoms of TB, but reported protocols are only moderately sensitive and somewhat cumbersome.[58,59] Consider immediate respiratory isolation for patients with high-risk chief complaints and those with hemoptysis, weight loss, or a prolonged cough. Also be aware of patients with HIV, with a history of TB, or from high-risk populations who have a cough or fever.[70] The best guideline is to initiate respiratory isolation as soon as TB is considered to be a possible diagnosis. Place masks on such patients before obtaining chest radiographs. Consider isolating patients with chest radiograph findings of an apical infiltrate, cavitary lesions, extensive hilar or mediastinal lymphadenopathy, or a miliary pattern.[70-73]

Postexposure Management

If health care workers are exposed to patients with active pulmonary TB, refer them to either employee health care or their primary care clinician for follow-up testing and treatment. To establish a health care worker's baseline PPD status, perform skin testing within days after exposure. If the baseline test is negative, perform a follow-up skin test 8 to 10 weeks later to determine whether PPD conversion has occurred. A positive baseline test (≥10-mm induration) indicates previous exposure or infection. A positive test consists of 5-mm induration after a negative baseline test or an increase to at least 10-mm induration after a baseline test of 1- to 9-mm induration.

Health care workers in whom PPD converts to positive after an exposure should undergo chest radiography to screen for active pulmonary TB.[19] If active disease is present, initiate treatment with at least four antituberculous medications. In PPD converters who do not have active disease, consider chemoprophylaxis. When deciding whether to initiate chemoprophylaxis, balance the potential benefit of TB prevention with the risk for medication-associated hepatitis. In general, give chemoprophylaxis in the case of a recent (≤2 years) PPD conversion, a known TB contact, a patient who is medically predisposed to TB, HIV-infected, intravenous drug users, or those younger than 35 years. For occupationally exposed health care workers who are PPD converters, give chemoprophylaxis, regardless of age. The preferred regimen for HIV-negative persons is daily isoniazid (INH) for 9 months, although acceptable alternative regimens can be considered.[74] Some health care workers may become exposed to strains of TB that are resistant to INH because of the continued emergence of multidrug-resistant and extensively drug-resistant strains of TB.[55,75] For exposure to multidrug-resistant TB, consult an expert when selecting an individualized chemoprophylaxis regimen. Baseline and serial liver function testing is not necessary for administration of chemoprophylaxis in most cases, but monitor closely for clinical symptoms suggestive of hepatotoxicity.

References are available at www.expertconsult.com

Educational Aspects of Emergency Department Procedures

Amita Sudhir and Jennifer Avegno

Learning to perform emergency department (ED) procedures is a complex and highly individualized educational process. No longer is the maxim of "see one, do one, teach one" an acceptable educational practice.[1] For many emergency medicine (EM) physicians, residency training may be the primary source of instruction on a wide range of common and uncommon procedures.[2] A variety of modalities and educational tools exist to aid medical educators in initial training and long-term skill retention.

CONCEPTS IN PROCEDURAL SKILL TRAINING

Trainees are often enthusiastic about performing procedures, which can provide an excellent opportunity for engaged learning. Teaching complex procedural skills remains a challenging task. Educators can be successful by thoroughly understanding the procedure before any attempt at teaching. A working understanding of the procedure's indications, contraindications, necessary equipment, detailed steps, complications, and critical actions is paramount. Procedures should be taught in a consistent and organized manner, with recognition that it is often challenging to teach adult learners a complicated psychomotor skill. As with any type of education, the lesson should be targeted to each individual's learning style. EM educators may use both formal and informal bedside techniques for procedural instruction.

Formal Education

Chapman described a set of eight steps to use as a framework for procedural learning (Box 69-1).[3] These steps incorporate the different stages of learning and are important to understand when teaching a procedural skill. This framework is best thought of as a longitudinal approach to teaching procedures over time. It includes focused preparation and memorization before any attempt at performance and progresses to actual practice with repeated feedback and assessment of competency. This outline is closely linked to theories of motor skill acquisition in which learners progress from cognition (understanding the task through explanation and demonstration) to integration (performing the task deliberately and with feedback) and finally to automation (increased speed, efficiency, and precision of the procedure).[4]

A practical synthesis of these theories for general practice has been described in a four-step process often used to teach procedural skills in a shorter time frame, such as in a simulation session or brief skills course.[5] In this approach, an expert teacher demonstrates the skill at regular speed without detailed explanation. Next, the educator performs the

procedure slowly and with detailed commentary. Third, the learner verbalizes the skill steps back to the teacher. Finally, the learner performs the procedure, with detailed discussion of each step before performing it.

Traditional lecture formats (small or large group) are often used for initial skill teaching (Figs. 69-1 and 69-2). However, there are other methods to introduce a skill concept. Using the four-step method, demonstration and deconstruction could be performed individually by the learner before a teaching session with standard texts, video, or other designated online resource.[5,6] Once the learner has progressed to actual practice of the skill, expert assistance and feedback are crucial to progression and mastery and may be the most important feature in some types of skill acquisition.[1] Feedback is not only informative but also motivational and should be directed externally (i.e., at the correct motor steps) rather than internally (i.e., at the individual's particular movements).[7] Learner-centered feedback should be delivered by expert tutors who slowly decrease their support as a trainee's proficiency increases.[8]

Procedural Training at the Bedside

Training at the bedside remains a common and important way to teach residents. Learners should go through formal training in the procedure before attempting it on a live patient. The clinical setting (Fig. 69-3B) should allow adequate time to discuss the procedure in detail. The teacher and learner should review the indications, contraindications, equipment, procedural steps, critical actions, and complications. The resident should be able to verbalize the steps involved in the procedure. This review may be provided either outside the patient's room or at the bedside, depending on the patient and the clinical scenario. The teacher should observe the learner as she or he performs the procedure and provide guidance and assistance when needed (see Fig. 69-3C). After the procedure, the teacher should examine the patient and assess the adequacy of the procedure, discuss problems that occurred during the procedure, offer suggestions for improvement, and provide a review of postprocedural care (see Fig. 69-3D).

The learner should be encouraged to engage the patient while practicing the procedure. In an article on bedside teaching, Monrouxe and colleagues suggested having students explain what they are doing to the patient in lay language because patients like to be involved in teaching so that they can learn more about their condition.[9] Explaining the procedure to the patient as it is performed can help consolidate the steps in the learner's mind and make the patient feel that he or she is an active part of the teaching process.

As part of bedside learning, newly deceased patients—those who have not expressly given consent for use of their bodies—have historically been used to practice procedures. In 1994, a survey of program directors of EM and critical care training programs found that 63% of EM programs allow procedures to be performed on newly dead patients.[10] Additionally, in a survey involving theoretical clinical scenarios, lay people responded that they would agree to after-death procedures on themselves in 75% of cases and on their relatives in 69% of cases with prior consent. Without prior consent, they would allow such procedures 40% of the time on themselves and 50% on their family members.[11]

Despite this apparent acceptance of performing invasive procedures on the newly dead by both educators and members

Eight Steps in Procedural Skill Learning

1. Identify an acceptable skill level.
2. Identify when to perform the procedure.
3. Select the instruments and equipment needed to perform the procedure.
4. Identify the critical steps in the procedure.
5. Memorize the sequential order of the steps.
6. Develop a mental image of performing the procedure.
7. Practice procedural movements with feedback.
8. Assess procedural competence.

Figure 69-1 Formal lecture to teach a new procedure.

Figure 69-2 Small-group review for free discussion between the teacher and fellow students.

of the public, this practice may be limited by certain debated ethical concerns.[12-16] There are many alternatives for procedural teaching if bedside teaching on a live, consenting patient is not feasible. Learning on newly deceased patients is not a necessary part of medical education and may, with its attendant ethical pitfalls, be easily avoided without detrimental effect on residents in training.

EDUCATIONAL ALTERNATIVES FOR PRACTICING PROCEDURES

For procedures that require a great deal of repetition to become proficient or for procedures that are less commonly encountered in the clinical setting, alternatives to bedside

teaching are essential. These methods are also useful for a resident's first introduction to a particular procedure. The following is a description of the currently available educational techniques. It is ideal to introduce the procedure via formal review before the learner practices the skill with one of the following procedural models. This may include listening to lectures, watching videotapes, using computerized instructional materials, and reading and reviewing procedural texts and atlases.

Volunteers

Human volunteers can be used for noninvasive procedures such as casting and splinting. Learners can also practice on each other for such procedures Volunteers are clearly not appropriate for most invasive procedures.

Simulation

We are now well into the information age, and medical simulation is taking an increasingly important role in medical education. An invaluable teaching tool, medical simulation can be used to improve a learner's competence and confidence, expose a learner to rare, but potentially lifesaving procedures, and decrease the rate of procedural errors. With a simulator, learners have the opportunity to practice every procedure that they need to know under a variety of different conditions. Modern human patient simulators have been developed or are currently under development for endotracheal intubation, chest compression, electrical cardioversion, cricothyroidotomy, chest tube insertion, pericardiocentesis, diagnostic peritoneal lavage, emergency thoracotomy, lumbar puncture, skin suturing, insertion of peripheral venous and arterial catheters, insertion of central venous lines, and more.[17] Many studies have demonstrated the efficacy and applicability of simulation with regard to procedural education.[18-20] A panel consisting of members from the Society for Academic Emergency Medicine (SAEM) Simulation Interest Group of the SAEM Technology in Medical Education Committee made the recommendation that "simulation-based training should prioritize procedures infrequently encountered in clinical practice and commonly performed procedures that possess a potential risk to a patient when performed by the less skilled practitioner." Two main types of simulators are in common use.

Task Trainers

Procedures can be simulated by using task trainers to teach procedures when available (Fig. 69-4). Each task trainer is a model designed to teach one specific procedure. Models are available for many procedures, including cardiopulmonary resuscitation, peripheral venipuncture, arterial puncture, intraosseous infusion, umbilical vessel catheterization, central line catheterization, lumbar puncture, endotracheal intubation, needle thoracostomy, urinary catheter placement, suturing, and emergency childbirth. They are limited by their inability to perfectly imitate the qualities of human tissue, to simulate force and tactile feedback, and to simulate complications. For example, chest tube task trainers do not bleed when the skin is cut into.

High-Fidelity Simulation

The educator can vary the difficulty of the situation according to the level of training of the learner. Complications can be simulated and the learner has the opportunity to learn how to avoid them or deal with the consequences should they arise. Debriefing is an important part of the simulator educational method.

High-fidelity simulation is designed to mimic a real-life medical scenario, including the procedures, decision-making skills, and possible permutations that may occur (Fig. 69-5).[21] This requires a high-fidelity mannequin, an instructor, a script, a scenario, and a debriefing. The instructor's responsibility is to create an environment that resembles reality as closely as possible.[17] Even though the script is standardized, the software and mannequin can take into account the unpredictable actions of participants, including simulating complications that would occur if certain decisions were made in a real-life scenario. The instructor may redirect participants to take an action that will result in a predetermined response. The debriefing process is also an important learning opportunity in which mistakes can be discussed and alternative courses of action can be explored.

In a review of simulation technology, Reznek and associates wrote that to be an effective teaching tool,[17] a simulator must provide both educationally sound and realistic feedback to a user's questions, decisions, and actions.

Cadaver Laboratories

Fresh cadavers are ideal for teaching procedures. To clarify, these are the bodies of individuals who have given consent for their bodies to be used for teaching. The advantage of using a fresh cadaver is that it more clearly resembles the tissue properties and pliability of a live human. The disadvantages are cost, limited availability, and potential risk for transmission of disease.[22]

Preserved cadavers are also an option if they are more readily available at your institution. A cadaver laboratory offers the advantage of a standardized reproducible laboratory experience under the guidance of an instructor and with no risk to the patient.[23] Disadvantages of preserved cadavers are that they do not bleed and they suffer from tissue adherence because of the preservation process, so though excellent for learning the anatomy of procedures, they may not completely simulate the in vivo experience.[24]

Figure 69-3 Procedural training at the bedside is an important part of learning a new skill. **A,** This ankle dislocation requires prompt relocation in the emergency department. **B,** The instructor first reviews the procedure with the trainee, including indications, contraindications, procedural steps, and complications. **C,** The trainee then performs the reduction while the instructor observes and provides guidance during the procedure. **D,** After the procedure, the instructor examines the patient and assesses the adequacy of reduction.

Long-Term Skill Retention and Uncommon Procedures

When teaching procedures, long-term skill retention is the goal because decay of procedural skills over time is natural. Information is lost from short-term memory through decay and interference, but fortunately, once committed to long-term memory, it is virtually permanent.[25,26] This is analogous to certain learned skills that are retained indefinitely, such as riding a bicycle. These skills are never forgotten because of a process called overlearning. Allowing learners to practice and execute movements actively during learning results in better recall than when they learn from a passive demonstration.[27,28] The exact number of times that a trainee must practice a particular skill is unknown, but certain factors have been shown to have an impact on skill retention: quality of the initial instruction, methodology of instruction and testing or evaluation, overlearning, retrieval conditions, length of the interval between training and actual practice, and individual learner and procedure qualities.[29]

Procedural learning curves are often steep, with novices showing the greatest improvement in skill initially and a plateau effect for more experienced practitioners.[29] A study of intubation skills using different task trainers and models found that learners had a success rate of only 50% when performing the skill for the first time on a new trainer but that after 10 to 12 trials on the same trainer, success levels reached a plateau of approximately 80%.[30] This same study also found that trainees learned more quickly after successful intubations than after failed ones, and the authors suggested that varying methods of practicing a skill slows learning but leads to increased retention and application to new settings.

Limited research has investigated the long-term practical retention of procedural skills. For most ED procedures, which are rarely overlearned, practice is required to maintain these skills.[3] Kovacs and colleagues demonstrated that airway management skills decline early after initial training but that performance may be maintained effectively with independent practice and periodic feedback.[31] A study of central line insertion found increased competence 3 months after a simulation-based training course, although there was a slight regression from the immediate posttest performance scores.[32] Similarly, Boet and coworkers found improved cricothyroidotomy skills at 6 and 12 months after simulator case instruction, although again there was regression from the immediate post-learning scores.[33] A chief limitation of these and other similar studies is that longitudinal skill retention is often not measured in actual clinical practice, but on simulators or task trainers, so the long-term effect of specific procedural skill teaching

Figure 69-4 Task trainers are available to teach many procedures, including endotracheal intubation.

Figure 69-5 Human patient medical simulator. **A,** In the control room, the educator is able to create and monitor clinical scenarios. **B,** The trainee manages a difficult airway on a human patient simulator. After the simulation, a debriefing is performed, which is an essential component of this teaching method.

sessions on translation to performance on patients in real clinical situations remains unclear.[29]

Training for Uncommon Procedures

The opportunity for learners to practice certain critical resuscitative procedures on human patients in the ED may be limited because they are performed so infrequently. With the advent of task trainers and simulators, these relatively rare procedures may be practiced frequently in a nonclinical setting. As noted earlier, it is unclear how this practice translates to real patient care settings.

The rate of performance of certain resuscitative procedures in recent years has declined because of several factors. For some procedures, such as ED thoracotomy, critical analyses of patient outcomes after ED thoracotomy have identified narrow conditions for decreased mortality (most notably penetrating trauma to the chest), which has virtually eliminated performing this procedure on victims of blunt trauma.[34,35] Chang and associates reported a significant decline in the rate of cricothyroidotomies performed on trauma patients following the beginning of a new EM residency training program.[36] They attributed this to several possible causes, including the widespread application of rapid-sequence intubation techniques, the presence of supervisory EM faculty 24 hours a day, and diminished concern regarding orotracheal intubation of patients whose cervical spines have not been radiographically cleared. Competition for procedures between EM residents and those from other specialties has increased; in fact, a survey of EM residency directors found that overall, emergency clinicians perform only 50% of 10 index procedures in the ED.[37,38]

Previous studies of EM residency trainees have confirmed the thought that certain emergency procedures are performed infrequently during the training years.[39-41] A 2008 paper on developing technical expertise in EM procedures via simulation identified several "high-risk, low-frequency" ED procedures: cricothyroidotomy, transvenous cardiac pacing, pericardiocentesis, vaginal delivery, and pediatric resuscitation (medical and trauma).[42] They suggested that because the correlation between simulator competence and actual practice ability is unknown, models or simulated scenarios that provide real-life situational learning should be encouraged and studied as bridges to actual practice. Wong and coworkers found that learners who participated in a cricothyroidotomy training session involving the use of video instruction and mannequin practice achieved 96% success rates within 40 seconds by the fifth attempt (with a skill and time plateau for all subsequent attempts).[43] Although the exercise was performed on a mannequin, adding a time constraint as part of the metric of success may be indicative of a more realistic situation. An animal procedure laboratory targeted to several uncommon procedures found that learners' confidence and willingness to perform these skills increased significantly, and use of live animals—though not applicable to all settings—may also enhance the realism of task performance (Fig. 69-6).[44]

TEACHING KEY ED PROCEDURES

Certain core lifesaving procedures are among the most commonly taught throughout emergency undergraduate and

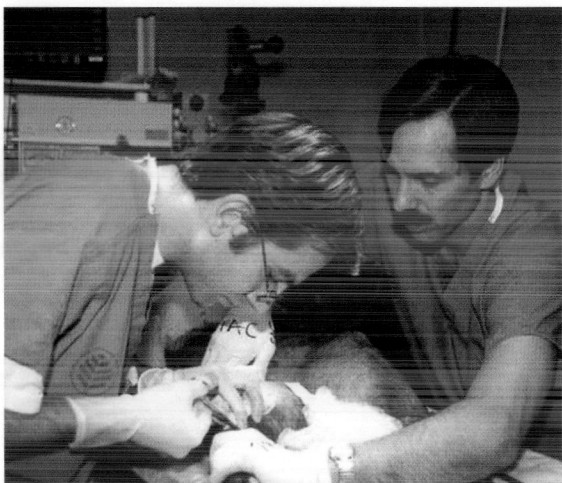

Figure 69-6 In the live animal laboratory, an instructor assists while the trainee performs a venous cutdown.

graduate medical education, and educational methods for each have been studied to various degrees.

Airway Management

Airway management is a frequently encountered procedure and critical skill to be mastered for any emergency physician (EP).[45] Both uncomplicated and difficult airway scenarios can be expected throughout the course of an EM residency and career. EPs must be taught to proficiently use a wide range of devices, from extraglottic tools to direct laryngoscopy and video-assisted or fiberoptic intubation equipment.

Much of the literature on methods of teaching airway management focuses on manikins or specific airway task trainers and more realistic patient simulators. No studies have proved the superiority of one specific type of manikin (high or low fidelity) for teaching intubation,[42] but they have been used to train learners on a wide variety of devices. A 1-year study of learners in a simulation center used manikins for initial stepwise teaching of uncomplicated intubations and then increased the difficulty of techniques and simulator scenarios.[46] The authors found that when using this method, the ideal ratio of learners to teachers was 2:1 and that it took each trainee approximately 75 to 90 minutes to achieve skill proficiency. Other researchers have found that simulator airway training improves performance on cadavers and recommended simulation for difficult or more realistic airway training.[47-49] Simulators have limitations in the teaching of airway skills. As one study noted, they were not effective in trainees' identification or management of esophageal intubation.[50]

The type of airway device used to train novice intubators has also been studied. Use of a video-assisted laryngoscope or flexible fiberoptic scope may provide an excellent teaching environment in that both the learner and teacher can watch the procedure in real time on a video screen (Fig. 69-7).[51] Educators can then give immediate feedback and guidance as the skill is being performed. Several studies have found superior acquisition and efficiency of intubating skills with video-assisted devices as compared with traditional direct laryngoscopy.[52-55]

Formal methods of instruction and feedback on airway management also have an impact on learners' experiences and

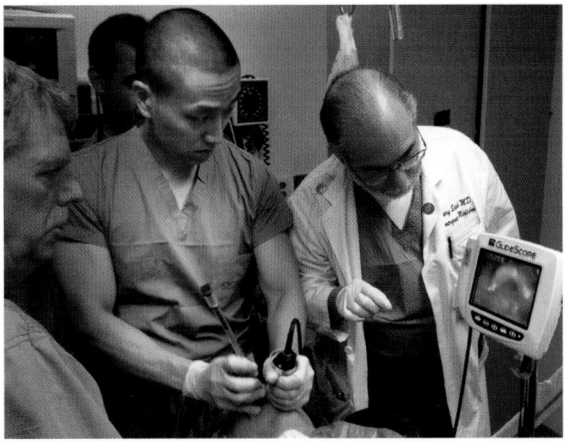

Figure 69-7 Use of a video-assisted laryngoscope provides an excellent opportunity for learning airway skills.

long-term skill retention. For simple airway techniques such as insertion of a laryngeal mask airway, the four-step method of skills teaching described earlier has not been found to be statistically different from the two-step ("see one, do one") approach.[56]

Learners who receive both regular feedback and dedicated airway practice at standard intervals have significantly higher and more stable procedural skill retention over time.[31] Another study of novice student learners found that an "experiential" group (trainees given autonomy to figure out the correct intubating technique on their own) had significantly higher long-term procedural success rates than did a group of students taught via a conventional stepwise approach.[57] Similarly, another study of novice intubators found that learners presented with a variety of manikins had low success rates on their initial attempt on each but quickly changed their technique to fit the particular model and had rapid progression to proficiency thereafter.[58]

Although the optimal method of teaching airway management for long-term skill retention and practical application is not known, several conclusions may be made. Mannikins and simulators are widely accepted methods of practice for this procedure, with simulators probably being best for providing realistic and dynamic scenarios. Use of video assists during training aids in direct feedback and may improve the learning environment. Regular practice and autonomy are crucial, and feedback should continue throughout the training period.

Lumbar Puncture

Although lumbar puncture is a common ED procedure, few trainees have a great deal of experience before residency.[59] As with other EM skills, task trainers and simulators are available to aid in teaching and practice of this skill. A training program for EM residents consisting of a traditional lecture, video demonstration, and simulator practice demonstrated competence initially after completion and additionally at 6 months.[60] A study of pediatric trainees demonstrated no difference at 7 months in lumbar puncture skills on a simulator or self-reported live-patient success after a dedicated procedure training program.[61] Because pediatric residents often perform a low number of clinical lumbar punctures,[62] it may be that EM trainees' skill retention is related to a higher volume of real-life procedural opportunities.

Cricothyroidotomy

Perhaps the most-feared ED procedure, cricothyroidotomy is established as a "high-risk, low-frequency" critical skill.[7] Because of obvious ethical issues and the rarity of the procedure—less than 1% of all airway interventions in a large trial—cricothyroidotomy has no opportunity for safe real-life practice while achieving competence.[63] Before the advent of manikins and simulators, cadaver and animal models were used for skill training and remain a part of cricothyroidotomy education. An anesthesia-based study recommended that based on learner experience and feedback, cadaveric practice be a mandatory part of any educational curriculum for cricothyroidotomy.[12] Anesthetized animals (or animal tracheas) are also used for training in this procedure, and animal practice has been shown to be accessible to novices and at least equivalent to conventional teaching in terms of speed, proficiency, and long-term (6-month) retention.[64,65]

With the ubiquity of nonliving models, much cricothyroidotomy training takes place on manikins or simulators. Animals and cadavers can be resource-intensive and are often limited by single use, whereas several different types of reusable synthetic "skins" allow multiple practice attempts on a simulator or task trainer. As with intubation, full-model, high-fidelity simulator scenarios, along with regular practice and feedback, are thought to best replicate real-life complex cases and promote long-term skill retention.[33,43,66] Whether the four-step or two-step method of skills training is superior for this procedure is unknown. A study of medical students demonstrated no significant difference between these approaches in terms of speed or proficiency.[6]

Ultrasound-Guided Procedures

A full description of teaching methods for the wide range of ultrasound-guided procedures is beyond the scope of this chapter. This group of skills has been identified as a "high-frequency, low-risk" domain of expected competence.[42] For a number of these procedures, simulators both specialized (i.e., a vaginal model with ectopic pregnancy or special trauma abdomen with free fluid) and general are of benefit for training. Learners express improved confidence and self-assessed skills after simulator-based ultrasound-guided invasive procedure education.[67] Web-based resources for ultrasound-guided skills—videos and online instructional modules—have also been used as alternatives to traditional lecture.[68]

Chest Tubes

In centers with a lower incidence of penetrating trauma, it may be necessary to use task trainers and other alternatives to live patients to ensure that learners are exposed to an adequate number of insertions. Although live animal laboratories were used extensively in the past, these are falling out of favor because of ethical concerns at many institutions. One alternative is to use animal cadavers sacrificed for unrelated research purposes—such cadavers can be obtained by communicating with professionals at one's home institution who do animal research. Another low-cost solution is to use grocery store pig ribs (Fig. 69-8). Lungs and pleura can be simulated with balloons or bags of saline. One group studied a model that they created and reported that proficiency by advanced trauma life support criteria was achieved by their learners.[69] A study of

Figure 69-8 An isolated pig's chest wall is a useful model to teach tube thoracostomy.

junior doctors in the United Kingdom using the "SuperAnnie" chest tube task trainer showed that the teaching program, designed to teach technical skill before a procedure was first carried out on a patient, was effective in improving confidence and objectively measured skill levels.[70]

Central Lines

Central line insertion can be taught well with task trainers. Although they cannot simulate complications, an extensive discussion about pneumothorax, wire embolization, and accidental arterial catheterization can be held during teaching of the procedure. In a study of medical residents, central line insertion was taught in a 2-hour session involving didactic instruction, discussion, and training on *Blue Phantom* task trainers. Learners had significantly improved skills immediately after the session, although the authors did find that the instruction conferred no advantage over traditional learning in the longer term.[71] Simulation can also be used to reinforce the use and steps of a central line–associated bloodstream infection prevention checklist to ensure that learning of the procedure is associated from the beginning with proper sterile technique and infection control measures such as hand washing.

Suturing

Even though suturing is one procedure that EM residents and students rotating through the department get plenty of exposure to, novice learners are often more comfortable throwing their first stitches in a simulated environment. Watching an instructional video alone can increase learners' confidence in their skills,[72] and using grocery store animal parts can be a very realistic simulation of human skin. Pigs' feet and ears are most commonly used, cheap, and widely available. There are also synthetic skin simulators that are especially helpful in teaching advanced suturing skills such as approximating the vermilion border. It is important to discuss wound cleaning, choice of suture, and possible complications in addition to providing technical instruction. Suturing is often taught to large groups of learners, and one interesting study determined the ideal teacher-to-student ratio for suturing to be 1:4.[73]

Incision and Drainage

Incision plus drainage of an abscess is a relatively simple procedure and can easily be taught at the bedside. Abscesses are common, and even an inexperienced operator can perform incision and drainage successfully with appropriate step-by-step guidance. It is helpful to practice on simulation modules, which allows learners to approach the procedure with more confidence. Most simulations involve low-cost models created by instructors out of food-based substances such as tapioca pudding to simulate purulent material under simulated skin. One such model involving a maple syrup– and mayonnaise-filled balloon embedded in a chicken breast was found to be both a sonographically and physically accurate approximation of a typical skin abscess.[74]

ASSESSING PROCEDURAL COMPETENCY

Developing the skills necessary to perform a procedure independently is different for everyone, and successful learning depends on both the quality of each procedural experience and the number of procedures performed.[75] If procedures have been taught or practiced incorrectly, experience is not a useful predictor of procedural competency. When a learner performs a manual skill incorrectly, even once, it is much more difficult to relearn the correct technique.[22] If procedures are learned incorrectly without the benefit of guidance and remediation, the learner may inevitably take the role of instructor and pass these mistakes on to other learners through the teaching process.[76] To avoid this, particularly in the beginning, learners should be observed closely and corrected when mistakes are made. In the words of Red Auerbach, the legendary coach of the Boston Celtics, "Practice does not make perfect; perfect practice makes perfect."[22]

The actual number of procedures necessary to ensure competency is unknown. In the case of thoracotomy, a study by Chapman and colleagues failed to show a significant correlation between the clinician's previous procedural experience and actual performance as assessed by written, computerized, or animal models. Similarly, knowledge of thoracotomy content and procedural steps did not predict procedural competency.[77] Typically, the number of procedures performed previously is taken as being predictive of procedural competency. The findings by Chapman and associates, however, suggest that procedural competency cannot be predicted by numbers. Despite these findings, many hospitals use the number of procedures previously performed as a criterion for hospital credentialing and for granting the privilege to perform procedures independently.[76] Some surgical residencies have adopted competency-based education and report success with the use of fresh cadavers as models to achieve rapid improvement in surgical skills.[78]

The EM Residency Review Committee and the Accreditation Council for Graduate Medical Education have devised a broad list of procedures for which competence should be achieved by all EM physicians, and it includes suggested numbers.[79,80] It is up to the individual program to choose how to demonstrate and document competency, and no guidelines for this have been outlined. Direct observation, procedure workshops, and simulations are all used, but it is difficult to come up with a reliable, objective method of assessing competency, especially for procedures in which a bad outcome may be delayed. For example, most instructors are aware when a learner has poor intubation skills. Every step of this procedure is visible to an instructor and standardized, and a bad outcome is identifiable immediately. For other procedures, such as incision and drainage or suturing, the instructor may not be present, especially when the learner is more advanced, and a bad outcome would not necessarily be obvious until follow-up, which often does not occur in the ED.

Currently, no competency criteria for emergency procedures and resuscitations have been set by the American Board of Emergency Medicine (ABEM), and a minimum number of procedures has not been established. Nor has the ABEM established a mechanism for testing procedural competency and must rely on residencies to provide the necessary training, evaluation, and assurance of competency.[81] Braen and Munger described the early efforts of the ABEM in evaluating procedural skills,[81] but these were not implemented, primarily because of a lack of reliable equipment and resources to examine large pools of candidates in a high-stakes national examination. To standardize testing, there must be an assurance that examiners will be able to reliably evaluate candidates. Bullock and colleagues demonstrated good interrater reliability by both expert and nonexpert observers when they were given structured checklists to assess procedural skills.[82] Custalow and associates likewise observed excellent interrater reliability among expert reviewers for the evaluation of critical step performance of saphenous vein cutdown, thoracotomy, and cricothyroidotomy.[64] Surgical specialties use a variety of scoring systems, including the well-studied Objective Structured Assessment of Technical Skills, to evaluate learners' proficiency, and perhaps the use of similar tools should be considered for EM.[83,84]

Ideally, a national procedural competency examination might incorporate animal, cadaver, and virtual reality simulation laboratories to evaluate candidates.[85]

ONLINE RESOURCES FOR PROCEDURAL EDUCATION

The Internet is an invaluable resource for educators and learners on EM procedures. Self-posting websites such as YouTube contain a wealth of videos on nearly every procedure imaginable, some with detailed step-by-step instructions. Many EM residency programs have developed their own bank of procedure websites for either internal or widespread consumption. Standard medical resources, such as the *New England Journal of Medicine* procedure videos or interactive texts and journal articles available through portals such as MDConsults, are widely available. Websites such as Procedures Consult (www.proceduresconsult.com) provide rich multimedia content that covers a wide variety of procedures and is intended to be used as a primary didactic source or as a refresher at the point of care. Other societies or groups dedicated to specific procedures, such as AirwayWorld (www.airwayworld.com), or general compendia, such as the online Multimedia Procedure Manual (emprocedures.com), are easily accessible at little or no cost. Since adult learners bring a variety of learning styles to each educational encounter, providing trainees with a list of appropriate online resources dedicated to the procedure being taught can lead to more frequent practice and self-directed education throughout the knowledge acquisition process.

CONCLUSION

Numerous educational alternatives are available for teaching ED procedures, each with advantages and disadvantages. Optimally, residencies will have the space and resources to use a combination of training techniques to ensure competent performance of procedures by EM graduates. Educators may find new ways to teach time-proven techniques, refine these techniques, or even develop new ones. Many questions remain unanswered regarding the best educational methods, but EM has the foundation for building a comprehensive instructional system to ensure the competency of trainees and maintenance of procedural skills throughout life. With repetition and reinforcement, these skills may then be committed to long-term memory for retrieval when they are most needed in the ED.

Until a national standard for procedural competency is established for most procedures, the approach that seems to make the most sense is to provide learners with a variety of alternatives to bedside teaching, constructive criticism during bedside teaching, and feedback in both practice and real-life settings to ensure optimal technique and consolidate learning.

References are available at www.expertconsult.com

CHAPTER 70

Physical and Chemical Restraint

J. Michael Kowalski and Adam K. Rowden

Emergency clinicians often face the challenge of caring for agitated, uncooperative, combative, and violent patients who are unable to participate in their care or make rational health care decisions or are a danger not only to themselves but to medical personnel as well.[1,2] Psychiatric illness, acute chemical intoxication or withdrawal, various stages of delirium, medical illness, uncontrolled rage, hypoxia, and rarely, central nervous system infection are causes of agitated or violent behavior in the emergency department (ED).[1] Excited delirium syndrome (EXDS), a variant of and the extreme form of agitated delirium, is a recently defined syndrome (http://www.ncbi.nlm.nih.gov/pubmed/21440403).[3] EXDS is at the far end of the spectrum of agitation. It appears to be a specific entity with unique characteristics. EXDS can be fatal, often as a result of severe physiologic and metabolic derangements from the combination of underlying agitation and continued violent exertion, coupled with physical restraint.[3] Causes of agitated delirium include manic-depressive disorder, psychosis, chronic schizophrenia, intoxication with sympathomimetics or anticholinergics, cocaine intoxication, alcohol withdrawal, hypoglycemia, the postictal state, or head trauma. Some causes are idiopathic, but many are due to a combination of underlying psychiatric illness and stimulant drugs or alcohol (or both). Because of the variety of causes, management of agitated and combative patients requires a systematic approach (Fig. 70-1).

Patients more likely to exhibit severe uncontrolled agitation are those who abuse alcohol; sympathomimetic agents such as cocaine or methamphetamines or designer drugs such as ecstasy (MDMA), mephedrone, or methylone (bath salts); and hallucinogenic drugs such as phencyclidine (PCP). Patients can also experience toxicity after accidental and intentional ingestion of medications. Drug-associated delirium may be related to anticholinergic toxicity, serotonin syndrome, or intoxication with sympathomimetics. Alcohol withdrawal may progress to delirium tremens, a condition typified by excessive agitation and confusion.

Schizophrenia, schizoaffective disorder, and the manic phase of bipolar disorder can all lead to an impaired perception of reality. Paranoid delusions, hallucinations, and hostile moods that can easily lead to severe agitation often develop in patients with these disorders.

Any medical condition that leads to brain dysfunction may also result in agitated, combative, or violent behavior (Box 70-1). Well-documented examples include hypoglycemia, hypoxia, medication intoxication, encephalitis, meningitis, intracranial hemorrhage, thyrotoxicosis, traumatic brain injury, febrile illnesses in the elderly, and dementia.[4]

It is essential to achieve control of an agitated patient as quickly as possible. Goals of management include preventing patients from harming themselves and others, identifying the underlying cause, and initiating medical treatment. Early intervention allows caregivers to implement appropriate monitoring, perform a physical examination, initiate diagnostic testing, and institute timely treatment. Successfully achieving these goals often necessitates physical and chemical restraint.

During the late 1980s and early 1990s, reports of restraint-associated deaths in psychiatric and extended care facilities[5] led lawmakers to pass legislation establishing regulations for the use of restraint.[6] Since then, the Joint Commission for Accreditation of Healthcare Organizations (JCAHO) and the Center for Medicare and Medicaid Services (CMS) have created standards governing the use of restraint in a variety of health care settings, including EDs and tertiary care facilities (Box 70-2).[7,8] The aforementioned standards allow the use of physical restraint for a limited period. A licensed practitioner must evaluate the patient and determine that less restrictive interventions have been ineffective and physical restraint is required to ensure the patient's well-being. The standards also include requirements for written policies and procedures governing the use of restraint that must address indications, staff training and education, patient assessment and reevaluation, appropriate documentation, and patient-focused issues such as maintaining dignity and respect. Hospitals and extended care facilities are required by law to report any death or adverse event related to the use of restraint.[8]

Some authors have advocated "restraint-free" environments in nursing homes, extended care facilities, and acute care hospitals.[9] Although this concept is laudable, mandating a restraint-free ED is impractical and potentially dangerous. Clinicians should recognize the risks associated with restraining a patient; however, *they should not be deterred from using either physical or chemical restraint when patients demonstrate dangerous behavior toward themselves or others.* Indeed, the American College of Emergency Physicians (ACEP) recently reaffirmed their policy statement in 2007 by supporting the careful and appropriate use of physical and chemical restraint or seclusion.[10]

EXDS

In September 2009, a task force of the ACEP published a multiauthored White Paper Report on EXDS. This was a landmark report because it legitimized a heretofore poorly defined serious medical scenario that was familiar to law enforcement, emergency medical services, and emergency physicians. In addition, it supported the aggressive and potentially lifesaving use of chemical restraint.

It was the consensus of the task force that EXDS is a unique syndrome that may be identified by the presence of a distinctive group of clinical and behavioral characteristics that can be recognized in the premortem state. EXDS, though potentially fatal, may be amenable to early therapeutic intervention in some cases.

The task force defined the existence of excited delirium as a true disease entity; described the signs, symptoms, and risk for death; and reviewed current and emerging methods of control and treatment. Before this report, agitated delirium and various poorly defined related terms were used to describe a serious form of agitated delirium that could culminate in death. Such deaths were often high-profile news events that inexplicably occurred in seemingly healthy

Figure 70-1 Approach to undifferentiated delirium in the emergency department. Intramuscular benzodiazepines and antipsychotic agents are used for the treatment of acute agitation or violence in the emergency department. *H&P,* history and physical examination. (*Adpated from Rund DA, Ewing JD, Mitzel K, et al. The use of intramuscular benzodiazepines and antipsychotic agents in the treatment of acute agitation or violence in the emergency department.* J Emerg Med. *2006;31:317-324.*)

BOX 70-1 **Conditions That May Cause Agitated and Violent Behavior**

ENDOCRINE
Hypoglycemia
Hyperglycemia
Thyrotoxicosis, thyroid storm
Myxedema

INFECTIOUS
Meningitis
Encephalitis
Sepsis
Urinary tract infection

TOXICOLOGIC
Acute alcohol intoxication
Sympathomimetic intoxication
Anticholinergic intoxication
Delirium tremens
Alcohol withdrawal
Benzodiazepine withdrawal
Narcotic withdrawal

TRAUMATIC
Intracranial hemorrhage
Diffuse axonal injury
Hypoxia
Low-flow states secondary to
  systemic hemorrhage

METABOLIC
Hypoxia
Hypercapnia
Hyponatremia
Hypernatremia

NEUROLOGIC
Status epilepticus
Postictal states
Acute delirium
Subarachnoid hemorrhage
Cerebral vascular accident

---

young males and often involved interactions with seriously deranged and violent individuals and law enforcement officers.

The majority of affected individuals are young males. Features of EXDS include uncontrolled aggression and agitation, tremendous pain tolerance, tachypnea, tachycardia, sweating, tactile hyperthermia, pacing, grunting, noncompliance with police orders, unusual and untiring strength, being inappropriately clothed, extreme paranoia, and having an attraction to mirror or glass. Individuals are unable to engage in rational discussion or understand or deescalate their abnormal aggressive, violent, and threatening behavior. A common fatal scenario is characterized by a period of extreme delirium, increasing agitation, and inability to reason or comply with efforts to control their agitated state, followed by a struggle with law enforcement that involves vigorous physical restraint (choke holds, hog-tying, prone positioning, knee to the throat), noxious chemicals, or use of a TASER. Intervention may be followed by a sudden cessation of struggling that may herald death by cardiopulmonary arrest.

BOX 70-2 **TJC Requirements for Patient Restraint Protocols and Documentation**

RESTRAINT PROTOCOLS SHOULD INCLUDE
- Guidelines for assessing the patient
- Criteria for applying restraint
- Criteria for monitoring the patient and reassessing the need for restraint
- Monitoring at least every 2 hours or sooner based on patient needs
- Criteria for terminating restraint

DOCUMENTATION SHOULD INCLUDE
- Relevant orders for use
- Results of patient monitoring
- Reassessment
- Significant changes in the patient's condition

TJC, The Joint Commission.

The exact cause of death is rarely identified at autopsy because the incidence of underlying pathology (such as cardiomyopathy, conduction abnormalities, and metabolic disturbances) is unknown. Lack of complete prior medical information, especially underlying cardiac abnormalities, hampers ascertainment of the actual cause of death when only the autopsy results are interpreted.

Stimulant drug use, including cocaine, methamphetamine, and PCP, has a well-established association with EXDS and is usually implicated as being closely linked to if not causative of death from EXDS. Persons with psychiatric illnesses represent the second largest, but distinctly smaller cohort of EXDS cases. The combination of drugs, alcohol, and psychiatric illness is well recognized. Some deaths are temporally related to the application of a conducted electrical weapon (CEW; e.g., a TASER), but there are well-documented cases of EXDS-associated deaths with minimal restraint such as handcuffs without TASER use.

No definitive diagnostic tests are available for EXDS. Currently, it must still be identified by clinical features, which renders it very difficult to ascertain the true incidence. Though not universally fatal, it is clear that a proportion of individuals with EXDS progress to cardiac arrest and death regardless of medical intervention.

Although the specific precipitants of fatal EXDS remain unclear, epidemiologic and clinical reports provide some understanding of the underlying pathophysiology. The clinical picture is one of an agitated and delirious state with severe autonomic dysregulation. When available, cardiac rhythm analysis demonstrates bradycardiac asystole; ventricular dysrhythmias are rare and have occurred in only a single patient in one study. Severe acidosis and hyperthermia appear to play a prominent role in lethal EXDS-associated cardiovascular collapse. One potential cause is thought to be excessive central dopamine stimulation.

Based on the available evidence, it was the consensus of the task force that EXDS is a real syndrome of uncertain etiology. It was also a consensus of the panel that rapid and appropriate, albeit limited physical restraint measures and immediate administration of benzodiazepines and ketamine intravenously (IV) or midazolam intranasally may be lifesaving.

Importantly, insufficient data were available to the task force to determine whether fatal EXDS is preventable or whether there is a point of no return after which the patient will die regardless of advanced life support interventions.

MEDICOLEGAL CONCERNS

Emergency clinicians need to be cognizant of the potential legal ramifications stemming from physically restraining patients. The risk for litigation may be mitigated by strict adherence to written institutional and departmental policies regarding the use of restraint and medications. Unfortunately, no one-size-fits-all protocol is realistic, and each case must be individualized by a clinician at the bedside, often with little data or background on which to base a specific intervention. Emphasis should be placed on timely and comprehensive assessment before restraint, regular patient reevaluation, limitations on the time spent in restraint, and detailed documentation in the ED record. Furthermore, clinicians need to recognize that *competent patients* do have the

legal right to refuse medical treatment even if the result of their refusal is death or serious bodily harm. Competence, however, may be difficult to evaluate or ascertain in the time frame required to make important clinical decisions. There are many gray areas that cannot simply be solved by attempting to obtain a formal psychiatric consultation. In fact, there are no data proving that a psychiatrist is any better than an emergency physician in determining competence in an ED patient within the time frame of the ED evaluation, when important decisions must be made. Individuals with true EXDS are clearly mentally incompetent, but coercive measures, including physical restraint or the threat of physical restraint, should not be used simply because a competent patient refuses treatment or as retaliation for perceived disruptive behavior.[11]

PATIENT ASSESSMENT

Emergency clinicians must avoid ascribing agitated or abusive behavior to drug or alcohol intoxication or underlying psychiatric disease before considering severe, life-threatening diagnoses (see Box 70-1). Every attempt should be made to obtain a detailed history of issues related to the patient's condition, as well as the patient's past medical and psychiatric history, including medications, drug and alcohol use, and previous similar events. In reality, *such information is rarely available or accurate, thus leaving only the clinician's clinical judgment to guide therapy.*

Five groups of patients have been identified as being at increased risk for an underlying medical problem: the elderly, those with a history of substance abuse, patients without a previous psychiatric disorder, those with preexisting or new medical complaints, and individuals from lower socioeconomic groups.[12,13] Of these, patients with new psychiatric symptoms are especially worrisome and require careful evaluation for underlying medical illness.[14]

Physical examination should be aimed at identifying organic causes of the patient's behavior such as trauma, infection, and metabolic derangements. Rapid beside serum glucose determination should be performed on any patient with agitated or combative behavior. Temperature measurements, preferably rectal, should be obtained as soon as possible because hyperthermia may be indicative of an underlying central nervous system infection or drug-induced toxidrome. Evidence of head trauma in a patient who appears intoxicated warrants further evaluation to exclude traumatic brain injury.

Once a patient has been restrained, frequent periodic reevaluation is paramount to the patient's safety and is required by the JCAHO (see Box 70-2).[15] Reevaluation of restrained patients should include a reassessment of vital signs, neurologic status, respiratory status, skin condition, and perfusion of the extremities (Box 70-3). Physical restraints should be removed as soon as the clinician has determined that patients are no longer a risk to themselves or others.

DEESCALATION TECHNIQUES

Coburn and Mycyk described three phases of escalating violence: anxiety, defensiveness, and finally, physical aggression.[16] Recognition of this somewhat predictable pattern may help

---

BOX 70-3 **Recommended Areas to Assess during Reevaluation of Restrained Patients**

NEUROLOGIC STATUS
- Level of alertness
- Degree of agitation
- Pupillary examination
- Motor examination
- Sensory examination

VASCULAR STATUS
- Capillary refill
- Distal pulses

VITAL SIGNS
- Blood pressure
- Heart rate

- Respiratory rate
- Oxygen saturation
- Temperature

PATIENT COMFORT
- Skin under and around the restraints
- Hydration
- Personal hygiene
- Toileting needs

ASSESSMENT FOR RESTRAINT REMOVAL

Figure 70-2 Leather extremity restraint. *(Courtesy of Posey Company, Inc., Arcadia, CA.)*

in defusing a difficult situation before physical or chemical restraint is necessary. Indeed, several deescalation techniques have been shown to assist in quelling agitated and violent patients.[2]

One simple, yet effective technique is verbally engaging the patient by asking, "how can we help you?" This display of compassion on the part of the treating clinician and staff may calm the patient. Similarly, offering food and drink will often soothe an agitated patient. Along with these displays of caring and empathy, it is important to impress on the patient that violent behavior will not be tolerated and will be dealt with quickly and firmly.[2] If the patient continues to demonstrate agitated or violent behavior, enlist the aid of a family member or a specially trained individual, such as a social worker, psychiatric counselor, or member of the clergy.

If these conservative measures fail, summon hospital security to ensure the safety of the patient and staff. In these situations, security staff should not rush to the patient's bedside but instead should gather outside the door or close by, within eye contact of the patient's room. *A strong show of force* may calm a potentially violent patient without the need for restraint.

TYPES OF PATIENT RESTRAINT

Seclusion

The utility of seclusion in psychiatric evaluation units and inpatient hospital wards is well documented in both adult and pediatric populations.[17-20] In the mid-1980s, seclusion was commonly used to calm combative and violent ED patients, but its popularity has declined since then.[1,21,22] Reasons for this decline are unclear but probably include lack of adequate space and concerns regarding provision of medical care and compliance with regulatory agencies.[22] Nevertheless, at institutions with adequate physical space and well-designed policies and procedures, experience has shown that seclusion is an effective ED practice for selected patients.[22,23]

Seclusion involves placing agitated and violent patients in an isolated space and confining them to dedicated hospital stretchers or beds that are secured in place to prevent injury. Seclusion is often used in conjunction with chemical sedation,

physical restraint, or both.[22] The seclusion room should be located near ED staff to allow continuous patient observation. Regularly reassess patients who are placed in seclusion, similar to physically restrained patients (see Box 70-3).

Physical Restraint

Research regarding the application of physical restraint in the ED is limited. In one prospective study of restraint-associated complications in 298 ED patients, minor complications occurred in only 7% of patients, and there were no serious complications or deaths.[24] The author of this study concluded that the dangers of ED patient restraint promulgated by professional organizations and health care regulators may be overstated.[24] Moreover, this study supports the safe use of restraint by emergency clinicians, who by virtue of their training and experience are experts in recognizing signs of deterioration and skilled in airway management and resuscitation. It should also be noted that JCAHO sentinel event tracking has demonstrated a decreased rate of complications when patients are restrained on their sides.[16,25]

Although the actual prevalence of patient restraint in EDs is unknown, it has been estimated that 25% of teaching hospitals physically restrain at least one person per day.[1]

Restraint Devices
Limb Holders (Restraints)
Restraining a patient's extremities is the primary method of physical restraint used in the ED. Limb restraints are constructed from a variety of materials, including leather, synthetic leather, cotton, and single-use foam material. These materials provide restraint that differs in strength, ease of removal, and cleaning.

Hard leather and synthetic leather limb holders are virtually impossible to break or tear but are difficult to sterilize if they become soiled with blood or body fluids (Fig. 70-2). They are more rigid than soft restraints, which also makes them somewhat more difficult and time-consuming to apply. More importantly, most leather limb holders require a key to unlock and, as a result, might take longer to remove after an adverse event such as vomiting or respiratory arrest. Leather limb holders are generally used to restrain combative and violent patients in whom the need for indestructible secure restraints outweighs the more time-consuming application and removal process.

Figure 70-3 Cotton extremity restraint. (*Courtesy of Posey Company, Inc., Arcadia, CA.*)

Figure 70-4 Fifth-point restraint. (*Courtesy of Posey Company, Inc., Arcadia, CA.*)

Figure 70-5 Restraint vest. (*Courtesy of Posey Company, Inc., Arcadia, CA.*)

Figure 70-6 Hobble leg restraint. (*Courtesy of Posey Company, Inc., Arcadia, CA.*)

Soft limb restraints are usually made from cotton or foam material, or both (Fig. 70-3). They are single-use devices, which obviates the need for cleaning and sterilization. Soft limb restraints are less rigid than leather limb restraints, which makes them easier to apply. In addition, because they are fastened without the use of a key, soft limb restraints are more easily removed. Soft restraints are typically used for agitated but less combative patients because they are not as secure as leather limb holders.

Belts/Fifth-Point Restraint
A fifth-point restraint is a belt apparatus used to supplement the use of four limb restraints by holding down the thighs, chest, or pelvis (Fig. 70-4). A fifth-point restraint is used on patients who continue to be at risk for harming themselves despite adequate limb restraint and whose continued combative behavior interferes with diagnostic or therapeutic interventions. When patients are restrained across the thighs, chest, or pelvis, they may not be able to sit up or turn onto their sides, thus placing them at higher risk for aspiration should vomiting occur. Keep the side rails of the stretcher in the upright position at all times and place the belt snugly enough to prevent the patient from slipping under the device and thereby increasing the risk for accidental suffocation.

Fifth-point restraints are usually made of synthetic material and are available with both quick-release and key-release locks.

Jackets and Vests
Jackets and vests are generally used on inpatient wards and extended care facilities for the prevention of falls; they have little utility in the ED (Fig. 70-5). Moreover, these products have been implicated in a number of restraint-associated deaths secondary to choking and suffocation. The use of restraint jackets and vests in the ED is not recommended.

Hobble Leg Restraints
Hobble leg restraints limit movement by securing the patient's ankles with connecting locking cuffs (Fig. 70-6). Hobble leg restraints are commonly used by law enforcement agencies because they impede running and kicking, which makes them an effective method of transporting potentially violent patients and those who pose a risk for flight. Hobble leg restraints are seldom used in the ED, but their use by law enforcement agencies and prison authorities means that most emergency

Figure 70-7 The "hog-tie" method of restraint. The combination of prone positioning, hobble leg restraints, and binding a patient's hand behind the back is commonly referred to as a *hog tie*. Although this was a common method of restraining prisoners and violent psychiatric patients in the past, the hog tie is no longer recommended. The exact physiologic and metabolic derangements from this position by itself are probably minimal, but the practice is strongly discouraged.

Figure 70-8 Show of force. A minimum of five well-trained individuals should be available to restrain a patient. This show of force may help discourage the patient from resisting and is an important part of the restraint process.

clinicians will encounter patients placed in these devices. The combination of prone positioning, hobble leg restraints, and binding a patient's hands behind the back, commonly referred to as *hog-tying*, was a common method of restraining prisoners and violent psychiatric patients (Fig. 70-7). However, this practice is no longer widely used because of the risk for suffocation (see "Positional Asphyxia," later).

Indications

Use limb restraints to prevent agitated, combative, or violent patients from harming themselves or others. Frequently, the use of restraints can be delayed while verbal deescalation techniques are attempted (see "Deescalation Techniques," earlier). However, if a patient is deemed an immediate threat to himself or others, restrain him without delay. Patients with altered mental status may require limb restraints so that diagnostic testing can be completed or appropriate treatment rendered, or both. Use limb restraints also to prevent patients from interfering with devices, such as endotracheal tubes, cardiac monitors, and indwelling intravenous lines and catheters.

Contraindications

When appropriate, delay physical restraint in favor of trying verbal deescalation techniques. Do not place limb restraints on extremities with fractures, open wounds, or acute skin and soft tissue infections. Use caution to avoid ischemia in patients who exhibit tenuous perfusion of extremities, such as those with peripheral vascular disease or previous arterial injury or surgery.

Avoid fifth-point restraint of the abdomen and pelvic region in patients with pelvic fractures, suprapubic tubes, ostomies, and percutaneous feeding tubes. In addition, it is important to note that patients with underlying pulmonary or cardiac disease may not tolerate restraint of their thorax.

Procedure

Use a minimum of five people, all trained in restraint techniques and patient safety, to restrain the patient if possible (Fig. 70-8). This show of force may help discourage the patient from resisting and is an important part of the restraint process. The individuals making up the restraint team may

include clinicians, nurses, technicians, and police or hospital security. When possible, undress and place the patient in a hospital gown before attempting to apply physical restraint. When this is not practical, restrain the patient, but promptly search for weapons and potentially harmful belongings. Confiscate these items and account for them in accordance with institutional policies.

Always restrain patients in the supine rather than the prone position because the prone position increases the risk for suffocation. Assign one person to hold each limb firmly against the stretcher by applying direct pressure proximal to the elbows and knees. The fifth member of the team places restraints around the wrists and ankles (Fig. 70-9). Control above the elbows and knees reduces the risk for injury to these joints and concentrates force closer to the patient's center of gravity for better control.

Apply the limb holders snugly enough to control movement and prevent escape, but not so tight that they cause pain or impair circulation. If necessary, place a fifth-point restraint across the patient's thighs, pelvis, or chest to further limit motion. Place a surgical mask temporarily over the patient's mouth to prevent the patient from spitting at members of the restraint team or ED staff. If leather restraints are used, keep a restraint key readily available in the event that the restraints need to be removed urgently.

If four-point rather than five-point restraints are applied (i.e., use of extremity restraints only), consider placing one arm up alongside the head and the opposite arm down along the side of the body. In this position it is less likely the patient will be able to overturn the stretcher.[16]

Once the patient has been safely restrained, frequently assess pulses, capillary refill, skin color and temperature, and motor and sensory function. Reevaluate frequently in accordance with your institution's policies and procedures because this is key to preventing complications. In general, restraints should have well-defined time limits and should be removed as soon as the patient's condition has changed sufficiently that the patient is no longer a threat to self or others. For further details regarding rules, regulations, and recommendations for restraint procedures and patient assessment, the reader is referred to the JCAHO website at www.jointcommission.org.

Figure 70-9 Technique to restrain a violent patient. **A,** Patients should always be restrained in the supine position. One person is assigned to each limb, which is held firmly against the stretcher by applying direct pressure proximal to the elbows and knees. **B,** The fifth member of the team places restraints around the wrists and ankles. The limb holders should be applied snugly enough to control movement and prevent escape, but not so tight that they cause pain or impair circulation. If necessary, a fifth-point restraint may be placed across the patient's thighs, pelvis, or chest to further limit motion.

Complications

Increased Agitation

For some patients, placement in physical restraints is so emotionally disturbing that it actually increases agitation and combative behavior. Patients who continue to struggle despite restraints are at risk for a number of potentially serious adverse events, including skin damage, ischemia, metabolic acidosis, rhabdomyolysis, hyperthermia, and even death (see "Other Complications," later). In these patients the addition of chemical sedation is highly recommended (see "Chemical Restraint," later). In contrast, the use of extremity restraints alone is often effective in an alcohol-intoxicated patient because the natural progression of alcohol intoxication is sedation and sleep. Intoxicated patients may benefit from a brief period of observation before a decision is made to administer chemical sedation. Most of these patients will fall asleep, thereby obviating the need for sedation and the accompanying risks.

Local Skin Complications

Restraints may cause skin irritation or breakdown. Risk factors include restraints that are too tight and those that have been left on for prolonged periods. Leather restraints are more likely than soft restraints to cause skin damage, particularly in patients who continue to struggle despite being placed in restraints. To help prevent skin complications, use soft restraints whenever possible, avoid overly tight restraints, limit restraint time, and reevaluate the patient frequently. In addition, use chemical restraint judiciously to help avoid skin damage in patients who continue to struggle. It is important to not ignore a patient's complaints of restraint pain without first evaluating the possibility of an adverse event.

Vascular Compromise

Restraints have the rare potential to impede blood flow to the hands and feet. In extreme cases, this could result in ischemia of the distal end of the extremity. Ischemia is more likely to occur in patients whose restraints are placed too tightly and in those in whom swelling develops as a result of an occult injury. Struggling against the restraints may further increase this risk. A thorough search for occult injuries, attention to proper fit, and limited restraint time will help avoid ischemia. Frequent assessment of pulses, capillary refill, skin color and temperature, and motor and sensory function is also extremely important. As mentioned previously, it is also important to not ignore a restrained patient's complaints regarding extremity pain without first evaluating for the possibility of ischemia.

Respiratory Compromise

Restraints may impair respiratory mechanics in some patients. This is more likely to occur in patients restrained in the prone or hog-tied positions and in those with underlying pulmonary disease.[26-30] Patients with chronic obstructive pulmonary disease (COPD) may not tolerate a fifth-point restraint across the chest. Avoid respiratory complications by not restraining patients in the prone or *hog-tied* position. In addition, use adequate chemical sedation to help negate the need for a supplemental restraint belt in patients with underlying COPD.

Positional Asphyxia

Positional asphyxia is a poorly elucidated respiratory complication often attributed to the use of restraints that results in asphyxia and eventually death. The specifics of respiratory embarrassment secondary to physical restraint are vague and unproven and have not been reproduced in volunteers, who do not experience severe pulmonary compromise from restraint. *Thus, though often implicated, the exact contribution of restraint to sudden death is unclear.* Obesity, underlying cardiac and pulmonary disease, prone positioning, and concurrent stimulant use are thought to be contributing factors.[26,28,30-33] The hog-tied position (see Fig. 70-7), in which a patient's hands and feet are bound behind the back, places a patient at theoretical risk for positional asphyxia and should therefore not be used in the ED.[26-28,33-36] Placing restrained patients in the supine position and frequently reevaluating them will help prevent positional asphyxia. Continuous monitoring of respiratory status, including oxygenation and tidal volume, is indicated in all physically restrained and chemically sedated patients, especially those with obesity, COPD, or intoxication from stimulant drugs.

Cocaine-Associated Agitated Delirium

Cocaine-associated agitated delirium is a syndrome consisting of hyperthermia with delirium and severe agitation that can progress to multisystem failure, coagulopathy, respiratory arrest, and death.[28,30,32,34,37] Much of the pathology may be due to cocaine alone, but restrained patients appear to be at particularly high risk for this syndrome. The syndrome was first described in 1985, but its incidence increased significantly in the 1990s because of the popularity of crack cocaine.[34,35]

The pathophysiology of cocaine-associated agitated delirium is a complex process involving downregulation of dopamine receptors with subsequent dopamine excess during times of cocaine binges.[34,38-40] When patients with cocaine-associated agitated delirium are restrained, especially in the prone position, interference with normal respiratory mechanics increases the likelihood of hypoventilation, hypercapnia, and hypoxemia and ultimately leads to asphyxia and death. It has also been suggested that the stress caused by the restraining process increases the risk for fatal cardiac arrhythmias secondary to catecholamine surge in an already cocaine-sensitized myocardium.[34] Chronic stimulant use leads to adrenergic-induced cardiomyopathy, which is often clinically silent until the individual is severely stressed. The potential for malignant arrhythmias is unknown, but they have been implicated in some cases of sudden death in restrained patients.

Metabolic Acidosis

In patients who have been restrained, continued agitation and struggling can lead to severe metabolic acidosis.[37] Their pH is often lower than 7.0. The etiology of this acidosis is unclear but probably involves the production of lactic acid from physical exertion compounded by sympathetic-induced vasoconstriction. Such vasoconstriction may result from agitation or cocaine (and other stimulant) use and is believed to enhance exercise-induced lactic acidosis by impeding clearance of lactate by the liver.[41,42] In some patients the buildup of lactate is further increased by the presence of psychosis and delirium, which may alter pain sensation and allow exertion far beyond normal physiologic limits.[37] In addition, some restraint positions (e.g., prone, hog-tied) may not allow adequate respiratory compensation, thereby resulting in further enhancement of the acidosis. A common scenario is an out-of-hospital cardiac arrest in which a severely agitated individual suddenly stops struggling and experiences a bradycardic, asystolic death that is not immediately recognized. Such patients may have been subdued by force, by TASER, or by mace or pepper spray, which has led to unproven speculation that these interventions may have caused the change in patient status.

Regardless of the etiology, profound metabolic acidosis has been associated with cardiovascular collapse and sudden and unexpected death in restrained patients.[37] Individuals suffer a bradycardic, pulseless electrical activity, asystolic cardiac arrest, and resuscitation is unlikely once cardiac arrest ensues. Patients who remain combative despite restraints, especially those who have used cocaine or other sympathomimetic agents, are at particularly high risk for death.[37] Clues to the presence of metabolic acidosis include severe agitation, abnormal vital signs (e.g., persistent tachycardia, tachypnea, and hyperpyrexia), and decreased or concentrated urine output despite adequate intravenous fluid administration. Laboratory testing, including arterial blood gas analysis, serum electrolytes, and serum creatine phosphokinase, is recommended in patients with signs and symptoms suggestive of metabolic acidosis and in those with potentially lethal co-ingestion (e.g., salicylates and toxic alcohols).

Restrained patients with severe metabolic acidosis should receive aggressive saline hydration and sedation with benzodiazepines to counteract the sympathetic hyperactivity.[37] The utility of sodium bicarbonate is unknown and it is probably best reserved for patients with a pH below 7.0.

Chemical Restraint

Agitation leading to delirium and culminating in EXDS is a continuum with no rigidly defined parameters. This chapter discusses the treatment of mild agitation, as well as life-threatening EXDS, but it is important to realize that the recommendations are subject to alteration or modification depending on the degree of impairment and the necessity of clinician to intervene differently in individuals with varying degrees of impairment. The exact role of chemical restraint will always be a clinical judgment call made at the bedside and based on the scenario at hand. It is, however, axiomatic that chemical restraint is mandated when physical restraint and other modalities have failed. *Medically compromised patients who appear mentally incompetent, are unable to comprehend or participate in the evaluation or treatment of a serious medical condition, or are otherwise unable to cooperate with required diagnostic or therapeutic medical interventions should be chemically restrained.*

Chemical restraint, more aptly termed chemical sedation, describes the act of quelling an agitated patient by the administration of approved sedative-hypnotic, antipsychotic, or dissociative medications. Early, liberal use of appropriate anxiolytic and sedating medications permits thorough evaluation of a patient's medical condition. In some cases, administration of anxiolytic drugs (e.g., benzodiazepines) may be the optimal treatment of a person with an undifferentiated delirious state such as delirium tremens.[43] This is supported by Khan and associates, who identified an association between the use of physical restraint and death in patients with delirium tremens.[44] Although a clear causal relationship between restraint and death is lacking, early use of chemical sedation may be safer than physical restraint for treatment of an undifferentiated delirium.

The CMS states that chemical restraint is "a medication used to control behavior or to restrict the patient's freedom of movement and is not a standard treatment for the patient's medical or psychiatric condition."[8] The JCAHO defines chemical restraint as "the inappropriate use of a sedating psychotropic drug to manage or control behavior."[15] These definitions lack perspective on the use of chemical sedation in the ED, where these medications are typically used after all other measures fail and the health and safety of the patient or staff are threatened. *Such statements do not reflect standard care in the ED and should not be interpreted as prohibition of the appropriate short-term use of chemical sedation.*

The pathogenesis of agitation is poorly understood; however, the advent of anxiolytic and antipsychotic medications has revolutionized the treatment of acute agitation. Not only has sedation become safer, but many of these new agents also have the added benefit of treating underlying psychotic states.[4] Benzodiazepines, with rare exception, have replaced barbiturates for the treatment of acute agitation. Recently, intramuscular preparations of "atypical antipsychotic" medications such as olanzapine, ziprasidone, and aripiprazole have provided additional treatment options for rapid control of acute psychosis.[45,46]

Oral administration of a medication implies consent on behalf of patients since they must cooperate to ingest it.

Previous reports have shown that patients prefer oral formulations of medications during the treatment of psychotic episodes.[47] Furthermore, patients may feel as though they are participating in their own care plan.[48] Oral lorazepam and oral risperidone have demonstrated increased efficacy when compared with the intramuscular administration of haloperidol.[49] However, in the ED setting, where rapid tranquilization is usually the goal, medications are typically administered IV or intramuscularly (IM). Obtaining early intravenous access allows titration of rapidly acting medications but may not be possible in some patients. When intravenous access is not possible, intramuscular administration is recommended and in some cases has been shown to be as efficacious and safe as intravenous administration.[50] Other routes (oral, transmucosal) may be used when parenteral administration is not practical or feasible.

An ideal drug for chemical sedation in the ED should have multiple routes of administration (e.g., intravenous, intramuscular, transmucosal), a rapid onset of action, negligible hemodynamic effects, and a good safety record with minimal adverse effects. Although no medication fits this profile perfectly, with proper patient assessment and careful drug selection, most ED patients can be rapidly and safely sedated. The remainder of this chapter discusses the safety, efficacy, side effect profile, and recommended dosages of the medications most commonly used for chemical sedation. Recommendations for drug selection are also discussed (Table 70-1).

Other Methods of Drug Delivery

Under most circumstances. sedative medications are best administered IV. A peripheral vein is adequate but may be difficult to access or maintain in a struggling patient. Although an indwelling catheter is preferable, to titrate escalating doses, the first dose may be directly administered into a peripheral vein via a syringe/needle, so-called mainlining (Fig 70-10). A large extremity vein in the arm or leg is usually available if the extremity can be adequately immobilized. The external jugular vein presents another route. The head can often be more easily stabilized than a muscular extremity, and the external jugular vein is usually quite prominent in a struggling patient. Note that some antipsychotics, such as olanzapine and ziprasidone, have indications only for use IM. Haloperidol is universally administered IV, although it has no formal indication for this route. Intranasal midazolam is another alternative route of administration that may have prehospital utility.

Indications

Chemical sedation is used to prevent patients from injuring themselves or others, attenuate psychosis, decrease the time spent in physical restraint, and calm patients enough to permit a medical history, physical examination, diagnostic testing, and procedures.

Contraindications and Adverse Effects

Absolute and relative contraindications, as well as adverse effects, vary by medication and are discussed separately for each drug.

Neuroleptic Agents

Neuroleptic medications or "typical antipsychotics" have been used safely and effectively for years to manage patients with undifferentiated agitated delirium in the ED. The antipsychotic effects of neuroleptic agents do not usually take place for 7 to 10 days, but the onset of sedation is rapid, thus making them useful to calm an acutely agitated patient. Potent neuroleptic agents such as haloperidol and droperidol are preferred because they lack tolerance after repeated uses, have a low addiction potential, and possess a high therapeutic index. Low-potency neuroleptics such as chlorpromazine are less desirable because of a higher incidence of hypotension, seizures, and anticholinergic effects.[51]

Contraindications

Haloperidol and droperidol are contraindicated in patients with thyrotoxicosis (neurotoxicity may develop), Parkinson's disease, or severe hepatic disease. These drugs can lower the seizure threshold, so they should be used with caution or be avoided altogether in patients with a history of seizures or those who may be at known risk for the development of seizures (i.e., meningitis, sympathomimetic intoxication). Nevertheless, droperidol has been used safely to manage patients with known seizure disorders.[52] In addition, like all neuroleptic agents, haloperidol and droperidol can cause QT prolongation. Therefore, they should be used with caution in patients at risk for QT prolongation and torsades de pointes (Box 70-4). Droperidol has also been associated with serotonin syndrome in patients taking lysergic acid diethylamide (LSD) and should be avoided in these patients.[51,53]

Adverse Effects

Adverse effects common to all neuroleptic agents include extrapyramidal symptoms (EPSs), QTc prolongation, neuroleptic malignant syndrome (NMS), hypotension, and cholinergic receptor antagonism.

EPSs include akathisia (restlessness), dystonia (muscular spasms of the neck, eyes [oculogyric crisis], tongue, or jaw), drug-induced parkinsonism (muscle stiffness, shuffling gait, drooling, tremor), and tardive dyskinesia. These effects are due to the drugs' antidopaminergic action and, though distressing to the patient, are seldom if ever life-threatening. Anticholinergic agents such as diphenhydramine (25 to 50 mg orally [PO], IM, or IV) and benztropine (1 to 2 mg PO, IM, or IV) are very effective in preventing or minimizing EPSs.

A potentially deadly, but exceedingly rare effect of neuroleptic drug use is prolongation of the QTc interval, which can lead to torsades de pointes, a polymorphic ventricular arrhythmia that can progress to ventricular fibrillation and sudden death.[4] Droperidol has been the most publicized agent associated with QTc prolongation. It is currently the only neuroleptic agent that has received a "black box warning" for its propensity to cause QTc prolongation and sudden death.[54] In addition, a number of case reports and small case series have documented QTc prolongation and torsades de pointes after the administration of haloperidol.[55] Risk factors for QTc prolongation and torsades de pointes are listed in Box 70-4.

Patients in whom symptoms of NMS develop exhibit autonomic instability, including rigidity of the extremities, hyperthermia, and delirium. Treatment includes cooling measures, sedation with benzodiazepines, and in severe cases, bromocriptine, dantrolene, neuromuscular paralysis, and endotracheal intubation.[51]

Hypotension is usually orthostatic in nature and tends to be more pronounced when the drugs are administered IV. In general, haloperidol and droperidol have a lower incidence of hypotension than do lower-potency neuroleptic agents.

TABLE 70-1   Drugs Used for Chemical Restraint in the ED

AGENT	DOSAGE	ONSET/DURATION OF ACTION	INDICATIONS	CONTRAINDICATIONS	ADVERSE EVENTS	COMMENTS*
Haloperidol	Adults: 5 mg IM/IV Children: 6-12 yr: 1-3 mg >12 yr: 2.5-5 mg	Onset: 30-45 min Duration: 4-24 hr	All forms of agitation	Patients with a history of QT prolongation, thyrotoxicosis, Parkinson's disease, and severe hepatic disease	EPSs, QTc prolongation, NMS, hypotension, cholinergic blockade	Can be given alone or in combination with a benzodiazepine; may lower the seizure threshold
Droperidol	Adults: 5 mg IM/IV Children: 0.03-0.07 mg/kg (maximum, 2.5 mg)	Onset: 3-10 min Duration: 2-12 hr	All forms of agitation	Patients with a history of QT prolongation, thyrotoxicosis, Parkinson's disease, severe hepatic disease, and intoxication with LSD	EPSs, QTc prolongation, NMS, hypotension, cholinergic blockade	Black box warning regarding QT prolongation and serious arrhythmias; rapid-onset IM; use with caution in children
Lorazepam	Adults: 2-4 mg IM/IV Children: 0.05-0.1 mg/kg	Onset: IV: 15-20 min Duration: 8-10 hr	All forms of agitation	Patients with respiratory depression and pregnant women	Respiratory depression, ataxia, hypotension	First-line therapy for children; use with caution in patients with alcohol intoxication because of the risk for respiratory depression
Diazepam	Adults: 5-10 mg IV Children: not indicated	Onset: IV: 1-5 min Duration: 15-60 min	All forms of agitation	Patients with respiratory depression and pregnant women	Respiratory depression, ataxia, hypotension	Use with caution in patients with alcohol intoxication because of the risk for respiratory depression
Midazolam	Adults: 5 mg IM/IV Children: 0.1-0.2 mg/kg	Onset: IV: 3 min IM: 5 min Duration: 30-120 min	All forms of agitation	Patients with respiratory depression and pregnant women	Respiratory depression, ataxia, hypotension	First-line therapy for children; rapid onset IM; use with caution in patients with alcohol intoxication because of the risk for respiratory depression
Ziprasidone	Adults: 10-20 mg IM Children: not indicated	Onset: 15-30 min Duration: 4 hr	Psychoses, intoxications	Patients with dementia	QT prolongation, somnolence, EPSs	Lower incidence of EPS than with haloperidol and droperidol; black box warning regarding use in elderly patients with dementia

Continued

TABLE 70-1   Drugs Used for Chemical Restraint in the ED—cont'd

AGENT	DOSAGE	ONSET/DURATION OF ACTION	INDICATIONS	CONTRAINDICATIONS	ADVERSE EVENTS	COMMENTS*
Olanzapine	Adults: 5-10 mg IM Children: not indicated	Onset: 15-30 min Duration: 2-24 hr	Psychiatric illness	Patients with dementia	Somnolence, EPSs	Lower incidence of EPS than with haloperidol and droperidol; black box warning regarding use in elderly patients with dementia
Aripiprazole	Adults: 5.25-9.75 mg IM (maximum, 30 mg/day) Children: not indicated	Onset: 15-30 min Duration: unknown	Psychiatric illness	Patients with dementia, leukopenia, or neutropenia	NMS, EPSs	Black box warning to avoid use for dementia-related psychosis; may cause or increase suicidal ideation
Ketamine	Adults/children: 1.5-2 mg/kg IV, 4-5 mg/kg IM	Onset: IV: 1 min IM: 3-5 min Duration IV: 15 min IM: 30 min The duration listed is for dissociation; full recovery takes longer	Acute agitation	Acute upper respiratory infection, children <3 mo of age	Emergence phenomenon, potential increased intracranial and intraocular pressure, hypertension, tachycardia, salivation, vomiting, laryngospasm	Doses provided are for achieving a dissociative state; use ketamine when rapid sedation is required for lifesaving interventions

ED, emergency department; *EPSs*, extrapyramidal symptoms; *IM*, intramuscularly; *IV*, intravenously; *NMS*, neuroleptic malignant syndrome; *LSD*, lysergic acid diethylamide.
*Many of the caveats concerning the safety and efficacy of long-term use cannot be equated to short-term ED use. These medications are currently often used in doses far exceeding those recommended by the manufacturer or under other clinical circumstances; safety and efficacy for short-term sedation have been demonstrated in clinical ED practice.

Figure 70-10 When intravenous (IV) access is problematic in a patient in urgent need of IV sedation, an alternative is to mainline medication into a large vein directly from a syringe. The external jugular vein (**A**) is usually prominent in a struggling patient, and the head and upper part of the torso are easier to control than an extremity. A finger occluding the distal end of the vein (arrow) allows better access. Other options include the antecubital fossa (**B**) and the greater saphenous ankle vein (**C**) if the respective extremity can be temporarily immobilized. Use a 23- to 25-gauge needle. When blood is aspirated, push the medication.

Likewise, the anticholinergic effects (e.g., confusion, dry mouth, blurred vision, urinary retention) of haloperidol and droperidol are much less severe than those of the lower-potency agents.

Haloperidol

Haloperidol is a neuroleptic and a butyrophenone. It is categorized as a high-potency neuroleptic because of its strong antidopaminergic activity. The antidopaminergic activity is

---

NONPHARMACOLOGIC

- Congenital long QT syndromes
- Cardiac disorders (ventricular hypertrophy, heart failure, bradycardia)
- Electrolyte imbalance (especially hypokalemia)
- Overdose of an antipsychotic drug
- Female sex
- Use of restraints and psychological stress
- Substance abuse
- Miscellaneous factors (obesity, hypothyroidism)
- Elderly patients
- Renal and hepatic impairment

PHARMACOLOGIC

Pharmacokinetic Factors

- Inhibition of specific cytochrome P-450 enzymes
- Competition for specific cytochrome P-450 enzymes

Pharmacodynamic Factors

- Independent QTc prolongation

---

responsible for both its intended effects against delusions, hallucinations, and psychomotor agitation and its unintended parkinsonian symptoms. Administration of haloperidol both alone and in combination with benzodiazepines has been evaluated in a large number of clinical trials.[56-61] *These studies have demonstrated the use of haloperidol IM to be both safe and effective for the management of acute agitation from virtually any cause.*

Dosage and Administration. Haloperidol can be administered PO, IV, and IM and has a low incidence of oversedation regardless of which route is chosen.[4] Despite a lack of U.S. Food and Drug Administration (FDA) approval for use IV, haloperidol is typically administered IV. The recommended starting dosage to achieve sedation is 5 mg IM or IV, titrated to effect. There is no absolute maximum dose, and in cases of severe EXDS, doses of 10 to 30 mg are common. Occasionally, extrapyramidal reactions occur but are easily treated. The dose should be halved when administered to elderly patients. In children 6 to 12 years of age, the dosage is 1 to 3 mg IM every 4 to 8 hours with a maximum of 0.15 mg/kg/day. Children older than 12 years can receive the adult dosage. Haloperidol administered IM has a peak clinical effect within 30 to 45 minutes and may last up to 24 hours when given for acute agitation. Haloperidol is metabolized by the liver and excreted by the kidneys.[62]

Droperidol

Droperidol, an analogue of haloperidol, is a high-potency butyrophenone with rapid sedating effects. It also possesses significant antidopaminergic activity. Droperidol acquired FDA approval in 1970 first as an antiemetic and antipsychotic agent. Soon thereafter, psychiatric EDs found it useful for chemical sedation.[63] Many physicians prefer droperidol to haloperidol because of its more rapid onset and shorter duration of action.

Use of droperidol as a chemical sedative continued until 2001, at which time the FDA issued a "black box" warning regarding the potential for fatal dysrhythmias.[64] Many hospitals and pharmacies subsequently sought to restrict or prohibit its use. However, two large retrospective studies encompassing more than 15,000 patients failed to demonstrate increased morbidity or mortality associated with the use of droperidol for the management of acute agitation.[52,63] This controversy prompted an independent review of the data submitted to the FDA that led to the black box warning. The authors of this review found a number of anomalies and duplicate reports. *They concluded that droperidol is a safe drug when used at the recommended dosage (i.e., 5 to 10 mg).*[65] Despite an apparent lack of evidence behind the black box warning, use of droperidol has declined dramatically.[66]

Studies comparing a variety of agents for rapid sedation have found that droperidol provides more rapid and effective control than do lorazepam,[67] haloperidol,[56] midazolam,[68,69] and ziprasidone.[68] In addition, droperidol has been proved to be safe in patients with head injuries, alcohol and cocaine intoxication, and seizure disorders.[52]

Dosage and Administration. The initial dosage used for sedation is 5 mg IV or IM. Its onset of action is 3 to 10 minutes with a peak clinical effect achieved in 30 minutes. The elimination half-life is 2 to 4 hours, but the sedative effects of droperidol may last up to 12 hours.[70]

Benzodiazepines

All benzodiazepines enhance the neurotransmission of γ-aminobutyric acid and thereby result in anxiolysis, sedation, hypnosis, and muscle relaxation. This combination makes them an excellent choice for tranquilization of agitated patients. *Because of an excellent safety profile, benzodiazepines are an excellent choice for sedating medically undifferentiated patients.* The differences in clinical effects (e.g., onset, duration, adverse effects) are primarily related to dosage, route of administration, and pharmacokinetics. Benzodiazepines can be used as single agents or in combination with an antipsychotic drug. Lorazepam and midazolam are the benzodiazepines most commonly used for chemical sedation. This is probably due to their rapid and predictable absorption when given IV or IM, as well as a long history of safety and efficacy. Unlike neuroleptics, benzodiazepines do not treat underlying psychiatric disorders. Some clinicians prefer to administer diazepam IV for the treatment of delirium related to sedative-hypnotic withdrawal.[43]

Contraindications

There are few contraindications to the use of benzodiazepines as a chemical sedating agent. Because of the possibility of respiratory depression, use benzodiazepines with caution in patients in respiratory distress.

Adverse Effects

As discussed previously, benzodiazepines may cause respiratory depression. Additionally, hypotension, deep sedation, and paradoxical agitation have been reported. However, when administered in the doses recommended for agitation, adverse events are rare, thus *making benzodiazepines the drugs of choice in most circumstances.*

Respiratory compromise is dose dependent and typically occurs only in the presence of other respiratory depressants.[71,72] Because of an increased risk for respiratory depression, administer benzodiazepines cautiously to elderly patients and those with chronic pulmonary diseases such as apnea and COPD. In healthy patients, particularly those suffering from agitated delirium, respiratory depression is very unlikely to occur, even when large doses of benzodiazepines are used. If available, end-tidal carbon dioxide monitoring (e.g., capnography) may assist the practitioner in detecting the onset of respiratory depression before it becomes clinically significant.[73,74]

The most appropriate benzodiazepine is the one that the clinician is most comfortable administering and that has a duration of action most appropriate for the clinical situation. Titrate all benzodiazepines administered IV until the desired level of sedation is reached. *In the setting of severe delirium, there is no maximum dose described for any benzodiazepine, and doses well in excess of the manufacturer's recommendation and even considered toxic under other circumstances are commonly used.* One difference that does bear mentioning is the use of propylene glycol, a solvent needed to keep non–water-soluble benzodiazepines (e.g., lorazepam, diazepam) in solution. In large doses, propylene glycol can cause an increased osmolar gap and metabolic acidosis and may precipitate or contribute to hypotension in some patients.

Lorazepam

Lorazepam is the benzodiazepine most frequently studied for the management of acute agitation. It enjoys popularity as part of the well-known "five and two" treatment regimen, which consists of haloperidol, 5 mg IM, and lorazepam, 2 mg IM.[75] In a number of clinical trials, lorazepam was shown to be an effective drug for rapid chemical sedation.[57,60,61,67] In these studies lorazepam had no extrapyramidal effects and was better tolerated than the neuroleptics. However, when compared with haloperidol, droperidol, midazolam, and a combination of haloperidol and lorazepam, the onset of sedation after administering lorazepam IM was more delayed.[57,60,67]

Dosage and Administration. When used alone, lorazepam is usually given in 2- to 4-mg doses and can be administered PO, sublingually, IM, IV, or rectally. No maximum dose has been established. Following an injection of lorazepam IM, adequate sedation is usually achieved in 30 to 45 minutes.[67] When given IV, sedation occurs in 15 to 20 minutes.[60] The elimination half-life is 12 to 15 hours, which produces a duration of effect of 8 to 10 hours. This makes lorazepam a better choice when long-term sedation is the goal. Lorazepam is rapidly conjugated to an inactive glucuronide. This does not require involvement of the cytochrome P-450 system, so lorazepam has few drug-drug interactions. Preparations of lorazepam intended for use IV or IM must be refrigerated, thus potentially limiting its use in underdeveloped countries and in the prehospital setting.[4]

Midazolam

Midazolam has been shown to be effective for rapid sedation.[59,60,68,69] It has a more rapid onset and shorter duration of action than other benzodiazepines do, which makes it a good choice when rapid short-term sedation is desired. Midazolam also compares favorably with haloperidol, droperidol, and ziprasidone for the treatment of acute agitation in the ED.[59,60,69] With the exception of droperidol, which had a similar time until onset (5 to 10 minutes), midazolam had a more rapid onset of sedation than the other drugs did in these studies. The studies also noted that midazolam, as expected, had a shorter duration of sedation.

Dosage and Administration. The initial dosage for an agitated adult is 5 mg IV or IM, and it may be repeated at 5- to

10-minute intervals. No maximum dose has been established. Nasal administration is also an option. The onset of sedation occurs approximately 3 minutes after intravenous administration, 5 minutes after an intramuscular injection, and 15 minutes after nasal administration. Midazolam is hydroxylated by the cytochrome P-450 system to its primary metabolite, α-hydroxymidazolam, which undergoes glucuronide conjugation before being excreted in urine. Its duration of action is between 30 and 120 minutes and does not vary significantly by route of administration.[60,76]

Diazepam

Diazepam has a long history of safe use in the management of agitated delirium, especially delirium tremens and alcohol withdrawal.[43,77] For patients experiencing delirium tremens the usual dose is 5 to 10 mg IV every 5 to 10 minutes until the desired level of sedation is achieved (lower doses are appropriate for less severe agitation or agitation from other causes). No maximum dose has been established, and doses of up to 2000 mg have been used safely over a 24-hour period in patients experiencing delirium tremons.[43,78] Because of erratic absorption, intramuscular administration of diazepam is not recommended. Following the administration of diazepam, peak sedation is reached in about 5 to 6 minutes, which allows additional titrated doses if the desired clinical effect is not achieved initially.

Atypical Antipsychotic Agents

Atypical antipsychotic agents have high affinity for 5-HT (serotonin) receptors and less affinity for D_1 and D_2 receptors. As a result, they have a lower incidence of EPSs than haloperidol and droperidol do.[62] In the past, medications in this class were available only in an oral formulation, thus limiting their use in the management of acute agitation. Recently, formulations of ziprasidone, olanzapine, and aripiprazole intended for administration IM have been developed. When administered IM, all three drugs are effective for the treatment of acute agitation.[79] Moreover, the combination of administration IM and the low incidence of EPSs makes these newer agents an attractive option for rapid sedation of ED patients with undifferentiated agitation. This is particularly true for patients with a history of mental illness, for whom this class of medications is now considered to be appropriate first-line management.[80]

Contraindications

In 2005, a metaanalysis of placebo-controlled trials demonstrated an increased risk for death associated with the atypical antipsychotic agents used to treat *elderly patients with dementia-related psychosis*.[81] This report led the FDA to issue a black box warning regarding the use of atypical antipsychotics for "behavioral disorders" in elderly patients with dementia. Such *warnings have not resulted in the prohibition of such agents for short-term use in the ED*. The FDA has also advised caution with ziprasidone because of its tendency to prolong the QTc interval, especially when used in patients taking other drugs or with medical conditions that increase the risk for prolongation of the QTc interval (see Box 70-4).[81] Ziprasidone prolongs the QTc interval more frequently than haloperidol, droperidol, and olanzapine do,[4] but the degree of prolongation is considered minor and is rarely greater than 500 msec.[82] To date, there have been no clinical reports of adverse events as a result of QTc prolongation with the short-term ED use of atypical antipsychotic agents. Experience with these agents

in undifferentiated acutely agitated patients in the ED is limited, but their use is increasing, and although initial reports are supportive, they are not yet definitive.

Adverse Effects

Atypical antipsychotic agents may cause somnolence, EPSs (though less often than with haloperidol and droperidol), QTc prolongation, and rarely, anticholinergic symptoms and NMS.

Ziprasidone

Ziprasidone is a benzylisothiazolylpiperazine antipsychotic agent whose effects are the result of dopamine and serotonin 5-HT$_{2A}$ receptor antagonism.[4,79,83] This was the first atypical antipsychotic agent available in a fast-acting preparation administered IM. In a double-blind, randomized study, Martel and coworkers[68] noted that ziprasidone was as effective as midazolam and droperidol in controlling acute agitation. Patients receiving ziprasidone and droperidol took longer to be sedated (30 minutes as compared with 15 minutes for midazolam) but were more deeply sedated at 60 and 120 minutes.[68] In a prospective, open-label study, ED patients receiving ziprasidone exhibited progressive improvement in anxiety, hostility, and cooperativeness starting at 15 minutes and continuing through the 90-minute study period.[46] In an observational study of agitated psychiatric ED patients with nonspecific psychosis, alcohol intoxication, or substance-induced psychosis, ziprasidone, 20 mg IM, was effective in sedating patients as early as 15 minutes.[84] Ziprasidone has not been approved by the FDA for the treatment of dementia-related psychosis.[83]

Dosage and Administration. The recommended dosage of ziprasidone is 10 mg IM, which can be repeated at 2 hours, or 20 mg IM, which may be repeated at 4 hours. The drug reaches peak plasma concentrations in 30 to 45 minutes and has an elimination half-life of 2 to 4 hours. Following an intramuscular injection, sedation usually begins within 15 to 30 minutes and peaks at around 2 hours. The clinical effects usually last at least 4 hours.[85]

Olanzapine

Olanzapine is a second-generation thienobenzodiazepine antipsychotic agent that is thought to exert its effects through antagonism of both dopamine and serotonin type 2 receptors. Olanzapine in an intramuscular formulation has recently been approved by the FDA for the treatment of agitation in acutely psychotic patients. Intramuscular olanzapine is comparable to haloperidol or lorazepam monotherapy for acute agitation associated with schizophrenia and dementia[58,86,87] and superior to lorazepam monotherapy in the management of agitation associated with bipolar disorder.[88] To date, there have been no clinical trials using intramuscular olanzapine for undifferentiated agitation in the ED, but its use is increasing.

Dosage and Administration. The recommended dosage is 5 to 10 mg IM. Additional doses may be considered 2 to 4 hours after the preceding dose with a maximum recommended dose of 30 mg/day IM. Olanzapine reaches peak plasma concentrations in 15 to 45 minutes and has an elimination half-life of 21 to 54 hours. The onset of sedation usually begins 15 to 30 minutes after intramuscular administration and typically lasts at least 2 hours. In some patients, the clinical effects have lasted as long as 24 hours. The drug is metabolized via direct glucuronidation and cytochrome P-450–mediated oxidation.[89]

Aripiprazole

Aripiprazole is an atypical antipsychotic that acts at both serotonin and dopamine receptors. Rates of EPSs are lower than with other antipsychotics, which may be a result of the drug's partial agonistic activity at dopamine receptors. Intramuscular administration has been approved for acute agitation related to schizophrenia and bipolar mania. To date, there have been no clinical trials using aripiprazole IM for undifferentiated agitation in the ED.

Dosage and Administration. The recommended dosage is 5.25 to 9.75 mg IM. Additional doses may be considered 2 to 4 hours after the preceding dose with a maximum recommended dose of 30 mg/day IM. Peak serum levels occur within 1 to 3 hours, with an elimination half-life of approximately 75 hours.

Dissociative Agents
Ketamine

Ketamine is a dissociative agent that has been used safely throughout the world for major surgery and with minimal monitoring.[90] Many clinicians are familiar with ketamine as a safe and rapidly effective dissociative agent for tracheal intubation and for children undergoing painful procedures in the ED, where its use has become standard practice. Ketamine has no significant adverse effects on blood pressure or respiration. It inhibits the reuptake of catecholamines promoting bronchodilation and increases in both heart rate and blood pressure. Commonly raised as a caution, there is no proven issue with ketamine causing harmful increased intracranial pressure.[91,92] Possible side effects of ketamine include salivation, vomiting, laryngospasm, and emergence phenomena consisting of nightmares, short-lived bizarre thoughts, and hallucinations. Fortunately, emergence phenomena have not been described as significant issues following ED use.

Although ketamine is not commonly used to control agitated and delirious patients, the drug's pharmacologic profile lends itself to use for acute agitation. For example, ketamine has been used successfully in aeromedical transport as a sedative agent for patients with agitation.[93] It has also been effective in the prehospital management and transport of patients with severe EXDS and in combative trauma patients (including those with head injury),[94] acutely agitated cocaine-intoxicated patients,[95] and agitated suicidal patients.[96]

Dosage and Administration. The dose of ketamine to produce profound dissociation is 1.5 to 2.0 mg/kg IV or 4 to 5 mg/kg IM. Intramuscular administration is ideal in the ED when access for intravenous administration is not readily available. The anterior aspect of the thigh is a preferred site of injection for rapid tranquilization. Time of onset may vary slightly, but both routes have a rapid onset of action (30 seconds IV, 3 to 5 minutes IM). At the current time, ketamine is undergoing resurgence in popularity among emergency physicians, and the role of ketamine for the chemical control of acutely agitated and delirious patients in the ED is evolving.

Choosing the Best Agent
Undifferentiated Agitation

The safest agent for undifferentiated agitation in the ED has traditionally been a benzodiazepine administered IV, often combined with judicious doses of haloperidol. Ketamine and newer atypical antipsychotics are gaining favor, but their track record is short. *Administering escalating doses of benzodiazepines seem to be a prudent choice in such circumstances when the clinician is comfortable prescribing a drug from this class.* There is little concern for respiratory or cardiovascular depression with the prudent use of carefully titrated intravenous benzodiazepines in the monitored setting. Figure 70-1 suggests a possible management approach to an acutely agitated patient in the emergency setting. It must be emphasized that benzodiazepine doses considered exceeding high or even toxic by other standards are routinely and safely administered in the ED when aggressive sedation and chemical control are mandated as clinical priorities. In severe cases, benzodiazepines alone will not be totally effective.

Agitation Caused by Alcohol and Drugs of Abuse

For patients who are suspected of intoxication from alcohol or other sedative agents, haloperidol, droperidol, or ziprasidone will provide rapid, safe, and effective tranquilization.[52,63,69] Benzodiazepines should be administered with caution to alcohol-intoxicated patients and those taking sedative agents because of the possibility of respiratory depression.[71,72] In contrast, benzodiazepines are the *drugs of choice* in patients who are agitated as a result of *alcohol or benzodiazepine withdrawal*. Large doses may be required, and the safety profile is wide. Patients who are agitated because of sympathomimetic agents such as cocaine or methamphetamines or hallucinogens such as PCP or LSD may be treated safely with large doses of benzodiazepines, butyrophenones, or a combination of the two.[52,57,67] Droperidol has been associated with serotonin syndrome in patients taking LSD and should be avoided in these patients.[51,53]

Agitation Caused by Medical Illness

In patients whose agitation is due to medical illness, treatment should be aimed at correcting the underlying pathology. If rapid sedation is required, typical antipsychotics or benzodiazepines should be used as first-line therapy. If the patient is frail or elderly or is known to have renal impairment, consider using smaller doses of a single agent.

Agitation Caused by an Underlying Psychiatric Disorder

Patients with an established psychiatric history and agitation attributed to schizophrenia, schizoaffective disorder, or the manic phase of bipolar disorder may be treated with typical antipsychotic agents, atypical antipsychotic agents, or benzodiazepines. However, a growing body of evidence seems to support the use of atypical antipsychotic agents in this circumstance.[46,58,68,84,86,87,95,97,98]

Agitation in Children

Because of years of experience and a proven safety record, benzodiazepines are considered first-line therapy for the management of agitation in children. The intramuscular dose of lorazepam is 0.05 to 0.1 mg/kg and the intramuscular dose of midazolam is 0.1 to 0.2 mg/kg. Neuroleptic agents have also been used to manage agitation in children. The intramuscular dose of haloperidol is 0.025 to 0.075 mg/kg, with a maximum dose of 2.5 mg. Children older than 12 years can receive the adult dose, usually 2.5 to 5.0 mg IM (see Table 70-1). Although droperidol is a highly effective drug for rapid sedation of adults, there is a paucity of literature supporting its use in children. The pediatric dose of droperidol is 0.03 to 0.07 mg/kg with a maximum initial dose of 2.5 mg.[51] Combination therapy is not generally recommended for children.[75]

Agitation in Pregnancy

Psychotropic and anxiolytic medications should be used during pregnancy only when the potential risk to the fetus from exposure is outweighed by the risk of not treating the disorder in the mother.[99] Based on years of accumulated clinical experience but very few scientific data, conventional antipsychotic agents such as haloperidol and droperidol (pregnancy class C) are recommended to control agitation in pregnant women.[100] In pregnancy, benzodiazepines (pregnancy class D) may be associated with teratogenicity (especially craniofacial abnormalities) when used for an extended period.[101] Although clear causation has not been proved, benzodiazepines are generally avoided during the first trimester to minimize the risk for fetal malformation.[102] Judicious benzodiazepine administration should be considered a viable option in the acute ED setting in the second and early third trimesters.

Agitation in Older Patients

Patients 65 years or older are particularly susceptible to adverse drug reactions because of coexisting medical illness, use of multiple prescription medications (which increase the risk for drug-drug interactions), and age-associated changes in pharmacokinetics and pharmacodynamics. Research suggests that conventional antipsychotic medications such as haloperidol and droperidol are safe and effective for both psychotic symptoms and nonpsychotic agitated behavior.[103] Low doses (e.g., half the usual dose) of benzodiazepines can also be used but require close observation for respiratory depression. Continued use (>8 to 10 weeks) of atypical antipsychotic agents has been associated with increased rates of death in cases of dementia-related psychosis.[81]

Conducted Electrical Weapons

CEWs, including TASERs (TASER International, Inc., Scottsdale, AZ) and stun guns, are used by law enforcement agencies throughout the world. These nonlethal weapons use a temporary high-voltage low-current electrical discharge to overcome a body's voluntary muscle-triggering mechanisms, which results in widespread involuntary muscle contractions that incapacitate the victim. The current is delivered by direct contact with a handheld device (i.e., electric shock prods) or via a small dart-like electrode fired from a gun using small gas charges (e.g., TASER) similar to some air rifle propellants. There are also electrical weapons that cause intense pain without incapacitating the target, so-called *drive stun devices*. Law enforcement and correctional personnel typically use drive stun devices as a pain compliance technique. A TASER may deliver approximately 1200 V but can reach up to 50,000 V across clothes without direct skin contact.[104]

The exact street scenario of EXDS, physical restraint, and a TASER-linked death will probably never be studied with unchallenged scientific accuracy, and hence one is left with animal and human volunteer data to intuit the cause and effect of untoward events. Despite claims of lethality in the press, emotional testimony and unscientific reports from human rights organizations, and poorly documented claims in case reports, there have been no documented deaths directly and indisputably attributable to a TASER discharge in humans.[105] Volunteer studies and animal models fail to provoke cardiac arrest or significant cardiopulmonary or metabolic derangements after standard electrical discharges, even when animal models include stimulant toxicity and human volunteers are

exercised to exhaustion.[104] Nevertheless, CEWs have been temporally linked to a number of fatalities.[104-106] The majority of these cases involved sympathomimetic drug intoxication (e.g., cocaine, methamphetamines), prolonged physical exertion, or both.[106] The role of severely altered metabolic and autonomic parameters, drug intoxication, or underlying comorbid conditions, including cardiomyopathy, obscures the exact contribution of CEW use in unexpected deaths. A complete discussion of this topic is beyond the scope of this chapter, but it has been well reviewed elsewhere.[107] The darts from a CEW often penetrate the skin and must be removed, so the remainder of this section focuses on the procedure for removing embedded TASER electrodes.

Electronic Control Devices

TASER is an acronym for "Thomas A. Swift's Electric Rifle" and has been in existence since the early 1990s (Fig. 70-11). More than 11,000 law enforcement, correctional, and military agencies in 44 countries deploy TASER devices, and many municipalities in the United States allow civilians to purchase and carry these weapons for personal protection.[108] A TASER uses compressed nitrogen to propel two electrode-tipped barbs at 180 ft/sec at the target. The electrode-tipped barbs are attached to the electric device via two thin 21-foot wires and are similar in size to a No. 8 fishhook measuring 4 mm in length (Fig. 70-12). The barbs may attach to clothing and fail to penetrate the skin, or they may become embedded in skin and must be removed.

Removal Techniques

Barbs embedded in soft tissue can easily be removed with direct pressure. Place one hand on the skin surrounding the barb to hold the skin taut and use the other hand to apply direct pressure to the barb[108,109] (Fig. 70-13). If the patient cannot tolerate the procedure, inject a small amount of local anesthetic near the barb and use a No. 11 scalpel blade to cut down through the soft tissue to the tip of the barb.[108] Because of the small size and linear shape of the barb, there is no need

Figure 70-11 TASER electrical control device.

Figure 70-12 TASER dart/electrode-tipped barb. *Note:* the groove in the shaft (*arrow*) lines up with the barb tip to aid in removal.

Figure 70-13 Removal of an electrode-tipped barb. Barbs embedded in soft tissue can easily be removed with direct pressure. Place one hand on the skin surrounding the barb to hold the skin taut and use the other hand to apply direct pressure to the barb.

to advance the barb through the skin to remove the tip as is commonly performed during the removal of fishhooks.[109] After removal, clean and dress the wound (see Chapter 34), but do not suture it. Analgesics (e.g., nonsteroidal antiinflammatory drugs, acetaminophen) may be administered.

After removing the barb, provide standard wound care. Advise the patient to watch for signs of infection; a 48-hour wound check may be prudent with contaminated wounds, when the barb was difficult to remove, and if there is concern for a retained foreign body. Significant infection after barb removal is rare, and prophylactic antibiotics are unnecessary. Following removal of a TASER dart, the disposition of the patient is based on the individual social scenario, and long-term ED observation is not required.

Complications

Because of the small size of the barb, the risk for significant injury to the heart, lungs, or bowel from a TASER device is small. Theoretical risk for injury to vascular structures and genitalia exists, although no cases have been reported in the literature. There have been case reports of serious intraocular and intracranial injuries resulting from a TASER barb, but these are rare.[110-113] A barb embedded in a vascular structure can probably be removed with manual traction followed by direct pressure on the wound because the size of the barb is similar to the size of devices used to obtain central venous access.[109] Consultation with a vascular surgeon may be required in complicated cases. Severe involuntary muscle contraction from the electrical discharge has been implicated as a cause of acute thoracic compression fractures.[114,115] Based on a literature review in 2011 by Vilke and colleagues, there is currently no indication for routine diagnostic or laboratory testing in asymptomatic patients following short-duration exposure (<15 seconds) to a CEW.[116]

TASER Use in the ED

While data are difficult to confirm, it has been estimated that about 150 hospitals allow hospital security guards to carry TASERS. Those equipped with TASERS should have specific training, and policies on the use of the TASER in the hospital setting should be in place and training periodically updated.

CMS regulations do not disallow TASERS in the hospital, but CMS and most states do not sanction the use of such devices *to restrain a patient or to make them comply with medical treatment.* Whenever possible, the least restrictive methods should be used to deescalate aggressive behavior, or calm agitated or disruptive individuals, such as a quiet and low-stimulation environment, reasonable bargaining, redirection of the patient, involvement of family, reality orientation, talk down, or a show of force. It is a gray area, indeed, as to when, or to what extent, any intervention is considered necessary to restrain a patient, or to protect a patient or medical personnel from harm. Every situation is somewhat unique so dogmatic approaches cannot be used. When a mentally incompetent or potentially suicidal patient wants to leave the ED against medical advice, and does not have insight into the adverse effects of such an egress, involuntary commitment is initiated. Effective measures are usually initiated by the emergency physician because psychiatric evaluation on such short notice is impractical or unavailable and important decisions must be made immediately with limited data. Such patients may assault those attempting to keep them from leaving the ED in their incompetent mental state, when medical consequences, suicide, or harm to others could be the ultimate outcome.

Per CMS guidelines, the use of weapons by security staff is considered a law enforcement action, not a health care intervention. CMS does not support the use of weapons by any hospital staff as a means of subduing a patient in order to place that patient in restraint or seclusion. CMS interpretive guidelines to section 482.13(e) of the State Operations Manual state: *"If a weapon is used by security or law enforcement personnel on a person in a hospital (patient, staff, or visitor) to protect people or hospital property from harm, we would expect the situation to be handled as a criminal activity and the perpetrator placed in the custody of local law enforcement."*

In one small nonvalidated study, Ho et al[117] concluded that the introduction of the TASER into the health care setting (a large urban tertiary care teaching hospital) demonstrated the ability to avert and control situations that could result in injury to medical personnel and patients, by simple TASER presentation or rarely actual use. In that study there was a reduction in personnel injury rates and the contention that one suicide was averted. Further study is required before definitive statements can be made. In summary, the use of the TASER in the ED has not yet been clarified, and there are advocates as well as critics. Any weapon, including the TASER, should not be used to force a patient to comply or to induce restraint in the absence of reasonable suspicion of impending harm or actual assault of medical personnel.

Acknowledgment

We would like to thank the previous authors Charles J. Fasano and Gregory Schneider for their work on earlier editions of this chapter.

References are available at www.expertconsult.com

CHAPTER 71

Noncardiac Implantable Devices

Paul Jhun and Eduardo Borquez

In addition to cardiac pacemakers and defibrillators, a number of noncardiac devices have been developed for electronic neuromodulation and drug delivery.[1,2] Although these devices are placed by a variety of subspecialists for the treatment of chronic illnesses, if the devices malfunction, patients may arrive at the emergency department in an acute state, thereby necessitating intervention by the emergency physician.

INSULIN INFUSION DEVICES

Background

External insulin infusion devices are becoming increasingly popular since their introduction in 1974. As of 2007, more than 375,000 external insulin infusion pumps are in use.[3]

Anatomy

An external insulin infusion pump device consists of a portable, programmable infusion pump connected to a subcutaneously implanted catheter maintained in place with adhesive tape (Fig. 71-1). The implanted catheter site varies, but it is commonly placed on the abdomen in adults and on the buttocks in young children. The thighs, hips, and upper part of the arms are other sites. It is recommended that the implanted catheter be replaced every 2 to 3 days.

Device Complications

In 2010, the Food and Drug Administration (FDA) published a panel report that highlighted problems associated with insulin infusion devices.[3] From the top five device manufacturers, the FDA noted 16,640 adverse events, including 310 deaths, 12,093 injuries, and 4,294 malfunctions. Box 71-1 lists the most frequently reported problems with devices in descending frequency. Box 71-2 lists the most frequently reported patient-oriented adverse reactions, which include hyperglycemia and hospitalization.

Of the 310 deaths reportedly related to insulin infusion pumps, the vast majority of problems with the device were not known to the patient or providers at the time and the root cause of failure of the device was not identified by the manufacturer. In 29 deaths, problems with the device identified included overinfusion, bent cannulas, disconnection, pump alarming, failure to deliver, suspected electromagnetic interference, and display failure.

Procedure

As with all patients seen in the emergency department, consider device malfunction as part of the differential diagnosis in patients with insulin infusion devices. In addition to medical management, troubleshoot the device and remove it in cases of uncertainty or emergency.

To remove the catheter, simply peel off the adhesive and embedded catheter together to discontinue the flow of injected medication into the patient. There are a variety of proprietary pump manufacturers, each with their own device programming. Call the appropriate manufacturer to troubleshoot the device, visit the manufacturer's website for an online troubleshooting manual, or simply instruct the patient to discontinue use of the device and return to a standard calculated insulin schedule by manual injection until the device-related complication is investigated and resolved.

INTRATHECAL DRUG DELIVERY SYSTEMS

Background

Intrathecal drug delivery systems (IDDSs) have been in clinical use since the 1980s. Although data are accumulating, very few robust clinical studies of IDDSs have been published.[4] The FDA approved the use of intrathecal baclofen in 1992 for severe spasticity secondary to spinal cord injury, multiple sclerosis, cerebral palsy, or stroke. In addition, the FDA approved the use of intrathecal morphine in 1995 for chronic pain refractory to traditional medical therapies. An IDDS is also used for the delivery of chemotherapeutic medications for specific oncologic conditions. Moreover, there are numerous off-label uses of various intrathecal medications.

Anatomy

Currently, Medtronic is the only IDDS manufacturer in the United States. Medtronic's SynchroMed II Programmable Infusion Pump consists of an infusion pump connected to an intrathecal catheter (Fig. 71-2A). The infusion pump is available with a refillable reservoir of either 20 or 40 mL. The pump is powered by a permanent lithium battery that cannot be recharged. The battery must be surgically replaced every 4 to 7 years. Normal refill intervals are usually between 2 and 3 months.

The pump is placed in a subcutaneous pocket, generally in the right lower abdominal region. The intrathecal catheter is inserted slightly lateral to the spinous process into an appropriate lower lumbar interspace and connects to the pump via a subcutaneous tract that wraps around the abdominal wall (see Fig. 71-2B).

Interrogation and programming of the device are conducted with a magnetic field–induced, external programming wand connected to a handheld computer.

Device Complications

Several studies have shown a significant rate of adverse effects in IDDS patients ranging anywhere from 2% to 50%.[5,6]

The most frequent and serious adverse events related to the device and implant procedures are catheter dislodgement from the intrathecal space, catheter fracture, implant site infection, and meningitis. Internal device programming errors that cause underdosing or overdosing are less common. If the drug supply is depleted, systemic symptoms related to acute drug withdrawal will occur. This is characteristic for the

Figure 71-1 External insulin infusion pump. Components include a subcutaneously implanted catheter (*A*) and a programmable infusion pump (*B*) (OneTouch Ping, Animas Corporation, West Chester, PA). To discontinue the flow of insulin into the patient, simply peel off the adhesive and embedded catheter together. Also shown is a wireless continuous glucose monitoring receiver (*C*), along with its sensor and transmitter (*D*) (exCom SEVEN PLUS, DexCom, Inc., San Diego, CA).

BOX 71-1 **Most Frequently Reported Problems with Insulin Infusion Pump Devices**

1. Unknown (19.7%)
2. Replace (9%)
3. Audible alarm (6%)
4. Use-of-device issue (5%)
5. Device displays error message (4.8%)
6. Not applicable (4%)
7. Failure to deliver (3%)
8. No information (3%)
9. Repair (3%)
10. Self-activation or keying (1.8%)

BOX 71-2 **Most Frequently Reported Patient Problems with Insulin Infusion Pump Devices**

1. Hyperglycemia (24.6%)
2. Hospitalization (21%)
3. Diabetic ketoacidosis (8%)
4. Treatment with medication (6%)
5. Blood glucose low (4.7%)
6. Therapy, nonsurgical management (4%)
7. No consequences to the patient (4%)
8. Unknown (3%)

Figure 71-2 A, The Medtronic SynchroMed II Programmable Infusion Pump. **B,** The pump is usually implanted in a subcutaneous pocket in the right lower quadrant, with the catheter tunneled subcutaneously to an appropriate lumbar interspace.

specific drug being delivered and should be anticipated. Opioid and baclofen withdrawal syndromes are unlikely.

Medications currently in use via IDDSs include clonidine, bupivacaine, morphine, hydromorphone, fentanyl, ziconotide, and baclofen.[7] Of these, bupivacaine and morphine have specific antidotes (Intralipid and naloxone, respectively). Medication overdoses, aside from standard emergency management, can also be treated by accessing the infusion pump reservoir.

A unique complication related to IDDSs that was identified by the FDA and issued as a warning is the formation of a granuloma at the tip of the intrathecal catheter. This can obstruct infusion of the medication and lead to withdrawal symptoms.[8,9]

Common adverse effects related to intrathecal baclofen include hypotonia, somnolence, headache, convulsions, dizziness, urinary retention, nausea, and paresthesias. Acute intrathecal baclofen withdrawal, which may resemble alcohol or benzodiazepine withdrawal, is also possible in cases of underdosing or inability to deliver medication.

With regard to intrathecal opioids, the degree of lipophilicity of the intrathecal opioid affects its pharmacokinetics.

BOX 71-3 Drainage of the Infusion Pump Reservoir

EQUIPMENT

Antiseptic agent
22-gauge needle
20-mL Luer-Lok syringe or syringes

PROCEDURE

1. Palpate and locate the pump on the patient (typically in the lower abdominal subcutaneous layer). The reservoir fill port is located in the center of the pump.
2. Cleanse the injection site with the antiseptic agent.
3. Attach the 20-mL syringe to the 22-gauge needle and insert the needle through the skin into the center of the reservoir fill port until the needle touches the metal needle stop (see Fig. 71-3).
4. Use negative pressure to withdraw fluid from the reservoir. Empty the reservoir until backflow has stopped. Depending on pump volume, more than one syringe may be needed. Intrathecal drug delivery systems vary in their reservoir capacity from 18 to 60 mL.[7]
5. Remove the needle from the reservoir fill port.
6. Record the amount of medication fluid removed from the reservoir.

Figure 71-3 The contents of the intrathecal pump reservoir can be removed with a syringe and 22-gauge needle (see Box 71-3).

Figure 71-4 Vagal nerve stimulator (Aspire HC, Cyberonics, Inc., Houston).

Fentanyl, with its high lipophilicity, is absorbed rapidly by the spinal cord and little is left to ascend in cerebrospinal fluid (CSF). Thus, it has a rapid onset and shorter duration with fewer adverse effects. Morphine, with its high hydrophilicity, penetrates the spinal cord slowly, which allows a considerable amount of the drug to ascend in CSF. This, in turn, results in a slower onset and longer duration with a higher incidence of adverse effects, including pruritus, nausea and vomiting, urinary retention, changes in mental status, and respiratory depression.[10,11]

Procedure

When there is concern for medication overdose secondary to malfunction of the device, in addition to emergency medical management, the emergency physician can empty the pump reservoir by using the steps outlined in Box 71-3.

Access the Medtronic online manual and review the steps necessary to remove the contents of the pump reservoir and thus prevent further infusion of intrathecal medication (Fig. 71-3).[12] Assuming no contraindications, withdraw an additional 30 to 40 mL of CSF by lumbar puncture to reduce the drug's concentration in CSF.

VNS

Background

Since the 1930s, numerous studies have shown the effects of vagal nerve stimulation on cerebral activity. In 1985, Zabara demonstrated the anticonvulsant effect of vagal nerve stimulation through animal studies.[13] In 1997 the FDA approved use of the vagal nerve stimulator (VNS) as an adjunctive treatment of medically refractory partial-onset epilepsy.[14] Subsequently, in 2005 the FDA approved use of the VNS as an adjunctive therapy for treatment-resistant depression.[15,16]

Anatomy

Currently, only one company in the United States, Cyberonics, manufactures the VNS under the brand name VNS Therapy System (formerly known as the NeuroCybernetic Prosthesis).

The device is composed of a generator attached to a bipolar VNS lead. The generator is approximately 4 cm long, 6 cm wide, and 7 mm thick and weighs 25 g. Figure 71-4 shows how the generator is implanted into subcutaneous tissue in the left upper part of the chest, with the electrode lead being attached to the left cervical vagus nerve trunk. Interrogation and programming of the device are conducted with a magnetic field–induced, external programming wand connected to a handheld computer. The variable settings that can be adjusted include current output, signal frequency, pulse width, and on/off stimulation times. When reset, the generator is *on* for 30 seconds, followed by 60 minutes *off*.[17,18]

Assuming normal parameters and output, the VNS generator has a projected battery life of approximately 10 years. Of note, VNS devices are implanted only on the left vagus nerve because the right vagus nerve directly innervates cardiac tissue and may have undesired cardiac effects if stimulated.

Device Complications

The device is typically turned on 10 to 14 days after implantation to allow adequate wound healing. Be aware that patients seen postoperatively during the first 2 weeks after implantation may not have had their device activated yet.

In addition to surgery-related risks and complications, if the patient complains of severe neck pain, worsening hoarseness, choking, or difficulty breathing, always consider device-specific complications. Voice alteration or hoarseness is the most common device-specific adverse effect, with more than 50% of patients being affected. Other common side effects include increased coughing, shortness of breath, and pharyngitis. Less common device-specific adverse effects reported during clinical studies include ataxia, dyspepsia, dysphagia, hypoesthesia, infection, insomnia, laryngismus, nausea, pain, paresthesia, and vomiting.[17,18]

Procedure

In cases of emergency, diagnostic uncertainty, or significant adverse effects, turn off the pulse generator temporarily by holding a magnet over the generator (Box 71-4). Pass the external VNS magnet over the generator to independently trigger it. This on-demand stimulation, if initiated at the onset of an aura or seizure, may abort the attack or, if initiated during a seizure, may halt its progression. Holding a magnet over the pulse generator causes a reed switch inside the generator to close. When the magnet closes the reed switch, the signal cannot be conducted and the pulse generator is temporarily turned *off*. When the magnet is removed, the switch opens and the generator is turned back *on*.[17,18]

Unlike the typical donut-shaped magnet of a cardiac pacemaker, the VNS magnet is bar shaped, as shown in Figure 71-5. Be aware that patients with VNSs are typically provided with two magnets: one fitted with a wristband and the other fitted with a belt clip.

ADDITIONAL IMPLANTABLE DEVICES

There are several additional noncardiac implantable devices that the emergency physician may encounter, which are outlined in Table 71-1. However, should these devices malfunction, there are no specific procedures to be aware of in the emergency setting beyond supportive treatment.

MRI AND IMPLANTABLE DEVICES

For patients with electrically, magnetically, or mechanically activated implants, the FDA requires labeling that magnetic resonance imaging (MRI) is contraindicated,[25] and indeed,

---

BOX 71-4 Vagal Nerve Magnet Applications

TO DELIVER ON-DEMAND STIMULATION

Place the magnet over the generator for longer than 1 second and then quickly remove it. The generator turns off and then immediately on again, thereby delivering a burst of vagal nerve stimulation based on the preprogrammed settings.

This maneuver can be repeated as needed.

TO TURN OFF THE STIMULATION

Hold and maintain the magnet over the pulse generator. If the device is properly turned off, the patient should notice loss of episodic adverse effects, such as stimulation-induced voice alteration or pain.[18,19]

TABLE 71-1 Additional Noncardiac Implantable Devices

DEVICE	DESCRIPTION	MALFUNCTION
Bladder stimulator or sacral nerve stimulator	Stimulator wire inserted into the S3 sacral foramen adjacent to the sacral nerve for the treatment of urinary incontinence in the setting of severe neurologic disease[20]	Hardware complications include infection, skin irritation, and wire migration[20]
Deep brain stimulator	Stimulator implanted into the thalamus for treatment of Parkinson's disease, tremor, and dystonia[1]	Hardware complications include infection and lead migration[21]
Gastric pacemaker	Neurostimulator with implanted leads into the gastric musculature to improve gastroparesis[22]	Gastric wall perforation, infection, and lead migration[22]
Phrenic nerve stimulator or diaphragmatic pacemaker	Electrodes implanted into each phrenic nerve with a receiver implanted into subcutaneous tissue. An external transmitter controls the receiver. Used to treat respiratory insufficiency secondary to upper motor neuron paralysis or respiratory drive dysfunction[23,24]	Pneumothoraces have been described immediately after implantation. Infection and wire migration have been described.[23,24] Failure of the pacemaker is treated by ventilatory support

Figure 71-5 Vagal nerve stimulator magnet.

manufacturers of gastric, urinary, diaphragmatic, and spinal cord stimulators list these devices as absolute contraindications to MRI.[21] However, there are a number of clinical series and case reports indicating the compatibility of certain devices with MRI. For VNSs, a 1.5-T magnet has been studied and deemed compatible with MRI by the manufacturer.[21,26,27] However, this compatibility is limited to MRI machines with transmit and receive head coils. MRI machines with transmit body coils and receive-only head coils may cause heat injury and damage the device. For deep brain stimulation, some studies have suggested that MRI is safe in certain circumstances,[28] but case reports of patient injury can be found in the literature.[29] For IDDSs, pumps have been shown to stop operating while in the magnetic field but resume functioning once removed.[25] Insulin pumps may easily be removed in the event that MRI is required.

In summary, the issue of MRI compatibility with implantable devices is very complex. In the event that MRI appears to be necessary, a case-by-case risk-benefit analysis involving the relevant subspecialist and radiologist is recommended.

References are available at www.expertconsult.com

CHAPTER 72

Radiation in Pregnancy and Clinical Issues of Radiocontrast Agents

Denis J. Dollard

Pregnant women are frequently evaluated in emergency departments (EDs) for complaints that may require diagnostic imaging. Their chief complaint may be related to pregnancy, an acute illness or injury, or a chronic condition diagnosed before pregnancy. Potential teratogenic effects in the developing fetus from diagnostic radiation and radionuclide procedures are more perceived than real. Clinicians should have a clear understanding of the actual risks and benefits associated with radiographic imaging during pregnancy.

The Joint Commission on Accreditation of Healthcare Organizations (JCAHO) published a sentinel alert[1] in August 2011 highlighting the radiation risks of diagnostic imaging in all patients, not just pregnant patients. This alert underscores the fact that x-rays are officially considered a carcinogen. Over the past 2 decades, total exposure to ionizing radiation has nearly doubled. Published reports estimate that the incidence of cancer secondary to radiation is 0.02% to 0.04%.

JACHO suggests that organizations can reduce the risk related to avoidable diagnostic radiation by raising awareness among staff and patients of the increased risk associated with cumulative doses and by providing the right test and the right dose (as low as reasonably achievable [ALARA]) through efficient processes, safe technology, and a culture of safety to make sure that doses are as low as possible while achieving the purpose of the study. Radiology departments should follow ALARA principles when imaging pregnant patients.

In utero exposure of the embryo or fetus to radiation generally causes great, but largely unnecessary anxiety in patients, their families, and the clinician. Much of this anxiety is secondary to a general misconception that any exposure to radiation is harmful and will result in an anomalous fetus. More often than not, clinicians themselves add to the confusion and fear by providing exposed women with erroneous information. Many clinicians, nurses, and even radiologists are ignorant of the qualitative and quantitative effects of ionizing radiation.[2] Multiple surveys in the literature reveal clinicians' dearth of knowledge about radiation exposure. This misinformation could lead to inappropriate abortions and litigation. For example, in Greece after the Chernobyl disaster, 23% of pregnancies were terminated because of unsubstantiated fears of teratogenicity.[3] A better understanding of the true risk estimates may help alleviate this fear.

It is widely held and published that concerns about the possible effects of exposure to ionizing radiation should not prevent medically indicated diagnostic procedures from being performed on the mother. It is not standard of care to withhold necessary radiologic studies because of fear of fetal injury from diagnostic studies. According to the American College of Radiology, "No single diagnostic x-ray procedure results in radiation exposure to the degree that would threaten the well being of the preembryo, embryo, or fetus."[4-6] This remarkable statement helps put into perspective the effects of diagnostic radiation exposure on pregnancy. Standard diagnostic radiologic procedures performed in the ED are not associated with significant proven fetal risks. A clear understanding of these risks enables clinicians to make an informed decision and knowingly counsel patients that radiologic procedures provide more benefit than harm.

Evaluation of a pregnant patient exposed to radiation should involve consideration of the type of radiation, types of examinations performed, gestational age, and radiation dose to determine an estimation of risk. The radiation dose of interest is the dose absorbed by the embryo or fetus and not by the mother. However, recent articles[7,8] have raised concern about exposure of maternal breast tissue to radiation and postulate a relationship to breast cancer decades later. The main goals of this chapter are to review the basic issues of pregnancy and radiation exposure and to provide a practical approach for clinicians in choosing a technique that entails the least risk and in counseling patients who have undergone or will undergo an emergency diagnostic procedure.

TYPES OF RADIATION

All imaging techniques involve radiation or transmission of energy from one body or source to another. Imaging modalities used for diagnosis during pregnancy can be subdivided into ionization techniques (radiographs, computed tomography [CT] scans, nuclear imaging) and nonionization techniques (magnetic resonance imaging [MRI] and ultrasonography [US]). The nonionization techniques have insufficient energy to ionize target cells. It is the ionization process and its sequelae that can induce health-related fetal effects.

Ionizing Radiation

Ionization is transfer of energy to a medium by either electromagnetic or particulate radiation that is sufficient to overcome the binding energy of an electron. The electron may be ejected from the atom. Both electromagnetic waves consisting of uncharged particles (x-rays and γ-rays) and charged particles (α and β) can produce radiation. Indirect ionization modalities such as x-rays release an electron from a source that interacts with the target. Direct ionization refers to charged particles, α and β, that strike the target directly.

UNITS OF RADIATION

The units used to measure the effects of x-rays can be confusing. Descriptive terms include the rad (radiation absorbed dose) and rem (roentgen equivalent man), along with the modern International System of Units (SI) of gray and sievert. In terms of radiation protection, the significant radiation quantity is the absorbed dose. The unit of absorbed radiation is the rad or gray (Gy) (1 Gy = 100 rad). Any risk associated with radiation is related to the amount of energy absorbed.

The dose equivalent, expressed in rem or sievert (Sv), is used to quantify the degree of biologic effect (1 Sv = 100 rem). This unit reflects the biologic response and can be used to compare the effects of different types of radiation. The dose equivalent is the product of the absorbed dose times a quality factor. The quality factor depends on the mass and charge of the radiated particle and is approximately 20 for an α-particle and 1 for x-rays and γ-rays. Therefore, for diagnostic radiographs, CT scans, and ^{99}Tc nuclear studies, the absorbed dose is equal to the dose equivalent; that is, an absorbed dose of 1 rad yields a dose equivalent of 1 rem (1 Gy = 1 Sv) (Table 72-1). All reference data have been converted into rad units for uniformity and comparison throughout the chapter.

TIMING OF RADIATION DURING PREGNANCY AND ITS EFFECTS

The effects of exposure to radiation on the conceptus depend on the gestational age and the amount of absorbed dose. The relationship between radiation-induced effects and stage of pregnancy is shown in Figure 72-1.[9] The harmful effects of ionizing radiation have the following principal biologic effects: intrauterine death, organ malformation, mental impairment, fetal growth retardation, cancer, and genetic mutation.[2]

Radiation-induced health effects are divided into two broad categories, stochastic and nonstochastic (Table 72-2). Stochastic effects, such as cancer or genetic mutation, can result from alterations produced in a single cell and are presumed to exist even at low exposure.[2] The probability of such an effect occurring increases with dose, and there is no identifiable threshold dose below which the chance is known to be zero. It is important to recognize that at low doses of radiation, the risks are far below the spontaneous incidence of carcinogenesis[10] or mutagenesis.[11]

The remaining harmful biologic effects mentioned earlier are nonstochastic effects. Nonstochastic effects require multicellular injury and have a threshold dose below which deleterious effects do not occur.[2] It is important to emphasize that the vast majority of embryopathologic effects are believed to be threshold phenomena; therefore, a dose of ionizing radiation below the threshold will not produce these effects.

The following section reviews in detail the timing of irradiation during pregnancy and its effects. In summary, the vast majority of embryonic and fetal pathologic effects are threshold phenomena. The imaging tests ordered in the ED yield levels far below these thresholds. Carcinogenesis and mutagenesis can occur at any radiation exposure level. However, the level of exposure from routine radiologic testing is very low; therefore, the number of radiation-induced cancers and mutations caused by irradiation of an embryo or fetus are very low.

Stages of Fetal Development

Development of an unborn child is expressed as postconceptional age and can be divided approximately into three major

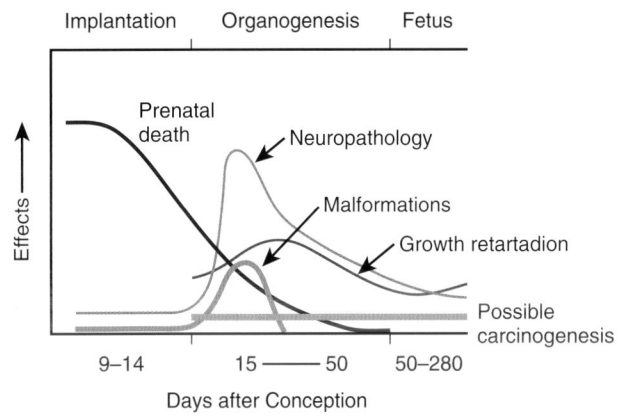

Figure 72-1 Schematic presentation of the various adverse effects associated with radiation and their relative incidence at different stages of gestation. (*Adapted from Mettler FA Jr, Upton A, eds. Medical Effects of Ionizing Radiation. 2nd ed. Philadelphia: Saunders; 1995.*)

TABLE 72-1 Units of Radiation

QUANTITY	UNIT	SI UNIT	RELATIONSHIP BETWEEN UNITS
Absorbed dose	Rad	Gray (Gy)	1 Gy = 100 rad 100 mGy = 10 rad 10 mGy = 1 rad 1 mGy = 100 mrad
Equivalent dose	Rem	Sievert (Sv)	1 Sv = 100 rem 100 mSv = 10 rem 10 mSv = 1 rem 1 mSv = 100 mrem

Absorbed dose (Gy) × quality factor = equivalent dose (Sv). The quality factor for radiographs = 1. Therefore, 1 rad = 1 rem; 1 Gy = 1 Sv.

TABLE 72-2 Stochastic and Nonstochastic (Threshold) Comparison

PHENOMENON	PATHOLOGY	DISEASES	RISK	DEFINITION
Stochastic	Damage to a single cell may result in disease	Cancer, germ cell mutation	Some risk exists at all dosages; at low doses the risk may be less than the spontaneous risk	The incidence of the disease increases, but the severity and nature of the disease remain the same
Nonstochastic (threshold)	Multicellular injury	Intrauterine death, organ malformations, mental impairment, growth retardation	No increased risk below the threshold dose	Both the severity and the incidence of the disease increase with the dose

Modified from Brent RL. Utilization of developmental basic science principles: the evaluation of reproductive risks from pre- and postconception environmental radiation exposures. *Teratology.* 1999;54:182.

TABLE 72-3 Risks and Threshold Doses of the Main Effects of Prenatal Irradiation

GESTATIONAL AGE	STAGE	POTENTIAL BIOLOGIC EFFECT	THRESHOLD	RISK
0-2 wk	Preimplantation/ implantation	Abortion Organ malformation	$>10^{2.8}$ rad $>5^{8}$; $>10^{2.9}$ rad	
3-7 wk 8-25 wk	Organogenesis Fetal	Growth retardation Growth retardation Mental impairment	$>10^{2.9}$ rad $>10^{2.9}$ rad $>10^{9.8}$ rad	
Whole pregnancy		Carcinogenesis Mutagenesis	None None	6×10^{-4} per rad 1×10^{-2} per rad

Modified from Fattibene P, Mazzei F, Nuccetelli C, et al. Prenatal exposure to ionizing radiation: sources, effects, and regulatory aspects. *Acta Paediatr.* 1999;88:693.

phases: (1) the preimplantation and implantation phase (0 to 2 weeks), from conception to implantation; (2) the phase of major organogenesis, which extends from the third to approximately the eighth week after conception; and (3) the phase of fetal development, which lasts from 9 weeks until birth.

Preimplantation and Implantation Phase

During the preimplantation and implantation phase, the principal radiation-induced health effect is abortion.[12] When the number of cells in the conceptus is small and their nature not yet specialized, the effect of damage to these cells is most likely to take the form of failure to implant or undeterminable death of the conceptus.[10] The no-effect threshold of an absorbed dose is quite high, estimated at 10 to 15 rad,[12] and not likely to be approached by diagnostic ED radiographs or radionuclide testing. By the time that the pregnancy is at term, the threshold for causing intrauterine mortality has risen to about 100 rad.[12] These estimates have been extrapolated from animal data. This period has been referred to as the "all-or-none period" because radiation is more likely to kill the embryo than result in a live malformed newborn.

Few human epidemiologic data are available for this period of gestation. Because many women are certainly unknowingly exposed to diagnostic radiation during this period, the lack of such data suggests no association between diagnostic radiation exposure and embryo death. Data from the Japanese atomic bomb experience have been cited for reference, but such a correlation is difficult to justify scientifically. Nonetheless, these data show a decrease in the number of offspring who retrospectively would have been 0 to 3 weeks' postconceptional age at the time of this significant radiation exposure, thus suggesting increased fetal loss caused by irradiation during preimplantation.[13] This decrease in the birth rate is probably multifactorial because stress, disease, and malnutrition were coexistent during this traumatic time. Importantly, fetal loss from exposure to an atomic bomb cannot be scientifically extrapolated to exposure to diagnostic radiation.

Any discussion concerning the potential adverse effects from diagnostic radiation must take into account the natural incidence of spontaneous abortion. Because the main effect of exposure to radiation during the first few weeks after fertilization is abortion as a result of death of the embryo, it is paramount to note that the normal incidence of spontaneous abortion in humans not exposed to radiation is in the 30% to 50% range.[2] Exposure to less than 10 rad yields no statistical change in the rate of preimplantation and early postimplantation spontaneous abortion from the expected baseline (Table 72-3).

Organogenesis

Exposure to very high-dose radiation, far greater than could be delivered by even aggressive diagnostic radiographs and radionuclide procedures, has been reported to result in teratogenesis. Such information is gleaned from women who were exposed to therapeutic radiation (in the range of 250 rad) during early pregnancy for conditions such as pelvic malignancies. Organ malformations are the main consequence of exposure to radiation during the organogenesis period (3 to 8 weeks). Abnormalities result from killing of cells during the active phase of proliferation and differentiation. Because the embryo is unable to completely replace damaged cells, malformations occur. The most common effects of exposure during organogenesis are malformations in the organs under development at the time of exposure and a reduction in skeletal development. Growth retardation and microcephaly are the predominant effects.[10,12,13] These effects have a reported threshold dose range of 5 to 20 rad or higher but are not generally observed unless the exposure is several orders of magnitude or higher.[10,12] This dose range is significantly higher than that attained in diagnostic radiology or diagnostic nuclear medicine procedures. Even though ocular abnormalities, developmental facial abnormalities, genital abnormalities, and physical deformities of the extremities have been reported after exposure of the embryo to very high doses, such abnormalities have not been linked to the amount of radiation that would be delivered from even multiple diagnostic radiographic procedures. Importantly, there are no reports of external radiation inducing morphologic malformations in humans unless the offspring also exhibited either growth retardation or a central nervous system (CNS) abnormality. Simply stated, isolated structural abnormalities will not develop in a fetus exposed to radiation. The fear of extra toes, cleft palate, or heart or kidney malformations from exposure to diagnostic radiation during pregnancy is simply unfounded, yet often believed by the general public.

Temporary growth retardation is likely with doses in the range of 10 to 25 rad.[13] Infants with low birth weight and length may recover fully and attain normal adult stature. The natural incidence of a live birth having a developmental anomaly is 2% to 4%,[9] and the incidence of intrauterine growth retardation is 2% to 3%.[9] Again, it is important to emphasize that exposure to less than 5 rad yields no change in the risk for occurrence of organ malformations or growth retardation[13] (see Table 72-3).

Fetal Period

The predominant observable effects of exposure to radiation during the fetal period are growth retardation, microencephaly, and severe mental retardation (SMR). The fetal stage has been subdivided into early fetal (8 to 15 weeks), midfetal (16 to 25 weeks), and late fetal (26-week term) because of identifiable periods of risk to the developing CNS.

Mental Impairment

From the 8th to the 15th week, there is a rapid increase in the number of neurons that migrate to their ultimate sites and lose their capacity to divide. At 15 to 25 weeks, there is more differentiation and architectural definition.[9] These embryologic changes make the fetus susceptible to damage to the CNS during the early fetal and midfetal periods.

In utero atomic bomb survivor data indicate that the risk for SMR per rad was higher if exposed during the early fetal versus the midfetal period.[13] In children exposed to greater than 50 rad between 8 and 15 weeks after conception, a drop in IQ score of 0.3 point per rad was estimated.[13] There is no documented increased risk for mental retardation in humans at a gestational age of less than 8 weeks or greater than 25 weeks when evaluated with doses of less than 50 rad.[14] The highest risk for SMR occurs during the early fetal period with fetal doses in the range of 100 rad. All clinical observations on significant reductions in IQ and SMR relate to fetal doses of about 50 rad and higher.[10] This dose range greatly exceeds the dosages used for diagnostic imaging.

It is important to relate the magnitude of radiation effects to abnormalities that occur spontaneously in the population. Multiple causes of mental retardation have been identified, including malnutrition, lead poisoning, rubella infection during pregnancy, and maternal alcoholism. Current prevalence figures indicate that the normal incidence of a person having an IQ below 70 is approximately 3%.[10] At fetal doses of 10 rad, the spontaneous incidence of mental retardation is much larger than any potential radiation effect on IQ reduction.[10] Regardless of the time of gestation, reduction in IQ cannot be clinically identified with fetal doses of less than 10 rad (see Table 72-3).[10]

Growth Retardation

The human data for Hiroshima and Nagasaki reveal that the major congenital anomaly observed was microencephaly.[13] Studies have not demonstrated any increased risk for microencephaly in the population exposed to less than 150 rad in Nagasaki; however, an increased risk in the Hiroshima population exposed to doses as low as 10 to 19 rad has been reported.[14] It is possible that the difference between the two cities is secondary to causes (e.g., trauma, stress, malnutrition) other than radiation. In experimental animal data, a dose of 10 to 20 rad did not increase the incidence of microencephaly.[15] The dose threshold for microencephaly, as well as other congenital anomalies, is generally accepted to be in the range of a few rad. Permanent growth retardation is not typically seen unless doses exceed 50 rad.[13] Irradiation of the human fetus at doses below 10 rad has not been observed to cause congenital malformations or growth retardation (see Table 72-3).[2,4,9]

Carcinogenesis

The magnitude of risk for carcinogenesis after low-dose radiation exposure and whether the risk changes throughout gestation have been the subject of many publications,[16-18] yet interpretation of the data remains open to date. Numerous studies[19-22] indicate a 1.3- to 3.0-fold higher incidence of leukemia in children exposed to diagnostic radiation in utero, although some studies fail to substantiate this association.[15,23] Excess cancer as a result of in utero exposure has not been clearly demonstrated in Japanese atomic bomb survivor studies even though the population has been monitored for about 50 years, but the number exposed is not large.[10] Identification and control of confounding factors make interpretation of radiation carcinogenesis studies difficult, if not impossible to interpret. Brent and coworkers[15] noted that most investigators agree that low doses of radiation present a carcinogenic risk to the embryo; however, findings of increased risk for cancer in children exposed in utero to low-dose diagnostic radiation must be reconciled with the fact that high-dose animal and human studies have not found a marked increase in the incidence of cancer.

Risk can be expressed in several ways, including relative risk and absolute risk. In relative risk, the risk is expressed as a function of the "background" risk. For example, a relative risk of 1.0 indicates that there is no effect of irradiation, whereas a relative risk of 1.5 for a given dose indicates that the radiation is associated with a 50% increase in cancer above background rates. The absolute risk estimate simply indicates the excess number of cancer cases expected in a population because of a certain radiation dose.[10]

The International Commission on Radiological Protection Publication 84[10] noted that a recent analysis of many of the epidemiologic studies conducted on prenatal x-ray exposure and childhood cancer are consistent with a relative risk of 1.4 (a 40% increase over the background risk) following a fetal dose of about 1 rad. The best methodologic studies, however, suggest that the risk is probably lower than this. Even if the relative risk were as high as 1.4, the individual probability of childhood cancer after in utero irradiation would be very low ($\approx$0.3% to 0.4%) because the background incidence of childhood cancer is so low ($\approx$0.2% to 0.3%). Absolute risk estimates for cancer from ages 0 to 15 after in utero irradiation have been estimated to be in the range of 600 per 10,000 persons each exposed to 100 rad, or 0.06%/rad.[10,12] If a fetus is exposed to 0.1 rad, the increased risk for carcinogenesis is 0.006%, or 3 in 50,000, as compared with the background incidence of 0.2% to 0.3%, or 100 to 150 per 50,000. The increased carcinogenic risk from exposure to 0.1 rad is approximately 50 times smaller than the already low natural incidence of cancer.

Mutagenesis

Investigating possible radiation-induced alterations in the human genome is exceedingly difficult. The geneticists who studied the irradiated populations in Japan are convinced that there were radiation-induced mutations. However, the calculated and confirmed risks were so small that the investigators were unable to demonstrate statistically significant genetic effects.[24]

The risk for radiation-induced hereditary disease in humans is reported to be around 1% per 100 rad.[13,15] If a fetus is exposed to 0.1 rad, the increased risk is approximately 0.001%, or 1 in 100,000. The natural frequency of genetic disease manifesting at birth is approximately 3%,[11] or 3000 per 100,000. For 0.1 rad, the increased genetic risk is minute in comparison to the natural incidence of genetic disease.

To put all risks into proper perspective, the range of fetal absorbed doses for diagnostic imaging must be reviewed. The vast majority of diagnostic radiographic studies are markedly less than 5 rad. A comparison of fetal absorbed doses for the more common ED radiographic procedures follows.

Radiation Exposure from Diagnostic Radiographs

Table 72-4 lists estimated fetal exposure for various diagnostic imaging modalities.[25-27] Multiple sources of estimated fetal exposure were reviewed, and the highest reported exposure from these sources is listed. The number of examinations required to reach a cumulative dose of 5 rad is calculated in the second column to underscore the order-of-magnitude difference between the dose considered to have negligible risk (5 rad) and the actual exposed fetal dose. For example, one would require 5000 radiographs of an upper or lower extremity, 12 pelvic radiographs, or more than 5000 two-view chest radiographs before the 5-rad limit is reached. This information is represented graphically in Figure 72-2.

Radiation Exposure from CT Scans

Many variables affect calculation of the fetal radiation dose from CT scans, especially slice thickness, number of cuts, distance of the target organ from the fetus, and gestational age. Table 72-4 summarizes the estimated maximal fetal radiation doses from CT scans. It should be noted that CT of the lumbar spine delivers radiation to the fetus that approaches the safe cutoff range. A CT scan of the abdomen exposes the fetus to less radiation than the 5-rad cutoff, but alternative methods of investigation such as US or MRI should be considered in early pregnancy if the clinical condition warrants.

Head CT is the most commonly requested CT scan in pregnancy. The expected fetal absorbed dose is less than 50 millirad (mrad), which is 100 times less than the dose with negligible risk. The estimated radiation dose to the fetus for CT of the chest is less than 0.100 rad. Spiral CT is commonplace in radiology departments and is a popular diagnostic tool used for suspected pulmonary embolism (PE) in pregnant patients. The dose with spiral CT of the chest is less because the duration of the procedure is much shorter.[28] Van der Molen[29] reported that using 16-slice versus 4-slice CT can equate to a reduction in radiation dose of 20% to 30%.

Ordering CT scans of the head, chest, abdomen, and pelvis is a daily occurrence for emergency medicine clinicians. With that in mind, it is sobering to realize that the seventh National Academy of Science report on the Biological Effects of Ionizing Radiation (BEIR VII) indicated that a 10-rad dose is associated with a lifetime attributable risk for development of a solid cancer or leukemia of 1 in 1000.[30,31] As data on the effects of ionized radiation accumulate and the technology of nonionizing techniques improves, our use of ionization-based modalities will diminish.

The American College of Radiology notes that iodinated low-osmolality contrast media (LOCM), most of which are nonionic agents, have been shown to be associated with less discomfort and a lower incidence of minor (1% versus 5% for high-osmolality contrast media [HOCM]) and severe reactions (0.015% versus 0.1% for HOCM). Many radiology departments routinely use LOCM.[32] Although authors have expressed concern over the possibility that iodinated contrast media may suppress fetal or neonatal thyroid function for a short period,[7] the added benefit of using nonionic contrast agents is that intravascular use of such agents has been reported to have no effect on neonatal thyroid function.[33] Postnatal screening for hypothyroidism is done routinely in the United States. The combination of increased use of iodinated contrast agents in pregnant women to rule out PE and the dearth of literature reporting increased fetal hypothyroidism in the United States supports the report that use of iodinated contrast agents does not affect fetal thyroid function.

Iodinated contrast material that is injected intravenously for CT scans and ingested orally for contrast enhancement does not emit radiation and is classified as pregnancy category B. The product insert for barium sulfate suspension used as an oral contrast agent for an abdominal CT scan (e.g., Redi-Cat) notes no adverse fetal reactions under the heading "Usage in Pregnancy." Barium preparations do not emit radiation.

NUCLEAR MEDICINE STUDIES

A common nuclear medicine procedure ordered from the ED is a ventilation-perfusion ($\dot{V}/\dot{Q}$) scan. The perfusion portion of the scan is performed by injecting a radioisotope intravenously. The isotope emits radiation and is detected by sensitive cameras. This requires that a radioisotope (e.g., ^{99}Tc) be tagged to a substrate, most commonly albumin. The albumin-technetium aggregate is temporarily trapped in arterioles and capillaries in the lung and its distribution can be identified. The principal photon that is useful for detection and imaging with technetium studies is the γ-ray.[34] When the radiotagged substrate is excreted into the maternal bladder, the fetus will receive additional radiation exposure because of the proximity of the maternal bladder. Patient hydration and frequent voiding or bladder catheterization after a $\dot{V}/\dot{Q}$ scan will lessen exposure of the fetus to radiation.

Measurement of a radioactive substance is based on its decay, and the units are the curie (Ci) and becquerel (Bq). Doses are usually expressed in millicurie (mCi). The usual dose of technetium for the lung perfusion portion of a $\dot{V}/\dot{Q}$ scan is 1 to 5 mCi of [99]Tc. Reduced doses, as low as 1 mCi, are often used in pregnancy.

Depending on the radioisotope and substrate used, average fetal exposures can be calculated. Commonly used radiopharmaceuticals and estimated fetal doses for $\dot{V}/\dot{Q}$ scans and other radionuclide studies are presented in Table 72-5.[14] A 5-mCi ^{99}Tc-albumin scan results in 175 mrad of fetal exposure. Reducing the dose to 2 mCi results in 70-mrad fetal exposure. ^{99}Tc-albumin is contraindicated in patients with severe pulmonary hypertension and is pregnancy category C.

Ten millicuries of ^{133}Xe is used for the ventilation portion of the $\dot{V}/\dot{Q}$ scan. [133]Xe has a short half-life and results in 40-mrad fetal exposure. Normal findings on the perfusion scan may obviate the need for the ventilation scan, and some centers routinely perform only the perfusion portion because most pregnant women have normal ventilation.

TABLE 72-4   Estimated Fetal Exposure from Various Diagnostic Imaging Methods

EXAMINATION TYPE	ESTIMATED FETAL DOSE PER EXAMINATION (rad)	NUMBER OF EXAMINATIONS REQUIRED FOR A CUMULATIVE 5-rad DOSE
Plain Films		
Skull	0.004	1,250
Dental	0.0001	50,000
Cervical spine	0.002	2,500
Upper or lower extremity	0.001	5,000
Chest (2 views)	<0.001	<5,000
Mammogram	0.020	250
Abdominal (multiple views)	0.420	12
Thoracic spine	0.009	555
Lumbosacral spine	1.0	13
Intravenous pyelogram	1.398	3
Pelvis	0.40	12
Hip (single view)	0.213	23
Computed Tomography Scans (Slice Thickness: 10 mm)		
Head (10 slices)	<0.050	>100
Chest (10 slices)	<0.100	>50
Abdomen (10 slices)	4.9	1
Lumbar spine (multiple views)	3.500	1
Pelvimetry (1 slice with a scout film)	0.250	20
Fluoroscopic Studies		
Upper gastrointestinal series	0.056	89
Barium swallow	0.006	833
Barium enema	3.986	1
Nuclear Medicine Studies		
Most studies using technetium (^{99m}Tc)	<0.500	>10
Hepatobiliary technetium HIDA scan	0.150	33

Ventilation-perfusion scan (total)
  Perfusion portion: technetium
  Ventilation portion: xenon (^{133}Xe)
	0.215
	0.175
	0.040
		23
		28
		125

Iodine (^{131}I) at fetal thyroid tissue	590.000	
Environmental Sources (for Comparison)		
Environmental background radiation (cumulative dose over 9 mo)	0.100	N/A

Reproduced from Toppenberg KS, Hill DA, Miller DP. Safety of radiographic imaging during pregnancy. *Am Fam Physician.* 1999;59:1813.
HIDA, hepatobiliary iminodiacetic acid; *rad,* unit of absorbed radiation.

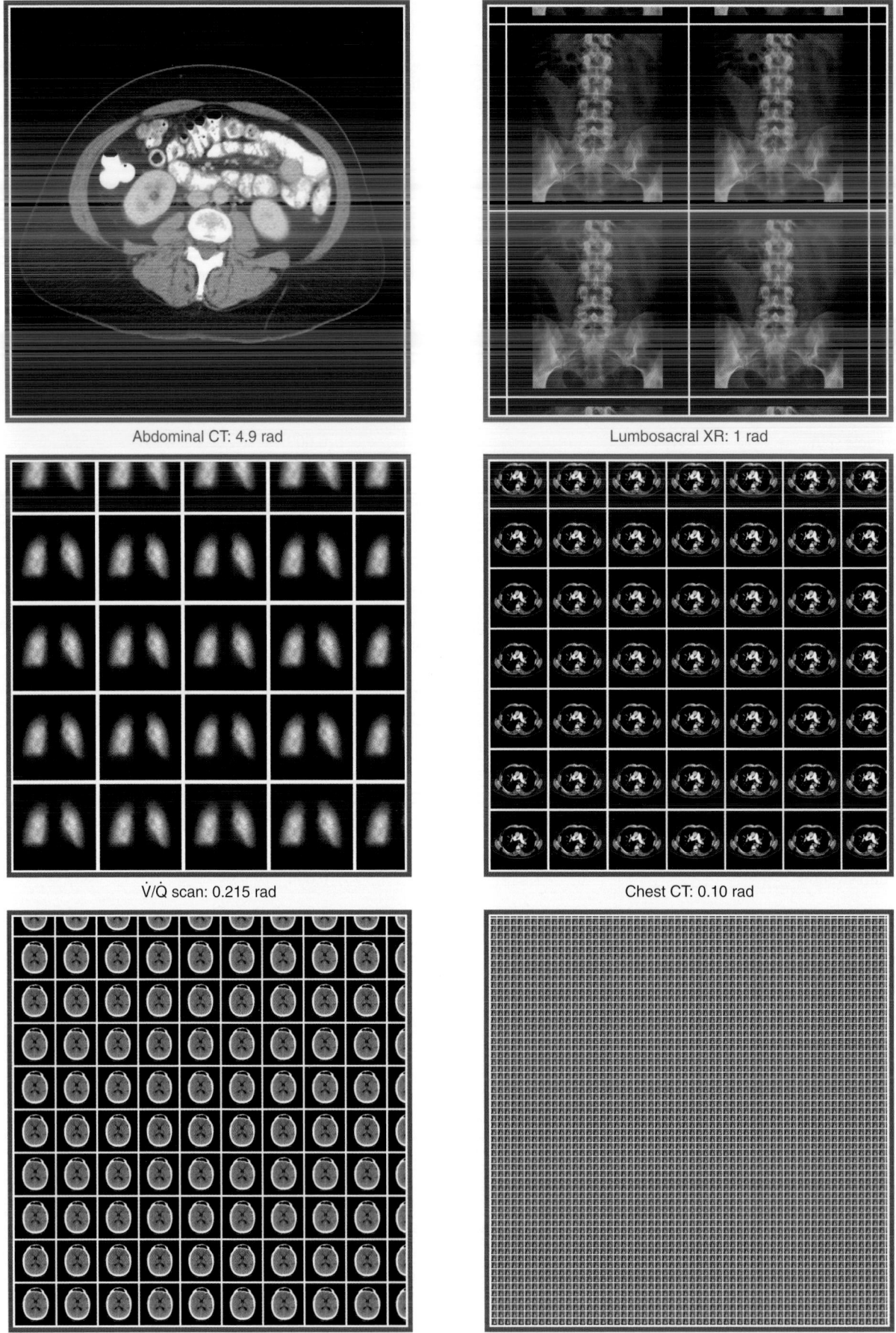

Abdominal CT: 4.9 rad

Lumbosacral XR: 1 rad

V̇/Q̇ scan: 0.215 rad

Chest CT: 0.10 rad

Head CT: 0.05 rad

Chest XR: 0.001 rad

Figure 72-2 Graphic representation of estimated fetal exposure for a variety of radiographic modalities. The area enclosed within each red box represents 5 rad, which is the dose considered to have negligible risk in pregnancy. The number of radiographic studies depicted in each red box represents the approximate number of such studies that could be obtained before exceeding the 5-rad limit. Note that for the chest radiograph, the print resolution of this book does not allow reproduction of the number of acceptable studies, which is higher than 5000. *CT,* computed tomography; *XR,* x-ray study.

TABLE 72-5   Radiopharmaceuticals Used in Nuclear Medicine Studies

EXAMINATION	ESTIMATED ACTIVITY ADMINISTERED PER EXAMINATION (mCi)	DOSE TO THE UTERUS/EMBRYO PER PHARMACEUTICAL (mrad)
Brain	20 mCi ^{99m}Tc-DTPA	700
	20 mCi ^{99m}Tc-O$_4$	960
Hepatobiliary	5 mCi ^{99m}Tc-sulfur colloid	55
	5 mCi ^{99m}Tc-HIDA	150
Bone	20 mCi ^{99m}Tc-phosphate	500
Respiratory		
Perfusion	5 mCi ^{99m}Tc-macroaggregated albumin	175
Ventilation	10 mCi ^{133}Xe gas	40
Renal	20 mCi ^{99m}Tc-DTPA	700
Abscess or tumor	3 mCi ^{67}Ga-citrate	840
Cardiovascular	20 mCi ^{99m}Tc-labeled red blood cells	120

Reproduced from Cunningham GF, ed. *Williams Obstetrics.* 21st ed. New York: McGraw-Hill; 2001.
DTPA, diethylenetriaminepentaacetic acid; *HIDA,* hepatobiliary iminodiacetic acid; *mCi,* millicurie; *mrad,* millirad.

DIAGNOSIS OF PE

The reported incidence of PE associated with pregnancy is equivalent to roughly 1 in every 2000 pregnancies.[7] The mortality rate of untreated acute PE is about 30%, as opposed to 2% to 10% with timely diagnosis and treatment.[35] Therefore, the potential morbidity of PE and the attendant risk associated with anticoagulant therapy in pregnant patients necessitate definitive diagnosis.

The radiologic modalities of choice for definitive diagnosis are $\dot{V}/\dot{Q}$ scanning versus CT pulmonary angiography. Although conventional pulmonary angiography was long considered the "gold standard" against which other imaging techniques were compared, it is now thought to be no more accurate than well-performed CT pulmonary angiography.[7]

The calculated radiation exposure of the fetus from both $\dot{V}/\dot{Q}$ scanning and CT of the chest confers minimal and essentially only theoretical fetal risk.[28] Fetal exposure from CT of the chest is less than 0.100 rad. Fetal exposure from CT has been reported to be as low as 0.026 rad with single–detector row helical CT and 0.013 rad for multidetector-row helical CT.[7] A 5-mCi ^{99}Tc perfusion scan and a 10-mCi ^{133}Xe ventilation scan summate to 0.225 rad.[25] The dose of fetal radiation from the perfusion scan can be altered and is often lowered in the evaluation of pregnant patients (Box 72-1). Lowering the dose by 60%, a level that will usually produce a suitable study, results in lowering fetal exposure to 0.110 rad. Recent articles state that the radiation dose to the fetus from CT angiography of the maternal chest is similar to or lower than that from a $\dot{V}/\dot{Q}$ scan.[36] Pulmonary angiography results in an estimated fetal exposure of 0.22 to 0.37 rad when done via the femoral route, but it can be lowered to less than 0.05 rad by using the brachial route.[28]

CT has supplanted $\dot{V}/\dot{Q}$ scanning as the standard diagnostic test in ruling out PE. Because the perfusion scan is being done on a relatively young healthy subset of the population, one would suspect that the percentage of nondiagnostic studies (low or intermediate probability) would be low. However, Chan and colleagues[37] reported that $\dot{V}/\dot{Q}$ scintigraphy is nondiagnostic in 25% of patients, with 73.5% of scans being read as normal and only 1.8% being read as high probability (113 patients in the study). Interestingly, 86% (24 of 28) of the patients who had a nondiagnostic finding did not receive anticoagulant therapy and were found to be free of a thromboembolic event for the following 20.6 months.

Recognizably, the utility of a test that does not answer your question 25% of the time is concerning but should be tempered by the fact that there is a 75% chance of getting a definitive diagnosis, along with published concerns that exposure of childbearing women's breasts to the higher level of radiation from CT may cause cancer decades later.[7,8] Remy-Jardin and Remy[38] and Scarsbrook and coworkers[7] reported that an exposure of 1 rad to the breasts of a woman aged 35 years increases her risk for breast cancer by approximately 14% over the background rate for the general population. Some authors[39] advocate that the breast radiation issue justifies the use of $\dot{V}/\dot{Q}$ scanning rather than CT angiography as the primary examination in a pregnant patient.

So which study does one order? Both modalities expose a fetus to low levels of radiation of similar magnitude (CT less than $\dot{V}/\dot{Q}$) with very low theoretical fetal risk. The advantages of CT pulmonary angiography include the speed with which one can obtain the study and the capability of delineating alternative causes of the symptoms. Scarsbrook and coworkers[7] presented an algorithm mindful of the radiation exposure to both the fetus and mother and provided convincing evidence for their recommendation (Fig. 72-3). They suggested that an echocardiogram is a good first step in critically ill pregnant patients in whom PE is being considered. All others should start with a chest radiograph with shielding of the fetus. If findings on the radiograph are normal, proceed with US of the lower extremities to evaluate for deep venous thrombosis. Although the combination may have lower diagnostic yield, it exposes the mother and fetus to minimal risk. If deep venous thrombosis is present, treatment can be instituted. If US is negative, proceed to a half-dose lung perfusion scan if the patient does not have a history of obstructive lung

BOX 72-1   The Technique of ($\dot{V}/\dot{Q}$) Scanning

This test uses both intravenous (perfusion) and aerosolized (ventilation) agents.

PERFUSION

1. Before injection, prepare the intravenous technetium. Mix sodium pertechnetate ^{99m}Tc with macroaggregated human albumin (MAA) to form ^{99m}Tc-MAA, the substance that is injected intravenously to investigate blood flow in the lungs. If the preparation is not used within 8 hours, discard it.
2. The usual dose is 1 to 5 mCi. Doses as low as 1 mCi are used in pregnancy.
3. Within 5 minutes of injection, more than 90% of the Tc-albumin aggregate is trapped in the arterioles and capillaries of the lung. The particle size determines where the ^{99m}Tc will be localized in the body.
4. Accumulation in the lung is temporary, and the fragile albumin aggregate quickly breaks down, thereby allowing Tc to enter the general circulation.
5. Once in the body, the half-life of ^{99m}Tc is 6 hours.
6. The majority of ^{99m}Tc is excreted in urine. If it remains in the urinary bladder, it is in close proximity to the fetus.
7. Tc in the bladder exposes the fetus to small amounts of radiation.
8. Frequent voiding or bladder catheterization after the study will lessen exposure of the fetus to radiation.
9. Tc is relatively contraindicated in patients with severe pulmonary hypertension (because ^{99m}Tc-MAA temporarily blocks blood flow in the lungs).
10. Allergic reactions to Tc and human serum albumin are extremely rare.
11. The radiation exposure to the total body from 2.5 mCi is extremely low: less than 0.1 rad.

VENTILATION

1. Some radiologists forgo the ventilation portion of the $\dot{V}/\dot{Q}$ scan in pregnancy to limit the total radiation exposure.
2. Most hospitals use ^{133}Xe for the ventilation portion of the $\dot{V}/\dot{Q}$ scan.
3. Fetal radiation exposure from xenon is extremely low, and the 5-rad cutoff is not reached until more than 125 scans have been performed.
4. The estimated dose to the fetus of the standard 10 mCi of xenon used in a $\dot{V}/\dot{Q}$ scan is 0.04 rad.
5. If Tc-based aerosol is the marker used for the ventilation portion, fetal exposure is higher than with xenon aerosol.

$\dot{V}/\dot{Q}$, *ventilation-perfusion.*

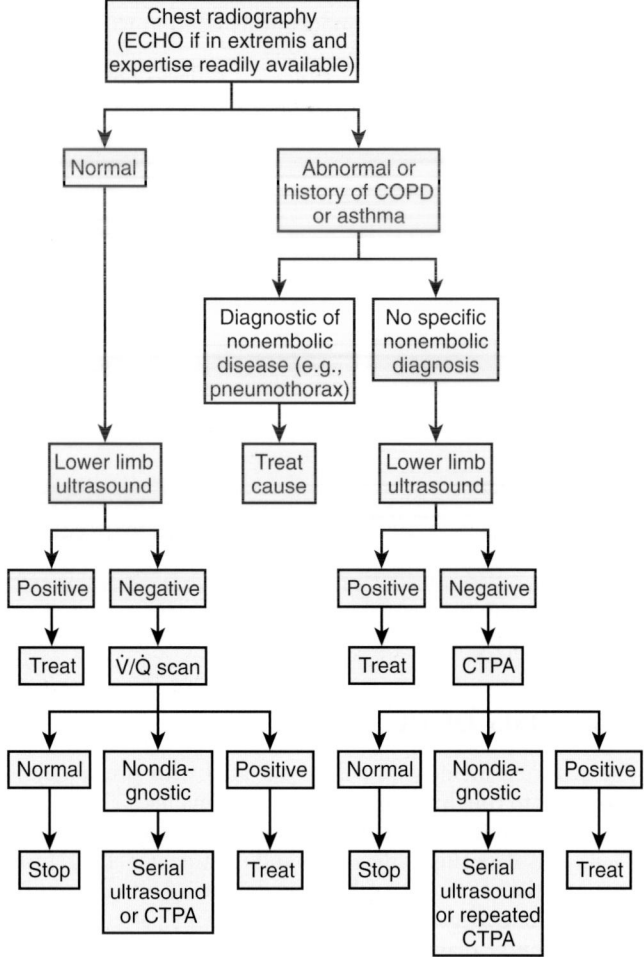

Figure 72-3 Suggested imaging algorithm for investigation of suspected pulmonary embolism in pregnancy. *COPD,* chronic obstructive pulmonary disease; *CTPA,* computed tomography pulmonary angiography; *ECHO,* echocardiography; *$\dot{V}/\dot{Q}$ scan,* ventilation-perfusion scan. *(Modified from Scarsbrook AF, Evans AL, Owen AR, et al. Diagnosis of suspected venous thromboembolic disease in pregnancy. Clin Radiol. 2006;61:1.)*

disease. The literature reports that findings in up to 75% of these scans are normal in the pregnant population. An important stipulation for using this algorithm is that one's hospital radiology team should have experience in reporting normal scans as opposed to low-probability ones, with the understanding that all nondiagnostic tests would lead to consideration of CT pulmonary angiography. The authors note that using this algorithm allows a definitive diagnosis in the vast majority of cases while minimizing risk to both the mother and fetus.

Scarsbrook and coworkers[7] recommended several dose reduction methods when using CT pulmonary angiography on pregnant patients. Although these methods do not fall into the realm of emergency medicine, it is worthwhile to raise these points with radiologists when developing a protocol to lower the radiation exposure to your patients (Box 72-2).

The role of D-dimer levels in the diagnosis of PE is evolving.[40,41] During pregnancy D-dimer levels increase, and such increases should be considered physiologic. D-dimer levels are similar to those in nonpregnant patients up to around 20 weeks and then are noted to increase throughout pregnancy to three times higher than the mean in a healthy nonpregnant patient.[42]

Recently, attempts have been made to establish a range of normal D-dimer values throughout pregnancy, which may be of great value, but as of yet have not been tested in clinical practice.[7]

BOX 72-2	Dose Reduction Methods When Using CT Pulmonary Angiography to Image Suspected Pulmonary Embolic Disease in Pregnancy

Reduce milliampere-second (mAs) settings.
Reduce kilovoltage (kVp).
Increase pitch.
Increase detector and beam collimation.
Reduce the field of view.

Reduce z-axis scan volume (caudal extent limited to the top of the diaphragm).
Eliminate frontal and lateral scout views.
Use circumferential shielding of the abdomen and pelvis.

From Scarsbrook AF, Evans AL, Owen AR, et al. Diagnosis of suspected venous thromboembolic disease in pregnancy. Clin Radiol. 2006;61:1.
CT, *computed tomography.*

Figure 72-4 Magnetic resonance imaging (MRI) for appendicitis in pregnancy. Right lower quadrant pain presents a diagnostic dilemma in pregnant patients, and abdominal computed tomography is generally eschewed in favor of modalities that do not use ionizing radiation. Ultrasound may be utilized but the appendix is often difficult to visualize, especially in the third trimester. **A,** MRI (fast spin echo, fat saturated) of a patient who is 33 weeks pregnant. A dilated appendix (12 mm) and periappendiceal edema are noted adjacent to the right psoas muscle (*arrow*), indicative of acute appendicitis. **B,** A coronal section from the same study reveals the fetus in a frank breech presentation. MRI is thought to present no risk to the fetus at any stage of pregnancy.

DIAGNOSIS OF APPENDICITIS

Acute appendicitis is the most common nonobstetric emergency requiring surgery during pregnancy. Appendicitis is associated with premature labor, fetal morbidity and mortality, and an increased rate of perforation. Concern for appendicitis in a pregnant patient warrants early surgical consultation and discussion of the need and type of imaging. Patel and coauthors[36] published an algorithm that uses US and MRI techniques before exposing patients to ionizing radiation. They recommended the use of graded-compression US followed by abdominal/pelvic US to search for other pathology if needed. If the US studies are negative, the authors recommend MRI of the abdomen and pelvis (Fig. 72-4). Notably, some authors[43] have found that using a non-ionic oral contrast agent (a mixture of ferumoxsil [category B] and barium sulfate) improved sensitivity and specificity in detecting appendicitis in pregnancy. The authors noted that US imaging of the appendix was more easily done during the first and early second trimester and that the left lateral decubitus position assisted in visualization of the appendix in third-trimester patients. Finally, if US and MRI are still inconclusive, CT of the abdomen and pelvis may be considered. Definitive surgical exploration should be discussed with a general surgeon before proceeding to ionizing radiation. If CT is required, the authors reported an estimate of about one cancer per 500 fetuses exposed to 3 rad.

DIAGNOSIS OF PREGNANCY AND CONSENT

If exposure to less than 5 rad does not measurably affect the exposed embryo, why should the clinician determine the pregnancy status of the patient? Brent[2] reported sound reasoning for diagnosing pregnancy before a radiographic study. The principle of informed consent must remain paramount. It is beneficial and ethically more sound to have the patient informed of her pregnancy status before imaging. An informative discussion about the risk-benefit aspects of the test before the study conveys concern for the patient and fetus.

Discussing the risk-benefit aspects of imaging after the study may be misconstrued as "backpedaling" and make the patient upset. Many lawsuits are stimulated by the factor of surprise. Frank discussion before imaging may prevent misguided litigation. More importantly, having patients both understand the problem (imaging in pregnancy) and take part in the management discussion can help them become more empowered and potentially reduce the anxiety associated with their condition and with their pregnancy.

Determination of pregnancy by the history and physical examination alone can be problematic. The menstrual history by itself may not be totally reliable in determining pregnancy. Amenorrhea and physical changes in the size and shape of the uterus may be consistent with pregnancy. A history of recent menstruation, use of an intrauterine device, tubal ligation, absence of coitus, or proper use of birth control pills can result in a suggestion of nonpregnant status more than 90% of the time, but these parameters are not 100% accurate. If the diagnosis of pregnancy is in the differential or imaging is ordered, or both, definitive determination of the patient's pregnancy status should be strongly considered if the clinical scenario is reasonable. A menstrual history and other information should be obtained whenever possible, and a confirmatory urine pregnancy test should be considered. Urine pregnancy tests to detect early pregnancy are quite sensitive and reliable, and it is not necessary to routinely order a quantitative serum test. Theoretically, there will be a few days' window between fertilization and implantation, a period when no method will confirm the presence or absence of early pregnancy.

A pregnant patient has the right to know the magnitude and type of risks that might result from in utero exposure to radiation. The Annals of the International Commission on Radiological Protection Publication 84[10] summarized the need for informed consent as follows:

> The need and degree of disclosure is usually measured by what a reasonable person believes is material to the mother's decision to be exposed to radiation. The level and degree of disclosure should be related to the level of risk. For low-dose procedures, such as chest x-rays, <100 mrad, the only information that may be needed is a verbal assurance that the risk is judged to be extremely low. When fetal doses are >100 mrad, usually a more detailed explanation is given. The information should include potential radiation risks and potential alternative modalities as well as the risk of harm from not having the medical procedure. The degree of documentation of such explanations and consent is variable but many clinicians will include a note of any such counseling or consent in the record of the patient.

PATIENT COUNSELING

When a pregnant patient requires an imaging study, be prepared to discuss the risk associated with the test. Counseling can be done after attempting to estimate the dose received by the conceptus from the procedure and comparing the radiation risk with other risks of pregnancy. It is important to use terminology that is easily understood by the patient. Figure 72-5 depicts three different strategies to inform the patient about the level of exposure from her study and established limits. Table 72-6 compares the level of exposure with established background risks.

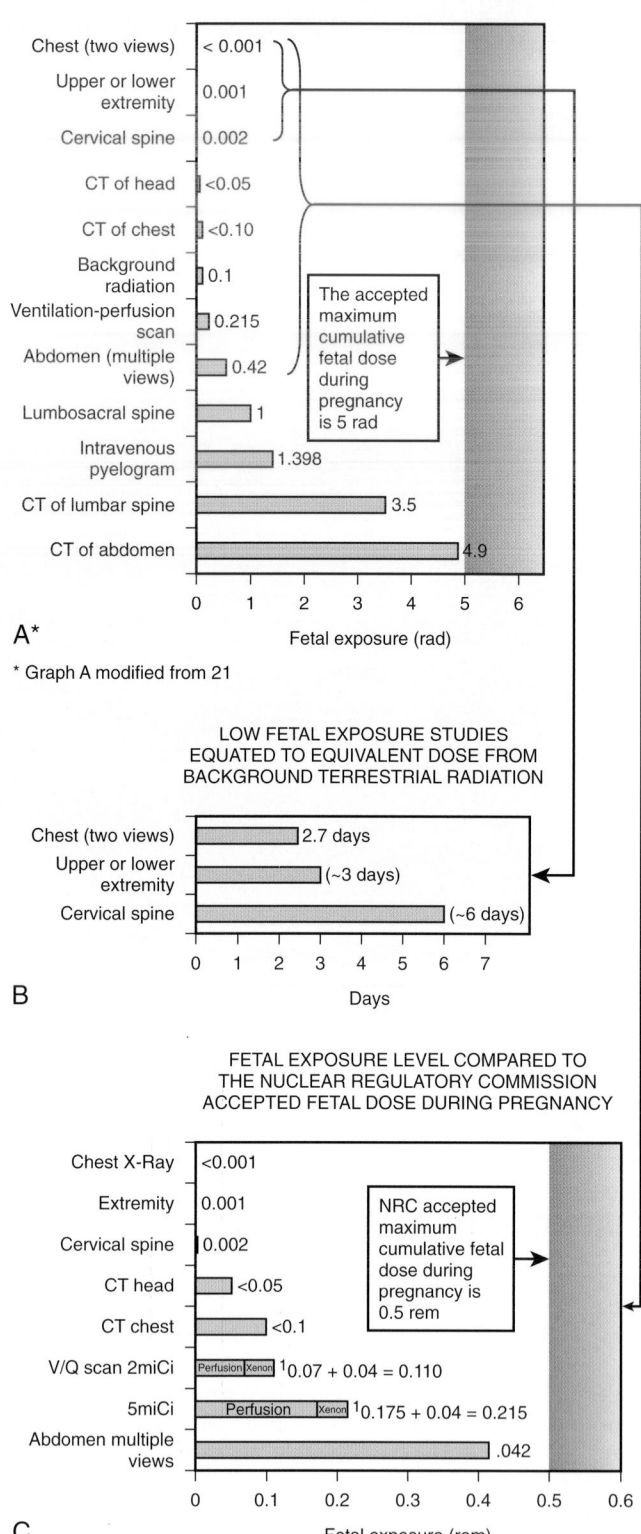

Figure 72-5 A, Comparison of common radiographic studies with the accepted 5-rad cumulative fetal exposure limit. **B,** Low–fetal exposure studies equated to the equivalent dose from background terrestrial radiation. **C,** Fetal exposure level compared with the fetal dose during pregnancy accepted by the Nuclear Regulatory Commission (NRC). *CT,* computed tomography; *V̇/Q̇ scan,* ventilation-perfusion scan.

TABLE 72-6 Probability of Bearing Healthy Children as a Function of Radiation Dose

RADIOGRAPHIC STUDY	FETAL EXPOSURE (rad)	INCREASED RISK FOR ABORTION, GROWTH RETARDATION, MENTAL IMPAIRMENT, AND MALFORMATION	PROBABILITY THAT A CHILD WILL HAVE NO MALFORMATION (%)	PROBABILITY THAT A CHILD WILL HAVE NO GENETIC DISEASE PRESENT AT BIRTH* (%)	PROBABILITY THAT CANCER WILL NOT DEVELOP IN A CHILD (AGE 0-19 yr)† (%)
No study	0	None	97	97	99.7
Chest radiograph (2 views)	0.0007	None	97	97	99.7
Extremity	0.001	None	97	97	99.7
Cervical spine	0.002	None	97	97	99.7
Head CT	<0.05	None	97	97	99.7
Chest CT	<0.10	None	97	97	99.7
V̇/Q̇ scan, 3 mCi	0.145	None	97	97	99.7
V̇/Q̇ scan, 5 mCi	0.215	None	97	97	99.7
Multiple studies	1	None	97	97	99.6
Multiple studies	5	None	97	97	99.4

Modified from International Commission on Radiological Protection. Publication 84: Pregnancy and medical radiation. *Ann ICRP.* 2000;30:iii, 1.
*Rounded values. The radiation risk for genetic mutation is assumed to be 0.01%/rad fetal dose with a linear dose-response relationship. The background rate for genetic mutation is estimated to be 3%. From Osie IK. Fetal doses from radiological examinations. *Br J Radiol.* 1999;72:773.
†Rounded values. The radiation risk for fatal cancer is assumed to be 0.06%/rad fetal dose with a linear dose-response relationship. Many epidemiologic studies suggest that the risk may be lower than that assumed here. The background risk for childhood cancer is calculated from NCI-SEER. *Surveillance, Epidemiology and End Results Cancer Statistics Review 1973-1991: Tables and Graphs.* Bethesda, MD: National Cancer Institute; 1994.

The main bar graph (*A*) in Figure 72-5 compares the fetal exposure level for various radiographic studies with the maximum accepted fetal dose during pregnancy (5 rad). A patient's particular study may be plotted on this graph to show the clear margin of safety that exists for all single diagnostic tests.

The middle graph (*B*) equates the exposure from low-level diagnostic studies to the number of hours needed to accumulate a similar exposure dose from background terrestrial radiation. One of the most commonly ordered studies in pregnancy is a chest radiograph. The potential risk to the fetus can be put into perspective for the patient by comparing the absorbed dose for the chest radiograph with the natural background radiation exposure. The environmental background radiation over a 9-month period results in a cumulative dose of 100 mrad,[44] or 0.015 mrad/hr. The fetal dose exposure for a chest radiograph (two views) is estimated to be less than 1 mrad. Therefore, the exposure dose to the fetus from a chest radiograph is equivalent to the same amount of naturally occurring background radiation to which the patient was exposed in the previous 2.7 days.

The lower graph (*C*) depicts the upper limit of the Nuclear Regulatory Commission (NRC) for cumulative gestational dose versus various diagnostic studies. The NRC has established occupational radiation dose limits for pregnancy. Its recommendation is that the dose to the fetus not be allowed to exceed 0.5 rem during gestation. Brent[2] noted that this factor-of-10 lowering of the widely accepted threshold is "extremely conservative." One can explain to the patient that the level of exposure from her radiograph is below the conservative cumulative acceptable dose for a pregnant employee at a nuclear facility in the United States.

Another useful approach is to indicate to the patient the probability of not having a child with either a malformation or cancer and how that probability is affected by radiation. Table 72-6 depicts the probability of bearing healthy children as a function of radiation dose. This discussion should be coupled with the fact that a nonexposed fetus has a baseline incidence of spontaneous abortion, multiple developmental abnormalities, and subsequent childhood cancer.

Numerous organizations have declared fetal exposure to less than 5 rad as being safe. Box 72-3 presents various conclusions from key organizations on the use of radiation and pregnancy. The International Commission on Radiological Protection concluded that fetal doses below 10 rad should not be considered a reason for terminating a pregnancy.[10] If a patient still has considerable concern or has possibly received greater than 5 rad, referral to a radiation physicist or genetic specialist for further counseling is reasonable.

NONIONIZING RADIATION: MRI AND US

The term *radiation* describes the transmission of energy from one body or source to another. Nonionizing radiation includes the portion of the electromagnetic spectrum in which the energy of emitted photons is insufficient to ionize atoms and molecules. MRI and US are forms of nonionizing radiation.

MRI

MRI is currently not approved by the U.S. Food and Drug Administration (FDA) for use in pregnant patients.[45] However, a body of data in this population is developing. MRI is

---

BOX 72-3   Key Statements on Diagnostic Imaging Modalities during Pregnancy

X-RAY IMAGING

"No single diagnostic procedure results in a radiation dose that threatens the well-being of the developing embryo and fetus." (American College of Radiology; from Hall EJ. Scientific view of low-level radiation risks. *Radiographics.* 1991;11:509.)

"[Fetal] risk is considered to be negligible at 5 rad or less when compared to the other risks of pregnancy, and the risk of malformations is significantly increased above control levels only at doses above 15 rad." (National Council on Radiation Protection and Measurements; from NCRPM. *Medical Radiation Exposure of Pregnant and Potentially Pregnant Women.* NCRPM Report No. 54. Bethesda, MD: NCRPM; 1977.)

"Women should be counseled that x-ray exposure from a single diagnostic procedure does not result in harmful fetal effects. Specifically, exposure to less than 5 rad has not been associated with an increase in fetal anomalies or pregnancy loss." (American College of Obstetricians and Gynecologists [ACOG], Committee on Obstetric Practice; from ACOG. *Guidelines for Diagnostic Imaging During Pregnancy.* ACOG Committee Opinion No. 299. Washington, DC: ACOG; September 2004.)

MRI

"Although there have been no documented adverse fetal effects reported, the National Radiological Protection Board arbitrarily advises against its use in the first trimester." (American College of Obstetricians and Gynecologists [ACOG], Committee on Obstetric Practice; from ACOG. *Guidelines for Diagnostic Imaging During Pregnancy.* ACOG Committee Opinion No. 158. Washington, DC: ACOG; 1995.)

US IMAGING

"There have been no reports of documented adverse fetal effects for diagnostic ultrasound procedures, including duplex Doppler imaging." "There are no contraindications to ultrasound procedures during pregnancy, and this modality has largely replaced x-ray as the primary method of fetal imaging during pregnancy." (American College of Obstetricians and Gynecologists [ACOG], Committee on Obstetric Practice; from ACOG. *Guidelines for Diagnostic Imaging During Pregnancy.* ACOG Committee Opinion No. 299. Washington, DC: ACOG; September, 2004.)

BOX 72-4   Summary of MRI during Pregnancy

1. MRI involves no ionizing radiation.
2. There are no known biologic risks associated with MRI, and no specific fetal abnormalities have been linked with standard low-intensity MRI.
3. Most obstetric problems can be evaluated adequately with ultrasound.
4. Contrast material is often avoided in conjunction with MRI during pregnancy.
5. Both maternal and fetal anatomy, including the fetal central nervous system, can be evaluated with MRI.
6. The FDA requires documented informed consent and cautions that the full effects of MRI during pregnancy have not yet been determined.
7. MRI is usually eschewed during the first trimester unless there is a clear risk-to-benefit indication, such as possible spinal cord compression.
8. Claustrophobia and a pregnant woman's inability to tolerate prolonged lying on her back can occasionally be problematic.
9. Fetal movement limits information on the fetus unless sedation is provided or ultrafast scans are available.

FDA, *U.S. Food and Drug Administration;* MRI, *magnetic resonance imaging.*

---

becoming a valuable complement to US when additional information is needed to make treatment decisions during pregnancy (see Fig. 72-4).[46,47] Recent advances in fast MRI techniques have helped eliminate previous obstacles of slow imaging times and fetal movement. Possible indications for the use of MRI in a pregnant patient include further evaluation for adnexal masses, placental status, hydronephrosis, pelvic vein thrombosis, appendicitis, and small bowel obstruction.[48]

Magnetic resonance direct thrombus imaging (MR-DTI) is a technique that allows direct visualization of PE and simultaneous imaging of the legs without the need for intravenous contrast media. Early data suggest that it is highly accurate in the detection of PE.[7] As more studies are conducted and the availability of MRI improves, MRI may replace ionizing techniques for the diagnosis of thromboembolism.

One of the most common reasons in the ED for MRI is evaluation of neurologic emergencies (e.g., spinal cord compression). In light of the serious sequelae of spinal cord compression along with a lack of data supporting adverse fetal effects, a pregnant patient exhibiting symptoms of cord compression should undergo MRI to establish a diagnosis.

The Safety Committee of the Society for Magnetic Resonance Imaging has stated that MRI procedures are indicated for use in pregnant women when other nonionizing diagnostic imaging methods are inadequate or when the examination will provide important information that would otherwise require exposure to ionizing radiation.[49] It is required that pregnant patients be informed that although to date there is *no indication that the use of clinical MRI procedures during pregnancy produces deleterious effects,* according to the FDA the safety of MRI procedures during pregnancy has not been definitively proved. It is advisable to obtain informed consent for MRI of a pregnant patient. In addition, because of limited data, most facilities avoid imaging patients in their first trimester. With inadvertent exposure in a wanted pregnancy, however, the present accumulated data would not warrant interruption of the pregnancy (Box 72-4).

Generally during pregnancy, non–contrast-enhanced MRI is performed. Fortunately, most maternal pelvic and fetal MRI does not require contrast media. Although no direct adverse effects on the fetus have been documented, gadolinium-based contrast material *is not recommended for use in pregnant patients.*[48,50] Gadolinium-based contrast material has been shown to cross the placenta and appear within the fetal bladder moments after intravenous administration.[51] It is then excreted into amniotic fluid and potentially reabsorbed from the gastrointestinal tract.[51] Because it is reabsorbed in the fetal gastrointestinal tract, the half-life of gadolinium-based contrast material in the fetal circulation is not known. Gadolinium is a class C drug.

There is concern about the use of gadolinium in any patient with renal insufficiency because of the development of a very rare gadolinium-related syndrome, nephrogenic systemic fibrosis.

US

US continues to be the screening modality of choice for evaluation of the maternal pelvis and the fetus because of its safety profile, relatively low cost, and real-time capability. Obstetric and gynecologic US accounts for more than half of the US imaging volume in the United States.[52] In the 40 years since its introduction into clinical practice, US has not been shown to convey any significant health risk to the fetus or mother,[53] although most safety data were collected before 1992, when the permissible power output of scanners was significantly lower than the power used in contemporary scanners.[54] Generally, the increasing power output raises concern for thermal and mechanical effects on developing tissue. These issues are small with standard B-mode imaging and more concerning with use of the Doppler modality. US societies have developed unitless output display standards, namely, a thermal index and mechanical index, to allow the operator to determine whether the study exceeds a generally accepted safe range.[55] The radiologic principle known as ALARA is generally supported and promotes a balance between obtaining the necessary medical information while using minimal settings and examination time. Human data accumulated over a 25-year period have revealed no consistent adverse effects from prenatal diagnostic US examination.[56,57] US in pregnancy is considered a safe procedure.

The American College of Obstetricians and Gynecologists has reviewed the effects of radiography, US, and MRI during pregnancy and suggested guidelines for radiographic examination during pregnancy (Box 72-5).[6]

SUMMARY

In summary, the threshold dose for the nonstochastic effects of radiation throughout the gestational period is greater than 5 rad. Prenatal doses of less than 5 rad present no measurable increased risk for prenatal death, malformation, growth retardation, or impairment of mental development over the background incidence of these entities. The risk for stochastic effects, carcinogenesis or mutagenesis, is related to the fetal absorbed dose and is very low in comparison to the natural background incidence of childhood cancer and genetic disease for most diagnostic procedures.

The vast majority of radiographic imaging obtained in the ED exposes the fetus to 100 times less than the threshold for adverse effects. The 5-rad threshold for onset of concern for adverse fetal effects is quite conservative, and any statistically

---

BOX 72-5   Guidelines for ED Diagnostic Imaging during Pregnancy

1. Women should be counseled that x-ray exposure from a single diagnostic procedure does not result in harmful fetal effects. Specifically, exposure to less than 5 rad has not been associated with an increase in fetal anomalies or loss of pregnancy.
2. Concern about the possible effects of exposure to high-dose ionizing radiation should not prevent medically indicated diagnostic x-ray procedures from being performed on a pregnant woman. During pregnancy, other imaging procedures not associated with ionizing radiation (ultrasonography and MRI) should be considered instead of x-ray studies when appropriate.
3. Ultrasonography and MRI are not associated with known adverse fetal effects.
4. Consultation with an expert in dosimetry calculations may be helpful in calculating the estimated fetal dose when multiple diagnostic radiographs are performed on a pregnant patient.
5. Radioactive isotopes of iodine are contraindicated for therapeutic use during pregnancy.
6. Radiopaque and paramagnetic contrast agents are unlikely to cause harm and may be of diagnostic benefit, but these agents should be used during pregnancy only if the benefit justifies the potential risk to the fetus.

Reproduced from American College of Obstetricians and Gynecologists (ACOG), Committee on Obstetric Practice. Guidelines for Diagnostic Imaging During Pregnancy. ACOG Committee Opinion No. 299. Washington, DC: ACOG; September 2004.
ED, *emergency department;* MRI, *magnetic resonance imaging.*

---

significant change in fetal outcome probably requires at least several times this dose. One of the methods put forth in this chapter can be used to counsel pregnant patients in need of diagnostic imaging. For women inadvertently exposed to radiation before pregnancy is recognized, open and frank discussion can help educate patients and alleviate their fear.

CLINICAL USE OF RADIOCONTRAST MATERIAL

Emergency clinicians must frequently initiate studies with the use of radiocontrast material. A full discussion of these procedures is not within the scope of this chapter, but basic issues of contrast material–induced nephropathy, the possible prevention thereof, and recent concern over the use of gadolinium for MRI studies have been included for completeness and ready reference (Table 72-7 and Box 72-6).

References are available at www.expertconsult.com

TABLE 72-7 Prevention of Contrast-Induced Nephropathy

Renal Failure: Radiocontrast Agents

Radiocontrast-induced acute renal failure is more likely to occur in the presence of advanced age, renal insufficiency, diabetes mellitus, severe congestive heart failure, multiple myeloma, volume depletion, low–cardiac output states, and high-dose contrast-enhanced studies (>125 mL). The incidence of nephrotoxicity depends on the underlying risk factors and the sensitivity of the measure used to determine nephrotoxicity. When a rather sensitive index of renal dysfunction (an increase in the level of serum creatinine to >0.3 mg/dL and >20% on day 1, 2, or 3 and day 5, 6, or 7) is used, the incidence of nephrotoxicity is about 2% in nondiabetic, nonazotemic patients and 16% in diabetic, nonazotemic patients. Diabetic patients with azotemia had about a 38% incidence of nephrotoxicity. In a study of 59 diabetic patients with advanced azotemia (mean serum creatinine level, 5.9 mg/dL) undergoing coronary angiography, contrast-related nephrotoxicity developed in 30 (51%), as defined by a serum creatinine level that was 25% above baseline 48 hr after angiography. Nine patients (15%) required hemodialysis.

Risk Factors for Radiocontrast Nephrotoxicity

Advanced age

Renal insufficiency

Decreased absolute and effective circulatory volume

Diabetes mellitus

Multiple myeloma

Coadministration of other nephrotoxic agents

From Brenner BM, ed. Brenner and Rector's The Kidneys. *7th ed. Philadelphia: Saunders; 2004, Table 34-3; from MD Consult.*
Note: *Renal failure may be oliguric or nonoliguric, with nonoliguric renal failure being more common in patients with previously nearly normal renal function. Most episodes of contrast-induced nephrotoxicity are mild and characterized by a reversible 1- to 3-mg/dL rise in serum creatinine; dialysis therapy is rarely needed and usually only in patients whose baseline serum creatinine level is high, for example, >3 mg/dL.*

Prevention of Radiocontrast Nephropathy

The development of acute renal failure significantly complicates the use of intravascular contrast medium (CM) and is linked with high morbidity and mortality. The increasing use of CM, an aging population, and an increase in chronic kidney disease (CKD) will result in an increased incidence of contrast-induced nephropathy (CIN)—unless preventive measures are used. *At the current time there is no universally accepted, agreed, or proven intervention to totally prevent CIN.* However, the Canadian Association of Radiologists has developed guidelines as a practical approach to risk stratification and potential prevention of CIN. The major risk factor predicting CIN is preexisting CKD, which can be predicted from the glomerular filtration rate (GFR). In terms of being an absolute measure, serum creatinine (SCr) is an unreliable measure of renal function. Patients with a GFR >60 mL/min have a very low risk for CIN, and preventive measures are generally unnecessary. With a GFR <60 mL/min, preventive measures should be instituted. The risk for CIN is greatest in patients with a GFR <30 mL/min. As preventive measures, alternative imaging that does not require CM should be considered. Fluid volume loading is the single most important protective measure. Nephrotoxic medications should be discontinued 48 hr before the study. CM volume and the frequency of administration should be minimized, but satisfactory image quality should still be maintained. High-osmolar CM should be avoided in patients with renal impairment. There is some evidence to suggest that isosmolar CM reduces the risk for CIN in patients with renal impairment, but further study is necessary to determine whether isosmolar CM is superior to low-osmolar CM. *N*-acetylcysteine (NAC) has been advocated to reduce the incidence of CIN; however, not all studies have shown a benefit, and it is difficult to formulate evidence-based recommendations at this time. Use of NAC may be considered in high-risk patients but is not thought to be mandatory.

Additional Caveats

1. Metformin use is not a contraindication to the use of CM, but metformin should be withheld for 48 hr after CM and after evaluation of renal function.

2. Although the GFR is the best way to predict renal dysfunction after CM, patients with normal creatinine are at minimal risk.

From Benko A. Canadian Association of radiologists: consensus guidelines for the prevention of contrast-induced nephropathy. Can Assoc Radiol J. *2007;58:79.*

Potential Prevention of Contrast-Induced Nephropathy*

NAC (N-Acetylcysteine)

Suggested regimen for **oral NAC:** 600 mg (3 mL of a 20% solution in liquid) twice a day for 24 hr before and 24 hr after procedure.

Suggested **IV NAC:** 150-mg/kg IV bolus over 30 min, followed by a 50-mg/kg infusion over 4 hr.[†]

Example in a 80-kg patient: 12,000 mg NAC in 500 mL normal saline over 30 min, followed by 4000 mg NAC in 500 mL normal saline over 4 hr.

TABLE 72-7 Prevention of Contrast-Induced Nephropathy—cont'd

Hydration

Suggested regimen for fluid therapy in elective cases: normal saline, at least 1 mL/kg/hr 12 hr before and 12 hr after the procedure.

Alternative if an emergency procedure is required: 5-mL/kg bolus of normal saline 1 hr before and 1 mL/kg/hr for 12 hr after the procedure.

Alternative fluid regimen with bicarbonate: add 154 mL of 1000 mEq/L sodium bicarbonate to 850 mL of 5% dextrose in water (D₅W) (or add 3 ampules of standard bicarbonate to 1 L D₅W). Initial bolus of 3 mL/kg for 1 hr before injection of contrast material, followed by 1 mL/kg/hr for 6 hr after the procedure.

From Merten GJ, Burgess P, Gray LV, et al. Prevention of contrast-induced nephropathology with sodium bicarbonate: a randomized controlled trial. JAMA. 2004;291:2328.
*Suggested but unproven, minimal downside.
†From Baker CS, Wragg A, Kumar S, et al. A rapid protocol for the prevention of contrast-induced renal dysfunction: the RAPPID study. J Am Coll Cardiol. 2003;41:2114.

Dispensing and Administration Guidelines for CIN (Contrast-Induced Nephropathy)

NAC (N-Acetylcysteine) + Hydration

ORAL NAC DOSING	ORAL NAC DOSING
Give NAC, 600 mg liquid (3 mL of a 20% solution) in 9 mL ginger ale or cola	0.9% sodium chloride IV fluid at 1 mL/kg/hr 12 hr before and after catheterization (normal saline preferred, but 0.45% has also been used with success)

IV Sodium Bicarbonate (154 mEq/L) Mixed in 1 L of D₅W

	3-mL/kg IV BOLUS OVER 1 hr	1 mL/kg/hr × 6 hr IV INFUSION	TOTAL mL INFUSED
60 kg	180 ml	360 mL (60 mL/hr)	540
70 kg	210 ml	420 mL (70 mL/hr)	630
80 kg	240 ml	480 mL (80 mL/hr)	720
90 kg	270 ml	540 mL (90 mL/hr)	810
100 kg	300 ml	600 mL (100 mL/hr)	900
≥110 kg	330 ml	660 mL (110 mL/hr)	990

From Merten GJ, Burgess WP, Gray LV, et al. Prevention of contrast-induced nephropathy with sodium bicarbonate: a randomized controlled trial. JAMA. 2004;291:2328.

IV N-Acetylcysteine

	150-mg/kg IV BOLUS OVER 30 min	50-mg/kg IV INFUSION OVER 4 hr
60 kg	9,000 mg/500 mL NS	3,000 mg/500 mL NS
70 kg	10,500 mg/500 mL NS	3,500 mg/500 mL NS
80 kg	12,000 mg/500 mL NS	4,000 mg/500 mL NS
90 kg	13,500 mg/500 mL NS	4,500 mg/500 mL NS
≥100 kg	15,000 mg/500 mL NS	5,000 mg/500 mL NS

From Baker CS, Wragg A, Kumar S, et al. A rapid protocol for the prevention of contrast-induced renal dysfunction: the RAPPID study. J Am Coll Cardiol. 2003;41:2114.
NS, normal saline.

UMMC Pharmacy Cost Comparisons with treatment regimens for CIN

REGIMENS	REGIMENS
600 mg NAC × 8 doses (oral)	$5.82
2 L NS	$1.60
Sodium bicarbonate, 154 mEq/L D₅W	$1.32 (drug only)
70-kg patient: 10,500 mg NAC/500 mL NS by IV bolus	$183.00 (drug only)
70-kg patient: 3500 mg NAC/500 mL NS by IV infusion	$61.00 (drug only)

BOX 72-6   MRI Contrast Agent Concerns and Contraindications

INFORMATION FOR HEALTH CARE PROFESSIONALS: GADOLINIUM-BASED CONTRAST AGENTS FOR MRI (MARKETED AS MAGNEVIST, MULTIHANCE, OMNISCAN, OPTIMARK, PROHANCE)

FDA ALERT (6/2006, updated 12/2006 and 5/23/2007): This updated alert highlights the FDA's request for the addition of a boxed warning and new warnings about the risk for nephrogenic systemic fibrosis (NSF) and full prescribing information for all gadolinium-based contrast agents (GBCAs) (Magnevist, Multi-Hance, Omniscan, OptiMARK, ProHance). This new labeling highlights and describes the risk for NSF following exposure to a GBCA in patients with acute or chronic severe renal insufficiency (glomerular filtration rate <30 mL/min/1.73 m^2) and patients with acute renal insufficiency of any severity as a result of hepatorenal syndrome or in the perioperative liver transplantation period. In these patients, avoid the use of a GBCA unless the diagnostic information is essential and not available with non–contrast-enhanced MRI. NSF may result in fatal or debilitating systemic fibrosis. The requested changes in GBCA product labeling are summarized below.

- Evaluate renal function in all patients before administering a GBCA.
- Whenever possible, avoid GBCAs for MRI and MRA in patients with moderate to end-stage renal failure. Contrast agents that contain gadolinium include Magnevist, MultiHance, Omniscan, OptiMARK, and ProHance.
- If GBCAs must be used, consider prompt dialysis after the procedure to eliminate circulating gadolinium. However, it is unknown whether dialysis can prevent or treat NSF/NFD.
- Encourage patients to contact their health care provider if they have signs of NSF/NFD.
- Report cases of NSF/NFD to the FDA's MedWatch program at www.fda.gov/medwatch/index.html or by calling 1-800-332-1088 (1-800-FDA-1088).

CONTRAINDICATIONS TO MRI

(Because this is an area of continuing change and there are rapid advancements in the technology to produce MRI-safe materials, consultation with the radiology department is suggested if any questions arise concerning the safety of MRI.)

Overview

There are few contraindications to MRI. Overall, no biologic adverse effects are associated with conventional MRI. Most contraindications to MRI are relative and essentially precautions related to the effect of MRI on devices and material within the body that may be affected by the magnetic field of MRI.

Implanted Devices and Foreign Bodies

Electronic devices and magnetizable material represent potential hazards to the patient. Titanium objects are safe for MRI.

- **Intracoronary stents:** It is considered safe to perform MRI at any time after placement of coronary artery stents of any type.
- **Sternal wires after sternotomy:** Sternal wire sutures are considered safe for MRI.

- **Mechanical cardiac valves:** It is safe to scan most prosthetic cardiac valves because at most, they experience only a mild torque. An exception involves the pre-6000 series Starr-Edwards caged ball valves, devices rarely used now.
- **Pacemakers, implantable defibrillators, and implanted electronic devices:** The risks of scanning patients with cardiac pacemakers are related to possible movement of the device, magnetically induced changes in programming, electromagnetic interference, and induced currents in lead wires leading to heating and/or cardiac stimulation. It is currently considered inadvisable for patients with pacemakers or other intracardiac wires to undergo MRI. Nerve stimulators, insulin pumps, cochlear implants, and other implanted electronic devices may also be affected by MRI and are considered unsafe.
- **Implanted vagal nerve stimulator:** Brain MRI performed at less than 2 T, with a send and receive head coil and the stimulator turned off, appears to be safe under guidelines published by the manufacturer. Other MRI studies are not known to be safe.
- **Aneurysm clips and magnetizable material:** Any ferromagnetic object within the body represents a potential hazard when exposed to the large magnetic field of an MRI system. The hazard primarily reflects the possibility of deflecting the foreign body sufficiently to injure vital structures. For example, certain older-model vascular clips used for cerebral aneurysms are ferromagnetic and could be moved by the magnetic field, with obviously dire consequences.
- **Intraorbital or intraocular metallic fragments,** such as might be acquired from machining, are a potential risk and generally a contraindication to MRI.
- **Cutaneous metal objects:** Although most metallic biomaterial is now nonferrous and nonmagnetizable, any metallic device within or connected to the patient needs to be evaluated for safety. Dental alloys, wires, splints, dental braces, and prostheses do not appear to pose a risk to the patient, although such material may result in artifactual changes. Cutaneous burns can result from contact of the skin with metal objects, including neurosurgical halo pins, pulse oximetry probes, and drug-eluting medical patches that contain metal foil (e.g., nicotine patch), although the mechanism of this injury is unclear.
- **Orthopedic/neurosurgical hardware:** It is safe to perform MRI in patients with titanium implants, screws, rods, and artificial joints.
- **Bullets/shrapnel:** These foreign objects within the body are relative contraindications to MRI. Many bullets are safe, but those with metal (specialized bullets, such as metal jackets) may pose a risk.
- **Tattoos:** The majority of professionally obtained tattoos are safe for MRI; however, tattoos containing lead, such as those obtained in prison, can burn the skin if exposed to MRI.
- **Oxygen cylinders:** Standard metal oxygen cylinders should not be used in the MRI suite. Safe oxygen cylinders are available.
- **Credit cards:** Credit card and other information-containing strips may be destroyed in the MRI scanner.

FDA, *U.S Food and Drug Administration*; MRA, *magnetic resonance angiography*; MRI, *magnetic resonance imaging*; NFD, *nephrogenic fibrosing deformity*.

Commonly Used Formulas and Calculations

Brian C. Kitamura, Eric D. Katz, and Brent E. Ruoff

INTRODUCTION

This appendix presents a list of calculations commonly used by emergency physicians. It is not all-inclusive and purposely does not include decision tools or scales that do not require algebraic calculations. These tools are very useful and can be found in other textbooks, as well as online; other calculators can be found on websites such as www.mdcalc.com and www.medcalc.com.

ENGLISH-TO-METRIC CONVERSIONS

Patients frequently express common figures such as weight, temperature, and volume in standard measurements. Please see Table A-1 for conversion factors and simple examples.

CALCULATION OF MAP

Calculation of mean arterial pressure (MAP) provides a weighted average of systolic blood pressure (SBP) and diastolic blood pressure (DBP). It is a determination of tissue perfusion pressure and is normally 70 to 100 mm Hg in adults. To determine MAP,

$$MAP = [SBP + (2 \times DBP)]/3$$

Example: A hypertensive emergency is diagnosed in an elderly, hypertensive patient. Current recommendations are to reduce MAP by 20% in the first hour. His blood pressure is 240/120. To calculate the current MAP,

$$MAP = [240 + (2 \times 120)]/3 = 160 \text{ mm Hg}$$

QT AND QTc INTERVALS

The QT interval on the electrocardiogram (ECG) represents the period of ventricular electrical activity from activation to repolarization. The most important determinant of the QT interval is the heart rate. As the heart rate increases, the QT interval shortens. Usually, this is calculated automatically; however, the presence of U waves or other ECG abnormalities can confuse the ECG machine. To calculate the rate-corrected QT interval (QTc), using Bazett's formula, divide the QT interval by the square root of the R-R interval (the interval between the R wave on two consecutive QRS complexes). The R-R interval may be measured from the ECG or calculated as 60 divided by the heart rate (in beats/min). The interval is represented in seconds or milliseconds:

$$QTc = QT/\sqrt{(R\text{-}R)}$$

The QTc is normally less than 0.46 second in men and 0.44 second in women.

The list of drugs that can cause QTc prolongation is quite lengthy. The clinical significance of QTc prolongation is often unclear. The following Internet websites offer up-to-date information on this ever-changing topic:

http://www.azcert.org/medical-pros/drug-lists/drug-lists.cfm
http://www.qtdrugs.org/
http://www.ncbi.nlm.nih.gov/pmc/articles/PMC1767957/

Table A-2 shows the normal range of the QT interval in adults.

Example: A 21-year-old man ingested a large quantity of amitriptyline (tricyclic antidepressant) tablets. His ECG revealed a QT interval of 0.37 second and a heart rate of 120 beats/min. The QTc is calculated as

$$R\text{-}R \text{ interval} = 60/120 = 0.50$$

$$QTc = 0.37/\sqrt{0.5} = 0.523 = 523 \text{ msec}$$

The patient's QTc is significantly prolonged for his heart rate and indicates significant cardiac effects from overdose of a tricyclic antidepressant.

PREDICTED PEFR

The peak expiratory flow rate (PEFR), measured in liters per minute, is a useful means of assessing airway obstruction. It is measured by having a patient exhale maximally through a peak-flow meter. Normal values range from 350 to 600 L/min. Comparison between the initial and posttreatment PEFR in patients with exacerbations of asthma helps determine the degree of severity. Patients with an initial PEFR of less than 20% of predicted or with a subsequent value of less than 60% of predicted after initial therapy may require further evaluation, treatment, or both. Many patients monitor PEFR on themselves and are able to state a personal best, which is the preferred standard for that individual. Other patients may be monitored with an estimated PEFR. Estimations are based primarily on a patient's gender, age, and height. Although graphs and tables are available to provide values across a range of ages and heights, the PEFR can also be approximated by using the following formulas:

$$\text{Adults: PEFR} = 13 \times (\text{Height [inches]} - 40) + 110$$

$$\text{Female children/adolescents: PEFR} = \text{Height (m)} \times 5.5 \times \text{Age (yr)} \times 0.03 - 1.11$$

$$\text{Male children/adolescents: PEFR} = \text{Height (m)} \times 6.14 - \text{Age (yr)} \times 0.043 + 0.15$$

ENDOTRACHEAL INTUBATION AND MECHANICAL VENTILATION

Patients with respiratory failure may require endotracheal intubation and mechanical ventilation in the emergency department (ED). The following are guidelines for choosing

TABLE A-1 Standard-to-Metric Calculations

Farenheit to Celsius $°C = (°F - 32)/1.8$	A patient's temperature is **100.4°F** $(100.4°F - 32)/1.8 = 38°C$
Pounds to kilograms $kg = lbs/2.2$	A patient reports his **weight to be 154 lb** $154\ lb/2.2 = 70\ kg$
Inches to centimeters $cm = inches \times 2.54$	The patient's height is 72 inches $72\ inches \times 2.54 = 182.9\ cm$
Fluid ounces to milliliters $mL = oz \times 30$	The child drinks 4 oz of formula at a sitting $4\ oz \times 30 = 120\ mL$

TABLE A-2 Normal Range of the QT Interval in Adults

HEART RATE (beats/min)	NORMAL QT RANGE (sec)
40	0.42-0.53
50	0.37-0.48
60	0.34-0.44
70	0.31-0.41
80	0.29-0.38
90	0.28-0.36
100	0.27-0.34
110	0.25-0.32
120	0.24-0.31
130	0.23-0.30
140	0.22-0.29
150	0.21-0.28

the size of endotracheal tube (ETT) and for calculating the initial ventilator settings.

Selecting the ETT

Adults. Select the largest-diameter ETT that can be tolerated for adults. A 7.5-mm cuffed ETT is well tolerated by most adult female patients. A 8.0-mm cuffed ETT is well tolerated by most adult male patients.

Pediatrics. An uncuffed ETT should be used for children younger than 8 years. A number of techniques are available for estimating the appropriate size of ETT in children. Commonly use formulas for estimating tube size and depth of insertion are as follows:

$$ETT\ size\ (mm) = (Age\ [yr] + 16)/4\ or\ 4 + age/4$$

To estimate depth of insertion for a child older than 2 years:

$$Depth\ of\ insertion = 3 \times Internal\ diameter\ of\ the\ ETT$$

Determining Initial Ventilator Settings

The recommended initial ventilator settings follow. Adjustments in these ventilator settings may be made according to the patient's clinical situation:

$$Tidal\ volume\ (V_T) = 6\text{-}12\ mL/kg *$$

V_T is often based on ideal body weight, and there is greater recognition that a lower V_T may be beneficial, such as 5 to 10 mL/kg.

Rate = 10 to 12 breaths/min for adults, 16 to 20 breaths/min for children, and 20 to 30 breaths/min for infants.
F_{IO_2} = 50% to 100% initially; reduce F_{IO_2} as quickly as possible to avoid oxygen toxicity.
Inspiratory-to-expiratory (I/E) ratio = 1:2. To allow complete exhalation, the I/E ratio should be at least 1:2.

$$Minute\ ventilation\ (\dot{V}_E) = Rate \times V_T$$

$\dot{V}_E$ will vary with the patient's mass and disease process; the normal adult range is approximately 7 to 10 L/min.

Example: A 6-year-old girl with asthma has respiratory distress and altered mental status and requires endotracheal intubation. Her weight is 20 kg. To prepare for intubation and mechanical ventilation, use the following equipment and settings:

ETT size (mm): $(6 + 16)/4 = 5.5$-mm ETT (uncuffed)
Depth of insertion: $3 \times 5.5 = 16.5$ cm
$V_T = 12\ mL/kg \times 20\ kg = 240\ mL$
Respiratory rate = 16 breaths/min
F_{IO_2} = 100%
I/E ratio = 1:2

RENAL FUNCTION

Creatinine clearance (Cr_{Cl}) occasionally needs to be calculated by emergency physicians to risk-stratify patients undergoing imaging studies requiring intravenous (IV) contrast material, as well as to determine the severity of renal failure in patients without a known baseline. Cr_{Cl} is best calculated from a collection of urine over a 24-hour period. However, if the patient's Cr_{Cl} is in steady state (i.e., without recent change), it is possible to estimate Cr_{Cl} by using a formula that incorporates serum creatinine, weight, age, and gender:

$$Cr_{Cl}\ (men) = [(140 - Age\ \{yr\}) \times (Lean\ body\ weight\ \{kg\})]/[72 \times Serum\ creatinine\ (mg/dL)]$$

$$Cr_{Cl}\ (women) = 0.85 \times [(140 - Age\ \{yr\}) \times (Lean\ body\ weight\ \{kg\})]/[72 \times Serum\ creatinine\ (mg/dL)]$$

Normal values: 74-160 mL/min
Mild renal impairment: 40-60 mL/min

*Adjust V_T to limit inflation or plateau pressures to 30 cm H_2O or lower.

Moderate renal impairment: 15-40 mL/min
Severe renal impairment: <15 mL/min indication for renal dialysis)

The following examples illustrate the importance of calculating Cr_{Cl}:

Example 1: A 71-year-old woman has upper abdominal tenderness. A computed tomography (CT) scan is planned, but the clinician is concerned about the risk for contrast-induced nephropathy. The patient's serum creatinine is 1.4 mg/dL and she weighs 55 kg. To calculate her Cr_{Cl}:

$$Cr_{Cl} \text{ (women)} = 0.85 \times [(140 - 71) \times (55 \text{ kg})/(72 \times 1.4)]$$
$$= 32.0 \text{ mL/min}$$

The patient has moderate renal impairment.

Example 2: A 21-year-old man has right lower quadrant tenderness. A CT scan is planned, but the radiologist is concerned about the risk for contrast-induced nephropathy. The patient's serum creatinine is 1.7 mg/dL, and he has a lean body weight of 100 kg. To calculate his Cr_{Cl}:

$$Cr_{Cl} \text{ (men)} = (140 - 21) \times (100 \text{ kg})/(72 \times 1.7)$$
$$= 97.2 \text{ mL/min}$$

The patient has adequate creatinine clearance.

ACID-BASE, FLUID, AND ELECTROLYTE BALANCE

The anion gap (AG) is an estimate of the amount of unmeasured negatively charged ions in serum that are not bicarbonate (HCO_3^-) and chloride (Cl^-). The AG is calculated by subtracting the sum of HCO_3^- and Cl^- values from sodium (Na^+), which is the major positive charge in serum. An elevated AG usually means that there is some unmeasured anion, toxin, or organic acid in the blood. Box A-1 lists many substances that can cause an AG acidosis. The AG is normally 8 to 12 mmol/L:

$$AG = Na^+ - (Cl^- + HCO_3^-) = 8\text{-}12 \text{ mmol/L}$$

Example: A suicidal young male drank an unknown amount of antifreeze. His electrolyte levels are Na^+, 144; K^+,

3.1; Cl^-, 108; and HCO_3^-, 14. The AG is calculated as follows:

$$AG = [144 - (108 + 14)] = 22 \text{ mmol/L}$$

His AG is abnormally elevated, presumably because of ingestion of ethylene glycol.

Calculating the Osmolal Gap

Serum osmolality can be measured in the laboratory by freezing point depression. The measured serum osmolality is usually higher than the calculated osmolality, and the difference is termed the *osmolal gap* (OG). The OG is normally 5 to 10 mOsm/kg. If there is a higher gap, the osmols unaccounted for may represent methanol, ethylene glycol, isopropyl alcohol, or other solutes (Table A-3). Large doses of medications such as lorazepam contain propylene glycol diluent that can raise the osmolal gap. To calculate serum osmolality (Osm_{calc}) and the OG:

$$Osm_{calc} = 2 \times Na^+ + [BUN \text{ (mg/dL)}/2.8]$$
$$+ [Glucose \text{ (mg/dL)}/18] = \text{Normally } 280\text{-}295$$

$$OG = Osm_{meas} - Osm_{calc}$$

where BUN indicates blood urea nitrogen.

Table A-3 shows the effect of some solutes on serum osmolality. The increase in osmolality caused by a solute can be calculated by dividing its serum concentration by the tabulated value.

BOX A-1	Substances Associated with a High Anion Gap*
Aspirin	Lactate (multiple causes)
Methanol, metformin	Ethylene glycol/propylene
Uremia	glycol (diluent)
Diabetic ketoacidosis	Carbon monoxide, cyanide
Paraldehyde, phenformin	Alcoholic ketoacidosis
Isoniazid, iron	Toluene

Follows the mnemonic A MUDPILE CAT.

TABLE A-3 Effect of Some Solutes on Serum Osmolality

EACH mg/dL OF	INCREASES SERUM mOsm/kg BY	FOR EACH SERUM mOsm/kg INCREASE DUE TO	THE CORRESPONDING mg/dL CHANGE IS (= Mol Wt/10)
Methanol	0.31	Methanol	3.2
Ethanol	0.22	Ethanol	4.6
Acetone	0.17	Acetone	5.8
Isopropyl alcohol	0.17	Isopropyl alcohol	6.0
Ethylene glycol	0.16	Ethylene glycol	6.2
Glycerol	0.11	Glycerol	9.2
Mannitol	0.05	Mannitol	18.2

Adapted from Kullig K, Duffy JP, Linden CH, et al. Toxic effects of methanol, ethylene glycol and isopropyl alcohol. *Top Emerg Med.* 1984;6(2):16.

Example: An intoxicated patient has serum chemistry results as follows: Na^+, 142; K^+, 4.5; Cl^-, 100; HCO_3^-, 22; glucose, 90; BUN, 14. His ethanol level is 240 and his measured serum osmolality is 354. You want to know whether he has ingested other osmotically active substances. His calculated serum osmolality is

$$Osm_{calc} = 2 \times 142 + (14/2.8) + (90/18) = 294$$

To evaluate for the effect of ethanol, refer to Table A-3 and add the alcohol level divided by 4.6:

$$240/4.6 = 52$$

$$Osm_{calc} = 294 + 52 = 346$$

Finally, calculate the OG:

$$OG = Osm_{meas} - Osm_{calc} = 354 - 346 = 8$$

His elevated osmolality is explained by the ethanol.

HYPONATREMIA

The following formula may be used to calculate the Na^+ deficit in hyponatremia:

$$Na^+ \text{ deficit} = 60\% \times \text{Weight (kg)} \times (\text{Desired } Na^+ - \text{Measured } Na^+)$$

Symptoms related to hyponatremia are variable, and the severity of symptoms should guide therapy. Sodium replacement is most commonly given as isotonic saline, which contains 154 mmol of Na^+/L. Patients who are severely symptomatic may require 3% saline solution, which contains 513 mmol of Na^+/L. The volume of solution needed to replace the Na^+ deficit (in millimoles) can be calculated by using the concentrations in the saline solutions listed earlier.

Example: A young man is seizing on arrival at the ED. He is known to have schizophrenia and compulsive water drinking. His Na^+ is 116 mmol/L. He weighs 65 kg. To determine his sodium deficit:

$$Na^+ \text{ deficit} = 0.6 \times 65 \text{ kg} \times (140 - 116) = 936 \text{ mmol of } Na^+$$

This amount of Na^+ deficit can be corrected by administering approximately 6 L of isotonic saline or 1.8 L of hypertonic saline. Na^+ should be replaced very slowly to avoid the possibility of inducing central pontine myelinolysis, which results from overaggressive correction of sodium.

Factitious hyponatremia may be due to hyperglycemia. In this hyperosmolal state, glucose tends to stay in extracellular fluid and draws water out of cells into extracellular fluid. Serum sodium is decreased by about 1.6 mmol/L for each 100 mg/dL of excess glucose. To calculate the corrected sodium:

$$Corrected \; Na^+ \text{ (mmol/L)} = \text{Measured } Na^+ \text{ (mmol/L)} + [1.6 \times (\text{Measured glucose [mg/dL]} - 100)/100]$$

Many laboratories automatically make this adjustment, so it is important to check with your laboratory to determine the necessity for this correction.

Example: An obtunded elderly man appears dehydrated. His sodium level is 126 mmol/L and his glucose is 1000 mg/dL.

$$Corrected \; Na^+ = 126 \text{ mmol/L } [1.6 \times (1000 - 100)/100]$$
$$= 126 + 14.4 = 140.4 \text{ mmol/L}$$

His corrected Na^+ suggests that he has factitious hyponatremia because of hyperglycemia.

HYPERNATREMIA

Elevation of the serum sodium concentration is proportionate to the free water deficit when volume is depleted. Because 60% of the adult body is water, the total-body free water deficit is calculated by using measured Na^+, desired Na^+, and body weight in kilograms. To calculate the free water deficit:

$$\text{Ideal total body water (TBW)} = 60\% \times \text{weight (kg)}$$

$$\text{TBW deficit} = [(\text{Measured } Na^+ - \text{Normal } Na^+)/ \text{Normal } Na^+] \times \text{TBW}$$

where normal Na^+ is assumed to be 140 mmol/L.

Example: An elderly man is brought to the ED in a coma. He has severe dehydration, his ideal body weight is 70 kg, and his serum Na^+ level is 165 mmol/L. To determine his free water deficit:

$$\text{Ideal TBW} = 0.6 \times 70 \text{ kg} = 42 \text{ L}$$

$$\text{Free water deficit} = [(165 - 140)/140] \times 42 = 7.5 \text{ L}$$

Fluid correction for hypernatremia should take place over a 48- to 72-hour period to avoid the potential for cerebral edema.

POTASSIUM

Serum potassium (K^+) levels change with acid-base status. In acidemic states, K^+ moves out of cells as H^+ moves in, thus raising serum K^+ levels. In alkalemic states, K^+ moves into cells as H^+ moves out, thus lowering serum K^+ levels. The change in K^+ varies inversely with pH at the following rates:

The serum K^+ concentration increases 0.6 mmol/L for each 0.1-unit decrease in pH.
The serum K^+ concentration decreases 0.6 mmol/L for each 0.1-unit increase in pH.

CALCIUM

Approximately 50% of serum calcium is bound to serum proteins (primarily albumin), 40% is in the free ionized state (the physiologically active form), and 10% is mixed with serum anions (phosphate, bicarbonate, citrate, and lactate). For this reason, serum calcium is lowered about 0.8 mg/dL for every decrease in albumin of 1 g/dL. To correct for decreased albumin (at levels <4 g/dL), the following formula can be used:

$$\text{Corrected Ca}^{2+} \text{ (mg/dL)} = \text{Serum Ca}^{2+} \text{ (mg/dL)} + (0.8 \times [4.0 - \text{serum albumin \{g/dL\}}])$$

Example: A malnourished man has a serum calcium level of 7.5 mg/dL and a serum albumin level of 2 g/dL. To calculate his corrected calcium level:

$$\text{Corrected Ca}^{2+} \text{ (mg/dL)} = 7.5 \text{ mg/dL} + [0.8 \times (4.0 - 2.0 \text{ g/dL})] = 9.1$$

MAINTENANCE IV FLUID RATE

To calculate maintenance IV fluids for a pediatric patient, use the following formula:

4 mL/kg/hr for the first 10 kg, plus
2 mL/kg/hr for the second 10 kg, plus
1 mL/kg/hr for each further kg

Example: A 5-year-old boy weighs 19 kg and requires maintenance IV fluids. To calculate his IV fluid rate:

4 mL/kg/hr for the first 10 kg: 4 × 10 kg = 40 mL/hr, plus

2 mL/kg/hr for the second 10 kg: 2 × 9 kg = 18 mL/hr

40 mL/hr + 18 mL/hr = 58 mL/hr

FLUID RESUSCITATION OF BURNED PATIENTS

Various formulas for IV fluid resuscitation in patients with burns have been recommended. The Parkland formula is commonly used and is calculated as follows:

$$\text{Replacement fluid} = 4 \text{ mL} \times (\text{Weight [kg]}) \times (\% \text{ Body surface area [BSA] burned}).$$

Count only second- and third-degree burns in calculating BSA.

The total volume should be administered in the first 24 hours with half the fluid given in the first 8 hours and the remaining half in the next 16 hours. Clinical parameters, including urine output, vital signs, and central venous pressure or pulmonary capillary wedge pressure, should be monitored carefully to assess the adequacy of resuscitation.

Example: A 65-kg woman has second- and third-degree burns covering 35% of her BSA. To determine her anticipated 24-hour fluid resuscitation needs:

Replacement fluid = 4 mL × 65 × 0.35 = 9100 mL

Half is given in the first 8 hours: 9100/2 = 4550 mL

4550 mL/8 hr = 569 mL/hr for the first 8 hours

Half is given in the second 16 hours: 284 mL/hr

Do not forget to add maintenance fluid rates to the results of the Parkland formula.

ACID-BASE BALANCE

By using the combination of an arterial blood gas (ABG) sample and serum electrolyte levels, a patient's acid-base status can be evaluated. A single acid-base disorder may be present as a primary disorder (respiratory acidosis, respiratory alkalosis, metabolic acidosis, or metabolic alkalosis), or several disorders may be present at the same time. When an acid-base disorder is present, the body will try to compensate to preserve the pH as close to normal as possible. The compensatory responses in relation to the primary disorder are as follows:

PRIMARY DISORDER	COMPENSATORY RESPONSE
Metabolic acidosis	Increased ventilation
Metabolic alkalosis	Decreased ventilation
Respiratory acidosis	Increased renal reabsorption of HCO_3^- in the proximal tubule. Increased renal excretion of H^+ in the distal tubule
Respiratory alkalosis	Decreased renal reabsorption of HCO_3^- in the proximal tubule. Decreased renal excretion of H^+ in the distal tubule

When interpreting acid-base disorders, the following basic steps are suggested:
Knowledge of normal values:

Normal serum pH = 7.40
Normal P_{CO_2} = 40 mm Hg

First, determine the patient's pH status. Acid-base changes are either metabolic or respiratory. Simple disturbances are categorized by examining pH, P_{CO_2}, and HCO_3^- (Table A-4). If pH is less than normal (<7.35), the patient is acidemic. If pH is above normal (>7.45), the patient is alkalemic. If the patient is acidemic and P_{CO_2} is elevated (>45 mm Hg) as a primary disorder, respiratory acidosis is present. If the patient is alkalemic and P_{CO_2} is decreased (<35 mm Hg) as a primary disorder, respiratory alkalosis is present. If the patient is acidemic and the arterial HCO_3^- level is less than normal (<22 mEq/L) as a primary disorder, metabolic acidosis is

TABLE A-4   Acidosis and Compensatory Response

PRIMARY DISTURBANCE	PREDICTED COMPENSATORY RESPONSE
Metabolic acidosis	$\downarrow$ in P_{CO_2} = 1.3 × $\downarrow$ in HCO_3^-
Metabolic acidosis	$\uparrow$ in P_{CO_2} = 0.6 × $\uparrow$ in HCO_3^-
Respiratory acidosis	*Acute:* For every P_{CO_2} $\uparrow$ of 10 mm Hg, $\uparrow$ by 1 mmol/L. *Chronic:* For every P_{CO_2} $\uparrow$ of 10 mm Hg, HCO_3^- $\uparrow$ by 4 mmol/L. *Acute:* For every P_{CO_2} $\downarrow$ of 10 mm Hg, HCO_3^- $\downarrow$ by 2 mmol/L. *Chronic:* For every P_{CO_2} $\downarrow$ of 10 mm Hg, HCO_3^- $\downarrow$ by 5 mmol/L

Adapted from Rutecki GW, Whittier FC. Acid-base interpretation. *Consultant.* November 1991, pp 44-59.

present. If the patient is alkalemic and the HCO_3^- level is greater than normal (>26 mEq/L) as a primary disorder, metabolic alkalosis is present.

Acid-base homeostasis is normally maintained because a change in pH will usually trigger a compensatory change to minimize the change in pH, although the compensation is never complete. The degree and timing of compensation are determined by the primary disturbance itself and by individual physiology. Respiratory compensation for metabolic disorders is more rapid and occurs through a change in the respiratory rate, which in turn adjusts the Pco_2. Metabolic compensation for a respiratory disturbance requires renal adjustment of HCO_3^- and can take 3 to 5 days. The predicted compensatory responses for the primary disturbances are shown in Table A-4. It is important to remember that physiologic compensatory mechanisms may themselves be compromised or overwhelmed by the acid-base disorder (Fig. A-1).

Figure A-1 Acid-base map.

Example 1: A 58-year-old woman has had profuse diarrhea for 1 week. Initial laboratory data include the following: Na^+, 133; K^+, 2.8; pH 7.26; Cl^-, 118; Pco_2, 13; HCO_3^-, 5.

1. Acidemia is present (pH < 7.40).
2. The primary process is metabolic (HCO_3^- < 22 mmoL, and Pco_2 is not increased).
3. Compensation: In primary metabolic acidemia, the formula that checks for compensation is

$$\Delta Pco_2 = 1.3 \times \Delta HCO_3^- \text{ (where } \Delta HCO_3^- \text{ is normal} - \text{current values)}$$

$$\Delta Pco_2 = 1.3 \times (25 - 5) = 26 \text{ mm Hg}$$

The predicted Pco_2 is the normal $Pco_2 - \Delta Pco_2 = 40 - 26 = 14$

The actual Pco_2 is 13 mm Hg

The respiratory compensation is predicted by the equation and suggests that no other acid-base disorder is present.

Example 2: A 74-year-old nursing home resident is admitted to the hospital with hypotension (96/70) and fever (39°C). He has had a positive urine culture for *Escherichia coli* and two positive blood cultures with the same organism. His laboratory values are as follows:

Sodium, 138 mmol/L
Potassium, 3.2 mmol/L
Chloride, 105 mmol/L
pH, 7.49
Pco_2, 25 mm Hg
HCO_3^-, 22 mmol/L

1. Alkalemia is present (pH > 7.44).
2. The primary process is respiratory (Pco_2 < 40 mm Hg and HCO_3^- was not increased).
3. Compensation: The decrease in Pco_2 is 40 − 25, or 15 mm Hg. The formula for an expected decrease in HCO_3^- is 2 mmol for every 10–mm Hg decrease in Pco_2. In this instance the expected decrease in HCO_3^- for the 15–mm Hg decrease in Pco_2 is 3 mmol/L, which is nearly identical to the actual decrease (i.e., 25 − 22). Therefore, only acute respiratory alkalemia is present with normal compensation.

WINTER'S FORMULA

In a pure primary metabolic acidosis, the body's normal response is a change (decrease) in Pco_2. The expected compensation can be predicted by Winter's formula:

$$\text{Expected } Pco_2 = 1.5 \times HCO_3^- + 8 \pm 2$$

Example: HCO_3^- calculated from ABG analysis is 10 mEq/L. With pure metabolic acidosis the expected Pco_2 is

$$\text{Expected } Pco_2 = 1.5 \times 10 + 8$$

$$\text{Expected } Pco_2 = 23 \text{ mm Hg (range, 21-25 mm Hg)}$$

If the measured Pco_2 is higher than the expected Pco_2, a concomitant respiratory acidosis is also present. Normocapnia or hypercapnia in the presence of severe metabolic acidosis may be a harbinger of impending respiratory failure and suggests the possible need for mechanical ventilation.

A lower Pco_2 would suggest a concomitant respiratory alkalosis, such as seen with salicylate poisoning.

Another useful tool in estimating Pco_2 in metabolic acidosis is the recognition that Pco_2 is approximately equal to the last 2 digits of the pH. In the above example, the expected pH should be 7.23.

GLASGOW COMA SCALE

For head-injured patients, the Glasgow Coma Scale (GCS) is a frequently referenced assessment of neurologic function. It is calculated by using best result of neurologic testing of eye opening, motor function, and verbal function. Each of the three subscores is determined by using verbal and painful stimuli. Point assessments are listed in Table A-5, with adjustments noted for pediatric patients. It is very important to remember to use the best score in each category when assigning points. For example, a person with right-sided motor deficits but otherwise normal function would have a normal GCS score because left-sided function is normal. Scores of 13 to 15 correlate with mild brain injury, 9 to 12 with moderate brain injury, and 3 to 8 with severe brain injury.

TABLE A-5   Glasgow Coma Scale Score (Adults/Children <5 yr When Different)

POINTS	BEST EYE RESPONSE	BEST VERBAL RESPONSE	BEST MOTOR RESPONSE
1	No eye opening	No verbal response	No motor response
2	Opens eyes to pain	Incomprehensible/Moans to pain	Extension to pain
3	Opens eyes to command/opens eyes to verbal cues	Inappropriate words/Cries to pain	Flexion to pain
4	Spontaneous eye opening	Confused/Decreased verbal ability, irritable crying	Withdrawal from pain
5	—	Orientated/Age-appropriate speech or cooing	Localizes pain/Localizes pain or withdraws from touch
6	—	—	Obeys commands/Normal spontaneous movements

Example: An intoxicated male is involved in a motor vehicle crash and is brought to your ED. He opens his eyes only to painful stimuli, is muttering incomprehensibly, and localizes pain on the left and withdraws from pain on the right. What is his GCS score, and what severity of injury does this score represent?

GCS = Eye opening + Verbal response + Motor response

Eye opening to pain = 2 points
Incomprehensible sounds = 2 points
Localizing pain is 5 points and withdrawal from pain is 4 points. The better score is used.

2 + 2 + 5 = 9 points

NIH STROKE SCORE

The full National Institutes of Health (NIH) stroke scale is shown in Table A-6. The scale includes directions for patient assessment, as well as recommended adjustments for special situations that might impair the ability of the patient to respond to the assessor. Training scenarios and the NIH stroke scale can be found at www.nihstrokescale.org.

The scale itself, in unedited format, is presented in Table A-6. Scores range from 0 (normal neurologic function) to 34 (maximal injury). Use of thrombolytics has been suggested for patients with scores between 8 and 26 who have no contraindications and can receive the intervention within a specified time of onset; for many sites the time of onset should be within 3 hours.

Example: A 74-year-old, left-handed woman arrives at the ED 90 minutes after the onset of left-sided arm and leg weakness. She has no headache. By 2 hours from symptom onset, she has confirmed normal findings on head CT and does not have contraindications to thrombolytics. Her symptoms have not changed in any way since onset. Using the NIH stroke scale, she is determined to have the following findings. On cognitive testing she is keenly responsive (0 points), knows her age and the current month (0 points), and can follow two-step commands with the unaffected side (0 points). She has a partial gaze palsy without forced deviation (1 point); partial hemianopia (1 point); unilateral, complete paralysis of her face (3 points); no drift on her right arm (0 points); no movement of her left arm (4 points); no drift on her right leg (0 points); and some effort of her left leg against gravity, although it falls to the bed within 2 seconds of elevation (2 points). She has no ataxia (0 points). Her sensation to pinprick is decreased, although she is aware of the testing (1 point). She has a mild expressive aphasia but is easily comprehensible (1 point), has some slurring of words but is still comprehensible (1 point), and exhibits no evidence of neglect (0 points). Her total NIH score is 14, and as a result she may be a candidate for thrombolytic therapy.

TABLE A-6   NIH Stroke Scale

Administer stroke scale items in the order listed. Record performance in each category after each subscale examination. Do not go back and change scores. Follow the directions provided for each examination technique. Scores should reflect what the patient does, not what the clinician thinks that the patient can do. The clinician should record answers while administering the examination and work quickly. Except when indicated, the patient should not be coached (i.e., repeated requests to patient to make a special effort).

IF ANY ITEM IS LEFT UNTESTED, A DETAILED EXPLANATION MUST BE CLEARLY WRITTEN ON THE FORM. ALL UNTESTED ITEMS WILL BE REVIEWED BY THE MEDICAL MONITOR AND DISCUSSED WITH THE EXAMINER BY TELEPHONE.

INSTRUCTIONS	SCALE DEFINITION	SCORE
1a. Level of Consciousness (LOC): The investigator must choose a response, even if a full evaluation is prevented by obstacles such as an endotracheal tube, language barrier, or orotracheal trauma or bandages. A 3 is scored only if the patient makes no movement (other than reflexive posturing) in response to noxious stimulation.	0 = Alert; keenly responsive 1 = Not alert but arousable by minor stimulation to obey, answer, or respond 2 = Not alert, requires repeated stimulation to attend, or is obtunded and requires strong or painful stimulation to make movements (not stereotyped) 3 = Responds only with reflex motor or autonomic effects or is totally unresponsive, flaccid, areflexic	_____
1b. LOC Questions: The patient is asked the month and his or her age. The answer must be correct—there is no partial credit for being close. Aphasic and stuporous patients who do not comprehend the questions will score 2. Patients unable to speak because of endotracheal intubation, orotracheal trauma, severe dysarthria from any cause, language barrier, or any other problem not secondary to aphasia are given a 1. It is important that only the initial answer be graded and that the examiner not "help" the patient with verbal or nonverbal cues.	0 = Answers both questions correctly 1 = Answers one question correctly 2 = Answers neither question correctly	_____

TABLE A-6 NIH Stroke Scale—cont'd

INSTRUCTIONS	SCALE DEFINITION	SCORE
1c. LOC Commands: The patient is asked to open and close the eyes and then to grip and release the nonparetic hand. Substitute another one-step command if the hands cannot be used. Credit is given if an unequivocal attempt is made but not completed because of weakness. If the patient does not respond to command, the task should be demonstrated (pantomime) and the result scored (i.e., follows none, one, or two commands). Patients with trauma, amputation, or other physical impediments should be given suitable one-step commands. Only the first attempt is scored.	0 = Performs both tasks correctly 1 = Performs one task correctly 2 = Performs neither task correctly	_____
2. Best Gaze: Only horizontal eye movements will be tested. Voluntary or reflexive (oculocephalic) eye movements will be scored, but caloric testing is not done. If the patient has a conjugate deviation of the eyes that can be overcome by voluntary or reflexive activity, the score will be 1. If a patient has an isolated peripheral nerve paresis (cranial nerve III, IV, or VI), score a 1. Gaze is testable in all aphasic patients. Patients with ocular trauma, bandages, preexisting blindness, or other disorders of visual acuity or fields should be tested with reflexive movements and a choice made by the investigator. Establishing eye contact and then moving about the patient from side to side will occasionally clarify the presence of a partial gaze palsy.	0 = Normal 1 = Partial gaze palsy. This score is given when gaze is abnormal in one or both eyes but forced deviation or total gaze paresis is not present 2 = Forced deviation or total gaze paresis not overcome by the oculocephalic maneuver	_____
3. Visual: Visual fields (upper and lower quadrants) are tested by confrontation, with finger counting or by visual threat used as appropriate. Patient must be encouraged, but if they look at the side of the moving fingers appropriately, this can be scored as normal. If there is unilateral blindness or enucleation, visual fields in the remaining eye are scored. Score 1 only if a clear-cut asymmetry, including quadrantanopia, is found. If the patient is blind from any cause, score 3. Double simultaneous stimulation is is extinction is present, the patient receives a 1 and the results are used to answer question 11.	0 = No visual loss 1 = Partial hemianopia 2 = Complete hemianopia 3 = Bilateral hemianopia (blind, including cortical blindness)	_____
4. Facial Palsy: Ask or use pantomime to encourage the patient to show his or her teeth or raise the eyebrows and close the eyes. Score the symmetry of grimace in response to noxious stimuli in a poorly responsive or noncomprehending patient. If facial trauma or bandages, an orotracheal tube, tape, or other physical barrier obscures the face, these impediments should be removed to the extent possible.	0 = Normal symmetric movement 1 = Minor paralysis (flattened nasolabial fold, asymmetry on smiling) 2 = Partial paralysis (total or nearly total paralysis of the lower part of the face) 3 = Complete paralysis of one or both sides (absence of facial movement in the upper and lower parts of the face)	_____

Continued

TABLE A-6 NIH Stroke Scale—cont'd

INSTRUCTIONS	SCALE DEFINITION	SCORE
5 and 6. Motor Arm and Leg: The limb is placed in the appropriate position: extend the arms (palms down) 90 degrees (if sitting) or 45 degrees (if supine) and the leg 30 degrees (always tested supine). Drift is scored if the arm falls before 10 seconds or the leg before 5 seconds. An aphasic patient is encouraged by using urgency in the voice and pantomime, but not noxious stimulation. Each limb is tested in turn, beginning with the nonparetic arm. Only in the case of amputation or joint fusion at the shoulder or hip may the score be "9," and the examiner must clearly write the explanation for scoring as a "9."	0 = No drift; the limb holds 90 (or 45) degrees for a full 10 seconds 1 = Drift; the limb holds 90 (or 45) degrees but drifts down before a full 10 seconds; does not hit the bed or other support 2 = Some effort against gravity; the limb cannot get to or maintain (if cued) 90 (or 45) degrees, drifts down to the bed, but has some effort against gravity 3 = No effort against gravity; the limb falls 4 = No movement 9 = Amputation, joint fusion; explain **5a. Left Arm** **5b. Right Arm** 0 = No drift; the leg holds a 30-degree position for a full 5 seconds 1 = Drift; the leg falls by the end of the 5-second period but does not hit the bed 2 = Some effort against gravity; the leg falls to the bed by 5 seconds but has some effort against gravity 3 = No effort against gravity; the leg falls to the bed immediately 4 = No movement 9 = Amputation, joint fusion; explain **6a. Left Leg** **6b. Right Leg**	_____ _____ _____ _____
7. Limb Ataxia: This item is aimed at finding evidence of a unilateral cerebellar lesion. Test with the eyes open. In case of a visual defect, ensure that testing is done in the intact visual field. The finger-nose-finger and heel-shin tests are performed on both sides, and ataxia is scored only if present out of proportion to weakness. Ataxia is absent in a patient who cannot understand or is paralyzed. Only in the case of amputation or joint fusion may the item be scored "9," and the examiner must clearly write the explanation for not scoring. In the case of blindness, test by touching the nose from an extended arm position.	0 = Absent 1 = Present in one limb 2 = Present in two limbs If present, is ataxia in the Right arm: 1 = Yes, 2 = No 9 = Amputation or joint fusion; explain Left arm: 1 = Yes, 2 = No 9 = Amputation or joint fusion; explain Right leg: 1 = Yes, 2 = No 9 = Amputation or joint fusion; explain Left leg: 1 = Yes, 2 = No 9 = Amputation or joint fusion; explain	 _____ _____ _____ _____
8. Sensory: Sensation or grimace in response to a pinprick when tested or withdrawal from a noxious stimulus in an obtunded or aphasic patient. Only sensory loss attributed to stroke is scored as abnormal, and the examiner should test as many body areas (arms [not hands], legs, trunk, face) as needed to accurately check for hemisensory loss. A score of 2, "severe or total," should be given only when severe or total loss of sensation can be clearly demonstrated. Stuporous and aphasic patients will therefore probably score 1 or 0. A patient with a brainstem stroke who has bilateral loss of sensation is scored 2. If the patient does not respond and is quadriplegic, score 2. Patients in coma (item 1a = 3) are arbitrarily given a 2 on this item.	0 = Normal; no sensory loss 1 = Mild to moderate sensory loss; the patient feels that a pinprick is less sharp or dull on the affected side or there is a loss of superficial pain with pinprick but the patient is aware of being touched 2 = Severe to total sensory loss; the patient is not aware of being touched on the face, arm, and leg	_____

TABLE A-6   NIH Stroke Scale—cont'd

INSTRUCTIONS	SCALE DEFINITION	SCORE
9. Best Language: A great deal of information about comprehension will be obtained during the preceding sections of the examination. The patient is asked to describe what is happening in the attached picture, to name the items on the attached naming sheet, and to read from the attached list of sentences. Comprehension is judged from responses here, as well as to all the commands in the preceding general neurologic examination. If visual loss interferes with the tests, ask the patient to identify objects placed in the hand, repeat, and produce speech. An intubated patient should be asked to write. A patient in coma (question 1a = 3) will arbitrarily score 3 on this item. The examiner must choose a score in a patient with stupor or limited cooperation, but a score of 3 should be used only if the patient is mute and follows no one-step commands.	0 = No aphasia; normal 1 = Mild to moderate aphasia; some obvious loss of fluency or facility of comprehension, without significant limitation in ideas expressed or form of expression. Reduction in speech and/or comprehension, however, makes conversation about the material provided difficult or impossible. For example, in conversation about the materials provided, the examiner can identify a picture or naming card from the patient's response 2 = Severe aphasia; all communication is through fragmentary expression; great need for inference, questioning, and guessing by the listener. The range of information that can be exchanged is limited; the listener carries the burden of communication. The examiner cannot identify materials provided from the patient's response 3 = Mute, global aphasia; no usable speech or auditory comprehension	_____
10. Dysarthria: If the patient is thought to be normal, an adequate sample of speech must be obtained by asking the patient to read or repeat words from the attached list. If the patient has severe aphasia, the clarity of articulation of spontaneous speech can be rated. Only if the patient is intubated or has another physical barrier to producing speech may the item be scored "9," and the examiner must clearly write an explanation for not scoring. Do not tell the patient why he or she is being tested.	0 = Normal 1 = Mild to moderate; the patient slurs at least some words and, at worst, can be understood with some difficulty 2 = Severe; the patient's speech is so slurred that it is unintelligible in the absence of or out of proportion to any dysphasia or is mute or anarthric 9 = Intubated or other physical barrier, explain	_____
11. Extinction and Inattention (Formerly Neglect): Sufficient information to identify neglect may be obtained during the prior testing. If the patient has a severe visual loss preventing visual double simultaneous stimulation and the cutaneous stimuli are normal, the score is normal. If the patient has aphasia but does appear to attend to both sides, the score is normal. The presence of visual spatial neglect or anosognosia may also be taken as evidence of abnormality. Since the abnormality is scored only if present, the item is never untestable. This is an additional item, not a part of the NIH Stroke Scale score.	0 = No abnormality 1 = Visual, tactile, auditory, spatial, or personal inattention or extinction to bilateral simultaneous stimulation in one of the sensory modalities 2 = Profound hemi-inattention or hemi-inattention to more than one modality. Does not recognize own hand or orients to only one side of space	_____
A. Distal Motor Function: The patient's hand is held up at the forearm by the examiner and patient is asked to extend the fingers as much as possible. If the patient cannot or does not extend the fingers, the examiner places the fingers in full extension and observes for any flexion movement for 5 seconds. The patient's first attempts only are graded. Repetition of the instructions or of the testing is prohibited.	0 = Normal (no flexion after 5 seconds) 1 = At least some extension after 5 seconds, but not fully extended. Any movement of the fingers that is not command is not scored 2 = No voluntary extension after 5 seconds. Movements of the fingers at another time are not scored **a. Left Arm** **b. Right Arm**	_____

NIH, National Institutes of Heath.

TABLE A-7   Definitions of Commonly Used Epidemiologic Terms

Prevalence	$= (a + c)/(a + b + c + d)$	$=$ Incidence of disease in the population tested
Sensitivity	$= a/(a + c)$	$=$ Probability of a positive test result, disease present
Specificity	$= d/(b + d)$	$=$ Probability of a negative test result, disease absent
False-negative rate	$= c/(a + c)$	$=$ Probability of a negative test result, disease present
False-positive rate	$= b/(b + d)$	$=$ Probability of a positive test result, disease absent
Positive predictive value	$= a/(a + b)$	$=$ Probability of a disease present, test positive
Negative predictive value	$= d/(c + d)$	$=$ Probability of a disease absent, test negative
Overall accuracy	$= (a + d)/(a + b + c + d)$	$=$ Probability of a "true" test result

	DISEASE STATE		
TEST RESULT	Present	Absent	
Positive	a (True positive)	b (False positive)	a + b = All positive tests
Negative	c (False negative) a + c = All patients with disease	d (True negative) b + d = All patients without disease	c + d = All negative tests a + b + c + d = All patients tested

Modified from Goldman L. Quantitative aspects of clinical reasoning. In: Isselbacher KJ, Braunwald E, Wilson JD, eds. *Harrison's Principles of Internal Medicine*. 13th ed. New York: McGraw-Hill; 1994:44.

DIAGNOSTIC PROBABILITY

The probability of obtaining a certain test result in the presence or absence of a particular disease entity for a given population with a given disease prevalence is presented in Table A-7.

No medical test is totally accurate. The parameters listed in Table A-7, when available, can help guide a clinician's test selection. When this information is not available, it may be difficult to identify random laboratory errors or detect failures. Knowledge of disease prevalence, combined with the sensitivity and specificity of the test, yields the positive (or negative) predictive value of that test. For a given sensitivity and specificity, predictive value is directly proportional to prevalence. Hence, even a test with high sensitivity and specificity may not detect a rare disease. This underscores the importance of pretest clinical evaluation.

Acknowledgment

The editors and authors wish to acknowledge the contributions of M. John Mendelsohn to this Appendix in previous editions.

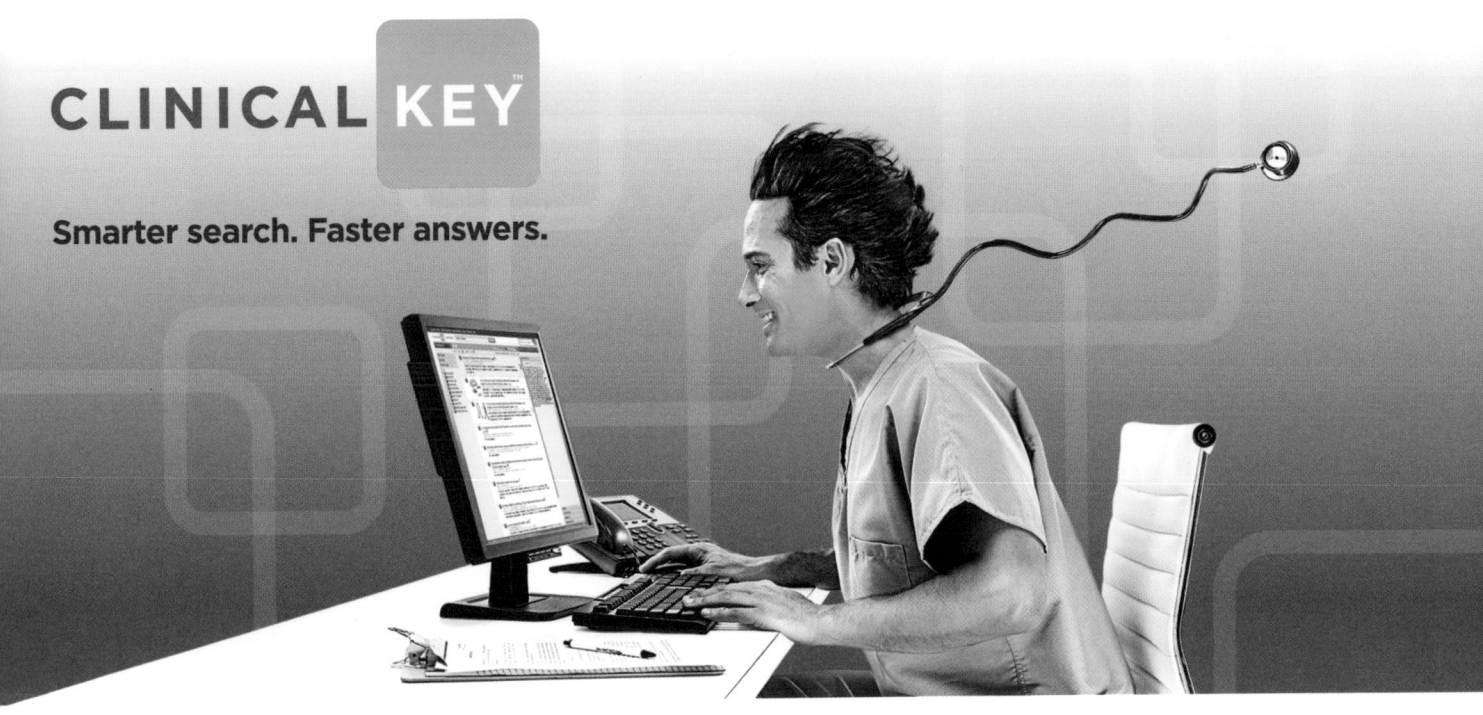

APPENDIX 2: Medications and Equipment for Resuscitation

Rapid Sequence Intubation (RSI) Medications		ADULT (70 kg)	ADULT (100 kg)	PREMIE (2 kg)	NB (3.5 kg)	2 mo (5 kg)	6 mo (8 kg)	1 yr (10 kg)
Pretreatment								
Atropine (pediatric)	0.02 mg/kg	N/A	N/A	0.1 mg	0.1 mg	0.1 mg	0.15 mg	0.2 mg
Lidocaine	1.5 mg/kg	105 mg	150 mg	3 mg	5 mg	7.5 mg	12 mg	15 mg
Vecuronium—defasciculating	0.01 mg/kg	0.7 mg	1 mg	N/A	N/A	N/A	N/A	N/A
Induction								
Fentanyl	5 µg/kg	350 µg	500 µg	10 µg	15 µg	25 µg	40 µg	50 µg
Etomidate	0.3 mg/kg	21 mg	30 mg	0.6 mg	1 mg	1.5 mg	2.5 mg	3 mg
Ketamine	2 mg/kg	140 mg	200 mg	4 mg	7 mg	10 mg	16 mg	20 mg
Propofol	2 mg/kg	140 mg	200 mg	4 mg	7 mg	10 mg	16 mg	20 mg
Paralytic								
Succinylcholine	1.5 mg/kg	105 mg	150 mg	3 mg	5 mg	7.5 mg	12 mg	15 mg
Vecuronium	0.1 mg/kg	7 mg	10 mg	0.2 mg	0.35 mg	0.5 mg	0.8 mg	1 mg
Rocuronium	1 mg/kg	70 mg	100 mg	2 mg	3.5 mg	5 mg	8 mg	10 mg
Pancuronium	0.1 mg/kg	7 mg	10 mg	0.2 mg	0.35 mg	0.5 mg	0.8 mg	1 mg
Crystalloid Fluids								
Resuscitation bolus	20 mL/kg	1.5 L	2 L	40 mL	70 mL	100 mL	160 mL	200 mL
Maintenance	4-2-1 mL/kg	110 mL/hr	140 mL/hr	8 mL/hr	14 mL/hr	20 mL/hr	32 mL/hr	40 mL/hr
Massive Transfusion Protocol (1:1:1)								
PRBCs (1 U = 250 mL)	20 mL/kg	6 U	6 U	40 mL	70 mL	100 mL	160 mL	200 mL
FFP	15 mL/kg	1500 mL	1500 mL	30 mL	50 mL	75 mL	120 mL	150 mL
Platelets	0.1 U/kg	6 U	6 U	0.2 U	0.4 U	0.5 U	0.8 U	1 U
Procedural Sedation								
Midazolam	0.05 mg/kg, titrate up	1 mg	1 mg	0.1 mg	0.2 mg	0.25 mg	0.4 mg	0.5 mg
Fentanyl	1 µg/kg/dose	50 µg	50 µg	2 µg	3.5 µg	5 µg	8 µg	10 µg
Ketamine	1 mg/kg, titrate up	70 mg	100 mg	2 mg	3.5 mg	5 mg	8 mg	10 mg
Propofol	0.5 mg/kg bolus prn	35 mg	50 mg	1 mg	2 mg	2.5 mg	4 mg	5 mg
Reversal Agents								
Naloxone	0.01 mg/kg/dose	0.4-2 mg	0.4-2 mg	0.02 mg	0.035 mg	0.05 mg	0.08 mg	0.1 mg
Flumazenil	0.02 mg/kg/dose to max of 0.2 mg/dose	0.2 mg	0.2 mg	0.1 mg	0.1 mg	0.1 mg	0.15 mg	0.2 mg
Tubes								
ET tube cuffed	(4 + Age*)/4	7.5-8	8-9	2.5	3	3.5	3.5	3.5-4
Blade		4	4	0s	1s	1s	1s	1s
cm to teeth	(Age*/2) + 12	21-23 cm	21-23 cm	8 cm	10 cm	10 cm	11 cm	12 cm
NG tube		18 Fr	18 Fr	5 Fr	5 Fr	8 Fr	8 Fr	10 Fr
Chest tube		42 Fr	42 Fr	8 Fr	10 Fr	10 Fr	12 Fr	16 Fr
Foley		16 Fr	16 Fr	5 Fr	5 Fr	5 Fr	8 Fr	8 Fr
Suction catheter		12 Fr	12 Fr	6 Fr	8 Fr	8 Fr	8 Fr	10 Fr
Percutaneous transtracheal jet ventilation	100% O_2	50 psi	50 psi	2-5 psi	2-5 psi	2-5 psi	5 psi	5 psi
Arrest								
Defibrillation (biphasic = ½ dose)	2-4 J/kg	200 J	200 J	4 J	7 J	10 J	16 J	20 J
Epinephrine 0.01 mg/kg of 1:10,000	0.1 mL/kg	1 amp	1 amp	0.2 mL	0.35 mL	0.5 mL	0.8 mL	1 mL
Amiodarone	5 mg/kg to max 300-mg bolus	300 mg	300 mg	10 mg	17.5 mg	25 mg	40 mg	50 mg
Procainamide	Load 30 mg/min	Max 1200 mg	Max 1700 mg	Max 20 mg	Max 35 mg	Max 50 mg	Max 80 mg	Max 100 mg
Lidocaine	1 mg/kg	70 mg	100 mg	2 mg	3.5 mg	5 mg	8 mg	10 mg
Atropine	0.02 mg/kg	1 mg	1 mg	0.1 mg	0.1 mg	0.1 mg	0.15 mg	0.2 mg
Adenosine	0.1 mg/kg, then double	6, 12 mg	6, 12 mg	0.2 mg	0.35 mg	0.5 mg	0.8 mg	1 mg
CaCl (100 mg/mL)	20 mg/kg	1 g	1 g	40 mg	70 mg	100 mg	160 mg	200 mg
$D_{25}W$	2-4 mL/kg of $D_{25}W$	1.5 amp $D_{50}W$	2 amp $D_{50}W$	4 mL	7 mL	10 mL	16 mL	20 mL
Bicarbonate 8.4% (1 mEq/mL)	1 mEq/kg	70 mL	100 mL	2 mL	3.5 mL	5 mL	8 mL	10 mL
Normal Vital Signs								
HR/RR/SBP		70/12/120	70/12/120	145/40/40	125/40/60	120/30/80	130/25/90	120/25/95

amp, ampule; $D_{25}W$, 25% dextrose in water; *ET*, endotracheal; *FFP*, fresh frozen plasma; *HR*, heart rate; *N/A*, not applicable; *NB*, newborn; *NG*, nasogastric; *PRBCs*, packed red blood cells; *premie*, premature; *prn*, as needed; *RR*, respiratory rate; *SBP*, systolic blood pressure.
*In years.